Dietary Reference Intakes (DRIs): Recommended Intakes for Individuals, Elements
Food and Nutrition Board, Institute of Medicine, National Academies

Life Stage Group	Calcium (mg/d)	Chromium (μg/d)	Copper (μg/d)	Fluoride (mg/d)	Iodine (μg/d)	Iron (mg/d)	Magnesium (mg/d)	Manganese (mg/d)	Molybdenum (μg/d)	Phosphorus (mg/d)	Selenium (μg/d)	Zinc (mg/d)
Infants												
0-6 mo	210*	0.2*	200*	0.01*	110*	0.27*	30*	0.003*	2*	100*	15*	2*
7-12 mo	270*	5.5*	220*	0.5*	130*	11	75*	0.6*	3*	275*	20*	3
Children												
1-3 y	500*	11*	340	0.7*	90	7	80	1.2*	17	460	20	3
4-8 y	800*	15*	440	1*	90	10	130	1.5*	22	500	30	5
Males												
9-13 y	1300*	25*	700	2*	120	8	240	1.9*	34	1250	40	8
14-18 y	1300*	35*	890	3*	150	11	410	2.2*	43	1250	55	11
19-30 y	1000*	35*	900	4*	150	8	400	2.3*	45	700	55	11
31-50 y	1000*	35*	900	4*	150	8	420	2.3*	45	700	55	11
51-70 y	1200*	30*	900	4*	150	8	420	2.3*	45	700	55	11
>70 y	1200*	30*	900	4*	150	8	420	2.3*	45	700	55	11
Females												
9-13 y	1300*	21*	700	2*	120	8	240	1.6*	34	1250	40	8
14-18 y	1300*	24*	890	3*	150	15	360	1.6*	43	1250	55	9
19-30 y	1000*	25*	900	3*	150	18	310	1.8*	45	700	55	8
31-50 y	1000*	25*	900	3*	150	18	320	1.8*	45	700	55	8
51-70 y	1200*	20*	900	3*	150	8	320	1.8*	45	700	55	8
>70 y	1200*	20*	900	3*	150	8	320	1.8*	45	700	55	8
Pregnancy												
≤18 y	1300*	29*	1000	3*	220	27	400	2.0*	50	1250	60	13
19-30 y	1000*	30*	1000	3*	220	27	350	2.0*	50	700	60	11
31-50 y	1000*	30*	1000	3*	220	27	360	2.0*	50	700	60	11
Lactation												
≤18 y	1300*	44*	1300	3*	290	10	360	2.6*	50	1250	70	14
19-30 y	1000*	45*	1300	3*	290	9	310	2.6*	50	700	70	12
31-50 y	1000*	45*	1300	3*	290	9	320	2.6*	50	700	70	12

SOURCES: Dietary Reference Intakes for Calcium, Phosphorous, Magnesium, Vitamin D, and Fluoride (1997); Dietary Reference Intakes for Thiamin, Riboflavin, Niacin, Vitamin B_6, Folate, Vitamin B_{12}, Pantothenic Acid, Biotin, and Choline (1998); Dietary Reference Intakes for Vitamin C, Vitamin E, Selenium, and Carotenoids (2000); and Dietary Reference Intakes for Vitamin A, Vitamin K, Arsenic, Boron, Chromium, Copper, Iodine, Iron, Manganese, Molybdenum, Nickel, Silicon, Vanadium, and Zinc (2001).

NOTE: This table presents Recommended Dietary Allowances (RDAs) in bold type and Adequate Intakes (AIs) in ordinary type followed by an asterisk (*). RDAs and AIs may both be used as goals for individual intake. RDAs are set to meet the needs of almost all (97 to 98 percent) individuals in a group. For healthy breastfed infants, the AI is the mean intake. The AI for other life stage and gender groups is believed to cover needs of all individuals in the group, but lack of data or uncertainty in the data prevent being able to specify with confidence the percentage of individuals covered by this intake.

Dietary Reference Intakes (DRIs): Tolerable Upper Intake Levels (UL[a]), Elements
Food and Nutrition Board, Institute of Medicine, National Academies

Life Stage Group	Arsenic[b]	Boron (mg/d)	Calcium (g/d)	Chromium	Copper (μg/d)	Fluoride (mg/d)	Iodine (μg/d)	Iron (mg/d)	Magnesium (mg/d)[c]	Manganese (mg/d)	Molybdenum (μg/d)	Nickel (mg/d)	Phosphorus (g/d)	Selenium (μg/d)	Silicon[d]	Vanadium (μg/d)[e]	Zinc (mg/d)
Infants																	
0-6 mo	ND[f]	ND	ND	ND	ND	0.7	ND	40	ND	ND	ND	ND	ND	45	ND	ND	4
7-12 mo	ND	ND	ND	ND	ND	0.9	ND	40	ND	ND	ND	ND	ND	60	ND	ND	5
Children																	
1-3 y	ND	3	2.5	ND	1000	1.3	200	40	65	2	300	0.2	3	90	ND	ND	7
4-8 y	ND	6	2.5	ND	3000	2.2	300	40	110	3	600	0.3	3	150	ND	ND	12
Males, Females																	
9-13 y	ND	11	2.5	ND	5000	10	600	40	350	6	1100	0.6	4	280	ND	ND	23
14-18 y	ND	17	2.5	ND	8000	10	900	45	350	9	1700	1.0	4	400	ND	ND	34
19-70 y	ND	20	2.5	ND	10,000	10	1100	45	350	11	2000	1.0	4	400	ND	1.8	40
>70 y	ND	20	2.5	ND	10,000	10	1100	45	350	11	2000	1.0	3	400	ND	1.8	40
Pregnancy																	
≤18 y	ND	17	2.5	ND	8000	10	900	45	350	9	1700	1.0	3.5	400	ND	ND	34
19-50 y	ND	20	2.5	ND	10,000	10	1100	45	350	11	2000	1.0	3.5	400	ND	ND	40
Lactation																	
≤18 y	ND	17	2.5	ND	8000	10	900	45	350	9	1700	1.0	4	400	ND	ND	34
19-50 y	ND	20	2.5	ND	10,000	10	1100	45	350	11	2000	1.0	4	400	ND	ND	40

SOURCES: Dietary Reference Intakes for Calcium, Phosphorous, Magnesium, Vitamin D, and Fluoride (1997); Dietary Reference Intakes for Thiamin, Riboflavin, Niacin, Vitamin B_6, Folate, Vitamin B_{12}, Pantothenic Acid, Biotin, and Choline (1998); Dietary Reference Intakes for Vitamin C, Vitamin E, Selenium, and Carotenoids (2000); and Dietary Reference Intakes for Vitamin A, Vitamin K, Arsenic, Boron, Chromium, Copper, Iodine, Iron, Manganese, Molybdenum, Nickel, Silicon, Vanadium, and Zinc (2001). These reports may be accessed via www.nap.edu.

[a]UL = The maximum level of daily nutrient intake that is likely to pose no risk of adverse effects. Unless otherwise specified, the UL represents total intake from food, water, and supplements. Due to lack of suitable data, ULs could not be established for arsenic, chromium, and silicon. In the absence of ULs, extra caution may be warranted in consuming levels above recommended intakes.

[b]Although the UL was not determined for arsenic, there is no justification for adding arsenic to food or supplements.

[c]The ULs for magnesium represent intake from a pharmacologic agent only and do not include intake from food and water.

[d]Although silicon has not been shown to cause adverse effects in humans, there is no justification for adding silicon to supplements.

[e]Although vanadium in food has not been shown to cause adverse effects in humans, there is no justification for adding vanadium to food and vanadium supplements should be used with caution. The UL is based on adverse effects in laboratory animals and this data could be used to set a UL for adults but not children and adolescents.

[f]ND = Not determinable due to lack of data of adverse effects in this age group and concern with regard to lack of ability to handle excess amounts. Source of intake should be from food only to prevent high levels of intake.

ESSENTIALS OF NUTRITION & DIET THERAPY

ESSENTIALS OF NUTRITION & DIET THERAPY

EIGHTH EDITION

Sue Rodwell Williams, PhD, MPH, RD
Davis, California

Eleanor D. Schlenker, PhD, RD
Professor, Department of Human Nutrition, Foods and Exercise
Associate Director for Family and Consumer Sciences and
Community Initiatives
Virginia Cooperative Extension
College of Human Resources and Education
Virginia Polytechnic Institute and State University
Blacksburg, Virginia

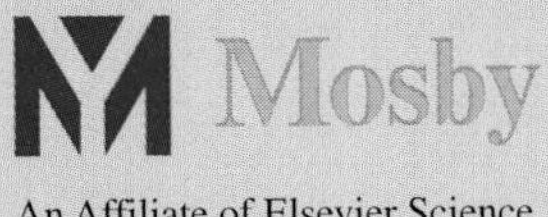

An Affiliate of Elsevier Science

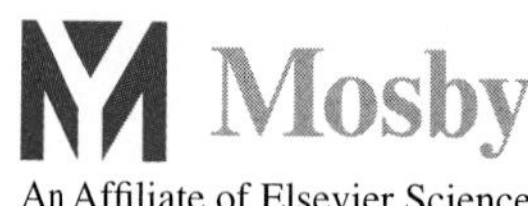

An Affiliate of Elsevier Science

11830 Westline Industrial Drive
St. Louis, Missouri 63146

ESSENTIALS OF NUTRITION AND DIET THERAPY
ISBN 0-323-01635-9

Notice

Nutrition is an ever-changing field. Standard safety precautions must be followed, but as new research and clinical experience broaden our knowledge, changes in treatment and drug therapy may become necessary or appropriate. Readers are advised to check the most current product information provided by the manufacturer of each drug to be administered to verify the recommended dose, the method and duration of administration, and contraindications. It is the responsibility of the licensed prescriber, relying on experience and knowledge of the patient, to determine dosages and the best treatment for each individual patient. Neither the publisher nor the editor assumes any liability for any injury and/or damage to persons or property arising from this publication.

Previous editions copyrighted 1974, 1978, 1982, 1986, 1990, 1994, 1999.

Library of Congress Cataloging in Publication Data

Williams, Sue Rodwell.
Essentials of nutrition and diet therapy / Sue Rodwell Williams, Eleanor D. Schlenker.—
8th ed.
p. cm.
Includes bibliographical references and index.
ISBN 0-323-01635-9 (alk. paper)
1. Diet therapy. 2. Nutrition. 3. Nursing. I. Schlenker, Eleanor D. II. Title.
RM216.W683 2002
613.2—dc21
2002037891

Vice President and Publishing Director, Nursing: Sally Schrefer
Acquisitions Editor: Yvonne Alexopoulos
Senior Developmental Editor: Melissa K. Boyle
Publishing Services Manager: Deborah L. Vogel
Project Manager: Kelley Barbarick
Design Manager: Bill Drone
Cover and Interior Designer: Lee Goldstein
Cover Photos: PhotoDisc and Digital Stock
Part and Chapter Opener Photos: PhotoDisc (except Chapter 18: Tony Stone Images, and Chapter 17)

Printed in the United States of America.

Last digit is the print number: 9 8 7 6 5 4 3 2 1

To my students
whose "whys" and "hows" and "so whats"
keep my feet to the fire of knowledge
and make the learning process exciting
and ever new.

Sue Rodwell Williams

To my parents, who taught me to appreciate
the opportunity to learn.

Eleanor D. Schlenker

Contributors

SARA LONG ANDERSON, PhD, RD
Associate Professor and Director, Didactic Program in Dietetics
Department of Animal Science, Food and Nutrition
Southern Illinois University, Carbondale
Carbondale, Illinois

GEORGIA CLARK-ALBERT, RD
Former Chair
Dietitians in General Clinical Practice Dietetic Practice Group
American Dietetic Association
Athens, Maine

DEBORAH A. COHEN, MMSc, RD
Clinical Faculty Associate
Southeast Missouri State University
Department of Human Environmental Studies
Cape Girardeau, Missouri

GAIL A. CRESCI, MS, RD, CNSD, LD
Assistant Clinical Professor of Surgery
Director, Surgical Nutrition Service
Medical College of Georgia
Department of Surgery
Augusta, Georgia

SUSAN EMERY, MS, RD
Dietitian
Thomas Jefferson University Hospital
Philadelphia, Pennsylvania

M. PATRICIA FUHRMAN, MS, RD, LD, FADA, CNSD
Chair of Dietetics/Assistant Professor
Jewish Hospital College of Nursing and Allied Health
St. Louis, Missouri

D. JORDI GOLDSTEIN-FUCHS, DSc, RD
Associate Research Professor
Nutrition Education and Research Program
School of Medicine
University of Nevada, Reno
Reno, Nevada

MARCIA SILKROSKI, RD, CNSD
Executive Director
Nutrition Advantage
Chester Springs, Pennsylvania

Reviewers

PETER L. BEYER, MS, RD
Associate Professor
Dietetics and Nutrition
University of Kansas Medical Center
Kansas City, Kansas

CARMEN BOYD, MS, LPC, RD
Instructor
Biomedical Sciences Department
Southwest Missouri State University
Springfield, Missouri

BONITA BROYLES, RN, BSN, EdD
Associate Degree Nursing Education Faculty
Piedmont Community College
Roxboro, North Carolina

EVELYN B. ENRIONE, PhD, RD
Associate Dean
College of Health and Urban Affairs
Florida International University
Miami, Florida

KATHY A. HAMMOND, MS, RN, CNSN, RD, LD, CNSD
Coordinator, Continuing Education
Clinical Nutrition Specialist
Chartwell Management Company
Atlanta, Georgia
Adjunct Assistant Professor
Department of Foods and Nutrition
University of Georgia
Athens, Georgia

JAIMETTE A. McCULLEY, MS, RD, CNSD
Instructor
Human Environmental Sciences Department
Fontbonne College
St. Louis, Missouri

PAULA F. SCHARF, PhD, RN
Associate Professor
Lienhard School of Nursing
Pace University
Pleasantville, New York

DIANE D. STADLER, PhD, RD, CD
Research Assistant Professor/Bionutritionist
General Clinical Research Center
Oregon Health Sciences University
Portland, Oregon

Preface

Through seven highly successful previous editions, this nutrition textbook has provided a sound basis for student learning and clinical practice in the health professions. It has always maintained both a strong research base and a person-centered approach to the study and application of nutrition in human health. I have been gratified by the contact I have had with users in colleges, community colleges, and clinical settings throughout the country and in other parts of the world and cherish their suggestions and expressions of appreciation.

In recent years, rapid changes have been occurring in nutrition. New regulations are being announced and debated. The science base in biology, biotechnology, and health is expanding. Social problems and structures are changing. Patient populations are more culturally diverse. Healthcare systems and practices are very different from a generation or even a decade ago. Public interest and concern with nutrition and healthcare are increasing. Nutrition has become more prominent in the marketplace of competing ideas and products. It is small wonder then that all of these changes are apparent in the field of nutrition education and professional practice because nutrition is fundamentally a very human applied science and art.

This new eighth edition reflects these far-reaching changes. As always, its guiding principle continues to be my own commitment and that of the publisher to the integrity of the textbook. Our goal is to build on the format that has evolved through previous editions and produce this new book, updated and rewritten, incorporating design and format with sound content to meet the expectations and changing needs of students, faculty, and practitioners in the health professions.

New To This Edition

With the intent of accommodating the demands of a rapidly developing science and society, a large part of the text has been updated and rewritten. Changes based on input from many teachers, students, and clinicians have been incorporated to increase the text's usefulness.

CHAPTER CHANGES

In this edition, Eleanor D. Schlenker, my co-author and good friend, has written the eight chapters in Part 1: *Introduction to Human Nutrition,* which provide an up-to-date sound understanding of the basic science of human nutrition, as well as Chapters 12 and 13, which together give insight into nutritional needs throughout the life cycle. She brings to the text a wealth of experience in nutrition education in academic and community settings, and I am pleased and proud that she is a major part of this edition.

In Part 3: *Introduction to Clinical Nutrition,* the chapters that deal with nutritional care needs within specific illnesses and clinical therapies have been revised for this edition by contributing authors experienced in current clinical nutrition practice. The topics of these chapters are drug-nutrient interactions; diseases of the heart, blood vessels, and lungs; and diabetes mellitus by Sara Long Anderson; nutrition support—enteral and parenteral nutrition by M. Patricia Fuhrman; gastrointestinal diseases by Georgia Clark-Albert; renal disease by D. Jordi Goldstein-Fuchs; nutritional care of surgery patients by Gail A. Cresci; nutrition and acquired immunodeficiency syndrome (AIDS) by Deborah A. Cohen; nutrition and cancer by Susan Emery; and nutrition therapy in chronic disabling conditions and rehabilitation by Marcia Silkroski.

New material is incorporated throughout the text of this edition and includes not only current scientific research findings and clinical treatment therapies but also coverage of significant nutrition-related developments in science and technology that are of wide and even controversial interest. For example, Chapter 9, "The Food Environment and Food Habits," includes a major new section discussing the growing presence of new biotechnology in the food supply, from farm fields to supermarket shelves, the controversies that have arisen over these changes, and the role of the scientific community and regulatory agencies.

In this edition, many of the *Issues & Answers, To Probe Further,* and *Practical Application* boxes are updated or new. In addition to those supplied by the authors of each chapter, contributor Meredith Catherine Williams has written new boxes on current issues such as mad cow disease, communication skills in nutrition interviews, the importance of folate in preventing spina bifida, and how pressures on female athletes can lead to eating disorders and low bone mass.

ILLUSTRATIONS AND DESIGN

Numerous illustrations—anatomic figures, graphic line drawings, and photographs—many in full color, enhance the overall design and help students better understand the concepts and clinical practices presented.

ENHANCED READABILITY AND STUDENT INTEREST

A great deal of attention has been given in this text to the issues of student interest and comprehension. Every effort has been made to enhance this text's readability and to enliven it stylistically. A large amount of the text has been rewritten as indicated to incorporate new material. Many new advances in basic and clinical science are explained and applied. Issues of student interest and public-professional controversy are discussed.

Learning Aids Within the Text

This new edition continues to use many learning aids throughout the text.

CHAPTER OPENERS

To alert students to the topic of each chapter and draw them into its study, each chapter opens with an illustration and a preview of the chapter topics.

CHAPTER OUTLINES

The major sections are listed at the beginning of each chapter and indicated by special type for ease in reading comprehension.

KEY TERMS

Key terms important to the student's understanding and application of the material in patient care are presented in three steps. They are first identified in blue type in the body of the text. These terms are then grouped and defined in boxes in the lower right corners of right-hand pages. Finally, all key terms are collected in a comprehensive glossary for easy reference at the end of the book. This three-level approach to vocabulary development greatly improves the overall study and use of the text.

PEDAGOGY BOXES: *ISSUES & ANSWERS, TO PROBE FURTHER,* AND *PRACTICAL APPLICATION*

Continuing special features in the chapters of this text are these supplemental material boxes, which present brief information on chapter-related issues or controversies, a deeper look at chapter topics, and illustrations of the practical application of nutrition concepts. These interesting and motivating studies help the student comprehend the importance of scientific thinking and develop sound judgment and openness to varied points of view.

CASE STUDIES

In many chapters, realistic case studies lead the student to apply the text material to related patient care problems. Each case is accompanied by questions for case analysis. These cases also help alert the student to applications of nutritional therapy for similar patient care needs in their own clinical assignments.

CHAPTER SUMMARIES

To help the student pull the chapter material together again as a whole, each chapter concludes with a summary of the key concepts presented and their significance or application. The student can then return to any part of the material for repeated study and clarification as needed.

REVIEW QUESTIONS

To help the student understand key parts of the chapter or apply it to patient problems, review questions are provided at the end of each chapter.

CHAPTER REFERENCES

A strength of this text is its updated range of current documentation for the topics presented, drawn from a wide selection of pertinent journals. To provide immediate access to all references cited in the chapter text, a full list of these key references is given at the end of each chapter rather than collected at the end of the book.

FURTHER READING

In addition to referenced material in the text, an annotated list of suggestions for further reading for added interest and study is provided at the end of each chapter. These selections extend or apply the material in the text according to student needs or areas of special interest. The annotations improve the student's ability to use them by identifying pertinent parts of the reference.

APPENDIXES

The revised appendixes include a number of materials for use as reference tools and guidelines in learning and practice. Food value tables include nutrient and energy references for a variety of basic foods. Appendix I presents the most current CDC growth charts. Appendix M, "Dietary Guidelines for Americans 2000," is completely rewritten in accordance with the most recent USDA guidelines and also connects them to related goals from the national *Healthy People 2010* program. A new Appendix R presents a table of energy expenditures for a variety of activities.

INDEX

The index extends the basic text cross-referencing and provides a quick reference to the book's content.

Supplementary Materials

Several available supplements enhance the teaching and learning process.

INSTRUCTOR'S RESOURCE

Prepared by Gill Robertson, MS, RD, this convenient electronic resource features chapter overviews, objectives, chapter outlines with teaching notes, individual/group activities, an extensive test bank of over 1250 multiple-choice questions, as well as an image collection of approximately 30 images from the text. This resource is available both on CD-ROM and online.

EVOLVE WEBSITE

Designed to provide supplemental online learning opportunities for students that complement the material in the book, this site offers students WebLinks to related sites, FAQs, and more. This site is also where faculty can access the online version of the Instructor's Resource.

NUTRITION AND DIET THERAPY NEWS

Published quarterly, this e-mail newsletter is written by a leading nutrition author, Michele Grodner, EdD, CHES. It provides information on the latest issues in the field of nutrition and is intended for all students, faculty, and professionals who use Elsevier Science's nutrition titles. Visit the Nutrition Resource Center at *http://www.us.elsevierhealth.com/MERLINSIMON/Nutrition* to learn more.

MOSBY'S NUTRITRAC NUTRITION ANALYSIS CD-ROM, VERSION III

This innovative program, packaged with every copy of this text, gives users the hands-on, interactive tools to perform a complete nutrition analysis of food intake, as well as calculate energy expenditure based on activity level and caloric intake. It generates helpful nutrient reports, calorie and fat content charts, DRI/RNI graphs, running tallies of energy expenditure, and much more. This latest version features a database of over 3000 foods in 18 different food categories, along with an expanded activities database of over 150 various daily/common, sporting, recreational, and occupational activities. A new Body Mass Index calculator has also been added.

Personal Approach

The person-centered approach that has been a hallmark of this book's previous editions remains in this new text. The authors and all contributors have followed throughout the book the principles of writing in a personal style, of using materials and examples from personal research and clinical experience, and of presenting scientific knowledge in human terms as a tool to find practical solutions to individual problems.

Acknowledgments

A textbook of this sort is never the work of just authors and contributors. It develops into the planned product through the committed hands and hearts of a number of persons. It would be impossible to name all of the individuals involved, but several groups deserve special recognition.

First of all, I am grateful to the reviewers who gave their valuable time and skills to strengthen the manuscript: Peter L. Beyer, Carmen Boyd, Bonita Broyles, Evelyn B. Enrione, Kathy A. Hammond, Jaimette A. McCulley, Paula F. Scharf, and Diane D. Stadler.

Second, I am indebted to Mosby and the many persons there who had a part in this extensive project. I especially thank my editor of nutrition publications, Yvonne Alexopoulos, whose skills and support have always been invaluable, and my senior developmental editor, Melissa Boyle, whose capable and energetic talents helped shape the book's pages. I also thank my production project manager, Kelley Barbarick, for essential guidance; the design manager, Bill Drone; and our director of publishing services, Peggy Fagen. To our marketing managers and the many fine Elsevier Science sales representatives throughout the country, I owe great appreciation for their help in ensuring the book's success with users.

I also thank my own staff during the various stages of preparing the manuscript, especially to my research assistant Mary Herbert, who gathered the comprehensive materials I requested. Most of all, I owe a special debt of gratitude to my author's editor, James C. Williams, for writing and editing assistance throughout. I also give special thanks to my many students, interns, colleagues, clients, and patients over the years, all of whom have taught me much; and to my family, who never cease to support all my efforts.

Sue Rodwell Williams
Davis, California

Contents in Brief

Part 1 Introduction to Human Nutrition

Part 2 Community Nutrition: The Life Cycle

PART 3 Introduction to Clinical Nutrition

Appendixes

Contents

PART 1 Introduction to Human Nutrition

PART 2 Community Nutrition: The Life Cycle

Appendixes

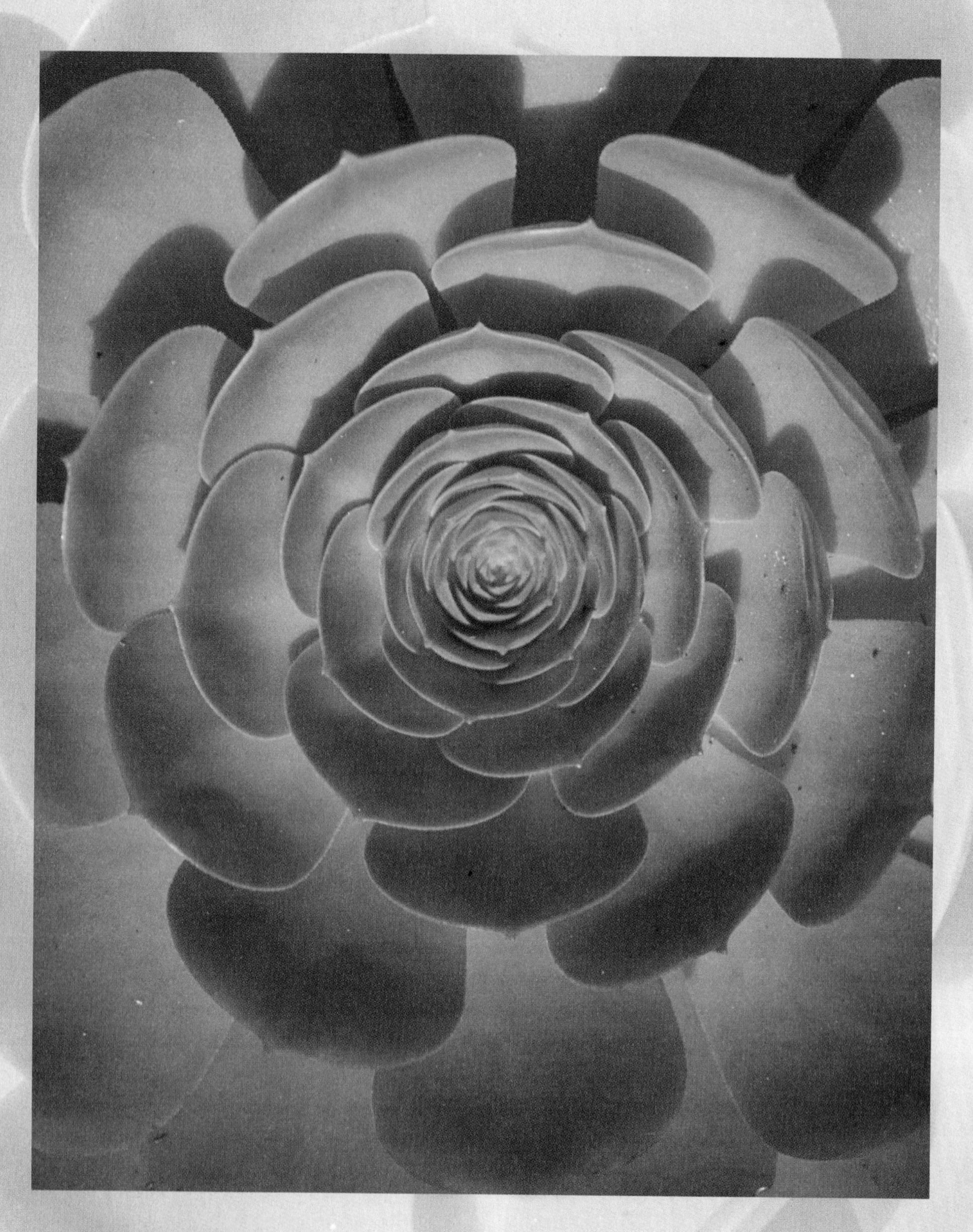

Part 1

INTRODUCTION TO HUMAN NUTRITION

Chapter 1

Nutrition and Health

Eleanor D. Schlenker

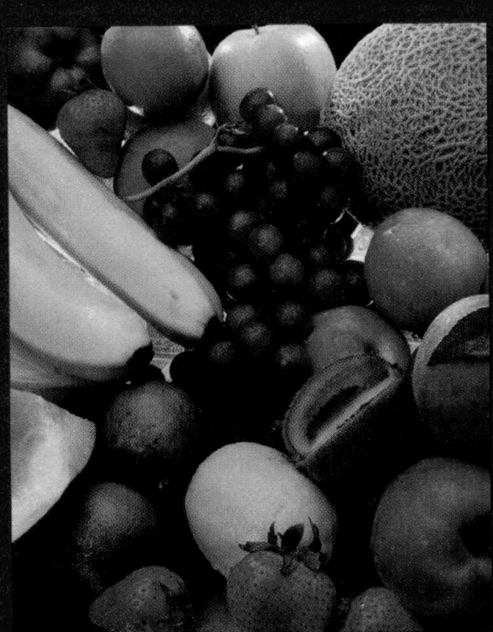

Chapter Outline

This chapter introduces the study of nutrition in human health and healthcare. Whether your future goals involve your personal health or your role as a health professional, a sound base of nutrition knowledge and skills is fundamental.

Current knowledge in nutrition and its basic science foundations reflects our rapidly changing world, including a changing food supply, a growing population, and an expanding scientific knowledge. Nutrition is rapidly emerging as a vital component in personal healthcare and in our national nutrition and health policies to meet human needs.

A primary means of promoting health and preventing disease rests on a wholesome food supply and the sound nutrition it provides. In this chapter we introduce a person-centered approach to nutrition and healthcare, an important focus throughout our study.

Nutrition and Human Health

NEW DIRECTIONS FOR NUTRITION

Biology and Agriculture

The twenty-first century promises a world of change, and this includes the field of nutrition. During the past 100 years, advances in nutrition have led to the discovery of more than 50 essential nutrients and their roles in preventing deficiency diseases. Much of this work evaluated changes that occur within the whole body or in particular tissues. New developments in the world of biology are making it possible for nutrition researchers to examine life at the molecular level and to begin to evaluate the interaction between nutrients and the genetic code.[1] We have identified certain gene types that have an increased need for particular nutrients, and in time we may be able to individualize diets based on one's genetic susceptibility to specific diseases. Advances in biotechnology also have influenced our food supply by enabling agricultural scientists to develop new varieties of crops that are resistant to particular insects or plant diseases. The introduction of genes that improve the nutritional quality of a particular food and are safe for human consumption is a topic of intense research among food scientists and nutritionists.[2] However, consumers are raising concerns about the use of genetically altered foods, with some groups seeking new legislation that would require special labeling of food products made from genetically altered plants. Current efforts to promote sustainable agricultural practices that conserve natural resources, while reducing air and water pollution and soil loss, demand the cooperation of nutrition professionals who will support farmers' markets and develop food guides that encourage the use of local agricultural products.[3]

Food and Health

Recent discoveries about the health-related aspects of certain foods have led to new government policies regulating food in the marketplace.[4] Food labels that describe the health benefits of food products provide important information for consumers but can lead to more questions about the relationship between food and health. The mass media carry articles about "functional foods," or foods that appear to have a health benefit over and above any known nutrients they contain. For example, researchers have found that phytoestrogens, which are found in soy products, may decrease one's risk of cardiovascular disease and bone loss in later years. (We talk more about food labels and health concerns in Chapter 9.)

Food and Lifestyle

Lifestyle patterns are bringing about changes in the types of foods and the nutrition information needed by consumers. A recent national survey reported that a growing proportion of men are doing the food shopping and meal preparation for their family,[5] suggesting that food and nutrition information, traditionally directed toward women in the household, should be formatted to appeal to men as well. The growing trend of eating more meals away from home shows no sign of decline and can have a detrimental effect on nutrient intake.[6] All-you-can-eat buffets and "portion distortion" (portions that greatly exceed food guide recommendations) are likely contributors to overweight, particularly in view of the finding that two thirds of all consumers eat everything on their restaurant plate.[7] Also, families are in a hurry for dinner and want recipes that can be prepared in 15 to 20 minutes.[8] Helping individuals learn to make better choices when eating out and to quickly prepare nutritionally appropriate and nutrient-dense meals at home remains a challenge for nutrition educators. The information explosion on the Internet has provided new sources of health and nutrition advice for the eager consumer. Unfortunately, many users are not able to evaluate the quality of information provided and may, for example, be particularly susceptible to the sale of herbs or supplements that make unfounded health claims.

NUTRITION AND HEALTH PROMOTION

A major goal for health professionals in this century will be the prevention and control of chronic diseases. Advances in sanitation and public health brought about a precipitous decline in the number of deaths from infectious diseases such as tuberculosis and pneumonia during the past 100 years. However, we have not made the same degree of progress in reducing death and disability from chronic diseases that increase as we age. Heart disease, cancer, and stroke have been the three leading causes of death in the United States and most industrialized nations for the past 50 years.[9] Sound nutrition and regular physical activity are well-recognized preventive behaviors for these conditions. No longer can we define health as simply the absence of overt disease; rather, we must direct our efforts toward helping individuals of all ages achieve optimum health status and delay chronic health problems. In this and succeeding chapters, we will gain perspective on how we can improve the life and health of those who come to be in our care.

THE SCIENCE OF NUTRITION

The study of nutrition builds on two fundamental areas of science. First, the physical sciences of biochemistry and physiology help us see how nutrition relates to our physical health and well-being. Second, the behavioral sciences help us better understand how nutrition is interwoven with our unique nature as human beings and what influences our food habits. Throughout our study, you will see both of these areas of learning at work in our lives.

The basic principles of biochemistry teach us that, in our physical being, human organisms are highly complex groupings of chemical compounds constantly at work in an array of reactions designed to sustain life. Nutrients, the basic currency of nutrition, are chemical compounds or elements that participate in these many chemical reactions. The integrating work of human physiology brings the beauty of order to the millions of individually functioning cells and organs, blending them into a total functioning whole. Physiologists call this highly sensitive level of internal control homeostasis.

However, if we were defined only by our physical and biologic components, we would not be fully human. We learn human aspects of being and nutrition from the behavioral sciences, which are rooted in our earliest awareness of psychosocial interactions and life experiences. Attitudes toward food and eating patterns develop throughout the lifespan from the acculturating influences of our primary family and relatives, friends, ethnic or cultural group, community, nation, and even the world. How we perceive ourselves and our food, what we choose to eat, why we eat what we do, and the manner in which we eat all become integral parts of human nutrition.

FOOD AND NUTRIENTS

The word nutrition refers to nourishment that sustains life. It centers on the food people eat and how it nourishes their lives, not only physically but also socially and personally. The science and art of human nutrition both focus on nourishing human life, and they do this in many ways. From the moment of conception until death, an appropriate diet supports optimum growth and maturation, mental and physical well-being, and resistance to disease. Nutrition and diet play a role in promoting health and reducing the risk of many adverse conditions, ranging from low birth weight to diabetes mellitus, cardiovascular disease, and cancer.[10] We need energy to carry out vital functions such as breathing, adapting to changes in our environment, and engaging in physical activity. We must constantly replenish our energy stores with food to sustain physical life. But food also nourishes the human spirit. We all have our particular "soul food," our comfort foods, that connect us to our family and provide a sense of psychological and spiritual well-being.

Nutrition is thus defined as the food people eat and how it nourishes their bodies. Nutritional science comprises the body of scientific knowledge that defines the nutritional requirements for body maintenance, growth, activity, and reproduction. Dietetics is the health profession that has primary responsibility for the practical application of nutritional science to persons and groups of persons in various conditions of health and disease. The registered dietitian (RD) is the nutrition expert on the healthcare team. The RD, in collaboration with the physician and nurse, carries the major responsibility for the nutritional care of patients. The public health nutritionist is responsible for nutritional care of groups of people in the community, especially those at high risk, such as pregnant teenagers or elderly persons, who require assessment of need and community programs to meet those needs. RDs working in the community may develop food and nutrition lessons for school health classes, help school food service managers develop lunch menus that are lower in fat, or assist clients at health clubs or fitness centers in planning diets consistent with improved body composition or athletic performance.

Functions of Food and Nutrients

The respective functions of food and nutrients in human nutrition need to be distinguished. First, we must dispense with the myth that any particular food or food combination is required by the body to ensure health. The human race has survived for centuries on wide varieties of foods, depending on what was available to eat and what the culture designated as human food. Various foods serve as important vehicles for taking nutrients into the body and for bringing human pleasure and comfort. It is the specific chemical compounds or elements—the nutrients—found in foods that the body requires.

dietetics Management of diet and the use of food; the science concerned with the nutritional planning and preparation of foods.

homeostasis State of relative dynamic equilibrium within the body's internal environment; a balance achieved through the operation of various interrelated physiologic mechanisms.

nutrients Substances in food that are essential for energy, growth, normal functioning of the body, and maintenance of life.

nutrition The sum of the processes involved in taking in food nutrients and in assimilating and using them to maintain body tissue and provide energy; a foundation for life and health.

nutritional science The body of scientific knowledge, developed through controlled research, that relates to the processes involved in nutrition—national, international, community, and clinical.

public health nutritionist A professional nutritionist who has completed an academic university program and special graduate study (MPH, DrPH) in a school of public health accredited by the American Association of Public Health and is responsible for nutrition components of public health programs in varied community settings—county, state, national, international.

registered dietitian (RD) A professional dietitian who has completed an accredited academic program and 900 hours of postbaccalaureate supervised professional practice and has passed the National Registration Examination for Dietitians administered by the American Dietetic Association.

Approximately 50 nutrients have been determined to be essential to human life and health, although countless other elements and molecules found in the human body are being researched and may in time be found to be essential. The identification of all possible essential nutrients is of particular concern to health professionals responsible for developing formulas for enteral and parenteral nutrition of the critically and chronically ill. Known essential nutrients include macronutrients—carbohydrates, fats, and proteins—whose constituent substances supply energy and build tissue, and micronutrients—vitamins and minerals—that the body uses in much smaller amounts to form specialized structures and to regulate and control body processes. Water is the often forgotten vital nutrient that sustains all of our life systems. The term metabolism refers to the sum of these chemical processes in the body that use nutrients to sustain life and health. The first part of this text will cover your study of these important nutrients. In later chapters we will look at the ways these nutrients participate in the growth and health of persons of various ages and at intervention strategies for those with acute or chronic disease.

Nutrient Interrelationships

An important concept that will continue to emerge in our study of nutrition is the fundamental principle of *nutrient interaction.* It consists of two parts.

1. Individual nutrients have many specific metabolic functions; in some functions, a nutrient will have a primary role, whereas in others, it will play a supporting role.
2. No nutrient ever works alone.

The human body is a fascinating whole made up of many parts and processes. Intimate metabolic relationships exist among all the basic nutrients and their metabolites. This key principle of nutrient interaction will be demonstrated more clearly in the following chapters. Remember, we may separate nutrients to simplify our study of nutrition, but they do not exist that way in the body. Nutrients are always interacting as a dynamic whole to produce and maintain the human body, providing energy, building and rebuilding tissue, and regulating metabolic processes. This synergy among nutrients likely plays a role in diet and health relationships and may impose a limitation on research studies that examine the effects of only one nutrient at a time.[11] In the next section, we briefly introduce the various classes of nutrients as a prelude to our detailed study of their roles and actions in the body.

ENERGY SOURCES

The energy-yielding nutrients—carbohydrates, fats, and proteins—provide primary and alternate sources of energy.

Carbohydrates

Dietary carbohydrates, the starches and sugars, are the body's primary source of fuel for heat and energy. One form of carbohydrate is the stored source of energy known as *glycogen.* Glycogen is sometimes called "animal starch" because its structure is so similar to that of plant starch. Each gram of carbohydrate, when metabolized in the body, yields 4 kilocalories (kcalories). This number is called the "fuel factor." A well-balanced diet for a healthy person usually supplies approximately 50% to 60% of the total kcalories from carbohydrates. The majority of these kcalories should be derived from complex carbohydrate foods (starches) and a smaller amount should be derived from simple carbohydrate foods (sugars).

Fats

Dietary fats from animal and plant sources provide the body's alternate, or storage, form of heat and energy. Fat is a more concentrated fuel, yielding 9 kcalories for each gram metabolized. The fuel factor of fats is therefore 9. It has been generally accepted that fats should supply no more than 25% to 30% of the total kcalories in a well-balanced diet. The majority of this fat, approximately two thirds, should consist of unsaturated fats, with only about one third coming from saturated fats.

Proteins

The body can draw on dietary or tissue protein to obtain needed energy when the fuel supply from carbohydrates and fats is insufficient. Protein yields 4 kcalories/g, making its fuel factor 4. Quality protein should provide approximately 15% to 20% of the total kcalories in a well-balanced diet of a healthy individual. Although protein's primary function is tissue building, some may be available for energy as needed.

TISSUE BUILDING

Protein is the primary nutrient used in tissue building; minerals, vitamins, and fatty acids also play important roles.

Proteins

The primary function of protein is tissue building. Dietary protein foods provide amino acids, the building units necessary for constructing and repairing body tissues. Body tissues undergo a constant, dynamic process of modeling and remodeling according to need that ensures growth and maintenance of a strong body structure and the production of vital substances for tissue functioning.

Minerals

Minerals have numerous functions in building tissues. For example, two of the major minerals, calcium and phosphorus, provide strength to bone tissue. An interesting structural example is that of the trace element cobalt, which is a central constituent of vitamin B_{12} (cobalamin) and thus functions as a component of this vitamin needed to form red blood cells.

Vitamins

Vitamins are complex molecules needed in very minute amounts; however, they fulfill very important roles in the formation of body tissues. Vitamin C helps form the cementing intercellular ground substance necessary for binding tissues together and preventing tissue bleeding. Vitamin A is found in the rods and cones in the eye that support vision in dim light.

METABOLIC REGULATION AND CONTROL

All of the multiple biochemical processes that make up body metabolism and are required to provide energy and build tissue must be controlled in perfect detail to maintain a smoothly running physiologic system. Otherwise there would be chaos within the body systems and death would eventually ensue. Life and health result from a dynamic balance, or state of homeostasis, among all of the body parts and processes. Vitamins and minerals are nutrients that play a vital role in this metabolic regulation and control; water provides the necessary fluid environment for these chemical reactions to take place.

Minerals

Minerals serve as coenzyme factors in cell metabolism. Iron is necessary for the action of enzymes in the mitochondria of cells that produce and store high-energy compounds for later use.

Vitamins

Many vitamins function as coenzyme factors, or components of cell enzyme systems, to govern chemical reactions in cell metabolism and the synthesis of important molecules. Thiamin, for example, helps govern the release of energy to carry on the work of the cell.

Water

Water functions as a regulatory agent, providing the essential solution base for all metabolic processes. Water also forms the blood, lymph, and intercellular fluids that transport needed nutrients to cells and remove waste.

LEVELS OF NUTRITIONAL STATUS

Nutritional status refers to the general nutritional health of an individual. It will vary depending on a person's living situation, available food supply, and health. You will be concerned with these varying levels as you assess your own nutritional status or that of others.

Ideal Nutrition

Ideal nutritional status, sometimes referred to as *optimum nutritional status,* should be our goal as health professionals. Evidence of optimum nutrition includes a well-developed body, ideal body weight for height with an appropriate body composition (ratio of muscle mass to fat), and good muscle development and tone. The skin is smooth and clear, the hair is glossy, and the eyes are clear and bright. Posture is good; the facial expression is alert. Appetite, digestion, and elimination are normal. Detailed characteristics of good and poor states of nutrition are given in Table 1-1. Begin to think about these signs as you progress in your study of nutrition and look for them as you become a more skilled observer. Well-nourished persons are much more likely to be alert, both mentally and physically. They are not only meeting their day-to-day needs but also maintaining essential nutrient reserves for resisting infectious diseases and extending their years of normal functioning.

Borderline Nutrition

As the descriptive label indicates, persons with only *borderline* or *marginal nutritional status* may be meeting their minimum day-to-day nutritional needs, but they lack nutrition reserves to meet any added physiologic or metabolic demand from injury or illness, to sustain fetal development during pregnancy, or to attain proper growth in childhood. A state of borderline nutrition may exist in persons with poor eating habits or in those who are living in stressed environments on low incomes.

Write Down

amino acid An acid containing the essential element nitrogen (in the chemical group NH_2). Amino acids are the structural units of protein and the basic building blocks of the body.

kilocalorie The general term *calorie* refers to a unit of heat measure and is used alone to designate the *small calorie.* The calorie used in nutritional science and the study of metabolism is the *large calorie,* 1000 calories, or kilocalorie, to be more accurate and to avoid use of very large numbers in calculations.

macronutrients The three large energy-yielding nutrients: carbohydrates, fats, and proteins.

metabolism Sum of all the various biochemical and physiologic processes by which the body grows and maintains itself (anabolism) and breaks down and reshapes tissue (catabolism) and transforms energy to do its work. Products of these various reactions are called *metabolites.*

metabolites Any substance produced by metabolism or by a metabolic process.

micronutrients The two classes of small non–energy-yielding elements and compounds: minerals and vitamins are essential for regulation and control functions in cell metabolism and for building certain body structures.

TABLE 1-1 Clinical Signs of Nutritional Status

Features	Good Nutritional Status	Poor Nutritional Status
General appearance	Alert, responsive	Listless, apathetic, cachectic
Hair	Shiny, lustrous, healthy scalp	Stringy, dull, brittle, dry, depigmented
Neck glands	No enlargement	Thyroid enlarged
Skin, face, neck	Smooth, slightly moist, good color, reddish pink mucous membranes	Greasy, discolored, scaly
Eyes	Bright, clear, no fatigue circles	Dryness, signs of infection, increased vascularity, glassiness, thickened conjunctivae
Lips	Good color, moist	Dry, scaly, swollen, angular lesions (stomatitis)
Tongue	Good pink color, surface papillae present, no lesions	Papillary atrophy, smooth appearance, swollen, red, beefy (glossitis)
Gums	Good pink color, no swelling or bleeding, firm	Marginal redness or swelling, receding, spongy
Teeth	Straight, no crowding, well-shaped jaw, clean, no discoloration	Unfilled cavities, absent teeth, worn surfaces, mottled, malpositioned
Skin, general	Smooth, slightly moist, good color	Rough, dry, scaly, pale, pigmented, irritated; petechiae, bruises
Abdomen	Flat	Swollen
Legs, feet	No tenderness, weakness, swelling, good color	Edema, tender calf, tingling, weakness
Skeleton	No malformations	Bowlegs, knock-knees, chest deformity at diaphragm, beaded ribs, prominent scapulas
Weight	Normal for height, age, body build	Overweight or underweight
Posture	Erect, arms and legs straight, abdomen in, chest out	Sagging shoulders, sunken chest, humped back
Muscles	Well-developed, firm	Flaccid, poor tone, undeveloped, tender
Nervous control	Good attention span for age, does not cry easily, not irritable or restless	Inattentive, irritable
Gastrointestinal function	Good appetite and digestion, normal, regular elimination	Anorexia, indigestion, constipation or diarrhea
General vitality	Endurance, energetic, sleeps well at night, vigorous	Easily fatigued, no energy, falls asleep in school, looks tired, apathetic

Other persons select poor-quality diets on the basis of taste or convenience, even though they may have the economic means to purchase a nutritionally adequate diet.[12] A U.S. survey found that some adults obtained 20% of their total kcalories from desserts and sugars, foods that are high in energy but low in vitamins and minerals. Those who obtained the most kcalories from these foods had lower blood levels of vitamin A, folate, and other important vitamins.[13] Individuals with poorer food habits, as just described, may not be undernourished; some persons can maintain general health on somewhat less than the optimal amounts of various nutrients. On the average, however, persons who do not receive the recommended amounts of nutrients have greater risk of physical illness than do persons who are well nourished. The human body has great capacity to adapt to such lowered nutritional states, but it can sustain only a given amount of physiologic stress before signs of malnutrition appear.

Malnutrition

Signs of *malnutrition* appear when nutritional reserves are depleted and nutrient and energy intake is not sufficient to meet day-to-day needs or an added metabolic stress. A large number of malnourished people live in high-risk conditions of poverty with diets that are lacking in both quantity and quality of food. Dietary surveys estimate that 4.2 million households in the United States, accounting for more than 11 million persons, have an inadequate supply of appropriate food because they do not have enough money to buy food, and in over 800,000 of these households hunger is severe.[14]

Conditions of hunger influence the health of all persons involved, but especially the lives of those who are most vulnerable—infants, children, pregnant women, and elderly adults. Prenatal care for many women who are poor, young, and lacking in education is often inadequate or nonexistent, resulting in poor pregnancy outcomes and higher infant mortality rates. Children who live in persistent poverty may experience stunted growth or deficiency diseases such as anemia, with lowered resistance to infections, impaired learning ability, and reduced activity levels. Chronically inadequate diets in the young child prevent catch-up growth after episodes of infection and can have lasting effects.[15] Hunger and malnutrition exist in the growing number of homeless persons, estimated to equal more than 500,000 in the United States.[16,17] Low socioeconomic status and physical disability are related to malnutrition in older adults.[18,19]

We also find malnutrition in hospital patients and residents of long-term care facilities. Hypermetabolic diseases or prolonged illness, especially among older persons with low nutrient reserves, can lead to debilitating weight loss and nutrient depletion. Many prescription medications used in the management of chronic diseases have an adverse effect on nutritional status. Nutrition assessment procedures, fundamental to appropriate clinical care, are described in Chapter 15.

Overnutrition

Some persons may be in a state of *overnutrition* with some degree of overweight and obesity resulting from excess energy intake and low levels of physical activity over time. We have come to recognize overnutrition as a form of malnutrition, especially when inappropriately high kcaloric intake produces excessive and harmful body weight and fatness. Childhood and adolescent obesity may set the stage for continuing adult obesity, increasing the risk for chronic disease. In the United States, almost one in five adults is obese, representing an increase of 61% in only 9 years.[20] In addition, nearly 60% of adults are considered overweight compared with only 45% ten years earlier, contributing to what healthcare professionals have described as the "obesity epidemic" that is occurring worldwide.[20,21] Of major concern is the growing overweight observed in children. More than 20% of U.S. children are above their recommended weight for height,[22] and this overweight coupled with a lack of physical activity is playing a role in the rapid increase in the diagnosis of type 2 diabetes among children and adolescents.[23]

Harmful overnutrition also occurs in persons who use excessive amounts of nutrient supplements that, over time, produce damaging effects on tissues. A recent report suggested that men eating 2 or 3 times the recommended serving size of highly fortified cereals could be taking in excess amounts of iron and folate, especially if they also use multivitamin or mineral supplements.[24] In addition, herbs are increasing in popularity as nutritional supplements, and interactions between nutrients and herbs are not well understood.

Nutrition Policy and National Health Problems

DIET, NUTRITION, AND CHRONIC DISEASE

Throughout the twentieth century, improvements in sanitation and the discovery of antibiotics and other valuable medicines led to a rapid decline in the number of deaths from infectious disease. The decline in infectious disease was paralleled by a steady rise in the prevalence of chronic diseases that develop as people age.[9] These chronic health problems include coronary heart disease, hypertension, cancer, diabetes mellitus, pulmonary disease, and obesity, which are contributing to the continued rise in healthcare costs. As we approached the new millennium, scientists, health professionals, and government policy-makers began to examine various lifestyle factors, including nutrition, that play a role in the prevention of chronic diseases that lead to death or disability.

Nutrition and Health

Research conducted in the 1960s and 1970s at universities, private research institutes, and government agencies began to provide a growing mass of evidence that dietary habits were a major influence on the development of heart disease, the number one cause of death in the United States. Congressional committees began to consider the role of the government in setting dietary guidelines for the general public in an effort to improve health. The first major policy report issued by the U.S. government linking nutrition and chronic disease was the *Surgeon General's Report on Nutrition and Health,*[25] released in 1988. This document reviewed the effects of the typical American diet on the incidence of cardiovascular disease and early death. Based on the evidence presented and the magnitude of the health problems involved, the American people were urged to reduce their use of foods high in fats and salt and to increase their use of foods high in complex carbohydrates and fiber.

Diet and Health

In 1989, the Diet and Health Committee of the Food and Nutrition Board, National Research Council, issued its extensive research report, *Diet and Health: Implications for*

anemia Blood condition characterized by decreased number of circulating red blood cells, hemoglobin, or both.

Reducing Chronic Disease Risk.[26] Their recommendations agreed with those of the Surgeon General and advised persons to (1) reduce total fat intake to 30% or less of total kcalories, with associated reductions in saturated fats and cholesterol; (2) increase intake of fiber and complex carbohydrates; (3) avoid excessive intakes of sodium and protein; and (4) maintain appropriate levels of calcium.

Healthy People 2010

In 1990, the U.S. Department of Health and Human Services (USDHHS) developed a public health initiative that addressed issues of diet, physical activity, and other health-related lifestyle factors with specific objectives and national health goals to be achieved by the year 2000.[27] Although some goals were achieved by the targeted date, others relating to the prevalence of obesity, intakes of appropriate foods, desirable levels of physical activity, and preventive healthcare practices fell short of their objectives. *Healthy People 2010* was developed to continue the work of *Healthy People 2000* with a new set of objectives and target indicators related to health and healthcare.[28,29] The overall goals for *Healthy People 2010* include (1) increasing the years of healthy life and (2) reducing the disparities in healthcare that exist among individuals of different races, ethnic groups, and income levels. As you continue your study of the nutrients and specific population groups, refer to the *Healthy People 2010* objectives that relate to our discussion.

Nutrition Guides for Health Promotion

Beginning in the early 1900s, a number of food and nutrient guides have been developed to help Americans meet their nutrition and health needs. A number of underlying assumptions about food, nutrition, and health have directed the design of these guides and have reflected not only developing nutritional science but also social, political, and economic events of the times including wars and national emergencies. Consistent with changing health problems, the focus of these guides has shifted from preventing primary deficiency diseases resulting from insufficient nutritional intake to controlling chronic diseases related to affluence and excess.

In general, these nutrition guides are classified into three groups: nutrition standards, food guides, and dietary guidelines, with each having a different purpose. They are reviewed briefly here for reference and guidance in your study.

NUTRIENT STANDARDS

U.S. Standards

Most of the developed countries of the world have set standards for the intake of major nutrients by healthy persons categorized by age and sex. These standards, based on current scientific knowledge, are not intended to indicate individual requirements or therapeutic needs related to illness or disease. Rather, they serve as a reference for intake levels of the essential nutrients judged to be adequate to meet the known nutritional needs of most healthy people. In the United States, these nutrient and energy standards have been called the Recommended Dietary Allowances (RDAs). Standards developed in other countries may vary somewhat according to their purpose and use. Nutrient standards are designed for use by professionals who make decisions regarding the nutritional health of individuals and groups.

Development of the RDAs

The first RDA standards grew out of a national nutrition conference held in 1941 during World War II.[30] These nutrient and energy recommendations, based on developing nutrition science, were first published in 1943 as a guide for nutrition workers in planning and obtaining food supplies for national defense and general population needs. After this first edition of the RDAs, a revised edition was published about every 4 to 5 years to reflect expanding scientific research. The tenth edition, issued in 1989, was the work of the Subcommittee on Dietary Allowances of the Food and Nutrition Board, National Research Council.[31]

During the 1990s, U.S. and Canadian nutrition experts recognized the need for an expanded framework for dietary standards that would (1) address the needs of the growing population of older adults, (2) apply new research findings that suggest beneficial effects of particular nutrient intake levels when there is insufficient research data available to establish an RDA (Adequate Intake [AI]), and (3) draw attention to the dangers of inappropriately high intakes of specific nutrients (Tolerable Upper Intake Level [UL]). This expanded framework of standards was given the working title of Dietary Reference Intakes (DRIs). The DRIs have highlighted the nutritional requirements of the growing numbers of older people in the United States and worldwide. The RDA age category that formerly included all persons aged 51 years and over was divided into two groups: 51 to 70 and 71 and over. This allows us to recognize the continuing changes in nutrient requirements that occur as people age.

The first set of DRIs released in 1997 provided us with new standards for calcium, phosphorus, magnesium, and vitamin D and emphasized the role of calcium and vitamin D in bone health.[32] Several reports have followed that reviewed new findings and recommendations for intake of the B complex vitamins (1998)[33]; provided new information regarding important antioxidant nutrients and carotenoids (2000)[34]; updated recommendations for vitamins A and K and the trace minerals (2001)[35]; and most recently set standards for the energy-supplying macronutrients, energy, and fiber (2002).[36] The new recommendations for carbohydrate, fat, and protein as percentages of total energy have been given the name *Acceptable Macronutrient Distribution Ranges (AMDRs)*. The AMDRs differ somewhat from the general guidelines for the U.S. population presented on p. 6. It is important for nutrition educators to review both sets of recommendations when developing meal plans for individuals. (The RDAs and DRIs can be found on the inside cover of your textbook.)

Other Standards

Canadian and British standards are similar to the U.S. standards. In less-developed countries where such factors as quality of available protein foods must be considered, workers usually look to standards set by the Food and Agriculture Organization (FAO) of the World Health Organization (WHO). All of these standards provide nutrient and energy guidelines to help health workers in a variety of locations promote physical well-being through sound nutrition.

FOOD GROUPS GUIDES

To interpret and apply sound nutrient standards, health workers need practical food guides to use in nutrition education and meal planning. Two such food guides developed for use by the general public are the basic food groups guide and the food exchange lists. As we will see these guides are very different in nature and serve different needs.

Basic Food Groups Guide

Probably the most familiar food group guide is the *Basic Four Food Groups Guide* issued by the U.S. Department of Agriculture (USDA). Over the years, the USDA has issued a succession of basic food guides, each reflecting the scientific understanding and nutritional concerns of the time. In 1991, the USDA issued a new edition, supporting current national goals for increasing energy intake from carbohydrates with foods from the fruit, vegetable, and grain groups. This revision also recommended controlling energy intake from fat by modifying food choices from the milk, meat, and fat groups.[37] This new approach, titled *The Guide to Daily Food Choices,* is summarized in Table 1-2.

To make these concepts come alive for the general public, the *Food Guide Pyramid* (FGP) (Figure 1-1) was developed to visually illustrate the relative amounts of each food group to be included in the daily diet.[38,39] The FGP has proved to be a useful educational tool that represents a total diet and is easy to understand. Nevertheless, critical issues remain for nutrition educators. At the time the FGP was developed in the early 1990s, it met the RDAs for all nutrients and age groups with the exception of the iron recommendation in pregnancy.[40] However, researchers suggest that to meet the current DRI for calcium, persons will require additional portions from the milk group or the use of calcium-containing dark-green leafy vegetables.[41] Also, a foundation of the FGP is the recommendation that an individual eat a variety of foods within each of the five groups to obtain all necessary nutrients. Eating a greater variety of healthful foods has been associated with lower mortality rates, most likely related to the simultaneous interplay of several nutrients and other substances. However, it must be made clear to consumers that we need to eat many different foods with a focus on the fruit, vegetable, and grain groups.[42] The inclusion of a variety of foods high in fat or sugars can contribute to unwanted weight gain.

To meet the needs of nutrition educators working with specific age groups, three new FGPs, *Food Guide Pyramid for Children Ages 2 to 6,*[43] *Modified Food Guide Pyramid for People Age 55 and Over,*[44] and *Modified Food Guide Pyramid for People Ages 70+,*[45] were developed. A variety of FGPs based on the eating patterns of various ethnic or cultural groups, such as the *Mexican-American Food Guide Pyramid,* the *Chinese Food Guide Pyramid,* and the *Vegetarian Food Guide Pyramid,* are also available to assist health professionals.

The *Exchange Lists* Food Guide

The *Exchange Lists for Meal Planning* was first introduced in 1950 by the American Diabetes Association and the American Dietetic Association as a meal-planning tool for assisting persons with diabetes. Although the FGP is organized according to food groups providing protein or specific vitamins and minerals, the *Exchange Lists for Meal Planning* groups foods on the basis of equivalent energy values. This guide is a useful tool for calculating and planning any diet, such as those for weight reduction, in which control of the energy-yielding nutrients—carbohydrate, fat, and protein—as well as total kcalories is the goal.

Because the foods in each group in the exchange system are equal to one another when eaten in the portions indicated, items can be freely exchanged within individual groups, thus maintaining consistent food values and kcalories. At the same time this freedom of exchange within groups allows a greater variety of foods and food

---

Adequate Intake (AI) Suggested daily intake of a nutrient to meet daily needs and support health; AIs have a more limited research base than do the RDAs but were developed to address current health concerns; the AI for calcium is expected to reduce the risk of bone loss and bone fractures in older adults.

Dietary Reference Intakes (DRIs) Term referring to the framework of nutrient standards now in place in the United States; this includes the Recommended Dietary Allowances, Adequate Intakes, and Tolerable Upper Intake Level.

Recommended Dietary Allowances (RDAs) Recommended daily allowances of nutrients and energy intake for population groups according to age and sex, with defined weight and height. The RDAs are established and reviewed periodically by a representative group of nutritional scientists in response to current research. These standards are very similar among the developed countries.

Tolerable Upper Intake Level (UL) The highest amount of a vitamin or mineral that can be consumed with safety; this standard was developed to advise people regarding inappropriate intakes of nutrient supplements.

TABLE 1-2 The Guide to Daily Food Choices: A Summary

Food Group	Number of Servings	Major Contributions	Foods and Serving Sizes*
Bread, cereals, rice, pasta	6-11	Starch Thiamin Riboflavin† Iron Niacin Folate Magnesium‡ Fiber‡ Zinc	1 slice of bread 1 oz ready-to-eat cereal ½-¾ cup cooked cereal, rice, pasta
Vegetables	3-5	Vitamin A Vitamin C Folate Magnesium Fiber	½ cup raw or cooked vegetables 1 cup raw leafy vegetables
Fruits	2-4	Vitamin C Fiber	¼ cup dried fruit ½ cup cooked fruit ¾ cup juice 1 whole piece of fruit 1 melon wedge
Milk, yogurt, cheese	2 (adults§) 3 (children, teenagers, young adults, pregnant or lactating women)	Calcium Riboflavin Protein Potassium Zinc	1 cup milk or fortified soy milk 1½ oz cheese 2 oz processed cheese 1 cup yogurt 2 cups cottage cheese 1 cup custard/pudding 1½ cups ice cream
Meat, poultry, fish, dry beans, eggs, nuts	2-3	Protein Niacin Iron Vitamin B_6 Zinc Thiamin Vitamin B_{12}‖	2-3 oz cooked meat, poultry, fish 1-1½ cups cooked dry beans 4 tbsp peanut butter 2 eggs ½-1 cup nuts
Fats, oils, sweets	Foods from this group should not replace any from the other groups. Amounts consumed should be determined by individual energy needs.		

From the U.S. Department of Agriculture, revised edition of former *Basic Four Food Groups Guide.*
*May be reduced for child servings.
†If enriched.
‡Whole grains especially.
§Age of at least 25 years.
‖Present only in animal food choices.

combinations to be used in planning meals and snacks. The six food groups included in the original exchange lists were starch/bread, fruit, vegetable, meat, milk, and fats. This food exchange group guide came to be widely used as a nutrition tool for meal planning, education, and counseling.

In 1986, the exchange lists were revised in accordance with new research and national dietary guidelines for the reduction of chronic disease. Meat and milk items were categorized according to their fat content, and saturated and unsaturated fat sources were described. Starch/bread items with added sugar were placed in a separate group, and food sources of sodium and fiber were flagged. Combination foods as well as lists of free foods and seasonings were added to assist in menu management.

The most recent revision of the *Exchange Lists for Meal Planning,* released in 1995, can be found in Appendix L.[46] Foods were arranged into three groups for easier use.

1. *Carbohydrate group.* This group includes the previous carbohydrate lists—starch (including bread), fruits,

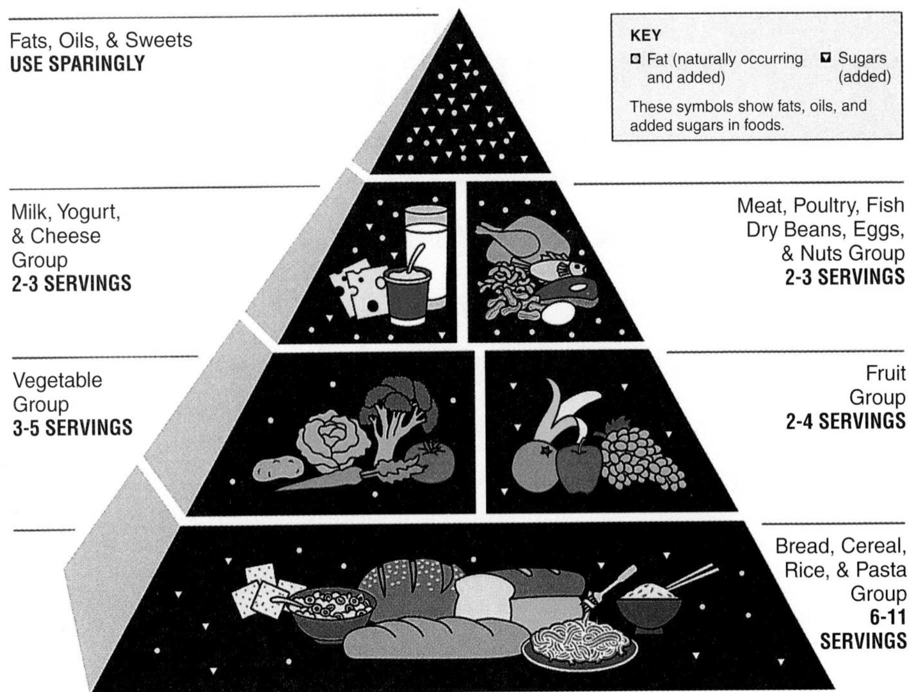

FIGURE 1-1 Eating right pyramid. A guide to daily food choices. *(Modified from the U.S. Department of Agriculture, 1992.)*

vegetables, milk—and a new list of other carbohydrates, such as cakes, cookies, and other sweets.

2. *Meat and meat substitutes group.* This group includes the protein foods previously in the meat list (lean, medium-fat, and high-fat) and a new list of very lean items and various meat substitutes.
3. *Fat group.* The fat foods are divided into three lists—monounsaturated, polyunsaturated, and saturated—to assist users in choosing smaller amounts of polyunsaturated and saturated fats and larger amounts of monounsaturated fats, while limiting total fat intake.

Other additions to help individuals plan an appropriate food pattern include lists of fat-modified, vegetarian, and fast-food items. The most recent edition of the exchange lists also provides tips on how to purchase and prepare certain foods. A booklet describing *Exchange Lists for Weight Management* is also available.[47]

DIETARY GUIDELINES

Dietary guidelines are intended for use by the general public but differ from food guides in two ways. First, dietary guidelines tend to be general in the advice they provide rather than quantifying food use as do food guides. Second, dietary guidelines are directed toward health concerns and call attention to proposed food habit changes that will reduce chronic disease risk and enhance health.

Beginning in 1980, several editions of the *Dietary Guidelines for Americans* have been issued in the United States in response to the growing health concerns of government agencies, professional groups, and the public.

U.S. Dietary Guidelines

Nutrition and Your Health: The Dietary Guidelines for Americans developed from public and professional concerns about our changing food environment and the chronic disease risk in our aging population. These publications represent a cooperative effort between the two federal government agencies concerned with food (USDA) and health (USDHHS). The statements emphasizing moderation and variety in food habits along with regular physical activity relate current scientific thinking to the leading U.S. health problems and the behavior changes needed to reduce the prevalence of these problems.[48] They are meant for healthy children aged 2 and older and adults of all ages.

In the most recent edition of the dietary guidelines, published in 2000, health messages are organized into three parts, the ABCs of good health,[48,49] to assist consumers in making food and lifestyle choices (Figure 1-2). First, there is increased emphasis on physical activity, based on the growing prevalence of obesity among Americans of all ages, and the association of overweight with increased risk of heart disease, stroke, diabetes mellitus, and cancer. In this edition, consumers are referred to the

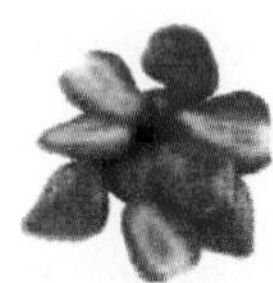

DIETARY GUIDELINES FOR AMERICANS

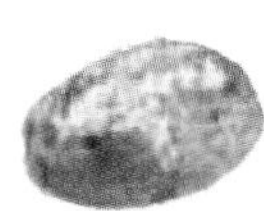

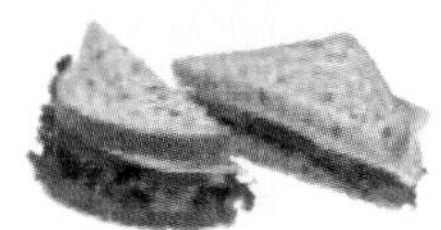

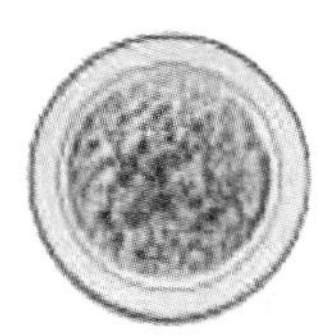

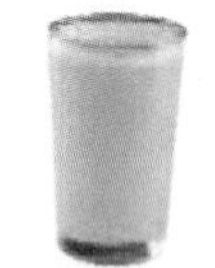

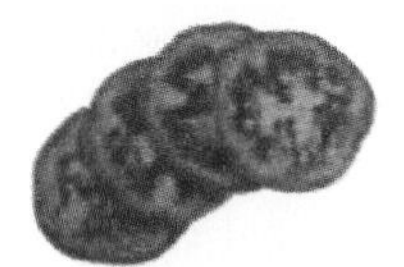

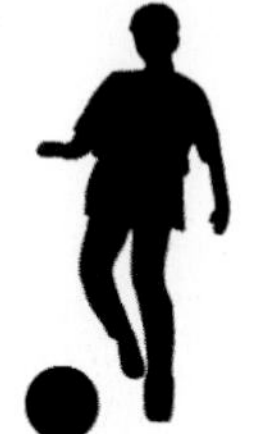

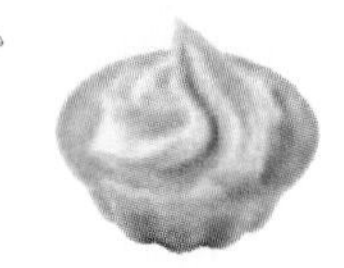

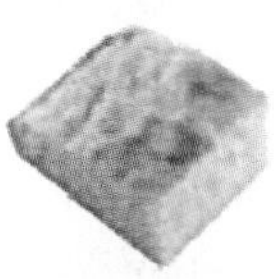

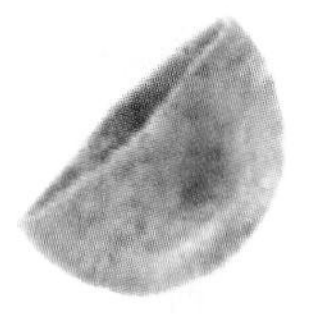

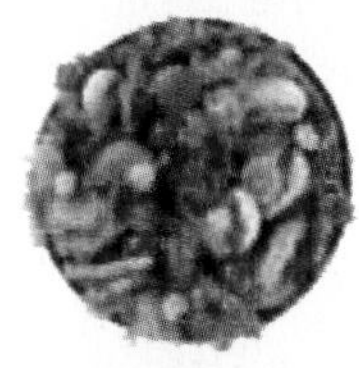

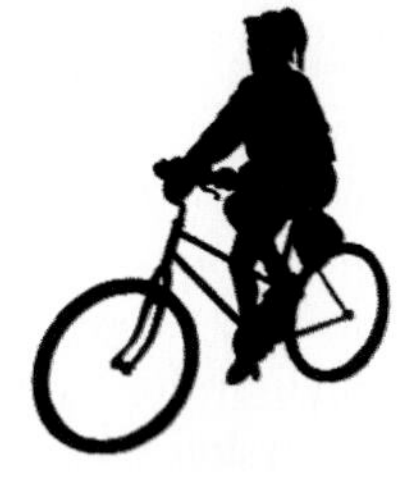

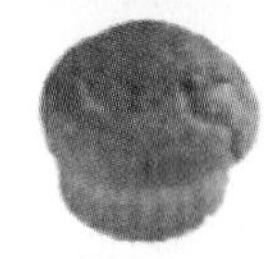

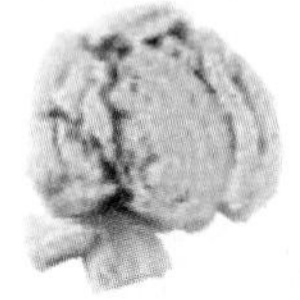

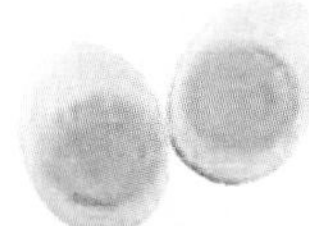

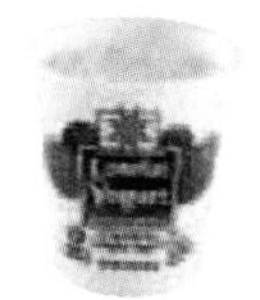

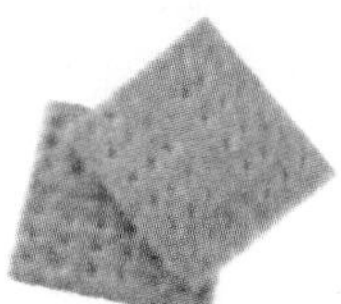

AIM FOR FITNESS...

- ▲ Aim for a healthy weight.
- ▲ Be physically active each day.

BUILD A HEALTHY BASE...

- ■ Let the Pyramid guide your food choices.
- ■ Choose a variety of grains daily, especially whole grains.
- ■ Choose a variety of fruits and vegetables daily.
- ■ Keep food safe to eat.

CHOOSE SENSIBLY...

- ● Choose a diet that is low in saturated fat and cholesterol and moderate in total fat.
- ● Choose beverages and foods to moderate your intake of sugars.
- ● Choose and prepare foods with less salt.
- ● If you drink alcoholic beverages, do so in moderation.

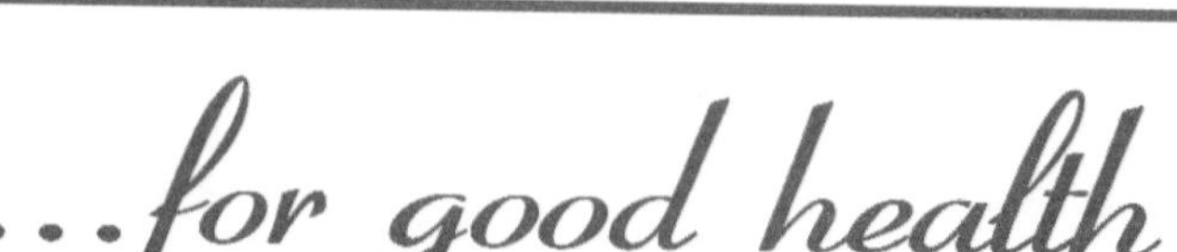

FIGURE 1-2 Dietary Guidelines for Americans. (*U.S. Department of Agriculture, U.S. Department of Health and Human Services:* Nutrition and your health: dietary guidelines for Americans, *ed 5, Home and Garden Bulletin No 232, Washington, DC, 2000, U.S. Government Printing Office* [*accessible at* http://www.usda.gov/cnpp].)

PRACTICAL APPLICATION

Nutrition and Your Health: Dietary Guidelines for Americans

Eating is one of life's greatest pleasures. Because there are many foods and many ways to build a healthy diet and lifestyle, there is lots of opportunity for choice. The suggestions included with the guidelines can help you and those you counsel find ways to enjoy food and physical activity as part of a healthy lifestyle.

The Dietary Guidelines for Americans carry three basic messages—the ABCs for good health.

Aim for fitness
Build a healthy base
Choose sensibly

Each of these messages includes important guidelines for building a healthy lifestyle.

AIM FOR FITNESS

- Aim for a healthy weight.
- Be physically active each day.

Following these two guidelines will help keep you healthy and fit.

Calculate your body mass index and talk with a health professional about reachable goals if you are not at a healthy weight. Regular physical exercise can prevent unwanted weight gain and assist in losing excess body fat. Daily physical activity enables people of all ages to work productively, enjoy life, and feel their best.

BUILD A HEALTHY BASE

- Let the Pyramid guide your food choices.
- Choose a variety of grains daily, especially whole grains.
- Choose a variety of fruits and vegetables daily.
- Keep food safe to eat.

Use the Food Guide Pyramid as a guide for healthy eating and to ensure that you get the nutrients your body needs each day. Make grains, fruits, and vegetables—the plant foods—the foundation of your meals. The plant foods form a solid base for good nutrition and good health, and can reduce your risk of certain chronic diseases. Be flexible and adventurous—choose new foods from these three groups to replace some of the less nutritious or higher kcalorie foods you usually eat. Always store foods under the appropriate conditions to prevent spoilage and the growth of harmful microorganisms. Remember that children and elderly persons are especially vulnerable to foodborne illness.

CHOOSE SENSIBLY

- Choose a diet that is low in saturated fat and cholesterol and moderate in total fat.
- Choose beverages and foods to moderate your intake of sugars.
- Choose and prepare foods with less salt.
- If you drink alcoholic beverages, do so in moderation.

These four guidelines can help you make sensible food choices that promote health. You can enjoy all foods as part of a healthy diet as long as you practice moderation. Excessive use of high-fat and high-sugar foods or alcohol can lead to unwanted weight gain and replace more nutrient-dense foods in the diet. Inappropriate intakes of fat, sodium, and alcohol also increase disease risk. Read nutrition labels to help you identify foods that are high in saturated fat, sugar, and sodium.

By following all of these guidelines you will improve your health and reduce your risk for cardiovascular disease, certain types of cancer, diabetes, stroke, and osteoporosis. These diseases are leading causes of death and disability among Americans of all ages. Good diets can also improve or prevent the major risk factors for chronic disease, such as obesity, hypertension, and inappropriate blood lipid and cholesterol patterns. Your food choices, your lifestyle, your environment, and your family history all affect your health and physical well-being. It is important for all persons to follow the Dietary Guidelines; however, if you are at higher risk for a chronic disease, it is especially important. So review your family history and identify any other existing conditions or risk factors for disease, to enable you to make more informed decisions about how to improve your health.

Reference

U.S. Department of Agriculture, U.S. Department of Health and Human Services: *Nutrition and your health: dietary guidelines for Americans,* ed 5, Washington, DC, 2000, U.S. Government Printing Office. The entire 40-page booklet can be accessed at *http://www.usda.gov/cnpp.*

FGP for assistance in achieving variety in their diets and including important sources of all major nutrients. Moreover, the FGP suggests both number of portions and portion sizes that may discourage overeating. Finally, the newest edition provides an important message about keeping food safe to eat. Foodborne illness is a growing and preventable public health problem, with particular dangers for the very young and the very old. (The general summary of the 2000 dietary guidelines can be found in the *Practical Application* box.)

Despite these efforts to simplify messages and to provide practical advice for food selection and physical activity, problems remain. Consumers still find it difficult to translate the sugar guideline into specific goals (e.g., how many servings of soft drinks are too many?).[50] For families with limited resources, the current guidelines that focus on recreational activities that require specific equipment or facilities are out of reach.[50] A respected nutrition educator has pointed out that the development of effective nutrition education guidelines requires the efforts of behavioral and communication scientists along with nutrition and biologic scientists.[51] When nutrition messages are not easily understood or implemented, they are more likely to be disregarded entirely.[52]

TO PROBE FURTHER
Personal Perceptions and Analysis of Food Patterns

What are your personal perceptions of your eating pattern? What are your food habits, attitudes, and values related to food? Do you eat regular meals or just snack most of the time? Do you make an effort to choose nutritious foods or eat mostly high-fat and high-sugar items? To find the answers, check yourself for a few days, using some of the procedures discussed here.

1. Keep a detailed record of everything you eat and drink for 3 days: 2 weekdays and 1 weekend day. Make it as complete as possible. Keep a small pocket pad with you and jot down what you eat or drink throughout the day and evening, while your memory is still clear on details. Be sure to note the type of food or ingredients, how much you ate using household measures such as cups or tablespoons, how the food was prepared, and brand name, if applicable. Be specific about the foods you eat; for example, was the milk you drank skim, 1%, 2%, or whole milk? Do not forget details such as butter or margarine on bread; fats, dressings, or salt added to foods in preparation or at the table; or additions to coffee or tea.

   Indicate the factors that influenced your food choices, such as where you ate and at what time. Did you eat alone or with someone, and how were you feeling at the time? Just this brief recording process alone is a good start because it may tell you some things about your eating habits that you were not aware of before. Remember that you are going to analyze this record; therefore make it as readable, accurate, and detailed as possible.
2. Using the Food Guide Pyramid, list the foods you ate or drank under their respective food group as best you can based on their content. For mixed dishes you may need to list ingredients separately, for example, spaghetti, tomato sauce, and meatballs. Compare what you ate with the numbers of servings and portion sizes recommended. Estimate how closely your choices fulfilled the recommended daily food choices and what you may fall short on.
3. Go through the same process of listing each food you ate in its respective food group, this time using the new food exchange lists (Appendix L). Total the amount of each macronutrient you consumed. Look particularly at your total amount of fat (g) and kcalories. How does your intake of fat compare with the recommended level of 25% to 30% of the total day's kcalories as suggested in the Dietary Guidelines? How closely do you match your RDA for kcalories?
4. Using the CD-ROM that came with your textbook, go to your college computer laboratory and enter your foods in the dietary analysis program. Calculate your intakes of both the macronutrients and important micronutrients. Are your kcalories partitioned appropriately? In other words, are you taking in 50% to 60% of your kcalories from carbohydrates, 15% to 20% of your kcalories from protein, and 25% to 30% of your kcalories from fat? How do your intakes compare with the DRIs for a person of your age and sex? If you are not meeting the Dietary Guidelines, suggest foods that you need to add or delete to bring your diet closer to the goals. If you are not consuming at least 70% of the DRI for important vitamins and minerals, suggest foods that you could add to your daily meal pattern that would supply these nutrients.
5. Compare your results using the three methods of dietary evaluation: the Food Guide Pyramid, the *Exchange Lists for Meal Planning*, and the dietary analysis program. Were you meeting your recommended amounts of food or nutrients by all three methods, one or two of the methods, or none of the methods? If your diet had a different level of adequacy when evaluated by one method versus another, what factors might have contributed to this difference? If you were a public health nutritionist working in a clinic serving pregnant women and their preschool children, which dietary assessment method would be most applicable to your work?

Now that you have thought about it, how do you see yourself as an eater? Are there any food behaviors that you may need or want to modify to promote good health? Also, give yourself a pat on the back for those categories where you are meeting current recommendations.

Personal Assessment of Food Patterns

PERSONAL PERCEPTIONS OF FOOD

Traditionally, each one of us develops food habits and ways of eating that are influenced by our ethnic background, cultural or religious beliefs, family habits, socioeconomic status, health status, available food, and personal likes and dislikes. However, the increasing ethnic diversity in our society has brought about a greater intermingling of a variety of foods and ideas about food. How persons perceive themselves in relation to food and food patterns plays an important role in developing their own attitudes toward food and personal eating behavior.

A simple way to get a basic idea of the general nutritional value of your own food pattern is to examine briefly what you actually eat. Keeping a record of everything you eat and drink for a few days, noting the time, place, activity, and persons with you, if any, can provide important insight into our true perceptions of food. Most of us eat by habit, usually according to where we are and what we are doing, and not because of any serious thought or plan. Evaluating what you have to eat and drink each day using the FGP (see Figure 1-1) will provide you with a rough estimate of your use of representative foods in each group. The food exchange lists provided in Appendix L will determine the energy-yielding values of the macronutrients involved in your food choices. The simple approach of analyzing food records by basic food groups and food exchange lists can increase awareness of our personal food patterns and is a rapid way to assess the food patterns of individuals that we counsel in community or healthcare settings. The FGP also has been useful in studies of population groups to provide meaningful information about the quality of their food habits (see *To Probe Further* box for a general outline to assist in evaluating your dietary intake).

NUTRITIONAL ANALYSIS BY NUTRIENTS AND ENERGY VALUES

A more comprehensive nutritional analysis of food intake records for specific macronutrients, micronutrients, and energy values can easily be accomplished using a nutrient analysis computer program. Most colleges and healthcare facilities have computer systems available for use by students and health professionals, respectively. If computer equipment is not available, a limited analysis can be completed by hand, using standard food value reference tables (see Appendix A). Based on the general concern about dietary fat as related to disease risk, an analysis that focuses on both total fat and the type of fat (saturated, monounsaturated, and polyunsaturated) in the diet would be useful for diet evaluation. This method of nutritional analysis is used by government agencies to evaluate dietary information obtained in national surveys and to make recommendations regarding nutritional problems related to specific vitamins, minerals, or macronutrients.

TO SUM UP

The role of nutrition in human health has been evolving in response to our changing society. The scientific base of nutrition is expanding in both its physical and behavioral foundations. Health goals and objectives have become more person centered, with a focus on health promotion. Health status in general has a fundamental nutritional base.

Nutrition assessment is an important activity for the nutrition and health professional. Clients may be categorized in several ways depending on their current nutritional intake and their nutrient reserves. Ideal or optimum nutrition describes those individuals who are consuming appropriate amounts and types of food, have an acceptable ratio of body weight to height and body composition, and have peak tissue reserves of important nutrients. Individuals whose nutritional state is borderline or marginal are consuming a sufficient amount of nutrients to meet day-to-day needs but have few or no reserves to draw on in a time of illness or physiologic stress. Malnourished individuals are not meeting daily needs and are vulnerable to infection, poor growth, and loss of mental and physical well-being. Overnutrition, a current public health problem, can indicate excessive kcaloric intake in respect to physical activity and energy output or the inappropriate use of high levels of nutritional supplements.

Various resources are available for use by health professionals and the general public in evaluating and planning diets. Nutrient standards or the DRIs are used by professionals in planning intervention programs and evaluating the current intakes of both individuals and groups. Food guides, including the FGP and *Exchange Lists for Meal Planning,* are designed to assist individuals in selecting a healthy diet. Dietary guidelines such as the *Dietary Guidelines for Americans* direct the attention of consumers to health-related aspects of nutrition. *Healthy People 2010,* a government public health initiative with the goals of extending years of healthy life and reducing the disparities in healthcare, provides a major opportunity for nutrition professionals to educate both consumers and other health workers about the contribution of nutrition to lifelong health and well-being.

■ Questions for Review

1. Describe the two major disciplines that are the foundations of nutrition science. What contributions does each make toward understanding human nutrition?
2. Define the terms *nutrition* and *dietetics.* Identify personal roles of professional practitioners in the field of human nutrition.

3. Compare the four levels of individual nutritional status: optimum nutrition, borderline nutrition, malnutrition, and overnutrition. Describe an individual or a situation to illustrate each level, and list the physical or clinical signs that you would use to identify it.
4. List and define each of the categories in the Dietary Reference Intakes.
5. Compare nutrient standards, food guides, and dietary guidelines, providing (a) an example of such a standard or guide currently being used, (b) the intended audience (professionals or consumers), (c) the type of information included, and (d) a professional situation in which you would use it.
6. Visit the *Healthy People 2010* website at *http://www.health.gov/healthypeople/*. List 10 measurable objectives that pertain to diet or nutrition.
7. Visit the U.S. Department of Agriculture's Center for Nutrition Policy and Promotion website at *http://www.usda.gov/cnpp* and follow the link to the ethnic food guides. Choose one of interest and research the food patterns of that group using the resources suggested in *Issues & Answers.* Develop a 1-day menu for a person belonging to that ethnic group.

■ References

1. Gilbride J: Genetics: brave new world, *J Am Diet Assoc* 100(9):996, 2000.
2. Greger JL: Biotechnology: mobilizing dietitians to be a resource, *J Am Diet Assoc* 100:1306, 2000.
3. Shanklin CW, Hackes BL: Position of the American Dietetic Association: dietetics professionals can implement practices to conserve natural resources and protect the environment, *J Am Diet Assoc* 101(10):1221, 2001.
4. Brecher SJ et al: Status of nutrition labeling, health claims, and nutrient content claims for processed foods: 1997 food label and package survey, *J Am Diet Assoc* 100(9):1057, 2000.
5. Harnack L et al: Guess who's cooking? The role of men in meal planning, shopping, and preparation in U.S. families, *J Am Diet Assoc* 98:995, 1998.
6. Eck-Clemens LH et al: The effect of eating out on quality of diet in premenopausal women, *J Am Diet Assoc* 99:442, 1999.
7. Pelegrin T: A super-sized problem: restaurant chains piling on the food, *J Am Diet Assoc* 101(6):620, 2001.
8. Grandgenett RS: Watching the trends helps focus nutrition education strategies, *J Am Diet Assoc* 98:1000, 1998.
9. Eberhardt MS et al: *Health, United States, 2001 with urban and rural health chartbook,* DHHS Publication No. (PHS) 01-1232, National Center for Health Statistics, Hyattsville, Md, 2001, U.S. Government Printing Office.
10. Anderson JV, Palombo RD, Earl R: Position of the American Dietetic Association: the role of nutrition in health promotion and disease prevention programs, *J Am Diet Assoc* 98:205, 1998.
11. Messina M et al: Reductionism and the narrowing nutrition perspective: time for reevaluation and emphasis on food synergy, *J Am Diet Assoc* 2001(12):1416, 2001.
12. Glanz K et al: Why Americans eat what they do: taste, nutrition, cost, convenience, and weight control concerns as influences on food consumption, *J Am Diet Assoc* 98:1118, 1998.
13. Kant AK: Consumption of energy-dense, nutrient-poor foods by adult Americans: nutrition and health implications. The Third National Health and Nutrition Examination Survey, 1988-1994, *Am J Clin Nutr* 72:929, 2000.
14. Klein BW: *Could there be hunger in America?* Washington, DC, September 1998, Nutrition Insight 8, Center for Nutrition Policy and Promotion, U.S. Dept of Agriculture (accessible at *http://www.usda.gov/cnpp*).
15. UNICEF: The state of the world's children 1998: A UNICEF report, *Nutr Rev* 56(4):115, 1998.
16. Kendall A, Kennedy E: Position of the American Dietetic Association: domestic food and nutrition security, *J Am Diet Assoc* 98:337, 1998.
17. Bell M, Wilbur L, Smith C: Nutritional status of persons using a local emergency food system program in middle America, *J Am Diet Assoc* 98:1031, 1998.
18. Marshall J et al: Indicators of nutritional risk in a rural elderly Hispanic and non-Hispanic white population: San Luis Valley Health and Aging Study, *J Am Diet Assoc* 99:315, 1999.
19. Kelsheimer HL, Hawkins ST: Older adult women find food preparation easier with specialized kitchen tools, *J Am Diet Assoc* 100:950, 2000.
20. Mokdad AH et al: The continuing epidemics of obesity and diabetes in the United States, *JAMA* 286:1195, 2001.
21. Popkin BM et al: Trends in diet, nutritional status, and diet-related noncommunicable diseases in China and India: the economic costs of the nutrition transition, *Nutr Rev* 59(12):379, 2001.
22. Hanley AJG et al: Overweight among children and adolescents in a native Canadian community: prevalence and associated factors, *Am J Clin Nutr* 71:693, 2000.
23. Ternand C: The new face of type 2 diabetes, *Nutr MD* 27(11):1, 2001.
24. Whittaker P, Tufaro PR, Rader JI: Iron and folate in fortified cereals, *J Am Coll Nutr* 20(3):247, 2001.
25. U.S. Department of Health and Human Services, Public Health Service: *The Surgeon General's report on nutrition and health,* PHS publication No. 88-50210, Washington, DC, 1988, U.S. Government Printing Office.
26. Food and Nutrition Board, Committee on Diet and Health: *Diet and health: implications for reducing chronic disease risk,* Washington, DC, 1989, National Academy Press.
27. U.S. Department of Health and Human Services, Public Health Service: *Healthy People 2000: national health promotion and disease prevention objectives,* Washington, DC, 1990, U.S. Government Printing Office.
28. U.S. Department of Health and Human Services: *Healthy People 2010: understanding and improving health,* Washington, DC, 2000, U.S. Government Printing Office (full report accessible at *http://www.health.gov/healthypeople/*).
29. Hahn NI: Setting the nation's health agenda: how ADA is helping shape Healthy People 2010, *J Am Diet Assoc* 99:415, 1999.
30. Mertz W: Three decades of dietary recommendations, *Nutr Rev* 58(10):324, 2000.

31. Food and Nutrition Board, National Research Council: *Recommended dietary allowances,* ed 10, Washington, DC, 1989, National Academy Press.
32. Food and Nutrition Board, National Research Council: *Dietary Reference Intakes for calcium, phosphorus, magnesium, vitamin D, and fluoride,* Washington, DC, 1997, National Academy Press.
33. Food and Nutrition Board: *Dietary Reference Intakes for thiamin, riboflavin, niacin, vitamin B_6, folate, vitamin B_{12}, pantothenic acid, biotin, and choline,* Washington, DC, 1998, National Academy Press.
34. Food and Nutrition Board, National Research Council: *Dietary Reference Intakes for vitamin C, vitamin E, selenium, and carotenoids,* Washington, DC, 2000, National Academy Press.
35. Food and Nutrition Board, National Research Council: *Dietary Reference Intakes for vitamin A, vitamin K, arsenic, chromium, copper, iodine, iron, manganese, molybdenum, nickel, silicon, vanadium, and zinc,* Washington, DC, 2001, National Academy Press.
36. Panel on Macronutrients, Panel on the Definition of Dietary Fiber, Subcommittee on Upper Reference Levels of Nutrients, Subcommittee on Interpretation and Uses of Dietary Reference Intakes, and the Standing Committee on the Scientific Evaluation of Dietary Reference Intakes: *Dietary reference intakes for energy, carbohydrate, fiber, fat, fatty acids, cholesterol, protein, and amino acids, parts 1 and 2,* Washington, DC, 2002, National Academy Press.
37. U.S. Department of Agriculture: *Guide to daily food choices,* Washington, DC, 1991, U.S. Government Printing Office.
38. Cronin FJ: Reflections on food guides and guidance systems, *Nutr Today* 33(5):186, 1998.
39. Nestle M: In defense of the USDA food guide pyramid, *Nutr Today* 33(5):189, 1998.
40. Welsh S: Nutrient standards, dietary guidelines, and food guides. In Ziegler EE, Filer LJ, eds: *Present knowledge in nutrition,* ed 7, Washington, DC, 1996, International Life Sciences Institute, Nutrition Foundation.
41. Shaw AM, Escobar AJ, Davis CA: Reassessing the Food Guide Pyramid: decision-making framework, *J Nutr Educ* 32:111, 2000.
42. Tucker KL: Eat a variety of healthful foods: old advice with new support, *Nutr Rev* 59(5):156, 2001.
43. U.S. Department of Agriculture: *Food Guide Pyramid for children age 2-6,* Washington, DC, 1996, Center for Nutrition Policy and Promotion (accessible at *http://www.usda.gov/cnpp*).
44. American Dietetic Association: *Food Guide Pyramid for persons fifty plus,* Chicago, 2001, American Dietetic Association (accessible at *http://www.eatright.org*).
45. Russell RM, Rasmussen H, Lichtenstein AH: Modified food guide pyramid for people over seventy years of age, *J Nutr* 129:751, 1999.
46. American Dietetic Association, American Diabetes Association: *Exchange lists for meal planning,* Chicago, 1995, American Dietetic Association.
47. American Dietetic Association, American Diabetes Association: *Exchange lists for weight management,* Chicago, 1995, American Dietetic Association.
48. U.S. Department of Agriculture, U.S. Department of Health and Human Services: *Nutrition and your health: dietary guidelines for Americans,* ed 5, Home and Garden Bulletin No 232, Washington, DC, 2000, U.S. Government Printing Office (accessible at *http://www.usda.gov/cnpp*).
49. Johnson R, Kennedy E: The 2000 Dietary Guidelines for Americans: what are the changes and why were they made? *J Am Diet Assoc* 100:769, 2000.
50. Keenan PK, Abusabha R: The fifth edition of the Dietary Guidelines for Americans: lessons learned along the way, *J Am Diet Assoc* 101(6):631, 2001.
51. Dwyer JT: Nutrition guidelines and education of the public, *J Nutr* 131:3074S, 2001.
52. Patterson RE et al: Is there a consumer backlash against the diet and health message? *J Am Diet Assoc* 101(1):37, 2001.

■ Further Reading

Kennedy E, Davis CA: Dietary Guidelines 2000—the opportunity and challenges for reaching the consumer, *J Am Diet Assoc* 100(12):1462, 2000.

Patterson RE et al: Is there a consumer backlash against the diet and health message? *J Am Diet Assoc* 101(1):37, 2001.

These articles give us some insight into how consumers interpret the dietary guidelines and how we can help them apply the guidelines to their personal lifestyles.

Partnership to Promote Healthy Eating and Active Living: Summit on promoting healthy eating and active living: developing a framework for progress, *Nutr Rev* 59(3, Part II), March 2001.

This supplement issue of *Nutrition Reviews* presents a series of articles on how individuals make food and activity decisions and provides suggestions on how we can bring about social change to support health.

Kennedy E, Offutt SE: Healthy lifestyles for healthy Americans: report on USDA's Year 2000 behavioral nutrition roundtable, *Nutr Today* 35(3):84, 2000.

The article reviews a government roundtable discussion about the gap that currently exists between what people know about healthy lifestyles and what they actually do on a day-to-day basis. Despite our efforts at health promotion, obesity and other chronic health problems are rising; this report tries to present some solutions.

Chinese Nutrition Society: Dietary guidelines and the Food Guide Pagoda, *J Am Diet Assoc* 100(8):886, 2000.

Ge K, McNutt KL: How the Chinese link dietary advice to their national plan of action for nutrition, *J Am Diet Assoc* 100(8):885, 2000.

These two articles provide an overview of how the Chinese developed a national nutrition plan for their country and developed a Food Guide Pagoda appropriate to their food supply and nutrition needs.

Issues & ANSWERS

Cross-Cultural Competence: A Goal for the Health Professional

Consider the following

You are working in a health clinic providing nutrition counseling and prenatal care to pregnant and lactating mothers. You are using the Food Guide Pyramid to evaluate the diet pattern of a pregnant Hmong (Vietnamese) mother. She tells you that she never eats bread and you are immediately concerned about her servings from the grain group.

You are working with an elderly African American man and he tells you that his favorite meal that his daughter cooks for him is Brunswick stew. What food groups are included in this dish?

Our population is becoming increasingly diverse; in fact by the year 2020, one of every three Americans will be an African American, Hispanic American, Asian American, Hmong American, Native American, or Pacific Islander American. Knowledge of and sensitivity to ethnic and cultural differences are expected by the general population and required of those in the helping professions. We cannot be effective as nutrition educators unless we are familiar with the food patterns of ethnic and cultural groups that differ from our own. Second, we need to recognize the patterns of family structure, health beliefs, and values that influence food choices and response to healthcare providers. For example, the Hmong mother described above is likely to have rice at every meal and to more than meet her recommended servings from the grain group. At the same time she may be reluctant to take the vitamin and mineral supplements that her doctor has recommended in the belief that they will cause her to have a large infant and difficult delivery. The elderly African American man will be eating some dark green and deep yellow vegetables in his Brunswick stew made with chicken, carrots, and greens. It is important that we learn as much as we can about not only what our patients enjoy eating but also what factors influence their decisions.

Cross-cultural situations

Cross-cultural situations, in which a health professional is a member of a different racial or ethnic group than the client or patient, are increasing as our population continues to change. Also, our philosophy regarding the role of cultural differences in our society is changing with striking implications for the delivery of healthcare. Over the years the United States has included a mix of people coming from many different countries and cultures and having different customs. The traditional image of our society was a "melting pot," in which newcomers were expected to blend their customs and beliefs with those of the mainstream white population. Healthcare professionals tended to impose their beliefs and values on other groups, as they considered their ideas and culture to be superior to those from other backgrounds.

In recent years we have moved beyond the narrow view of the "melting pot" to the image of the "salad bowl." This suggests that individual differences are important and need to be valued and preserved. Each individual adds a special quality to the mix that enhances the lives of those around them. Health professionals should respect the customs and ideals of others and provide counseling and support in a manner that is consistent with the goals of the patient or client. Recognizing rather than ignoring the reliance on alternative medical practices such as the use of herbs will allow the development of an effective nutritional care plan that is more likely to be successful.

The health professional working with diverse population groups must be attentive to the differences in communication patterns that exist among various groups. Both verbal and nonverbal communication becomes important in the counseling situation. Gestures, eye contact, and touching may have very different meanings for individuals who practice more formal behaviors than the majority of Americans. Family structures that expect the approval of the male head of the family before visiting a health professional or initiating a recommended treatment are found in many traditional cultures. One's locus of control or the individual's perception of the degree of control that he or she has over what will happen differs strikingly among cultures and has important implications for health. A man with an external locus of control who perceives life as predetermined is less likely to change his food habits in an effort to reduce his risk of a heart attack. An internal locus of control in which a person feels that he or she can change the outcome is supportive of behavior change toward the goal of good health.

You can begin to develop competence in cross-cultural situations in the following ways.

1. Learn about other cultures by reading, observing, and sharing experiences with members of different ethnic and cultural groups.

2. Examine your own beliefs and feelings about other cultures; identify and resolve any stereotypes that you may have about certain ethnic or culture groups.
3. Assess how other cultures view you and make an effort to present yourself in a positive light.
4. Value the differences among people; avoid the expression that your way is best.

REFERENCES

Curry KR: Multicultural competence in dietetics and nutrition, *J Am Diet Assoc* 100:1142, 2000.

Owen A et al: *Nutrition in the community: the art and science of delivering services,* ed 4, Dubuque, Iowa, 1998, WCB/McGraw-Hill.

OTHER RESOURCES

American Diabetes Association and American Dietetic Association: *Ethnic and regional food practices: a series,* Chicago, American Dietetic Association.

Alaska Native Food Practices, Customs, and Holidays, 1998.

Chinese American Food Practices, Customs, and Holidays, 1998.

Filipino American Food Practices, Customs, and Holidays, 1994.

Hmong American Food Practices, Customs, and Holidays, 1999.

Indian and Pakistani Food Practices, Customs, and Holidays, 2000.

Jewish Food Practices, Customs, and Holidays, 1998.

Mexican American Food Practices, Customs, and Holidays, 1998.

Navajo Food Practices, Customs, and Holidays, 1998.

Soul and Traditional Southern Food Practices, Customs, and Holidays, 1995.

Kittler PG, Sucher K: *Food and culture in America,* ed 2, New York, 2000, Van Nostrand Reinhold.

Chapter

2

Digestion, Absorption, and Metabolism

Eleanor D. Schlenker

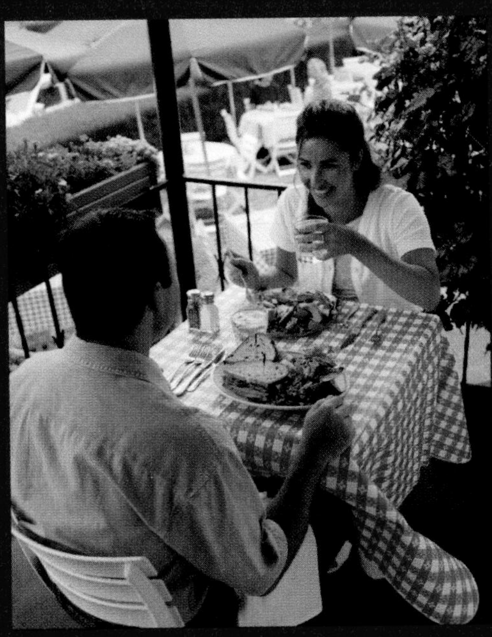

Chapter Outline

In this chapter, we begin our story of what happens to the foods we eat and their general fate in the body. We look first at the integrated overall body systems that handle them. Once the body receives the foods we eat, unique structures and functions transform them for our use.

The overall physiologic and biochemical process that turns the food we eat into energy and body tissues has three integrated parts: digestion, absorption, and metabolism. We begin with a look at the gastrointestinal tract and then follow the path of the nutrients to the cells where they nourish and sustain our lives. We see how each part of the system makes its own special contribution to the integrated whole.

The Human Body: Role of Nutrition

FOOD: CHANGE AND TRANSFORMATION

The foods we eat contain the necessary nutrients for our survival, but these life-sustaining nutrients must first be released and transformed into units the body can use. Through a successive interrelated system, the foods we eat are transformed into simpler substances and then into other, still simpler, substances that our cells can use to sustain life. All of these many changes prepare food for use by the body; however, the parts of this overall process of change do not act separately. Each is unique, but together they compose one continuous integrated *whole.* Clinical problems involving organs of the gastrointestinal tract are usually the result of a breakdown in this integrated process.

IMPORTANCE OF THIS HUMAN LIFE SYSTEM

Why is this intricate complex of activities so necessary to human life? Two reasons are apparent: (1) *Food,* as it occurs naturally and as we eat it, is not a single substance but a mixture of chemical substances or nutrients. If these substances are to release their stored energy and building materials for our use, they must be separated into their respective components so that the body may handle each one as a separate unit. (2) *Nutrients* released from food may still remain unavailable to the body, and some additional means of changing their forms may need to follow. The intermediate units must be broken down, simplified, regrouped, and rerouted.

This complex chemical work must take place because the human being, whose life is developed and sustained in a dynamic internal chemical environment, is the most highly organized and intricately balanced of all organisms. This high level of internal body control and balance is called homeostasis, and it is achieved through the effectiveness of the body's control mechanisms that keep the various functional systems operating in harmony with one another.[1] This view of the human body as an integrated physiochemical organism is basic to an understanding of human nutrition, both in health and in disease.

The Gastrointestinal Tract

COMPONENT PARTS

The gastrointestinal tract, sometimes referred to as the alimentary canal, is a long hollow tube that begins at the mouth and ends at the anus. The specific parts that make up the gastrointestinal tract are the mouth, esophagus, stomach, small intestine, large intestine or colon, and rectum. Other organs that lie outside of the gastrointestinal tract but support its work through their secretion of important enzymes and digestive fluids are the pancreas, the gallbladder, and the liver. Look carefully at the respective components of the gastrointestinal tract and their relative position in this overall body system (Figure 2-1). The incredible organization of this fundamental body system is evident in its estimated capacity to break down and absorb daily several kilograms of carbohydrate, a half kilogram of fat, a half kilogram of protein, and 20 or more liters of water.[1] Follow the fate of these food components as they travel *together* through the successive parts of the gastrointestinal tract and into the body cells.

GENERAL FUNCTIONS

The gastrointestinal tract has several specific functions in preparing nutrients for absorption and use by body cells.

1. *Receiving food.* The mouth is the entrance to the gastrointestinal tract. Here food is chewed, softened,

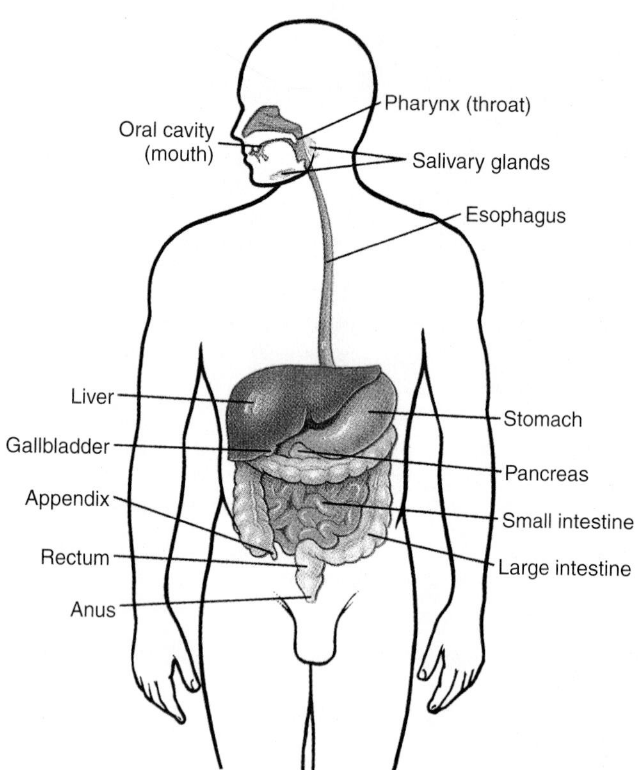

FIGURE 2-1 The gastrointestinal system. Through the successive parts of the system, multiple activities of digestion liberate and reform food nutrients for our use. (*From Seeley RR, Stephens TD, Tate PP:* Anatomy and physiology, *ed 2, New York, 1992, McGraw-Hill. Reproduced with permission of The McGraw-Hill Companies.*)

and mixed with saliva before being transported to the stomach.

2. *Breaking down food into its component nutrients.* On reaching the stomach, digestion is begun and continues as food is slowly transferred to the small intestine, where digestion is completed.
3. *Absorbing nutrients into the blood.* In the small intestine, absorbing structures called microvilli complete the process of transferring the nutrients across the mucosal cells and into the portal blood (fats first enter the lymph and then are transferred into the blood); water is absorbed mostly in the large intestine or colon.
4. *Excreting nondigestible food parts from the body.* The large intestine transports the remaining fecal mass to the rectum, where it is stored until excreted.

Both chemical processes and physical actions by the muscles participate in accomplishing these tasks.

SENSORY STIMULATION AND GASTROINTESTINAL FUNCTION

Digestive functions are controlled by both physical and psychologic factors. The presence of food in the mouth, stomach, or small intestine initiates a variety of controlled responses that coordinate the muscular movements and chemical secretions that bring about the breakdown and absorption of nutrients. However, sensory stimulation—visual, olfactory, auditory, and tactile—can bring about the secretion of digestive juices and muscle motility. Smelling the aroma of cookies baking, hearing the sizzling of foods on an outdoor grill, or picking a fresh berry can begin to evoke the physiologic processes of digestion. Even thinking about food acts as a stimulus to the gastrointestinal tract. In the same way, apprehension related to an unpleasant-tasting medication or recall of the stomach upset that occurred after a treatment such as chemotherapy can inhibit appetite or the desire for food. Positive associations with food or mealtime promote both appropriate food intake and efficient digestion and absorption of nutrients.

Basic Principles of Digestion

Digestion is the first step in preparing food for use by the body. We will examine each of the two types of actions involved—muscular and chemical.

GASTROINTESTINAL MOTILITY: MUSCLES AND MOVEMENT

The digestion of food involves mechanical mixing and propulsive movement that take place through a number of neuromuscular, self-regulating processes. These actions work together to move the food mass along the alimentary tract at the best rate for digestion and absorption of the nutrients.

Types of Muscles

Organized muscle layers of the gastrointestinal wall, shown in Figure 2-2, provide the necessary motility for digestion. From the outside surface inward, the layers are (1) the serosa, (2) a *longitudinal muscle layer,* (3) a *circular muscle layer,* (4) the *submucosa,* and (5) the mucosa. Imbedded in the deeper layers of the mucosa are thin bundles of smooth muscle fibers called the *muscularis mucosae.* The coordinated interaction of all of these smooth muscle layers makes possible four necessary types of movement (Figure 2-3).

1. *Longitudinal muscles.* These long, smooth muscles, arranged in fiber bundles that extend lengthwise along the gastrointestinal tract, help propel the food mass forward along the tract.
2. *Circular contractile muscles.* In the circular muscle layer, smooth muscle fibers extend around the gut. They form rhythmic contractile rings that cause sweeping waves along the digestive tract and push forward the food mass. These regularly occurring propulsive movements are called peristalsis.
3. *Sphincter muscles.* More defined circular muscles occur at strategic points to provide muscle sphincters that act as valves—pyloric, ileocecal, and anal—to prevent reflux or backflow, and thereby control the movement of the food mass in a forward direction.
4. *Mucosal muscles.* This imbedded thin layer of smooth muscle produces *local constrictive contractions* that occur every few centimeters. These contractions mix and chop the food mass as it moves along the tract, effectively churning the mass and mixing it with secretions to form a semiliquid called chyme that is ready for digestion and absorption.

---

digestion The process of breaking down food to release its nutrients for absorption and transport to the cells for use in body functions.

chyme Semifluid food mass in the gastrointestinal tract after gastric digestion.

homeostasis State of relative dynamic equilibrium within the body's internal environment; a balance achieved through the operation of various interrelated physiologic mechanisms.

mucosa The mucous membrane comprising the inner surface layer of the gastrointestinal tract, providing extensive nutrient absorption and transport functions.

peristalsis A wavelike progression of alternate contraction and relaxation of the muscle fibers of the gastrointestinal tract.

serosa Outer surface layer of the intestines interfacing with the blood vessels of the portal system going to the liver.

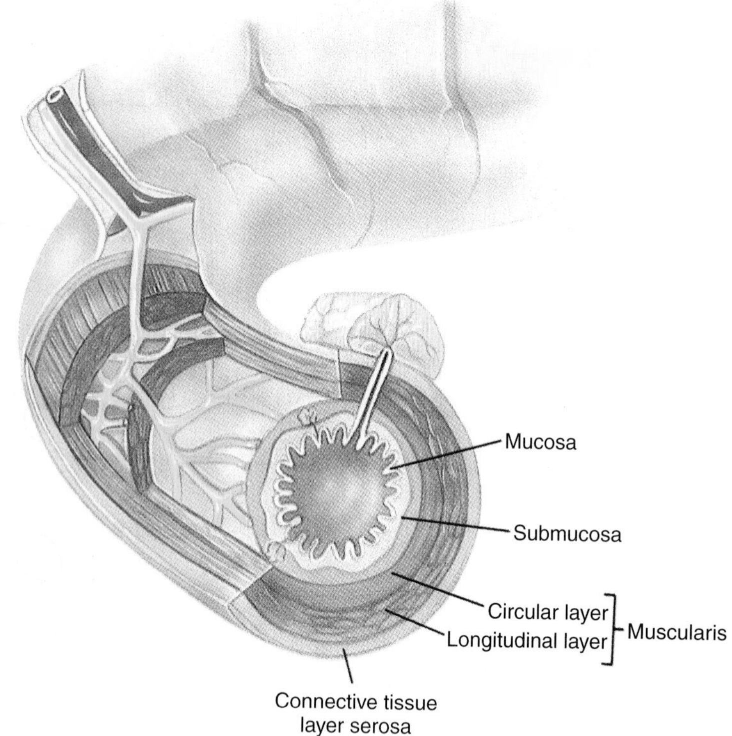

FIGURE 2-2 Muscle layers of the intestinal wall. (*From Raven P, Johnson G:* Biology, *ed 3, New York, 1992, McGraw-Hill. Reproduced with permission of The McGraw-Hill Companies.*)

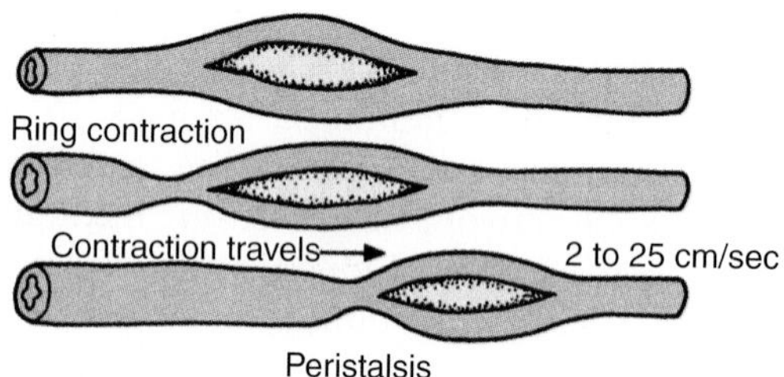

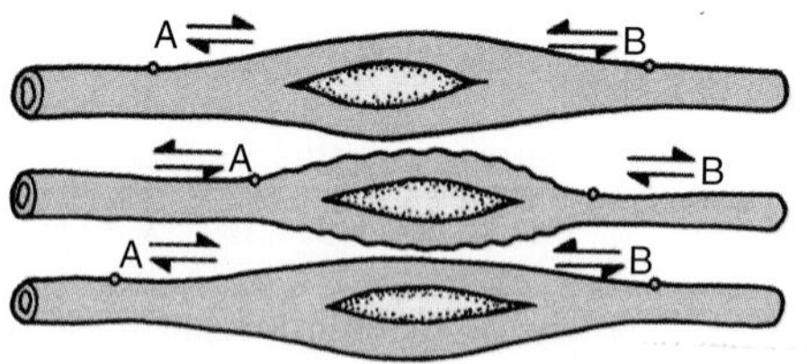

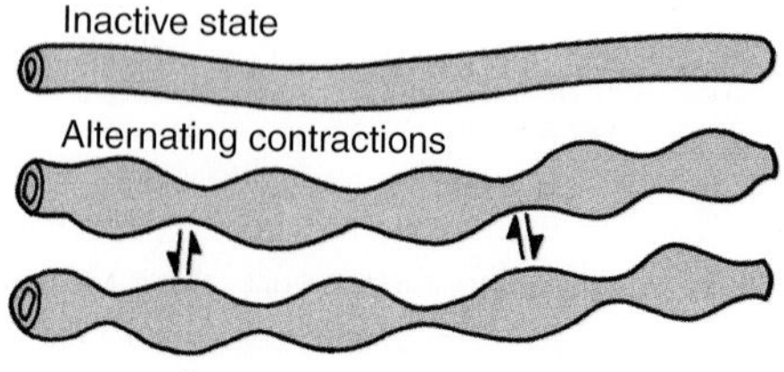

FIGURE 2-3 Types of movement produced by muscles of the intestine: peristaltic waves from contraction of deep circular muscle, pendular movements from small local muscles, and segmentation rings formed by alternate contraction and relaxation of circular muscle.

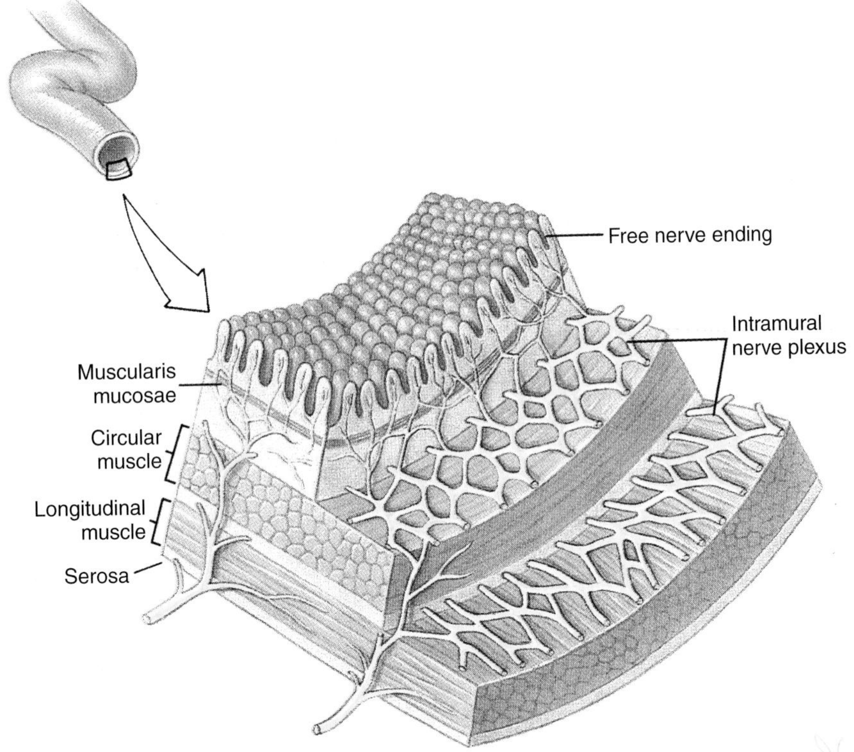

FIGURE 2-4 Innervation of the intestine by intramural nerve plexus. *(Medical and Scientific Illustration.)*

In summary, the interaction of the gastrointestinal muscles produces two basic types of action.

1. General muscle tone or tonic contraction that ensures continuous passage and valve control
2. Periodic, rhythmic contractions that mix and propel the food mass

These alternating muscular contractions and relaxations force the contents forward and facilitate specific digestion and absorption.

NERVOUS SYSTEM CONTROL

Throughout the gastrointestinal tract, specific nerves regulate these muscular actions. An interrelated network of nerves within the gastrointestinal wall, called the intramural nerve plexus (Figure 2-4), extends from the esophagus to the anus. This network of about 100 million nerve fibers regulates the rate and intensity of muscle contractions, controls the speed at which the food mass moves along the tract, and coordinates the digestive process, including the secretion of enzymes and digestive juices.[2]

GASTROINTESTINAL SECRETIONS

Food is digested chemically through the combined action of a number of secretions. Generally, these secretions are of four types.

1. *Enzymes.* Specific kinds and quantities split designated chemical bonds within the structure of specific nutrient compounds, freeing their component parts.
2. *Hydrochloric acid and buffer ions.* These agents produce the necessary pH for the activity of certain enzymes.
3. *Mucus.* This agent lubricates and protects the tissues along the inside wall of the gastrointestinal tract and facilitates food mass passage.
4. *Water and electrolytes.* These agents provide a balanced solution base in sufficient volumes to circulate the organic substances released in the digestive process.

Special cells in the mucosal tissue of the gastrointestinal tract or in adjacent accessory organs, especially the pancreas, produce these secretions. The secretory action of these cells or glands is stimulated by the presence of food in the gastrointestinal tract; by the sensory nerve network of sight, taste, or smell; or by hormones specific for certain nutrients.

---

intramural nerve plexus Network of nerves in the walls of the intestine that make up the intramural nervous system, controlling muscle action and secretions for digestion and absorption.

Mouth and Esophagus: Preparation and Delivery

Up to this point, we have viewed the gastrointestinal tract in terms of the integrated muscular-secretory functions that govern its operation as a whole. Here we begin to follow this process through its successive parts to see what happens when we eat food. Actually, eating starts a remarkable physiologic event. It prepares food for entry into a complex system that radically changes its form and finally nourishes the body with its contents. Each step of the way requires motility and secretions. In this first step, highly synchronized actions prepare food in the mouth, control the intricate act of swallowing, and deliver the food to the stomach by way of the esophagus.

TASTE AND SMELL

Taste buds located on the tongue, roof of the mouth, and pharynx contain chemical receptors that respond to food and produce the four sensations of taste: *salty, sweet, sour,* or *bitter.* Some individuals have a stronger perception of one taste over another, and this can influence food intake. Certain medications bring about a change in taste, and some older individuals experience a loss of taste, although this is not true for all.[3] The volatile elements in food can move from the back of the mouth up into the nasal cavity, where they act on olfactory receptors that produce the sensations of smell associated with particular foods. In fact, much of what we perceive as the taste of a certain food may actually be its odor. Persons who have been treated with radiation therapy in the head or neck and patients with Parkinson's disease or Alzheimer's disease often undergo olfactory losses, which adversely affects their enjoyment of food.

MASTICATION

Initial biting and chewing begin to break food down into smaller particles. The teeth and other oral structures are particularly suited for this function. The incisors cut; the molars grind. Tremendous force is supplied by the jaw muscles: 55 lb of muscular pressure is applied through the incisors, and 200 lb is applied through the molars. Because digestive enzymes can act only on the surface of food particles, sufficient chewing to prepare an enlarged surface area to receive constant enzyme action is an important step in preparing food for digestion. Also, the fineness of the food particles eases the continued passage of material into the esophagus and on through the gastrointestinal tract.

An appropriate amount of chewing is particularly important in preparing fruits, vegetables, and whole grains that contain undigestible fiber for digestion. Loss of teeth and gingivitis and periodontal disease that can lead to oral infections, mouth pain, and further loss of teeth can restrict food intake and contribute to malnutrition.

SWALLOWING

The process of swallowing involves both the mouth and the pharynx. It is intricately controlled by the swallowing center in the brain stem,[4] and damage to these nerves through radiation therapy, aging, or disease can make swallowing a difficult process. The tongue initiates the swallowing process by pressing the food upward and backward against the palate. At that point, swallowing proceeds as an involuntary reflex, and once begun, it usually cannot be interrupted. Swallowing is extremely rapid, taking less than 1 second, but involves an intricate series of events, including (1) the closing of the larynx to prevent food from entering the trachea and moving into the lungs and (2) the raising of the soft palate to prevent food from entering the nasal cavity. Individuals should never be fed in a supine position, which increases the risk of food aspiration.

ESOPHAGUS

The esophagus is a muscular tube that connects the mouth and pharynx with the stomach and serves as a channel to carry the food mass into the body for processing and absorption. Functionally, it may be divided into three main parts.[4]

1. *Upper esophageal sphincter (UES).* The UES controls the passage of food into the esophagus. At rest, between intakes of food, the UES muscle is closed. Within 0.2 to 0.3 second after a swallow of food or drink, nerve stimuli immediately open the sphincter to receive the nourishment.
2. *Esophageal body.* A mixed bolus of food particles passes immediately down the esophagus, moved along by peristaltic waves controlled by nerve reflexes. A decrease in the size and frequency of these peristaltic waves sometimes occurs in elderly persons, resulting in difficult passage of the food down the esophagus and discomfort in eating.[5] Gravity aids the movement of food when the person is in the upright position.
3. *Lower esophageal sphincter (LES).* The LES controls the passage of the food mass from the esophagus into the stomach for continuing digestion. When the LES muscles maintain an excessively high degree of muscle tone, even while resting, the muscles may fail to open when the person swallows, preventing the passage of food into the stomach. This condition is called achalasia, meaning unrelaxed muscle state (see Chapter 18).

ENTRY INTO THE STOMACH

At the point of entry into the stomach, the gastroesophageal constrictor muscle relaxes to allow food to pass from the esophagus into the stomach. Then it contracts again to prevent regurgitation or reflux of the now acidic stomach contents up into the esophagus. When regurgitation does occur, through failure of this mechanism, the person feels it as "heartburn." A Gallup poll estimated that 50% of the adult population in the United States experience heartburn at least once a month, and over $8 billion a year is spent on over-the-counter and prescription drugs to relieve this condition. Gastroesophageal reflux disease (GERD) has been defined as a gastrointestinal disorder, although for some individuals heartburn is an occasional rather than a chronic condition.[6]

Two clinical problems may hinder normal food passage into the stomach: (1) cardiospasm, caused by failure of the constrictor muscle to relax properly, or (2) hiatal hernia, caused by protrusion of the upper part of the stomach into the thorax through an abnormal opening in the diaphragm.

CHEMICAL DIGESTION

In the mouth, three pairs of salivary glands—parotid, submaxillary, and sublingual—secrete serous material containing salivary amylase. This is an enzyme specific for starch. Mucus also is secreted to lubricate and bind the food particles. Stimuli such as sight, smell, taste, and touch—and even thoughts of likes and dislikes in food—greatly influence these secretions. The normal daily secretion of saliva ranges between 800 and 1500 ml, with a pH range of 6.0 to 7.4 (approximately neutral) (Table 2-1). Food remains in the mouth for only a short time; therefore starch digestion here is brief. However, salivary amylase, when bound to starch molecules, is resistant to inactivation by stomach acid, and significant breakdown of the starch molecules continues in the stomach.[2] Smoking appears to influence the composition of juices from the salivary gland. This change in salivary fluids may play a part in the loss of taste that occurs in smokers and the increased taste that returns when persons stop smoking.[7]

Although the actual digestion occurring in the mouth is limited, the fluids produced by the salivary glands still have very important functions: (1) they moisten the food particles so they will bind together to form a bolus that will move easily down the esophagus, and (2) they lubricate and cleanse the teeth and tissues of the mouth, destroying harmful bacteria or other microorganisms and neutralizing toxic substances entering the mouth. Reduced secretion of saliva (dry mouth) or the more serious condition of xerostomia adds to problems in swallowing as individual particles of food can get separated in the esophagus. Also, infections and ulcers in the mouth, along with tooth decay, are serious outcomes of this condition. Various medications contribute to dry mouth.[8]

TABLE 2-1 Comparative pH Values and Approximate Daily Volumes of Gastrointestinal Secretions

Secretion	pH	Daily Volume (ml)
Salivary	6.0-7.4	1000
Gastric	1.0-3.5	1500
Pancreatic	8.0-8.3	1000
Small intestinal	7.5-8.0	1800
Brunner's gland	8.0-8.9	200
Bile	7.5-7.8	1000
Large intestinal	7.5-8.0	200
TOTAL		6700

Modified from Guyton AC, Hall JC: *Textbook of medical physiology*, ed 9, Philadelphia, 1996, WB Saunders.

Stomach: Storage and Initial Digestion

MOTILITY

The major parts of the stomach are shown in Figure 2-5. Muscles in the stomach wall provide three basic motor functions: storage, mixing, and controlled emptying. As the food mass enters the stomach, it lies against the stomach walls, which stretch outward to store as much as 1 L. Local tonic muscle waves gradually increase their kneading and mixing action as the mass of food and secretions moves on toward the pyloric valve at the distal end of the stomach. Here waves of peristaltic contractions reduce the food mass to a semifluid chyme. Finally, with each wave, small amounts of chyme are forced through the pyloric valve and enter the duodenum. This sphincter muscle periodically constricts and relaxes and then constricts again to control the emptying of the stomach contents into the upper end of the small intestine. This control releases the acid chyme slowly enough to be buffered by the alkaline intestinal secretions.

The kilocaloric (kcaloric) density of a meal, in addition to its particular volume and composition, influences the rate of stomach emptying. The rate at which food moves from the antrum to the distal end of the stomach and on into the small intestine also influences food intake, as messages to the brain signal the arrival of food and increase feelings of satiety (we discuss this influence on appetite in Chapter 6).

bolus Rounded mass of food formed in the mouth and ready to be swallowed.

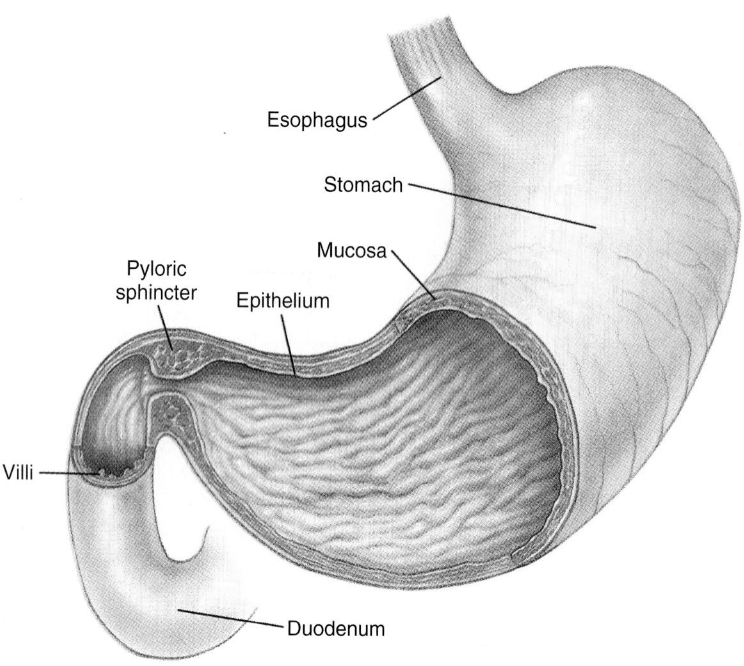

FIGURE 2-5 Stomach. (*From Raven P, Johnson G:* Biology, *ed 3, New York, 1992, McGraw-Hill. Reproduced with permission of The McGraw-Hill Companies.*)

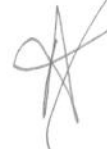

CHEMICAL DIGESTION

Types of Secretion

Secretions produced in the stomach contain three types of materials: acid, mucus, and enzymes.

1. *Acid.* Hydrochloric acid prepares certain enzymes and materials for digestion and absorption by creating the necessary degree of acidity for particular enzymes to work. For example, the range of pH necessary for the enzyme pepsin to act on protein is 1.8 to 3.5; at a pH of 5.0 or above there is little or no pepsin activity (see *Practical Application* box).
2. *Mucus.* Special mucous secretions protect the stomach lining from the eroding effect of the acid. This mucus also binds and mixes the food mass and helps move it along.
3. *Enzymes.* The main enzyme in the stomach is pepsin, which begins the breakdown of protein. It is first secreted in the inactive form of pepsinogen, which is then activated by the hydrochloric acid that is present. A small amount of gastric lipase (tributyrase) is present in the stomach, but it acts only on butterfat and has a relatively minor role in overall digestion. In childhood, an enzyme called rennin (not to be confused with the vital lifelong renal enzyme renin) is also present in gastric secretions and aids in the coagulation of milk. Rennin is absent in adults.

Control of Secretion

Stimuli for these gastric secretions come from two sources.

1. *Nerve stimulus* is produced in response to the visual and chemical senses, ingested food, and emotions. Anger and hostility increase gastric secretions; fear and depression decrease secretions and inhibit blood flow and motility.
2. *Hormonal stimulus* is produced in response to the entrance of food into the stomach. Certain stimulants, especially caffeine, alcohol, and meat extracts, cause the release of a local gastrointestinal hormone, gastrin, from the mucosal cells in the antrum, which in turn stimulates the secretion of more hydrochloric acid. When the pH falls below 3, a feedback mechanism stops further secretion of gastrin to prevent excess acid formation.[2] Another local gastrointestinal hormone, enterogastrone, is produced by glands in the mucosa of the duodenum. This hormone counteracts excessive gastric activity by inhibiting hydrochloric acid secretion, pepsin secretion, and gastric motility.

Small Intestine: Major Digestion, Absorption, and Transport

MOTILITY

Intestinal Muscle Layers

Note the complex structural arrangement of the intestinal wall shown in Figure 2-2. Finely coordinated intestinal motility is achieved by the three layers of muscle: (1) the thin layer of smooth muscle imbedded in the mucosa, the muscularis mucosae, with fibers extending up into the villi;

PRACTICAL APPLICATION
Not Enough Stomach Acid: Is This a Problem?

Recent nutrition surveys tell us that many young adults and older adults have lower blood levels of vitamin B_{12} than expected and their vitamin B_{12} status is marginal to poor. As we will learn in our continuing study of nutrition, vitamin B_{12} is necessary to produce mature red blood cells, and, also, to maintain the nerves in the brain and spinal cord. Vitamin B_{12} is found only in animal foods, but it seems unlikely that persons other than vegans, who consume no animal foods, would develop a vitamin B_{12} deficiency. A very small number of individuals have a condition called pernicious anemia which means they are not able to produce the protein molecule known as intrinsic factor needed to absorb vitamin B_{12} in the small intestine.

Researchers have now discovered another reason why some adults are less able to absorb vitamin B_{12}. Some persons, especially older persons, do not secrete normal levels of hydrochloric acid because of changes in the mucosal lining and acid-producing cells in the stomach. This condition of producing less hydrochloric acid than normal is referred to as hypochlorhydria. Those who secrete no hydrochloric acid are said to have achlorhydria. The vitamin B_{12} found in meats is strongly bound to the protein fibers and a normal amount of gastric acid is needed to release the vitamin so it can be absorbed. Consequently, persons who secrete only low amounts of hydrochloric acid are not able to absorb sufficient amounts of vitamin B_{12} even though they have the needed intrinsic factor. We are not sure why some younger persons who do not have pernicious anemia and eat generous amounts of animal protein also have low blood vitamin B_{12} levels.

There are some recommendations that we can make to both younger and older adults to increase their absorption of vitamin B_{12} and promote good vitamin B_{12} status. First, the form of vitamin B_{12} found in fortified breads and cereals, and other fortified foods does not require hydrochloric acid for digestion and release from its food component. Therefore it is available for absorption even if gastric acid is limited. Adults, especially older adults, should be encouraged to have a vitamin B_{12}-fortified food several times a week. Researchers also have found that vitamin B_{12} is more easily released from dairy foods than from muscle foods such as meat. This is another good reason to consume dairy products regularly (see Chapter 8). We can no longer take for granted that persons who eat animal foods regularly have good vitamin B_{12} nutrition.

References

Baik HW, Russell RM: Vitamin B-12 deficiency in the elderly, *Annu Rev Nutr* 19:357, 1999.

Russell RM: Factors in aging that effect the bioavailability of nutrients, *J Nutr* 131:1359S, 2001.

Russell RM, Baik H, Kehayias JJ: Older men and women efficiently absorb vitamin B-12 from milk and fortified bread, *J Nutr* 131:291, 2001.

Tucker KL et al: Plasma vitamin B-12 concentrations relate to intake source in the Framingham Offspring study, *Am J Clin Nutr* 71:514, 2000.

(2) the circular muscle layer; and (3) the longitudinal muscle lying next to the outer serosa.

Types of Intestinal Muscle Actions

Under the control of the intramural nerve plexus of the enteric nervous system, wall-stretch pressure from food or hormonal stimuli will produce two different types of muscle movement to aid digestion.

1. *Propulsive movements.* Peristalsis produced by waves of contracting deep circular muscle propels the food mass slowly forward. The intensity of the wave may be increased by food intake or by the presence of irritants, causing in some cases long sweeping waves over the entire intestine. A series of local segmental contractions also aid the forward movement of the food mass. The presence of fiber or undigestible materials from plant foods supports this process, providing bulk for the action of these muscles.
2. *Mixing movements.* Peristalsis and local constrictive contractions that occur every few centimeters in the muscle wall mix and chop the food mass as it moves along the gastrointestinal tract. This combined action effectively churns the food mass, gradually mixing it with secretions to form the semiliquid chyme.

Thus the interaction of the muscles in the small intestine produces two basic types of action: (1) a general muscle tone or tonic contraction that ensures continuous passage and valve control and (2) periodic, rhythmic contractions that mix and propel the food mass. These alternating muscular contractions and relaxations force the contents forward and facilitate appropriate digestive and absorptive processes.

enterogastrone A duodenal peptide hormone that inhibits gastric hydrochloric acid secretion and motility.

gastrin Hormone secreted by mucosal cells in the antrum of the stomach that stimulates the parietal cells to produce hydrochloric acid. Gastrin is released into the stomach in response to stimulants, especially coffee, alcohol, and meat extracts. When the gastric pH falls below 3, a feedback mechanism cuts off gastrin secretion and prevents excess acid formation.

TABLE 2-2 Summary of Digestive Processes

Nutrient	Mouth	Stomach	Small Intestine
Carbohydrate	Starch $\xrightarrow{\text{Alpha-amylase}}$ Dextrins		Pancreas Starch $\xrightarrow{\text{Amylase}}$ Maltose and sucrose (Disaccharides) Intestine Lactose $\xrightarrow{\text{Lactase}}$ Glucose and galactose (Monosaccharides) Sucrose $\xrightarrow{\text{Sucrase}}$ Glucose and fructose Maltose $\xrightarrow{\text{Maltase}}$ Glucose and glucose
Protein		Protein $\xrightarrow{\text{Pepsin HCl}}$ Polypeptides	Pancreas Proteins, Polypeptides $\xrightarrow{\text{Trypsin}}$ Dipeptides Proteins, Polypeptides $\xrightarrow{\text{Chymotrypsin}}$ Dipeptides Polypeptides, Dipeptides $\xrightarrow{\text{Carboxypeptidase}}$ Amino acids Intestine Polypeptides, Dipeptides $\xrightarrow{\text{Aminopeptidase}}$ Amino acids Dipeptides $\xrightarrow{\text{Dipeptidase}}$ Amino acids
Fat		Tributyrin (butterfat) $\xrightarrow{\text{Tributyrinase}}$ Glycerol and Fatty acids	Pancreas Fats $\xrightarrow{\text{Lipase}}$ Glycerol and Glycerides (di-, mono-) and Fatty acids Intestine Fats $\xrightarrow{\text{Lipase}}$ Glycerol and Glycerides (di-, mono-) and Fatty acids Liver and gallbladder Fats $\xrightarrow{\text{Bile}}$ Emulsified fat

CHEMICAL DIGESTION

Major Role of Small Intestine

More than any other part of the gastrointestinal tract, the small intestine carries the major burden of chemical digestion. This area secretes a large number of enzymes, each specific for one of the macronutrients—carbohydrates, fats, and proteins. These specific enzymes are secreted from both the intestinal glands and the pancreas (Table 2-2). The small intestine acts as a regulatory center that senses the nutrient content, pH, and osmolarity of its contents and controls enzyme secretions accordingly.[2]

Types of Secretions

Four types of digestive secretions complete this final process of chemical breakdown in the small intestine.

1. *Enzymes.* A number of specific enzymes (see Table 2-2) act on specific macronutrients in food to cause a final breakdown of the nutrient materials to forms the body can absorb and use.
2. *Mucus.* Intestinal glands located immediately inside the duodenum secrete large quantities of mucus. This secretion protects the mucosa from irritation and digestion by the highly acid gastric juices in the chyme entering the duodenum. Additional mucous cells along the intestinal surface continue to secrete mucus when touched by the moving food mass. This secretion lubricates and protects the tissues from abrasion.
3. *Hormones.* In response to the presence of acid in the entering food mass, mucosal cells in the upper part of the small intestine produce the local gastrointestinal hormone secretin.[9] In turn, secretin stimulates the pancreas to send alkaline pancreatic juices into the duodenum to buffer the entering gastric acid chyme. The unprotected intestinal mucosa in the upper duodenum could not withstand this high degree of acidity from the entering chyme without the bicarbonate-containing pancreatic juice.
4. *Bile.* Another important aid to digestion and absorption in the small intestine is bile, an emulsifying agent for fats. A large volume of bile is produced in the liver as a dilute watery solution. It is then concentrated and stored by the gallbladder (Figure 2-6). When fat enters the duodenum, the local gastrointestinal hormone cholecystokinin (CCK) is secreted by glands in the intestinal mucosa and stimulates the gallbladder to contract and release the needed bile. The bile-conserving *enterohepatic circulation* of bile (see Figure 2-6), which involves the liver, gallbladder, and gastrointestinal tract, serves the needs of all organs involved.[10] In this way molecules of bile can be returned to the liver and gallbladder and used over and over again. CCK likely acts on the pancreas to also stimulate the release of enzymes for the breakdown of fats, proteins, and carbohydrates.[2]

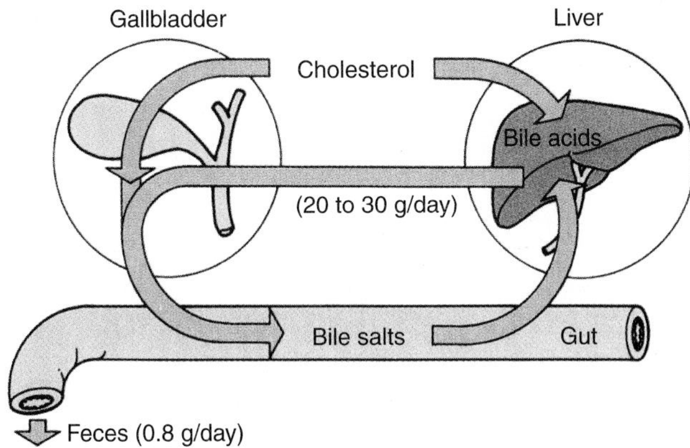

FIGURE 2-6 Enterohepatic circulation of bile salts.

Factors Influencing Secretions

In the small intestine, as well as in other parts of the gastrointestinal system, many factors influence the release of various secretions. These factors include controls from hormones and nerve systems stimulated by physical contact with food materials and stimulated by emotions. These influencing factors are summarized in Figure 2-7.

ABSORPTION

End Products of Digestion

After digestion of the food nutrients is complete, the simplified end products are ready for absorption. These end products include the *monosaccharides:* glucose, fructose, and galactose from carbohydrates; *fatty acids* and *glycerides* from fats; and *amino acids* from proteins. In some cases, incompletely digested nutrients remain in the small intestine and cause gas.[11] For example, in persons lacking lactase, the disaccharide lactose remains in the intestine and causes problems[12] (see *Issues & Answers*). Some small peptides made up of several amino acids may be absorbed intact and finally broken down within the mucosal absorptive cells to yield their amino acids. Vitamins and minerals are also liberated. Finally, with a water base for solution and transport, plus necessary electrolytes, the total fluid food mass is now prepared for absorption, the next phase of the gastrointestinal process (Table 2-3).

Surface Structures

Viewed from the outside, the small intestine appears smooth, but the inner mucosal surface lining is quite different. Note carefully in Figure 2-8 the three types of convolutions and projections that greatly enhance the absorbing surface area.

1. *Mucosal folds.* Large mucosal folds, similar to hills and valleys in a mountain range, can easily be seen by the naked eye.
2. *Villi.* Fingerlike projections on these folds, called villi, can be seen through a simple microscope.
3. *Microvilli.* These extremely small projections on each villus can be seen only with an electron microscope. The array of microvilli covering the edge of each villus is called the *brush border* because it looks like bristles on a brush. Each villus has an ample network of blood capillaries for the absorption of monosaccharides and amino acids, as well as a central lymph vessel called a *lacteal* for the absorption of fat substances that have a creamy, milklike appearance at this point.

Absorbing Surface Area

The three structures of the small intestine—mucosal folds, villi, and microvilli—increase the inner absorbing surface area about 1000 times over that of the outside serosa.[1] These special structures, plus the contracted length of the live organ—630 to 660 cm (21 to 22 ft)—produce a tremendously large absorbing surface. This inner surface of the small intestine, if stretched out flat, would be as large or larger than a tennis or basketball court! All three of these mucosal structures serve as a unit for the absorption of nutrients. Although the intestine is often referred to as the gut, it is actually one of the most highly developed, exquisitely fashioned, specialized tissues in the human body.

Mechanisms of Absorption

Absorption of the finely dispersed, water-based nutrient solution is accomplished through the wall of the small intestine by means of a number of transport processes. The particular transport process used depends on the nature of the nutrient and the prevailing electrochemical fluid pressure gradient.

---

absorption Transport of digested nutrients across the intestinal wall into the body circulation.

cholecystokinin (CCK) A peptide hormone secreted by the mucosa of the duodenum in response to the presence of fat. Cholecystokinin causes the gallbladder to contract and propel bile into the duodenum, where it is needed to emulsify the fat. The fat is thus prepared for digestion and absorption.

microvilli Minute vascular structures protruding from the surface of villi covering the inner surface of the small intestine, forming a "brush border" that facilitates absorption of nutrients.

mucus Viscous fluid secreted by mucous membranes and glands, consisting mainly of mucin (a glycoprotein), inorganic salts, and water. Mucus lubricates and protects the gastrointestinal mucosa and helps move the food mass along the digestive tract.

secretin Hormone produced in the mucous membrane of the duodenum in response to the entrance of acid contents from the stomach into the duodenum. Secretin in turn stimulates the flow of pancreatic juices, providing needed enzymes and the proper alkalinity for their action.

villi Small protrusions from the surface of a membrane; fingerlike projections covering mucosal surfaces of the small intestine.

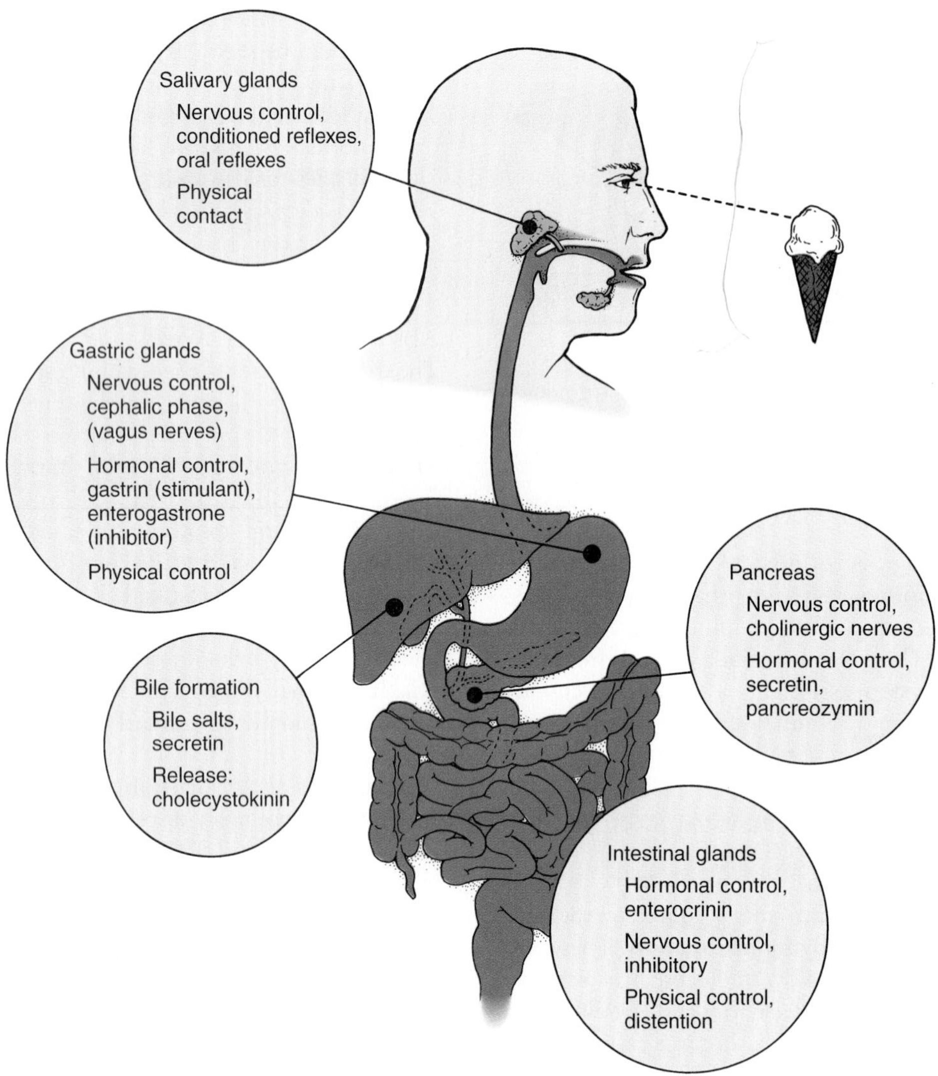

FIGURE 2-7 Summary of factors influencing secretions of the gastrointestinal tract.

TABLE 2-3 Daily Absorption Volume in Gastrointestinal System

	Intake (L)	Intestinal Absorption (L)	Elimination (L)
Food ingested	1.5		
Gastrointestinal secretions	8.5		
TOTAL	10.0		
Fluid absorbed in small intestine		9.5	
Fluid absorbed in large intestine		0.4	
TOTAL		9.9	
Feces			0.1

1. *Passive diffusion and osmosis.* When no opposing pressure exists, molecules small enough to pass through the capillary membranes diffuse easily into the capillaries of the villi in the direction of the pressure flow and in quantities that depend on their solute concentration (Figure 2-9). This varying solute concentration determines the electrochemical gradient based on the degree and direction of the osmotic pressure[1] (see Chapter 8).
2. *Facilitated diffusion.* Even though the pressure gradient is favorably flowing from greater to lesser concentration, which characterizes the process of diffusion, some particular molecules may be too large to easily go through the membrane pores and require assistance. In such cases a specific protein located in the membrane facilitates passage by carrying the particular nutrient molecule across the membrane.
3. *Energy-dependent active transport.* Nutrient molecules must cross the intestinal epithelial membrane to feed

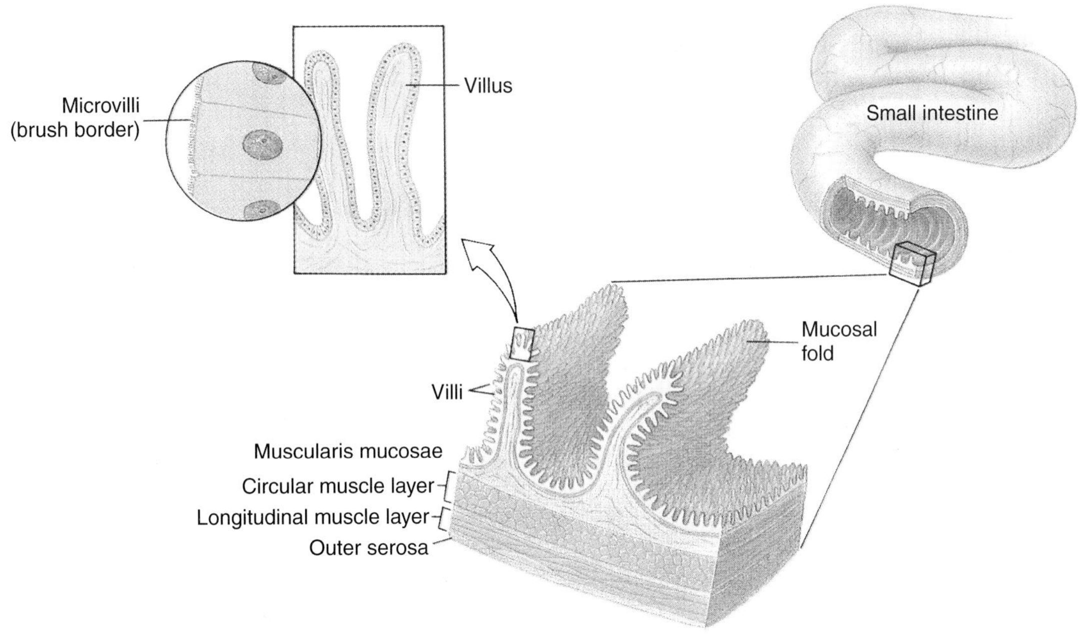

FIGURE 2-8 Intestinal wall. Note the arrangement of muscle layers and the structures of the mucosa that increase the surface area for absorption: mucosal folds, villi, and microvilli. *(Medical and Scientific Illustration.)*

hungry tissue cells even when the fluid flow pressures are against them. Such active work requires extra energy supplied by the metabolism of the cell and a pumping mechanism. A special membrane protein carrier, coupled with the active transport of sodium, assists the process. The active sodium-coupled transport of glucose is an example of this action. An important enzyme, *sodium- and potassium-dependent adenosine triphosphatase* (Na^+-, K^+-ATPase), which is present in the cell membrane, supplies the energy for this interesting pumping action.

4. *Engulfing pinocytosis.* At times, fluid and nutrient molecules use pinocytosis, still another means of reaching the tissue circulation outposts in the villi. In these instances, when the particular particle touches the absorbing cell membrane, the membrane dips inward around the fluid and nutrient material, surrounding it to form a vacuole, and then engulfs it. The materials are then conveyed through the cell cytoplasm and discharged into the circulation. Occasionally, smaller whole proteins, as well as neutral fat droplets, are absorbed through pinocytosis (Figure 2-10).

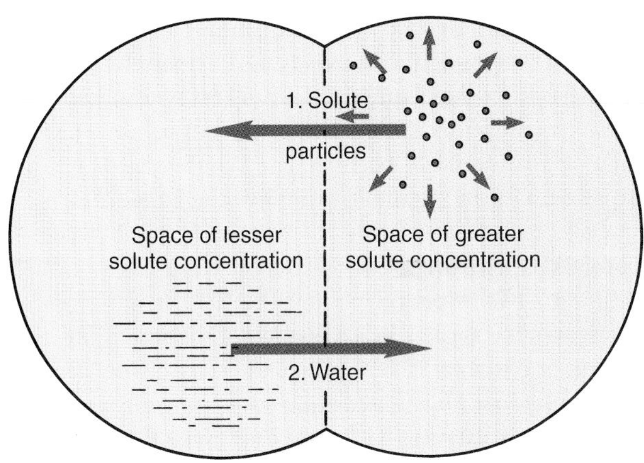

FIGURE 2-9 Movement of molecules, water, and solutes through osmosis and diffusion.

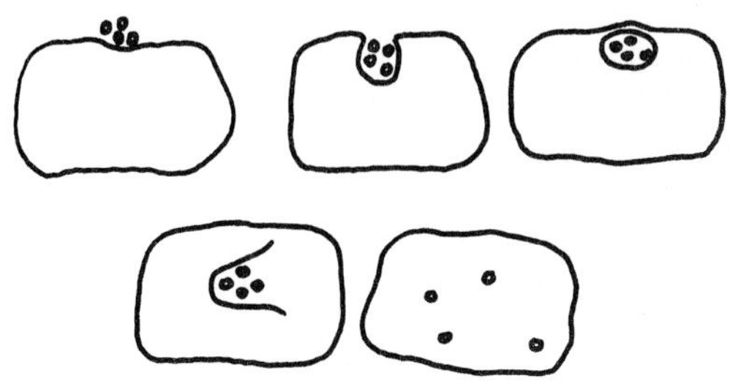

FIGURE 2-10 Pinocytosis, or engulfing of large molecules by the cell.

Routes of Absorption

After their absorption by one of these processes, the nutrients from carbohydrates and proteins, being water soluble, enter directly into the portal bloodstream and travel to the liver and other body tissues. Only fat, which is not water soluble, is unique in its route. Fats are carried in a bile complex into the cells of the intestinal wall, processed by enzymes to human lipid compounds, converted to a complex with protein as a carrier, and packaged as lipoproteins (we talk about this process in detail in Chapter 4). These packages of fat flow into the lymph; empty into the cisterna chyli, the major central abdominal collecting vessel of the lymphatic system of the body; travel upward into the chest through the thoracic duct; and finally flow into the venous blood at the left subclavian vein. These initial lipoproteins, called chylomicrons, are then rapidly cleared from the blood by the special fat enzyme, lipoprotein lipase. Exceptions to this route of fat absorption are the shorter chain fatty acids with 10 or fewer carbons, which are water soluble; hence, they are absorbed directly into the blood circulation, as are nutrients from carbohydrates and protein. However, most fats in the human diet are made of long-chain fatty acids, are not water soluble, and must travel via the lacteal lymphatic route.

Large Intestine: Final Absorption and Waste Elimination

ROLE IN ABSORPTION

The absorption of water is the main task remaining for the large intestine. The actual capacity of the colon for water absorption is great; the net daily maximum is approximately 5 to 8 L.[1] In daily function, however, approximately 1 to 1.5 L is received from the ileum and 95% of that is absorbed.[2] Related nutrient factors, such as electrolytes, minerals, vitamins, amino acids, intestinal bacteria, and nondigestible residue, also remain in the chyme delivered to the large intestine.

Water Absorption

Within a 24-hour period, about 500 ml of remaining food mass leaves the *ileum,* the last portion of the small intestine, and enters the *cecum,* the pouch at the start of the large intestine or colon. Here the *ileocecal valve* controls passage of the semiliquid chyme. Normally the valve remains closed, but each peristaltic wave relaxes the valve and squirts a small amount of chyme into the cecum. This mechanism holds the food mass in the small intestine long enough to ensure digestion and maximum absorption of vital nutrients.

The watery chyme continues to move slowly through the large intestine, aided by muscle contractions and the mucus secreted by the mucosal glands along this passage. The major portion of the water in the chyme, 350 to 400 ml, is absorbed in the first half of the colon. Only about 100 to 150 ml remains to form the feces.[1] The reabsorption of water in the colon is important in the regulation of water balance and in the elimination of fecal waste. When the chyme first enters the colon, it is a semiliquid, but the water reabsorption that takes place during its passage through the colon changes it to the semisolid nature of normal feces.

The degree of water absorbed is dependent on the motility and rate of passage. Poor motility and a slow passage rate, often related to diets low in fiber and low fecal mass, result in greater absorption of water and hard stools that are difficult to pass and in constipation. Excess motility and too rapid passage of the chyme through the colon limit the reabsorption of water and important electrolytes, producing a high volume of loose, watery stool (diarrhea). Severe, extended diarrhea leads to dehydration and serious loss of electrolytes. Diarrhea can result from a disease condition, a microbial infection or irritant as in foodborne illness, or the presence of a large amount of undigested sugar such as lactose that exerts osmotic pressure and holds large amounts of fluid (see *Issues & Answers*).

Mineral Absorption

Electrolytes, mainly sodium, are transported into the bloodstream from the colon. Intestinal absorption is a major balance control point for many of the minerals, and much of the dietary intake remains unabsorbed for elimination in the feces. For example, 20% to 70% of the calcium and 80% to 85% of the iron ingested are eliminated. The bioavailability of nutrients, especially minerals and vitamins, is largely reflected by their relative overall absorption during their passage through the gastrointestinal system.[13] This is an important aspect of nutrient balance and dietary evaluation.

Vitamin Absorption

Intestinal absorption also serves as a balance control point for some of the vitamins, determining how much the body will keep and how much it will excrete.[11] In addition, bacteria in the colon can be a source of particular vitamins. Colon bacteria synthesize vitamin K and biotin, which can be absorbed from the colon to help meet daily needs.

BACTERIAL ACTION

At birth the colon is sterile, but intestinal bacterial flora soon become well established. The adult colon contains large numbers of bacteria. One species receiving much attention is *Escherichia coli*[9] because great masses of this bacteria are passed in the stool. Secretions from the immune system help to protect the mucosal lining of the stomach and intestines from any harmful effects of normal intestinal bacteria and environmental pathogens entering the body through the gastrointestinal tract[14] (see *To Probe Further* box).

Intestinal bacteria also affect the color and odor of the stool. The brown color is a result of bile pigments formed by the colon bacteria from bilirubin. Thus in conditions that hinder bile flow, the feces may become clay colored or white. The characteristic odor results from amines, especially *indole* and *skatole,* which are formed from amino acids by bacterial enzymes.

Intestinal gas, or *flatus,* contains hydrogen sulfide and methane produced by these bacteria. Gas formation, a common complaint, is not necessarily the result of specific foods but rather the result of individual conditions in the body that receives them. Many foods have been labeled "gas formers," but in reality these effects are highly

TABLE 2-4 Intestinal Absorption of Some Major Nutrients

Nutrient	Form	Means of Absorption	Control Agent or Required Cofactor	Route
Carbohydrate	Monosaccharides (glucose and galactose)	Competitive	—	Blood
		Selective	—	
		Active transport via sodium pump	Sodium	
Protein	Amino acids	Selective	—	Blood
	Whole protein (rare)	Pinocytosis	—	Blood
	Some dipeptides	Carrier transport systems	Pyridoxine (pyridoxal phosphate)	Blood
Fat	Fatty acids	Fatty acid–bile complex (micelles)	Bile	
	Glycerides (mono-, di-)		—	Lymph
	Few triglycerides (neutral fat)	Pinocytosis	—	Lymph
Vitamins	B_{12}	Carrier transport	Intrinsic factor (IF)	Blood
	A	Bile complex	Bile	Blood
	K	Bile complex	Bile	From large intestine to blood
Minerals	Sodium	Active transport via sodium pump	—	Blood
	Calcium	Active transport	Vitamin D	Blood
	Iron	Active transport	Ferritin mechanism	Blood (as transferritin)
Water	Water	Osmosis	—	Blood, lymph, interstitial fluid

variable from one person to another, and such classifications have little or no scientific basis.[11,15]

ROLE OF DIETARY FIBER

Because humans have no microorganisms or enzymes that break down dietary fiber, this residue from plant foods remains after nutrient digestion and absorption have been completed. Undigested fiber contributes important bulk to the diet and helps form the feces. As we will learn in Chapter 3, a high-fiber diet can help prevent constipation, diverticulitis, and other problems of the colon.[16,17] Fully formed and ready for elimination, normal feces contain about 75% water and 25% solids.[1] The solids include fiber, bacteria, inorganic matter such as minerals, a small amount of fat and its derivatives, some mucus, and sloughed-off mucosal cells.

Some major aspects of nutrient absorption are summarized in Table 2-4.

WASTE ELIMINATION

This mass of food residue now begins to slow its passage. A meal, having traveled the 630 to 660 cm (21 to 22 ft) of the small intestine, starts to enter the cecum about 4 hours after it is consumed. About 8 hours later it reaches the sigmoid colon, having traveled about 90 cm (3 ft) through the large intestine. In the sigmoid colon the residue descends still more slowly toward the rectum.

bilirubin A reddish bile pigment resulting from the degradation of heme by reticuloendothelial cells in the liver; a high level in the blood produces the yellow skin symptomatic of jaundice.

cisterna chyli Cistern or receptacle of the chyle; a dilated sac at the origin of the thoracic duct, which is the common trunk that receives all the lymphatic vessels. The cisterna chyli lies in the abdomen between the second lumbar vertebra and the aorta. It receives the lymph from the intestinal trunk, the right and left lumbar lymphatic trunks, and two descending lymphatic trunks. The chyle, after passing through the cisterna chyli, is carried upward into the chest through the thoracic duct and empties into the venous blood at the point where the left subclavian vein joins the left internal jugular vein. This is the way absorbed fats enter the general circulation.

colon The large intestine extending from the cecum to the rectum.

TO PROBE FURTHER
Intestinal Microflora: Friend or Foe?

Over 400 different species of bacteria normally reside in the human gastrointestinal tract, and most are found in the large intestine. In fact the contents of the large intestine may contain as many as 1 billion bacteria/g. In the human the microflora begins to establish itself in the gastrointestinal tract shortly after birth. The intestinal microflora play many different roles, with both positive and negative outcomes. Particular microflora produce excessive and bothersome gas for the host or increase the risk of gastrointestinal disease. Other species synthesize important vitamins or help protect the body against pathogens that enter the gastrointestinal tract. Here we examine these outcomes in greater detail.

PRODUCTION OF INTESTINAL GAS

Intestinal bacteria are the major contributors to gas production in the gastrointestinal tract, producing CO_2, H_2, and methane. These gases are produced from undigested or incompletely absorbed carbohydrate, and in some individuals, gas production is excessive. Even persons with normal digestion can have carbohydrate remaining in their intestine that is fermented by bacteria. For example, fructose is not completely absorbed by most people, and highly sweetened soft drinks or fruit drinks contain up to 23 g of fructose per can. Apple juice is high in sorbitol, a naturally occurring sugar that is not absorbed, and can cause diarrhea and abdominal discomfort in young children. No humans possess the enzymes necessary to digest the oligosaccharides raffinose and stachyose. These substances are found in legumes and lead to the excessive intestinal gas sometimes associated with these foods.

Certain starches found in grains, fruits, and vegetables, referred to as resistant starch, are resistant to pancreatic amylase and thus cannot be broken down and absorbed in the small intestine. When we encourage persons to increase their intakes of foods known to be high in resistant starch and fiber (also fermentable in the large intestine), we need to make them aware that they may experience increased intestinal gas. In most cases individuals adjust easily as they continue to consume these foods on a regular basis.

Some individuals have a problem with excessive gas production that has social implications. Although the gases noted above—CO_2, H_2, and methane—have no odor, hydrogen sulfide gases produce a striking odor. Hydrogen sulfide is more likely to be present when persons consume many servings of cruciferous vegetables such as cabbage, cauliflower, or broccoli or large amounts of beer, because these foods are high in sulfur. However, some endogenous substances, such as mucin, also supply sulfur in the gut. Bismuth subsalicylate (Pepto Bismol) has been successfully used in research experiments to bind sulfides and to eliminate odor; however, we need to caution clients about the risks involved with frequent and long-term use of bismuth-containing compounds.

FORMATION OF ULCERS

Specific microflora in the stomach may be involved in the etiology of peptic and duodenal ulcers. Ulcers can result from (1) excessive secretion of gastric acid that destroys the mucosal lining of the stomach or duodenum or (2) a reduced ability of the mucosal tissues to protect themselves against the harmful effects of gastric acid. In past years ulcer treatment focused on the use of drugs that inhibited gastric acid production. More recently, the bacterium *Helicobacter pylori* has been implicated in the formation of ulcers. *H. pylori* is able to burrow into the mucosal lining of the stomach or duodenum and to destroy the mucus-producing cells that are normally protective, thus leaving the sensitive tissues beneath exposed to the digestive action of gastric acid. It appears that 75% of persons with peptic ulcers have chronic infections of *H. pylori.* Treatment with antibiotics, as well as with acid-reducing drugs, is now part of most ulcer protocols.

Some persons who do not have ulcers experience the pain and gastric distress often associated with ulcers, and this condition is sometimes referred to as nonulcer dyspepsia. Individuals with stomach pain often resort to self-medication, and drugs that inhibit acid secretion in the stomach have become available for sale without a prescription. It is important that these drugs not be used habitually, because the reduction of gastric acid could over time induce a deficiency of vitamin B_{12} or important minerals (see *Practical Application* box).

SYNTHESIS OF PARTICULAR VITAMINS

Intestinal microflora also bring positive effects to their hosts. Certain bacteria produce both vitamin K and biotin. It is likely that the vitamin K produced and absorbed in the large intestine plays a vital role in meeting the vitamin K requirement. With new research identifying vitamin K as a necessary participant in bone remodeling and formation, the bacteria-produced supplies of vitamin K may be especially important to postmenopausal women and older men.

TO PROBE FURTHER
Intestinal Microflora: Friend or Foe?—cont'd

PROBIOTICS IN HUMAN HEALTH

Probiotics, live microbial food supplements that benefit their host by improving the balance of microbes in the gastrointestinal tract, are receiving attention as new alternatives for treating chronic problems and improving health. Several distinct species of bacteria, *Lactobacilli* and *Bifidobacteria,* have beneficial effects in the human colon. *Lactobacilli* stimulate antibody production and immune function in both infants and adults. *Lactobacilli* and *Bifidobacteria* work together to lower the production of microbial enzymes that can activate carcinogens found in the lower bowel. Certain forms of *Lactobacilli* have proved to be effective treatments for virus-based diarrhea in children and appear to have promise for preventing traveler's diarrhea in adults. Lactic acid bacteria are effective in reducing the symptoms of lactose intolerance in lactase-deficient individuals, and the use of this treatment increases their intake of dairy products. Researchers are looking for mechanisms by which the growth or activity of these helpful species of bacteria can be enhanced while the growth of harmful bacteria can be reduced.

Certain nondigestible carbohydrates that serve as a source of nutrition for the growth of *Lactobacilli* and *Bifidobacilli* have now been termed prebiotics and are being studied for their potential usefulness in human health. Prebiotics can increase fecal mass and improve bowel habits in the elderly, although these improvements may be accompanied by an increase in flatulence. The positive effects of prebiotics will need to be weighed against the less desirable side effects of increased production of intestinal gas.

We are continuing to learn more about the actions, both beneficial and detrimental, of gastrointestinal microflora. Bacteria residing in the human intestine may play a role in preventing or alleviating chronic nutrition and health problems. As probiotics continue to be recognized for their health benefits, we must begin to establish standards of identity and safety for their addition to food products and regulations for their addition to over-the-counter drugs and products for self-care. Health professionals should provide appropriate advice regarding the benefits and potential deterrents to use of products claiming to improve gastrointestinal health.

References

Brody T: *Nutritional biochemistry,* ed 2, New York, 1999, Academic Press.

Guyton AC, Hall JE: *Textbook of medical physiology,* ed 10, Philadelphia, 2000, WB Saunders.

Kopp-Hoolihyan L: Prophylactic and therapeutic uses of probiotics: a review, *J Am Diet Assoc* 101:229, 2001.

Roberfroid MB: Prebiotics and probiotics: are they functional foods? *Am J Clin Nutr* 71(suppl):1682S, 2000.

Saavedra JM: Clinical applications of probiotic agents, *Am J Clin Nutr* 73(suppl):1147S, 2001.

Suarez FL: Managing intestinal gas, *Nutr MD* 26:1, 2000.

The rectum begins at the end of the large intestine, immediately following the descending colon, and ends at the anus. Feces are usually stored in the descending colon; however, when this becomes full, feces pass into the rectum, leading to an urge to defecate. Anal sphincters, under voluntary control, regulate the elimination of feces from the body. As much as 25% of a meal may remain in the rectum for up to 72 hours.

Clinical Problems and Gastrointestinal Function

For most individuals, the gastrointestinal tract is a smoothly working system that supports food intake and effectively handles digestion, absorption, and the elimination of waste with scant attention. For others, gastrointestinal discomfort and distress are daily occurrences, related to side effects of prescription drugs, chronic disease, or unexplained causes. Interventions for medical conditions such as duodenal ulcers and diverticular disease or for constipation related to diet or lifestyle will be discussed in later chapters. Unfortunately, both children[18] and adults[19] experience functional dyspepsia with abdominal pain, nausea, vomiting, and anorexia, for which no specific cause or disease can be found.[20] Medical researchers have discovered that a microorganism found in the gastrointestinal tract, *Helicobacter pylori,* attacks the mucosal lining of the stomach and duodenum and is a major cause of ulcers. Recent studies have tried to learn if this organism may also cause chronic dyspepsia in some persons, but at this time we do not know the answer.[21]

Mental and emotional stress, depression, and chronic disease can all influence gastrointestinal function. It is important that we listen carefully to our clients and patients when they tell us about gastrointestinal problems that interfere with eating and the enjoyment of food.[20,22] Health education that focuses on self-care should point to the dangers of special supplements such as food enzymes advertised to enhance digestion, inappropriate laxatives, or ill-advised procedures such as colonic irrigation. Chronic digestive problems require medical assessment and intervention.

Metabolism

The various absorbed nutrients, including water and electrolytes, are carried to the cells and used to produce many substances the body needs to sustain life. Cell metabolism encompasses the total continuous complex of chemical changes that determine the final use of the individual nutrients.

CARBOHYDRATE METABOLISM

Glucose is an immediate and important source of energy for all cells in the body, but it is the energy nutrient of choice for the brain and nervous system. Consequently, blood glucose is important to sustain life and is carefully regulated by a series of metabolic control systems.

Sources of Blood Glucose

Both carbohydrate and noncarbohydrate substances are sources of blood glucose.

1. *Carbohydrate sources.* Three carbohydrate sources provide blood glucose: (1) dietary starches and sugars, (2) glycogen stored in liver and muscle tissue, and (3) products of intermediary carbohydrate metabolism, such as lactic acid and pyruvic acid. (The hydrolysis of glycogen to form glucose is called glycogenolysis.)
2. *Noncarbohydrate sources.* Both protein and fat provide additional indirect sources of glucose. Certain amino acids from protein are called *glucogenic amino acids* because they form glucose after they are broken down. About 58% of the protein in a mixed diet is composed of glucogenic amino acids. Thus more than half of dietary protein may ultimately be used for energy if sufficient carbohydrates and fat are not available for fuel. After the breakdown of fat into fatty acids and *glycerol,* the small glycerol portion (about 10% of the fat) can be converted to glycogen in the liver and made available for glucose formation. The production of glucose from protein, glycerol (from fat), and intermediary carbohydrate metabolites is called gluconeogenesis.

Uses of Blood Glucose

Three uses of glucose serve to regulate the blood glucose within a normal range of 70 to 140 mg/dl (3.9 to 7.8 mmol/L).

1. *Energy production.* The primary function of glucose is to supply energy to meet the body's constant demand. A vast array of interacting metabolic pathways that use many specific and successive cell enzymes accomplish this task in a highly efficient manner.
2. *Energy storage.* There are two storage forms for glucose: (a) *glycogen*—glucose may be converted to glycogen and stored in limited amounts in the liver and muscle tissue; only a small supply of glycogen is present at any one time and it turns over rapidly; and (b) *fat*—after energy demands have been fulfilled, any excess glucose is converted to fat and stored as adipose tissue.
3. *Glucose products.* Small amounts of glucose are used in the production of various carbohydrate compounds that have significant roles in overall body metabolism. Examples include DNA and RNA, galactose, and certain amino acids.

These sources and uses of glucose act as checks and balances to maintain normal blood glucose levels by adding glucose to the blood or removing it as needed.

Hormonal Controls

A number of hormones directly and indirectly influence the metabolism of glucose and regulate the blood glucose level.

1. *Blood glucose–lowering hormone.* Only one hormone, insulin, acts to lower blood glucose. It is produced by special beta cells in the pancreas. These cells are scattered in cell clusters, forming "islands" in the pancreas—thus the name *islets of Langerhans,* after the scientist Paul Langerhans (1847-1888), who as a young German medical student first discovered and studied them. Insulin regulates blood glucose through several actions: (1) *glycogenesis* stimulates the conversion of glucose to glycogen in the liver for constant energy reserve; (2) *lipoprotein lipase* stimulates conversion of glucose to fat for storage in adipose tissue; and (3) *cell permeability* to glucose is increased, allowing it to pass into the cells for oxidation to supply needed energy.
2. *Blood glucose–raising hormones.* A number of hormones effectively raise blood glucose levels.
   - *Glucagon,* produced by pancreatic islet alpha cells, acts opposite to insulin, increasing breakdown of liver glycogen to glucose and maintaining blood glucose during fasting sleep hours.
   - *Somatostatin,* produced in the pancreatic delta cells and in the hypothalamus, suppresses insulin and glucagon and acts as a general modulator of related metabolic activities.
   - *Steroid hormones,* secreted by the adrenal cortex, release glucose-forming carbon units from protein and act as insulin antagonists.
   - *Epinephrine,* originating from the adrenal medulla, stimulates the breakdown of liver glycogen and quick release of immediate glucose.
   - *Growth hormone (GH)* and *adrenocorticotropic hormone (ACTH),* released from the anterior pituitary gland, act as insulin antagonists.

- *Thyroxine,* originating from the thyroid gland, increases the rate of insulin breakdown, increases glucose absorption from the small intestine and liberates epinephrine.

LIPID METABOLISM

Lipid Synthesis and Breakdown

Two organ tissues, the liver and adipose tissue, form a balanced axis of lipid metabolism. Both function in lipid synthesis and breakdown. The fatty acids released from lipids are used by body cells as concentrated fuel to produce energy.

Lipoproteins

These lipid-protein complexes provide the major transport form of lipids in the blood. An excess amount of lipoproteins in the blood produces a clinical condition called *hyperlipoproteinemia.* Lipoproteins are produced (1) in the intestinal wall after initial absorption of dietary lipids and (2) in the liver for constant recirculation to and from cells.

Hormonal Controls

Because lipid and carbohydrate metabolism are closely interrelated, the same hormones are involved.

- *GH, ACTH,* and *thyroid-stimulating hormone (TSH),* all from the pituitary gland, increase the release of free fatty acids from stored body lipids when energy demands are imposed.
- *Cortisol* and *corticosterone,* from the adrenal gland, cause the release of free fatty acids.
- *Epinephrine* and *norepinephrine* stimulate the breakdown of lipids and release of free fatty acids.
- *Insulin,* from the pancreas, promotes lipid synthesis and storage, whereas glucagon has the opposite effect of breaking down lipid stores to release free fatty acids.
- *Thyroxine,* from the thyroid gland, stimulates lipid tissue release of free fatty acids and also lowers blood cholesterol levels.

PROTEIN METABOLISM

Anabolism, or Tissue Building

Protein metabolism centers on the essential balance between anabolism (tissue building) and catabolism (tissue breakdown). The process of anabolism builds protein tissue through the synthesis of new protein. This tissue building is governed by a definite pattern—a specific "blueprint" provided by DNA in the cell nucleus—that requires specific amino acids. A particular selection and supply of amino acids are necessary. Control agents include specific cell enzymes and coenzymes. Also, particular hormones—GH, gonadotropins, and thyroxine—control or stimulate the building of tissue protein.

Catabolism, or Tissue Breakdown

Amino acids released by tissue breakdown, if not reused in new tissue synthesis, are further broken down and used for other purposes. Two main parts of these amino acids result from this breakdown: the nitrogen-containing group and the remaining non-nitrogen residue.

1. *Nitrogen group.* The nitrogen portion is first split off from the amino acid, a process called deamination. The nitrogen is converted to ammonia and excreted in the urine or retained for use in making other nitrogen compounds.
2. *Non-nitrogen residue.* The non-nitrogen residues are called keto acids. They can be used to form either carbohydrates or fats. They also can be reaminated to form a new amino acid.

As in the case of tissue building, cell enzymes and coenzymes, as well as hormones, influence tissue catabolism. In health there is a dynamic equilibrium between the two processes of anabolism and catabolism to sustain growth and maintain sound tissue.

METABOLIC INTERRELATIONSHIPS

Each of the chemical processes of body metabolism is purposeful, and all are interdependent. They are designed to fill two essential needs: production of energy and growth and maintenance of healthy tissue. The controlling agents in the cells that are necessary for all of these intricately balanced processes to proceed in an orderly fashion are the cell enzymes, their coenzymes (many of which involve key vitamins and minerals), and special hormones. Overall, human metabolism is an exciting biochemical process, designed to develop, sustain, and protect our most precious possession—life itself.

TO SUM UP

Nutrients present in the foods we eat are converted into forms that the body can use through the process of digestion and absorption. Metabolism is the series of chemical reactions by which the body uses these nutrients to produce energy, build and rebuild body tissues, and maintain normal body functions.

---

deamination Removal of an amino group (NH_2) from an amino acid.

glycogenolysis Specific term for conversion of glycogen into glucose in the liver; chemical process of enzymatic hydrolysis or breakdown by which this conversion is accomplished.

gluconeogenesis Production of glucose from keto acid carbon skeletons from deaminated amino acids and the glycerol portion of fatty acids.

keto acid Amino acid residue after deamination. The glycogenic keto acids are used to form carbohydrates.

Digestion consists of two basic activities: mechanical and chemical. Muscular activity is responsible for the mechanical breakdown of food through such actions as mastication and the movement of food along the gastrointestinal tract by the motion of peristalsis. Chemical activity involves enzymatic action that degrades food into smaller and smaller components for absorption.

Absorption is the passage of nutrients across the intestinal wall into the bloodstream. This occurs mainly in the small intestine via a number of mechanisms, including diffusion, facilitated diffusion, active transport, and pinocytosis. Monosaccharides resulting from the breakdown of carbohydrates and amino acids from proteins are water soluble and pass directly from the mucosal cells of the small intestine into the portal blood circulation. Long-chain fatty acids, which are not water soluble, are packaged in lipid-protein complexes called lipoproteins, enter the lymph, and pass through the thoracic duct into the blood. Water absorption takes place primarily in the large intestine or colon.

Cell metabolism makes use of the absorbed nutrients. This metabolic work is accomplished by a large number of biochemical reactions that produce energy and maintain a dynamic balance between tissue breakdown and rebuilding.

■ Questions for Review

1. List the muscle types and their locations in the walls of the gastrointestinal tract. What types of motions or movements do they provide in each major section of the gastrointestinal tract? What is the role of the intramural nervous system in controlling gastrointestinal muscle function?
2. You are working with an elderly person who had a stroke that resulted in damage to the nerves in the swallowing center of the hypothalamus. What are the implications for his food intake or nutritional well-being?
3. Make a chart of the chemical actions of digestion that occur in each major section of the gastrointestinal tract. List across the top of your page the mouth, esophagus, stomach, and small intestine. List along the side of your page (a) the enzymes or fluids that act on the food mass in that location, (b) the sources of those enzymes or fluids, (c) the factors that stimulate their release, and (d) the factors that inhibit their activity.
4. Describe what happens in absorption. Explain the four mechanisms by which nutrients are absorbed from the small intestine.
5. You have just eaten a lunch that included a hamburger on a whole wheat bun, a glass of low-fat milk, and a bunch of grapes. Trace the digestion and final destination of each of the macronutrients present in your lunch. Indicate (a) the enzymes, locations, and breakdown products formed in the complete digestion of these foods; (b) the routes taken by the breakdown products after absorption (be sure to note the difference between the route followed by carbohydrates and proteins versus that followed by lipids; and (c) one possible destination for each breakdown product, either a type of body tissue or molecule.
6. Describe in detail two important activities that occur in the large intestine.
7. Visit your local supermarket or drug store and examine several over-the-counter medications that make claims to reduce stomach acid or alleviate intestinal gas. Make a table that includes each product and list the active ingredients as given on the product label. Using the *Physicians Desk Reference* or other drug index, identify the specific actions of the active ingredients. Based on your study of the process of digestion and absorption, explain the mechanism by which each active ingredient is believed to bring about the desired effect.

■ References

1. Guyton AC, Hall JE: *Textbook of medical physiology,* ed 10, Philadelphia, 2000, WB Saunders.
2. Klein S, Cohn SM, Alpers DH: The alimentary tract in nutrition. In Shils MA et al, eds: *Modern nutrition in health and disease,* ed 9, Philadelphia, 1999, Lippincott Williams & Wilkins.
3. Mattes RD: The chemical senses and nutrition in aging: challenging old assumptions, *J Am Diet Assoc* 102:192, 2002.
4. Clouse RE, Diamant NE: Motor physiology and motor disorders of the esophagus. In Feldman M, Scharschmidt BF, Sleisenger MH, eds: *Gastrointestinal and liver disease,* vol 2, ed 6, Philadelphia, 1998, WB Saunders.
5. Grande L et al: Deterioration of esophageal motility with age: a manometric study of 79 healthy subjects, *Am J Gastroenterol* 94:1795, 1999.
6. Eisen G: The epidemiology of gastroesophageal reflux disease: what we know and what we need to know, *Am J Gastroenterol* 96:S16, 2001.
7. Ma L et al: Cigarette smoke increases apoptosis in the gastric mucosa: role of epidermal growth factor, *Digestion* 60:461, 1999.
8. Ship JA, Pillemer SR, Baum BJ: Xerostomia and the geriatric patient, *J Am Geriatr Soc* 50:535, 2002.
9. Brody T: *Nutritional biochemistry,* ed 2, New York, 1999, Academic Press.
10. Hofmann AF: Bile secretion and the enterohepatic circulation of bile acids. In Feldman M, Scharschmidt BF, Sleisenger MH, eds: *Gastrointestinal and liver disease,* vol 1, ed 6, Philadelphia, 1998, WB Saunders.
11. Strocchi A, Levitt MD: Intestinal gas. In Feldman M, Scharschmidt BF, Sleisenger MH, eds: *Gastrointestinal and liver disease,* vol 1, ed 6, Philadelphia, 1998, WB Saunders.
12. Vesa TH, Marteau P, Korpela R: Lactose intolerance, *J Am Coll Nutr* 19:165S, 2000.
13. Marsh MN, Riley SA: Digestion and absorption of nutrients and vitamins. In Feldman M, Scharschmidt BF, Sleisenger MH, eds: *Gastrointestinal and liver disease,* vol 2, ed 6, Philadelphia, 1998, WB Saunders.

14. Mestecky JH, Russell MW, Elson CO: Intestinal IgA: novel views on its function in the defence of the largest mucosal surface, *Gut* 44:2, 1999.
15. Serra J, Azpiroz F, Malagelada JR: Intestinal gas dynamics and tolerance in humans, *Gastroenterology* 115:542, 1998.
16. Slavin JL: Epidemiologic and clinical studies on whole grains, *Nutr Today* 36:61, 2001.
17. Mceligot AJ et al: High dietary fiber consumption is not associated with gastrointestinal discomfort in a diet intervention trial, *J Am Diet Assoc* 102:549, 2002.
18. Papadopoulou A et al: Nutritional implications of chronic dyspepsia in childhood, *Dig Dis Sci* 47:32, 2002.
19. Rabeneck L et al: Sociodemographics, general health, and psychologic health in uninvestigated dyspepsia: a comparison of public and private patients, *J Clin Gastroenterol* 34:516, 2002.
20. Spiller RC: ABC of the upper gastrointestinal tract: anorexia, nausea, vomiting, and pain, *BMJ* 323:1354, 2001.
21. Froehlich F et al: Helicobacter pylori eradication treatment does not benefit patients with nonulcer dyspepsia, *Am J Gastroenterol* 96:2329, 2001.
22. Beyer PL: Gastrointestinal disorders: roles of nutrition and the dietetics practitioner, *J Am Diet Assoc* 98:272, 1998.

■ Further Reading

Duffy VB, Bartoshuk LM: Food acceptance and genetic variation in taste, *J Am Diet Assoc* 100:647, 2000.

Mattes RD: The chemical senses and nutrition in aging: challenging old assumptions, *J Am Diet Assoc* 102:192, 2002.

These authors tell us about the genetic factors that influence taste and their relationships to food preferences in individuals of all ages. Genetic differences in taste may influence one's preference for sweet, high-fat, or bitter foods.

Velazquez A, Bourges H: Implications of the Human Genome Project for understanding gene-environment interactions, *Nutr Rev* 57:S39, 1999.

This article presents an overview of how genes influence our health or dietary needs based on the presence or absence of particular digestive enzymes or susceptibility to certain chronic diseases.

Beyer PL: Gastrointestinal disorders: roles of nutrition and the dietetics practitioner, *J Am Diet Assoc* 98:272, 1998.

Kopp-Hoolihyan L: Prophylactic and therapeutic uses of probiotics: a review, *J Am Diet Assoc* 101:229, 2001.

These clinicians describe issues and new opportunities for the prevention and treatment of gastrointestinal problems.

Issues & ANSWERS

Lactose Intolerance: Common Problem Worldwide

Consider this: a natural disaster strikes an underdeveloped nation, leaving thousands homeless and with very little food. CARE, UNICEF, and other international organizations work quickly to collect and ship foodstuffs to the area. Yet the recipients of this food now have an additional problem—gastrointestinal distress.

One of the most common foodstuffs shipped from the United States to impoverished areas is dry milk. And one of the most common digestive problems throughout the world is lactose intolerance, a condition that results in abdominal cramps, nausea, bloating, and diarrhea when milk is consumed. The problem stems from a deficiency of lactase. Lactase is a digestive enzyme found in the microvilli of the small intestine that hydrolyzes lactose, the sugar in milk, into its component monosaccharides, glucose and galactose, for absorption. Because lactose cannot be absorbed, it remains in the intestines and exerts an osmotic pressure that attracts fluid into the lower gastrointestinal tract, resulting in diarrhea. Bacteria present in the small intestine and the colon act on the lactose to produce gas and bloating.

All mammals are born with sufficient amounts of lactase to accommodate the high lactose levels in mother's milk. In animal species lactase enzyme activity drops off significantly shortly after birth. In humans this fall in lactase activity usually occurs between the ages of 2 and 20 years and is genetically determined. Only a few population groups do not experience this significant childhood drop in the enzyme lactase. Lactase levels tend to remain high among northern Europeans but fall to lower levels in most other groups, including Africans, Asians, and Latinos. Some individuals experience symptoms after drinking even 1 cup of milk.

Many lactose-intolerant persons can digest cultured or fermented milk products such as buttermilk, yogurt, or cheese and can use these foods as their primary source of calcium. However, it is usually not possible to supply items that require refrigeration to disaster areas. Cheese can be too expensive to completely satisfy the calcium needs of American school children through school breakfast and lunch programs, and many cheeses add significant amounts of fat to the diet. At the same time the nutritional benefits of lactose-rich foods may become crucial in offsetting protein, calcium, and some vitamin deficiencies among those in need.

Continuing study seems to cloud the lactose-calcium issue even further. Sensitive tests used to measure lactase status and calcium absorption indicate that lactase-deficient persons may absorb calcium even better than persons who are lactase sufficient. Also, there seem to be subjective issues associated with the appearance of symptoms after the ingestion of lactose-containing foods. When persons believed to be lactose intolerant were given lactose-free or lactose-containing milk and not told which milk they were drinking, about one third did not experience abdominal distress even when drinking the lactose-containing beverage. This suggests that the abdominal symptoms that persons believed to be associated with milk may actually be related to other foods, food ingredients, or conditions.

Individuals who are lactose intolerant are less likely to experience symptoms if they (1) drink 1 cup of milk at a time along with a meal and (2) use milk with some fat content. This will allow the milk to move more slowly into the intestine and diminish the production of gas. In a recent study with adolescent African American girls, a gradual increase in milk intake over a 3-week period brought about an adaptation in the large intestine, reducing symptoms and increasing acceptability.

So what do we tell persons who are lactase deficient about supplementing their dietary intake of calcium? They have several options, all of which may have drawbacks for some: (1) using low-lactose milk that has been treated with lactase products such as Lactaid or taking lactase tablets with meals; (2) using cultured or fermented forms of milk such as yogurt or buttermilk; (3) trying small amounts of milk at a time and only with meals; and (4) using other calcium-fortified food items such as fortified soy milk, cereals, and juice. The low-lactose milks are sweeter than regular milk but have proved to be both acceptable and more effective at reducing symptoms than the alternate product, sweet acidophilus milk. Processing of the low-lactose product involves incubation with yeast, which breaks down the lactose but slightly increases the cost.

Premenopausal women who maldigest lactose and avoid dairy products can have calcium intakes that are less than half those of women who can consume milk comfortably, and in some lactose-intolerant women, calcium intakes are less than 40% of the current Dietary Reference Intake. This places these women at high risk of osteoporosis and poor bone health in later life. The inclusion of dairy foods on a daily basis may help to enhance the digestion and metabolism of lactose.

REFERENCES

Buchowski MS, Semenya J, Johnson AO: Dietary calcium intake in lactose maldigesting intolerant and tolerant African-American women, *J Am Coll Nutr* 21:47, 2002.

Jackson KA, Savaiano DA: Lactose maldigestion, calcium intake and osteoporosis in African- Asian-, and Hispanic-Americans, *J Am Coll Nutr* 20(2 suppl):198S, 2001.

McBean LD, Miller GD: Allaying fears and fallacies about lactose intolerance, *J Am Diet Assoc* 98:671, 1998.

Pribla BA et al: Improved lactose digestion and intolerance among African-American adolescent girls fed a dairy-rich diet, *J Am Diet Assoc* 100:524, 2000.

Strocchi A, Levitt MD: Intestinal gas. In Feldman M, Scharschmidt BF, Sleisenger MH, eds: *Gastrointestinal and liver disease,* ed 6, vol 1, Philadelphia, 1998, WB Saunders.

Chapter 3

Carbohydrates

Eleanor D. Schlenker

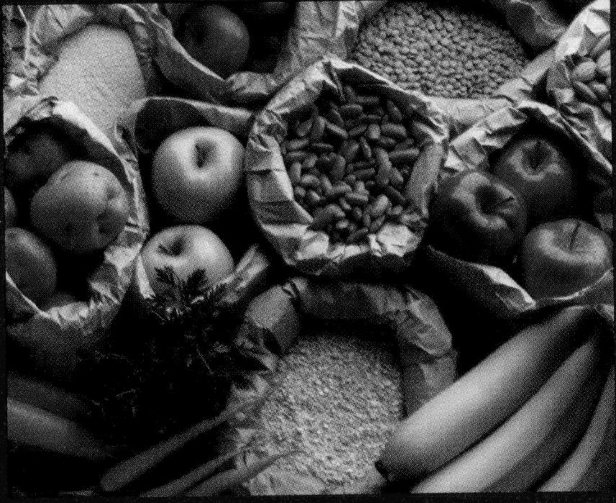

Chapter Outline

With this chapter, we begin a three-chapter sequence on the macronutrients: carbohydrates, fats, and proteins. Among all the nutrients, these three share a unique capacity, the ability to yield energy.

Carbohydrates have long been of prime importance in the human diet as the primary source of energy. They are the most important fuel source in the body. Over the ages they have nurtured cultures throughout the world, providing the major energy source to sustain work and growth.

In this chapter we look first at the nature of this major macronutrient and then its function as the basic body fuel.

The Nature of Carbohydrates

BASIC FUELS: STARCHES AND SUGARS

The basic fuel forms of carbohydrate are the starches and sugars that occur naturally in our foods. Energy on the planet Earth comes ultimately from the sun and its extraordinary action on plants. In the presence of this life-giving sunlight, plants use their internal process of photosynthesis to transform the sun's energy into the stored plant fuel form of carbohydrate (Figure 3-1). In this important process, plants use carbon dioxide from the air and water from the soil—along with the plant pigment *chlorophyll* in their green leaves, which serves as a chemical catalyst—to manufacture starches and sugars. The starch that plants store in reserve for their future energy needs becomes an important source of fuel for humans, who eat those plants and break down that starch to provide glucose for immediate energy and body metabolism. Because the human body can rapidly break down various forms of starches and sugars to yield body energy, carbohydrates are called "quick energy" foods. They provide our major source of energy.

DIETARY IMPORTANCE

There are practical reasons for the large quantities of carbohydrates in diets all over the world. First, carbohydrates are widely available, easily grown in plants as grains, vegetables, and fruits. In some countries, carbohydrate foods make up 85% of the diet.[1] For the typical American about half of the total kilocalories (kcalories) in the diet are consumed in the form of carbohydrates. Second, carbohydrates are relatively low in cost. And third, they can be stored easily. Compared with other types of foods, carbohydrate foods can be kept in dry storage for relatively long periods without spoilage. Modern processing and packaging further extend the shelf life of carbohydrate products almost indefinitely.

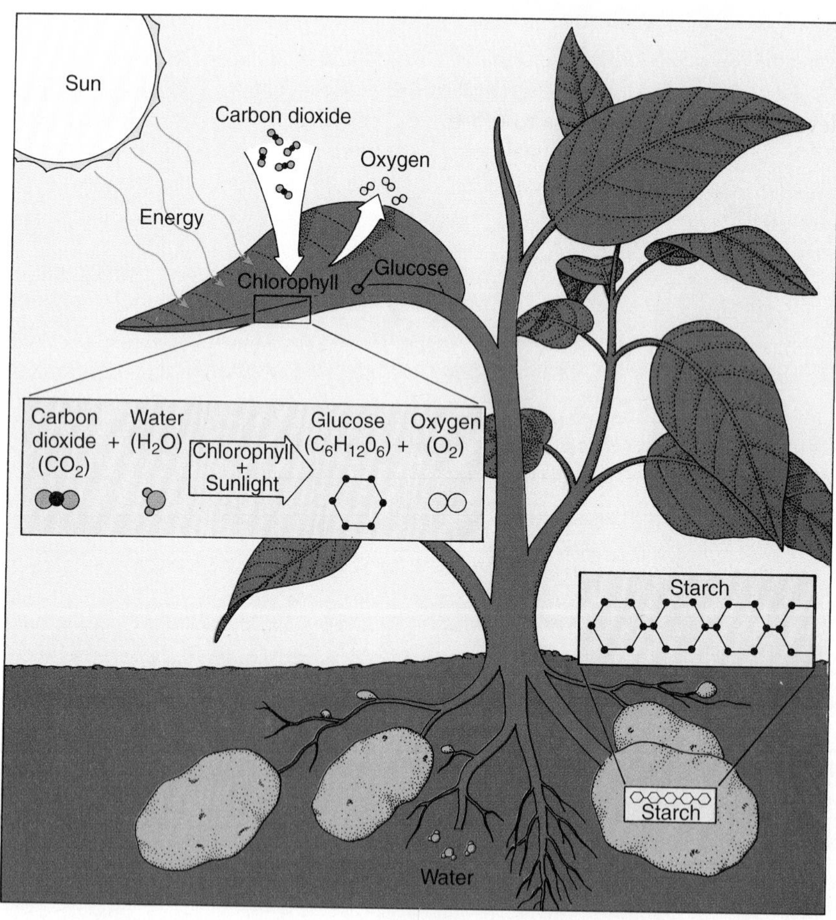

FIGURE 3-1 Photosynthesis. In the presence of sunlight and the green leaf pigment chlorophyll, green plants use the raw materials water and carbon dioxide to produce glucose and starch by capturing the sun's energy and transforming it into chemical energy in the food products stored in roots, stems, and leaves and returning oxygen to the atmosphere. *(Medical and Scientific Illustration.)*

Classification of Carbohydrates

The term carbohydrate comes from the chemical nature of the molecule. A carbohydrate is composed of the elements carbon, hydrogen, and oxygen, with the hydrogen/oxygen ratio usually that of water—CH_2O. Carbohydrates are classified according to the number of basic sugar, or saccharide, units that make up their structure.

MONOSACCHARIDES

The simplest form of carbohydrate is the monosaccharide, often called a simple (single) sugar. The three main monosaccharides important in human nutrition are glucose, fructose, and galactose.

Glucose

A moderately sweet sugar, glucose is found naturally in only a few foods, such as corn syrup. It is mainly created in the body from the digestion of starch. In human metabolism, all other types of sugar are converted into glucose. Glucose, called by its older name, dextrose, in hospital intravenous solutions, is the form in which carbohydrates circulate in the bloodstream. Blood glucose levels in adults normally range from about 3.9 to 5.8 mmol/L (70 to 105 mg/dl). After a high-carbohydrate meal, blood glucose levels may temporarily rise to 6.5 to 7.2 mmol/L (115 to 130 mg/dl).[2] The term *hyperglycemia* refers to an elevated blood glucose level, and the term *hypoglycemia* refers to blood glucose levels that fall below the normal range. In recent years, there has been public attention to the condition of hypoglycemia (see *Practical Application* box). Glucose is the common refined body fuel that is oxidized in the cells to give energy.

Fructose

The sweetest of the simple sugars, fructose is found in fruits and other naturally occurring substances such as honey. However, honey should not be given to infants younger than 1 year because of the possibility of botulism. Fructose intake has greatly increased in the United States since 1970 when high-fructose corn syrup was first introduced for use in food processing. High-fructose corn syrup is now the major sweetening agent in commercial baked products, dessert mixes, fruit drinks, and soft drinks.[2] In human metabolism fructose is converted to glucose to be burned for energy. Fructose can cause gastrointestinal distress if present in the intestines in too large an amount.

Galactose

The simple sugar galactose is not found free in foods but is produced in human digestion from lactose (milk sugar) and then converted to glucose in the liver. This reaction is reversible, and during lactation glucose can be reconverted to galactose for use in milk production.

The general physiologic and nutritional importance of these major monosaccharides (called *hexoses* because of their basic six-carbon structure) is summarized in Table 3-1. Their chemical structures are described in Figure 3-2.

DISACCHARIDES

The disaccharides are double sugars composed of two monosaccharides that are linked together. The three main disaccharides of physiologic importance are sucrose, lactose, and maltose. Their respective monosaccharide components are as follows.

Sucrose = one glucose + one fructose
Lactose = one glucose + one galactose
Maltose = one glucose + one glucose

Notice that glucose is a major component in each of these disaccharides.

Sucrose

Sucrose is the common "table sugar" made commercially from sugar cane and sugar beets. It is the most prevalent disaccharide. With the increasing use of processed foods containing added sugars, sucrose contributes some 30% of the total kcalories in the American diet.[2] Sucrose is found in all forms of common sugar, in molasses, and in some fruits and vegetables such as peaches and carrots.

Lactose

The sugar in milk is called *lactose* because of its source. It is formed in the body from glucose to supply the needed sugar component of milk during lactation. It is the least sweet of the disaccharides, about one sixth as sweet as sucrose. When milk sours, as in the initial stages of cheese making, the lactose changes its form and dissolves in the liquid whey, which separates from the solid curd. The curd is then processed for cheese, but the whey is discarded. Thus although milk has a relatively high carbohydrate content in the form of

---

carbohydrate Compound of carbon, hydrogen, and oxygen; starches, sugars, and dietary fiber made and stored in plants; major energy source in the human diet.
disaccharides Class of compound sugars composed of two molecules of monosaccharide. The three most common are sucrose, lactose, and maltose.
monosaccharide Simple single sugar; a carbohydrate containing a single saccharide (sugar) unit.
photosynthesis Process by which plants containing chlorophyll are able to manufacture carbohydrate by combining CO_2 from air and water from soil. Sunlight is used as energy; chlorophyll is a catalyst.

$$6\,CO_2 + 6\,H_2O + \text{Energy} + \text{Chlorophyll} \rightarrow C_6H_{12}O_6 + 6\,O_2$$

PRACTICAL APPLICATION
Hypoglycemia: Fact or Fiction?

Practitioners who promote alternative nutrition therapies often diagnose hypoglycemia, the condition of low blood glucose, in patients who have symptoms of nervousness or fatigue. As a result some controversy has developed regarding the actual incidence of hypoglycemia. Is it fact or fiction? Probably some of both. The lay public associates hypoglycemia with excessive sugar intake, which causes blood glucose levels to rise rapidly and then drop quickly as glucose moves into the cells. A number of symptoms—ranging from hunger and headache to depression and unbalanced behavior—have been attributed to this condition. On the other hand, members of the medical community consider the condition to be quite rare.

Clinically, hypoglycemia is usually defined on the basis of a blood glucose level below 45 mg/dl, 2 to 4 hours after eating. Physicians and consumers alike agree on some of the symptoms, such as, nervousness, anxiety, hunger, heart palpitations, and headache. But they disagree about the causes of the problem, methods of diagnosis, and treatment.

CAUSE

Clinicians have specifically identified two types of hypoglycemia and their causes.

1. Reactive hypoglycemia occurs after a meal and most frequently affects persons who recently had gastric surgery, have dumping syndrome related to peptic ulcer surgery, or have diabetes.
2. Fasting hypoglycemia occurs after extended periods without adequate food intake or as a result of poor eating habits. It may also be caused by several drugs: (1) alcohol, which blocks glucose production by the liver; (2) hypoglycemic medications used to treat diabetes; and (3) salicylate in aspirin. More serious conditions that may lead to hypoglycemia include (1) tumors of the pancreas that stimulate excessive insulin secretion and (2) adrenal insufficiency, a rare condition that prevents the adrenal glands from responding to certain body needs, especially under stress. Unrelieved general stress, regardless of the cause, increases metabolic demands on the body and can contribute to hypoglycemia.

DIAGNOSIS

A normal blood glucose range is about 3.9 to 7.8 mmol/L (70 to 140 mg/dl); for comparison, the current cutoff point for the diagnosis of diabetes is 7.8 mmol/L (140 ml/dl). The traditional basis for the medical diagnosis of hypoglycemia has been the oral glucose tolerance test in which the patient is given a beverage containing 75 to 100 g of glucose and the blood glucose levels are measured at half-hour intervals for up to 3 hours. However, this test situation itself is unrealistic and can actually induce an abnormal response. In current practice, physicians use blood tests to determine the glucose level at the time the person is experiencing the characteristic symptoms; in true hypoglycemia, the symptoms should be relieved immediately when the blood sugar level is raised.

TREATMENT

Practitioners who recommend alternative nutrition therapies and the lay public often believe that hypoglycemia should be treated with a very low-carbohydrate, high-protein diet. However, a very low-carbohydrate diet will make it difficult for the body to obtain sufficient amounts of glucose to achieve and to maintain normal blood glucose levels. It has become evident from current carbohydrate research that a diet of frequent small meals, rich in complex carbohydrates and dietary fiber and limited in simple carbohydrates and sugars, will maintain a more stable blood glucose level and prevent periods of low blood glucose. Pectin, in particular (see Table 3-3), appears to slow gastric emptying and carbohydrate absorption, thus supporting a consistent release of glucose into the portal vein.

SOUND APPROACHES

The simple procedure for home blood glucose monitoring developed for persons with diabetes can be used by persons with hypoglycemic symptoms to test their blood glucose levels at the time they are exhibiting symptoms. They should keep a record of their results, which will provide an accurate profile of their blood glucose levels in the free home environment. This procedure can provide a therapeutic tool for use in counseling and teaching. If the record shows no documented hypoglycemic periods, a sensitive counselor can help the person gain more insight into the problem, exploring other reasons such as stress that might be the cause of the symptoms. On the other hand, if the record documents actual hypoglycemia, further diagnostic evaluation is required. This technique is simple, accurate, and effective for persons being evaluated for reactive or postprandial hypoglycemia.

References

Bloch AS, Shils ME: Postgastrectomy diet. In Shils ME et al, eds: *Modern nutrition in health and disease,* ed 9, Philadelphia, 1999, Lippincott Williams & Wilkins.

Greenberg LW et al: Grand rounds: clinicopathologic exercise: hypoglycemia in a young woman with amenorrhea, *J Pediatr* 136:818, 2000.

Guyton AC, Hall JE: *Textbook of medical physiology,* ed 10, Philadelphia, 2000, WB Saunders.

Herbert V, Barrett S: Alternative nutrition therapies. In Shils ME et al, eds: *Modern nutrition in health and disease,* ed 9, Philadelphia, 1999, Lippincott Williams & Wilkins.

Jensen RT, Norton JA: Endocrine tumors of the pancreas. In Feldman M, Scharschmidt BF, Sleisenger MH, eds: *Gastrointestinal and liver disease,* ed 6, vol 1, Philadelphia, 1998, WB Saunders.

TABLE 3-1 Summary of Physiologic and Nutritional Significance of Selected Monosaccharides

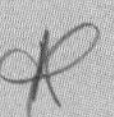

Hexose	Source	Significance
D-Glucose	Fruit juices; hydrolysis of starch, cane sugar, maltose, and lactose	Body "sugar"; found in blood and tissue fluids; cell fuel
D-Fructose	Fruit, juices, honey; hydrolysis of sucrose from cane sugar	Changed to glucose in the liver and intestine to serve as basic body fuel
D-Galactose	Hydrolysis of lactose (milk sugar)	Changed to glucose in the liver; cell fuel; synthesized in mammary gland to make lactose of milk; constituent of glycolipids and glycoproteins

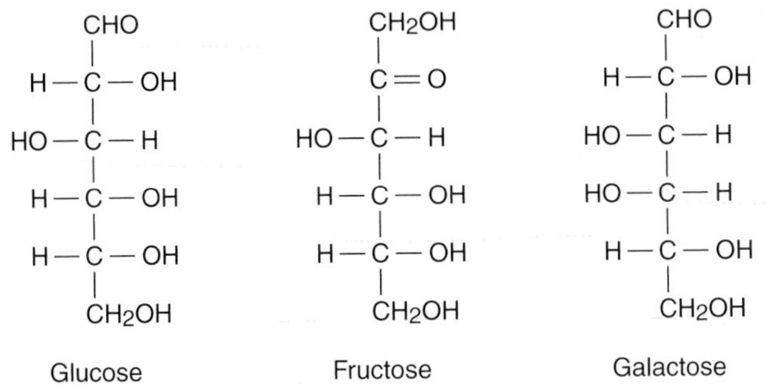

Glucose	Fructose	Galactose
CHO	CH_2OH	CHO
H—C—OH	C=O	H—C—OH
HO—C—H	HO—C—H	HO—C—H
H—C—OH	H—C—OH	HO—C—H
H—C—OH	H—C—OH	H—C—OH
CH_2OH	CH_2OH	CH_2OH

FIGURE 3-2 Glucose, fructose, and galactose. These three simple sugars are all hexoses with six carbon atoms forming their basic structure. They differ in the placement of hydroxyl (OH) groups and oxygen bonds.

lactose, one of its main products—cheese—has very little or none. Approximately one third to one half of adults worldwide are lactose intolerant but can tolerate such lactose-free milk products as cheese.[3] Also, the use of commonly marketed lactase enzyme supplements with lactose-containing meals prevents the discomfort of symptoms such as gas, cramping, bloating, stomach rumbling (borborygmi), altered bowel habits, and diarrhea.

Maltose

Maltose occurs in commercial malt products formed by the breakdown of starch and in germinating cereal grains. As such, it is a negligible *dietary* carbohydrate, but it is a highly significant *metabolic* carbohydrate as an intermediate product of starch digestion.

The general physiologic and nutritional significance of the disaccharides is summarized in Table 3-2. The U.S. Department of Agriculture (USDA) Continuing Survey of Food Intake by Individuals (CSFII) indicates that in the U.S. population, the proportion of energy intake contributed by added sweeteners such as sucrose or high-fructose corn syrup is nearly 16%, with the highest intake (20%) occurring among teenagers 12 to 17 years old[4] (see *Issues & Answers*).

TABLE 3-2 Summary of Physiologic and Nutritional Significance of Selected Disaccharides

	Source	Significance
Maltose	Starch digestion by amylase or commercial hydrolysis; malt and germinating cereals	Hydrolyzed to D-glucose; basic body fuel and metabolite; fermentable
Sucrose	Cane and beet sugar, sorghum cane, carrots, pineapple	Hydrolyzed to glucose and fructose; body fuel
Lactose	Milk	Hydrolyzed to glucose and galactose; body fuel; constituent for milk production during lactation

SUGAR ALCOHOLS

Another form of carbohydrate that is receiving increased attention in human nutrition is the sugar alcohols such as sorbitol and xylitol. These carbohydrate substances are found in nature and also are prepared commercially for use by the food industry.[1] They have become very attractive to food processors because (1) they are not attacked by bacteria in the mouth and thus do not promote the formation of dental caries and (2) they are not well digested or absorbed and sweeten a product without adding many additional kcalories. The sugar alcohols are added to many low-fat items such as ice cream or baked goods that are advertised as lower-calorie foods.

POLYSACCHARIDES

The more complex carbohydrates are called polysaccharides because they are made up of *many* single glucose

polysaccharides Class of complex carbohydrates composed of many monosaccharide units. Common members are starch, dextrins, dietary fiber, and glycogen.

(saccharide) units. The most important polysaccharide in human nutrition is starch; other forms are glycogen and dextrins. The nondigestible forms of dietary fiber, cellulose, and other noncellulose polysaccharides provide important bulk in the diet.

Starch

In human nutrition, starch is by far the most significant polysaccharide. It is a relatively large complex compound made up of many coiled or branching chains of single glucose units. It yields only glucose on digestion. The cooking of starch not only improves its flavor but also softens and ruptures the starch cells, which makes digestion easier. Starch mixtures thicken when cooked because the portion that encases the starch granules has a gel-like quality that thickens the mixture in the same way that pectin causes jelly to set.

Resistant Starch

Until recently starch was thought to be completely digested and absorbed in the small intestine. However, studies have shown that starch from various sources, including cereals, potatoes, bananas, and legumes, is not completely broken down in the small intestine and passes on to the large intestine generally intact.[2,5,6] The extent of starch breakdown within the small intestine varies, depending on the physical form of the food; therefore a substantial amount of the total starch, called *resistant starch,* can escape digestion in the small intestine and enter the colon. Resistant starch may equal 2% to 5% of the total starch eaten in the typical Western diet.[2] Three main types of resistant starch occur naturally in the human diet: (1) physically trapped starch, found in coarsely ground or chewed cereals; (2) ungelatinized starch granules, which are highly resistant to digestion by the starch enzyme alpha-amylase until gelatinized (these granules are found in uncooked potato and green banana); and (3) starch polymers, mainly amylose, which are produced when starch is cooled after gelatinization (as in cooled cooked potato).[2]

This undigested or resistant starch, passing through the small intestine into the colon, plays an important role in health.[2] In the large intestine, mostly in the colon, energy is salvaged from resistant starch through bacterial fermentation. The principal products of this fermentation are short-chain fatty acids, especially butyrate. Resistant starch may promote health in several ways.

1. *Effect on the gastrointestinal tract.* The short-chain fatty acids formed by bacterial fermentation provide a valuable energy source for the cells forming the colonic epithelium and may help protect against cancer of the large intestine.[7,8]
2. *Effect on appetite.* Diets containing higher amounts of these starch molecules that are not broken down to produce energy until they reach the colon appear to suppress feelings of hunger for longer periods than do diets with few or none of these compounds. Thus, diets rich in cereals, legumes, and potatoes that release glucose into the bloodstream at a slower rate, over a longer period, may assist in the regulation of food intake.[9]
3. *Effect on blood glucose levels.* The delayed release of glucose into the bloodstream from foods containing resistant starch helps to moderate the rapid rise in blood glucose levels that can occur after a meal high in simple sugars or rapidly digested carbohydrate. A slower rise in blood glucose level supports the more efficient movement of glucose into cells and may prevent elevated blood insulin levels, which can contribute to the development of diabetes.[10]

Based on the health-related benefits of resistant starch, food industry researchers are looking for new ways of processing grain foods that will maximize the amount of these molecules.[6]

Starch is by far the most important source of dietary carbohydrate worldwide. Plant-based diets are recognized as a significant factor in human nutrition and health. For example, the U.S. *Dietary Guidelines* and the *Food Guide Pyramid,* outlined in Chapter 1, recommend that grain foods form the foundation of the daily diet. The major form of dietary carbohydrate should be complex carbohydrate obtained from starch foods, with a more limited amount coming from added sugar. For those following a plant-based diet, starch is the staple food material, and carbohydrate may compose an even greater portion of the daily kcalories. The major food sources of starch include cereal grains, legumes, potatoes, and other vegetables.

Glycogen

The storage form of carbohydrate in animals is glycogen; in plants, it is starch. Glycogen is formed during cell metabolism and is stored in relatively small amounts in the liver and muscle. Liver stores help sustain normal blood glucose levels during fasting periods such as sleep hours, and muscle stores provide immediate fuel for muscle action, especially during athletic activity. Sometimes athletes practice pregame "glycogen loading" to provide added fuel stores for use during athletic events (see Chapter 14). Dietary carbohydrate is essential to maintain these needed glycogen stores and to prevent the stress symptoms of low carbohydrate intake—fatigue, dehydration, and energy loss—as well as other undesirable metabolic effects such as *ketoacidosis* (see Chapter 20). The lack of dietary carbohydrate will also result in excessive protein breakdown and the conversion of amino acids to an energy form. A carbohydrate intake of at least 100 g/day will prevent these symptoms.[11] Most diets provide well over 200 g/day, with the average diet containing 300 g or more.[12]

Dextrins

Dextrins are polysaccharide compounds formed as intermediate products in the breakdown of starch. This starch breakdown occurs constantly in the process of digestion.

Starch + water → soluble starch + maltose
Soluble starch + water → dextrins + maltose
Dextrins + water → maltose
Maltose + water → glucose + glucose

Oligosaccharides

These carbohydrates are small fragments of partially digested starch, ranging in size from 3 to 10 glucose molecules. They form either naturally through the process of digestion or commercially through acid hydrolysis. Oligosaccharides are irregular in form and, when digested, yield their constituent monosaccharides. These small starch molecules are used extensively in special formulas for infants or persons with gastrointestinal problems because they are so easily digested. These smaller starch fragments are also used in sports drinks, in which they may contribute almost half of the total glucose in the solution (see Chapter 14).

Some naturally occurring oligosaccharides are constructed with bonds that cannot be broken by human enzymes; therefore they are indigestible. Two of these—stachyose and raffinose—are found in legumes such as beans, peas, and soybeans. These small starch fragments provide a feast for bacterial flora in the intestines, producing a large amount of gas that can bring discomfort and embarrassment (see *Issues & Answers,* Chapter 2).

GLYCEMIC INDEX

As we noted in our discussion of the various types of carbohydrate, different food carbohydrates are broken down and enter the bloodstream at different rates. These differences become important in the management of diabetes, hypoglycemia, or other conditions in which it is important to prevent rapid elevations or falls in blood glucose levels. The rate at which glucose rises in the bloodstream after an individual has consumed a particular food is called its glycemic index, and using this measure foods have been compared as to their effect on blood glucose levels. We have come to realize that not only the type of carbohydrate but also home cooking methods or commercial food processing influence its rate of digestion and absorption. Highly processed grain foods may be similar to sugar-containing foods in their ability to bring about rapid elevations in blood glucose. Other substances present in the food, such as fiber, can slow the glycemic response.[10] It is best for all persons to select a diet that contains a variety of plant-based foods that will help to prevent wide fluctuations in blood glucose levels.

DIETARY FIBER

Dietary fiber may be classified into three major categories according to structure and properties, with one of these categories having five different members.

Cellulose

This dietary fiber is the chief constituent of the framework of plants. Humans cannot digest cellulose because they lack the necessary digestive enzymes. Therefore, it remains in the digestive tract and contributes important bulk to the diet. This bulk helps move the food mass along and stimulates *peristalsis* (see Chapter 2). Cellulose makes up the principal structural material in plant cell walls, and major food sources are the stems and leaves of vegetables, coverings of seeds and grains, skins, and hulls. Cellulose is present in higher amounts in vegetables than in fruits and cereals.[5]

Noncellulose Polysaccharides

The noncellulose polysaccharides, also forms of carbohydrate, include five members: hemicellulose, pectins, gums, mucilages, and algal substances. They absorb water and slow gastric emptying time. With the exception of hemicellulose, all are gumlike water-soluble substances that aid in binding cholesterol and controlling its absorption. They also regulate colon pressure by providing bulk for normal intestinal muscle action.

Lignin

This substance is the only noncarbohydrate type of dietary fiber. It is a large compound that forms the woody part of plants. In the intestine it combines with bile acids to form insoluble compounds, thus preventing their absorption. Lignin contributes the sandy texture of pears and lima beans.

A summary of these dietary fiber classes is given in Table 3-3, and a comparison of their solubility groupings

---

dietary fiber Nondigestible carbohydrates and lignin found in plants; the plant foods supplying fiber also contain other macronutrients and vitamins and minerals; plant foods containing dietary fiber have nutritional benefits such as preventing gastrointestinal disease like diverticulosis or reducing serum lipid and glucose levels that are related to the chronic conditions of heart disease and diabetes.

glycogen A polysaccharide, that is, a large compound of many saccharide (i.e., sugar) units. It is the main body storage form of carbohydrate, largely stored in the liver, with lesser amounts stored in muscle tissue.

oligosaccharides Intermediate products of polysaccharide breakdown that contain a small number (from 3 to 10) of single sugar units of the monosaccharide glucose.

raffinose A colorless crystalline trisaccharide found in legumes, composed of galactose and sucrose connected by bonds that human enzymes cannot break; thus it remains whole in the intestines and produces gas as bacteria attack it.

TABLE 3-3 Summary of Dietary Fiber Classes

Dietary Fiber Class	Plant Parts	Functions
Cellulose	Main cell wall constituent	Insoluble; holds water, functions as laxative, reduces elevated colonic intraluminal pressure; binds minerals
Noncellulose Polysaccharides		
Hemicellulose	Secretions, cell wall material	Mostly insoluble; holds water, increases stool bulk, reduces colonic pressure; binds bile acids
Pectins	Intracellular cement material	Soluble; binds cholesterol and bile acids
Gums	Special cell secretions	Soluble; binds cholesterol and bile acids; slows gastric emptying; provides fermentable material for colonic bacteria with production of volatile fatty acids and gas
Mucilages	Cell secretions	Soluble; slows gastric emptying time; fermentable substrate for colonic bacteria; binds bile acids
Algal substances	Algae, seaweeds	Soluble; slows gastric emptying time; fermentable substrate for colonic bacteria; binds bile acids
Noncarbohydrate		
Lignin	Woody part of plants	Insoluble; antioxidant; binds bile acids and metals

TABLE 3-4 Summary of Soluble and Insoluble Fibers in Total Dietary Fiber

Insoluble	Soluble
Cellulose	Gums
Most hemicelluloses	Mucilages
Lignin	Algal polysaccharides
	Most pectins

is given in Table 3-4. Some major food sources of the various types of dietary fiber are presented in Table 3-5. Also, note in the food exchange lists (Appendix L) that the high-fiber foods in each food category are indicated. Comparisons of dietary fiber content of some selected foods are given in Table 3-6.

Physiologic Effects of Fiber

In general, dietary fiber produces various effects on the food mix consumed and its fate in the body. Most of these effects are caused by its physiologic properties.

1. *Water absorption.* The capacity of dietary fiber to absorb water contributes to its bulk-forming laxative effect. As a result, the food mass moves more rapidly through the small intestine. This decrease in transit time of the food mass through the digestive tract allows less time for absorption to occur and can lower the absorption of the various nutrients.[13]
2. *Binding effect.* Such fibers as the noncellulose substances influence blood lipid levels through a binding effect—the capacity to bind cholesterol and bile salts and to prevent their absorption. However, excessive dietary fiber can have the undesirable effect of binding such minerals as iron, zinc, or calcium, thus preventing needed absorption and creating an unbalanced diet effect.
3. *Colon bacteria effect.* Undigestible dietary fiber serves as a substrate for fermentation by bacteria residing in the colon. This fermentation produces gas and volatile fatty acids, which are important sources of energy for the cells lining the colon.[5]

Various clinical applications of dietary fiber have centered on diabetes mellitus, coronary heart disease, colon cancer, and other intestinal problems such as diverticulosis.[14-17] Some of these clinical associations between dietary fiber and various chronic health problems are summarized in Table 3-7 and in *Issues & Answers.* A more recent application of dietary fiber is its effect on appetite and satiety. Diets low in fat and high in fiber may be the most effective means for promoting weight loss or avoiding unwanted weight gain.[18]

Although numerous research studies have shown a relationship between eating foods high in dietary fiber and the health benefits described previously, we still cannot be sure that other nutrients or substances present in these foods did not exert an effect on the results that were observed. To address this question, research scientists have isolated from natural foods various fiber-type substances and added them to foods or to a person's diet to see if there were any physiologic benefits. Some of these fiber components have also been manufactured by pharmaceutical companies and tested to observe any positive effects on human health. The new Dietary Reference Intakes (DRIs) refer to these isolated fiber substances that have health

Text continues on p. 57.

TABLE 3-5 Selected Food Sources of Various Classes of Dietary Fiber

Dietary Fiber Class	Grains	Fruits	Vegetables
Cellulose	Bran Whole wheat Whole rye	Apples Pears	Beans, peas Cabbage family Root vegetables Tomatoes, fresh
Noncellulose Polysaccharides			
Hemicellulose	Bran Cereals Whole grains		
Pectins		Apples Citrus fruits Berries, especially strawberries	Green beans Carrots
Gums	Oatmeal	Food products thickener, stabilizer	Dried beans, other legumes Vegetable gums used in food processing
Mucilages		Food products thickener, stabilizer	
Algal substances		Food products thickener, stabilizer	
Noncarbohydrate			
Lignins	Whole wheat Whole rye	Strawberries Peaches Pears Plums	Mature vegetables

TABLE 3-6 Dietary Fiber and Kcalorie Values for Selected Foods

Foods	Serving Size	Dietary Fiber (g)	Kcalories
Breads and Cereals			
All Bran	½ cup	8.5	70
Bran (100%)	½ cup	8.4	75
Bran Buds	⅓ cup	7.9	75
Corn Bran	⅔ cup	5.4	100
Bran Chex	⅔ cup	4.6	90
Cracklin' Oat Bran	⅓ cup	4.3	110
Bran Flakes	¾ cup	4.0	90
Air-popped popcorn	1 cup	2.2	25
Oatmeal	1 cup	2.5	144
Grapenuts	¼ cup	1.4	100
Whole-wheat bread	1 slice	1.4	60
Legumes, Cooked			
Kidney beans	½ cup	7.3	110
Lima beans	½ cup	4.5	130
Vegetables, Cooked			
Green peas	½ cup	3.6	55
Corn	½ cup	2.9	70
Parsnip	½ cup	2.7	50
Potato, with skin	1 medium	2.5	95
Brussels sprouts	½ cup	2.3	30
Carrots	½ cup	2.3	25
Broccoli	½ cup	2.2	20
Vegetables, Cooked—cont'd			
Beans, green	½ cup	1.6	15
Tomato, chopped	½ cup	1.5	17
Cabbage, red and white	½ cup	1.4	15
Kale	½ cup	1.4	20
Cauliflower	½ cup	1.1	15
Lettuce, fresh	1 cup	0.8	7
Fruits			
Apple	1 medium	3.5	80
Raisins	¼ cup	3.1	110
Prunes, dried	3	3.0	60
Strawberries	1 cup	3.0	45
Orange	1 medium	2.6	60
Banana	1 medium	2.4	105
Blueberries	½ cup	2.0	40
Dates, dried	3	1.9	70
Peach	1 medium	1.9	35
Apricot, fresh	3 medium	1.8	50
Grapefruit	½ cup	1.6	40
Apricot, dried	5 halves	1.4	40
Cherries	10	1.2	50
Pineapple	½ cup	1.1	40

Adapted from Lanza E, Butrum RR: A critical review of food fiber analysis and data, *J Am Diet Assoc* 86:732, 1986.

TABLE 3-7 Relationship Between Fiber Intake and Various Health Problems

Problem	Effect of Fiber	Possible Mode of Action	Future Research Needs
Diabetes mellitus	Reduces fasting blood sugar levels Reduces glycosuria Reduces insulin requirements Increases insulin sensitivity	Slows carbohydrate absorption by Delaying gastric emptying time Forming gels with pectin or guar gum in the intestine, thus impeding carbohydrate absorption "Protecting" carbohydrates from enzymatic activity with a fibrous coat Allowing "protected" carbohydrates to escape into the colon where they are digested by bacteria	Influence on short-chain fatty acid production or metabolism of glucose and fats in the liver Exact mechanisms by which fiber influences glucose metabolism
	Inhibits postprandial (after meals) hyperglycemia	Alters gut hormones (for example, glucagon) to enhance glucose metabolism in the liver	
Obesity	Increases satiety rate	Prolongs chewing and swallowing movements	Cause of increased satiety rate reported by subjects
	Reduces nutrient bioavailability	Increases fecal fat content	Effect of nutrient binding on nutritional status
	Reduces energy density	Inhibits absorption of carbohydrates in high-fiber foods	Studies based on food composition and kcaloric density instead of fiber content alone
		Decreases transit time	Effects of different types of fiber on gastric, small intestine, and colonic emptying time
	Alters hormonal response	Alters action of insulin, gut glucagon, and other intestinal hormones	
	Alters thermogenesis		
Coronary heart disease	Inhibits recirculation of bile acids	Alters bacterial metabolism of bile acids	Influence of fiber on cholesterol content of specific lipoprotein fractions (see Chapter 19)
		Alters bacterial flora, resulting in a change in metabolic activity	Influence on production of short-chain fatty acids
		Forms gels that bind bile acids	Role of dietary fiber as an independent variable in reducing risk of heart disease
		Alters the function of pancreatic and intestinal enzymes	
	Reduces triglyceride and cholesterol levels*	Reduces insulin levels†	Relationship between lipoprotein turnover and glucose turnover/sensitivity to insulin
		Binds cholesterol, preventing its absorption	Effect of higher concentration of bile salts on colon function
		Slows fat absorption by forming gel matrices in the intestine	
Colon cancer	Reduces incidence of disease‡	Bile acids or their bacterial metabolites may affect the structure of the colon, its cell turnover rate, and function	Testing of current hypotheses regarding the effects of dietary factors on the structure of the colon and cell turnover rate
Other gastrointestinal disorders Diverticular disease Constipation Hiatal hernia Hemorrhoids	Reduces pressure from within the intestinal lumen Increases diameter of the intestinal lumen, thus allowing intestinal tract to contract more, propelling contents more rapidly and inhibiting segmentation§	Decreases transit time Increases water absorption, resulting in a larger, softer stool	

*This effect is based on epidemiologic studies, usually observed in combination with reduced fat intake.
†Insulin is required for fat synthesis.
‡Preventive effect of fiber is assumed from epidemiologic studies that associate low-fiber, high-fat diets with an increased incidence of disease.
§Segmentation increases pressure and weakness along the walls of the intestinal tract.

benefits and are added to foods as functional fiber to distinguish them from the intact dietary fiber that we consume when we eat plant foods.[19]

Recommendations for Fiber Intake

Sufficient evidence exists to suggest that Americans should increase their intake of total fiber by consuming more whole grain foods, fruits, and vegetables (see *To Probe Further* box). Fiber supplements are neither needed nor appropriate for healthy persons. Recent studies indicate that the average dietary fiber intake of American adults is only about 15 g/day.[12] This intake meets only half or less of the Adequate Intake (AI) for total fiber set at 38 g/day for men ages 19 to 50 years 30 g/day for those ages 51 years and over. The AI for younger women and older women are 25 g/day and 21 g/day, respectively.[19] These AIs for total fiber are based on the amounts of fiber needed to protect against coronary heart disease. The American Heart Association proposed that meeting the *Food Guide Pyramid* guidelines of at least five servings of fruits and vegetables and six servings of grains, including whole grains, on a daily basis will provide at least 25 g of fiber and support heart health.[20] The indiscriminate use of bran is not justified.

COMPLEX CARBOHYDRATES

The term *complex carbohydrate* refers to large molecular forms of carbohydrate such as starch and dietary fiber. These foods make up a large part of the diet, and since the 1970s they have been an important component of various dietary guidelines. The most recent update of the *Dietary Guidelines for Americans* released in 2000 (see Chapter 1) emphasized the importance of complex carbohydrates by establishing separate guidelines for the use of fruits and vegetables and grain foods. The current food label provides consumers with some information about the carbohydrate content of foods. Although the content of complex carbohydrate is not included, the current nutrition label does contain the amount of fiber

functional fiber Nondigestible carbohydrates isolated from plant foods or manufactured that have been individually tested and found to have beneficial physiologic effects in the body; these substances may be added to natural foods to increase their fiber content.

total fiber Dietary fiber plus functional fiber; the total amount of fiber in an individual's diet from all sources.

TO PROBE FURTHER

Does All Fiber Work the Same: How Do We Advise Consumers?

As government agencies and health organizations such as the American Heart Association and the American Cancer Society encourage us to increase our intakes of fiber to protect against heart disease, colon cancer, and other problems of the gastrointestinal tract, questions arise as to what foods best meet our fiber needs. Fruits, vegetables, legumes, nuts, seeds, and whole grains are all good sources of fiber. Do we need a variety of sources or will one or another do? Some of the confusion concerning dietary fiber centers on semantics. No term has been fully acceptable to cover all the different types of fiber or their various roles. The older word "roughage" and the current term "fiber" suggest a rough, abrasive, woody type of material as observed in plant stems containing cellulose. However, a number of the indigestible materials in food, also classified as fiber, have a soft, amorphous, and gel-like character and are more soluble in their physical nature; hence they also have different properties and functions. These differences in physical properties add to the problem nutritionists and clinicians have in determining the precise nutritional and physiologic significance of fiber in the human diet and the particular food substances involved. Further problems have been encountered in developing appropriate and precise methods for measuring these substances in food sources.

Dietary fiber refers to the total amount of naturally occurring carbohydrate and lignin materials from plant foods that is not digested. This includes dietary fiber from such foods as whole grains, legumes, vegetables, fruits, seeds, and nuts. Particular undigestable carbohydrate substances that have been chemically isolated from plant foods or manufactured by pharmaceutical companies and found to have beneficial properties in the body have been given the new term of functional fiber.

Fibers from different sources have been classified on the basis of their solubility in water. The insoluble fibers include cellulose, hemicellulose, and lignin, whereas the soluble fibers (sometimes referred to as the viscous fibers) include pectin, gums, and mucilage. Both the specific food sources and physiologic effects differ between the insoluble and soluble fibers, although most foods contain a certain amount of both types.

INSOLUBLE FIBER

Insoluble fiber found in bran, vegetables, wheat, and most other grain products is most effective in preventing or relieving problems of the lower gastrointestinal tract. Cellulose, lignin, and the hemicelluloses increase fecal bulk and help to achieve a large, soft stool. Insoluble fibers decrease transit time for the

Continued

TO PROBE FURTHER

Does All Fiber Work the Same: How Do We Advise Consumers?—cont'd

passage of the fecal mass through the large intestine and colon and thus prevent excessive reabsorption of water that results in a hard stool. Increasing the intake of insoluble fiber with the use of whole grain breads and cereals and vegetables is often used clinically to help prevent or relieve constipation. Insoluble fiber also provides bulk, which relieves excessive pressure build-up in the colon that can lead to diverticulosis. In recent years insoluble fiber has been found to assist in the management of irritable bowel syndrome in some individuals.

Intakes of foods high in cellulose have been associated with a lower risk of colon cancer. The decreased transit time that occurs with higher intakes of insoluble fiber decreases the length of time that colon tissues are exposed to potential cancer-promoting substances in the feces. Another explanation given for the protective role of fiber against colon cancer is the fermenting action of colon bacteria on cellulose, producing short-chain fatty acids that create a more acid environment and discouraging the growth of microorganisms that promote the development of cancers.

SOLUBLE FIBER

Soluble fibers such as pectin, guar gum, and mucilage have been shown to assist in the management of heart disease, hyperlipidemia, and diabetes mellitus. Soluble fibers are found in fruits, many vegetables, legumes, and other plant foods such as oats and psyllium seeds (psyllium is the major ingredient in the laxative Metamucil). Legumes high in soluble fiber have been shown to decrease blood cholesterol levels. In fact, oat products containing the viscous fiber beta-glucan have been approved by the Food and Drug Administration to carry a health claim on their nutrition label indicating their usefulness in preventing heart disease. Soluble fibers assist in lowering blood low-density lipoprotein (LDL) cholesterol levels but do not reduce important high-density lipoprotein (HDL) cholesterol, which helps to remove excess cholesterol from the body. Soluble fiber acts in two different ways to reduce blood LDL cholesterol levels: (1) it prevents the reabsorption of bile acids, resulting in a lower pool of body cholesterol, and (2) it may reduce body synthesis of new cholesterol. An analysis of studies that compared the effect of cellulose (an insoluble fiber) with that of psyllium (a soluble fiber) found that LDL cholesterol levels dropped by 7% in persons with elevated serum cholesterol levels who were consuming psyllium. Psyllium is now added to many ready-to-eat cereals, and those products also have been approved to carry a nutrition label health claim indicating their value in preventing heart disease and cancer. Soluble fiber from fruits, vegetables, and grain foods, including apples, cantaloupe, oranges, raisins, peaches, lima beans, peas, sweet potatoes, and whole wheat bread, helped to lower blood glucose levels in patients with type 2 diabetes mellitus (Chandalia et al, 2000). It is important to note that this effect was accomplished with the use of real food, not bran supplements. Fiber is believed to slow the absorption of carbohydrates, resulting in less fluctuation and better control of blood glucose levels. An adequate fiber intake may also assist in preventing the onset of type 2 diabetes in later life. Older individuals who regularly ate three servings of whole grain foods each day lowered their risk of developing this chronic disease. Despite the many positive effects of fiber, there is concern about the ability of fiber substances to trap nutrients such as trace minerals and prevent their absorption. We will learn more about that in Chapter 8 when we discuss the essential minerals and their important roles in the body.

Fiber is an important constituent of the diet that plays an important role in maintaining health and preventing disease. There are various types of fiber, and each has a specific purpose in the body. It is important that consumers obtain their fiber from a variety of foods, including fruits, vegetables, legumes, nuts, and whole grain breads and cereals.

References

Anderson JW et al: Cholesterol-lowering effects of psyllium intake adjunctive to diet therapy in men and women with hypercholesterolemia: meta-analysis of 8 controlled trials, *Am J Clin Nutr* 71:472, 2000.

Chandalia M et al: Beneficial effects of high dietary fiber intake in patients with type 2 diabetes, *N Engl J Med* 342:1392, 2000.

Jenkins DJA, Kendall CWC, Vuksan V: Viscous fibers, health claims, and strategies to reduce cardiovascular disease risk, *Am J Clin Nutr* 71:401, 2000.

Jenkins DJA, Wolever TMS, Jenkins AL: Fiber and other dietary factors affecting nutrient absorption and metabolism. In Shils ME et al, eds: *Modern nutrition in health and disease,* ed 9, Philadelphia, 1999, Lippincott Williams & Wilkins.

Marsh MN, Riley SA: Digestion and absorption of nutrients and vitamins. In Feldman M, Scharschmidt BF, Sleisenger MH, eds: *Gastrointestinal and liver disease,* ed 6, vol 2, Philadelphia, 1998, WB Saunders.

Meyer KA et al: Carbohydrates, dietary fiber, and incident type 2 diabetes in older women, *Am J Clin Nutr* 71:921, 2000.

Schneeman BO: Building scientific consensus: the importance of dietary fiber, *Am J Clin Nutr* 69:1, 1999.

TABLE 3-8 Postabsorptive Carbohydrate Storage in Normal Adult Man (70 kg [154 lb])

	Glycogen (g)	Glucose (g)
Liver (weight 1800 g)	72	
Muscles (mass weight 35 kg [77 lb])	245	
Extracellular fluids (10 L)		10
Component totals	317	10
TOTAL STORAGE	327	

in a serving and recommends an intake of 25 g of fiber in a 2000 kcalorie/day diet. This level is considerably lower than the recently released DRI.

Functions of Carbohydrates

ENERGY

The primary function of carbohydrates in nutrition is to provide fuel for energy production. Fat is also a fuel, but the body needs only a small amount of dietary fat, mainly to supply the essential fatty acids. To function properly, however, the body tissues require a daily dietary supply of carbohydrates sufficient to provide a major portion of the total kcalories.

The amount of carbohydrates in the body, although relatively small, is important to maintain energy reserves. For example, in a man about 300 to 350 g of carbohydrate is "stored" in the liver and muscle tissues as glycogen and about 10 g is present as circulating blood glucose (Table 3-8). This total amount of available glycogen and glucose will provide sufficient energy for only about half a day of moderate activity. Thus carbohydrate foods must be eaten regularly and at moderately frequent intervals to meet the constant energy demands of the body.

SPECIAL FUNCTIONS OF CARBOHYDRATES IN BODY TISSUES

As part of their general function as the body's main energy source, carbohydrates also serve special functions in many body tissues.

Glycogen Reserves

As noted earlier, the liver and muscle glycogen reserves provide a constant interchange with the body's overall energy balance system. Thus these reserves protect cells from depressed metabolic function and injury.

Protein-Sparing Action

Carbohydrates help regulate protein metabolism. The presence of sufficient carbohydrates to meet the energy demands of the body prevents the channeling of protein for this purpose. This protein-sparing action of carbohydrates allows the major portion of protein to be used for its structural purpose of tissue building and repair.

Antiketogenic Effect

Carbohydrates also relate to fat metabolism. The amount of carbohydrates present in the diet determines how much fat will be broken down, thus affecting the formation and disposal rates of *ketones*. Ketones are intermediate products of fat metabolism, which normally are produced at low levels during fat oxidation. However, in such extreme conditions as starvation or uncontrolled diabetes, or with the unwise use of very low-carbohydrate diets, carbohydrates are inadequate or unavailable for energy needs so that too much fat is oxidized. Ketones accumulate, and the result is *ketoacidosis* (see Chapter 20). Sufficient amounts of dietary carbohydrate prevent this damaging excess of ketones.

Heart Action

Heart action is a life-sustaining muscular exercise. Although fatty acids are the preferred regular fuel for the heart muscle, the glycogen reserves in cardiac muscle are an important emergency source of contractile energy. In congestive heart failure energy needs are elevated but at the same time dietary fat is less well absorbed, pointing to the importance of carbohydrate for this patient.[21]

Central Nervous System Function

A constant supply of carbohydrates is necessary for the proper functioning of the central nervous system (CNS). The usual energy source for the CNS is glucose; however, the CNS regulatory center, the brain, contains no stored supply of glucose and is therefore especially dependent on a minute-to-minute supply of glucose from the blood. Sustained and profound hypoglycemic shock may cause irreversible brain damage. In all nerve tissue, carbohydrates are indispensable for functional integrity. A practical application of the need for a constant supply of glucose to the brain is the finding that individuals who eat breakfast have better memory and are in a better mood in mid-morning than are those who skip breakfast.[22]

RECOMMENDED INTAKE OF CARBOHYDRATE

Attention to the relative amounts of carbohydrate and fat in the diet has been spurred by the associations of these nutrients with health and chronic disease. A diet high in plant-based foods and fiber appears to lower the risk of heart disease and some cancers, but it is not necessarily beneficial for individuals to take in a disproportionate amount of carbohydrate, just as it is not a good idea to severely limit carbohydrate intake.

The DRIs released in 2002 were the first to set a specific Recommended Dietary Allowance (RDA) for carbohydrate.[19] It is recommended that all persons from the age of 1 year and throughout adulthood consume 130 g/day of carbohydrate. This recommendation is based on the average minimum amount of glucose needed to supply the energy needs of the brain for 1 day. Some individuals may eat a greater amount of carbohydrate to meet their overall energy requirements and keep fat and protein intakes at acceptable levels.

High-Carbohydrate Diets

The recommended intake of carbohydrate as a percentage of total kcalories as given in the Acceptable Macronutrient Distribution Range (AMDR) is 45% to 60% of total kcalories. However, in an effort to lower intake of dietary fat and to achieve reductions in blood lipoprotein levels, diets containing as much as 65% to 75% carbohydrate have been evaluated. It appears that the benefits of increasing carbohydrate intake above the generally recommended level varies among individuals.[23] Dietary intake, lifestyle, and, in particular, genetic factors appear to influence how our bodies use carbohydrate. In some persons, diets containing more than 55% carbohydrate lead to an actual increase in blood lipid (triglyceride) levels,[24] and a diet moderate in both carbohydrate and fat is most appropriate.

Low-Carbohydrate Diets

Diets containing 20% or fewer kcalories from carbohydrate have been advocated in various books and articles in the popular press as an efficient means of achieving weight loss. Such diets are not effective in bringing about long-term success in weight reduction and carry both nutritional and physiologic risks. Individuals studied in the CSFII who were following low-carbohydrate diets did not meet the minimum servings of fruits, vegetables, and grains from the *Food Guide Pyramid* and consumed a low variety of foods.[25] Also, diets low in carbohydrate are likely to be high in fat; in fact the persons participating in this study who were following low-carbohydrate diets obtained 46% of their kcalories from fat. Low-carbohydrate diets often lead to a rapid, initial weight loss, but this loss of weight is related to a shift in body water compartments and a general loss of body water, not a loss of body fat. When carbohydrate intake falls below 100 g, it becomes necessary for the body to synthesize glucose from amino acids, the building block of proteins, forcing the kidneys to excrete the nitrogen byproducts from this conversion. The added burden on the kidneys can lead to further water loss. Finally, if insufficient amounts of carbohydrate are available to metabolize the fat being mobilized for energy, the excessive production of ketones results in further metabolic complications with disturbance of acid-base balance.[26] Establishing a kcaloric deficit between energy intake and energy expenditure using a combination of foods that support nutritional well-being and can be continued after achieving a healthy weight is the only effective means of long-term weight management.

Although a more detailed and integrated discussion of digestion, absorption, and metabolism of the macronutrients is given in Chapter 2, a brief summary of these aspects for each individual macronutrient is presented at the end of each macronutrient chapter, to set the scene for the larger picture that follows. Here we provide that summary outline for carbohydrates.

Digestion-Absorption-Metabolism Summary

DIGESTION

Most carbohydrate foods, starches and sugars, cannot be used immediately by the cells to produce energy. They must first be changed into the refined fuel for which the cell is designed—glucose. The process by which these vital changes are made is digestion. The digestion of carbohydrate foods proceeds through the successive parts of the gastrointestinal tract and is accomplished by two types of actions: (1) mechanical or muscle functions that render the food mass into smaller particles and (2) chemical processes by which specific enzymes break down food nutrients into smaller, usable metabolic products.[27]

Mouth

Mastication breaks food into fine particles and mixes it with the salivary secretions. During this process, a salivary amylase (ptyalin) is secreted by the parotid gland. It acts on starch to begin its breakdown into dextrins and maltose.

Stomach

Successive wavelike contractions of the muscle fibers of the stomach wall continue the mechanical digestive process. This action is called peristalsis. It further mixes food particles with gastric secretions to allow chemical digestion to take place more readily. The gastric secretions contain no specific enzyme for the breakdown of carbohydrates, and the hydrochloric acid in the stomach stops the action of salivary amylase. Before the food mixes completely with the gastric acid secretion, as much as 20% to 30% of the starch may have been changed to maltose. Muscle actions continue to move the food mass to the lower part of the stomach. The food mass is now a thick creamy chyme, ready for its controlled emptying through the pyloric valve into the duodenum, the first portion of the small intestine.

Small Intestine

Peristalsis continues to aid digestion in the small intestine by mixing and moving the chyme along the lumen for the length of the tube. Chemical digestion of carbohydrates is completed in the small intestine by specific enzymes from two sources: the pancreas and the intestine.

Pancreatic secretions. Secretions from the pancreas enter the duodenum through the common bile duct. They contain a pancreatic amylase, which continues the breakdown of starch to maltose.

Intestinal secretions. Intestinal secretions contain three disaccharidases—sucrase, lactase, and maltase. These enzymes act on their respective disaccharides to render the monosaccharides—glucose, galactose, and fructose—ready for absorption. These specific disaccharidases are integral proteins of the brush border of the small intestine that break down the disaccharides as absorption takes place. The digestive products, the monosaccharides, are then immediately absorbed into the portal blood circulation.

A summary of the major aspects of carbohydrate digestion through these successive parts of the gastrointestinal tract is given in Table 3-9.

ABSORPTION

The refined fuel glucose is now ready to be carried to the individual cells to be stored or "burned" to produce energy. The body rapidly absorbs glucose, the basic end product of carbohydrate digestion, and transports it to the cells throughout the body. The major glucose absorption mechanism is an active transport "pumping" system, requiring sodium as a carrier substance. Of the total carbohydrates absorbed, 80% is in the form of glucose and is absorbed by the sodium cotransport mechanism; the remaining 20% is absorbed in the form of galactose coming from milk and some fructose.[27]

Absorbing Structures

The absorbing surface area of the small intestine is uniquely enhanced by its three basic structures (mucosal folds, villi, and microvilli) which are described in detail in Chapter 2. Together, these structures provide a greatly increased absorbing surface that allows 90% of the digested food material to be absorbed in the small intestine. Only water absorption remains for the large intestine.

Route of Absorption

Via the capillaries of the villi, the simple sugars—glucose, galactose, and fructose—enter the portal circulation and are transported to the liver. Here fructose and galactose are converted to glucose, which is either used immediately for fuel or converted to glycogen for brief storage. This glycogen constantly reconverts to glucose as needed by the body.

METABOLISM

Definition

The general term metabolism refers to the sum of the various chemical processes in a living organism by which energy is made available for the functioning of the entire organism. It includes all the processes by which basic structures are built and maintained, carry out their function, and then are broken down to be rebuilt. Products of specific metabolic processes are called metabolites.

Cell Metabolism of Carbohydrate Products

Cells are the functional units of life in the human body. In cell nutrition the most important end product of carbohydrate digestion is glucose, because the other two monosaccharides—fructose and galactose—are eventually converted to glucose. The liver is the major site of the intricate machinery that handles glucose. However, en-

TABLE 3-9 Summary of Carbohydrate Digestion

	Enzyme	Action
Mouth	Salivary amylase: ptyalin	Starch → dextrins → maltose
Stomach	None	Starch hydrolysis continued briefly
Small intestine	Pancreatic amylase: amylopsin	Starch → dextrins → maltose
	Intestinal disaccharidases:	
	sucrase	Sucrose → glucose + fructose
	lactase	Lactose → glucose + galactose
	maltose	Maltose → glucose + glucose

lactase Enzyme that splits the disaccharide lactose into its two monosaccharides: glucose and galactose.
lumen The cavity or channel within a tube or tubular organ, such as the intestines.
maltase Enzyme that breaks down the disaccharide maltose into two units of glucose; a monosaccharide.
metabolism Sum of all the various biochemical and physiologic processes by which the body grows and maintains itself (anabolism), breaks down and reshapes tissue (catabolism), and transforms energy to do its work. Products of these various reactions are called *metabolites.*
portal An entryway, usually referring to the portal circulation of blood through the liver. Blood is brought into the liver via the portal vein and out via the hepatic vein.
sucrase Enzyme splitting the disaccharide sucrose into its two monosaccharides of glucose and fructose.

ergy metabolism occurs in all cells. In each individual cell, glucose is burned to produce energy through a series of chemical reactions involving specific cell enzymes. The final energy produced is then available to the cell to do its work. Extra glucose not immediately needed for energy may also be converted to adipose tissue and stored as a reserve fuel. Review details of the interactive metabolic activities among the nutrients provided in Chapter 2.

Metabolic Concept of Unity

Here and in following discussions of other nutrients, a central significant scientific principle will emerge—the unity of the human organism. The human body is a whole made up of many parts and processes that possess unequaled specificity and flexibility. Intimate metabolic relationships exist among all the basic nutrients and metabolites. Thus it is impossible to understand any one of the body's many metabolic processes without viewing it in relation to the whole.

Therefore, in all your study and work with patients and clients, remember this important fact: all nutrients do their best work in partnership with other nutrients. From this fundamental fact you can draw two practical conclusions: (1) the emphasis in health teaching and nutrition education should be on achieving an overall sound, balanced nutritional program, and (2) deficiency states may be related to an illness and its medical treatment, may originate from an inappropriate diet adopted to achieve weight loss or another reason, or may be caused by long-term, overzealous emphasis on one particular nutrient to the exclusion of other equally essential nutrients.

TO SUM UP

Carbohydrates supply most of the world's population with its primary source of energy. A product of photosynthesis, carbohydrate is widely distributed in nature and its food products are easy to store and generally low in cost.

There are two basic types of carbohydrates: simple and complex. Simple carbohydrates consist of single- and double-sugar units (monosaccharides and disaccharides), which are easily digested and provide quick energy. Complex carbohydrates, or polysaccharides, are less easily prepared for use. Although they vary somewhat in their effect on blood sugar, in general, they provide energy more slowly and prevent large fluctuations in blood glucose levels.

In addition to providing general body energy, carbohydrates maintain liver, heart, brain, and nerve tissue function. They prevent the rapid breakdown of lipids for energy, which can result in excessive production of toxic metabolic byproducts, and spare protein for tissue building and repair. Dietary fiber, a complex carbohydrate that forms the indigestible part of plants, also affects the digestion and absorption of foods in ways that have proved beneficial to good health.

■ Questions for Review

1. Differentiate among the terms *monosaccharide, disaccharide,* and *polysaccharide.* List two common examples of each in the general food supply.
2. What is a resistant starch? Where are these compounds found and how are they formed? What is a health benefit of resistant starch?
3. For breakfast you have a piece of whole grain bread with jelly, a banana, and a glass of milk. List all of the forms of carbohydrate that are included in this meal. Make a table showing the digestion of these carbohydrates, indicating the site of digestion and the products formed.
4. Refer to the Recommended Daily Allowance table to determine the daily energy need of a 25-year-old woman who is 5 ft 4 in tall and weighs 125 lb. How many kcalories should be provided by carbohydrates in her diet? How much fiber is recommended? Develop a 3-day menu plan that will provide the appropriate amount of dietary fiber.
5. Describe briefly the clinical effects of fiber in the prevention or treatment of the following disease states: diverticular disease, hyperlipidemia, diabetes mellitus, and colon cancer.
6. Your client, Mr. B, wants to lose 20 lb before his high school reunion next month. He has decided to eat only meat, fish, poultry, or other protein foods for the next 4 weeks because he believes a very low-carbohydrate diet will help him lose weight. He is adamant about not eating any starches or sweets. Based on your readings, how would you explain the effects of a very low-carbohydrate diet on body metabolism so that he will understand why carbohydrates are important even in a weight-loss program?
7. Briefly describe five special functions of carbohydrate in the body and why they are important.
8. Visit your local grocery store and make a list of the fruit juices, fruit drinks, and carbonated beverages available in single-serving, easy-to-carry containers. Check the nutrition labels for the amount of sugar, fiber, vitamins, and minerals found in each. Which of these beverages are appropriate for daily use; which should be used on a more limited basis?

■ References

1. Englyst HN, Hudson GJ: Carbohydrates. In Garrow JS, James WPT, Ralph A, eds: *Human nutrition and dietetics,* ed 10, Edinburgh, 2000, Churchill Livingstone.
2. Levin RJ: Carbohydrates. In Shils ME et al, eds: *Modern nutrition in health and disease,* ed 9, Philadelphia, 1999, Lippincott Williams & Wilkins.
3. Tolstoi LG: Adult-type lactase deficiency, *Nutr Today* 35(4):134, 2000.
4. Guthrie JF, Morton JF: Food sources of added sweeteners in the diets of Americans, *J Am Diet Assoc* 100(1):43, 2000.

5. Brody T: *Nutritional biochemistry,* ed 2, New York, 1999, Academic Press.
6. Wolf BW, Bauer LL, Fahey GC: Effects of chemical modification on in vitro rate and extent of food starch digestion: an attempt to discover a slowly digested starch, *J Agric Food Chem* 47:4178, 1999.
7. Hylla S et al: Effects of resistant starch on the colon in healthy volunteers: possible implications for cancer prevention, *Am J Clin Nutr* 67:136, 1998.
8. Ahmed R, Segal I, Haswsan H: Fermentation of dietary starch in humans, *Am J Gastroenterol* 95:17, 2000.
9. Sparti A et al: Effects of diets high or low in unavailable and slowly digestible carbohydrates on the pattern of 24-h substrate oxidation and feelings of hunger in humans, *Am J Clin Nutr* 72:1461, 2000.
10. American Diabetes Association Task Force for Writing Nutrition Principles and Recommendations for the Management of Diabetes and Related Complications: American Diabetes Association Position Statement: evidence-based nutrition principles and recommendations for the treatment and prevention of diabetes and related complications, *J Am Diet Assoc* 102:109, 2002.
11. Food and Nutrition Board, National Research Council: *Recommended dietary allowances,* ed 10, Washington, DC, 1989, National Academy of Sciences.
12. U.S. Department of Agriculture: *Continuing survey of food intake by individuals 1994-1996,* can be accessed at *http://www.barc.usda.gov/bhnrc/foodsurvey/Products9496.html#anchor164107.*
13. Jenkins DJA, Wolever TMS, Jenkins AL: Fiber and other dietary factors affecting nutrient absorption and metabolism. In Shils ME et al, eds: *Modern nutrition in health and disease,* ed 9, Philadelphia, 1999, Lippincott Williams & Wilkins.
14. Liu S et al: Fruit and vegetable intake and risk of cardiovascular disease: the Women's Health Study, *Am J Clin Nutr* 72:922, 2000.
15. Jacobs DR, Murtaugh MA: It's more than an apple a day: an appropriately processed plant-centered dietary pattern may be good for your health, *Am J Clin Nutr* 72:899, 2000.
16. Kushi LH, Meyer KA, Jacobs DR: Cereals, legumes, and chronic disease risk reduction: evidence from epidemiologic studies, *Am J Clin Nutr* 70(suppl):451S, 1999.
17. Slavin JL: Mechanisms for the impact of whole grain foods on cancer risk, *J Am Coll Nutr* 19(3 suppl):300S, 2000.
18. Yao M, Roberts SB: Dietary energy density and weight regulation, *Nutr Rev* 59(8):247, 2001.
19. Panel on Macronutrients, Panel on the Definition of Dietary Fiber, Subcommittee on Upper Reference Levels of Nutrients, Subcommittee on Interpretation and Uses of Dietary Reference Intakes, and the Standing Committee on the Scientific Evaluation of Dietary Reference Intakes: *Dietary reference intakes for energy, carbohydrate, fiber, fat, fatty acids, cholesterol, protein, and amino acids, parts 1 and 2,* Washington, DC, 2002, National Academy Press.
20. Krauss RM et al: Revision 2000: a statement for healthcare professionals from the nutrition committee of the American Heart Association, *J Nutr* 131:132, 2001.
21. Hughes C, Kostka P: Chronic congestive heart failure. In Shils ME et al, eds: *Modern nutrition in health and disease,* ed 9, Philadelphia, 1999, Lippincott Williams & Wilkins.
22. Benton D: The impact of the supply of glucose to the brain on mood and memory, *Nutr Rev* 59(1 pt 2):S20, 2001.
23. Schneeman BO: Carbohydrate: friend or foe? Summary of research needs, *J Nutr* 131:2764S, 2001.
24. Parks EJ: Effect of dietary carbohydrate on triglyceride metabolism in humans, *J Nutr* 131:2772S, 2001.
25. Kennedy ET et al: Popular diets: correlation to health, nutrition, and obesity, *J Am Diet Assoc* 101(4):411, 2001.
26. Guyton AC, Hall JE: *Textbook of medical physiology,* ed 10, Philadelphia, 2000, WB Saunders.
27. Marsh MN, Riley SA: Digestion and absorption of nutrients and vitamins. In Feldman M, Scharschmidt BF, Sleisenger MH, eds: *Gastrointestinal and liver disease,* ed 6, vol 2, Philadelphia, 1998, WB Saunders.

■ Further Reading

Slavin JL et al: The role of whole grains in disease prevention, *J Am Diet Assoc* 101(7):780, 2001.

Dr. Slavin and her coauthors describe the nutritional differences between whole grains and refined grains and help us understand the process that brings about these changes in nutrient and fiber content.

Geiger CJ: Health claims: history, current regulatory status, and consumer research, *J Am Diet Assoc* 98:1312, 1998.

This article outlines the process by which the Food and Drug Administration evaluates and approves foods to carry a label with a health claim. Several foods rich in particular types of fiber now carry such health claims.

Duffy VB, Anderson GH: Use of nutritive and nonnutritive sweeteners: Position of the American Dietetic Association, *J Am Diet Assoc* 98:580, 1998 (reaffirmed until 2001).

McNutt K: What clients need to know about sugar replacers, *J Am Diet Assoc* 100:466, 2000.

These two articles help us evaluate nonnutritive sweeteners and provide information to guide us in educating our patients about their appropriate use in a balanced diet.

Johnson RK, Frary C: Choose beverages and foods to moderate your intake of sugars: The 2000 Dietary Guidelines for Americans—what's all the fuss about? *J Nutr* 131:2766S, 2001.

Kantor LS et al: Choose a variety of grains daily, especially whole grains: a challenge for consumers, *J Nutr* 131:473S, 2001.

The 2000 edition of the *Dietary Guidelines for Americans* emphasizes the importance of plant foods. These two articles provide us with information regarding current use of sugars and grains, and how we might guide our clients in choosing carbohydrate foods.

Issues & ANSWERS

Carbohydrates in the Diets of Children: Too High or Too Low?

High-sugar foods in the diets of children

Over the years we have improved the health of our nation's children by eliminating many serious childhood diseases such as polio and measles, through the development of new vaccines and prevention programs. In the past 10 years, however, the number of children who are overweight has doubled, and many others have eating patterns that put them at nutritional risk. More than 70% of youth aged 2 to 19 do not eat the recommended number of servings from the fruit and grains groups of the *Food Guide Pyramid,* and 64% do not eat the suggested number of servings of vegetables. Soft drinks and fruit drinks high in added sugar are replacing fruit juice and milk in the diets of many children and teenagers. Fiber intakes have not increased among U.S. children since 1976, despite our attention to fiber in nutrition education for all age groups. How has this occurred, and what can we do to correct this imbalance of overconsumption of carbohydrate foods high in sugar and underconsumption of carbohydrate foods high in complex carbohydrates?

Children aged 6 to 17 have the highest intakes of added sweeteners as a proportion of their total kcalories of any age group, getting close to 20% of their energy from added sugars. For children aged 2 to 5, 16% of their kcalories come from added sugars. Fruit drinks, soft drinks, and sweetened grain products such as cookies, along with table sugar, syrups, candy, and jelly, are major sources of added sugars in the diets of children. Fruit juice containing naturally occurring sugars, breakfast cereals, and milk products contribute much smaller amounts of sugar. Substituting soft drinks and fruit drinks for milk or fruit juice changes the quality of the diet in several ways. First, children who drink soft drinks tend to have higher energy intakes. In a recent national survey children who drank at least 9 oz (1.1 cups) of a soft drink every day had energy intakes about 200 kcalories above those who did not have a soft drink. Over time these additional kcalories can add to weight gain in children who are physically inactive. The use of soft drinks also lowered children's intakes of important nutrients that they would have received from fruit juice or milk. Those who had soft drinks regularly had lower intakes of riboflavin, folate, vitamins A and C, and calcium. Fruit juice can supply a portion of the two to four fruit servings recommended in the *Food Guide Pyramid* but should not exceed 12 fluid oz/day. Adding servings of fresh or canned fruits will supply dietary fiber.

Complex carbohydrate foods in the diets of children

The AI for total fiber is 25 g/day for children ages 4 to 8 years, 31 g/day for boys ages 9 to 13 years, and 26 g/day for girls ages 9 to 13 years. This AI for fiber rises to 38 g/day in boys ages 14 to 18 years but remains at 26 g/day for girls ages 14 to 18 years. A review of the food intake of 1400 children between the ages of 4 and 10 years told us that 55% in the 4- to 6-year-old age group consumed less than 11 g of fiber on a daily basis, and fewer than one third of the children in the 7- to 10-year-old age group had even 15 g/day, or half of the current recommendation (Panel on Macronutrients et al, 2002). These results are easily understood when we look at servings from the *Food Guide Pyramid* groups that supply our fiber. Although children regularly consume about seven servings a day from the grain group, only one of these servings is a whole grain. Looking at fruits and vegetables, children averaged fewer than two servings of fruit (including juice) and fewer than three servings of vegetables every day. These intakes do not meet even the minimum number of servings in each of these groups.

Goals for intervention

What can we do to improve this situation? First we might look at the items available in vending machines in locations frequented by children. Fruit juices should be an option, and parents and school authorities need to be educated on the value of fruit juice versus soft drinks. High-fiber grain snacks such as popcorn might replace some of the high-sugar, high-fat cookies and cakes. Whole grain flour might be used in children's favorite foods, including pizza crusts and pasta. School programs should incorporate whole grain, high-fiber products in their breakfast programs that serve cereals and muffins. Both parents and nutritionists should work together to influence food industry advertising that now promotes cereals high in sugar and low in fiber.

Vegetables containing fiber need to be made more attractive to children of all ages. Raw carrots or other vegetables that are finger food might be encouraged as snacks, and vegetables already popular with children, such as potatoes, might be prepared with less added fat. Legumes and rice add both fiber and important vitamins and minerals and are ingredients in many popular ethnic foods that children enjoy. A noted researcher on children's diets commented that "children eat what their parents eat" (Doucette and Dwyer, 2000). As nutrition educators we need to work with all age groups to reverse the current carbohydrate pattern that emphasizes high-sugar rather than complex carbohydrate foods.

REFERENCES

Doucette RE, Dwyer JT: Is fruit juice a "no-no" in children's diets, *Nutr Rev* 58:180, 2000.

Guthrie JF, Morton JF: Food sources of added sweeteners in the diets of Americans, *J Am Diet Assoc* 100:43, 2000.

Hampl JS, Betts NM, Benes BA: The 'age + 5' rule: comparisons of dietary fiber intake among 4- to 10-year-old children, *J Am Diet Assoc* 98:1412, 1998.

Harnack L, Stang J, Story M: Soft drink consumption among US children and adolescents: nutritional consequences, *J Am Diet Assoc* 99:436, 1999.

Kantor LS et al: Choose a variety of grains daily, especially whole grains: a challenge for consumers, *J Nutr* 131 (suppl):473S, 2001.

Krebs-Smith SM, Kantor LS: Choose a variety of fruits and vegetables daily: understanding the complexities, *J Nutr* 131(suppl):487S, 2001.

Panel on Macronutrients, Panel on the Definition of Dietary Fiber, Subcommittee on Upper Reference Levels of Nutrients, Subcommittee on Interpretation and Uses of Dietary Reference Intakes, and the Standing Committee on the Scientific Evaluation of Dietary Reference Intakes: *Dietary reference intakes for energy, carbohydrate, fiber, fat, fatty acids, cholesterol, protein, and amino acids, parts 1 and 2,* Washington, DC, 2002, National Academy Press.

Chapter

4

Lipids

Eleanor D. Schlenker

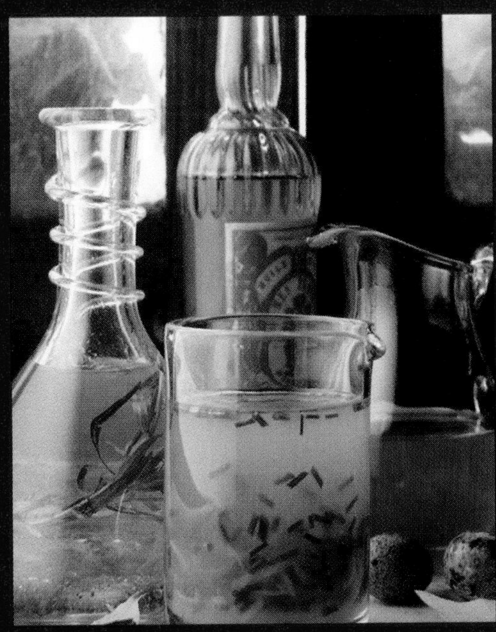

Chapter Outline

Lipids, the second of our energy-yielding macronutrients, have for the most part received negative reporting for the past few years because of their association with a number of chronic diseases. This is especially true for heart disease. But the real culprit, as with many things, is the excessive amount of fat we eat. Fat itself is an essential nutrient.

Traditionally, fat has held a prominent place in the American diet. However, spurred by our justified health concerns, our attitudes and habits regarding dietary lipids have changed.

Our goal is to achieve some balance in our food choices and our use of dietary fats. As health professionals we need to focus on the total diet, not on a single nutrient.[1] *Based on the information provided about the nature of lipids and their role in nutrition, we will see why we need a moderate amount of fat for energy and overall good health.*

Lipids in Nutrition and Health

HEALTH NEEDS FOR LIPIDS

We need some lipids in our food and in our bodies to keep us in good health. This need is indicated by the number of functions lipids perform in nutrition, in providing fuel for energy, in maintaining our body structure, and in supporting our overall body metabolism.

Food Lipids

The lipids in our food provide energy, essential nutrients, and satiety, as the following list explains.

- *Fuel source for energy.* Food lipids supply a concentrated source of fuel for the body to store and utilize as needed for energy. Food lipids yield 9 kilocalories (kcalories)/g when oxidized in the body in comparison with carbohydrates and protein, which yield only 4 kcalories/g.
- *Essential nutrient supply.* Food lipids supply the essential fatty acids (EFAs), linoleic acid, and linolenic acid. Food lipids from animal sources also supply cholesterol supplementing the body's endogenous supply.
- *Food palatability.* Lipids in the diet supply flavor to food and a certain mouth feel, which contributes to a feeling of satisfaction that lasts longer than does the feeling of satisfaction after eating carbohydrates and protein. Our food choices are strongly influenced by taste and texture, much of which lipids contribute, thus enhancing our eating pleasure.[2] The fuller texture and body that fat contribute to food mixtures and the slower gastric emptying time it brings may play a role in satiety.

Body Lipids

The body stores energy as adipose tissue. These lipid tissue reserves serve a number of vital functions that are essential to health and life itself.

- *Energy.* A major function of lipids in nutrition is to supply an efficient fuel to all tissues, although the central nervous system and brain depend on a steady supply of glucose.
- *Thermal insulation.* The layer of lipid deposits directly underneath the skin controls body temperature within the range necessary for life.
- *Vital organ protection.* A weblike padding of adipose tissue surrounds vital organs such as the kidneys, protecting them from mechanical shock and providing a structure for support.
- *Nerve impulse transmission.* Lipid layers surrounding nerve fibers provide electrical insulation and transmit nerve impulses.
- *Tissue membrane structure.* Lipids serve as vital constituents in cell membranes, helping transport nutrient materials, metabolites, and waste molecules across cell membranes.
- *Cell metabolism.* Combinations of lipids and protein, known as lipoproteins, carry lipids in the blood to all cells.
- *Essential precursor substances.* Lipids supply necessary components, such as fatty acids and cholesterol, for the synthesis of many materials required for metabolic functions and tissue integrity. For example, tissues in the brain and the retina of the eye contain many fatty acids.
- *Carriers of fat-soluble vitamins.* Lipids provide essential transport for carrying the fat-soluble vitamins, A, D, E, and K, to the cells for vital metabolic needs.

HEALTH PROBLEMS AND LIPIDS

From lists such as the one given earlier and world health reports, it is evident that lipids make up an essential nutrient class. If lipids are as vital to human health as indicated, why are there so many questions about the amount and type of fat in our diet?[3,4] As with so many things, the old maxim holds true: you need what you need, but you don't need more than you need. In general, health problems related to lipids focus on two main issues: too much dietary fat reflected in excessive body fat, and too much of the dietary fat coming from animal food sources. As we will learn in future sections, different types of fat have very different effects on body tissues and functions.

Amount of Fat

Too much fat in the diet provides excess kcalories, more than required for immediate energy needs. Excess kcalories are stored as excess adipose tissue, thereby increasing body weight. This increased body weight—more precisely, an increased proportion of body fat making up the total body composition—has been associated with such health problems as diabetes, hypertension, and heart disease.[5] Look for specific relationships between increased body weight (and body fat) and these health problems in later chapters on these topics.

Type of Fat

Current research has shown a clear relation between a diet containing excess saturated fat and cholesterol, which come from animal sources, and atherosclerosis. *Atherosclerosis* is a blood vessel disease characterized by fatty plaques that build up on the interior walls of the major blood vessels and, over time, can fill the vessel and cut off blood circulation (see Chapter 19). This disease process contributes to heart attacks and strokes. On the other hand, certain lipids such as those found in fatty fish[6] or olive oil[7] may actually reduce our risk of heart disease and stroke. So it is important to help persons learn to recognize the different sources and types of lipids and how they affect health.

The Physical and Chemical Nature of Lipids

PHYSICAL CHARACTERISTICS

Lipids include such substances as fat, oil, and related compounds that are greasy to the touch and insoluble in water. Some food forms of lipids are easily recognized as fat, such as butter, margarine, or cooking oil. At the same time foods that appear to be high carbohydrate and low fat, such as grain or bakery foods, may contain significant amounts of fat, often referred to as hidden fat.[8]

CHEMICAL CHARACTERISTICS

The chemical class name for fats and fat-related compounds is lipids. By chemical definition, these are all organic compounds, consisting mainly of a chain of the basic element carbon as a "backbone," with attached hydrogen and oxygen atoms and other radicals or groups of elements. All lipids have in common a relation to the fatty acids. The same basic chemical elements that make up carbohydrates—carbon, hydrogen, and oxygen—also make up the fatty acids and their related lipids. It is important to remember that these two nutrients differ in two main ways: (1) lipids are more complex in structure, with more carbon (C) and hydrogen (H) and less oxygen (O) and (2) the common structural units of lipids are fatty acids, whereas the common structural units of carbohydrates are simple sugars. Fatty acids are also refined fuel forms that some cells, such as those making up the heart muscle, prefer over glucose. In our discussion here, we look first at the basic structural units, the fatty acids, and their unique characteristics of saturation, essentiality, and chain length. Then we focus on the nature of the basic lipids, known as triglycerides, that are built from fatty acids.

Basic Lipids: Fatty Acids and Triglycerides

CHARACTERISTICS OF THE FATTY ACIDS: SATURATION

The state of saturation or unsaturation gives lipids their varying textural characteristics. Saturated lipids are harder, less saturated ones are softer, and unsaturated ones are usually liquid oils at room temperature. These differing physical states result from the ratio of hydrogen to carbon in the structures of the respective fatty acids that make up a particular lipid. If a given fatty acid is filled with as much hydrogen as can be attached, the fatty acid is said to be completely saturated with hydrogen. If, however, the fatty acid has fewer hydrogens attached with some hydrogen spaces unfilled, it is obviously less saturated. Three terms designate the varying degree of saturation.

1. *Saturated.* Food lipids composed of saturated fatty acids are called *saturated fats.* The most saturated forms of lipid are found in tropical oils such as coconut and palm kernel oils (88% and 80% saturated, respectively).[9] Other sources of saturated fats are mainly of animal origin, for example, meats and whole milk dairy products.
2. *Monounsaturated.* Food lipids composed mainly of fatty acids with one hydrogen space unfilled, creating one double bond, are called *monounsaturated fats.* These lipids are mostly from plant sources, for example, olive oil and canola oil, which is derived from a variety of rapeseed.
3. *Polyunsaturated.* Food lipids composed mainly of unsaturated fatty acids with two or more places unfilled with hydrogen, creating two or more double bonds, are called *polyunsaturated fats.* These lipids come from plant sources. Common polyunsaturated fats are corn oil and safflower seed oil. Notable exceptions are coconut oil, palm oil, and cocoa butter, which are saturated plant oils.

Polyunsaturated fatty acids are sometimes referred to as n-3 or n-6 fatty acids. This refers to the position in the carbon chain where the first double bond appears. A common n-6 fatty acid is linoleic acid, the essential fatty acid that is described later. It is found in common vegetable oils such as corn or safflower oil. The n-3 fatty acids are most commonly found in fatty fish and appear to play a role in preventing heart disease.[9]

CHARACTERISTICS OF THE FATTY ACIDS: ESSENTIALITY

The terms *essential* and *nonessential* are applied to nutrients according to their relative necessity in the diet. A particular nutrient is essential if the body cannot

adipose Fat present in cells of adipose (fatty) tissue.

fatty acid The structural components of fats.

lipids Chemical group name for fats and fat-related compounds such as cholesterol, lipoproteins, and phospholipids; general group name for organic substances of a fatty nature, including fats, oils, waxes, and related compounds.

organic Carbon-based chemical compounds.

saturated Term used for a substance that is united with the greatest possible amount of another substance through solution, chemical combination, or the like. A saturated fat, for example, is one in which the component fatty acids are filled with hydrogen atoms. A fatty acid is said to be saturated if all available chemical bonds of its carbon chain are filled with hydrogen. If one bond remains unfilled, it is a monounsaturated fatty acid. If two or more bonds remain unfilled, it is a polyunsaturated fatty acid. Fats of animal sources are more saturated. Fats of plant sources are unsaturated.

TO PROBE FURTHER

Health Benefits of Unsaturated Fatty Acids: What's in a Double Bond?

Over the past 30 years, evidence has been mounting that saturated fatty acids or fatty acids that have the maximum number of hydrogen atoms attached to their carbon core have detrimental effects on health. Dietary intakes high in saturated fatty acids have been associated with greater risk of heart disease, stroke, and damage to the coronary arteries, and these findings led to the recommendation that saturated fats provide less than 10% of total dietary kcalories. At the same time we are learning that monounsaturated fatty acids that have one double bond and polyunsaturated fatty acids with two or more double bonds have very different effects on health. Not only do unsaturated fatty acids not increase cardiovascular risk when consumed in moderation, but also they may help to prevent heart attacks or stroke through their effects on blood lipoproteins and blood clotting factors.

MONOUNSATURATED FATTY ACIDS

Monounsaturated fatty acids, especially oleic acid, are plentiful in certain plant-based foods, including olive oil, canola oil, and nuts. Individuals whose primary sources of fat are olive oil and nuts appear to experience important health benefits. In fact olive oil and its constituent fatty acid, oleic acid, have been credited with bringing about some of the positive effects associated with the Mediterranean diet, an eating pattern based on plant foods, especially legumes and grains. Olive oil also contains important polyphenols (chemical substances in plants) that may contribute to its healthful effects. Monounsaturated fatty acids decrease low-density lipoprotein (LDL) cholesterol levels and other blood fats while raising the high-density lipoprotein (HDL) cholesterol levels. Monounsaturated fatty acids have this favorable effect on blood fats even in diets containing as much as 34% fat, as long as one third or more of the fat is monounsaturated.

POLYUNSATURATED FATTY ACIDS

We are also learning more about the polyunsaturated fatty acids that contain at least two double bonds. These include the n-6 fatty acids such as linoleic acid and arachidonic acid and the n-3 fatty acids such as linolenic acid, eicosapentaenoic acid, and docosahexaenoic acid. The n-6 fatty acids, when replacing saturated fatty acids in the diet, lower LDL cholesterol levels but also lower HDL cholesterol, which helps to excrete cholesterol from the body. Thus, the positive effects of lowering LDL cholesterol levels need to be balanced with the undesirable change in HDL cholesterol levels. On the other hand, the n-3 fatty acids, obtained primarily from fatty fish and also found in canola oil, have many positive effects. The n-3 fatty acids eicosapentaenoic acid and docosahexaenoic acid were first identified in the diets of Eskimos from Greenland, who had low rates of heart disease despite their high fat intakes from fish. These fatty acids found in fish prevent cardiovascular problems in several ways. First, they decrease the ability of blood platelets to form a clot, thus reducing the risk of an unwanted clot in the coronary arteries or arteries of the brain. Second, HDL cholesterol levels rise when fish is consumed regularly, and although LDL cholesterol molecules increase in size, there is no increase in number. The n-3 fatty acids also appear to lower blood pressure, which likely plays a role in lowering the risk of heart attack or stroke. This effect on blood pressure relates to the ability of the eicosanoids to act on the major arteries and cause them to dilate.

Fish oils can benefit those who already have heart disease. Among patients who had survived one heart attack and then began to eat fish twice a week, the mortality rate over the next 2 years was 29% lower than in those who were not eating fish regularly. The n-3 fatty acids may be important for heart transplant recipients because of their ability to dilate the major arteries and thus reduce the workload of the heart as a pump. Based on their action in reducing inflammation, n-3 and n-6 fatty acids are being studied for the treatment of rheumatoid arthritis.

Despite the positive health benefits of some polyunsaturated fatty acids, there is a risk of adverse health effects if these fatty acids are consumed in very high amounts. As we will learn in Chapter 7, fatty acids and other molecules containing double bonds are vulnerable to oxidation reactions that change their structure. These changes not only reduce their ability to carry out their normal functions in the body but also cause reactions against other molecules with double bonds. Thus it is suggested that polyunsaturated fatty acids make up no more than 10% of total energy.

• • •

Vegetable oils such as corn oil, safflower oil, and soybean oil, as well as seeds and nuts, are good sources of n-6 fatty acids. Two servings of fish a week will provide adequate but not excessive levels of n-3 fatty acids. The use of olive and canola oils in cooking and

TO PROBE FURTHER
Health Benefits of Unsaturated Fatty Acids: What's in a Double Bond?—cont'd

the addition of peanuts or other nuts to the diet on a regular basis will supply appropriate levels of oleic and other monounsaturated fats. In a diet containing 30% fat, monounsaturated fats should provide at least 10% to 12% of the total fat consumed.

Attention to the benefits of both monounsaturated and polyunsaturated fatty acids has led to the manufacture of a variety of supplements designed to meet our dietary needs for these nutrients. It is always best to obtain our nutrients from real food that will supply a variety of important nutrients. We should encourage our clients to include good sources of the unsaturated fatty acids in their regular dietary patterns.

References

Dewailly E et al: Relations between n-3 fatty acid status and cardiovascular disease risk factors among Quebecers, *Am J Clin Nutr* 74:603, 2001.

Eritsland J: Safety considerations of polyunsaturated fatty acids, *Am J Clin Nutr* 71(suppl):197S, 2000.

Feldman EB: Assorted monounsaturated fatty acids promote healthy hearts, *Am J Clin Nutr* 70:953, 1999.

Visioli F, Galli C: The effect of minor constituents of olive oil on cardiovascular disease: new findings, *Nutr Rev* 56(5):142, 1998.

Von Schacky C: n-3 fatty acids and the prevention of coronary atherosclerosis, *Am J Clin Nutr* 71(suppl):224S, 2000.

manufacture it and therefore must obtain it from the diet; a failure to do so would result in a deficiency disease. Two fatty acids—linoleic acid and linolenic acid—are the only fatty acids known to be essential for the complete nutrition of humans, and Adequate Intake (AI) levels have been set for both of these nutrients.[10] Arachidonic acid, an important fatty acid in human nutrition, can be synthesized from linolenic acid; however, if lipids make up only 10% or less of the diet's daily kcalories, it is likely that the body will not obtain adequate amounts of the essential fatty acids. These fatty acids, linoleic and linolenic, serve important body functions.

- *Membrane structure.* Linoleic acid strengthens cell membranes, helping to prevent a harmful increase in skin and membrane permeability. A linoleic acid deficiency leads to a breakdown in skin integrity, resulting in characteristic eczema and skin lesions. A similar effect also occurs in other tissue membranes throughout the body.
- *Cholesterol transport.* Like other fatty acids, linoleic acid combines with cholesterol to form cholesterol esters for transport in the blood.
- *Serum cholesterol.* As do other unsaturated fatty acids, linoleic acid helps lower serum cholesterol levels. It plays a key role in both transport and metabolism of cholesterol.
- *Blood clotting.* Along with linolenic acid, linoleic acid helps prolong blood clotting time and increases fibrinolytic activity.
- *Local hormone-like effects.* Linoleic acid is a major metabolic precursor of a group of physiologically and pharmacologically active compounds known as *prostaglandins, prostacyclins, thromboxanes,* and *leukotrienes.* This family of compounds is called the eicosanoids because of their structure (see *To Probe Further* box). They are synthesized in the body from arachidonic acid, which is derived from the essential linoleic acid. The synthesis of these highly active, important compounds is diagrammed in Figure 4-1; the eicosanoid compounds have extensive local hormone-like effects,[11,12] with many significant physiologic functions and sites. Other eicosanoid products, the fatty acids eicosapentaenoic acid and docosahexaenoic acid (n-3 fatty acids), can be made from linolenic acid or supplied in the diet by fatty fish such as herring or salmon and eggs.[13]

Prostaglandins

Of these groups of *eicosanoid* compounds related to the essential fatty acids, perhaps the most familiar is the group known as prostaglandins because of their extensive functions. They were first discovered by Swedish investigators in their study of reproductive physiology. They were identified initially in human semen, and

eicosanoids Long-chain fatty acids composed of 20 carbon atoms.

essential fatty acid A fatty acid required in the diet because the body cannot synthesize it or synthesize it in adequate amounts.

linoleic acid An essential fatty acid for humans; an n-6 polyunsaturated fatty acid.

linolenic acid An essential fatty acid for humans; an n-3 polyunsaturated fatty acid.

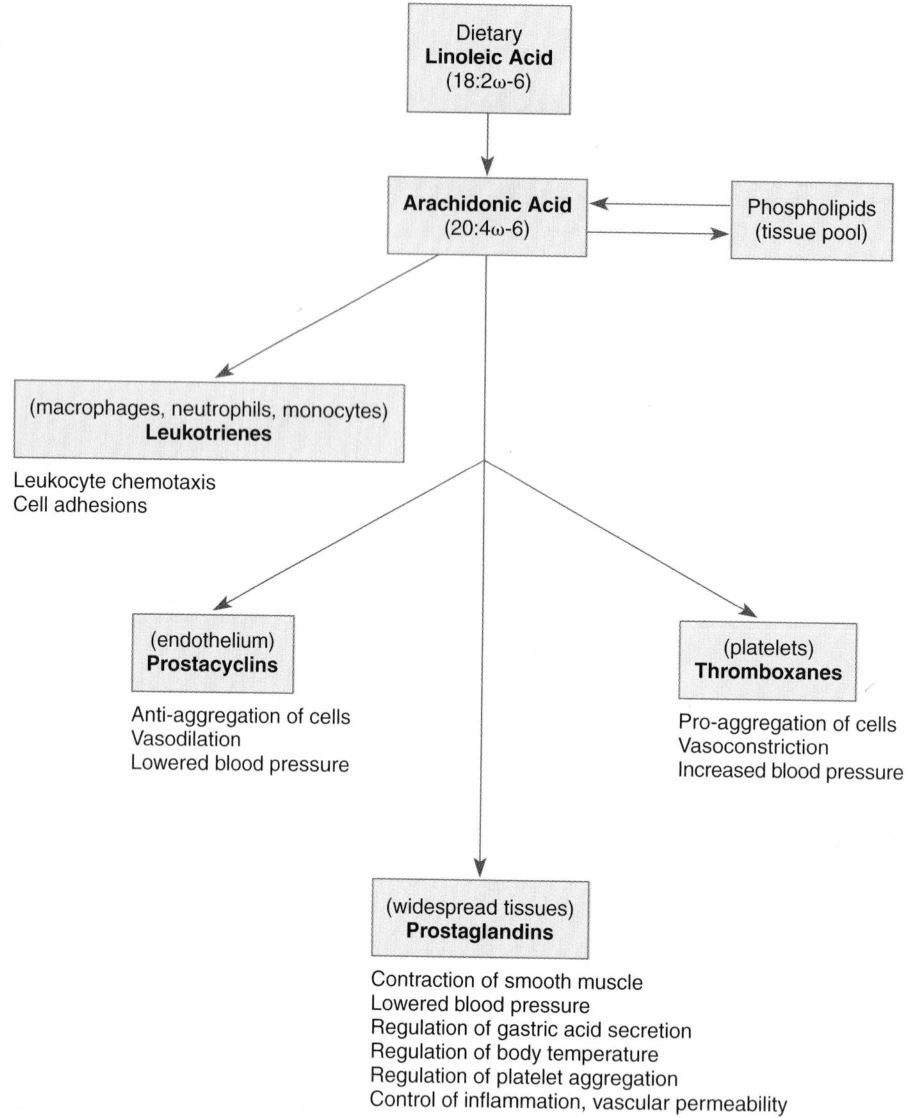

FIGURE 4-1 Synthesis, sites, and functions of eicosanoids.

named prostaglandins because they were thought to originate in the prostate gland. They are now known to exist in virtually all body tissues, acting as local hormones to direct and coordinate important biologic functions. For example, they have been shown to be powerful modulators of vascular smooth muscle tone and platelet aggregation and hence have a significant relationship to blood pressure, blood clotting, and cardiovascular disease.[11,12]

Recommended Intake of Essential Fatty Acids

The most recent edition of the Dietary Reference Intakes set AI levels for linoleic and linolenic acids. The AI for linoleic acid (an n-6 acid) is 17 g/day for men and 12 g/day for women ages 19 to 50 years. Men ages 51 years and over should take in 14 g/day of linoleic acid and women of that age should take in 11 g/day. The AI for linolenic acid (an n-3 acid) is 1.6 g/day for men and 1.1 g/day for women.[10] We will talk more about the essential fatty acids and their importance in development of the brain and nervous system when we discuss the nutrient needs of infants and young children.

CHARACTERISTICS OF FATTY ACIDS: CHAIN LENGTH

Another characteristic of fatty acids, important in their absorption, is the length of the carbon chain forming their structure. Fatty acids in food range from 4 carbons to 22 carbons in length. Those made up of 4 to 6 carbons are referred to as short-chain fatty acids; those with 8, 10, or 12 carbons are the medium-chain fatty acids;

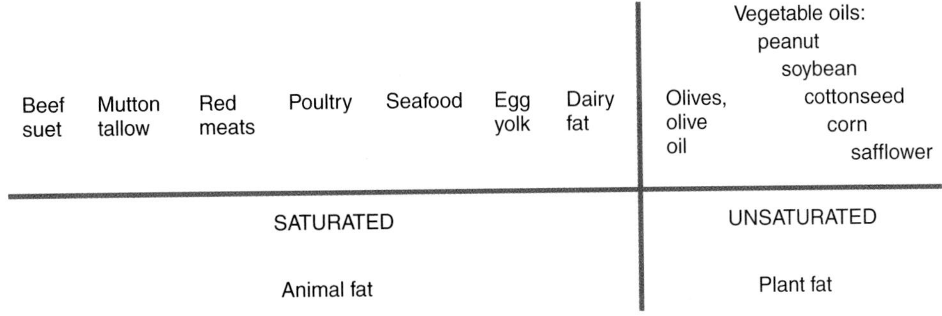

FIGURE 4-2 Spectrum of food fats according to degree of saturation of component fatty acids.

and those with 14, 16, 18, or more carbons are the long-chain fatty acids. The long-chain fatty acids are more difficult to absorb and require a helping carrier. The short- and medium-chain fatty acids are more soluble in water and therefore easier to absorb directly into the bloodstream. In intestinal malabsorption diseases, when the absorbing mucosal surface is inflamed or infected, short- or medium-chain fatty acid products are preferred. A commercial product called MCT (medium-chain triglycerides) is an oil made of short- and medium-chain fatty acids that can be used in the diet just as any ordinary vegetable oil.

TRIGLYCERIDES

Basic Structure

Triglycerides are the storage form of fatty acids. The name indicates the basic chemical structure: three fatty acids attached to a glycerol base. Thus lipids are glycerides composed of glycerol and fatty acids. When glycerol is combined with one fatty acid, it is called a *monoglyceride;* with two fatty acids, a *diglyceride;* and with three fatty acids, a *triglyceride.* Whether in food or in the body, fatty acids combine with glycerol to form glycerides. Most natural lipids, from either animal or plant sources, are triglycerides. These lipids, the triglycerides, occur in body cells as oily droplets. They circulate in the water-based blood serum encased in a covering of water-soluble protein. These lipid-protein complexes are called *lipoproteins.* They serve multiple functions throughout the body.

Nature of Food Lipids

Food lipids, as well as body lipids, are composed of saturated and unsaturated fatty acids. If the food lipid is made up mainly of saturated fatty acids, it is called a saturated fat. Foods from animal sources—such as meat, milk, and eggs—contain saturated fats. Conversely, food from plant sources such as the vegetable oils are usually unsaturated. A general saturated-unsaturated spectrum of food lipids is shown in Figure 4-2. The animal food lipids on the saturated end of the spectrum are solid at room temperature; those toward the center become somewhat less saturated and are softer. The plant lipids on the unsaturated end are free-flowing oils that do not solidify even at low temperatures. Exceptions to the usual pattern of plant oils containing unsaturated fatty acids are tropical oils such as coconut oil and palm oil, which *are* saturated lipids. These saturated plant fats are used extensively in commercial products such as nondairy creamers because they are usually cheaper oils.

As the availability of processed food items higher in fat continues to increase in the marketplace, it becomes increasingly important for consumers to read food labels carefully. The current food label on processed foods indicates the number of grams of saturated and unsaturated fatty acids per serving. Both the general distinction in saturation between animal and plant foods (see Figure 4-2), as well as food labels on processed foods, can be helpful in assisting persons in making wise choices of food fats.

---

glyceride Group name for fats; any of a group of esters obtained from glycerol by the replacement of one, two, or three hydroxyl (OH) groups with a fatty acid. Monoglycerides contain one fatty acid; diglycerides contain two fatty acids; and triglycerides contain three fatty acids. Glycerides are the principal constituent of adipose tissue and are found in animal and vegetable fats and oils.

glycerol A colorless, odorless, syrupy, sweet liquid; a constituent of fats usually obtained by the hydrolysis of fats. Chemically, glycerol is an alcohol; it is esterified with fatty acids to produce fats.

prostaglandins Group of naturally occurring substances, first discovered in semen, derived from long-chain fatty acids that have multiple local hormone-like actions; these include regulation of gastric acid secretion, blood platelet aggregation, body temperature, and tissue inflammation.

triglyceride Chemical name for fat, indicating structure; attachment of three fatty acids to a glycerol base. A neutral fat, synthesized from carbohydrate and stored in adipose tissue, it releases free fatty acids into the blood when hydrolyzed by enzymes.

The *Cis* and *Trans* Unsaturated Fatty Acid Products

Unsaturated liquid plant oils can be hardened to form products such as margarine and shortening by the injection of hydrogen gas, causing hydrogen ions to attach at available double bonds and resulting in a more saturated fat. This process is called hydrogenation. Recently, health professionals have become concerned about a particular form of unsaturated fatty acid (a *trans* fatty acid) that is formed in this process and seems to have a detrimental effect on health. First, let's compare the various possible structures of the commonly occurring monounsaturated fatty acid, oleic acid, which has one unsaturated double bond occurring in the middle of its chain of 18 carbon atoms.

When double bonds occur naturally in food lipids, the fatty acid chain usually bends in such a way that the two remaining parts of the structure are on the same side of the bond. In this case the fatty acid is called *cis* ("same side") (Figure 4-3). All fatty acids that occur naturally in vegetable oils are in the *cis* form. However, when vegetable oils are partially hydrogenated to make food products, the normal bend is changed so that the remaining parts are on opposite sides of the bond. In this case the form is called *trans* ("opposite side"). Commercially hydrogenated lipids found in soft margarine and many other food products are in the *trans* form. It appears that the *trans-cis* structure of fatty acids can influence their effect on human health, as does their degree of saturation. Human studies tell us that *trans* fatty acids increase blood low-density lipoprotein (LDL) cholesterol levels even more than do saturated fats.[14,15] The problem for consumers and health educators extends beyond just a simple choice of margarine because fats high in *trans* fatty acids are used extensively in baked products such as doughnuts and in commercial frying at fast food restaurants.[8] The requirement to include the *trans* fatty acid content on the nutrition label is now being reviewed by the Food and Drug Administration.[16]

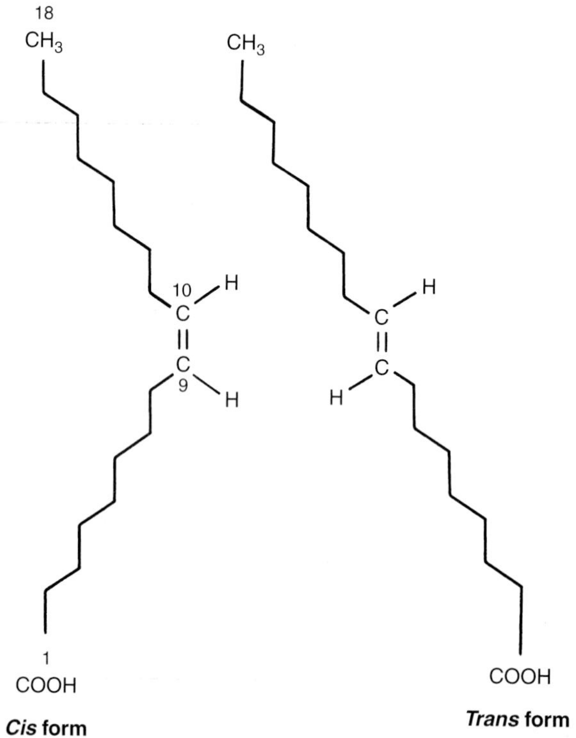

FIGURE 4-3 The *cis* and *trans* forms of a fatty acid.

VISIBLE AND HIDDEN FOOD FAT

As mentioned earlier, food fats are sometimes called "visible" or "hidden" fats according to how obvious they are in food. In many cases food fat is quite evident, such as in butter, margarine, oil, salad dressing, bacon, and cream, which account for about 40% of the fat in the American diet.[17] However, less obvious hidden fats in foods such as meat, milk (unless it is a nonfat form), eggs (only in the yolk; the white is pure protein), nuts, seeds, olives, and avocados also contribute to our fat intake.

A large part of the hidden fat in the American diet comes from our relatively high consumption of meat. Even when all the obvious fat is trimmed from a cut of meat, its lean portion still contains 4% to 12% hidden fat from the "marbling"—tiny fat deposits within the muscle tissue. This is especially true of beef, the most popular meat in the United States. Food items included in the tip of the *Food Guide Pyramid* (the "Other" group), which includes grain foods with added fat, such as pastries and desserts, and fats added in food preparation or at the table, account for 25% of all kcalories consumed by both men and women in the United States. Fat supplied by the other five food groups in the *Food Guide Pyramid* makes up 8% to 9% of the total kcalories in the American diet.[17] (For a review of the *Food Guide Pyramid*, see Chapter 1.)

The new *Dietary Guidelines for Americans* (see Chapter 1) recommend that all persons above 2 years of age choose a diet providing no more than 30% of kcalories from total fat and less than 10% of kcalories from saturated fat. The Acceptable Macronutrient Distribution Range (AMDR) for fat is 20% to 30% of total kcalories.[10] In future chapters we will consider situations in which a fat intake above or below 30% might be appropriate.

The public health campaigns urging Americans to reduce their fat intake have led many consumers to make changes in their diet. A review of the food choices of over 3700 participants in the Continuing Survey of Food Intake by Individuals (CSFII) identified three different strategies for reducing dietary fat: (1) choosing a lower-fat milk, (2) choosing a lower-fat meat, or (3) choosing a fat-modified product such as a salad dressing, dessert, or yogurt.[18] Some consumers combined all three strategies. The men and women who used at least one strategy obtained no more than 32% of their total kcalories from fat and no more than 10% of their kcalories from saturated fat. Those who used two or three strategies lowered their fat intakes to 25% of total kcalories. In contrast, those who adopted no strategy for controlling their fat intake consumed 36% of their kcalories from fat and 12% of their kcalories from saturated fat, and intakes of other necessary nutrients were generally inadequate.

It is important that we assist persons in taking appropriate actions to lower their dietary fat. Individuals who lower their dietary fat intake by substituting fat-modified foods for higher fat foods also lower their energy intake by 400 to 500 kcalories and have higher intakes of other important nutrients compared with those who substitute high-carbohydrate foods, including soft drinks for high-fat foods.[19] Efforts of food technologists to improve the texture and taste of fat-modified foods have increased their attractiveness to the health conscious consumer.[20] Balancing your diet to include a variety of both higher-fat and lower-fat foods is the best strategy for achieving a healthy diet (see *Issues & Answers* for more information on fat-reduced foods).

SPECIAL LIPID-RELATED COMPOUND: CHOLESTEROL

Structure

Although cholesterol is often discussed in connection with dietary lipids, it is not a fat or triglyceride itself. Many people confuse cholesterol with saturated fat. Cholesterol is a lipid-related compound that is quite different from triglycerides in structure. Generally, cholesterol travels in the bloodstream attached to long-chain fatty acids, forming cholesterol esters.

Functions

Cholesterol is a vital substance in human metabolism. It belongs to a family of substances called steroids, or sterols, and is a precursor to all steroid hormones. A cholesterol compound in the skin, *7-dehydrocholesterol,* is irradiated by the ultraviolet rays of sunlight and is activated in the body to produce vitamin D hormone. Cholesterol is also essential in the formation of bile acids, which emulsify fats for enzymatic digestion and then serve as carriers for fat absorption. Cholesterol is widely distributed in all cells of the body and is found in large amounts in brain and nerve tissue. It is an essential component of cell membranes. It is no wonder therefore that a constant supply of so vital a material for body processes would be made in body tissues, mainly in the liver. If a person consumed no cholesterol at all, the body would still synthesize an adequate supply.

Food Sources

Cholesterol occurs naturally in all animal foods but not in plant foods. The main food sources of cholesterol are egg yolks and organ meats such as liver and kidneys. Animal fats, but *not* plant fats, are rich sources of cholesterol. Plant or vegetable oils may vary in degree of saturation, but none of them contain cholesterol.

Health Concerns

Cholesterol has been increasingly implicated in vascular disease as a major risk factor in the development of *atherosclerosis,* the underlying pathology in coronary heart disease. In atherosclerosis cholesterol-containing fatty plaques build up on blood vessel walls. If this plaque forms a blood clot and narrows the major arteries serving the heart muscle, a heart attack is triggered. If this plaque initiates a clot that finally lodges in an artery in the brain, it causes a stroke or cerebral hemorrhage. Elevated serum cholesterol levels have been associated with more rapid progression of atherosclerosis (see Chapter 19). Thus government health officials and health professionals have recommended that Americans reduce their dietary cholesterol to no more than 300 mg/day, an intake associated with appropriate serum cholesterol levels.[5] Genetic selection within the agricultural industry to produce eggs and meat lower in cholesterol content and efforts by food technologists to develop modified fat products that can be marketed as cholesterol free have contributed to keeping cholesterol intake within recommended levels. In the United States, men making no effort to reduce their dietary fat intakes still have average intakes of only 302 mg of cholesterol, and women average 204 mg.[18]

Increasing your intake of soluble types of dietary fiber—described in Chapter 3—helps to control blood cholesterol levels because such fibers bind bile acids and dietary cholesterol, and thus help eliminate excess cholesterol from the body.[21] Certain plant sterols, now being added to particular margarines, can assist in lowering serum cholesterol levels[22,23] (see *Practical Application* box). Further research is needed to determine the possible effect of plant sterols on absorption of the fat-soluble vitamins. For those individuals with high blood cholesterol levels for whom dietary intervention does not prove effective, drugs that prevent the synthesis of endogenous cholesterol by the body are often prescribed.[24]

cholesterol A fat-related compound, a sterol ($C_{27}H_{45}OH$). It is a normal constituent of bile and a principal constituent of gallstones. In body metabolism cholesterol is important as a precursor of various steroid hormones, such as sex hormones and adrenal corticoids. Cholesterol is synthesized by the liver. It is widely distributed in nature, especially in animal tissue such as glandular meats and egg yolk.

ester A compound produced by the reaction between an acid and an alcohol with elimination of a molecule of water. This process is called esterification. For example, a triglyceride is a glycerol ester. Cholesterol esters are formed in the mucosal cells by combination with fatty acids, largely linoleic acid.

hydrogenation Process of hardening liquid vegetable oils by injecting hydrogen gas to produce margarines and shortenings.

steroids Group name for lipid-based sterols, including hormones, bile acids, and cholesterol.

PRACTICAL APPLICATION
Plant Sterols: New Weapon for Lowering Serum Cholesterol Levels

Plant sterols, also known as phytosterols, are found in small quantities in various plant foods, including vegetable oils and grains such as corn, rye, and wheat. The molecular structure of plant sterols is similar to the structure of cholesterol. Because of this similarity, certain plant sterols compete with cholesterol for absorption sites in the small intestine. Many years ago researchers recognized that plant sterols would lower the amount of cholesterol that could be absorbed in the small intestine and delivered to the liver. When less cholesterol is delivered, the liver produces fewer lipoproteins, and serum levels of both total cholesterol and low-density lipoprotein (LDL) cholesterol are reduced.

Although we have known for some time that plant sterols could assist in the clinical management of serum cholesterol, the amount of these compounds naturally occurring in foods was too low to have any measurable effect on the proportion of dietary cholesterol absorbed. Recently, researchers in Finland discovered a way to incorporate the plant sterol sitostanol into fat products, making it possible to increase the level of sterols in the diet. Table fats containing sterols are now available in the United States under the trade name of Benecol, and their effect on serum cholesterol levels has been tested. Under normal circumstances, about 50% of dietary cholesterol is actually absorbed. When individuals with high serum cholesterol levels had sterol-enriched margarine 3 times a day (used as a table spread on a slice of bread), they absorbed only 20% of the cholesterol they consumed that day. Because they absorbed less of the cholesterol in their food, their total serum cholesterol level dropped by 10% and their LDL cholesterol level dropped by 14%. Plant sterols lower serum cholesterol levels even further when used in conjunction with a low-fat diet. Plant sterols that behave in a way similar to sitostanol in lowering cholesterol absorption have been identified in soy protein and may contribute to the heart-healthy effect of that food. (We discuss other important components of soy protein in Chapter 7.)

The use of sterol-fortified fats along with a prudent diet that does not exceed 30% of total kcalories from fat offers an important dietary intervention for individuals at risk of heart disease.

References

Hallikainen MA, Uusitupa MIJ: Effects of 2 low-fat stanol ester-containing margarines on serum cholesterol concentrations as part of a low-fat diet in hypercholesterolemic subjects, *Am J Clin Nutr* 69:403, 1999.

Levine BS, Cooper C: Plant stanol esters. A new tool in the dietary management of cholesterol, *Nutr Today* 35(2):61, 2000.

Maki KC et al: Lipid responses to plant-sterol-enriched reduced-fat spreads incorporated into a National Cholesterol Education Program Step 1 diet, *Am J Clin Nutr* 74:33, 2001.

Normen L et al: Soy sterol esters and B-sitostanol esters as inhibitors of cholesterol absorption in human small bowel, *Am J Clin Nutr* 71:908, 2000.

SPECIAL LIPID-RELATED COMPOUNDS: LIPOPROTEINS

Function

The liver serves as the center for (1) receiving fatty acids and cholesterol either absorbed from the diet or released from body tissues, (2) packaging them into lipoproteins, and (3) releasing them into the circulation.[25] The lipoproteins are important combinations of lipids with protein and other lipid-related components and are highly significant in human nutrition. Chemically, the lipoproteins are not true lipids but are really *complexes* (noncovalent structures) of lipids surrounded by protein. The lipoproteins—together with their attached apolipoprotein—serve as the major vehicle for lipid transport in the bloodstream (see Chapter 19).

Lipid Transport

Lipids are insoluble in water. This simple characteristic poses a problem in carrying lipids to cells in a water-based circulatory system. The body has solved this problem through the development of the lipoproteins, packages of lipids wrapped in water-soluble protein. These plasma lipoproteins contain fatty acids, triglycerides, cholesterol, phospholipids, and traces of other materials such as fat-soluble vitamins and steroid hormones. The high or low density of the lipoprotein is determined by its relative loads of lipids and protein. The higher the protein ratio, the higher is the density.

Thus the lipoproteins are usually classified according to density and by their relative lipid and cholesterol content.[26]

1. *Chylomicrons.* These are formed in the intestinal wall after a meal and carry the fat load from the meal just consumed to liver cells for initial conversion to other transport lipoproteins.
2. *Very low-density lipoproteins (VLDLs).* These are formed in the liver during the fasting intervals between meals. When there is no food in the digestive tract and chylomicrons are not being formed, VLDLs serve as the major transporters of triglycerides in the continuing

process of lipid transport and metabolism, and deliver endogenous triglycerides to tissue cells.

3. *Intermediate low-density lipoproteins (ILDLs).* These are formed from VLDLs and continue the delivery of endogenous triglycerides to tissue cells.
4. *Low-density lipoproteins (LDLs).* These are formed from VLDLs and ILDLs and carry cholesterol to the peripheral tissue cells.
5. *High-density lipoproteins (HDLs).* These are formed in cell metabolism and carry cholesterol from the cells to the liver for breakdown and elimination from the body.

There continues to be intensive research regarding the influence of particular fatty acids on the various classes of lipoproteins.

The relative amounts of the various lipoproteins in the blood are influenced by the types of fats in the diet. Both the number and position of double bonds in the fatty acid carbon chain influence the positive or negative effects of fatty acids on blood lipid levels. (For a discussion of these differences, see the *To Probe Further* box.)

Digestion-Absorption-Metabolism Summary

DIGESTION

The basic lipid fuels—the various animal and plant lipids (triglycerides) that naturally occur in food—are taken into the body with food. Then the task is to change these basic fuel lipids into a refined fuel form that the cells can burn for energy. This key refined fuel is the individual *fatty acid*. The body accomplishes this task through the process of lipid digestion.

Mouth

No major chemical lipid breakdown takes place in the mouth. In this first section of the gastrointestinal tract, the main action is mechanical as lipids are broken up into smaller particles through chewing and are moistened for passage into the stomach with the general food mass.

Stomach

Little, if any, chemical lipid digestion takes place in the stomach. General peristalsis continues the mechanical mixing of lipids with the stomach contents. No significant enzymes specific for lipids are present in the gastric secretions except for gastric lipase (tributyrinase), which acts on emulsified butterfat. As the main gastric enzymes act on other specific nutrients in the food mix, lipids are separated from the general food mix and made readily accessible to their own specific enzymes that bring about chemical breakdown in the small intestine.

Small Intestine

Not until lipids reach the small intestine do the chemical changes necessary for lipid digestion occur. Digestive agents for lipid breakdown come from three major sources: the biliary tract—consisting of the liver and gallbladder—which contributes a preparation agent, and the pancreas and the small intestine, which both release specific enzymes for lipid digestion.

1. *Bile from the liver and gallbladder.* The presence of lipids in the duodenum stimulates the secretion of cholecystokinin (CCK), a local hormone secreted by glands in the intestinal walls. In turn, cholecystokinin causes contraction of the gallbladder, relaxation of the sphincter muscle, and the subsequent flow of bile into the intestine via the common bile duct. The liver produces a large amount of dilute bile, then the gallbladder concentrates and stores it, ready for use with lipids as needed. The function of bile is that of an emulsifier. The process of *emulsification* is not a chemical digestive action itself, but it is an important first preparation step for the chemical digestion of lipids. This preparation process accomplishes two important tasks: (1) it breaks the lipids into small particles, or globules, which greatly enlarges the total surface area available for action of the digestive

---

apolipoprotein A separate protein compound that attaches to its specific receptor site on a particular lipoprotein and activates certain functions, such as synthesis of a related enzyme. An example is apolipoprotein C II, an apolipoprotein of chylomicrons and very low-density lipoprotein that functions to activate the enzyme lipoprotein lipase.

bile A fluid secreted by the liver and transported to the gallbladder for concentration and storage. It is released into the duodenum on entry of fat to facilitate enzymatic fat digestion by acting as an emulsifying agent.

cholecystokinin (CCK) A peptide hormone secreted by the duodenal mucosa in the presence of fat. The cholecystokinin causes the gallbladder to contract and propel bile into the duodenum, where it is needed to emulsify the fat. The fat is thus prepared for digestion and absorption.

emulsifier An agent that breaks down large fat globules to smaller, uniformly distributed particles. This action is accomplished in the intestine chiefly by the bile acids, which lower surface tension of the fat particles. Emulsification greatly increases the surface area of fat, facilitating contact with fat-digesting enzymes.

lipase Group of fat enzymes that cut the ester linkages between the fatty acids and glycerol of triglycerides (fats).

lipoprotein Noncovalent complexes of fat with protein. The lipoproteins function as major carriers of lipids in the plasma because most of the plasma fat is associated with them. Such a combination makes possible the transport of fatty substances in a water medium such as plasma.

phospholipid Any of a class of fat-related substances that contain phosphorus, fatty acids, and a nitrogenous base. The phospholipids are essential elements in every cell.

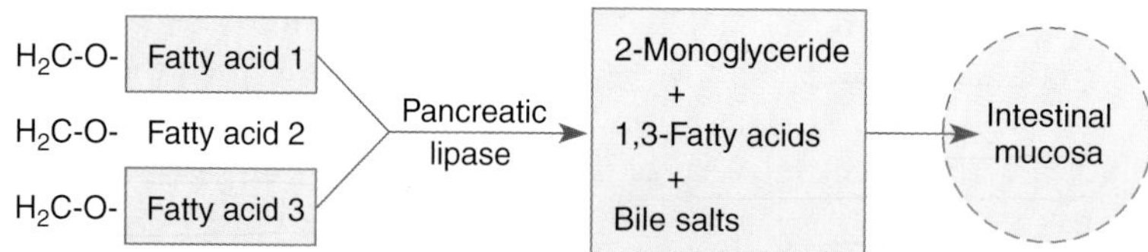

FIGURE 4-4 Micellar complex of fats with bile salts for transport of fats into intestinal mucosa.

TABLE 4-1 Summary of Fat Digestion

Organ	Enzyme	Activity
Mouth	None	Mechanical, mastication
Stomach	No major enzyme	Mechanical separation of fats as protein and starch are digested out
	Small amount of gastric lipase tributyrinase	Tributyrin (butterfat) to fatty acids and glycerol
Small intestine	Gallbladder bile salts (emulsifier)	Emulsifies fats
	Pancreatic lipase (steapsin)	Triglycerides to diglycerides and monoglycerides in turn, then fatty acids and glycerol

enzymes, and (2) it lowers the surface tension of the finely dispersed and suspended lipid globules, which allows the enzymes to penetrate more easily. This process is similar to the wetting action of detergents. The bile also provides an alkaline medium for the action of the lipid lipase enzyme. When bile secretion is limited, as in gallbladder disease, fat cannot be digested and absorbed efficiently. In that situation as much as 40% of the fat in food is lost in the feces.[12]

2. *Enzymes from the pancreas.* Pancreatic juice contains an enzyme for lipids and one for cholesterol. First, *pancreatic lipase,* a powerful lipid enzyme, breaks off one fatty acid at a time from the glycerol base of lipids. The initial action on a triglyceride yields one fatty acid plus a diglyceride, and continuing action produces in turn another fatty acid plus a monoglyceride. Each successive step in this breakdown occurs with increasing difficulty. In fact, separation of the final fatty acid from the remaining monoglyceride is such a slow process that less than one third of the total fat present actually breaks down completely. The final products of lipid digestion to be absorbed are fatty acids, diglycerides, monoglycerides, and glycerol. Some remaining lipids may pass into the large intestine for fecal elimination. Another enzyme secreted by the pancreas is *cholesterol esterase.* Cholesterol esterase acts on free cholesterol to form cholesterol esters by combining free cholesterol and fatty acids in preparation for absorption.
3. *Enzyme from the small intestine.* The small intestine secretes an enzyme in the intestinal juice called lecithinase. As its name indicates, it acts on lecithin, a *phospholipid,* to break it down into its components for absorption.

A summary of lipid digestion in the successive parts of the gastrointestinal tract is given in Table 4-1.

ABSORPTION

The task of lipid absorption is not easy. The problem is that lipids are not soluble in water and blood is basically water. Hence lipids always require some type of solvent carrier. To accomplish this task of transporting lipids from the small intestine into the bloodstream, the body has three basic stages of operation.

Stage I: Initial Lipid Absorption

In the small intestine, bile combines with products of lipid digestion to form a micellar bile-lipid complex. This unique carrier system, shown in Figure 4-4, moves the products of lipid digestion along the initial passage into the intestinal wall.

Stage II: Absorption Within the Intestinal Wall

Once inside the wall of the small intestine, the bile separates from the lipid complex, is absorbed, and returns to the liver via the *enterohepatic circulation* to accomplish its task over and over again. Two important actions on the lipid digestion products occur inside the intestinal wall: (1) *enteric lipase action:* an enteric lipase within the cells of the intestinal wall completes the digestion of the remaining diglycerides and monoglycerides releasing fatty acids and glycerol, and (2) *triglyceride synthesis:* with the resulting fatty acids and glycerol, new human triglyc-

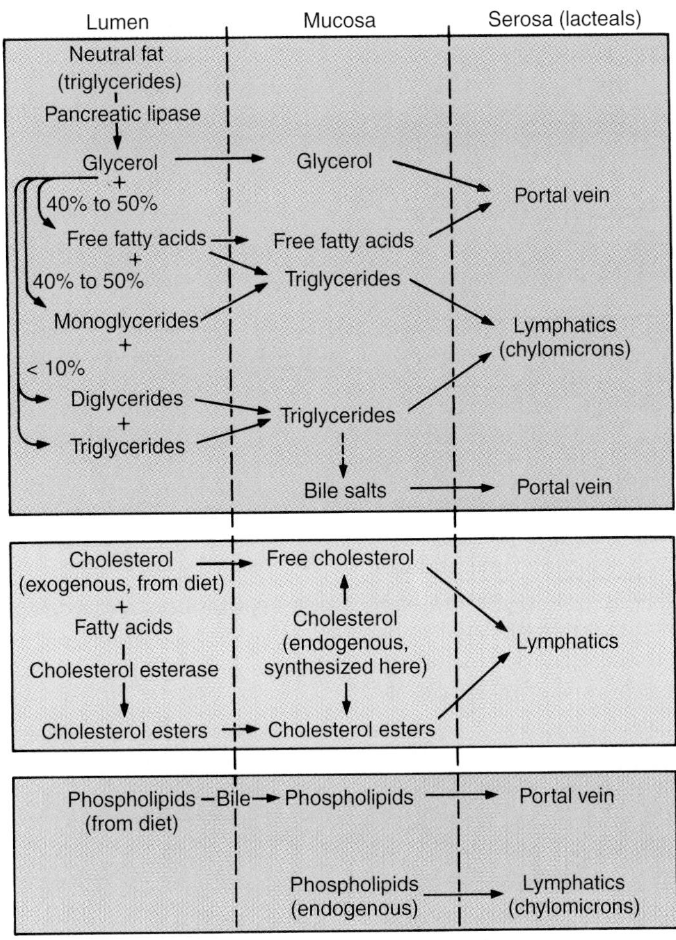

FIGURE 4-5 Absorption of fat, cholesterol, and phospholipids.

erides are formed as body lipids, ready now for final absorption and circulation.

Stage III: Final Lipid Absorption and Transport

These newly formed human lipids—triglycerides—along with other lipid materials present are combined with a small amount of protein covering to form lipoproteins called chylomicrons. These packages of lipids, in a milklike liquid called *chyle,* cross the cell membrane into the lymphatic system and then into the portal blood. Here a final lipid-clearing enzyme, *lipoprotein lipase,* helps clear the large meal load of dietary lipids from circulation. In the liver the lipids are converted to other lipoproteins for transport to the body cells for energy and other structural functions.

Because of the association of dietary fat and saturated fatty acids with cardiovascular disease, attention has been directed toward means of preventing the absorption of dietary fat. Increasing intakes of soluble fiber (see Chapter 3) and plant sterols (see *Practical Application* box) have been promoted as dietary means of lowering fat absorption. A drug that inhibits the activity of pancreatic lipase and thereby prevents fat digestion, has also been used successfully to increase loss of dietary fat through the feces.[26]

Figure 4-5 illustrates the general process of lipid absorption through its three stages.

METABOLISM

In the body cells, fatty acids are utilized as concentrated fuel to produce energy. These lipid units have about twice the energy value of glucose products. As seen in the broad picture of metabolism discussed in Chapter 2, cell metabolism of lipids is closely interrelated with that of the other nutrients.

---

chylomicrons Initial lipoproteins formed in the intestinal wall after a meal for absorption of the food fats into circulation.

micellar bile-lipid complex A combination of bile and fat in which the bile emulsifies fat into very minute globules or particles that can be absorbed easily into the small intestine wall in preparation for the final stage of absorption into circulation to the cells.

TO SUM UP

Lipids make up an essential nutrient class that not only supplies the highest density of energy among the energy nutrients, but also insulates the body against low temperatures and protects vital organs from damage. Lipids aid in the transmission of nerve impulses, production of metabolic precursors for important body molecules, formation of cell membranes and other structures, and transport of other molecules such as fat-soluble vitamins.

Lipids are composed of glycerol and attached fatty acids of varying lengths and degrees of saturation. Essential fatty acids are long-chain polyunsaturated fatty acids that cannot be manufactured by the body. The essential fatty acids are linoleic acid and linolenic acid. Their functions include maintaining skin integrity, lowering serum cholesterol levels, prolonging blood clotting time, and developing a group of special substances called *ecosanoids*—including *prostaglandins.* Ecosanoids and their related compounds are involved in many tissue activities including maintenance of the smooth muscle tone of blood vessels and controlling platelet aggregation.

Both the type and amount of dietary lipids can affect health. Large amounts of saturated lipids and cholesterol increase the risk for cardiovascular disease and other general health problems. Too small an amount of lipids can result in a deficiency of the essential fatty acid, linoleic acid, and inadequate absorption of the fat soluble vitamins. Americans over the age of 20 get 32% to 34% of their total kcalories from lipids depending on their sex and race. The *Dietary Guidelines for Americans* recommend a limit of 30%. When lipids provide 10% or less of total kcalories, supplies of linoleic acid and absorption of the fat soluble vitamins may not be adequate to meet body needs.

■ Questions for Review

1. What is a lipid? Name several members of this nutrient class that are normally found in the diet of humans.
2. Compare saturated, monounsaturated, and polyunsaturated fatty acids in terms of their (a) chemical composition, (b) effects on health, and (c) usual food sources.
3. Name several molecules important to human nutrition that are derived from the eicosanoids. What is the role of each in human health?
4. Name the essential fatty acids. Why are they called essential? What happens when the essential fatty acids are in short supply? What are the suggested AIs?
5. What are potential problems associated with eating large amounts of fat-replaced foods? You are counseling a patient who has been told that he should lose 10 to 15 pounds. He tells you that it will not be difficult because all of his favorite snack foods are available in reduced-fat forms. What would you tell him?
6. Two persons with strong family histories of cardiovascular disease are concerned about avoiding heart problems. Both reduce their cholesterol intake and avoid butter. The first person replaces butter with stick margarine made from corn oil, the second with a soft corn oil margarine. Which person has made the better choice? Identify and describe two characteristics of a dietary lipid that may influence cardiovascular disease.
7. A woman runner concerned about her health dropped her total lipid intake to an amount supplying less than 10% of her total energy intake. What health problems might she encounter?

■ References

1. Freeland-Graves J, Nitzke S: Position of the American Dietetic Association: total diet approach to communicating food and nutrition information, *J Am Diet Assoc* 102(1): 100, 2002.
2. Drewnowski A: Energy density, palatability, and satiety: implications for weight control, *Nutr Rev* 56(12):347, 1998.
3. 1998 International Conference on the Mediterranean Diet: Dietary fat: how much? what type? reaching for consensus, *Nutr Today* 33(4):173, 1998.
4. Hu FB, Manson JAE, Willett WC: Types of dietary fat and risk of coronary heart disease: a critical review, *J Am Coll Nutr* 20(1):5, 2001.
5. Krauss RM et al: Revision 2000: a statement for healthcare professionals from the Nutrition Committee of the American Heart Association, *J Nutr* 131:132, 2001.
6. Iso H et al: Intake of fish and omega-3 fatty acids and risk of stroke in women, *JAMA* 285:304, 2001.
7. Van Horn L, Ernst N: A summary of the science supporting the new National Cholesterol Education Program dietary recommendations: what dietitians should know, *J Am Diet Assoc* 101(10):1148, 2001.
8. Elias SL, Innis SM: Bakery foods are the major dietary source of trans-fatty acids among pregnant women with diets providing 30% energy from fat, *J Am Diet Assoc* 102(1): 46, 2002.
9. Jones PJH, Papamandjaris AA: Lipids: cellular metabolism. In Bowman BA, Russell RM eds: *Present knowledge in nutrition,* ed 8, Washington, DC, 2001, International Life Sciences Institute.
10. Panel on Macronutrients, Panel on the Definition of Dietary Fiber, Subcommittee on Upper Reference Levels of Nutrients, Subcommittee on Interpretation and Uses of Dietary Reference Intakes, and the Standing Committee on the Scientific Evaluation of Dietary Reference Intakes: *Dietary reference intakes for energy, carbohydrate, fiber, fat, fatty acids, cholesterol, protein, and amino acids, parts 1 and 2,* Washington, DC, 2002, National Academy Press.
11. Sellin JH: Intestinal electrolyte absorption and secretion. In Feldman M, Scharschmidt BF, Sleisenger MH, eds: *Gastrointestinal and liver disease,* ed 6, vol 2, Philadelphia, 1998, WB Saunders.

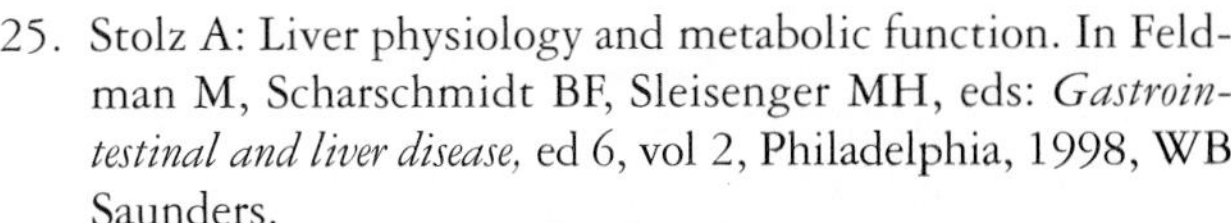

12. Guyton AC, Hall JE: *Textbook of medical physiology,* ed 10, Philadelphia, 2000, WB Saunders.
13. Kris-Etherton PM et al: Polyunsaturated fatty acids in the food chain in the United States, *Am J Clin Nutr* 71 (suppl):179S, 2000.
14. Lichtenstein AH et al. Effects of different forms of dietary hydrogenated fats on serum lipoprotein cholesterol levels, *N Engl J Med* 340:1933, 1999.
15. Ascherio A et al: Trans fatty acids and coronary heart disease, *N Engl J Med* 340:1994, 1999.
16. Dausch J: Trans-fatty acids: a regulatory update, *J Am Diet Assoc* 102(1):18, 2002.
17. U.S. Department of Agriculture: Continuing Survey of Food Intake by Individuals, 1994-1996; may be accessed at *http://www.barc.usda.gov/bhnrc/foodsurvey/Products9496.html#anchor164107.*
18. Peterson S et al: Impact of adopting lower-fat food choices on energy and nutrient intakes of American adults, *J Am Diet Assoc* 99:177, 1999.
19. Kennedy E, Bowman S: Assessment of the effect of fat-modified foods on diet quality in adults, 19 to 50 years, using data from the Continuing Survey of Food Intake by Individuals, *J Am Diet Assoc* 101(4):455, 2001.
20. Campbell AD, Bell ln: Acceptability of low-fat, sugar-free cakes: effect of providing compositional information during taste-testing, *J Am Diet Assoc* 101(3):354, 2001.
21. Ballesteros MN et al: Dietary fiber and lifestyle influence serum lipids in free living adult men, *J Am Coll Nutr* 20(6):649, 2001.
22. Maki KC et al: Lipid responses to plant-sterol-enriched reduced-fat spreads incorporated into a National Cholesterol Education Program Step I diet, *Am J Clin Nutr* 74:33, 2001.
23. Davidson MH et al: Safety and tolerability of esterified phytosterols administered in reduced-fat spread and salad dressing to healthy adult men and women, *J Am Coll Nutr* 20(4):307, 2001.
24. Jula A et al: Effects of diet and simvastatin on serum lipids, insulin, and antioxidants in hypercholesterolemic men, *JAMA* 287:598, 2002.
25. Stolz A: Liver physiology and metabolic function. In Feldman M, Scharschmidt BF, Sleisenger MH, eds: *Gastrointestinal and liver disease,* ed 6, vol 2, Philadelphia, 1998, WB Saunders.
26. Lichtenstein A, Jones PJH: Lipids: absorption and transport. In Bowman BA, Russell RM eds: *Present knowledge in nutrition,* ed 8, Washington, DC, 2001, International Life Sciences Institute.

■ Further Reading

Abusabha R, Hsieh K-H, Achterberg C: Dietary fat reduction strategies used by a group of adults aged 50 years and older, *J Am Diet Assoc* 101(9):1024, 2001.

Anttolainen M et al: Characteristics of users and nonusers of plant stanol ester margarine in Finland: an approach to study functional foods, *J Am Diet Assoc* 101(11):1365, 2001.

Callaway CW: The role of fat-modified foods in the American diet, *Nutr Today* 33:(4):156, 1998.

Neuhouser M, Kristal AR, Patterson RE: Use of food nutrition labels is associated with lower fat intake, *J Am Diet Assoc* 99:45, 1999.

Neumark-Sztainer D et al: Early adopters of Olestra-containing foods: who are they? *J Am Diet Assoc* 100(2):198, 2000.

These articles address several aspects of the controversy relating to fat intake and fat-reduced foods, including an appropriate role for fat-reduced foods in the total diet and successful nutrition education strategies for helping people reduce their fat intake.

Dixon LB, Ernst ND: Choose a diet that is low in saturated fat and cholesterol and moderate in total fat: subtle changes to a familiar message, *J Nutr* 131:510, 2001.

This article describes the major sources of fat in the diets of different age groups in the United States. If we understand what foods persons are now eating, we can help them make better choices that will be consistent with their lifestyle and food preferences.

Issues & ANSWERS

Fat Replacers: Do They Help Prevent Obesity?

Two major goals of the *Healthy People 2000 Disease Prevention and Health Promotion Objectives* were to reduce dietary fat intakes and the prevalence of obesity in the U.S. population. Although dietary fat intake as a percentage of total kcalories declined from 36% to 34% in the 1990s, this change did not lower the prevalence of obesity. In fact, obesity increased by 8% over this same period and continues to rise in persons of all ages. In a survey conducted in 1996, 88% of adults reported using low-fat, reduced-fat, or fat-free foods and beverages. Their reason for selecting these foods was to improve their health and to reduce their intakes of total fat and kcalories. What has gone wrong?

Various types of ingredients have been developed that can replace fats in food. These ingredients can be used to replace all of the fat or part of the fat in a food product, and they provide the sensory and mouth feel associated with natural fats but fewer of the kcalories. Although some fat replacers add as much as 5 kcalories/g to the food product (still less than the 9 kcalories/g supplied by natural fats), others are not metabolized and carry no energy value.

Fat replacers are sometimes classified by their primary component—carbohydrate, protein, or fat. The majority of fat replacers are carbohydrates, plant polysaccharides, celluloses, or gums. As food ingredients they act as thickeners and emulsifiers, presenting the mouth feel associated with fat. Fat replacers made from protein form gels that give structure to products and contribute amino acids to the diet. The newest fat replacers are composed of fatty acids mixed with carbohydrate compounds.

Major questions have surrounded the increasing use of fat replacers. Consumer groups and nutritionists have asked about their long-term safety and their influence on overall nutritional well-being. All fat replacers must be approved by the Food and Drug Administration (FDA), which evaluates all food additives in terms of their known safety and intended use. The FDA also requires that consumers be informed of possible adverse reactions related to such ingredients. Fat replacers that are not digested or absorbed have been reported to cause gastrointestinal distress, including diarrhea, and this possible side effect must be indicated on the food label. Another concern about nonabsorbed fat replacers is their potential to rob the body of fat-soluble vitamins. Fat-soluble vitamins, dissolved in these lipids, are carried into the colon and lost in the feces. To address this problem snack foods containing the fat replacer Olestra, a sucrose polyester that is not absorbed, are fortified with fat-soluble vitamins to counter such dietary losses.

Noting that the growing use of reduced-fat snack foods has paralleled the growing prevalence of obesity in the U.S. population, one clinician has suggested that the low-fat message promoted by health professionals has been distorted. Instead of choosing healthier lower-fat foods such as fruits, vegetables, whole grains, or low-fat dairy products, consumers are eating more of the reduced-fat snack products now available in the grocery store. Unfortunately, many of these low-fat products contain the same number of kcalories or even more kcalories than their higher-fat counterparts. Consequently, those individuals who feel empowered to eat greater amounts of these foods because they are lower in fat are consuming even more kcalories than before, even though their fat intake has been reduced. This erroneous interpretation of the benefits of reduced-fat foods has likely contributed to the growing obesity problem despite the small downward shift in fat intake.

As health professionals we need to evaluate carefully the advice that we give to others. Persons who replace higher fat foods with fat-replaced foods but do not increase their number of portions will benefit by lowering their intake of total fat and, in some cases, saturated fat. Among adults who followed such a pattern, total serum cholesterol dropped by 10% over the study period of 1 year. On the other hand, persons who previously avoided high-fat snacks will see no benefit from starting to consume the lower-fat varieties. Think about substituting snacks low to moderate in fat such as fruits, vegetables, dairy foods, or whole grain crackers in place of fat-containing or fat-replaced snacks that are still high in kcalories.

REFERENCES

Blackburn G: Reduced-fat fallacy. The physician's perspective, *Health News* 6(11):4, 2000.

Mattess RD: Position of the American Dietetic Association: fat replacers, *J Am Diet Assoc* 98:463, 1998.

Paterson RE et al: Changes in diet, weight, and serum lipid levels associated with Olestra consumption, *Arch Intern Med* 160(17):2600, 2000.

Willett W: Is dietary fat a major determinant of body fat? *Am J Clin Nutr* 67(suppl):556S, 1998.

Chapter

5

Proteins

Eleanor D. Schlenker

Chapter Outline

In this chapter, which completes our introductory sequence on the macronutrients, we look at protein. It is quite different from its partners, carbohydrate and fat. Although protein also yields energy as needed, its main job is building and rebuilding body tissue. It is the body's major provider of nitrogen, the essential element for all living beings.

Here, then, we focus primarily on the body's builder. We see how protein accomplishes this unique task through its marvelous building units, the amino acids.

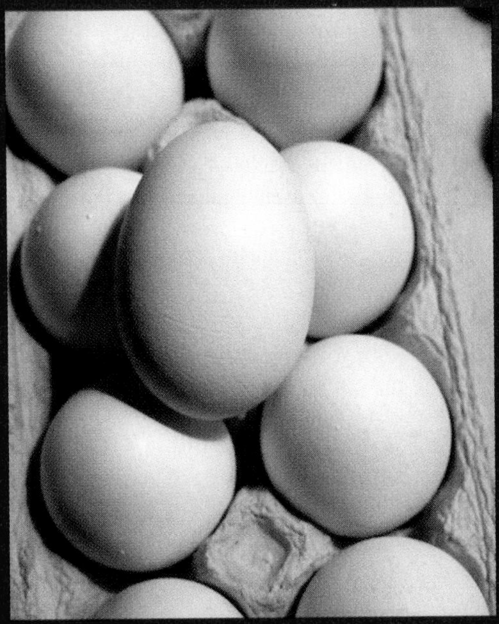

PHYSICAL AND CHEMICAL NATURE OF PROTEINS

GENERAL DEFINITION

When Dutch chemist Johann Mulder (1802-1880) first classified protein in 1838 as a prime substance of all life forms, he could scarcely guess how far-reaching his work would become. Proteins are associated with all forms of life, and much of the effort to determine how life began has centered on how proteins were first produced.[1]

In many ways, proteins act to shape our lives. They act as structural units to build our bodies. As enzymes, they change our food into nutrients our cells can use. As antibodies, they shield us from disease. As peptide hormones, they send messages that coordinate continuous body activity. Proteins also do much more: they guide our growth during childhood and then maintain our bodies throughout adulthood. They ensure our nutritional well-being. They make us the unique individuals that we are.

CHEMICAL NATURE

The proteins we eat do none of this wonderful work as proteins. Their specific structural chemical units—the *amino acids* released at initial digestion—provide the living, working currency of our body cells. These unique units are composed of the basic elements carbon, hydrogen, oxygen, and the special element of all living matter—nitrogen. It is with these basic units of the substance of life that we begin this chapter.

The Nature of Amino Acids

The story of protein must begin with its unique building materials, the amino acids. A major life-sustaining task of the human body is the constant building and rebuilding of all its individual tissues. The name of these building units, the "amino acids," indicates that they have a dual nature. The word "amino" refers to "base (alkaline) substance," so we at once confront a paradox. How can a chemical material be both a base and an acid at the same time, and why is this important here? Consider the significance of this fact as you first examine the structure of amino acids.

GENERAL PATTERN AND SPECIFIC STRUCTURE

A common baseline pattern holds for all amino acids. First, look carefully at the characteristic common pattern built around a central *alpha*-carbon and the significant parts of the amino acid structure.

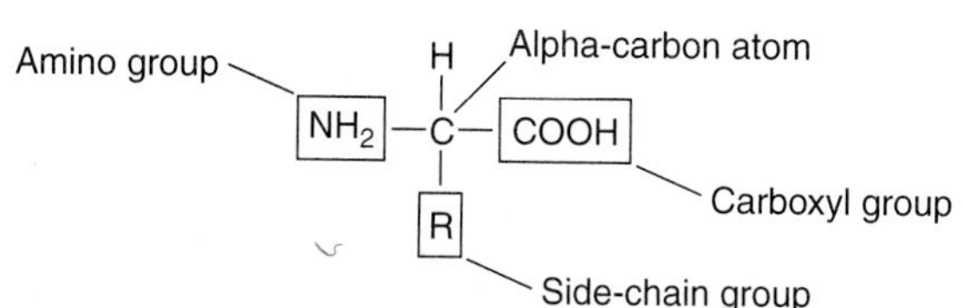

1. *Amino (base, NH_2) group.* This part of the molecule carries the essential nitrogen and, in its ionic form, the positive charge.
2. *Carboxyl (acid, COOH) group.* This part of the molecule is the characteristic acid group found in all acids and, in the amino acid ionic form, carries the negative charge.
3. *Varying attached radical.* The *R* stands for *radical,* a general term for parts of a chemical compound. In the common core pattern it stands for the varying attached side chains on amino acids, each one different. The distinctive side chain of each amino acid gives it a distinctive size, shape, and set of properties.[2] Note the structure of the two simplest amino acids, glycine and alanine, based on the core amino acid pattern.

H, NH_2—C—COOH, H

Glycine

H, NH_2—C—COOH, CH_3

Alanine

Now, compare a larger amino acid, for example, the amino acid *arginine* (see p. 85), which has an extended carbon chain and three additional nitrogen radicals.

Thus it is the unique side group radical (R) attached to the common base pattern that makes each of the amino acids that constitute protein unique. Amino acids are made of the same three elements—carbon, hydrogen, and oxygen—that make up carbohydrates and fats. But amino acids and their proteins have an additional important element—*nitrogen*—as the base (alkaline [NH_2]) portion of their structure. Twenty amino acids are used to build body proteins.[1,2] They all have the same basic core pattern, but each is unique because it has a specific and different side group attached.

ESSENTIAL AMINO ACIDS

All amino acids are necessary for building our various body tissue proteins. We know that 9 of the 20 amino acids used to build body proteins cannot be synthesized by the body or cannot be synthesized in sufficient amounts and thus must be supplied by foods. These amino acids have been referred to as the essential amino acids, and the 5 amino acids that can be synthesized by the body in adequate amounts have been referred to as nonessential amino acids. Six amino acids have been classified as conditionally essential amino acids. These molecules can be synthesized by humans, but under certain conditions, when tissues needs are escalated or the supply of precursors is inadequate, synthesis cannot keep pace with body needs. Arginine is one of the amino acids classified as conditionally indispensable. Although it can be synthesized in large amounts in the liver, in periods of high demand, such as in catch-up growth in infants or children, the amount produced by the body may not be sufficient to meet tissue needs.[2]

Recently, nutrition experts suggested that we change the current designations of essential amino acids and nonessential amino acids because the term *nonessential* implies that these amino acids are not really necessary for human health. The recently released Dietary Reference Intakes (DRIs) for protein are using the terms indispensable (essential) amino acids for those amino acids that must be supplied in the diet, *dispensable amino acids* for those that can be synthesized by the body in sufficient amounts, and *conditionally indispensable amino acids* for those that must be supplied by the diet under particular conditions.[3] We will use these new terms for the remainder of our study of proteins, although you will likely see amino acids referred to as essential or nonessential in other readings. However, the concept of *dietary* essentiality for these so-designated 9 amino acids is important to remember in assessing protein quality.

$$
\begin{array}{c}
\text{H} \\
| \\
\boxed{\text{NH}_2}-\text{C}-\boxed{\text{COOH}} \\
| \\
\text{CH}_2 \\
| \\
\text{CH}_2 \\
| \\
\text{CH}_2 \\
| \\
\text{NH} \\
| \\
\text{C}=\text{NH} \\
| \\
\text{NH}_2
\end{array}
$$

Arginine

Arginine modulates the bioavailability of nitrous oxide (NO), a powerful vasodilator in the blood vessels that inhibits atherogenesis (see Chapter 19). Increasingly, the biochemical mystique and complexity of the NO molecule extend to the amino acid arginine from which it is derived.[4] The 9 indispensable amino acids are listed in Box 5-1 along with the 5 dispensable amino acids and the 6 conditionally indispensable amino acids.[3] The remaining amino acids—13 of them, which we can synthesize in our own bodies in adequate amounts—are then labeled *"nonessential" amino acids.* Actually this is a poor choice of label in the sense that all 22 of the amino acids are necessary for building the various body tissue proteins. For this reason some nutritionists have suggested we change these designations to "indispensable" for the essential amino acids and "dispensable" for the nonessential amino acids. However, the concept of *dietary* essentiality for these so-designated 9 amino acids is important to remember in assessing protein quality.

BOX 5-1 Amino Acids Required in Human Nutrition, Grouped According to Nutritional Dietary Essentiality

Indispensable Amino Acids	Conditionally Indispensable Amino Acids	Dispensable Amino Acids
Histidine	Arginine	Alanine
Isoleucine	Cysteine	Asparagine
Leucine	Glutamine	Aspartic acid
Lysine	Glycine	Glutamic acid
Methionine	Proline	Serine
Phenylalanine	Tyrosine	
Threonine		
Tryptophan		
Valine		

From Panel on Macronutrients, Panel on the Definition of Dietary Fiber, Subcommittee on Upper Reference Levels of Nutrients, Subcommittee on Interpretation and Uses of Dietary Reference Intakes, and the Standing Committee on the Scientific Evaluation of Dietary Reference Intakes: *Dietary reference intakes for energy, carbohydrate, fiber, fat, fatty acids, cholesterol, protein, and amino acids, parts 1 and 2,* Washington, DC, 2002, National Academy Press. Source: Laidlaw SA, Kopple JD: Newer concepts of the indispensable amino acids, *Am J Clin Nutr* 46:593, 1987.

Some researchers are asking whether amino acid requirements are the same for populations around the world, or if individuals from developing countries where protein intakes tend to be lower have adapted to lower intakes and thus have lower amino acid requirements. Studies of healthy individuals from Asian nations with traditionally low protein intakes indicate that their requirements for individual amino acids do not differ from those of healthy persons accustomed to higher amino acid intakes.[5]

The dual chemical structure of amino acids, combining both acid (carboxyl [COOH]) and base (amino

---

amino acid An acid containing the essential element nitrogen (in the chemical group NH_2). Amino acids are the structural units of protein and are the basic building blocks of the body.

carboxyl (COOH) The monovalent radical, COOH, occurring in those organic acids termed carboxylic acids.

indispensable (essential) amino acid Any one of nine amino acids that the body cannot synthesize at all or in sufficient amounts to meet body needs and that therefore must be supplied by the diet and is hence a *dietary* essential. These nine specific amino acids are histidine, isoleucine, leucine, lysine, methionine, phenylalanine, threonine, tryptophan, and valine. Two amino acids—cysteine and tyrosine—are called conditionally indispensable amino acids because the body cannot synthesize sufficient amounts under certain conditions.

[NH_2]) components, gives them a unique amphoteric nature. As a result, an amino acid in solution can behave either as an acid or a base, depending on the pH of the solution. This means that amino acids have a buffer capacity, which is an important clinical characteristic.

The Building of Proteins

The building units, amino acids, are used by the body to construct specific tissue proteins. This process is made possible by the nature of amino acids, which enables them to form peptide linkages and to arrange themselves into peptide chains.

TISSUE PROTEIN STRUCTURE

Peptide Bond

The dual chemical nature of amino acids—the presence of a base (amino [NH_2]) group containing nitrogen on one end and an acid (carboxyl [COOH]) group on the other—enables them to join in the distinguishing chain structure of proteins. The end amino group of one amino acid joins the end carboxyl group of another amino acid beside it. This characteristic joining of amino acids is called a peptide bond. Specific amino acids are joined in a specific sequence to form long chains of amino acids called *polypeptides,* and specific peptides form proteins. These peptides may vary in chain length from relatively short chains of 3 to 15 amino acids, called *oligopeptides,* to medium-sized polypeptides, such as insulin, with chains of 21 to 30 amino acids.

Large Complex Proteins

Larger still are complex proteins of several hundred amino acids that require special techniques to study. Exciting new technology, such as nuclear magnetic resonance (NMR) spectroscopy and special radiographic techniques, allows scientists to view polypeptides in four dimensions of space, enabling them to examine closely much larger and more complex proteins. This new view enables researchers to learn how long protein chains fold and twist in space and how they interact with other body molecules. This knowledge helps us understand how enzymes and other regulatory proteins work, as well as aiding scientists in developing new drugs or understanding how genes can influence risk of certain diseases.

To make a compact structure, the long polypeptide chains coil or fold back on themselves in a spiral shape called a helix, or "pleated sheet," arrangement. They are held together in some instances by additional strengthening cross-links of sulfur and hydrogen bonds.

TYPES OF PROTEINS

The proteins illustrate a huge diversity of compounds produced by specific amino acid linkages. Tissue proteins perform many vital roles in body structure and metabolism, controlled by their specific construction of amino acids. Consider several examples.

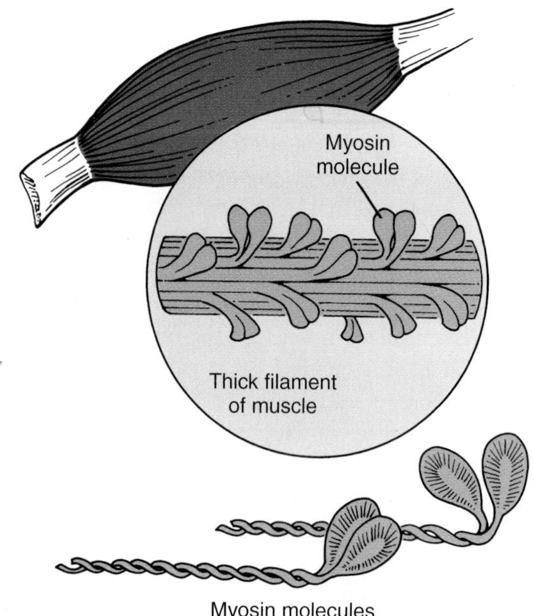

FIGURE 5-1 Myosin is a globulin in muscle that, in combination with actin, forms actomyosin, the fundamental contractile unit of muscle active with ATP.

Myosin

This fibrous type of protein found in muscle fiber, shown in Figure 5-1, is composed of 153 amino acid long chains that coil and unfold on contraction and relaxation. Shaped into long rods, these fibers end in two-headed bundles so they can change their shape and bend, making it possible to tighten and contract muscles and then relax them.

Collagen

This structural protein, shown in Figure 5-2, is made up of three separate polypeptide chains wound around each other to produce a triple helix. Thus strengthened, the collagen is shaped into long rods and bundled into stiff fibers because its job is to strengthen bone, cartilage, skin, and other body structures and to maintain their form.

Hemoglobin

This globular-type protein, shown in Figure 5-3, is made up of four globin polypeptide chains in a molecule of hemoglobin. Each chain has several hundred amino acids, conjugated with a nonprotein portion—an oxygen-carrying pigment, *heme*—which attaches to iron. The globin, in a compact globular shape, wraps around the heme and forms protective pockets to secure the iron and facilitate its exposure to oxygen as it travels in circulating red blood cells.

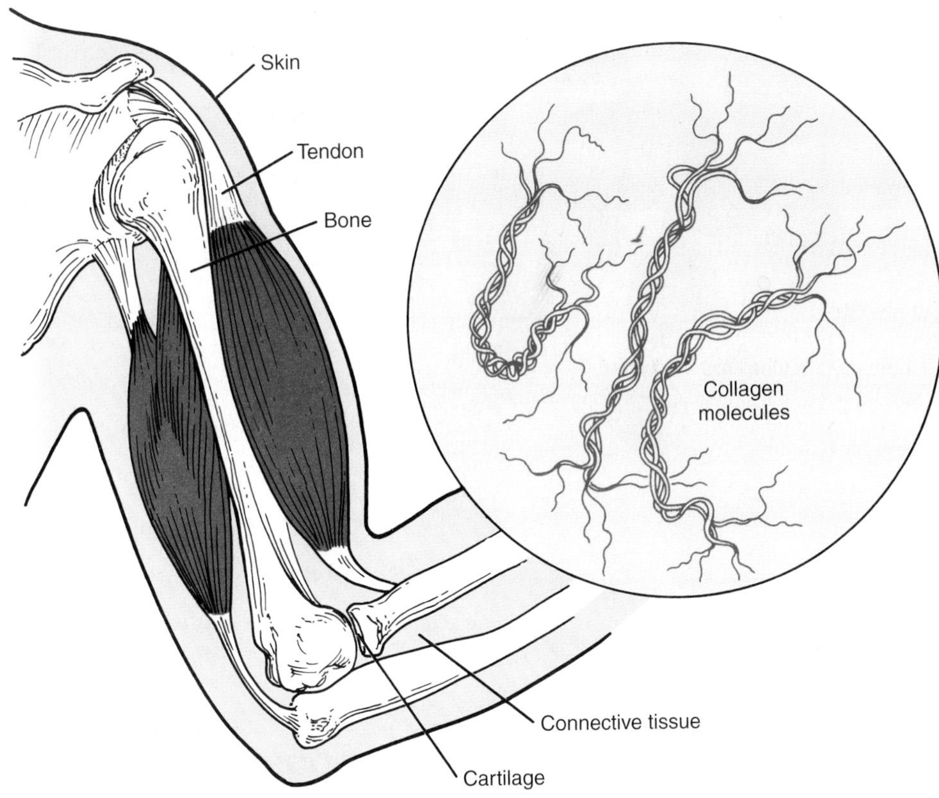

FIGURE 5-2 Tissues that contain collagen, the basic structural material forming connective tissue throughout the body.

Albumin

This major plasma protein is made up of similar compact globular shapes. It consists of a single polypeptide chain of 584 amino acids, twisted and coiled into helixes held together by 17 disulfide bridges.[6] Albumin plays an important role in fluid balance by providing colloidal pressure in the capillaries that assists in the flow of fluid and nutrients into the cells and in the return of fluid and waste out of the cells for transport to the kidney. Albumin also is easily broken down to supply amino acids for the synthesis of new proteins in times of body stress.

Other Proteins With Special Roles

Other examples of tissue proteins shaped for special structural or metabolic roles in the body include antibodies of the immune system, such as gamma globulin; the blood protein fibrinogen, important in blood clotting; some regulating hormones, such as insulin, thyroxin, and the gastrointestinal peptides; and all of the enzymes that regulate our day-to-day metabolic activities.

COMPLETE AND INCOMPLETE FOOD PROTEINS

A common way of designating the quality of protein foods is whether they are complete or incomplete in terms of the amounts of indispensable or essential amino acids they contain.

Complete Protein Foods

Foods called *complete protein foods* are those that contain all the indispensable amino acids in sufficient quantity and ratio to meet the body's needs. These proteins are of animal origin: eggs, milk, cheese, and meat, including poultry and fish. Another protein of animal origin, gelatin, does not qualify because it lacks three indispensable amino acids—tryptophan, valine, and isoleucine—and has only small amounts of leucine.

---

amphoteric Having opposite characteristics; capable of acting either as an acid or a base, combining with both acids and bases.

buffer Mixture of acidic and alkaline components that, when added to a solution, is able to protect the solution against wide variations in its pH, even when strong acids and bases are added to it. If an acid is added, the alkaline partner reacts to counteract the acidic effect. If a base is added, the acid partner reacts to counteract the alkalizing effect. A solution to which a buffer has been added is called a buffered solution.

helix A coiled structure as found in protein. Some are simple chain coils; others are made of several coils, as in a triple helix.

peptide bond The characteristic joining of amino acids to form proteins. Such a chain of amino acids is termed a peptide. Depending on its size, it may be a dipeptide fragment of protein or a large polypeptide.

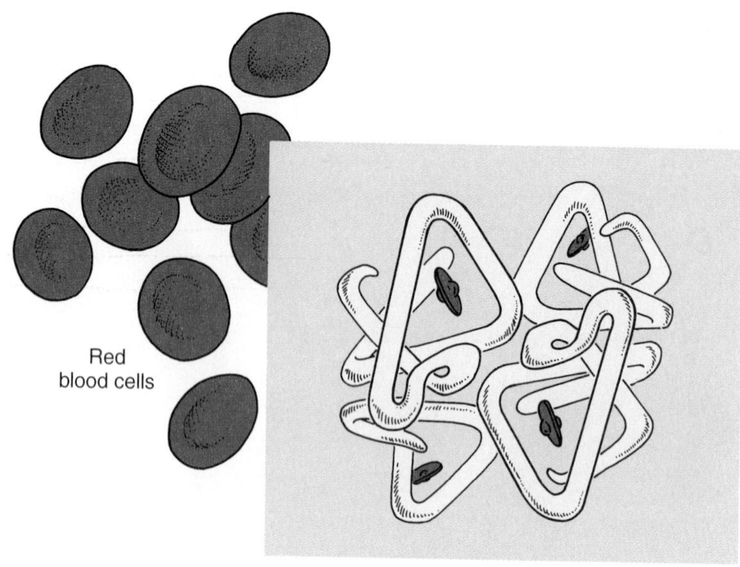

FIGURE 5-3 Hemoglobin is an oxygen-carrying protein of red blood cells.

Incomplete Protein Foods

Foods called incomplete protein foods are those deficient in one or more of the indispensable amino acids. These proteins are mostly of plant origin: grains, legumes, nuts, and seeds. In a mixed diet, however, animal and plant proteins complement one another. Even a mixture of plant proteins alone can provide adequate amounts of amino acids when our basic use of various grains is expanded to include soy protein and other dried legume storage proteins (beans and peas). Legumes and soy are good sources of quality protein, being relatively low in only the sulfur-containing amino acids, methionine and cysteine.[7]

Both the type of protein and the amount that we eat may influence our risk of chronic diseases. As we will learn a bit later in our study of nutrition, high protein intakes have been associated with loss of bone calcium, but animal rather than vegetable protein may be responsible for this effect.[8,9] Soy protein exerts a protective effect against the development of heart disease[10,11] and lowers the risk of bone loss. Thus, the value of obtaining our protein from a *variety* of dietary sources is evident.

In the final analysis, the most significant measure of the protein quality of the diet is the variety of foods in the total food mix. When we eat a variety of protein foods, the amino acid patterns of the various food components, both complete and incomplete food proteins, complement one another and the total protein intake is sufficient to meet the body's total need.[12] A sound diet is the best way to obtain needed protein, eliminating any need for protein or amino acid supplements (see *Practical Application* box).

Functions of Protein

GROWTH, TISSUE-BUILDING, AND MAINTENANCE

The primary function of dietary protein is to supply building material for growth and maintenance of body tissue. It does this by furnishing amino acids in the appropriate amounts and types for efficient synthesis of specific cellular tissue proteins. Nitrogen, in its key position in amino acids and hence in building body tissues, is the vital element in our body's structure. Without it, we—and life as we know it on our planet—would not exist. Unlike carbohydrates and fats, which contain no nitrogen, protein is about 16% nitrogen. Protein also supplies amino acids for making other essential nitrogen-containing substances such as enzymes and hormones.

SPECIFIC PHYSIOLOGIC ROLES

All amino acids supplied by dietary protein participate in growth and tissue maintenance. But some also perform other important physiologic and metabolic roles. For example, *methionine* is an agent in the formation of choline, which is a precursor of acetylcholine, one of the major neurotransmitters in the brain. In addition, methionine is the precursor of the conditionally indispensable amino acid *cysteine,* along with the less well known amino acids carnitine and taurine, which are now recognized to have widespread metabolic functions. *Carnitine* plays an important role in transporting long-chain fatty acids into the mitochondria for energy production. *Taurine* is a constituent in bile salts and may also control fluid pressure in the cells,

PRACTICAL APPLICATION

Increase Your Variety: Exploring Complementary Proteins

Over the centuries populations have been surviving and thriving on diets based on complementary proteins. In many parts of the world animal protein is generally not as plentiful as it is in the United States and some European nations. Traditional diets the world over have been plant based, emphasizing cereals, pulses, legumes, vegetables, and fruit. In many countries the main dish served at mealtime is a stew that contains a variety of plant foods. Some recipes are based on plant foods with a small amount of added animal protein in the form of meat, fish, poultry, eggs, or cheese. In Chapter 1 we discussed the need to become familiar with the food patterns of different cultural and ethnic groups. Exploring complementary protein dishes is a perfect way to do that. Visit your local library and review some ethnic cookbooks. Or visit a website that provides ethnic recipes. Better yet, seek out a member of a cultural or ethnic group different from your own and learn more about their food and the customs that it represents. Try a new recipe that may be unfamiliar to you and calculate the protein content coming from both animal and vegetable sources.

Some traditional food patterns based on plant proteins that can help you get started are described here.

Mexican: The traditional Mexican diet is founded on beans, corn, and rice. Corn tortillas combined with beans and vegetables provide a complete protein, as do beans and rice. The addition of cheese to stews or tortillas adds some complete animal protein to complement the incomplete proteins of the grain foods. Eggs accompanied by beans are a favorite Mexican breakfast.

East Indian: The Hindu religion forbids the slaying of animals for meat; thus many East Indians are vegetarians, although they may eat eggs, yogurt, and cheese. Traditional East Indian meals are based on stews with a variety of accompaniments. A stew containing rice, vegetables, and beans might be served with yogurt, cheese, and peanuts. Bread may contain wheat flour as well as flour made from ground peas or beans, which add good-quality protein.

Hmong (Vietnamese): The traditional pattern of this family emphasizes rice and vegetables; in fact, rice is served at every meal including breakfast. Rice mixed with green vegetables and small amounts of added fish and peanuts are typical of this region of the world. Rice rather than bread is the basic grain in this dietary pattern.

African-American Soul Food: *Soul food* is the term used to refer to the food patterns that developed among the African slaves brought to America. Food played an important role in preserving their traditions and nourishing their spirits. Beans and rice provided some protein in that diet along with the corn used to make a variety of breads, including corn bread or hoe cakes. Fish, pork, and chicken were popular sources of animal protein when available and were used to flavor both stews and cooked vegetables.

Traditional American: Don't forget some of the typical American dishes that represent the use of complementary proteins. A peanut butter sandwich, a ready-to-eat cereal and milk, macaroni and cheese, and pinto beans and cornbread all represent the concept of complementary proteins.

References

American Dietetic Association: *Hmong American food practices, customs, and holidays,* Chicago, 1999, American Dietetic Association.

American Dietetic Association: *Indian and Pakistani food practices, customs, and holidays,* Chicago, 1996, American Dietetic Association.

American Dietetic Association: *Mexican American food practices, customs, and holidays,* Chicago, 1998, American Dietetic Association.

American Dietetic Association: *Soul and traditional southern food practices, customs, and holidays,* Chicago, 1995, American Dietetic Association.

Kittler P, Sucher K: *Food and culture in America,* ed 2, New York, 2000, Van Nostrand Reinhold.

including pressure in the cells of the eye.[13] *Tryptophan* is the precursor of the B vitamin niacin and of the neurotransmitter serotonin. *Tyrosine* is needed for the synthesis of dopamine and norepinephrine, other neurotransmitters vital to the function of the central nervous system. When intakes of these amino acids are inadequate, function of the nervous system is impaired.[14] *Phenylalanine* is the precursor of the conditionally indispensable amino acid tyrosine, leading to formation of the hormones thyroxine and epinephrine. In addition, protein antibodies are essential components of the body's immune system, and plasma proteins guard water balance.

carnitine A naturally occurring amino acid ($C_{17}H_{15}NO_3$) formed from methionine and lysine, required for transport of long-chain fatty acids across the mitochondrial membrane, where they are oxidized as fuel substrate for metabolic energy.

incomplete protein food A protein food having a ratio of amino acids different from that of the average body protein and therefore less valuable for nutrition than a complete protein food.

taurine A sulfur-containing amino acid, $NH_2(CH_2)_2 \cdot SO_2OH$, formed from the indispensable amino acid methionine. It is found in various body tissues, such as lungs and muscles, and in bile and breast milk.

Glutamine, the most abundant free amino acid in the human body, is receiving increased attention as a potential addition to enteral or parenteral nutrition formulas for critically ill patients.[15] Glutamine, derived from the dispensable amino acid *glutamic acid,* has two amino (NH_2) groups and can serve two roles. It can be a donor of an amino group for the synthesis of other amino acids or, when its amino groups are removed, it can be an important energy source for liver cells, intestinal mucosal cells, and immune cells. In patients with extensive trauma or burns, major surgery, sepsis, or acquired immunodeficiency syndrome, all conditions in which skeletal muscle is rapidly broken down to meet energy and amino acid needs, glutamine may be a means of reducing nitrogen loss.[16]

In the extreme metabolic stress of malnutrition in childhood, evident in the conditions of kwashiorkor and marasmus, decreased protein synthesis and rapid tissue breakdown give stark evidence to these constant protein needs for normal growth, development, and resistance to disease.[17,18] Providing sufficient amounts of high-quality protein and amino acids is also important in helping low birth weight infants achieve normal growth.[19]

AVAILABLE ENERGY

Protein also contributes to the body's overall energy metabolism. This occurs as needed in the fasting state or during extended physical effort such as marathon running, but not in the fed state.[20] After the removal of the nitrogen-containing portion of the constituent amino acid, the amino acid residue—a carbon skeleton now called a *keto*-acid—may be converted to either glucose or fat. On the average, 58% of the total dietary protein can become available if needed to be burned for energy. Thus sufficient amounts of nonprotein kilocalories (kcalories) from carbohydrates are always needed to spare protein for its primary building purpose and to prevent unnecessary protein breakdown to provide energy.

Digestion-Absorption-Metabolism Summary

After the source of basic body building materials—the food protein—is secured, it must be changed into the needed ready-to-use building units—the amino acids. This work is accomplished throughout the successive parts of the gastrointestinal tract by the mechanical and chemical processes of digestion.

MOUTH

In the mouth, the only digestive action on protein foods is the mechanical breaking up of the foods by chewing. Here the food particles are mixed with saliva and passed on as a semisolid mass into the stomach.

STOMACH

Because proteins are such large complex structures, a series of reactions is necessary to finally break them down to release the amino acids. These chemical changes, through a system of enzymes, begin in the stomach. In fact, the stomach's chief digestive function in relation to all foods is the initial partial enzymatic breakdown of protein. Three agents in the gastric secretions help with this task: pepsin, hydrochloric acid, and rennin.

1. *Pepsin.* The main gastric enzyme, specific for proteins, is pepsin. It is first produced as the inactive proenzyme, *pepsinogen,* by a single layer of cells (the chief cells) in the mucosa of the stomach wall. Pepsinogen then requires hydrochloric acid to be transformed into the enzyme pepsin. The active pepsin then begins splitting the peptide linkages between the protein's amino acids, breaking the large polypeptides into successively smaller peptides. If the protein were held in the stomach longer, pepsin could continue the breakdown until individual amino acids resulted. However, with normal gastric emptying time, only the beginning stage is completed by the action of pepsin.
2. *Hydrochloric acid.* Gastric hydrochloride is an important catalyst in gastric protein digestion. It provides the acid medium necessary to convert pepsinogen to pepsin. Clinical problems result from lack of the normal secretion of hydrochloric acid (see Chapter 2).
3. *Rennin.* This gastric enzyme (not to be confused with the renal enzyme renin) is present only in infancy and childhood and disappears in adulthood. It is especially important in the infant's digestion of milk. Rennin and calcium act on the casein of milk to produce a curd. By coagulating milk, rennin prevents too rapid a passage of the food from the infant's stomach.

SMALL INTESTINE

Protein digestion begins in the acid medium of the stomach and is completed in the alkaline medium of the small intestine. A number of enzymes, from secretions of both the pancreas and the intestine, take part in protein digestion.

1. *Pancreatic secretions.* Three enzymes produced by the pancreas continue breaking down proteins to simpler and simpler substances.
   - *Trypsin* is secreted first as inactive trypsinogen and is then activated by the hormone enterokinase, which is produced by glands in the duodenal wall. The active enzyme trypsin then acts on protein and large polypeptide fragments carried over from the stomach, producing smaller polypeptides and dipeptides.
   - *Chymotrypsin* is produced by special cells in the pancreas as inactive chymotrypsinogen and is then activated by the trypsin already present. Chymotrypsin continues the same protein-splitting action of trypsin.
   - *Carboxypeptidase,* as its name indicates, attacks the carboxyl end (acid [COOH]) of the peptide chain.

TABLE 5-1 Summary of Protein Digestion

Organ	Enzyme: Inactive Precursor	Enzyme: Activator	Enzyme: Active Enzyme	Digestive Action
Mouth			None	Mechanical only
Stomach (acidic)	Pepsinogen	Hydrochloric acid	Pepsin	Protein → polypeptides
			Rennin (infants) (calcium necessary for activity)	Casein → coagulated curd
Intestine (alkaline)				
Pancreatic secretions	Trypsinogen	Enterokinase	Trypsin	Protein, polypeptides → polypeptides, dipeptides
	Chymotrypsinogen	Active trypsin	Chymotrypsin	Protein, polypeptides → polypeptides, dipeptides
			Carboxypeptidase	Polypeptides → simpler peptides, dipeptides, amino acids
Intestinal secretions			Aminopeptidase	Polypeptides → peptides, dipeptides, amino acids
			Dipeptidase	Dipeptides → amino acids

This action of carboxypeptidase in turn produces smaller peptides and some free amino acids.

2. *Intestinal secretions.* Glands in the intestinal wall produce two more protein-splitting enzymes in the peptidase group.
   - *Aminopeptidase* releases amino acids one at a time from the nitrogen-containing amino end (base [NH_2]) of the peptide chain. Through this cleavage, aminopeptidase produces smaller short-chain peptides and free amino acids.
   - *Dipeptidase* is the final enzyme in this protein-splitting system. Dipeptidase breaks the remaining dipeptides into their two, now free, amino acids.

Through this total system of protein-splitting enzymes, the large complex proteins are broken down into progressively smaller peptide chains and finally into free amino acids, now ready for absorption by the intestinal mucosa. A summary of these steps in protein digestion is given in Table 5-1.

ABSORPTION

Absorption of Amino Acids

The end products of protein digestion are the amino acids. They are water soluble; therefore their absorption directly into the water-based bloodstream poses no problem. These building units are rapidly absorbed from the small intestine through the fine network of villus capillaries by means of competitive active transport, and enter the portal blood.

1. *Active transport system.* Most of the amino acid absorption takes place in the first section of the small intestine, the duodenum. An energy-dependent active transport process, coupled with sodium transport, moves the amino acids into the blood circulation, delivering them to the cells for eventual metabolism.

---

aminopeptidase Protein-splitting enzyme that cuts the peptide bond (linkage) at the amino end of amino acids, splitting off the amino group NH_2.

carboxypeptidase A protein enzyme that splits off the chemical group *carboxyl* (COOH) at the end of peptide chains, acting on the peptide bond of the terminal amino acid having a free-end carboxyl group.

chymotrypsin One of the protein-splitting and milk-curdling pancreatic enzymes, activated in the intestine from precursor chymotrypsinogen. It breaks peptide linkages of the amino acids phenylalanine and tyrosine.

dipeptidase Final enzyme in the protein-splitting series that cleaves the one remaining amino acid bond in dipeptides.

pepsin The main gastric enzyme specific for proteins. Pepsin begins breaking large protein molecules into shorter chain polypeptides, proteases, and peptones. Gastric hydrochloric acid is necessary to activate pepsin.

proenzyme An inactive precursor converted to the active enzyme by the action of an acid, another enzyme, or other means. Also called zymogen.

trypsin A protein-splitting enzyme formed in the intestine by action of enterokinase on the inactive precursor trypsinogen.

2. *Competition for absorption.* When we eat a mixed diet containing a variety of different amino acids, the amino acids compete with each other for absorption. The amino acid present in the largest quantity retards the absorption of the others. In plasma, circulating amino acids also compete for the entry receptor sites on cell membranes that control transport into the cell.

Absorption of Peptides and Whole Proteins

A few larger fragments of short-chain peptides or smaller intact proteins are absorbed as such and then by hydrolysis within the absorbing cells yield their amino acids. These whole protein molecules may play a part in the development of immunity and sensitivity. For example, antibodies in the mother's colostrum, the premilk breast secretion, are passed on to her nursing infant.

METABOLISM

The construction sites in the body for building necessary specific tissue proteins are in the cells. Each cell, depending on its particular nature and function, has a specific job to perform and requires a unique mix of amino acids to build the specific proteins needed. In human nutrition the amino acids are the "metabolic currency" of protein. It is with the fate of these vital compounds that the metabolism of protein is ultimately concerned. Protein's fascinating array of complex metabolic activities are intricately interwoven with those of carbohydrates and fats. Here we will look briefly at the fundamental metabolic concept of protein and nitrogen balance. This will provide a base for relating the tissue-building processes of anabolism with those of the breaking-down processes of catabolism, necessary to maintain these important protein balances.

The Concept of Balance

Many interdependent checks and balances exist throughout the body to keep it in working order. There is a constant ebb and flow of materials, a building up and breaking down of parts, and a depositing and taking up of components. The body has built-in controls that operate as finely tuned coordinated responses to meet any situation that disturbs its normal condition or function. This resulting state of dynamic equilibrium is called homeostasis, and the various mechanisms designed to preserve it are called *homeostatic mechanisms.* This highly sensitive balance between body parts and functions is life sustaining. As more and more is learned about human nutrition and physiology, older ideas of a rigid body structure are giving way to this important concept of dynamic equilibrium—balance amid constant change. All body constituents are in a constant state of flux, although some tissues are more actively engaged than others. This dynamic concept can be seen in all metabolism. It is especially striking in protein metabolism.

Protein Balance

Overall protein balance involves concepts of protein turnover, protein compartments, amino acid pool, and nitrogen balance.

1. *Protein turnover.* The use of radioactive isotopes has clearly demonstrated that the body's protein tissues are continuously being broken down into amino acids and then resynthesized into tissue proteins. When amino acids labeled with a radioactive carbon atom are fed, they can be traced—that is, we can follow them in their journey as they are rapidly incorporated into various body tissue proteins, and then, some time later, when these tissues are broken down, used again to produce yet another tissue protein. The rate of this protein turnover varies in different tissues. It is highest in the intestinal mucosa, liver, pancreas, kidney, and plasma, tissues that tend to be more metabolically active. It is lower in muscle, brain, and skin. It is much slower in structural tissues such as collagen and bone.
2. *Protein compartments.* Body protein exists in a balance between two compartments—tissue protein and plasma protein. These stores are further balanced with dietary protein intake. Protein from one compartment may be drawn to supply a need in the other. For example, during fasting, resources from the body protein stores may be used for tissue synthesis. But even when the intake of protein and other nutrients is adequate, the tissue proteins are still being constantly broken down, reshaped, and reformed according to body need. Such a dynamic state is necessary to life and growth because the body is an open system. It must sustain a dynamic balance not only within its own internal environment but also with its larger and extended external environment.

   The body's steady state is the result of tissue protein balance between the rates of protein breakdown *(catabolism)* and protein synthesis *(anabolism).* In periods of growth the synthesis rate is higher so that new tissue can be formed. In conditions of starvation, wasting disease, and more gradually as aging continues in elderly persons, tissue breakdown exceeds that of synthesis, and the body gradually deteriorates.
3. *Metabolic amino acid pool.* Amino acids derived from tissue breakdown and amino acids from dietary protein digestion and absorption both contribute to a common collective metabolic "pool" of amino acids held throughout the body that are available for use (Figure 5-4). A balance of amino acids is thus maintained to supply the body's constant needs. Shifts in balances between tissue breakdown and dietary protein intake ensure a balanced mixture of amino acids. From this reserve pool, specific amino acids are supplied to synthesize specific body proteins.
4. *Nitrogen balance.* Another useful reference for indicating a person's state of protein balance is nitrogen balance. Total nitrogen balance involves all sources of nitrogen

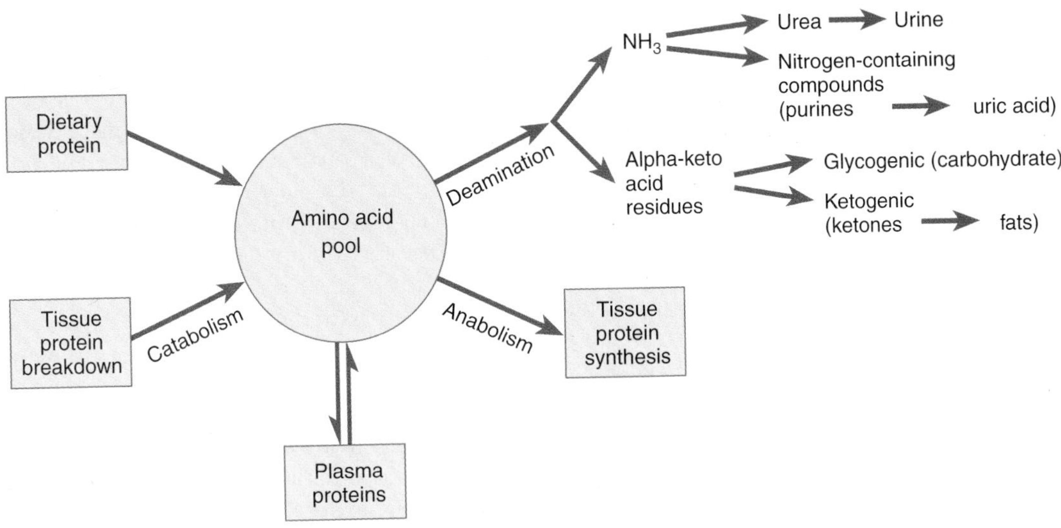

FIGURE 5-4 Balance between protein compartments and amino acid pool.

in the body—protein nitrogen as well as nonprotein nitrogen present in other compounds, such as urea, uric acid, ammonia, and other body tissues and fluids. It is the net result of nitrogen gains and losses in all the body protein. A person is in a harmful state of negative nitrogen balance when the loss of body protein exceeds the input of food protein; such a state exists in conditions of long-term illness, hypermetabolic wasting disease, or starvation.

Protein Requirements

PROTEIN INTAKE

Type of Protein

It is clear that protein is an essential nutrient. But just how much and what kind of protein do we actually need? We know that some people get far less than they need. On a worldwide basis, protein-energy malnutrition is a major health concern, especially in developing countries. In contrast, protein deficiency is generally not a problem in the United States and most other Western societies. Actually, most persons in America eat 2 or 3 times as much protein as they really need, and most of this protein comes from animal sources, largely as a result of the extensive role of meat and dairy products in traditional food patterns. U.S. surveys indicate that foods of animal origin contribute 69% of the daily protein intake, with 42% coming from meat, including poultry and fish; 20% from dairy products; and the remainder from eggs.[21] As for plant protein, 18% is supplied by grains and only 4% by legumes, soy, and nuts.

Legumes are a source of not only good-quality protein but also fiber and resistant starch (see Chapter 3), and nuts add both protein and important monounsaturated fatty acids to the diet (see Chapter 4). Substitution of up to 30% of the animal protein with soy protein in hamburgers, tacos, and lasagna served in school lunch programs resulted in a decrease in kcalories, total fat, and saturated fat.[22] Soy and legumes also appear to assist in lowering serum blood lipoprotein levels in men and women. The substitution of soy foods for animal foods higher in fat plays a role in bringing about this effect; however, plant chemicals called isoflavones,

anabolism Metabolic process by which body tissues are built.

catabolism The breaking-down phase of metabolism, the opposite of anabolism. Catabolism includes all the processes in which complex substances are progressively broken down into simpler ones. Catabolism usually involves the release of energy. Together, anabolism and catabolism constitute metabolism, which is the coordinated operation of anabolic and catabolic processes into a dynamic balance of energy and substance.

homeostasis State of relative dynamic equilibrium within the body's internal environment; a balance achieved through the operation of various interrelated physiologic mechanisms.

hydrolysis Process by which a chemical compound is split into other simpler compounds by taking up the elements of water, as in the manufacture of infant formulas to produce easier-to-digest derivatives of the main protein casein, the cow's milk base. This process occurs naturally in digestion.

nitrogen balance The metabolic balance between nitrogen intake in dietary protein and output in urinary nitrogen compounds such as urea and creatinine. For every 6.25 g dietary protein consumed, 1 g nitrogen is excreted.

protein balance Body tissue protein balance between building up tissue (anabolism) and breaking down tissue (catabolism) to maintain healthy body growth and maintenance.

found in soy, may assist in the control of blood lipid levels. A 19-year follow-up of 9600 men and women with varied diets who participated in a national dietary survey found that individuals who ate legumes at least 4 times a week had a 22% lower risk of cardiovascular disease than did those who ate legumes less than once a week.[23] Regular use of legumes even benefited those with higher intakes of saturated fat, or lower levels of physical activity, or who smoked. All persons, regardless of their dietary preferences, will benefit from increased intakes of these plant foods. Nutrition education should emphasize ways of adding vegetable proteins to the daily dietary pattern.

Because protein foods such as meat, fish, poultry, and dairy foods tend to be among the more costly foods in the food supply, it follows that individuals identified to be food insufficient, meaning they do not always have enough food, might be lacking in protein. Surprisingly, in a national survey young adults classified as food insufficient had protein intakes that were 145% of the Recommended Dietary Allowance (RDA) and food insufficient older adults met 101% of their protein RDA.[24]

High-Protein Diets

Excess protein intake often creates other problems. First, excessive intake of animal protein items high in saturated fat can contribute to obesity and vascular health problems. Second, the excessive protein load can place accumulative burden on the kidneys for nitrogen excretion. Clinicians have begun to raise questions about the long-term effects of habitual excess protein intake on the human kidney, designed in earlier ages to handle a different supply of protein. Finally, excessive protein intake appears to increase serum insulin levels and may contribute to the development of type 2 diabetes.[25] Another controversy regarding high protein intakes is their effect on bone health. Women with higher proportions of their protein coming from animal sources and lesser amounts from vegetable sources lose bone more rapidly, although effects differ among studies and the various sites of bone loss.[8,9]

In recent years diets promoted in the popular press as effective weight loss diets have advocated intakes of protein that reach 20% to 30% of total energy, thus raising protein intake to levels of 225 g/day or higher.[26] Such diets also tend to raise fat intake and limit carbohydrate intake and restrict the use of plant foods that not only provide important macronutrients but also help control blood pressure. We will discuss these issues of weight loss and the role of micronutrients in the control of blood pressure in later chapters.

Although recent DRIs for protein did not set a Tolerable Upper Intake Level (UL), it was recommended that total daily protein not exceed 30% of total kcalories.[3] It would seem prudent for nutrition experts to reinforce that recommendation in light of current protein intakes.

Low-Protein Diets

In the United States, we associate low-protein diets with the severe malnutrition observed in underfed children and adults in developing countries; however, those individuals lack not only protein but also energy and important micronutrients. There are clinical situations in which it is beneficial to limit protein intake. In patients with Parkinson's disease it is important that protein intake be controlled to ensure that excess amounts of amino acids will not compete with the treatment drug levodopa in crossing the blood-brain barrier.[27] In chronic renal failure, lowering dietary protein intake, and thus the levels of nitrogen-containing waste such as urea and ammonia that must be removed from the blood, may reduce the symptoms of metabolic acidosis and slow the progression of renal failure, thus delaying the need for or frequency of dialysis. Weight training can assist in supporting protein utilization and maintenance of muscle mass in renal patients.[28]

FACTORS INFLUENCING PROTEIN REQUIREMENTS

Tissue Growth

The primary purpose of protein in the diet is to supply amino acids in the quantity and proportions necessary for tissue growth and maintenance. Thus any period of growth increases the need for protein. Growth-related factors include age, body size, and general physical state. Also, special periods of rapid growth—such as the growth of the fetus and maternal tissue during pregnancy—require added protein.

Diet

Another factor that influences protein requirements is the nature of the protein in the diet and its ratio or pattern of amino acids. Also, there must be a sufficient supply of nonprotein foods in the diet to have a protein-sparing effect; in other words, there must be an adequate amount of carbohydrate and fat available so the total amount of dietary protein can be used for tissue building and not for meeting energy requirements. The digestibility and absorption of protein can be affected by food preparation methods; heat can cause chemical bonding between some sugars and amino acids, forming compounds that cannot be digested. Digestibility and absorption can be influenced by the time interval between meals; increased time intervals between eating protein foods lowers the competition for available enzymes and absorption sites.

State of Health

Any illness or disease will usually increase the protein requirement. Diseases accompanied by fever increase the need for protein because of the increase in basal metabolic rate and the general breaking down of tissue. Traumatic injury requires extensive tissue rebuilding. Postsurgical states need protein for wound healing, to replenish losses, and to support production of immune cells to fight infec-

TABLE 5-2 Estimates of Amino Acid Requirements

Amino Acid	Requirements, mg/kg/day, by Age Group				
			Children, Age 9-13 yr		
	Infants, Age 0-6 mo	Children, Age 4-8 yr	Boys	Girls	Adults
Histidine	23	16	17	15	14
Isoleucine	88	22	22	21	19
Leucine	156	49	49	47	42
Lysine	107	46	46	43	38
Methionine plus cysteine	59	22	22	21	19
Phenylalanine plus tyrosine	135	41	41	38	33
Threonine	73	24	24	22	20
Tryptophan	28	6	6	6	5
Valine	87	28	28	27	24

Compiled from Panel on Macronutrients, Panel on the Definition of Dietary Fiber, Subcommittee on Upper Reference Levels of Nutrients, Subcommittee on Interpretation and Uses of Dietary Reference Intakes, and the Standing Committee on the Scientific Evaluation of Dietary Reference Intakes: *Dietary reference intakes for energy, carbohydrate, fiber, fat, fatty acids, cholesterol, protein, and amino acids, parts 1 and 2,* Washington, DC, 2002, National Academy Press.

tion. Extensive tissue destruction, as occurs with burns, requires a substantial increase in protein intake for the healing process (see Chapter 22). A current clinical concern is the low protein and energy intake that can occur in hospitalized elderly patients.[29] Critical illness, anorexia, and immobilization all lead to deteriorating nutritional status and, in the elderly, accelerate the loss of muscle mass and muscle strength that contributes to further disability. Optimum energy and protein intakes during the rehabilitation period can reverse these trends with the synthesis of new muscle protein and an increase in muscle strength.[30]

As persons of all ages are encouraged to increase their physical activity, the influence of exercise on protein needs will continue to be an area of interest and study. Among a group of healthy, normal weight 8- to 10-year-olds, nitrogen retention increased during a 6-week walking program, indicating a change in body protein metabolism over this period.[31]

MEASUREMENT OF PROTEIN REQUIREMENTS

Both quantity and quality must be considered when measuring the protein requirement.

Recommended Dietary Allowance

The quantity of protein needed is the basis for establishing the total protein requirement. Some people will require less than the recommended level because the standard allows for a margin of safety to cover the variety of needs in a given population. (Review the concept of nutrition standards as discussed in Chapter 1.) The current RDA for adults, released in 2002, is 0.8 g/kg of body weight.[3] For adults aged 19 years and older, this standard amounts to 56 g/day for a man weighing 70 kg (154 lb) and 46 g/day for a woman weighing 57 kg (125 lb). An additional 25 g of protein/day is needed during pregnancy, and lactation. The needs of infants and children vary according to age and growth patterns.

Protein Quality

The value of a protein depends on its content of indispensable amino acids, or, to put it another way, its relative content of indispensable amino acids compared with the total amount of nitrogen-containing substances present.[32] Guidelines for protein needs, based on nitrogen balance studies that determined specific amino acid requirements, have been developed (Table 5-2).

Comparative Quality of Food Proteins

The nutritive value of a food protein is often expressed in terms of its *chemical score,* a value derived from its amino acid composition. Using the amino acid pattern of a high-quality protein food—such as egg—and giving it a value of 100, other foods are compared according to their ratios of indispensable amino acids. Of the indispensable amino acids, the one showing the greatest deficit in that particular food is called the limiting amino acid because when it is used up in making a specific protein, it limits the ability of the body to make more of that protein.

Other measures also are used by researchers to determine protein quality.

limiting amino acid The amino acid in foods occurring in the smallest amount, thus limiting its availability for tissue structure.

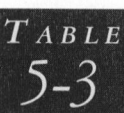

Table 5-3 Comparative Protein Quality of Selected Foods According to Chemical (Amino Acid) Score, Biologic Value (BV), Net Protein Utilization (NPU), and Protein Efficiency Ratio (PER)

Food	Chemical Score	BV	NPU	PER	Food	Chemical Score	BV	NPU	PER
Egg	100	100	94	3.92	Polished rice	57	64	57	2.18
Cow's milk	95	93	82	3.09	Whole wheat	53	65	49	1.53
Fish	71	76	—	3.55	Corn	49	72	36	—
Beef	69	74	67	2.30	Soybeans	47	73	61	2.32
Unpolished rice	67	86	59	—	Sesame seeds	42	62	53	1.77
Peanuts	65	55	55	1.65	Peas	37	64	55	1.57
Oats	57	65	—	2.19					

Data adapted from Food and Nutrition Board, National Academy of Sciences—National Research Council: *Recommended dietary allowances,* ed 10, Washington, DC, 1989, National Academy Press.

TO PROBE FURTHER

Will Protein Supplements Help Build Muscle?

As the mass media continue to promote the benefits of body-building and strength training for all age groups, supplement manufacturers have responded with the development of a myriad of products designed to catch the consumer's attention. Many of these products contain protein or amino acids, the building blocks for muscle protein. However, can these products, often high in cost, provide a better source of protein than real food? This is a question that you, as a practicing health professional, are likely to be asked by future clients.

At present there are differing opinions regarding the protein needs of both young adults and the elderly who are lifting weights to build muscle. A generally held view is that resistance training or strength training does increase the need for protein above the general requirement; however, the energy intakes of individuals engaged in regular physical activity can provide the protein needed without resorting to supplements. High doses of selected amino acids are not only expensive, but also do not improve muscle mass. Moreover, amino acid supplements can lead to harmful side effects ranging from stomach cramps and diarrhea, to blocking the absorption of other important amino acids, to toxicity.

Recently, whey protein has been touted as a protein having a specific ability to increase muscle mass and enhance performance. Whey comprises about 20% of milk protein, and casein makes up the remaining 80%. Whey protein separates from the casein in cheese-making, and is either discarded or made into protein powder. Some proponents claim that whey protein is superior to other proteins in supporting an increase in muscle mass, although most of the experimental work used to support these claims was carried out in animals, not humans. Although whey protein does appear to enhance immune function, there is no evidence to support a beneficial effect on muscle mass in athletes, apart from general protein needs.

The American Dietetic Association suggests that endurance athletes take in 1.2 to 1.4 g of protein/kg of body weight, whereas those performing resistance training such as lifting weights may need intakes of 1.6 to 1.7 g/kg of body weight. More protein is needed at the beginning of a weight training program, for as training continues muscle cells become more efficient in their use of protein. For most people the additional protein needed to support muscle growth can be obtained by adding 2 to 4 oz of meat, fish, or poultry or 1 to 2 cups of legumes or 1 to 2 cups of milk to the diet. Protein intakes above 2.0 g/kg of body weight can result in dehydration because the body must produce more urine to excrete the high levels of nitrogen-containing waste that accumulate from the excess protein. Intakes of this level should be avoided unless supervised by a physician. Excessive protein intakes are more problematic for women, as increasing dietary protein can increase bone calcium loss, and women of all ages are at risk for low bone mass.

While the nutrition experts quoted above recommend an increased protein intake for individuals performing endurance or weight training, the Expert Panels (2002) setting the DRIs for protein did not see a need for additional protein over and above the RDA. We will discuss this topic further in Chapter 14.

References

Clarkson PM, Rawson ES: Nutritional supplements to increase muscle mass, *Crit Rev Food Sci Nutr* 39(4):317, 1999.

Coleman E: Does whey protein enhance performance, Special Supplement on Sports Nutrition, *Nutr MD* 27(6), 2001.

Manore MM, Barr SI, Butterfield GE: Position of the American Dietetic Association, dietitians of Canada, and the American College of Sports Medicine: nutrition and athletic performance, *J Am Diet Assoc* 100(12):1543, 2000.

Panel on Macronutrients, Panel on the Definition of Dietary Fiber, Subcommittee on Upper Reference Levels of Nutrients, Subcommittee on Interpretation and Uses of Dietary Reference Intakes, and the Standing Committee on the Scientific Evaluation of Dietary Reference Intakes: *Dietary reference intakes for energy, carbohydrate, fiber, fat, fatty acids, cholesterol, protein, and amino acids, parts 1 and 2,* Washington, DC, 2002, National Academy Press.

Wolfe RR: Protein supplements and exercise, *Am J Clin Nutr* 72(suppl):551S, 2000.

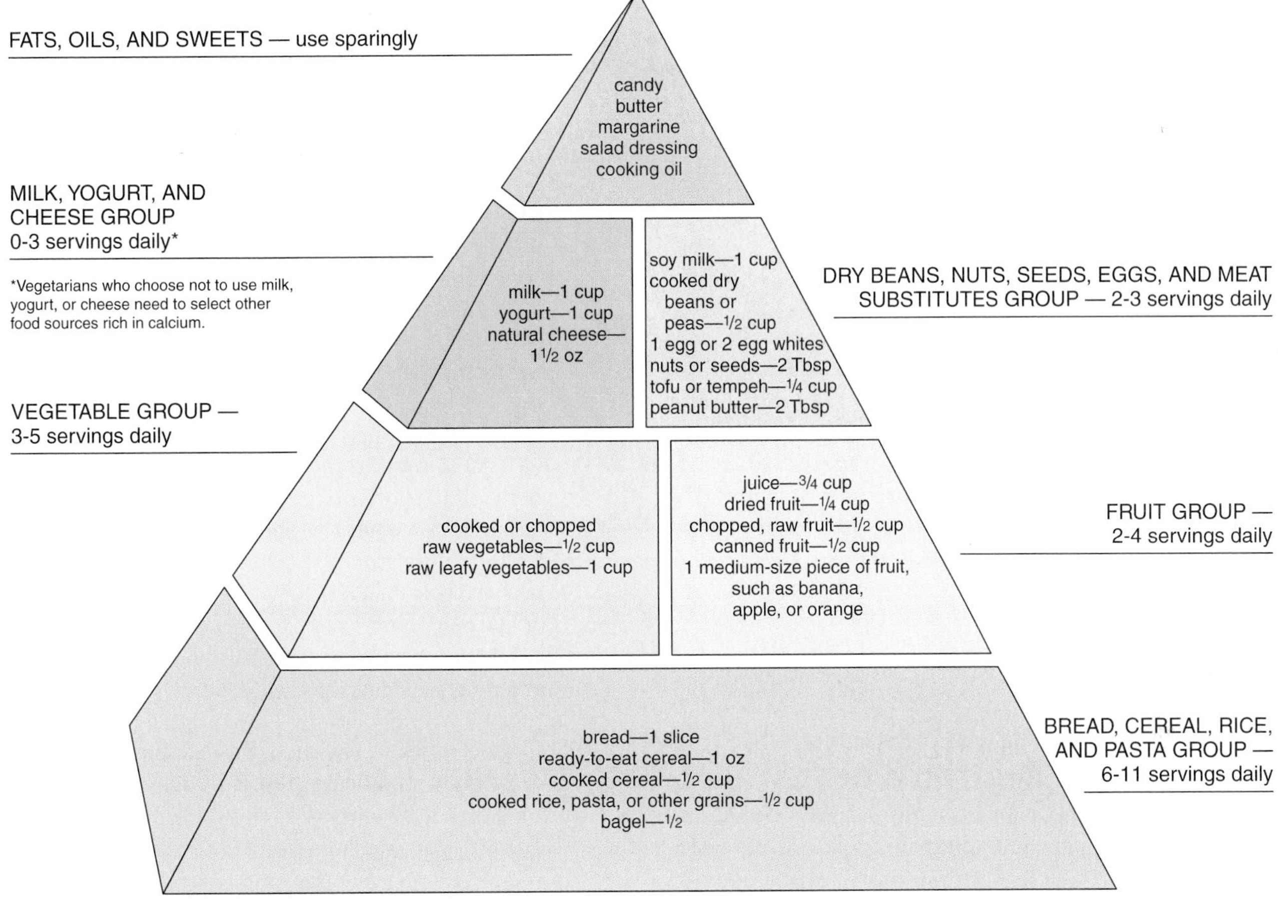

FIGURE 5-5 Food Guide Pyramid for Vegetarian Meal Planning. *(From Messina VK, Burke KI: Vegetarian diets: position of the American Dietetic Association. Copyright by the American Dietetic Association. Reprinted with permission from* J Am Diet Assoc *97:1320, 1997.)*

1. *Biologic value (BV)* is based on nitrogen balance and the ability of that protein to replace daily protein losses or support growth.
2. *Net protein utilization (NPU)* is based on biologic value and degree of digestibility.
3. *Protein efficiency ratio (PER)* is based on weight gain of a growing test animal divided by its protein intake.

A comparison of the scores of various protein foods with their nutritive values based on these measures is shown in Table 5-3. Food is the best way to obtain needed protein. There is no need for amino acid supplements even for those with added protein requirements related to rapid growth or weight training. Amino acid supplements are both costly and inefficient (see *To Probe Further* box).

VEGETARIAN DIETS

On the basis of religious or cultural beliefs, concern for animals, desire to preserve the natural environment, or support of a healthy lifestyle, some persons choose to follow a diet concentrated on plant foods and to limit their intakes of meat, fish, and poultry or other animal foods. Such diets are generally referred to as vegetarian diets despite the fact that this term does not take into consideration the many variations that exist among diets generally focused on plant foods.[33] There are three general types of vegetarian diets: (1) ovolactovegetarian (including dairy foods and eggs), (2) lactovegetarian (including dairy foods), and (3) vegan (no animal foods). Others who consider themselves to be vegetarians eat fish occasionally, and some may eat poultry. Vegetarian diets, involving particular deletions or combinations of foods, are planned as any diet is planned, to secure needed nutrients and sufficient energy kcalories (see *Issues & Answers*). The American Dietetic Association has developed a *Food Guide Pyramid for Vegetarian Meal Planning* to assist in planning nutritionally sound diets based on plant foods (Figure 5-5). Current thought regarding vegetarian diets suggests that the conscious combining of complementary plant proteins within a given meal is unnecessary,[12] as long as an individual consumes various sources of amino acids over the course of a day.

Various health benefits appear to accompany a vegetarian diet. Vegetarians are less likely to develop high blood pressure and have a lower risk of coronary heart disease. Plant-based diets are high in vitamins, minerals, and phytochemicals that offer some protection against these chronic problems. Colorectal cancer is lower among vegetarians, likely related to their relatively high fiber intake, and a well-planned vegetarian diet has been used successfully to manage renal disease.[12]

Interesting recipes for preparing nutritionally appropriate vegetarian meals are widely available as increased public interest has given rise to many popular cookbooks with tasty and easy to prepare dishes. In comparison to animal protein sources, it is generally necessary to consume larger amounts of vegetable protein foods to obtain comparable amounts of amino acids.

TO SUM UP

Proteins build tissue, assist in carrying out various physiologic functions, and provide energy. Amino acids are the structural components that make up proteins. There are 20 amino acids important to human nutrition; the body cannot synthesize 9 of these at all or in sufficient amounts, and 6 cannot be synthesized in adequate amounts under conditions of stress or accelerated growth. The 9 amino acids that must be supplied by food are called indispensable or essential amino acids. Food proteins are considered complete when they contain all 9 indispensable amino acids in appropriate amounts. Animal proteins are complete proteins. Vegetable proteins are incomplete but can be mixed with complete proteins or with each other to provide all 9 indispensable amino acids in the proportions necessary to support tissue maintenance and growth.

Amino acids participate in protein building (anabolism) and breakdown (catabolism). Both processes are dictated by genetic information and hormonal influences. Anabolism occurs when the specific amino acids required for each protein are present. If one is missing, the protein is not formed—the law of "all or none." Catabolism occurs when a body tissue is broken down and its constituent amino acids are released. An amino acid can be split apart to yield its nitrogen group, which can be used to make another amino acid or nitrogen compound, and its nonnitrogen carbon skeleton that can be used to form carbohydrates for energy or fat for storage. In the unfed state, proteins are broken down for energy if carbohydrate is not available. Thus dietary carbohydrates have a protein-sparing effect.

Protein requirements are influenced by growth needs and rates of protein synthesis, food protein quality, and dietary carbohydrate and fat levels. Clinical factors affecting protein needs include fever, disease, surgery, or other trauma to body tissues.

■ Questions for Review

1. What is the difference between an indispensable and a dispensable amino acid? List the names of the indispensable amino acids as well as those that are indispensable under certain conditions.
2. What is meant by nitrogen balance? How does it relate to protein turnover?
3. Distinguish between protein anabolism and protein catabolism. Describe a situation in which you would expect to see each of these actions.
4. Describe the process of protein digestion and absorption, including the (a) site in the gastrointestinal tract where each action occurs, (b) the enzymes responsible and their source, and (c) the resulting products.
5. Explain the term *protein-sparing effect.* Which nutrients have this effect?
6. List and describe factors that affect dietary protein needs.
7. Visit a grocery store or drugstore and review the high-protein supplements for sale. Make a chart that includes (a) the number of grams of protein provided in the container, (b) the cost of the container, and (c) the calculated cost for 8 g of protein from this product. How does each product compare with the cost of 1 cup (8 oz) of milk or ½ cup of beans, which provide about 8 g of high-quality protein? Are there other nutrients in addition to protein provided by these products compared with the additional nutrients provided by milk or beans?
8. A vegetarian couple decides to raise their 2-year-old daughter on a strict vegan diet. As often occurs with young children, she does not always finish meals and snacks on fruits and whole grain biscuits. Eventually, they notice that she is falling behind in her growth rate and becoming thin. What dietary factor may be involved in the child's poor growth? What advice would you offer these parents to improve their child's nutritional status? Plan 1 day of meals for this family, indicating amounts for the child that would meet her protein needs, while still adhering to a typical vegan meal pattern.
9. You are working with a teenager who is dieting and restricting her kcalorie intake to no more than 1000 kcalories/day. When you express concerns about her protein status she assures you that she is meeting her RDA for protein. What would you tell her about her body need for and utilization of protein?
10. Nutrition experts have expressed concern about the excessive protein intakes of many persons of all ages. Using the food values in Appendix A or a computer nutrient analysis program, calculate both the kcalorie value and the number of grams of protein in a fast food meal that consists of a double-patty cheeseburger,

a serving of French fries, and a milkshake. Compare the total grams of protein and the total kcalories with the protein and energy RDAs for a 16-year-old boy. What proportion of his daily protein and energy needs are provided by this one meal?

■ References

1. Matthews DE: Proteins and amino acids. In Shils ME et al, eds: *Modern nutrition in health and disease,* ed 9, Philadelphia, 1999, Lippincott Williams & Wilkins.
2. Rucker RR, Kosenen T: Structure and properties of proteins and amino acids. In Stipanuk MH, ed: *Biochemical and physiological aspects of human nutrition,* Philadelphia, 2000, WB Saunders.
3. Panel on Macronutrients, Panel on the Definition of Dietary Fiber, Subcommittee on Upper Reference Levels of Nutrients, Subcommittee on Interpretation and Uses of Dietary Reference Intakes, and the Standing Committee on the Scientific Evaluation of Dietary Reference Intakes: *Dietary reference intakes for energy, carbohydrate, fiber, fat, fatty acids, cholesterol, protein, and amino acids, parts 1 and 2,* Washington, DC, 2002, National Academy Press.
4. Stipanuk MH, Watford M: Amino acid metabolism. In Stipanuk MH, ed: *Biochemical and physiological aspects of human nutrition,* Philadelphia, 2000, WB Saunders.
5. Kurpad AV et al: Daily requirement for and splanchnic uptake of leucine in healthy adult Indians, *Am J Clin Nutr* 74:747, 2001.
6. Guyton AC, Hall JE: *Textbook of medical physiology,* ed 10, Philadelphia, 2000, WB Saunders.
7. Messina MJ: Legumes and soybeans: overview of their nutritional profiles and health effects, *Am J Clin Nutr* 70(suppl):439S, 1999.
8. Heaney RP: Protein intake and bone health: the influence of belief systems on the conduct of nutritional science, *Am J Clin Nutr* 73:5, 2001.
9. Sellmeyer DE et al: A high ratio of dietary animal to vegetable protein increases the rate of bone loss and the risk of fracture in postmenopausal women, *Am J Clin Nutr* 73:118, 2001.
10. Anderson JW, Smith BM, Washnock CS: Cardiovascular benefits of dry bean and soybean intake, *Am J Clin Nutr* 70(suppl):464S, 1999.
11. Wangen KE et al: Soy isoflavones improve plasma lipids in normocholesterolemic and mildly hypercholesterolemic postmenopausal women, *Am J Clin Nutr* 73:225, 2001.
12. Messina VK, Burke KI: Position of the American Dietetic Association: vegetarian diets, *J Am Diet Assoc* 47 (11):1317, 1997. (Reaffirmed until December, 2001.)
13. Young VR: Protein and amino acids. In Bowman BA, Russell RM, eds: *Present knowledge in nutrition,* ed 8, Washington, DC, 2001, International Life Sciences Institute.
14. Fernstrom D, Fernstrom MH: Monoamines and protein intake: are control mechanisms designed to monitor a threshold intake or a set point? *Nutr Rev* 59(8 suppl):S60, 2001.
15. Boelens PG et al: Glutamine alimentation in catabolic state, *J Nutr* 131:2569S, 2001.
16. Buchman AL: Glutamine: commercially essential or conditionally essential? A critical appraisal of the human data, *Am J Clin Nutr* 74:25, 2001.
17. Khanum S, Ashworth A, Huttly SRA: Growth, morbidity, and mortality of children in Dhaka after treatment for severe malnutrition: a prospective study, *Am J Clin Nutr* 67:940, 1998.
18. Thissen, JP, Underwood LE, Ketelslegers JM: Regulation of insulin-like growth factor-I in starvation and injury, *Nutr Rev* 57:167, 1999.
19. Kennedy TS, Oakland MJ, Shaw RD: Growth patterns and nutritional factors associated with increased head circumferences at 18 months in normally developing, low-birth-weight infants, *J Am Diet Assoc* 99:1522, 1999.
20. Colombani PC et al: Metabolic effects of a protein-supplemented carbohydrate drink in marathon runners, *Int J Sport Nutr* 9:181, 1999.
21. Smit E et al: Estimates of animal and plant protein intake in US adults: Results from the Third National Health and Nutrition Examination Survey, 1988-1991, *J Am Diet Assoc* 99:813, 1999.
22. Thomas JN, Lutz SF: Soy protein lowers fat and saturated fat in school lunch beef and pork entrees, *J Am Diet Assoc* 101:461, 2001.
23. Bazzano LA et al: Legume consumption and risk of coronary heart disease in US men and women. NHANES I Epidemiologic Follow-up Study, *Arch Intern Med* 161:2573, 2001.
24. Dixon LB, Winkleby MA, Radimer KL: Dietary intakes and serum nutrients differ between adults from food-insufficient and food-sufficient families: Third National Health and Nutrition Examination Survey, 1988-1994, *J Nutr* 131: 1232, 2001.
25. Metges C, Barth CA: Metabolic consequences of a high dietary-protein intake in adulthood: assessment of the available evidence, *J Nutr* 130:886, 2000.
26. St Joer ST et al: Dietary protein and weight reduction: a statement for healthcare professionals from the Nutrition Committee of the Council on Nutrition, Physical Activity, and Metabolism of the American Heart Association, *Circulation* 104(15):1869, 2001.
27. Holdern K: Reducing fracture risk in patients with Parkinson disease, *Nutr MD* 27(4):1, 2001.
28. Castaneda C et al: Resistance training to counteract the catabolism of a low-protein diet in patients with chronic renal insufficiency. A randomized, controlled trial, *Ann Intern Med* 135(11):999, 2001.
29. Barrocas A: Nutrition support of the hospitalized elderly, *Nutr MD* 27(9):1, 2001.
30. Bourdel-Marchasson I et al: Functional and metabolic early changes in calf muscle occurring during nutritional repletion in malnourished elderly patients, *Am J Clin Nutr* 73: 832, 2001.
31. Bolster DR et al: Exercise affects protein utilization in healthy children, *J Nutr* 131:2659, 2001.
32. Yates AA: Overview of key nutrients: energy and macronutrient aspects, *Nutr Rev* 56:S29, 1998.
33. Weinsier R: Use of the term vegetarian, *Am J Clin Nutr* 71(5):1211, 2000.

Further Reading

Kwon T-W et al: The relative constancy of protein as percent of calories in world food supplies, *Nutr Today* 35:129, 2000.

This article looks at the relative supply of protein in countries around the world and suggests how food patterns are changing as people adopt diets that are higher in fat.

Skinner JD et al: Longitudinal study of nutrient and food intakes of white preschool children aged 24 to 60 months, *J Am Diet Assoc* 99:1514, 1999.

Dr. Skinner and her coworkers followed the food patterns of preschoolers for 3 years and tell us about the foods these children ate regularly and the nutrients these foods contributed to the diet. You will see that although the protein intakes of these children were meeting the recommended levels, they were not choosing protein foods that also contribute other important vitamins and minerals to the diet.

Messina VK, Burke KI: Position of the American Dietetic Association: vegetarian diets, *J Am Diet Assoc* 47(11):1317, 1997. (Reaffirmed until December, 2001.)

This article provides practical advice for planning a vegetarian diet that provides appropriate amounts of protein, vitamins, and minerals for body growth and maintenance.

Grivetti LE, Corlett JL, Lockett CT: Food in American history, part 3: beans, *Nutr Today* 36(3):172, 2001.

Vegetable protein in the form of legumes has played an important role in the food history of the United States. Dr. Grivetti, a noted food historian, and his coauthors tell us about the use of legumes among various cultural groups in the early years of the American colonies.

Issues & ANSWERS

Vegetarian Diets: Implications for Nutrition and Health

Since ancient times vegetarian diets have been advocated for a variety of reasons. The ancient Greeks are considered to be the founders of the vegetarian diet, and Benjamin Franklin, the famous American inventor in the eighteenth century, was a vegetarian. Over the past decade the number of persons in the United States following vegetarian diets has about doubled, and it is estimated that currently 10% of all Americans consider themselves to be vegetarians. As we mentioned on p. 97, many different food patterns are included within the general term of vegetarian. It is important when counseling a person who is a vegetarian that you give particular attention to the foods that are eaten and the foods that are avoided by that individual. For example, a recent survey found that 20% of the vegetarians ate meat at least once a month. On the other hand, vegan diets contain only plant foods including grains, vegetables, fruits, legumes, nuts, seeds, and vegetable fats. Thus, we cannot make generalizations that apply to all vegetarian diets. In general, the more restrictive the diet, the more likely that nutrient deficiencies may occur; however, even vegan diets can be adequate with appropriate planning.

Why choose a vegetarian diet?

There are many reasons why an individual may choose to be a vegetarian. The three major ones include religious beliefs, concerns relating to sustainability of the food supply, and personal health goals. Several major world religions, including Hinduism and Buddhism, advocate the avoidance of meat and the preservation of animal life. Many members of the Seventh Day Adventist church avoid eating meat, fish, or poultry but include dairy products and eggs in their meal plans. Sustainability of the food supply is a growing concern in the developed nations and has led many persons to center their diet on plant foods. About 40% of the world's supply of grain is used to feed animals to be sold for meat; thus some persons have adopted plant-based diets with the intent that direct consumption of grains might assist in reducing the food shortages that exist in many parts of the world. Finally, well-planned vegetarian diets support good health and diminish the risk of many chronic diseases. Individuals who eat more grains, fruits, and vegetables and less meat have a lower risk of heart disease and cancer. A major research question is how does a vegetarian diet promote health? First, are there factors in meat, such as saturated fats, that exert a negative effect on health so that excessive intakes increase health risks? Or, does a higher intake of plant foods that add important phytochemicals, vitamins, and fiber to the diet help to prevent the development of chronic disease? It is likely that both of these factors play a role in the observed positive effect on health.

Nutritional implications of a vegetarian diet

Vegetarian diets, including vegan diets that exclude all animal foods, will support nutritional needs throughout the life cycle *if* they are well planned. In fact recent studies suggest that vegan children had higher intakes of fiber and all nutrients except for calcium compared with omnivore children, and the growing availability of fortified vegan foods is enabling the provision of adequate nutrients for all ages. Population groups with elevated nutrient needs such as pregnant women, young children, and adolescents require special attention regardless of dietary preference.

For those vegetarians who consume some animal foods, such as eggs or dairy products, protein, calcium, vitamin D, and vitamin B_{12} are not a problem. If eggs are used regularly, they will help to supply the n-3 fatty acid docosahexaenoic acid. However, these nutrients listed above demand special attention in the vegan diet. Although iron and zinc are found in many plant foods, they are less well absorbed from plants than from animal sources and are nutrients of concern for all vegetarians with high iron needs. Sufficient carbohydrate and fat must be included in the diet to spare protein and to allow all amino acids to be used for growth and maintenance of body tissues, but fat intake should still remain within the guidelines of 30% of total energy in both children and adults.

The American Dietetic Association has developed a Food Guide Pyramid for Vegetarian Meal Planning that can assist professionals and families in developing diets that will meet nutritional needs and support personal goals. The foundation of the pyramid is the bread and cereals group, and recommended servings are the equivalent of the *Food Guide Pyramid* developed for the general population. Similarly, fruit and vegetable servings do not differ between the two food guide pyramids. Protein is a critical nutrient for individuals experiencing a rapid expansion of body tissues, and important sources are included in the dry bean, nuts, seeds, eggs, and meat substitutes group and the milk, yogurt, and cheese group. Ovolactovegetarians who consume eggs and dairy products will have no problem obtaining sufficient amounts of protein with several daily servings of these foods. Vegans can meet their requirements with two or three servings of soy milk, cooked dry beans or peas, peanut butter or nuts, seeds, or tofu. The two amino acids of particular concern for vegans are lysine and methionine.

Lysine is the limiting amino acid in cereals, and methionine is the limiting amino acid in soy and legumes. Regardless, soy protein has been used successfully as the sole source of protein for children and adults. Meat analogues such as vegetarian lunch meat, sausage, or hamburgers prepared from soy also provide an opportunity for variety in the diet. Soy protein isolates are comparable to milk protein in supporting growth and nutritional well-being in young children and in rehabilitation of children who were malnourished earlier; however, it may be necessary to add methionine to infant formulas to ensure sufficient amounts of that amino acid.

A nutrient normally obtained only from animal sources, vitamin B_{12}, requires special attention in a vegan diet. Currently, many soy and other meat analogues sold in the United States have added vitamin B_{12}. Also, various brands of soy milk are fortified with this vitamin. Recent attention to vitamin B_{12} fortification of breakfast cereals and other grain foods to help meet the vitamin needs of older adults (see Chapter 2) has provided options for those eating only plant foods. Supplementation with vitamin B_{12} is also an important alternative. Although some vitamin B_{12} may find its way into plant foods through exposure to soils containing vitamin B_{12}, this should not be depended on as a reliable source.

Calcium and vitamin D can be problematic in the vegan diet. Dark green vegetables help supply calcium, as do some nuts and dried figs, although calcium from plant sources may be less well absorbed. Legumes supply some calcium to the diet, but it is important that vegans choose soy milk that has been fortified with both calcium and vitamin D and look for juices and other foods with added calcium. Vitamin D may be difficult to obtain, especially for older people who cannot manufacture vitamin D as well in their skin. Calcium and vitamin D supplements may be necessary to meet recommended levels of both nutrients for those following vegan diets.

In the typical U.S. diet, iron and zinc are most likely supplied by red meat; therefore alternative sources must be recommended for both ovolactovegetarians and vegans. Overall, vegetarians have higher iron intakes than do omnivores, although the iron found naturally in whole grain cereals, legumes, and many vegetables is less easily absorbed than the heme iron found in red meat, poultry, or fish. Providing a vitamin C source at the same meal as the iron-rich plant food can help facilitate the absorption of nonheme iron. Also, fortified breads and cereals will be important in meeting the iron requirement of children, adolescents, and women of child-bearing age. It is interesting to note, however, that the prevalence of anemia is no higher in vegetarian women than in nonvegetarian women in the United States, despite the difference in the consumption of meat. Dietary zinc can be obtained from cereals, legumes, wheat germ, corn, and peas. Dairy foods will supply some zinc for those who use these items.

Recent attention to the role of the n-3 fatty acids in important body functions makes sources of these nutrients an important consideration. For vegans or ovolactovegetarians who do not eat fish, good intakes of linolenic acid, a precursor of eicosapentaenoic acid and docosahexaenoic acid, may help to meet this need, although conversion is slow. Canola and linseed oils, soybeans and soybean oil, walnuts, and flaxseed are good sources of linolenic acid. The *trans* fatty acids, formed in the hydrogenation of liquid vegetable oils to form solid fats, are thought to interfere with the synthesis of the long-chain n-3 fatty acids. Thus, vegetable oils or tub margarines rather than solid stick margarines are better food sources (see Chapter 4 for a review of this topic). Vegans tend to have higher intakes of linoleic acid than of linolenic acid.

A noted expert on both child and adult nutrition commented recently that we have had a paradigm shift in our thinking about the healthfulness of vegetarian diets. As we have come to recognize the benefits of plant-based foods in preventing chronic disease, we have begun to encourage use of more cereals, legumes, fruits, and vegetables. It is possible to plan both plant-rich and plant-only diets that will support nutrient needs at all stages of the lifecycle. The increased availability of fortified foods makes dietary planning a bit easier for those consuming plant-only diets. We need to make our clients aware of all alternatives for obtaining a nutritionally adequate diet.*

*Practical advice for vegetarian meal planning can be found in Duyff RL: *The American Dietetic Association's complete food and nutrition guide,* Minneapolis, 1998, Chronimed Publishing.

REFERENCES

Dwyer J: Convergence of plant-rich and plant-only diets, *Am J Clin Nutr* 70(suppl):620S, 1999.

Hebbelinch M, Clarys P, DeMalsche A: Growth, development, and physical fitness of Flemish vegetarian children, adolescents, and young adults, *Am J Clin Nutr* 70(suppl):579S, 1999.

Hokin BD, Butler T: Cyanocobalamin (vitamin B-12) status in Seventh-Day Adventist ministers in Australia, *Am J Clin Nutr* 70(suppl):576S, 1999.

Johnson PK: Nutritional implications of vegetarian diets. In Shils ME et al, eds: *Modern nutrition in health and disease,* ed 9, Philadelphia, 1999, Lippincott Williams & Wilkins.

Messina V, Burke KI: Vegetarian diets: position of the American Dietetic Association, *J Am Diet Assoc* 97:1317, 1997 (reaffirmed until December 31, 2001).

Messina V, Mangels AR: Considerations in planning vegan diets: children, *J Am Diet Assoc* 101:661, 2001.

Peregrin T: A successful diet for vegan children nourishes the child, *J Am Diet Assoc* 101:669, 2001.

Willett WC: Convergence of philosophy and science: the third international conference on vegetarian nutrition, *Am J Clin Nutr* 70(suppl):434S, 1999.

Chapter

6

Energy Balance and Weight Management

Eleanor D. Schlenker

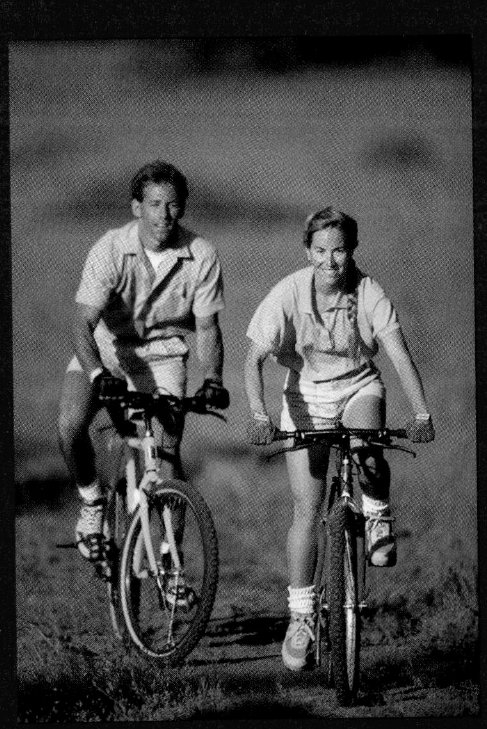

Chapter Outline

In Chapters 3, 4, and 5 we reviewed the three energy nutrients—carbohydrate, fat, and protein. In this chapter we consider the relationship between body energy balance and body weight, problems of overweight and underweight, and their effects on health.

We will find, however, that energy balance is not a simple matter. We are not all alike, and our energy needs vary under different circumstances and for different body types. Each of us is unique, and our varying body weights reflect this fact. This individual view of weight patterns is difficult for modern society to accept, and the social norm of thinness creates undue pressure for many whose natural weight cannot conform.

Here we will seek an improved goal of weight management based on sound nutrition, physical and emotional health, and physical fitness. This approach is important for all persons, but especially for those with health risks related to excess body weight.

The Human Energy System

ENERGY CYCLE AND ENERGY TRANSFORMATION

Forms of Human Energy

It is clear that in our physical world, energy, like matter, is neither created nor destroyed. When we speak of energy "production," what we really mean is energy is being *transformed.* Energy is being changed in form and cycled throughout a system. In the human body the various metabolic processes convert the stored chemical energy in our food to other forms of energy for the body's work. In our bodies, energy is available in four basic forms for life processes: *chemical, electrical, mechanical,* and *thermal.* Our ultimate source of power is the sun with its vast reservoir of heat and light (Figure 6-1). Then through the process of photosynthesis, described in the discussion on carbohydrates in Chapter 3 (see Figure 3-1), plants use water and carbon dioxide as raw materials to transform the sun's energy into food storage forms of chemical energy. In the body these stored food fuels are converted to the basic energy unit glucose, which together with fatty acids is metabolized to release its energy to be transformed and cycled through body systems. Water and carbon dioxide, the initial materials used by plants, are retrieved as end products of this process of oxidation in the body. And so the cycle goes on and on.

Transformation of Energy

After the stored chemical energy in food is taken into the body, it undergoes the many processes of metabolism that convert it further to other metabolic products containing stored chemical energy to do the body's work. This chemical energy is then changed still further to other forms of energy as body work is performed. For example, chemical energy is changed to electrical energy in brain and nerve activity. It is changed to mechanical energy in muscle contraction. It is changed to thermal energy in the regulation of body temperature. It is changed to still other types of chemical energy in the synthesis of new compounds. In all of these work activities of the body, heat is given off to the surrounding atmosphere and larger biosphere.

In human *metabolism,* as in any energy system, energy is always present as either *free energy* or *potential energy.* Free energy is the energy involved at any given moment in the performance of a task. It is unbound and in motion. Potential energy is the energy that is stored or bound in the various chemical compounds available for conversion to free energy as needed for work. For example, energy stored in sugar is potential energy. When we eat it and it is metabolized, free energy is released and body work is accomplished. As work is done, energy in the form of heat is released.

Energy Balance: Input and Output

Whether the energy system is electrical, mechanical, thermal, or chemical, the supply of free energy is decreased

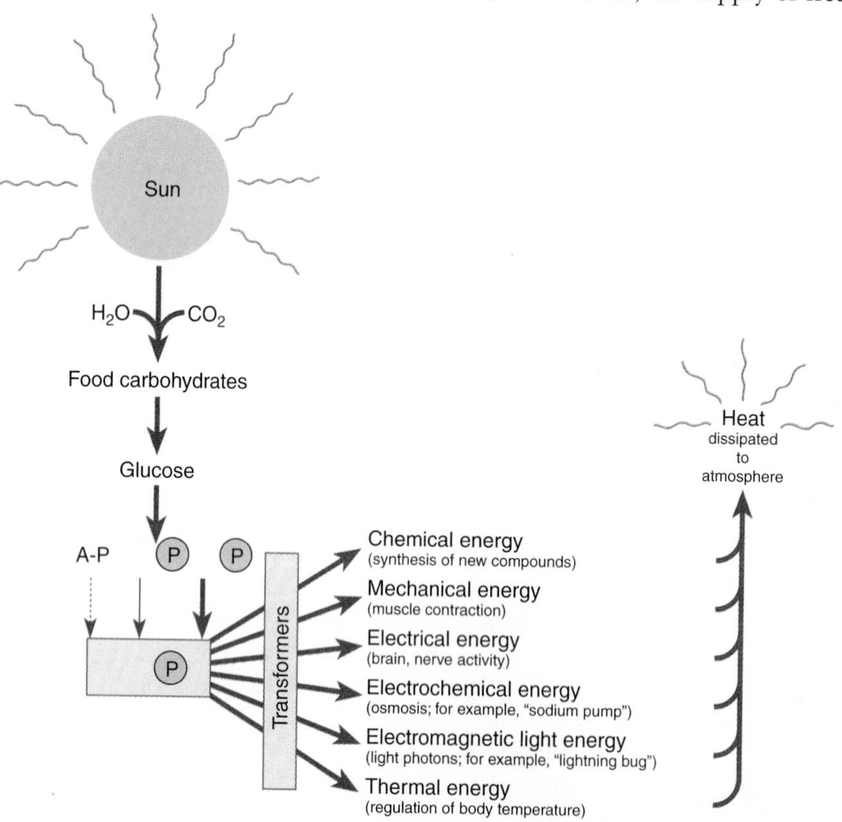

FIGURE 6-1 Transformation of energy from its primary source (the sun) to various forms for biologic work by means of metabolic processes ("transformers").

and the reservoir of potential energy is secondarily diminished through the course of the many reactions and essential work that comprise the body's internal operation. Therefore the system must be constantly refueled from some outside source; in the human energy system, this basic input of fuel is our food.

The energy demands of the body require a constant supply of available energy. Energy is needed to support the body's basal metabolic needs and to meet physical activity requirements. In the human energy system this physical energy output is evident in our activities. But energy output to an even larger degree is also going on internally at all times to meet our basal or resting energy needs.

ENERGY CONTROL IN HUMAN METABOLISM

In the human body the energy produced in its many chemical reactions, if "exploded" all at once, would be destructive. Therefore some mechanism by which energy release is controlled in the human system must exist so that it may support life and not destroy it. Two basic means of control—chemical bonding and controlled reaction rates—accomplish this task.

Chemical Bonding

The main mechanism controlling energy in the human system is chemical bonding. The chemical bonds that hold the elements in compounds together are energy bonds. As long as the compound remains constant, energy is being exerted to maintain it. When the compound is taken into the body and broken into its parts, this energy is released and available for body work. Three basic types of chemical bonds transfer energy in the body.

1. *Covalent bonds.* These are regular bonds, based on relative valence of constituent elements, that link the elements of a chemical compound together—for example, those that hold carbon atoms together in the core of an organic compound such as glucose.
2. *Hydrogen bonds.* Weaker than covalent bonds, these bonds are nonetheless significant because they can be formed in large numbers. Also, the very fact that they are less strong and can be broken easily makes them important because they can be transferred or passed readily from one substance to another to help form still another substance. The hydrogen attached to the oxygen molecule in the carboxyl group of amino or fatty acids is an example of this type of bond.
3. *High-energy phosphate bonds.* A main example of these high-energy phosphate bonds at work is the compound adenosine triphosphate (ATP), which is the unique compound the human body uses to store energy for its cell work. Like storage batteries for electrical energy, these bonds become the controlling force for ongoing energy needs.

Controlled Reaction Rates

The many chemical reactions that make up the body's energy system must have controls. Some of the reactions that break down proteins, if left to themselves—for example, as in sterile decomposition of plants—would span several years. Such reactions must be accelerated, or getting the needed energy from eating a meal would take years. At the same time, these chemical reactions must be regulated so that too fast a reaction will not produce a burst of energy in a single "explosion." Control agents that regulate these cell activities are the enzymes, coenzymes, and hormones.

1. *Enzymes.* Specific enzymes in every cell control specific cell reactions. All enzymes are protein compounds. They are produced in the cells under the control of specific genes. One specific gene controls the making of one specific enzyme, and there are thousands of enzymes in each cell. Each enzyme works on its own particular

---

adenosine triphosphate (ATP) The high-energy compound formed in the cell and called the "energy currency" of the cell because of the binding of energy in its high-energy phosphate bonds for release for cell work as these bonds are split. A compound of adenosine (a nucleotide containing adenine and ribose) that has three phosphoric acid groups. ATP is a high-energy phosphate compound important in energy exchange for cellular activity. The splitting off of the terminal phosphate bond (PO_4) of ATP to produce adenosine diphosphate (ADP) releases bound energy and transfers it to free energy available for body work. The reforming of ATP in cell oxidation again stores energy in high-energy phosphate bonds for use as needed.

chemical bonding Process of linking the radicals, chemical elements, or groups of a chemical compound.

energy The capacity of a system for doing work; available power. Energy is manifest in various forms—motion, position, light, heat, and sound. Energy is interchangeable among these various forms and is constantly being transformed and transferred among them.

enzyme Various complex proteins produced by living cells that act independently of these cells. Enzymes are capable of producing certain chemical changes in other substances without themselves being changed in the process. Their action is therefore that of a catalyst. Digestive enzymes of the gastrointestinal secretions act on food substances to break them down into simpler compounds and greatly accelerate the speed of these chemical reactions. An enzyme is usually named according to the substance (substrate) on which it acts, with the common suffix *-ase;* for example, sucrase is the specific enzyme for sucrose and breaks it down to glucose and fructose.

valence Power of an element or a radical to combine with or to replace other elements or radicals. Atoms of various elements combine in definite proportions. The valence number of an element is the number of atoms of hydrogen with which one atom of the element can combine.

substance, which is called its substrate. The enzyme and its substrate lock together to produce a new reaction product, and the original enzyme remains unchanged, ready to do its specific work over and over again (Figure 6-2).

2. *Coenzymes.* Many reactions require a partner to assist the enzyme in completing the reaction. These coenzyme partners in many instances are vitamins, especially the B-complex vitamins, or a particular mineral. It may be helpful to think of the coenzyme as another substrate, because in receiving the material transferred, the coenzyme is changed or reduced.
3. *Hormones.* In energy metabolism hormones act as messengers to trigger or control enzyme action. For example, the rate of oxidative reactions in the tissues—the body's metabolic rate—is controlled by the *thyroid-stimulating hormone (TSH)* from the anterior pituitary gland. Another familiar example is the controlling action of insulin from the beta cells of the pancreas on the rate of glucose utilization in the tissues. Steroid hormones also have the capacity to regulate the cell's ability to synthesize enzymes.

Types of Metabolic Reactions

The two types of reactions constantly going on in energy metabolism are anabolism and catabolism. Each requires energy. The process of *anabolism* synthesizes new and more complex substances. The process of *catabolism* breaks down more complex substances to simpler ones. These processes release free energy, but the work also uses up some free energy. Therefore there is a constant energy deficit, which must be supplied by food.

Sources of Stored Energy

When food is not available, as in periods of fasting or starvation, the body must draw on its own stores for energy:

1. *Glycogen.* Only a 12- to 36-hour reserve of glycogen exists in liver and muscle, and it is quickly depleted.
2. *Muscle mass.* Storage of energy as protein exists in limited amounts in muscle mass but in greater volume than in glycogen stores.
3. *Adipose fat tissue.* Although fat storage may be larger, the supply varies from person to person and from circumstance to circumstance.

MEASUREMENT OF ENERGY BALANCE

Kilocalorie

Because the body performs work only as energy is released by chemical reactions and because all work takes the form of heat production, energy may be measured in terms of heat equivalents. Such a heat measure is the calorie. To avoid using large numbers, the professional nutritionist and biochemist use the term kilocalorie (1000 calories), abbreviated kcalorie or kcal. This is the amount of heat required to raise 1 kg of water 1° C.

Joule

The international (*Système International d'Unités* [SI]) unit of energy measurement is the joule. It expresses the amount of energy expended when 1 kg of a substance is moved 1 m by a force of 1 Newton (N). It was named for James Prescott Joule (1818-1889), an English physicist who discovered the first law of thermodynamics. The conversion factor for changing kcalories to kilojoules (kJ) is 4.184—1 kcalorie equals 4.184 kJ. Because the energy values of diets expressed in kilojoules are very large numbers, a simpler term is the megajoule (MJ)—1 MJ equals 239 kcalories. Many nutrition and dietetics research journals now describe the results of energy metabolism studies in kJ rather than in kcalories; therefore it is important that you keep these conversion factors in mind.

FOOD ENERGY MEASUREMENT

The energy value of a particular food can be measured in two ways: calorimetry and calculation of the approximate composition.

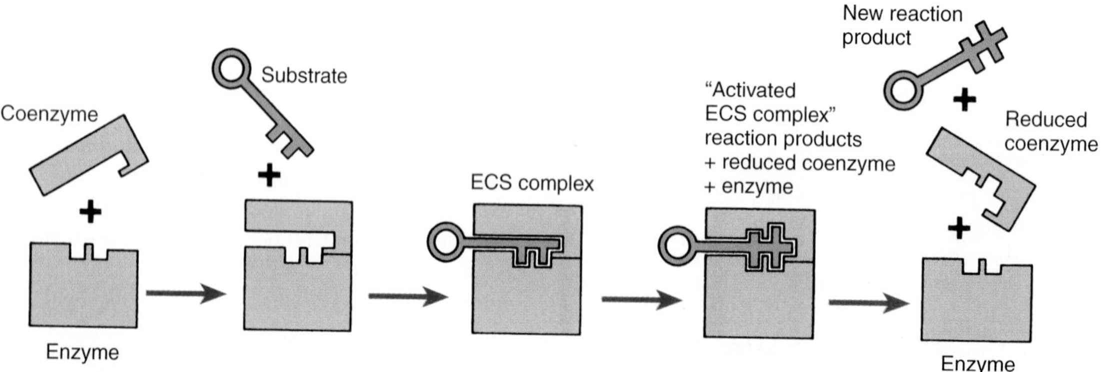

FIGURE 6-2 Lock-and-key concept of the action of enzyme, coenzyme, and substrate to produce a new reaction product.

Calorimetry

The kcalorie values of various foods expressed in food tables (as found in Appendix A) have usually been determined by a method called direct calorimetry.[1] This method uses a metal container called a *bomb calorimeter.* The name comes from its long tubular shape. A weighed amount of food is placed inside, and the instrument is immersed in water. The food is then ignited by an electric spark in the presence of oxygen and burned. The increase in the temperature of the surrounding water indicates the number of kcalories given off by the oxidation of the food. You must remember when you use food value tables, however, that these values represent averages from a number of samples of the given food tested. The value of a particular serving of that food varies around that average.

Approximate Composition

An alternate method of measuring food energy is by calculating the kcalorie contribution of the carbohydrate, fat, and protein contents given in the approximate nutrient composition of the food in food tables. These calculations are based on the average kcalorie value per gram of each of the three energy-yielding macronutrients. These values are known as their respective fuel factors: 1 g of carbohydrate yields 4 kcalories, 1 g of fat yields 9 kcalories, and 1 g of protein yields 4 kcalories. In comparison, 1 g of beverage alcohol yields 7 kcalories.

Total Energy Requirements

The total energy expended by an individual supports three essential energy needs: (1) basal metabolic rate, (2) food intake effect, and (3) physical activity.

BASAL METABOLIC NEEDS

Basal Metabolic Rate (BMR)

The sum of all the internal chemical activities that maintain the body at rest comprise its basal metabolism. The basal metabolic rate (BMR) is a measure of the energy required by these activities of resting tissue. Certain small but vitally active tissues—brain, liver, gastrointestinal tract, heart, and kidneys—together make up less than 5% of the total body weight, yet they contribute about 60% of the total basal metabolic activity. The BMR is the largest component of energy expenditure in humans, making up about 60% to 75% of the daily energy expenditure of most persons.[2] The basal energy metabolism is influenced by not only the physical characteristics of the individual but also the pretesting environment.[1,2] For the measurement of BMR, the individual must be (1) in a postabsorptive state (12 to 16 hours after food intake), (2) reclining but awake (½ to 1 hour of rest prior), (3) relaxed, (4) at normal body temperature, and (5) in a comfortable room temperature (neither hot nor cold). In practice the BMR is seldom measured because of the practical problems involved. Instead, the resting metabolic rate (RMR) is most often used in the clinical setting, because it does not require the subject to be in a fasting state. The RMR may be slightly higher than the BMR,

basal metabolic rate (BMR) Amount of energy required to maintain the resting body's internal activities after an overnight fast with the subject awake. See also **resting metabolic rate (RMR)**.

calorie A unit of heat energy. The calorie used in the study of metabolism is the large calorie, or kilocalorie, defined as the amount of heat required to raise the temperature of 1 kg of water 1° Celsius (centigrade).

calorimetry Measurement of amounts of heat absorbed or given out. *Direct method:* measurement of amount of heat produced by a subject enclosed in a small chamber. *Indirect method:* measurement of amount of heat produced by a subject by the quantity of nitrogen and carbon dioxide eliminated.

fuel factor The kilocalorie value (energy potential) of food nutrients; that is, the number of kilocalories that 1 g of the nutrient yields when oxidized. The kilocalorie fuel factor for carbohydrate is 4; for protein, 4; and for fat, 9. The basic figures are used in computing diets and energy values of foods. (For example, 10 g of fat yields 90 kcalories.)

hormones Various internally secreted substances from the endocrine organs, which are conveyed by the blood to another organ or tissue on which they act to stimulate increased functional activity or secretion. This tissue or substance is called its target organ or substance.

joule The international (SI) unit of energy and heat, defined as the work done by the force of 1 N acting over the distance of 1 m. A Newton (named for Sir Isaac Newton, 1643-1727, English mathematician, physicist, and astronomer) is the international unit of force, defined as the amount of force that, when applied in a vacuum to a body having a mass of 1 kg, accelerates it at the rate of 1 m/s. These are examples of the exactness with which terms and values used by the world's scientific community must be defined, as illustrated in the *Système International d'Unités* (SI).

kilocalorie The general term *calorie* refers to a unit of heat measure and is used alone to designate the *small calorie.* The calorie used in nutritional science and the study of metabolism is the *large calorie,* 1000 calories, or kilocalorie, to be more accurate and to avoid the use of very large numbers in calculations.

resting metabolic rate (RMR) Amount of energy required to maintain the resting body's internal activities when in a normal environmental temperature and awake. Because of small differences in measuring techniques, RMR may be slightly different from the same person's **basal metabolic rate (BMR)**. In practice, however, RMR and BMR measurements may be used interchangeably.

substrate The specific organic substance on which a particular enzyme acts to produce new metabolic products.

because it likely includes energy being expended in the digestion, absorption, or metabolism of food.

Measuring Basal Metabolic Rate

The BMR can be measured by both direct and indirect methods of calorimetry.

1. *Direct calorimetry.* With the direct method, a person is placed in a large chamber and the body's heat production at rest is measured. This instrument is large and costly and therefore is limited to research studies.[1]
2. *Indirect calorimetry.* With the indirect method, a portable instrument called a *respirometer* is brought to the side of the bed or chair on a cart. In the clinical situation this complete apparatus is often called the *metabolic cart.* The person breathes into the instrument through a mouthpiece or by means of a ventilated hood, and the exchange of gases in respiration, the *respiratory quotient* (CO_2/O_2), is measured with the subject at rest. The metabolic rate can be calculated with a high degree of accuracy from the rate of oxygen utilization, because more than 95% of the energy expended by the body is derived from metabolic reactions with oxygen.[3] The energy expenditure (BMR) measured in this manner is equivalent to the heat released by the body.
3. *Indirect laboratory tests.* Because the thyroid hormone thyroxin regulates BMR, thyroid function tests are used in clinical practice to serve as indirect measures of BMR and thyroid function. These tests include measures of serum TSH and thyroxin levels, both triiodothyronine (T_3) and thyroxin (T_4), as well as the radioactive iodine uptake test. T_3 and T_4 are produced in the final two stages of thyroid hormone synthesis and reflect the relative functioning of the thyroid gland and the amount of hormone activity influencing the BMR.

Factors Influencing Basal Metabolic Rate

The four main factors influencing BMR are lean body mass (LBM), growth, fever or disease, and climate.

1. *Lean body mass.* LBM, including muscle cells and vital body organs, is the major factor influencing BMR because of its greater level of metabolic activity compared with the less active tissues of fat and bones. For example, differences in metabolic requirements between women and men are primarily related to the generally lower amount of muscle mass and higher amount of body fat in women compared with those in men. The lower BMR of elderly people is related to the loss of lean tissue that occurs as we age.
2. *Growth.* Growth during childhood and pregnancy and milk production during lactation require anabolic work under the influence of growth hormone.
3. *Fever and disease.* Fever increases BMR about 7% for each 0.83° C (1° F) rise in body temperature. In addition, diseases involving increased cell activity—such as cancer, certain anemias, cardiac failure, hypertension, and respiratory problems such as chronic obstructive pulmonary disease—usually increase BMR. The involuntary muscle tremors occurring in Parkinson's disease appear to increase metabolic energy needs in these patients.[2] Conversely, the abnormal states of starvation and protein-energy malnutrition lower BMR because the LBM is diminished.
4. *Climate.* BMR rises in response to lower temperatures as a compensatory mechanism to produce heat and maintain body temperature. An opposite action occurs in those living in the tropics, and they have a decreased BMR.

FOOD INTAKE EFFECT

Food ingestion stimulates metabolism and requires energy to meet the multiple activities of digestion, absorption, metabolism, and storage of nutrients. This overall metabolic stimulation is called the thermic effect of food (TEF). About 10% of the body's total energy needs are used in activities related to metabolizing food.

PHYSICAL ACTIVITY NEEDS

Exercise performed in work and recreation or in physical training and competition accounts for wide individual variations in energy requirements (see Chapter 14). The effects of various activities on energy metabolism have been measured by the oxygen consumption method of indirect calorimetry. Some of these representative kcalorie expenditures in various types of work and recreation are given in Table 6-1. The feelings of fatigue after periods of mental concentration or study are not caused by the cerebral activity that has taken place but by the muscle tension or moving about that is involved. Heightened emotional states alone do not increase metabolic activity, but they may bring additional energy needs because they lead to increased muscle tension, restlessness, and agitated movements.

TOTAL ENERGY EXPENDITURE

In summary, the basic components of energy expenditure when body weight is remaining constant are (1) the BMR, the energy demands of the involuntary processes of the body—about 70% of the total; (2) the TEF—about 10% of the total; and (3) the variable requirements of *physical activity.* Another factor called *adaptive thermogenesis* is sometimes added. This is defined as the

TABLE 6-1 Energy Expenditure/Hour During Various Activities*

Light Activities (120-150 kcalories/hr)	Light to Moderate Activities (150-300 kcalories/hr)	Moderate Activities (300-400 kcalories/hr)	Heavy Activities (420-600 kcalories/hr)
Personal Care Dressing Shaving Washing ***Sitting*** Peeling potatoes Playing cards Playing piano Rocking Sewing Typing Writing ***Standing or Slowly Moving Around*** ***Billiards***	***Domestic Work*** Ironing Making beds Sweeping floors Washing clothes ***Yard Work*** Light gardening Mowing (power mower) ***Light Work*** Auto repair Painting Shoe repair Store clerk Washing car ***Walking*** 2-3 mph on level surface or down stairs ***Recreation*** Archery Bicycling 5½ mph on level surface Bowling Canoeing 2½-3 mph	***Yard Work*** Digging Mowing lawns (not motorized) Pulling weeds ***Walking*** 3½-4 mph on level surface Up and down small hills ***Recreation*** Badminton Ballet exercises Calisthenics Canoeing 4 mph Dancing (waltz, square) Golf (no cart) Ping-pong Tennis (doubles) Volleyball	***Yard Work*** Chopping wood Digging holes Shoveling snow ***Walking*** 5 mph Up stairs Up hills Climbing ***Recreation*** Bicycling 11-12 mph or up and down hills Cross-country skiing Jogging 5 mph Swimming Tennis (singles) Waterskiing

*Energy expenditure depends on the physical fitness (i.e., amount of lean body mass) of the individual and continuing of exercise. Note that some of these activities can be used as aerobic activities to promote cardiovascular fitness.

change in RMR associated with adaptation to environmental stress, such as changes in dietary intake, area temperature, or emotional state.

In the traditional sense a condition of overweight represents an energy imbalance resulting from an excess of energy input (fuel from food) over energy output (energy requirement or expenditure). However, investigators are continuing to learn more about genetic-related characteristics that influence weight gain and body weight. An exceptionally low RMR, characteristic of an inherited obesity disorder, has been identified in certain persons and population groups.[4,5] Characteristic fidgeting-like activity, sometimes referred to as nonexercise activity thermogenesis, appears to prevent weight gain in particular individuals.[6] Obese persons seem to be more efficient in metabolizing and storing absorbed nutrients and expend less energy in the TEF.[7] Some medical conditions may contribute to body weight gain.

Weight loss results from a deficit of energy intake to meet the body's energy requirement, as fat stores or muscle is broken down to provide the necessary energy. Uncontrolled weight loss may result from a hypermetabolic disease such as cancer or from a psychologic problem leading to self-starvation as occurs in anorexia nervosa (see *Issues & Answers*).

Where do you stand in your own energy balance? Try estimating your energy requirement based on your (1) total energy output per day, (2) body mass index (BMI), and (3) height-weight tables (see *Practical Application* box). Compare your estimate with your general energy needs as indicated in the Recommended Dietary Allowance (RDA) standards printed inside the back cover of this book.

thermic effect of food (TEF) Body heat produced by food; amount of energy required to digest and absorb food and transport nutrients to the cells. This basic preparatory work accounts for about 10% of the day's total energy (kcalories) requirement.

PRACTICAL APPLICATION
Evaluating Your Energy Expenditure and Body Weight

As a health professional you will be assisting others in defining their energy expenditure and evaluating their current body weight according to established standards. This exercise will give you experience in carrying out these activities and help you assess your own energy expenditure and weight status. Remember: a status of underweight presents as urgent a need for intervention as does a status of overweight or obesity.

A. CALCULATE YOUR TOTAL ENERGY OUTPUT PER DAY

Your total energy output in kcalories per day is the sum of your body's three uses of energy.

1. Resting metabolic rate (RMR)
2. Thermic effect of food (TEF)
3. Physical activity

1. RMR

Use the general formula.

Women: 0.9 kcalories/kg/hr
Men: 1.0 kcalories/kg/hr

Convert your body weight (lb) to kg: 1 kg = 2.2 lb. Multiply by the following formula.

RMR (kcalories) = 0.9 or 1.0 × kg body weight × 24 (hours in day) = ________

2. TEF Intake

The TEF is the energy the body uses in the process of digestion and absorption. It averages 10% of the energy in the food.

Record your food intake for 1 day (24 hours) and calculate the approximate energy value in kcalories, using either the table of food values in Appendix A or a simple computer program. If you completed the *Practical Application* in Chapter 1, you might want to use the average energy intake calculated from that dietary record.

Find the energy cost of TEF.

TEF (kcalories) = 0.10 × total food intake (kcalories)
TEF (kcalories) = ______

3. Physical Activity

Estimate your average level of physical activity. Energy expended in physical activity can be approximated from your RMR and varies with the level or amount of physical activity. Use the following to select your activity level.

Average Activity Level	Energy Cost (% of RMR)
Sedentary	20
Very light	30
Moderate	40
Heavy	50

Calculate the energy cost of your physical activity.

Your RMR × your activity (%) = ______

For example, if you are sedentary (mostly sitting), you would multiply your RMR × 0.20.

4. Calculate Your Total Energy Output

Total energy output (kcalories) = ____ (RMR) + ____ (TEF) + ____ (physical activity)

Total energy output (kcalories) = ____

Example 1

A woman weighs 130 lb (59 kg) and eats an average of 1800 kcalories per day. She has begun and has maintained a regular physical exercise program.

RMR = 0.9 × 59 × 24 = 1274 kcalories
TEF = 1800 × 0.10 = 180 kcalories
Activity = 1274 × 0.40 = 510 kcalories
Total energy output = 1964 kcalories

Result: Her energy output exceeds her energy intake by about 150 kcalories per day. Is this woman gaining or losing weight? In general, 1 lb of body weight equals approximately 3500 kcalories. What would be her approximate rate of weight gain or weight loss if she continues to follow this diet and exercise pattern?

Example 2

A man weighs 180 lb (82 kg), eats an average of 2700 kcalories per day, and has a sedentary lifestyle.

RMR = 1 × 82 × 24 = 1968 kcalories
TEF = 2700 × 0.10 = 270 kcalories
Activity = 1968 × 0.20 = 394 kcalories
Total energy output = 2632 kcalories

Result: This man will tend to gain weight slowly over time. What would be his approximate weight gain per month? What would be your clinical advice to him?

B. EVALUATE YOUR BODY WEIGHT STATUS ACCORDING TO THE BODY MASS INDEX (BMI)

1. Calculate Your BMI

BMI is usually calculated in metric terms as follows.

$$\text{BMI} = \text{weight (kg)} \div \text{height (m)}^2$$

BMI may also be calculated using weight in pounds and height in inches, using a mathematical calculation factor as follows.

Step 1: Multiply your body weight (lb) × 705 = ______

PRACTICAL APPLICATION
Evaluating Your Energy Expenditure and Body Weight—cont'd

Step 2: Divide your result from Step 1 by your height (in) = ______

Step 3: Divide your result from Step 2 by your height (in) = ______

Your BMI = ______

Most adults have a BMI in the 20s. Health risks associated with overweight begin at a BMI above 25, and individuals with a BMI of 30 or above are considered obese (see p. 113).

What is your assessment of your body weight status using the BMI? Are you seriously underweight, overweight, or in a healthful range? Based on the chart in Figure 6-3, are you at health risk related to your current BMI? If you are not in the healthful range, how would you go about improving your situation?

Example 3

The man described below has come to you for a health assessment. He currently weighs 160 lb and he is 62 inches tall. First, you will need to calculate his BMI.

Step 1:	160 × 705 =	112,800
Step 2:	112,800 ÷ 62 =	819
Step 3:	1819 ÷ 62 =	29
	His BMI =	29

What is your assessment of this man's health risk? What type of program would you develop for him?

C. EVALUATE YOUR BODY WEIGHT USING A WEIGHT-FOR-HEIGHT TABLE

Using Table 6-2 in your text, find the average weight and weight range for a person of your age and sex. Does your body weight fall within the body weight range given? Are you underweight, overweight, or in the appropriate weight range according to this table?

Example 4

A young woman who is 34 years of age is 5 ft 3 in tall and weighs 113 lb. The weight range for this woman is 107 to 141 lb and the average weight is 124 lb. How would you advise her regarding her body weight. What is her BMI?

COMPARISON OF METHODS

How did your assessment of your body weight status compare using the two methods above? In other words, were you underweight, overweight, or in an appropriate weight range by both methods? If your assessment was not the same, what are some reasons why this might have occurred?

Body Composition: Fatness and Leanness

BODY WEIGHT VERSUS BODY FAT

Sometimes the common terms obesity and *overweight* are used without the necessary attention to body composition. It is important to consider first the distinct meanings and concepts embodied in each of these terms.

Obesity

As used in the traditional medical model, the word *obesity* is a clinical term for excess body weight, defined in the sense of a disease. It is generally applied to a person who is 20% or more above a so-called *standard weight,* displayed in a height-weight table. The first height-weight tables were constructed many years ago by the Metropolitan Life Insurance Company from information obtained from their life insurance holders, largely white middle-aged men. Desirable weights were based on the body weights of the individuals who lived the longest. The Metropolitan Life Insurance Standards, last updated in 1983, are still in use in many healthcare facilities. Unfortunately, these standards suggest that body weight should not increase beyond age 20 to 30, which may not be appropriate for the evaluation of elderly individuals.[8] Also, traditional height-weight tables are not appropriate for all racial and ethnic groups in whom body build and weight patterns may differ.[9] Thus, they tell us little about particular individuals.

Another problem lies in use of the word *standard.* Standard weight is the average weight of an individual of a particular sex, height, and frame. But every person is an individual, a unique and complex human being, and *normal* values in healthy persons vary over a relatively wide range. Age also plays a large role in this variance. Later in this chapter we will discuss the concept of *healthy weight,*

---

body composition The relative sizes of the four basic body compartments that make up the total body: lean body mass (muscle mass), fat, water, and bone.

obesity Fatness; an excessive accumulation of fat in the body.

a more appropriate term for helping our clients manage their body weight.

Overweight Versus Overfat

We often use the term *overweight* as a synonym for obese, but the two terms are not interchangeable, and the distinction is important. A football player in peak condition can be markedly "overweight" according to standard height-weight charts. That is, he can weigh considerably more than the average man of the same height, but his body tissues may be very different. A sedentary individual above average weight likely has an excess amount of body fat adding to his total body weight. In contrast, the athlete above average weight likely has an exceptionally high amount of body muscle adding to his body weight. In clinical use, the term *overweight* refers to a person with a body weight about 10% above the desirable weight given in the height-weight table.[8] For those individuals for whom this overweight is related to excessive body fat rather than greater amounts of lean tissue, the term *overfat* would be a more correct designation. Individuals who are more than 20% above desirable weight are considered to be obese, and the excessive amount of fat associated with this condition presents a significant health risk.

Body Composition

The critical element in determining a reasonable body weight is body composition. In relation to body weight and health, what we really need to know is how much of the body weight is fat and how much is LBM. It is much more precise to talk in terms of *fatness* and *leanness* than in terms of body weight or overweight. When speaking of body weight, we need to ask for whom, under what circumstances, and by what measures. We need to consider individual body composition and use some practical means of determining it as a guideline for planning individual care. On the basis of metabolic activity—energy (kcalories) demand—and comparative size, the four-compartment model of body composition is commonly used. The four compartments include LBM, body fat, body water, and mineral mass (mainly bone). Based on laboratory studies with adults, in this model approximately 50% of the body weight is water, 25% is fat, 20% is LBM, and 5% is mineral mass.

1. *Lean body mass.* This major body component, composed of active fat-free cell mass, largely determines the BMR and energy and nutrient needs. It changes through the life cycle and in adulthood accounts for 30% to 65% of the total body weight. In sedentary people it accounts for almost the entire energy requirement. When persons lose body weight from changes in their diet, the weight loss reflects changes not only in body fat but also in LBM. Physical activity and exercise are essential for developing and maintaining the relative size of the LBM across the adult years.
2. *Body fat.* Total body fat varies widely with individual degrees of fatness or leanness. These differences reflect both the number and the size of fat cells (the adipocytes) that make up the adipose tissue. In an adult man of average weight, fat accounts for a range of 14% to 28% of total body weight. In a woman, it is somewhat greater, about 15% to 29% of body weight. These amounts vary with age, climate, exercise, and fitness. About half the body fat is found in the subcutaneous fat layers under the skin, where it serves as insulation. In younger people the subcutaneous fat provides a useful measure—the triceps skinfold—for estimating body fat in relation to LBM. In older individuals more of the body fat is deposited on the trunk, and abdominal and hip circumferences may be better measures of health risk.
3. *Body water.* The body water content varies with relative leanness or fatness and with age, hydration status, and health status. Generally water makes up about 50% to 65% of body weight. Lean persons have a somewhat larger proportion of body water because lean muscle tissue contains more water than any other body tissue except blood. Adipose tissue is rather low in water content.
4. *Bone.* The remaining mineral mass, found largely in the skeleton, accounts for only about 4% to 6% of the total body weight. The major mineral component is calcium, as you would expect, which constitutes about 75% of the body mineral mass in bone and other body cells and fluids.

In free-living populations, however, individuals vary widely around these general body composition proportions. A number of factors influence these variances.[9]

- *Gender.* Women have more fat tissue, and men have more muscle mass.
- *Age.* Younger adults have more LBM and less fat than older adults.
- *Physical exercise.* Persons who are physically fit from daily work or other physical activities have less fat and more LBM than do persons who lead sedentary lives.
- *Race.* Black men and women have higher bone mineral mass than do white men and women, respectively.
- *Climate.* Individuals living in cold climates have somewhat more subcutaneous fat to protect body temperature than do those living in hot tropical areas.
- *Weight extremes.* Obese persons have excess fat in relation to LBM.

Measuring Body Composition

Various indirect methods of measuring body composition have been developed; these include such classic means as water displacement (weighing under water) or measuring amounts of naturally occurring radioactive isotopes in the body using a whole body counter. Newer methods include x-ray absorption and reflection, electrical conductivity and resistance, magnetic resonance, and other research techniques that can differentiate among muscle, fat, and bone.[10] In clinical practice estimates of body composition can be made from measurements of body circumferences and skinfold thicknesses. (We will discuss these methods in detail in Chapter 15.)

STANDARD WEIGHT-FOR-HEIGHT MEASUREMENTS

Despite the limitations associated with weight-for-height standards, they continue to be used in the clinical setting as a means of estimating body composition and body fat and relating these findings to health status. Several approaches can be used to evaluate body weight: (1) height-weight tables from insurance data, (2) National Research Council height-weight tables, and (3) BMI.

Height-Weight Tables From Insurance Data

The height-weight tables used in many healthcare settings are based on the Metropolitan Life Insurance Company's so-called ideal weight-for-height charts, derived from life expectancy data gathered by the company since the 1930s. As noted earlier, however, this information base is not adequate for today's diverse population. Also, researchers have found that health risks are as great in the very low-weight range as in the very high-weight range. Within each age group, extremely thin—as well as extremely obese—persons have higher mortality rates, although high mortality rates among extremely thin persons may be related to smoking.[11] The most appropriate message is that persons should strive to be neither excessively overweight nor excessively underweight. Increased mortality rates become most apparent at body weights that are 20% below average weight or 20% or more above average weight.[11,12]

Age is also a factor when considering the risk associated with increasing body weight. Moderate obesity increases the risk of cardiovascular disease in younger men; however, excessive body fat does not add substantially to mortality risk in the elderly.[13]

National Research Council Tables From Population Surveys

The Food and Nutrition Board of the National Research Council has developed height-weight standards based on the average weights of Americans measured in national dietary surveys. These guides, found in Table 6-2, relate height and adult age to good ranges of body weight, as well as to BMI.[14] It is important to remember, however, that these average weights, based on actual measurements of the current population, are higher than the body weights set forth as desirable weights in the Metropolitan Life Insurance Standards. Unfortunately, Americans of all ages are becoming heavier, and average weights are increasing.

Body Mass Index

The BMI, first developed by Quetelet in 1871, provides a better estimate of body fat than standard height-weight tables and has become the medical standard to define obesity. Based on a body weight and body height measurement, this index correlates well with estimates of total body fat obtained from laboratory research studies. Moreover, in population studies the BMI was an effective predictor of excessive fat-related increases in health risk. The BMI can be calculated as follows.

$$\text{BMI} = \text{Weight (kg)} \div \text{height (m)}^2$$

The metric conversion factors involved are (1) 1 kg equals 2.2 lb and (2) 1 m equals 39.37 in. The desirable BMI range for health maintenance in adults is 20 to 25 kg/m^2. Health risks associated with obesity begin at about 25 kg/m^2 and become apparent at 30 kg/m^2. Values above 40 kg/m^2 indicate severe obesity. The healthy weight chart included in the 2000 edition of the *Dietary Guidelines for Americans* is based on the BMI[14] (Figure 6-3).

INDIVIDUAL VARIATION

Ideal Weight Versus Healthy Weight

The basic problem with the concept of an ideal weight is that it really cannot be defined for most people. An appropriate body weight depends on many factors, including age, body shape, metabolic rate, genetic makeup, gender, and physical activity, among many others. Persons can carry different amounts of body weight in good health based on their age, sex, and race. A cycle involving a rapid loss of weight brought about by a poorly designed low-kcalorie diet followed by an equal or even greater weight gain is undesirable for health and well-being. According to the American Dietetic Association, goals for successful weight management are based on the development of healthy eating and exercise patterns that are tolerable and enjoyable and can be maintained for a lifetime.[15] Goals for the obese individual may include halting further weight gain and reducing health risks, keeping in mind that a weight loss as low as 10 lb can lead to functional improvements in blood pressure or glucose tolerance. Programs should focus on healthy weight goals and functional improvements that can be achieved and maintained, rather than an ideal body weight that cannot be realized, leading to further frustration and self-doubt.

---

adipocyte A fat cell. All cell names end in the suffix *-cyte,* with the type of cell indicated by the root word to which it is added.

TABLE 6-2 Good Body Weights-for-Height for Adults, Expressed in Pounds (for Height, in feet and inches) and in Kilograms (for Height, in Centimeters) and Related to Body Mass Index (BMI)*

	Age (yr)					Age (yr)			
	19-34		35+			19-34		35+	
Height (ft, in)†	Average Weight (lb)	Weight Range (lb)	Average Weight (lb)	Weight Range (lb)	Height (cm)	Average Weight (kg)	Weight Range (kg)	Average Weight (kg)	Weight Range (kg)
5'0"	112	97-128	123	108-138	152	51	44-58	55	49-62
5'1"	116	101-132	127	111-143	155	53	46-60	58	50-65
5'2"	120	104-137	131	115-148	157	54	47-62	59	52-67
5'3"	124	107-141	135	119-152	160	56	49-64	61	54-69
5'4"	128	111-146	140	122-157	163	58	51-66	64	56-72
5'5"	132	114-150	144	126-162	165	60	52-68	65	57-74
5'6"	136	118-155	148	130-167	168	62	54-71	68	59-76
5'7"	140	121-160	153	134-172	170	64	55-72	69	61-78
5'8"	144	125-164	158	138-178	173	66	57-75	72	63-81
5'9"	149	129-169	162	142-183	175	67	58-77	74	64-83
5'10"	153	132-174	167	146-188	178	70	60-79	76	67-86
5'11"	157	136-179	172	151-194	180	71	62-81	78	68-88
6'0"	162	140-184	177	155-199	183	74	64-84	80	70-90
6'1"	166	144-189	182	159-205	185	75	65-86	82	72-92
6'2"	171	148-195	187	164-210	188	78	67-88	85	74-95
6'3"	176	152-200	192	168-216	191	80	69-91	88	77-99
6'4"	180	156-205	197	173-222	193	82	71-93	89	78-101
6'5"	185	160-211	202	177-228	196	85	73-96	92	81-104
6'6"	190	164-216	208	182-234	198	86	75-98	94	82-106
					BMI (kg/m^2)	22	19-25	24	21-27

Data from U.S. Department of Agriculture, Department of Health and Human Services: *Nutrition and your health: dietary guidelines for Americans,* ed 3, Washington, DC, 1990, U.S. Government Printing Office; and from Bray GA: Pathophysiology of obesity, *Am J Clin Nutr* 55:448S, 1992.
*Without clothes.
†Without shoes.

Need for Body Fat

Some body fat is necessary for survival. This has been demonstrated in times of human starvation. Such victims die of fat loss, not of protein depletion. For mere survival, men require about 3% body fat and women require about 12%. However, we need to do more than just stay alive. For the human race to continue, we must be able to work and reproduce. The additional body fat carried by women has evolved to enable them to bear children. For reproductive capacity, women require about 20% body fat. The initiation of menstruation, or menarche, occurs when the female body reaches a certain size or, more precisely, when the young girl's body fat reaches this critical proportion of body weight (about 20%). Approximately this amount is needed for ovulation and thus for eventual pregnancy. Most women gain body fat during pregnancy. This fat storage is important for lactation because the production of breast milk has a high energy cost. Usually the lactation period brings about a gradual loss of these body fat stores. Ill-advised dieting during pregnancy in an attempt to avoid normal weight gain can interfere with the development of the fetus and lead to a low-birth-weight infant at risk for various health problems.

Health, Obesity, and Social Image

OBESITY AND HEALTH

Common Beliefs

General opinion regarding obesity and health has undergone many changes over the years. In colonial times obesity was a sign of economic well-being and identified a family that was prosperous. In recent years the general public has come to see obesity as "bad for you," and the unfortunate media reports that glamorize the very thin body image have reinforced these concerns about body weight. Health professionals have added to this preoccupation with body weight with the traditional medical opinion that obesity is an illness, and the news media saturates the public with reports relating obesity to a wide variety of health problems.[11,15,16] Individuals with excessive body fat are at greater risk of hyperlipidemia, diabetes, hypertension, and complications with surgery or pregnancy. This broad "medicalization" of obesity views all fatness as an unhealthy condition that must be prevented, controlled, or treated indefinitely, with drugs if

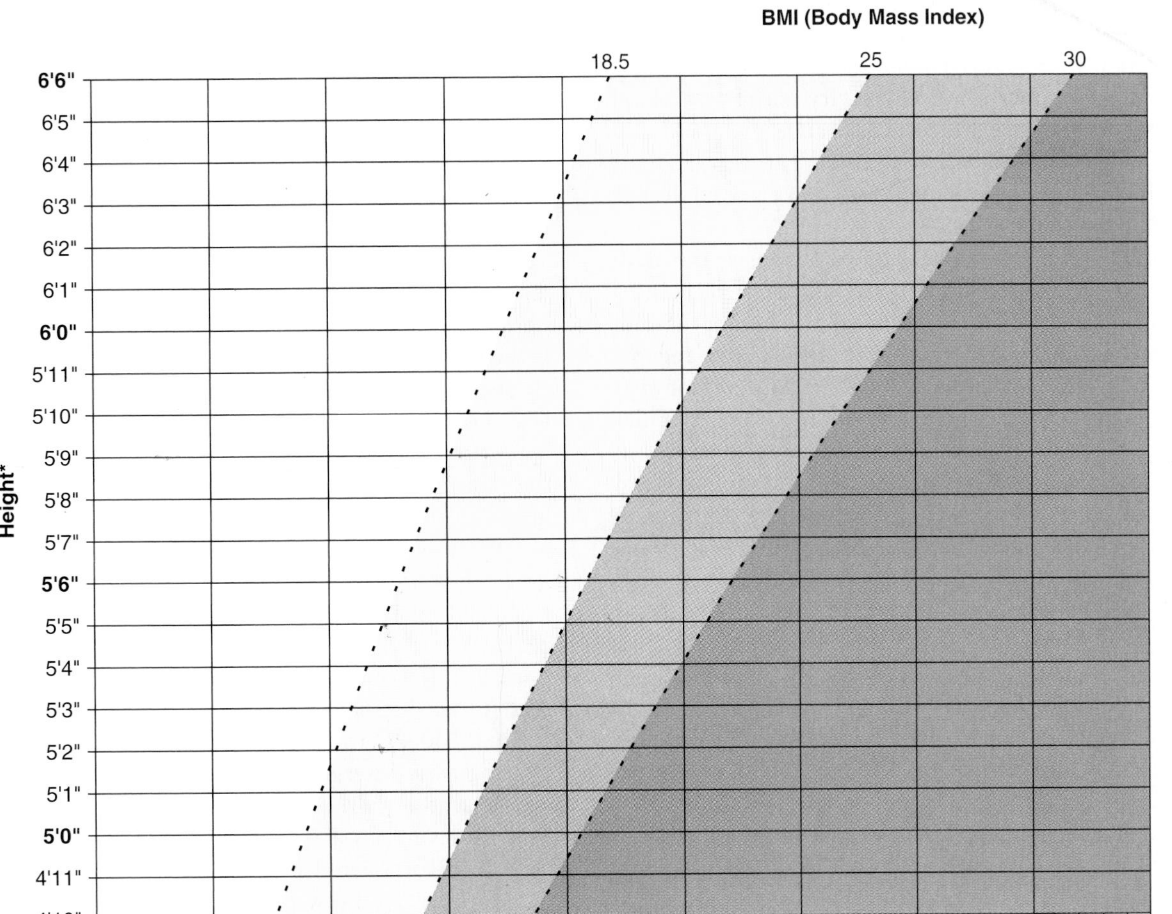

BMI measures weight in relation to height. The BMI ranges shown above are for adults. They are not exact ranges of healthy and unhealthy weights. However, they show that health risk increases at higher levels of overweight and obesity. Even within the healthy BMI range, weight gains can carry health risks for adults.

Directions: Find your weight on the bottom of the graph. Go straight up from that point until you come to the line that matches your height. Then look to find your weight group.

Healthy Weight BMI from 18.5 up to 25 refers to healthy weight.

Overweight BMI from 25 up to 30 refers to overweight.

Obese BMI 30 or higher refers to obesity. Obese persons are also overweight.

FIGURE 6-3 Chart for evaluating body mass index (BMI). Based on measurements of body height and body weight, this chart will provide an indication of an individual's body mass index and relative health risk. (*From U.S. Department of Agriculture, U.S. Department of Health and Human Services:* Nutrition and your health: dietary guidelines for Americans, *ed 5, Washington, DC, 2000, USDA/USDHHS.*)

necessary.[17,18] Such publicity has led individuals to adopt weight loss regimens that can inflict long-term damage to their overall health, result in regain of any weight lost, and lead to further loss of self-esteem.

Obesity as defined by a BMI of greater than 25 carries health risks.[14,16] However, it is important to remember that other factors associated with overweight populations also contribute to health risk. Overweight persons are more likely to belong to limited-resource families[19] and to have increased health risk as a result of less access to healthy food, hazardous environmental conditions, and inadequate healthcare. African Americans carry greater risk of developing diabetes than do Caucasians, regardless of weight status.[20] Finally, we need to

menarche The beginning of first menstruation with the onset of puberty.

look at fitness level and not merely body weight. Two overweight persons with similar body weights may differ markedly in fitness level if one walks for 30 minutes 3 times each week and the other does not. Implementing a program of regular physical activity may lower blood pressure or improve glucose tolerance even if body weight does not change. We need to learn more about the influence of fitness on health risk in the overweight or obese individual.

Public emphasis on the dangers of obesity can have negative consequences in the behaviors adopted by individuals in their attempts to achieve a more appropriate weight. Although a body weight 20% above recommended weight carries health risks, it is important that persons do not adopt eating behaviors or resort to popular drugs carrying health risks that may equal or even exceed the risk associated with their overweight. As one medical writer has pointed out, "We don't know if a person who loses 20 lb will acquire the same reduced risk as someone who started out 20 lb lighter."[16] In future sections we will discuss both appropriate and inappropriate interventions for the obese client.

Health Implications of Obesity

Obesity does carry important implications for health. Researchers have identified several adverse effects of obesity on health.

- *Hypertension, hypercholesterolemia, and diabetes.*[18,20,21] For the three health problems of essential hypertension, elevated serum cholesterol levels, and type 2 diabetes mellitus, the evidence indicates a strong association with obesity. The risk of these conditions varies directly with the extent of the obesity, and risk is lowered with weight reduction. There is also a genetic factor related to each of these chronic conditions. Thus early intervention will be of benefit, especially in high-risk families. Intervention begun as early as childhood can support fitness and a healthy weight.
- *Coronary heart disease.* Data from many studies indicate an association between degree of obesity and coronary heart disease (CHD), independent of other risk factors. This relationship starts to appear in men about age 40.[11,13] The primary conditions of hypertension, elevated blood cholesterol, and diabetes also are strong risk factors for CHD; thus obesity appears to influence the development of CHD both directly and indirectly.[18,21]
- *Cancer.* Research studies suggest a relationship between some types of cancer and obesity.[11] Obese individuals, regardless of smoking habits, have a higher cancer risk, particularly for cancers of the esophagus, stomach, and colon.[22,23] Lifestyle factors that heighten a person's risk of obesity and diabetes may also influence the development of colon cancer.[24]

Evaluations from the National Health and Nutrition Examination Survey indicated that participants with a BMI of 27 or higher had a 70% chance of an obesity-related health problem such as CHD, hypertension, diabetes, or musculoskeletal impairments.[24] Even small amounts of weight loss—5% to 10% of body weight—have been shown to improve these conditions.[18]

Emerging Attitudes About Obesity and its Treatment

A major shift, one that promotes a philosophy of trust rather than *control,* is emerging among health professionals as we develop a deeper understanding of the psychologic and social factors surrounding fatness.[15] This new philosophy supports an unrestrictive approach to eating based on internal regulation of hunger and satiety. Included in such a program is the need for options that allow choices compatible with a person's lifestyle and the opportunity for the client to participate in setting goals that are realistic and support both physical and psychologic health.

Wise professionals are evaluating the role of the medical community in not only treating but also taking a leadership role in preventing obesity.[25] This involves decisions on when individuals should first be counseled to make adjustments in their food patterns and physical activity levels: should this occur after they have gained 10 lb or added 2 in to their waist circumference, demonstrating early intervention, or after body fat has continued to accrue?[26] Trial programs offering weight reduction classes in physicians' offices to overweight patients have been successful in retention, with 65% of the participants remaining with the program for 1 year.[27] The concept of a healthy weight, a new paradigm introduced in the 2000 edition of the *Dietary Guidelines for Americans,* recognizes that not only a person's relative leanness/fatness but also the position of fat on the body and family history need to be considered when determining health risk.[14]

SOCIAL IMAGES: FEAR OF FATNESS AND EATING DISORDERS

The Thinness Model

A model of thinness, especially directed toward women, has pervaded American society. Fueled by advertising dollars from the corporate sector, an exaggerated image of thinness has been the drive for marketing many products, especially to teenagers and young adults. This ideal of thinness is impossible for most women to attain, resulting in depression and loss of self-esteem. The appearance of the somewhat emaciated models adorning the covers of many glamour magazines seem to mock most women's attempts to feel good about themselves and their bodies. Social pressures have created a fear of fatness that leads to a persistent pursuit of the abnormally thin and unrealistic ideal to the point that even fashion models express dissatisfaction with their overall body shapes.[28] These fears of fatness develop early, as observed among children in elementary and middle school. Children as young as 6 years of age report "feeling bad" after eating a high-kcalorie snack such as ice cream or a candy bar.[29] In a group of 10-year-old girls, 29% were trying to lose weight.[30] Guilt feelings after eating certain foods and inappropriate perceptions about one's body weight often form the basis for serious eating disorders that threaten both nutritional and physical health. School programs, voluntary community programs for youth such as The Girl Scouts, or sports programs can be effective environments for providing appropriate information and primary prevention for disordered eating.[30]

Chronic Dieting

The ongoing quest for the perfect body has given rise to the chronic dieter, who is constantly attempting to restrict food intake[31] although body weight often does not change. This pattern of restrained eating is most common among young women who seek to lose weight, although dieting appears to be a concern for both sexes. Among a representative sample of 16,000 U.S. adolescents, 58% of the girls and 25% of the boys were dieting.[32] While concerns regarding chronic dieting have tended to focus on weight-loss behaviors, it is important to recognize the inappropriate eating patterns being used by adolescent boys attempting to gain weight or increase muscle mass. Such diets have emphasized the use of cakes, pies, butter, fried foods, or alcohol or nighttime eating.[33]

Evolutionary Conflict and Social Pressure

The extreme degree of thinness now popular in America, however, goes against evolutionary body wisdom. It took the human species thousands of years to evolve the greater fat-carrying capacity of women for reproductive purposes. The largely futile and often dangerous attempts to drastically lower body weight have damaged the self-image of many women and men alike. Strong prejudice can exist against obese persons, regardless of their age, sex, race, or socioeconomic status. Try as they might, some persons simply cannot and do not lose weight, or they live with a perpetual cycling of ups and downs of weight, which may pose an even greater threat to their physical and emotional health.[12] They do not and cannot conform to the social norms and are blamed for their condition. Persons sometimes see obese individuals as (1) gluttonous—they eat more than they should; (2) lazy—if they wanted to, they could lose weight; (3) neurotic—they have an oral fixation on food; or (4) unhappy—they eat because they are depressed. There is no evidence for any of these stereotyped beliefs about overweight persons.

Eating Disorders

The American Psychiatric Association has described specific eating disorders, their characteristics, and the criteria for diagnosis. The most common eating disorders include anorexia nervosa, bulimia nervosa, and binge eating disorder.[34,35]

- *Anorexia nervosa,* a form of self-induced starvation, is more common in adolescent girls than in boys. Individuals with anorexia nervosa become terrified of gaining weight and refuse to eat, even though they may be hungry. They often perceive themselves to be fat, even when they are severely underweight or emaciated. This condition can become life-threatening, inducing malnutrition and requiring hospitalization (see *Issues & Answers*). A small percentage of these young victims eventually die from this disorder.
- *Bulimia nervosa,* a gorging-purging syndrome, also involves both emotional and physical problems. It is being reported more frequently, particularly by adolescent girls. Among students in grades 7 to 12, 30% of the girls reported binge eating, with 14% inducing vomiting or using laxatives. Bulimia nervosa appears to occur less frequently among boys, as only 13% engaged in binge eating and only 6% in self-induced vomiting.[36]
- *Eating disorders not otherwise specified (EDNOS).* Some individuals develop eating disorders that do not meet the criteria for any specific one. For example, the person's eating behavior may be similar to that observed in anorexia nervosa, but despite substantial weight loss, the current weight remains in the normal range and, in females, regular menses continue.[34]
- *Binge eating disorder,* an EDNOS, is characterized by recurrent episodes of eating large amounts of food in a short period. It differs from bulimia nervosa in that the recurrent episodes of binge eating are not followed by compensatory behaviors such as purging by self-induced vomiting or laxative use. The person eats rapidly and usually eats alone because of embarrassment. He or she quickly consumes large amounts of food until feeling uncomfortably full and afterward has a deep sense of guilt. These feelings of guilt make it difficult

---

anorexia nervosa Extreme psychophysiologic aversion to food, resulting in life-threatening weight loss. A psychiatric eating disorder caused by a morbid fear of fat, in which the person's distorted body image is reflected as fat when the body is actually malnourished and extremely thin from self-starvation.

binge eating An eating disorder that includes binge eating episodes but without the purging behavior of persons with bulimia nervosa. This is an emotional, reactive eating pattern occurring in response to stress or anxiety and used to soothe painful feelings.

bulimia nervosa A psychiatric eating disorder in which cycles of gorging on large quantities of food are followed by self-induced vomiting and use of diuretics and laxatives to maintain a "normal" body weight.

to obtain accurate reports of typical food intakes from patients entering a treatment program.[37]

Successful assessment and intervention for individuals with eating disorders require a team approach that includes a nurse, physician, dentist, dietitian, psychologist, and psychiatrist. These patients need not only treatment for their medical and nutrition conditions related to the eating disorder but also help with the emotional and psychologic issues that led to the problem.[35] Extensive and specialized training and experience are necessary before planning a nutrition intervention program for a patient with an eating disorder.

The Problem of Weight Management

Efforts to control body weight are common; in the United States, we spend $33 billion annually on a wide range of weight loss diets, products, and services.[15] In a recent survey of over 14,000 persons aged 18 and older, 45% of the women and 29% of the men were trying to lose weight,[38] although data collected from the *Healthy People 2000* evaluations indicate that fewer people are dieting than in previous years.[39] This change may indicate that the public is tiring of the constant barrage of health directives coming from the mass media and is paying less attention to health.[40] Nevertheless an important role for health professionals is to assist in preventing inappropriate weight gain and in managing previously gained excess weight or, more correctly, excess fat. Using an energy balance sheet, it is simple to predict that when energy taken in does not equal energy expended the difference is reflected in weight either gained or lost; 3500 kcalories has been determined to be the equivalent of 0.45 kg (1 lb) of body fat. That is part of the answer, but, unfortunately, it is not quite that simple. Many individual factors combine to make weight loss a tenuous process, and for some individuals, metabolic actions can make long-term weight loss extremely difficult, if not impossible.

INDIVIDUAL VARIANCE

Energy Balance Factors

Keeping an energy balance score as described above is not that easy. First, it is difficult to know precisely how many kcalories are in the food you are eating. Second, it is even more difficult to know how many kcalories you are burning up. This depends on your BMR or RMR, TEF, body size, amount of LBM, age, gender, and physical activity. An Expert Panel on dietary requirements has defined the Estimated Energy Requirement (EER) as the dietary energy intake predicted to maintain energy balance in a healthy adult of a defined age, gender, weight, height, and level of physical activity consistent with good health.[41] Table 6-3 indicates the wide variation in EER among individuals of different ages and levels of physical activity with the same height, weight, and BMI. Differences in body dimensions, BMI, and proportion of fat versus muscle will influence the EER. Individuals with a high body fat content will likely need fewer kcalories than estimated based on their body weight.

Metabolic Efficiency

Some persons have proclaimed for years, "It's not fair! She can eat twice as much as I can and never gains an ounce." Until recently, we assumed that individuals who gained weight exercised less than those who did not. That may be true in some cases, but not all. Some persons have a low metabolic rate—especially a low TEF that contributes to their overweight state.[7] Researchers have also compiled considerable evidence that human obesity can have a significant genetic component, in youth as well as in middle age.[20] Researchers have identified obesity genes (*ob* genes) that may cause some individuals to take in greater amounts of food or convert more of their ingested food to fat. One way by which obesity genes may exert their influence on body weight is through control of the hormone leptin,[5,8] a hormone that appears to control food intake. To conform to society's thinness values, they are often consigned to a lifetime battle against biologic mechanisms that operate within their bodies to return them to their natural weight or metabolic set-point—a high price for false hope.[12]

TABLE 6-3 Estimated Energy Requirement (EER) Based on Height, Weight, Gender, Age, and Physical Activity Level

	Male (178 lb, 71 in) Kcalories*		Female (132 lb, 61 in) Kcalories*	
Physical Activity Level	Age 25	Age 65	Age 25	Age 65
Very sedentary	2685	2285	1869	1589
Low active	2934	2534	2072	1792
Active	3250	2850	2325	2045
Very active	3770	3370	2628	2348

Calculations based on data presented in Panel on Macronutrients, Panel on the Definition of Dietary Fiber, Subcommittee on Upper Reference Levels of Nutrients, Subcommittee on Interpretation and Uses of Dietary Reference Intakes, and the Standing Committee on the Scientific Evaluation of Dietary Reference Intakes: *Dietary reference intakes for energy, carbohydrate, fiber, fat, fatty acids, cholesterol, protein, and amino acids, parts 1 and 2,* Washington, DC, 2002, National Academy Press.

*An individual of this height and weight has a BMI of approximately 25 kg/m^2.

Diet Composition

The fat, carbohydrate, fiber, and water contents of the diet influence both energy metabolism and appetite regulation and may be a factor in obesity. Diets high in fat contribute to weight gain in several ways. First, fat is easily stored; in fact, fatty acids, converted to triglycerides in the intestinal mucosa and carried to the adipose cells via the lymph and the portal blood, can be immediately stored with almost no associated energy cost. In contrast, complex carbohydrates, after their breakdown into glucose in the digestive tract, require a complicated energy-requiring process to be converted into storage fat, thus a diet equal in kcalories but higher in fat results in more available kcalories for storage as fat.[42,43] Foods high in fat are also highly palatable, and persons may eat more of foods that taste good to them.[44] High-fat foods are likely to be energy dense and provide a meal that is high in kcalories but may be low in volume. Distention of the stomach after a meal sends signals to the brain that triggers fullness and satiety and encourages the person to stop eating.[44] It has been suggested that the volume of the food in the stomach plays an important role in regulating food intake, and this may be why complex carbohydrates that are high in fiber and water content may assist in energy regulation. Consider the volume of food supplied by one small chocolate bar versus three medium apples—both foods contain about 350 kcalories. In fact increasing fiber intake by 14 g led to a 10% decrease in energy intake, and the effect of fiber was even greater in obese compared with normal weight persons.[45]

Comparisons of weight management diets containing various proportions of fat, sugars, and complex carbohydrates indicate that a food pattern low in fat and high in complex carbohydrates and fiber is of greatest benefit in weight loss or avoidance of weight gain.[45] Such diets are also likely to be high in nutrient quality based on use of fruits, vegetables, and grains.[46]

APPROACHES TO WEIGHT LOSS

Overweight and many normal weight persons endure rather incredible experiences in their constant struggle to lose weight. Advertisements for weight loss books, appetite suppressants, drugs to enhance body metabolism, and supplements that will interfere with nutrient absorption abound in the media. Government agencies such as the Federal Trade Commission (FTC) and the Food and Drug Administration (FDA) are charged with the responsibility of preventing false claims in the advertising of weight loss products and removing from the market products found to carry risk of dangerous side effects or death. Unfortunately, the multitude of products introduced for sale and the limited staff of these agencies make it difficult to effectively monitor the marketplace.

Popular Diets

A constant array of diet books flood the American market. They usually sell briefly and then fade away, largely because their guaranteed quick fix does not work. Weight loss is a long-term and difficult process requiring modification of lifestyle patterns. These diets often present simple answers to a far more complex problem, recommending that you limit your food intake to one or two food items or eat little or no carbohydrates. Most popular diets fail on three counts: (1) they are based on scientific inaccuracies and misinformation, hence they are often nutritionally inadequate; (2) they do not address the basic physiologic and behavioral problems involved in weight management and the lifelong changes in food and exercise patterns that will be required to maintain a healthy weight once it is achieved; and (3) they do not recognize that some persons' natural healthy weight may exceed existing and rigid parameters. Individuals who are desperate to lose weight may continue a diet that is nutritionally or medically unsound to the point of inducing medical complications or deficiency diseases. In many cases the degree of energy restriction advocated for weight loss places impossible demands, and dieters find themselves caught in the chronic dieting syndrome with its harmful physical and psychologic effects. Severe energy restriction or fasting can result in feelings of fatigue that limit physical activity, an essential component of lifelong weight control.[47]

Fasting and Liquid Diets

Fasting as a means of weight loss takes many forms from literal fasting to use of very-low-calorie diets or special formulas. Effects may be those of semistarvation: acidosis, postural hypotension, increase in urinary loss of important electrolytes, increase in serum uric acid, constipation, and decrease in BMR. Very-low-energy diets (VLEDs), providing 400 to 800 kcalories daily, have been used under medical supervision with morbidly obese patients and have enabled individuals to lose weight rapidly, but they are not appropriate for individuals to try on their own. Follow-up of patients placed on VLEDs indicates that long-term maintenance of weight loss equals that of individuals following more conventional diets[48]; however, as with any weight reduction regimen, persons must learn new eating patterns that will maintain their lower weight when normal feeding is resumed.

Liquid meal replacements, nutritionally planned to substitute for a food meal, have been used to take the place of one or two meals a day in combination with normal food meals. Such a program can assist individuals who find it difficult to plan or stay within lower-kcalorie meals throughout the day.[49] Liquid meal replacements are often milk based and may not be suitable for those who are lactose intolerant.[50]

Special Gimmicks

Special sauna suits are claimed to bring about weight loss in specific areas of the body or to remove cellulite tissue. *Cellulite,* a word often used in advertisements for weight loss products, has no factual basis. Suits that cause excessive perspiration result in temporary water loss, but any perceived weight loss is promptly regained when rehydration is achieved. This method of weight loss, sometimes used by high school or college wrestlers to reach their preferred weight class, is dangerous and can lead to death.

Over-the-Counter Weight Loss Preparations

Various drugs and dietary supplements have been marketed as weight loss treatments. *Phenylpropanolamine hydrochloride (PPA),* a metabolic stimulant similar to amphetamine, was sold in over-the-counter preparations until removed from the market by the FDA because of its risk for hemorrhagic stroke.[38,51] Similarly, a potent thyroid hormone derivative, triiodothyroacetic acid, may no longer be formulated in weight loss products.[52] *Ephedra (ephedrine alkaloids),* found in nonprescription weight loss products and advertised to increase thermogenesis and reduce appetite, is particularly dangerous for individuals with heart disease, hypertension, or diabetes who also are taking prescription drugs. It was reported recently that 11 of 20 ephedra-containing products evaluated did not even mention the presence of this ingredient on the label.[38] Chitosan, an indigestible polysaccharide found in the skeleton of shellfish, is being marketed as a product that produces rapid weight loss by binding fat in the stomach and preventing its digestion and absorption.[53] As a dietary supplement chitosan is not regulated for purity or safety, and evaluation by university researchers indicates that it does not bring about weight loss as advertised.

Pharmacologic Approaches

The alarming increase in obesity with its high risk for chronic disease has renewed medical interest in drug research for its treatment. Drugs that suppress appetite (anorectic drugs) by acting directly on the central nervous system have been available for more than 40 years but were seldom prescribed until the mid-1990s. Two drugs, fenfluramine and phentermine, commonly called "fen-phen," that decrease appetite by acting on the neurotransmitter serotonin were found to contribute to heart valve defects and primary pulmonary hypertension in some users and were removed from the market in the late 1990s.[17] Sibutramine, which acts on both norepinephrine and serotonin, was introduced in 1997 and is generally well tolerated. Orlistat, approved by the FDA in 1999, inhibits the release of pancreatic lipase and blocks the digestion and absorption of dietary fat. About 30% of ingested fat is lost through the feces with the use of this drug.[17] It is important, however, for patients to recognize that diet drugs are not a quick fix but an adjunct to a program that also addresses lifestyle changes in food behavior, daily walking, or other exercise patterns.

Surgery

Surgical intervention is usually reserved for medical treatment of severely obese persons after more traditional methods have failed. Gastroplasty (Figure 6-4), which reduces the stomach volume and influences the neurohormonal regulation of appetite, leads to early satiety and loss of 30% to 40% of excess weight.[17] Gastric and jejunal bypass procedures reduce the absorption of the energy-yielding macronutrients and lead to significant weight loss. These operations require skilled team management, including nutritional care.[54] They are usually reserved for individuals whose BMI exceeds 40 kg/m² who have medical complications relating to their obesity and for whom other weight management methods have failed.

Cosmetic surgery involving fat removal or lipectomy, commonly called *liposuction,* is used to remove fat deposits under the skin in places such as the hip and thigh. This procedure is intended to improve appearance and body shape and is not a means of weight loss. For liposuction a thin tube is inserted through a small incision in the skin, and a desired amount of the fat deposit is suctioned away. However, this procedure carries risks of infection, can

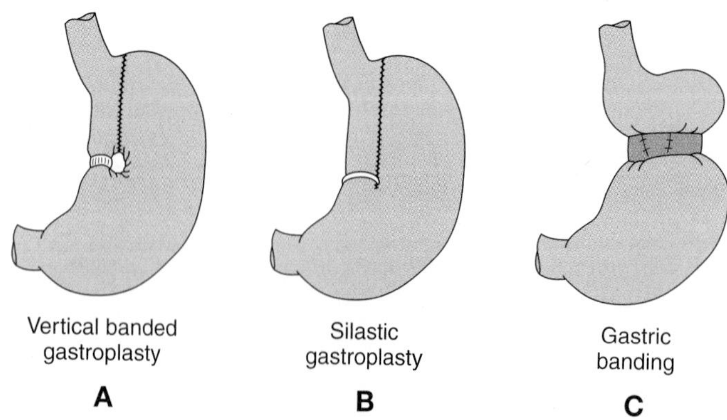

FIGURE 6-4 Simple gastric-restriction procedures for treatment of obesity in order of frequency in current practice. **A**, Vertical banded gastroplasty—50%. **B**, Silastic ring gastroplasty—5%. **C**, Gastric banding—4%. More complex procedures that bypass part of the digestive tract are reserved for treating severe, massive obesity. (*Adapted from Grace DM: Gastric restriction procedures for treating severe obesity,* Am J Clin Nutr *55:556S; 1992; and Mason EE et al: Perioperative risks and safety of surgery for severe obesity,* Am J Clin Nutr *55:573S, 1992.*)

leave large disfiguring skin depressions, or can result in blood clots with dangerous circulatory problems and possible kidney failure. Any surgical procedure carries risk and may lead to other medical problems.

TYPES AND CAUSES OF OBESITY

Theories about the cause of obesity have been a subject of discussion for many years. Although at one time the cause of overweight and overfat was believed to be a simple matter of excessive food intake, we have come to recognize this condition as multifactorial with no simple explanation. We are beginning to understand that there are different forms of obesity, which vary in extent, body fat distribution, and underlying genetic-metabolic factors. This knowledge provides a more realistic individual approach to nutritional care. Four basic factors contribute to this condition: genetic-metabolic, physiologic, psychologic, and social.

Genetic-Metabolic Factors

Genetic inheritance linked to family traits strongly influences a person's likelihood of becoming obese. A genetic base may disrupt the normal balance between energy intake and expenditure by acting to enhance fat storage or promote energy intake. A gene-controlled low RMR is a contributor to obesity, not a result; offspring with an obese parent were found to have an RMR that was 6% lower than offspring of two lean parents.[20] The semistarvation of rigorous dieting reduces the RMR even further as an adaptive response to dietary restriction and body effort to conserve nutrients. Total energy expenditure and energy expended in physical activity may actually be higher in certain individuals at risk for obesity than in lean individuals. The concept of the "thrifty genotype" that leads to weight gain and predisposes one to diabetes refers to the individual who efficiently stores energy nutrients.[55] This genetic trait likely contributed to survival through periods of famine or food uncertainty. Once stored, the body vigorously defends its adipose tissue, which makes it difficult to sustain successful weight loss. This characteristic provides some evidence for the existence of a metabolic set-point for adipocyte fat content or total body fat that predisposes an individual to a particular natural weight level.

Leptin and other hormones secreted by the adipose tissue that act on the brain to control appetite and satiety play a major role in the regulation of body fat content (see *To Probe Further* box). Although high levels of blood leptin, reflecting high levels of adipose tissue, would be expected to reduce feeding behavior, many obese individuals with high fat stores have low leptin levels, which promote sensations of hunger and repress satiety. Other obese individuals with high leptin levels appear to be resistant to the normal actions of leptin.[56] This genetic-metabolic variability should not lead persons with a greater likelihood of weight gain to adopt inadequate diets, but instead guide them into developing wise dietary and exercise habits that promote fitness regardless of body weight. Genetic-metabolic factors that contribute to obesity are of special importance in children, for whom wise food practices may help prevent rapid weight gain that contributes to chronic disease.

Psychologic Factors

We sometimes perceive overweight persons as having less control over their appetites or being more responsive to external cues. Some individuals may have been conditioned through family patterns to eat when it is mealtime or by the clock, instead of when they are really hungry. Being surrounded by tasty foods may carry a greater influence to eat in some persons. Others may eat when they are depressed or because as children they were given food as a reward and were encouraged to eat more than they needed. It is true that reactive eating from stress or anxiety may contribute to obesity, but these factors cannot be applied to all overweight persons as a group. They have no more tendency to these actions and feelings than anyone else, but there is no question about the role that psychology must play in any wise weight management program.

Food insecurity may be linked with overweight in women. In a national study carried out by the U.S. Department of Agriculture, 52% of those women identified to be moderately food insecure were also overweight, and it may be that individuals who are concerned about having enough food tend to eat more when food is available.[57] Among food insecure families, food stamps can be a major resource for obtaining food, and food may be more plentiful during the first weeks of the month and less plentiful during the last weeks, representing a sequence of substantial kcalorie intake followed by a period of food restriction.

Our cultural ideal of the thin body type and social discrimination against obese persons have created psychologic problems in many individuals. Psychosocial support—in the form of a counselor, support group, friends, or family—is critical for a successful weight management program.

Social Factors

The class values placed on the obese state by different social groups also influence its frequency. As a person moves upward in socioeconomic class, there is greater social pressure to maintain a lower body weight. In lower socioeconomic groups obesity is more prevalent and carries less stigma. The length of exposure to these values and their pressure on individuals in any social class determines reactions to them. Other social and environmental factors associated with body weight issues include cultural and family food patterns, job environments, recreational eating that encourages the use of high-kcalorie foods, and the social role of eating. Individuals employed in a food-related facility may find it difficult to avoid constant snacking throughout the day. The current expectation that social events include food and the pressure on guests to eat make it difficult for individuals to limit food intake. The strong sense within certain cultural groups that an offer of food is an essential component of welcoming

TO PROBE FURTHER

Appetite and Body Weight: How Do We Know When to Stop Eating?

Over the years researchers have asked the question, Why do some individuals maintain a normal and consistent body weight throughout their adult life while others gain excessive amounts of body fat? We know there is tremendous variation in the amounts of food persons normally consume and their average capacity for food intake. Some individuals feel full very quickly even though they may have consumed a very small amount of food. Others seem to have an almost unlimited capacity for food intake.

In recent years we have learned more about the body hormones and regulators that control food intake and help us adjust to periods of lower or higher energy expenditure. These regulators work with other body systems to maintain an appropriate body weight. However, sometimes these regulators do not carry out this task appropriately, and weight imbalances, either severe underweight or severe overweight, result. Some regulators act on a short-term basis and control food intake from meal to meal. We have identified other hormonal regulators that may control food intake and body weight on a long-term basis. We will look at both of these groups of control agents and see how they influence food intake.

SHORT-TERM REGULATION OF FOOD INTAKE

Food intake from meal to meal is controlled by the hypothalamus in the brain, which sends and receives messages from the various organs in the gastrointestinal tract.

1. *Hypothalamus.* The part of the brain called the hypothalamus helps to control our appetite and the amount of food that we eat. Certain cells in the hypothalamus, sometimes called the *hunger center,* are very alert to food intake. Because continuing food intake is essential for life, these cells send out strong signals that bring about feelings of hunger and encourage us to eat. These cells are also very sensitive to glucose levels, and feelings of hunger result when blood glucose drops to fasting levels, about 3 to 4 hours after your last meal. These cells also respond to messages from other parts of the brain that receive stimuli from the sensory organs that report the taste, smell, or sight of food. Brain peptides called *orexins* that originate in the hypothalamus and act under genetic control stimulate appetite and food intake.

   In another section of the hypothalamus are cells referred to as the *satiety center.* These cells respond to messages from the gastrointestinal tract as food moves along the digestive path and tell us when to stop eating. The formation of larger or smaller amounts of orexins in the hypothalamus, causing us to eat more or less food, may be one way by which our genes influence our body weight.
2. *Stomach.* The fundus of the stomach—which receives the food when it passes through the sphincter leading from the esophagus to the stomach—has sensors that cause the muscle fibers to stretch when food is received. This stretching of the muscle fibers allows more food to move into the stomach without causing discomfort. As the stomach fills with food, the food slowly moves from the fundus to the lower region of the stomach called the *antrum,* and from here small squirts of the food bolus will begin to enter the small intestine. Receptors in the antrum send messages back to the hypothalamus, telling the brain that food is arriving, and these messages help to bring about the feelings of satiety telling us that we have eaten enough. Problems with these regulators in the stomach contribute to the early satiety and weight loss that sometimes occur in older people. In some older people the fundus does not stretch in size; therefore these people feel full very quickly after eating even very small amounts of food. Also, the lack of stretch in the fundus causes food to move more quickly into the antrum, sending early signals to the brain that it is time to stop eating. Conversely, if the fundus stretches excessively, it may delay the continued movement of the food and delay feelings of satiety, resulting in additional food intake.
3. *Small intestine.* Receptors in the small intestine tell the hypothalamus when food is being delivered from the stomach, and these messages also help to produce satiety. Cells in the duodenum produce increased amounts of the gastrointestinal hormone *cholecystokinin* in response to the arrival of food, and this hormone sends messages to the hypothalamus that tell us we have eaten enough.

LONG-TERM REGULATION OF FOOD INTAKE

Although we have identified the feedback loop between parts of the digestive tract and the brain that seem to control food intake on a meal-to-meal basis, researchers are anxiously looking for the master control that links

TO PROBE FURTHER

Appetite and Body Weight: How Do We Know When to Stop Eating?—cont'd

food intake and body weight. Several years ago workers discovered a hormone called *leptin* that is produced in the adipose cells, and, in general, blood levels of leptin are proportional to the relative amount of body fat. Leptin and now several other newly discovered control agents, including *neuropeptide Y,* found in the hypothalamus, and *resistin,* another protein secreted by the adipose cells, are being studied to determine their possible role in regulating body fat and energy metabolism. Leptin can act on the hunger center in the hypothalamus to reduce hunger and appetite and thereby lower food intake. According to this idea, increased amounts of adipose tissue would produce higher levels of leptin, which would repress appetite and prevent additional weight gain. Individuals who lack the gene to produce leptin become obese, and their body weight and fat are reduced when they are treated with recombinant leptin. However, in other obese individuals treatment with leptin decreases feelings of hunger but has no effect on body weight or body fat.

Many persons with similar amounts of body fat have different blood leptin levels; therefore other factors in addition to amount of adipose tissue must also influence leptin secretion. It is interesting to note that both high-fat diets and physical activity seem to have independent effects on leptin levels. In overweight men, those who ate less fat and exercised 3 times a week had a greater drop in their blood leptin levels than was expected based on their loss of body fat. These changes in this body regulator suggest that keeping fat intake within 25% to 30% of total kcalories and emphasizing regular physical activity may be important goals in long-term body weight management.

References

Arioglu Oral E et al: Leptin-replacement therapy for lipodystrophy, *N Engl J Med* 346:570, 2002.

Friedman J: Leptin, receptors, and the control of body weight, *Nutr Rev* 56(suppl):S38, 1998.

Morley JE: Management of nutritional problems in subacute care, *Clin Geriatr Med* 16(4):817, 2000.

Reseland JE et al: Effect of long-term changes in diet and exercise on plasma leptin concentrations, *Am J Clin Nutr* 73:240, 2001.

Schwartz MW et al: Model for the regulation of energy balance and adiposity by the central nervous system, *Am J Clin Nutr* 69:584, 1999.

Trayhurn P, Beattie JH: Physiological role of adipose tissue: white adipose tissue as an endocrine and secretory organ, *Proc Nutr Soc* 60:329, 2001.

Westerterp-Plantenga MS et al: Effects of weekly administration of pegylated recombinant human OB protein on appetite profile and energy metabolism in obese men, *Am J Clin Nutr* 74:426, 2001.

visitors to your home can increase the number of eating events of the day. Sedentary patterns of recreation and employment, time spent in computer games or on the Internet, and television viewing time, with its inactivity and constant snacking, are all likely major contributors to unwanted weight gain. Obesity in children has been related to their number of hours of television viewing.[28] The popular pastime of "surfing the web" no doubt contributes to the sedentary patterns of both children and adults.

Physiologic Factors

Normal physiology during the growth years contributes to the accumulation of fat deposits. Critical periods during growth for the development of obesity are early childhood and early stages of puberty.[20] Early and middle adulthood are also potential periods of excess fat accumulation. In women inappropriate weight gain may occur during pregnancy or in the period after menopause as a result of hormonal changes. For men a critical period is early to middle adulthood, when physical activity declines but food habits formed during adolescence, a period of peak energy needs, are continued. Both men and women tend to gain weight after age 50 because of their lower RMR, decreased physical exercise, and failure to adjust food habits accordingly.

Study of the physiologic aspects of obesity has focused on the number and size of adipose cells. Normally, the full genetic complement of fat cells is reached by puberty and then remains constant. After puberty, these fat cells may increase in size within limits but do not usually increase in number. However, if excessive kcalorie intake continues after the fat cells have reached their maximal capacity, cell proliferation is triggered again. Once this increase in cell number has occurred, it is not reversed. In extreme obesity, for example, the number of fat cells may increase from a norm of about 30 billion to approximately 120 billion, and each one is also increased in size. Once the body has added fat cells to accommodate extra fuel storage, these cells remain and store varying amounts of fat. The only means of weight reduction then is to diminish individual cell size. This similar harmful pattern of increased fat storage also occurs in individuals whose natural metabolic set-point for body weight is higher than the cultural ideal of thinness. Obesity research is also looking at the fetal origins hypothesis, as we try to learn if nutrition in prenatal life influences body weight and fat mass in adult life.[58]

Increased fat cell formation also affects body fat distribution. A form of localized fat cell increase occurs in women over the lower body areas of thighs and hips, called *gynecoid,* or lower body, obesity. This form of obesity leads to fewer metabolic complications of obesity. However, a second type of fat distribution, central abdominal fat deposition—called *android* because it is the usual pattern of adult male fat distribution—also occurs in women and is associated with metabolic complications in both males and females. Excessive abdominal fat appears to have metabolic consequences related to hyperlipidemia and the development of diabetes. For this reason the waist-to-hip ratio and abdominal circumference measurements are receiving increasing attention in clinical assessment. A small decrease in abdominal fat can lower health risk in an obese individual even if weight loss is limited. Body fat redistribution leading to greater fat on the trunk and an increase in the waist-to-hip ratio has been reported in patients infected with the human immunodeficiency virus being treated with protease inhibitors and appears to contribute to changes in glucose tolerance and elevated cholesterol levels.[59]

The Health Model for Weight Management: A Positive Personal Approach

GENERAL COMPONENTS

Healthful adult weight management is based on combined wisdom from both nutrition and behavioral research. A well-balanced, individually tailored food plan, together with a gradually increased exercise program and supportive behavioral change measures, can be effective and personally rewarding. In healthcare practice, the general approach to weight management is based on sound nutrition and energy balance and the client's personal situation. It focuses on two main aspects: (1) motivation and support and (2) a personalized program.

Motivation and Support

The degree of personal motivation is a prime factor. Through initial interviews, the nutrition counselor—usually a specially trained registered dietitian (RD)—seeks to determine lifestyle patterns related to food and exercise, attitudes toward food and weight, and the meaning food has for the client. Recognition is given to the emotional factors involved, and support is provided by the nutritionist, together with the nurse and the physician, to meet the client's particular needs. Throughout this process the emphasis should be placed on improved fitness and health, not merely weight loss.

Personal Program

To be successful, a weight management program must meet personal needs and goals. Such a program includes to some extent suggestions from each of the following sections.

1. *Food behavior.* Note the quantity of food served and eaten. Use moderate to small portions, attractively served. Take time to eat slowly and savor the food taste and texture. Reduce hidden kcalories added in food preparation, mainly fat. Increase fiber content. When eating out, recognize expanded portion size and ask to take remaining food home or share an entrée with a companion. Choose a variety of foods from a basic food guide, as a focus for sound realistic nutrition education. Emphasize whole primary foods and a minimum of processed foods. Plan a fairly even food distribution throughout the day. Plan for snacks if that has been a regular part of the dietary pattern. Attention to portion control and education on appropriate portion sizes are essential for the success of a weight loss program.[60]
2. *Exercise behavior.* Plan for regular daily exercise. Start with walking, building to a brisk aerobic pace continuing for about 30 minutes at least 3 times a week or, if possible, every day. Aerobic exercise benefits a person in a weight-management program because it (1) lowers the body-weight set-point, (2) suppresses appetite, (3) reduces body fat including abdominal fat, (4) increases BMR, and (5) increases energy expenditure. Exercise that increases the heart rate to the highest level appropriate for the particular individual is especially effective in burning body fat. If possible, gradually increase the time of the exercise period to 45 to 60 minutes, and add other activities that have aerobic value, such as swimming. Adults of all ages will benefit from a routine of body exercises for strength training that support the retention and building of muscle and general fitness as well as increasing energy expenditure. Set occasional goals and keep a record of progress. Use variety in the program that will add to personal enjoyment. If possible, set up a buddy system to offer companionship and to keep both persons on track.
3. *Stress reduction exercises.* Practice progressive muscle relaxation and stress-reduction exercises. Learn an appropriate pattern as a guide, using imagery as a mental focusing device, or use tapes of environmental recordings if they are helpful. Start with a brief 10-minute period and increase as desired. Select a suitable time and stay with it for daily practice. In our stress-filled modern environment, many persons really do not know how to relax.
4. *Personal interest area.* Develop some creative interest area for intellectual stimulation, personal enjoyment, and fulfillment. Explore various community groups or resources to support such activities.

5. *Follow-up program.* A follow-up schedule of appointments with the nutrition counselor should be outlined, and its values discussed with the client. On subsequent visits, progress can be reviewed, problems discussed, and solutions explored. Continuing support can be provided. Practical suggestions for dealing with such things as realistic goals, food and exercise behaviors, meals at home and away from home, and any other special situations can be discussed. This follow-up support helps the client anticipate changing needs or new situations, reinforce new learning, sustain motivation, and deal positively with periods of frustration. Computer programs can successfully enhance education, goal-setting, and reinforcement for individuals in a weight loss program.[61]

BEHAVIORAL ASPECTS

Behavioral change in respect to food and exercise is an important component of long-term weight management. It requires family, individual, or group support. Experienced and sensitive practitioners in healthcare settings have come to recognize that ongoing training and support that empower a client to modify any undesirable food behaviors or sedentary habits that may have contributed to a body weight problem is essential to long-range success. Such support may be provided on an individual basis, although peer support is also valuable as clients can support each other. Food behavior is rooted in many human experiences, associations, and environmental situations. These experiences often produce addictive forms of eating response. Behavior-oriented therapies are designed to help the person change those lifestyle patterns that contribute to the adding of unwanted body fat. These strategies help to increase insight, awareness, and understanding of present behaviors; provide motivation toward positive change; and recondition old behaviors into new ones that will help reach personal goals. When a person changes past associations with undesirable habit patterns, he or she can then plan a means of constructive action. Supportive behavioral change activities are directed toward (1) self-management of eating behavior—the when, what, why, where, how, and how much, and (2) promotion of physical activity and increased energy output, providing a better total energy balance as well as an added means of reducing stress.

PRINCIPLES OF A SOUND FOOD PLAN

On the basis of careful interviewing, body composition measures, and evaluation of available laboratory data, the nutritionist makes a comprehensive assessment of nutritional and health status, food and physical activity habits and behaviors, and living situation. Details for such a full assessment are described in Chapter 15. Then, on the basis of this individual assessment, personal needs and goals can be established in conversation with the client. An appropriate food plan is developed cooperatively by the counselor and the client to meet normal nutritional needs and any therapeutic modification indicated for health problems that are present. Such a personal plan has several basic parts.

Energy Balance

The energy intake level is adjusted to meet individual weight management needs. A moderate personal eating pattern is outlined. This gradual process is best for long-term success and health. On the average, for women, a sound plan for energy needs is based on about 1200 to 1500 kcalories/day. For larger women and for men, a plan of about 1500 to 1800 kcalories/day would meet gradual weight adjustment energy needs. It may be helpful to some persons to determine what their basal and activity needs are as a basis for understanding their overall energy expenditure (see Table 6-3). Energy intake should be adjusted to allow a weight loss of no more than 1 to 2 lb per week.

Nutrient Balance

Basic energy nutrients are outlined to achieve the following nutrient balance.

1. *Carbohydrate.* About 50% to 55% of total kcalories, with emphasis on complex forms such as starches with fiber and limited amounts of sugars.
2. *Protein.* Approximately 20% of total kcalories, with emphasis on lean food choices and small portions to curtail fat.
3. *Fat.* About 25% to 30% of total kcalories, with emphasis on plant fats, scant use, and alternate seasonings.

In general, this nutrient balance approximates the recommendations of the U.S. *Dietary Guidelines for Americans.* Review these guidelines in Chapter 1. They are helpful as a basic nutrition education tool.

Distribution Balance

Spread food fairly evenly throughout the day to meet energy needs. Consider any daily "problem times" and plan simple snacks to meet such needs.

Food Guide

Use some type of general food reference list from which the client can make a variety of food choices to fulfill the basic personal food plan. The *Food Exchange List for Meal Planning* is such a guide. It draws on a broad database to provide a general reference guide with comparative food values and portions that allow the client to develop a variety and to include personal choices in basic meal planning. Food items can easily be combined into desired dishes. To lower fat in food preparation, use alternate seasonings such as herbs and spices, onion and garlic, lemon and other fruit juices, vinegar, wine, fat-free broth, mustard, and other condiments.

PERSONAL NEEDS

Individual Adaptations

Throughout the planning, remember to focus on the individual client and personal needs. If the plan is unrealistic, whatever its form or basis, it will not be followed. Some persons find it helpful to keep a daily journal, which can include notes of food intake, environmental food cues, feelings, physical symptoms, and any stress factors related to food behavior. It may also include notes about other activities such as physical exercise or stress-reduction practices. A periodic review of such notes may help in making general observations, determining problem areas, monitoring progress, and gaining insights for readjusting goals to achieve desired health and fitness behavior changes. Essential parts of all programs are nutrition counseling and education—for limiting total fat, selecting protein and carbohydrate foods to optimize nutrient intake, increasing physical activity, and providing ongoing support for behavioral change.

In the United States, there is a growing awareness that the modern phenomenon of constant restrictive dieting is counterproductive and, in the long run, harmful to many persons. This is especially true for growing children and adolescents and women whose natural body weight levels do not match the society norm.[15] As a result, health professionals are developing alternative approaches based on a health and fitness model that emphasizes regular exercise and gradual dietary changes that control fat and kcalories and promote healthy choices. Success should be measured by changes in diet and lifestyle that support health, rather than in pounds lost. The American Dietetic Association has developed two concepts for the treatment of obesity: (1) that the goal be weight management and not weight loss, keeping in mind that not all clients will be able to lose weight, and (2) that achievement of the best weight possible be considered in the context of overall health.[15] Individual weight management programs must emphasize the gradual development of a healthful eating style with the increased use of whole grains, fruits, and vegetables and a nonrestrictive approach to eating based on internal regulation of hunger and satiety. Favorite foods or comfort foods should be included in the diet occasionally, regardless of their kcalories. Such health and fitness models provide needed help with positive behavioral changes through ongoing counseling and peer group support.

WEIGHT MANAGEMENT FOR CHILDREN

Weight management for children should center on trust and building self-esteem and responsibility as children experience normal growth and develop behaviors that will prevent inappropriate weight gain. Second, it is important that the family as a whole adopt new food patterns to provide support and appropriate food patterns for the child.[62] A smart goal is to maintain a healthy balance between energy intake through wise food choices and control of portion size and energy output in enjoyable physical exercise, recognizing all the while that fatness is a normal condition for some people. Early nutrition education, positive food and fitness behavior, and habit formation in the family—with support and guidance for young parents and children before an obese condition develops—will help prevent problems in later adulthood.

The Problem of Underweight

We have discussed at length the major problem of excess body weight and body fat. Conversely, what about the state of less-than-adequate weight? Excluding the self-imposed eating disorders, what dangers lie in being generally underweight? What are some of its causes and approaches to treatment?

DEFINITION

Extremes in underweight, just as in overweight, bring or accompany serious health problems.[63] Although general underweight is less common in the American population than is overweight, it does occur in a small percentage. It is estimated that somewhat less than 10% of persons have trouble gaining and maintaining weight. Some seem to lack control over how much they eat at a meal and reach a full feeling with less food than do persons of normal weight (see *To Probe Further* box). Underweight may be associated with poverty, poor living conditions, or long-term disease. A person more than 10% below the average weight for height and age is considered underweight; 20% or more below is cause for concern. Serious problems may result in these persons, especially young children who may experience long-term growth retardation or failure to thrive. Resistance to infection is lowered, general health is poor, malnutrition develops, and strength is reduced in seriously underweight individuals. Elderly persons experiencing changes in appetite regulation are at risk of underweight.[64]

GENERAL CAUSES

In general, underweight is associated with conditions that cause basic malnutrition, such as the following.

- *Wasting disease.* Long-term hypermetabolic diseases such as cancer, acquired immunodeficiency syndrome (AIDS), or short- or long-term infection and fever place metabolic demands on the body that drain the body's resources.
- *Poor food intake.* Diminished food intake can result from (1) psychologic factors that cause a person to refuse to eat, (2) loss of appetite related to imbalance in the brain's hunger-satiety centers, (3) anorexia related to use of certain medications such as digoxin, or (4) personal poverty and limited food supply.

- *Malabsorption.* Poor nutrient absorption results from (1) prolonged diarrhea, (2) gastrointestinal disease, or (3) abuse of laxatives.
- *Hormonal imbalance.* Hyperthyroidism or other abnormalities may increase the nutrient needs of the body.
- *Energy imbalance.* Greatly increased physical activity without a corresponding increase in food intake creates an energy balance deficit.
- *Poor living situation.* An unhealthy home environment or no home at all results in irregular and inadequate meals or, in some persons, an indifferent or defeated attitude toward food.

NUTRITIONAL CARE

Underweight persons require special nutritional care to rebuild their body tissues and nutrient stores and regain their health. Any food plan needs to be adapted for each person's unique situation, whether it involves personal or economic needs, living situation, or underlying disease. The dietary goal, according to each person's tolerance, is to increase energy and nutrient intake in a diet that is (1) high in kcalories, at least 50% above standard needs; (2) high in protein, to rebuild tissue; (3) high in carbohydrates, to provide a primary energy source in easily digested form; (4) moderate in fat, to add kcalories but not exceed toleration limits; and (5) optimum in vitamins and minerals, including individual supplements where deficiencies require them. Good food of wide variety, well prepared and seasoned, and attractively presented helps revive lagging appetites and increases the desire to eat. Frequent, small nourishing meals and snacks spread through the day, including favorite foods, stimulate interest in eating and increase the optimal use of foods and their nutrients. To achieve the desired increase in kcalories, use (1) food seasonings, such as margarine or butter, sauces, and dressings, and (2) liquid nutritional supplements to add kcalories and key nutrients.

A basic aim is to help build the best food habits possible, within any limitations that may exist; therefore the improved nutritional status and weight will be maintained once they are regained. This rehabilitation process requires much creative counseling with each individual and family, with attention to the underlying socioeconomic or disease conditions. Practical personal guides and ongoing support are needed to counteract root causes of the malnutrition. In some extreme cases, tube feeding or total parenteral nutrition (TPN) may be necessary (see Chapter 17).

TO SUM UP

Energy is that force or power that enables the body to maintain its life-sustaining metabolic work, as well as all of its physical work and activity. The energy provided by food is measured in kilocalories or joules. Body energy moves among various basic forms such as chemical, electrical, mechanical, and thermal. Metabolism is the body's way of changing the chemical energy of food into these cycling forms of energy according to body needs. When food is not available, the body draws on its own stores to meet energy needs: glycogen from carbohydrate stores, fatty acids from adipose tissue, and amino acids from lean body mass.

Total energy needs are a sum of basal (maintenance) and nonbasal (exercise) requirements. The BMR (the amount of energy required to maintain the body at rest after a 12-hour fast) along with the TEF compose the body's metabolic energy needs; added to this are variable needs for work and other physical activities. The four main compartments of body composition are LBM, body fat, body water, and mineral mass. LBM, including both muscle cells and vital organs, is a major contributor to the basal metabolism. Body composition is measured by a number of methods developed for research, population surveys, and clinical practice.

Body weight has traditionally been used as an indicator of obesity, a condition that raises the risk of health problems. But it is the composition of the body weight, lean versus fat tissue, that is the most important aspect. Weight-management programs have traditionally been designed for persons with excessive amounts of body fat. However, the current obsession with thinness has created a new weight-management problem, the chronic dieting syndrome, which leads to ever-increasing cycles of dieting with the regain of lost weight and a decrease in self-esteem. Growing numbers of adolescents have unhealthy body images that lead to eating disorders such as anorexia nervosa, bulimia nervosa, or binge eating.

The health and fitness model of weight management is based on personal motivation and individual support. Aspects of such a program include changing food attitudes and behaviors, increasing physical activity, learning and practicing relaxation techniques, and developing personal interests that can divert attention from eating. Behavioral strategies, with counselor and group support, help the individual examine the effect of life situations on eating habits and change those situations that encourage overeating. An adjusted energy intake is developed based on individual needs with an emphasis on decreasing fat intake and increasing exercise. This model allows for (1) a gradual small to moderate rate of weight loss or, in some instances, a more healthful holding pattern that recognizes individual natural weight levels, (2) optimum intake of all required nutrients, and (3) support for food and exercise behavior changes.

The opposite problem of underweight also requires nutrition intervention. It results from physiologic, psychosocial, economic, or disease causes. A nutrient- and energy-rich diet supplied through multiple small meals is indicated, with ongoing counseling to help with the underlying causes and rehabilitation process.

Questions for Review

1. What does the term *fuel factor* mean? What is the fuel value for each of the three energy-yielding nutrients?
2. Define *basal metabolic rate.* What factors influence this rate? Which body tissues contribute most to basal metabolic needs and what approximate percentage of the total energy expenditure do these basal metabolic needs require?
3. What factors influence nonbasal energy needs?
4. Calculate your own energy balance for 1 day based on your energy input (food) and your energy output (RMR + TEF + physical activity) (see *Practical Application* box).
5. Describe the major eating disorders associated with America's growing obsession with thinness. What social factors contribute to this obsession? Compare these with the factors that contribute to the growing tendency of overweight.
6. Describe four general causes for obesity.
7. Describe the five components of the health model for weight management. How does it differ from the traditional medical model?
8. What are the basic principles of a sound food-exercise plan for weight management programs?
9. You are working with a single mother and her 3-year-old daughter, and both are underweight. They live in a small apartment in a dilapidated building in the inner city. Their electricity was disconnected; therefore they have no working equipment for cooking and no refrigeration. They receive a noon and supper meal at a nearby food program for the homeless. Plan a series of snacks and food supplements for them that could increase their kcalorie intake. (Remember all foods you suggest must be safely stored at room temperature.)
10. Visit your local library and review the magazines directed toward the teen audience. Look for three articles that suggest regimens for weight loss or weight control. Evaluate each article in terms of (a) nutritional implications, (b) overall health implications, (c) use of commercial weight-loss products or supplements, and (d) safety for long-term use.

References

1. Brody T: *Nutritional biochemistry,* ed 2, New York, 1999, Academic Press.
2. Poehlman ET, Horton ES: Energy needs: assessment and requirements in humans. In Shils ME et al, eds: *Modern nutrition in health and disease,* ed 9, Philadelphia, 1999, Lippincott Williams & Wilkins.
3. Guyton AC, Hall JE: *Textbook of medical physiology,* ed 10, Philadelphia, 2000, WB Saunders.
4. Fox CS et al: Is a low leptin concentration, a low resting metabolic rate, or both the expression of the "thrifty genotype"? Results from Mexican Pima Indians, *Am J Clin Nutr* 68:1053, 1998.
5. Schwartz MW et al: Model for the regulation of energy balance and adiposity by the central nervous system, *Am J Clin Nutr* 69:584, 1999.
6. Levine JA, Schleusner SJ, Jensen MD: Energy expenditure of nonexercise activity, *Am J Clin Nutr* 72:1451, 2000.
7. Schoeller DA: The importance of clinical research: the role of thermogenesis in human obesity, *Am J Clin Nutr* 73:511, 2001.
8. Pi-Sunyer FX: Obesity. In Shils ME et al, eds: *Modern nutrition in health and disease,* ed 9, Philadelphia, 1999, Lippincott Williams & Wilkins.
9. Brandon LJ: Comparison of existing skinfold equations for estimating body fat in African American and white women, *Am J Clin Nutr* 67:1155, 1998.
10. Forbes GB: Body composition: role of nutrition, growth, physical activity, and aging. In Shils ME et al, eds: *Modern nutrition in health and disease,* ed 9, Philadelphia, 1999, Lippincott Williams & Wilkins.
11. Calle EE et al: Body-mass index and mortality in a prospective cohort of U.S. adults, *N Engl J Med* 341:1097, 1999.
12. Phinney SD, Halsted CH: Obesity, anorexia nervosa, and bulimia. In Feldman M, Scharschmidt BF, Sleisenger MH, eds: *Gastrointestinal and liver disease,* ed 6, vol 1, Philadelphia, 1998, WB Saunders.
13. Stevens J: Impact of age on associations between weight and mortality, *Nutr Rev* 58:129, 2000.
14. Flegal KM, Troiano RP, Ballard-Barbash R: Aim for a healthy weight: what is the target? *J Nutr* 131:440S, 2001.
15. Cummings SM, Goodrick GK, Foreyt JP: Position of the American Dietetic Association: weight management, *J Am Diet Assoc* 97:71, 1997.
16. Kassirer JP, Angell M: Losing weight—an ill-fated New Year's resolution, *N Engl J Med* 338:52, 1998.
17. Glazer G: Long-term pharmacotherapy of obesity 2000. A review of efficacy and safety, *Arch Intern Med* 161:1814, 2001.
18. Rippe JM, Crossley S, Ringer R: Obesity as a chronic disease: modern medical and lifestyle management, *J Am Diet Assoc* 98(suppl 2):S9, 1998.
19. Townsend MS et al: Food insecurity is positively related to overweight in women, *J Nutr* 131:1738, 2001.
20. Goran MI: Metabolic precursors and effects of obesity in children: a decade of progress, 1990-1999, *Am J Clin Nutr* 73:158, 2001.
21. Franz MJ: Managing obesity in patients with comorbidities, *J Am Diet Assoc* 98(suppl 2):S39, 1998.
22. David S, Mobarhan S: Association between body mass index and adenocarcinoma of the esophagus and gastric cardia, *Nutr Rev* 58:54, 2000.
23. Kim Y-I: Diet, lifestyle, and colorectal cancer: is hyperinsulinemia the missing link? *Nutr Rev* 56:275, 1998.
24. Wolf AM: What is the economic case for treating obesity? *Obes Res* 6:2S, 1998.
25. Williamson DF: The prevention of obesity, *N Engl J Med* 341:1140, 1999.
26. Willett WC, Dietz WH, Colditz GA: Guidelines for healthy weight, *N Engl J Med* 341:427, 1999.
27. Ashley JM et al: Weight reduction in the physician's office, *Arch Intern Med* 161:1599, 2001.
28. Grivetti L: Psychology and cultural aspects of energy, *Nutr Rev* 59:S5, 2001.

29. Fisher JO, Birch LL: Parents' restrictive feeding practices are associated with young girls' negative self-evaluation of eating, *J Am Diet Assoc* 100:1341, 2000.
30. Neumark-Sztainer D et al: Primary prevention of disordered eating among adolescent girls: feasibility and short-term effect of a community-based intervention, *J Am Diet Assoc* 100:1466, 2000.
31. Bellisle F, Dalix AM: Cognitive restraint can be offset by distraction, leading to increased meal intake in women, *Am J Clin Nutr* 74:197, 2001.
32. Story M et al: Dieting status and its relationship to eating and physical activity behaviors in a representative sample of US adolescents, *J Am Diet Assoc* 98:1127, 1998.
33. O'Dea JA, Rawstorne PR: Male adolescents identify their weight gain practices, reasons for desired weight gain, and sources of weight gain information, *J Am Diet Assoc* 101:105, 2001.
34. American Psychiatric Association: *Diagnostic criteria for eating disorders,* ed 4 revised (DSM IV-R), Washington, DC, 1994, American Psychiatric Association.
35. Spear BA, Stellefson-Myers E: Position of the American Dietetic Association: nutrition intervention in the treatment of anorexia nervosa, bulimia nervosa, and eating disorders not otherwise specified (EDNOS), *J Am Diet Assoc* 101:810, 2001.
36. Neumark-Sztainer D et al: Lessons learned about adolescent nutrition from the Minnesota Adolescent Health Survey, *J Am Diet Assoc* 98:1449, 1998.
37. Reeves RS et al: Nutrient intake of obese female binge eaters, *J Am Diet Assoc* 101:209, 2001.
38. Blanck HM, Khan LK, Serdula MK: Use of nonprescription weight loss products. Results from a multistate survey, *JAMA* 286:930, 2001.
39. Crane NT, Hubbard VS, Lewis CJ: National nutrition objectives and the dietary guidelines for Americans, *Nutr Today* 33:49, 1998.
40. Patterson RE et al: Is there a consumer backlash against the diet and health message? *J Am Diet Assoc* 101:37, 2001.
41. Panel on Marcronutrients, Panel on the Definition of Dietary Fiber, Subcommittee on Upper Reference Levels of Nutrients, Subcommittee on Interpretation and Uses of Dietary Reference Intakes, and the Standing Committee on the Scientific Evaluation of Dietary Reference Intakes: *Dietary reference intakes for energy, carbohydrate, fiber, fat, fatty acids, cholesterol, protein, and amino acids, parts 1 and 2,* Washington, DC, 2002, National Academy Press.
42. Shepard TY et al: Occasional physical inactivity combined with a high-fat diet may be important in the development and maintenance of obesity in human subjects, *Am J Clin Nutr* 73:703, 2001.
43. Poppitt S et al: Long-term effects of ad libitum low-fat high-carbohydrate diets on body weight and serum lipids in overweight subjects with metabolic syndrome, *Am J Clin Nutr* 75:11, 2002.
44. Yao M, Roberts SB: Dietary energy density and weight regulation, *Nutr Rev* 59:247, 2001.
45. Howarth NC, Saltzman E, Roberts SB: Dietary fiber and weight regulation, *Nutr Rev* 59:129, 2001.
46. Kennedy ET et al: Popular diets: Correlation to health, nutrition, and obesity, *J Am Diet Assoc* 101:411, 2001.
47. Foreyt JP, Goodrick GK: Dietary intake and weight loss: the energy perspective, *Nutr Rev* 59:S25, 2001.
48. Anderson JW et al: Long-term weight-loss maintenance: a meta analysis of US studies, *Am J Clin Nutr* 74:579, 2001.
49. Rothacker DQ, Staniszewski BA, Ellis PK: Liquid meal replacement vs traditional food: a potential model for women who cannot maintain eating habit change, *J Am Diet Assoc* 101:345, 2001.
50. Suarez FL et al: Nutritional supplements used in weight-reduction programs increase intestinal gas in persons who malabsorb lactose, *J Am Diet Assoc* 101:1447, 2001.
51. Food and Drug Administration: Phenylpropanolamine (PPA) information page, access at *http://www.fda.gov/cder/drug/infopage/ppa/default.htm,* Nov 21, 2000.
52. Food and Drug Administration: Risky "weight loss" product prompts warning from FDA, *FDA Consumer* 34:3, 2000.
53. Coleman E: Is chitosan a fat magnet? Special Supplement on Sports Nutrition, *Nutr MD* 27(6), 2001.
54. Kushner R: Managing the obese patient after bariatric surgery: a case report of severe malnutrition and review of the literature, *JPEN* 24:126, 2000.
55. Neel JV: The "thrifty genotype" in 1998, *Nutr Rev* 57(suppl):S2, 1998.
56. Ruhl CE, Everhart JE: Leptin concentrations in the United States: relations with demographic and anthropometric measures, *Am J Clin Nutr* 74:295, 2001.
57. Townsend MS et al: Food insecurity is positively related to overweight in women, *J Nutr* 131:1738, 2001.
58. Martorell R, Stein AD, Schroeder DG: Early nutrition and later adiposity, *J Nutr* 131:874S, 2001.
59. Gerrior JUL et al: The fat redistribution syndrome in patients infected with HIV: measurements of body shape abnormalities, *J Am Diet Assoc* 101:1175, 2001.
60. Chambers EIV et al: Cognitive strategies for reporting portion sizes using dietary recall procedures, *J Am Diet Assoc* 100(8):891, 2000.
61. Tate DF, Wing RR, Winett RA: Using Internet technology to deliver a behavioral weight loss program, *JAMA* 285:1172, 2001.
62. Golan M et al: Parents as the exclusive agents of change in the treatment of childhood obesity, *Am J Clin Nutr* 67:1130, 1998.
63. Klein S, Jeejeebhoy KN: The malnourished patient: nutritional assessment and management. In Feldman M, Scharschmidt BF, Sleisenger MH, eds: *Gastrointestinal and liver disease,* ed 6, vol 1, Philadelphia, 1998, WB Saunders.
64. Marcus EL, Berry EM: Refusal to eat in the elderly, *Nutr Rev* 56:163, 1998.

■ Further Reading

Flegal KM, Troiano RP, Ballard-Barbash R: Aim for a healthy weight: what is the target? *J Nutr* 131(suppl):440S, 2001.

This article reviews the evolution of weight control and healthy weight advice included in the *Dietary Guidelines for Americans* since the first edition was developed in 1980. It also gives us some background for the development of the expanded goal for exercise included in the 2000 edition.

Lake AJ, Staiger PK, Glowinski H: Effect of western culture on women's attitudes to eating and perceptions of body shape, *Int J Eat Disord* 27:83, 2000.

This article explores the cultural differences in perceptions of the ideal body shape among young women and how this can affect the development of disordered eating.

Anderson JW, Konz EC, Jenkins DJA: Health advantages and disadvantages of weight-reducing diets: a computer analysis and critical review, *J Am Coll Nutr* 19:578, 2000.

Dr. Anderson and his colleagues performed computer analyses to determine the nutrient content of a series of popular weight-loss regimens and evaluated their safety and potential effect on nutritional status.

Grivetti L: Psychology and cultural aspects of energy, *Nutr Rev* 59:S5, 2001.

This article provides an excellent overview of the social and cultural issues that contribute to the development of obesity in our society.

Bren L: Losing weight: more than counting calories, *FDA Consumer* 36:18, 2002.

This article appearing in the publication of the U.S. Food and Drug Administration gives us a perspective on both the appropriate and inappropriate treatments for obesity.

Blanck HM, Khan LK, Serdula MK: Use of nonprescription weight loss products. Results from a multistate survey, *JAMA* 286:930, 2001.

These researchers tell us about the findings of a survey across five states that explored the use of over-the-counter drugs by adults who were trying to lose weight. We also learn about some of the health dangers and problems associated with these products.

CASE STUDY The obese patient with hypertension

Mrs. Giovanni is a 45-year-old woman who is the mother of three children and was first seen in the clinic 6 months ago for a routine checkup. At that time she weighed 90 kg (200 lb) and had a blood pressure reading of 152/88 mm Hg. She is 155 cm (5 ft 2 in) tall. At the initial visit she had no serious complaints other than a bad cold. Her physician warned her that her blood pressure was somewhat elevated and scheduled a return visit for another reading the next week. After two more readings of 160/95 and 155/89 mm Hg consecutively, Mrs. Giovanni was told that she had hypertension. No medication was prescribed. However, she was referred to the nutritionist to begin weight management and sodium control.

During the assessment interview the clinic nutritionist discovered that Mrs. Giovanni ate two meals at home and one at work. Breakfast usually consisted of scraps of food left on plates by her school-age children. Lunch was a hot meal with dessert purchased in the cafeteria of the hospital where she worked part-time as an admissions clerk. Dinner was almost always an Italian-style meal, often including pasta with rich sauces and cheese or filled with meat, plus a variety of vegetables and salads. Desserts, usually made from scratch, were served with every dinner.

Mrs. Giovanni was very interested in gradually losing some weight to avoid taking antihypertensive medication if possible. However, she was apprehensive about the possibility of having to give up her favorite foods to do so. The nutritionist reassured her. With Mrs. Giovanni, the nutritionist helped with a food preparation plan to reduce fat and salt by using a number of alternative seasonings in the family recipes. Then she arranged for Mrs. Giovanni to join one of the clinic's peer support groups where she could experience some stress reduction exercises and new ways of looking at food.

Three months later Mrs. Giovanni had lost 8 kg (18 lb). She reported feeling much better and said her family was very supportive of her efforts. As a result of new cooking methods, her overweight husband had finally started to lose weight as well. She continued to lose an average of 0.7 kg (1.4 lb) per week for another month, but suddenly she gained 2.5 kg (5 lb) in a 2-week period. At a nutrition interview conducted shortly after that time, she revealed that her husband had recently been hospitalized with a stroke. Apparently he also had hypertension but had refused to see a physician for many years. The effects of the stroke were very mild; however, Mrs. Giovanni continued to worry about her husband's health. She began to eat desserts with lunch again and kept nuts, candies, and other snack foods at home for "nibbling." The nutritionist provided personal support in the office and suggested adding exercise to the routine as a good form of healthy weight and stress management. Mrs. Giovanni resisted the idea at first, saying that she could not fit it into her current schedule of caring for three children and her husband and working part-time at the hospital. However, after bringing the subject up in her weight management group meeting, she gained positive feedback and practical ideas for fitting some aerobic activities into her busy schedule.

During the next 3 months, Mrs. Giovanni resumed her previous weight loss pattern and has begun to feel better. The exercise routine has also helped her to look better and to feel better about herself. She informed the nutritionist that, aside from her appearance, she is most proud of the effect of her healthy diet program on her family. Her children have reduced their junk food intake, and her husband has even begun exercising with her almost every day.

QUESTIONS FOR ANALYSIS

1. How do you think Mrs. Giovanni's lifestyle, meal pattern, food habits, and food preparation methods influenced her weight status?
2. What is hypertension? What role does weight management play in controlling it? Why did Mrs. Giovanni's physician recommend nondrug methods of control through diet?
3. In developing a meal plan with Mrs. Giovanni, what advice would you offer to help her retain the cultural flavor of her meals while reducing her kcalorie intake?
4. What are some ways that Mrs. Giovanni may strengthen her behavioral changes toward food and exercise? What other behavioral approaches may be useful?
5. What is aerobic exercise? Why is it effective for a weight management program?
6. What practical suggestions would you offer to Mrs. Giovanni for helping her incorporate exercise time into her busy routine? Why?

Issues & ANSWERS

Eating Disorders: The High Price of Our Drive for Thinness

More than 5 million Americans have eating disorders. Although eating disorders are considered to be psychiatric disorders, they are characterized by abnormal eating patterns that lead to nutritional deficiencies and medical complications and, if pursued in an unrelenting fashion, disability and death. Although we associate eating disorders with the drive for thinness that pervades our society, references to a condition similar to anorexia nervosa can be found in the medical literature from many centuries ago. Physicians in Great Britain and France formally described this disorder in the 1800s.

What leads to eating disorders?

Eating disorders are believed to have multiple causes that interact to produce the behavior that we associate with these problems. Biologic, psychologic, and social forces all seem to play a role. Hormonal changes occurring at puberty along with genetic components contribute to the development of eating disorders, but at this time we do not understand exactly how this occurs. Family dysfunction and family conflict can contribute to disordered eating, but no one family model has been identified that exists in all cases. Social pressures and expectations on young women today play a major role. Prior history of substance abuse is a risk factor for eating disorders. For each individual who develops an eating disorder, a particular factor may be more important or less important. For example, because of innate biologic factors some girls may develop an eating disorder despite a very supportive family environment, whereas others are more strongly influenced by society expectations. Eating disorders can be found in all social classes and demographic groups. Adolescent females are especially vulnerable to these conditions.

The growing interest in athletics among children in middle school and beyond can increase risk or help to prevent eating disorders. Elite athletes in sports such as gymnastics or dance in which thinness is expected are at higher risk for developing an eating disorder. Students who take part in school sports as a recreational activity are less likely to develop an eating disorder than are students who do not participate in athletics. Young women who select a sport that does not require a thin body have less risk of an eating problem. Good self-esteem helps protect adolescents against acquiring an eating disorder; thus participation in athletics or other activities that help young people feel good about themselves and their accomplishments should be encouraged.

The major characteristics of eating disorders are (1) a disturbed body image in which an individual perceives himself or herself as fat, even though body weight is normal or even below normal; (2) an intense fear of gaining weight or becoming fat; and (3) an unrelenting desire to become thinner. Cultural background influences a person's level of satisfaction or dissatisfaction with his or her body shape. Among African American, Latino American, and Caucasian college students, large differences existed in their level of satisfaction with their physical appearance. The African American students were the most satisfied with their appearance and the least likely to overestimate their current body weight. The Caucasian students were the most dissatisfied with their appearance and tended to estimate their body weight as being much higher than it actually was. The Latino American students fell in between the other two groups. The women were more concerned about their body weight than were the men.

How do we prevent these distorted images of personal appearance from getting started? Children as young as kindergarten age are beginning to be concerned about their body weight and to avoid foods that they perceive to be high in kcalories and fat. Primary prevention must begin in the school. One school program carried out with boys and girls aged 11 to 14 was entitled Everyone's Different and emphasized a positive image of self, how to value and accept differences, and how to follow good food and exercise behaviors. After 1 year those children considered to be at risk of developing an eating disorder at the beginning of the program had actually gained weight and were following positive eating behaviors. Health professionals need to join forces with teachers, psychologists, counselors, and parents to support the development of such intervention programs.

Criteria for diagnosis. Three forms of eating disorders are now recognized and described by the American Psychiatric Association (APA) in its guidelines for medical therapy teams. These diagnoses are based on psychologic, behavioral, and physiologic characteristics and include anorexia nervosa (AN), bulimia nervosa (BN), and eating disorder not otherwise specified (EDNOS). Binge eating disorder is included under the heading of EDNOS. Each has distinctive characteristics based on the APA diagnostic criteria and symptoms.

Anorexia nervosa

The term *anorexia nervosa (AN)* means "appetite loss from nervous disease." AN leads to starvation with excessive weight loss, self-imposed at great physical and psychologic cost. These patients may have a body weight less than 85% of average body weight or a BMI of less than 17.5. With their distorted body image, those with AN have an intense fear of gaining weight, becoming fat, or eating food items containing fat. They do not see themselves as underweight and emaciated but rather as always fat, and this distorted body image can persist during recovery as well.

AN can lead to sudden death from severe hypoglycemia and cardiac arrest, and the mortality rate may be as high as 21%. Low bone mass is a frequent complication of AN, increasing the risk of bone fractures in these individuals. Many of these persons take vitamin and mineral supplements; therefore obvious deficiencies seldom occur even though they eat very little food. With treatment one third of patients with AN will experience a full recovery, one third will be able to return to a productive level of function but continue to struggle with issues of body weight, and one third will require repeated hospitalizations.

Diagnostic criteria. *DSM-IV-TR Diagnostic and Statistical Manual of Mental Disorders, Fourth Edition, Text Revision (DSM-IV-TR)* describes the following conditions as diagnostic for AN.

1. Refusal to eat sufficient food to maintain a body weight at least 85% of average.
2. Intense fear of gaining weight or becoming fat, even though current weight is below average.
3. Disturbed perception of one's body weight, size, or shape; the patient claims to be fat even if emaciated and refuses to recognize the seriousness of the underweight or emaciated condition.
4. In females, the absence of at least three consecutive menstrual cycles when otherwise expected to occur.

Bulimia nervosa

Bulimia, from the word meaning "ox-hunger," is descriptive of the massive amounts of food sometimes consumed by persons with this condition. BN also has been called the binge-and-purge syndrome. Because this individual is eating, body weight is usually normal or may even be higher than normal; therefore the underlying problem is a guilt-ridden secret. BN is often associated with depression or he or she may find it difficult to meet social or role expectations. In some cases weight loss is viewed as a solution. When large amounts of food are consumed, the eating episode is followed by purging through self-induced vomiting, excessive exercise, or use of laxatives or diuretics. The emotional and physical cost of this behavior is great.

Diagnostic criteria. The *DSM-IV-TR* describes the following conditions as diagnostic for BN.

1. Recurrent episodes of binge eating—rapid consumption of a large amount of food in a single and relatively short period.
2. Lack of control over eating behavior during the binges; feeling that one cannot stop eating or control how much is being eaten.
3. Regular self-induced vomiting, use of laxatives or diuretics, strict dieting or fasting, or vigorous exercise as compensatory behavior to prevent weight gain.
4. Minimum average of two binge eating episodes a week for at least 3 months.
5. Persistent overconcern with body shape and weight.

Eating disorder not otherwise specified

About 50% of the persons with eating disorders fall under the category of EDNOS. If their problems remain untreated, and this behavior continues, they may progress to the conditions of either AN or BN. EDNOS includes binge-eating disorder.

Diagnostic criteria. This eating disorder category, as its name indicates, includes eating behaviors that do not meet the conditions for other eating disorders.

1. It is like AN except that regular menses continue and, despite substantial weight loss, current body weight is normal.
2. It is like BN except that binges occur less often than twice a week and the pattern lasts less than 3 months.
3. The person maintains a normal weight by self-induced vomiting after eating even small amounts of food such as two cookies, or by chewing and then spitting out the food, but not swallowing.

Binge eating disorder

This eating disorder includes binge eating episodes without the purging behavior of BN. Binge eating may occur in response to stress or anxiety or to soothe or relieve painful feelings. Many of these patients are overweight and have the same medical problems as obese individuals who do not binge eat.

Diagnostic criteria. The *DSM-IV-TR* describes these conditions as diagnostic for binge eating disorder.

1. Recurrent episodes of binge eating—rapid consumption of a large amount of food in a single, relatively short period of time to the point of feeling uncomfortably full.
2. Lack of control over eating behavior during the binges; feeling that one cannot stop eating or control how much is being eaten.
3. Eating large amounts of food when not feeling hungry and eating alone as a result of feeling embarrassed by the amount.
4. Feelings of self-disgust, depression, or guilt after a bingeing episode, which occurs at least 2 days a week.

5. Marked distress about the binge eating, but no compensatory behaviors such as purging, fasting, or excessive exercise.

Treatment approaches

Eating disorders take a high toll on both the physical and psychologic health of many adolescents and young women and men, and they require individualized care. The best chance for success in improving their condition lies with team care by a sensitive, experienced group of health professionals including a physician, clinical psychologist, clinical nutritionist, and nurse. Outpatient services may provide needed care for less advanced cases, but for life-threatening AN, more intense inpatient care is essential.

Treatment must focus on nutritional, medical, and cognitive therapy. A meal plan that provides a framework for meals, snacks, and food choices, and supplements, if indicated, must be implemented on a gradual basis to address the issues of underweight or overweight. Medical complications arising from severe malnutrition, dehydration, habitual vomiting, and excessive use of diuretics or laxatives must be addressed. Cognitive therapy including the counseling technique of cognitive-behavioral therapy (CBT; challenging erroneous beliefs and thought patterns) can lead to appropriate interpretations about nutrition, diet, and body weight. The psychologist or psychiatrist on the healthcare team can focus on those personal or family issues that may have led to the distorted body image and eating disorder, and assist in the development of healthy behavior patterns that will sustain the nutritional and medical recovery.

Eating disorders are serious health matters. How long can we pay this heavy price for distorted societal images of personal worth based on how we look instead of who we are? Change in any area is difficult, but it rests on a foundation of awareness and knowledge of the problem that can lead to changes in attitude. Certainly, we need to practice ethical behavior and respect individual differences in our own work, as well as seek reforms in the diet industry. More realistic individualized approaches to help persons with weight and health issues can reduce the risks for serious eating disorders.

REFERENCES

American Psychiatric Association: *Diagnostic and statistical manual of mental disorders,* ed 4, Text Revision, Washington, DC, 2000, The American Psychiatric Association. (Diagnostic criteria reprinted with permission from the *Diagnostic and statistical manual of mental health disorders,* ed 4, Text Revision. Copyright 2000, American Psychiatric Association.)

Hadigan CM et al: Assessment of macronutrient and micronutrient intake in women with anorexia nervosa, *Int J Eat Disord* 28:284, 2000.)

Huse DM, Lucas AR: Behavioral disorders affecting food intake: anorexia nervosa, bulimia nervosa, and other psychiatric conditions. In Shils ME et al, eds: *Modern nutrition in health and disease,* ed 9, Philadelphia, 1999, Lippincott Williams & Wilkins.

Mayer L: Body composition and anorexia nervosa: does physiology explain psychology? *Am J Clin Nutr* 73:851, 2001.

Miller KJ et al: Comparisons of body image dimensions by race/ethnicity and gender in a university population, *Int J Eat Disord* 27:310, 2000.

O'Dea JA, Abraham S: Improving the body image, eating attitudes, and behaviors of young male and female adolescents: a new educational approach that focuses on self-esteem, *Int J Eat Disord* 28:43, 2000.

Polivy J, Herman PC: Causes of eating disorders, *Annu Rev Psychol* 53:187, 2002.

Spear B, Stellefson-Myers E: Position of the American Dietetic Association: nutrition intervention in the treatment of anorexia nervosa, bulimia nervosa, and eating disorders not otherwise specified (EDNOS), *J Am Diet Assoc* 101:810, 2001.

Winston AP et al: Prevalence of thiamin deficiency in anorexia nervosa, *Int J Eat Disord* 28:451, 2000.

Chapter 7

Vitamins

Eleanor D. Schlenker

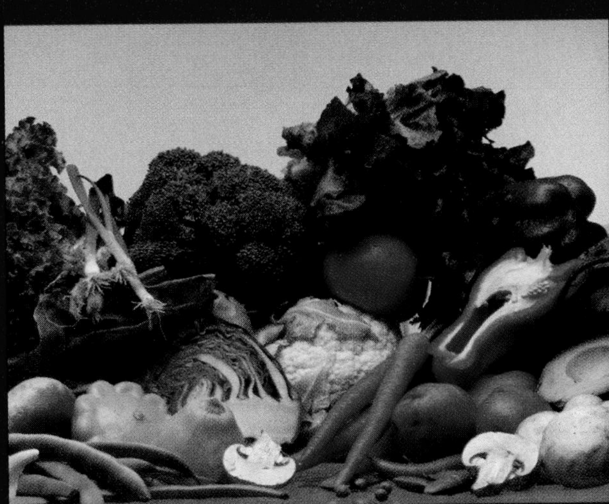

Chapter Outline

Now we begin a two-chapter sequence on the non–energy-yielding micronutrients: the vitamins and minerals. First, we look at the vitamins.

Probably no other group of nutritional elements has so captured the interest of scientists, health professionals, and the general public as the vitamins. Both scientific journals and the popular press have printed articles describing how vitamins may help to prevent chronic disease in ways over and above their usual roles in body functions. Attitudes about the need for vitamins have varied widely, running the gamut from wise functional use to wild flagrant abuse.

In this chapter we review both fat-soluble and water-soluble vitamins. We focus on why we need them and how we may obtain them.

THE STUDY OF VITAMINS: ESSENTIAL NUTRIENTS

GENERAL NATURE AND CLASSIFICATION

During the years of rapid vitamin discovery from 1900 to 1950, the remarkable nature of these vital molecules became increasingly apparent. Three key characteristics became evident: (1) they were not metabolized to yield energy as were carbohydrate, fat, and sometimes protein; (2) they were vital to life; and (3) often not a single substance but a group of related substances turned out to have the particular metabolic activity. The name vitamin developed during the early research years when one of the scientists working with a nitrogen-containing chemical substance called an amine thought this was the common nature of all of these vital molecules. So he named his discovery vitamine ("vital amine"). Later the final "e" was dropped when other similarly vital substances turned out to have different organic structures, but the name vitamin has been retained to designate compounds of this class of essential substances. At first, letter names were given to individual vitamins as they were discovered. But as the number of known vitamins increased rapidly, this practice created confusion. Thus in recent years more specific scientific names based on structure or function were developed. However, for the fat-soluble vitamins, their letter names have been retained for clarity because in each case a number of closely related compounds with similar properties and structures are well known.[1]

DEFINITION OF A VITAMIN

As the vitamins were discovered one by one and the list of them grew, several basic characteristics clearly emerged to define a compound as a vitamin.

1. It must be a vital organic dietary substance that is not an energy-producing carbohydrate, fat, or protein.
2. It is usually necessary in only very small quantities to perform a particular metabolic function or to prevent an associated deficiency disease.
3. It cannot be manufactured by the body and therefore must be supplied in food.

These criteria are the basis for identifying a vitamin as essential; however, new research showing associations between intakes of some vitamin-like substances and increased resistance to chronic diseases such as cancer or heart disease has raised questions about the definition of "essential nutrient." Should a substance that appears to promote health be considered "essential" even if no specific deficiency disease has been identified? For the present such molecules continue to be referred to as desirable rather than "essential," with the decision about essentiality awaiting further research.[2]

CLASSIFICATION

As the vitamins were first discovered they were grouped and distinguished according to their solubility in either fat or water and this classification has continued.

Fat-Soluble Vitamins

The fat-soluble vitamins are A, D, E, and K. They are closely associated with lipids in the body. They can be stored, and their functions are generally related to proteins involved in structural activities.

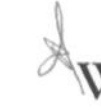

Water-Soluble Vitamins

The water-soluble vitamins are C and the B-complex family. These vitamins are more easily absorbed and transported. They cannot be stored except in the general sense of tissue saturation. The B vitamins function mainly as coenzyme factors in cell metabolism. Vitamin C is a vital structural agent.

CURRENT CONCEPTS AND KEY QUESTIONS

To clarify current knowledge concerning each known vitamin, consider these key questions as the basis for your study.

- *Nature.* What is the vitamin's general structure?
- *Absorption and transport.* How does the body handle this particular vitamin?
- *Function.* What does this vitamin do? This is, perhaps, the most significant question.
- *Related deficiency symptoms or disease.* What occurs when this vitamin is absent or not available in sufficient amounts?
- *Clinical role in health.* How is this vitamin related to the prevention of chronic disease?
- *Requirement and possible toxicity.* How much of this vitamin do we need but how much is too much? What are the consequences of excessive intake?
- *Food sources.* Where can we obtain this vitamin?

We will briefly review each of the vitamins in turn—the four fat-soluble (A, D, E, K) and the nine water-soluble (C and B complex vitamins). For each we will identify the specific chemical name and the more common term now in use and review answers to the key questions just given. In some cases, a group of similar substances all have the vitamin activity, not just a single substance bearing the specific name.

FAT-SOLUBLE VITAMINS

Vitamin A

CHEMICAL AND PHYSICAL NATURE

Vitamin A is a generic term for a group of compounds having similar biologic activity. These compounds include retinol, retinal, and retinoic acid. The term *retinoids* refers to both the natural forms of retinol and its synthetic copies. Chemically, retinol is a primary alcohol of high molecular weight ($C_{20}H_{29}OH$). Because it has a specific function in the retina of the eye and is an alcohol, vitamin A has been given the specific chemical name retinol. It is soluble in fat and in ordinary fat solvents. Because it is insoluble in water, it is fairly stable in cooking.

FORMS

There are two basic dietary forms of vitamin A.

1. *Preformed vitamin A: retinol.* This is the natural form of vitamin A, found only in animal food sources and usually associated with fats. Vitamin A compounds are deposited primarily in the liver but also in small amounts in the kidneys, lungs, and fat tissue. In this form, its dietary sources are mainly the fat portion of dairy products, egg yolk, fish, and animal storage organs such as liver.
2. *Provitamin A: beta-carotene.* Plants cannot synthesize vitamin A but instead produce a family of compounds called carotenoids. These substances found in plants that animals have eaten are then converted to vitamin A. Thus humans can obtain their vitamin A directly from eating animal tissues or by converting the carotenoids obtained from plant foods. The original plant source, beta-carotene ($C_{40}H_{56}$), is found in plant pigments and was called carotene because one of its main sources is the yellow and orange pigment of carrots and other vegetables and fruits. In recent years numerous other carotenoids have been identified, including beta-cryptoxanthin, lutein, and zeaxanthin. The carotenoids are significant in human nutrition and contribute 26% of the vitamin A in the diets of men and 34% in the diets of women. Beta-carotene is the carotenoid that is most efficiently converted to vitamin A in the body and provides about 21% of the total vitamin A intake in the United States.[3] Enzymes that can split the carotenoid molecules to yield retinol are found in the mucosal cells lining the small intestine and in the liver. The yellow and red carotenoid pigments, which occur in abundance in many fruits and vegetables, are major sources of vitamin A for many of the world's population.[4]

ABSORPTION, TRANSPORT, AND STORAGE

Substances That Aid Absorption

Vitamin A enters the body as the preformed vitamin A from animal sources and the precursor beta-carotene from plant sources. Several substances are needed for the absorption of vitamin A and beta-carotene by the body.

1. *Bile salts.* Bile salts transport vitamin A joined with fat and other fat-related compounds in micelles. Micelles are minute fat globules formed in the small intestine after initial digestion and then carried into the intestinal wall for further breakdown. Clinical conditions affecting the biliary system, such as obstruction of the bile ducts, infectious hepatitis, and liver cirrhosis, hinder vitamin A absorption.
2. *Pancreatic lipase.* This fat-splitting enzyme released into the upper small intestine is necessary for initial hydrolysis of fat emulsions or oil solutions of vitamin A. Water-based preparations of retinol are available for use in conditions where secretion of pancreatic lipase or absorption of fat is curtailed, such as in cystic fibrosis or pancreatitis.[1]
3. *Dietary fat.* Some fat in the food mix, simultaneously absorbed along with the vitamin, stimulates bile release for effective absorption of vitamin A. Vitamin A is absorbed most efficiently when fat intake is more than 10 g/day.[5]

Beta-Carotene Conversion

Some of the beta-carotene is converted to vitamin A as it passes through the intestinal wall during absorption. The remainder is absorbed and transported as beta-carotene, dissolved in the fat portion of lipoproteins. At one time it was believed that the only biologic importance of beta-carotene or other carotenoids was in their role as precursors to vitamin A. Recent research has established that the carotenoids perform roles in human health that are completely unrelated to the actions of vitamin A. Carotenoids are included in the broad category of phytochemicals or plant chemicals that have beneficial effects in promoting health and preventing disease. Phytochemicals are discussed in greater detail in the *Issues & Answers* at the end of this chapter.

Transport and Storage

The route of absorption of both vitamin A and the carotenes parallels that of fat. In the intestinal mucosa all the retinol, from both preformed animal sources and from plant carotene conversion, is incorporated into the chylomicrons.[1] In this form it enters the bloodstream via the lymphatic system and is carried to the liver for storage or distribution to the cells. The liver, by far the most efficient

---

amine An organic compound containing nitrogen. Amino acids and pyridoxine are examples of amines.

precursor Something that precedes; in biology, a substance from which another substance is derived.

retinal Organic compound that is the aldehyde form of retinol, derived by the enzymatic splitting of absorbed carotene. It performs vitamin A activity. In the retina of the eye, retinal combines with opsins to form visual pigments. In the rods it combines with scotopsin to form rhodopsin (visual purple). In the cones it combines with photopsin to form the three pigments responsible for color vision.

retinol Chemical name for vitamin A derived from its function relating to the retina of the eye and light-dark adaptation. Daily RDA standards are stated in retinol equivalents (RE) to account for sources of the preformed vitamin A and its precursor provitamin A, beta-carotene.

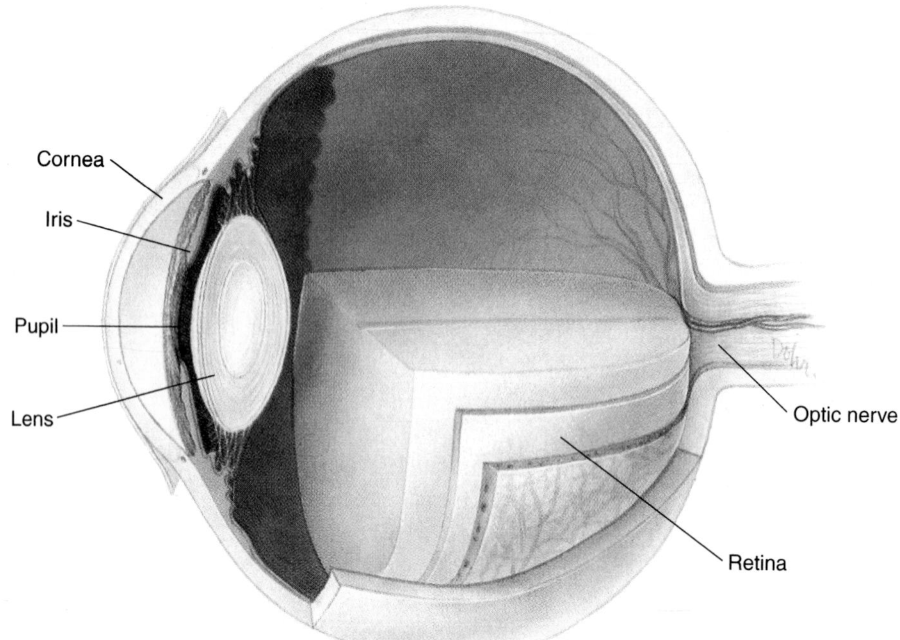

FIGURE 7-1 Structure of the eye. (*From Seeley RR, Stephens TD, Tate PP:* Anatomy and physiology, *ed 2, New York, 1992, McGraw-Hill. Reproduced with permission of The McGraw-Hill Companies.*)

storage organ for vitamin A, contains up to 85% of the body's total supply. This amount is sufficient to supply the body's needs for about 6 to 12 months, and some persons have been known to store as much as a 4-year supply. These stores are reduced, however, during infectious disease, especially in childhood infections such as measles. For example, among malnourished children in many parts of the world, measles has become a leading killer disease and is now designated by the World Health Organization (WHO) Expanded Program on Immunization as a target for both vitamin A supplementation and immunization. Age is also a factor in absorption. In the newborn, especially the premature infant, absorption is poor. With advancing age, elderly persons using mineral oil as a laxative will reduce vitamin A absorption.

FUNCTIONS OF VITAMIN A

The role of vitamin A in visual adaptation to light and darkness has been well established. This vitamin also has a number of more generalized functions that influence vision, the health of body coverings and linings (epithelial tissue), the process of growth, the immune system, and reproductive function.

VITAMIN A DEFICIENCY AND CLINICAL PROBLEMS

Vision

The ability of the eye to adapt to changes in light depends on a light-sensitive pigment, rhodopsin—commonly known as visual purple—in the rods of the retina (Figure 7-1). Rhodopsin is composed of the vitamin A substance retinal and the protein opsin (Figure 7-2). When the body is deficient in vitamin A, the normal rhodopsin cannot be made and the rods and cones of the retina become increasingly sensitive to light changes, causing night blindness. This condition can usually be cured in about 30 minutes by an injection of vitamin A (retinol), which is readily converted into retinal and then into rhodopsin.

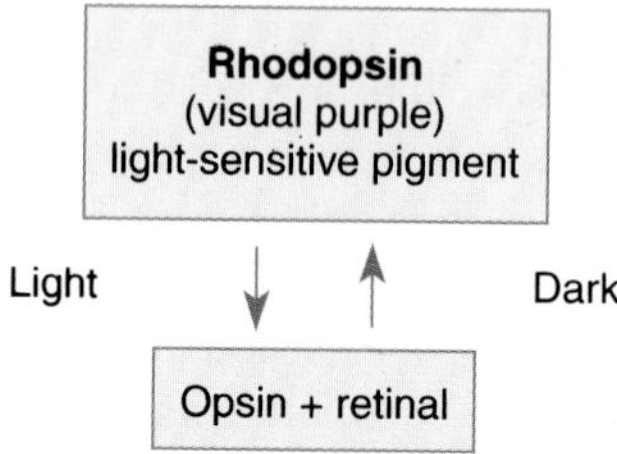

FIGURE 7-2 The vision cycle: light-dark adaptation role of vitamin A.

Cell Differentiation

Vitamin A controls the differentiation of cells, or in other words, the types of cells that are formed from basic tissues. Vitamin A is necessary to build and maintain healthy epithelial tissue, which provides our primary barrier to infections. The epithelium includes not only the outer skin but also the inner mucous membranes of many body structures. Without vitamin A, we form cells that are dry and flat rather than soft and moist. These dry, flat cells gradually harden to form keratin, a process called keratinization. Keratin is a protein that forms dry, scaly tissue, normal in the case of nails and hair but abnormal in the case of skin and mu-

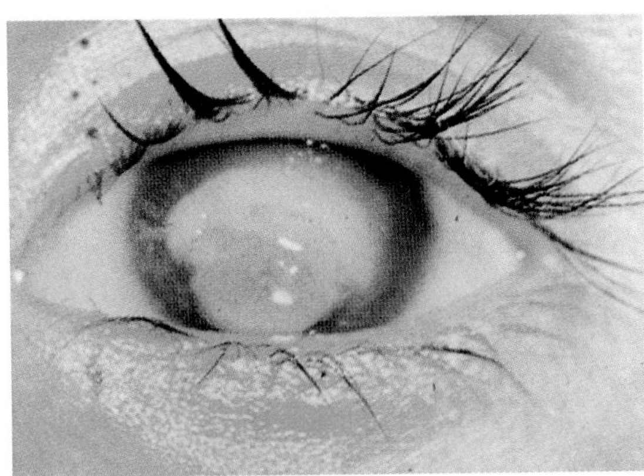

FIGURE 7-3 Xerophthalmia. (*From McLaren DS:* A colour atlas and text of diet-related disorders, *ed 2, London, 1992, Mosby–Year Book Europe Limited.*)

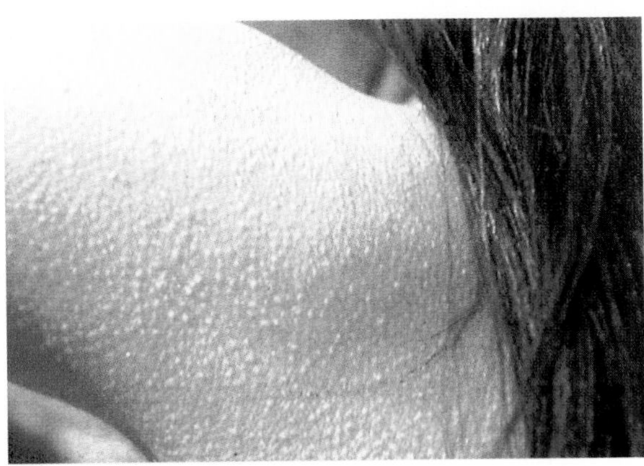

FIGURE 7-4 Follicular hyperkeratosis caused by vitamin A deficiency. (*From McLaren DS:* A colour atlas and text of diet-related disorders, *ed 2, London, 1992, Mosby–Year Book Europe Limited.*)

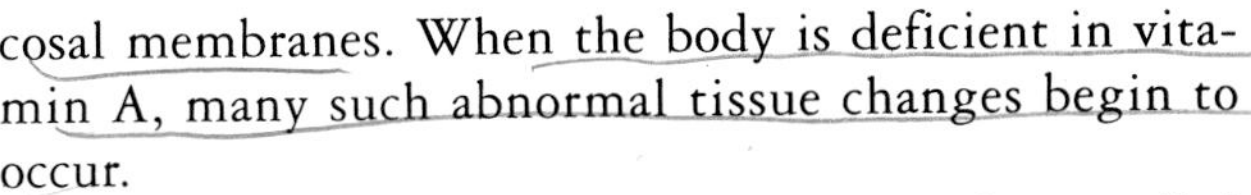

cosal membranes. When the body is deficient in vitamin A, many such abnormal tissue changes begin to occur.

1. *Eye.* The cornea dries and hardens, a condition called xerophthalmia (Figure 7-3). In extreme deficiency it progresses to blindness. This progressive blindness resulting from vitamin A deficiency is a serious world public health problem; each year more than 350,000 preschool children lose their sight.[5] The tear ducts dry, robbing the eye of its cleansing and lubricating fluid, and infection follows easily.
2. *Respiratory tract.* Ciliated epithelium in the nasal passages dries and the cilia are lost, thus removing a barrier to entry of infectious organisms. The salivary glands dry, and the mouth becomes dry and cracked, open to invading bacteria.
3. *Gastrointestinal tract.* Mucosal membrane secretions decrease so that tissues dry and slough off, affecting digestion and absorption.
4. *Genitourinary tract.* As epithelial tissue breaks down, problems such as urinary tract infections, formation of calculi, and vaginal infections increase.
5. *Skin.* As skin becomes dry and scaly, small pustules or hardened, pigmented, papular eruptions appear around hair follicles, a condition called follicular hyperkeratosis (Figure 7-4).
6. *Tooth formation.* Specific epithelial cells surrounding tooth buds in fetal gum tissue that normally become specialized cup-shaped organs called ameloblasts may not develop properly. These little organs form the enamel of the developing tooth.

Growth

Vitamin A is essential for the growth of bones and soft tissues. This effect is likely caused by the influence of vitamin A on protein synthesis, *mitosis* (cell division), differentiation of cells, and stability of cell membranes. Growth and maintenance of bone require constant remodeling of the bone tissue according to growth and repair needs. To accomplish this constant reshaping and balance, continuous growth of new bone and removal of old bone must occur. Vitamin A participates in the important job of tunneling out old bone to make way for new bone; then the tunnels are filled in to accommodate growth needs, all the while maintaining the precise pattern set in the initial embryonic cartilage model. Although appropriate levels of vitamin A support bone health, excess intakes of vitamin A promote bone loss and may contribute to thinning bone in older people.[6]

As noted earlier, vitamin A deficiency causes changes in the mucosal lining of the gastrointestinal tract that can result in poor absorption of other nutrients important to growth. Vitamin A supplementation was associated with catch-up growth of stunted preschool children in the Sudan.[7]

Reproduction

The retinoids, except for retinoic acid, are necessary to support normal sexual maturation and function. Vitamin A appears to participate in gene expression and plays an important role in fetal development, including development of the central nervous system.[8] It also is required for successful milk production and lactation. Vitamin A deficiency leads to glandular degeneration and sterility.

---

keratinization The process of creating the protein keratin, which is the principal constituent of skin, hair, nails, and the organizing matrix of the enamel of the teeth. It is a very insoluble protein.

night blindness Inability to see well at night in diminished light, resulting from lack of required vitamin A.

Immunity

Poor vitamin A status results in reduced resistance to infection not only through its effect on epithelial and mucosal tissue but also through its direct effect on the immune system. Both cell-mediated immunity and antibody-mediated immunity are affected. Vitamin A–deficient children are less able to resist infectious diseases such as measles than are well-nourished children. Immune response returns to normal quite rapidly when vitamin A is provided; therefore it would seem that the cell machinery is intact, but the signal to produce the needed proteins for immune cells and antibodies is missing.[9]

VITAMIN A REQUIREMENT

Influencing Factors

A number of variables modify vitamin A needs. In a given individual the need for vitamin A may be altered by (1) amount stored in the liver, (2) form in which it is eaten (beta-carotene or preformed vitamin A), (3) illness, and (4) gastrointestinal or hepatic defects. Vitamin A deficiency may occur as a result of (1) inadequate dietary intake, (2) poor absorption resulting from lack of bile, lack of dietary fat, or defective absorbing surface, and (3) inadequate conversion of beta-carotene because of liver or intestinal disease.

Dietary Reference Intakes

The Recommended Dietary Allowance (RDA) for vitamin A was based on the amount of the vitamin required to maintain optimum liver stores. At one time vitamin A was measured in international units (IU) and retinol equivalents (RE); however, the RDA released in 2001 is given in μg.[3] The new RDA presented in μg also reflects new research indicating that the conversion of beta-carotene and other carotenoids to retinol is less efficient than previously thought, although most food composition tables still report vitamin A content using RE. The RDA for men ages 19 and over is set at 900 μg and the RDA for women in this age group is 700 μg. To ensure a sufficient supply of the vitamin to support a successful pregnancy and the production of milk with an appropriate content of vitamin A, the RDA is raised to 770 μg in pregnancy and 1300 μg during lactation.

VITAMIN A TOXICITY

Hypervitaminosis A

Because the liver can store large amounts of vitamin A, it is clearly possible for persons taking high-potency supplements to consume a potentially toxic amount. Hypervitaminosis A is manifested by joint pain, thickening of the long bones, loss of hair, and jaundice. Excess vitamin A may cause liver injury with resulting portal hypertension and ascites. Daily intakes above the established Tolerable Upper Intake Level (UL) of 3000 μg of preformed vitamin A are particularly dangerous for pregnant women because they can lead to congenital malformations of the fetus.[10]

FOOD SOURCES OF VITAMIN A

There are few animal sources of preformed vitamin A: liver, kidney, whole milk, butter, and egg yolk. In addition, commercial products such as margarine and some cereal products are fortified with vitamin A. Skim and low-fat milk is fortified with vitamin A to the level usually found in whole milk. Dark yellow, orange, and green vegetables and fruits containing a variety of carotenoids make a major contribution toward meeting the vitamin A requirement. Carotenoids are more easily broken away from other plant components and available for absorption by the body when vegetables are eaten cooked rather than raw.[3] Although a person may enjoy eating raw vegetables at times, it may be of benefit to include a variety of cooked vegetables as well. The vitamin A values of selected foods are given in Table 7-1.

Vitamin D

CHEMICAL AND PHYSICAL NATURE

Early investigators wrongly classified this substance as a vitamin. It is now clear that vitamin D is really a prohormone of a sterol type and in its active form is viewed as a hormone. The precursor of vitamin D found in human skin is the lipid cholesterol molecule 7-dehydrocholesterol. All forms of the compounds with vitamin D activity are soluble in fat but not in water. They are heat stable and not easily oxidized.

FORMS

Two substances with vitamin D activity are involved in nutrition: ergocalciferol (vitamin D_2) and cholecalciferol (vitamin D_3). Vitamin D_2 is formed by irradiating ergosterol, which is found in ergot (a fungus growing on rye and other cereal grains) and yeast. The more significant form of the vitamin in human nutrition is D_3, cholecalciferol, which is formed by irradiating 7-dehydrocholesterol in the skin. D_3 also is found in fish liver oils, and it is added to fortified milk and dairy products.

ABSORPTION, TRANSPORT, AND STORAGE

Absorption

The absorption of dietary vitamin D_3 occurs in the small intestine with the aid of bile. It mixes with the intestinal bile-fat complex and is absorbed in these fat packets called *micelles*. Malabsorption diseases such as celiac syn-

TABLE 7-1 Food Sources of Vitamin A

Food Source	Quantity	Vitamin A (μg RE)
Bread, Cereal, Rice, Pasta		
This food group is not an important source of vitamin A		
Vegetables		
Asparagus	½ cup	196
Beet greens	½ cup	1110
Bok choy cabbage	½ cup	790
Broccoli (fresh)	1 med stalk	1350
Broccoli (frozen)	½ cup (chopped)	721
Brussels sprouts	½ cup (4 sprouts)	121
Carrots (raw)	½ cup (1 med)	2379
Collard greens	½ cup	2223
Corn	1 sm cob	93
Dandelion greens	½ cup	1843
Green beans	½ cup	102
Green peas	½ cup	144
Kale	½ cup	1369
Lima beans	½ cup	60
Mustard greens	½ cup	1218
Pumpkin (canned)	½ cup	2352
Romaine lettuce	½ cup (chopped)	157
Spinach	½ cup	2187
Summer squash	½ cup	123
Sweet potato (baked, in skin)	1 med	2769
Tomato (cooked)	½ cup	325
Winter squash	½ cup	1021
Fruits		
Apricot (dried)	4 halves	490
Apricot (fresh)	3 med	867
Avocado	1 med	189
Banana	1 med	69
Fruits—cont'd		
Cantaloupe	½ med	1386
Grapefruit (pink)	½ med	162
Orange juice	½ cup	75
Papaya	1 cup (cubes)	735
Peach	1 med	399
Prunes (dried)	4 prunes	207
Tangerine	1 med	108
Watermelon	1 wedge (4 × 8 in)	753
Meat, Poultry, Fish, Dried Beans, Eggs, Nuts		
Clams (canned)	3 oz	144
Egg, whole	1 large	78
Liver, beef	3.5 oz	10,831
Liver, chicken	3.5 oz	4912
Salmon, pink (raw)	3 oz	30
Milk, Dairy Products		
Cheddar cheese	1 oz	90
Milk, low fat 2% (fortified)	8 fl oz	150
Milk, skim (fortified)	8 fl oz	150
Milk, whole (unfortified)	8 fl oz	101
Soy milk (fortified)	8 fl oz	150
Ricotta cheese, whole milk	½ cup	182
Swiss cheese	1 oz	72
Yogurt, whole milk	8 fl oz	84
Fats, Oils, Sugar		
Butter	1 tbsp	138
Margarine	1 tbsp	141

Recommended Dietary Allowance for adults: women, 700 μg; men, 900 μg.

drome, colitis, and Crohn's disease hinder vitamin D absorption.

Active Hormone Synthesis

The active hormonal form of vitamin D is 1,25-dihydroxycholecalciferol [$1,25(OH)_2D_3$], usually referred to as calcitriol. The production of calcitriol is accomplished by the combined action of the skin, liver, and kidneys, an overall process now called the vitamin D endocrine system.[11]

1. *Skin.* In the skin, 7-dehydrocholesterol, the precursor cholesterol compound, when irradiated by the ultraviolet rays of the sun, is transformed into vitamin D_3. The amount of D_3 produced by this irradiation reaction in the skin depends on a number of variables, including length and intensity of sunlight exposure and pigment in the skin. For example, heavily pigmented skin can prevent more than 95% of ultraviolet radiation from reaching the deeper layer of the skin where

calcitriol Activated hormone form of vitamin D [$1,25(OH)_2D_3$]—1,25-dihydroxycholecalciferol.

cholecalciferol Chemical name for vitamin D in its inactive dietary form (D_3). When the inactive cholecalciferol is consumed or its counterpart cholesterol compound is developed in the skin, its first stage of activation occurs in the liver and then is completed in the kidney to form the active vitamin D hormone *calcitriol,* 1,25-dihydroxycholecalciferol, or $1,25(OH)_2D_3$.

7-dehydrocholesterol A precursor cholesterol compound in the skin that is irradiated by sunlight to produce cholecalciferol (D_3).

retinol equivalent (RE) Unit of measure for dietary sources of vitamin A, both preformed vitamin, retinol, and the precursor provitamin, beta-carotene. 1 RE = 1 μg retinol or 6 μg beta-carotene.

the synthesis of vitamin D_3 occurs.[12] Also, persons who lack exposure to sunlight—housebound elderly persons and those living in nursing homes and confined indoors, or individuals residing in crowded city areas with high air pollution rates—fail to receive adequate skin irradiation as needed to synthesize vitamin D. The use of sunscreen to reduce skin cancer risk also dramatically decreases the production of vitamin D_3. More than half of adult sunscreen users were found to have low blood vitamin D levels.[12]

2. *Liver.* Vitamin D_3, whether produced in the skin or absorbed from dietary sources, is transported by a globulin protein carrier to the liver. Here a special liver enzyme converts D_3 to 25-hydroxycholecalciferol [25(OH)D_3], the intermediate product in the vitamin D endocrine system. This intermediate product is then transported by the same blood protein carrier to the kidney for final activation.
3. *Kidneys.* In the kidneys a special renal enzyme, 1-alpha-hydroxylase, completes the last step in forming the physiologically active vitamin D hormone, 1,25-dihydroxycholecalciferol [1,25$(OH)_2D_3$]. As noted earlier, the chemical name given to the active vitamin D hormone is calcitriol.

FUNCTIONS OF VITAMIN D HORMONE

Vitamin D is predominantly associated with calcium and phosphorus metabolism. It influences both the absorption of these minerals and their deposit in bone tissue.

Control of Bone and Blood Calcium and Phosphorus Levels

The vitamin D endocrine system based in the kidneys in balance with parathyroid hormone and calcitonin (1) stimulates the active transport of calcium and phosphorus in the small intestine, (2) promotes normal bone mineralization, and (3) maintains blood calcium at an appropriate level. Each of these hormones—vitamin D, parathyroid hormone, and calcitonin—has a specific role in controlling bone and blood calcium levels. Vitamin D acts primarily on the intestine to stimulate calcium and phosphorus absorption and then facilitates their deposit in bone tissue. Parathyroid hormone and calcitonin are responsible for maintaining blood calcium and phosphorus levels in the normal range. The level of blood calcium must be maintained within very narrow limits to ensure proper function of the heart and nervous system. When blood calcium levels begin to fall, parathyroid hormone stimulates calcium withdrawal from the bone and excretion of phosphorus in the urine to help raise the calcium-phosphorus ratio to normal. If blood calcium levels become too high, calcitonin, a polypeptide hormone secreted by connective tissue cells in the thyroid gland, increases calcium excretion to lower blood calcium. For the most part, both parathyroid hormone and calcitonin are constantly secreted at low levels to prevent rapid fluctuations in blood calcium levels.

An optimum intake of calcium and supply of vitamin D ensures the absorption of sufficient amounts of calcium and phosphorus to maintain normal blood calcium/phosphorus levels and to prevent the rise in parathyroid hormone levels and mobilization of bone calcium. The lack of sunlight in northern climates during winter months can have a detrimental effect on vitamin D status and bone health in all age groups, including adolescents in periods of peak bone growth.[13]

New Roles for Vitamin D

Beyond this role in bone and mineral metabolism, growing evidence indicates that the vitamin D hormone system is involved in widespread cell processes in a number of organ tissues. Vitamin D binds to cells in the brain, kidney, liver, skin, and reproductive tissues and to certain cells of the immune system. Vitamin D may play an active hormonal role in controlling cell reproduction and multiplication, and cell differentiation.[14] These discoveries could lead to possible use of vitamin D analogs in treating some types of leukemia and persistent skin disorders such as psoriasis.

VITAMIN D DEFICIENCY AND CLINICAL PROBLEMS

Role in Bone Disease

When the body does not have sufficient vitamin D, it cannot build normal bones. In children this vitamin D deficiency disease is called rickets. In the growing child the condition is characterized by malformation of skeletal tissue (Figure 7-5). In adults the disease is called osteomalacia; previously deposited bone mineral is rapidly mobilized from bone, resulting in bone pain and weak, brittle bones. Osteomalacia occurs mostly in women of childbearing age who receive little exposure to sunlight, have diets low in calcium and vitamin D, or have frequent pregnancies followed by periods of lactation. Older people who use antacids containing aluminum are at risk of osteomalacia because the aluminum binds phosphorus and causes its excretion from the body.

The widespread use of vitamin D–fortified foods, especially milk, has nearly eliminated common vitamin D deficiency rickets in developed countries, but it does still occur. Increasing cases have been reported in the United States among breast-fed infants, especially African American breast-fed infants who were not receiving the recommended vitamin D supplements and whose mothers have low vitamin D intake and limited sun exposure.[15,16] It occurs more often in northern regions with limited winter sunlight or in individuals whose skin pigmentation inhibits passage of the ultraviolet rays of the sun. Another problem relates to lactose intolerance and avoidance of vi-

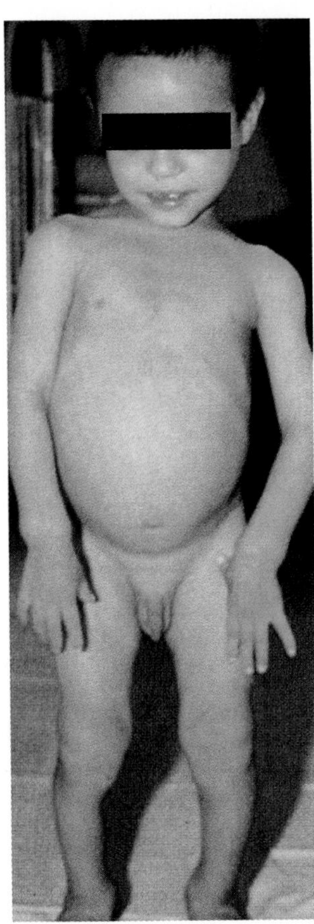

FIGURE 7-5 Bowlegs in rickets. (*From McLaren DS:* A colour atlas and text of diet-related disorders, *ed 2, London, 1992, Mosby–Year Book Europe Limited.*)

tamin D–fortified dairy products. African Americans with greater skin pigmentation that interferes with the formation of vitamin D from 7-dehydrocholesterol in the skin are also less likely to consume dairy products as a result of lactose intolerance.

Because of the active regulatory role of vitamin D in balancing bone mineral absorption and deposition, it has been used to treat the bone disease renal osteodystrophy. This condition occurs secondary to renal failure and is characterized by defective bone formation. Vitamin D also assists in the treatment of osteoporosis, a bone loss disease common in older women and men that leads to bone fractures. Older persons who increased their servings of vitamin D–fortified milk and dairy foods from 1.5 to 3 servings a day reduced their bone mineral loss.[17]

VITAMIN D REQUIREMENT

Influencing Factors

Many difficulties exist in setting dietary recommendations for vitamin D, including the limited number of food sources available, lack of knowledge of precise body needs, and differing degrees of skin synthesis by irradiation. Needs vary between winter and summer in northern climates. Also, a person's lifestyle and work pattern influence the degree of sunlight exposure and thus influence individual need. Persons living and working indoors need more vitamin D from dietary sources than someone who works outside all day. Regular use of sunscreen dramatically reduces skin synthesis. Elderly people are less able to synthesize vitamin D regardless of sun exposure because of aging changes in the skin.[11] Growth demands in childhood and in pregnancy and lactation necessitate increased intake.

Dietary Reference Intake

In light of the increased attention to bone health among all adults and the importance of developing optimum bone mass during the formative years, the Food and Nutrition Board has set an Adequate Intake (AI) for vitamin D (see Chapter 1). The AI was based on the amount of dietary vitamin D needed to maintain an appropriate vitamin D blood level in the absence of sun exposure. The suggested intake for persons from 6 months to 50 years of age is the same: 5 μg (200 IU). For adults aged 51 to 70 years the AI is raised to 10 μg (400 IU), and for those aged 71 and older it increases to 15 μg (600 IU).[18] The elevated AI for persons aged 71 and older addresses the critical need for elderly people to maintain bone mass and their limited ability to synthesize vitamin D in their skin. We will learn more about bone health in older people in Chapter 8.

VITAMIN D TOXICITY

Toxic amounts of vitamin D build up in the body easily because vitamin D is stored in adipose tissue and is released slowly. Toxic intakes of vitamin D usually result from self-administered doses of a vitamin supplement. Adults taking continued megadoses of 1000 μg (40,000 IU) or more daily have shown signs of severe intoxication.[19] Hypervitaminosis D in adults results in progressive weakness, bone pain, and hypercalcemia. Symptoms in young children include failure to thrive and calcium deposits in soft tissues such as the kidney nephrons. General infant feeding poses special problems. Excess intake is possible in infant feeding if fortified milk, fortified cereal, and varying vitamin supplements are used simultaneously. The infant needs only

25-hydroxycholecalciferol [25,(OH)D_3] Initial product formed in the liver in the process of developing the active vitamin D hormone.

osteodystrophy Defective bone formation.

osteoporosis Abnormal thinning of bone, producing a porous, fragile bone tissue of enlarged spaces, prone to fracture or deformity, associated with the aging process in older men and women.

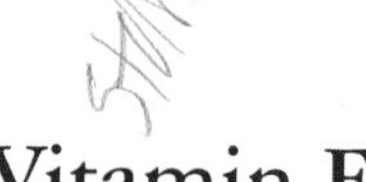

5 μg (200 IU) daily, but the amount in all of these items together could reach above that level.

Consuming excess vitamin D in food products is not a far-reaching problem, however; the increased use of tanning beds by some groups raises the question of hypervitaminosis D arising from prolonged exposure to high-intensity ultraviolet lamps. Vitamin D toxicity has not been known to occur from exposure to normal sunlight.

FOOD SOURCES OF VITAMIN D

Few natural food sources of vitamin D exist. The two basic substances with vitamin D activity, D_2 and D_3, occur only in yeast and fish liver oils. The main food sources are those to which crystalline vitamin D has been added. Milk, because it is commonly used, has proved to be the most practical carrier. The added vitamin D content of milk has been standardized at 10 μg (400 IU)/qt. Milk is also a good carrier for the vitamin because it contains calcium and phosphorus as well, and the addition of D_3 to this food has largely eradicated rickets in the United States. Margarines are fortified with 37.5 μg (1500 IU)/lb to serve as butter substitutes. Certain brands of yogurt and some cereals are now fortified with vitamin D. A summary of food sources is given in Table 7-2.

Vitamin E

CHEMICAL AND PHYSICAL NATURE

Vitamin E was discovered as a necessary dietary component in studies looking at the reproductive responses of laboratory animals and was identified as an alcohol. Because of its association with reproductive function and its chemical nature as an alcohol, it was named tocopherol from the Greek word *tokos,* meaning "childbirth." Since then, tocopherol has come to be known as the antisterility vitamin, but this effect has been demonstrated only in laboratory rats and not in humans, despite advertising claims for its contribution to sexual performance.

CHEMICAL FORMS

Vitamin E is the generic name for a group of compounds with similar physiologic activity. It is the collective term for eight fat-soluble, 6-hydroxychroman compounds that show some degree of the biologic activity of alpha-tocopherol, the most significant in human nutrition.[20] Vitamin E is a pale yellow oil, stable to acids and heat and insoluble in water. It oxidizes very slowly, which gives it an important role as an antioxidant to "neutralize" free cell radicals and prevent oxidation of the unsaturated fats.

TABLE 7-2 Food Sources of Vitamin D

Food Source	Quantity	Vitamin D (μg)
Bread, Cereal, Rice, Pasta		
Corn flakes	1 cup (1 oz)/28 g	1.00
Granola	¼ cup (1 oz)/28 g	1.23
Raisin bran	½ cup (1 oz)/28 g	1.23
Vegetables		
This food group is not an important source of vitamin D		
Fruits		
This food group is not an important source of vitamin D		
Meat, Poultry, Fish, Dried Beans, Nuts		
This food group is not an important source of vitamin D		
Eggs		
Egg, whole	1 large/50 g	0.68
Egg yolk	Yolk of 1 large egg/17 g	0.68
Milk, Dairy Products		
Cheddar cheese	1 oz/28 g	0.08
Cream cheese	1 oz/28 g	0.05
Evaporated milk (vitamin D fortified)	½ cup (4 fl oz)/126 g	2.50
Milk, Dairy Products—cont'd		
Milk, whole or nonfat (vitamin D fortified)	1 qt/960 g	10.00
Milk, whole or nonfat (vitamin D fortified)	1 cup (8 fl oz)/240 g	2.50
Soy milk (vitamin D fortified)	1 cup (8 fl oz)/240 g	2.50
Fats, Oils, Sugar		
Margarine	1 tbsp	1.50

Adequate Intake for adults: 19-50 years, 5 μg (200 IU); 51-70 years, 10 μg (400 IU); and ≥71 years, 15 μg (600 IU).

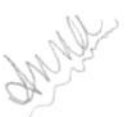

This capacity to serve as an antioxidant gives vitamin E widespread clinical application.[20]

ABSORPTION, TRANSPORT, AND STORAGE

Vitamin E is absorbed with the aid of bile. With other lipids in the chylomicrons, it is transported out of the intestinal wall into the lymph and then into body circulation as part of the blood plasma lipoproteins. Vitamin E is stored in the liver and in fat tissue. In adipose tissue, it is held in bulk liquid droplets, and mobilization of alpha-tocopherol from these droplets is slow.

FUNCTIONS OF VITAMIN E

Antioxidant

Vitamin E acts as nature's most potent fat-soluble antioxidant. The polyunsaturated fatty acids in the structural lipid membranes of cells are particularly vulnerable to oxidative breakdown by free radicals in the cell. The tocopherols can interrupt this oxidation process, protecting the cell membrane fatty acids from oxidative damage. Damage to the cell membrane changes its ability to allow passage of appropriate substances into the cell and prevent passage of harmful substances. Vitamin E has been shown to stimulate immune function in elderly people, which may be related to its antioxidant effects.[21] (See *To Probe Further* box for more information as to how antioxidants protect tissues.)

Selenium Relationship

Even with adequate vitamin E intake, some damaging cell peroxides may be formed; therefore a second line of defense is needed to destroy them before they can damage the cell membrane. The agent providing this added defense is a selenium-containing enzyme. Thus the trace element selenium spares vitamin E and reduces the vitamin E requirement. Similarly, in this partnership role, vitamin E helps reduce the selenium requirement.

New Roles for Vitamin E

Recent population studies have linked dietary vitamin E intake and reduced risk of cardiovascular disease and stroke.[22] Vitamin E prevents the oxidation of low-density lipoprotein (LDL) cholesterol, which promotes the deposit of lipids in the coronary arteries. Vitamin E also protects the arterial lining from inflammation that can promote atherosclerosis.[23] (The relationship between vitamin E and heart disease will be discussed again in Chapter 19.) There also are similarities between the changes in neural tissues that occur in vitamin E deficiency and the changes observed in brain diseases of older people such as Alzheimer's disease and other types of age-related dementia.[24] Vitamin E supplements were found to slow the downhill course of Alzheimer's disease in one group of patients; however, more studies are needed to confirm that vitamin E was the active agent causing this response.[25] Vitamin E through its protective effect against atherosclerosis and damage to the arteries may help to prevent dementias caused by changes in these blood vessels that supply blood and oxygen to the brain.[24] Most recently, researchers have begun to examine a possible therapeutic role for vitamin E in the treatment of rheumatoid arthritis.[26]

VITAMIN E DEFICIENCY AND CLINICAL PROBLEMS

When adequate vitamin E is not available, the cells are more vulnerable to oxidative attack and damage. For example, when vitamin E is lacking, the polyunsaturated fatty acids in the lipid membranes of red blood cells are exposed to oxidation, the membranes are broken, the cell contents are lost, and the cell is destroyed. The continued loss of red blood cells leads to anemia; this vitamin E deficiency disease is called hemolytic anemia. Premature infants are especially vulnerable to hemolytic anemia because they missed the last month or two of fetal life, when vitamin E stores are normally built up.

In older children and adults, vitamin E deficiency can present a different set of symptoms.[27] These symptoms are associated with functions of the nervous system. The main nerves involved are (1) the spinal cord fibers that affect physical activity such as walking and (2) the retina of the eye, which affects vision. This group of neurologic problems was recognized in children with chronic defective absorption of fats and fat-soluble vitamins, such as those with cystic fibrosis and pancreatic insufficiency. The loss of the pancreatic fat-digesting enzyme lipase and its associated emulsifying agent bile leads to a chronic fatty diarrhea and inability to absorb fat and fat-soluble nutrients such as vitamin E. This vitamin E deficiency disrupts the making of myelin, the protective lipid covering for the long axons of nerve cells that helps pass messages along to muscles they serve. This neurologic disorder from lack of vitamin E also causes pigment degeneration of the rods and cones of the retina. These light-sensitive cell membranes are rich in polyunsaturated fatty acids, and vitamin E is critical for preventing oxidation damage.

---

antioxidant A substance that inhibits oxidation of polyunsaturated fatty acids and formation of free radicals in the cells.

hemolytic anemia An anemia (reduced number of red blood cells) caused by breakdown of the outer membrane of red blood cells and loss of their hemoglobin.

myelin Substance with a high lipid-to-protein composition forming a fatty sheath to insulate and protect neuron axons and facilitate their neuromuscular impulses.

tocopherol Chemical name for vitamin E. In humans it functions as a strong antioxidant to preserve structural membranes, such as cell walls.

TO PROBE FURTHER

What is an Antioxidant: Why are They Important?

A new word has been added to the vocabulary of both the general public and health professionals. This word is "antioxidant." We know that we need more of these substances in our diet but we are still learning what they do. In chemistry class you learned about molecules called free radicals. These high-energy molecules have an unpaired electron and are on the lookout for other molecules with an unpaired electron. Free radicals are highly reactive and can be very damaging to various tissues in the body.

Free radicals such as free oxygen or other compounds are formed in the body as byproducts of normal metabolism in cells. They also result from environmental exposure to tobacco smoke, car exhaust fumes, the ozone, x-rays, or other air pollutants. Free radicals can damage the cell nucleus, cell membranes, and cell metabolites or kill the cell outright. These effects accumulate and are believed to accelerate the aging process and contribute to the development of chronic degenerative changes. Antioxidant substances such as vitamin E join with the unpaired electron of free radicals and break the chain of oxidation reactions that continues across the tissues.

Oxidation reactions are especially harmful to lipid molecules. Both cell membranes and the membranes of the organ machinery within the cell, such as the mitochondria, have a high content of unsaturated fatty acids that contain at least one double bond. Remember that each of these double bonds has an unpaired electron that is vulnerable to oxidation by a free radical. Brain cells and nerve fibers have a high proportion of polyunsaturated fatty acids. Proteins and DNA in the cell nucleus can be changed by inappropriate oxidation reactions. Changes in DNA result in the production of proteins that are not effective in carrying out body functions or in replacing worn out structural proteins. All cells are exposed to free radicals arising from within the body or from the environment; the issue is whether any damage occurs. This depends on the level of antioxidants or protective compounds available to the cell. Oxidative stress refers to the situation in which there are insufficient amounts of antioxidant compounds available to neutralize the free radicals attacking the cells.

Damage that occurs through these unwanted oxidation reactions may contribute to the development of various chronic diseases.

1. *Cancer.* Oxidation reactions can produce mutations in the cellular DNA that cause a cell to begin uncontrolled growth and to form a carcinoma. Populations who have diets high in plant foods and naturally occurring antioxidants have less oxidative damage to their DNA and experience fewer cancers.
2. *Cardiovascular disease.* Free radicals cause the oxidation of blood LDL cholesterol. Oxidized LDL cholesterol is more likely to be deposited in the vascular lining of the coronary arteries and to form atherosclerotic deposits that narrow the arteries and impede blood flow.
3. *Aging changes.* Several complications of aging, including cataracts, age-related macular degeneration, and Alzheimer's disease, are associated with protein and lipid oxidation products in the tissues.

Vitamin C, vitamin E, and the carotenoids, along with the mineral selenium, act as biologic antioxidants. Meeting the recommended intakes of these nutrients and eating plant foods regularly may help prevent oxidative stress.

Reference

Food and Nutrition Board, National Research Council: *Dietary reference intakes for vitamin C, vitamin E, selenium, and carotenoids,* Washington, DC, 2000, National Academy Press.

VITAMIN E REQUIREMENT

Dietary Reference Intake

The requirements for vitamin E vary with the amount of polyunsaturated fatty acids in the diet. The new RDA standards are expressed as mg of alpha-tocopherol because it appears that other forms of tocopherol are not well utilized by the body. The current RDA is 15 mg for both males and females aged 14 and older. Needs during childhood growth years range from 6 to 11 mg. These stated allowances estimate that 80% of the vitamin E in the diet will be alpha-tocopherol and 20% will come from other tocopherol forms, including those used in vitamin supplements and fortified foods.[20] Although it is believed that alpha-tocopherol is the most important form of vitamin E in human nutrition, other forms of the vitamin, plentiful in the U.S. diet, may also have distinctive roles in the health benefits associated with vitamin E.[28]

Special Clinical Needs

Because vitamin E protects cellular and subcellular membranes and hence supports tissue health, it is an important nutrient in the diets of pregnant and lactating women, and especially urgent for newborn infants. Hemolytic anemia, a medical problem found in infants, particularly premature ones, responds positively to vitamin E therapy[27] and can be avoided by increasing the vitamin E intake of these infants.

TABLE 7-3 Food Sources of Vitamin E as Alpha-Tocopherol

Food Source	Quantity	Vitamin E (mg Alpha-Tocopherol)	Food Source	Quantity	Vitamin E (mg Alpha-Tocopherol)
Bread, Cereal, Rice, Pasta			***Meat, Poultry, Fish, Dried Beans, Eggs***		
This food group is not an important source of vitamin E			This food group is not an important source of vitamin E		
Vegetables			***Nuts***		
Asparagus (raw)	4 spears/58 g	1.15	Almonds (dried)	1 oz (24 nuts)/28 g	6.72
Avocado (raw)	1 med/173 g	2.32	Hazelnuts (dried)	1 oz/28 g	6.70
Brussels sprouts (boiled)	½ cup (4 sprouts)/78 g	0.66	Peanut butter	1 tbsp/16 g	3.00
Cabbage, green (raw)	½ cup shredded/35 g	0.58	Peanuts (dried)	1 oz/28 g	2.56
Carrot (raw)	1 med/72 g	0.32	Walnuts (dried)	1 oz (14 halves)/28 g	0.73
Lettuce, iceberg (raw)	¼ head/135 g	0.54	***Milk, Dairy Products***		
Spinach (raw)	½ cup chopped/28 g	0.53	This food group is not an important source of vitamin E		
Sweet potato (raw)	1 med/130 g	5.93	***Fats, Oils, Sugar***		
Fruits			Corn oil	1 tbsp/14 g	1.90
Apple (raw, with skin)	1 med/138 g	0.81	Cottonseed oil	1 tbsp/14 g	4.80
Apricot (canned)	4 halves/90 g	0.80	Olive oil	1 tbsp/14 g	1.60
Banana (raw)	1 med/114 g	0.31	Palm oil	1 tbsp/14 g	2.60
Mango (raw)	1 med/207 g	2.32	Peanut oil	1 tbsp/14 g	1.60
Pear (raw)	1 med/166 g	0.83	Safflower oil	1 tbsp/14 g	4.60
			Soybean oil	1 tbsp/14 g	1.50

Recommended Dietary Allowance for adults: 15 mg.

In the general population there are wide variations in vitamin E intake. In a study of 1500 eighth graders, supplement users were consuming more than 3 times the RDA for vitamin E.[29] On the other hand, adults who were food insecure, meaning they did not always have an available supply of nutritious and safe foods, were meeting less than 50% of their RDA for this vitamin.[30] Regular vitamin E replacement therapy is needed for those with chronic pancreatic insufficiency and other fat malabsorption conditions.

VITAMIN E TOXICITY

Vitamin E is the only one of the fat-soluble vitamins for which no toxic effects have been identified in humans. Its use as a supplement has shown no harmful effects at intake levels of 268 to 567 mg of alpha-tocopherol/day. However, individuals with intakes of 1600 mg to 3000 mg of vitamin E/day reported side effects of fatigue, gastrointestinal disturbances, altered blood lipoprotein patterns, and changes in thyroid function. Based on the information available, the Food and Nutrition Board established the UL of 1000 mg of alpha-tocopherol/day.[20]

Current interest in vitamin E and its role in reducing the adhesiveness of blood platelets, thus preventing the formation of unwanted blood clots and cerebrovascular disease, has led some researchers to recommend use of vitamin E supplements at a level of 2 times the RDA by middle-aged and older adults.[31] Other studies have evaluated the effects of as much as 400 mg to 800 mg/day in preventing heart disease.[20] At high intakes, however, vitamin E can seriously interfere with the action of the blood platelets and prevent normal blood clotting; thus individuals should consult their physician before beginning such use. This is especially important for persons with low intakes of vitamin K or for patients receiving medications to prevent unwanted blood clotting.

FOOD SOURCES OF VITAMIN E

The richest dietary sources of vitamin E are the vegetable oils. Safflower oil and olive oil contain the highest proportion of alpha-tocopherol, followed by soybean oil.[5] Curiously enough, these oils are also the richest sources of polyunsaturated fatty acids, which vitamin E protects from oxidation. Other food sources include nuts and certain vegetables and fruits, with only small amounts found in cereals, dairy products, and meats. A summary of major food sources of vitamin E is given in Table 7-3.

Vitamin K

CHEMICAL AND PHYSICAL NATURE

The studies of Henrik Dam, a biochemist at the University of Copenhagen, working with a hemorrhagic disease in chicks that were fed a fat-free diet led to the discovery of vitamin K. He found that the absent factor responsible was a fat-soluble, blood-clotting vitamin. Because of its blood clotting function, he called it the *koagulations vitamin,* or vitamin K, from this Swedish word for its physiologic action. Later he succeeded in isolating and identifying the compound from alfalfa, for which he received the Nobel Prize in physiology and medicine.

Chemical Nature

The major form of vitamin K found in plants was named phylloquinone for its chemical structure. This is the major dietary form of vitamin K, being widely distributed in both animal and vegetable foods. Menaquinones, another form of the vitamin, are synthesized by intestinal bacterial flora. Both forms can be used by the body to meet the need for vitamin K. The water-soluble vitamin K analog menadione does not require bile for absorption but goes directly into the portal blood system,[32] thus making it an important source for individuals with pancreatic insufficiency.

ABSORPTION, TRANSPORT, AND STORAGE

Both naturally occurring forms of vitamin K require bile salts and pancreatic secretions for absorption, as do the other fat-soluble vitamins.[1,32] They are packaged in the intestinal chylomicrons and travel via the lymphatic system and then the portal blood in transport to the liver. In the liver, vitamin K is stored in small amounts and excreted rapidly after administration of therapeutic doses.

FUNCTIONAL ROLES OF VITAMIN K AND CLINICAL PROBLEMS

Blood Clotting

A major function of vitamin K is to catalyze the synthesis of blood-clotting factors by the liver. Vitamin K is essential for maintaining normal levels of four blood-clotting factors: (1) factor II (prothrombin), (2) factor VII, (3) factor IX, and (4) factor X.[32] Each of these specific clotting factors is a protein synthesized by the liver in the form of an inactive precursor dependent on vitamin K for activation. Vitamin K acts as an essential cofactor with a carboxylase enzyme to produce the active form of these precursors, mainly prothrombin. This activation involves adding a carboxyl (COOH) radical to the amino acid glutamic acid (Glu). This process converts specific glutamic acid residues in vitamin K–dependent proteins to gamma-carboxyglutamic acid (Gla). The activated clotting factors can then combine with calcium (factor IV), an element essential to the clotting process.

Vitamin K requires a functioning liver to carry out its tasks. When liver damage has caused decreased blood levels of prothrombin, and this problem in turn has led to hemorrhage, vitamin K is ineffective as a therapeutic agent. Vitamin K is also required for the liver synthesis of three proteins labeled protein C, S, and Z, which act as feedback proteins and regulate the speed and duration of the coagulation process. This feedback mechanism prevents the development of dangerous blood clots or thrombosis.[32]

Skeletal Metabolism

Numerous vitamin K–dependent proteins have been found in bone, including osteocalcin and other matrix Gla proteins.[33] Bone is constantly being remodeled (see Chapter 8) and vitamin K–dependent proteins are essential to the formation of bone matrix and its subsequent mineralization. Individuals with higher intakes of vitamin K are less likely to experience a hip fracture. Among middle-aged and older women, lettuce was the food that contributed the most to vitamin K intake, and those women who ate one serving of lettuce a day were only half as likely to have a hip fracture as were those who ate lettuce only once a week or less often.[34]

Neonatology

The sterile intestinal tract of the newborn can supply no vitamin K during the first few days of life until normal bacterial flora develop. Consequently, during this immediate postnatal period hemorrhagic disease of the newborn can occur. To prevent this from happening, a prophylactic dose of vitamin K is usually given to each infant soon after birth.

Malabsorption Disease

Any defect in fat absorption will cause a failure in vitamin K absorption, resulting in prolonged blood clotting time. Thus there are various clinical situations in which supplemental vitamin K is required. For example, patients with bile duct obstruction are usually given vitamin K before surgery. Also, after a cholecystectomy, which hinders normal bile release, vitamin K is not readily absorbed. Children with cystic fibrosis who have fat malabsorption can become deficient in vitamin K.

Drug Therapy

Several drug-nutrient interactions involve vitamin K. An anticlotting drug such as bishydroxycoumarin (Dicumarol) or warfarin, which acts as an antimetabolite, prevents the liver from making the proteins needed to form blood clots, and thus inhibits the action of vitamin K. When a drug of this nature is used to treat conditions such as blood clots in the lung or blood vessels, the dietary intake of vitamin K must be monitored closely. Too much vitamin K will oppose the action of the drug and neutralize its effect; on the other hand, too little vitamin K could lead to serious hemorrhage. Individuals receiving these drugs require help in choosing foods that will help maintain a constant intake of 65 to 85 μg/day.[35] Dark green leafy vegetables are rich sources of naturally occurring vitamin K, but patients need also to be alerted to the vitamin K added to processed foods. For example, snack foods made with Olestra, a noncaloric fat substitute, are fortified with 80 μg of vitamin K per 1-oz serving (see Chapter 4).[36] Vitamin K is also included in many multivitamin supplements, and patients must be alerted to this potential source. After the extended use of antibiotics, the intestinal bacterial flora is diminished, thus reducing one of the body's main sources of vitamin K.

VITAMIN K REQUIREMENT

It has been difficult to determine a specific dietary recommendation for vitamin K for several reasons: (1) part of the body's apparent need may be supplied by bacterial synthesis, (2) our body reserves are small and turn over rapidly, (3) biologic measures for evaluating vitamin K status are just being developed, and (4) we lack reliable information as to food content of vitamin K and its bioavailability. Based on these uncertainties the Food and Nutrition Board has established an AI rather than an RDA for this nutrient. The AI for men aged 19 and over is 120 μg/day and the equivalent AI for women is 90 μg/day.[3] These values were based on the median intakes of nearly 20,000 men and women participating in a national nutrition and health survey between 1988 and 1994. Although this level appears adequate to preserve the blood clotting mechanism, further research is needed to determine the optimum level of vitamin K to preserve bone health.

The average daily intake of vitamin K in the United States seems to relate to age. Although children and adults aged 45 and over are eating foods supplying at least 1 μg/kg body weight, persons aged 18 to 44 are falling below that amount.[37] Groups with particular needs include newborns, who require a vitamin K injection shortly after birth. Persons who are taking antibiotics, who are being fed by enteral or parenteral nutrition for extended periods, or who have biliary obstruction or chronic malabsorption disease should be monitored and may require therapeutic supplementation. Toxicity from vitamin K, even with large amounts taken over extended periods, has not been observed.

TABLE 7-4 Food Sources of Vitamin K

Food Source	Quantity	Vitamin K (μg)
Bread, Cereal, Rice, Pasta		
Oats (dry)	100 g	63
Wheat bran	100 g	83
Whole wheat flour	100 g	30
Vegetables		
Broccoli (raw)	100 g	132
Cabbage (raw)	100 g	149
Cauliflower (raw)	100 g	191
Lentils (dry)	100 g	223
Lettuce, iceberg (raw)	100 g	112
Spinach (raw)	100 g	266
Turnip greens (raw)	100 g	650
Fruits		
This food group is not an important source of vitamin K		
Meat, Poultry, Fish, Dried Beans, Eggs, Nuts		
Beef liver	100 g	104
Chicken liver	100 g	80
Pork liver	100 g	88
Milk, Dairy Products		
This food group is not an important source of vitamin K		
Fats, Oils, Sugar		
Corn oil	100 g	60
Soybean oil	100 g	540

Adequate Intake for adults: women, 90 μg; men, 120 μg.

FOOD SOURCES OF VITAMIN K

Dietary vitamin K, phylloquinone, is present to some extent in most vegetables but is highest in green vegetables and in liver. Menaquinones are found in liver and certain cheeses.[32] A summary of main food sources is given in Table 7-4.

A complete summary of the fat-soluble vitamins can be found in Table 7-5.

antimetabolite A substance bearing a close structural resemblance to one required for normal physiologic functioning that exerts its effect by interfering with the utilization of the essential metabolite.
menadione The parent compound of vitamin K in the body; also called *vitamin K_3*.
menaquinone Form of vitamin K synthesized by intestinal bacteria; also called *vitamin K_2*.
phylloquinone A fat-soluble vitamin of the K group (K_1), $C_3H_{46}O_2$, found in green plants or prepared synthetically.
prothrombin Blood-clotting factor (number II) synthesized in the liver from glutamic acid and CO_2, catalyzed by vitamin K.

TABLE 7-5 Summary of Fat-Soluble Vitamins

Vitamin	Physiologic Functions	Results of Deficiency	Dietary Reference Intake	Food Sources
Vitamin A Provitamin: beta-carotene Vitamin: retinol	Production of rhodopsin and other light-receptor pigments Formation and maintenance of epithelial tissue Growth Reproduction Toxic in large amounts	Poor dark adaptation, night blindness, xerosis, xerophthalmia Keratinization of epithelium Growth failure Reproductive failure	Adults: Males aged ≥19: 900 μg Females aged ≥19: 700 μg Pregnancy: Aged ≤18: 750 μg Aged ≥19: 770 μg Lactation: Aged ≤18: 1200 μg Aged ≥19: 1300 μg	Butter; fortified margarine Whole, fortified low-fat, and fortified nonfat cow's milk Fortified soy milk Egg yolk Liver Green, yellow, and orange vegetables Yellow and orange fruits
Vitamin D Provitamins: ergosterol (plants); 7-dehydrocholesterol (skin) Vitamins: D_2 (ergocalciferol) and D_3 (cholecalciferol)	Calcitriol a major hormone regulator of bone mineral (calcium and phosphorus) metabolism Calcium and phosphorus absorption Toxic in large amounts	Faulty bone growth; rickets, osteomalacia	Adult males/females: Aged 19-50: 5 μg Aged 51-70: 10 μg Aged ≥71: 15 μg Pregnancy: All ages: 5 μg Lactation: All ages: 5 μg	Fortified cow's milk Fortified soy milk Fortified yogurt Fortified margarine Fish oils Sunlight on the skin
Vitamin E Tocopherols	Antioxidant Hemopoiesis Related to action of selenium	Anemia in premature infants	Adults: Males/females aged ≥19: 15 mg Pregnancy: All ages: 15 mg Lactation: All ages: 19 mg	Vegetable oils
Vitamin K K_1 (phylloquinone) K_2 (menaquinone) Analog: K_3 (menadione)	Activates blood-clotting factors (e.g., prothrombin) by alpha-carboxylating glutamic acid residues Toxicity can be induced by water-soluble analogs	Hemorrhagic disease of the newborn Defective blood clotting Deficiency symptoms are produced by coumarin anticoagulants and by antibiotic therapy	Adults: Males aged ≥19: 120 μg Females aged ≥19: 90 μg Pregnancy: Aged ≤18: 75 μg Aged ≥19: 90 μg Lactation: Aged ≤18: 75 μg Aged ≥19: 90 μg	Cheese, egg yolk, liver Green leafy vegetables Synthesized by intestinal bacteria

WATER-SOLUBLE VITAMINS

Vitamin C

CHEMICAL AND PHYSICAL NATURE

The recognition of vitamin C is associated with the history of an unrelenting search for the cause of the ancient hemorrhagic disease scurvy. Early observations, mostly among British sailors and explorers, led to the American discovery of an acid in lemon juice that prevented or cured scurvy. The specific chemical name of vitamin C is ascorbic acid, given to this substance because of its antiscorbutic or antiscurvy properties. The structure of vitamin C is similar to that of glucose, its metabolic precursor in most animals, but humans lack the specific enzyme needed to change glucose to ascorbic acid. Thus human scurvy can be called a disease of distant genetic origin, an inherited metabolic defect.

Vitamin C is an unstable, easily oxidized acid. It is destroyed by oxygen, alkalis, and high temperatures.

ABSORPTION, TRANSPORT, AND STORAGE

Vitamin C is easily absorbed from the small intestine, but absorption is hindered by a lack of hydrochloric acid or by bleeding from the gastrointestinal tract. After it is absorbed vitamin C is not stored in a single tissue deposit as is vitamin A; rather it is more generally distributed throughout the body tissues, maintaining a tissue saturation level. Any excess is excreted in the urine. Tissue levels relate to intake, and the size of the total body pool adjusts to maintain balances. The total amount in adults varies from about 2 g to as little as 0.3 g.[20] Tissue levels diminish slowly; therefore with no intake, deficiency symptoms do not appear for approximately 3 months. This explains why generally healthy people in more isolated living situations can survive the winter without eating many fresh fruits and vegetables. Sufficient vitamin C for early infancy needs is present in breast milk if the mother has a good lactation diet. Cow's milk, however, contains very little vitamin C; remember that these animals have the enzymes to make their own vitamin C from glucose. Thus, human infant formulas made from cow's milk are supplemented with ascorbic acid.

FUNCTIONS OF VITAMIN C AND DEFICIENCY CONDITIONS

General Antioxidant Capacity

Along with vitamin E and the carotenoids, vitamin C is an antioxidant. This means that vitamin C takes up free oxygen in the cells resulting from cell metabolism. This action prevents oxygen from feeding oxygen-hungry free radicals that also result from normal cell metabolism but damage or destroy cells if they are not defused. This action may define a role for vitamin C in the prevention of chronic disease.

Intercellular Cement Substance

Vitamin C is needed to build and maintain body tissues in general, including bone matrix, cartilage, dentin, collagen, and connective tissue. Collagen is a protein substance that exists in many body tissues, such as the white fibers of connective tissue. When vitamin C is absent, the important ground substance does not develop into collagen and the collagen fibers formed in most body tissues remain defective and weak.[38] Blood vessel tissue requires the cementing substance from the metabolic action of vitamin C that helps provide firm capillary walls. Thus vitamin C deficiency is characterized by fragile capillaries, easily ruptured by blood pressure or trauma, resulting in diffuse tissue bleeding. Deficiency signs include easy bruising, pinpoint hemorrhages of the skin, bone and joints, easy bone fracture, poor wound healing, and soft bleeding gums, a condition called *gingivitis*. When vitamin C is given, the formation of collagen tissue follows quickly. Vitamin C may be acting at the level of the gene to initiate the synthesis of these molecules.[38,39]

General Body Metabolism

The concentration of vitamin C is greater in more metabolically active tissues, such as the adrenal and pituitary glands, brain, eye tissues, and leukocytes, than in less active tissues. More vitamin C is present in a child's actively multiplying tissue than in adult tissue. Vitamin C also helps in the formation of hemoglobin and the development of red blood cells. It does this in two ways: (1) it aids in the absorption of iron, overcoming the action of known iron absorption inhibitors such as phytate,[40] and (2) it assists in the removal of iron from ferritin, the protein-iron-phosphorus complex in which iron is stored so that more iron is made available to tissues producing the hemoglobin.

Vitamin C participates in many other processes that have clinical implications. For example, in addition to its role in collagen formation, vitamin C is needed for the synthesis of carnitine, an amino acid that transports long-chain fatty acids into cell mitochondria, where they are used to produce energy. Also, vitamin C is necessary for synthesis of many peptide hormones, including the hormone norepinephrine, and receptors for the neurotransmitter acetylcholine. Vitamin C participates in the mixed-function oxidase system that metabolizes drugs and breaks down carcinogens and other molecules foreign to the body. It may offer some protection against lead poisoning in children and adults exposed to this hazard.[41]

VITAMIN C REQUIREMENTS

Clinical Problems and Normal Growth

Some basic clinical problems, as well as normal growth, require additional vitamin C.

1. *Wound healing*. The significant role of vitamin C in cementing the ground substance of supporting tissues makes it an important agent in wound healing. This creates added demands for vitamin C in traumatic injury or surgery, especially where extensive tissue

---

collagen The protein substance of the white collagen fibers of skin, tendon, bone, cartilage, and all other connective tissue.

scurvy A hemorrhagic disease caused by lack of vitamin C. Diffuse tissue bleeding occurs, limbs and joints are painful and swollen, bones thicken because of subperiosteal hemorrhage, ecchymoses (large, irregular, discolored skin areas resulting from tissue hemorrhages) form, bones fracture easily, wounds do not heal well, gums are swollen and bleeding, and teeth loosen.

regeneration is involved. Formulas for parenteral feeding generally provide 100 mg of vitamin C daily. Protocols for burn patients with a high need for tissue growth and who must fight infection include 1000 mg/day given in two divided doses.[42]

2. *Fevers and infections.* Infectious processes deplete tissue stores of vitamin C. Optimal tissue stores help maintain resistance to infection. Just how large an amount of vitamin C may be required to maintain this protection is not known. Fevers also deplete tissue stores of vitamin C, as they accompany the infectious process and produce a catabolic effect.
3. *Growth periods.* Additional vitamin C is required during the growth periods of infancy and childhood. It is also important during pregnancy to supply demands for rapid fetal growth and development of maternal tissues.
4. *Stress and body defense.* Body stress from injury, fracture, general illness, or psychologic loss or shock calls on vitamin C stored in tissues. A large amount of vitamin C is present in the adrenal glands, which play a primary role in the stress response pattern.
5. *Prevention of chronic disease.* Current research is looking at a role for vitamin C in the prevention of cardiovascular disease and cancer, possibly through its action as an antioxidant.[43] Also, the high concentration of vitamin C in the eye suggests an action in the prevention of cataract or macular degeneration (an age-related change in the macula that leads to blindness).[39] A national study reported that low blood ascorbic acid levels increased mortality risk from all causes in men but did not increase risk in women, regardless of smoking habits.[44] Further research may help us learn if men have greater needs for vitamin C than women.

Dietary Reference Intake

Difficulties in establishing recommended intakes for vitamin C involve questions about individual tissue needs and whether minimum or optimum intakes are desirable.[43] In men maximum tissue saturation and antioxidant protection to body tissues are achieved with an RDA of 90 mg.[20] Based on their lower lean body mass and body size, the RDA for women is 75 mg. Cigarette smokers need an additional 35 mg of vitamin C each day. Amounts are added for pregnancy and lactation needs with gradual increases during childhood to support growth.

VITAMIN C TOXICITY

A long-time controversy has existed regarding the efficacy of vitamin C in preventing or curing the common cold. Although pharmacologic doses of 1 g or more daily have been reported to reduce the frequency and severity of symptoms of the common cold and other respiratory problems, controlled trials have not supported this claim. Such amounts are not recommended for the entire population. Nonetheless, many persons do habitually ingest such a dose of vitamin C daily with no toxic effects. The UL is set at 2 g, based on the appearance of gastrointestinal symptoms and diarrhea at higher levels.[20]

FOOD SOURCES OF VITAMIN C

Vitamin C can be oxidized easily. Thus the handling, preparation, cooking, and processing of any food source must be considered in evaluating the actual contribution by that food of vitamin C to the diet. It is best to cook vitamin C foods in as little water as possible for brief periods with the pan covered. Do not cut vegetables into small pieces until time of use, to curtail cut surface exposure to the air. Store juices in tightly closed containers. Well known sources include citrus fruit and tomatoes, as vitamin C is quite stable in an acid solution. Less regarded but good additional sources include white potatoes, sweet potatoes, cabbage, broccoli, and other green and yellow vegetables and fruits. A summary of food sources of vitamin C is given in Table 7-6.

A summary of vitamin C and its role in the body can be found in Table 7-7.

B Vitamins

DEFICIENCY DISEASES AND VITAMIN DISCOVERIES

The story of the B vitamins is a compelling one. It is a story of persons dying of a puzzling, age-old disease for which there was no cure. It was eventually learned that common, everyday food held the answer. The paralyzing disease was beriberi, which had plagued the Orient for centuries and caused persons in many places to search for its solution (Figure 7-6). Early observations and studies provided important clues, but application of the "vitamine" connection to this human sickness was needed. This was finally achieved when an American chemist, R.R. Williams, and his associates with the Philippine Bureau of Science used extracts of rice polishings and cured the epidemic infantile beriberi. This condition of paralysis was named by the repeated native words, "I can't, I can't," describing its crippling effects. The food factor was named water-soluble B because it was thought to be a single vitamin. Now we know it as a large group of individual B vitamins, all water soluble but each having unique metabolic functions in human health. The original letter-naming scheme has long since become meaningless, and we are now accustomed to calling the B vitamins by their specific chemical names.

VITAL COENZYME ROLE

The B vitamins, originally believed to be important only in preventing the deficiency diseases that led to their dis-

TABLE 7-6 Food Sources of Vitamin C

Food Source	Quantity	Vitamin C (mg)	Food Source	Quantity	Vitamin C (mg)
Bread, Cereal, Rice, Pasta			***Fruits—cont'd***		
This food group is not an important source of vitamin C			Orange, navel	1 med	80
Vegetables			Papaya (raw)	1 med	188
Asparagus (boiled)	½ cup (6 spears)	18	Pineapple (raw)	½ cup	12
Avocado (raw)	1 med	14	Raspberries (raw)	½ cup	15
Broccoli (raw)	½ cup	41	Strawberries (raw)	½ cup	44
Brussels sprouts (boiled)	½ cup (4 sprouts)	48	Tangerine (raw)	1 med	26
			Meat, Poultry, Fish, Dried Beans, Eggs, Nuts		
Cauliflower (raw)	½ cup, pieces	38	Beef liver (fried)	3.6 oz	23
Green pepper (raw)	½ cup, chopped	64	Ham, lean (canned; vitamin C added)	3.5 oz	27
Kale (boiled)	½ cup	27			
Potato (baked, with skin)	1 med	26	Lentils (boiled)	1 cup	3
			Soybeans (boiled)	1 cup	3
Sweet potato (baked)	1 med	28	***Milk, Dairy Products***		
Tomato (raw)	1 med	22	Milk, skim	8 fl oz	2
Fruits			Milk, whole	8 fl oz	4
Cantaloupe (raw)	½ cup, pieces	34	***Fats, Oils, Sugar***		
Grapefruit, white	½ med	39	This food group is not an important source of vitamin C		
Kiwi (raw)	1 med	75	***Other***		
Lemon	1 med	31	Fruit drinks (vitamin C fortified)	8 fl oz	85
Lemon juice (fresh)	8 fl oz	112			
Orange juice (fresh)	8 fl oz	124			

Recommended Dietary Allowance for adults: women, 75 mg; men, 90 mg.

TABLE 7-7 Summary of Vitamin C (Ascorbic Acid)

Physiologic Functions	Clinical Applications	Dietary Reference Intake	Food Sources
Antioxidation Collagen biosynthesis General metabolism Makes iron available for hemoglobin synthesis Influences conversion of folic acid to folinic acid Oxidation-reduction of the amino acids phenylalanine and tyrosine	Scurvy (deficiency) Wound healing, tissue formation Fevers and infections Stress reactions Growth	Adults: Males aged ≥19: 90 mg Females aged ≥ 19: 75 mg Pregnancy: Aged ≤18: 80 mg Aged ≥19: 85 mg Lactation: Aged ≤18: 115 mg Aged ≥19: 120 mg	Fresh fruits, especially citrus Vegetables, such as tomatoes, cabbage, potatoes, chili peppers, and broccoli

covery, have now been identified in relation to many important metabolic functions. As vital control agents, they serve as coenzyme partners with key cell enzymes in many specific reactions controlling energy metabolism and tissue building.

We will review briefly the eight vitamins in this group of water-soluble compounds. First we will look at the three classic deficiency disease factors—thiamin, riboflavin, and niacin. Then we will explore more recently

beriberi A disease of the peripheral nerves caused by a deficiency of thiamin (vitamin B_1). It is characterized by pain (neuritis) and paralysis of the extremities, cardiovascular changes, and edema. Beriberi is common in the Orient, where diets consist largely of milled rice with little protein.
coenzyme A major metabolic role of the micronutrients, vitamins and minerals, as essential partners with cell enzymes in a variety of reactions in energy, lipid, and protein metabolism.

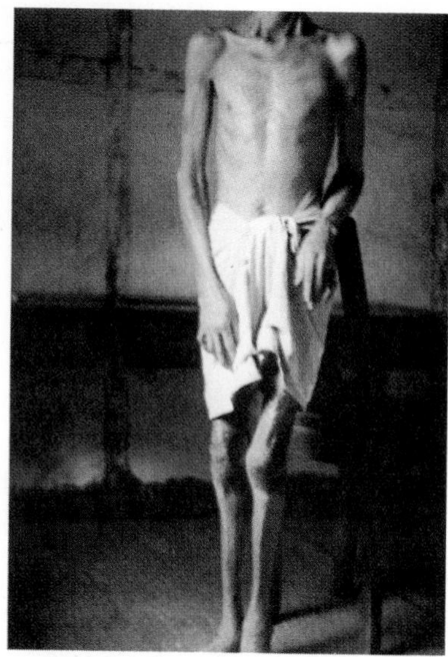

FIGURE 7-6 Beriberi is a thiamin deficiency characterized by extreme weakness, paralysis, anemia, and wasting away (e.g., decreased metabolic function in the liver). *(From McLaren DS:* A colour atlas and text of diet-related disorders, *ed 2, London, 1992, Mosby–Year Book Europe Limited.)*

discovered coenzyme factors—pyridoxine (vitamin B_6), pantothenic acid, and biotin. Finally, we will examine the important blood-forming factors—folate and cobalamin (vitamin B_{12}).

Thiamin

The search by many persons for the cause of beriberi led eventually to a successful conclusion with the identification of thiamin as the control agent involved. Its basic nature and metabolic function were then clarified in the early 1930s.

CHEMICAL AND PHYSICAL NATURE

Thiamin is a water-soluble, fairly stable vitamin. However, it is destroyed by alkalis. Its name comes from its chemical ringlike structure; one of its major parts is a thiazole ring.

ABSORPTION AND STORAGE

Thiamin is absorbed more readily in the acid medium of the upper small intestine before the acidity of the food mass is buffered by the alkaline intestinal secretions. Thiamin is not stored in large quantities in the tissues; thus a continuous supply is necessary.[45] Tissue thiamin content is highly responsive to increased metabolic demand, as in fever, increased muscular activity, pregnancy, and lactation. The tissue stores also depend on the adequacy of the diet and on its general composition. For example, carbohydrate increases the need for thiamin, whereas fat and protein spare thiamin. When tissues are saturated, unused thiamin is constantly excreted in the urine.

FUNCTION OF THIAMIN

Basic Coenzyme Role

The main function of thiamin as a metabolic control agent is related to energy metabolism. When actively combined with phosphorus as the coenzyme thiamin pyrophosphate (TPP), thiamin serves as a coenzyme in key reactions that produce energy from glucose or convert glucose to fat for energy storage. About 90% of the body's total thiamin is in the coenzyme form.[46] Thus the symptoms of beriberi—muscle weakness, gastrointestinal disturbances, and neuritis—can be traced to problems related to the basic energy functions of thiamin.

THIAMIN DEFICIENCY AND CLINICAL PROBLEMS

When thiamin levels are inadequate to provide the key energizing coenzyme factor in cells, broad clinical effects become apparent.

1. *Gastrointestinal system.* Various symptoms such as anorexia, indigestion, constipation, gastric atony, and deficient hydrochloric acid secretion can result from thiamin deficiency. When the cells of the smooth muscles and the secretory glands do not receive sufficient energy from glucose, they cannot do their work in digestion to provide still more glucose to meet body needs. A vicious cycle ensues as the deficiency continues.
2. *Nervous system.* The central nervous system depends on glucose to do its work. Without sufficient thiamin to help provide this constant fuel, nerve activity is impaired, alertness and reflex responses are diminished, and general apathy and fatigue result. If the deficiency continues, lipogenesis is hindered; damage and degeneration of the myelin sheaths—lipid tissue covering the nerve fibers—follow. This causes increasing nerve irritation, pain, and prickly or deadening sensations. Paralysis results if the process continues unchecked, as in the classic thiamin deficiency disease beriberi.
3. *Cardiovascular system.* With continuing thiamin deficiency, the heart muscle weakens, leading to cardiac failure. Also, the smooth muscle of the vascular system may become involved, causing dilation of the peripheral blood vessels. As a result of cardiac failure, edema appears in the lower legs.
4. *Musculoskeletal system.* A chronic painful musculoskeletal condition results from inadequate amounts of TPP in muscle tissue. The widespread muscle pain responds to TPP therapy. The biochemical response to thiamin therapy can measured by the activity of a key related

enzyme, transketolase, in red blood cells. This is a common test for individual thiamin status.[46]

THIAMIN REQUIREMENT

Dietary Reference Intake

The thiamin requirement in human nutrition is based on energy intake as expressed in kilocalories (kcalories). It is estimated that the minimum requirement is 0.3 mg of thiamin/1000 kcalories. Based on this value and the need for a margin of safety the new RDAs were set at 1.2 mg of thiamin for adult men and 1.1 mg thiamin for adult women.[45] An intake of 1.4 mg/day is needed during pregnancy, and an intake of 1.5 mg/day is needed for lactation. Because excess thiamin is easily cleared by the kidneys, there have been no reports of toxicity from oral doses up to 50 mg. However, there has been no systematic study of large intakes of thiamin; therefore no UL can be established.

Special Needs

Several important conditions influence thiamin requirements.

1. *Alcoholism.* Thiamin is most important in nutritional therapy for persons who abuse alcohol.[45] Both a primary deficiency (lack of adequate diet) and a conditioned deficiency (effect of alcohol itself) lead to malnutrition and bring about serious neurologic disorders. Alcohol interferes with the active transport of thiamin across the intestinal wall.
2. *Other disease.* Fever and infection increase cellular energy requirements. Persons with chronic illness, especially older adults, and patients on dialysis because of renal failure require particular attention to prevent deficiencies.
3. *Normal growth and development.* An increase in the thiamin requirement accompanies pregnancy and lactation, demanded by the rapid fetal growth, the increased metabolic rate during pregnancy, and the production of milk. Continuing growth during infancy, childhood, and adolescence requires attention to thiamin needs. At any point in the life cycle, the larger the body and its tissue volume, the greater are cellular energy requirements and thus thiamin needs.
4. *Patients on diuretics.* Diuretic drugs are commonly used in the treatment of hypertension and cardiac failure. All diuretics cause increased urinary loss of thiamin. If thiamin intake is low, these patients can, over time, develop a thiamin deficiency that could worsen their cardiac symptoms.[47]

FOOD SOURCES OF THIAMIN

Although thiamin is widespread in almost all plant and animal tissues commonly used as food, the content in each food is usually small. Deficiency of thiamin is a distinct possibility when kcalories are markedly curtailed, as in alcoholism or anorexia, and when persons are following some highly inadequate special diet. Good food sources include lean pork, beef, and liver, but major sources are seeds of plants, including whole and enriched grains and legumes.[1] Thiamin is extremely water soluble and thus is readily lost in cooking water. Table 7-8 provides some comparative food sources of thiamin.

Riboflavin

DISCOVERY

As early as 1897 a London chemist observed in milk whey a water-soluble pigment with peculiar yellow-green fluorescence, but it was not until 1932 that riboflavin was actually discovered by researchers in Germany.[48] The vitamin was given the chemical group name *flavins* from the Latin word for "yellow." Later, when the vitamin was found to contain a sugar named ribose, the name riboflavin was officially adopted.

CHEMICAL AND PHYSICAL NATURE

Riboflavin is a yellow-green fluorescent pigment that forms yellowish brown, needle-like crystals. It is water soluble and relatively stable to heat but easily destroyed by light and irradiation.

ABSORPTION AND STORAGE

Absorption of riboflavin occurs readily in the upper section of the small intestine. Long-term laxative use of bulk fiber supplements such as psyllium gum, especially when taken with milk or near meals, can hinder riboflavin absorption and contribute to its deficiency. Storage is limited, although small amounts are found in liver and kidney. Day-to-day tissue turnover needs must be supplied in the diet.

FUNCTIONS OF RIBOFLAVIN

Basic Coenzyme Role

The cell enzymes in which riboflavin is an important part are called flavoproteins. Riboflavin-containing enzymes flavin mononucleotide (FMN) and flavin adenine

---

pantothenic acid A B vitamin found widely distributed in nature and occurring throughout the body tissues. Pantothenic acid is an essential constituent of coenzyme A, which has extensive metabolic responsibility as an activating agent of a number of compounds in many tissues.

thiamin pyrophosphate (TPP) Activating coenzyme form of thiamin that plays a key role in carbohydrate metabolism.

TABLE 7-8 Food Sources of Thiamin

Food Source	Quantity	Thiamin (mg)
Bread, Cereal, Rice, Pasta		
Bran flakes	1 cup	0.46
Bread, whole wheat	1 slice	0.10
Corn muffin	1 muffin	0.10
Egg noodles, enriched	1 cup	0.20
Pasta, enriched	1 cup	0.23
Rice, enriched	1 cup	0.23
Wheat flakes	1 cup	0.40
Vegetables		
Asparagus (boiled)	½ cup (6 spears)	0.09
Avocado (raw)	1 med	0.19
Brussels sprouts (boiled)	½ cup (4 sprouts)	0.08
Corn, yellow (boiled)	½ cup	0.18
Green peas (boiled)	½ cup	0.21
Potato (baked, with skin)	1 med	0.22
Fruits		
Figs (dried)	10 figs	0.13
Orange juice (fresh)	8 fl oz	0.22
Orange, navel (raw)	1 med	0.13
Raisins, seedless	⅔ cup	0.16
Meat, Poultry, Fish, Dried Beans, Eggs, Nuts		
Beef liver (fried)	3.5 oz	0.21
Black-eyed peas (boiled)	1 cup	0.35
Cashews (roasted)	1 oz	0.12
Chicken, light and dark (roasted, without skin)	3.5 oz	0.07
Chicken liver (simmered)	3.5 oz	0.18
Ham (canned)	3.5 oz	0.88
Kidney beans (boiled)	1 cup	0.28
Lentils (boiled)	1 cup	0.34
Lima beans (boiled)	1 cup	0.30
Navy beans (boiled)	1 cup	0.37
Peanuts (roasted)	1 oz	0.12
Pecans (dried)	1 oz	0.24
Pinto beans (boiled)	1 cup	0.32
Sirloin steak (broiled)	3.5 oz	0.13
Soybeans (boiled)	1 cup	0.27
Top round (broiled)	3.5 oz	0.12
Tuna (baked)	3 oz	0.24
Milk, Dairy Products		
Milk, skim	8 fl oz	0.09
Milk, whole	8 fl oz	0.09
Fats, Oils, Sugar		
This food group is not an important source of thiamin		

Recommended Dietary Allowance for adults: women, 1.1 mg; men, 1.2 mg.

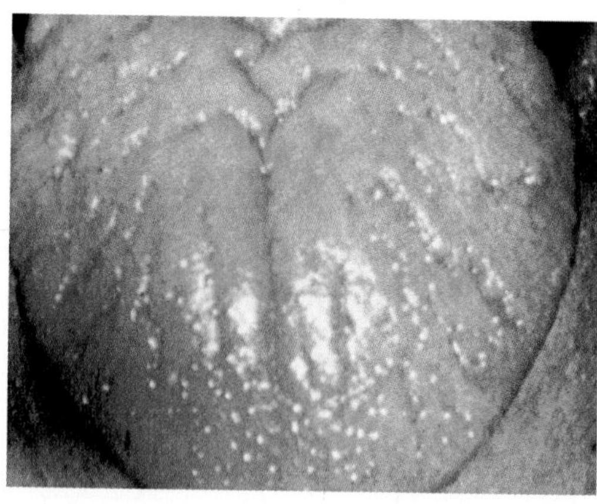

FIGURE 7-7 Glossitis. (*From McLaren DS:* A colour atlas and text of diet-related disorders, *ed 2, London, 1992, Mosby–Year Book Europe Limited.*)

dinucleotide (FAD) operate at vital reaction points in the process of energy metabolism and in deamination. *Deamination* is the key reaction that removes the nitrogen-containing amino group from certain amino acids so that new amino acids can be formed. Thus riboflavin acts as a control agent in both energy production and tissue building. In its important coenzyme role in FMN and FAD, riboflavin acts as an antioxidant.[45]

RIBOFLAVIN DEFICIENCY AND CLINICAL PROBLEMS

Problems associated with riboflavin deficiency include the following two conditions.

1. *Ariboflavinosis.* A deficiency of riboflavin, or ariboflavinosis, brings a combination of symptoms that center on tissue inflammation and breakdown and poor wound healing. Even minor injuries become aggravated and do not heal easily. The lips become swollen, cracking easily, and characteristic cracks develop at the corners of the mouth, a condition called *cheilosis.* Cracks and irritation develop at nasal angles. The tongue becomes swollen and reddened, a condition called glossitis (Figure 7-7). Extra blood vessels develop in the cornea, creating corneal vascularization, and the eyes burn, itch, and tear. A scaly, greasy skin condition, seborrheic dermatitis, may develop, especially in skin folds. Because nutritional deficiencies are usually multiple rather than single, riboflavin deficiencies seldom occur alone; they are especially likely to occur in conjunction with deficiencies of other B vitamins.
2. *Deficiency in newborns.* Because riboflavin is light sensitive, newborn infants with elevated blood levels of bilirubin who are treated with phototherapy may require additional riboflavin.

RIBOFLAVIN REQUIREMENT

Influencing Factors

The body's riboflavin requirement is determined by total energy needs, body size, metabolic rate, and rate of growth—all of which are related to protein intake. People who engage in regular physical activity seem to have a greater need for riboflavin, likely related to increased energy metabolism, adaptation to training, and muscle maintenance and repair.[49]

Dietary Reference Intake

The new RDA for riboflavin is based on the amount of riboflavin necessary to maintain appropriate levels of the flavoproteins in healthy persons. The allowance was set at 1.3 mg/day for adolescent and adult men and 1.1 mg/day for adolescent and adult women.[45] The differences between men and women are based on their different body size and kcalorie intakes. No UL has been set for riboflavin, but this does not mean that there is no danger in consuming high-potency supplements.

Risk Groups

Persons in certain risk groups or clinical situations may require increased riboflavin. Kidney patients on dialysis are likely to require extra riboflavin.[45] This also applies to those with gastrointestinal disease or chronic illness where poor appetite and malabsorption exist. Individuals who have poor wound healing and those in growth stages such as in childhood, pregnancy, and lactation have greater need for riboflavin.

FOOD SOURCES OF RIBOFLAVIN

The most important source of riboflavin is milk; thus individuals who are lactose intolerant may have poor intake. Each quart of milk contains 2 mg of riboflavin, which is more than the daily requirement. Other good sources are organ meats such as liver, kidney, and heart; whole or enriched grains; and vegetables. Because riboflavin is destroyed by light, milk is now sold in cardboard or opaque plastic containers. It is stable to heat and not easily destroyed in proper cooking. Table 7-9 lists some food sources of riboflavin.

Niacin

The age-old disease related to niacin (nicotinic acid) is pellagra (Figure 7-8). It is characterized by a typical dermatitis and often has fatal effects on the nervous system.[50] Pellagra was first observed in eighteenth-century Europe, where it was endemic in populations subsisting largely on corn. Later the American physician Goldberger, who made his observations while studying the problem in the southern region of the United States, found further clues among children in an orphanage. He noticed that although the majority of the children had pellagra to some degree, a few of them did not. He discovered that the few who were free of pellagra were sneaking into the pantries at night and eating the orphanage's limited supply of milk and meat. His investigation established the relation of the disease to a certain food factor, but it was not until 1937 that University of Wisconsin scientist Elvehjem definitely associated niacin with pellagra by using it to cure a related disease—black tongue—in dogs. Correlation between human pellagra and niacin deficiency was then rapidly secured.[50]

CHEMICAL AND PHYSICAL NATURE

Further study of niacin and pellagra made clear a close connection of niacin to the essential amino acid tryptophan.

1. *Precursor role of tryptophan.* Curious observations made by early investigators raised puzzling questions. Why was pellagra rare in some population groups whose diets were actually low in niacin, whereas the disease was common in other groups whose diets were higher in niacin? And why did milk, which is low in niacin, cure or prevent pellagra? Furthermore, why was pellagra so common in groups subsisting on diets high in corn? In 1945, scientists at the University of Wisconsin made the key discovery—tryptophan can be used by the body to make niacin; in other words, tryptophan is a precursor of niacin. Milk prevents pellagra because it is high in tryptophan. A diet based on corn and little else contributes to pellagra because it is low in both tryptophan and niacin (the bound niacin found in corn is not available for absorption). But some populations with diets low in niacin may never have pellagra because they happen also to be consuming adequate amounts of tryptophan in animal protein foods. It is interesting to note that Mexican families with a corn-based diet who soaked their corn in lime (alkali) when preparing tortillas did not get pellagra because the lime treatment released the bound niacin in the corn and made it available to be absorbed.[50]
2. *Niacin equivalent.* This tryptophan-niacin relation led to the development of the unit of measure called a niacin equivalent (NE). In persons with average

ariboflavinosis Group of clinical manifestations of riboflavin deficiency.

glossitis Swollen, reddened tongue; riboflavin deficiency symptom.

niacin equivalent (NE) A measure of the total dietary sources of niacin equivalent to 1 mg of niacin. Thus an NE is 1 mg of niacin or 60 mg of tryptophan.

TABLE 7-9 Food Sources of Riboflavin

Food Source	Quantity	Riboflavin (mg)
Bread, Cereal, Rice, Pasta		
Bran flakes	1 cup	0.40
Bread, whole wheat	1 slice	0.05
English muffin, plain	1 muffin	0.18
Noodles, enriched	1 cup	0.18
Spaghetti, enriched	1 cup	0.11
Wheat flakes	1 cup	0.42
Vegetables		
Asparagus (boiled)	½ cup (6 spears)	0.11
Avocado (raw)	1 med	0.21
Mushrooms (boiled)	½ cup (pieces)	0.23
Spinach (boiled)	½ cup	0.21
Sweet potato (baked)	1 med	0.15
Fruits		
Blueberries (raw)	1 cup	0.07
Figs (dried)	10 figs	0.17
Pear (raw)	1 med	0.07
Prunes (dried)	10 prunes	0.14
Raspberries (raw)	1 cup	0.11
Meat, Poultry, Fish, Dried Beans, Eggs, Nuts		
Almonds (oil roasted)	1 oz	0.28
Beef liver (fried)	3.5 oz	4.14
Chicken, dark (roasted, without skin)	3.5 oz	0.23
Chicken, light (roasted, without skin)	3.5 oz	0.12
Chicken liver (simmered)	3.5 oz	1.76
Clams (baked)	3 oz (9 small)	0.36
Egg, fresh	1 large	0.18
Ground beef, regular (baked)	3.5 oz	0.19
Ham loin, lean (baked)	3.5 oz	0.31
Kidney beans (boiled)	1 cup	0.10
Lentils (boiled)	1 cup	0.18
Lima beans (boiled)	1 cup	0.10
Mackerel (baked)	3 oz	0.35
Rainbow trout (baked)	3 oz	0.19
Sirloin steak (broiled)	3.5 oz	0.30
Soybeans (boiled)	1 cup	0.49
Top round (broiled)	3.5 oz	0.27
Milk, Dairy Products		
Brie cheese	1 oz	0.15
Buttermilk	8 fl oz	0.38
Cheddar cheese	1 oz	0.11
Cottage cheese, creamed	1 cup	0.34
Cottage cheese, 2% fat	1 cup	0.42
Milk, skim	8 fl oz	0.34
Milk, whole	8 fl oz	0.39
Ricotta cheese, whole milk	1 cup	0.48
Yogurt, whole milk	8 fl oz	0.32
Fats, Oils, Sugar		
This food group is not an important source of riboflavin		

Recommended Dietary Allowance for adults: women, 1.1 mg; men, 1.3 mg.

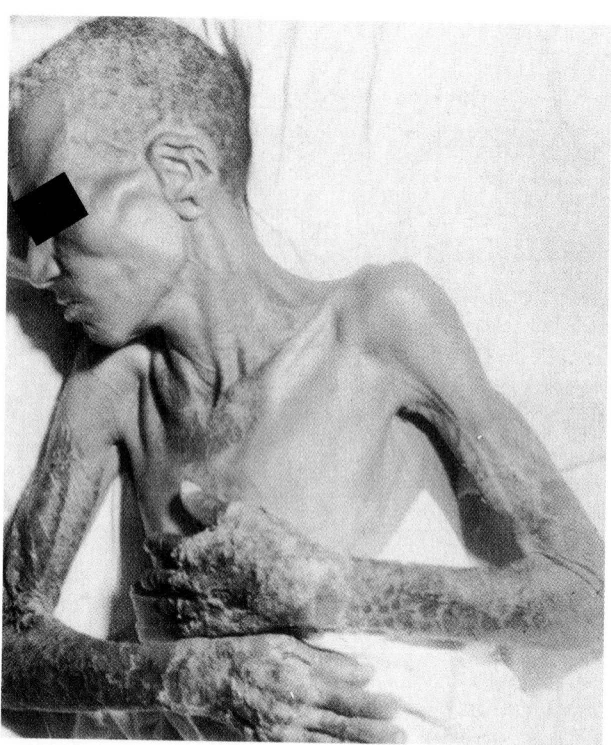

FIGURE 7-8 Pellagra results from a niacin deficiency. (*From McLaren DS:* A colour atlas and text of diet-related disorders, *ed 2, London, 1992, Mosby–Year Book Europe Limited.*)

physiologic needs, approximately 60 mg of tryptophan produces 1 mg of niacin, the amount designated as an NE. Dietary recommendations are now given in terms of total milligrams of NE.[45]

FORMS

Two forms of niacin exist: nicotinic acid and nicotinamide. Niacin (nicotinic acid) is easily converted to its amide form, nicotinamide, which is water soluble, stable to acid and heat, and forms a white powder when crystallized.

FUNCTIONS OF NIACIN

Basic Coenzyme Role

Niacin has two coenzyme forms: nicotinamide-adenine dinucleotide (NAD) and nicotinamide-adenine dinucleotide phosphate (NADP). In these forms, niacin is a partner with riboflavin in the cellular coenzyme systems that convert proteins and glycerol to glucose and then oxidize the glucose to release energy. (Recall that glycerol comes from the hydrolysis of triglycerides.)

Drug Therapy

High doses of niacin act as vasodilators and cause skin flushing, gastrointestinal distress, and itching. Such dosages have been effective in lowering serum cholesterol

TABLE 7-10 Food Sources of Niacin

Food Source	Quantity	Niacin (mg)
Bread, Cereal, Rice, Pasta		
Bread, whole wheat	1 slice	1.0
Corn meal, yellow, enriched	1 cup	4.8
Cream of wheat (regular, cooked)	¾ cup	1.1
Oatmeal (cooked)	¾ cup (⅓ cup dry)	0.2
Rice, white, enriched (cooked)	½ cup	1.1
Wheat flour, all-purpose, enriched	1 cup	4.8
Vegetables		
Asparagus (boiled)	½ cup (6 spears)	0.9
Avocado (raw)	1 med	3.3
Broccoli (raw)	½ cup (chopped)	0.3
Carrot (raw)	1 med	0.7
Corn, yellow (boiled)	½ cup	1.3
Mushrooms (raw)	½ cup (pieces)	1.4
Peas, green (boiled)	½ cup	1.8
Potato (baked, with skin)	1 med	3.3
Tomato (boiled)	½ cup	0.9
Tomato juice	6 fl oz	1.2
Fruits		
Banana (raw)	1 med	0.8
Figs (dried)	10 figs	1.3
Mango (raw)	1 med	1.2
Raspberries (raw)	1 cup	1.1
Meat, Poultry, Fish, Dried Beans, Eggs, Nuts		
Beef liver (fried)	3.5 oz	14.4
Chicken liver (simmered)	3.5 oz	4.6
Ground beef, regular (broiled)	3.5 oz	6.8
Ham, cured, regular	3.5 oz	4.8
Peanut butter	1 tbsp	2.2
Peanuts (dry roasted)	1 oz	3.8
Salmon (baked)	3 oz	5.7
Sirloin steak (lean, broiled)	3.5 oz	4.3
Swordfish (baked)	3 oz	10.0
Top round, lean (broiled)	3.5 oz	6.0
Milk, Dairy Products		
Milk, skim	8 fl oz	0.2
Milk, whole	8 fl oz	0.2
Fats, Oils, Sugar		
This food group is not an important source of niacin		

Recommended Dietary Allowance for adults: women, 14 mg NE; men, 16 mg NE.

levels in some patients; however, the long-term use of high doses of niacin carries the danger of liver damage.

NIACIN DEFICIENCY AND CLINICAL PROBLEMS

Generally niacin deficiency results in muscle weakness, anorexia, and indigestion. More specific symptoms involve the skin and nervous system. Skin areas exposed to sunlight develop a dark, scaly dermatitis. If deficiency continues, the central nervous system is affected, and confusion, apathy, disorientation, neuritis, and eventually death, occur.

NIACIN REQUIREMENT

Influencing Factors

Factors such as age and growth periods, pregnancy and lactation, illness, tissue trauma, body size, and physical activity affect the niacin requirement.

Dietary Reference Intake

The current RDAs are 16 mg of NE/day for adolescent and adult men and 14 mg of NE/day for adolescent and adult women.[45] These recommendations allow for differences in energy intake and adjust for the availability and relative efficiency of converting tryptophan to niacin.

FOOD SOURCES OF NIACIN

Meat and dairy products are major sources of niacin. Good sources include peanuts and dried beans and peas. Enriched grain products are good sources; otherwise corn and rice are poor niacin sources because they are low in tryptophan. Table 7-10 describes some comparative food sources of niacin.

Pyridoxine (Vitamin B_6)

CHEMICAL AND PHYSICAL NATURE

The chemical structure of pyridoxine, a pyridine ring, accounts for its specific name. It is water soluble and heat stable but sensitive to light and alkalis.

FORMS

Vitamin B_6 is a generic term for a group of vitamins with a similar function. Three forms occur in nature: pyridoxine, pyridoxal, and pyridoxamine. In the body all three forms are equally active as precursors of the potent pyridoxine coenzyme pyridoxal phosphate (B_6-PO_4)—PLP.[45]

ABSORPTION AND STORAGE

Pyridoxine is well absorbed in the upper portion of the small intestine. It is stored in the muscle but found throughout the body, evidence of its many essential metabolic activities involving protein.

FUNCTIONS OF PYRIDOXINE

Coenzyme in Protein Metabolism

In its active phosphate form (PLP), pyridoxine is a coenzyme in more than 100 amino acid reactions.

1. *Neurotransmitters.* Converts glutamic acid to gamma-aminobutyric acid (GABA), a substance found in the gray matter of the brain, and converts the essential amino acid tryptophan to serotonin, a potent regulatory substance in brain activity.
2. *New amino acids.* Transfers nitrogen from amino acids to form new ones and releases carbon residues for energy.
3. *Sulfur transfer.* Moves sulfur from an essential sulfur-containing amino acid (methionine) to form other sulfur compounds.
4. *Niacin.* Controls formation of niacin from tryptophan.
5. *Hemoglobin.* Incorporates amino acids into heme, the essential nonprotein core of hemoglobin.
6. *Immune function.* Plays a role in the production and release of antibodies and immune cells.

Coenzyme in Carbohydrate and Fat Metabolism

PLP provides metabolites for energy-producing fuel. It also converts the essential fatty acid linoleic acid to another fatty acid, arachidonic acid.

PYRIDOXINE DEFICIENCY AND CLINICAL PROBLEMS

It is evident from this list of metabolic activities that pyridoxine holds a key to a number of clinical problems.

1. *Anemia.* A hypochromic type of anemia is related to the role of pyridoxine in heme formation. It can occur even in the presence of a high serum iron level. Such deficiency of pyridoxine has been demonstrated and the anemia cured by supplying the deficient vitamin.
2. *Central nervous system problems.* Through its role in the formation of the two regulatory compounds in brain activity, serotonin and GABA, pyridoxine controls related neurologic function. In infants deprived of pyridoxine, as occurred when a batch of hospital formula was mistakenly autoclaved at high temperature, there is increased irritability progressing to convulsions. Immediate supplementation with the vitamin restored their normal function.
3. *Physiologic demands in pregnancy.* Pyridoxine deficiencies during pregnancy have been identified in mothers with preeclampsia (hypertension with edema and proteinuria) and eclampsia (convulsions).[45] Fetal growth creates greater maternal metabolic needs and increases the pyridoxine requirement.
4. *Oral contraceptive use.* Women taking estrogen-progesterone oral contraceptives with high concentrations of estrogen, as were common in past years, require additional pyridoxine. This is less of a problem currently.
5. *Blood homocysteine levels.* Homocysteine is an intermediate product when the body converts methionine (an essential amino acid) to cysteine (a nonessential amino acid). Vitamin B_6 is required for the last step in this reaction—the conversion of homocysteine to cysteine—and when it is in short supply, the process stops and homocysteine accumulates in the blood. Folate is also required for the metabolism of homocysteine, and low folate levels also influence plasma homocysteine levels. High homocysteine levels increase the severity of lipid deposits in the arteries and increase the risk of heart disease beginning in childhood.[51]
6. *Drug therapy.* The drug isoniazid (isonicotinic acid hydrazide [INH]), used as a chemotherapeutic agent in treating tuberculosis, is an antagonist to pyridoxine. Treatment with large doses of pyridoxine, 50 to 100 mg/day, prevents this effect. Levodopa, a therapeutic agent that the body can convert to dopamine, is being used to ease the symptoms of Parkinson's disease. This drug also lowers blood PLP levels.[45]

PYRIDOXINE REQUIREMENT

Dietary Reference Intake

The RDA released in 1998 was based on studies that told us what dietary level of vitamin B_6 was needed to maintain adequate blood PLP levels.[45] The influence of high intakes of protein on the need for vitamin B_6 was also considered in developing this recommendation. The RDA for men and women aged 19 to 50 years is the same, 1.3 mg/day. However, older men and women require higher intakes of pyridoxine to maintain optimum blood levels than younger men and women, and older men require higher intakes than older women. Thus the RDA for men aged 51 years and over was set at 1.7 mg/day, and the RDA for women aged 51 and over was set at 1.5 mg/day. The recommended intakes for infants, children, and adolescents may be found in the Dietary Reference Intake tables on the front inside cover of this book.

PYRIDOXINE TOXICITY

Acute toxicity of pyridoxine is rare. However, pyridoxine intakes from supplements that are several thousand-fold higher than the RDA, amounts in the range of 2 to 4 g, disturb muscular coordination, and severe nerve damage can occur.[45] This has happened in women taking this level of vitamin B_6 for premenstrual tension. Symptoms disappeared over time in most of the women when the large supplements were discontinued, but permanent damage could occur with long-term use. Women need to be warned about this danger.

FOOD SOURCES OF PYRIDOXINE

Pyridoxine is widespread in foods, but many sources provide only very small amounts. Good sources include grains, seeds, legumes, and liver and other meats. Table 7-11 provides some comparative food sources of pyridoxine.

TABLE 7-11 Food Sources of Pyridoxine (Vitamin B_6)

Food Source	Quantity	Pyridoxine (mg)
Bread, Cereal, Rice, Pasta		
Wheat germ (toasted)	¼ cup (1 oz)	0.28
Vegetables		
Avocado (raw)	1 med	0.48
Asparagus (boiled)	1 med	0.13
Broccoli (boiled)	½ cup	0.15
Carrot (raw)	1 med	0.11
Potato (baked, with skin)	1 med	0.70
Fruits		
Apple (raw, with skin)	1 med	0.07
Banana (raw)	1 med	0.66
Figs (dried)	10 figs	0.42
Grape juice (bottled)	8 fl oz	0.16
Meat, Poultry, Fish, Dried Beans, Eggs, Nuts		
Beef liver (fried)	3.5 oz	0.27
Cashews (roasted)	1 oz	0.07
Chicken light meat (roasted, without skin)	3.5 oz	0.60
Chicken liver (simmered)	3.5 oz	0.68
Ground beef, regular (broiled)	3.5 oz	0.27
Ham (canned)	3.5 oz	0.48
Kidney beans (boiled)	1 cup	0.21
Lentils (boiled)	1 cup	0.35
Lima beans (boiled)	1 cup	0.30
Navy beans (boiled)	1 cup	0.30
Peanut butter (chunk style)	1 tbsp	0.14
Peanut butter (creamy)	1 tbsp	0.06
Peanuts (roasted)	1 oz	0.07
Pinto beans (boiled)	1 cup	0.27
Sirloin steak (broiled)	3.5 oz	0.45
Soybeans (boiled)	3 oz	0.40
Swordfish (baked)	3 oz	0.32
Top round (broiled)	3.5 oz	0.61
Walnuts (dried)	1 oz	0.18
Milk, Dairy Products		
Milk, skim	8 fl oz	0.10
Milk, whole	8 fl oz	0.10
Fats, Oils, Sugar		
This food group is not an important source of pyridoxine		

Recommended Dietary Allowance for adults: men and women aged 19-50 years, 1.3 mg; men ≥51 years, 1.7 mg; women ≥51 years, 1.5 mg.

Pantothenic Acid

DISCOVERY

Pantothenic acid was first isolated from yeast by researchers looking for a growth factor that prevented dermatitis.[45] Because it occurs in all forms of living things and is an acid, it was named pantothenic acid. True to its name, it is widespread in nature and in body functions. Intestinal bacteria synthesize considerable amounts. This source, together with its natural occurrence in a wide variety of foods, makes deficiencies unlikely.

CHEMICAL AND PHYSICAL NATURE

Pantothenic acid is a white crystalline compound. It is readily absorbed in the intestine, and combines with phosphorus to form the active molecule acetyl coenzyme A (CoA). It is in this key controlling compound of CoA that pantothenic acid has such broad metabolic presence and use throughout the body. There is no known toxicity or natural deficiency.

FUNCTIONS OF PANTOTHENIC ACID

In its one basic role as an essential constituent of the body's key activating agent CoA, pantothenic acid is vital to metabolic reactions involving carbohydrate, fat, and protein metabolism.[45]

PANTOTHENIC ACID REQUIREMENTS

Dietary Reference Intake

Because we have limited knowledge about the dietary requirement for pantothenic acid, the Food and Nutrition Board has set an AI rather than an RDA.[45] The AI of 5 mg/day for all adults is estimated to replace the amount of vitamin lost daily in the urine. There is no available information at this time to warrant a UL for this nutrient.

FOOD SOURCES OF PANTOTHENIC ACID

Pantothenic acid is widespread in both plant and animal foods. Rich sources include metabolically active tissue such as liver, egg yolk, and milk. Broccoli is a good source. Table 7-12 notes some food sources of pantothenic acid.

TABLE 7-12 Food Sources of Pantothenic Acid

Food Source	Quantity	Pantothenic Acid (mg)
Bread, Cereal, Rice, Pasta		
All-bran	⅓ cup (1 oz)	0.49
Bagel	1 bagel	0.20
Bread, whole wheat	1 slice	0.18
English muffin, plain	1 muffin	0.29
Oatmeal, regular (quick)	¾ cup (1 oz)	0.35
Shredded wheat	1 oz	0.24
Soybean flour (defatted)	½ cup	1.00
Wheat germ (toasted)	¼ cup (1 oz)	0.39
Vegetables		
Avocado (raw)	1 med	1.68
Broccoli (raw)	½ cup, chopped	0.24
Corn, yellow (boiled)	½ cup	0.72
Potato (baked, with skin)	1 med	1.12
Squash, winter, all varieties (baked)	½ cup	0.36
Sweet potato (boiled)	½ cup, mashed	0.87
Tomato (boiled)	½ cup	0.35
Fruits		
Apricots (raw)	3 med	0.25
Banana (raw)	1 med	0.30
Figs (dried)	10 figs	0.81
Orange juice (fresh)	8 fl oz	0.47
Orange, navel (raw)	1 med	0.35
Papaya (raw)	1 med	0.86
Pomegranate (raw)	1 med	0.92
Meat, Poultry, Fish, Dried Beans, Eggs, Nuts		
Almonds (dried)	1 oz (24 nuts)	0.13
Beef liver (fried)	3.5 oz	5.92
Black beans (boiled)	½ cup	0.24
Black-eyed peas (boiled)	½ cup	0.35
Cashews (roasted)	1 oz (16 med nuts)	0.34
Chicken, dark meat (roasted without skin)	3.5 oz	1.21
Meat, Poultry, Fish, Dried Beans, Eggs, Nuts—cont'd		
Chicken, light meat (roasted without skin)	3.5 oz	0.97
Chicken liver (simmered)	3.5 oz	5.41
Egg, fresh	1 large	0.85
Egg yolk, fresh	Yolk of 1 large egg	0.76
Garbanzo beans (boiled)	½ cup	0.24
Ground beef, regular (boiled)	3.5 oz	0.38
Ham, cured, regular	3.5 oz	0.50
Lentils (boiled)	½ cup	0.83
Lima beans (boiled)	½ cup	0.36
Peanut butter (chunk style)	2 tbsp	0.31
Peanuts (roasted)	1 oz	0.39
Pinto beans (boiled)	½ cup	0.26
Salmon (smoked)	3 oz	0.74
Sirloin steak (broiled)	3.5 oz	0.35
Top round (broiled)	3.5 oz	0.48
Turkey, light meat (roasted without skin)	3.5 oz	0.63
Milk, Dairy Products		
American cheese, processed	1 oz	0.14
Blue cheese	1 oz	0.49
Cheddar cheese	1 oz	0.12
Milk, skim	8 fl oz	0.81
Milk, whole	8 fl oz	0.76
Yogurt, whole milk	8 fl oz	0.88
Fats, Oils, Sugar		
This food group is not an important source of pantothenic acid		

Adequate Intake for adults: 5 mg.

Biotin

GENERAL NATURE OF BIOTIN

Biotin is an essential sulfur-containing vitamin. The minute traces of biotin in the body perform multiple metabolic tasks. Its potency is great, and natural deficiency is unknown. However, some cases of induced deficiency have occurred in patients on long-term total parenteral nutrition (TPN) that did not include biotin. Also, several inborn errors of biotin metabolism have been defined according to the specific enzyme that is lacking.[52] Raw egg whites contain a protein avidin that binds biotin, and, if eaten regularly over time, can induce a biotin deficiency. (Raw eggs can also result in food-borne illness that is sometimes fatal in the very young, the very old, or those with compromised immune function.) Cooking eggs denatures this protein and destroys its ability to bind biotin. There is no known toxicity for this nutrient.

FUNCTIONS OF BIOTIN

Biotin functions as a partner with acetyl-CoA in reactions that transfer carbon dioxide from one compound and fix it onto another. Examples of this combination of cofactors at work include (1) initial steps in the synthesis of some fatty acids, (2) conversion reactions involved in synthesis of some amino acids, and (3) carbon dioxide fixation to form purines.

BIOTIN REQUIREMENT

Dietary Reference Intake

Because the amount of biotin needed for metabolism is so small, the AI for this nutrient has been set at 30 μg/day for all adults.[45] Intestinal bacterial synthesis contributes to the body's supply of biotin, and the amount may be significant. Crystalline biotin appears to be well absorbed; when given in pharmacologic doses to individuals with inborn errors of biotin-containing enzymes, it is completely absorbed regardless of the magnitude of the dose.[53]

FOOD SOURCES OF BIOTIN

Biotin is widely distributed in natural foods, but its bioavailability is highly variable in different foods. For example, the biotin in corn and soy foods is completely available, whereas that in wheat is almost completely unavailable. Excellent food sources include egg yolk, liver, tomatoes, and yeast. Fruit and meat are poor sources.

Folate

DISCOVERY

Folate is the generic name for a group of substances that have similar nutritional properties and chemical structures. Early studies investigating the anemia that developed among poor Indian women during pregnancy were the basis for the discovery of folic acid.[46] One of the substances in the folate group was first extracted from dark green, leafy vegetables and given the name folic acid from the Latin word for "leaf."

CHEMICAL AND PHYSICAL NATURE

Folic acid forms yellow crystals and is a conjugated substance made up of three acids: (1) pteroic acid, (2) *para*-aminobenzoic acid (PABA), and (3) glutamic acid (an amino acid). The chemical name for folic acid, taken from its structure, is pteroylmonoglutamic acid. Folic acid is rarely found naturally in food but is the form most often used in vitamin supplements and fortified foods. Naturally occurring folate or food folate is the compound pteroylpolyglutamate, which contains additional glutamic acid molecules.[45]

PABA is sometimes touted by nutrition supplement makers as a separate essential factor in human nutrition, but it is not. Its only role is as a component of the vitamin folate. Dietary folate, preformed by plants, is the essential substance in human nutrition.

FUNCTIONS OF FOLATE

Basic Coenzyme Role

Folates function as necessary coenzyme agents in the important task of attaching single carbons to many metabolic compounds. Several key compounds are examples.

1. *Purines.* Nitrogen-containing compounds found in genetic material and essential to all living cells; involved in cell division and in the transmission of inherited traits.
2. *Thymine.* Essential compound forming a key part of deoxyribonucleic acid (DNA), the important material in the cell nucleus that controls and transmits genetic characteristics.
3. *Hemoglobin.* Heme, the iron-containing nonprotein portion of hemoglobin, important for transporting oxygen and carbon dioxide in the blood.

FOLATE DEFICIENCY AND CLINICAL PROBLEMS

1. *Anemia.* A nutritional megaloblastic anemia often occurs in simple folate deficiency. Because tissue growth requires additional folate, this folate deficiency anemia is a special risk in pregnant women, growing infants, and young children. It also occurs in adolescent girls who severely limit their food intake; those who also smoke are at greater risk.[54]
2. *Chemotherapy.* The drug amethopterin (Methotrexate), used in cancer chemotherapy, acts as a folate antagonist to reduce tumor growth. The effect of this action is to prevent the synthesis of DNA and purines.
3. *Anticonvulsant medications.* High intakes of folate interfere with some drugs such as phenobarbital used in the control of epilepsy.[45]
4. *Acid environment in the stomach and intestine.* An acid environment is needed to support the release of folate from its food source and its absorption into the blood. Low secretion of hydrochloric acid in the stomach, a common problem in older people, and use of prescription drugs that raise the pH in the gastrointestinal tract can adversely affect folate status.[55]

---

megaloblastic anemia Anemia resulting from faulty production of abnormally large immature red blood cells, caused by a deficiency of vitamin B_{12} or folate.

PRACTICAL APPLICATION

Folate Intake and the Prevention of Neural Tube Defects

In recent decades health professionals worldwide have tried to learn the cause and possible prevention of neural tube defects (NTDs). NTDs are the most common birth defects affecting the central nervous system. Neural tissues and their coverings fail to develop normally as a result of some disturbance in embryonic development. In some cases part of the brain is absent; these children are likely to die shortly after birth. In other children with an NTD, the spinal cord may be located on the outside of the body as a result of the failure of the neural tube to close at this location. In the less severe cases, a child may be otherwise normal and live a productive life if surgical and medical intervention is effective. For many children, however, a normal life cannot be achieved.

Scientists have focused on two possible causes of NTDs. First, there appears to be a genetic link to the birth of a child with an NTD. Some individuals have a genetic trait that alters their metabolism of folate and homocysteine and lowers the amount of folate in their red blood cells. Elevated blood homocysteine levels may be a potential screening tool for women at risk of an NTD pregnancy or other congenital abnormality such as club foot. There also appears to be a nutritional relationship to NTDs, as women with daily folate intakes below 400 μg are more likely to give birth to an infant with an NTD. The current incidence of NTDs in the United States is 1:1000 births, and it has been estimated that about half of these cases are related to inadequate folate intake.

There is national concern for improving the intake of folate among women of childbearing age. Development of the fetal nervous system occurs early in pregnancy, between day 21 and day 28 of gestation, before a woman is even aware that she might be pregnant. Consequently, it is critical that a mother be in good folate status at the time of conception—the problem of NTDs cannot be solved with folate supplements after a pregnancy has been confirmed. To improve folate intake among all population groups, the U.S. government set standards requiring folate fortification of all grain products, effective in 1998. Folate now joins iron, thiamin, riboflavin, and niacin as mandatory additions to all ready-to-eat and cooked cereals, flour and cornmeal, rice, pasta, and breads prepared from milled grains. The level of fortification required is 1.4 mg of folic acid/kg of grain. In practical terms, one slice of fortified bread and one serving of fortified pasta add 136 μg to the diet or about one third of the recommended intake (the RDA for women of childbearing age is 400 μg). Five servings from the bread and cereal group, depending on the portion size, could come close to meeting the RDA.

A recalculation of folate intakes from a 1996 national study using the new folate fortification levels for all servings of bread, cereal, and grains indicated that more than 80% of women between the ages of 20 and 49 would have consumed at least 320 μg of folate from bread and cereal products alone. In a group of low-income minority mothers participating in a food distribution program, average intakes from the grain group, including bread, cereal, rice, and pasta, totaled 11 servings a day, contributing over 700 μg of folic acid. Mexican American, Vietnamese American, and East Indian American women, for whom rice is a diet staple, should be urged to use rice processed in the United States with added folate rather than imported rice that does not have added folate.

Although health professionals know that folate is important for women of childbearing age, a recent nutrition education survey reported that only 30% of a group of low-income women could identify a food source rich in folate. As health educators we need to make all women aware of good food sources of folate, including fortified breads and cereals, oranges and orange juice, dark green leafy vegetables, and tomatoes. The potential contribution of grain products to the total folate intake underscores the need to encourage all women to eat 6 to 11 servings of grain products every day as recommended in the *Food Guide Pyramid.*

References

Food and Nutrition Board, National Research Council: *Dietary reference intakes for thiamin, riboflavin, niacin, vitamin B_6, folate, vitamin B_{12}, pantothenic acid, biotin, and choline*, Washington, DC, 1998, National Academy Press.

Lewis CJ et al: Estimated folate intakes: data updated to reflect food fortification, increased bioavailability, and dietary supplement use, *Am J Clin Nutr* 70:198, 1999.

Loeblen AS: Folate knowledge, intake from fortified grain products, and periconceptional supplementation patterns of a sample of low-income pregnant women according to the Health Belief Model, *J Am Diet Assoc* 99:33, 1999.

Vollet SE et al: Plasma total homocysteine, pregnancy complications, and adverse pregnancy outcomes: the Hordaland Homocysteine Study, *Am J Clin Nutr* 71:962, 2000.

FOLATE REQUIREMENT

Clinical Considerations

Heart disease and folate. Observations of men and women with low or high folate intakes found that those with lower intakes of folate, including intake from both food and supplements, were more likely to have serious heart disease.[56] High plasma homocysteine levels, found in persons with lower folate intakes, increase both atherosclerotic damage to the arteries and the formation of blood clots. Many factors contribute to heart disease, but low blood folate levels resulting from low folate intake seem to play a role, and low levels of vitamins B_6 and B_{12} also seem to be involved.[57] Recent steps to fortify grain products with folate have raised folate intakes in the general population; however, adults may still benefit from a folate supplement of 400 μg/day to help lower plasma homocysteine levels.[58] Men and women aged 40 and over who have higher plasma homocysteine levels are more than twice as likely to have a heart attack or stroke.[59]

Folate and birth defects. Folate plays an essential role in the formation and closure of the neural tube in the early weeks of fetal development. The neural tube eventually develops into the brain and spinal cord as growth and maturation continue before birth. Infants born to mothers with poor folate status before their pregnancy are more likely to have a neural tube defect (NTD) with accompanying physical and developmental disabilities.[60] Folate and the incidence of NTDs are *discussed in greater detail in the* Practical Application box.

Dietary Reference Intake

The absorption of folate is greatly influenced by its source. About 50% of the folate occurring naturally in plant foods can be absorbed. In contrast, about 85% of the folate added to fortified foods such as grains and cereals is absorbed. Conversion factors were developed by the Food and Nutrition Board to allow professionals to consider these differences when calculating folate intake.[61] The current folate RDA for adolescents and adults of all ages is 400 μg/day.[45] The RDA increases to 600 μg/day for women during pregnancy to meet increased needs for fetal and maternal tissue growth.

The U.S. Public Health Service recently expanded fortification rules that require the addition of folate to flour, grain, and cereal foods to help ensure that all women of childbearing age have a dietary folate intake of at least 400 μg/day.[45] This level should protect against the risk of a pregnancy with spina bifida or other NTD and may also offer some protection against atherosclerosis and heart disease (see *Practical Application* box).

FOLATE TOXICITY

The UL established for folate is 1000 μg folic acid/day.[45] Persons should not use a folate supplement that exceeds the RDA without the supervision of a physician. Another important reason for not exceeding recommended intakes of folate is the interrelationship between folate and vitamin B_{12}. If vitamin B_{12} levels are low but folate levels are very high, folate can substitute for vitamin B_{12} in preventing the development of a megaloblastic anemia. This can be dangerous for a person deficient in vitamin B_{12}, for as we will learn in the next section, vitamin B_{12} also has an important function in maintaining nerve tissues. The appearance of a megaloblastic anemia is often the first sign that alerts the health professional to the vitamin B_{12} deficiency. If high intakes of folate "mask" this deficiency, serious damage to the nervous system will continue with no intervention.

FOOD SOURCES OF FOLATE

Folate is widely distributed in food. Good sources include green leafy vegetables, legumes, tomatoes, and various fruits such as oranges, orange juice, and cantaloupe. All flour and grain products produced in the United States, including bread, cereals, and other baked products and mixes, are fortified with folate. Table 7-13 gives a summary of food sources of folate.

Cobalamin (Vitamin B_{12})

DISCOVERY

The discovery of cobalamin (vitamin B_{12}) coincided with the search for the agent needed to control pernicious anemia.[62] At first this disease was thought to be related to a deficiency of folate. However, although folate helped to initiate the regeneration of red blood cells, it was not permanently effective and did not control the nerve problems associated with the disease.

In 1948 two groups of workers, one in America and one in England, crystallized a red compound from liver, which they numbered B_{12}. That year it was clearly shown that this new vitamin could control both the blood-forming defect and the neurologic involvement in pernicious anemia. The scientists named their vitamin discovery cobalamin because of its unique structure with a single red atom of the trace element cobalt at its center.

CHEMICAL AND PHYSICAL NATURE

Vitamin B_{12} is a complex red crystalline compound of high molecular weight, with a single cobalt atom at its

---

pernicious anemia A chronic macrocytic anemia occurring most commonly after age 40. It is caused by absence of the intrinsic factor normally present in the gastric juices and necessary for the absorption of cobalamin (B_{12}) and is controlled by intramuscular injections of vitamin B_{12}.

TABLE 7-13 Food Sources of Folate

Food Source	Quantity	Folate (μg)
Bread, Cereal, Rice, Pasta		
Bread, whole wheat	1 slice	14
Wheat germ (toasted)	¼ cup (1 oz)	100
Vegetables		
Asparagus (boiled)	½ cup (6 spears)	88
Avocado (raw)	1 med	113
Peas, green (boiled)	1 cup	51
Spinach (boiled)	1 cup	262
Fruits		
Banana (raw)	1 med	22
Figs (dried)	10 figs	14
Orange (raw)	1 med	47
Strawberries (raw)	1 cup	26
Meat, Poultry, Fish, Dried Beans, Eggs, Nuts		
Beef liver (fried)	3.5 oz	220
Black beans (boiled)	1 cup	256
Black-eyed peas (boiled)	1 cup	358
Chicken liver (simmered)	3.5 oz	770
Chick-peas (boiled)	1 cup	282
Egg, whole	1 large	32
Green beans (boiled)	1 cup	42
Kidney beans (boiled)	1 cup	229
Lima beans, baby (boiled)	1 cup	273
Navy beans (boiled)	1 cup	255
Peanut butter	1 tbsp	13
Peanuts (dry roasted)	1 oz	41
Pinto beans (boiled)	1 cup	794
Milk, Dairy Products		
Milk, whole	8 fl oz	12
Yogurt, whole milk	8 fl oz	17
Fats, Oils, Sugar		
This food group is not an important source of folate		

Recommended Dietary Allowance for adults: 400 μg.

core. It occurs as a protein complex in foods of animal origin only. The ultimate source, however, is the synthesizing bacteria in the intestinal tract of herbivorous animals. Some synthesis also occurs by human intestinal bacteria.

ABSORPTION, TRANSPORT, AND STORAGE

Absorption

Intestinal absorption takes place in the ileum. Vitamin B_{12} is first split from its protein complex by the hydrochloric acid in the stomach and then bound to a specific glycoprotein called intrinsic factor, secreted by the gastric mucosal cells. This vitamin B_{12}–intrinsic factor complex then moves into the intestine, where it is absorbed by special receptors in the ileal mucosa.

Storage

About 50% of body vitamin B_{12} is stored in the liver, with the remainder distributed among active tissues. These amounts are minute, but the body holds them tenaciously and stores are only slowly depleted. For example, after a gastrectomy, a megaloblastic anemia does not become apparent for 3 to 5 years after removal of the organ and subsequent loss of its secretions.

FUNCTIONS OF VITAMIN B_{12}

Basic Coenzyme Role

As an essential coenzyme factor, vitamin B_{12} is closely related to amino acid metabolism and the formation of the heme portion of hemoglobin. It also participates in the synthesis of important lipids and proteins that form the myelin sheath covering nerves of the brain and spinal cord.

VITAMIN B_{12} DEFICIENCY AND CLINICAL PROBLEMS

Special needs for vitamin B_{12} occur in several problems related to blood formation.

1. *Pernicious anemia.* In the absence of intrinsic factor—the specific component of gastric secretion required for vitamin B_{12} absorption—deficiency begins to develop. B_{12} deficiency results in a megaloblastic anemia usually referred to as pernicious anemia because of the dangerous consequences if left untreated. B_{12} supports the formation of red blood cells in two ways. First, the vitamin has a key role in heme formation, and in its absence, adequate hemoglobin cannot be synthesized. Second, vitamin B_{12} indirectly affects blood formation by providing an activated form of folate that also assists in the process.

   A person with defective vitamin B_{12} absorption, and hence pernicious anemia, can be adequately maintained with monthly intramuscular injections of 1000 μg of this vitamin.[46] This treatment controls both the blood-forming disorder and prevents the degenerative effects on the nervous system.
2. *Cognitive function in the elderly.* Because of the function of vitamin B_{12} in maintaining neural tissues, researchers have been looking at the role of this vitamin and the changes in personality, judgment, and cognitive abilities that sometimes occur with aging.[63,64] It appears that some older people with low levels of gastric acid have difficulty absorbing vitamin B_{12} from animal foods, and over time they can become deficient. Unfortunately, in older people nerve damage and changes in brain function can occur before the characteristic megaloblastic anemia

TABLE 7-14 Food Sources of Vitamin B_{12}

Food Source	Quantity	Vitamin B_{12} (μg)
Bread, Cereal, Rice, Pasta		
This food group is not a source of vitamin B_{12} unless cereals are fortified with this vitamin		
Vegetables		
This food group is not a source of vitamin B_{12}		
Fruits		
This food group is not a source of vitamin B_{12}		
Meat, Poultry, Fish, Dried Beans, Eggs, Nuts		
Beef liver (fried)	3.5 oz	111.80
Chicken liver (simmered)	3.5 oz	19.39
Chicken, white meat (roasted)	3.5 oz	0.34
Clams (steamed)	3 oz (9 small)	84.05
Egg, fresh	1 large	0.77
Ground beef, regular (broiled)	3.5 oz	2.93
Ham, cured, regular	3.5 oz	0.80
Mackerel (baked)	3 oz	16.18
Oysters (steamed)	3 oz (12 med)	32.63
Salmon (baked)	3 oz	4.93
Sirloin steak (lean, (broiled)	3.5 oz	2.86
Swordfish (baked)	3 oz	1.72
Top round, lean (broiled)	3.5 oz	2.48
Milk, Dairy Products		
Cheddar cheese	1.5 oz	0.23
Milk, skim	8 fl oz	0.83
Milk, whole	8 fl oz	0.87
Swiss cheese	1.5 oz	0.48
Yogurt, whole milk	8 fl oz	0.84
Fats, Oils, Sugar		
This food group is not a source of vitamin B_{12}		

Recommended Dietary Allowance for adults: 2.4 μg.

appears as a visible sign of B_{12} deficiency. Older persons might try to obtain some of their vitamin B_{12} from fortified foods as this form of the vitamin is more easily absorbed (review *Practical Application* box in Chapter 2).

VITAMIN B_{12} REQUIREMENT

Dietary Reference Intake

The amount of vitamin B_{12} needed for normal human metabolism is very minute. The RDA for vitamin B_{12} is 2.4 μg for both younger and older adults.[45] See the inside book cover for recommended levels for other age groups.

FOOD SOURCES OF VITAMIN B_{12}

Vitamin B_{12} is supplied by animal foods; rich sources include lean meat, milk, egg, and cheese. For individuals consuming any animal foods, the recommended amount can be obtained easily. Vegans who consume no animal foods or individuals with low gastric acid levels can obtain their needed amounts from fortified cereal and grain products. Vitamin B_{12} supplements are also available. Table 7-14 lists food sources of vitamin B_{12}.

A summary of the water-soluble B vitamins can be found in Table 7-15.

TO SUM UP

A vitamin is an organic, noncaloric food substance that is (1) required in very small amounts, (2) participates in certain metabolic functions, and (3) cannot be manufactured by the body. Vitamins may be fat or water soluble, and their solubility affects their absorption and mode of transport to target tissues.

The fat-soluble vitamins are A, D, E, and K. Their metabolic tasks focus on the synthesis of important proteins, the development and differentiation of cells and tissues, and the protection of structural membranes. Their absorption and transport in the body are associated with lipids. The possibility of toxicity is enhanced for fat-soluble vitamins because the body has a high storage capacity for these nutrients. Such toxicity can occur with the overuse of supplements containing concentrated levels of vitamins A and D.

The water-soluble vitamins include ascorbic acid (vitamin C) and the B-complex vitamins. These vitamins share three characteristics: (1) they are synthesized by plants and thus (with the exception of vitamin B_{12}) are supplied to the diet by both plant and animal foods; (2) body stores are limited so they must be provided regularly in the diet; and (3) they function as coenzyme factors in cell metabolism and synthesis of vital molecules. Toxicity levels do not usually occur with water-soluble vitamins because any excess is easily excreted in the urine. However, two vitamins have shown toxic effects when taken in gram amounts: pyridoxine (vitamin B_6) can result in severe nerve damage and ascorbic acid (vitamin C), has been associated with gastrointestinal disturbances, renal calculi, and lowered resistance to infection. All water-soluble vitamins, especially vitamin C and folate, are easily oxidized, and care must be taken in food storage and preparation practices to preserve them. A number of recently discovered *phytochemicals* (plant chemicals) in foods have important functions in the body, particularly as related to the prevention or delay of chronic disease.

TABLE 7-15 Summary of B-Complex Vitamins

Vitamin	Coenzyme: Physiologic Functions	Clinical Applications	Dietary Reference Intake	Food Sources
Thiamin	Carbohydrate metabolism Thiamin pyrophosphate (TPP): oxidative decarboxylation	Beriberi (deficiency) Neuropathy Wernicke-Korsakoff syndrome (alcoholism) Depressed muscular and secretory symptoms	Adults: Males aged ≥19: 1.2 mg Females aged ≥19: 1.1 mg Pregnancy: All ages: 1.4 mg Lactation: All ages: 1.5 mg	Pork, beef, organ meats Whole or enriched grains and cereals Legumes
Riboflavin	General metabolism Flavin adenine dinucleotide (FAD) Flavin mononucleotide (FMN)	Cheilosis, glossitis, seborrheic dermatitis	Adults: Males aged ≥19: 1.3 mg Females aged ≥19: 1.1 mg Pregnancy: All ages: 1.4 mg Lactation: All ages: 1.6 mg	Milk products, organ meats Enriched grains and cereals
Niacin (nicotinic acid, nicotinamide)	General metabolism Nicotinamide adenine dinucleotide (NAD) Nicotinamide adenine dinucleotide phosphate (NADP)	Pellagra (deficiency) Weakness, anorexia Scaly dermatitis Neuritis	Adults: Males aged ≥19: 16 NE Females aged ≥19: 14 NE Pregnancy: All ages: 18 NE Lactation: All ages: 17 NE	Meat, protein foods containing tryptophan Peanuts Enriched grains and cereals
Vitamin B_6 (pyridoxine, pyridoxal, pyridoxamine)	General metabolism Pyridoxal phosphate (PLP): transamination and decarboxylation	Reduced serum levels associated with pregnancy and use of certain oral contraceptives Antagonized by isoniazid, penicillamine, and other drugs	Adult males: Aged 19-50: 1.3 mg Aged ≥51: 1.7 mg Adult females: Aged 19-50: 1.3 mg Aged ≥51: 1.5 mg Pregnancy: All ages: 1.9 mg Lactation: All ages: 2.0 mg	Meat, organ meats Whole grains and cereals Legumes Bananas
Pantothenic acid	General metabolism CoA (coenzyme A): acetylation	Many roles through acyl transfer reactions (for example, lipogenesis, amino acid activation, and formation of cholesterol, steroid hormones, heme)	Adults: Males/females aged ≥19: 5 mg Pregnancy: All ages: 6 mg Lactation: All ages: 7 mg	Egg, milk, liver

TABLE 7-15 Summary of B-Complex Vitamins—cont'd

Vitamin	Coenzyme: Physiologic Functions	Clinical Applications	Dietary Reference Intake	Food Sources
Biotin	General metabolism *N*-Carboxybiotinyl lysine: CO_2 transfer reactions	Deficiency induced by avidin (a protein in raw egg white) and by antibiotics Synthesis of some fatty acids and amino acids	Adults: Males/females aged ≥19: 30 μg Pregnancy: All ages: 30 μg Lactation: All ages: 35 μg	Egg yolk, liver Synthesized by intestinal microorganisms
Folate (folic acid, folacin)	General metabolism Single carbon transfer reactions (for example, purine nucleotide, thymine, heme synthesis)	Megaloblastic anemia Elevated blood homocysteine levels	Adults: Males/females aged ≥19: 400 μg Pregnancy: All ages: 600 μg Lactation: All ages: 500 μg	Green leafy vegetables Oranges, orange juice, tomatoes Liver and organ meats Fortified breads and cereals
Vitamin B_{12} (cobalamin)	General metabolism Methylcobalamin: methylation reactions (for example, synthesis of amino acids, heme)	Pernicious anemia induced by lack of intrinsic factor Megaloblastic anemia Methylmalonic aciduria Homocystinuria Peripheral neuropathy (strict vegetarian diet)	Adults: Males/females aged ≥19: 2.4 μg Pregnancy: All ages: 2.6 μg Lactation: All ages: 2.8 μg	Meat, milk, cheese, egg, liver (all animal foods) Fortified cereals

Questions for Review

1. How do the absorption and storage of a vitamin affect its potential deficiency or toxicity? Provide several examples to illustrate this concept.
2. List and describe three health problems caused by a vitamin A deficiency. Give three possible causes of a vitamin A deficiency.
3. Describe the formation and function of the vitamin D hormone calcitriol. Who is at risk for developing a deficiency? Why?
4. Vitamin E plays an important role in the body as an antioxidant. What is an antioxidant? How does vitamin E protect body tissues? A woman tells you that she is taking 1000 mg of vitamin E to prevent signs of aging—what do you tell her?
5. List three conditions or situations that increase the risk for vitamin K deficiency. How do these deficiencies develop?
6. What three characteristics are shared by most water-soluble vitamins? Identify an exception to each and explain the reason.
7. Define the term *coenzyme factor* as applied to the role of vitamins, especially water-soluble vitamins. Give several examples to illustrate.
8. Which water-soluble vitamins are potentially toxic? Why? What signs of toxicity have been observed for each?
9. Which B vitamins play significant roles in blood formation? Describe their roles and interactions.
10. You have been asked to speak at a senior citizens center and they have asked about phytochemicals. Outline your presentation describing (a) what a phytochemical is, (b) why they are important, and (c) good food sources to include in your diet. The senior center director has given you some money for groceries to provide taste treats to serve with your program. What foods or recipes will you prepare?
11. Visit a nearby grocery store and check the food label to determine the folate content of (a) five different breads, (b) five different ready-to-eat cereals, (c) five types of rice or rice-containing dishes, and (d) five types of pasta or pasta-containing dishes. Rice and

pasta dishes may be dry mixes or frozen entrees. Develop menus for 3 days that include a daily minimum of six servings from the grains group and provide at least 400 μg of folate.

References

1. Marsh MN, Riley SA: Digestion and absorption of nutrients and vitamins. In Feldman M, Scharschmidt BF, Sleisenger MH, eds: *Gastrointestinal and liver disease,* ed 6, vol 2, Philadelphia, 1998, WB Saunders.
2. Harper AE: Defining the essentiality of nutrients. In Shils ME et al, eds: *Modern nutrition in health and disease,* ed 9, Philadelphia, 1999, Lippincott Williams & Wilkins.
3. Food and Nutrition Board: *Dietary reference intakes for vitamin A, vitamin K, arsenic, boron, chromium, copper, iodine, iron, manganese, molybdenum, nickel, silicon, vanadium, and zinc,* Washington, DC, 2001, National Academy Press.
4. Tang G et al: Green and yellow vegetables can maintain body stores of vitamin A in Chinese children, *Am J Clin Nutr* 70:1069, 1999.
5. Olson JA et al: Fat-soluble vitamins. In Garrow GS, James WPT, Ralph A, eds: *Human nutrition and dietetics,* ed 10, Edinburgh, 2000, Churchill Livingstone.
6. Binkley N, Krueger K: Hypervitaminosis A and bone, *Nutr Rev* 58:138, 2000.
7. Sedgh G et al: Dietary vitamin A intake and nondietary factors are associated with reversal of stunting in children, *J Nutr* 130:2520, 2000.
8. Wolf G: Vitamin A functions in the regulation of the dopaminergic system in the brain and pituitary gland, *Nutr Rev* 56:354, 1998.
9. Ross AC: Vitamin A. In Shils ME et al, eds: *Modern nutrition in health and disease,* ed 9, Philadelphia, 1999, Lippincott Williams & Wilkins.
10. Azais-Braesco V, Pascal G: Vitamin A in pregnancy: requirements and safety limits, *Am J Clin Nutr* 71(suppl): 1325S, 2000.
11. Norman AW: Sunlight, season, skin pigmentation, vitamin D, and 25-hydroxyvitamin D: integral components of the vitamin D endocrine system, *Am J Clin Nutr* 67:1108, 1998.
12. Holick MF: Vitamin D. In Shils ME et al, eds: *Modern nutrition in health and disease,* ed 9, Philadelphia, 1999, Lippincott Williams & Wilkins.
13. Outila TA, Karkkainen MUM, Lamberg-Allardt CJE: Vitamin D status affects serum parathyroid hormone concentrations during winter in female adolescents: associations with forearm bone mineral density, *Am J Clin Nutr* 74:206, 2001.
14. DeLuca HF, Zierold C: Mechanisms and functions of vitamin D, *Nutr Rev* 56(2, Part II):S4, 1998.
15. Sills IN: Nutritional rickets: a preventable disease, *Top Clin Nutr* 17:36, 2001.
16. Fitzpatrick S et al: Vitamin D-deficient rickets: a multifactorial disease, *Nutr Rev* 58:218, 2000.
17. Heaney RP et al: Dietary changes favorably affect bone remodeling in older adults, *J Am Diet Assoc* 99:1228, 1999.
18. Food and Nutrition Board, National Research Council: *Dietary reference intakes for calcium, phosphorus, magnesium, vitamin D, and fluoride,* Washington, DC, 1997, National Academy Press.
19. Vieth R: Vitamin D supplementation, 25-dihydroxyvitamin D concentrations, and safety, *Am J Clin Nutr* 69:842, 1999.
20. Food and Nutrition Board, National Research Council: *Dietary reference intakes for vitamin C, vitamin E, selenium, and carotenoids,* Washington, DC, 2000, National Academy Press.
21. Meydani S et al: Assessment of the safety of supplementation with different amounts of vitamin E in healthy older adults, *Am J Clin Nutr* 68:311, 1998.
22. Yochum LA, Folsom AR, Kushi LK: Intake of antioxidant vitamins and risk of death from stroke in postmenopausal women, *Am J Clin Nutr* 72:476, 2000.
23. Meydani M: Vitamin E and atherosclerosis: beyond prevention of LDL oxidation, *J Nutr* 131:366S, 2001.
24. Meydani M: Antioxidants and cognitive function, *Nutr Rev* 59(8, Part II):75S, 2001.
25. Grundman M: Vitamin E and Alzheimer disease: the basis for additional clinical trials, *Am J Clin Nutr* 71(suppl): 630S, 2000.
26. Tidow-Kebritchi S, Mobarhan S: Effects of diets containing fish oil and vitamin E on rheumatoid arthritis, *Nutr Rev* 59:335, 2001.
27. Traber MG: Vitamin E. In Shils ME et al, eds: *Modern nutrition in health and disease,* ed 9, Philadelphia, 1999, Lippincott Williams & Wilkins.
28. Jiang Q et al: Gamma tocopherol, the major form of vitamin E in the US diet, deserves more attention, *Am J Clin Nutr* 74:714, 2001.
29. Dwyer JT et al: Do adolescent vitamin-mineral supplement users have better nutrient intakes than nonusers? Observations from the CATCH tracking study, *J Am Diet Assoc* 101:1340, 2001.
30. Dixon LB, Winkleby MA, Radimer KL: Dietary intakes and serum nutrients differ between adults from food-insufficient and food-sufficient families: Third National Health and Nutrition Examination Survey, 1988-1994, *J Nutr* 131:1232, 2001.
31. Steiner M: Vitamin E, a modifier of platelet function: rationale and use in cardiovascular and cerebrovascular disease, *Nutr Rev* 57:306, 1999.
32. Olson RE: Vitamin K. In Shils ME et al, eds: *Modern nutrition in health and disease,* ed 9, Philadelphia, 1999, Lippincott Williams & Wilkins.
33. Olson RE: Osteoporosis and vitamin K intake, *Am J Clin Nutr* 71:1031, 2000.
34. Feskanich D et al: Vitamin K intake and hip fractures in women: a prospective study, *Am J Clin Nutr* 69:74, 1999.
35. Booth SL, Centurelli MA: Vitamin K: a practical guide to the dietary management of patients on warfarin, *Nutr Rev* 57:288, 1999.
36. Harrell CC, Kline SS: Vitamin K-supplemented snacks containing Olestra: implications for patients taking warfarin, *JAMA* 282:1133, 1999.
37. Booth SL, Webb DR, Peters JC: Assessment of phylloquinone and dihydrophylloquinone dietary intakes among a nationally representative sample of US consumers using 14-day food diaries, *J Am Diet Assoc* 99:1072, 1999.
38. Guyton AC, Hall JE: *Textbook of medical physiology,* ed 10, Philadelphia, 2000, WB Saunders.
39. Jacob RA: Vitamin C. In Shils ME et al, eds: *Modern nutrition in health and disease,* ed 9, Philadelphia, 1999, Lippincott Williams & Wilkins.

40. Davidsson L et al: Influence of ascorbic acid on iron absorption from an iron-fortified, chocolate-flavored milk drink in Jamaican children, *Am J Clin Nutr* 67:873, 1998.
41. Houston DK, Johnson MA: Does vitamin C intake protect against lead toxicity? *Nutr Rev* 58:73, 2000.
42. Winkler MA, Manchester S: Medical nutrition therapy for metabolic stress, sepsis, trauma, burns, and surgery. In Mahan KL, Escott-Stump S, eds: *Krause's food, nutrition, & diet therapy*, ed 10, Philadelphia, 2000, WB Saunders.
43. Levine M et al: Criteria and recommendations for vitamin C intake, *JAMA* 281:1415, 1999.
44. Loria CM et al: Vitamin C status and mortality in US adults, *Am J Clin Nutr* 72:139, 2000.
45. Food and Nutrition Board, National Research Council: *Dietary reference intakes for thiamin, riboflavin, niacin, vitamin B_6, folate, vitamin B_{12}, pantothenic acid, biotin, and choline*, Washington, DC, 1998, National Academy Press.
46. Thurnham DI et al: Water-soluble vitamins. In Garrow GS, James WPT, Ralph A, eds: *Human nutrition and dietetics*, ed 10, Edinburgh, 2000, Churchill Livingstone.
47. Suter PM, Vetter W: Diuretics and vitamin B1: are diuretics a risk factor for thiamin malnutrition? *Nutr Rev* 58:319, 2000.
48. McCormick D: Riboflavin. In Shils ME et al, eds: *Modern nutrition in health and disease*, ed 9, Philadelphia, 1999, Lippincott Williams & Wilkins.
49. Manore MM: Effect of physical activity on thiamine, riboflavin, and vitamin B-6 requirements, *Am J Clin Nutr* 72(suppl):598S, 2000.
50. Cervantes-Laurean D, McElvaney NG, Moss J: Niacin. In Shils ME et al, eds: *Modern nutrition in health and disease*, ed 9, Philadelphia, 1999, Lippincott Williams & Wilkins.
51. Ueland PE et al: The controversy over homocysteine and cardiovascular risk, *Am J Clin Nutr* 72:324, 2000.
52. Mock DM: Biotin. In Shils ME et al, eds: *Modern nutrition in health and disease*, ed 9, Philadelphia, 1999, Lippincott Williams & Wilkins.
53. Zempleni J, Mock DM: Bioavailability of biotin given orally to humans in pharmacologic doses, *Am J Clin Nutr* 69:504, 1999.
54. Green TJ et al: Oral contraceptives did not affect biochemical folate indexes and homocysteine concentrations in adolescent females, *J Am Diet Assoc* 98:49, 1998.
55. Gregory JF: Case study: folate bioavailability, *J Nutr* 131:1376S, 2001.
56. Rimm EB et al: Folate and vitamin B6 from diet and supplements in relation to risk of coronary heart disease among women, *JAMA* 279;359, 1998.
57. Jacques PF: Determinants of plasma total homocysteine concentration in the Framingham Offspring cohort, *Am J Clin Nutr* 73:613, 2001.
58. McKay DL et al: Multivitamin/mineral supplementation improves plasma B-vitamin status and homocysteine concentration in healthy older adults consuming a folate-fortified diet, *J Nutr* 130:3090, 2000.
59. Morris MS et al: Serum total homocysteine concentration is related to self-reported heart attack or stroke history among men and women in the NHANES III, *J Nutr* 130:3073, 2000.
60. Moyers S, Bailey LB: Fetal malformations and folate metabolism: review of recent evidence, *Nutr Rev* 59:215, 2001.
61. Suitor CD, Bailey LB: Dietary folate equivalents: interpretation and application, *J Am Diet Assoc* 100(1):81, 2000.
62. Weir DG, Scott JM: Vitamin B_{12} "Cobalamin." In Shils ME et al, eds: *Modern nutrition in health and disease*, ed 9, Philadelphia, 1999, Lippincott Williams & Wilkins.
63. Selhub J et al: B vitamins, homocysteine, and neurocognitive function in the elderly, *Am J Clin Nutr* 71:614S, 2000.
64. Nourhashemi F et al: Alzheimers disease: protective factors, *Am J Clin Nutr* 71(suppl):643S, 2000.

Further Reading

Ho C, Kauwell GPA, Bailey LB: Practitioners' guide to meeting the vitamin B_{12} Recommended Dietary Allowance for people aged 51 years and older, *J Am Diet Assoc* 99:725, 1999.

This article offers suggestions on how we can assist older people with low gastric acid levels in obtaining the recommended levels of vitamin B_{12}.

The following three articles focus on factors that influence fruit and vegetable intakes in various groups and nutrition outcomes.

Hampl JS, Betts NM: Cigarette use during adolescence: effects on nutritional status, *Nutr Rev* 57:215, 1999.

This article tells us about the effects of smoking on the health of adolescents, especially as related to their dietary intake and risk of future chronic disease based on their level of oxidative stress.

Quan T et al: Behaviors of low-income mothers related to fruit and vegetable consumption, *J Am Diet Assoc* 100:567, 2000.

This article provides us with suggestions on how to help mothers learn behaviors that will increase their intakes of fruits and vegetables.

Cullen et al: The effect of a la carte/snack bar foods at school on children's lunchtime intake of fruits and vegetables, *J Am Diet Assoc* 100:1482, 2000.

Children who have access to a snack bar in their school may not consume as many fruits and vegetables at lunchtime. This article helps us think about school food service issues and their influence on nutrient intake.

Issues & ANSWERS

Phytochemicals and Functional Foods: What's the Connection?

The term *phytochemical* comes from the Greek word *phyton* meaning "plant" and refers to the chemicals found in plants. Phytochemicals include hundreds of naturally occurring substances in plants that are incurring increasing attention based on their potential effects on human health. Phytochemicals participate in the normal biochemical and physiologic functions of plants, and plants produce these substances to protect themselves against bacteria and viruses. When eaten, these substances in plants are absorbed and can act as protective factors in humans. Growing numbers of research studies tell us that phytochemicals play an important role in preventing chronic disease.

Widespread interest in the idea that particular foods might promote health led to the new term "functional food." A functional food is a food that carries a health benefit beyond that provided by the traditional nutrients it contains. Functional foods and the naturally occurring substances found in them are being studied in relation to the prevention of cardiovascular disease, cancer, cataracts, and osteoporosis.

Fruits, vegetables, and whole grains are receiving new attention as functional foods. Several categories of phytochemicals found in these foods have important roles in human health; many of these substances act as antioxidants.

Carotenoids

The term *carotenoids* describes a group of pigments that contribute to the rich yellow, orange, green, and red pigments in fruits and vegetables. We learned earlier that beta-carotene can be split in the human intestine to form a molecule of vitamin A. It is important to understand that the physiologic actions of the carotenoids are completely separate from the actions of vitamin A. Individuals who eat five or more fruits and vegetables a day are less likely to develop cancer or experience a myocardial infarction than those who eat fewer servings. Vitamin A supplements or supplements of the antioxidant vitamins C and E cannot take the place of plant foods in providing this protection. Although vitamins can be lost from food by inappropriate cooking practices, it is interesting to note that carotenoids are better absorbed from cooked vegetables than fresh vegetables. Lycopene, a carotenoid found in tomatoes that may help to prevent both cancer and cardiovascular disease, is absorbed best from cooked tomato products such as catsup and pizza sauce.

Some major carotenoids in the U.S. diet and their food sources include the following examples.

- *Alpha-carotene:* carrots
- *Beta-carotene:* broccoli, cantaloupe, carrots, spinach
- *Beta-cryptoxanthin:* oranges and orange juice, peaches, tangerines
- *Lutein:* broccoli, corn, green beans, green peas, spinach, and other greens
- *Lycopene:* tomatoes and tomato products

Phytoestrogens

Phytoestrogens (a type of polyphenol) have estrogen-like effects in the human body. They support bone health in postmenopausal women by exercising the protective effect of the hormone estrogen on bone. Phytoestrogens appear to lower plasma levels of total cholesterol, LDL cholesterol, and triglycerides in both men and women. The major phytoestrogens are genistein, daidzein, and other isoflavones found in soybeans and soy foods.

Other polyphenols

More than 4000 polyphenols have been identified in plants, and many appear to have biologic action in humans. They are widely distributed in plant foods, including cereals, vegetables, fruits, nuts, tea, and wine. The formation of polyphenols is light dependent; therefore the highest concentration of these compounds is usually found in the leaves and outer parts of the plant. Polyphenols have many actions in the body such as preventing the oxidation of LDL cholesterol. They attack potential carcinogens and interfere with the steps that lead to development of tumors. Some polyphenols are not absorbed and exert their effects in the gastrointestinal tract, protecting proteins, lipids, and carbohydrates from oxidative damage during digestion. Several important polyphenols are listed here.

- *Phenolic acid and flavonoids:* wine, apples, citrus fruit
- *Anthocyanins:* cocoa beans, berries, red wine
- *Tannins:* nuts, cocoa beans
- *Catechins:* grapes, green tea
- *Sulforaphane and other isothiocyanates:* cruciferous vegetables such as broccoli, cabbage, and cauliflower
- *Diallyl disulfide and allicin:* garlic, onions

Some of these substances have been extracted from their plant sources and are now being sold as supplements. It is important to help people understand that these health-promoting substances as well as others we may not know about are best supplied in the foods we eat. Choosing a variety of fruits, vegetables, and grains will provide us with an ample supply of important phytochemicals.

REFERENCES

Arab L, Steck S: Lycopene and cardiovascular disease, *Am J Clin Nutr* 71(suppl):1691S, 2000.

Bagchi D: Bioflavonoids and polyphenols in human health and disease prevention, *Nutr MD* 25:1, 1999.

Bidlack WR, Wang W: Designing functional foods. In Shils ME et al, eds: *Modern nutrition in health and disease,* ed 9, Philadelphia, 1999, Lippincott Williams & Wilkins.

Milner JA: Functional foods: the US perspective, *Am J Clin Nutr* 71(suppl):1654S, 2000.

Chapter

8

Minerals

Eleanor D. Schlenker

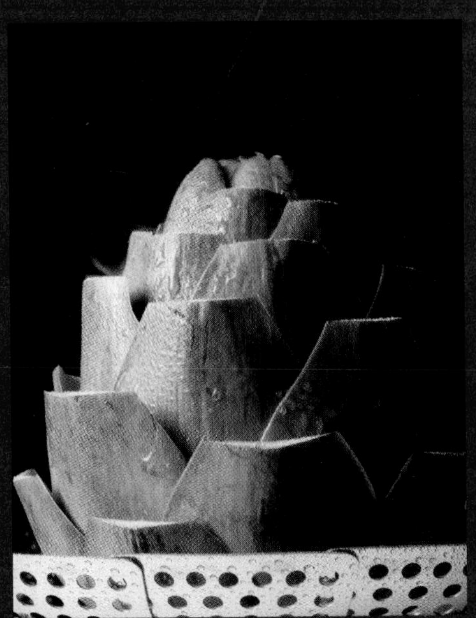

Chapter Outline

In this chapter we look at the remaining micronutrients, the minerals. They may seem simple in comparison to the complex organic vitamin compounds, but they fulfill a variety of structural and metabolic functions.

Elements for which the requirement is greater than 100 mg/day are called major minerals, *not because they are more important but because there are more of them in the body. Those needed in much smaller amounts are called* trace elements, *and a few that are needed in only minute amounts are sometimes called* ultratrace elements. *For some of the trace elements we are still unsure of the amount that is needed.*

Here we will review each of these groups of minerals. As with the vitamins, we will focus on why we need them and how we may obtain them.

MINERALS IN HUMAN NUTRITION

OUR CYCLE OF MINERALS

On Earth, we live within a vast slow-motion cycle of minerals essential to our existence as humans. Elements initially present in the water have found their way into rocks and soils, and through plants, to animals and humans.[1] Until recent times our access to some of these elements in sufficient measure for health depended on luck—where we happened to live. But over time, with more knowledge of how they can be processed, transported, and used in agriculture, persons living in all parts of the country or the world can be supplied with adequate mineral nutrition.

METABOLIC ROLES

Variety in Function

Minerals are inorganic elements widely distributed in nature. They have vital roles in human metabolism that are as varied as the minerals themselves. These substances, which appear so inert in comparison to the complex organic vitamin compounds, fulfill an impressive variety of metabolic functions: building, activating, regulating, transmitting, and controlling. For example, ionized sodium and potassium exercise all-important control over shifts in body water. Calcium and phosphorus provide structure for the body's framework. Oxygen-hungry iron gives a core to *heme* in hemoglobin. Brilliant red cobalt is the atom at the center of the cobalamin (vitamin B_{12}) molecule. Iodine is a necessary constituent of the thyroid hormones, which in turn control the rate of body metabolism. Far from being static and inert, minerals are active participants, helping to control many of the metabolic processes in the body.

Variety in Amount Needed

Minerals also differ from vitamins in another way. As we learned in the previous chapter, vitamins are all required in very small amounts to do their metabolic jobs. Minerals, however, are required in varying amounts, from the relatively large amounts of the major minerals to the exceedingly small amounts of the trace elements. For example, the major mineral calcium makes up a relatively large amount of body weight—about 2%. Most of this calcium is in skeletal tissue. Thus a man weighing 150 lb has about 3 lb of calcium in his body. On the other hand, the trace element iron is present in small amounts. This same adult has only about 3 g (about 1/10 oz) of iron in his body, mostly in the hemoglobin of red blood cells.

Concept of Bioavailability

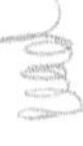

In general, absorption of minerals is less efficient than absorption of vitamins and macronutrients. Unfortunately, the amount of a mineral found in a food as determined by analysis in a laboratory may not be the amount that is actually available and absorbed by an individual. The term bioavailability refers to the degree to which the body can absorb and use a particular nutrient to carry out normal functions.[2] Bioavailability depends on many factors that influence the absorption-excretion balance of a mineral or its balance in body tissues. For example, the minerals in some plant foods are less available for absorption because they are bound to other substances in the plant and are not easily released. Oxalates found in some green leafy vegetables and phytates in grains can bind minerals and prevent their absorption. The amount of hydrochloric acid produced in the stomach affects bioavailability, as many minerals are better absorbed in an acid medium. Bioavailability is also influenced by body need; the absorption rate of various minerals increases during periods of growth, pregnancy, and lactation. Issues of bioavailability make it difficult to set precise dietary recommendations for these nutrients.

CLASSIFICATION

For our study we will group these important mineral elements into three main sections: major minerals, trace elements that are known to be essential, and trace elements that are probably essential. These commonly used divisions are based on (1) how much of the mineral is required by the body and (2) how much we know at this point about its essentiality (as for some of the trace elements).

Major Minerals

Seven minerals present in the body in large amounts are called the major minerals; these include calcium, phosphorus, magnesium, sodium, potassium, sulfur, and chloride.

Trace Elements

The remaining minerals are present in smaller amounts and are called trace elements. The essential nature of 10 of these has been determined. For the remaining 8, their precise function in the body is not yet clear.

In Table 8-1, you will find a listing of the minerals in each group. We will review each, looking at (1) balance controls that maintain the body's needed amount, (2) physiologic function, (3) associated clinical problems, (4) daily requirement, and (5) food sources.

MAJOR MINERALS

Calcium

Of all the minerals in the body, calcium by far occurs in the largest amount. The total amount of body calcium is in constant balance with food sources from the outside as well as with tissue calcium within the body and its various

TABLE 8-1 Major Minerals and Trace Elements in Human Nutrition

Major Minerals (Required Intake >100 mg/day)	Trace Elements: Essential (Required Intake <100 mg/day)	Trace Elements: Essentiality Unclear
Calcium (Ca)	Iron (Fe)	Silicon (Si)
Phosphorus (P)	Iodine (I)	Vanadium (V)
Magnesium (Mg)	Zinc (Zn)	Nickel (Ni)
Sodium (Na)	Copper (Cu)	Tin (Sn)
Potassium (K)	Manganese (Mn)	Cadmium (Cd)
Chloride (Cl)	Chromium (Cr)	Arsenic (As)
Sulfur (S)	Cobalt (Co)	Aluminum (Al)
	Selenium (Se)	Boron (B)
	Molybdenum (Mo)	
	Fluoride (F)	

parts. A number of dynamic mechanisms are constantly at work to maintain these levels within normal ranges. The balance concept, therefore, can be applied at three levels: (1) the intake-absorption-excretion balance, (2) the bone-blood balance, and (3) the calcium-phosphorus blood serum balance.

INTAKE-ABSORPTION-EXCRETION BALANCE

Calcium Intake

The average adult woman in the United States consumes about 650 mg of calcium/day, whereas the average adult man consumes about 900 mg.[3] Most of this is derived from dairy products, and some is derived from green leafy vegetables and grains. Unfortunately, the calcium found in dark green leafy vegetables is often bound to substances called *oxalates* and not well absorbed compared with the more bioavailable calcium in dairy foods.

Skeletal growth during childhood and adolescence makes tremendous calcium demands.[4-6] This skeletal bone growth demand for calcium is especially evident during the adolescent growth spurt, particularly in boys.[7] If intake of calcium is low or if the primary sources of calcium in the diet have low bioavailability, skeletal demands may not be met and bone growth will be compromised.

Absorption of Calcium

Calcium absorption can range from 10% to 60% but decreases with age.[1,8] Most food calcium occurs in complexes with other dietary components. These complexes must be broken down and the calcium released in a soluble form before it can be absorbed. Absorption takes place in the small intestine, chiefly in the first section, the duodenum. Here the gastric acidity is still effective, rather than farther along in the intestine, as the acid food mass is buffered by pancreatic juices and becomes more alkaline.

Factors Increasing Calcium Absorption

The following factors increase calcium absorption.

1. *Vitamin D hormone.* An optimal amount of this control agent is necessary for calcium absorption. The active form of vitamin D, *calcitriol,* controls the synthesis of a calcium-binding protein carrier in the duodenum that transports the mineral across the mucosal cells and into the blood circulation.[1]
2. *Body need.* During periods of greater body demand, such as growth or depletion states, more calcium is absorbed. Physiologic states in the life cycle—growth, pregnancy, lactation, and older age—have a strong influence on the rate of absorption. Absorption is highest in times of most need, such as the adolescent growth spurt or lactation period. In elderly persons in general and in postmenopausal women in particular, the ability to absorb calcium is reduced.[1,8]
3. *Dietary protein and carbohydrate.* A greater percentage of calcium appears to be absorbed when the diet is high in protein, although this effect is not consistent among all persons. Regardless of the effect on absorption, larger amounts of dietary protein result in increased calcium excretion in the urine.[9] Thus, in essence, high-protein diets induce increased calcium requirements to maintain calcium balance. Soy protein, however, may have a favorable effect on calcium balance because of its isoflavones, which have estrogen-like activity.[10] Lactose (the major carbohydrate found in milk) may enhance calcium absorption through the action of the lactobacilli, which produce lactic acid and lower intestinal pH.
4. *Acidity.* Lower pH (increased acidity) favors solubility of calcium and thereby enhances its absorption.

Factors Decreasing Calcium Absorption

The following factors decrease calcium absorption.

1. *Vitamin D deficiency.* Vitamin D hormone, along with parathyroid hormone, is essential for calcium absorption.
2. *Dietary fat.* Poor absorption of fats or a high fat intake results in an excess of fat in the intestine. This fat can combine with calcium to form insoluble soaps that cannot be absorbed. These insoluble soaps are excreted, with consequent loss of the incorporated calcium.

bioavailability Amount of a nutrient ingested in food that is absorbed and thus available to the body for metabolic use.

hemoglobin Oxygen-carrying pigment in red blood cells; a conjugated protein containing four heme groups combined with iron and four long polypeptide chains forming the protein globin, named for its ball-like form; made by the developing red blood cells in bone marrow, hemoglobin carries oxygen in the blood to body cells.

3. *Fiber and other binding agents.* An excess of dietary fiber binds calcium and hinders its absorption. Other binding agents include *oxalic acid,* which combines with calcium to produce calcium oxalate, and *phytic acid,* which forms calcium phytate. Oxalic acid is a constituent of green leafy vegetables, but the amount of oxalates in them varies, making some better sources of calcium than others. Phytic acid is found in the outer hull of many cereal grains, especially wheat.
4. *Alkalinity.* Calcium is insoluble at a higher pH or alkaline medium and is poorly absorbed.

Calcium Output

The overall body calcium balance is controlled first at the point of absorption. A large unabsorbed amount—up to 90% of total intake depending on body need—remains to be eliminated in the feces. A small amount of calcium is also excreted in the urine, about 200 mg/day, to maintain normal levels in the body fluids.

BONE-BLOOD BALANCE

Calcium in the Bones

In a healthy person the body maintains a constant turnover of the calcium in bone, which is the major site of calcium storage. Calcium in the bones and teeth is about 99% of that in the entire body. However, this is not a static storage. Bone tissue is constantly being built and reshaped according to various body needs and stresses (Figure 8-1). As much as 700 mg of calcium enters and leaves the bones each day, maintaining a dynamic equilibrium. In certain conditions or disease, however, withdrawals may exceed deposits and a state of calcium imbalance occurs. For example, conditions such as immobility from a body cast or diseases such as osteoporosis cause excess bone calcium withdrawals.

Calcium in the Blood

The remaining small amount of body calcium that is not in bone tissue—about 1%—circulates in the blood and other body fluids. Despite its small amount, however, this serum calcium plays a vital role in controlling body functions. Calcium in the blood occurs in two main forms.

1. *Bound calcium.* About half the calcium in the blood is bound to plasma proteins; hence it is not free or *diffusible,* that is, able to move into cells or enter into other activities.
2. *Free ionized calcium.* Free particles of calcium, carrying electrical charges and hence in an active ionized form, move about freely and diffuse through membranes to control a number of body functions. These functions include blood clotting, transmission of nerve impulses,

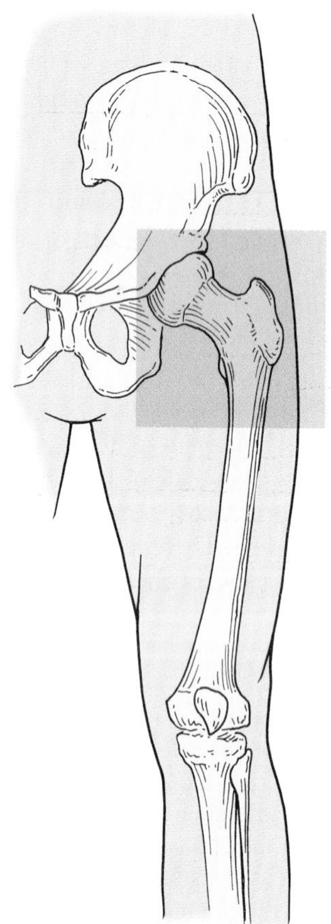

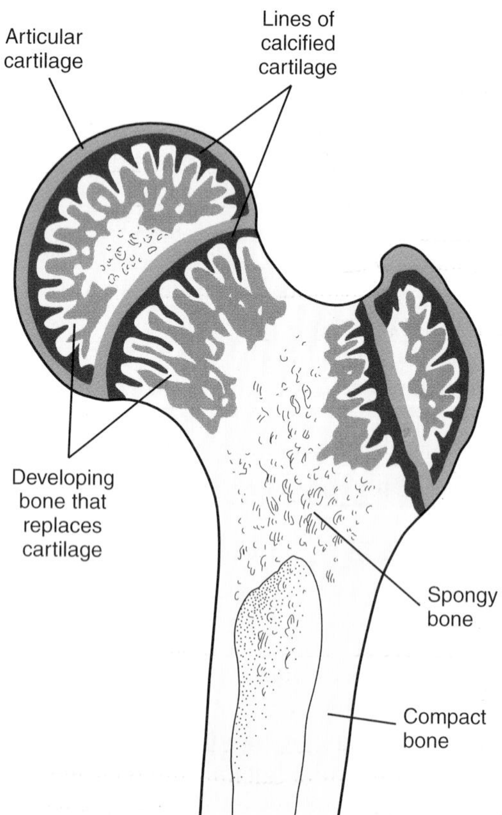

FIGURE 8-1 Bone and cartilage development.

muscle contraction and relaxation, membrane permeability, and enzyme activation. This is a good illustration of a small amount of a nutrient doing a great deal of metabolic work because it is in an activated form.

CALCIUM-PHOSPHORUS SERUM BALANCE

A final level of calcium balance is the balance that calcium maintains with phosphorus in the blood serum. The amounts of these two minerals in the blood are normally maintained in a definite relationship because of their relative solubility. This relationship is called the calcium-phosphorus serum balance. The serum balance is the solubility product of calcium and phosphorus, expressed in milligrams per deciliter (mg/dl) of each mineral. Normal serum levels are 10 mg/dl of calcium in children and adults, and 4 mg/dl of phosphorus in adults and 5 mg/dl in children. Thus the normal serum calcium-phosphorus solubility products are $10 \times 4 = 40$ for adults and $10 \times 5 = 50$ for children. Any situation that causes an increase in the serum phosphorus level would cause a decrease in the serum calcium level to hold the calcium-phosphorus solubility product constant. A decrease in serum calcium can lead to signs of tetany from lack of neuromuscular control. At one time it was believed that calcium and phosphorus should be consumed in a specific ratio to promote calcium balance; however, it appears that the calcium/phosphorus ratio is not an important issue across the general range of intakes.[11]

Control Agents for Calcium Balance

Three main control agents work together to maintain these vital levels of calcium balance in the body: parathyroid hormone, vitamin D hormone (calcitriol), and the hormone calcitonin. The cooperative action of these three control agents is a good example of the synergistic behavior of metabolic controls. Consider the interdependent relationship of the following agents.

1. *Parathyroid hormone.* The parathyroid glands, lying adjacent to the thyroid glands, are particularly sensitive to changes in the circulating blood level of free ionized calcium. When this level drops, the parathyroid gland releases its hormone, which then acts in three ways to restore the normal blood calcium level: (1) it stimulates the intestinal mucosa to absorb more calcium, (2) it rapidly withdraws more calcium from the bone compartment, and (3) it causes the kidneys to reabsorb more calcium and to excrete more phosphate. These combined activities restore calcium and phosphorus to their correct balance in the blood.
2. *Vitamin D hormone (calcitriol).* Along with parathyroid hormone, vitamin D hormone controls absorption of calcium. It also, with the help of parathyroid hormone, regulates the deposit of calcium and phosphorus in bone tissue. Thus these two agents balance each other, with vitamin D hormone acting more to control calcium absorption and bone deposit and parathyroid hormone acting more to control calcium withdrawal from bone and kidney excretion of its partner phosphorus.
3. *Calcitonin.* A third hormonal agent, calcitonin, is also involved in calcium balance. Produced by special C cells in the thyroid gland, it prevents abnormal rises in serum calcium by modulating the release of bone calcium. Thus its action counterbalances that of parathyroid hormone to help keep serum calcium at normal levels in balance with bone calcium.

The overall relationship of the various factors involved in calcium balance and metabolism is illustrated in Figure 8-2.

PHYSIOLOGIC FUNCTIONS OF CALCIUM

Bone Formation

The physiologic function of 99% of the body calcium is to build and maintain skeletal tissue. This is done by special types of cells that maintain a balance between deposits and withdrawals of bone calcium.

Tooth Formation

Special tooth-forming organs in the gums deposit calcium to form teeth, and the mineral exchange continues as in bone. This calcium exchange in dental tissue occurs mainly in the dentin and cementum. Very little deposit occurs in the enamel once the tooth is formed.

General Metabolic Functions

The remaining 1% of the body's calcium performs a number of vital physiologic functions.

1. *Blood clotting.* In the blood clotting process, serum calcium ions are required for cross-linking of fibrin, giving stability to the fibrin threads.
2. *Nerve transmission.* Normal transmission of nerve impulses along axons requires calcium. A current of calcium ions triggers the flow of signals from one nerve cell to another and on to the waiting target muscles.
3. *Muscle contraction and relaxation.* Ionized serum calcium helps initiate the contraction of muscle fibers and controls the return to steady state after the contraction. This catalyzing action of calcium ions on the muscle protein filaments allows the sliding contraction between them to occur (see Chapter 14). This action of

---

calcitonin A polypeptide hormone secreted by the thyroid gland in response to hypercalcemia, which acts to lower both calcium and phosphate in the blood.

compartment The collective quantity of material of a given type in the body. The four body compartments are *lean body mass* (muscle and vital organs), *bone, fat,* and *water.*

osteoporosis Abnormal thinning of bone, producing a porous, fragile bone tissue of enlarged spaces prone to fracture or deformity, associated with the aging process in older men and women.

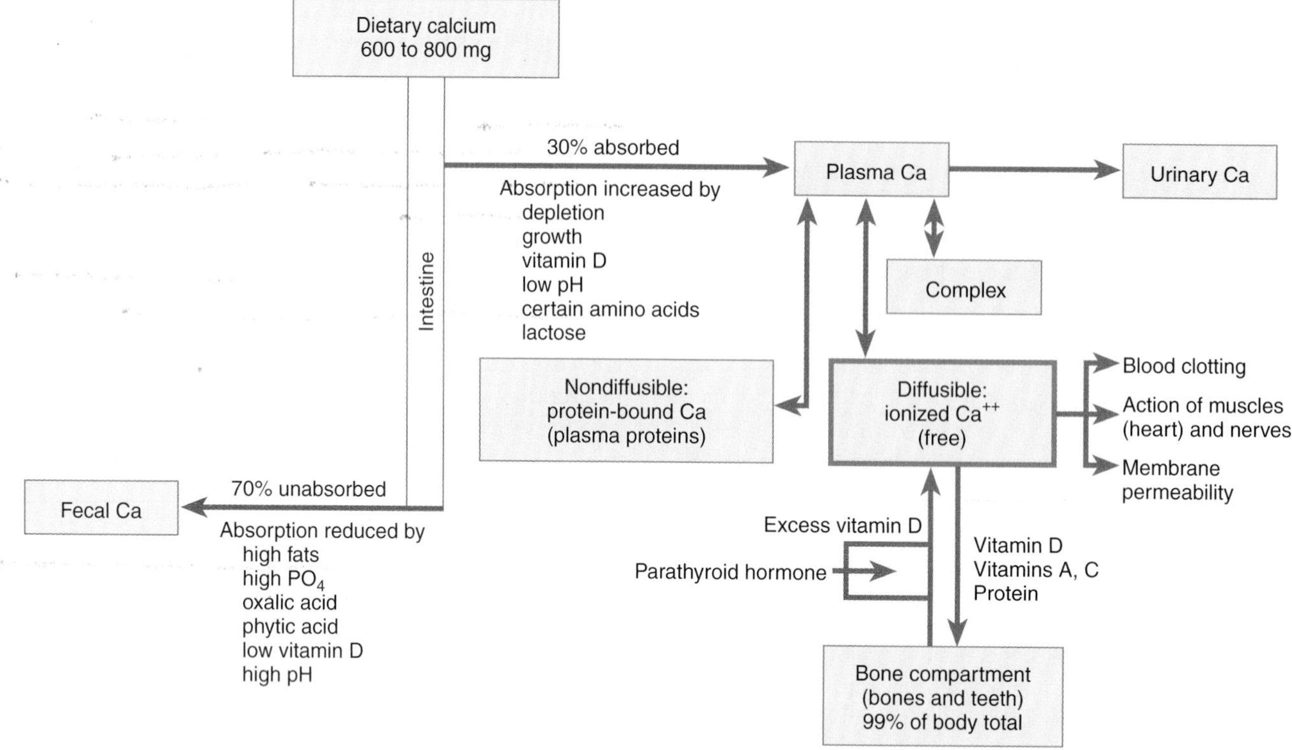

FIGURE 8-2 Calcium metabolism. Note the relative distribution of calcium in the body.

calcium is particularly vital in the constant contraction-relaxation cycle of the heart muscle.

4. *Cell membrane permeability.* Ionized calcium controls the passage of fluids and solutes through cell membranes by affecting membrane permeability. It influences the integrity of the intercellular cement substance.
5. *Enzyme activation.* Calcium ions are important activators of specific cell enzymes, especially ones that release energy for muscle contraction. They play a similar role with other enzymes, including lipase, which digests fat, and with some members of the protein-splitting enzyme system.
6. *Control of blood pressure.* Several researchers have reported that individuals with higher levels of dietary calcium have lower blood pressure than do people similar in age, sex, and state of health who do not take in as much calcium.[12-14] In both African American adolescents[12] and African American and Caucasian middle-age and older adults,[13,14] those who had more calcium-rich foods in their diet had lower blood pressure. The greater intake of calcium may have caused more sodium to be excreted and thus lowered blood pressure levels. Another explanation for the observed benefit of dairy foods in controlling blood pressure could be the combination of minerals found in these foods.[15] Calcium, magnesium, and potassium are all present in dairy foods in substantial amounts, and both potassium and magnesium also appear to influence blood pressure. This is another example of the synergism among nutrients that we discussed in Chapter 1.

CALCIUM AND CLINICAL PROBLEMS

A number of clinical problems can develop from imbalances that interfere with the various physiologic and metabolic functions of calcium.

Tetany

A decrease in ionized serum calcium causes *tetany,* a state marked by severe, intermittent spastic contractions of the muscles and by muscular pain.

Rickets and Osteomalacia

A deficiency of vitamin D hormone results in a bone disorder called *rickets* in growing children and *osteomalacia* in adults. When there is inadequate exposure to sunlight or deficient dietary intake of vitamin D, proper bone formation cannot take place.

Osteoporosis

The usual form of *osteoporosis,* characterized by bone mineral loss, occurs mainly in older persons, especially postmenopausal women. Osteoporosis carries with it the increased risk of bone fracture and physical disability. In the women affected, the most rapid rate of bone loss occurs in the first few years immediately after menopause.

This on-going negative calcium balance leads to loss of the outer bone layer—the cortex—of the long bones such as the femur, and the delicate needlelike projections of bone—the trabecula—in the spine. About 5 years after menopause the rate of bone loss falls to about 1% a year and stays at that level for the remainder of the life span. Once a large amount of bone has been lost, increased dietary calcium, even if accompanied by exercise and optimum vitamin D, may not be sufficient to reduce the risk of bone fracture.[16] Hormone replacement therapy that can inhibit further bone loss, or several newly discovered drugs that can help to replace lost bone are being used to treat osteoporotic patients. Nutrition education for young and middle-age women should focus on the need for an adequate calcium intake and lifestyle practices that support bone health and help prevent bone loss.[17]

Resorptive Hypercalciuria and Renal Calculi

These two conditions can tilt the usually fine-tuned calcium deposition-mobilization balance maintained by the controlling hormones. When this normal balance is disturbed, resorption of calcium from bone and its excretion in the urine are accelerated. A main factor leading to such a condition is prolonged immobilization. This can occur from a full body cast made necessary by orthopedic surgery or a spinal cord injury, or with a body brace after a back injury. In such cases, the normal muscle tension on bones that is necessary to maintain calcium bone mass is lessened, and the risk of renal stones from increased urinary calcium is increased.

CALCIUM REQUIREMENT

Dietary Reference Intake

Increased concern about the amount of dietary calcium required for optimum development and lifetime maintenance of healthy bones has led to new Dietary Reference Intakes for nutrients that play important roles in bone. In Chapter 7 we learned about the Adequate Intake (AI) established for vitamin D. The expert panel evaluating current dietary intake standards also established an AI for calcium.[11] (To review the differences between a Recommended Dietary Allowance [RDA] and an AI, see Chapter 1.) Youth aged 9 through 18 years should have intakes of 1300 mg of calcium/day to support maximum deposit of bone calcium, important in this stage of growth. Men and women aged 19 to 50 are urged to take in 1000 mg of calcium/day to maintain positive calcium balance. For persons above age 50, 1200 mg of calcium/day is needed to support bone health and prevent bone loss. Women aged 19 and over who are pregnant or lactating should obtain at least 1000 mg of calcium each day. At the same time, it is important that persons not exceed the Tolerable Upper Intake Level (UL) of 2500 mg/day.

FOOD SOURCES OF CALCIUM

Dairy products are the best sources of calcium in the American diet, making up 73% of the calcium intake.[18] One quart of milk contains about 1.2 g (1200 mg) of calcium. Cheese is also a major source. Other sources, including eggs, green leafy vegetables, broccoli, legumes, nuts, and whole grains, contribute smaller amounts. For individuals who are lactose intolerant, calcium-fortified soy milk or calcium-fortified juices will supply calcium. Hard cheeses or yogurt may be possible sources for those who are lactase deficient. Individuals should be encouraged to obtain at least half of their calcium from food sources that will provide other important nutrients as well and to not rely on supplements alone to supply this nutrient. It is especially important that we emphasize dairy foods that are low in fat and kilocalories (kcalories) because fear of gaining weight and increasing their cholesterol intake were mentioned by younger women as reasons why they do not eat dairy foods.[18] Table 8-2 provides some comparative food sources of calcium.

Phosphorus

Phosphorus makes up about 1% of total body weight. It is closely associated with calcium in human nutrition and has been called its metabolic twin. However, it has some unique characteristics and functions of its own.

ABSORPTION-EXCRETION BALANCE

Absorption

Free phosphate is absorbed throughout the length of the small intestine and is regulated by the vitamin D hormone and some phosphate carrier proteins.[19] Because phosphorus occurs in food as a phosphate compound, mainly with calcium, the first step for its absorption is its splitting off as the free mineral. Factors similar to those that influence calcium absorption also affect phosphorus absorption. For example, an excess of calcium or other binding material, such as aluminum or iron, and the phytic acid found in whole grains inhibit phosphorus absorption.

Excretion

The kidneys provide the main excretion route for regulation of the serum phosphorus level. Usually, 85% to 95% of plasma phosphate is filtered by the renal glomeruli and reabsorbed in the renal tubules

solutes Particles of a substance in solution; a solution consists of a substance and a dissolving medium (solvent), usually a liquid.

synergism The joint action of separate agents in which the total effect of their combined action is greater than the sum of their separate actions (adjective: synergistic).

TABLE 8-2 Food Sources of Calcium

Food Source	Quantity	Calcium (mg)
Bread, Cereal, Rice, Pasta		
Bran muffin, homemade	1 muffin	54
Bread, whole wheat	1 slice	18
Corn muffin, from mix	1 muffin	96
Cream of wheat (cooked)	¾ cup	38
Pasta, enriched (cooked)	1 cup	16
Rice, enriched	1 cup	21
Wheat flakes	1 cup	43
Vegetables		
Artichoke (boiled)	1 med	47
Asparagus (boiled)	½ cup (6 spears)	22
Avocado (raw)	1 med	19
Broccoli (raw)	½ cup	21
Brussels sprouts (boiled)	½ cup (4 sprouts)	28
Carrots (raw)	1 med	19
Collards (boiled)	1 cup	148
Corn, yellow (boiled)	½ cup	2
Kale (chopped)	½ cup	47
Peas, green (boiled)	½ cup	19
Potato (baked, with skin)	1 med	115
Tomato (raw)	1 med	8
Vegetable juice (fortified)	8 fl oz	300
Fruits		
Apricots (raw)	3 med	15
Banana (raw)	1 med	7
Cantaloupe (raw)	½ cup	8
Figs (dried)	10 figs	269
Orange juice (fresh)	8 fl oz	27
Orange juice (fortified)	8 fl oz	300
Fruits—cont'd		
Orange, navel (raw)	1 med	56
Papaya (raw)	1 med	72
Raspberries (raw)	½ cup	14
Strawberries (raw)	½ cup	11
Tangerine (raw)	1 med	12
Meat, Poultry, Fish, Dried Beans, Eggs, Nuts		
Almonds (roasted)	1 oz	148
Beef liver (fried)	3.5 oz	11
Cashews (roasted)	1 oz	13
Chicken, dark (roasted, without skin)	3.5 oz	179
Chicken, light (roasted, without skin)	3.5 oz	216
Egg, whole	1 large	90
Ham (canned)	3.5 oz	6
Kidney beans (boiled)	1 cup	50
Lentils (boiled)	1 cup	37
Lima beans (boiled)	1 cup	32
Peanuts (roasted)	1 oz	15
Soybeans (boiled)	1 cup	175
Milk, Dairy Products		
Milk, skim	8 fl oz	302
Milk, whole	8 fl oz	290
Yogurt, whole milk	8 fl oz	355
Soy milk fortified with calcium	8 fl oz	300
Fats, Oils		
This food group is not an important source of calcium		
Sugar		
Brown sugar	1 cup	123
Molasses, barbados	1 tbsp	49

Adequate Intakes for adults: aged 19-50, 1000 mg; aged ≥ 51, 1200 mg.

along with calcium, under the influence of vitamin D hormone. But when increased phosphate excretion is needed to maintain the normal serum calcium-phosphorus balance, parathyroid hormone acts to override the effect of vitamin D hormone and to raise excretion levels. The amount of phosphorus excreted in the urine of a person ingesting an average diet is 600 to 1800 mg/day.

BONE-BLOOD-CELL BALANCE

Bone

From 80% to 90% of the body's phosphorus is in the skeleton, including the teeth, compounded with calcium. This bone compartment of phosphorus is in constant interchange with the rest of the body's phosphorus, which is circulating in the blood and other body fluids.

Blood

The serum phosphorus level normally ranges from 3.0 to 4.5 mg/dl in adults, and is somewhat higher, 4 to 7 mg/dl, in children. The higher range during the growth years is a significant clue to its role in cell metabolism.

Cells

In its active phosphate form, phosphorus plays a major role in the structure and function of all living cells. Here it works with proteins, lipids, and carbohydrates to produce energy, build and repair tissues, and act as a buffer.

Hormonal Controls

Because calcium and phosphorus work closely together, phosphorus balance is under the direct control of the same two hormones controlling calcium—vitamin D hormone and parathyroid hormone. A deficiency or depletion of phosphate occurs from (1) low intake, (2) diminished absorption from the intestine usually as a result of an interfering substance such as phytic acid or aluminum, or (3) excessive wasting through the kidney. (Aluminum is found in several over-the-counter antacids.)

PHYSIOLOGIC FUNCTIONS OF PHOSPHORUS

The normal adult plasma concentration of phosphorus ranges from 3.0 to 4.5 mg/dl; levels below 2.5 or above 5.0 mg/dl require immediate medical attention.[19] High phosphorus intakes leading to high serum levels can stimulate parathyroid hormone release and mobilization of bone calcium. On the opposite side, continued use of phosphorus-binding antacids can lower serum phosphorus.[16] Body phosphorus serves many diverse roles, both inside and outside of cells, and enters practically every cell metabolic pathway.

Bone and Tooth Formation

About 80% to 90% of the body phosphorus helps make bones and teeth. As a component of calcium phosphate, it is constantly being deposited and resorbed in the process of bone formation.

General Metabolic Activities

Far out of proportion to its relatively small amount, the phosphorus outside the bone is intimately involved in overall human metabolism in every living cell. It has several vital roles.

1. *Absorption of glucose and glycerol.* Phosphorus combines with glucose and glycerol to assist in their intestinal absorption. It also promotes renal tubular reabsorption of glucose to return this sugar to the blood.
2. *Transport of fatty acids.* Phospholipids provide a form of fat transport.
3. *Energy metabolism.* Phosphorus-containing compounds, for example, adenosine triphosphate (ATP), are key cell substances in energy metabolism.
4. *Buffer system.* The phosphate buffer system of phosphoric acid and phosphate helps control acid-base balance in the blood.

Physiologic Changes

Situations involving physiologic and clinical changes in serum phosphorus level include the following.

1. *Recovery from diabetic acidosis.* Active carbohydrate absorption and metabolism use much phosphorus, depositing it with glycogen and causing temporary hypophosphatemia.
2. *Growth.* Growing children usually have higher serum phosphate levels, resulting from high levels of growth hormone.
3. *Hypophosphatemia.* Low serum phosphorus occurs in intestinal diseases such as sprue and celiac disease, which hinder phosphorus absorption; in bone disease such as rickets or osteomalacia, which upset the calcium-phosphorus serum balance; and in primary hyperparathyroidism, in which the excess secretion of parathyroid hormone causes excess renal tubular excretion of phosphorus. Hypophosphatemia can also occur as part of the refeeding syndrome, sometimes seen during the first days of nutritional repletion of a severely wasted patient. Phosphorus is required for the storage of glycogen that follows refeeding with high levels of carbohydrate, resulting in lowered blood levels. Symptoms of hypophosphatemia include muscle weakness because the cells are deprived of phosphorus, which is essential for energy metabolism.
4. *Hyperphosphatemia.* Both renal insufficiency and hypoparathyroidism cause excess accumulation of serum phosphate. As a result, the calcium side of the serum calcium-phosphorus balance becomes low, causing tetany.

PHOSPHORUS REQUIREMENT

Dietary Ratio

In past years much attention was given to the ratio between calcium and phosphorus intakes. It was believed that an ideal ratio, often reported to be in the range of 1:1, was an important factor in formation and maintenance of bone. Intakes higher in phosphorus than calcium were thought to be detrimental to bone mineral deposition. Our current thinking is that having available the needed amounts of each nutrient is more important than their ratio to each other.[11] Because these two minerals are found in many of the same food sources, if calcium needs are met, adequate phosphorus is also likely.

Dietary Reference Intake

The current RDA standard for phosphorus is 500 mg/day for children 4 to 8 years of age, 1250 mg/day for those aged 9 to 18 years, and 700 mg/day for all adults beyond the age of 18.[11] For formula-fed infants the Food and Nutrition Board has set AIs of 100 mg/day from birth to 6 months of age and 275 mg/day from 6 to 12 months.

FOOD SOURCES OF PHOSPHORUS

Milk and milk products are significant sources of phosphorus, as they are for calcium. However, because phosphorus plays such a large role in cell metabolism, it is also found in lean meats. The use of phosphorus-containing additives in food processing and the high phosphorus content of soft drinks are also adding phosphorus to the American diet. Table 8-3 provides a list of food sources of phosphorus.

TABLE 8-3 Food Sources of Phosphorus

Food Source	Quantity	Phosphorus (mg)
Bread, Cereal, Rice, Pasta		
Bran flakes	¾ cup	158
Bran muffin, homemade	1 muffin	111
Bread, whole wheat	1 slice	65
Cream of wheat (cooked)	¾ cup	31
English muffin, plain	1 muffin	64
Oatmeal (cooked)	¾ cup	133
Pasta, enriched (cooked)	1 cup	70
Rice, enriched (cooked)	1 cup	57
Wheat flakes	1 cup	98
Vegetables		
Artichoke (boiled)	1 med	72
Avocado (raw)	1 med	73
Brussels sprouts (boiled)	½ cup (4 sprouts)	44
Carrots (raw)	1 med	32
Corn, yellow (boiled)	½ cup	84
Peas, green (boiled)	½ cup	94
Potato (baked, with skin)	1 med	115
Spinach (boiled)	½ cup	50
Sweet potato (baked)	1 med	62
Fruits		
Figs (dried)	10 figs	128
Kiwi fruit (raw)	1 med	31
Orange juice (fresh)	8 fl oz	42
Orange, navel (raw)	1 med	27
Raisins, seedless	⅔ cup	97
Meat, Poultry, Fish, Dried Beans, Eggs, Nuts		
Almonds (roasted)	1 oz (22 nuts)	156
Bacon (fried)	3 med	64
Beef liver (fried)	3.5 oz	461
Beef top round, lean (broiled)	3.5 oz	246
Black-eyed peas (broiled)	1 cup	266
Chicken, dark (roasted, without skin)	3.5 oz	179
Meat, Poultry, Fish, Dried Beans, Eggs, Nuts—cont'd		
Chicken, light (roasted, without skin)	3.5 oz	216
Chick-peas (boiled)	1 cup	275
Clams, canned	3 oz	287
Cod (baked)	3 oz	117
Crab, Alaska king (steamed)	3 oz	238
Egg, whole	1 large	90
Ground beef, regular (broiled)	3.5 oz	170
Halibut (baked)	3 oz	242
Ham, canned (lean)	3.5 oz	224
Lentils (boiled)	1 cup	356
Lobster (steamed)	3 oz	157
Oysters (steamed)	3 oz (12 med)	236
Peanut butter, creamy	1 tbsp	60
Peanuts (roasted)	1 oz	100
Pinto beans (boiled)	1 cup	273
Sirloin steak, lean (broiled)	3.5 oz	244
Sole (baked)	3.5 oz	344
Soybeans (boiled)	1 cup	421
Trout, rainbow (baked)	3 oz	272
Tuna, light, canned in water	3 oz	158
Walnuts, dried	1 oz	132
Milk, Dairy Products		
Cheddar cheese	1.5 oz	145
Cottage cheese, creamed	1 cup	277
Milk, skim	8 fl oz	247
Milk, whole	8 fl oz	227
Swiss cheese	1 oz	171
Yogurt, whole milk	8 fl oz	215
Fats, Oils, Sugar		
This food group is not an important source of phosphorus		

Recommended Dietary Allowances for adults: 700 mg.

Sodium

As the major cation in the extracellular body fluid, sodium is one of the most plentiful minerals in the body. About 120 g (4 oz) is in the body of an adult, with one third in the skeleton as inorganic bound material. The remaining two thirds are in the form of free ionized sodium.

ABSORPTION-EXCRETION BALANCE

Absorption

Sodium is readily absorbed from the intestine; normally only about 5% remains for elimination in the feces. Larger amounts are lost in abnormal states such as diarrhea.

Excretion

The major route of excretion is through the kidney, under the powerful hormonal control of aldosterone, the sodium-conserving hormone from the adrenal glands.

PHYSIOLOGIC FUNCTIONS OF SODIUM

Water Balance

Ionized sodium is the major guardian of body water outside of cells. Variations in the sodium concentrations of body fluids largely determine the distribution of water via osmosis from one body area to another.

Acid-Base Balance

In association with chloride and bicarbonate ions, ionized sodium helps regulate acid-base balance.

Cell Permeability

The sodium pump in all cell membranes helps exchange sodium and potassium and other cellular materials. A major substance carried into cells via this active transport system is glucose.

Muscle Action

Sodium ions play a large role in transmitting electrochemical impulses along nerve and muscle membranes and in helping to maintain normal muscle action. Potassium and sodium ions balance the response of nerves to stimulation, the travel of nerve impulses to muscles, and the resulting contraction of the muscle fibers.

Hypertension

Several large studies, including a worldwide epidemiologic study (the international INTERSALT study) with a sample size of 10,079 subjects from 32 countries, have evaluated the influence of sodium intake on blood pressure.[20] These results clearly related an increasing dietary salt (NaCl) intake, primarily from the increasing use of processed foods, to the increasing incidence of hypertension. Nonetheless, the sodium-blood pressure link remains controversial. Some experts believe that reducing dietary salt plays a role in reducing blood pressure only in those individuals who are salt sensitive and that other factors in the diet also play an important role in controlling blood pressure.[21] African Americans appear to be particularly sensitive to the blood pressure–raising effect of sodium.[22]

A recent study that evaluated the relationship between diet and blood pressure (Dietary Approaches to Stop Hypertension [DASH]) used a diet rich in vegetables, fruits, and low-fat dairy products and did not restrict dietary salt. The participants took in an average of about 3000 mg/day of sodium[23] (the current recommendation is 2400 mg/day or less[24]). After 8 weeks on the intervention diet, blood pressure fell in those with elevated blood pressure and those with normal blood pressure.[23] In a second study participants followed the DASH diet *and* limited their sodium intake to 2300 mg or less.[25] Their blood pressure fell by even more than with the DASH diet alone. The drop in both systolic and diastolic blood pressure was greater in those with hypertension, telling us that diet and lifestyle interventions can play a role in the management of high blood pressure. It is likely that the phytochemicals present in the DASH diet also contributed to the results observed (see *Issues & Answers,* Chapter 7). Dietary intervention may also assist in controlling blood pressure in older persons. Individuals aged 65 and over who successfully reduced their intakes of sodium were more able to control their blood pressure without using antihypertensive drugs.[26]

SODIUM REQUIREMENT

Standard of Intake

The body can adjust to a rather wide range of dietary sodium by mechanisms designed to conserve or excrete this mineral. Thus there is no specific stated requirement. However, the Food and Nutrition Board has set an estimated minimum requirement for healthy persons for the three minerals—sodium, chloride, and potassium—that are major electrolytes in body fluids.[24] The estimated minimum requirement for sodium is 500 mg/day for

---

aldosterone Potent hormone of the cortex of the adrenal glands, which acts on the distal renal tubule to cause reabsorption of sodium in an ion exchange with potassium. The aldosterone mechanism is essentially a sodium-conserving mechanism but indirectly also conserves water because water absorption follows the sodium reabsorption.

electrolytes A chemical element or compound, which in solution dissociates as ions carrying a positive or negative charge (e.g., H^+, Na^+, K^+, Ca^{2+}, and Mg^{2+} and Cl^-, HCO_3^-, HPO_4^{2-}, and SO_4^{2-}). Electrolytes constitute a major force controlling fluid balances within the body through their concentrations and shifts from one place to another to restore and maintain balance—*homeostasis.*

healthy persons over age 18. To cover wide variations in individual patterns of physical activity and climate, which influence relative losses in perspiration, the upper limit for sodium in adults has been set at 2400 mg/day or less. Higher intakes carry no health benefits and may actually be detrimental in raising blood pressure in salt-sensitive persons.

General Dietary Intake

Sodium in the average American diet, supplied mainly by processed foods, tends to far exceed the suggested intake, even excluding any amount of salt added at the table. Caucasian men between the ages of 20 and 59 have the highest daily intakes of sodium, with 95% exceeding the maximum suggested intake of 2400 mg. Women and African Americans consume the least amount of sodium.[27] There is about 4 g (4000 mg) of sodium in the average 10 g of table salt (NaCl) consumed daily. Lowering the intake of table salt to about 5 g (1 teaspoon) would bring sodium intake down to 2 g (2000 mg), well within the recommended range.

FOOD SOURCES OF SODIUM

The main dietary source of sodium is common salt (NaCl) used in cooking, seasoning, and processing of foods. Natural food sources include milk, meat, eggs, and certain vegetables such as carrots, beets, leafy greens, and celery.

Some comparative food sources of sodium are listed in Table 8-4.

TABLE 8-4 Food Sources of Sodium

Food Source	Quantity	Sodium (mg)
Bread, Cereal, Rice, Pasta		
Bran flakes	¾ cup	264
Bran muffin, homemade	1 muffin	168
Bread, whole wheat	1 slice	159
Corn flakes	1 cup	310
Wheat flakes	1 cup	270
Vegetables		
Artichoke (boiled)	1 med	79
Broccoli (boiled)	½ cup	12
Brussels sprouts (boiled)	½ cup	17
Carrot (raw)	1 med	25
Potato (baked, with skin)	1 med	16
Spinach (boiled)	½ cup	63
Tomato (raw)	1 med	10
Fruits		
This food group is not an important source of sodium		
Meat, Poultry, Fish, Dried Beans, Eggs, Nuts		
Almonds (roasted, unsalted)	1 oz (22 nuts)	3
Bacon (broiled/fried)	3 med pieces	303
Beef liver (fried)	3.5 oz	106
Beef top round, lean (broiled)	3.5 oz	61
Black-eyed peas (boiled)	1 cup	6
Chicken, dark (roasted, without skin)	3.5 oz	93
Chicken, light (roasted, without skin)	3.5 oz	77
Clams (steamed)	3 oz (9 small)	95
Crab, blue (steamed)	3 oz	237
Egg, whole	1 large	69
Ground beef, regular (broiled)	3.5 oz	83
Meat, Poultry, Fish, Dried Beans, Eggs, Nuts—cont'd		
Halibut (baked)	3 oz	59
Ham, canned (lean)	3.5 oz	1255
Lentils (boiled)	1 cup	4
Lobster (steamed)	3 oz	323
Mackerel (baked)	3 oz	71
Oysters (steamed)	3 oz (12 med)	190
Peanut butter, creamy (unsalted)	1 tbsp	3
Peanut butter, creamy (with salt)	1 tbsp	131
Shrimp (steamed)	3 oz (15 large)	190
Sirloin steak, lean (broiled)	3.5 oz	66
Soybeans (boiled)	1 cup	1
Tuna, light, canned in water (with salt)	3 oz	303
Milk, Dairy Products		
Cheddar cheese	1 oz	176
Cottage cheese, creamed	1 cup	850
Milk, skim	8 fl oz	126
Milk, whole	8 fl oz	119
Swiss cheese	1 oz	74
Yogurt, whole milk	8 fl oz	105
Fats, Oils, Sugar		
Butter (salted)	1 tbsp	123
Butter (unsalted)	1 tbsp	2
Margarine, stick, corn oil (salted)	1 tbsp	132
Margarine, stick corn oil (unsalted)	1 tbsp	3
Molasses, black	1 tbsp	19
Sugar, brown	1 cup	44

Estimated minimum requirement for adults: 500 mg; a maximum daily intake of 2400 mg is a health-related goal.

Potassium

Potassium is about twice as plentiful as sodium in the body. An adult body contains about 270 g (9 oz, or 4000 *milliequivalents (mEq)*). The greater portion by far is found inside the cells because potassium is the major guardian of the body water inside cells. However, the relatively small amount in fluid outside cells has a significant effect on muscle activity, especially heart muscle.

ABSORPTION-EXCRETION BALANCE

Absorption

Dietary potassium is easily absorbed in the small intestine. Potassium also circulates in the gastrointestinal secretions and is reabsorbed in the digestive process. However, conditions such as prolonged diarrhea cause dangerous losses.

Excretion

Urinary excretion is the principal route of potassium loss. There is excess loss with some diuretic drugs. Because the maintenance of serum potassium within the narrow normal range is vital to heart muscle action and electrolyte balance, the kidneys guard potassium carefully. However, they cannot guard potassium as effectively as sodium. Aldosterone acts in the kidney to conserve sodium, but by this mechanism potassium is lost in exchange for sodium. The normal obligatory potassium loss is about 160 mg/day.

PHYSIOLOGIC FUNCTIONS OF POTASSIUM

Water and Acid-Base Balance

As the major guardian of cell water, potassium inside the cells balances with sodium outside the cells to maintain normal osmotic pressures and to protect cellular fluid. Potassium also works with sodium and hydrogen to maintain acid-base balance.

Muscle Activity

Potassium plays a significant role in the activity of skeletal and cardiac muscle. Together with sodium and calcium, potassium regulates neuromuscular stimulation, transmission of electrochemical impulses, and contraction of muscle fibers. This effect is particularly notable in the action of the heart muscle. Even small variations in serum potassium are reflected in electrocardiographic (ECG) changes. Variations in serum levels or low serum potassium may cause muscle irritability and paralysis. The heart may even develop a gallop rhythm, ending in cardiac arrest.

Carbohydrate Metabolism

When blood glucose is converted to glycogen for storage, 0.36 mmol of potassium is stored for each 1 g of glycogen. When a patient in diabetic acidosis is treated with insulin and glucose, rapid glycogen production draws potassium from the serum. Serious hypokalemia can result unless adequate potassium replacement accompanies treatment.

Protein Synthesis

Potassium is required for the storage of nitrogen in muscle protein and general cell protein. When tissue is broken down, potassium is lost together with the nitrogen. Amino acid replacement includes potassium to ensure nitrogen retention.

Control of Blood Pressure

Potassium seems to play a role in controlling blood pressure.[15,28] It may dilate the major arteries, thereby lowering blood pressure, or act by limiting the release of *renin,* the important kidney enzyme that triggers a chain of reactions leading to the reabsorption of sodium and water in the kidney tubule.

POTASSIUM REQUIREMENT

As with sodium, no specific dietary requirement is given for potassium. However, based on the amount needed to replace losses and to maintain normal body stores and plasma levels, a minimum daily intake for adults is approximately 1600 to 2000 mg.[24] In light of growing evidence that dietary potassium has a beneficial effect in controlling blood pressure, the National Research Council recommends that persons increase their potassium intake by eating more fruits and vegetables, and optimum potassium intake may be 3500 mg or higher. A suitable range for potassium in adults is 2000 to 5625 mg.[24] The diet used in the DASH study, which encouraged participants to eat at least five fruits and vegetables every day, provided about 5000 mg of potassium.[29]

FOOD SOURCES OF POTASSIUM

Potassium is widely distributed in natural foods because it is an essential constituent of all living cells. Legumes, whole grains, fruits such as oranges and bananas, leafy green vegetables, broccoli, potatoes, meats, and milk products supply considerable amounts. People who eat many servings of fruits and vegetables have a high potassium intake of about 8 to 11 g/day, well above the minimum level of the ESADDI.[24] Table 8-5 gives some comparative food sources of potassium.

Other Major Minerals

Three additional minerals are assigned to the major minerals group because of the extent of their occurrence in the body—magnesium, chloride, and sulfur.

TABLE 8-5 Food Sources of Potassium

Food Source	Quantity	Potassium (mg)
Bread, Cereal, Rice, Pasta		
Bran flakes	½ cup	184
Bran muffin, homemade	1 muffin	99
Bread, whole wheat	1 slice	44
Oatmeal (cooked)	¾ cup	99
Pasta, enriched (cooked)	1 cup	85
Rice, white, enriched	1 cup	57
Wheat flakes	1 cup	110
Wheat germ, toasted	¼ cup (1 oz)	268
Vegetables		
Artichoke (boiled)	1 med	316
Asparagus (boiled)	½ cup (6 spears)	279
Avocado (raw)	1 med	1097
Broccoli (raw)	½ cup, chopped	143
Brussels sprouts (boiled)	½ cup (4 sprouts)	247
Carrot (raw)	1 med	233
Corn, yellow (boiled)	½ cup	204
Mushrooms (boiled)	½ cup, pieces	277
Potato (baked, with skin)	1 med	844
Spinach (boiled)	½ cup	419
Sweet potato (baked)	1 med	397
Tomato (raw)	1 med	254
Fruits		
Apple (raw, with skin)	1 med	159
Banana	1 med	451
Cantaloupe	1 cup, pieces	494
Dates (dried)	10 dates	541
Figs (dried)	10 figs	1332
Orange juice (fresh)	8 fl oz	486
Orange, navel	1 med	250
Prunes (dried)	10 prunes	626
Prune juice (canned)	8 fl oz	706
Raisins, seedless	⅔ cup	751
Meat, Poultry, Fish, Dried Beans, Eggs, Nuts		
Almonds (dry roasted)	1 oz (22 nuts)	219
Beef liver (fried)	3.5 oz	364
Meat, Poultry, Fish, Dried Beans, Eggs, Nuts—cont'd		
Beef top round, lean (broiled)	3.5 oz	442
Black-eyed peas (boiled)	1 cup	476
Chicken, dark (roasted, without skin)	3.5 oz	240
Chicken, light (roasted, without skin)	3.5 oz	247
Clams (steamed)	3 oz (9 small)	534
Crab, blue (steamed)	3 oz	275
Egg, whole	1 large	65
Ground beef, regular (broiled)	3.5 oz	292
Halibut (baked)	3 oz	490
Ham, canned (lean)	3.5 oz	364
Lentils (boiled)	1 cup	731
Lima beans (boiled)	1 cup	955
Lobster (steamed)	3 oz	299
Mackerel (baked)	3 oz	341
Oysters (steamed)	3 oz (12 med)	389
Peanut butter, creamy	1 tbsp	110
Peanuts (dry roasted)	1 oz	184
Pinto beans (boiled)	1 cup	800
Salmon (baked)	3 oz	319
Sirloin steak, lean (broiled)	3.5 oz	403
Soybeans (boiled)	1 cup	886
Trout, rainbow (baked)	3 oz	539
Tuna, light, canned in water (with salt)	3 oz	267
Milk, Dairy Products		
Cottage cheese, creamed	1 cup	177
Milk, skim	8 fl oz	406
Milk, whole	8 fl oz	368
Yogurt, whole milk	8 fl oz	351
Fats, Oils		
This food group is not an important source of potassium		
Sugar		
Molasses, black	1 tbsp	585
Sugar, brown	1 cup	499

Estimated minimum requirement for adults: 2000 mg. Optimum intake may be 3500 mg or above.

MAGNESIUM

Magnesium has widespread metabolic functions and is present in all body cells. An adult body contains about 25 g of magnesium, or a little less than an ounce. About two thirds of this small but vital amount is combined with calcium and phosphorus in bone.[30] The remainder is distributed in muscle and other tissues and fluids, where it has widespread metabolic use in all cells as a control agent. Magnesium acts as an enzyme activator for energy production and building tissue protein. It also aids in normal muscle action. Because so much of body magnesium is found in bone, researchers are trying to learn more about magnesium and bone health.

TABLE 8-6 Food Sources of Magnesium

Food Source	Quantity	Magnesium (mg)	Food Source	Quantity	Magnesium (mg)
Bread, Cereal, Rice, Pasta			***Meat, Poultry, Fish, Dried Beans, Eggs, Nuts—cont'd***		
Bran flakes	¾ cup	68	Cod (baked)	3 oz	36
Bran muffin, homemade	1 muffin	35	Crab, blue (steamed)	3 oz	28
Bread, whole wheat	1 slice	23	Egg, whole	1 large	6
Oatmeal (cooked)	¾ cup	42	Ground beef, regular (broiled)	3.5 oz	20
Pasta, enriched (cooked)	1 cup	28	Halibut (baked)	3 oz	91
Wheat flakes	1 cup	31	Ham, canned (lean)	3.5 oz	17
Vegetables			Lentils (boiled)	1 cup	71
Artichoke (boiled)	1 med	47	Lobster (steamed)	3 oz	30
Avocado (raw)	1 med	70	Mackerel (baked)	3 oz	83
Corn, yellow (boiled)	½ med	26	Oysters (steamed)	3 oz (12 med)	92
Okra (boiled)	½ cup	46	Peanut butter, creamy	1 tbsp	28
Peas, green (boiled)	½ cup	31	Peanuts (roasted)	1 oz	49
Potato (baked, with skin)	1 med	55	Pinto beans (boiled)	1 cup	95
Spinach (boiled)	½ cup	79	Sirloin steak, lean (broiled)	3.5 oz	32
Sweet potato (baked)	1 med	23	Soybeans (boiled)	1 cup	95
Fruits			Trout, rainbow (baked)	3 oz	33
Figs (dried)	10 figs	111	Tuna, light, canned in water	3 oz	25
Kiwi (raw)	1 med	23	Walnuts, dried	1 oz	57
Orange juice (fresh)	8 fl oz	27	***Milk, Dairy Products***		
Raisins, seedless	⅔ cup	33	Cheddar cheese	1 oz	8
Meat, Poultry, Fish, Dried Beans, Eggs, Nuts			Cottage cheese, creamed	1 cup	11
Almonds (roasted)	1 oz (22 nuts)	86	Milk, skim	8 fl oz	28
Beef liver (fried)	3.5 oz	23	Milk, whole	8 fl oz	33
Beef top round, lean (broiled)	3.5 oz	31	Swiss cheese	1 oz	10
Black-eyed peas (boiled)	1 cup	91	Yogurt, whole milk	8 fl oz	26
Chicken, dark (roasted, without skin)	3.5 oz	23	***Fats, Oils, Sugar***		
Chicken, light (roasted without skin)	3.5 oz	27	This food group is not an important source of magnesium		
Chick-peas (boiled)	1 cup	78			

Recommended Dietary Allowances for adults: women aged 19-30, 310 mg; men aged 19-30, 400 mg; women ≥31, 320 mg; men ≥31, 420 mg.

They have found that older people who have higher intakes of magnesium do not lose bone mineral as rapidly as those who have lower intakes.[31] The RDA standard for individuals aged 19 to 30 is 400 mg/day for men and 310 mg for women.[11] To allow for changes in kidney function as individuals age, leading to greater loss of magnesium, the RDAs for individuals above age 30 are raised to 420 mg/day for men and 320 mg/day for women.

Magnesium is relatively widespread in nature and thus in unprocessed foods. For example, large concentrations of magnesium occur in unmilled grains, but more than 80% is lost by removal of the germ and outer layers of the grain. The main food sources include nuts, soybeans, cocoa, seafood, whole grains, dried beans and peas, and green vegetables. Most fruits, except bananas, are relatively poor sources, as are meat and fish. Milk provides some magnesium in the American diet. On the whole, diets rich in vegetables and unrefined grains are much higher in magnesium than are diets made up mostly of refined foods and meat. Table 8-6 provides some comparative food sources of magnesium.

CHLORINE (CHLORIDE)

Chlorine appears in the body as the chloride ion (Cl^-). Chlorine accounts for about 3% of the body's total mineral content and is found in the fluid outside of cells, where it helps control water and acid-base balances. Spinal fluid has the highest concentration. A relatively large amount of ionized chloride is found in the gastrointestinal secretions, especially as a component of gastric hydrochloric acid (HCl).

SULFUR

Sulfur is present in all body cells, usually as a constituent of cell protein. Elemental sulfur occurs in sulfate compounds with sodium, potassium, and magnesium. Organic forms occur mainly with other protein compounds: (1) sulfur-containing amino acids, such as methionine and cysteine; (2) glycoproteins in cartilage, tendons, and bone matrix; (3) detoxification products formed in part by bacteria in the intestine; (4) other organic compounds such as heparin, insulin, coenzyme A, lipoic acid, thiamin, and biotin; and (5) keratin in hair and nails.

The major minerals are summarized in Table 8-7.

TABLE 8-7 Summary of Major Minerals

Mineral	Metabolism	Physiologic Functions	Clinical Applications	DRI/ESADDI	Food Sources
Calcium (Ca)	Absorption according to body need; requires Ca-binding protein and regulated by vitamin D, parathyroid hormone, and calcitonin; absorption favored by protein, lactose, acidity Excretion chiefly in feces: 70%-90% of amount ingested Deposition-mobilization in bone tissue is constant, regulated by vitamin D and parathyroid hormone	Constituent of bones and teeth Participates in blood clotting, nerve transmission, muscle action, cell membrane permeability, enzyme activation	Tetany (decrease in serum Ca) Rickets, osteomalacia Osteoporosis Resorptive hypercalciuria, renal calculi Hyperparathyroidism and hypoparathyroidism	Male/female adults: Aged 19-50: 1000 mg Aged ≥51: 1200 mg Pregnancy: Aged ≤ 18: 1300 mg Aged ≥ 19: 1000 mg Lactation: Aged ≤18: 1300 mg Aged ≥19: 1000 mg	Milk, cheese, yogurt Green leafy vegetables Whole grains Legumes, nuts Fortified soy foods
Phosphorus (P)	Absorption with Ca aided by vitamin D and parathyroid hormone as for calcium; hindered by binding agents Excretion chiefly by kidney according to serum level, regulated by parathyroid hormone Deposition-mobilization in bone compartment is constant	Constituent of bones and teeth, ATP, phosphorylated intermediary metabolites Participates in absorption of glucose and glycerol, transport of fatty acids, energy metabolism, and buffer system	Growth Recovery from diabetic acidosis Hypophosphatemia: bone disease, malabsorption syndromes, primary hyperparathyroidism Hyperphosphatemia: renal insufficiency, hypoparathyroidism, tetany	Male/female adults: Aged ≥19: 700 mg Pregnancy: Aged ≤18: 1250 mg Aged ≥19: 700 mg Lactation: Aged ≤18: 1250 mg Aged ≥19: 700 mg	Milk, cheese Meat, egg yolk Whole grains Legumes, nuts Soft drinks
Magnesium (Mg)	Absorption according to intake load; hindered by excess fat, phosphate, calcium, protein Excretion (regulated by kidney)	Constituent of bones and teeth Coenzyme in general metabolism, smooth muscle action, neuromuscular irritability	Low serum level following gastrointestinal losses Tremor, spasm in deficiency induced by malnutrition, alcoholism	Adults: Males aged 19-30: 400 mg Males aged ≥31: 420 mg Females aged 19-30: 310 mg Females aged ≥31: 320 mg	Milk, cheese Meat, seafood Whole grains Legumes, nuts

TABLE 8-7 Summary of Major Minerals—cont'd

Mineral	Metabolism	Physiologic Functions	Clinical Applications	DRI/ESADDI	Food Sources
Magnesium (Mg) —cont'd		Cation in intracellular fluid		Pregnancy: Aged ≤18: 400 mg Aged 19-30: 350 mg Aged 31-50: 360 mg Lactation: Aged ≤18: 360 mg Aged 19-30: 310 mg Aged 31-50: 320 mg	
Sodium (Na)	Readily absorbed Excretion chiefly by kidney, controlled by aldosterone	Major cation in extracellular fluid, water balance, acid-base balance Cell membrane permeability, absorption of glucose Normal muscle irritability	Losses in gastrointestinal disorders, diarrhea Fluid-electrolyte and acid-base balance problems Muscle action	Adults: Minimum intake: 500 mg Recommended intake: not to exceed 2400 mg	Salt (NaCl) Sodium compounds used in baking and food processing Milk, cheese Carrots, spinach, beets, celery
Potassium (K)	Readily absorbed Secreted and reabsorbed in gastrointestinal circulation Excretion chiefly by kidney, regulated by aldosterone	Major cation in intracellular fluid, water balance, acid-base balance Normal muscle irritability Glycogen formation Protein synthesis	Losses in gastrointestinal disorders, diarrhea Fluid-electrolyte, acid-base balance problems Muscle action, especially heart action Losses in tissue catabolism Treatment of diabetic acidosis: rapid glycogen production reduces serum potassium level Losses with diuretic therapy	Adults: Minimum intake: 2000 mg Optimum intake: ≥3500 mg	Fruits Vegetables Legumes, nuts Whole grains Meat
Chloride (Cl)	Readily absorbed Excretion controlled by kidney	Major anion in extracellular fluid, water balance, acid-base balance, chloride-bicarbonate shift Gastric hydrochloride—digestion	Losses in gastrointestinal disorders, vomiting, diarrhea, tube drainage Hypochloremic alkalosis	Adults: Minimum intake: 750 mg	Salt (NaCl)
Sulfur (S)	Elemental form absorbed as such; split from amino acid sources (methionine and cysteine) in digestion and absorbed into portal circulation Excreted by kidney in relation to protein intake and tissue catabolism	Essential constituent of protein structure Enzyme activity and energy metabolism through free sulfhydryl group (–SH) Detoxification reactions	Cystine renal calculi Cystinuria	Adults: No specific recommendation: diets adequate in protein are usually adequate in sulfur	Meat, eggs Milk, cheese Legumes, nuts

PRACTICAL APPLICATION

Do You Need a Mineral Supplement?

The U.S. population is constantly barraged by advertisements urging them to purchase nutritional supplements, including mineral supplements, to prevent real or imagined nutrient deficiencies. We know that it is possible for most of us to obtain all of the minerals we need from food by choosing a balanced diet that conforms to the *Food Guide Pyramid.* One exception to this general guideline is the pregnant woman, who will likely need to rely on an iron supplement provided by her physician to obtain the 27 mg/day that is recommended. As we will learn in Chapter 13, it is imperative that adults of all ages take in a sufficient amount of calcium to promote bone health, and, for individuals whose food sources of calcium are limited, supplements may be necessary. Women or children who develop an iron deficiency anemia are treated with iron supplements, but this must be carried out under medical supervision. Persons who must follow severely restricted diets in the treatment of a specific medical problem or elderly persons with very low food intake and energy expenditure may require a multivitamin-mineral supplement to ensure that all essential micronutrients are provided in adequate amounts. But are there other circumstances that might suggest the need for a mineral supplement?

Health professionals are urging us to increase our intakes of dietary fiber. The *Dietary Guidelines for Americans* (see Chapter 1) continue to emphasize the importance of fiber, and the nutrition label suggests an intake of 25 g of fiber for persons consuming about 2000 kcalories/day. Fiber intakes of 50 g or higher are being tested for their ability to help control blood glucose levels in patients with diabetes and thus reduce their dependence on medication. If we continue to increase our dietary fiber, what will be the effect on trace mineral status? Phytates, substances found in whole grains, and oxalates, substances found in many fruits and vegetables, bind trace minerals and inhibit their absorption.

The long-term effects of dietary fiber on trace mineral status are being evaluated by many researchers. Calcium is less effectively absorbed from vegetables than from dairy products because of the interference of oxalates. A lower proportion of the iron and zinc in whole grains and legumes is absorbed compared with the proportion absorbed from animal foods. For individuals who obtain their minerals from a variety of food sources, the effect of phytates and oxalates is likely not a problem. However, individuals whose food intake is primarily from plant sources may be at risk for poor mineral nutrition. Vegetarian women whose sole food sources of iron and zinc were vegetables and grains were found to have low body stores of these minerals. A fiber intake of 25 to 35 g/day obtained from a variety of food sources does not appear to compromise the mineral status of individuals eating the recommended servings of mineral-rich foods. It will be important, however, to monitor the mineral status of individuals consuming higher levels of fiber daily as a therapeutic measure for controlling blood glucose and lipid levels or based on individual food patterns. It is also best to obtain fiber from food, which will also supply minerals and other important nutrients. Fiber supplements are costly and, if used in excessive amounts, can lead to fecal impaction.

For those persons who are concerned about their intake of minerals and are considering adding a dietary supplement, how much is too much? It is unlikely that an individual could take in too much of a particular mineral from food sources. On the other hand, mineral supplements, some of which exceed the recently published ULs, hold the potential for inducing not only a toxicity but also a possible deficiency of other minerals or trace elements. In naturally occurring foods, trace elements are present in balanced proportions so that one is unlikely to interfere with another. This becomes important for absorption in the small intestine because several trace minerals can be absorbed by the same receptor sites and an exaggerated amount of one of these minerals can effectively monopolize the receptor site and crowd out the others. If this happens regularly, as in the case of someone who is consistently taking in high amounts of a certain mineral, a serious deficiency can arise. Concentrated iron supplements can induce a copper deficiency if continued over an extended period. And we are still investigating the long-term effect of calcium supplements on the absorption of zinc.

Over-the-counter medications can add significantly to mineral intake or potential toxicity. Various antacids are advertised as inexpensive sources of calcium, but others have as a major ingredient aluminum hydroxide, and aluminum can enhance bone mineral loss. Excessive use of magnesium-containing products sold as antacids or laxatives can lead to magnesium intoxication, particularly in older individuals with impaired renal function, with serious effects on nerve and cardiac function. Magnesium intoxication has not been known to occur as a result of food intake.

If circumstances preclude an individual from obtaining the recommended levels of minerals from food alone, consider the following guidelines.

- Use supplements in addition to, not in place of, real food. A poor diet with added supplements is still a poor diet. Make an effort to obtain all needed nutrients with appropriate meal planning.
- Choose a multimineral or multivitamin-mineral supplement that contains each of the needed minerals and/or vitamins in the amount recommended by the RDA or AI; this will ensure that these nutrients are present in the appropriate pro-

PRACTICAL APPLICATION
Do You Need a Mineral Supplement?—cont'd

portions and that no one mineral is present in an excessive amount.
- Avoid individual supplements of particular vitamins or minerals because these often contain excessive amounts in comparison with the DRI. (Possible exceptions may be iron or calcium and a physician's advice is needed.)
- Choose supplements that do not exceed 100% of the RDA or AI. It is especially important that no mineral be present at a level that approaches or exceeds the UL for that nutrient.
- If you are already using a highly fortified cereal that supplies 100% of the recommended levels of most minerals and/or vitamins, it is best not to take a supplement that provides additional amounts without seeking the advice of a physician.
- Take your mineral supplement with meals because other foods in the digestive tract will enhance absorption.

References

Food and Nutrition Board, National Academy of Sciences: *Dietary reference intakes for vitamin A, vitamin K, arsenic, boron, chromium, copper, iodine, iron, manganese, molybdenum, nickel, silicon, vanadium, and zinc,* Washington, DC, 2001, National Academy Press.

Hunt J, Dwyer J: Position of the American Dietetic Association: food fortification and dietary supplements, *J Am Diet Assoc* 101(1):115, 2001.

King JC, Keen CL: Zinc. In Shils ME et al, eds: *Modern nutrition in health and disease,* ed 9, Philadelphia, 1999, Lippincott Williams & Wilkins.

Marsh MN, Riley SA: Digestion and absorption of nutrients and vitamins. In Feldman M, Scharschmidt BF, Sleisenger MH, eds: *Gastrointestinal and liver disease,* ed 6, vol 2, Philadelphia, 1998, WB Saunders.

Nielsen FH: Ultratrace minerals. In Shils ME et al, eds: *Modern nutrition in health and disease,* ed 9, Philadelphia, 1999, Lippincott Williams & Wilkins.

TRACE ELEMENTS: THE CONCEPT OF ESSENTIALITY

By the simplest definition, an essential element is one required for existence; conversely, its absence brings death. For major elements that occur in relatively large amounts in the body, such determinations can be made fairly easily because the quantity present is sufficiently available for study. However, for elements that occur in very small amounts, this determination of essentiality is not easy to make. For example, of the 54 known chemical elements in the major part of the periodic table, 27 have been determined to be essential to human life and function. By far, most living matter as we know it is made up of five fundamental elements: hydrogen (H), carbon (C), nitrogen (N), oxygen (O), and sulfur (S). We know these elements well because their concentrations are relatively large and more easily studied, and their requirements for human function can be stated in multiples of grams per kilogram of body weight. This is a recognizable quantity with which we can be comfortable. Also, we have methods for analysis of such quantities and can easily see that these are essential elements. The major minerals we have just reviewed occur in respectable amounts in the body; therefore their essentiality has been more easily studied and determined.

A much larger number of elements—microelements or trace elements—occur in biologic matter in such small amounts that measurement and analysis are exceedingly difficult. In many cases we know little about them and understand even less. It is much harder to determine the essentiality of these trace elements because we apparently require so little of them. In general, trace elements have been defined as those having a required intake of less than 100 mg/day, yet some of them exist in fairly large amounts in our diet and our environment.

ESSENTIAL FUNCTION

Despite difficulties in determining the essentiality of these very small amounts of trace minerals in our bodies, we have acquired enough important information to help us make appropriate intake recommendations based on their function and deficiency effects. At the same time we must avoid intakes resulting from inappropriate use of supplements (see *Practical Application* box) that lead to toxicity or adverse health effects. Mertz, a leading researcher who has taught us much about the trace minerals, cautions us about the appearance of precision or accuracy, meaning that our current recommendations are based on judgments and assumptions that may not be correct.[32] As research continues, we may acquire new information telling us that some of these recommendations need to be revised or that a particular function may be based on the actions of several rather than one nutrient.

An element is considered essential when a deficiency causes an impairment of function and when supplementation with that element, but not with others, prevents or cures this impairment. So far researchers have identified two basic functions of trace elements: (1) as catalysts of chemical reactions and (2) as structural components of larger molecules.

ESSENTIAL TRACE ELEMENTS: DEFINITE AND PROBABLE

On the basis of current knowledge, these small trace elements may be separated into two groups: those that are definitely essential and those that are probably essential.

Definite Essential Elements

Ten trace elements have been assigned essential roles in human nutrition based on defined function and need determined from research. This group includes iron (Fe), iodine (I), zinc (Zn), copper (Cu), manganese (Mn), chromium (Cr), cobalt (Co), selenium (Se), molybdenum (Mo), and fluoride (Fl).

Probable Essential Elements

The remaining eight trace elements are known to perform a metabolic function in animals but at this time have not been shown to play a role in *human* health.[33] As we develop better means of analysis and tests for function that are appropriate for human studies, we will learn more about their roles in the human body. These elements include silicon (Si), vanadium (V), nickel (Ni), tin (Sn), cadmium (Cd), arsenic (As), aluminum (Al), and boron (B).

We look first at iron and iodine because of their long history and clearly defined specific functions in humans. Then we will briefly review the remainder. These essential elements are summarized in Table 8-8.

Iron

Of all the micronutrients, iron has the longest and best described history, and its mechanisms for body regulation to avoid both iron overload and iron deficiency have been well described.

FORMS OF IRON IN THE BODY

The human body contains only about 40 to 50 mg iron/kg body weight. This iron is distributed in four forms that point to its basic metabolic function.

TABLE 8-8 Summary of Trace Elements

Element	Metabolism	Physiologic Functions	Clinical Applications	DRI	Food Sources
Iron (Fe)	Absorption controls bioavailability; favored by body need, acidity, and reduction agents such as vitamins; hindered by binding agents, reduced gastric HCl, infection, gastrointestinal losses Transported as transferrin, stored as ferritin or hemosiderin Excreted in sloughed cells, bleeding	Hemoglobin synthesis, oxygen transport Cell oxidation, heme enzymes	Anemia (hypochromic, microcytic) Excess: hemosiderosis, hemochromatosis Growth and pregnancy needs	Adults: Males aged ≥19: 8 mg Females aged 19-50: 18 mg Females aged ≥51: 8 mg Pregnancy: All ages: 27 mg Lactation: Aged ≤18: 10 mg Aged ≥19: 9 mg	Meat, eggs, liver Whole grain and enriched breads and cereals Dark green vegetables Legumes, nuts Acid foods cooked in iron utensils
Iodine (I)	Absorbed as iodides, taken up by thyroid gland under control of thyroid-stimulating hormone (TSH) Excretion by kidney	Synthesis of thyroxin, which regulates cell metabolism, basal metabolic rate (BMR)	Endemic colloid goiter, cretinism Hypothyroidism and hyperthyroidism	Adults: Males/females aged ≥19: 150 μg Pregnancy: All ages: 220 μg Lactation: All ages: 290 μg	Iodized salt Seafood
Zinc (Zn)	Absorbed with zinc-binding ligand (ZBL) from pancreas Transported in blood by albumin; stored in many sites Excretion largely intestinal	Essential coenzyme constituent: carbonic anhydrase, carboxypeptid ase, lactic dehydrogenase	Growth: hypogonadism Sensory impairment: taste and smell Wound healing Malabsorption disease	Adults: Males aged ≥19: 11 mg Females aged ≥19: 8 mg Pregnancy: Aged ≤18: 13 mg Aged ≥19: 11 mg Lactation: Aged ≤18: 14 mg Aged ≥19: 12 mg	Beef and other meats; liver Oysters, seafood Milk, cheese, eggs Whole grains Widely distributed in food

TABLE 8-8 Summary of Trace Elements—cont'd

Element	Metabolism	Physiologic Functions	Clinical Applications	DRI	Food Sources
Copper (Cu)	Absorbed with copper-binding protein metallothionein Transported in blood by histidine and albumin Stored in many tissues	Associated with iron in enzyme systems, hemoglobin synthesis Metalloprotein enzyme constituent	Hypocupremia: nephrosis and malabsorption Wilson's disease, excess copper storage	Adults: Males/females aged ≥19: 900 μg Pregnancy: All ages: 1000 μg Lactation: All ages: 1300 mg	Meat, liver, seafood Whole grains Legumes, nuts Widely distributed in food
Manganese (Mn)	Absorbed poorly Excretion mainly by intestine	Enzyme component in general metabolism	Low serum levels in diabetes, protein-energy malnutrition Inhalation toxicity	Adults: Males aged ≥19: 2.3 mg Females aged ≥19: 1.8 mg Pregnancy: All ages: 2.0 mg Lactation: All ages: 2.6 mg	Whole grains and cereals Legumes, soybeans Green leafy vegetables
Chromium (Cr)	Absorbed in association with zinc Excretion mainly by kidney	Associated with glucose metabolism; improves faulty glucose uptake by tissues	Potentiates action of insulin in persons with diabetes May lower serum cholesterol, low-density lipoprotein cholesterol and raise high-density lipoprotein cholesterol	Adults: Males aged 19-50: 35 μg Males aged ≥51: 30 μg Females aged 19-50: 25 μg Females aged ≥51: 20 μg Pregnancy: Aged ≤18: 29 μg Aged ≥19: 30 μg Lactation: Aged ≤18: 44 μg Aged ≥19: 45 μg	Whole grains and cereals Brewer's yeast Animal protein foods
Cobalt (Co)	Absorbed as component of food source, vitamin B_{12} Elemental form shares transport with iron Stored in liver	Constituent of vitamin B_{12}, functions with vitamin	Deficiency associated only with deficiency of vitamin B_{12}	Unknown (usually consumed as part of the vitamin B_{12} molecule	Animal foods containing vitamin B_{12}
Selenium (Se)	Absorption depends on solubility of compound form Excreted mainly by kidney	Constituent of enzyme glutathione peroxidase Synergistic antioxidant with vitamin E Structural component of teeth	Marginal deficiency when soil content is low Deficiency secondary to parenteral nutrition (TPN), malnutrition Toxicity observed in livestock	Adults: Males/females aged ≥19: 55 μg Pregnancy: All ages: 60 μg Lactation: All ages: 70 μg	Seafood Legumes Whole grains Vegetables Low-fat meats and dairy foods Varies with soil content
Molybdenum (Mo)	Readily absorbed Excreted rapidly by kidney Small amount excreted in bile	Constituent of oxidase enzymes, xanthine oxidase	Deficiency unknown in humans	Adults: Males/females aged ≥19: 45 μg Pregnancy: All ages 50 μg Lactation: All ages: 50 μg	Legumes Whole grains Milk Organ meats Leafy vegetables

Continued

TABLE 8-8 Summary of Trace Elements—cont'd

Element	Metabolism	Physiologic Functions	Clinical Applications	DRI	Food Sources
Fluoride (F)	Absorption in small intestine; little known of bioavailability Excreted by kidney—80%	Accumulates in bones and teeth, increasing hardness	Dental caries inhibited Osteoporosis: may reduce bone loss Excess: dental fluorosis	Adults: Males aged ≥19: 4 mg Females aged ≥19: 3 mg Pregnancy: All ages: 3 mg Lactation: All ages: 3 mg	Fish and fish products Tea Drinking water (fluoridated) Foods cooked in fluoridated water

Transport Iron

A trace of iron, 0.05 to 0.18 mg/dl, is in blood plasma and bound to its transport carrier protein transferrin.

Hemoglobin

Most of the body's iron, about 70%, occurs in red blood cells as a vital constituent of the heme portion of hemoglobin. Another 5% is a part of the muscle oxygen-carrying molecule myoglobin.

Storage Iron

About 20% of the body iron is stored as the protein-iron compound ferritin, mainly in the liver, spleen, and bone marrow. Excess iron is stored in the body as hemosiderin, interchanging with ferritin as needed.

Cellular Tissue Iron

The remaining 5% of body iron is distributed throughout all cells as a major component of oxidative enzyme systems for the production of energy.

TABLE 8-9 Characteristics of Heme and Nonheme Portions of Dietary Iron

	Dietary Iron	
	Heme (Smallest Portion)	Nonheme (Largest Portion)
Food sources	None in plant sources; 40% of iron in animal sources	All plant sources of iron; 60% of iron in animal sources
Absorption rate	Rapid; transported and absorbed intact	Slow; tightly bound in organic molecules

ABSORPTION-TRANSPORT-STORAGE-EXCRETION BALANCE

Iron follows a unique system of interrelated absorption-transport-storage-excretion. Optimal levels of body iron are not regulated by urinary excretion as is the case with most plasma constituents. Rather, the mechanisms of iron control lie in the absorption-transport-storage complex.

Absorption

The main control of the body's iron balance is at the site of intestinal absorption. Dietary iron enters the body in two forms: heme iron and nonheme iron (Table 8-9). By far the larger portion is nonheme—all plant sources plus 60% of animal sources.[33] But nonheme iron is absorbed at a much slower rate than the smaller heme portion because nonheme iron is tightly bound in its food sources to organic molecules in the form of ferric iron (Fe^{3+}). In the acid medium of the stomach, ferric iron must be disassociated and reduced to the more soluble ferrous iron (Fe^{2+}) before it can be absorbed. This is a source of nutritional concern because nonheme iron is found in greater quantities in the diet.

Control of iron distribution and transfer in the absorbing cell of the intestinal mucosa involves several receiving substances. Iron is never allowed to travel about the body unescorted. First, the iron, all now in the ferrous form, is bound by an intracellular protein carrier. This protein carrier leaves a portion of the iron to serve the needs of the mitochondria of the absorbing cell and then delivers specific proportions to its regular receptors and carriers. These two carriers are (1) apoferritin, the cell's special protein receptor, which combines with iron to form the intermediate iron-holding compound, epithelial ferritin, and (2) apotransferrin, the blood's special protein receptor, which combines with iron to form the circulating iron-carrier compound, serum transferrin.

The amount of ferritin already present in the intestinal mucosa determines the amount of ingested iron that is absorbed or rejected. When all available apoferritin has been bound to iron to form ferritin, any additional iron that arrives at the binding site is rejected, returned to the lumen of the intestine, and passed on for excretion in the feces. About 1% to 15% of nonheme iron is absorbed compared with 15% to 45% of heme iron.[34] The remaining amounts are eliminated. Most absorption takes place in the upper small intestine.

The following factors favor absorption.

1. *Body need.* In deficiency states or in periods of extra demand, as in growth or pregnancy, mucosal ferritin is lower and more iron is absorbed. When tissue reserves are ample or saturated, iron is rejected and excreted.
2. *Ascorbic acid or other acid agents.* Vitamin C (ascorbic acid) and other acids increase iron absorption by their reducing action and ability to create an acid environment. These reducing agents act on dietary ferric iron to reduce it to ferrous iron, the soluble form that can be absorbed. Adding 50 mg of ascorbic acid in the form of orange juice or other food can triple the absorption of nonheme iron.[33] Gastric hydrochloric acid provides the optimal acid medium for preparing iron for use.
3. *Animal tissues.* Meat, fish, and poultry improve iron absorption by providing some iron in the heme form that is well absorbed. It has been learned that animal tissues also improve the absorption of nonheme iron eaten at the same meal. It appears that peptides, released from meat, fish, and poultry during digestion, enhance the absorption of iron from other sources.[33]

The following factors hinder absorption.

1. *Binding agents.* Substances such as phosphate, phytate, and oxalate bind iron and remove it from the body. Some vegetable proteins, including soy protein, decrease iron absorption independent of the effect of phytates. Substances in tea and coffee also can decrease nonheme iron absorption.
2. *Reduced gastric acid secretion.* Surgical removal of stomach tissue (gastrectomy) reduces the number of cells that secrete hydrochloric acid, thus limiting the acid needed for reducing ferric iron to ferrous iron. Persons who abuse antacids and thereby decrease available acid may have trouble absorbing their dietary iron.
3. *Infection.* Severe infection hinders iron absorption.
4. *Gastrointestinal disease.* Malabsorption or any disturbance that causes diarrhea or steatorrhea (fatty diarrhea) hinders iron absorption.
5. *Calcium.* Large amounts of calcium can inhibit the absorption of both heme and nonheme iron eaten at the same meal. This interaction could affect the iron status of persons who take calcium supplements with meals; however, a group of breastfeeding mothers taking 500 mg calcium supplements twice a day with meals did not lower their body iron stores.[35]

The bioavailability of iron essentially depends on its absorption, which in turn depends on a number of influencing factors in the body. This is a unique and precarious arrangement.

Transport

As mentioned earlier, in the mucosal cells of the duodenum and proximal jejunum, iron is oxidized and bound with the protein transferrin for transport to body cells. Normally, only about 20% to 35% of the iron-binding capacity of transferrin is filled. The remaining capacity forms an unsaturated plasma reserve for handling variances in iron intake.

Storage

Bound to plasma transferrin, iron is delivered to its storage sites in bone marrow and liver. Here it is transferred again to apoferritin to form ferritin for storage and use as needed in synthesizing hemoglobin for red blood cells. This binding with apoferritin provides a stable, exchangeable storage form for the body needs. A second, less soluble storage compound, hemosiderin, provides reserve storage in the liver. From these storage compounds, iron is mobilized for hemoglobin synthesis as needed. In the average adult, 20 to 25 mg of iron/day is used in hemoglobin synthesis. However, the body avidly conserves the iron in hemoglobin, recycling the iron when red blood cells are destroyed. The average life span of a red blood cell is about 120 days. These interrelationships of body iron absorption-transport-storage mechanisms are diagrammed in Figure 8-3.

Excretion

Because the main regulatory mechanism controlling iron levels in the body occurs at the point of absorption, only minute amounts are lost by renal excretion. This is quite different from other circulating minerals, which are

---

ferritin Protein-iron compound in which iron is stored in tissues; the storage form of iron in the body.

heme iron Dietary iron from animal sources, from the heme portion of hemoglobin in red blood cells. Heme iron is more easily absorbed and transported in the body than nonheme iron from plant sources, but it supplies the smaller portion of the body's total dietary iron intake.

hemosiderin Insoluble iron oxide–protein compound in which iron is stored in the liver if the amount of iron in the blood exceeds the storage capacity of ferritin, such as during rapid destruction of red blood cells (malaria, hemolytic anemia).

nonheme iron The larger portion of dietary iron, including all the plant food sources and 60% of the animal food sources. This form of iron is not part of a heme complex and is less easily absorbed.

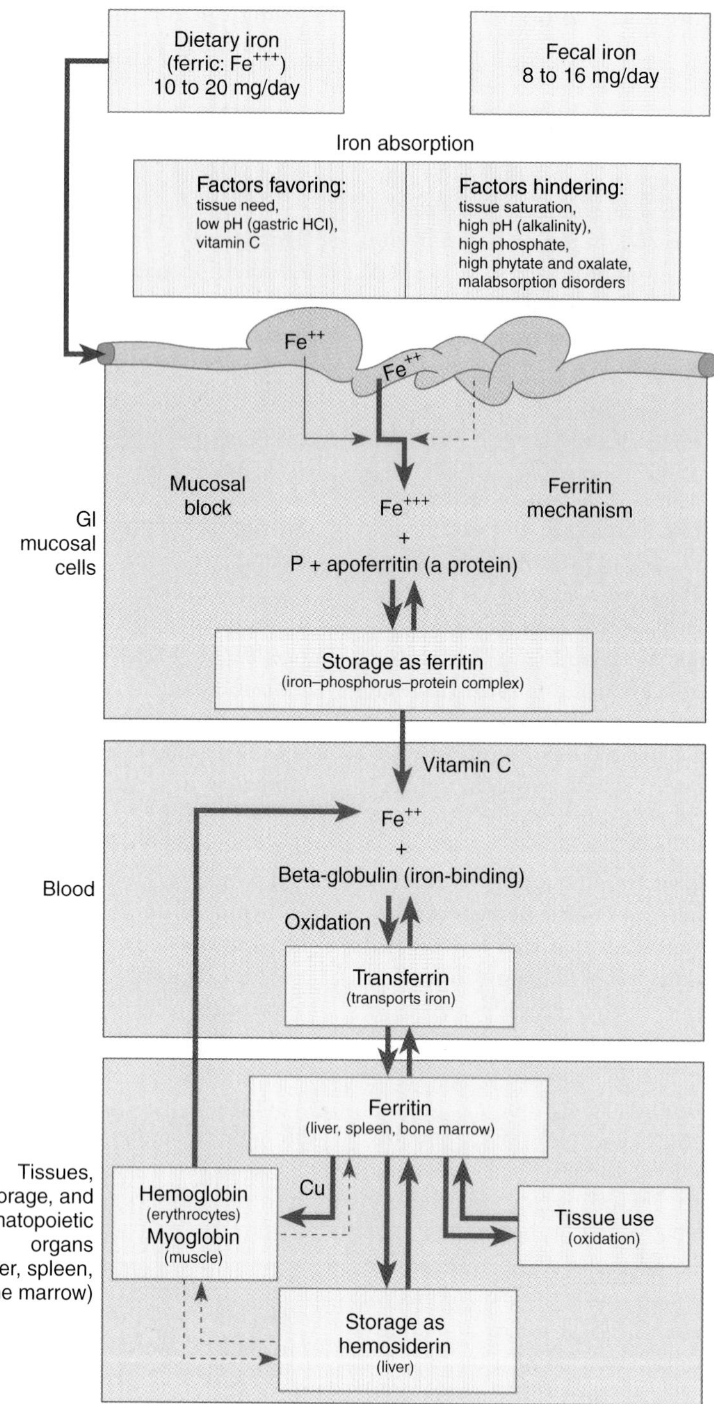

FIGURE 8-3 Summary of iron metabolism, showing its absorption, transport, main use in hemoglobin formation, and storage forms (ferritin and hemosiderin).

often excreted in the urine. Body iron is lost through the sloughing off of skin cells and gastrointestinal cells and through normal gastrointestinal and menstrual blood loss. Unusual blood loss such as that from heavy menstrual flow, childbirth, surgery, acute and chronic hemorrhage, gastrointestinal disease, or parasitic infestation may bring severe iron loss and depletion of body iron stores.

PHYSIOLOGIC FUNCTIONS OF IRON

Oxygen Transport

Iron is "pocketed" within the heme molecule, which is the nonprotein part of hemoglobin in the red blood cells. As such, iron functions as a major transporter of vital oxygen to the cells for respiration and metabolism. Iron is also a constituent of the similar compound, myoglobin, which delivers oxygen within muscle tissue.

Cellular Oxidation

Although present in small amounts, iron functions in the cells as a vital component of enzyme systems that oxidize glucose to produce energy.

Growth Needs

During growth, positive iron balance is imperative. At birth, the infant has a small 4- to 6-month supply of iron stored in the liver from fetal development. Breastfed infants obtain some iron in breast milk. However, because cow's milk does not supply iron, iron is added to commercial infant formulas. Supplementary iron-rich and fortified foods are added to the diet at about 4 to 6 months of age.[7] In this way the classic milk anemia of young children is prevented. Iron is also needed for continued growth and to build up reserves for the physiologic stress of adolescence, especially the onset of menses in girls. The woman's need for iron increases greatly during pregnancy to maintain the increased number of red blood cells in an expanded circulating blood volume and to supply the iron needed for storage in the developing fetal liver. Normal blood loss during delivery also reduces iron stores.

Brain and Cognitive Function

Iron has an important role in the function of nerve cells. Having a sufficient amount of available iron is important for infants and young children, whose brain and other nerve cells are growing rapidly[36,37] (see *To Probe Further* box).

IRON DEFICIENCY AND CLINICAL PROBLEMS

Because of the unique physiologic control of the body's iron content, clinical abnormalities may result from either a deficiency or an excess of iron.

Iron Deficiency Anemia

Surprisingly, iron deficiency occurs in both developed and underdeveloped countries for two main reasons: (1) the modest dietary supply is not readily absorbed, and (2) iron is lost through various avenues despite the efforts of the body to prevent the loss of absorbed iron. Iron deficiency results in a hypochromic microcytic anemia. This deficiency may stem from several causes.[33]

1. *Low iron intake.* Nutritional anemia occurs from an inadequate dietary supply of iron and other nutrients needed for hemoglobin and red blood cell production. The role of hemoglobin in providing oxygen to the cells is important in understanding the symptoms of anemia.
2. *Blood loss.* Hemorrhagic anemia occurs when there is excessive blood iron loss from uncontrolled bleeding. Aspirin causes small amounts of blood loss through the gastrointestinal tract; as a result, long-term use of aspirin in large amounts by older people for relief of pain can lower body iron stores.[38]
3. *Gastrectomy.* Postgastrectomy anemia occurs because of the lack of gastric hydrochloric acid necessary to liberate iron for absorption.
4. *Malabsorption.* Anemia can occur because of iron-binding agents that prevent absorption of iron or as a result of mucosal lesions that damage the absorbing surface.
5. *Chronic disease.* Anemia of chronic disease is caused by abnormalities in the recycling of iron from the hemoglobin of old red blood cells. It is associated with infections, inflammatory disorders, connective tissue diseases such as arthritis, and renal disease. This anemia occurs mostly in older persons.

Worldwide Problem of Iron-Deficiency Anemia

Nutritional anemias, with iron-deficiency anemia being the most common, are second only to protein-energy malnutrition as the most prevalent nutritional deficiency in the world. It is estimated that more than 2 billion persons around the world are anemic or iron deficient, with women and children most likely to be affected.[39] Iron deficiency anemia respects neither social class nor geographic situation; general iron balance in many places is precarious. Vulnerable periods in the life cycle include infancy and early childhood, adolescence, the reproductive years of women from menses to menopause, and pregnancy.

IRON REQUIREMENT

Dietary Reference Intake

Body iron stores vary widely, from about 300 mg or even less in women to 1000 mg in men. Iron losses in healthy men average about 1 mg/day; in women of child-bearing age, loss is about 1.5 mg/day. The addition for women is based on usual menstrual losses averaged over the month. When setting the RDA for iron, the expert panel took

TO PROBE FURTHER

Iron, Zinc and Iodine: Collaborators in Brain Development and Function

Does what we eat influence our ability to think, observe, remember, or decide? Although we know that protein-energy malnutrition, a condition involving deficiencies of many important nutrients, affects brain development in children and their ability to learn, we have come to recognize that several minerals—iron, zinc, and iodine—individually affect the brain and nervous system. Some of what we have learned has come from studies with animals; unfortunately, natural disasters involving famine or mothers and children deprived of important nutrients as a result of poverty have also provided evidence of the devastating effects of poor mineral nutrition. Deficiencies of these minerals have their greatest impact if they occur at a time of rapid brain growth in the fetus and during the first years of life, and damage occurring during these periods may not be reversible. Inadequate intakes of iron, zinc, and iodine affect cognitive performance and the ability to learn in older children and adults, but normal patterns are usually restored when appropriate nutrient levels are provided.

Consider the role of each of these minerals in the development and function of brain and nerve cells. High concentrations of iron are found in various parts of the brain that control mental activities that involve thinking and behavior as well as motor function. If less iron is available when these brain cells are growing, their iron concentration will be lower. Also, these brain cells have fewer receptors where important neurotransmitters, the chemical messengers necessary for the transmission of brain impulses, must attach.

Zinc is found in the highest amounts in the cerebral cortex of the brain, which handles higher thinking and reasoning skills. In zinc deficiency there are lower amounts of neurotransmitters available to send brain messages. Also, nerve cells do not grow as they should. A study in Egypt compared infants born to mothers who had adequate zinc during pregnancy with infants whose mothers had poor intakes of zinc during their pregnancy. The babies born to the well-nourished mothers had better scores on attention tests, although other factors such as the economic status or level of education of the parents or the amount of stimulation provided to the infants in the home could have influenced this outcome.

Iodine deficiency in fetal life or infancy results in the classic deficiency disease of cretinism with mental retardation, deaf-mutism, and neuromuscular problems. Iodine deficiency is considered by the World Health Organization to be the most common preventable cause of brain damage in the world. Iodine deficiency during the critical period of brain development results in a lower brain weight, fewer brain cells, and lower amounts of DNA in existing cells. Older children and adults who are iodine deficient tend to have poor school performance or work performance and general lethargy, likely caused by low thyroxin levels. In a village population with endemic iodine deficiency, intervention with iodine led to better school work and improved activity levels and well-being among all members of the community. That author noted that even the village dogs became more active.

A priority for researchers today is the effect of marginal iron and zinc deficiency on children and adults. Adolescents with poor iron status had improved learning and memory skills after receiving increased amounts of dietary iron. The Women-Infant-Children Supplementary Food Program (WIC) has evaluated the effect of iron intervention with anemic children and noted an improvement in their activity levels and general health. Poor zinc status also results in decreased activity levels in children, suggesting that evaluation of activity should be included in routine nutritional assessments. Intakes of both iron and zinc are low to marginal in many low-income children and adults in the United States, making this an important area for public health intervention.

References

Hetzel BS: Iodine and neuropsychological development, *J Nutr* 130(suppl):493S, 2000.

Pollitt F: Developmental sequel from early nutritional deficiencies: conclusive and probability judgments, *J Nutr* 130(suppl):350S, 2000.

Sandstead HH: Causes of iron and zinc deficiencies and their effects on brain, *J Nutr* 130(suppl):347S, 2000.

into consideration available iron balance studies, the estimated iron absorption rate of 18% from the U.S. food supply, and the need to maintain adequate iron reserves. The new RDAs for iron have been set at 18 mg/day for women aged 19 to 50 and 8 mg/day for men aged 19 and over.[33] Young women who consciously restrict their energy intakes in an effort to maintain low body weight are likely to have low iron intakes. For postmenopausal women whose menses have ceased, the RDA for iron is the same as that for adult men: 8 mg/day. Pregnancy has a "high iron cost," and the daily allowance increases to 27 mg/day. Iron needs fall during lactation because the menses are usually absent during this period; thus the RDA has been set at 9 mg/day for lactating mothers aged 19 and over.[33] Children's growth needs for iron are indicated in the Dietary Reference Intake table inside the front book cover.

Vegetarians who do not eat any meat and obtain all of their dietary iron from plant foods are at increased risk of iron deficiency. Not only is the bioavailability of iron lower in plant foods, but also heme iron is not present to enhance the absorption of iron from plant sources. It has been suggested that iron absorption from vegetarian diets may be only 10% compared with 18% for the typical American diet. For these reasons the Food and Nutrition Board recommends that vegetarian adult men take in 14 mg of iron/day and vegetarian premenopausal women take in 33 mg/day. Vegetarian adolescent girls need 26 mg/day. Note that these recommendations are about twice the RDAs for persons of comparable age who consume a mixed diet containing meat, fish, or poultry.[33]

IRON TOXICITY

Iron toxicity has not been observed as a result of normal food intake except among individuals in Southern Africa who consumed foods cooked in iron vessels and who also had a genetic tendency to absorb and store abnormally high amounts of iron.[33] However, there are cases of iron poisoning every year in the United States, especially among young children. In fact accidental iron overdose is the most common cause of poisoning death among children under the age of 6. At all times, caution concerning iron supplements is vital. The other cause of iron overload is the genetic disease hemochromatosis, which is present in 3 to 5:1000 persons in the United States but is often undiagnosed. Researchers recently identified the gene that causes this disease.[39]

Although iron is absolutely necessary, it becomes toxic at high levels. The UL for iron intake in all persons aged 14 and over is 45 mg/day.[33] Although it would seem unlikely that a person could reach such an intake level from food alone, current iron fortification practices, developed to meet the iron needs of women in the child-bearing years, add considerable amounts of iron to the diet. Persons who eat generous servings of cereals containing 15 to 18 mg of iron per serving, along with other iron-containing foods, and possibly supplements, will have intakes well above the RDA. A study of 1014 older people living in the community found that nearly 13% had body iron stores above the normal range.[40] Iron overload does appear to increase a person's risk of cancer, particularly colorectal cancer.[41] Young men and older men and women who have lower body requirements for iron need to be aware of the number of servings of iron-fortified foods they eat each day and avoid extremely high intakes. Iron supplements should never be taken unless supervised by a physician.

FOOD SOURCES OF IRON

The typical Western diet provides about 5 to 7 mg of iron per 1000 kcalories of energy.[39] Heme iron is an important dietary source of iron because it is more effectively absorbed than nonheme iron. Thus although heme iron usually supplies a smaller portion of the total dietary iron, it may supply a greater portion of the total absorbed iron. Nonheme iron makes up 60% of the iron from animal sources and 100% of the iron found in plant sources.[33]

Iron is widespread in the U.S. food supply, especially in meats (particularly organ meats such as liver), eggs, dried peas and beans, vegetables, and whole grain and fortified cereal products. Fortified cereals and grain products such as breakfast bars can contain from 1 mg to as much as 24 mg of iron per serving. Fortified breads and cereals provide about half of the iron intake of the U.S. population.[33] Heme iron provides less than 10% of the iron intake of girls and women and less than 12% of the iron intake of boys and men. Table 8-10 lists some comparative food sources of iron.

Iodine

Iodine shares with iron a longer history of study than the other trace minerals. Its function and requirement are clearly defined. The basic function of iodine is as a component of the hormone thyroxin, which controls the rate of energy metabolism in cells.

The body of the average adult contains a small amount of the trace element iodine, from 15 to 20 mg. Approximately 70% to 80% is in the thyroid gland, which has a remarkable ability to concentrate iodine.[42] Here, iodine participates in the synthesis of the thyroid hormone thyroxine.

ABSORPTION-EXCRETION BALANCE

Absorption

Dietary iodine is absorbed in the small intestine in the form of iodides. These are loosely bound with proteins and carried by the blood to the thyroid gland, which takes up as much as it needs to maintain an adequate

TABLE 8-10 Food Sources of Iron

Food Source	Quantity	Iron (mg)
Bread, Cereal, Rice, Pasta		
Bran flakes	¾ cup	4.50
Bran muffin, homemade	1 muffin	1.26
Bread, whole wheat	1 slice	0.86
Cream of wheat, regular (cooked)	¾ cup	7.70
Oatmeal (cooked)	¾ cup	1.19
Pasta, enriched (cooked)	1 cup	2.40
Rice, white, enriched (cooked)	1 cup	1.80
Wheat flakes	1 cup	4.45
Vegetables		
Artichoke (boiled)	1 med	1.62
Avocado (raw)	1 med	2.04
Broccoli (boiled)	½ cup	0.89
Brussels sprouts (boiled)	½ cup	0.94
Peas, green (boiled)	½ cup	1.24
Potato (baked, with skin)	1 med	2.75
Spinach (boiled)	½ cup	3.21
Fruits		
Dates (dried)	10 dates	0.96
Figs (dried)	10 figs	4.18
Prune juice (canned)	8 fl oz	3.03
Prunes (dried)	10 prunes	2.08
Raisins, seedless	⅔ cup	2.08
Meat, Poultry, Fish, Dried Beans, Eggs, Nuts		
Almonds (roasted)	1 oz (22 nuts)	1.08
Beef liver (fried)	3.5 oz	6.28
Beef top round, lean (broiled)	3.5 oz	2.88
Black-eyed peas (boiled)	1 cup	4.29
Cashews (roasted)	1 oz	1.70
Chicken, dark (roasted, without skin)	3.5 oz	1.33
Meat, Poultry, Fish, Dried Beans, Eggs, Nuts—cont'd		
Chicken, light (roasted, without skin)	3.5 oz	1.06
Chick-peas (boiled)	1 cup	4.74
Clams (steamed)	3 oz (9 small)	7.9
Crab, blue (steamed)	3 oz	0.77
Egg, whole	1 large	1.04
Ground beef, regular (broiled)	3.5 oz	2.44
Halibut (baked)	3 oz	0.91
Ham, canned (lean)	3.5 oz	0.94
Lentils (boiled)	1 cup	6.59
Lima beans (boiled)	1 cup	4.50
Mackerel (baked)	3 oz	1.33
Oysters (steamed)	3 oz (12 med)	1.9
Pinto beans (boiled)	1 cup	4.47
Shrimp (steamed)	3 oz (15 large)	2.62
Sirloin steak, lean (broiled)	3.5 oz	3.36
Sole (baked)	3.5 oz	1.40
Soybeans (boiled)	1 cup	8.84
Trout, rainbow (baked)	3 oz	2.07
Tuna, light, canned in water	3 oz	2.07
Milk, Dairy Products		
Cheddar cheese	1 oz	0.19
Cottage cheese, creamed	1 cup	0.29
Milk, skim	8 fl oz	0.10
Milk, whole	8 fl oz	0.12
Yogurt, whole milk	8 fl oz	0.11
Fats, Oils		
This food group is not an important source of iron		
Sugar		
Molasses, black	1 tbsp	3.20
Sugar, brown	1 cup	4.90

Recommended Dietary Allowances for adults: women aged 19-50, 18 mg; women aged ≥51, 8 mg; men, 8 mg.

level of hormone synthesis. About one third of this iodide is used to produce active thyroid hormone, and the remainder is used to form hormone precursors that are held for later use.

Excretion

Absorbed iodide not needed by the thyroid gland is excreted in the urine. More than 90% of dietary iodine appears in the urine.

Hormonal Control

A pituitary hormone, thyroid-stimulating hormone (TSH), stimulates the uptake of iodine by the thyroid cells in direct feedback response to the plasma levels of thyroid hormone. This normal physiologic feedback mechanism maintains a healthy circular balance between supply and demand. This is a characteristic pattern for governing all the hormones from the several endocrine glands that are controlled by the pituitary master gland.

PHYSIOLOGIC FUNCTION OF IODINE

Thyroid Hormone Synthesis

The major function of iodine in human metabolism is its participation in the synthesis of the thyroid hormone thyroxine. The hormone thyroxine in turn stimulates

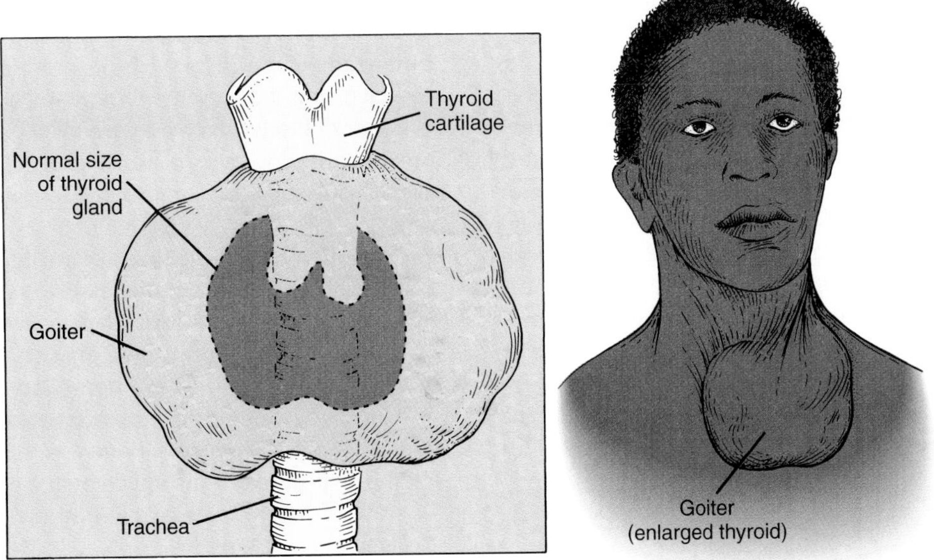

FIGURE 8-4 Goiter. The extreme enlargement shown here is a result of extended duration of iodine deficiency.

cell oxidation and regulates basal metabolic rate (BMR), apparently by increasing oxygen uptake and the reaction rates of enzyme systems handling glucose. In this role iodine indirectly exerts tremendous control on the body's total metabolism. Thyroid hormone also may regulate protein synthesis in the developing brain and other organs.[42]

Plasma Thyroxine

Free thyroxine, with its associated iodine, is secreted into the bloodstream and bound to plasma protein for transport to body cells as needed. After being used to stimulate oxidation in the cell, the hormone is degraded in the liver and the iodine is excreted in bile as inorganic iodine.

IODINE DEFICIENCY AND CLINICAL PROBLEMS

Abnormal Thyroid Function

Both hyperthyroidism and hypothyroidism affect the rate of iodine uptake and use and thereby influence the body's overall metabolic rate.

Iodine Deficiency Disorder: Goiter

Endemic goiter, characterized by great enlargement of the thyroid gland, occurs in persons living where water and soil, and thus locally grown foods, contain little iodine. Some 800 million persons live in iodine-deficient areas in underdeveloped countries of the world where endemic goiter is a large health problem. In such situations the iodine-starved thyroid gland cannot produce a normal quantity of thyroxine. The low blood level of thyroid hormone causes secretion of TSH by the pituitary gland. The pituitary gland continues putting out TSH, and these large quantities of TSH continue to stimulate the thyroid gland, calling on it to produce the thyroxine that it cannot supply. In this iodine-deficient state, the only response that the thyroid can make is to increase the amount of thyroglobulin (colloid), which then accumulates in the thyroid follicles. Such a gland becomes increasingly engorged and may attain a tremendous size, weighing 500 to 700 g (1 to 1½ lb) or more (Figure 8-4). Some areas of the world have severe iodine deficiency, with related disease and mortality rates. In the West African goiter belt of New Guinea, Zaire, and the Sudan, iodized rapeseed oil and iodine added to the drinking water have eradicated severe endemic goiter.[42,43]

Goiter may also be caused by the use of foods that contain substances that inhibit important steps in the synthesis of thyroxin by the thyroid gland. Pearl millet, a cereal grain used by many people in the Sudan region of Africa, was found to be the cause of goiter in some preschool children.[44] Iodine deficiency has been referred to as the leading cause of preventable mental retardation in the world, and breastfed infants of iodine-deficient mothers are especially at risk during periods of rapid brain development.[45]

---

goiter Enlargement of the thyroid gland caused by lack of sufficient available iodine to produce the thyroid hormone thyroxine.

IODINE REQUIREMENT

Dietary Reference Intake

Tests for urinary iodide excretion can be used to indicate iodine intake and status, as well as risk for goiter or other iodine deficiency disorders. These disorders can range from severe cretinism with mental retardation to barely visible enlargement of the thyroid gland. Using information from balance studies, the new RDA for iodine for both men and women was set at 150 μg/day.[33] To meet the needs of both mother and developing fetus, the RDA in pregnancy is raised to 220 μg/day. To ensure a sufficient amount of iodine in breast milk to meet infant growth needs, the RDA for lactating mothers is 290 μg/day. The demand for iodine is increased during periods of accelerated adolescent growth. Thus the allowance for youth aged 14 to 18 is set at 150 μg/day, the same as that for adults.

IODINE OVERLOAD

Incidental dietary intake of iodine may occur through methods used in dairy farming. These dairy farm sources include iodized salt licks for the animals and the use of iodophors, iodine-containing chemicals, for sanitizing udders, milking machines, and milk tanks. Other iodine-containing compounds that find their way into the human food supply are the iodates used as dough conditioners in breads, erythrosine used as food coloring, and derivatives of iodine supplements added to animal feeds. Various case reports of iodine toxicity have indicated that levels of iodine obtained through foods, dietary supplements, or topical medications may exceed by many times the RDA.

FOOD SOURCES OF IODINE

Seafood provides a considerable amount of iodine. The quantity in other food sources varies widely depending on the iodine content of the soil and the iodine compounds used in food processing. The commercial iodizing of table salt (1 mg to every 10 g of salt) provides a main dietary source. Processed foods may contain higher levels of iodine than the natural ingredients, based on the use of various iodine-containing additives such as calcium iodate and potassium iodate.[46] Some iodine deficiencies have been observed in persons who avoid salt.

Other Essential Trace Elements

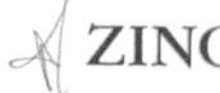

ZINC

Zinc has risen to nutritional prominence based on its clinical significance. Its wide tissue distribution reflects its broad metabolic activity as a component of key cell enzymes and its strong influence on growth. An adult's total zinc content ranges from about 2.3 mmol (1.5 g) in women to 3.8 mmol (2.5 g) in men.[47] It is present in minute quantities in all body organs, tissues, fluids, and secretions. Although it is vital throughout life, it is especially important through growth periods such as pregnancy and lactation, infancy and childhood, and adolescence.[48-50] Zinc is closely involved with DNA and RNA metabolism and protein synthesis, and if deficient, tissue growth and metabolism cannot progress at normal rates.

Zinc Deficiency and Clinical Problems

Because of its widespread metabolic use, a number of clinical problems caused by zinc deficiency can occur.

1. *Hypogonadism.* Diminished function of the gonads and dwarfism can result from pronounced human zinc deficiency during critical growth periods.
2. *Taste and smell defects.* Hypogeusia (diminished taste) and hyposmia (diminished smell) sometimes improve with zinc supplementation in individuals who are zinc deficient.
3. *Wound healing.* The healing of wounds or tissue injury from physiologic stress, inflammation, or other causes are retarded in zinc-deficient persons. Older persons with pressure sores can sometimes benefit from zinc supplementation. Frequently, hospital and institutional diets, especially when combined with poor food intake by chronically ill persons, provide inadequate amounts of dietary zinc.
4. *Growth, development, and life cycle needs.* Periods of rapid growth among infants, children, and adolescents carry special needs for zinc. Young children with inadequate zinc have stunted growth because proteins necessary for the linear growth of the long bones are not produced.[51] Sexual maturation is delayed in male adolescents deprived of adequate zinc. Poor zinc intake during pregnancy can result in congenital malformations and low birth weight. During pregnancy a greater proportion of dietary zinc is absorbed by the intestine, which may be a response to increased body need.[2] Older persons with poor appetites who subsist on marginal diets are vulnerable to zinc deficiency that results in impaired immune function.[52]
5. *Malabsorption disease.* Zinc deficiency occurs with malabsorption diseases such as Crohn's disease. The ulcerative lesions in the mucosal surface hinder the absorption of zinc, and zinc intake is also likely to be low as a result of anorexia or selection of foods low in zinc.

ZINC REQUIREMENT

Dietary Reference Intake

As with the trace element iron, optimal zinc intake cannot be assumed among the U.S. population. The adult RDAs are set at 11 mg for men and 8 mg for women[33]; the requirement for women is lower because of their generally lower body weight. To ensure sufficient zinc for optimum growth and development, RDAs for the adolescent years of 14 to 18 are 11 and 9 mg for boys and girls, respectively.

TABLE 8-11 Food Sources of Zinc

Food Source	Quantity	Zinc (mg)
Bread, Cereal, Rice, Pasta		
Bran muffin, homemade	1 muffin	1.08
Bread, whole wheat	1 slice	0.42
Cream of wheat (cooked)	¾ cup	0.24
English muffin, plain	1 muffin	0.41
Oatmeal (cooked)	¾ cup	0.86
Pasta, enriched (cooked)	1 cup	0.70
Wheat flakes	1 cup	0.63
Vegetables		
Artichoke (boiled)	1 med	0.43
Asparagus (boiled)	½ cup (6 spears)	0.43
Avocado (raw)	1 med	0.73
Broccoli (raw)	½ cup	0.18
Brussels sprouts (boiled)	½ cup (4 sprouts)	0.25
Carrots (raw)	1 med	0.14
Collards (boiled)	½ cup	0.23
Kale (boiled, chopped)	½ cup	0.15
Peas, green (boiled)	½ cup	0.95
Potato (baked, with skin)	1 med	0.65
Tomato (raw)	1 med	0.13
Fruits		
Apricots (raw)	3 med	0.28
Banana (raw)	1 med	0.19
Cantaloupe (raw)	½ cup	0.25
Figs (dried)	10 figs	0.94
Orange juice (fresh)	8 fl oz	0.13
Orange, navel (raw)	1 med	0.08
Meat, Poultry, Fish, Dried Beans, Eggs, Nuts		
Almonds (roasted)	1 oz (22 nuts)	1.39
Beef liver (fried)	3.5 oz	6.07
Cashews (roasted)	1 oz	1.59
Chicken, dark (roasted, without skin)	3.5 oz	2.80
Chicken, light (roasted without skin)	3.5 oz	1.23
Chick-peas (boiled)	1 cup	2.51
Clams, canned	3 oz	2.32
Crab, Alaska king (steamed)	3 oz	6.48
Egg, whole	1 large	0.72
Ham, canned (lean)	3.5 oz	1.93
Kidney beans (boiled)	1 cup	1.89
Lentils (boiled)	1 cup	2.50
Lima beans (boiled)	1 cup	1.79
Lobster (steamed)	3 oz	2.48
Oysters (steamed)	3 oz (12 med)	25.8
Peanuts (roasted)	1 oz	0.93
Soybeans (boiled)	1 cup	1.98
Milk, Dairy Products		
Milk, skim	8 fl oz	0.98
Milk, whole	8 fl oz	0.93
Yogurt, whole milk	8 fl oz	1.34
Fats, Oils, Sugar		
This food group is not an important source of zinc		

Recommended Dietary Allowances for adults: women, 8 mg; men, 11 mg.

Food Sources of Zinc

The best sources of dietary zinc are seafood (especially oysters), meat, and eggs. Less rich sources are legumes and whole grains. Because meat and seafood supply a major portion of the zinc in the American diet, vegetarians (especially women) may be at particular risk for development of marginal zinc deficiency. Many grain and legume foods that are the principal sources of dietary zinc in the vegetarian diet contain phytates that bind zinc and interfere with its absorption.[47] Although zinc deficiency must be avoided, excess zinc interferes with the absorption of copper, the next trace element we will discuss. Table 8-11 lists some comparative food sources of zinc.

COPPER

This trace element has frequently been called the "iron twin." The two elements are metabolized in much the same way and share functions as cell enzyme components. Both are related to energy production and hemoglobin synthesis. Copper is widely distributed in natural foods; therefore a general dietary deficiency is rare.[33] Copper deficiency has been observed only under special circumstances such as unsupplemented total parenteral nutrition (TPN) feeding, high levels of zinc intake, or premature infants who are fed only cow's milk, which is low in copper. Until recent studies became available the Food and Nutrition Board was unable to determine an RDA for copper. It is now recommended that adults take in 900 μg/day (0.9 mg/day) of copper.[33] In a Maryland study of adults, more than half of the participants had copper intakes below this level, but copper intake varies widely from day to day; therefore it is necessary to evaluate food intake over a long period to find a person's true intake.[53] Copper is widely distributed in natural foods but, like

cretinism A congenital disease resulting from absence or deficiency of normal thyroid secretion, characterized by physical deformity, dwarfism, mental retardation, and often goiters.

many of the trace elements, can be lost in food processing. Its richest sources are organ meats (especially liver), seafood (especially oysters), nuts, and seeds; smaller amounts are found in whole grains and legumes.

MANGANESE

The total adult body content of manganese is about 20 mg, found mainly in the liver, bones, pancreas, and pituitary gland. Although it is considered a dietary essential, manganese is toxic at high levels.[54] It functions like other trace elements as an essential part of cell enzymes that catalyze a number of important metabolic reactions. Manganese deficiency, indicated by low serum levels, has been reported in diabetes and pancreatic insufficiency, as well as in kwashiorkor and protein-energy malnutrition. Toxicity has occurred as an industrial disease syndrome in miners and other workers who had prolonged exposure to manganese dust. In these cases excess manganese accumulated in the liver and central nervous system, producing psychiatric disturbances and severe neuromuscular symptoms that resemble those of Parkinson's disease. The AI for manganese is 2.3 mg/day for men and 1.8 mg/day for women.[33] The typical American diet supplies manganese at a level of 1.6 mg/1000 kcalories. The best food sources are plant foods—cereal grains, legumes, seeds, nuts, leafy vegetables, tea, and coffee. Animal foods are relatively poor sources.

CHROMIUM

The precise amount of chromium present in body tissues is not well defined because of difficulties in analysis, but total body content is small, less than 6 mg. Chromium is a bone-seeking element and accumulates in the bone, spleen, liver, and kidney.[55] It functions as an essential component of a low-molecular-weight chromium complex,[56] previously referred to as the GTF (glucose tolerance factor), which facilitates the action of insulin. At one time the proposed GTF was believed to actively control glucose transport, but such a molecule has not been identified. Moreover, the glucose intolerance associated with diabetes mellitus does not appear to be related to chromium deficiency. Various researchers have tested the effect of chromium supplementation on reducing the high blood glucose levels that occur in diabetes; however, such efforts have been unsuccessful. The amount of chromium needed for optimum health is controversial, especially with the current interest in chromium picolinate as a potential ergogenic aid for body-builders.[57]

Because research describing the general body need for chromium is limited, an AI rather than an RDA has been developed for this nutrient. The AI for men aged 19 to 50 is 35 μg/day, and that for women in this age range is 25 μg/day.[33] Because persons above age 50 have lower energy intakes, their AIs are lower: 30 and 20 μg/day for men and women, respectively. Brewer's yeast is a rich source of chromium. Good food sources include liver, cheddar cheese, and wheat germ. Most grain products, especially whole grains, also provide this nutrient.

COBALT

Cobalt occurs in only minute traces in body tissues, and the main storage area is the liver. As an essential component of cobalamin (vitamin B_{12}), the known functions of cobalt are associated with red blood cell formation and support of the myelin sheath surrounding nerve fibers in the central nervous system. The normal cobalt blood level, including cobalt in transit and in red blood cells, is exceedingly small, about 1 μg/dl. Cobalt is provided in the human diet only by vitamin B_{12}. The human requirement is unknown but is evidently minute. For example, as little as 0.045 to 0.09 μg/day maintains bone marrow function in patients with pernicious anemia. Cobalt is widely distributed in nature. However, humans obtain their cobalt in preformed vitamin B_{12}, synthesized in animals by intestinal bacterial flora.

SELENIUM

Selenium is deposited in all body tissues except fat. Highest concentrations occur in the liver, kidney, heart, and spleen. Selenium functions as an integral component of an antioxidant enzyme that protects cells and lipid membranes against oxidative damage. In this role, selenium balances with tocopherol (vitamin E), each sparing the other.[58] This protective function is widespread, as this important selenium-containing enzyme is found in most body tissues. The importance of selenium in even the early stages of life is suggested by the discovery of highly bioavailable selenium compounds in breast milk.[54] The RDA for all adults aged 19 and over is 55 μg/day.[59] Food sources vary with the selenium soil content; usually good sources include seafood, legumes, whole grains, low-fat meats, and dairy products, with smaller amounts occurring in vegetables.

MOLYBDENUM

Molybdenum functions as an enzyme cofactor in numerous metabolic activities involving the hydroxylation of various molecules.[33] The precise occurrence of molybdenum in human tissues and its clear coenzyme roles are still being investigated. The RDA has been set at 45 μg/day for men and women. The amounts of molybdenum in foods vary considerably, depending on the soil content in which the food is grown. In general, however, the richest sources include legumes, whole grains, and nuts. The poorer sources include animal products, fruit, and many vegetables.

FLUORIDE

The trace element fluoride accumulates in the calcified tissues in the body. In human nutrition, fluoride protects against the loss of mineral in bones and teeth. When fluoride is present at the time of formation of the calcium-phosphorus crystals in bones and teeth, a fluoride ion (F^-) replaces a hydroxyl ion (OH^-) in the crystal, resulting in a substance that is more resistant to resorption (resorption is the breaking down of bone mineral crystals and release of the minerals into solution). The principal cause of dental caries is the action of acid in dissolving the tooth enamel. This acid is produced by microorganisms feeding on fermentable carbohydrates adhering to the teeth after a meal or snack. Fluoride-containing crystals are more resistant to the erosive effect of the bacterial acid.[60]

Based on its ability to protect against dental caries, an AI for fluoride has been set at 2 mg/day for children aged 9 to 13 and 3 mg/day for adolescents aged 14 through 18. The AI for adult men is 4 mg/day, and that for adult women is 3 mg/day.[11] Fish, fish products, and tea contain the highest concentration of fluoride. Cooking in fluoridated water raises the level in many foods. Fluoridated dental products also contribute to fluoride intake. The public health measure of adding fluoride to public water supplies in the amount of 1 part per million (p.p.m.) provides adequate amounts and has contributed to a significant decline in dental caries in those communities. We will discuss fluoride in relation to its role in the treatment of osteoporosis in Chapter 13.

Probable Essential Trace Elements

The metabolic functions of the remaining trace elements that have been detected in human tissue are less well understood. However, they have been found to be essential in animal nutrition and are probably essential in human nutrition in a similar manner, as cofactors for cell enzymes in key metabolic reactions and as structural components in special tissues. Such an example is the apparent role of boron with calcium in bone building. These eight trace elements are silicon (Si), vanadium (V), nickel (Ni), tin (Sn), cadmium (Cd), arsenic (As), aluminum (Al), and boron (B). Apparently most of these trace elements are needed in such minute amounts that primary dietary deficiency is highly unlikely. However, with increased use of long-term TPN therapy, induced deficiencies are increasing in clinical importance.

WATER-ELECTROLYTE BALANCE

A number of the major minerals just described function as electrolytes in controlling the body's vital water balance. This collective function is fundamental to health and often a vital part of patient care. In this section we will look at the three basic interdependent factors that control this balance: (1) the water itself (the *solvent* base for solutions), (2) the various particles (solutes) in solution in the water, and (3) the separating membranes that control the flow.

WATER BALANCE

Body Water Distribution

If you are a woman, your body is about 50% to 55% water. If you are a man, your body is about 55% to 60% water. Men have a higher water content because they have a greater proportion of muscle mass and a smaller proportion of fat. Striated muscle contains more water than any body tissue other than blood. The remaining 40% of a man's weight is about 18% protein and related substances, 15% fat, and 7% minerals. A woman's remaining body composition is about the same except for a somewhat smaller muscle mass and a larger fat deposit. Body fat has a low water content compared with body muscle.

Water Functions

Body water performs three essential functions: (1) it helps give structure and form to the body through the *turgor* it provides for tissues, (2) it creates the water-based environment necessary for the vast array of chemical actions and reactions that comprise the body's metabolism and sustain life, and (3) it provides the means for maintaining a stable body temperature.

Water Compartments

Consider the water in your body in two compartments, as shown in Figure 8-5: (1) the total water outside of cells—the *extracellular fluid compartment* and (2) the total water inside of cells—the *intracellular fluid compartment.*

1. *Extracellular fluid* (*ECF*). Water outside of cells makes up about 20% of the total body weight. It consists of four parts: (1) blood plasma, which accounts for about 25% of the ECF and 5% of body weight; (2) interstitial fluid, the water surrounding the cells; (3) secretory fluid, the water circulating in transit; and (4) dense tissue fluid, water in dense connective tissue, cartilage, and bone.
2. *Intracellular fluid* (*ICF*). Water inside cells makes up about 40% to 45% of the total body weight. Because the body cells handle our vast metabolic activity, it is no surprise that the total water inside the cells is about twice the amount outside the cells.

---

low-molecular-weight chromium complex (previously referred to as glucose tolerance factor [GTF]) A biologically active complex of chromium that facilitates the reaction of insulin with receptor sites on tissues.

interstitial fluid The fluid situated between parts or in the interspaces of a tissue.

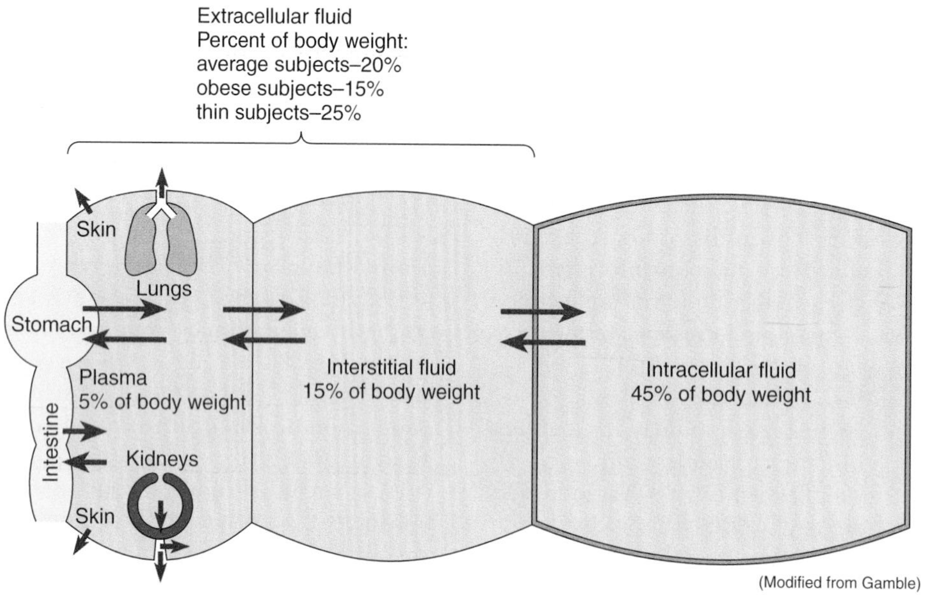

(Modified from Gamble)

FIGURE 8-5 Body fluid compartments. Note the relative total quantities of water in the intracellular compartment and in the extracellular compartment. (*Data from Gamble JL:* Chemical anatomy, physiology, and pathology of extracellular fluid, *Cambridge, Mass, 1964, Harvard University Press.*)

TABLE 8-12 Approximate Daily Adult Intake and Output of Water

	Intake (Replacement) ml/day		Output (Loss) (ml/day) Obligatory (Insensible) ml/day	Output (Loss) (ml/day) Additional (According to Need) ml/day
Preformed		Lungs	350	
Liquids	1200-1500	Skin		
In foods	700-1000	Diffusion	350	
Metabolism	200-300	Sweat	100	±250
(oxidation of food)				
		Kidneys	900	±500
		Feces	150	
TOTAL	2100-2800 (≈2600 ml/day)	TOTAL	1850 (≈2600 ml/day)	750

OVERALL WATER BALANCE: INTAKE AND OUTPUT

The average adult metabolizes from 2.5 to 3 L of water per day in a constant turnover balanced between intake and output. This water enters and leaves the body via various routes, controlled by the basic mechanisms of thirst and hormonal activity.

Water enters the body in three main forms: (1) preformed water taken in as water and in other beverages that are consumed, (2) preformed water in foods that are eaten, and (3) metabolic water, a product of cell oxidation.

Water leaves the body through the kidneys, skin, and lungs and through fecal elimination via the large intestine.

These routes of intake and output must be in constant balance. This balance is summarized in Table 8-12. Abnormal conditions, such as diarrhea or dysentery, produce much greater losses, causing serious clinical problems if prolonged. Extensive loss of body fluids can be especially dangerous in infants and children. Their bodies contain a greater percentage of total body water, and much more of the water is outside of the cells and easily available for loss.

FORCES CONTROLLING WATER DISTRIBUTION

Forces that influence and control the distribution of body water revolve around two factors: (1) the solutes or particles in solution in body water and (2) the separating membranes between water compartments.

Solutes

A variety of particles occur in body water at varying concentrations. Two main types—electrolytes and plasma proteins—control water balance.

Electrolytes. Several minerals provide major electrolytes for the body. In this role, these small inorganic elements are called electrolytes because they are free in solution and carry an electrical charge. These free, charged forms are called *ions,* that is, atoms, elements, or groups of atoms that, in solution, carry either a positive or negative electrical charge. An ion carrying a positive charge is called a *cation;* examples are sodium (Na^+)—major cation of water outside cells, potassium (K^+)—major cation of water inside cells, calcium (Ca^{2+}), and magnesium (Mg^{2+}). Conversely, an ion carrying a negative charge is called an *anion;* examples are chloride (Cl^-), bicarbonate (HCO_3^-), phosphate (HPO_4^{2-}), and sulfate (SO_4^{2-}). Because of their small size, these ions or electrolytes can diffuse freely across body membranes; thus they produce a major force controlling movement of water within the body.

Plasma proteins. Organic substances of large molecular size, mainly albumin and globulin of the plasma proteins, influence the shift of water in and out of capillaries in balance with their surrounding water. In this function, these plasma proteins are called *colloids* (from the Greek word *kolla* for "glue") and form colloidal solutions. Because of their large size, these particles or molecules do not pass readily through separating capillary membranes. Therefore they normally remain in the blood vessels, where they exert colloidal osmotic pressure (COP) to maintain the vascular blood volume.

Organic compounds of small molecular size. Other organic compounds of small size, such as glucose, urea, and amino acids, diffuse freely but do not influence shifts of water unless they occur in abnormally large concentrations. For example, the large amount of glucose in the urine of a patient with uncontrolled diabetes mellitus causes an abnormal osmotic diuresis or excess water output.

Water and solutes move across the body's separating membranes via the basic physiologic mechanisms that handle fluid balances according to body need. These mechanisms include osmosis, diffusion, filtration, active transport, and pinocytosis.

INFLUENCE OF ELECTROLYTES ON WATER BALANCE

Measurement of Electrolytes

The concentration of electrolytes in a given solution determines the chemical activity of that solution. It is the number of particles in a solution that is the important factor in determining chemical combining power. Thus electrolytes are measured according to the total number of particles in solution. Each particle contributes chemical combining power according to its valence, rather than according to the total weight of the particle. The unit of measure commonly used is an *equivalent.* Because small amounts are usually in question, most physiologic measurements are expressed in terms of milliequivalents (mEq). The term refers to the number of ions—cations and anions—in solution, as determined by their concentration in a given volume. This measure is expressed as the number of milliequivalents per liter *(mEq/L).*

Electrolyte Balance

Electrolytes are distributed in the body water compartments in a definite pattern, which has physiologic significance. This distribution pattern maintains stable electrochemical neutrality in body fluid solutions. According to biochemical and electrochemical laws, a stable solution must have equal numbers of positive and negative particles. It must be electrically neutral. When shifts and losses occur, compensating shifts and gains follow to maintain this dynamic balance, *essential electroneutrality.*

Electrolyte Control of Body Hydration

As mentioned earlier, ionized sodium is the chief cation of ECF, and ionized potassium is the chief cation of ICF. These two electrolytes control the amount of water retained in any given compartment. The usual bases for shifts in water from one compartment to the other are ECF changes in concentration of these electrolytes. The terms *hypertonic* and *hypotonic dehydration* refer to the

---

colloidal osmotic pressure (COP) Pressure produced by the protein molecules in the plasma and in the cell. Because proteins are large molecules, they do not pass through the separating membranes of the capillary cells. Thus they remain in their respective compartments, exerting a constant osmotic pull that protects vital plasma and cell fluid volumes in these compartments.

---

electrolyte concentration of the water outside the cell, which in turn causes a shift of water into or out of the cell to maintain balance, respectively.

INFLUENCE OF PLASMA PROTEIN ON WATER BALANCE

Capillary Fluid Shift Mechanism

Water is constantly circulated throughout the body by the blood vessels. However, fluid must get out of the vessels to service the tissues and then be drawn back into the vessels to maintain the normal transporting flow. Two main opposing pressures—COP from plasma protein (mainly albumin) and the hydrostatic pressure (blood pressure) of the capillary blood flow—provide balanced control of water and solute movement across capillary membranes. The body maintains this constant flow of water and the materials it is carrying to and from the cell by means of a shifting balance of these two pressures. It is a filtration process operating according to the differences in osmotic pressure on either side of the capillary membrane.

When blood first enters the capillary system, the greater blood pressure forces water and small solutes (glucose, for example) out into the tissues to bathe and nourish the cells. The plasma protein particles, however, are too large to go through the pores of capillary membranes. Hence the protein remains in the vessel and exerts the now greater COP that draws the returning fluid and its materials back into circulation from the cells. This process is called the capillary fluid shift mechanism. It provides one of the most important and widespread homeostatic mechanisms in the body to maintain water balance, without which cells would die.

Cell Fluid Control

Much as plasma protein provides COP to maintain the volume of extracellular fluid, cell protein helps to provide the osmotic pressure that maintains the volume of fluid inside the cell. Also, ionized potassium within the cell guards cell water in balance with ionized sodium guarding water outside the cell. This balance supports the flow of water, nutrients, and metabolites in and out of cells to sustain life.

INFLUENCE OF HORMONES ON WATER BALANCE

Antidiuretic Hormone Mechanism

The antidiuretic hormone (ADH), also called vasopressin, is secreted by the posterior lobe of the pituitary gland. It causes reabsorption of water by the kidneys according to body need; thus it is a water-conserving mechanism. In any stress situation with threatened or real loss of body water, this hormone is triggered to hold on to precious body water.

Aldosterone Mechanism

Aldosterone is primarily a sodium-conserving hormone, related in its operation to the renin-angiotensin system, but in doing this job it also exerts a secondary control over water loss. The full name of this mechanism is the renin-angiotensin-aldosterone mechanism because renin, an enzyme from the kidney, and angiotensin, the active product of its substrate (angiotensinogen) from the liver, are the intermediate substances used to trigger the adrenal glands to produce the aldosterone hormone. Both aldosterone and ADH are activated by stress situations such as injury or surgery.

TO SUM UP

Minerals are inorganic substances that are widely distributed in nature. They build body tissues; activate, regulate, and control metabolic processes; and help transmit messages across nerve fibers.

Minerals are classified as (1) major minerals and (2) trace elements. Major minerals are required in relatively large quantities and make up 60% to 80% of all the inorganic material in the body. Trace elements, required in quantities as small as a microgram (μg), make up less than 1% of the body's inorganic material. Seven major minerals and 10 trace minerals are known to be essential in human nutrition; another 8 trace elements are probably essential and their possible roles in the body are being studied. The major minerals include calcium and phosphorus, which play important roles in bone health, energy metabolism, and nerve transmission; magnesium, found in bone and a participant in many metabolic reactions; sodium, potassium and chloride, particles in body fluids that control water balance; and sulfur, found in the amino acids methionine and cysteine and other organic compounds. Essential trace elements include iron, necessary for the formation of hemoglobin and energy metabolism within the cell mitochondria; iodine, a component of thyroxin that controls basal metabolism; zinc, vital for normal growth and maturation; chromium, necessary for the binding of insulin to cell membranes; selenium, an important antioxidant; fluoride, a protector of mineral crystals in the bones and teeth; cobalt, a component of vitamin B_{12}; and molybdenum and manganese, active enzyme cofactors.

Overall water balance in the body is regulated by fluid intake and output. The distribution of body fluids is mainly controlled by two types of solutes: (1) electrolytes, which are charged mineral elements and other particles derived from inorganic compounds, and (2) plasma proteins, mainly albumin, that are too large to pass through capillary membranes but influence the flow of fluid from one compartment to another. These solute particles influence the distribution of fluid passing across cell or capillary membranes to maintain normal fluid levels in the intracellular and extracellular compartments. ADH acts on the kidney to reabsorb water as needed, and aldosterone hormone, secreted by the adrenal gland, acts in a similar way to conserve body sodium.

■ Questions for Review

1. List the seven major minerals and describe their (a) physiologic function, (b) clinical and metabolic problems created by dietary deficiency or excess, and (c) dietary sources.
2. List the 10 trace elements with proven essentiality for humans. Which have established Dietary Reference Intake (DRI) standards? Which have estimated minimum daily intakes? Why has it been difficult to establish DRIs for all nutrients?
3. The AI for calcium for people over age 50 is 1200 mg/day. Develop a menu for a frail 83-year-old woman that will provide this level of calcium.
4. You are working with a teenage woman who does not eat meat, fish, or poultry. She is concerned about her weight and eats only the minimum number of portions listed in the *Food Guide Pyramid* (two milks, two fruits, three vegetables, two meats, and six grains). Based on this *Food Guide Pyramid* pattern, list the foods with portion sizes that you would select to provide her RDA of 18 mg of iron. When making your selections, consider other factors in the diet that will enhance or impede the absorption of the iron you provide.
5. What causes the edema in protein-energy malnutrition?
6. Why does prolonged diarrhea lead to potassium depletion?
7. Go to a nearby grocery store or drug store that sells mineral supplements. Check five supplements marketed for children (use the DRI of the age group noted on the label) and five supplements marketed for adults. Prepare a table that lists each brand and include (a) the percent of the DRI of each mineral provided and (b) the cost of a 1-day supply of the supplement. Did any of the supplements you examined exceed the UL for any nutrient, and, if so, what is the danger of toxicity? Based on cost and content, would an individual be better off spending that extra amount of money for food?

capillary fluid shift mechanism Process that controls the movement of water and small molecules in solution (electrolytes, nutrients) between the blood in the capillary and the surrounding interstitial area. Filtration of water and solutes out of the capillary at the arteriole end and reabsorption at the venule end are accomplished by shifts in balance between the intracapillary hydrostatic blood pressure and the colloidal osmotic pressure exerted by the plasma proteins.

renin-angiotensin-aldosterone mechanism Three-stage system of sodium conservation, hence control of water loss, in response to diminished filtration pressure in the kidney nephrons: (1) pressure loss causes kidney to secrete the enzyme renin, which combines with and activates angiotensinogen from the liver; (2) active angiotensin stimulates the adjacent adrenal gland to release the hormone aldosterone; and (3) aldosterone causes reabsorption of sodium from the kidney nephrons and water follows.

■ References

1. Weaver CM, Heaney RP: Calcium. In Shils ME et al, eds: *Modern nutrition in health and disease,* ed 9, Philadelphia, 1999, Lippincott Williams & Wilkins.
2. King JC: Effect of reproduction on the bioavailability of calcium, zinc and selenium, *J Nutr* 131:1355S, 2001.
3. U.S. Department of Agriculture: Continuing Survey of Food Intake by Individuals, 1994-1996 (accessible at *http://www.barc.usda.gov/bhnrc/foodsurvey/Products9496.html*).
4. Wosje KS, Specker BL: Role of calcium in bone health during childhood, *Nutr Rev* 58(9):253, 2000.
5. Weaver CM: Calcium and the prevention of osteoporosis, *Nutr MD* 26(9):1, 2000.
6. Teegarden D et al: Previous milk consumption is associated with greater bone density in young women, *Am J Clin Nutr* 69:1014, 1999.
7. Kleinman RE, ed: *Pediatric nutrition handbook,* ed 4, Elk Grove Village, Ill, 1998, American Academy of Pediatrics.
8. Wolf RL et al: Factors associated with calcium absorption efficiency in pre- and perimenopausal women, *Am J Clin Nutr* 72:466, 2000.
9. Heaney RP: Dietary protein and phosphorus do not affect calcium absorption, *Am J Clin Nutr* 72:758, 2000.
10. Erdman JW, Stillman RJ, Boileau RA: Provocative relation between soy and bone maintenance, *Am J Clin Nutr* 72:679, 2000.
11. Food and Nutrition Board, National Academy of Sciences: *Dietary reference intakes for calcium, phosphorus, magnesium, vitamin D, and fluoride,* Washington, DC, 1997, National Academy Press.
12. Dwyer JT et al: Dietary calcium, calcium supplementation, and blood pressure in African American adolescents, *Am J Clin Nutr* 68:648, 1998.
13. McCarron DA, Metz JA, Hatton DC: Mineral intake and blood pressure in African Americans, *Am J Clin Nutr* 68:517, 1998.
14. Jorde R, Bonaa KH: Calcium from dairy products, vitamin D intake, and blood pressure: the Tromso study, *J Am Diet Assoc* 71:1530, 2000.
15. Massey LK: Dairy food consumption, blood pressure and stroke, *J Nutr* 131:1875, 2001.
16. Krall EA, Dawson-Hughes B: Osteoporosis. In Shils ME et al, eds: *Modern nutrition in health and disease,* ed 9, Philadelphia, 1999, Lippincott Williams & Wilkins.
17. Tepper BJ, Nayga RM: Awareness of the link between bone disease and calcium intake is associated with higher dietary calcium intake in women aged 50 years and older: results of the 1991 CSFII-DHKS, *J Am Diet Assoc* 98(2):196, 1998.

18. Gulliver P, Horwath CC: Assessing women's perceived benefits, barriers, and stage of change for meeting milk product consumption recommendations, *J Am Diet Assoc* 101(11): 1354, 2001.
19. Knochelk JP: Phosphorus. In Shils ME et al, eds: *Modern nutrition in health and disease,* ed 9, Philadelphia, 1999, Lippincott Williams & Wilkins.
20. Kaplan NM: The dietary guideline for sodium: should we shake it up? No, *Am J Clin Nutr* 71:1020, 2000.
21. McCarron DA: The dietary guideline for sodium: should we shake it up? Yes! *Am J Clin Nutr* 71:1013, 2000.
22. Kumanyika SK et al: Outcomes of a cardiovascular nutrition counseling program in African-Americans with elevated blood pressure or cholesterol level, *J Am Diet Assoc* 99:1380, 1999.
23. Harsha DW et al: Dietary Approaches to Stop Hypertension: a summary of study results, *J Am Diet Assoc* 99:(8 suppl):S35, 1999.
24. Food and Nutrition Board, National Academy of Sciences: *Recommended dietary allowances,* ed 10, Washington, DC, 1989, National Academy Press.
25. Sacks FM et al: Effects on blood pressure of reduced dietary sodium and the Dietary Approaches to Stop Hypertension (DASH) diet, *N Engl J Med* 344:3, 2001.
26. Whelton PK et al: Sodium reduction and weight loss in the treatment of hypertension in older persons. A randomized controlled trial of nonpharmacologic interventions in the elderly (TONE), *JAMA* 279:839, 1998.
27. Loria CM, Obarzanek E, Ernst ND: Choose and prepare food with less salt: dietary advice for all Americans, *J Nutr* 131:536S, 2001.
28. Suter PM: Potassium and hypertension, *Nutr Rev* 56:151, 1998.
29. Karanja NM et al: Descriptive characteristics of the dietary patterns used in the Dietary Approaches to Stop Hypertension trial, *J Am Diet Assoc* 99(suppl):S19, 1999.
30. Martini MA: Magnesium supplementation and bone turnover, *Nutr Rev* 57:227, 1999.
31. Tucker KL et al: Potassium, magnesium, and fruit and vegetable intakes are associated with greater bone mineral density in elderly men and women, *Am J Clin Nutr* 69:727, 1999.
32. Mertz W: Three decades of dietary recommendations, *Nutr Rev* 58:324, 2000.
33. Food and Nutrition Board, National Academy of Sciences: *Dietary reference intakes for vitamin A, vitamin K, arsenic, boron, chromium, copper, iodine, iron, manganese, molybdenum, nickel, silicon, vanadium, and zinc,* Washington, DC, 2001, National Academy Press.
34. Hunt JR, Roughead ZK: Adaptation of iron absorption in men consuming diets with high or low iron availability, *Am J Clin Nutr* 71:94, 2000.
35. Kalwarf HJ, Harrast SD: Effects of calcium supplementation and lactation on iron status, *Am J Clin Nutr* 67:1244, 1998.
36. Beard JL: Iron biology in immune function, muscle metabolism, and neuronal functioning, *J Nutr* 131(suppl): 568S, 2001.
37. Grantham-McGregor S, Ani C: A review of studies on the effect of iron deficiency on cognitive development in children, *J Nutr* 131(suppl):649S, 2001.
38. Fleming DJ et al: Aspirin and the use of serum ferritin as a measure of iron status, *Am J Clin Nutr* 74:219, 2001.
39. Fairbanks VF: Iron in medicine and nutrition. In Shils ME et al, eds: *Modern nutrition in health and disease,* ed 9, Philadelphia, 1999, Lippincott Williams & Wilkins.
40. Fleming DJ et al: Iron status of the free-living, elderly Framingham Heart Study cohort: an iron-replete population with a high prevalence of elevated iron stores, *Am J Clin Nutr* 73:638, 2001.
41. Nelson RL: Iron and colorectal cancer risk: human studies, *Nutr Rev* 59(5):140, 2001.
42. Hetzel BS, Clugston GA: Iodine. In Shils ME et al, eds: *Modern nutrition in health and disease,* ed 9, Philadelphia, 1999, Lippincott Williams & Wilkins.
43. Solomons NW: Slow-release iodine in local water supplies reverses iodine deficiency disorders: is it worth its salt? *Nutr Rev* 56:280, 1998.
44. Elnour A et al: Endemic goiter with iodine sufficiency: a possible role for the consumption of pearl millet in the etiology of endemic goiter, *Am J Clin Nutr* 71:59, 2000.
45. Semba RD, Delange F: Iodine in human milk: perspectives for infant health, *Nutr Rev* 59(8):269, 2001.
46. Lee K et al: Too much vs too little: the implications of current iodine intake in the United States, *Nutr Rev* 57:177, 1999.
47. King JC, Keen CL: Zinc. In Shils ME et al, eds: *Modern nutrition in health and disease,* ed 9, Philadelphia, 1999, Lippincott Williams & Wilkins.
48. King JC: Determinants of maternal zinc during pregnancy, *Am J Clin Nutr* 71(suppl):1334S, 2000.
49. Black MM: Zinc deficiency and child development, *Am J Clin Nutr* 68(suppl):464S, 1998.
50. Krebs NF: Zinc supplementation during lactation, *Am J Clin Nutr* 68(suppl):509S, 1998.
51. Hotz C, Brown KH: Identifying populations at risk of zinc deficiency: the use of supplementation trials, *Nutr Rev* 59(3):80, 2001.
52. Shankar AH, Prasad AS: Zinc and immune function: the biological basis of altered resistance to infection, *Am J Clin Nutr* 68(suppl):447S, 1998.
53. Pang Y, MacIntosh DL, Ryan PB: A longitudinal investigation of aggregate oral intake of copper, *J Nutr* 131:2171, 2001.
54. Nielsen FH: Ultratrace minerals. In Shils ME et al, eds: *Modern Nutrition in Health and Disease,* ed 9, Philadelphia, 1999, Lippincott Williams & Wilkins.
55. Stoecker B: Chromium. In Shils ME et al, eds: *Modern nutrition in health and disease,* ed 9, Philadelphia, 1999, Lippincott Williams & Wilkins.
56. Jeejeebhoy KN: The role of chromium in nutrition and therapeutics and as a potential toxin, *Nutr Rev* 57:329, 1999.
57. Anderson RA: Effects of chromium on body composition and weight loss, *Nutr Rev* 56:266, 1998.
58. Holben DH, Smith AM: The diverse role of selenium within selenoproteins: a review, *J Am Diet Assoc* 99:836, 1999.
59. Food and Nutrition Board, National Academy of Sciences: *Dietary reference intakes for vitamin C, vitamin E, selenium, and carotenoids,* Washington, DC, 2000, National Academy Press.

60. Palmer CA, Anderson JJB: Position of the American Dietetic Association: the impact of fluoride on health, *J Am Diet Assoc* 101(1):126, 2001.

■ Further Reading

Kleiner SM: Water: an essential but overlooked nutrient, *J Am Diet Assoc* 99:200, 1999.

Wagner DR: Hyperhydrating with glycerol: implications for athletic performance, *J Am Diet Assoc* 99:207, 1999.

These two articles help us understand the importance of proper fluid intake for individuals in various states of health and levels of physical activity. We will review the many roles of water in the body and learn more about the development of new fluid products designed to enhance athletic performance.

Gulliver P, Horwath C: Assessing women's perceived benefits, barriers, and stage of change for meeting milk product consumption recommendations, *J Am Diet Assoc* 101(11):1354, 2001.

Hunt CD, Meacham SL: Aluminum, boron, calcium, copper, iron, magnesium, manganese, molybdenum, phosphorus, potassium, sodium, and zinc: concentrations in common Western foods and estimated daily intakes by infants; toddlers; and male and female adolescents, adults, and seniors in the United States, *J Am Diet Assoc* 101(9):1058, 2001.

Retslaff BM et al: Iron and zinc status of women and men who followed cholesterol-lowering diets, *J Am Diet Assoc* 98:149, 1998.

Trumbo P et al: Dietary Reference Intakes: vitamin A, vitamin K, arsenic, boron, chromium, copper, iodine, iron, manganese, molybdenum, nickel, silicon, vanadium, and zinc, *J Am Diet Assoc* 101(3):294, 2001.

These articles describe the dietary needs and intakes of important minerals in several population groups. The first article helps us understand how perceived benefits and barriers can influence food decision-making and calcium intake in women and how nutrition educators can use this information in developing program strategies. The second article provides some insight as to the current mineral intakes of various age groups in the United States and the food categories that contributed the most to their intake. The third article describes the effect of cholesterol-lowering diets on mineral intakes and suggests how a diet designed to limit one nutritional component will also influence others. The last article reviews the most recent report issued by the Food and Nutrition Board of the National Academy of Sciences that presents the DRI for the trace minerals.

Korrick SA et al: Lead and hypertension in a sample of middle-aged women, *Am J Public Health* 89:330, 1999.

Stanek K et al: Lead consumption of 18- to 36-month-old children as determined from duplicate diet collections: nutrient intakes, blood lead levels, and effects on growth, *J Am Diet Assoc* 98:155, 1998.

The presence of the trace mineral lead as a contaminant in food and in the environment is a health matter of great concern in the United States. These two articles address this issue in children and as a possible contributor to chronic disease in adults.

Center for Food Safety and Applied Nutrition: Tips for the savvy supplement user, *FDA Consumer* 36(2):17, 2002.

Hunt J, Dwyer J: Position of the American Dietetic Association: Food fortification and dietary supplements, *J Am Diet Assoc* 101(1):115, 2001.

Steindel SJ, Howanitz PJ: The uncertainty of hair analysis for trace minerals, *JAMA* 285(1):67, 2001.

The public media carries many advertisements for dietary supplements including vitamins, minerals, and plant and herbal preparations. Unscrupulous entrepreneurs often resort to false claims about their products or try to make persons believe that they have a nutritional or health deficiency that can be relieved by the use of a particular product. Hair analysis is a frequent advertising ploy to make individuals believe that they may have a deficiency (see *Issues & Answers*). These three articles by health professionals address the problems associated with hair analysis and the appropriate circumstances and cautions for use of dietary supplements.

Issues & ANSWERS

Hair Analysis: What Can It Tell Us About Mineral Status?

Many Americans, at one time or another, have spent a great deal of money getting their hair analyzed. For a few strands of hair and a sizable fee, they have been told they can find out if their potassium levels are low, their lead levels are high, or their sodium levels are just right. Or can they?

Hair is dead tissue. It starts out as living cells, full of the same vitamins and minerals found in the rest of the body. The dead cells are "glued" together with a sulfur-rich protein called keratin, and, as more are added, they continue to grow in length as a single strand of hair. Vitamins disappear when the cells die so no vitamins are found in hair, but most of the inorganic minerals remain behind. Yet even with the detection of minerals there are problems.

- Some minerals are lost when hair cells die. The keratin is so rich in sulfur that it masks the presence of some minerals and attracts others in levels that exceed those found in other parts of the body.
- Hair can be contaminated by shampoos, hard or soft water, dyes, or even air pollution, thereby skewing laboratory calculations.
- For certain nutrients we do not know the relationship between hair levels and blood levels.
- Some hair samples become contaminated with certain minerals in the process of preparing them for chemical analysis; therefore large amounts of mineral contaminants also get included in the results reported to the client.
- There are no standard laboratory values for the mineral content of hair. Laboratories simply state that levels are higher, lower, or the same as those seen previously in other people.

But hair analysis is not totally worthless. Coroners use it all the time to find out if a person has died from arsenic, lead, or other poisons. Public health workers use it to compare mineral levels in populations from different parts of a country if they suspect that soil depletion, water contamination, or other environmental changes have affected nutrient levels in local food supplies. Czech researchers are using hair analysis to determine those regions of their country that have low soil selenium concentrations, putting the local population at risk of selenium deficiency. Also, hair analysis can help researchers and health professionals monitor changing nutrient levels over time. Increasing hair concentrations of calcium, iron, and zinc demonstrated the effectiveness of a mineral supplementation program for malnourished women in China, and the hair mineral measurements were confirmed by blood mineral measurements taken in the same population. Hair analysis might have some benefit as a screening tool where conditions make it difficult to obtain or preserve biochemical samples such as blood or in communities where the population objects to such procedures. In one study hair zinc levels were lower in women whose diets were high in phytate or who had multiple pregnancies. However, before hair sampling can be used routinely, it will be necessary to establish the relationship between mineral levels in hair samples and the mineral content of biological fluids such as blood.

The usefulness of hair analysis in general practice, however, is not recommended by health professionals. This negative response comes not only because of the shortcomings of hair analysis as a diagnostic tool for measuring the mineral status of a particular individual but also because mail-order hair analysis companies often diagnose conditions that do not exist and suggest treatment with a variety of supplements. Also, such companies may not practice quality control standards. In a recent evaluation a split hair sample from a healthy volunteer was sent to six different laboratories for analysis. For nearly half of the minerals analyzed, laboratory results differed by more than 10-fold between the highest value reported and the lowest value reported.

It is important that we discourage persons from wasting their money and possibly taking dangerous levels of minerals based on a hair analysis obtained through commercial advertising.

REFERENCES

Barrett S, Herbert V: Fads, frauds, and quackery. In Shils ME et al, eds: *Modern nutrition in health and disease,* ed 9, Philadelphia, 1999, Lippincott Williams & Wilkins.

Gibson RS, Huddle JM: Suboptimal zinc status in pregnant Malawian women: its association with low intakes of poorly available zinc, frequent reproductive cycling, and malaria, *Am J Clin Nutr* 67(4):702, 1998.

Kvicala J, Zamrazil V, Jiranek V: Characterization of selenium status of inhabitants in the region Usti and Orlici, Czech Republic by INAA of blood serum and hair and fluorimetric analysis of urine, *Biol Trace Elem Res* 71-72:31, 1999.

Leung PL et al: Hair concentrations of calcium, iron, and zinc in pregnant women and effects of supplementation, *Biol Trace Elem Res* 69:269, 1999.

Steindel SJ, Howanitz PJ: The uncertainty of hair analysis for trace minerals, *JAMA* 285(1):67, 2001.

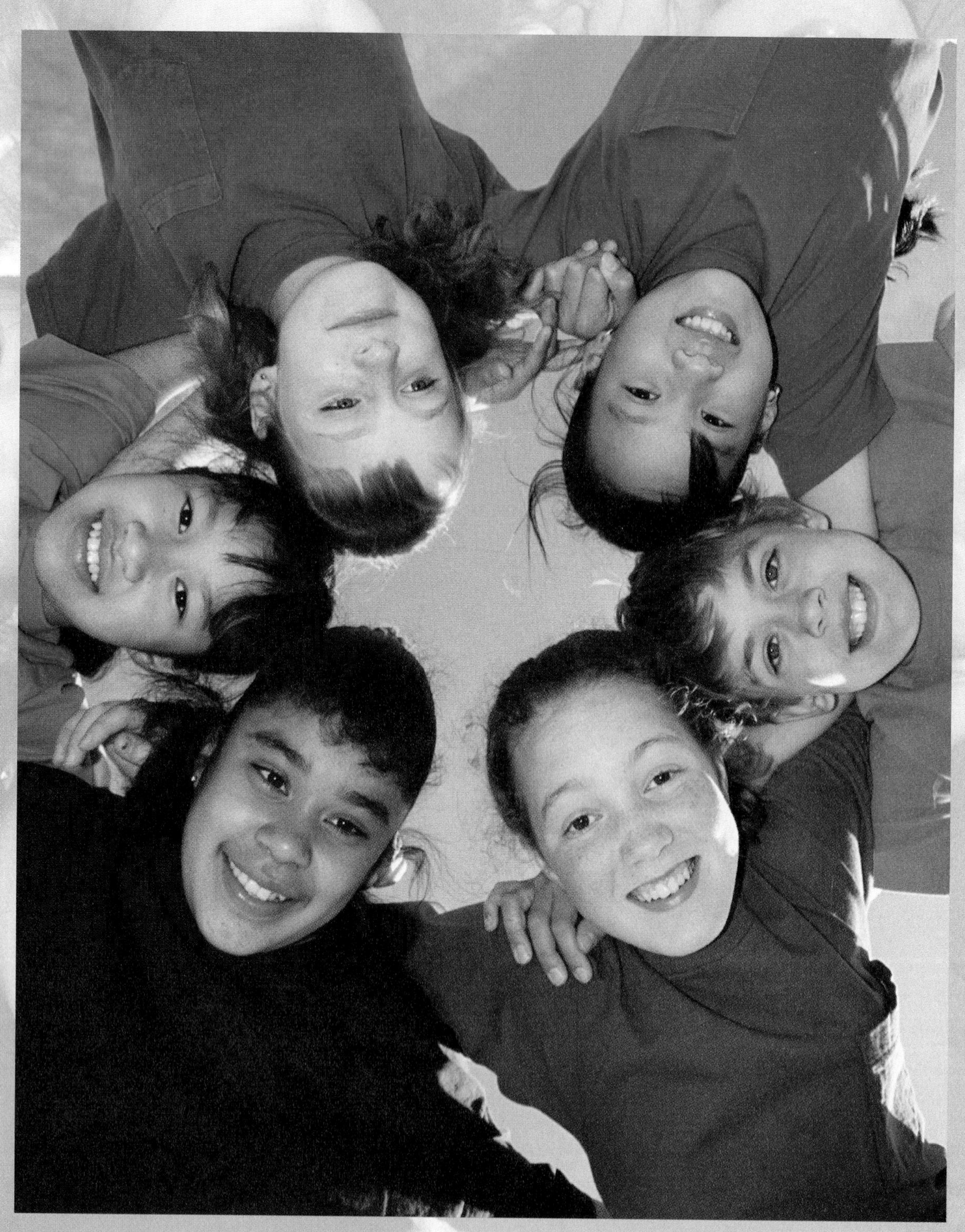

Part 2

COMMUNITY NUTRITION: THE LIFE CYCLE

Chapter

9

The Food Environment and Food Habits

Sue Rodwell Williams

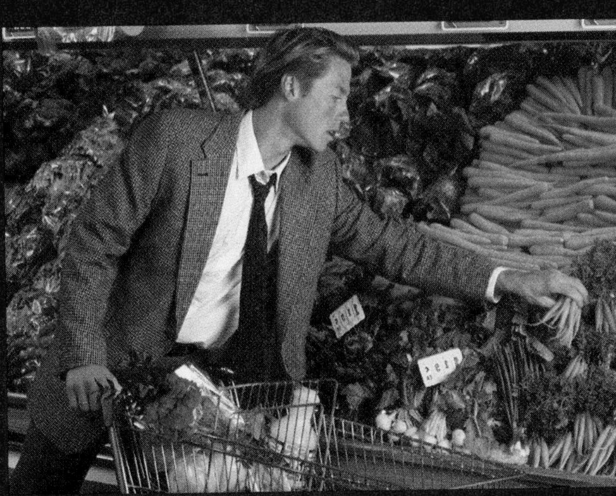

Chapter Outline

This chapter begins the second part of your study of nutrition with a two-chapter sequence on food habits and family nutrition counseling. Here we seek to apply the nutritional science principles you have learned to personal and family needs.

The science of human nutrition comes alive only in terms of personal need. Human compassion and concern are as necessary as practical guides and skills to apply knowledge in a useful and helpful manner.

Here we begin with a look at our changing food environment and the web of influences that determine personal food choices and habits.

The Development of Food Habits

In addition to the factors of poverty and politics, other aspects of our lives influence our food patterns. Food habits, like other forms of human behavior, do not develop in a vacuum. They result from many personal, cultural, social, and psychologic influences. For each of us these factors are interwoven to develop a unique individual.

CULTURAL INFLUENCES

Strength of Personal Culture

Often the most significant thing about a society's culture is what it takes for granted in daily life. Culture involves not only the more obvious and historical aspects of a person's communal life, that is, language, religion, politics, technology, and so on, but also all the little habits of everyday living, such as preparing and serving food and caring for children, feeding them, and lulling them to sleep. These many facets of a person's culture are learned gradually as a child grows up in a society. Through a slow process of conscious and unconscious learning, we take on our culture's values, attitudes, habits, and practices through the influence of our parents, teachers, and others. Whatever is invented, transmitted, and perpetuated—socially acquired knowledge and habits—we learn as part of our culture. These elements become internalized and entrenched.[1]

Food in a Culture

Food habits are among the oldest and most deeply rooted aspects of many cultures, and they exert a deep influence on the behavior of the people. The cultural and subcultural background determines what shall be eaten as well as when and how it shall be eaten.[2] There is, of course, considerable variation. Rational and irrational, beneficial and injurious customs are found in every part of the world. Nevertheless, food habits are primarily based on food availability, economics, and personal food meanings and beliefs. Included among these influential factors are the geography of the land, the agriculture practiced by the people, their economic and marketing practices, their view about healthy or safe food, and their history and traditions. Within every culture certain foods are deeply infused with symbolic meaning. These symbolic foods are related to major life experiences from birth through death, to religion, to politics, and to general social organization. From early times, ceremonies and religious rites have surrounded certain events and seasons. Food gathering, preparing, and serving have followed specific customs and commemorated special events of religious and national significance and heritage. Many of these customs remain today.[3]

SOCIAL INFLUENCES

Social Organization

The study of human group behavior reveals numerous activities, processes, and structures by which social life goes on. Human behavior can be understood in terms of social phenomena and problems, such as social change, urbanism, rural life, the family, the community, race relations, delinquency, drugs, and crime. These social problems carry nutritional implications. Two aspects of social organization concern health professionals: class structure and value systems.

1. *Class structure.* The structure of a society is largely formed by groupings according to factors such as economic status, education, residence, occupation, or family. Within a given society many of these groups exist, and their values and habits vary widely. Subgroups develop on the basis of region, religion, age, sex, social class, health concerns, occupation, or political affiliation. Within these subgroups there may be still smaller groupings with distinct attitudes, values, and habits. A person may be a member of several subcultural groups, each of which influences values, attitudes, and habits. Our democratic philosophy and the humanitarian ideals on which the health professions have been nurtured combine to make the reality of class differences difficult for us to accept.
2. *Value systems.* A society's value systems develop as a result of its history and heritage. Traditionally, four basic premises have influenced American value systems and have affected attitudes toward healthcare and food habits.
   - *Equality.* A high value on equality leads healthcare workers to establish quality healthcare standards for all people, although in reality this does not always occur.
   - *Sociality.* The high respect accorded to a social nature builds peer group pressures and status seeking within social groups. Foods may be accepted because they are high-status foods or rejected because they are low-prestige foods. Even the use of dietary supplements has been associated with the desire for prestige, along with health concerns.
   - *Success.* The esteem in which success is held often leads persons to measure life in terms of competitive superlatives. They want to set the best table, provide the most abundant supply of food for the family, or have the biggest eater and the fattest baby of any in the neighborhood.
   - *Change.* The value placed on change leads families and individuals to seek constant variety in their diets, to be geared for action, to be a mobile society, and to seek quick-cooking, conveniently prepared foods. In response to such marketing demands, food technologists continually produce an array of new food products.

Food and Social Factors

Food habits in any setting are highly socialized. These habits perform significant social functions, some of which may not always be evident. First, within social relationships, food is a symbol of social acceptance, warmth, and friendliness. People tend to accept food more readily from those persons they view as friends or allies. They accept advice about food from persons they consider to be authorities or with whom they can feel warm relationships.

Second, within family relationships, the primary social unit, strong food patterns develop. Food habits that are most closely associated with family sentiments are the most tenacious throughout life. Long into adulthood, certain foods trigger a flood of childhood memories and are valued for reasons totally apart from any nutritional value. Strong religious factors associated with food tend to have their origin and reinforcement within the family meal circle. Also, family income, community sources of food, and market conditions influence food habits and ultimately food choices. Persons eat foods that are readily available to them and that they have the money to buy.

PSYCHOLOGIC INFLUENCES

Social Psychology

Social psychology is concerned with (1) social interaction in terms of its effect on individual behavior and (2) the social influences of individual perception, motivation, and action. How does a particular individual perceive a given situation? What basic needs motivate action and response? What social factors surround a particular action? Issues of particular concern include the effect of culture on personality, the socialization of the child, differences in individuals in groups, group dynamics, group attitudes and opinions, and leadership. The methods of social psychology have made important contributions to nutrition, medicine, nursing, and allied healthcare, especially to problems of human behavior under stress.

Food and Psychologic Factors

Individual behavior patterns, especially those related to eating, result from many interrelated psychosocial influences. Factors that are particularly pertinent to the shaping of food habits are motivation and perception.

1. *Motivation.* People are not the same the world over. Those of differing cultures are not motivated by the same needs and goals. Even primary biologic drives such as hunger and sex are modified in their interpretation, expression, and fulfillment by many cultural, social, and personal influences. The kinds of food sought, prized, or accepted by one individual at one time and place may be rejected by another living in different circumstances. For persons existing in a state of basic hunger or semistarvation, food is the whole perception and motivation. Such a person thinks, talks, and dreams about food. Under less severe circumstances, however, the concern for food may be on a relatively abstract level and may involve symbolism that is associated with other needs. For example, Maslow's classic hierarchy of human needs illustrates these human strivings.[4] He described five levels of need that operate in turn, each building on the previous ones.
   - *Basic physiologic needs.* Hunger, thirst.
   - *Safety needs.* Physical comfort, security, protection.
   - *"Belongingness" needs.* Love, giving and receiving affection.
   - *Recognition needs.* Self-esteem, status, sense of self-worth, strength, self-confidence, capability, adequacy.
   - *Self-actualization needs.* Self-fulfillment, creative growth.

   Of course, these levels of need overlap and vary with time and circumstance, but we can use them to help us understand the needs of our clients and to plan care accordingly.
2. *Perception.* To make sense out of an otherwise chaotic assortment of impressions, we perceive our environment in different ways. These perceptions enable us to live in an environment that feels relatively stable. However, perception also limits understanding. Every phenomenon that the outer world offers is filtered through our own social and personal lenses. In every experience of our lives, we perceive a blend of three facets: (1) the external reality, (2) the message of the stimulus that is conveyed by the nervous system to the integrative centers of the brain where thinking and evaluation go on, and (3) the interpretation that we put on every part of our personal experience. A host of subjective elements—hunger, thirst, hate, fear, love, self-interest, values, temperament—influence our response to the outer world's phenomena.

On the basis, then, of personal motivation and perception, personal learning takes place. In the final analysis, each person must learn in his or her own way according to need. It is this personal human dimension that makes a health professional's work profound. Persons learn because they have an urgent need to know. They learn because their curiosity is aroused. They learn because they want to make meaning out of their lives. They learn by exploring, making mistakes and correcting them, testing, verifying. All of these things individuals must do for themselves. This is true of everyone's learning. It is true of the learning we desire for our clients. It is true of our own learning.

FOOD MISINFORMATION

Unscientific statements about food and nutrition often mislead the public and contribute to poor food habits. Persons have often surrounded their cultural eating habits with myths of various sorts. Some scientifically unsubstantiated beliefs about certain foods may be harmless, but others may have more serious implications for health and well-being. Claims about foods or supplements that are not based on scientific evidence, such as heavy use of vitamin supplements for general health maintenance, often mislead the public and contribute to poor food habits. False information may come from folklore, or it may be built on half-truths, innuendoes, and outright deception, as in cases of fraud.

In contrast, nutritional science is a growing body of knowledge built on vigorously examined scientific evidence. Concern for food safety and wholesomeness clearly existed long before the scientific method was known. Nonetheless, in this rapidly changing world, it is only on the sound basis of scientific knowledge that we may make wise food choices and recognize misinformation as such.

Types of Food Faddist Claims

Food faddists make exaggerated claims for certain types of food. These claims fall into four basic groups: (1) certain foods will cure specific conditions, (2) certain foods are harmful and should be avoided, (3) special food combinations are very effective as reducing diets or have special therapeutic effects, and (4) other "natural" foods can meet body needs and prevent disease. A basic error can be found when we examine these claims carefully. Notice that each one focuses on foods as such, not on the chemical components, the nutrients that are the actual physiologic agents of life and health. It is true, of course, that certain individuals may be allergic to specific foods and obviously should avoid them. It is also true that certain foods have particularly high concentrations of certain nutrients and are therefore good sources of such nutrients. But it is the nutrients, not the specific foods, that have specific functions in the body. Furthermore, each of these nutrients may be found in a number of different foods. Persons require specific nutrients, never specific foods.

Why should the health worker be concerned about food faddism and its effects on food habits? What harm may food faddism do? Essentially, food fads involve three basic dangers that concern all members of the healthcare team.

1. *Dangers to health.* Responsibility for one's health is fundamental. However, self-diagnosis and self-treatment can be dangerous, especially where health problems are concerned. When such action is based on questionable sources, the dangers are multiplied. By following such a course, a person with a real illness may fail to seek appropriate medical care. Many anxious patients who have cancer, diabetes, or arthritis have been misled by fraudulent claims of cures and postponed effective therapy. Superstitions that are perpetuated counteract scientific progress and sound health teaching.
2. *Money spent needlessly.* Some of the foods and supplements used by faddists are harmless, but most are expensive. As much as $2.5 billion per year has been spent by consumers on nutrient supplements. Such money may be wasted. When dollars are scarce, the family may neglect to buy foods that fill its basic needs, opting instead to purchase a "guaranteed cure."
3. *Distrust of the food market.* Our food environment is rapidly changing. We need intelligent concern and rational problem solving to meet nutritional requirements. A wise course is to select a variety of primary foods "closer to the source," having minimal processing, and add a few carefully selected processed items for specific uses. Blanket erroneous teaching concerning food and health breeds public suspicion and distrust of the common food market and of food technology and agriculture in general. Each food product must be evaluated on its own merits in terms of individual needs. These needs include nutrient contribution, aesthetic values, safety, and cost.

Groups Vulnerable to Food Fads

Food fads appeal especially to certain groups of people with particular needs and concerns; among these are older adults, adolescents, obese persons, athletes, and those whose living depends on their physical appearance.

- *Older persons.* Fear of changes that come as youth and potency wane leads many middle-aged persons to grasp at exaggerated claims that some product will restore their youthful vigor. Elderly persons in pain and discomfort, perhaps living alone with chronic illness, may respond to the hope that the special supplement holds a sure cure. Desperately ill and lonely individuals are easy prey for exaggerated health claims.
- *Young persons.* Figure-conscious adolescent girls and muscle-minded rapidly growing boys frequently respond to advertisements for crash programs to attain the perfect body. Young people, particularly those who are lonely or have exaggerated ideas of glamour, hope to achieve peer-group acceptance by these means.
- *Obese persons.* One of the most disturbing and frustrating health problems in America is obesity. Obese persons, faced with a bewildering barrage of propaganda advocating diets, pills, and devices, are likely to respond to the fad of the moment "to solve everything."
- *Athletes and coaches.* Athletes and their coaches are prime targets for those who push supplements. Always looking for the added something to give them the competitive edge, athletes can be lured by nutrition myths and hoaxes.[5-7]
- *Entertainers.* Persons in the public eye, such as entertainers, may look for certain foods, drugs, or dietary combinations that will help them retain the physical appearance and strength on which their careers depend; they may easily believe false claims about these foods.

These various groups are vulnerable for obvious reasons. No segment of the population, however, seems to be completely free from the appeal of food faddism. Particularly in metropolitan areas, "health food," with its attendant supplements, is a large industry, bigger in the United States than in any other country.

The Answer

How do we respond to food habits associated with food faddism, misinformation, or even deception? What can health professionals do? What should they do? Several things merit consideration.

1. *Assess your own attitudes and habits.* We cannot counsel or teach others until we have first examined our own position. Instruction based on personal conviction, practice, and enthusiasm will achieve far more than teaching that says, in effect, "Do as I say, not as I do."
2. *Use reliable sources.* Two types of background knowledge are vital: (1) knowledge of the product and the persons behind it and (2) knowledge of human nutritional physiology and the scientific method of problem solving.
3. *Recognize human needs.* Observe these needs in yourselves and in others to understand how psychologic and cultural factors affect food habits. Consider the emotional needs that are symbolically fulfilled by foods, by the eating of foods, and by the rituals surrounding the process. Respect personal needs. Welcome the positive power that food and eating rituals possess for filling these needs. Even when there is reason to believe that the client is using food as a crutch for emotional adjustment, the value of such an adjustment must be considered. To aid the client in letting go of such an emotional crutch, alternative support must be provided with care and sensitivity.
4. *Be alert to community opportunities.* Grasp any opportunity that arises to present sound health information to groups or individuals, formally or informally. Learn of available community resources and use them. Develop communication skills. Avoid monotony. Use a well-disciplined imagination. Without these things, the message will not convince.
5. *Think scientifically.* We can teach young children to use the problem-solving approach to everyday situations. Children are naturally curious. With their eternal "Why?" they often seek evidence to support statements made to them. We need to teach them and ourselves the value of asking three significant questions: "What do you mean?" "How do you know?" and "What is your evidence?"
6. *Know responsible authorities.* The Food and Drug Administration (FDA) has the legal responsibility of controlling the quality and safety of food and drug products marketed in the United States. However, it needs the vigilance of consumers to help fulfill so large a task. Other government, professional, and private organizations also provide resources for consumer education. The American Dietetic Association has provided guidance for a U.S. national policy on enrichment and fortification of the food supply that protects against nutrient insufficiencies and toxicities.

Ethnic Diversity in American Food Patterns

In the area of good food, the increasing ethnic diversity in the U.S. population is cause for celebration. Our taste buds celebrate the spice such ethnic diversity brings to American food patterns. Older American traditions from a variety of cultures mingle with more recent arrivals to provide a smorgasbord of ethnic experiences. Each reflects the culture in which it developed, based on both religious laws and regional influences.[8]

RELIGIOUS DIETARY LAWS

Jewish

The observance of Jewish food laws differs among the three basic groups within Judaism: (1) Orthodox—strict observance, (2) conservative—less strict, and (3) reform—less ceremonial emphasis and minimum general use.[9] The basic body of dietary laws is called the Rules of Kashruth. Foods selected and prepared according to these rules are called *kosher,* from the Hebrew word meaning "fit, proper." Originally these laws had special ritual significance. Present Jewish dietary laws apply this significance to laws governing the slaughter, preparation, and serving of the meat, to the combining of meat and milk, to fish, and to eggs. Various food restrictions exist.

1. *Meat.* No pork is used. Forequarters of other meats are allowed, as well as all commonly used forms of poultry. All forms of meat that are used are rigidly cleansed of all blood. Rabbinical supervision certifies proper preparation throughout the process.
2. *Meat and milk.* No combining of meat and milk is allowed. Orthodox homes maintain two sets of dishes—one for serving meat and the other for meals using dairy products. Separate sets of cooking pots, pans, and utensils should be maintained as well. The dishes and cookware must be washed and stored separately also.
3. *Fish.* Only fish with fins and scales are allowed. These may be eaten with either meat or dairy meals. No shellfish or eels may be used.
4. *Eggs.* No egg with a blood spot may be eaten. Eggs may be used with either meat or dairy meals.

Many of the traditional Jewish foods relate to festivals of the Jewish calendar that commemorate significant events in Jewish history. Often special Sabbath foods are used. A few representative foods include the following.

- *Bagels.* Doughnut-shaped, hard yeast rolls.
- *Blintzes.* Thin filled and rolled pancakes.
- *Borscht (borsch).* Soup of meat stock, mixed with beaten egg or sour cream, beets, cabbage, or spinach. Served hot or cold.

- *Challah.* Sabbath loaf of white bread, shaped as a twist or coil, used at the beginning of the meal after the kiddush, the blessing over wine.
- *Gefullte (gefilte fish).* From a German word meaning "stuffed fish," usually the first course of Sabbath evening meal, made of fish fillet, chopped, seasoned, and stuffed back into the skin or rolled into balls.
- *Kasha.* Buckwheat groats (hulled kernels), used as a cooked cereal or as a potato substitute with gravy.
- *Knishes.* Pastry filled with ground meat or cheese.
- *Lox.* Smoked, salted salmon.
- *Matzo.* Flat unleavened bread.
- *Strudel.* Thin pastry filled with fruit and nuts, rolled and baked.

Moslem

Moslem dietary laws are based on restrictions or prohibitions of some foods and promotion of others, derived from Islamic teachings in the Koran. The laws are binding and must be followed at all times, even during pregnancy, hospitalization, or travel. The general rule is that "all foods are permitted" unless specifically conditioned or prohibited.[10]

- *Milk products.* Permitted at all times.
- *Fruits and vegetable.* Except if fermented or poisonous.
- *Breads and cereals.* Unless contaminated or harmful.
- *Meats.* Seafood, including fish, shellfish, eels, and sea animals, and land animals except swine; pork is strictly prohibited.
- *Alcohol.* Strictly prohibited.

Any food combinations are used as long as no prohibited items are included. Milk and meat may be eaten together, in contrast to Jewish kosher laws. The Koran mentions certain foods as being of special value: figs, olives, dates, honey, milk, and buttermilk. Prohibited foods in the Moslem dietary laws may be eaten when no other sources of food are available.

Among the Moslem people, a 30-day period of daylight fasting is required during Ramadan, the ninth month of the Islamic lunar calendar, thus rotating through all seasons. The fourth pillar of Islam commanded by the Koran is fasting. Ramadan was chosen for the sacred fast because it is the month in which Mohammed received the first of the revelations that were subsequently compiled to form the Koran and also the month in which his followers first drove their enemies from Mecca in 624 AD. During the month of Ramadan, Moslems throughout the world observe daily fasting, taking no food or drink from dawn to sunset. Nights, however, are often spent in special feasts. First, an appetizer is taken, such as dates or a fruit drink, followed by the family's "evening breakfast," the *iftar.* At the end of Ramadan a traditional feast lasting up to 3 days climaxes the observance. Special dishes mark this occasion, including delicacies such as thin pancakes dipped in powdered sugar, savory buns, and dried fruits.

SPANISH (HISPANIC) AND NATIVE AMERICAN INFLUENCES

Mexican

Food habits of early Spanish settlers and Indian nations form the basis of present food patterns of persons of Mexican (Hispanic) heritage who now live in the United States, chiefly in the Southwest. Three foods are basic to this pattern: dried beans, chili peppers, and corn. Variations and additions may be found in different places or among those of different income levels. Relatively small amounts of meat and occasionally eggs are used. Fruit such as oranges, apples, bananas, papayas, and mangos are used, depending on availability. For centuries corn has been the basic grain used as bread in the form of tortillas, which are flat cakes baked on a hot griddle. Some wheat is used in making tortillas; rice and oat are added cereals. Coffee is a main beverage. Major seasonings are chili peppers, onions, and garlic; the basic fat is lard.

Puerto Rican

The Puerto Rican people share a common heritage with the Mexicans, so much of their food pattern is similar.[11] They add tropical fruits and vegetables, many of which are available in their neighborhood markets in the United States. A main type of food is *viandas,* starchy vegetables and fruits such as plantain and green bananas. Two other staples of the diet are rice and beans. Milk, meat, yellow and green vegetables, and other fruits are used in limited quantities, but dried codfish is a staple food. Coffee is a main beverage. Lard is the main cooking fat.

Native American

The Native American population, Indian and Alaskan Natives, is composed mainly of more than 500 federally recognized diverse groups living on reservations, in small rural communities, or in metropolitan areas.[12] Despite their individual diversity, the various groups share a spiritual attachment to the land and a determination to retain their culture. Food has great religious and social significance and is an integral part not only of celebrations and ceremonies but also of everyday hospitality, which includes a serious obligation for serving food. Foods may be prepared and used in different ways from region to region and vary according to what can be grown locally, harvested or hunted on the land or fished from its rivers, or is available in food markets. Among the Native American groups of the southwest United States, the food pattern of the Navajo people, whose reservations extend over a 25,000 square mile area at the junction of the three states New Mexico, Arizona, and Utah, may serve as an example.[12]

Historically, the Navajos learned farming from the early Pueblo people, establishing corn and other crops as staples. Later they learned herding from the Spaniards, making sheep and goats available for food and wool. Some families also raised chickens, pigs, and cattle. Currently, Navajo food habits combine traditional dietary staples with modern food products available from supermarkets and fast-food restaurants. Meat is eaten daily, including fresh mutton, beef, pork, and chicken or smoked or processed meat. Other staples include bread tortillas or fry bread, blue cornbread, and cornmeal mush; beverages of coffee, soft drinks, and fruit-flavored drinks; eggs; vegetables of corn, potatoes, green beans, and tomatoes; and some fresh or canned fruit. Frying is a common method of food preparation; lard and shortening are main cooking fats. There is an increased use of modern snack foods that are high in fat, sugar, calories, and sodium, especially among children and teenagers.

SOUTHERN UNITED STATES INFLUENCES

African Americans

The black populations, especially in the Southern states, have contributed a rich heritage of American food patterns, particularly to Southern cooking as a whole. Like their moving original music of spirituals, blues, gospel, and jazz, Southern black food patterns were born of hard times, and developed through a creative ability to turn any basic staples at hand into memorable food. Although regional differences occur as with any basic food pattern, surveys indicate representative use of foods from basic food groups.

1. *Breads/cereals.* Traditional breads include hot breads such as biscuits, spoonbread (a souffle-like dish of cornmeal mush with beaten eggs), cornmeal muffins, and skillet cornbread. Commonly used cereals are cooked cereals such as cornmeal mush, hominy grits (ground corn), and oatmeal. In general, more cooked cereal is used than ready-to-eat dry cereals.
2. *Eggs/dairy products.* Eggs are used and some cheese, but little milk, probably as a result of the greater prevalence of lactose intolerance among blacks than among whites.
3. *Vegetables.* A common type of vegetable is leafy greens—turnip greens, collards, mustard greens, and spinach—usually cooked with bacon or salt pork. Cabbage is used boiled or chopped raw with a salad dressing (cole slaw). Other vegetables include okra (coated with cornmeal and fried), sweet potatoes (baked whole or sliced and candied with added sugar), green beans, tomatoes, potatoes, corn, butterbeans (lima), and dried beans such as black-eyed peas or red beans cooked with smoked ham hocks and served over rice. Black-eyed peas served over rice is a dish called Hopping John, traditionally served on New Year's Day for good luck in the new year.
4. *Fruits.* Commonly used fruits include apples, peaches, berries, oranges, bananas, and juices.
5. *Meat.* Pork is a common meat, including fresh cuts and ribs, sausage, and smoked ham. Some beef is used, mainly ground for meat loaf or hamburgers. Poultry is used frequently, mainly fried chicken and baked holiday turkey. Organ meats such as liver, heart, intestines (chitterlings), or poultry giblets (gizzard and heart) are used. When it is available, fish includes catfish, some flounder, and shellfish such as crab and shrimp. Frying is a common method of cooking; fats used are lard, shortening, or vegetable oils.
6. *Desserts.* Favorites include pies (pecan, sweet potato, pumpkin, and deep-dish peach or berry cobblers), cakes (coconut and chocolate), and bread pudding, which uses leftover bread.
7. *Beverages.* Coffee, apple cider, fruit juices, lemonade, iced tea, carbonated soft drinks, and buttermilk, a better-tolerated form of milk.

French Americans

The Cajun people of the southwestern coastal waterways in southern Louisiana have contributed a unique cuisine and food pattern to America's rich and varied fare. It provides a model for learning about rapidly expanding forms of American ethnic food.[13] The Cajuns are descendants of the early French colonists of Acadia, a peninsula on the eastern coast of Canada now known as Nova Scotia. In the pre-Revolutionary wars between France and Britain, both countries contended for the area of Acadia. However, after Britain finally gained control of all of Canada, fear of an Acadian revolt led to a forcible deportation of French colonists in 1755. After a long and difficult journey down the Atlantic coast and then westward along the Gulf of Mexico, a group of the impoverished Acadians finally settled along the bayou country of what is now Louisiana. To support themselves, they developed their unique food pattern from seafood at hand and what they could grow and harvest. Over time they blended their own French culinary background with the Creole cookery they found in their new homeland around New Orleans, which had descended from classic French cuisine combined with other European, American Indian, and African dishes.

The unique Cajun food pattern of the southern United States represents an ethnic blending of cultures using basic foods available in the area. Cajun foods are strong-flavored and spicy, with the abundant seafood as a base, usually cooked as stew and served over rice. The well-known hot chili sauce, made of crushed and fermented red chili peppers blended with spices and vinegar and sold worldwide under the trade name of Tabasco sauce, is still made by generations of a Cajun family on Avery Island on the coastal waterway of southern Louisiana. The most popular shellfish native to the region is the crawfish, now grown commercially in the fertile rice paddies of the bayou area. Other seafood that is used includes catfish, red snapper, shrimp, blue crab, and oysters. Cajun dishes usually start with a roux made from heated oil and flour mixed with liquid to form a sauce base, to which vegetables and then meat or seafood and seasonings are added to form a stew. Vegetables include onions, bell peppers, parsley, shallots, and tomatoes; seasonings are cayenne (red) pepper, hot pepper sauce (Tabasco), crushed black pepper, white pepper, bay leaves, thyme, and filé powder. Filé powder is made from ground sassafras leaves and serves both to season and to thicken the dish being made. Some typical Cajun dishes include seafood or chicken gumbo, jambalaya (dish of Creole origin, combining rice, chicken, ham, pork, sausage, broth, vegetables, and seasonings), red beans and rice, blackened catfish or red snapper (blackened with pepper and seasonings and seared in a hot pan), barbecued shrimp, breaded catfish with Creole sauce, and boiled crawfish. Breads and starches include French bread, hush puppies (fried cornbread-mixture balls), cornbread muffins, cush-cush (cornmeal mush cooked with milk), grits (hominy, ground corn), rice, and yams. Vegetables include okra, squash, onions, bell peppers, and tomatoes. Desserts include ambrosia (fresh fruits such as oranges and bananas with grated coconut), sweet potato pie, pecan pie, berry pie, bread pudding, and pecan pralines.

ASIAN FOOD PATTERNS

Chinese

Chinese cooks believe that refrigeration diminishes natural flavors. Therefore they select the freshest foods possible, hold them the shortest time possible, and then cook them quickly at a high temperature in a wok with only small amounts of fat and liquid. This basic round-bottom pan allows control of heat in a quick stir-frying method that preserves natural flavor, color, and texture. Vegetables cooked just before serving are still crisp and flavorful when served. Meat is used in small amounts in combined dishes rather than as a single main entree. Little milk is used, but eggs and soybean products such as tofu add protein. Foods that have been dried, salted, pickled, spiced, candied, or canned may be added as garnishes or relishes to mask some flavors or textures or to enhance other. Fruits are usually eaten fresh. Rice is the staple grain used at most meals. The traditional beverage is unsweetened green tea. Seasonings include soy sauce, ginger, almonds, and sesame seed. Peanut oil is a main cooking fat.[14]

Japanese

Japanese food patterns share some general similarities with Chinese cooking: both use rice as a basic grain and both emphasize fresh ingredients. However, Japanese food has many distinctive differences. The Japanese use paddy rice, whereas the Chinese cultivate primarily upland rice. More important are differences in cooking methods. Japanese cooking uses typically less oil than its Chinese counterpart because there is much less use of oil-based wok-style cooking. The usual vegetable dish is boiled or shredded fresh vegetables with vinegar and soy sauce. The Japanese food pattern contains steamed rice, along with grilled, broiled, or pan-cooked fish or shellfish, and a wide variety of cooked vegetables. Poultry, pork, and beef are also often in the diet. A large bowl of noodles combined with some meat and vegetables is popular as a quick and easy meal during the day. Soy sauce and rice vinegar are often used as flavorings. Japanese cooking has become popular in the United States, especially the sushi and sashimi dishes with various kinds of very fresh, carefully prepared raw fish and the tempura dishes of battered and deep-fried shrimp and vegetables.

Southeast Asian

Since 1971, in the wake of the war in Vietnam, more than 340,000 Southeast Asians have come to the United States as refugees. The largest group are Vietnamese; others have come from the adjacent war-torn countries of Laos and Cambodia. They have settled mainly in California, with other groups in Florida, Texas, Illinois, and Pennsylvania. Their basic food patterns are similar. They are making an impact on the American diet and agriculture, and Asian grocery stores stock many traditional Indo-Chinese food items. Rice, both long-grain and glutinous, forms the basis of the Indonesian food pattern, and it is eaten at most meals. The Vietnamese usually eat rice plain in a separate rice bowl and not mixed with other foods, whereas other Southeast Asians may eat rice in mixed dishes. Soups are also commonly used at meals. Many fresh fruits and vegetables are used along with fresh herbs and other seasonings such as chives, spring onions, chili peppers, ginger root, coriander, turmeric, and fish sauce. Many kinds of fish and shellfish are used, as well as chicken, duck, pork, and beef. Stir-frying in a wok-type pan with a small amount of lard or peanut oil is a common method of cooking. A variety of vegetables and seasonings are used, with small amounts of seafood or meat added. Since coming to the United States, the Indonesians have made some diet changes that reflect American influence. These include the use of more eggs, beef, and pork but less seafood and more candy and other sweet snacks, bread, fast foods, soft drinks, butter and margarine, and coffee.

MEDITERRANEAN INFLUENCES

Italian

The sharing of food is an important part of Italian life. Meals are associated with warmth and fellowship, and special occasions are shared with families and friends. Bread and pasta are basic foods. Milk, seldom used alone, is typically mixed with coffee in equal portions. Cheese is a favorite food, with many popular varieties. Meats, poultry, and fish are used in many ways, and the varied Italian sausages and cold cuts are famous. Vegetables are used alone, in mixed main dishes or soups, in sauces, and in salads. Seasonings include herbs and spices, garlic, wine, olive oil, tomato puree, and salt pork. Main dishes are prepared by initially browning vegetables and seasonings in olive oil; adding meat or fish for browning as well; covering with such liquids as wine, broth, or tomato sauce; and simmering slowly on low heat for several hours. Fresh fruit is often the dessert or a snack.[15]

Greek

Everyday meals are simple, but Greek holiday meals are occasions for serving many delicacies. Bread is always the center of every meal, with other foods considered accompaniments. Milk is seldom used as a beverage, but rather as the cultured form of yogurt. Cheese is a favorite food, especially feta, a white cheese made from the sheep's milk and preserved in brine. Lamb is a favorite meat, but others, especially fish, are also used. Eggs are sometimes a main dish, never a breakfast food. Many vegetables are used, often as a main entree, cooked with broth, tomato sauce, onions, olive oil, and parsley. A typical salad of thinly sliced raw vegetables and feta cheese, dressed with olive oil and vinegar, is often served with meals. Rice is a main grain in many dishes. Fruit is an everyday dessert, but rich pastries, such as baklava, are served on special occasions.[15]

Biotechnology and Food: Promise and Controversy

Each era in human history seems to be characterized by a dominant science, whose breakthroughs in understanding lead to new products and opportunities, as well as revolutionary changes and challenges for society. From this viewpoint, the twentieth century was the century of physics. During the twentieth century, advances in the physical sciences gave us wonders such as nuclear power, airplanes, automobiles, television, and computers; they also gave us atomic bombs, toxic wastes, smog, and traffic jams. But a new dominant science is arising. The twenty-first century will be the century of biology—more specifically, the century of biotechnology.[16] Advances in the biologic sciences will lead to equally profound wonders and new challenges and dangers for society. Already astonishing biologic technologies are advancing rapidly. New wonders are upon us, such as recombinant DNA bioengineering, the mapping of the human genome showing us the complete sequence of all 30,000-plus genes in the human DNA molecule, the mapping of the genomes of important animal and plant species, the successful cloning of animals such as sheep, and the prospect of human cloning in the not-too-distant future. These developments cause everyone in society—scientists, educators, consumers, government officials, industry leaders—to debate questions of how best to enjoy the benefits and minimize the dangers as humans learn to control biology in ways that were never before possible.

Two trends are certain: (1) biotechnology will continue to bring profound changes to food production and (2) these new food-related technologies will continue to generate in the scientific, political, and public arenas much discussion and even controversy over which techniques are safe and how to regulate them. Many new technologies are genuine scientific advances and should be freely used. At the same time, the public is rightly skeptical when new techniques appear to be introduced too quickly for primarily commercial reasons.

Regarding biotechnology—as in all areas of science—practitioners and consumers alike benefit from paying attention to serious scientific investigations as reported in peer-reviewed scientific journals. These journals present the research findings that over time produce society's growing body of trustworthy scientific knowledge. For the general public, the quality and accuracy of science news reporting in the major national newspapers and news magazines are usually very good, although more depth and consistent follow-up are always desirable. Unfortunately, however, the public is often left confused by exaggerated reports in other parts of the media that combine a small dose of science with a large dose of unfounded fearful claims. It is also true that the answers to many questions are simply not known at present and must await further scientific study. Sometimes both the consumer in the supermarket and the government regulation writer must make decisions based on partial knowledge. Keeping informed with the advances of tested science is the best way to sort out opposing viewpoints and to avoid falling for hype and exaggeration.

Each area of debate should be examined on its own merits. Sometimes an informed judgment can be made relatively easily, whereas in other cases it will be more appropriate to take a cautious approach to a new biotechnology, pending further investigations. These concerns are illustrated by a closer look at three food-related developments from biotechnology that have generated controversy—the uses of irradiation, growth hormones in dairy cows, and genetic engineering in agriculture.

FOOD IRRADIATION

Irradiation is a technique that kills bacteria in food—in effect, pasteurizing the food—by passing through it short-wavelength gamma rays, similar to microwaves. Because gamma rays do not emit neutrons, the food is not made radioactive. Unlike with pasteurization, because the food is not heated, there is almost no loss of nutrients. The process of irradiation has had more than 40 years of scientific testing and is approved by the FDA for use in wheat and wheat flour, fruits, vegetables, potatoes, poultry, and red meat. The U.S. Department of Agriculture (USDA) has instituted procedures allowing the increased use of irradiation in red meat production.

Hospitals use irradiation for patients who need completely germ-free food, such as those receiving bone marrow transplants, and NASA uses irradiation on the food consumed in space by astronauts. The U.S. Postal Service uses irradiation on mail to kill potentially dangerous biologic organisms. Irradiation has been approved as safe by a long list of scientific organizations, including the American Medical Association, the American Dietetic Association, the World Health Organization, and the United Nations Food and Agriculture Organization.

Despite its benefits, irradiation has been only slowly adopted. One drawback has simply been the word itself; people associate the name with the dangers of radiation. Studies have shown, though, that the public will purchase irradiated food when adequately informed of the benefits. Some consumer concerns have raised worries since irradiation produces free radical (radiolytic) compounds, which are considered by some to be linked with an increased risk of cancer and other diseases. However, as the American Dietetic Association has pointed out, the same free radicals are produced to a much greater extent by the act of cooking, and extensive scientific testing has failed to show any health risk from radiolytic compounds.[17] Because the overall benefits of irradiation outweigh any potential risks by a wide margin, this technique is likely to continue to be adopted in food production. Informed judgment in this case favors the use of irradiation when done in accordance with the USDA guidelines.

BOVINE GROWTH HORMONE AND DAIRY COWS

The FDA approved in 1993 the use of recombinant bovine growth hormone (rBGH) in dairy cows to increase milk production. This hormone has become widely used in the dairy industry, and approximately 3 million of the dairy cows in the United States (about 30% of the total) have been treated with rBGH. The commercial product rBGH is a genetically engineered protein molecule that is identical to the natural protein found in cows.

Growth hormone is a protein that is secreted naturally in the pituitary gland of animals, including humans and cows. It plays an essential role in growth, development, and health maintenance. BGH extracted from cattle pituitary glands had been used for more than 60 years in the dairy industry as a means to boost milk production, although the supply was limited. In the 1980s, it became technically and economically possible to use recombinant DNA processes to make large quantities of BGH. The FDA issued its approval of the use of rBGH after its review of experimental test data led to the finding that there is no significant absorption of the hormone by the gastrointestinal tract and that there is no appreciable risk to humans from milk produced by cows given rBGH. The FDA in its 1993 approval did not require long-term testing of the effects of rBGH on either cows or humans.

During the 1990s, many dairies began using rBGH, whereas others did not. Critics of the FDA said that the agency had not thoroughly investigated rBGH. Public controversy over rBGH was renewed in 1999 when Health Canada, the Canadian counterpart to the FDA, decided not to approve rBGH for use in Canada. Health Canada reviewed the original test data, including a 90-day study of possible absorption of the hormone by rats, and concluded that there could be possible adverse health effects on humans because the FDA had not conducted long-term studies on humans of the safety of milk from cows treated with rBGH. The Canadian action led to criticism of the FDA within the U.S. Congress that the FDA was not handling its regulatory responsibilities properly and to formal petitions to the FDA that it reverse its approval of rBGH.

In the face of controversy, the FDA acted responsibly, both as a government agency and as a scientific body. The FDA went back to the origins of its 1993 approval and conducted a comprehensive audit and reexamination of all data concerning rBGH and of all the concerns expressed by the Canadian study and by other critics. The FDA has issued detailed reports that present the scientific evidence from the original test data as well as from the scientific literature on all questions raised about rBGH. The concerns over possible health risks involved four main areas.

1. *Absorption of rBGH.* One concern is that rBGH might be absorbed into the body from the gastrointestinal tract, with potential adverse biologic effects, such as on the liver. Proteins consumed orally, such as from milk, are normally broken down by the body's digestive enzymes and are not absorbed into the body. In tests on rats, over both 28 days and 90 days, oral administration of rBGH at over 50 times the daily dose given to dairy cattle resulted in no biologic effects on the rats.[18]
2. *Antibody response.* The Canadian analysis cited concern over evidence from the rat study that very high oral doses of rBGH appeared to produce an antibody response measurable in the rats' blood. The FDA's reexamination of all relevant studies concludes that the antibody response is not significant for several reasons: the level of antibodies present is very low; the dose of rBGH needed to elicit an antibody response is several hundred times higher than a human adult or child could reasonably consume on a daily basis; and the same antibody response is produced by a number of food proteins and is therefore not in itself an indication of the absorption of intact rBGH.
3. *Thyroid cysts.* Another concern involved the data showing that some of the test rats developed thyroid cysts, which are noncancerous. The detailed reexamination, however, revealed that a similar percentage of rats developed such cysts in both the group given doses of rBGH and the untested control group.
4. *Insulin-like growth factor-1 (IGF-1).* The Canadian report also expressed the concern that milk from rBGH-treated cows sometimes contains higher levels of insulin-like growth factor-1 (IGF-1), which could raise safety concerns in humans. The FDA examined in de-

tail the question of IGF-1 levels in milk and found no scientific support for the viewpoint that it is a significant risk. IGF-1 is a protein normally produced by the body and found in human blood, and it is not typically harmful; it is similar to insulin and is not biologically active when taken orally. IGF-1 is a normal component of cow's milk, and its concentration varies considerably within a normal dairy herd. Several comprehensive studies show that the range of IGF-1 in milk from rBGH-treated herds is within the range of that found normally in untreated herds. In addition, there is no definitive evidence that biologically active IGF-1 from milk is absorbed into the body. There also is no clear evidence to support claims that IGF-1 is a causative agent in either breast cancer or prostate cancer.

rBGH is now used regularly by a sizable portion of the dairy industry. It is generally considered by most observers to be a safe product coming from applied biotechnology. The controversies that flowed around rBGH in the 1990s illustrate how different observers can reach different conclusions about policy from essentially the same body of experimental data. Risk assessment in science involves weighing numerous, often subtle, variables. Risk assessment is inherently never able to be a completely exact science. This case also shows how the main body of science accumulates evidence over time and thereby allows both scientists and policymakers to make progressively better judgments. The FDA has served the public interest well in addressing questions concerning rBGH and in basing its policy conclusions on the accumulated weight of the best science available.

GENETICALLY MODIFIED FOODS

Genetically modified (GM) foods are agricultural crops that have been genetically engineered by altering or replacing some of the plant's original, natural genetic DNA material. The biotechnologies that enable this process have developed tremendously during the past 25 years since the birth of the science of molecular biology in the 1970s, when the first gene-splicing techniques were invented.[16] The initial applications of molecular biology were in the field of pharmaceuticals, and genetically engineered drugs are widely used today, with more than 150 products on the market. GM bacteria, for example, have been producing human insulin since 1978, a product used today by 3.3 million people with diabetes.[19] Bioengineered food crops began to be introduced in the mid-1990s, and their use has increased dramatically since then. Today more than 100 million acres worldwide are planted with GM crops. The United States by far leads the world in growing GM crops, accounting for 68% of all worldwide GM crops in 2000.[20] More than 40 new GM crop products have been approved by the Environmental Protection Agency (EPA) for sale in the United States. Regulatory oversight of GM crops, and food products made from GM crops, is shared by the EPA, the FDA, and the USDA.

By 2000, 52% of all soybeans, 25% of all corn, and 12% of all cotton grown in the United States were grown from GM seeds.[19] Indeed, food products made from GM crops are already everywhere in the American supermarket. Corn, potatoes, and soy products may contain a gene from a bacterium to be pest resistant; they may also have had genes inserted in them that allow these crops to withstand herbicides. Summer squash, melons, and papayas may contain GM protein that makes the plant resistant to viruses. Tomatoes may be modified to resist herbicides and to have a longer shelf-life. The canola oil plant may be modified to produce oil that is low in saturated fat. About 70% of processed foods and soft drinks contain ingredients that are from GM crops.[21] Strawberries may contain a gene from a fish, the Arctic flounder, that gives the berries frost resistance and enables them to be grown in more northern climates.[19] GM foods entered the American food marketplace as food producers sought ways to reduce crop losses and extend the life of products. Food labels are not required to give information about the GM content of food products. The regulatory agencies of the government, with the support of the scientific community, have generally followed the position that food produced using both conventional methods and genetic engineering are safe and do not need specific content labeling.

Much of genetic engineering can be seen as essentially an extension of classic plant cross-breeding techniques—called hybridization—that farmers and scientists have used formally since the nineteenth century and informally for thousands of years. With new techniques it is possible to breed new varieties with desirable traits much faster than the many months or years needed using classic plant cross-breeding. Often the insertion of just one gene will produce a new desired trait. New varieties of crops are now being developed using genetic engineering to do more of what the plant normally does—such as increase the yield of the crop or enhance its nutritional content.

Genetic engineering of crops, however, can do much more than enhance natural characteristics. More dramatic, and also more controversial, is engineering a plant to have new characteristics that the crop could never have had naturally, such as being able to tolerate weed-killing herbicide treatments, carrying a protein within it that acts as a built-in insecticide, or being able to grow in extreme environmental conditions. This form of genetic modification uses gene-splicing and recombinant DNA techniques to put into a plant's genetic material pieces of new DNA that come from nonplant species, such as from bacteria or from fish. The goal is for the new GM plant to have desirable characteristics that are not found in nature. It may seem odd to use a gene from a bacterium in a plant. The focus, however, should be more on a gene's function, rather than on its origin. Thus the gene inserted into strawberries is more properly viewed as a cold-tolerance gene than as simply an Arctic flounder gene. It is also true that the same genes are found in many different species. Human beings, for example, share about 7000 genes with a worm named *Caenorhabditis elegans.*[22]

For agricultural crops, two traits are very highly desirable: the ability to resist insects and the ability to tolerate herbicides. With these traits in the crops, farmers can reduce their use of toxic chemical pesticides—insect-killing insecticides and weed-killing herbicides. Environmentalists have long worried about the very large amount of harsh chemical pesticides sprayed every year on food crops, which total more than 970 million pounds annually in the United States. Although the pesticides kill insects, weeds, and fungi, and thereby enable America's high agricultural productivity, they also linger in the soil and on crops, seep into groundwater, and get into the food chain of other wildlife. In addition, the high cost of spraying lowers farm income. In the mid-1990s, agribusiness companies began selling to farmers GM seeds that produce crops that are insect resistant, herbicide tolerant, or both. The benefits to farmers were reduced pesticide spraying and higher income. As the use of GM crops has spread, the reduction in chemical pesticide use, and accompanying environmental impact, has been dramatic in many places. American soybean farmers nationally are saving more than $200 million per year with GM crops due to a reduced need for herbicide spraying to control weed growth.[19] The growing of GM cotton has led to a greater than 20% reduction in insecticide spraying in many states.[20] Many cotton farmers have been able to reduce spraying for bollworm and budworm from seven times per season to none. Cotton farmers in developing countries, such as in China, have enthusiastically embraced the introduction of pest-resistant cotton. Many Chinese farmers say their personal health has improved now that they do not have to spray by hand large quantities of strong pesticide.[23]

The genetically engineered crops that would provide the greatest benefit to the largest number of people are those that would be better sources of essential nutrients. The potential health benefits are enormous. Especially in developing countries, the affordable basic food crops need to be as nutritious as possible. Rice is eaten as the staple food by half the world's population, but it is a poor source of many essential micronutrients and vitamins, especially vitamin A. Vitamin A deficiency afflicts millions of people in regions where rice is usually the only staple food available, and children are especially vulnerable. As a result, in Southeast Asia, 70% of children have vitamin A deficiency, leading to vision impairment and lower resistance to disease. The World Health Organization and UNICEF (United Nations Children's Fund) estimate that worldwide, approximately 500,000 children become blind each year and that 1 to 2 million children die from vitamin A deficiency.[24] An international team of genetic scientists in Switzerland has succeeded in bioengineering rice to produce beta-carotene (which converts to vitamin A in the body) and iron.[25] This type of rice has become known as "golden rice," so named because the beta-carotene it contains gives the rice grains a slight yellowish color. International efforts are under way to overcome legal and cultural barriers and to introduce golden rice to farmers in these areas and promote its consumption. Although some of the biotechnology that went into creating golden rice is proprietary, an international agreement has been reached that will allow the free distribution of golden rice seeds and genetic materials to poor farmers in developing countries. This program is expected to serve as a model of how proprietary biotechnology can be shared in noncommercial ways in areas of the world that need it the most.

Insect-resistant and herbicide-tolerant crops owe their remarkable abilities to a gene in a lowly bacterium common in soil, the *Bacillus thuringiensis* (Bt). These bioengineered crops are referred to as Bt corn, Bt cotton, and so on. This bacterium contains a gene that directs cells to create a protein that is toxic to insects such as caterpillars and beetles that try to eat the plant but is normally harmless to other organisms. Using genetic engineering techniques, this specific Bt gene is inserted into the genetic makeup of seeds, and crops grown from these seeds will contain this insect-killing protein. Bt plants in essence produce their own insecticide. In a similar fashion, crops are developed that tolerate herbicides, thus allowing farmers to spray less often and to use lesser-strength herbicides.

What are the potential risks that have caused worry and controversy over GM crops and foods made from them, especially in light of their significant environmental and economic benefits? Also, what is the current state of research concerning these risks? There are several main areas of concern.[20,26]

1. *Other life will be harmed.* The insect-killing compound built into many GM crops has the potential of harming innocent species. The monarch butterfly became the symbol of this concern when laboratory studies reported that monarch caterpillars died after eating pollen from Bt corn. International concern ensued, and a large number of researchers went into the cornfields to study the issue. Initial findings are that the overall risk to the monarch butterfly in its habitats is small from Bt corn. An international scientific conference on the issue concluded that we are far from knowing enough about the complex ecologic interactions involved to be able to make judgments about what the long-term effects of GM organisms might be.[27] The EPA continues to review studies of the monarch butterfly and other nontarget species.[28]
2. *Superweeds will be created.* Observers are concerned that pollen from GM crops that are insect resistant and herbicide tolerant could find its way to weed plants in a neighboring field. If the weeds are genetically close enough relatives to the GM plant, the weeds could be-

come fertilized by the GM pollen. The result would be a superweed that would be very hard to control and could spread widely. This process is called *gene flow,* and it is a real possibility. No one knows, however, how likely any widespread effect might be. Studies have not found superweeds thus far. A 10-year study in England found no weedlike developments around GM corn, canola, potatoes, or beets in that country.[29] Regulations in the United States prohibit planting GM crops in areas where there are closely related plants nearby. Traveling GM pollen may turn out to be more of a problem in developing countries than in temperate climates because many cultivated crops in tropical regions have weedy close relatives.

3. *GM crops will eventually fail to perform.* Agriculture has been described as a race between plant protection and pests. The tendency for insects to develop resistance to insecticides, and of weeds to develop resistance to herbicides, has been an increasing long-term problem for many years in agriculture. Biotechnology will inevitably be subject to the same evolutionary pressures. To slow the development of insect resistance to Bt crops, the EPA requires farmers to set aside a portion of their fields to grow crops that have not been genetically modified. In these areas, insects that have acquired some degree of Bt resistance interbreed with those that have not, thereby slowing the spread of resistance.[20] Eventually, resistant beetles will happily munch away on Bt crops. In the long run our food supply will likely also make greater use of organic farming techniques, which do not rely on pesticides.
4. *Foods with GM ingredients pose a higher risk of allergic reaction.* This is the primary concern about foods with GM ingredients. The possibility of allergic reaction was behind the recall in the fall of 2000 of taco shells by Kraft Foods that were discovered to contain a variety of Bt corn (StarLink) that had not been approved for human consumption by the FDA.[30] The FDA had noted the allergy connection when it had approved StarLink as an animal feed only. The recall pulled taco and tortilla products off grocery shelves across America, cost StarLink's maker Aventis an estimated $500 million, and was used by critics of GM foods as an example of how easily intermingling of ingredients can happen. Biotechnology manufacturers have a good record of voluntarily doing extensive tests for possible allergic reactions before putting GM foods on the market. New FDA rules in 2001 make such premarket reviews a requirement.[31]

GM crops and foods containing them will likely remain a source of concern for a long time. Public skepticism about GM foods has been particularly strong in Europe, where they have been branded with the derogatory name "Frankenfoods." After 3 years of refusing to allow imports of GM seeds and foods, the European Union Parliament in 2001 responded to public concerns and passed legislation controlling the testing, planting, and sale of GM crops and food, with labeling requirements to follow.[32] In the United States, GM food products have not been labeled. Eventually, some form of informational labeling on foods with GM ingredients is likely. This will be part of the larger process of putting in place a regulatory framework for the twenty-first century that will ease public concerns by maintaining the benefits and controlling the risks of these new food technologies.

Our expanding knowledge of genetics will allow further technical advances with less potential risk. A very important advance is that the complete genome of important food plants is being decoded, starting with rice, which in 2001 became the first major crop to have its genetic code fully sequenced.[33] Knowledge of the genes in rice can speed the development of improved varieties with higher yields, better nutrition, and a greater ability to withstand drought, pests, and poor soils. Improved rice, such as the "golden rice" with beta-carotene, can directly benefit half the world's population, who depend on rice as their staple food.

Another application of advanced genetic knowledge will be more effective conventional breeding of crops and livestock, without using the recombinant DNA techniques of genetic engineering. This enhanced breeding approach is also called *marker-assisted breeding* because it uses known genes as markers to guide the process. Enhanced breeding does not require review by government regulators and is more acceptable in the marketplace to a public skeptical of genetic engineering. The first step in this process uses genetic tests to determine which genes are in a plant or animal and where they are on the genome. By doing this, research scientists are able to select more easily and accurately which genes to cross-breed and are able to reduce by years the time it takes to breed a new variety. These new techniques can identify genes in cattle and other livestock that are associated with higher milk production, more tender meat, and other desirable traits. The knowledge of the location and function of these genes will be used to guide conventional breeding, not to create genetically altered herds. Better understanding of genetic science will also help organic farming. Enhanced breeding will not be able to replace genetic engineering completely because it does not have the precision needed to transfer only an individual gene with a desired trait. The new "golden rice," for example, could only have been created using genetic engineering because the genes in it that provide the vitamin A originated in daffodils and bacteria. Marker-assisted breeding brings together classic breeders and molecular geneticists using modern genome knowledge.

As this century of biotechnology unfolds, the two trends noted earlier about biotechnology—that it brings both revolutionary changes and ongoing debates about safety—will continue. A third major trend will join them: an increasing emphasis on ecology. Being ecology-minded means being aware of the complex interconnectedness of all life. The debates over the risks of biotechnology will generate in coming years a great deal of scientific study, both in the laboratory and in the field. As our knowledge expands, our awareness also rises of the importance of basing technical, political, and personal decisions on an ecologic perspective. Genetic engineering, with its power and promise, will have its greatest benefit when used within a knowledge of the larger ecologic framework. Approaches such as the new enhanced breeding that relies on scientific knowledge will undoubtedly play a major role in agriculture and food production during the twenty-first century. Biotechnology is here to stay. Its benefits and its risks are here to stay also.

Food Safety

America's food supply has radically changed during the past years. These changes, which have swept the food-marketing system, are rooted in widespread social change and scientific advance. The agricultural and food processing industries have developed a wide variety of technologies to increase and preserve our food supply and to create new products. These advances are accompanied by concerns that these changes have positive effects on food safety, food habits, and the overall environment.

AGRICULTURAL PESTICIDES AND ORGANIC FARMING

American agriculture during the past few decades has developed into a modern mechanized business structure. As a whole, it has brought large crop yields to feed a growing population. Large American agricultural corporations, as well as individual farmers, typically use a number of chemicals to advance food production. Agricultural chemicals are used for a variety of reasons to control destructive insects, kill weeds, control plant diseases, stop fruit from dropping prematurely, cause leaves to fall and thus facilitate harvesting, make seeds sprout, keep seeds from rotting before they sprout, increase yield, and improve marketing quality. Over time, however, problems from the frequent use of pesticides have developed in four main areas: (1) pesticide residues on food, (2) leaching of the chemicals into ground water and surrounding wells, (3) increased exposure of farm workers to the strong chemicals, and (4) increased amount of chemicals required as insect tolerance for pesticides develops. The FDA has the difficult task of assessing health risks for the thousands of pesticides in use or being developed.

Organic farming—the agricultural methods that grow crops without the use of pesticides and herbicides—has grown in popularity in recent years. Organic farming can include organically grown fruits and vegetables as well as organically raised beef and poultry. Organic farmers, with help from soil scientists, are developing systems of sustainable agriculture that do not rely on heavy pesticide use. Instead, they combine pesticide-free farming practices and appropriate modern technology. An increasing numbers of consumers are willing to pay a premium for organically produced food. The USDA in October 2002, following criteria set by Congress, issued national standards that both domestic and imported food labeled "organic" must meet. Both farms and food processors must follow strict growing and production standards and must be certified by the USDA before a food can be labeled "organic." New labeling rules include a new *USDA Organic seal* for products that are at least 95% organic.[34] Despite the economic trends toward food globalization, a growing willingness among consumers to support local farmers and to consume a diet based on locally produced food has many advantages, both for the environment and for health: local farmland is retained, the environmental damage from food production and transport is minimized, the food supply becomes more sustainable, and our exposure to foodborne contamination and illness is reduced.[35]

FOOD PROCESSING ADDITIVES

During the past few decades, chemicals added to foods during processing have become an integral part of our food supply. Our present variety of food market items would be impossible without them. For example, additives enrich food with added nutrients, produce uniform qualities of food products, standardize functional factors such as thickening and stabilization, preserve foods, and improve flavor and texture. Table 9-1 lists some examples of these additives. A number of micronutrients and antioxidants are being added to processed foods, not for increasing the nutrient content but for their technical effects.

FOOD SAFETY LAWS: FOODS, ADDITIVES, SUPPLEMENTS, AND DRUGS

The legal framework in federal law regulating what may legally be in food, additives, supplements, and drugs has evolved through the years. The initial control of food and drug ingredients for safety began in 1938 with the passage of the Federal Food, Drug, and Cosmetic Act (FFDCA). The category of pharmaceutical drugs has always been the most highly regulated legally because drugs can have such great benefits when used properly and such great dangers when misused. While a new drug is in development, extensive testing must be done, often over a period of years, and the drug must pass a high legal standard that it be both "safe and effective." Convincing scientific evidence must be presented to the FDA by the manufacturer, and the FDA must give its formal approval before the drug can be sold.

TABLE 9-1 Some Examples of Intentional Food Additives

Function	Chemical Compounds	Common Food Uses
Acids, alkalis, buffers	Sodium bicarbonate	Baking powder
	Tartaric acid	Fruit sherbets
		Cheese spreads
Antibiotics	Chlortetracycline	Dip for dressed poultry
Anticaking agents	Aluminum calcium silicate	Table salt
Antimycotics	Calcium propionate	Bread
	Sodium propionate	Bread
	Sorbic acid	Cheese
Antioxidants	Butylated hydroxyanisole (BHA)	Fats
	Butylated hydroxytoluene (BHT)	Fats
Bleaching agents	Benzoyl peroxide	Wheat flour
	Chlorine dioxide	
	Oxides of nitrogen	
Color preservative	Sodium benzoate	Green peas
		Maraschino cherries
Coloring agents	Annotto	Butter, margarine
	Carotene	
Emulsifiers	Lecithin	Bakery goods
	Monoglycerides, diglycerides	Dairy products
	Propylene glycol alginate	Confections
Flavoring agents	Amyl acetate	Soft drinks
	Benzaldehyde	Bakery goods
	Methyl salicylate	Candy, ice cream
	Essential oils, natural extracts	Canned meats
	Monosodium glutamate	
Nonnutritive sweeteners	Saccharin	Diet packed canned fruit
	Aspartame	Low-kcalorie soft drinks and other foods
Nutrient supplements	Potassium iodide	Iodized salt
	Vitamin C	Fruit juices
	Vitamin D	Milk
	Vitamin A	Margarine
	B vitamins, iron	Bread and cereal
	Calcium	Orange juice
Sequestrants	Sodium citrate	Dairy products
	Calcium pyrophosphoric acid	
Stabilizers and thickeners	Pectin	Jellies
	Vegetable gums (carob bean, carrageenan, guar)	Dairy desserts and chocolate milk
	Gelatin	Confections
	Agar-agar	Low-kcalorie salad dressings
Yeast foods and dough conditioners	Ammonium chloride	Bread, rolls
	Calcium sulfate	Bread, rolls
	Calcium phosphate	Bread, rolls

The legal structure is complex for foods, food additives, and dietary supplements. The makers of all foods are legally obligated to assure the public that their products are safe. For conventional foods, the safety standard under the FFDCA is that the food, including all ingredients, must not be "ordinarily injurious." Safety is assumed to exist for ingredients with a long history of use. These food products may be marketed without prior approval of the FDA. For example, a package of cookies whose ingredients include flour, brown sugar, eggs, butter, baking soda, etc. meets this standard.

In 1960, further regulatory legislation extended the FFDCA and created two legal classes of food additives. The first group encompassed all food additives that had

ecology Relations between organisms and their environments.

been marketed before 1958. These additives were "grandfathered" in under the law and placed in a category known as Generally Recognized as Safe (GRAS) ingredients. There are thousands of additives on the GRAS list. An example is the coloring added to margarine to make it yellow, which has been in use since the 1930s. The safety standard under the FFDCA is that the food is unsafe if the additive "may render injurious" the food product. Additives on the GRAS list are assumed under the law to be acceptable under that standard. Food makers are not required to obtain FDA approval to use additives on the GRAS list. Safety was claimed for GRAS additives based on wide prior use, but testing to determine their true safety, however, was lacking. In 1977 Congress directed the FDA to test the thousands of GRAS items; this testing is ongoing. The second legal category of additives includes any additive developed since 1958. These additives are not on the GRAS list. The same legal standard of "may render injurious" applies, but these newer additives must have rigid testing for safety under FDA scrutiny. FDA approval must be obtained before any food product containing a new additive may be legally sold.[36] An example of a new additive is aspartame, the artificial sweetener marketed under the brand name NutraSweet. Aspartame received FDA approval after extensive testing, and today is the sweetener ingredient in virtually all sugar-free soft drinks sold worldwide.

Dietary supplements have received special favorable legal treatment. In 1994 Congress passed the Dietary Supplement Health and Education Act (DSHEA), which effectively deregulated the entire supplements industry. All additive ingredients marketed as supplements before October 1994 were "grandfathered" in under this law as safe, in the same manner as the GRAS food additives. This category includes almost all of the thousands of products containing vitamins, minerals, herbal preparations, therapeutic botanical compounds, Asian medicinal herbals, and similar products. Under this law, supplements are legally classified as neither foods nor drugs. No scientific testing to demonstrate either product safety or the effectiveness of product claims is required of supplement manufacturers, and no FDA approval is required. For newer supplement ingredients developed after 1994, the safety standard is simply that there is no "unreasonable risk." The maker must notify the FDA before marketing the product, but no FDA approval is required.

The DSHEA has been a controversial law. The marketing of dietary supplements has grown enormously into a major industry with large advertising budgets and a wide range of products, from single vitamins to complex compounds. Claims of supplements benefits are everywhere, but reliable, scientifically supported evidence is usually lacking. Under the law, a claim cannot be made that a supplement product cures a disease. However, statements concerning how the human body will respond to the supplement, such as a claim that it makes your body burn fat faster, are completely unregulated and require no proof. The supplements industry believes in self-regulation, but many consumer advocates and scientific groups believe that the lack of effective FDA supervision of this growing part of the American diet is a flaw in the law. As the supplements market has grown, dietary supplements and the active ingredients within them are coming under increasing scrutiny by scientists, the FDA, and Congress. Consumer advocates and the makers of dietary supplements are increasingly coming to agreement over the desirability of further scientific study of supplements and botanicals, as well of taking steps to increase consumer confidence in supplement safety, appropriate uses, labeling truthfulness, and recommended dosage sizes.

FDA FOOD RESEARCH

Research has always been a large part of the FDA's work. Along with the USDA Agricultural Research Service, FDA scientists continually evaluate foods and food components through their own research. In the past, FDA views and policies have varied with administrators and sometimes have left much to be desired. Nevertheless, broader views more in tune with current needs prevail now. Today people want to know more than just that a given food will not kill them. They want to know whether it has any positive nutritional value. Thus for a more health-conscious public and a changed marketplace, the FDA has developed expanded nutrition guidelines for food labels on a variety of food products.

FDA FOOD LABELING REGULATIONS

Prior Nutrition Label Information

In the mid 1970s, the FDA began describing general nutrition information on food labels, and some producers added limited information on their own in response to increasing market demand. Nutrients and food constituents that consumer groups wanted listed on labels included the macronutrients (carbohydrates, fat, and protein) and their total energy value (kilocalories [kcalories]), key micronutrients (vitamins and minerals), sodium, cholesterol, and saturated fat.

Current FDA Food Label Regulations

The nutrition labels that are now familiar on products on supermarket shelves were created as a requirement under the Nutrition Labeling and Education Act of 1990 (NLEA). This law enacted a major improvement in conveying nutritional information about food products to consumers. The NLEA requires mandatory labeling of most processed foods under the jurisdiction of the FDA and forms the core of the FDA's reform effort. It also includes voluntary labeling of fresh fruits, vegetables, and seafood. The USDA is responsible for standards and consumer information concerning other meat and poultry, as well as dairy products. During a 3-year process that involved consumers, producers, and health professionals, the new food labels emerged. Basic features of the revised labeling regulations now include guidelines to define the following items: kcalories and nutrients, descriptive terms, serving sizes and number of servings per container, health claims, and a standardized label format based on results of consumer research.

Major Food Label Changes

Consumers began seeing the new nutrition label on food products in 1994 (Figure 9-1). The most visible changes now in practice are how food is advertised and marketed. For example, manufacturers no longer can claim that a product does not contain an ingredient that has never been contained in that product. This means that products that never contained cholesterol cannot make the claim "no cholesterol." Descriptors such as "light," "low fat," and "reduced kcalories" now have legal definitions that are universal to all products.

The current Nutrition Facts label (see Figure 9-1), now familiar on food products in all food markets and grocery stores, uses the term Daily Reference Value (DRV) rather than the former outdated values. DRVs are now listed for carbohydrates, proteins, total fat, saturated fat, fiber, cholesterol, sodium, and potassium. DRVs for energy sources (fats, carbohydrates, protein) are based on percentages of 2000- and 2500-kcalorie diets, and DRVs for other food components represent the uppermost limit that is considered desirable. FDA guidelines for these nutrient labeling regulations are defined in the *To Probe Further* box. In August 1996, the FDA completed and published final regulations for the nutrition labeling of raw fruits, vegetables, and fish.[37] In 1994 the trilateral North American Free Trade Agreement (NAFTA) was enacted, committing Canada, the United States, and Mexico to work toward harmonized consumer labeling standards.[38]

Nutrition Facts

Serving Size: 1/2 cup (114 g)
Servings Per Container: 4

Amount per Serving	
Calories 260	
Calories from Fat 120	
	% Daily Value*
Total Fat 13 g	20%
Saturated Fat 5 g	25%
Cholesterol 30 mg	10%
Sodium 660 mg	28%
Total Carbohydrate 31 g	11%
Dietary Fiber 0 g	0%
Sugars 5 g	
Protein 5 g	

Vitamin A 4% • Vitamin C 1%
Calcium 15% • Iron 4%

*Percents (%) of a Daily Value are based on a 2,000 calorie diet. Your Daily Values may vary higher or lower depending on your calorie needs.

Nutrient	2,000 calories	2,500 calories
Total Fat	<65 g	<80 g
Saturated Fat	<20 g	<25 g
Cholesterol	<300 mg	<300 mg
Sodium	<2,400 mg	<2,400 mg
Total Carbohydrate	300 g	375 g
Dietary Fiber	25 g	30 g

1 g Fat = 9 calories
1 g Carbohydrate = 4 calories
1 g Protein = 4 calories

FIGURE 9-1 Example of a current food label. *(From Food and Drug Administration, Washington, DC.)*

GOVERNMENT FOOD SAFETY CONTROL AGENCIES

A Shared Regulatory System: USDA and FDA

The current regulatory system for food safety in the United States began in 1906, when Congress gave responsibility for keeping the nation's food supply safe to the USDA. The USDA instituted the system, still in force today, of continuous on-site inspection of beef carcasses in packing plants, as well as daily inspections of poultry processing plants, an enormous job that is done by thousands of USDA inspectors nationwide. The FDA was originally a part of the USDA. Later Congress moved the FDA out of the USDA and made it part of the Department of Health and Human Services (DHHS). The FDA was given responsibility for ensuring the safety of all food except for meat and poultry, which remained in the jurisdiction of the USDA's well-established inspection system. These agencies work together to ensure that pesticide residue levels in food do not exceed the tolerance standards set by the EPA. Interagency cooperation is increasingly recognized as essential in responding effectively to new food-related threats to health. The USDA and the Centers for Disease Control and Prevention (CDC) have worked closely together to prevent the spread of mad cow disease and the related human disease from Great Britain and Europe to the United States (see *Issues & Answers*).

Food and Drug Administration

The FDA is a law enforcement agency charged by Congress to ensure, among other things, that our food supply is safe, pure, and wholesome. The agency enforces federal food safety regulations through various activities, including (1) food sanitation and quality control, (2) control of chemical contaminants and pesticides, (3) control of food additives, (4) regulation of movement of food across state lines, (5) nutrition and nutrition labeling of foods, (6) safety of public food service, and (7) safety of meat and milk. The most common means of enforcement is the use of recalls and seizures of contaminated food.

The FDA is committed to its role in food safety law enforcement, but outside observers and the FDA itself admit that its inspection ability is inadequate in today's global food economy. The FDA has fewer than one-tenth

TO PROBE FURTHER

Food and Drug Administration Guidelines for Nutrition Labeling Regulations

Implementation of the 1990 Nutrition Labeling and Education Act (NLEA) has changed the way consumers look at food labels. This law, NLEA, was developed by the FDA through a painstaking public process with the input of consumers, the food industry, and health professionals. It now empowers the FDA to enforce these regulations for the food industry and the public to help consumers make wise food choices.

The FDA label guidelines cover five main areas: (1) nutrients and energy (as kcalories), (2) serving sizes, (3) definitions for terms used, (4) label format, and (5) health claims.

NUTRIENTS AND KCALORIES

The NLEA requires a food product to provide nutrient and energy information for the following.

- Protein (in terms of amino acid quality)
- Energy (as kcalories)
- Fat-soluble vitamins A, D, E, and K
- Water-soluble vitamins C, thiamin, riboflavin, niacin, pyridoxine (B_6), folate, and cobalamin (B_{12})
- Calcium, phosphorus, magnesium, iron, zinc, iodine, and selenium

On the revised label, new reference nutrient values have replaced the outdated and confusing term *U.S. RDAs*. Instead, the terms now used are Reference Daily Intake (RDI) and Daily Reference Value (DRV). The RDIs are derived from RDAs and are population-based averages for all age and sex groups (excluding pregnant and lactating women). The DRV of a given nutrient in a food product is its content in that product expressed as a percentage of the RDI for that nutrient.

SERVING SIZES

Under the revised label rules, a standardized reference serving size is set for a large number of food categories in quantities customarily eaten. These portions are expressed in common household measures. The USDA has standardized serving sizes of meat and poultry products.

DESCRIPTORS

To improve communication between producers and consumers, everyone must work from the same FDA-supplied "dictionary." In this "dictionary" nine core terms have been defined: free, low, light or lite, less, high, source of, more, fresh, and reduced. The following are examples.

- *Fat free*—less than 0.5 g of fat per serving.
- *Low cholesterol*—20 mg of cholesterol or less per serving and per 100 g; 2 g saturated fat or less per serving. Any label claim about cholesterol is prohibited for all foods that contain more than 2 g of saturated fat per serving.
- *Light or lite*—at least a one-third reduction in kcalories (40 kcalories with minimum fat reduction of 3 g; if fat contributes 50% or more of kcalories, fat content must be reduced by 50% compared with the reference food).
- *Less sodium*—at least a 25% reduction or more than 140 mg per serving.
- *High*—20% or more of the RDI or DRV per serving.
- *Reduced saturated fat*—saturated fat content reduced by 50% or more, with a minimum reduction of more than 1 g/serving.

NUTRITION LABEL FORMAT

The standardized nutrition labeling format provided by the FDA is mandatory for all food producers and marketing agents. This format resulted from consumer research for developing sound nutrition information the consumers want and readily understand. It continues to serve as an important vehicle for nutrition education, as the law (NLEA) mandated.

The FDA guidelines indicate that any label health claim must be supported by substantial scientific evidence and has found that only four health relationships meet this test and can be used; these involve the relation of (1) sodium to hypertension, (2) calcium to osteoporosis, (3) lipids to cancer, and (4) lipids to cardiovascular disease.

References

FDA staff: The new food label: your guide to better nutrition, *Nutr Today* 25(1):37, 1992.

Legislative News: Terms on food labels: ADA comments on proposals from FDA and USDA, *J Am Diet Assoc* 2(3):543, 1992.

Pennington JAT, Wilkening VL: Final regulations for the nutrition labeling of raw fruits, vegetables, and fish, *J Am Diet Assoc* 97(11):1299, 1997.

Salton E et al: The new food label as a tool for healthy eating, *Nutr Today* 29(3):18, 1994.

the number of inspectors that the USDA has, with only about 400 inspectors to check more than 57,000 food manufacturing plants nationwide. In addition, the source of danger in food today is much wider than simply the tainted beef and poultry that the public already knows. A study by the General Accounting Office of the U.S. Congress estimates that as many as 85% of food poisoning cases are from the fruit, vegetables, seafood, and cheeses that are under the FDA's inspection jurisdiction. In addition, the quantity of imported food is rising faster than the FDA's capabilities, from 2.7 million items in 1997 to 4.1 million items in 2000.[39] Given the impossibility today of adequately inspecting food products before they are sold, the FDA relies on the food industry's own safety, surveillance, and recall programs and on regulations requiring industry to use more scientific risk assessment techniques.

In 1995 the FDA began introducing a major change in food protection strategy. Both regulators and industry alike are now increasing the use of risk assessment programs, instead of relying solely on direct inspection.[40] In use in industry since the 1960s, these programs, called HACCP (Hazard Analysis and Critical Control Points), aim to identify contamination hazards systematically in advance and provide plant managers ways to control them during the production process. HACCP recognized advances in bacterial testing and placed for the first time into federal food safety regulations a requirement for actual testing for the presence of dangerous microbes. The previous method of "poke and sniff" had not been updated since its inception in 1906. Both the FDA and the USDA are seeking to expand HACCP regulations; the FDA has done so in the seafood and fruit juice industries, and the USDA is expanding such programs among meat and poultry processors.[17] The HACCP program appears to be working. It is credited with helping to reduce the percentage of chickens contaminated with *Salmonella* by 50%.

The FDA Division of Consumer Education conducts an active program of protection through public education and general information. Special attention is given to nutrition misinformation. Materials are prepared and distributed to individuals, students, and community groups. Consumer specialists work through all FDA district offices.

FOODBORNE DISEASE

Prevalence and Costs

Foodborne disease continues to be a major public health problem. Many disease-bearing organisms inhabit our environment and can contaminate our food and water. With advances in regulation and technology, there have been major improvements in food handling and food safety, from inspection to refrigerated trucks to freeze-drying. Yet food poisoning in America is at least as common today as it was 50 years ago. According to the CDC, the rate of serious gastrointestinal illness, which is often seen as a measure of the prevalence of food poisoning, is now 34% higher than it was in 1948. Better reporting of cases may account for part of this change, but foodborne disease remains widespread. The CDC reports that every year 5000 deaths, 325,000 hospitalizations, and 76 million illnesses are caused by food poisoning.[39]

Two trends in recent decades—in how our food is produced and how we consume it—give disease microbes new opportunities. Changes in the way that food is produced and distributed have increased the possibilities of spreading contamination. The thousands of small family farms of the past have given way increasingly to large factory farms and giant food corporations that ship both fresh and processed food products worldwide. Disease pathogens can now be transported quickly across wide areas. Another change contributing to food contamination involves contemporary eating habits. Fruits and vegetables are more often eaten without cooking them, which increases the chances of infection. In today's fast-paced life, people are also eating more precooked foods, such as seafood salads, deli meats, and food kept warm for extended periods until being purchased, which are more dangerous than traditional meals eaten directly from the stove or oven. There also has been in supermarkets a huge increase in the variety of foods available, with many imported from around the world. With budget constraints, the FDA is able to inspect only a tiny proportion of food products.[39] When food poisoning outbreaks do occur, the food industry's surveillance and recall systems work to limit their spread. The total yearly economic cost of food-related illness in the United States is estimated to be from $8 to $10 billion. The most economically significant diseases are *Salmonella* and staphylococcal poisoning, costing annually about $4 and $1.5 billion, respectively. Other costly types include listeriosis, trichinosis, *Clostridium perfringens* enteritis, and botulism. Although a healthy person can withstand most foodborne infections, older persons have weaker immune systems and the national population is aging, making Americans overall more susceptible to foodborne diseases.

Food Sanitation

Strict sanitation measures and rigid personal hygiene are essential. Throughout all preparation, the food and everything that touches it must be scrupulously clean. Cooking procedures and temperature standards must be followed, all serving equipment must be kept clean, leftover food must be stored and reused appropriately or discarded, and garbage must be contained and disposed of in a sanitary manner. We know all these measures, but some persons do not always practice them. These rules are especially important for food handlers working in any phase of public food service operations, food processing and packaging plants, public markets, or delicatessen shops or counters.

Also, persons with any infectious disease or any hand injury, however small, should not work with food.

Bacterial Food Infections

Bacterial food infections result from eating food contaminated by large colonies of bacteria. Specific bacteria cause specific diseases. Examples of illness-causing bacteria that contaminate food are *Escherichia coli* O157:H7, *Salmonella, Campylobacter, Shigella,* and *Listeria.*

1. *Escherichia coli* O157:H7. Microorganisms inhabit the intestines of animals and humans. Most types of *E. coli* intestinal bacteria are benign; some even do nutritionally important tasks such as bacterial fermentation of resistant starch. Some strains, however, such as *E. coli serotype* O157:H7, produce toxins that cause serious disease. This *E. coli* strain was first recognized as a source of food poisoning in 1982. Over the past decade, *E. coli* O157:H7 has emerged as a major cause of individual cases and large outbreaks of diarrhea, both bloody and nonbloody.

   The Foodborne and Diarrheal Diseases Branch of the CDC in Atlanta reports that from a public health standpoint *E. coli* O157:H7 is by far the most important *E. coli* strain in North America. In the United States alone, it is estimated to cause more than 25,000 illnesses and as many as 500 deaths each year.[41] Major outbreaks have resulted from eating beef, mainly undercooked ground beef. The largest North American outbreak was in the Northwest in 1993; this killed four children and made more than 700 persons ill, some of whom were left with permanent kidney damage. The outbreak was traced to a meat processing plant in southern California that produced ground beef containing *E. coli,* which was shipped to four Northwest states and then to fast-food restaurants that did not cook the hamburger meat sufficiently to kill the *E. coli.*[42] The lesson learned from this incident is that all parties throughout the entire food chain are responsible for food safety. Consumers directly learned the need for adequate cooking of ground beef patties to ensure safety against *E. coli.*[43]
2. *Salmonella.* The bacterium *Salmonella* is named for the American veterinarian-pathologist Daniel Salmon (1850-1914), who first isolated and identified the species commonly causing human foodborne infections, *Salmonella typhi* and *Salmonella paratyphi.* These organisms grow readily in common foods such as milk, custards, egg dishes, salad dressings, and sandwich fillings. Seafood, especially shellfish such as oysters and clams, from polluted waters may also be a source of infection. The contamination of eggs with *Salmonella enteritidis* has become a worldwide problem in recent years. *Salmonella* continues to be one of the main causes of foodborne disease worldwide. The single largest outbreak of food poisoning in U.S. history occurred in 1994, when *Salmonella*-tainted milk was delivered to an ice cream factory in Minnesota. The source was traced to a contaminated truck that had carried a previous shipment of raw eggs. The ice cream made with that milk was shipped to stores in several states and made an estimated 224,000 people ill.[41] Unsanitary handling of foods and utensils can spread the bacteria. Resulting cases of gastroenteritis may vary in intensity from mild diarrhea to severe attacks. Practices of immunization, pasteurization, and sanitary regulations involving community water and food supplies as well as food handlers help to control such outbreaks. Incubation and multiplication of the bacteria take time after the food is eaten, so symptoms of food infection develop slowly, usually 12 to 24 hours after ingestion.
3. *Campylobacter.* The *Campylobacter jejuni* bacterium was long known as a pathogen in animals but was identified as a cause of human disease only in the 1980s through the use of better detection methods. *Campylobacter* is now recognized as the single most common reason for acute diarrhea caused by bacteria in America and many other countries. As few as 400 bacteria can be an infective dose. *Campylobacter* is found in raw and undercooked beef, poultry, and seafood; raw milk; and untreated water. *Campylobacter* contained in oysters that were eaten raw was the cause of food poisoning in Washington State in 1998.[44]
4. *Shigella.* The bacterium *Shigella* is named for the Japanese physician Kiyoshi Shiga (1870-1957), who first discovered a main species of the organism *Shigella dysenteriae* during a dysentery epidemic in Japan in 1898. Food poisoning from *Shigella* is usually confined to the large intestine and may vary from a mild transient disturbance in adults to fatal dysentery in young children. The bacteria grow easily in foods, especially in milk, a common carrier to infants and children. Reported outbreaks have been traced to uncooked tofu salad and to shredded lettuce and cabbage packaged for restaurants and the retail market. The boiling of water or the pasteurization of milk kills the organisms, but the food or milk can easily be reinfected by unsanitary handling by a carrier. The bacterium is spread in much the same way as *Salmonella* is transmitted—by unsanitary handling of food.
5. *Listeria.* The bacterium *Listeria* is named for the English surgeon Baron Joseph Lister (1827-1912), who first applied knowledge of bacterial infection to principles of antiseptic surgery in a benchmark 1867 publication that led to "clean" operations and the development of modern surgery. Only within the past few decades, however, has the major species causing human illness, *Listeria monocytogenes,* been identified and linked with foodborne disease in humans.[45] Before 1981 *Listeria* was thought to be a disease organism only in animals. Now we know that these organisms occur widely in the environment. In high-risk individuals such as elderly persons, pregnant women, infants, or

persons with suppressed immune systems, the organisms can produce a rare but often fatal illness, with severe symptoms such as diarrhea, flulike fever and headache, pneumonia, sepsis, meningitis, and endocarditis. Foodborne disease has been traced to a variety of foods, including raw milk, raw eggs, seafood, chicken, turkey, meat, and meat products. According to the CDC, *Listeria* causes at least 1850 illnesses and 425 deaths each year in the United States.[17]

Bacterial Food Poisonings

Food poisoning is caused by the ingestion of bacterial toxins that have been produced in foods by the growth of specific kinds of bacteria before the food is eaten. The powerful toxin is ingested directly, and symptoms therefore develop rapidly, usually within 1 to 6 hours after the food is eaten. Two types of bacterial food poisoning are most commonly responsible—staphylococcal and clostridial.

1. *Staphylococcal food poisoning.* Named for the shape of the main causative organism, *Staphylococcus aureus,* staphylococcal food poisoning is by far the most common form of bacterial poisoning observed in the United States. Powerful preformed toxins contaminate the food, producing rapid illness within 1 to 6 hours after ingestion. Symptoms come on suddenly and consist of severe cramping and abdominal pain with vomiting and diarrhea, usually accompanied by sweating, headache, and fever. In some cases there may be shock and prostration. Recovery is fairly rapid, however, depending on the amount of toxin ingested. The source of contamination is usually an infection on the hand of a worker preparing the food, often minor or unnoticed. Foods that are particularly effective culture beds include custard- and cream-filled bakery goods, chicken and ham salads, processed meats, cheese, sauces, and combination dishes. The toxin makes no change in the normal odor, taste, or appearance of the food, so the person eating it is not warned.
2. *Clostridial food poisoning.* Named for the shape of the bacterium *Clostridium,* mainly *Clostridium perfringens* and *Clostridium botulinum,* clostridial food poisoning is caused by powerful toxins in contaminated foods. The *C. perfringens* spores are in soil, water, dust, and refuse—virtually everywhere. The organism multiplies in cooked meat and meat dishes and develops its toxin in foods held for extended periods at warming or room temperatures. Thus many reported outbreaks occur from food eaten in school cafeterias, college dining rooms, and restaurants. In each case, cooked meat was improperly handled in preparation and refrigeration. Control rests mainly on careful preparation and adequate cooking of meats, prompt service, and immediate refrigeration at sufficiently low temperatures. *C. botulinum* causes far more serious, often fatal food poisoning from eating food containing its powerful toxin. Depending on the dose of toxin taken and the individual response, the illness may vary from mild discomfort to death within 24 hours. Mortality rates are high. Vomiting, weakness, and dizziness are initial complaints. Progressively, the toxin irritates motor nerve cells and blocks transmission of neural impulses at the nerve terminals, causing gradual paralysis. Sudden respiratory paralysis with airway obstruction is the major cause of death, especially in infants and young children.

   C. botulinum spores are widespread in soil throughout the world and may be carried on harvested food to the canning process. Like all clostridia, this species is anaerobic (develops in the absence of air) or nearly so. The relatively air-free can and the canning temperatures (above 27° C [80° F]) provide good conditions for toxin production. The development of high standards in the commercial canning industry has eliminated this source of botulism, but cases still result each year, mainly from eating carelessly home-canned foods. Boiling for 10 minutes destroys the toxin (not the spore), so all home-canned food, no matter how well preserved, should be boiled at least 10 minutes before eating. In the United States, Alaska and Washington have the highest incidence. Alaska has the greater number of botulism cases because of the native habits of eating uncooked or partially cooked meat that has been fermented, dried, or frozen.

Table 9-2 summarizes these bacterial sources of food contamination.

Viruses

Illnesses caused by viral contamination are few compared with those caused by bacterial contamination. Illnesses caused by viruses include upper respiratory infections, such as colds and influenza, and infections from hepatitis A virus. Explosive epidemics of infectious hepatitis have occurred in schools, towns, and other communities after fecal contamination of water, milk, or food. Contaminated shellfish from polluted waters have caused several outbreaks. Again, stringent control of community water and food supplies, as well as personal hygiene and sanitary practices of food handlers, are essential for the prevention of disease.

---

dysentery A general term given to a number of disorders marked by inflammation of the intestines, especially of the colon, and attended by abdominal pain and frequent stools containing blood and mucus. The causative agent may be chemical irritants, bacteria, protozoa, or parasites.

endocarditis Inflammation of the *endocardium,* the serous membrane that lines the cavities of the heart.

meningitis Inflammation of the *meninges,* the three membranes that envelop the brain and spinal cord, caused by a bacterial or viral infection and characterized by high fever, severe headache, and stiff neck or back muscles.

sepsis Presence in the blood or other tissues of pathogenic microorganisms or their toxins; conditions associated with such pathogens.

TABLE 9-2 Selected Examples of Bacterial Foodborne Disease

Foodborne Disease	Causative Organisms (Genus and Species)	Food Source	Symptoms and Course
Bacterial Food Infections			
Salmonellosis	Salmonella *S. typhi* *S. paratyphi*	Milk, custards, egg dishes, salad dressings, sandwich fillings, polluted shellfish	Mild to severe diarrhea, cramps, vomiting; appears ≥12-24 hr after eating; lasts 1-7 days
Shigellosis	Shigella *S. dysenteriae*	Milk and milk products, seafood, salads	Mild diarrhea to fatal dysentery (especially in young children); appears 7-36 hr after eating; lasts 3-14 days
Listeriosis	Listeria *L. monocytogenes*	Soft cheese, poultry, seafood, raw milk, meat products (pâté)	Severe diarrhea, fever, headache, pneumonia, meningitis, endocarditis; symptoms begin after 3-21 days
Bacterial Food Poisoning			
Enterotoxins			
Staphylococcal	Staphylococcus *S. aureus*	Custards, cream fillings, processed meats, ham, cheese, ice cream, potato salad, sauces, casseroles	Severe abdominal pain, cramps, vomiting, diarrhea, perspiration, headache, fever, prostration; appears suddenly 1-6 hr after eating; symptoms subside generally within 24 hr
Clostridial	Clostridium		
Perfringens enteritis	*C. perfringens*	Cooked meats, meat dishes held at warm or room temperature	Mild diarrhea, vomiting; appears 8-24 hr after eating; lasts ≤1 day
Botulism	*C. botulinum*	Improperly home-canned foods; smoked and salted fish, ham, sausage, shellfish	Symptoms range from mild discomfort to death within 24 hr; initial nausea, vomiting, weakness, dizziness, progressing to motor and sometimes fatal breathing paralysis

Changes in Personal Food Habits

BASIC DETERMINANTS OF FOOD CHOICE

We have discussed the broad areas of environment, culture, and psychosocial development, as well as modern food safety concerns, in terms of their influence on food habits. Clearly, some of the basic determinants of food choice focus on a variety of interacting physical, social, and physiologic factors, as summarized in Table 9-3. It is difficult to change some of our own eating patterns for health needs or personal desires. It is even more difficult to help our healthcare clients modify some of their habits, even when we understand their cultural patterns. We need to understand just how complex the factors are that influence the food choices persons make when they eat what they do (see *Practical Application* box).

NEW FACTORS INFLUENCING FOOD CHOICES

Family and ethnic patterns and regional cultural habits are strong influences in our lives. They establish our early food habits and make changing those habits difficult. On the other hand, our technology-based and media-saturated contemporary American society puts old influences in conflict with new forces. As society evolves, newer factors influence changes in our food habits.[46]

- *Income.* The generally improved economic situation of society provides sufficient income in most cases to give us more choice and time. Many people are able to purchase and enjoy a wider variety of foods than those they grew up eating.
- *Technology.* Expansion in the fields of science and technology increases the number and variety of food items available. The globalization of the food industry combined with modern transportation brings foods from around the world to the neighborhood supermarket.
- *Environment.* Our rapidly changing environment results in increased consumer awareness of food and health issues. Food safety and healthy nutrition concerns prompt many persons to prefer organically grown foods.
- *Vision.* Our expanding mass media, especially television, stimulates many options for new items and changes our expectations and desires. The current market target for television advertisements is younger children, who then influence the family's buying habits.

TABLE 9-3 Factors Determining Food Choices

Physical Factors	Social Factors	Physiologic Factors
Food supply available	Advertising	Allergy
Food technology	Culture	Disability
Geography, agriculture, distribution	Education, nutrition, and general	Health-disease status
Personal economics, income	Political and economic policies	Personal food acceptance
Sanitation, housing	Religion and social customs	Needs, energy, or nutrients
Season, climate	Social class role	Therapeutic diets
Storage and cooking facilities	Social problems, poverty, or alcoholism	

IMMIGRATION AND ETHNIC DIVERSITY

The story of immigration to the United States and our growing ethnic diversity is hardly a new one; it is one of the fundamental themes of this country's development. We have discussed the importance of these ethnic, cultural, and religious identities. In the United States we have many cultures and subcultures that have remained distinct or have become assimilated in varying degrees. Every group has contributed parts of its food habits to the general culture. In turn, American food patterns have infused into these new cultures, so that lines of difference are less distinct.

Americans of many different ethnic backgrounds have enriched our overall cultural patterns. We find varied and intermingling foods and food patterns blending with those of our own particular background. Sometimes, however, this intermingling of different cuisine has both a nutritional and a financial cost. A study of the food consumption patterns of immigrants from Central America living in Los Angeles revealed a complex cross-cultural blending of traditional Central American foods and mainstream American foods. The Central American foods were purchased in specialty markets, even though they were higher in cost than American or Mexican foods. Although most people in this immigrant group believed that the overall quality of their diet had improved, most of the foods added to their diet were high in fat or sugar and the diet was still low in milk products, vegetables, and fruits.[47] Immigrant groups show a strong desire for a healthy and affordable diet, while also wanting to maintain contact with their traditional foods. This food acculturation process does not occur without difficulty and cultural dislocation. Ethnic groups within the United States encounter a new world. Their lifestyles often undergo dramatic alterations, and the cultural integrity of the group can be severely shaken. Every group adapts in a unique way specific to its original culture and to the historic circumstances in which it undergoes the change.

CHANGING AMERICAN FOOD AND POPULATION PATTERNS

Traditional American food patterns are changing along with shifts in the structure of the national population. The stereotype of the all-American family with parents and two children eating three meals a day with a ban on snacking is no longer the common pattern. During the past two decades, we have experienced far-reaching changes in our way of living and, subsequently, in our food patterns.

The number of households is gradually increasing with population growth. An increasing proportion of new households are "nontraditional" households, which in population statistics are persons living alone or groups of unrelated persons. The U.S. Census Bureau projects that from 2000 to 2010 the number of these non-"family" households will increase 17%, whereas "family" households will increase 9%. Households are also gradually getting smaller, primarily because more people are living alone. The average size of American households is projected to decline from 2.59 persons in 2000 to 2.53 persons in 2010. Married couple households as a percentage of all households will decline from 54% in 2000 to 52% in 2010, as one-person households continue to rise. These changes reflect the increasing variety of living options in American society. The U.S. population will continue to become older during the next several decades, with its median age increasing from 36 years in 2000 to 37 years in 2010. The older segments of the population will grow significantly during this period; people over age 65 will increase from 35 to 40 million, and those over 85 will increase from 4.3 to 5.8 million. By 2010, life expectancy will rise to 78 years on average: 74 years for men and 81 years for women.[48]

The racial and ethnic makeup of the American population is also changing, characterized by increasing ethnic diversity. According to the 2000 census, America's total population in 2000 was 281 million people, an overall increase of 13% from the 249 million in 1990. The fastest growing population group is the Hispanics. The total number of Hispanics listed in the 2000 census was 35 million, an increase of 58% from their total of 22 million in the 1990 census. Black Americans, including those who declared mixed backgrounds, total 36 million persons, an increase of 21% since the 1990 figure of 30 million. During the decade of 2000 to 2010, Hispanics will surpass blacks and become the second largest ethnic group in the country. People of Asian background are also a fast-growing group. The numbers of other racial groups, including Native Americans, Alaskan natives, and Pacific

PRACTICAL APPLICATION

Cultural Sensitivity in Nutritional Care in a Multicultural Society

Traditional folk wisdom gives rise to the common saying that you do not really know another person until you have walked a mile in that person's shoes. This traditional wisdom conveys a deep truth and is needed today more than ever. American health workers of all kinds need high cultural sensitivity to do their work in an increasingly multicultural society.

Too often, pressures of time and circumstance mean that a health professional's individual culture may conflict with professional community nutrition health services or clinical medical nutrition therapy for persons of another culture. To apply the principles of cultural sensitivity, we need to understand and incorporate cultural awareness in all of our nutrition work. This opportunity comes first in nutrition assessment, always the necessary basis for the nutritional care that is developed together with the client or family.

NUTRITION ASSESSMENT

Cultural knowledge is a needed foundation for sound nutritional care. We need to gather basic information about the client's culture, foods most frequently used, and how the culture influences food environment and behavior. Aspects of the family and community food environment that must be understood to provide relevant individual medical nutrition therapy and family guidance include the following.

- Types of food available
- Which foods are accepted and/or preferred
- Safety of food supply and related health problems
- Energy and nutrient quality of major foods chosen

Aspects of family and community food behaviors that must also be understood include the following.

- Most commonly used foods, who selects them, how and where they are obtained
- Food preparation, how divided among family/community
- Food eaten, how much, when, with whom, where
- Food storage, facilities and methods, food safety, garbage disposal

SKILLS NEEDED FOR CULTURALLY SENSITIVE CARE

Discovering special cultural knowledge is no small task. It may begin with regular library research, but it must broaden with techniques such as observation, participant observation, and informal interviewing.

Observation

Observe the neighborhood and homes in which clients live as well as where they shop for foods and the types of food available. If possible, a home visit may be planned, where facilities for food storage, food preparation, and eating may be informally discussed.

Participant Observation

Learn more about the client group by participating in their activities. For example, read the same newspaper, listen to the same radio stations, go to the same community meetings, and shop in the same food markets that clients use.

Informal Interviewing

Learn more about the client group by interviewing individuals from or closely associated with the client group. Ask relevant questions about food and health behaviors, or ask other healthcare professionals who serve the cultural group, any community leaders among the group, and any other members of the group.

As the contemporary societal and demographic environment for healthcare continues to change, public health leaders nationwide recognize that all health practitioners need cultural sensitivity knowledge and skills to effectively serve a more multicultural patient population. Such skills enable culturally relevant programs and services to be developed and implemented. Bilingual practitioners are important in patient care in both urban and rural settings.

References

Cassidy CM: Walk a mile in my shoes: culturally sensitive food-habit research, *Am J Clin Nutr* 59(suppl 1S):190S, 1994.

Pobocik RS, Shovic AC: Development of a nutrition exchange booklet for Guam using culturally accepted foods, *J Am Diet Assoc* 96(3):285, 1996.

Shovic AC: Development of a Samoan nutrition exchange list using culturally accepted foods, *J Am Diet Assoc* 94(5):541, 1994.

Terry RD: Needed: a new appreciation of culture and food behavior, *J Am Diet Assoc* 94(5):501, 1994.

Islanders, are also increasing.[48] These continuing trends indicate significant changes in the American social picture, part of a dynamic and rapidly changing society.

WORKING WOMEN AND COUPLES

The number of working women continues to increase. The largest group of new entrants into the labor force will continue to be women of all racial and ethnic backgrounds, who will make up 50% of the total work force by 2005, up from 46% in 2000. Women are participating in the rise of technology in the economy. By the year 2010, more than 50% of all jobs will be in information industries or require technical skills. There is a correlation between the education of women and their presence in the labor force, with about 51% of college undergraduates being women.

In general, women account for 30% of the enrollment in law schools, 25% in medical schools, 30% in business schools, and 12% in technical graduate schools.

These trends mean that the number of working couples will also continue to increase. This phenomenon of working couples is not restricted to one social, economic, or ethnic group. It is a widespread societal change, bringing with it changes in the functioning of the family. It is natural that working parents rely on food items and cooking methods that save time and labor.

FAMILY MEALS

Family meals are less common. Many persons rarely eat breakfast and lunch in the family setting, but family dinners occur about 75% of the time. Often both parents work or the single parent works, and many late afternoon sports or other activities among the children curtail the time available for meal preparation and having the whole family sit down to eat at the same time. The habits of both adults and children have changed dramatically as to when we eat and whether we eat with our families. Midmorning and midafternoon breaks at work usually involve food, beverage, or both. Evening television snacks plus a midnight refrigerator raid are common. Nutrition hardliners of the old school may denounce this snacking behavior, but they are out of step. Americans are moving toward a concept of *balanced days* instead of *balanced meals.* They are increasing the number of times a day they eat to as many as 11 "eating occasions," a pattern recently termed *grazing.* This shift is not necessarily bad, depending on the nature of the periodic snacking or more constant "grazing." Frequent small meals can be better for the body than three larger meals per day, especially when healthy snacking and grazing contribute to needed nutrient and energy intake. Rather than condemn all snacking, we need to promote snack foods that enhance nutritional well-being.

HEALTH CONSCIOUSNESS

The interest of Americans in physical fitness continues. This has taken primarily two forms. First, there is more general nutrition awareness. Consumers have an increased interest in the nutrition content of their food, an expressed concern about a wholesome and safe food supply, and a strong support of the new nutrition labeling regulations. Interest in health claims on food products has increased, but there is some uncertainty about how to evaluate them. Second, there is more attention to weight watching, although not always through a healthy approach that includes regular meals with less fat combined with moderate regular physical exercise. More than half of the American population at any given time is on a weight-reducing diet. Consumers are interested in "light" foods perceived to be lower in kcalories.

ECONOMY

More and more Americans are economizing on food. Many supermarket shoppers are changing their diets primarily to save money. Consumers are stocking up on bargains and cutting back on expensive convenience foods. They are buying items in larger packages and in bulk and doing much less store hopping for bargains, staying with the store they consider to have the lowest overall prices. Brand loyalty has declined, and the purchase of generic products has increased. Consumers look more carefully at labels to gain information about comparative products.

GOURMET COOKING

The use of gourmet foods and specialty ethnic dishes has risen, and food specialty shops have sprung up in every shopping center. Gourmet cooking has become a popular hobby, and entertaining guests at home over a gourmet meal often displays the chef's skills in the elegance and quality of the food. This phenomenon parallels the general trend toward meals that are easy to fix, take little time, and fulfill the consumers' nutrition needs. Supermarkets are establishing special gourmet deli shops and specialty fast foods, take-out picnic baskets, and other creative items.

FAST FOODS

The typical American today consumes about three hamburgers and four orders of French fries each week. More than 35% of all food that Americans eat today is eaten away from home, at restaurants, schools, and other public places. More than 15% of our total calories are from fast-food restaurants, and more than 50 million people eat at a fast-food restaurant each day, accounting for about 1 of every 10 meals. Americans spent about $6 billion on fast food in 1970. By the year 2000, the total was more than $110 billion.[49] Fast foods are especially a major component for those people who have very poor diets. The National Health and Nutrition Examination Survey (NHANES) revealed that one third of American adults get almost half of their total calories from high-calorie, low-nutrition foods such as soft drinks, desserts, chips, candy, and ice cream.[50] Several factors have contributed to this phenomenal increase in the use of fast foods, including a greater number of working women, dual-career families, more diverse schedules of family members, an aging population, and an increasing number of one- and two-person households. Fast foods meet the needs of many people because they are quick, reasonably priced, and readily available. The concern over the impact of this trend on our national health is that when restaurants do the cooking, the food is frequently less healthy, with more fat, saturated fat, sodium, and refined carbohydrates and less calcium than food prepared at home. With the exception of the lettuce and the tomatoes, much of modern fast food, although it may look familiar, has in fact been completely reformulated and is the end product of a complex technological system of mass production.[49] The fast-food restaurant does not cook food; it is simply the final heating-up point of processed food products that have been manufactured elsewhere. To their credit, however, fast-food restaurants will respond when customers express health concerns. Change is coming to some of their practices: there is increasing use of vegetable oils instead of animal fats for frying, an increase in the number of low-fat menu items, and more fruits and vegetables available at salad bars. Consumer's choices for quick and easy meals are widening. Today high-quality meals that are fast also come from home delivery services, high-quality vending machine foods, and easy-to-prepare and ready-to-microwave dinner packages sold at supermarkets.

TO SUM UP

We all grow up and live our lives in a social context. We each inherit at least one cultural background and live in our particular society's social structure, complete with food habits and attitudes about eating. It is from a social perspective that we can best examine changes in food habits. We need to understand the effects on health that are associated with major social and economic shifts. We also need to understand current social forces to best help persons make new dietary changes that will benefit their health. We must meet concerns about food misinformation and food safety.

The United States has a long history of immigration. Every new group has adjusted to life in the new country in its own way. They have contributed a unique ethnic diversity to American life and food patterns.

Traditional American food patterns are changing in a number of ways. We increasingly rely on food technology in our fast, complex life. More women are employed, households are getting smaller, more and more persons are living alone, and our meal patterns are different. We search for less-fancy, lower-cost food items and for creative gourmet cooking for special occasions. In general we are more nutrition and health conscious. At the same, however, in response to the pace and structure of modern society, fast-food outlets have increased and become a large factor in our changing food patterns.

Questions for Review

1. Describe some ways in which environmental factors interact to produce malnutrition and give examples.
2. What is the meaning of culture? How does it affect our food patterns?
3. What are some social and psychologic factors that influence our food habits? Give examples of personal meanings related to food.
4. Why does the public tend to accept nutrition misinformation so easily? What groups are more susceptible? Select one such group and give some effective approaches you might use in reaching them with sound nutrition information.
5. How do food misinformation and concerns about food safety affect food habits?
6. What is the basis of concern about food additives and pesticide residues?
7. In what ways does ethnic diversity enrich American food patterns? Give several examples.
8. Name several trends in America's changing food patterns and discuss their implications for nutrition and health.

References

1. Kittler PG, Sucher KP: *Food and culture in America,* ed 2, New York, 1998, The West Group.
2. Griffiths S, Wallace J: *Consuming passions: food in an age of anxiety,* New York, 1998, Manchester University Press.
3. Counihan C, Van Esterik P: *Food and culture: a reader,* New York, 1997, Routledge.
4. Maslow AH: *Motivation and personality,* New York, 1954, Harper & Row.
5. Juhn MS, O'Kane JW, Vincent DM: Oral creatine supplement in male collegiate athletics: a survey of dosing habits and side effects, *J Am Diet Assoc* 99(5):593, 1999.
6. Nmakwe N: Anabolic steroids and cardiovascular risk in athletes, *Nutr Today,* 31(5):206, 1996.
7. Wagner DR: Hyperhydrating with glycerol: implications for athletic performance, *J Am Diet Assoc* 99(2):207, 1999.
8. Bell D, Valentine G: *Consuming geographies: we are what we eat,* New York, 1997, Routledge.
9. Kittler PG, Sucher KP: *Cultural foods: traditions and trends,* New York, 1999, Wadsworth Publishing Co.
10. Zubila S, Tapper R: *Culinary cultures of the Middle East,* New York, 1995, IB Tauris.
11. Sanjur D: *Hispanic foodways, nutrition, and health,* Boston, 1995, Allyn & Bacon.
12. Barer-Stein T: *You eat what you are: people, culture, and food traditions,* ed 2, New York, 1999, Culture Concepts.
13. Gabacia DR: *We are what we eat: ethnic food and the making of Americans,* Cambridge, Mass, 1998, Harvard University Press.
14. Davidson A: *The Oxford companion to food,* New York, 1999, Oxford University Press.
15. Fieldhouse P: *Food and nutrition: customs and culture,* ed 2, New York, 1995, Chapman and Hall USA.
16. Rifkin J: *The biotech century: harnessing the gene and remaking the world,* New York, 1998, Tarcher/Putnam.
17. Schmidt CW: Safe food: an all-consuming issue, *Environ Health Perspect* 107(3):A144, 1999.
18. Food and Drug Administration, Center for Veterinary Medicine: *Bovine somatropin (BST),* can be accessed at *http://www.fda.gov/cvm/index/bst/bst.htm.*
19. Brody JE: Gene altered foods: a case against panic, *New York Times* Dec 5, 2000.
20. Brown K: Seeds of concern, *Sci Am* 284(4):52, 2001.

21. Slobin S, Chen A: The genetic market basket, *New York Times* Jan 25, 2001.
22. McHughen A: *Pandora's picnic basket: the potential and hazards of genetically modified foods,* New York, 2001, Oxford University Press.
23. Smith CS: China rushes to adopt genetically modified crops, *New York Times* Oct 7, 2000.
24. Guerinot ML: The green revolution strikes gold, *Science* 287(5451):241, 2000.
25. Ye X et al: Engineering the provitamin A (beta-carotene) biosynthetic pathway into (carotenoid-free) rice endosperm, *Science* 287(5451):303, 2000.
26. Wolfenbarger LL, Phifer PR: The ecological risks and benefits of genetically engineered plants, *Science* 290:2088, 2000.
27. Yoon CK: What's next for biotech crops? *New York Times* Dec 19, 2000.
28. National Research Council: *Genetically modified pest-protected plants: science and regulation,* Washington, DC, 2000, National Academy Press.
29. Crawley MJ et al: Transgenic crops in natural habitats, *Nature* 409:682, 2001.
30. Biochips down on the farm, *Economist* 358(8214):13, 2001.
31. Hopkin K: The risks on the table, *Sci Am* 284(4):60, 2001.
32. McNeil DG: Europe approves new genetically modified food control, *New York Times* Feb 15, 2001.
33. Pollack A, Yoon CK: Rice genome called a crop breakthrough, *New York Times* Jan 27, 2001.
34. U.S. Department of Agriculture, Agricultural Marketing Service: *The National Organic Program,* can be accessed at *http://www.ams.usda.gov/nop.*
35. Gussow JD: Is local vs. global the next environmental imperative? *Nutr Today* 35(1):29, 2000.
36. Hathcock JN: Safety of physiologically active components, *Nutr Today* 35(5):193, 2000.
37. Pennington JAT, Wilkening VL: Final regulations for the nutrition labeling of raw fruits, vegetables, and fish, *J Am Diet Assoc* 97(11):1299, 1997.
38. Food labeling: a Canadian and international perspective, *Nutr Rev* 53(4):103, 1995.
39. Winter G: Contaminated food makes millions ill despite advances, *New York Times* Mar 18, 2001.
40. Food and Nutrition Board, Institute of Medicine: *Food safety policy, science, and risk assessment: strengthening the connection,* Washington, DC, 2001, National Academy Press.
41. Liebman B, Schardt D: Diet and health: ten megatrends, *Nutr Action Health Letter* 28(1):9, 2001.
42. Buchanan RL, Doyle MP: Foodborne disease significance of *Escherichia coli* O157:H7 and other enterohemorrhagic *E. coli, Food Technol* 51(10):69, 1997.
43. Juneja VK et al: Thermal destruction of *Escherichia coli* O157:H7 in hamburger, *J Food Protection* 60(10):1163, 1997.
44. Walter PK: Home for the holidays: preventing foodborne illness at family gatherings, *FDA Consumer* p 9, Nov 2000.
45. Armstrong D: *Listeria monocytogenes.* In Mandel GL, Bennett JE, eds: *Principles and practice of infectious diseases,* ed 4, New York, 1995, Churchill Livingstone.
46. Southgate DAT: Dietary change: changing patterns of eating. In Meiselman HL, MacFie HJH, eds: *Food choices, acceptance, and consumption,* London, 1999, Chapman and Hall.
47. Romero-Gwynn E et al: Dietary patterns and acculturation among immigrants from El Salvador, *Nutr Today* 35(6):233, 2000.
48. U.S. Census Bureau, U.S. Department of Commerce: *Statistical abstract of the United States 2002,* ed 122, Washington, DC, 2002, Government Printing Office.
49. Schlosser E: *Fast food nation: the dark side of the all-American meal,* Boston, 2001, Houghton Mifflin Company.
50. Kant A: Junk diets: damage report, *Am J Clin Nutr* 72:929, 2000.

■ Further Reading

Angulo FJ et al: A community waterborne outbreak of Salmonellosis and the effectiveness of a boil water order, *Am J Public Health* 87(4):580, 1997.

Cieslak PR et al: Hamburger-associated *Escherichia coli* O157:H7 infection in Las Vegas: a hidden epidemic, *Am J Public Health* 87(2):176, 1997.

Tilden J Jr et al: A new route of transmission for *Escherichia coli:* infection from dry fermented salami, *Am J Public Health* 86(8):1142, 1996.

These three reports of community disease outbreaks describe the intense investigations of infection sources—two with meat hamburgers and salami and one with a community water source. Rapid public response in the meat cases helped investigators stop further spread quickly. But in the case of the contaminated water supply, even after immediate and continuous warnings via local radio stations to boil all drinking water, a number of persons became seriously ill. Their excuses for not complying with the warnings were "I forgot" and "I didn't believe it."

Ingham S, Thies ML: Position of the American Dietetic Association: food and water safety, *J Am Diet Assoc* 97(2):184, 1997.

This professional statement outlines the responsibility of all collaborating healthcare workers to maintain a safe food and water supply and describes ways in which all persons involved can work together to ensure this safety level at all times. A current list of food safety education resources for professionals is provided.

Issues & ANSWERS

Mad Cow Disease: How Dangerous Is It?

Meredith Catherine Williams

Mad cow disease first gained international attention in the mid 1990s when several people in the United Kingdom died from a new form of a rare brain disease. Researchers discovered that this new human disease was apparently connected with eating beef from cattle afflicted with the "mad cow disease" that had been seen in British cattle since 1986. Since then, more than 170,000 cattle, most in the United Kingdom and some in western Europe, have been slaughtered in an attempt to prevent even more infected meat from reaching the public. Scientists are now working to understand how mad cow disease causes brain damage, how it infects herds of sheep and cattle, and if the United States is at risk of importing the disease from overseas.[1]

Mad cow disease is the name given by the press for bovine spongiform encephalopathy (BSE). It is a rare neurologic disorder in cattle that causes the cows to be disorientated, stare at imaginary objects, and kick and paw at the ground. This disease is unique in that it is caused not by bacteria, viruses, or even genetic inheritance, but by a malformed version of a protein called a prion. Normal prions are present in lymph and brain tissue, and their three-dimensional coiled-helix shape helps maintain the integrity of nerve cells. Diseased prions uncoil in certain sections to form straight protein sheets that destroy brain tissue. Lacking DNA, diseased prions only proliferate by inducing other healthy prion proteins to change to the harmful shape. Deformed prions can incubate in lymph tissue before moving to the brain for up to 10 years according to some estimates. Once in the brain, if there is a great enough build up of diseased proteins, lethal gaps or holes in neurologic tissue will form.[2]

Cow populations contracted the abnormal prions from their feed. In a process known as rendering, unused ground-up pieces of meat, bone, glands, and spinal cord from sheep and cattle are processed and become cattle feed. It is suspected that cows contracted BSE from eating parts infected with scrapie, a sheep version of the fatal brain disorder. Rendering does not destroy the malformed prions, and the more virulent strains will resist being destroyed by partial heat-inactivation or consumed by enzymes in the stomach. After each cycle of consumption and rendering, the prions that are able to replicate quickly, resist the acidic stomach environment, and infect other tissues can survive and become highly concentrated in the extremely processed feed. It is theorized that the rendering process may have also selected for prions that were more capable of jumping the species barrier from sheep to cow, as only the most virulent forms were able to survive. This process, although now outlawed in Europe and the United States, occurred for years until whole cattle populations became infected with mad cow disease.[3]

The same prions that cause BSE in cows cause a variant of Creutzfeldt-Jakob disease (vCJD) in humans. The original and extremely rare CJD strikes persons in their 50s or older and causes dementia, uncoordinated movements, sleep disorders, and eventual death in approximately 4 months. However, the variant form that surfaced in the mid 1990s affects people in their 20s and causes death in an average of 14 months. Until then, there had been no strong indication linking BSE to CJD. Even now there is no completely conclusive evidence to prove that infection stems from eating beef, but that is the most widely accepted theory, for it is clear that the prions are more able to cross species barriers than previously thought. By the time symptoms appear, the damage to the brain is too extensive to be countered. Some researchers have identified little pieces of protein that can impede mutant prions and slow damage to the brain, thereby extending the life of an infected person. Others seek to design a diagnostic test that would scan for mutant prions in the blood and amplify any located prions to allow for earlier identification.[4]

There are several factors that impede the speedy development of a treatment. One problem with studying vCJD is the necessity of working with infected brain tissues, which are hard to obtain. The lethal dose of prions needed to develop vCJD is also relatively unknown. It is assumed that the more you eat, the greater the risk of developing the disease, but the type of beef that is eaten is also a factor. Processed or ground meats, such as sausage, salami, bologna, or ground beef, are more likely than pure steak to contain bits of brain or spinal cord, which have a high concentration of prions. There may also be a genetic component, for all those who have contracted vCJD have had a specific variation of their prion gene, a variation that occurs in 40% of the Caucasian population in Great Britain. It is possible that some people are immune to vCJD, but if not, then the infection rate will rise.

Although more than 95% of all BSE-infected cattle since 1986 have been in Great Britain, mad cow disease has spread from cattle populations in England to most other European countries, with the exception of Austria and Finland. Political pressure is mounting from both a concerned population that fears infection and from farmers and cattlemen who are having to slaughter their means of income with little federal recompense. Fear is spreading that other meats, such as lamb, pork, or even fish in some cases, have been infected. Some in Europe blame the current epidemic on lazy politicians who turned a blind eye to the practices of remnant feeding. However, the threat of vCJD is still extremely low everywhere in Europe. There have been only about 80 cases of human vCJD since it was first identified. Even though there is never a completely risk-free situation, people have a many times greater chance of being afflicted by the deadly form of *E. coli* bacteria than they do of encountering mad cow disease.

Officials in the United States hope to avoid infection of U.S. cattle and keep herds healthy. Since 1985, a full year before the first reported cases in British cows, the United States has had a ban on all beef imports from Great Britain. That import ban was expanded in 1989 to include all live cattle and bovine products such as tallow and bone meal. The United States has expanded the ban to other countries, such as Ireland, Switzerland, France, and Portugal, where mad cow disease has been detected. In 1997, the United States, like the European Union, instituted a countrywide ban on the manufacture and use of cattle feed that contains rendered parts from other cattle and sheep. Violators can face seizures of feed, company closures, or criminal prosecution. In addition, the CDC established a surveillance system to continuously monitor national health trends and statistics to detect any cases of vCJD. As part of this effort, thousands of cow brains have been examined for signs of infection or neurologic degradation. So far, there have been no reported cases of either mad cow disease or vCJD in the United States.[5]

In the light of all the alarming publicity about mad cow disease, some consumers fear that all beef is contaminated and advocate the extreme measure of avoiding meat entirely. These fears appear to be unfounded. A major study done in 2001 for the USDA by the Harvard Center for Risk Analysis examined what would happen if BSE were introduced into the United States.[6] Using dozens of projected scenarios and assumptions, this analysis found that there would be little real threat to the American cattle herd or to public health. In all projected cases, even with very pessimistic assumptions, BSE would fail to take hold and spread widely, and the disease would die out within a few years at most and would affect only small numbers of cattle. The critical control mechanism is the ban on cattle feed containing rendered parts from other cattle. This prohibition, in place since 1997, breaks the cycle by which BSE is spread among cattle and thus keeps any future outbreak in check, even with incomplete compliance with the regulations. The USDA is expanding its inspection and enforcement of cattle feed regulations.[7]

Both BSE in cattle and vCJD in people are dramatic, frightening, and terrible diseases. It is easy to understand the fear that many people experience. In response, government authorities in all countries have become focused on stopping any further spread of this disease and on restoring public confidence in the food supply, especially meat. These efforts, which will be ongoing, appear likely to succeed.

REFERENCES

1. Is mad-cow disease a threat in the U.S.? *Tufts Univ Health Nutr Lett* 18(12):1, 2001.
2. Yam P: Mad cow's human toll, *Sci Am* 284(5):12, 2001.
3. U.S. Department of Agriculture, Animal and Plant Health Inspection Service: *Bovine spongiform encephalopathy (BSE),* can be accessed at *http://www.aphis.usda.gov/oa/bse.*
4. Caughey B: A sane look at mad cows, *Discover* 22(3):16, 2001.
5. Enserink M: Is the U.S. doing enough to prevent mad cow disease? *Science* 292:1639, 2001.
6. Harvard Center for Risk Analysis: *Risk analysis of transmissible spongiform encephalopathies in cattle and the potential for entry of the etiologic agent(s) into the U.S. food supply,* can be accessed at *http://www.hcra.harvard.edu/cattle.html.*
7. Newman L: Risk of BSE in USA is low, *Lancet* 358(9298):2053, 2001.

Chapter

10

Family Nutrition Counseling: Food Needs and Costs

Sue Rodwell Williams

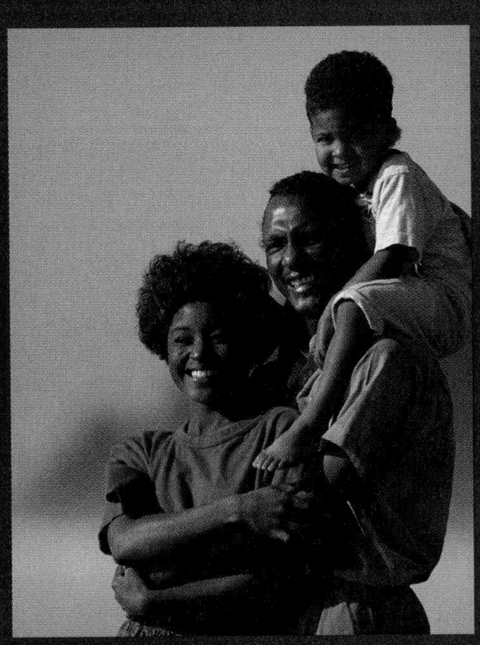

Chapter Outline

This chapter continues the two-chapter opening sequence on food habits and family nutrition counseling that introduces Part 2 of your study on Community Nutrition and the Life Cycle.

In the previous chapter we considered the food environment and influences that shape food habits. Here we continue with family counseling and education approaches to meeting health problems, often in the face of economic hardships. Knowledge of the ecology of the food environment, global, local, and individual, and the problem of malnutrition that can occur in many settings provides a context for sensitive counseling when needed.

Often in our clinics and communities, we must interpret complex information in a variety of settings to meet numerous family health and nutrition needs. Here, then, we seek approaches and resources to help meet these needs.

Family Nutrition Counseling

Community healthcare workers often need to apply the principles of health teaching in family nutrition counseling. Health and nutrition are inseparable, and the term *counseling* is appropriate. If we work with the family on the basis of counseling principles, various members are led to explore their own situation, to express their needs, and to find ways of meeting those needs that are best suited to their particular life situation. It has long been evident that societies shape their own patterns of disease; sociodemographic factors largely determine health at all ages.[1,2] With American society becoming increasingly diverse, nutrition counselors need an increased knowledge of and sensitivity to the diet patterns of people coming from a variety of ethnic and national backgrounds, as well as the acculturation difficulties that recent immigrants may face as they adapt to a new food and cultural environment.[3] Our job is to help persons and families explore their options and make decisions in the light of knowledge and personal support.

PERSON-CENTERED GOALS

Realistic family diet counseling must be person-centered. It involves close attention to personal and family needs, nutrition and health problems, and food choices and costs. In our work we have three main goals: (1) to obtain basic information about the client and the living situation that relates to nutrition and health needs, (2) to provide basic health teaching to help meet these needs, and (3) to support the client and family in all personal efforts to meet needs through encouragement, reinforcement, general caring and concern, and practical resources. A basic skill that all healthcare workers must learn, therefore, is the skill of talking with clients in a helpful manner.

INTERVIEWING

Skills in interviewing are essential in healthcare. Interviewing does not necessarily mean only the more formal or structured history-taking activity; commonly it means a purposeful planned conversation in either the hospital, clinic, or home. It may be a simple telephone call to the home to determine ongoing needs or progress. General principles of interviewing should guide these activities, including the purpose or focus, means used to achieve the purpose, and measuring results.

Focus and Purpose

As indicated, the focus of all healthcare is the individual client and personal health needs. It may be a small intermediate goal relating to some aspect of the overall care, or it may be a long-term goal. Our ultimate purpose is to provide whatever help the individual or family may need to determine personal health needs and goals and to work with the person or family in finding ways of meeting these needs and goals.

Means Used to Achieve Purpose

Healthcare workers use various means of accomplishing these purposes—building a helping relationship, creating a comfortable climate, and developing positive attitudes.

1. *Relationship.* Counseling is a dynamic person-centered process built on a helping relationship. This is reflected in the common use of the word *services* for all healthcare-related activities. The most important means of helping a person is establishing a relationship of mutual trust and respect. The most significant tool we ever have for helping others is ourselves. Our role is that of a helping vehicle. Within this kind of relationship, true healing can take place.
2. *Climate.* The kind of climate we create involves both the physical setting and the psychologic feelings involved. The physical setting should be as comfortable as possible in relation to space, ventilation, heating, lighting, and sitting or lying down. Other important factors include providing sufficient time for the interview in a quiet setting free from interruptions and with sufficient privacy to ensure confidentiality. If it is in an office setting, the desk should be to the side, not between the therapist and client.
3. *Attitudes.* The word *attitude* refers to that aspect of personality that accounts for a consistent behavior toward persons, situations, or objects. Our attitudes are learned. Hence they develop from life experiences and influences. Because they are learned, they can be examined. We can become more aware of them. We can try to strengthen those attitudes that are desirable and constructive and at the same time seek to change or modify those attitudes that are less desirable and more destructive. If a healthcare worker is to be able to help meet clients' needs, certain attitudes are necessary components of behavior.
   - *Warmth.* A genuine concern for the client or patient is displayed by interest, friendliness, and kindness; we convey warmth by being thoughtful.
   - *Acceptance.* We must meet clients as they are and where they are. To accept the client does not necessarily mean approval of behavior. It does mean a realization that clients or patients usually regard their behavior as purposeful and meaningful. It may be a means of handling stress. An attitude of acceptance conveys that a person's thoughts, ideas, and actions are important and worth attention simply because a human being has the right to be treated as having worth and dignity.
   - *Objectivity.* To be objective is to be free of bias. It is having a nonjudgmental attitude. Of course, complete objectivity is impossible, but reasonable objectivity is certainly a goal that can be attained. We must be aware of our own feelings and biases, and

we should attempt to control them. The evaluation of a situation must be based on what is actually happening, that is, the facts as we perceive them, not on mere opinions, assumptions, or inferences.

- *Compassion.* An attitude of compassion enables us to feel with and for another person or oneself. It means accepting the impact of an emotion, holding it long enough to absorb its meaning, and entering into a kind of fellowship of feeling with the person who is moved by the emotion. There is nothing easy in developing the attitude of compassion; it requires emotional maturity.

Measuring Results

Continuous and terminal evaluation of our interviews is an ongoing part of our activity. Evaluation is measuring how behavioral changes in the client and in ourselves are related to the needs and goals that have been identified. In summary, therefore, healthcare workers will always be dealing with the following sequence of questions in interviewing.

1. *Need.* What is wrong? What is the health problem or need of the client or patient?
2. *Goal.* What does the client want to do about it? What is the client's immediate goal? What is the long-range goal?
3. *Information.* What information do I need to know to help the client? What does the client need to know to help take care of personal needs? What knowledge and skills are necessary to solve the health problem?
4. *Action.* What has to be done to help meet the need? What plan of action is best for solving the health problem and meeting the client's personal needs?
5. *Result.* What happened? What was the result of the action planned and carried out? Did it solve the problem or meet the need? If not, why not? What change in plan is indicated?

IMPORTANT ACTIONS OF THE INTERVIEW

Five important actions of an interview can be identified: observing, listening, responding, terminating, and recording. Each of these requires study, practice, and development of skills.

Observing

Ordinarily we do not deliberately and minutely look at all the persons we meet. However, in the care of persons with health needs, the helping role requires such behavior. Our purpose is to gather information that will guide us in understanding clients and their environment. Valid observation is a skill that is developed through concentration, study, and practice. Areas of such needed observation include the following.

1. *Physiologic functioning and features.* Refer to Table 1-1 in the first chapter and review the clinical signs of nutritional status. Such features as these may be used as a basis for making detailed observations of physical features. Learning to take an organized look at the person may help develop greater accuracy and objectivity. We tend to see what we have the mindset, sensitivity, or awareness to see. Therefore, we need to develop certain sensitivities to detect pertinent details that can provide important clues to real needs.
2. *Behavior patterns.* Observe closely not only the physical features but also the immediate behavior of the client or patient in the healthcare situation. Attempt to look at the behavior in terms of its meaning to the person in relation to self-concept and the illness. From these observations, certain assumptions or educated guesses can be made. But realize all the while that these are only assumptions and hence need to be validated and clarified with the client to determine whether they are indeed factual. This action helps us to understand our own feelings and to rule out our own biases, prejudices, or distortions of the situation.
3. *Environment.* Observing the client's immediate environment in an organized manner is also helpful. This may be the home and community environment on a visit, or it may be the immediate environment in a clinic or hospital setting.

Listening

Hearing and listening are not the same thing. *Hearing* is purely a physiologic function, only the first phase of the listening process. The function of *listening* is to hear, to identify the sound, to understand its meaning, and to learn by it.

Although the senses have amazing powers of perception, they are limited. The nervous system must constantly select and discriminate among the millions of bits of information it confronts. Listening is also limited. A large part of communication time is spent in listening, but the average person without special training has only about 25% listening efficiency. In other words, one hears only a small percent of the total surrounding communication.

The task of the healthcare worker is to learn the art of creative listening. First, we must learn to be comfortable as a listener. Usually our lives are so filled with activity and noise that to sit and listen quietly is often difficult. Actually, most of us have had little experience during our own development of being listened to and therefore listening to others must be learned. We practice listening by staying close by, assuming a comfortable position, and giving our full attention to the person who is speaking. We show genuine interest by indicating agreement or understanding with a nod of the head or making such sounds as "Uh-huh," "I see," or "And then?" at the appropriate moments in the conversation. We must learn to remain silent when the other person's comment jogs some personal memory or parallel experience of our own. We learn to listen not only for the words the patient uses but also for the repetition of key words, the rise and fall of the tone

TABLE 10-1 Verbal Responses Used by the Helping Professions

Purpose of Response	Type of Response	Description
Clarification	Content	Counselor summarizes content of conversation up to that point
	Affective	Counselor paraphrases or defines concern that client has implied but not actually stated
Leading	Closed question	Question that can be answered with "yes" or "no" or with very few words
	Open question	Question that cannot be answered briefly; often triggers discussion or a flow of information
	Advice	Provision of an alternative type of behavior by counselor for client; may be an activity or thought
	Teaching	Information presented by counselor with intention of helping client acquire knowledge and skills to perform appropriate nutrition-related behaviors
Self-revealing	Self-involving	Response made to client's statements that reflects the personal feelings of counselor
	Self-disclosing	Response made to client's statements that reflects factual information about counselor
	Aside	Statement counselor makes to self

of voice, hesitant or aggressive expression of words and ideas, and the softness or harshness of tone. We listen to the overall content of what is being said, to the main ideas being expressed, and to the topics chosen for discussion. We listen for the feelings, needs, and goals that are being stated. We learn to listen to the silences and to be comfortable with them, giving the person time to frame thoughts and express them.

Responding

The responses we give to the client or patient may be verbal or nonverbal. Nonverbal responses include signs and actions, such as gestures and movements, silences, facial expressions, nods of the head, and touch. Verbal responses make use of language—words and meanings (Table 10-1). But we must remember that we give our own meanings to the words we use. A word is only a symbol, not the thing itself. Thus we must give attention to our choice of words—we must "begin where the person is." And all the while we must provide a supportive environment for responses (see *Practical Application* box). Also, we must watch the level and pace of our speaking. Questions should be clear, concise, free from bias, and always nonthreatening. Sometimes a verbal response may be a simple restatement of what the client has said. This enables the person to hear the statement again, think about it, and thus reinforce, expand, or correct it. At other times the response may be a reflection of what the expressed feelings seem to be. This enables the client to respond, to verify or to deny that this was indeed the feeling. We must never act on our assumptions about the client's feelings without verifying them first.

Terminating the Interview

The close of the interview should meet several needs. It may be used to summarize the main points covered or to reinforce learning. If contact with the client is to continue, it can include plans for the follow-up visits or activities. It should always leave the person with the sense that the healthcare worker's concern has been sincere and that the door is always open for further communication, should the person so desire.

Recording

Some means of recording the important points of the interview should be arranged. This should be as unobtrusive as possible, with little note taking, if any, during the interview itself and completion of the record immediately afterward. If some recording device is used, the client's permission must always be obtained. Give full assurance that identity will be erased and that the recording will only be used for a specific purpose, such as to help the healthcare worker improve interviewing skills or to learn the health needs of a particular group of people, as in gathering research data.

Various members of the healthcare team contribute information about the client or patient and the health problem in a system of written reports. This is the patient's chart, a legal document, which, in case of litigation, could be used in court. There is an obligation to the client or patient to respect confidentiality and to determine what and how much information is shared and with whom. At the same time healthcare workers have a responsibility for relaying to other healthcare team members pertinent information to aid in the total planning of care.

What aspects of the interview should be recorded? Data from two basic areas of communication are needed: (1) a description of the client's or patient's general physical and emotional status and concerns, followed in some instances by judgment of the immediate and ongoing care needs, and (2) a description of whatever care and teaching

PRACTICAL APPLICATION
Creating a Supportive Nutrition Counseling Environment

More than 50 years ago, a sensitive physician named Dr. Henderson expressed truths about the client interview in a healing environment; his thoughts are as applicable today as they were then. Perhaps they are even more true in today's far more complex world. He reminds us anew that we must truly listen to our clients and patients every day if we are to help them.

LISTENING
On naval ships the phrase "Now hear this" from the loudspeaker would direct everyone's attention to listen for an important message. Dr. Henderson similarly directs us to listen carefully. "We must listen," he said, "for what the client wants to tell us, for what he does not want to tell us, and for what he cannot tell us. He does not want to tell things that are shameful or painful. And he cannot tell us his implicit assumptions that even he does not know."[1] It sounds like the "creative listening" that a more modern philosopher and counselor, Carl Rogers, used to call it.[2] This is no passive activity; it is an active counseling skill. Only by using it can we really hear and respond wisely.

Also, nutrition counselors may inadvertently close communication channels by failing to ask questions or otherwise verbally discouraging the client from expressing real concerns and expectations or by using body language that is distracting, inappropriate, or misinterpreted by the client because of cultural differences.[3]

QUESTIONS AND REFLECTIONS
Questions or statements that reflect what the client says or feels and that encourage further expression are usually open-ended, making a simple yes-or-no response inadequate, or they are affective, reflecting feelings that the client may have implied but not expressed directly. Closed questions and self-directed statements do little to encourage the person to "open up" (see Table 10-1).

BODY LANGUAGE
Body language can be distracting or intimidating, or it can make the client feel at home. The key is to understand the client's concept of the following communication factors.[3]

- *Personal space.* Americans like a lot of room. Try sitting next to the only passenger on a city bus and note the amount of anxiety created! In other cultures, such as the Middle East, closeness, even to the point of pushing and shoving, is considered acceptable behavior. Thus we must understand that our distance from our clients may affect their sense of comfort.
- *Eye contact.* Americans show respect by looking at each other straight in the eye. Asians, for example, show the same respect by looking downward. Attempts to interchange these behaviors can be interpreted as being rude.
- *Speech inflection.* The tone of voice and its loudness and inflection may be interpreted as threatening or comforting depending on the region or country of origin of the listener.

You cannot always be aware of your clients' attitudes toward body language ahead of time. However, you can take note of any signs of uneasiness and at least invite them to discuss anything about the interview that may be causing concern.

Yes, Dr. Henderson, we still hear you. We can—and must—listen.

References

1. Henderson L: Physician and patient as a social system, *N Engl J Med* 212: 819, 1935.
2. Heppner PP et al: Carl Rogers: reflections on his life, *J Counsel Dev* 63:14, 1984.
3. Jerome NW: Culture-specific strategies for capturing local dietary intake patterns, *Am J Clin Nutr* 65(suppl):1166S, 1997.

were provided and the results that were observed. In addition, we sometimes include follow-up plans made with the patient and the family or notes concerning needs that were passed on to other healthcare team members or to other agencies. Similar information is often communicated through oral team reports and various case conferences.

NUTRITION HISTORY AND ANALYSIS

Personal Life Situation and Food Patterns
Working closely with the nutritionist on the healthcare team, learn the family's situation and values and identify health and nutrition needs through a general nutrition history and analysis. Several methods for such interviewing may be used, either separately or in combination, depending on the circumstances and the need.

1. *24-Hour recall.* Ask the person to recall all food and drink consumed during the previous day, noting the nature and amount of each item.[4] This method has disadvantages with some persons whose memory may be limited, such as elderly people or young children, and it does not reveal long-term food habits. Simple food models in pictorial form can be used successfully to help quantify the reported food intake.
2. *Food records.* Persons are asked to record their food intake for a brief period, usually about 3 days. Each

person is taught how to describe the food items used singly or in combination and how to measure amounts consumed. Often a 3-day record is used after an initial diet history as a periodic monitoring tool.

3. *Food frequency.* Use a structured questionnaire that lists common food items or food groups to obtain information about quantity and frequency of use. This tool may be helpful in relation to a particular disease risk or incidence by helping to determine the use of specific groups of foods over an extended period.
4. *Diet history.* At the initial individual or family contact, a nutrition interview provides needed information for planning continuing care. Professional nutritionists and dietitians use a comprehensive form of this approach in a variety of clinical and community settings, usually evaluating their findings by detailed computer analysis. Other healthcare team members working with the dietitian may contribute helpful nutrition information through the use of a simplified version, such as the activity-associated general day's food pattern given in Figure 10-1. Most people eat in relation to activity or work throughout the day, where they are, what they are doing, and whom they are with at the time. Using such an activity-associated guide throughout the day gives both interviewer and client a structure and provides a series of memory jogs to flesh out the information in greater detail to permit constructive counseling. With respect to each item, questions are asked in terms of general habits—nature of food items, form, frequency, preparation, portion, seasoning—not in terms of a specific day's intake. Through such an interview, important clues to food attitudes and values can be communicated. Note these for later thought and exploration. An added practical method that may be helpful is a brief informal household food inventory, such as, a short checklist of high-fat foods, in conjunction with assessment of how often each item is eaten.[5] If your manner is interested and accepting, the information should be valid and straightforward. Conversely, if you are judgmental and authoritarian, people will probably tell you only what they think you want to hear.

Food intake records are a very helpful and time-tested tool in nutrition counseling. However, nutritionists have long known that the underreporting of food intake is a pervasive problem, especially affecting studies of the relationships between diet patterns and disease risk. In surveys, underreporting involves from 10% to 45% of the total, and is most prevalent among children, women, and the obese. Recent advances in nutrition science overcome

Name ______________________________ Date __________

Height __________ Weight (lb) __________ (kg) __________ Age __________

Ideal weight __________

Referral
Diagnosis
Diet order
Members of household
Occupation
Recreation, physical activity

Present food intake	Place	Hour	Frequency, form, and amount checklist
Morning			Milk Cheese Meat Fish Poultry
Noon			Eggs Cream Butter, margarine Other fats
Evening			Vegetables, green Vegetables, other Fruits (citrus) Legumes Potato Bread–kind Sugar Desserts Beverages
Summary			Alcohol Vitamins Candy

FIGURE 10-1 Nutrition history: activity-associated general day's food pattern. Also record general activity pattern throughout the day.

this problem through the use of biomarkers, which are measurements in body fluids or tissues that reflect the true intake of a food component. Biomarker applications, such as the "doubly-labeled water" technique, allow the measurement of total energy expenditure as a check on the accuracy of self-reported energy intakes. In the future, the use of biologic samples to validate estimates of dietary intake should become routine.[6]

Changing American Eating Behavior

A basic reason for using an activity-associated general day's food intake as the structure for a diet history is that Americans' eating behavior is changing from traditional patterns. Surveys indicate that current eating behavior has become much more fragmented into frequent light feedings—called "grazing" by many observers—than the traditional family meals. Actually, studies of American eating patterns during the past 20 years have consistently found that the smallest and fastest shrinking population segment (only about 15%) is composed of those who still cook three regular meals a day, and the largest and most rapidly growing group is composed of those who eat easily portable items that do not take much time to cook or consume.

Plan of Care

On the basis of the diet history and review of any health problems requiring diet modification, a realistic personal food plan can be developed with the individual and family. Then any related follow-up care that is needed can be developed. This may take the form of return visits to the clinic, home visits, consultation and referral with other members of the healthcare team, or use of community resources. Follow-up work requires patience and a steady focus on the goal, knowing that there are various ways of reaching it. Imagination and good humor are invaluable. Take one step at a time; guide the client and family in applied nutrition principles, give support as needed, help with adjustments of the plan, provide reinforcement of prior learning, and continue to add new learning opportunities as the family's needs develop.

The Teaching-Learning Process

LEARNING AND CHANGED BEHAVIOR

There is far more to teaching and learning than merely dispensing information, but the myth still prevails in much of health education that if enough information is provided, harmful health practices will be changed. This is not always the case. There is a vast difference between a person who has learned and a person who has only been informed. Learning must ultimately be measured in terms of changed behavior. As with counseling, valid education focuses not on the practitioner or teacher or the content but on the learner. The health teacher's major task is to create situations in which clients and their families can learn, succeed, and develop self-direction, self-motivation, and self-care. These learning goals are especially important in dealing with adult patients and clients[7] (see *To Probe Further* box).

ASPECTS OF HUMAN PERSONALITY INVOLVED IN LEARNING

The teaching-learning experience involves three fundamental aspects of the human personality—thinking, feeling, and the will to act.

Thinking

We grasp information through our personal thinking process. We take in information selectively and then process and shape it according to our needs. The total thought process provides the background knowledge that is the basis for reasoning and analysis. The learner senses the contribution of this thinking to the learning process as "I know how to do it."

Feeling

In each of us, specific feelings and responses are associated with given items of knowledge and situations. These emotions reflect desires and needs that are aroused. Emotions provide impetus, creating the tensions that spur us to act. The learner senses the contribution of emotion to the learning process as "I want to do it."

Will to Act

The will to act arises from the conviction that the knowledge discovered can fulfill the felt need and relieve the symptoms of tension. The will focuses the decision to act on the knowledge received so that attitude, value, thought, or pattern of behavior can be changed. The learner senses the contribution of the will to the learning process as "I will do it."

PRINCIPLES OF LEARNING

Learning follows three basic laws: (1) learning is *personal,* occurring in relation to perceived personal needs; (2) learning is *developmental,* building on prior knowledge and experience; and (3) learning means *change,* resulting in some form of changed behavior.

Individuality

Learning can only be individual. We must all learn for ourselves, according to our own needs, in our own way and time, and for our own purpose. The teacher must discover who the learner is by asking questions that clarify the learner's relationship to the problem. New approaches to realistic nutrition education can help teachers vary teaching-learning strategies to meet the differing needs of learners and learning situations.

TO PROBE FURTHER

Effective Communication in the Nutrition Interview

Meredith Catherine Williams

Effective communication between clients and nutrition counselors is essential, especially when changes in dietary habits are needed to preserve health. The ability of a practitioner to impart information or to teach an adult can be affected by the type of words used and by the attitude displayed. Three models of communication styles—prescription, persuasion, and interaction—describe ways in which an adult patient can be approached.

In the prescription model, medical information is imparted in a highly cognitive manner. Remember that clients want to be treated as adults and not "talked down to." Often an objective and business-like approach can be conducive to a fruitful counseling session. The use of titles and surnames can add a degree of formality to the meeting, thus creating a professional and structured environment to which most working adults are accustomed.

However, a completely informational approach will not work for everyone. Some people respond better with the persuasion approach. Here nonrational outlooks and fears are taken into consideration. This approach accepts that there is some barrier put up by the client that will not be surpassed by pure information. Clients often resist change and can perceive it as threatening, especially when it involves eating habits, which are influenced by culture, media, and other social sources. Many have been exposed to years of out-of-date or incorrect information, and client education levels can vary widely. A noncondescending and patient approach can help convince the patient that your information is reliable and trustworthy. This approach, when used with tact and genuine care, will accomplish more than a firm insistence on change. Some clients lack confidence in their ability to follow diet plans, and the goal is the make the client feel comfortable and unafraid to ask questions and to verbalize concerns.

Some patients will want to discuss their health and plans for change. With these patients, the interactive model is ideal. This provides a give-and-take between both parties, where the counselor tries to become familiar with the patient's values, experiences, and what the patient see as the causes of the problem. Isolated facts are hard to remember; therefore if the client can personally relate to nutrition concepts, they will be more meaningful. The person's lay knowledge about food receives a more prominent place in this method. What the client thinks about healthy food, how he or she discusses food issues, and how the person approaches and considers different information sessions are important topics for discussion. Often the setting of realistic goals can help a client become more accustomed to the idea of change. Some clients will be overconfident and set for themselves an extreme alteration in diet or lifestyle. This can be used to cover real fears of failure. If small steps are established, the likelihood of failure and disappointment is reduced. In this effort, clients need positive reinforcement and feedback, especially if they express fear or anxiety.

There are sometimes physical factors, such as impaired sight or hearing, that can interfere with effective communication. Limited literacy or a language barrier can also make a presentation more difficult. The use of a variety of methods or helpful audiovisuals can facilitate learning. The presence of a family member or friend to support or interpret can also aid in communication. There may also be economic considerations if the client believes that the change in food habits will be expensive. It is important to stress the relative cost of a change in diet versus the expense of continued healthcare. Again, a supportive and nonintimidating manner will help the client to overcome anxiety. If cost does present a serious barrier, the counselor can refer the client to a social worker or a social service organization.

Above all, clients want to be treated as individuals. A combination of all three communication models will probably be used in a nutrition interview. It is up to the practitioner or counselor to determine what mix will be the most effective. Each client wants to be treated as if his or her problem presents a unique need and wants to feel that the counselor is giving the appropriate attention. At the beginning of a session, the counselor strives to achieve a rapport with the client and to establish an environment conducive to effective communication. Wise practitioners develop approaches that encourage thinking, problem solving, and self-confidence on the part of the client. Nutrition counseling must start where the client is and then work to establish both short- and long-term goals and to match these steps with stages of intervention to help motivate each individual.

Reference

Truswell AS: Family physicians and patients: is effective nutrition interaction possible? *Am J Clin Nutr* 71:6, 2000.

Need Fulfillment

An important initial force in learning is personal motivation. Persons learn only what they believe will be useful to them, and they retain only what they think they need. The more immediately that a person can put new learning to use, the more readily he or she can grasp it. The more it satisfies his or her immediate goal, the more effective the learning will be.

Contact

Learning starts from a point of contact between prior experience and knowledge, an overlap of the new with the familiar. Find out what the individual already knows and to what past experiences the present situation can be related. Start the process of learning at this point. Search for the areas of association that are present and then relate your teaching to that point of contact.

Active Participation

Because learning is an active process through which behavior can change, learners must become personally involved. They must participate actively. Indeed, effective teaching strategies require active participation of learners to bring about desired changes in attitudes and behaviors. One means of securing participation is through planned feedback. Feedback may take several forms.

1. Ask questions that require more than a "yes" or "no" answer and that reveal a degree of understanding and motivation, such as those in Table 10-1.
2. Use guided return demonstrations, which are brief periods in which procedures are practiced and skills discussed. Such guided practice develops ability, self-confidence, and security. It enables the learner to clarify the principles involved as a basis for decision-making about particular situations and actions.
3. Have the learner try out the new learning in personal experiences outside the teacher-directed situation. Alternate such trials with return visits to review these experiences. Answer, or help the person to answer, any questions raised and provide continued support and reinforcement.

Appraisal

At appropriate intervals, take stock of the changes that your clients have made in outlook, attitude, and actions toward their specific goals in health and nutrition care and education. Careful, sympathetic questioning may reveal any blocks to learning. In addition to speeding the learning process, such concern will show you whether you are communicating clearly, making contact, or choosing the best method. It may help you to recall principles that you may have glossed over. In the final analysis, the measure of success in teaching lies not in the number of facts transferred but rather in the change for the better that has been initiated in your client.

In all, the nutrition educator who builds on clients' needs and goals imparts a strong knowledge and interest in the subject, shows respect and concern for each individual in the program, and projects self-confidence has the greatest chance for success. In the long run, clients who follow a personal goal-setting approach in their nutrition counseling and education will have more opportunity to develop self-care responsibility and personal choice than will those who follow a purely diet-prescription approach (see *Issues & Answers*). Initially the personal goal-setting approach may take longer, but it achieves far greater long-term results.

In its position paper on nutrition education for the public, the American Dietetic Association summed up its key education philosophy in four brief statements concerning food choices to maintain good nutrition: (1) the focus should be on total diet rather than on individual foods, (2) there are no good or bad foods, (3) the keys to a good diet are balance, variety, and moderation, and (4) a positive approach to foods should be emphasized.[8] Nutrition educators using these approaches and a sound knowledge of science can also help clients avoid confusion in the face of the multitude of often conflicting media reports about research in nutrition. The truth is that good science progresses slowly, and its advance is seldom steady. Nutrition education is most effective when it focuses on easy-to-understand basic principles: follow the *Food Guide Pyramid,* eat a lot of fruits, vegetables, and grains, practice portion size control, and exercise regularly.[9]

The Ecology of Human Nutrition and Malnutrition

THE FOOD ENVIRONMENT AND MALNUTRITION

Out of necessity our food habits are inevitably linked to our environment. As a result, our rapidly changing human environment, with its problems of imbalance, such as pollution and malnutrition, often threatens health. The word *ecology* comes from the Greek word *oikos,* which means "house." Just as many factors and forces within a family interact to influence its members, so even greater forces in our physical environment and social system can interact to produce disease.

The public health significance of malnutrition, local and worldwide, continues to grow. Globally, unequal distribution of income leaves a fifth of the world's population, a billion people, living in absolute poverty.[10] It is

motivation Forces that affect individual goal-directed behavior toward satisfying needs or achieving personal goals.

estimated that each day 35,000 persons (14 million per year) die of hunger, malnutrition, and its preventable burden of disease.[11] Protein-energy malnutrition continues to rank first among the world's nutritional deficiency diseases. Observation and experience have brought deepened awareness of two important interrelated facts: (1) having adequate food alone is not the complete answer, although it fulfills a fundamental need for all persons, and (2) a national high standard of living does not necessarily eliminate the problem of malnutrition. Even in the midst of plenty in America, malnutrition exists.[12] Many malnourished people live in high-risk conditions of poverty, which influences the health of everyone involved. Among young pregnant women, malnutrition brings rising infant mortality rates. It occurs among vulnerable groups such as elderly and hospitalized persons. It is found among persons with alcoholism and drug addition. Malnutrition is associated with poverty and homelessness. In other cases, it is partner to a distorted obsession with thinness. Human misery and human waste of life from malnutrition, more prevalent in some regions of our country and regions of the world than in others, occur in both world hemispheres. The extent of this human suffering is impossible to quantify.

At its fundamental biologic level, malnutrition results from an inadequate supply of nutrients to the cells. However, this lack of essential nutrients at the cell level is by no means a simple problem. It is caused by a complex web of factors: physical, psychologic, personal, social, cultural, economic, political, and educational. Each of these factors is more or less important at a given time and place for a given individual. If these factors are only temporarily adverse, the malnutrition may be short term, alleviated rapidly, and cause no longstanding results or harm to life. But if malnutrition continues unrelieved, it becomes chronic. Irreparable harm to life follows, and eventually death ensues. For the epidemiologist a triad of variables influences disease: (1) agent, (2) host, and (3) environment. These three factors describe malnutrition.

Agent

The fundamental agent in malnutrition is lack of food. Because of this lack, certain food nutrients that are essential to maintaining cell activity are missing. As indicated, many factors may interact to cause or modify this lack of food: inadequate quantity and quality of food; insufficient amounts for children during critical growth periods; loss of supply through famine, poverty, war, or unequal distribution; or unwise choices made from foods available.

Host

The host is the person, the infant, child, or adult who has malnutrition. Various personal characteristics may influence the disease: presence of other diseases; increased need for food during times of growth, pregnancy, or heavy labor; congenital defects or prematurity; and personal factors such as emotional problems and poverty.

Environment

Many environmental factors influence malnutrition; these include sanitation, social problems, culture, economic and political structure, and agriculture.

The classic interactive and tangled web of some of these factors leading to malnutrition, as experienced by pioneer British pediatrician Cecily Williams in her early work in Africa with kwashiorkor, is shown in Figure 10-2. This debilitating web of malnutrition factors, in one combination or another, is still being experienced in numerous places around the world everyday.

ECONOMIC AND POLITICAL ENVIRONMENT

Food Availability and Use

In any society, at both government and personal levels, food availability and use involve both money and politics. It is plainly evident that money is a basic necessity for obtaining an adequate food supply. Sometimes, however, the role of politics and government structure and policies is not always as evident. Nonetheless, both are always intertwined in securing human nutrition.

Government Food and Agriculture Programs

In any country, food and agricultural programs at any level of government influence food availability and distribution. A number of factors may be involved, such as land management practices and erosion, water distribution, water pollution from long-term use of questionable pesticides, food production and distribution policies, and food assistance programs for persons in need.

THE PROBLEM OF POVERTY

We are all made increasingly aware through the daily news that malnutrition, even famine and death, exists in many countries that are hard-pressed by social conditions such as war, inequity, and desperate poverty. But even in the United States, one of the wealthiest world nations, many studies document widespread hunger and malnutrition among the poor, especially among minority groups, with increasing numbers of infants and young children involved.[13] For example, African American infants in the United States still have twice the chance of dying in their first year as do Caucasian infants, one of five U.S. children under age 18 lives in poverty, and African American and Hispanic children are nearly 3 times more likely to live in poverty as are Caucasian children.

Tremendous problems exist among the poor, and at times they seem almost insurmountable. Often a culture of poverty develops and is reinforced and perpetuated by society's values and attitudes, which wall off such persons more completely than do physical barriers. As a result of extreme pressures caused by living conditions, poverty-stricken persons become victims of negative attitudes and

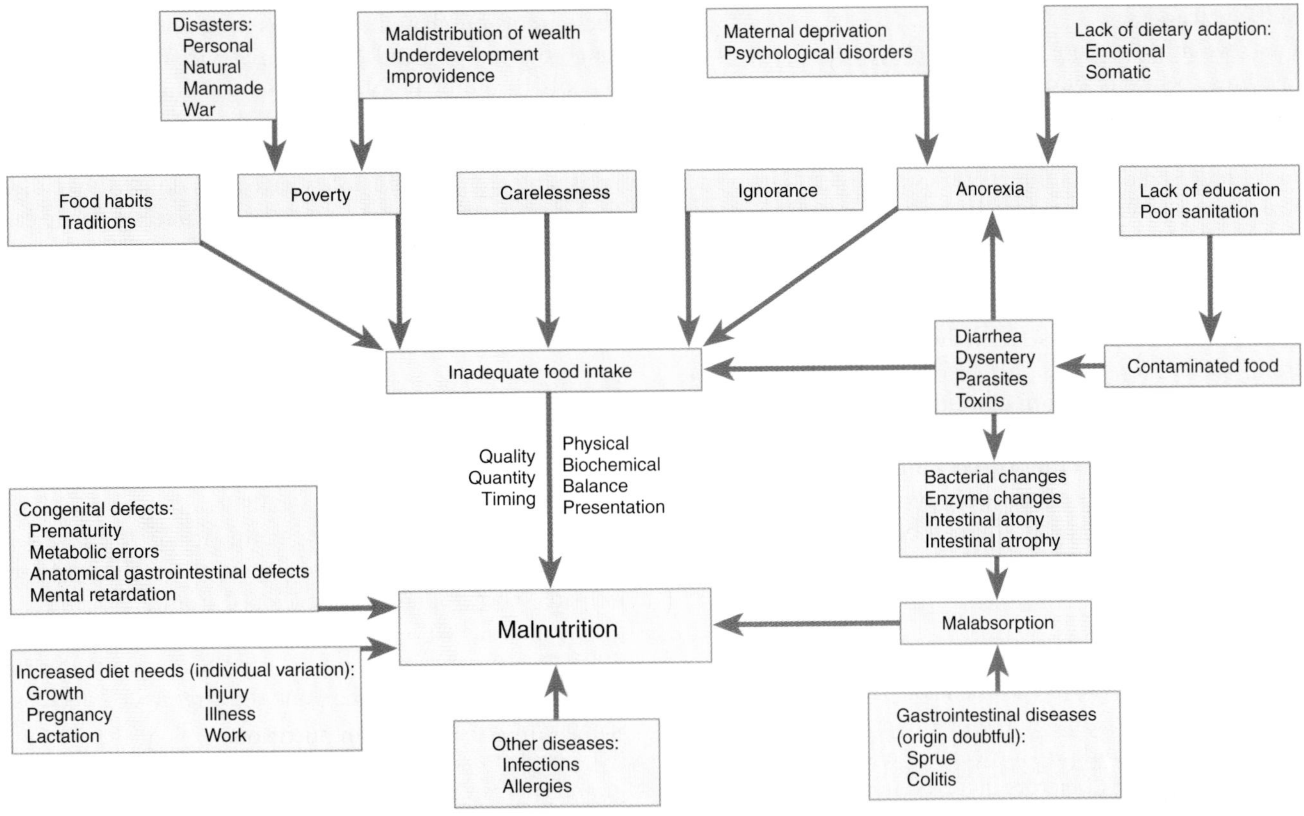

FIGURE 10-2 The multiple etiology of malnutrition. (*Modified from Williams CD: Malnutrition,* Lancet *2:342, 1962.*)

characteristics, feeling isolated, powerless, and insecure—feelings that influence their use of community health services.

Isolation

Strong feelings of alienation from mainstream society are common among the poor. In many communities, few, if any, channels of communications are open between the lowest-income groups and the rest of society. In most instances a poor person responds to such feelings of alienation by further withdrawal. Each person feels isolated and alone and concludes that no one is concerned. Hazards to health are inherent in poor housing and poor nutrition and are often compounded by distance from the sources of healthcare.

Powerlessness

It is ironic that often those persons most exposed to risks and emergencies have the fewest coping resources. Extreme frustration is inevitable and persons become overwhelmed. Why try, they conclude, if they have no control over the situation? Why plan, if there is no future different from today? In such a day-to-day struggle to exist, poor persons often see little value in long-range preventive health measures.

Insecurity

Subjected to forces outside their control, poor individuals and families have little or no security. Insecurity and anxiety often incapacitate them. In such a setting, where hunger may be a constant companion, food, which has the same deep psychologic and emotional meaning for poor people that it has for all people, assumes even greater meaning than it has for persons who rarely know hunger. The U.S. Department of Agriculture (USDA) defines food security as "access by all people at all times to enough food for an active, healthy life."[14] Minimally, this means ready availability of nutritionally adequate and safe foods in socially accepted ways.[15]

ROLE OF THE HEALTHCARE WORKER

How can concerned healthcare workers help individuals and families conditioned by years of poverty or crushed by new poverty? In the face of such overpowering feelings of isolation, helplessness, and insecurity, what attitudes are necessary to be of real help? What methods and approaches are most likely to reach our clients and patients and to supply their needs? Some basic principles can help.

Self-awareness

First, we must explore our own feelings about the poor. We must be aware of our own distorted vision, our own class values and attitudes. If we are to be agents of constructive change, true helping vehicles, we must first have some understanding of the person's situation and its broad social setting. We must also better understand ourselves and confront our cultural conditioning and biases.

Rapport

Genuine warmth, interest, friendliness, and kindness grow from within. *Rapport* is that feeling of relationship between persons that is born of mutual respect, regard, and trust. This sense of relationship gives both the helper and the helped a deep feeling of working together. Its most basic ingredient is a concern for people and persons—a positive orientation toward human beings in general and concern for individuals in particular. It is born of a deep knowledge of what it means to be human.

Client Focus

One must begin where the client or patient is situated. Each person's concerns should be the primary consideration. Often we work with other team specialists to cut through the maze of factors involved in a given situation before the client or patient is ready to accept or even to consider the health practice or diet counsel that is needed or desired. Much time may have to be spent, for example, in coming to understand the meaning of food to this person before practical dietary matters can begin to be explored.

Family Economic Needs: Food Assistance Programs

In your counseling you will discover economic stress among many clients and their families. Some may need financial help. In such situations you will need to discuss available food assistance programs and to make appropriate referrals, through your team nutritionist and social worker or directly to community agencies and programs.

COMMODITY DISTRIBUTION PROGRAM

In the post-Depression years, legislation was initiated to stabilize agricultural prices. This legislation provided for the federal government to purchase market surpluses of perishable goods. Later the resulting accumulation of food stocks led to the creation of distribution programs as a means of disposing of the stored products. Such surplus has been defined as either *physical* (exceeding requirements) or *economic* (prices below desired levels). Foods coming under these regulations include meat and poultry, fruits and vegetables, eggs, dried beans, and peas. Most of these items purchased under this program have been donated by the Food and Nutrition Service of the USDA to schools through the National School Lunch and School Breakfast Programs. Foods accumulated through other aspects of the legislation are price-supported basic and nonperishable items. These foods have been donated to child-feeding programs, summer camps, Native American reservations, trust territories, nutrition programs for the elderly, charities, disaster-feeding programs, and the Commodities Supplemental Food Program.

FOOD STAMP PROGRAM

Also growing out of the post-Depression years, the Food Stamp Program was founded to help low-income families purchase needed food. The program became part of permanent legislation by the Food Stamp Act of 1964, which made the program available to all counties wishing to participate. The program has developed from a $13 million program in 1961 to a nearly $18 billion program in 2001.[16] Although it has experienced budget cuts during the past two decades, it remains the largest U.S. food assistance program. In 2001, the program helped 17.3 million people in 7.4 million households every day.[17] The program is operated by the Food and Nutrition Service of the U.S. Department of Agriculture. A participating household is defined by the program as a group of people living in the same house who buy, store, and eat food together. Benefit allotments are supposed to be sufficient to cover the household's food needs for 1 month. Under this program participants have historically been issued coupons or food stamps, but the actual coupons have been phased out by 2002. Congress mandated that all 50 states convert their coupon programs to new electronic benefit transfer (EBT) card systems. The EBT client uses a plastic card that is similar to a bank debit card when buying groceries. Funds are transferred from the client's food stamp benefit account to the retailer's account automatically, thus controlling program costs and helping to eliminate fraud.[17] Participating households must meet the program's eligibility requirements to qualify. Eligibility and benefit allotments are based on several factors, such as household income, household size, assets, work registration requirements, and other factors. The eligible income is adjusted annually. For the federal fiscal year ending September 30, 2003, the net monthly income limit for a four-person household is set at $1509.[18] This limit is quite low, and usually families who qualify simply are not making enough money to buy food. Over 50% of all food stamp program participants are children, and almost 10% are elderly. Women account for 70% of the nonelderly adult participants.

CHILD NUTRITION PROGRAMS

After the Surplus Commodities Program was initiated, the government faced a glut of accumulated food items and needed a means of disposing of them. During World War II, the military discovered a distressing rate of nutrition-related disorders that prevented a number of its draftees from serving in the army. From these two situations, the National School Lunch Program of 1946 was born. From this initial program came all of today's child nutrition programs.

National School Lunch and Breakfast Programs

These programs of the Food and Nutrition Service of the U.S. Department of Agriculture provide financial assistance to schools to enable them to provide nutritious lunches and breakfasts to their students. In 2001, the National School Lunch Program served on average every day 27.5 million children in more than 98,000 schools, while the School Breakfast Program served daily an average of 7.8 million children in almost 74,000 schools.[17] The program allows poor children to eat free meals or meals at reduced prices, and other students pay somewhat less than the full cost of the meal. Commodity foods, as described previously, are available to participating schools, and the programs usually entail minimal costs to the school district. All public and private nonprofit schools are eligible to participate in the program if their average tuition per student does not exceed $1500. Children's residential institutions, preschools, and the Head Start programs run as part of a school system are also eligible. Lunches served must fulfill approximately one third of the child's daily nutrient needs.

Child Care Food Program

This program provides USDA food commodities, cash equivalents, and meal reimbursements for most or all of the meal and administration costs of feeding children up to 12 years of age who are enrolled in organized child care programs. These settings include daycare centers, recreation centers, settlement houses, homeless shelters, and some Head Start programs. The children's eligibility for free and reduced-price meals is the same as for the school lunch and breakfast programs.

WOMEN, INFANTS, AND CHILDREN PROGRAM

The Special Supplemental Food Program for Women, Infants, and Children (commonly called WIC) provides nutritious foods to low-income women who are pregnant or breastfeeding and to their infants and children under the age of 5 years. The goal of the program is to improve the health of participating mothers and infants by providing supplemental foods, nutrition education, and access to health services.[17] Food is either distributed free or purchased with free vouchers. It is designed to supplement the diet with rich sources of iron, protein, and certain vitamins. The vouchers are good for such foods as milk, eggs, cheese, juice, fortified cereals, and infant formulas. The program includes funding to cover clinic visits for medical checkups and for nutrition education and counseling by public health nutritionists. It is administered by the USDA's Food and Nutrition Service through state health departments and Native American tribes, bands, or groups and is operated locally by public health facilities or organizations.

WIC participants must be pregnant or postpartum mothers (up to 6 months), lactating mothers (up to 12 months), or women with children under the age of 5 years. They must be at nutritional risk and must have an income under the reduced-price guidelines for the school lunch program. Factors indicating nutritional risk include evidence of an inadequate diet, poor growth patterns, a lack of nutrition understanding, or a medical history of nutrition-related problems, such as low birth weight or premature infants, pregnancy-induced hypertension (toxemia), spontaneous abortions (miscarriages), and anemia. The prevalence of anemia among infants and children in low-income families has steadily declined during the past 10 years. The decline is largely a result of the positive impact of public health programs such as WIC, which includes both food support and continuing nutrition education. A specially developed "Simple-Easy" education plan provides WIC clients with personalized action plans they need to achieve needed behavior change. WIC prenatal supplementation has helped reduce the incidence of low birth weight and raise the mean birth weight. WIC nutrition education programs have also supported the national health goals for all Americans to eat at least five servings of fruits or vegetables a day. Nutrition interventions, such as education campaigns, neighborhood-focused cooking events, and distribution of coupons to improve affordability, have successfully promoted increased awareness and consumption of fruits and vegetables among low-income families.[19,20]

Since its legislation by the U.S. Congress in 1972, the WIC program has served the needs of millions of women and children who have received benefits at more than 1000 clinics across the United States.[21] Unlike the food stamp or school lunch programs, however, WIC is not an "entitlement" program. This means that eligibility does not automatically entitle one to benefits. There is an absolute ceiling each year on funding and therefore on participation.

NUTRITION PROGRAM FOR ELDERLY PERSONS

Congress has provided two types of food programs to benefit the growing numbers of elderly citizens in the United States. Regardless of their income level, all persons over 60 years of age are eligible to receive meals from the Congregate Meals Program or the Home-Delivered Meals Program. Elderly persons often face many social, physical, and economic difficulties and do not eat adequately to fulfill their nutritional needs. Many of them experience isolation and social deprivation. The main difference in these two programs is their setting and social aspect. The Congregate Meals Program provides ambulatory elderly persons with a hot nourishing noon meal at a community center where they can share food once a day, 5 days a week, with a group of their peers at no charge. Free transportation is often provided. Social events and nutrition information accompany the meals. The nutrition education component often includes, for example, one of a special series of brief 10-statement self-check reviews of true-false questions, each designed to correct misconceptions about the relationship between diet and one of the common chronic diseases among the elderly. In comparison, the Home-Delivered Meals Program, sometimes called Meals-on-Wheels, provides homebound elderly persons who have difficulty preparing their own meals with at least one nutritious meal delivered to them in their home Monday through Friday. A special concern in this program centers on the very frail elderly persons being served who are most needy. Both programs may accept voluntary contributions for meals from those who are able to do so. The National Institutes of Health continues to support research into developing effective means of combating the causes and consequences of malnutrition among the elderly, especially those who are homebound.[22]

All of the food assistance programs reviewed here provide a base of food security for many low-income families. However, studies indicate that family food shortages in general have increased during the past decade among low-income families who are barely subsisting, as well as among participants in these government assistance programs who also experience food shortages, especially during the last week of each monthly cycle of stamps, coupons, or vouchers. U.S. populations most at risk for these food shortages include the elderly, single-parent families, and children.

Food Buying Guides

General family nutrition counseling may also involve guidance in planning for control of family food costs.

U.S. DEPARTMENT OF AGRICULTURE FOOD PLANS

The USDA periodically issues low-cost food plans to serve as guides for food assistance programs. These plans are called liberal, moderate, low, and thrifty or very low-cost food plans, but in comparison to modern consumer food costs in general they are all low-cost plans. These very low-cost food plans are developed by nutritionists, economists, and computer experts at USDA on the basis of a predetermined level of spending appropriate to the prevailing policy identifying the poverty threshold. The lowest of all these low-cost plans is used to determine allotments of food stamp program benefits to poor households.

FAMILY FOOD COSTS

A number of factors influence the way a family divides its food dollar. Some of these factors as listed here can help your client's family work out their household food plan.

1. Family income
2. Number, sex, ages, and general activities of family members
3. Any family food produced or preserved at home
4. Likes and dislikes of family members and special family dishes
5. Special dietary needs of any family member
6. Time, transportation, and energy for food shopping and preparation
7. Skill and experience in food management: planning, buying, cooking
8. Storing and cooking facilities in the home
9. Amount and kind of entertaining, if any
10. Meals eaten away from home
11. Value family places on food and eating

GOOD SHOPPING AND FOOD-HANDLING PRACTICES

Today's American family spends more time shopping for food than cooking it. Food marketing is big business, and buying food for a family may seem to be a more complex affair than the preparation of food at home. A large American supermarket may stock some 8000 or more different food items, and more are being added daily.[23,24] A single food item may be marketed in a dozen different ways at as many different prices. Commonly client families ask for more help with food buying than with any other aspect of fulfilling their diet needs, in terms of both cost and nutrition. The following four food handling practices will help to control costs and maintain healthy eating.

Plan Ahead

Use market guides in newspapers, plan general menus, keep a kitchen supply checklist, and make out a market list ahead of time according to location of items in a regularly visited market. Such planning helps avoid impulse buying and extra trips.

Buy Wisely

Know the market, market items, packaging, grades, brands, portion yields, measures, and food value in a market unit. Read food labels for nutrition information.[25] Watch for sale items and buy in quantity if it results in savings and the food can be adequately stored or used. Be cautious in selecting convenience foods. The added time-saving may not be worth the added cost. Be aware that new food products come on the market all the time, many involving new food technologies. They should be evaluated as much for their price value as for improvements in shelf-life or ease of preparation.[26]

Store Food Safely

The kitchen waste that results from food spoilage and misuse can be controlled. Conserve food by storing items according to their nature and use, using dry storage, covered containers, and refrigeration as needed. Keep opened and partly used food packages at the front of the shelf for early use. Avoid plate waste by preparing only the amount needed by the family and use leftovers intelligently and creatively.

Cook Food Well

Retain maximum food value in cooking processes and prepare food with imagination and good sense. Give zest and appeal to dishes by using a variety of seasonings and combinations.

In all family nutrition counseling, however, we must remember that as much as the family may have learned about nutrition, this is not always a primary factor. Family members usually eat because they are hungry or because the food looks and tastes good, not necessarily because it is nutritious.

THE BEST FOOD BUYS

Vegetables and Fruits

In addition to minerals, vegetables and fruits supply vitamins A and C, two nutrients found in surveys to be most often lacking in the average American diet. Give your clients the following guidelines.

1. Buy fresh items in season to avoid costs of out-of-season foods transported in from warmer, distant places.
2. Select fresh produce that is firm, crisp, and heavy for size. Medium-size items are usually better buys than large items, most of which may need to be discarded in preparation.
3. Distinguish between types of fresh produce defects. Small surface defects do not affect quality or food value and may cost less. Many or deep defects cause more waste, as does decay that is even slightly evident.
4. Compare costs of fresh produce sold by weight or count. The resulting price per item can be computed by each method of sale to make the best choice.
5. Avoid fancy grades in canned vegetables and fruits. Grading is based on shape, size, and perfection of pieces. Lower grades contain small, broken, or imperfect pieces, but they are equal in taste and food value and thus are good buys.
6. Buy vegetable and fruits in large cans, if family size warrants it.
7. Select low-cost dried foods. Dehydrated foods vary in price. Dried beans, peas, and lentils are excellent food buys, but specialty dried foods, such as potatoes or dried fruits, are usually more expensive than fresh ones.
8. Compare the costs of frozen, canned, and fresh vegetable and fruit items. Frozen items are usually more expensive. However, specials and family-sized packages can be compared on a weight-for-weight basis with canned or fresh items in season.
9. Cook vegetables with care. Excess cooking water and time destroy or eliminate vitamins and minerals and rob the vegetable of color, texture, and taste. Such unappetizing food often goes uneaten and causes costly waste.

Breads and Cereals

Most bread and cereal products are well liked and inexpensive and fit easily into meal plans. This group of foods, along with potatoes and other vegetables, provides complex carbohydrates, which on nutritionists' advice should be the staple food of most persons' diets. Whole-grain foods are good sources of dietary fiber and are high in important vitamins and minerals. They are also important sources of amino acids and, in combination with other grains and legumes, form complete proteins. Many foods in this group can be excellent bargains.

1. *Whole-grain or enriched products* are much more nutritious than refined grains and products and are usually no more expensive.
2. *Enriched specialty breads,* such as French or Italian, cost up to 3 times more than whole-grain bread with similar or better nutritive value.
3. *Precooked rice* is much more expensive than unprocessed and often lacks many of the nutrients lost in processing.
4. Many *cereals* have nutrients added. Cereals that advertise 100% of the Recommended Dietary Allowance for vitamins and minerals are usually more expensive. If the diet is adequate, such levels of supplementation are unnecessary.
5. *Ready-to-eat cereals, instant hot cereals, and those packaged for individual servings* are usually much more expensive. Buy grains in bulk if adequate storage can be provided.
6. *Baked goods* made at home, from scratch or even from some mixes, are usually much cheaper than bakery goods.
7. A *large loaf of bread* may not weigh more than a small loaf. Compare prices of equal weights of bread to find the better buy.
8. Try *unusual forms of grains.* For example, bulgur, buckwheat groats (hulled kernels), barley, and millet are excellent grains and can be used in many meals. Bulgur, which is cooked like rice, has a toastlike color, is rich in wheat flavor, and is equal in food value to whole wheat.

PROTEIN FOODS

Plant Proteins

Dried beans and peas, grains, nuts, and seeds are inexpensive sources of proteins. Legumes and grains contribute needed amino acids to provide food sources of protein.

These foods store well and are versatile in preparation, low in fat, and free of cholesterol, which is purely an animal product. They are also good sources of vitamins and minerals, including iron, zinc, and the B vitamins. For example, tofu, a curd made from soybean milk, has been the low-cost protein backbone of the East Asian diet for more than 2000 years. Today tofu is well known in the American diet. Soy protein is also consumed as a common ingredient in processed foods such as chips, pasta, chili, and trail mix.[26]

Eggs

Eggs provide high-quality complete protein and are sold according to grade and size, neither of which is related to food value. Egg grades are based on qualities such as firmness of egg white, appearance, and delicacy of flavor, not on food value or quality. Shell color varies with species of chicken and has no effect on quality.

Milk and Cheese

Dairy products are good sources of high-quality complete protein. However, whole milk products carry saturated fat; therefore distinguish among them those that are lower in fat as well as lower in price.

1. *Fluid nonfat milk, buttermilk, and canned evaporated milk* cost less than whole, fluid milk. Low-fat milks may be 1% or 2% butterfat; whole milk is 4%. To produce these lower-fat milks, part of the butterfat is removed and dry milk solids are added. For example, whole milk contains 170 kcalories/cup, 2% milk contains 135 kcalories/cup, and nonfat milk contains 80 kcalories/cup.
2. *Nonfat dried milk* is the best bargain of all forms of milk. Reconstituted with water, it provides a fluid nonfat milk at less than half the cost of the fresh form. It can also be used in many ways in cooking to add valuable nutrition, as well as the base for making yogurt.
3. If family size warrants it, buy *milk in bulk containers.*
4. If *cheese* is used often, buy it in bulk. It costs less per unit of weight and keeps better. Cheese standards set by the Food and Drug Administration (FDA) are based on percentage of fat and moisture. The most commonly used, cheddar cheese (American, Daisy, Longhorn), is 50% fat and 30% moisture. Spread cheeses and imported cheeses are much more expensive.
5. *Cottage cheese* is an unripened, soft curd (80% moisture) and hence a rapidly perishable item. Buy it only as used to avoid waste from spoilage.
6. *Butter* is a fat made from milk. Because it is an animal product, it contains both saturated fat and cholesterol. Margarine, made from vegetable oil, contains no cholesterol and is usually lower in price. For people who are trying to lower their cholesterol levels to reduce their risk of heart disease, the FDA in 2000 gave approval to food makers to add certain plant extracts (plant sterol and stanol esters, which work by blocking the absorption of cholesterol) to margarine-type spreads and to label these products as helping to reduce cholesterol.[27] Consumers will have to judge, however, whether the potential benefits outweigh the high cost of these spreads.

Poultry

Buy poultry by the whole bird. Usually the larger, more mature birds cost less than the young broilers and fryers, and they can be made equally tender with longer, moist cooking methods, such as braising, stewing, or pressure cooking.

Organ Meats

Liver, kidney, and heart carry many nutrients, especially iron, although liver is high in cholesterol. However, in some areas they may actually be more expensive than some other boneless cuts of meat. A good cookbook will have appetizing ways of cooking them for family acceptance.

Fish

This is sometimes a fairly expensive food in many areas, depending on the season and the kind. Shellfish is more costly. Less expensive packed styles of canned fish may be available. For example, tuna is packed according to sizes of pieces, with fancy or solid pack (large pieces) being most expensive. Fish consumption is part of the diet pattern called the Mediterranean diet (rich in fish, canola oil, fruits, cereals, and beans) that research indicates can reduce the risk of heart disease.[28]

Red Meats

Because meat is commonly one of the most costly food items, learn how it is graded, cut, processed, and marketed. Excellent learning material is available through the local county home advisor of the USDA Extension Service. Avoid cuts with large amounts of gristle, bone, and fat. The lower grades provide good quality and less fat, and they cost less.

ADDITIONAL RESOURCES

Farmers' Markets

In community farmers' markets, local produce is made available directly to consumers. This outlet has the advantage of fresh produce at prices lower than those found in the supermarket. It also offers opportunities for socializing experiences between growers and consumers and provides a sense of community cohesion. The public considers local fruits and vegetables to be fresher and to look and taste better. Buying local produce can be an effective way to support a sustainable local agricultural economy.[29]

Consumer Cooperatives

Consumer cooperatives focus on the economics of food marketing as well as on the issues of nutrition and ecology.

The newer food cooperatives usually deal in bulk sales of whole or minimally processed foods. Belonging to a food cooperative increases personal responsibility and individual choice and brings food issues into the hands of the consumer. Many of these food cooperatives stress the purchase of locally grown foods, thus strengthening local farmers while providing very fresh foods for consumers.

Home Gardens

With a little effort, any extra yard space may be turned into a home garden. Many persons are now turning to their backyards, interspacing vegetable plants among flowers and shrubbery in front yards, using allotted community spaces, window boxes, planter boxes on porches, and even indoor potted plots to grow at least a portion of their own produce.

TO SUM UP

A major role of healthcare professionals is to translate the large amount of nutrition information available so that it can meet the needs of clients and families. They must present it in such a way that it is easily understood, is retained and applied by the learner, and can be evaluated to improve its effectiveness and ability to meet continuing care needs. Valid health and nutrition education must focus on the needs of the learner. Goals for planning counseling and educational activities and the methods for meeting these goals must be based on identifiable client and family needs.

Families and individuals under economic stress need counseling concerning financial assistance. Various U.S. food assistance programs operate to help families in need. Referrals to appropriate agencies may be made. The nutrition counselor may also need to assist the family in planning the most economic and nutritious meals possible within their limited circumstances. The family may need help in learning good shopping and food handling practices—planning ahead, buying wisely, storing safely, and cooking appropriately to preserve nutritional values and to make food appetizing.

Questions for Review

1. Identify and describe the skills necessary for an effective nutrition counseling session.
2. Identify the basic principles of learning and describe how they may be used in planning nutrition education for one of your clients and his or her family.
3. What government food assistance programs are available to help low-income families? What other local food resources are available in your community?
4. List and discuss the "best food buys" described in this chapter. How many of the recommended practices do you follow in selecting, storing, and preparing foods?

References

1. Link BG, Phelan JC: Understanding sociodemographic differences in health—the role of fundamental social causes, *Am J Public Health* 86(4):471, 1996.
2. Jefferys M: Social inequalities in health—do they diminish with age? *Am J Public Health* 86(4):474, 1996.
3. Romero-Gwynn et al: Dietary patterns and acculturation among immigrants from El Salvador, *Nutr Today* 35(6):233, 2000.
4. Smith GJ et al: Survey of the diet of Pima Indians using quantitative food frequency assessment and 24-hour recall, *J Am Diet Assoc* 96(8):778, 1996.
5. Patterson RE et al: Using a brief household inventory as an environmental indicator of individual dietary practices, *Am J Public Health* 87(2):272, 1997.
6. Johnson RK: What are people really eating and why does it matter? *Nutr Today* 35(2):40, 2000.
7. Kicklighter JR: Characteristics of older adult learners: a guide for dietetics practitioners, *J Am Diet Assoc* 91(11):1418, 1991.
8. Shafer L et al: Position of the American Dietetic Association: nutrition education for the public, *J Am Diet Assoc* 96(11):1183, 1996.
9. Kulman L: Food news can get you dizzy, so know what to swallow, *US News & World Report* 129(19):68, 2000.
10. Godal T: Fighting the parasites of poverty: public research, private industry, and tropical diseases, *Science* 264(5167): 1864, 1994.
11. Beckman D et al: Position of the American Dietetic Association: world hunger, *J Am Diet Assoc* 95(10):1160, 1995.
12. Vozenilek GP: Dietetics in the fight against domestic hunger, *J Am Diet Assoc* 98(3):266, 1998.
13. Singh GK, Yu SM: Infant mortality in the United States: trends, differentials, and projections, 1950 through 2010, *Am J Public Health* 85(7):957, 1995.
14. Staff report: Public policy news: ADA action on food security and proposed federal regulations, *J Am Diet Assoc* 97(9):952, 1997.
15. Kendall A, Kennedy E: Position of the American Dietetic Association: Domestic food and nutrition security, *J Am Diet Assoc* 98(3):337, 1998.
16. U.S. Department of Agriculture, Food and Nutrition Service: *Food Stamp Program participation and costs*, accessible at *http://www.fns.usda.gov/pd/fssummar.htm.*
17. U.S. Department of Agriculture, Food and Nutrition Service: *FNS Online: Food and Nutrition Service program data*, accessible at *http://www.fns.usda.gov/pd.*
18. U.S. Department of Agriculture, Food and Nutrition Service: *FNS Online: Food Stamp Program income eligibility standards*, accessible at *http://www.fns.usda.gov/fsp.*
19. Anderson J et al: 5 A Day fruit and vegetable intervention improves consumption in a low income population, *J Am Diet Assoc* 101(2):195, 2001.
20. Weaver M, Poehlitz M, Hutchison S: 5 A Day for low-income families: evaluation of an advertising campaign and cooking events, *J Nutr Educ* 31(3):161, 1999.
21. Owen AL, Owen GM: Twenty years of WIC: a review of some effects of the program, *J Am Diet Assoc* 97(7):777, 1997.

22. Pennington JAT et al: Diet-related observational studies supported by the National Institutes of Health: causes/consequences of malnutrition in homebound elderly, *Nutr Today* 34(1):29, 1999.
23. Glanz K et al: Why Americans eat what they do: taste, nutrition, cost, convenience, and weight concerns as influences on food consumption, *J Am Diet Assoc* 98(10):1118, 1998.
24. Southgate DAT: Dietary change: changing patterns of eating. In Meiselman HL, MacFie HJH, editors: *Food choices, acceptance, and consumption,* London, 1999, Chapman & Hall.
25. Neuhouser ML et al: Use of food nutrition labels is associated with lower fat intake, *J Am Diet Assoc* 99(1):45, 1999.
26. Lemley B: Future food, *Discover* 21(12): 82, 2000.
27. Lewis C: Health claim for foods that could lower heart disease risk, *FDA Consumer* Nov/Dec 2000, p 11.
28. Seppa N: Mediterranean diet proves value again, *Science News* 155(8):119, 1999.
29. Wilkins JL, Bowdish E, Sobal J: University student perceptions of seasonal and local foods, *J Nutr Educ* 32(5):261, 2000.

■ Further Reading

Coulston AM et al: Meals-on-Wheels applicants are a population at risk for poor nutritional status, *J Am Diet Assoc* 96(6):570, 1996.

Shovic A, Geoghegan P: Assessment of meal portion, food temperature, and select nutrient content of the Hawaii Meals-on-Wheels program, *J Am Diet Assoc* 97(5):530, 1997.

These two articles describe current services of the Meals-on-Wheels program for homebound elderly persons, who are often frail and malnourished.

Kendall A et al: Relationship of hunger and food insecurity to food availability and consumption, *J Am Diet Assoc* 96(10):1019, 1996.

Lee JD et al: Implementing the community-university model: dietetics students collaborate with Volunteers of America, *J Am Diet Assoc* 97(3):297, 1997.

These two articles describe the severe problems of hunger in a rural community and the hands-on experience of nutrition students with congregate meal sites for older adults.

Issues & ANSWERS

A Person-Centered Model Applied to Diabetes Education

A paradigm for nutrition education called *holistic education* can well apply to teaching good self-care practices to clients with chronic disorders such as diabetes.

This approach draws from good management and good medicine: (1) it varies its style to meet the situation, and (2) it focuses on the whole person—mind-body-spirit, well-being, and wellness. Holistic education regards clients or patients as active partners in the mutual goal of good healthcare. And further, it teaches persons to use their "boxes and their bubbles"—an excellent thinking model. Our "box" is our rational left side of the brain. Our "bubbles" emerge from our intuitive right side of the brain. We need both. We need to combine rational processes and intuitive ones to build creative thinking skills. Activity that just provides information or shows techniques does not help clients build creative thinking skills for themselves.

Investigations of national patient education programs indicate that many of them provide information and skills training without incorporating learning theories in the design of the program. They also lack a systematic way of assessing and influencing learner attitudes.

Learning theories are usually based on the psychosocial needs of the persons involved as well as their educational needs. In this instance, the person with diabetes has the major responsibility for the day-to-day management of the disease to maintain health and to avoid complications. Thus diabetes education serves as a model for all good nutrition education and counseling in healthcare. With approximately 75% of all treated persons with diabetes failing to some degree to follow their prescribed diets, we should examine what we are doing in designing instruction for the person with diabetes. Ask yourself the following questions.

Is the teaching process effective?

Does the teaching process take into account the following.

- How do people learn?
- What is worth learning?
- Who really is responsible for a person's health?
- What responsibilities for learning lie within the learner versus the instructor?

Is the learning process effective?

Does the learning process consider the following.

- How significant is the condition to the person at that point in his or her life?
- Does the person have a sense of psychologic safety; that is, does the person feel well enough accepted to discuss diabetes control problems openly and honestly?
- How will the instructor know if the person's attitude has changed toward receiving or using new information?

These questions are important reminders to consider factors that influence learning behavior when planning any healthcare and education program. Although this may seem to be immediately beyond the realm of nutrition, it is extremely important in any aspect of the care plan and learning process precisely because self-care control of any chronic disease lies primarily in the hands of the person with the disease. This is especially true in diabetes care. No matter how much information is provided, it is ultimately up to the individual to decide what foods are selected, how much is eaten, and when it is consumed.

Diabetes educators, for example, often fail to consider major aspects of the person's individual and unique personal life that may influence these decisions, such as family finances, work situation, or social activities. They may also fail to recognize the effect of these activities on the individual's sense of personal responsibility for his or her own health. This may also influence the type of instruction provided or even the decision to provide instruction at that time at all.

The educator must be able to assess the person's sense of responsibility and capacity for continuing self-care daily and to use this information to develop or revise instruction and counseling that leads to positive behaviors. Dietitians and other healthcare workers may benefit from

paradigm A pattern or model serving as an example; a standard or ideal practice or behavior based on a fundamental value or theme.

TABLE 10-2 Levels of Personal Responsibility and Relevant Intervention Methods—Diabetes as an Example Case

Level of Personal Responsibility	Client Characteristics	Intervention Method
1. Being diabetic is a disaster	Feels hopeless, helpless, defeated; self-care may be impossible	Educate family member or other caregivers
2. Being diabetic is a burden	Blames problem on others; expects others to feel sorry for him or her; feels angry, threatened	Provide emotional support; help client accept anger to move on
3. Being diabetic is a problem	Blames self as often as others; personal growth is possible	Reinforce attitudes that reflect sense of responsibility; examine irresponsibility; examine irresponsible attitude in nonjudgmental way
4. Being diabetic is a challenge	Rarely blames others for problem; recognizes responsibility, but does not act on it; good self-care expected	Point out discrepancies between stated need and actual behavior
5. Being diabetic is an opportunity	Takes total responsibility for the problem; acts positively on decisions; optimal self-care is expected	Provide tools required for good self-care

the systematic methods of assessment that have already been developed in the field of clinical psychology. Therapists have identified five levels of responsibility and client characteristics, with possible intervention methods for each level, as shown in Table 10-2.

Such a system for assessing client attitudes has specific benefits. These benefits can guide client education in good self-care involving food habits not only in diabetes but also in other chronic conditions in families, such as hypertension and cardiovascular disease. Benefits of such a system include the following.

1. It recognizes, and reinforces in the instructor, that the client is ultimately responsible for his or her health.
2. It gives the instructor an objective, measurable way of assessing client attitudes that can be compared and evaluated for progress.
3. It serves as a basis for selecting appropriate teaching methods or counseling techniques, which can then be changed to match the client's current level of responsibility.

REFERENCES

American Medical Association Council on Scientific Education for Health: Education for health: a role for physicians and the efficacy of health education efforts, *JAMA* 263:1816, 1990.

Johnson CC et al: Behavioral counseling and contracting as methods for promoting cardiovascular health in families, *J Am Diet Assoc* 92(4):479, 1992.

Leontos C et al: National Diabetes Education Program: opportunities and challenges, *J Am Diet Assoc* 98(1):73, 1998.

McNutt K: Why some consumers don't believe some nutrition claims, *Nutr Today* 32(6):252, 1997.

Rinke WJ: Holistic education: a new paradigm for nutrition education, *J Nutr Educ* 18(4):151, 1986.

Chapter

11

Nutrition During Pregnancy and Lactation

Sue Rodwell Williams

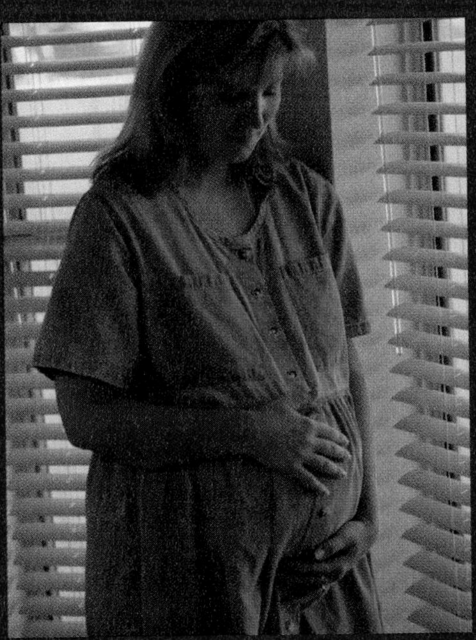

Chapter Outline

In this chapter we begin a three-chapter sequence on nutrition in health care throughout the life cycle. In each chapter, we will relate principles of nutrition to the remarkable process of human growth and development.

As we focus first on the beginning of new life, we examine the prenatal nutritional demands of the pregnant mother and her developing child. Mother and child possess great powers of adaptation to meet these demands.

Here we explore these tremendous physiologic changes during pregnancy and some possible complications. You will see how vital a role nutritional support plays in a successful course and outcome.

Maternal Nutrition and the Outcome of Pregnancy

EARLY MEDICAL PRACTICE

For centuries, in all cultures, a great body of folklore has surrounded pregnancy. Various traditional practices and diets have been followed, many of which have had little basis in fact, and much clinical advice has been based only on supposition. For example, early obstetricians even held the notion that semistarvation of the mother was really a blessing in disguise because it produced a small baby of light weight who would be easier to deliver. To this end they used diets restricted in kilocalories (kcalories), protein, water, and salt. Despite the lack of any scientific evidence to support such ideas, two assumptions, now known to be false, governed practice: (1) the *parasite theory:* whatever the fetus needs it draws from the stores of the mother despite the maternal diet, and (2) the *maternal instinct theory:* whatever the fetus needs, the mother instinctively craves and consumes.

HEALTHY PREGNANCY

It is clear now that until recently much of the counsel given to pregnant women over the past few decades has been based more on tradition than on scientific fact. Increasing evidence indicates that positive nutritional support of pregnancy, rather than past negative restrictions born of limited knowledge and false assumptions, promotes a positive successful outcome with increased health and vigor of mothers and infants alike. This struggle over the past few decades, particularly to define the "healthy pregnancy," has not been easy. Now a healthy pregnancy is described in broader terms of mother and infant and family. We are beginning to understand more about what this really means, especially as we see around us the current fetal damages from malnutrition and drug abuse. We know that we must assess and support more fully the quality of life of each mother and her family if we are to approach the healthy pregnancy we desire for all mothers.

DIRECTIONS FOR CURRENT PRACTICE

Clinical observations and developing science in both nutrition and medicine have provided directions for healthier pregnancies. They have long refuted previous false ideas and laid a sound base for our current practice. A classic report of the National Research Council (NRC) first reflected this applied scientific base and led the way. This report, *Maternal Nutrition and the Course of Human Pregnancy,* was a clear turning point and provided undeniable direction for a new positive approach to the management of pregnancy.[1] Indeed, continuing research has reinforced this positive direction. On the basis of the significant NRC findings, guidelines for the nutritional care of pregnant women were then issued by the American College of Obstetrics and Gynecology and the American Dietetic Association.[2,3] These reports continue to provide useful guidelines for physicians, nutritionists, dietitians, and nurses in their prenatal care. Nutritional guidelines for pregnancy and lactation for all nutrients are also included in the Dietary Reference Intake (DRI) recommendations published by the National Academy of Sciences.[4-7] We are reminded by these guides that a child is nutritionally 9 months old at birth, even older when we consider the significance of the mother's preconception status.

FACTORS DETERMINING NUTRITIONAL NEEDS

It is evident from increased knowledge and the wide experience of many clinicians that maternal nutrition is critically important to both the mother and the child. It lays the fundamental foundation for the successful outcome of pregnancy—a healthy and happy mother and child.[8] Several vital considerations emerge as factors that determine the nutritional requirements of the mother during her pregnancy.

Age, Gravida, and Parity

Age plays a major role in pregnancy; the teenage mother adds her own immaturity and growth needs to those imposed by pregnancy. At the other end of the reproductive cycle, hazards increase with age. Also, the number of pregnancies (gravida) and the number of viable offspring (parity), as well as the time intervals between them, greatly influence the mother's nutrient reserves, her increased nutritional needs, and the outcome of the pregnancy.

Preconception Nutrition

The mother brings to each pregnancy all of her previous life experiences, including her diet and eating habits. Her general health and fitness and her state of nutrition at the time of conception are products of her lifelong dietary habits and her genetic heritage.

Complex Physiologic Interactions of Gestation

Three distinct biologic entities are involved during gestation: the mother, the fetus, and the placenta, which nourishes fetal growth. Together they form a unique biologic whole. Constant metabolic interactions occur among them. Their functions, although unique, are at the same time interdependent. It is this unique biologic synergism that nourishes and sustains the pregnancy.

BASIC CONCEPTS INVOLVED

As a result of our increased knowledge of pregnancy and nutrition, we can provide better nutritional guidance. Three basic concepts form a fundamental framework for assessing maternal nutrition needs and for planning supportive prenatal care for both parents.

Perinatal Concept

The prefix *peri-* comes from the Greek root meaning "around, about, or surrounding." Thus the word *perinatal* refers more broadly to the scope of factors that surround a birth than merely the 9 months of the physical gestation. Certainly, as nutrition knowledge and understanding have increased, health professionals realize that all of a woman's life experiences surrounding her pregnancy need to be considered. Her nutritional status and food patterns, which have developed over a number of years, and the degree to which she has established and maintained nutritional reserves are all important factors. Cultural and social influences have shaped beliefs and values of both parents about pregnancy. All of these influences come to bear on any pregnancy.

Synergism Concept

The word *synergism* is a term used to describe biologic systems in which the cooperative action of two or more factors produces a total effect greater than and different from the mere sum of the parts. In short, a new whole is created by the unified, joint effort of blending the parts in which each part makes more powerful the action of the others. Of the many biologic and physiologic examples of synergism, pregnancy is a prime case in point. Maternal organism, fetus, and placenta combine to produce a new whole, a system not existing before and producing a total effect greater than and different from the sum of the parts, all for the sole purpose of sustaining and nurturing the pregnancy and its offspring. Physiologic measures change. Blood volume increases, cardiac output increases, ventilation rate and tidal volume of breathing increase, and basal metabolic rate increases. The physiologic norms of the nonpregnant woman do not apply.

Thus the normal physiologic adjustments of pregnancy cannot be viewed as pathologic with application of treatment procedures for that same type of response in the nonpregnant state. For example, a normal physiologic generalized edema of pregnancy is a protective response. It reflects the normal increase in total body water necessary to support the increased metabolic work of pregnancy and is associated with enhanced reproductive performance.

Life Continuum Concept

In a real sense, throughout her life a woman is providing for the ongoing continuum of life through food that she eats. Each child obviously becomes a part of this continuing process during the pregnancy when the mother's diet directly sustains growth. But in the broader sense, both parents carry over their nutritional heritage, practices, and beliefs in the teaching of their growing children, who in the next generation pass on this heritage both genetically and culturally.

Positive Nutritional Demands of Pregnancy

BASIC NUTRIENT ALLOWANCES AND INDIVIDUAL VARIATION

The period of gestation is an exceedingly rapid growth period. During this brief 9 months, the human life grows from a single fertilized egg cell (ovum) to a fully developed infant weighing about 3 kg (7 lb). On the basis of this intense physiologic growth and development of the fetus, what nutrients must the mother supply? What must her diet provide to meet the nutritional demands of the fetus and of her own changing body during this critical period of human growth?

Throughout the pregnancy there is an increased need for most of the basic nutrients, as indicated by the DRI guidelines from the National Academy of Sciences[4-7] (Table 11-1). However, it is important to remember that these are guidelines, and individual variances in need must be examined for each pregnancy. Individual variations such as body size, activity, and multiple pregnancy need to be considered. Also, the quantitative need for nourishment of pregnant adolescents must be noted. The need for individual counseling and for correct use of nutrition guidelines has been clearly stated by the National Research Council: "They are not called 'requirements,' because they are not intended to represent merely literal (minimal) requirements of average individuals, but to cover substantially the individual variations in the requirements of healthy people."[9] In considering the needs of the healthy pregnant woman, we will review here the nutrient elements in terms of general amounts of increased intake indicated, why this increase is recommended, and how it may be obtained in basic foods.

ENERGY NEEDS

The kcalories must be sufficient to (1) supply the increased energy and nutrient demands created by the increased metabolic workload, including some maternal fat storage

---

fetus The unborn offspring in the postembryonic period, after major structures have been outlined; in humans the growing offspring from 7 to 8 weeks after fertilization until birth.

gestation The period of embryonic and fetal development from fertilization to birth; pregnancy.

gravida A pregnant woman.

parity The condition of a woman with respect to having borne viable offspring.

placenta Special organ developed in early pregnancy that provides nutrients to the fetus and removes metabolic waste.

synergism The joint action of separate agents in which the total effect of their combined action is greater than the sum of their separate actions.

TABLE 11-1 Dietary Reference Intakes Per Day of Some Selected Nutrients for Pregnancy and Lactation

Nutrients	Nonpregnant Girl 9-13 yr 46 kg 101 lb	Nonpregnant Girl 14-18 yr 55 kg 120 lb	Nonpregnant Woman 19-50 yr 63 kg 138 lb	During Pregnancy 19-50 yr	Lactation (600 ml/day) First 6 mo	Lactation (750 ml/day) Second 6 mo
Kcalories	2000-2200	2200	2200	No change in the first trimester; add 300 kcalories/day for second and third trimesters	2700	2700
Protein (g)	46	44	50	60	65	62
Calcium (mg)	1300	1300	1000	1000 mg throughout	1000 mg throughout	
Iron (mg)	8	15	18	27 mg throughout	15 mg throughout	
Vitamin A (μg RAE)*	600	700	700	770 μg RAE throughout	1300 μg throughout	
Thiamin (mg)	0.9	1.0	1.1	1.4 mg throughout	1.4 mg throughout	
Riboflavin (mg)	0.9	1.0	1.1	1.4 mg throughout	1.6 mg throughout	
Niacin (mg NE)	12	14	14	18 mg NE throughout	17 mg NE throughout	
Vitamin C (mg)	45	65	75	85 mg throughout	120 mg throughout	
Vitamin D (μg)	5	5	5	5 μg throughout	5 μg throughout	
Folic acid (μg)†	300	400	400	600 μg throughout	500 μg throughout	

*As retinal activity equivalents (RAEs). One RAE is equal to 1 μg all-*trans* retinal or 12 μg beta-carotene.

†As dietary folate equivalents (DFEs). One DFE is equal to 1 μg food folate or 0.6 μg of folic acid from fortified food or as a supplement consumed with food or 0.5 μg of a supplement taken on an empty stomach.

From Food and Nutrition Board, Institute of Medicine, *Dietary reference intakes, vol 1-4,* Washington, DC, 1998-2002, National Academy Press; National Research Council: *Recommended dietary allowances,* ed 10, Washington, DC, 1989, National Academy Press.

and fetal fat storage to ensure an optimal newborn size for survival, and (2) spare protein for tissue building. A minimum of about 36 kcalories/kg is required for efficient use of protein during pregnancy. The DRI standard recommends an additional amount of energy, 300 kcalories/day during the second and third trimesters of pregnancy, to supply needs during this time of rapid growth, making a total of about 2200 to 2500 kcalories, about a 10% to 15% increase over the mother's general prepregnancy need. This amount may be insufficient for active, large, or nutritionally deficient women, who may need as much as 2500 to 3000 kcalories/day. Remember that for most women, a minimum of 1800 kcalories is required just to avoid negative nitrogen balance, to say nothing of the added pregnancy and activity needs. This primary positive emphasis on sufficient kcalories is critical to ensure nutrient and energy needs to support the pregnancy. Appropriate weight gain during the pregnancy indicates whether sufficient kcalories are being provided.

PROTEIN AND FAT NEEDS

The total amount of protein recommended for a pregnant woman is about 60 g/day, an increase of about 10 to 15 g/day. Protein, with its essential nitrogen, is the nutrient basic to tissue growth. Nitrogen balance studies provide some indication of the large amounts of nitrogen used by the mother and child during pregnancy and emphasize the importance of maternal reserves to meet initial needs even before the pregnancy is confirmed. More protein is necessary to meet tissue demands posed by (1) rapid growth of the fetus, (2) enlargement of the uterus, mammary glands, and placenta, (3) increase in maternal circulating blood volume and subsequent demand for increased plasma proteins to maintain colloidal osmotic pressure and circulation of tissue fluids to nourish cells, and (4) formation of amniotic fluid and storage reserves for labor, delivery, and lactation. Milk, egg, cheese, and meat are complete protein foods of high biologic value. Protein-rich foods also contribute other nutrients, such as calcium, iron, and B vitamins. Additional protein may be obtained from legumes and whole grains, with lesser amounts in other plant sources.

An adequate supply of essential fatty acids is also vital throughout pregnancy. Tissue growth, especially the proper development of cell membranes in nerve and brain tissue, requires that essential fatty acids in sufficient amounts reach the developing fetus. Depending on individual needs, supplementation of the mother's essential fatty acid intake may be useful to maintain adequate levels.[10,11]

MINERAL NEEDS

All of the major and trace minerals play roles in maternal health. Two that have special functions in relation to pregnancy—calcium and iron—deserve particular attention.

Calcium

The pregnant woman's DRI recommendation is 1000 mg of calcium/day, the same as the general recommendation for all women aged 19 to 50. Calcium is the essential element for the construction and maintenance of bones and teeth. It is also an important factor in the blood-clotting mechanism and is used in normal muscle action and other essential metabolic activities. Improved absorption of calcium supplies the needs arising from the rapid fetal mineralization of skeletal tissue during the final period of rapid growth. Dairy products are a primary source of calcium. Some increase in the consumption of milk or equivalent milk foods (cheese or nonfat milk powder used in cooking) is recommended. Additional calcium is obtained in whole or fortified cereal grains and in green leafy vegetables.

Iron

The pregnant woman needs 27 mg of iron/day, a 33% increase over her general DRI needs.[7] Some pregnant women may need supplementary iron in addition to increased dietary sources to meet the additional requirement of pregnancy. The iron cost of pregnancy is high. With increased demands for iron, often insufficient maternal stores, and inadequate provision through the usual diet, a daily supplement of 30 to 60 mg of iron may be prescribed. If the woman is anemic at conception, a larger therapeutic amount of 120 to 200 mg of iron is recommended.

To obtain the needed amount of iron, check the percentage of elemental iron in the iron preparation being used. For example, the commonly used compound ferrous sulfate is a hydrated salt ($FeSO_4\ 7H_2O$), which contains 20% iron. It is usually dispensed in tablets containing 195, 300, or 325 mg of the ferrous sulfate compound. Each tablet, then, would contain 39, 60, or 65 mg of iron, respectively. Thus to supply a regular daily supplement of 60 mg of iron, one 300-mg tablet of ferrous sulfate is required, and for a therapeutic dose of 120 mg iron, two 300-mg tablets are required.

However, there are problems with routine iron supplementation for all pregnant women, such as unpleasant gastrointestinal side effects and less motivation to maintain a good diet. Also, there may be imbalances with other trace elements, such as zinc, which competes with iron for absorption. Actually, excess iron intake, when not needed, may mask inadequate pregnancy-induced hemodilution, a normal pregnancy adaptation that puts less strain on the maternal heart, minimizes hemoglobin loss with blood loss at delivery, and increases nutrient flow to the fetus. Thus some prenatal clinics follow protocols that prescribe regular prenatal vitamins with iron at the first clinic visit. Then individual additional iron supplementation is used only if hemoglobin falls to 10.5 g/dl or less at any time during the pregnancy.

During pregnancy, the maternal circulating blood volume normally increases from 40% to 50% and may increase more with multiple births. An individual mother's iron supplement need must be assessed accordingly. Maternal iron is also needed to supply iron stores for the developing fetal liver. Adequate maternal iron stores help fortify the mother against iron losses related to blood loss at delivery.

It is no surprise, then, that our major food source of iron is liver. Its use can be encouraged by suggesting appetizing ways of preparing it. Other food sources include meat, legumes, dried fruit, green leafy vegetables, eggs, and enriched bread and cereals (see list of iron-containing foods in Chapter 8).

VITAMIN NEEDS

Increased amounts of vitamins A, B complex, C, and D are needed during pregnancy. If these needs are met, sufficient amounts of vitamins E and K are also available.

Vitamin A

The daily amount of vitamin A recommended for pregnancy is 770 μg of retinol activity equivalents (RAE), a slight increase over the woman's regular need.[7] For most women in the United States, no extra amount is needed. However, malnourished, underweight women, and those with multiple pregnancies need more. Vitamin A is an essential factor in cell development, maintenance of strong epithelial tissue, tooth formation, and normal bone growth. Liver, egg yolk, butter and fortified margarine, dark green and yellow vegetables, and fruits are good food sources.

B Vitamins

There is a special need for the various B vitamins during pregnancy. These are usually supplied by a well-balanced diet that is increased in quantity and quality to supply needed energy and nutrients. The B vitamins are important as coenzyme factors in a number of metabolic activities related to energy production, tissue protein synthesis, and function of muscle and nerve tissue; therefore they play key roles in the increased metabolic work of pregnancy.[12]

---

amniotic fluid The watery fluid within the membrane enveloping the fetus, in which the fetus is suspended.

There is a special increased metabolic need for the B vitamin folate during pregnancy. Folate deficiency usually occurs in conjunction with general malnutrition, making the pregnant woman in low-socioeconomic conditions especially vulnerable. A specific megaloblastic anemia caused by maternal folate deficiency sometimes occurs and warrants supplementation of the diet with folic acid. This added amount is particularly needed where such demands are greater, as in a multiple pregnancy.

Folic acid taken before conception has been shown in randomized clinical trials to greatly reduce a woman's risk of bearing a child with a neural tube defect, which is the source of the serious defects of spina bifida and anencephaly. These congenital defects in the formation of the spine develop in early embryonic life, when the neural tube, which forms the spinal cord, does not close completely, leaving part of one or more vertebrae of the spinal cord exposed at birth (see Chapter 25). Each year in the United States approximately 2500 infants are born with spina bifida and anencephaly, and an estimated 1500 affected fetuses are aborted.[13] Since 1992, the U.S. Public Health Service has recommended that all women of childbearing age who are capable of becoming pregnant consume from food or supplementation 400 μg of folic acid/day to prevent such deficiencies. This recommendation continues in the latest DRI guidelines, which recommend 400 μg/day for nonpregnant women, rising to 600 μg/day during pregnancy and 500 μg/day during lactation.[5] The Food and Drug Administration, acting to increase folic acid consumption nationally, began requiring in 1996 that enriched cereal grain products be fortified with folic acid.[14-16]

Vitamin C

Special emphasis must be given to the pregnant woman's need for ascorbic acid. Vitamin C is essential to the formation of intercellular cement substance in developing connective tissues and vascular systems. It also increases the absorption of iron that is needed for the increasing quantities of hemoglobin. The DRI standard recommends 85 mg/day for the pregnant women, an increase of 10 mg/day over the regular adult female need of 75 mg/day.[6] Additional food sources such as citrus fruit and other vegetables and fruits should be included in the mother's diet.

Vitamin D

Adults who lead active lives involving adequate exposure to sunlight probably need little additional vitamin D. During pregnancy, because of the need for calcium and phosphorus presented by the developing fetal skeletal tissue, vitamin D is used to promote the absorption and utilization of these minerals. The DRI recommended amount for pregnancy is 5 μg cholecalciferol (200 IU/day), which is the same as for the nonpregnant woman. Food sources include fortified milk, liver, egg yolk, and fortified margarine.

DIETARY PATTERNS: GENERAL AND ALTERNATIVE

General Daily Food Pattern

Two useful general principles concerning eating habits for all persons also apply during pregnancy: (1) eat a sufficient quantity of food and (2) eat regularly, avoiding fasting or skipping meals, especially breakfast. During pregnancy, a variety of familiar foods usually supply the mother's need for added nutrients and make eating a pleasure. The increased quantities of essential nutrients needed during pregnancy may be met in many ways by planning around a daily food pattern and using key types of suggested core foods. A general daily food pattern that meets basic nutrient needs is suggested in Table 11-2. Compare the increases in each food group suggested for the pregnant or lactating adolescent or woman during the reproductive cycle with the basic amounts for the nonpregnant woman. The comparison indicates the need for increased amounts of basic foods during pregnancy to meet increased key nutrient needs. It may be used as a guide, with additional foods added according to individual energy needs and personal desires. This pattern represents the "orthodox middle-class American diet." It has been labeled the "biomedically recommended prenatal diet," which is generally used worldwide by most health professionals in industrialized, affluent countries.

Alternative Food Patterns

With the increasing ethnic diversity in our American culture, it is especially important to use the mother's personal cultural food patterns in dietary counseling. We are ethnocentric if we rigidly adhere to the orthodox pattern previously discussed as the pattern for all pregnant women. It is but one alternative diet pattern among many others from different cultures, belief systems, and lifestyles. We need to remind ourselves that an extreme, unquestioning pursuit of "science versus magic" may lead us to label any alternative practice as unscientific and unreasonable, thus closing our minds to some possibly fruitful avenues of scientific exploration. We must always remember that specific nutrients, not specific foods, are required for a successful pregnancy and that these nutrients are found in a wide variety of food choices. If we are wise, we will encourage our clients to use foods that serve their nutritional needs, whatever those foods might be. A number of resources are available as guides for cultural, religious, and vegetarian food patterns.

General Dietary Problems

FUNCTIONAL GASTROINTESTINAL PROBLEMS

Nausea and Vomiting

Symptoms of nausea and vomiting are usually mild and short term, the so-called morning sickness of early pregnancy because it occurs more often on arising than later in the day. At least 50% of all pregnant women, most of

TABLE 11-2 Daily Food Guide for Women

Food Group	One Serving Equals		Recommended Minimum Servings		
			Nonpregnant		Pregnant/ Lactating
			11-24 yr	25+ yr	
Protein Foods	*Animal Protein*	*Vegetable Protein*			
Provide protein, iron, zinc, and B vitamins for growth of muscles, bone, blood, and nerves; vegetable protein provides fiber to prevent constipation	1 oz cooked chicken or turkey 1 oz cooked lean beef, lamb, or pork 1 oz or ¼ cup fish or other seafood 1 egg 2 fish sticks or hot dogs 2 slices luncheon meat	½ cup cooked dry beans, lentils, or split peas 3 oz tofu 1 oz or ¼ cup peanuts, pumpkin seeds, or sunflower seeds 1½ oz or ⅓ cup other nuts 2 tbsp peanut butter	5 ½ serving of vegetable protein daily	5 ½ serving of vegtable protein daily	7 1 serving of vegetable protein daily
Milk Products					
Provide protein and calcium to build strong bones, teeth, and healthy nerves and muscles and to promote normal blood clotting	8 oz milk 8 oz yogurt 1 cup milk shake ½ cup cream soup (made with milk) 1½ oz or ⅓ cup grated cheese (like cheddar, Monterey, mozzarella, or Swiss)	1½-2 slices presliced American cheese 4 tbsp Parmesan cheese 2 cups cottage cheese 1 cup pudding 1 cup custard or flan 1½ cups ice milk, ice cream, or frozen yogurt	3	2	3
Breads, Cereals, Grains					
Provide carbohydrates and B vitamins for energy and healthy nerves; also provide iron for healthy blood; whole grains provide fiber to prevent constipation	1 slice bread 1 dinner roll ½ bun or bagel ½ English muffin or pita 1 small tortilla ¾ cup dry cereal ½ cup granola ½ cup cooked cereal	½ cup rice ½ cup noodles or spaghetti ¼ cup wheat germ 1 4-in pancake or waffle 1 small muffin 8 medium crackers 4 graham cracker squares 3 cups popcorn	7 4 servings of whole grain products daily	6	7
Vitamin C–Rich Fruits and Vegetables					
Provide vitamin C to prevent infection and to promote healing and iron absorption; also provide fiber to prevent constipation	6 oz orange, grapefruit, or fruit juice enriched with vitamin C 6 oz tomato juice or vegetable juice cocktail 1 orange, kiwi, or mango ½ grapefruit or cantaloupe ½ cup papaya 2 tangerines	½ cup strawberries ½ cup cooked or 1 cup raw cabbage ½ cup broccoli, Brussels sprouts, or cauliflower ½ cup snow peas, sweet peppers, or tomato puree 2 tomatoes	1	1	1
Vitamin A–Rich Fruits and Vegetables					
Provide beta-carotene and vitamin A to prevent infection and to promote wound healing and night vision; also provide fiber to prevent constipation	6 oz apricot nectar or vegetable juice cocktail 3 raw or ¼ cup dried apricots ¼ cantaloupe or mango 1 small or ½ cup sliced carrots 2 tomatoes	½ cup cooked or 1 cup raw spinach ½ cup cooked greens (beet, chard, collards, dandelion, kale, mustard) ½ cup pumpkin, sweet potato, winter squash, or yams	1	1	1

References: California Department of Health Services, Maternal and Child Health: *Nutrition during pregnancy and postpartum period: a manual for health care professionals,* Sacramento, 1990, CDHS; California Department of Health Services, BabyCal Campaign 2001: *BabyCal nutrition tips for pregnant/breastfeeding women,* Sacramento, 2001, CDHS.

NOTE: The Daily Food Guide for Women may not provide all of the kcalories you require. The best way to increase your intake is to include more than the minimum servings recommended.

Continued

TABLE 11-2 Daily Food Guide for Women—cont'd

Food Group	One Serving Equals		Recommended Minimum Servings: Nonpregnant 11-24 yr	Nonpregnant 25+ yr	Pregnant/Lactating
Other Fruits and Vegetables					
Provide carbohydrates for energy and fiber to prevent constipation	6 oz fruit juice (if not listed previously) 1 medium or ½ cup sliced fruit (apple, banana, peach, pear) ½ cup berries (other than strawberries) ½ cup cherries or grapes ½ cup pineapple ½ cup watermelon	½ cup dried fruit ½ cup sliced vegetable (asparagus, beets, green beans, celery, corn, eggplant, mushrooms, onion, peas, potato, summer squash, zucchini) ½ artichoke 1 cup lettuce	3	3	3
Unsaturated Fats					
Provide vitamin E to protect tissue 1 tsp margarine 1 tsp mayonnaise 1 tsp vegetable oil	⅛ medium avocado	2 tsp salad dressing (mayonnaise-based) 1 tbsp salad dressing (oil-based)	3	3	3

References: California Department of Health Services, Maternal and Child Health: *Nutrition during pregnancy and postpartum period: a manual for health care professionals,* Sacramento, 1990, CDHS; California Department of Health Services, BabyCal Campaign 2001: *BabyCal nutrition tips for pregnant/breastfeeding women,* Sacramento, 2001, CDHS.

NOTE: The Daily Food Guide for Women may not provide all of the kcalories you require. The best way to increase your intake is to include more than the minimum servings recommended.

them in their first pregnancy, experience this condition, beginning during the fifth or sixth week of the pregnancy and usually ending about the fourteenth to sixteenth week. A number of factors may contribute to the situation. Some are physiologic, with causal factors based on hormonal changes that occur early in pregnancy or on low blood sugar, which can be relieved by carbohydrate foods but *which will* return within 2 to 3 hours after a meal. Others may be psychologic, based on situational tensions or anxieties about the pregnancy itself. Still others may be dietary problems, based on poor food habits. Simple treatment generally improves food tolerance. Frequent small low-fat meals and snacks, which are fairly dry and consisting chiefly of easily digested energy-yielding foods such as carbohydrates (mainly starches), are usually more readily tolerated. Also, it may help to avoid cooking odors as much as possible. Liquids are best taken between meals instead of with meals.

Hyperemesis

In a small number of pregnant women, about 3.5:1000 pregnancies, a severe form of persistent nausea and vomiting occurs that does not respond to usual treatment. This condition, *hyperemesis,* begins early in the pregnancy and may last throughout. It may develop into the more serious pernicious form of hyperemesis gravidarum. This persistent condition causes severe alterations in fluids and electrolytes, weight loss, and nutritional deficits, sometimes requiring alternative feeding by enteral or parenteral methods to sustain the pregnancy (see Chapter 17). If the condition is unchecked, the mother is usually hospitalized and receives peripheral parenteral nutrition, followed by careful oral refeeding or tube feeding. In any case, continued personal support and reassurance are important.

Constipation

The complaint of constipation is seldom more than minor, but it contributes to discomfort and concern. Placental hormones relax the gastrointestinal muscles, and the pressure of the enlarging uterus on the lower portion of the intestine may make elimination somewhat difficult. Increased fluid intake and the use of naturally laxative foods containing dietary fiber, such as whole grains, fruits and vegetables, dried fruits (especially prunes and figs), and other fruits and juices, generally promote regularity. Laxatives should be avoided. Appropriate daily exercise is essential for overall health during pregnancy.

Hemorrhoids

A fairly common complaint during the latter part of pregnancy is that of hemorrhoids. These are enlarged veins in the anus, often protruding through the anal sphincter. This vein enlargement is usually caused by the increased weight of the fetus and its downward pressure. The hemorrhoids may cause considerable discomfort, burning, and itching. Occasionally, they may rupture and bleed under pressure of a bowel movement, causing the mother still more anxiety. The problem is usually controlled by the dietary suggestions given for constipation. Also, sufficient rest during the latter part of the day may help relieve some of the downward pressure of the uterus on the lower intestine.

Heartburn or Gastric Pressure

The related complaints of heartburn or a full feeling are sometimes voiced by pregnant women. These discomforts occur especially after meals and are usually caused by the pressure of the enlarging uterus crowding the stomach. Gastric reflux of some of the food mass, now a liquid chyme mixed with stomach acid, may occur in the lower esophagus, causing an irritation and a burning sensation. Obviously, this common complaint has nothing to do with heart action but is so called because of the close proximity of the lower esophagus to the heart. The full feeling comes from general gastric pressure, lack of normal space in the area, a large meal, or gas formation. These complaints are usually remedied by dividing the day's food into a series of small meals, avoiding eating large meals at any time, and not lying down after a meal. Comfort is also improved by wearing loose-fitting clothing.

Effects of Iron Supplements

During pregnancy an iron supplement in the form of ferrous sulfate may be given to counteract the physiologic dilution anemia of pregnancy because of the increased circulating blood volume. The effects of added iron medication include gray or black stools and sometimes nausea, constipation, or diarrhea. To help avoid food-related effects, the iron supplement should be taken 1 hour before a meal or 2 hours after with liquid such as water or orange juice but not with milk or tea. The iron effect in the body is increased with vitamin C and decreased with milk, other dairy foods, eggs, whole grain bread and cereal, and tea.

WEIGHT GAIN DURING PREGNANCY

General Amount of Weight Gain

Healthy women produce healthy babies over a wide range of total weight gain. During pregnancy, therefore, the nutritional focus should always be on an individualized assessment of need and the quality of the weight gain. Optimal weight gain from a quality diet throughout pregnancy makes an important contribution to a successful course and outcome. It should not be a problem or a source of contention. An average weight gain during normal pregnancy is about 11 to 16 kg (25 to 35 lb).[17] Around this average many individual variations occur. There is no specific rigid norm or restriction to which all women should be held regardless of individual needs; such a course is obviously unwise and unscientific. Current recommendations are therefore usually stated in terms of ranges to accommodate variances in needs. An initial base for evaluation, however, may be the average weight of the products of pregnancy as shown in Table 11-3. In addition to the components of growth and development usually attributed to a pregnancy, an important part is maternal stores. This laying down of extra adipose fat tissue is necessary for maternal energy reserves to sustain rapid fetal growth during the latter half of pregnancy and for labor and delivery and maintaining lactation after birth. About 2 to 3.5 kg (4 to 8 lb) of adipose tissue is commonly deposited for these needs. A report of the National Academy of Sciences, *Nutrition During Pregnancy,* recommends setting weight gain goals together with the pregnant woman according to her prepregnancy nutritional status and weight-for-height.[17]

1. *Normal weight women:* 11.5 to 16 kg (25 to 35 lb)
2. *Underweight women:* 13 to 18 kg (28 to 40 lb)
3. *Overweight women:* 7 to 11.5 kg (15 to 25 lb)

The recommendation for adolescent mothers is that they should strive for the upper end of the range: 16 kg (35 lb). The recommendation for a woman carrying twins to avoid complications is a target weight gain of 16 to 20.5 kg (35 to 45 lb).[17] Compared with single-birth infants, twin-birth infants are 5 times more likely to be born premature (<37 weeks' gestation), 9.5 times more likely to be very low birth weight (<1500 g), and 8.5 times more likely to be low birth weight (<2500 g).[18]

TABLE 11-3 Approximate Weight of Products of Normal Pregnancy

Products	Weight
Fetus	3400 g (7.5 lb)
Placenta	450 g (1 lb)
Amniotic fluid	900 g (2 lb)
Uterus (weight increase)	1100 g (2.5 lb)
Breast tissue (weight increase)	1400 g (3 lb)
Blood volume (weight increase)	1800 g (4 lb) (1500 ml)
Maternal stores	1800-3600 g (4-8 lb)
TOTAL	10,850-12,650 g (10.8-12.7 kg; 24-28 lb)

hyperemesis gravidarum Severe vomiting during pregnancy, which is potentially fatal.

PRACTICAL APPLICATION

Preventing Spina Bifida: The Importance of Folate

Meredith Catherine Williams

The Centers for Disease Control and Prevention estimates that in the United States, about 2500 infants are born every year with a neural tube defect (NTD), with the most common defects being anencephaly and spina bifida. Babies with anencephaly do not develop any brain tissue, and most are stillborn or die soon after birth. Spina bifida is caused by a defect in the development of the spinal column where the vertebrae surrounding the spinal cord do not close properly in early development. In the mild form, *spina bifida occulta,* there is only a small gap between two vertebrae of the spine. This usually produces no symptoms, and the only sign may be a small dimple in the skin covering the gap. The severe form is *spina bifida aperta,* where a larger space develops in the spine. There is a visible sac, called a meningocele, on the infant's back where spinal fluid bulges out, most commonly in the lower back. This causes little to no muscle paralysis once repaired by surgery. Yet in the majority of cases of spina bifida aperta, part of the undeveloped spinal cord sticks through the gap and into the protruding sac on the baby's back. This undeveloped or damaged spinal cord that extends beyond the vertebrae, called a *myelocele* or *meningomyelocele,* causes the most acute cases of paralysis, bladder or bowel incontinence, scoliosis (a sideways bending of the spine), and mental retardation. Again surgery can help reduce these symptoms, and 85% to 90% percent of infants with spina bifida are able to survive into adulthood.

However, a woman can reduce the risk of her baby being born with an NTD by increasing her consumption of folate. Folate is often consumed in the form of folic acid from a fortified food or from a food supplement. Folic acid helps to ensure normal embryonic tissue growth and to prevent malformation of the neural tube. Folic acid is the synthetic version of the B vitamin folate, and slightly easier for the body to absorb. Recommended intakes are expressed in units of dietary folate equivalents (DFE). One DFE equals 1 μg of food folate or 0.6 μg of folic acid from fortified foods or from a supplement consumed with food or 0.5 μg of a supplement taken on an empty stomach.

Folic acid is also recommended for women who are not pregnant because the beneficial effect of folic acid must be present in the first 2 weeks of pregnancy, a time when the woman typically does not know she is pregnant. Neurulation, and the possibility for defects, occurs in humans from approximately day 21 through day 28 of development. More than half of all pregnancies are unexpected; therefore the U.S. Public Health Service recommends that all women capable of becoming pregnant consume 400 μg of folate/day, to ensure an adequate supply for the fetus.

To achieve the recommended 400 μg DFE/day, women can take a vitamin supplement that contains folic acid; eat a variety of folate-rich foods, such as dark green leafy vegetables, fruits, and dried beans and peas; or eat folic acid–fortified enriched products. As part of the public health effort to increase folic acid consumption, the Food and Drug Administration has mandated that all manufacturers of grain products, including cereals, breads, flours, corn meals, and pastas, include 0.43 to 1.4 mg of folic acid in each pound of product. This addition will not harm males and nonpregnant women and is a benefit for women who are pregnant. The goal in fortifying food for an entire population is to increase general intake levels of folic acid while remaining below the upper limit of 1 mg/day so as to be safe for everyone. Although the effects of high folic acid consumption are not generally well known, there is evidence to suggest that high intake can interfere with the diagnosis of a vitamin B_{12} deficiency. It is recommended that women consume 600 μg of folate/day when pregnant to ensure that the fetus is completely supplied. During lactation, the recommended folate intake daily is 500 μg.

Reference

1. Food and Nutrition Board, Institute of Medicine: *Dietary reference intakes for thiamin, riboflavin, niacin, vitamin B_6, folate, vitamin B_{12}, pantothenic acid, biotin, and choline,* Washington, DC, 1999, National Academy Press.

BOX 11-1 Nutritional Risk Factors in Pregnancy

Risk Factors Present at the Onset of Pregnancy

- Age: ≤15 yr or ≥35 yr
- Frequent pregnancies: 3 or more during a 2-yr period
- Poor obstetric history or poor fetal performance
- Poverty
- Bizarre or faddist food habits
- Abuse of nicotine, alcohol, or drugs
- Therapeutic diet required for a chronic disorder
- Weight: <85% or >120% of standard weight

Risk Factors Occurring During Pregnancy

- Low hemoglobin or hematocrit: Hgb <12 g; Hct <35 mg/dl
- Inadequate weight gain: Any weight loss *or* weight gain of <1 kg (2 lb)/mo after the first trimester
- Excessive weight gain: >1 kg (2 lb)/wk after the first trimester

From American College of Obstetrics and Gynecologists and American Dietetic Association Task Force on Nutrition: *Assessment of maternal nutrition,* Chicago, 1978, The College and Association.

Quality of Weight Gain

The important consideration, as indicated, lies in the nutritional quality of the gain. Specifically, the foods consumed should be nutrient dense. They should be nutritious foods to meet the nutrient requirements, not foods contributing only empty kcalories. Also, there has been failure in some cases to distinguish between weight gained as a result of edema and that as a result of deposition of fat—maternal stores for energy to sustain rapid fetal growth during the latter part of pregnancy and energy for lactation to follow. Analysis of the total tissue gained in an average pregnancy shows that the largest component, 62%, is water. Fat accounts for 31% and protein for 7%. Water is also the most variable component of the tissue gained, accounting for a range of 8 kg (18 lb) to as much as 11 kg (24 lb). Of the 8 kg of water usually gained, about 5.5 kg (12 lb) is associated with fetal tissue and other tissues gained in pregnancy. The remaining 2.5 kg (6 lb) accumulates in the maternal interstitial tissues.[18] Gravity causes the maternal tissue fluids to pool more in the lower extremities, leading to general swelling of the ankles, which is seen routinely in pregnant women. This fluid retention is a normal adaptive phenomenon designed to support the pregnancy and to exert a positive effect on fetal growth. The connective tissue becomes more hygroscopic as a result of the estrogen-induced changes in the ground substance. The connective tissue thus becomes softer and more easily distended to facilitate delivery through the cervix and the vaginal canal. Also, the increased tissue fluid during pregnancy provides a means for handling the increased metabolic work and circulation of numerous metabolites necessary for fetal growth.

Clearly, severe kcaloric restriction is harmful to the developing fetus and the mother. It is inevitably accompanied by restriction of the vitally needed nutrients essential to the growth process.[19] Thus *weight reduction should never be undertaken during pregnancy.* To the contrary, sufficient weight gain should be encouraged with the use of a nourishing diet.

Rate of Weight Gain

On the whole, about 1 to 2.3 kg (2 to 5 lb) is an average weight gain during the first trimester. Thereafter, an average weight gain of about 0.5 kg (1 lb)/week during the remainder of the pregnancy is usual, although some women may need to gain more. There is no scientific justification for routinely limiting weight gain to lesser amounts. Moreover, an individual woman who needs to gain more should not have unrealistic grid patterns imposed on her. It is only unusual patterns of gain, such as a sudden sharp increase in weight after the twentieth week of pregnancy, that may signal abnormal water retention, which should be monitored closely, especially if it occurs in conjunction with blood pressure elevation and proteinuria. On the other hand, an insufficient or low maternal weight gain during the second or third trimester increases the risk for intrauterine growth retardation.[19,20]

Weight Gain and Sodium Intake

In relation to weight gain, questions are sometimes raised about the use of salt during pregnancy. A moderate amount of dietary sodium is needed for two essential reasons: (1) it is the major mineral required to control the extracellular fluid compartment and (2) this vital body water is increased during pregnancy to support its successful outcome. Current practice usually follows a regular diet with moderate sodium intake, 2 to 3 g/day, with light use of salt to taste. Limiting sodium beyond this general use is contrary to physiologic need in pregnancy and is unfounded. The NRC and professional obstetric guidelines have labeled routine salt-free diets and diuretics as potentially dangerous.[1-3] Maintaining the needed increase in circulating blood volume during pregnancy requires adequate amounts of sodium and protein, as well as adequate fluid intake throughout to prevent dehydration and possible premature contractions.

High-Risk Mothers and Infants

IDENTIFY RISK FACTORS INVOLVED

To avoid the consequences of poor nutrition during pregnancy, a first procedure is to identify mothers at risk (see *Practical Application* box). In a joint report, the American College of Obstetrics and Gynecology and the American Dietetic Association issued a set of risk factors, as shown in Box 11-1, that identify women with special nutritional needs during pregnancy.[3] These nutrition-related factors are based on clinical evidence of inadequate nutrition. However, rather than waiting for clinical symptoms of poor nutrition to appear, a better approach would be to identify poor food patterns that will bring on nutritional problems and to prevent these problems from developing. On this basis, three types of dietary patterns predict failure to support optimal maternal and fetal nutrition: (1) insufficient food intake, (2) poor food selection, and (3) poor food distribution throughout the day. These patterns, added to the list of risk factors in Box 11-1, are much more sensitive for nutritional risk.

PLAN PERSONAL CARE

Once early assessment identifies risk factors, practitioners can then give more careful attention to these women. By working closely with each mother and her personal food pattern and living situation, a food plan can be developed with her to ensure an optimal intake of energy and nutrients to support her pregnancy and its successful outcome.

---

hygroscopic Taking up and retaining moisture readily.

RECOGNIZE SPECIAL COUNSELING NEEDS

Several special needs require sensitive counseling. These areas of need include the age and parity of the mother; any use of harmful agents such as alcohol, cigarettes, drugs, or pica; and socioeconomic problems.

Age and Parity

Pregnancies at either age extreme of the reproductive cycle pose special problems. The adolescent pregnancy carries many social and nutrition-related risks. Imposed onto a still immature teenage body are the additional demands of the pregnancy. The obstetric history of a woman is expressed in terms of number and order of pregnancies, or her gravida status. A nulligravida (no prior pregnancy) who is 15 years of age or younger is especially at risk because her own growth is incomplete; therefore sufficient weight gain and the quality of her diet are particularly important.[18] Sensitive counseling provides both information and emotional support; it should involve family members or other persons significant to the young mother. On the other hand, the older primigravida (first pregnancy), older than 35 years, also requires special attention. She may be more at risk for hypertension, either preexisting or pregnancy induced, and may need more attention to the rate of weight gain and amount of sodium used, as well as any drug therapy prescribed. In addition, several pregnancies within a limited number of years leave a mother drained of nutritional resources and entering each successive pregnancy at a higher risk.

Social Habits: Alcohol, Cigarettes, and Drugs

These three personal habits cause fetal damage and are contraindicated during pregnancy. Even moderate prenatal alcohol exposure is associated with low birth weight and has effects on a child's psychomotor development.[21] Extensive or habitual alcohol use leads to the well-described and documented *fetal alcohol syndrome (FAS),* which is currently a leading cause of mental retardation.[22] Cigarette smoking during pregnancy is also contraindicated.[23] Harmful substances in tobacco cause fetal damage and special problems of placental abnormalities, leading to greater risk of spontaneous abortion (miscarriage) and prematurity and low birth weight[24] (see *Practical Application* box), largely as a result of impaired oxygen transport. Counseling with mothers who smoke should stress the importance of quitting.

Drug use, both recreational and medicinal, also poses numerous problems.[24] Self-medication with over-the-counter drugs carries potential adverse effects. The use of street drugs is especially hazardous, exposing the developing fetus to the risks of addiction and possibly AIDS from the mother's use of contaminated needles in her drug injections. Dangers come not only from the drug itself or contaminated needles but also from the impurities contained by such street drugs. In addition, drug abuse from megadosing with basic nutrients such as vitamin A during pregnancy may cause fetal damage. Especially dangerous are drugs made from vitamin A compounds, retinoids such as Accutane or etretinate, prescribed for severe acne, which have caused spontaneous abortion of malformed infants by women who conceived during such acne treatment. Thus the use of these drugs without contraception is definitely contraindicated (see *Issues & Answers*).

Caffeine

Although milder in its effect (depending on the extent of use) than the agents just discussed, caffeine remains a widely used drug that can cross the placenta and enter fetal circulation.[25] Its use at pharmacologic levels has been associated with first-trimester spontaneous abortion (miscarriage) and with low birth weight.[26,27] A pharmacologic dose of caffeine—250 mg—is contained in 2 cups of coffee, 3.5 cups of tea, or 5 12-oz colas; therefore such use is not recommended. Most health agencies have recommended that pregnant women avoid caffeine-containing beverages and that products containing caffeine be plainly labeled to inform consumers.

Pica

Pica is the craving and consumption of unusual nonfood substances such as laundry starch, clay, dirt, or ice. This practice during pregnancy is more widespread than health care workers have believed. The eating of clay or dirt may indicate an iron deficiency anemia.[28,29] Where these unusual practices exist, they must be understood as deep-rooted cultural patterns that require a respectful approach by health workers who seek to negotiate appropriate behavior changes.[28]

Socioeconomic Problems

Special counseling is required for women and young girls living in low-income situations or extreme poverty. Numerous studies and clinical observations indicate that lack of prenatal care, often associated with racial prejudices and fears as well as poverty, places the expectant mother in grave difficulty. Special counseling that is sensitive to personal needs is needed to help plan resources for care and financial assistance. Resources include programs such as the federally funded Women-Infant-Children Supplementary Food Program (WIC), described in Chapter 10, as well as numerous state and local programs. An example of a successful state-sponsored program promoting prenatal care is BabyCal, a public awareness and education campaign launched in 1991 by the California Department of Health Services. The BabyCal outreach program uses a statewide network of community-based support organizations, along with a focused media campaign involving pop music and television personalities, to reach low-income expectant mothers with messages stressing prenatal care, a healthy lifestyle during pregnancy, and the importance of infant immunization. The result has been greatly increased rates of participation in prenatal care programs and a 15% reduction in statewide infant mortality over the past decade.

Complications of Pregnancy

ANEMIA

Anemia is common during pregnancy. It is often associated with a normal maternal blood volume increase of about 50% and a disproportionate increase in red cell mass of about 20%. About 10% of all women in large prenatal clinics in the United States have hemoglobin concentrations of less than 10 g/dl and a hematocrit reading below 32%. Anemia is far more prevalent among the poor, many of whom live on diets barely adequate for subsistence. However, anemia is by no means restricted to lower economic groups.

Iron-Deficiency Anemia

A deficiency of iron is by far the most common cause of anemia in pregnancy. The total cost of a single normal pregnancy in iron stores is large—about 500 to 800 mg. Of this amount nearly 300 mg is used by the fetus. The remainder is used in the expanded maternal blood volume and its increased red blood cells and hemoglobin mass. This iron requirement typically exceeds the available reserves in the average woman. Thus in addition to including iron-rich foods in the diet, a daily supplement of 30 to 60 mg may be recommended. Treatment of highly deficient states requires daily therapeutic doses of 120 to 200 mg, which is usually continued for 3 to 6 months after the anemia has been corrected to replenish the depleted stores.

Folate-Deficiency Anemia

A less common megaloblastic anemia of pregnancy results from folate deficiency. During pregnancy, the fetus is sensitive to folate inhibitors and therefore has increased metabolic requirements for folate. To prevent this anemia, the DRI standard recommends 600 μg of folate/day during pregnancy. Women with poor diets will need supplementation to reach this intake goal.

Hemorrhagic Anemia

Anemia caused by blood loss is more likely to occur during labor and delivery than during pregnancy. Blood loss may occur earlier, as a result of abortion or ruptured tubular pregnancy. Most patients undergoing these physiologic problems receive blood via transfusion, and iron therapy may be indicated for adequate replacement hemoglobin formation.

PREGNANCY-INDUCED HYPERTENSION

Relation to Nutrition

A number of clinicians have presented clinical and laboratory evidence that *pregnancy-induced hypertension* (PIH [formerly labeled toxemia]) is a disease that principally affects young women with their first pregnancy. It is especially related to diets poor in protein, kcalories, calcium, and salt. Such malnutrition affects the liver and its metabolic activities. Regardless of the underlying causes and multiorgan effects, nutritional support of the pregnancy is, as always, a primary concern. Certainly, as many practitioners have observed, PIH is classically associated with poverty, inadequate diet, and little or no prenatal care. Much of the PIH problem, which seems to develop early from the time of implantation of the fertilized ovum into the uterine lining, may be reduced by good prenatal care from the beginning of the pregnancy, which inherently includes attention to sound nutrition. It is this sound nutritional status, which a woman brings to her pregnancy and maintains throughout, that provides her with optimal resources for adapting to the physiologic stress of gestation. Her fitness during pregnancy is a direct function of her past state of nutrition and her optimal nutrition throughout pregnancy.

Clinical Symptoms

PIH is defined according to its manifestations, which generally occur in the third trimester toward term. These symptoms are hypertension, abnormal and excessive edema, albuminuria, and, in severe cases, convulsions or coma, a state called eclampsia.

Treatment

Specific treatment varies according to the individual patient's symptoms and needs. Optimal nutrition is a fundamental aspect of therapy in any case. Emphasis is given to a regular diet with adequate dietary protein and calcium. Correction of plasma protein deficits stimulates the capillary fluid shift mechanism and increases circulation of tissue fluids, with subsequent correction of the hypovolemia.

---

eclampsia Advanced pregnancy-induced hypertension (PIH), manifested by convulsions.

hypovolemia Abnormally decreased volume of circulating blood in the body.

nulligravida A woman who has never been pregnant.

primigravida A woman who is pregnant for the first time.

In addition, adequate salt and sources of vitamins and minerals are needed for correction and maintenance of metabolic balance.

MATERNAL DISEASE CONDITIONS

Preexisting clinical conditions in the mother further complicate pregnancy. In each case, management of these conditions is based on general principles of care related to both pregnancy and the particular disease involved. Examples of such maternal conditions are reviewed here; they are hypertension, diabetes mellitus, phenylketonuria, and AIDS.

Hypertension

Preexisting hypertension in the pregnant woman can cause considerable maternal and fetal consequences. Many of these problems can be prevented by initial screening and continued monitoring by the prenatal nurse, with referral to the clinical nutritionist for a plan of care. The hypertensive disease process begins long before signs and symptoms appear, and later symptoms are inconsistent. Risk factors for hypertension before and during pregnancy are given in Box 11-2. Nutritional therapy centers on the (1) prevention of weight extremes, underweight or obesity; (2) correction of any dietary deficiencies and maintenance of optimal nutritional status during pregnancy; and (3) management of any related preexisting disease such as diabetes mellitus or hyperlipidemia. Sodium intake may be moderate but should not be unduly restricted because of its relation to fluid and electrolyte balances during pregnancy and its controversial therapy in hypertension in general. Initial and continuing client education and a close relationship with the nurse-nutritionist care team contribute to successful management of the hypertension and prevent problems that may occur.

Diabetes Mellitus

The management of preexisting diabetes in pregnancy presents special problems. Today, however, improved expectations for the diabetic mother's pregnancy constitute one of the success stories of modern medicine.[30] Contributing factors to this improved outlook include advances in technology for monitoring fetal development, increased knowledge of nutrition and diabetes, and management refinements in tight blood glucose control through self-monitoring.[31,32] Routine screening protocols are used during pregnancy to detect gestational diabetes, and team management is required for preexisting insulin-dependent diabetes mellitus.[33,34] During pregnancy, glycosuria is not uncommon because of the increased circulating blood volume and its load of metabolites.[35] Gestational diabetes occurs in 2% to 13% of the pregnant population, but only 20% to 30% of these women showing this pregnancy-induced abnormal glucose tolerance subsequently develop diabetes. Nonetheless, follow-up is important because of the higher risk these women carry for fetal damage during this gestational period.[36] Refer to Chapter 20 for a detailed discussion of diabetes care.

Maternal Phenylketonuria

The successful detection and management of phenylketonuria (PKU) infants through U.S. newborn screening programs in all states have ensured their normal growth and development to adulthood. PKU is a genetic metabolic disease caused by a missing enzyme for the metabolism of the essential amino acid phenylalanine. It is controlled by a special low-phenylalanine diet initiated at birth. Now a new generation of young women with PKU since birth are beginning to have children of their own. However, maternal PKU presents potential fetal hazards. Experience has shown how crucial it is for the mother to follow a strict low-phenylalanine diet before conception, whenever possible, to minimize risks of fe-

BOX 11-2 Risk Factors in Pregnancy-Induced Hypertension

Before Pregnancy

- Nulligravida
- Diabetes
- Preexisting condition (hypertension, renal or vascular disease)
- Family history of hypertension or vascular disease
- Diagnoses of pregnancy-induced hypertension in a previous pregnancy
- Dietary deficiencies
- Age extremes
  - ≤20 yr
  - ≥35 yr

During Pregnancy

- Primigravida
- Large fetus
- Glomerulonephritis
- Fetal hydrops
- Hydramnios
- Multiple gestation
- Hydatidiform mole

tal damage in the early cell differentiation weeks of pregnancy.

AIDS

Carefully monitored care throughout pregnancy and after birth is essential for pregnant women who are infected by the human immunodeficiency virus (HIV). Two goals are most important: (1) to reduce the rate of the disease progression in the mother through nutritional support and (2) to minimize the chance of HIV vertical transmission from mother to child either in the womb or after birth via breastfeeding. Nutrient deficiencies are often found in HIV-positive patients. Although specific nutrient requirements for HIV-infected pregnant women have not been established, these patients may need up to 150% of normal pregnancy intakes of both macronutrients and micronutrients. Continual individual monitoring and adjustment are essential. Babies can be infected by HIV from the mother during labor and delivery and through breast milk. Where safe alternatives to breast milk are available, such as commercial formula or banked human milk, a decision on breastfeeding depends on the HIV status of the newborn infant. In the United States, both the Centers for Disease Control and Prevention (CDC) and the American Academy of Pediatrics recommend HIV-positive mothers do not breastfeed when the infant is not infected.[37,38]

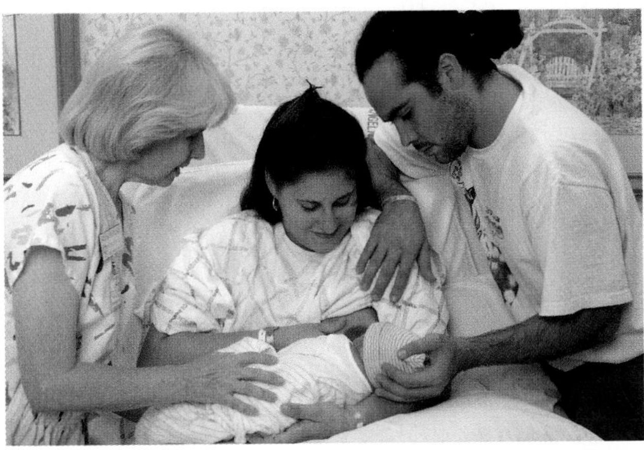

FIGURE 11-1 By teaching about the newborn and family, the nurse helps parents develop confidence in their ability to provide care for the infant. (*From McKinney ES et al:* Maternal-child nursing, *Philadelphia, 2000, WB Saunders.*)

Nutrition During Lactation

CURRENT BREASTFEEDING TRENDS

An increasing number of mothers in the United States and other developed countries are choosing breastfeeding for their infants[39] (see *To Probe Further* box). Several factors have contributed to this choice: (1) more mothers are informed about the benefits of breastfeeding[40] (Figure 11-1), (2) practitioners recognize the ability of human milk to meet infant needs (Table 11-4) and boost immunity,[41,42] (3) maternity wards and alternative birth centers are being modified to facilitate successful lactation, (4) community support is increasingly available, even in workplaces,[43,44] and (5) programs that promote breastfeeding are increasingly responsive to a wider range of maternal income levels and cultural backgrounds.[45-52] Exclusive breastfeeding by well-nourished mothers can be adequate for periods ranging from 2 to 15 months.[53-57] Solid foods are usually added to the baby's diet at about 6 months of age.

TABLE 11-4 Nutritional Components of Human Milk (per 100 ml)

Milk Component	Colostrum	Transitional	Mature	Cow's Milk
Kcalories	57.0	63.0	65.0	65.0
Vitamins, fat-soluble				
A (μg)	151.0	88.0	75.0	41.0
D (IU)	—	—	5.0	2.5
E (mg)	1.5	0.9	0.25	0.07
K (μg)	—	—	1.5	6.0
Vitamins, water-soluble				
Thiamin (μg)	1.9	5.9	14.0	43.0
Riboflavin (μg)	30.0	37.0	40.0	145.0
Niacin (μg)	75.0	175.0	160.0	82.0
Pantothenic acid (μg)	183.0	288.0	246.0	340.0
Biotin (μg)	0.06	0.35	0.6	2.8
Vitamin B_{12} (μg)	0.05	0.04	0.1	1.1
Vitamin C (mg)	5.9	7.1	5.0	1.1

TO PROBE FURTHER

Breastfeeding: The Dynamic Nature of Human Milk

There is no question that human milk is the ideal first food for human infants. Its dynamic nature changes to match growth needs. The mother's choice to breastfeed her infant depends on a number of factors, however, especially for new mothers, who often need information and counseling from early pregnancy.

Even premature infants can thrive on human milk. Mothers and physicians have sometimes been reluctant to consider breastfeeding for babies born prematurely or delivered by cesarean section, fearing that there may be some negative effect on the quantity or quality of human milk. This uncertainty about the nutritional quality of mother's milk has also led them to encourage adding formula and/or solid foods to the diet to make sure the baby is well fed. These practices are usually unnecessary. They often contribute to allergies, obesity, and digestive problems because of the extra stress placed on an immature gut.

BREAST MILK FOR THE PRETERM INFANT

Levels of nutrients in mother's milk shift according to the gestational age of the infant at birth. The preterm infant is often denied its mother's milk by some hospital workers because they think of it as mature milk having too little protein and too much lactose to meet the child's needs. An analysis of the nutritional quality of preterm milk, however, reveals energy and fat concentrations that are 20% to 30% higher, protein levels 15% to 20% higher, and lactose levels 10% lower than those found in mature milk. Premature milk can meet the preterm infant's needs.

BREAST MILK DURING WEANING

Nutrient levels continue to change with time to match changing growth patterns and developing digestive abilities. Mother's milk does provide sufficient kcalories and nutrients to keep babies well fed without supplemental formula or food. Even when the infant is being weaned, the nature of human milk ensures adequate nutrients, just in case the new, solid-food diet cannot meet the child's needs. Human milk collected during gradual weaning has been found to have higher concentrations of protein, sodium, and iron. Lactose levels are lower, possibly so that higher amounts of kcalories can be supplied by fats, a more concentrated source.

BREAST MILK AND THE CESAREAN SECTION INFANT

The quality of human milk is not influenced by the way the baby comes into the world. Many women fear that a baby born by cesarean section cannot be nursed because they think that this method of delivery delays or prevents the production of mature milk. Milk production is stimulated by the release of the placenta, which occurs regardless of whether the delivery is vaginal. Studies confirm that there is no significant difference in the length of time it takes for mature milk to come in after vaginal or cesarean deliveries.

Thus premature or cesarean deliveries should not discourage women from breastfeeding. Mothers should not underestimate the nutritive quality of their milk simply because it does not appear as rich and thick as cow's milk. After all, cow's milk is made for young calves, who are up and running around after birth and have a much shorter, faster growth period. For the human infant, in both nutritional and immunologic terms, breast milk remains the best milk.

MOTHERS' FACT AND FANCY ABOUT BREASTFEEDING

In early counseling, mothers express a variety of concerns about breastfeeding. These are a few such statements.

"My breasts aren't big enough." When it comes to breastfeeding, all women are created equal. The only parts of the breast that participate in milk production are the glandular and nervous tissue and the nipple; these are basically the same in healthy women. The only difference between a size 32A and a size 42DD is the amount of fat the breast contains.

"Breastfeeding causes cancer." Actually, in recent years, investigators have been looking to breastfeeding as a possible means of preventing breast cancer. At this point, however, no studies exist that convincingly show that breastfeeding either helps or hinders a woman from the development of this disease.

"Breastfeeding will ruin my figure." Breastfeeding might actually help a woman regain her figure more quickly. Because the caloric demand of breastfeeding exceeds that of the nonpregnant woman by about 500 kcalories, a slightly faster rate of weight loss may be expected. Furthermore, oxytocin, the hormone manufactured to stimulate milk production, also stimulates uterine contractions, helping reduce the uterus to its prepregnancy size more rapidly.

"Breastfeeding is painful." It can be painful if the baby is nursed infrequently or the mother's hygienic practices leave much to be desired. However, if milk is not allowed to collect in the breast

TO PROBE FURTHER
Breastfeeding: The Dynamic Nature of Human Milk—cont'd

to the point of engorgement, if the nipples are kept clean and dry, and if proper latch-on techniques are used while nursing, the chances of having a painful experience will be relatively small.

"Breast milk isn't nutritious." The thin, bluish appearance of breast milk has some women convinced that it is no more nourishing than water. Let them look at Table 11-4; they will be pleasantly surprised at how well breast milk meets the nutritional needs of the infant.

"I can't go to work or school if I breastfeed." Breast milk can be stored for 24 hours in the refrigerator or several months in the freezer. Many working mothers take advantage of this by expressing their milk and storing it for use by a babysitter. In fact, women often express milk on their breaks at school or work. (Some employers even provide breast pumps at the workplace.) Not only does this relieve the pressure of buildup, but it also allows the milk to be stored for later use at home.

Other women would like to breastfeed but are worried about special "what if" situations, such as the following.

"What if I need a cesarean section?" The method of delivery does not affect the quality or quantity of milk produced. The baby can be held in such a way (the "football hold") that he or she does not rest on the mother's abdominal stitches.

"What if the baby is premature?" Mother's milk changes to meet the infant's needs at all stages of development.

"What if the baby has a birth defect such as Down syndrome?" This baby can be nursed; however, it does require time, patience, and the use of slightly different nursing techniques. The mother should be told about the special nursing needs of this infant to avoid disappointment or a feeling of failure in case breastfeeding becomes impractical for her particular living situation.

"What if I have twins?" Believe it or not, it has been done. It takes time, patience, and good coordination, but it can be done. Triplets, however, are another matter altogether. Women have successfully nursed triplets, but often they did very little else until the babies were weaned. This mother will need emotional support whether she attempts to nurse or, finding the amount of time and patience required overwhelming, is forced to bottle-feed.

Some women may purposefully choose to breastfeed to avoid pregnancy, but this is by no means a dependable contraception method. The more well-nourished women of the world tend to be more fertile and have been surprised to find themselves pregnant and breastfeeding at the same time. Women who breastfeed must understand that the lack of a menstrual period during lactation does not mean they cannot become pregnant. Contraceptives, preferably barrier types, may be required if another pregnancy is not desired at that time.

ADVANTAGES AND BARRIERS TO BREASTFEEDING

These factors need to be reviewed with each individual mother in her particular situation. Only on this basis can she make the informed decision that is best for the baby and for herself.

There are many nutritional, physiologic, psychologic, and practical advantages to breastfeeding.

1. *Human milk changes* to meet changing nutrient and energy needs of both the newborn and the maturing infant during the first months of life. It is always there in the correct form to meet the growing infant's needs.
2. Infants experience *fewer infections* because the mother transfers certain antibodies or immune properties in human milk to her nursing infant. Also, there is no exposure of the infant to infectious organisms in the environment that can contaminate preparation and equipment for bottle-feeding, especially in poorer living situations.
3. *Fewer allergies and intolerances occur,* especially in allergy-prone infants, because cow's milk contains a number of potentially allergy-causing proteins that human milk does not have.
4. *Ease of digestion* is greater with breast milk because human milk forms a softer curd in the gastrointestinal tract that is easier for the infant to digest.
5. *The convenience and economy* of breast milk are greater because the mother is free from the time and expense involved in buying and preparing formula, and her breast milk is always ready and sterile.
6. Breastfeeding provides *psychologic bonding* because the mother and infant relate to one another during feeding, regular times of rest and enjoyment, cuddling and fulfillment.

Despite the advantages of breastfeeding, some women do have to deal with perceived barriers associated with misinformation, personal feelings of modesty, family pressures, or outside employment.

Continued

TO PROBE FURTHER
Breastfeeding: The Dynamic Nature of Human Milk—cont'd

1. *Misinformation,* a major barrier, creates negative impressions and ideas. Women in today's world often lack positive role models in extended families or experienced friends with whom they can discuss their feelings and obtain much practical guidance. Experienced breastfeeding mothers can fill this need, especially for young first-time mothers.
2. *Personal modesty and anxiety,* or a fear of appearing immodest in breast exposure, may hinder some young mothers from breastfeeding. Sensitive counseling, especially with a positive role model as described, can help to allay some of these personal fears. Most of women's breastfeeding is done in the privacy of the home rather than around others; therefore early support during initial experiences would be helpful.
3. *Family pressures,* especially from the husband, not to breastfeed have strong influences on the young first-time mother, even though she may want to do so. Initial counseling and education about breastfeeding should include both parents whenever possible. Reasons for negative attitudes can be explored and misinformation clarified with sound education.
4. *Outside employment,* with a limited maternity leave and job loss if the mother does not return to work at that time, can complicate the mother's decision, even though she may want to breastfeed her baby. However, if the mother does have the will, there are ways to do both. After breastfeeding is well established during her maternity leave, she can regularly express milk by hand or with a breast pump into sterile disposal nursing bags to use with disposal holder, cap, and nipple ensemble. Rapid chilling and strict sanitation are required, but it can be planned, given the commitment. Some companies provide child care facilities for their employees, recognizing this modern need as good business. The mother can plan occasional formula feeds to fill in with the sustained breastfeeding.

All of these approaches to breastfeeding have real rewards for the infant. In addition, they can strengthen the mother's confidence in her maternal capabilities. The importance even of these intangible benefits should not be underestimated.

References

American Academy of Pediatrics Work Group on Breast-feeding: Policy statement on breast-feeding, *Pediatrics* 100(Dec):1035, 1997.

Armotrading DC et al: Impact of WIC utilization rate on breast-feeding among international students at a large university, *J Am Diet Assoc* 92(3):352, 1992.

Ghaemi-Ahmadi S: Attitudes toward breast-feeding among Iranian, Afghan, and Southeast Asian immigrant women in the United States: implications for health and nutrition education, *J Am Diet Assoc* 92(3):354, 1992.

Krebs NF, Murtaugh MA: Position of the American Dietetic Association: promotion of breast feeding, *J Am Diet Assoc* 97(6):662, 1997.

NUTRITIONAL NEEDS

The physiologic needs of lactation are greater than those of pregnancy, and they demand adequate nutritional support (see Tables 11-1 and 11-2). The basic nutritional needs for lactation include the following additions to the mother's prepregnancy needs.

Protein

The Recommended Dietary Allowance (RDA) standard for protein needs during lactation is 65 g/day during the first 6 months and 62 g/day during the second 6 months. This is an increase of about 15 to 20 g/day from the regular needs of the adolescent girl (44 to 46 g/day) and the adult woman (46 to 50 g/day).

Energy

The recommended kcaloric increase is 500 kcalories more than the usual adult allowance. This makes a daily total of about 2500 to 2700 kcalories. This additional energy need for the overall total lactation process is based on three factors.

1. *Milk content.* An average daily milk production for lactating women is 850 ml (30 oz). Human milk has a kcalorie range of 20 to 70 kcalories/oz, or an average of 24 kcalories/oz. Thus 30 oz of milk has a value of about 700 kcalories.
2. *Milk production.* The metabolic work involved in producing this amount of milk requires from 400 to 450 kcalories. During pregnancy the breast is developed for this purpose, stimulated by hormones from the placenta, and forms special milk-producing cells called *lobules* (Figure 11-2). After birth the mother's production of the hormone *prolactin* continues this milk-production process, which the suckling infant stimulates. Thus milk production depends on the demand of the infant. The suckling infant stimulates the brain's release of the hormone *oxytocin* from the pituitary gland to initiate the letdown reflex for the release of the milk

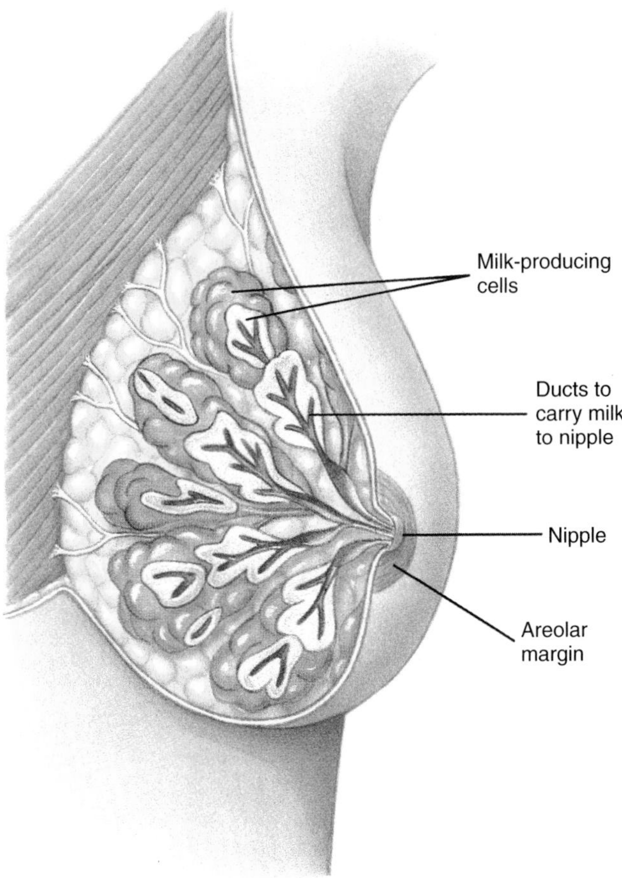

FIGURE 11-2 Anatomy of the breast. (*From Wardlaw G, Insel P:* Perspectives in nutrition, *ed 2, New York, 1993, McGraw-Hill. Reproduced with permission of the McGraw-Hill Companies.*)

from storage cells to travel down to the nipple. This reflex is easily inhibited by the mother's fatigue, tension, or lack of confidence, a particular source of anxiety in the new mother. She may be reassured that a comfortable and satisfying feeding routine is usually established in 2 to 3 weeks (Figure 11-3).

3. *Maternal adipose tissue storage.* The additional energy need for lactation is drawn from maternal adipose tissue stores deposited during pregnancy in normal preparation for lactation to follow in the maternal cycle. Depending on the adequacy of these stores, additional energy input may be needed in the lactating woman's daily diet.

In some women, the weight gained during pregnancy may be largely retained and contribute to obesity. Such overweight women who are breastfeeding have concerns regarding whether a weight loss program might endanger the growth of their infants. Recent research with overweight women who are exclusively breastfeeding shows that a diet and exercise program that leads to a weight loss of around 0.5 kg/week (approximately 1 lb/week) from 4 to 14 weeks postpartum should not affect infant growth.[58] Both the mother and the child who are involved in any

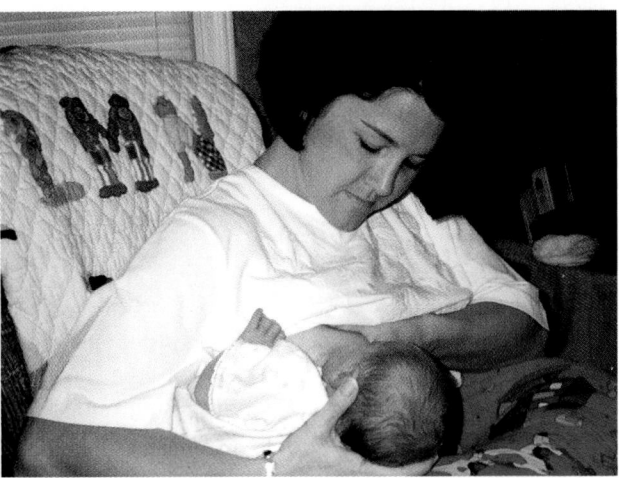

FIGURE 11-3 Breastfeeding infant and mother. (*From Lowdermilk DL, Perry SE, Bobak IM:* Maternity & women's health care, *ed 7, St Louis, 2000, Mosby.*)

specific weight loss program during lactation need to be monitored closely.[59]

Minerals

The DRI standard for calcium during lactation is 1000 mg/day, the same as for the nonpregnant adult woman. The calcium needs of the breastfeeding mother are not greater than those during pregnancy. The increased amount of calcium that was required during gestation for the mineralization of the fetal skeleton is now diverted into the mother's milk production. Iron, because it is not a major mineral component of milk, need not be increased for the production of milk.

In addition, for the breastfeeding infant, the American Academy of Pediatrics recommends a fluoride supplement of 0.25 mg/day because lactating mothers produce milk that is low in fluoride (about 16 μg/L).

Vitamins

The DRI standard for vitamin C during lactation is 120 mg/day. This is a considerable increase from the regular 75 mg/day for adult women. Increases over the mother's prenatal intake are also recommended for vitamin A because it is a constituent of milk and for the B-complex vitamins because they are involved as coenzyme factors in energy metabolism. The quantities of vitamins needed therefore invariably increase as the kcalorie intake increases.

Fluids

Ample fluid intake is needed before and during lactation—8 to 10 glasses/day consumed throughout the day. Also, the critical factor necessary for successful milk production is the increased energy intake. The basis for this increased caloric need is described in the previous discussion. Additional beverages such as juices and milk contribute both fluid and kcalories.

REST AND RELAXATION

In addition to the increased diet, the nursing mother requires rest, moderate exercise, and relaxation. Both parents may benefit from counseling focused on reducing the stresses of their new family situation, as well as meeting their own personal needs.

TO SUM UP

Pregnancy involves synergistic interactions among three distinct biologic entities: the fetus, the placenta, and the mother. Maternal needs reflect the increasing nutritional needs of the fetus and the placenta, as well as the need to meet maternal needs and to prepare for lactation. An optimal weight gain of about 11 kg (25 lb), or more as needed, is recommended during pregnancy to accommodate the rapid growth taking place. Even more significant than the actual weight gain is the quality of the diet.

Common problems occurring during pregnancy include nausea and vomiting, heartburn, or constipation. In most cases they are easily relieved without medication by simple, often temporary, changes in the diet. Serious problems with pregnancy may be associated with preexisting chronic maternal conditions, such as diabetes mellitus, or conditions arising as a result of the physical or metabolic demands of pregnancy, such as iron- deficiency anemia and PIH. Unusual or erratic eating habits, age, parity, prepartum weight status, and low income are among the many related factors that also place the mother at risk for complications.

The American Dietetic Association strongly encourages public health and clinical efforts that promote breastfeeding to optimize the indisputable nutritional, immunologic, psychologic, and economic benefits. The ultimate goal of prenatal care is a healthy infant and a mother physically capable of breastfeeding her child, should she choose to do so. Human milk provides essential nutrients in quantities required for optimal infant growth and development. It also supplies immunologic factors that offer protection against infection. Lactation requires an increase in kcalories beyond the needs of pregnancy. Adequate fluid intake is guided by the mother's natural thirst.

■ Questions for Review

1. List and discuss five factors that influence the nutritional needs of the woman during pregnancy. Which factors would place a woman in a high-risk category? Why?
2. List six nutrients that are required in larger amounts during pregnancy. Describe their special role during this period. Identify four food sources of each.
3. Identify two common problems associated with pregnancy, and describe the dietary management of each.
4. List and describe the screening indicators and risk factors for hypertension and diabetes mellitus during pregnancy.
5. List and discuss five major nutritional factors of lactation.

■ References

1. Food and Nutrition Board Committee on Maternal Nutrition, National Research Council National Academy of Sciences: *Maternal nutrition and the course of human pregnancy,* Washington, DC, 1970, National Academy Press.
2. American College of Obstetricians and Gynecologists, Committee on Nutrition: *Nutrition in maternal health care,* Chicago, 1974, The College.
3. American College of Obstetrics and Gynecologists and American Dietetic Association Task Force on Nutrition: *Assessment of maternal nutrition,* Chicago, 1978, The College and Association.
4. Food and Nutrition Board, Institute of Medicine: *Dietary reference intakes for calcium, phosphorus, magnesium, vitamin D, and fluoride,* Washington, DC, 1998, National Academy Press.
5. Food and Nutrition Board, Institute of Medicine: *Dietary reference intakes for thiamin, riboflavin, niacin, vitamin B_6, folate, vitamin B_{12}, pantothenic acid, biotin, and choline,* Washington, DC, 1999, National Academy Press.
6. Food and Nutrition Board, Institute of Medicine: *Dietary reference intakes for vitamin C, vitamin E, selenium, and carotenoids,* Washington, DC, 2000, National Academy Press.
7. Food and Nutrition Board, Institute of Medicine: *Dietary reference intakes for vitamin A, vitamin K, arsenic, boron, chromium, copper, iodine, iron, manganese, molybdenum, nickel, silicon, vanadium, and zinc,* Washington, DC, 2002, National Academy Press.
8. Nutrition-Cognition National Advisory Committee: *Statement on the link between nutrition and cognitive development in children,* Medford, MA, 1998, Center on Hunger, Poverty, and Nutrition Policy, Tufts University.
9. National Research Council, Food and Nutrition Board: *Recommended dietary allowances,* ed 10, Washington, DC, 1989, National Academy Press.
10. Al MDM et al: Long-chain polyunsaturated fatty acids, pregnancy, and pregnancy outcome, *Am J Clin Nutr* 71(suppl): 285S, 2000.
11. Uauy R, Hoffman DR: Essential fat requirements of preterm infants, *Am J Clin Nutr* 71(suppl):245S, 2000.
12. Reynolds RD: Perinatal vitamin B_6 deficiency and poverty: is there a link? *Nutr Today* 35(6):222, 2000.
13. Worthington-Roberts B: The role of maternal nutrition in the prevention of birth defects, *J Am Diet Assoc* 97(10, suppl 2):S184, 1997.
14. Mills JL: Fortification of foods with folic acid: how much is enough? *N Engl J Med* 342(19):1442, 2000.
15. Kloeben AS: Folate knowledge, intake from fortified grain products, and periconceptional supplementation patterns of a sample of low-income pregnant women according to the Health Belief Model, *J Am Diet Assoc* 99(1):33, 1999.
16. Mackey AD, Picciano MF: Maternal folate status during extended lactation and the effect of supplemental folic acid, *Am J Clin Nutr* 69(1):285, 1999.
17. Food and Nutrition Board, Institute of Medicine: *Nutrition during pregnancy,* Washington, DC, 1990, National Academy Press.
18. Luke B, Leurgans S: Maternal weight gains in ideal twins outcomes, *J Am Diet Assoc* 96(2):178, 1996.
19. Strauss RS, Dietz WH: Low maternal weight gain in the second or third trimester increases the risk for intrauterine growth retardation, *J Nutr* 129(5):988, 1999.

20. Butte NF: Adjustments in energy expenditure and substrate utilization during late pregnancy and lactation, *Am J Clin Nutr* 69(1):299, 1999.
21. Barinaga M: A new clue to how alcohol damages brains, *Science* 287(5455):947, 2000.
22. Ikonomidou C et al: Ethanol-induced apoptotic neurodegeneration and fetal alcohol syndrome, *Science* 287(5455): 1056, 2000.
23. Hellerstadt WL et al: The effects of cigarette smoking and gestational weight change on birth outcome in obese and normal weight women, *Am J Public Health* 87(4):591, 1997.
24. Ness RB et al: Cocaine and tobacco use and the risk of spontaneous abortion, *N Engl J Med* 340:333, 1999.
25. Eskenazi B: Caffeine: filtering the facts, *N Engl J Med* 341:1688, 1999.
26. Cnattingius S et al: Caffeine intake and the risk of first-trimester spontaneous abortion, *N Engl J Med* 343(25): 1839, 2000.
27. Hinds TS et al: The effect of caffeine on pregnancy outcome variables, *Nutr Rev* 54(7):203, 1996.
28. Kolasa KM, Weismiller DG: Nutrition during pregnancy, *Am Fam Physician* 56(1):205, 1997.
29. Rainville AJ: Pica practices of pregnant women are associated with lower maternal hemoglobin level at delivery, *J Am Diet Assoc* 98(3):293, 1998.
30. American Diabetes Association: Gestational diabetes mellitus, *Diabetes Care* 21(suppl 1):S60, 1998.
31. Langer O et al: A comparison of glyburide and insulin in women with gestational diabetes mellitus, *N Engl J Med* 343(16):1134, 2000.
32. Pasui K, McFarland KF: Management of diabetes in pregnancy, *Am Fam Physician* 55(8):2731, 1997.
33. Naylor CD et al: Selective screening for gestational diabetes mellitus, *N Engl J Med* 337(22):1591, 1997.
34. Green MF: Screening for gestational diabetes mellitus, *N Engl J Med* 337(22):1625, 1997.
35. Tepper BJ, Seldner AC: Sweet taste and intake of sweet foods in normal pregnancy and pregnancy complicated by gestational diabetes mellitus, *Am J Clin Nutr* 70:277, 1999.
36. Jovanovic L: Time to reassess the optimal dietary prescription for women with gestational diabetes, *Am J Clin Nutr* 70(1):3, 1999.
37. Wunderlich SM: Nutritional assessment and support of HIV-positive pregnant women and their children, *Nutr Today* 35(3):107, 2000.
38. Taren D: The infant feeding and HIV transmission controversy impacts public health services, *Nutr Today* 35(3):103, 2000.
39. Ryan AS: The resurgence of breast-feeding in the United States, *Pediatrics* 99:E12, 1997.
40. World Health Organization: WHO advises: ten steps to successful breast-feeding, *World Health* 2:28, 1997.
41. Schanler RJ et al: Pediatricians' practices and attitudes regarding breastfeeding promotion, *Pediatrics* 103:E35, 1999.
42. Lawrence R: *Breastfeeding: a guide for the medical profession,* St Louis, 1999, Mosby.
43. Chezem J, Friesen C: Attendance at breast-feeding support meetings: relationship to demographic characteristics and duration of lactation in women planning postpartum employment, *J Am Diet Assoc* 99(1):83, 1999.
44. Wright AL et al: Increasing breast-feeding rates to reduce infant illness at the community level, *Pediatrics* 101:837, 1998.
45. Carmichael SL et al: Breast-feeding practices among WIC participants in Hawaii, *J Am Diet Assoc* 101(1):57, 2001.
46. Beshgetor D: Attitudes toward breast-feeding among WIC employees in San Diego County, *J Am Diet Assoc* 99(1):86, 1999.
47. Caulfield LE et al: WIC-based interventions to promote breastfeeding among African-American women in Baltimore: effects on breastfeeding initiation and continuation, *J Hum Lact* 14:15, 1998.
48. Misra R, James DCS: Breast-feeding practices among adolescent and adult mothers in the Missouri WIC population, *J Am Diet Assoc* 100(9):1071, 2000.
49. Pobocik RS et al: Effect of a breastfeeding education and support program on breastfeeding initiation and duration in a culturally diverse group of adolescents, *J Nutr Educ* 32(3):139, 2000.
50. Schmidt MM, Sigman-Grant M: Perspectives of low-income fathers' support of breastfeeding: an exploratory study, *J Nutr Educ* 32(1):31, 2000.
51. Sharma M, Petos R: Impact of expectant fathers in breast-feeding decisions, *J Am Diet Assoc* 11:1311, 1997.
52. Kannan S et al: Cultural influences on infant feeding beliefs of mothers, *J Am Diet Assoc* 99(1):88, 1999.
53. Murtaugh M: Optimal breast-feeding duration, *J Am Diet Assoc* 97:1252, 1997.
54. American Academy of Pediatrics: Breast-feeding and the use of human milk: policy statement on breast-feeding, *Pediatrics* 100(12):1035, 1997.
55. Howard CR et al: The effects of early pacifier use on breast-feeding duration, *Pediatrics* 103:E33, 1999.
56. Kitzman H et al: Enduring effects of nurse home visitation on maternal life course, *JAMA* 283(15):1983, 2000.
57. Jornsay DL: Pumps and pregnancy, *Diabetes Forecast* 53(9):68, 2000.
58. Lovelady CA et al: The effect of weight loss in overweight, lactating women on the growth of their infants, *N Engl J Med* 342(7):449, 2000.
59. Butte NF: Dieting and exercise in overweight, lactating women, *N Engl J Med* 342(7):502, 2000.

■ Further Reading

Gord C: Nutrition for a healthy pregnancy: national guidelines for the childbearing years, *Can J Diet Pract Res* 60(2):Summer, 1999.

This excellent resource provides helpful guidance for healthy pregnancies, as well as important information for identifying women at nutritional risk.

Vozenilek GP: What they don't know could hurt them: increasing public awareness of folic acid and neural tube defects, *J Am Diet Assoc* 99(1):20, 1999.

This informative article draws a clear picture of the cloud of ignorance that still hangs over the general population about the devastating results of neural tube defects in an affected child from birth because of the mother's folic acid deficiency early in pregnancy.

CASE STUDY A baby for the Delgados

Mrs. Delgado is a 19-year-old married primigravida who tested positive for urinary human chorionic gonadotropin (hCG) 2 weeks earlier. Mrs. Delgado is 160 cm (5 ft 4 in) tall with an average pregravid weight of 57 kg (125 lb). Her current gestational age is 6 weeks. Her history for chronic disorders and other serious health problems is negative.

During her initial nutrition interview, Mrs. Delgado indicated that the pregnancy was unplanned. She seemed especially worried about the effects of her irregular diet on the baby. As college students, she and her 21-year-old husband had erratic meals, dominated by junk food. Mrs. Delgado's 24-hour diet history revealed an inadequate intake of dark green or yellow vegetables and milk products, as well as meat or eggs and citrus fruits. The couple realized that these types of foods were an important part of a nutritious diet but felt inexperienced as cooks and lacked the time and money to prepare healthful meals every day.

At the end of the initial counseling session, the nutritionist told the couple about a series of prenatal group discussions conducted by members of the clinic's perinatal health team, including sessions on pregnancy, labor and delivery, and the care and feeding of the infant. These are attended primarily by a mixture of experienced parents and young, first-time parents-to-be and are offered as a means of introducing practical aspects of pregnancy and parenting.

The Delgados attended every prenatal group meeting and kept all consequent diet-counseling sessions. Their food choices improved in time, and Mrs. Delgado's weight gain progressed normally, to a total of 12 kg (28 lb) by the time of delivery. The Delgados had a healthy 4 kg (8 lb 2 oz) baby girl.

QUESTIONS FOR ANALYSIS

1. What health professional ideally should be included on the health care team caring for Mrs. Delgado? Describe the significance of each role to the outcome of her pregnancy. What are the roles of Mr. and Mrs. Delgado?
2. What nutritional deficiencies would you expect in Mrs. Delgado's diet? What practical problems would you expect her to encounter in attempting to improve her diet?
3. Write a 1-day meal plan for Mrs. Delgado, taking into account her lifestyle and schedule, as well as the amounts of nutrients considered adequate for pregnancy.
4. Write a lesson plan for a group session on nutrition during pregnancy. Include a general description, behavioral objectives, content outline, teaching methods and materials, and evaluation tool(s) you would use.
5. Would you encourage Mrs. Delgado to breastfeed? If so, why? What factors would you expect might discourage her from trying? How would you discuss these factors?
6. Write a lesson plan for an infant feeding session, addressing breastfeeding and bottle-feeding methods. Include the components listed in Questions 3 and 4.

Issues & ANSWERS

Drug Use and the Outcome of Pregnancy

Since the tragic discovery a number of years ago of the teratogenic effects of thalidomide, the interest in the effects of drugs used during pregnancy has risen dramatically among healthcare workers and the general public. The tragic consequences of inappropriate drug use make it of quintessential importance that the nutritionist or nurse, while obtaining a dietary history, also gather a complete history of drug use, both licit and illicit, to warn the mother of the potential dangers involved and have the mother discuss in detail any prescribed drugs with her physician. Listed here are descriptions of the effects of a variety of common drugs on the pregnant woman, the fetus, and the outcome of pregnancy.

Alcohol

No safe level of alcohol consumption has yet been found for pregnant women, despite a recent claim that pregnant women can safely have up to two drinks a day. Even moderate social drinking has been associated with subclinical signs of fetal alcohol syndrome (FAS). This disorder is characterized by growth retardation, malformed facial features, joint and limb abnormalities, cardiac defects, mental retardation, and, in serious cases, death. FAS signs have been seen in tests with rats as early as the human equivalent of the third week of gestation, when most women are unaware of their pregnancies. Thus moderate-to-heavy drinking among sexually active women of childbearing age may carry potential danger.

The nutritional problems of FAS are similar to those seen in chronic alcoholism. A zinc deficiency has specifically been associated with congenital defects and impaired immune function among children born to alcohol abusers. Alcohol has also induced signs of secondary hyperparathyroidism in pregnant animals, thus potentially affecting serum calcium levels.

Psychotropic drugs

A number of drugs are often prescribed for female patients to treat a variety of psychologic and mental health disorders. However, if taken during pregnancy, they exhibit teratogenic effects. If any of these drugs are being taken on a long-term basis for the treatment of serious conditions, such as clinical depression, bipolar disorder, or schizophrenia, comprehensive medical and psychologic assessment and follow-up is needed throughout the pregnancy.

Lithium has recently been associated with an increased risk for Epstein's anomaly (a rare cardiovascular abnormality), goiter, and diabetes insipidus, as well as neonatal toxic disturbances such as cyanosis, hypothermia, and bradycardia. A diminished suck reflex will impede attempts to nourish the infant exposed to lithium in utero.

Diazepam (Valium) is associated with an abnormal fetal heart rate. The neonate risks delivery by cesarean section, with oral-facial malformations, a depressed Apgar score, and a reluctance to feed. Rats exposed to diazepam in utero have exhibited abnormal motor skills and arousal processes.

Tricyclic antidepressants (e.g., imipramine) have led to morphologic and behavioral abnormalities in rats.

Anticonvulsants

Phenytoin (Dilantin, Hydantoin) is prescribed to control seizures caused by epilepsy and other conditions. Even though this drug has caused malformations in the offspring of rats, physicians are reluctant to discontinue it for their patients with epilepsy during pregnancy. Because only 7% of children born to mothers using the drug develop malformations, and significantly more develop malformations and developmental disabilities when the mother's epilepsy is untreated, this may be one case in which prenatal drug use is more beneficial than not using it.

Caffeine

It is wise to avoid this very commonly used stimulant, at least during pregnancy. Pregnant women who are heavy coffee drinkers are considered at risk for miscarriages, premature deliveries, and small-for-gestational age infants. Therefore intake of caffeinated foods, beverages (coffee, tea, cocoa, cola), and medications should be avoided.

Marijuana

Evaluation of the effects of street drugs (marijuana, cocaine, heroin, methadone) on nutritional status is difficult because of multiple drug use, uncertain purity, unknown dosage and timing, and inadequate nutritional status of many drug users. A 1982 report on a study of marijuana use in 35 pregnancies revealed a higher incidence of meconium staining (which could relate to fetal damage), poor prenatal weight gain, very short (<3 hours) or prolonged labor, operative delivery (cesarean, forceps), and other perinatal problems among marijuana users. Although the researchers admitted flaws in their study (e.g., the use of subjects who chose to participate or not), the outcome indicates a need to further investigate these potentially fatal effects.

Nicotine

Cigarette smoking has been well documented for its association with low birth weight infants, impairment of mental and physical growth, and increased potential mortality. The dietary implications of prenatal smoking are presented in at least one study showing that although the smokers may eat more than nonsmokers, they still deliver smaller babies. In addition, the ability of nicotine to increase heart rate, blood pressure, and fat breakdown compromises the health and nutritional status of mother and infant alike.

Thus with the exception of drugs used to treat individuals with seizure disorders or natural replacement therapy (e.g., insulin for persons with type 1 diabetes), drugs should be avoided at all costs during pregnancy to ensure the health of the mother and a safe and healthy outcome of the pregnancy. The nutrition counselor is well advised to keep up with the most recent findings regarding medications (prescribed, over-the-counter, and street drugs) to evaluate the nutritional status of the mother using them and warn her of the potential harm they may pose for her and her baby.

REFERENCES

Frank DA et al: Cocaine and marijuana use during pregnancy by women intending and not intending to breast-feed, *J Am Diet Assoc* 92(2):215, 1992.

Hellerstedt WL et al: The effects of cigarette smoking and gestational weight change on birth outcomes in obese and normal-weight women, *Am J Public Health* 87(4):591, 1997.

Hinds TS et al: The effect of caffeine on pregnancy outcome variables, *Nutr Rev* 54(7):203, 1996.

Larroque B et al: Moderate prenatal alcohol exposure and psychomotor development at preschool age, *Am J Public Health* 85(12):1654, 1995.

Chapter

12

Nutrition for Growth and Development

Eleanor D. Schlenker

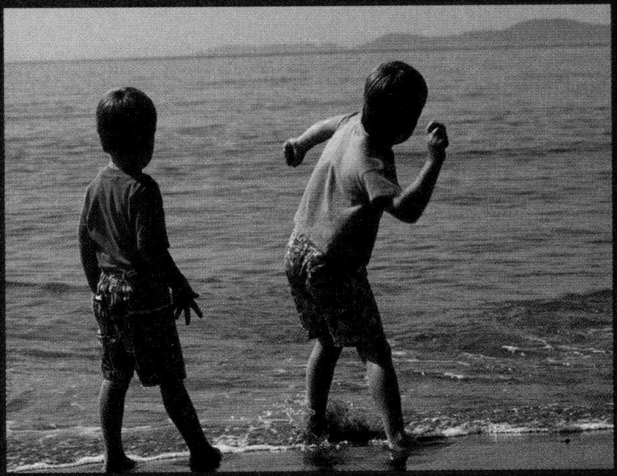

Chapter Outline

In this second chapter in our life cycle series, we look at growing infants, children, and adolescents. We consider their physical growth and their inseparable psychosocial development at each progressive stage. This unified growth and development nurture the integrated progression of the child into the adult.

Within this dual framework of physical and psychosocial development, we consider food and feeding and their vital roles in the development of the whole child. In each age group, we relate nutritional needs and the food that supplies them to the normal physical maturation and psychosocial development achieved in each stage.

Human Growth and Development

INDIVIDUAL NEEDS OF CHILDREN

Growth may be defined as an increase in body size. Biologic growth of an organism occurs through cell multiplication and cell enlargement. *Development* is the associated process by which growing tissues and organs take on a more complex function. Both of these processes are part of one whole, forming a unified and inseparable sequence of growth and development. Through these changes a small dependent newborn is transformed into a fully functioning independent adult. However, each child is a unique individual with individual needs. This is a paramount principle in working with children. Thus we must always seek to discover these individual human needs if we are to help each child reach his or her greatest growth and development potential.[1]

Normal Life Cycle Growth Pattern

The normal human life cycle includes four general stages of overall growth and development: infancy, childhood, adolescence, and adulthood.

1. *Infancy.* Growth velocity is rapid during the first year of life, with the rate tapering off in the latter half of the year. At the age of 6 months, an infant has probably doubled its birth weight, and at 1 year, he or she may have tripled it.
2. *Childhood.* During the latent period of childhood between infancy and adolescence, the growth rate slows and becomes erratic. During some periods there are plateaus. At other times small spurts of growth occur. This overall growth deceleration affects appetite accordingly. At times children will have little or no appetite, and at other times they will eat voraciously. Parents who know that this is a normal pattern can relax and avoid making eating a battleground with their children.
3. *Adolescence.* With the beginning of puberty, the second period of growth acceleration occurs. Because of the hormonal influences involved, enormous physical changes take place, including the development of the long bones, the sex characteristics, and fat and muscle mass.
4. *Adulthood.* In the final stage of a normal life cycle, growth levels off on the adult plateau. Then it gradually declines during old age—the period of senescence.

MEASURING CHILDHOOD PHYSICAL GROWTH

Growth Charts

Children grow at widely varying individual rates. In clinical practice a child's pattern of growth is compared with percentile growth curves derived from measurements of large numbers of children throughout the growth years. Contemporary growth chart grids, developed by the National Center for Health Statistics (NCHS), were recently revised to reflect the growth patterns of both breastfed and formula-fed infants and to provide a broad baseline for evaluating growth patterns in children today.[2] These charts are based on data from a nationally representative sample of children that includes various racial and ethnic groups. Two age intervals are presented: birth to 3 years and 2 to 20 years, with separate curves for boys and girls (see Appendix I, CDC Growth Charts: United States).

Anthropometry

Practitioners use anthropometry to monitor a child's growth, with growth charts and other clinical standards as points of reference. A number of methods and measures may be used.

1. *Body weight and height.* These are common general measures of physical growth. They provide a basic measure of change in body size but give only a crude index of growth without the finer details of individual variations in body fat or muscle or bone. They are used mainly to monitor patterns of growth over time, as the individual child's pattern is plotted on the growth chart for that age group. The recumbent length of infants and small children is measured initially and then standing height is measured as they grow older.
2. *Body circumferences and skinfolds.* The head circumference is a valuable measure in infants, but it is seldom measured routinely after 3 years of age. Circumference measures of abdomen, chest, and leg at its maximal girth of the calf are usually included at periodic intervals. Other measures for monitoring muscle mass growth and body composition include the midarm circumference and the triceps skinfold taken at the same point. Using these two measures, the midarm muscle circumference can be calculated easily (see Chapter 15). Skinfold measures, taken at a number of body sites, are performed with special calipers and require skill and practice for accuracy. Longitudinal growth studies in research centers use many measures of development in addition to these basic ones to monitor growth in general practice. Because national statistics inform us of the growing prevalence of fatness among children of all ages,[3] the use of skinfold thicknesses or other measures to monitor the relative increase in muscle versus fat should be incorporated into regular physical examinations.

Clinical Signs

Various clinical signs of optimal growth can be observed as indicators of a child's nutritional status. These include such indicators as general vitality; sense of well-being; good posture; healthy gums, teeth, skin, hair, and eyes; appropriate muscle development; and nervous control. Refer to Table 1-1 for a review of these general signs and observations.

Laboratory Tests

Other measures of growth can be obtained with various laboratory tests, including studies of blood and urine to determine levels of hemoglobin, vitamins, and similar substances (see Appendix K, Normal Constituents of Blood and Urine in Adults). Radiographs of the hand and wrist measure degrees of bone development.

Nutritional Analysis

A nutritional analysis of general eating habits (see Chapter 10) provides helpful information for assessing the adequacy of the diet for meeting growth needs. A diet history form (see Figure 10-1) and food value tables (see Appendix A) may be used. In clinical practice, diet evaluations and nutrient intake calculations are usually completed using computer analysis. The nutritionist puts together information obtained from a variety of methods to complete a food intake analysis to use in diet counseling with the parents.

MENTAL AND PSYCHOSOCIAL DEVELOPMENT

Mental Growth

Measures of mental growth usually involve abilities in speech and other forms of communication, as well as the ability to handle abstract and symbolic material in thinking. Young children think in very literal terms. As they develop in mental capacity, they can handle more than single ideas, and they can form constructive concepts.

Emotional Growth

Emotional growth is measured in the capacity for love and affection, as well as the ability to handle frustration and its anxieties. It also involves the child's ability to control aggressive impulses and to channel hostility from destructive to constructive activities.

Social and Cultural Growth

The social development of a child is measured as the ability to relate to others and to participate in group living and cultural activities. These social and cultural behaviors are first learned through relationships with parents and family, and these relationships greatly influence food habits and feeding patterns. As the child's horizon broadens, relationships are developed with those outside the family, with friends, and with others in the community at school or at religious or other social gatherings. For this reason a child's play during the early years is a highly purposeful activity.

Nutritional Requirements for Growth

ENERGY NEEDS

During childhood the demand for kilocalories (kcalories) is relatively great. However, there is much variation in need with age and condition. For example, the total daily kcaloric intake of a 5-year-old child is spent in the following way: (1) about 50% supplies basal metabolic requirements (BMR), (2) 5% is used in the thermic effect of food (TEF), (3) 25% goes toward daily physical activity, (4) 12% is needed for tissue growth, and (5) about 8% is lost in the feces. Of these kcalories, carbohydrates are the primary energy source and are important in sparing protein for its essential role in tissue formation.

ESSENTIAL FATTY ACID NEEDS

Fat kcalories are important as backup energy sources but are particularly needed to supply the essential fatty acids—linoleic and linolenic acids. Linoleic acid is required for the synthesis of brain and nerve tissue and normal mental development. However, an excess of fat, especially from animal sources, should be avoided.

PROTEIN NEEDS

Protein provides amino acids, the essential building materials for tissue growth. As a child grows, the protein requirements per unit of body weight gradually decrease. For example, during the first 6 months of life an infant requires 1.52 g of protein/kg.[4] This amount gradually decreases throughout childhood until adulthood, when protein needs are only about 0.8 g/kg.[4] Usually, the healthy, active, growing child will consume the necessary amounts of kcalories and protein if a variety of food is provided.

WATER REQUIREMENTS

The infant's relative need for water is greater than that of the adult. The infant's body content of water is about 70% to 75% of total body weight, whereas in the adult, water makes up only about 60% to 65% of total body weight. Also, a large amount of the infant's total body water is outside the

anthropometry The science of measuring the size, weight, and proportions of the human body.
body composition The relative sizes of the four basic body compartments that make up the total body: lean body mass (muscle and vital organs), fat, water, and bone.
growth acceleration Period of increased speed of growth at different points of childhood development.
growth chart grids Grids comparing stature (length), weight, and age of children by percentile; used for nutritional assessment to determine how their growth is progressing. The most commonly used grids are those of the National Center for Health Statistics (NCHS).
growth deceleration Period of decreased speed of growth at different points of childhood development.
growth velocity Rapidity of motion or movement; rate of childhood growth over normal periods of development compared with a population standard.
percentile One of 100 equal parts of measured series of values; rate or proportion per hundred.

cell and more easily lost. Thus prolonged water loss because of diarrhea, as occurs among infants in developing countries given formula prepared from contaminated water, is a serious threat to life and requires immediate oral hydration therapy.[5] The child's water need is related to kcaloric intake and urine concentration. Generally an infant drinks daily an amount of water equivalent to 10% to 15% of body weight, whereas the adult's daily water intake equals 2% to 4% of body weight. A summary of approximate daily fluid needs during the growth years is given in Table 12-1.

MINERAL AND VITAMIN NEEDS

In our previous study of minerals and vitamins, we learned of their essential roles in tissue growth and maintenance and in overall energy metabolism. Positive childhood growth and development depend on an adequate amount of these essential substances. For example, rapidly growing young bones require calcium and phosphorus. A radiograph of a newborn's body would reveal a skeleton appearing as a collection of disconnected, separate bones requiring mineralization. Calcium is also needed for tooth development, muscle contraction, nerve irritability, blood coagulation, and heart muscle action. Another mineral of concern is iron, essential for hemoglobin formation and mental and psychomotor development.[6,7] The infant's fetal iron stores are depleted in 4 to 6 months after birth. Thus solid food additions at that time help supply needed iron. Such foods as iron-fortified cereal and egg, and later meat, accomplish this. The use of iron-fortified formulas and other foods by high-risk children enrolled in the Women-Infant-Children Supplementary Food Program (WIC) assist in reducing the incidence of iron-deficiency anemia among infants and young children from limited-resource families such as the homeless.[8,9]

Excess amounts of particular micronutrients are also of concern in feeding children. Excess intake is usually the result of inappropriate use of vitamin or mineral supplements and may occur because of misunderstanding, ignorance, or carelessness. When supplements are indicated because of a specific and defined medical or nutrition condition, parents must be carefully instructed to use only the amount directed and no more. Two nutrients that pose particular hazards when consumed in excessive amounts are the following.

1. *Vitamin A.* Symptoms of toxicity from excess vitamin A include lack of appetite, slow growth, drying and cracking of the skin, enlargement of the liver and spleen, swelling and pain in the long bones, and bone fragility.
2. *Vitamin D.* Symptoms of toxicity from excess vitamin D include nausea, diarrhea, weight loss, excess urination (especially at night), and eventual calcification of soft tissues, including the renal tubules, blood vessels, bronchi, stomach, and heart.

A summary of the Dietary Reference Intakes (DRIs) for overall nutritional needs and growth, developed by the National Research Council, is given in Tables 12-2, 12-3, and 12-4.

TABLE 12-1 Approximate Daily Fluid Needs During Growth Years

Age	ml/kg
0-3 months	120
3-6 months	115
6-12 months	100
1-4 years	100
4-7 years	95
7-11 years	90
11-19 years	50
>19 years	30

TABLE 12-2 Recommended Dietary Allowances for Energy and Protein (2002)

	Age (yr)	Weight (kg)	Weight (lb)	Height (cm)	Height (in)	Energy* (kcalories)	Protein (g)
Infants	0-0.5	6	13	62	24	438-645	9.1
	0.5-1	9	20	71	28	608-844	13.5
Children	1-3	12	27	86	34	837-1683	13
	4-8	20	44	115	45	1133-2225	19
Males	9-13	36	79	144	57	1530-3038	34
	14-18	61	134	174	68	2090-3804	52
Females	9-13	37	81	144	57	1415-2762	34
	14-18	54	119	163	64	1690-2883	46

From Panel on Macronutrients, Panel on the Definition of Dietary Fiber, Subcommittee on Upper Reference Levels of Nutrients, Subcommittee on Interpretation and Uses of Dietary Reference Intakes, and the Standing Committee on the Scientific Evaluation of Dietary Reference Intakes: *Dietary reference intakes for energy, carbohydrate, fiber, fat, fatty acids, cholesterol, protein, and amino acids, parts 1 and 2,* Washington, DC, 2002, National Academy Press.

* Varies according to body size, age, and level of physical activity.

Stages of Growth and Development: Age Group Needs

THE STAGES OF HUMAN LIFE

Throughout the human life cycle, food and feeding not only supply nutrients for physical growth but also play a role in personal and psychosocial development. The nutritional age group needs of children cannot be understood apart from the child's overall maturation as a unique person. A leading American psychoanalyst, Erikson,[10] has contributed to our understanding of human personality and growth throughout critical periods of development. His theory of human development has come to play a significant role in our view of the human life cycle.

PSYCHOSOCIAL DEVELOPMENT

Erikson identified eight stages in human growth and a basic psychosocial developmental problem with which the individual struggles at each stage.[10] The developmental problem at each stage has a positive ego value and a conflicting negative counterpart, as given here.

1. *Infancy:* trust versus distrust
2. *Toddler:* autonomy versus shame and doubt
3. *Preschooler:* initiative versus guilt

TABLE 12-3 Dietary Reference Intakes for Vitamins

Age (yr)	Vitamin A (μg)	Vitamin D (μg)	Vitamin E (mg TE)	Vitamin K (μg)	Vitamin C (mg)	Thiamin (mg)	Riboflavin (mg)	Niacin (mg NE)	Vitamin B_6 (mg)	Folate (μg)	Vitamin B_{12} (μg)
Infants 0-0.5	400	5	4	2	40	0.2	0.3	2	0.1	65	0.4
Infants 0.6-1.0	500	5	5	2.5	50	0.3	0.4	4	0.3	80	0.5
Children 1-3	300	5	6	30	15	0.5	0.5	6	0.5	150	0.9
Children 4-8	400	5	7	55	25	0.6	0.6	8	0.6	200	1.2
Boys 9-13	600	5	11	60	45	0.9	0.9	12	1	300	1.8
Boys 14-18	900	5	15	75	75	1.2	1.3	16	1.3	400	2.4
Girls 9-13	600	5	11	60	45	0.9	0.9	12	1	300	1.8
Girls 14-18	700	5	15	75	65	1.0	1.0	14	1.2	400	2.4

Data compiled from Food and Nutrition Board, National Research Council: *Dietary reference intakes for calcium, phosphorus, magnesium, vitamin D, and fluoride,* Washington, DC, 1997, National Academy Press; Food and Nutrition Board, National Research Council: *Dietary reference intakes for thiamin, riboflavin, niacin, vitamin B_6, folate, vitamin B_{12}, pantothenic acid, biotin, and choline,* Washington, DC, 1998, National Academy Press; Food and Nutrition Board, National Research Council: *Dietary reference intakes for vitamin C, vitamin E, selenium, and carotenoids,* Washington, DC, 2000, National Academy Press; Food and Nutrition Board, National Research Council: *Dietary reference intakes for vitamin A, vitamin K, arsenic, boron, chromium, copper, iodine, iron, manganese, molybdenum, nickel, silicon, vanadium, and zinc,* Washington, DC, 2001, National Academy Press.

TABLE 12-4 Dietary Reference Intakes for Minerals

Age (yr)	Calcium (mg)	Phosphorus (mg)	Magnesium (mg)	Iron (mg)	Zinc (mg)	Iodine (μg)	Selenium (μg)	Fluoride (mg)
Infants 0-0.5	210	100	30	0.27	2	110	15	0.01
Infants 0.6-1.0	270	275	75	11	3	130	20	0.5
Children 1-3	500	460	80	7	3	90	20	0.7
Children 4-8	800	500	130	10	5	90	30	1
Boys 9-13	1300	1250	240	8	8	120	40	2
Boys 14-18	1300	1250	410	11	11	150	55	3
Girls 9-13	1300	1250	240	8	8	120	40	2
Girls 14-18	1300	1250	360	15	9	150	55	3

Data compiled from Food and Nutrition Board, National Research Council: *Dietary reference intakes for calcium, phosphorus, magnesium, vitamin D, and fluoride,* Washington, DC, 1997, National Academy Press; Food and Nutrition Board, National Research Council: *Dietary reference intakes for thiamin, riboflavin, niacin, vitamin B_6, folate, vitamin B_{12}, pantothenic acid, biotin, and choline,* Washington, DC, 1998, National Academy Press; Food and Nutrition Board, National Research Council: *Dietary reference intakes for vitamin C, vitamin E, selenium, and carotenoids,* Washington, DC, 2000, National Academy Press; Food and Nutrition Board, National Research Council: *Dietary reference intakes for vitamin A, vitamin K, arsenic, boron, chromium, copper, iodine, iron, manganese, molybdenum, nickel, silicon, vanadium, and zinc,* Washington, DC, 2001, National Academy Press.

4. *School-age child:* industry versus inferiority
5. *Adolescent:* identity versus role confusion
6. *Young adult:* intimacy versus isolation
7. *Adult:* generativity versus stagnation
8. *Older adult:* ego integrity versus despair

Given favorable circumstances, a growing child develops positive ego strength at each life stage and builds increasing inner resources and strengths to meet the next life crisis. The struggle at any age, however, is not forever won at this point. A residue of the negative remains, and in periods of stress, such as an illness, some regression is likely to occur. But as the child gains mastery at each stage of development, assisted by significant positive and supportive relationships, integration of self-controls takes place. Changes occurring at each stage influence both food intake and the interaction of the child with family members, peers, and counselors.[11]

1. *Infant.* Infants require appropriate stimulation to thrive—they enjoy seeing different colors, talking, and being physically held. Activities such as looking at pictures or hearing nursery rhymes support cognitive development. The attention span is short, which can create problems at feeding time.
2. *Toddler.* Toddlers grow rapidly and begin to demonstrate autonomy with display of temper tantrums or negative behavior. They begin to develop language skills and can recall past experiences. Play is an important medium for self-expression and allows the child to express some control over his or her environment.
3. *Preschooler.* The preschool years are a time for increasing social experiences, and children begin to interact more with other children. Preschoolers have an increased ability to express themselves and may try to exert control through demands for or refusal of certain foods (food jags).
4. *School-age child.* The school-age child enters a formal learning environment and attention span increases. At this age children are more selective in choosing friends, and the influence of peers becomes more obvious. As the environment becomes more structured, physical activity may decline.
5. *Adolescent.* Adolescents become more autonomous in their actions and attempt to exert independence from parental control. Teens perceive themselves to be invulnerable to illness or injury, and risk-taking behaviors involving drugs or alcohol may begin. Obsession with body image may result in inappropriate nutrition practices.

Various related developmental tasks surround each of these stages. These learnings, when accomplished, contribute to successful resolution of the core problem.

PHYSICAL GROWTH

The developmental tasks of choosing and consuming food do not develop in a vacuum. They flow as an integral part of physical and psychosocial development. In this section we discuss food and feeding practices at each of the stages of childhood and their relationship to normal physical and psychosocial maturation. Developing neuromuscular motor skills enable the child to accomplish related physical activities involved with food. Psychosocial development influences food attitudes, behavior, patterns, and habits.

INFANT (BIRTH TO 1 YEAR)

Physical Characteristics of a Full-Term Infant

The full-term infant is born after successful growth and development during a normal gestation period of about 40 weeks (280 days). During the first year of life, the infant about triples in weight, growing rapidly from an average birth weight of 3.2 kg (7 lb) to a 1-year-old child ready to walk and weighing about 9 kg (20 lb). Thus energy requirements during this first year of tremendous growth are high.

Full-term infants have the ability to digest and absorb protein, a moderate amount of fat, and simple carbohydrates. They have some difficulty with starch because amylase, the starch-splitting enzyme, is not being produced at birth. However, as starch is introduced, this enzyme begins to function. The renal system functions well in infancy, but more water relative to body size is needed than in the adult to manage urinary excretion. The first baby teeth do not erupt until about the fourth month; therefore initially food must be liquid or semiliquid.

Nutrition for the Full-Term Infant

The first food for infants, breast milk or infant formula, generally provides all the nutrients required by a healthy infant for the first 5 to 6 months of life. All infants born in a hospital receive an injection of vitamin K shortly after birth to ensure an adequate level of this nutrient, and it is important that infants born at home also receive supplemental vitamin K. It is necessary to provide vitamin D supplements to breastfed infants because breast milk may not supply adequate vitamin D to prevent deficiency and the development of rickets. This is especially critical in the case of African American mothers, who are less able to synthesize vitamin D in their skin, or for mothers who wear special garb for religious reasons that limits their skin exposure to the sun.[12] Fomon, a noted pediatrician specializing in infant nutrition, recommends that breastfed infants who receive no feedings of iron-fortified formula be supplemented with iron to the level of 5 mg/day, to make up for the limited amount of iron in breast milk.[13] It has been suggested that fluoride supplements be provided for breastfed infants or formula-fed infants above 6 months of age in geographic regions where the water is low in fluoride, but not all nutritionists agree on this matter.[5,14] It is important that nursing mothers be well nourished to supply adequate levels of vitamins and minerals in their milk.

Infants have limited nutritional stores from gestation, and this is especially true for iron. By the age of 6 months, semisolid foods such as iron-fortified cereals must be added to the diet to help meet increasing nutritional needs.

Psychosocial Development

The core psychosocial developmental task during infancy is the establishment of trust in others. Much of the infant's early psychosocial development is tactile in nature from touching and holding, especially with feeding. Feeding is the infant's primary means of establishing human relationships. The close mother-infant bonding in the feeding process fills the basic need to build trust. The need for sucking and the development of the oral organs, the lips and mouth, as sensory organs represent adaptations that ensure an adequate early food intake for survival. As a result, food becomes the infant's general means of exploring the environment and is one of the early means of communication. The infant has additional "nonnutritive" sucking need that is satisfied especially with the extra effort required in sucking while breastfeeding. As muscular coordination involving the tongue and the swallowing reflex develops, infants gradually learn to eat a variety of semisolid foods, beginning about 6 months of age. As physical and motor maturation proceed, infants begin to show a desire for self-feeding. When these stages of development occur, the exploration of new powers should be encouraged. If their needs for food and love are fulfilled in this early relationship with the mother, father, other caregivers, or family members, trust is developed. They evidence this trust by an increasing capacity to wait a few minutes for feedings until they are prepared.

Breastfeeding

The ideal food for the human infant is human milk. It has specific characteristics that match the infant's nutritional requirements during the first year of life. The process of breastfeeding today, as in the past, is successfully initiated and maintained by most mothers who try. However, sometimes there are problems when getting started, as well as a high degree of variability among nursing mothers as to frequency of feedings, intake per feeding, and infant growth. Thus in providing support for mothers who want to breastfeed their babies, experienced nutritionists and nurses, many of whom are certified professional lactation counselors, advise flexibility rather than a rigid approach.

The mother's breasts, or mammary glands, are highly specialized secretory organs, as indicated in Chapter 11 and illustrated in Figure 11-2. They are composed of glandular tissue, fat, and connective tissue. The secreting glandular tissue has 15 to 24 lobes, each containing many smaller units called *lobules.* In the lobules secretory cells called *alveoli* or *acini* form milk from the nutrient material supplied to them via a rich capillary system. During pregnancy the breasts are prepared for lactation. The alveoli enlarge and multiply, and toward the end of the prenatal period they secrete a thin, yellowish fluid called colostrum, which contains important antibodies and proteins. Hormonal components in breast milk also enhance the maturation of the gastrointestinal tract. As the infant grows, the breast milk develops, adapting in composition to meet growth needs.

A topic of current research is the nutritional benefit of the substantial amounts of the long-chain fatty acids *arachidonic acid* and *docosahexaenoic acid* provided in breast milk.[15] These fatty acids appear to play a special role in development of the brain and tissue of the retina,[16] and it has been suggested that the addition of these fatty acids to formula would be beneficial to formula-fed infants. However, such an addition to infant formula would require extensive testing and the approval of the Food and Drug Administration.[15]

Breast milk is produced under the stimulating influence of the hormone *prolactin* from the anterior pituitary gland. After the milk is formed in the mammary lobules by the clusters of secretory cells (alveoli or acini), it is carried through converging branches of the lactiferous ducts to reservoir spaces called ampullae located under the areola, the pigmented area of skin surrounding the nipple. Another pituitary hormone, *oxytocin,* stimulates the ejection of the milk from the alveoli to the ducts, releasing it to the baby. This is commonly called the *let-down reflex.* It causes a tingling sensation in the breast and the flow of milk. The initial sucking of the baby stimulates this reflex. The newborn rooting reflex, oral needs for sucking, and basic hunger drive usually induce and maintain normal relaxed breastfeeding for the healthy mother.

---

ampullae A general term for a flasklike wider portion of a tubular structure; spaces under the nipple of the breast for storing milk.

areola A defined space; a circular area of different color surrounding a central point, such as the darkened pigmented ring surrounding the nipple of the breast.

autonomy The state of functioning independently, without extraneous influence.

colostrum Thin yellow fluid first secreted by the mammary gland a few days before and after childbirth, preceding the mature breast milk. It contains up to 20% protein including a large amount of lactalbumin, more minerals and less lactose and fat than in mature milk, and immunoglobulins representing the antibodies found in maternal blood.

lactiferous ducts Branching channels in the mammary gland that carry breast milk to holding spaces near the nipple ready for the infant's feeding.

rooting reflex A reflex in a newborn in which stimulation of the side of the cheek or the upper or lower lip causes the infant to turn its mouth and face to the stimulus.

tactile Pertaining to the touch.

The mother should follow the baby's lead with an on-demand schedule. The baby's continuing rhythm of need establishes feedings, usually about every 2 to 3 hours in the first few weeks after birth.[5,14] The newborn's rooting reflex and somewhat recessed lower jaw are natural adaptations for feeding at the breast. The mother can feed the baby for about 5 to 10 minutes on each breast, burping the baby gently between each period of sucking to expel swallowed air. When the baby is satisfied, he or she can be removed from the breast. The nipple should air dry to prevent irritation and soreness. Interval use of a pacifier provides more sucking if needed.

The mother's diet and rest are important factors in establishing lactation and breastfeeding. Table 11-2 suggests a balanced diet to support ample milk production, including food choices from various food groups for meals and snacks. Natural thirst guides adequate fluid intake. Sufficient rest and relaxation for the mother are essential. An adequate energy intake is especially important in the early weeks to establish regular milk production. A gradual weight loss occurs naturally as maternal fat stores are slowly depleted, but the mother should not expect a rapid return to her prepregnancy weight. Overweight mothers with a body mass index between 25 and 30 kg/m^2 lost about 1 lb a week while successfully breastfeeding their infants.[17] These infants were fed on demand and grew normally; however, rigorous dieting should not be undertaken by breastfeeding mothers.

Breastfeeding may influence feeding behavior on into childhood.[18-20] A recent study suggested that breastfed infants are less likely to become obese as children as are infants who are formula-fed, although more studies are needed to affirm this finding.[20] Infants who develop a pattern of eating in moderation are less likely to become obese, and breastfed infants have more control over the amount of milk they consume than do formula-fed infants.[13] Formula-fed infants may be urged to empty their bottle even though they may turn away when they are satisfied. Force-feeding is less likely to occur in the breastfed infant but should be avoided in all infants. Feeding should be discontinued at the first sign that the infant has had enough. Children who gain weight more rapidly during the first 4 months of life are more likely to be overweight at age 7.[21] A breastfeeding mother needs to be aware that her infant will likely gain weight more slowly than bottle-fed infants, but this should not be a concern.[22]

A growing public health issue in the United States and worldwide is the advisability of breastfeeding by human immunodeficiency virus (HIV)-positive mothers, as breastfeeding can be a route of HIV transmission to an infant.[23] In African countries where formula is very expensive and clean water is not readily available, the risks of bottle feeding may still outweigh the risk of HIV transmission for breastfed infants. For the premature and low-birth-weight baby, feeding through the first year of life poses more problems.

Bottle-Feeding

Formula feeding by bottle may be preferred by some mothers. If the mother does not choose to breastfeed or stops breastfeeding before her infant reaches the age of 1 year, bottle-feeding of an appropriate formula is an acceptable alternative. A variety of commercial formulas that attempt to approximate the composition of human milk are available. Some of the cow's milk–based formulas are adjusted with whey protein to more nearly approximate the protein ratio in human milk.

Special formulas have been developed for infants with allergies, lactose intolerance, diarrhea, fat malabsorption, or other problems,[24] and several types of constituent proteins and carbohydrates are used. These include cow's milk protein, soy protein, casein hydrolysate, or elemental formulas (amino acids) (Table 12-5). Hypoallergenic formulas have been developed for infants who are allergic to cow's milk or commercial formulas based on cow's milk and have existing symptoms of that allergy.[20] Even partially hydrolyzed proteins can provoke an allergic response in infants with hypersensitivity to cow's milk. In the preparation of hypoallergenic formulas, all proteins are completely hydrolyzed to free amino acids. Although soy formulas are tolerated by some infants allergic to cow's milk, they are not hypoallergenic.

In recent years there has been growing use of soy protein–based infant formulas, and it is estimated that by 6 months of age, 16% of formula-fed infants in the United States are on this type of formula.[25] At one time soy protein–based formula was used primarily to feed infants who could not tolerate the protein from cow's milk or the lactose found in standard formulas, but the use of soy protein–based formulas has been growing among parents who wish to feed their infants vegetarian diets. Also, soy protein–based formulas have been effective in the management of babies with acute diarrhea. To ensure an appropriate complement of amino acids, soy protein–based formulas are supplemented with methionine, one of the sulfur-containing essential amino acids.

Standards for the levels of nutrients required in infant formulas are based on recommendations from the American Academy of Pediatrics. Minimum levels have been established for protein, fat, and 27 micronutrients. Maximum levels have been set for 9 nutrients including vitamins A and D and iron.[5]

When feeding formula, the baby should be cradled by the arm, as in breastfeeding, keeping the baby's head upright as much as possible to avoid milk running into the ear canals and resulting in an ear infection. The close human touch and warmth are important. When the infant is obviously satisfied, extra milk should not be forced, regardless of the amount remaining in the bottle. Any remaining formula should be thrown away and not refrigerated for reuse. Infants usually take the amount of formula they need. Today most infants are fed on a so-called demand schedule, which works out to

TABLE 12-5 A Comparison of Types of Formulas Manufactured for Full-Term Infants

Type of Formula Used		Protein Content	Fat Content	Carbohydrate Content
Milk-based routine	Source:	Nonfat cow's milk	Vegetable oils	Lactose
	g/100 kcalories:	2.2-2.3	5.4-5.5	10.5-10.8
	% kcalories:	9	48-50	41-43
Whey-adjusted routine	Source:	Nonfat cow's milk plus demineralized whey	Vegetable and oleo oils	Lactose
	g/100 kcalories:	2.2	5.4	10.8
	% kcalories:	9	48	43
Soy isolate (cow's milk sensitivity)	Source:	Soy isolate	Vegetable oils	Corn syrup solids and/or sucrose
	g/100 kcalories:	2.5	5.3-5.5	10.3-10.6
	% kcalories:	10	47-50	41-42
Casein hydrolysate (protein sensitivity, galactosemia)	Source:	Casein hydrolysate	Corn oil, other vegetable oils and MCT	Tapioca starch and glucose, sucrose, or corn syrup solids
	g/100 kcalories:	2.8	5.0-5.6	10.2-11.0
	% kcalories:	11	45-50	41-44
Meat-based (cow's milk sensitivity, galactosemia)	Source:	Beef hearts	Sesame oil and beef heart fat	Tapioca starch and sucrose
	g/100 kcalories:	4.0	4.8	9
	% kcalories:	16	47	37

MCT, Medium-chain triglycerides.

be about every 2 to 3 hours. A healthy infant will soon establish an individual pattern according to growth requirements.

Cow's Milk

Regular unmodified cow's milk is not suitable for infants for several reasons.

1. It causes gastrointestinal bleeding.
2. Its renal solute load is too heavy for the infant's renal system to handle; this leaves too small a margin of safety for maintaining water balance, especially during illness, diarrhea, or hot weather.
3. Early exposure to cow's milk increases the risk of developing allergies to milk proteins.
4. It adversely affects nutritional status.[13,14] Not only is cow's milk low in iron but, also, iron status in the infant is lowered even further by the associated gastrointestinal bleeding and blood loss caused by this milk. In addition cow's milk is a poor source of vitamins C and E and essential fatty acids. Infants have need for fat; thus they should not be fed reduced fat milks such as nonfat or 2% fat. Low or nonfat milks do not provide (1) sufficient energy to support growth requirements, leading the infant to consume increased volumes of milk and excessive protein, and (2) sufficient linoleic acid, the essential fatty acid needed for growth and development of body tissues found in the fat portion of milk.[14] A specific form of eczema has been observed in infants deficient in linoleic acid, and a low-fat diet in infancy may impair physical and intellectual development.

To meet the special needs of infants, the American Academy of Pediatrics recommends breast milk or formula as the major food source up to 1 year of age, with a gradual addition of appropriate foods beginning at 4 to 6 months.[5,13] There is no need for special formulas for older infants; such formulas also present an added expense to the family.

The Premature Infant

Infants born too small or too early have many food-related difficulties to overcome and present a special

casein hydrolysate formula Infant formula composed of hydrolyzed casein, a major milk protein, produced by partially breaking down the casein into smaller peptide fragments, making a product that is more easily digested.

elemental formula A nutrition support formula composed of single elemental nutrient components that require no further digestive breakdown and thus are readily absorbed. Infant formula produced with elemental, ready-to-be-absorbed components of free amino acids and carbohydrate as simple sugars.

renal solute load Collective number and concentration of solute particles in a solution carried by the blood to the kidney nephrons for excretion in the urine. The particles are usually nitrogenous products from protein metabolism and the electrolyte sodium.

TABLE 12-6 Nutritional Value of Special Formulas and Human Milk for the Preterm Infant

Nutritional Component	Advisable Intake for Birth Weight 1.0 kg (2.2 lb)	Advisable Intake for Birth Weight 1.5 kg (3.3 lb)	Human Milk Content Preterm	Human Milk Content Mature	Standard Formulas Enfamil* Similac† SMA‡	Special Premature Formulas Enfamil* Premature with whey*	Special Premature Formulas Similac Special Care†	Special Premature Formulas "Preemie" SMA‡
Kcalories/dl			73	73.0	67.0	81.0	81.0	81.0
Protein (g/200 kcalories)	3.1	2.7	2.6§	1.5	2.2	3.0	2.7	2.5
Vitamins, Fat-Soluble								
D (IU/120 kcalories/kg/day)	600.0	600.0	—	4.0	70-75	75.0	180.0	76.0
E (IU/120 kcalories/kg/day)	30.0	30.0	—	0.3	2-3	2.0	4.0	2.0
Vitamins, Water-Soluble								
Folic acid (μg/120 kcalories/kg/day)	60.0	60.0	—	8.0	9-19	36.0	45.0	14.0
Vitamin C (mg/120 kcalories/kg/day)	60.0	60.0	—	7.0	10.0	10.0	45.0	10.0
Minerals								
Calcium (mg/100 kcalories)	160.0	140.0	40.0	43.0	66-68	117.0	178.0	92.0
Phosphorus (mg/100 kcalories)	108.0	95.0	18.0	20.0	49-66	58.0	89.0	49.0
Sodium (mEq/100 kcalories)	2.7	2.3	1.5‖	0.8	1.0-1.8	1.78	1.9	1.7

*Mead Johnson Nutritional Division, Evansville, Ind.
†Ross Laboratories, Columbus, Ohio.
‡Wyeth Laboratories, Philadelphia, Pa.
§Range: 1.9-2.8 g/100 kcalories.
‖Range: 0.9-2.3 mEq/100 kcalories.

challenge in feeding. A poor sucking reflex, difficulty in swallowing, small gastric capacity, reduced intestinal motility, tiring easily from eating and being handled, and increased nutrient requirements for catch-up growth all need to be considered. The health team involved in the care of premature and small-for-gestational-age infants is faced with a myriad of decisions to overcome these feeding difficulties. Whenever possible these infants are fed breast milk, usually fortified with additional protein, vitamins, and minerals to the levels found in special formulas developed to meet the particular needs of premature infants. Delivery of breast milk or formula using tube feeding (enteral feeding) carries less risk of complications than the delivery of nutrients through the veins (parenteral feeding).

A comparison of the nutrient content of breast milk and special formulas for the premature infant is presented in Table 12-6. Formulas developed for the premature infant may have as much as 30% more protein per fluid volume than those developed for the normal infant, as well as higher amounts of calcium, zinc, and the B-complex vitamins. This enriched formula also supports catch-up growth in term infants who are small-for-gestational-age.[26] Nutritional support of the high-risk infant requires a team approach that includes the pediatrician, the nurse, the dietitian, and a lactation counselor who can assist the mother in developing a routine for expressing and safely storing her milk to feed her infant.

Beikost: Solid Food Additions

Beikost feeding begins the transition from a predominantly liquid diet to a predominantly solid food diet. Nutritional and medical authorities agree that for the first 4 to 6 months of life the optimal single food for the infant is human milk or an appropriate formula. There is no nutritional basis for introducing solid foods to infants earlier than 4 to 6 months of age, and before this age it may contribute to overfeeding.[13] Until then the infant does not need any additional food and is not able to adequately handle other foods. In addition to nutritional reasons, there are developmental reasons for delaying the addition of solid foods until the age of 4 to 6 months. The following developmental tasks must have been mastered before the infant is prepared to receive solid foods.

1. The infant can communicate desire and interest in food by opening his or her mouth and leaning forward or, conversely, leaning back or turning away, participating in the feeding process.
2. The infant can sit up with support and has good control of the trunk and neck.

TABLE 12-7 Guideline for Adding Solid Foods to Infant's Diet During the First Year*

When to Start	Foods Added	Feeding
Months 5-6	Cereal and strained cooked fruit	10 AM and 6 PM
	Egg yolk (at first, hard cooked and sieved; soft boiled or poached later)	
	Strained, cooked vegetable and strained meat	2 PM
	Zwieback or hard toast	At any feeding
Months 7-9	Meat: beef, lamb, or liver (broiled or baked and finely chopped)	10 AM and 6 PM
	Potato: baked or boiled and mashed or sieved	
Suggested Meal Plan for 8 Months to 1 Year or Older		
7 AM	Milk	240 ml (8 oz)
	Cereal	2-3 tbsp
	Strained fruit	2-3 tbsp
	Zwieback or dry toast	
12 NOON	Milk	240 ml (8 oz)
	Vegetables	2-3 tbsp
	Chopped meat or one whole egg	
	Puddings or cooked fruit	2-3 tbsp
3 PM	Milk	120 ml (4 oz)
	Toast, zwieback, or crackers	
6 PM	Milk	240 ml (8 oz)
	Whole egg or chopped meat	
	Potato: baked or mashed	2 tbsp
	Pudding or cooked fruit	2-3 tbsp
	Zwieback or toast	

*Semisolid foods should be given immediately before milk feeding. One or 2 tsp should be given first. If food is accepted and tolerated well, the amount should be increased to 1 to 2 tbsp per feeding.

NOTE: Banana or cottage cheese may be used as substitution for any meal.

3. The infant has developed the ability to move food to the back of the mouth for swallowing.

Developmental abilities to use the hands and fingers are required before self-feeding can be initiated. Self-feeding efforts begin first with a whole hand (palmar) grasp and then move to a more refined finger (pincer) grasp by the end of the first year. The first item for self-feeding may be a piece of Melba toast that can be grasped with the whole hand. As solid food is gradually added, the amount of breast milk or formula consumed is reduced accordingly.

Both cultural patterns and the age and educational level of the mother influence infant-feeding practices. Some of these practices, such as adding cereal to the infant's bottle to help the baby sleep through the night, are related more to the convenience of the mother than to the benefit of the infant.[27,28] It may not be in the infant's best interests to sleep through the night at a very early age or to adapt as early as possible to three meals a day. Smaller amounts of food, eaten on a more frequent basis, may contribute to the pattern of eating in moderation.[13]

The traditional transition food is fortified infant cereal—specifically, infant rice cereal mixed with a little milk or formula, because rice cereal has the least potential for allergic reaction. Fruits, vegetables, egg yolk, potato, and finally meat can be added to the diet in a gradual sequence. No one sequence of food additions must be followed. A general guide is given in Table 12-7. Single foods are given first, one at a time in small amounts; in this way, adverse reactions can be identified. These foods are usually offered before the milk feeding. Individual responses and needs can be a basis for choice, as food becomes a source of enjoyment and a new means of bonding warm family relationships. A basic goal during this time is to have the infant learn to enjoy many different foods. This is the perfect time to introduce a wide variety of foods because infants appear to be more willing to taste new foods than are toddlers; in fact, the greater the variety of foods presented when the addition of solid food is begun, the greater the number of foods the infant will accept when first presented.[29] Breastfed infants seem to be more receptive to new foods with new flavors, and it has been suggested that exposure to a variety of flavors in

palmar grasp Early grasp of the young infant, clasping an object in the palm and wrapping the whole hand around it.

pincer grasp Later digital grasp of the older infant, usually picking up smaller objects with a precise grip between thumb and forefinger.

breast milk, the result of the mother's varied diet, helps prepare an infant to accept new flavors and foods.[30]

Many commercial baby foods are available and are prepared without the formerly used ingredients of sugar, salt, or monosodium glutamate. Some mothers prefer preparing their own baby food. This can be done by cooking and straining vegetables and fruits and forming a puree using a blender, food processor, or Foley mill. These foods can be frozen in ice cube trays or in 1-tablespoon amounts on a cookie sheet. The cubes or individual portions are easily stored in plastic bags in the freezer. Then a single portion can be reheated conveniently for use at a feeding. When working with mothers it is important to stress the need for a clean environment when preparing infant foods to avoid the danger of foodborne illness.

Two foods that require special attention in infant feeding are honey and fruit juices. Honey should never be given to an infant who is younger than 1 year because it can lead to botulism, a fatal condition in infants. Some fruit juices, including apple, pear, and prune, contain sorbitol, which can lead to diarrhea in infants and toddlers.

Two basic principles should guide the feeding process: (1) it is nutrients that are needed, not specific foods; and (2) food is a main basis of early learning. Food not only provides for physical sustenance but also fulfills other personal development and cultural needs. Good food habits are formed early in life and continue to develop as a child grows older. By the time infants are about 8 or 9 months old, they should be able to eat family foods that are cooked, chopped, or mashed and simply seasoned, without the need for special infant foods. Throughout the first year of life the infant's needs for physical growth and psychosocial development will be met by breast milk or formula, a variety of solid food additions, and a loving, trusting relationship between parents and child (Figure 12-1).

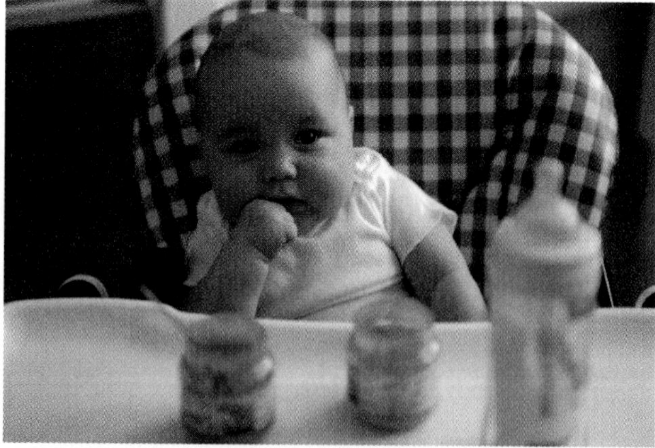

FIGURE 12-1 This child is taking a variety of solid food additions and developing wide tastes. Here, feeding serves as a source not only of physical growth but also of psychosocial development. Optimal physical development and security are evident, the result of sound nutrition and loving care. (*Credit: PhotoDisc.*)

TODDLER (1 TO 3 YEARS)

Physical Characteristics and Growth

After the rapid growth of the first year, the growth rate of children slows. But although the rate of gain is less, the pattern of growth produces significant changes in body form. The legs become longer, and the child begins losing baby fat. There is less total body water and more of the remaining water is inside the cells. The young child begins to look and feel less like a baby and more like a child. Energy demands are lower because of the slackened growth rate. However, important muscle development is taking place. In fact, muscle mass development accounts for about one half of the total weight gain during this period. As the child begins to walk and stand erect, more muscle is needed to strengthen the body and support these movements. For example, there is special need for big muscles in the back, the buttocks, and the thighs. The overall rate of skeletal growth slows, with greater deposits of mineral in existing bone rather than a lengthening of the bones. The increased mineralization strengthens the bones to support the increasing body weight. The child has six to eight teeth at the beginning of the toddler period. By 3 years of age the remainder of the deciduous teeth have erupted.

Psychosocial Development

The psychosocial development of the toddler is pronounced. The core developmental problem they struggle with is the desire for autonomy. Each child has a profound increasing sense of self—of being a distinct and individual person apart from the parents, not just an extension of them. As physical mobility increases, the sense of autonomy and independence grows. An expanding curiosity leads to much exploration of the environment, and increasingly the mouth is used as a means of exploring. Touch is important, providing the means of learning what objects are like. The constant use of "no" reflects the significant struggle with newly emerging ego needs in conflict with the caregiver's control efforts. The child wants to do more and more, but the attention span is fairly short and interest shifts quickly from one thing to another.

Food and Feeding

Physical growth and psychosocial development during the toddler period influence nutrient needs (see Tables 12-2 to 12-4) and food patterns (see *Practical Application* box).

1. *Energy.* The need for kcalories is not high because of the relative decrease in growth rate after the first year of life. The energy requirement now increases very slowly in small spurts. At about 1 year of age, children need approximately 850 kcalories/day, and this rises to 1200 kcalories by age 3.[4] From age 1 to 2, some children do not eat as much as they did in the second half of infancy. Caregivers will avoid conflict with their toddler about eating if they remember this decrease in need for kcalories is normal, resulting from

PRACTICAL APPLICATION
Feeding Toddlers and Preschoolers: Nutrition is a Family Affair

No matter what their age, children need the same nutrients as adults but in different amounts. The challenge for parents and caregivers is to make available appropriate and appealing foods and to set the time and place for eating. Young children must learn how to make food choices and to decide how much food they need to consume.

We can help parents and caregivers develop child-feeding strategies based on the developmental needs of their young children. First we must remind them that their children are not growing as fast as they did during the first year of life; it follows that they need less food. Also, a child's energy needs are sporadic; therefore periods of greater food intake will vary with periods of smaller intake. Forcing food during periods of low intake may encourage overeating or food aversion, leading to food intake problems later in life.

AMOUNT OF FOOD

Children are not ready for adult-size portions and may be overwhelmed by large amounts of food on their plate. It is better to serve less food than they are likely to eat and to have them ask for more. In planning portion sizes, a good rule of thumb is 1 tablespoon of food for every year of age. When the child begins to play with the food on the plate or seems to lose interest in eating, remove the plate and provide another activity.

FEEDING FREQUENCY

Children do best with a regular feeding schedule; try to keep meals and snacks at regular times. Young children have small stomachs and it is difficult for them to consume enough food at one meal to last them until the next meal. They may need to eat 5 or 6 times a day. Try to allow at least 1½ or 2 hours between snacks and meals. When choosing between-meal snacks, look to foods that will provide not only additional kcalories but also protein and important vitamins and minerals. Fruit, crackers, raw vegetables (as appropriate), cheese, milk, and cereal are good snacks. It is best if children are not overtired at mealtime; if possible, plan a short rest period immediately before a meal.

WHAT FOODS

Over time it is important for the young child to learn to eat a variety of foods, although it may be necessary to offer a new food 8 to 10 times, each including at least a taste, before it will be accepted. The child should learn to eat what other family members are eating and not be provided with special foods. But when planning meals, be sure to have one item that the child likes and will eat. Also, children are more willing to try a new food if it is accompanied by a favorite food; try to pair such foods at the same meal. Serve dessert, if any, with the main meal rather than later; it should not assume special importance in relation to other foods. Do allow your toddler or preschooler to make some choices about foods for meals or snacks just as older children are able to do. This develops skills in making food choices.

Avoid Forbidding Certain Foods

All foods, including sweets, can be included in a healthy diet for young children if limited in frequency and amount. It is important that children learn how to moderate their intakes of such foods. Excluding certain foods makes them more attractive and ultimately leads to increased intake when they do become available.

FOOD SAFETY

Two major safety considerations in feeding children are avoidance of foodborne illness and the possibility of choking. Young children are very vulnerable to foodborne illness resulting from (1) foods that are not fully cooked, such as hamburger or eggs, (2) foods that became contaminated by contact with an unwholesome food or other source of bacteria, or (3) improperly stored food with bacterial growth. Eating such foods can lead to serious illness or even death in the young child, as occurred when preschoolers ate improperly cooked hamburger at a fast food restaurant. Children must be taught at a young age to wash their hands thoroughly after they use the bathroom and before they touch a food. Parents should ask about food handling and other sanitary practices when evaluating the suitability of a caregiver or a care facility.

Children younger than 4 years are at greatest risk for choking and death by asphyxiation. Foods most likely to cause choking are those that are round and hard and do not dissolve in saliva. Typical items that cause choking are hot dogs, grapes, peanut butter in globs, hard pieces of raw fruits and vegetables, hard candy, or popcorn. Young children should always be supervised when eating and should eat sitting down.

SOCIAL ENVIRONMENT AT MEAL TIME

Try to keep mealtime as pleasant as possible. Allow enough time for the young child to eat. Having to hurry adds stress to mealtime and takes away the pleasure of eating, especially for the child who is still learning to self-feed. Be patient about spills or accidents; it takes time to develop feeding skills. Choose appropriate utensils that are unbreakable and easy for the child to grasp. Children are less likely to accept a food that was first introduced in

Continued

PRACTICAL APPLICATION

Feeding Toddlers and Preschoolers: Nutrition is a Family Affair—cont'd

a negative meal situation; therefore make mealtime an enjoyable family time that reinforces positive eating behaviors. Parental modeling is an important influence in encouraging children to try new foods. Toddlers are more likely to taste a new food if they see an adult, especially a familiar adult or parent, eating it. Children model the eating behavior of parents and caregivers; be sure that others at the table are eating vegetables and drinking milk. Parental modeling is as important in the choice of snacks as it is at mealtime.

NOTE: You may wish to visit the website of the U.S. Department of Agriculture Center for Nutrition Policy and Promotion at *http://www.usda.gov/cnpp/* to view the *Food Guide Pyramid for Young Children* and tips for its use.

References

Duyff RL: *The American Dietetic Association's complete food & nutrition guide,* Minneapolis, Minn, 1998, Chronimed Publishing.

Fisher JO, Birch LL: Restricting access to palatable foods affects children's behavioral response, food selection, and intake, *Am J Clin Nutr* 69:1264, 1999.

Kleinman RE, ed: *Pediatric nutrition handbook,* ed 4, Elk Grove Village, Ill, 1998, American Academy of Pediatrics.

Nicklas TA et al: Family and child-care provider influences on preschool children's fruit, juice, and vegetable consumption, *Nutr Rev* 59(7):224, 2001.

Thorpe M: Parents as role models: nutrition is a family affair, *J Am Diet Assoc* 102(1):64, 2002.

Tibbs T et al: The relationship between parental modeling, eating patterns, and dietary intake among African-American parents, *J Am Diet Assoc* 101(5):535, 2001.

a slowing in the growth rate and the child's necessary struggle for autonomy and selfhood, which often involves refusal of food. Appetite varies in the toddler; therefore food intake may be irregular with periods of good appetite and periods of disinterest in food. Encouragement is needed from caregivers, but constant conflict with the child about eating serves no useful purpose. A small plate of snacks, including finger food pieces of raw fruit and cheese kept in the refrigerator or a few crackers on a special colorful plate, can give the child a measure of positive control when hungry. Toddlers will eat when they are hungry. Positive early experiences help develop appropriate food acceptance patterns.[1]

2. *Protein.* In relation to energy (kcalorie) needs, protein needs are relatively increased during this stage of life. The toddler requires about 13 g of protein/day.[4] Muscle and other body tissues are growing rapidly. At least half of this protein should be of animal origin because animal protein has high biologic value. This does not mean that meat, poultry, or fish is necessary. Children who follow a balanced and well-planned ovolactovegetarian diet grow just as well and attain similar heights as their nonvegetarian counterparts.[5]

   Diets planned for vegan children will need to incorporate soy and legume protein and build on the complementarity of plant proteins (see Chapter 5).
3. *Minerals.* Calcium and phosphorus are needed for bone mineralization. The bones are strengthening to keep pace with muscle development and increasing activity. Iron is needed to maintain adequate hemoglobin levels as the increase in body size requires an increasing blood volume. Adequate levels of zinc are necessary to support protein synthesis and cell division. The principle of increasing iron absorption from nonheme sources such as vegetables by including a small amount of heme iron from meat at the same meal, as discussed in Chapter 8, holds true for feeding the toddler.
4. *Food choices.* About 2 to 3 cups of milk daily is sufficient for the young child's needs. Sometimes excessive milk intake, a habit carried over from infancy, excludes many solid foods from the diet. As a result, the child may lack iron and develop a so-called milk anemia. On the other hand, if a child dislikes milk as a beverage, replacement can be made with cheese, creamed soups, puddings, or custards, or nonfat dry milk can be used in cooked cereals, mashed potatoes, meatloaf, and casseroles. Calcium-fortified foods can assist in adding calcium to the diet. Offering the child an increasing variety of foods will help to develop good food habits because food habits are learned and there is little opportunity for learning if a child is not exposed to a wide variety of foods. Refined sweets are best avoided, reserving them for special occasions, not for habitual use or to bribe a child to eat.

Another important consideration when selecting food for the toddler is the risk of choking and death by asphyxiation. Foods that are round, hard, and not easily dissolved can cause choking. Such food items include hot dogs, grapes, peanut butter in globs, hard pieces of raw fruits and vegetables, hard candy, and popcorn. Young children should always be supervised when eating and should eat sitting down. Running when eating can lead to choking. It is best that children not eat in a moving car unless a second adult, in addition to the driver, is available to assist if needed.

Summary Principles

Two important principles to be emphasized when working with caregivers should guide feeding practices during this period.

1. The child needs fewer kcalories but relatively more protein and minerals for physical growth; therefore a variety of foods should be offered in smaller amounts to provide key nutrients. As more children are entering day care, it is important that day care providers and parents work cooperatively to support the development of good food patterns.[31]
2. The child is struggling for selfhood as part of normal psychosocial development. This struggle is expressed in refusing food and the desire to do things for self before being fully able to do them efficiently. If caregivers are patient, offer a variety of foods in small amounts, and encourage some degree of food choice and self-feeding in the child's own ceremonial manner, eating can be a happy, positive means of development.

If we are to achieve the goal of establishing good food patterns for life, it is especially important to introduce a variety of fruits and vegetables along with grains and meats during this stage of development. A study of 72 children from 2 to 5 years of age found that they ate rather few fruits and vegetables and that their food choices changed very little over the 3 years.[32] Only three fruits (apples, bananas, and grapes) and four vegetables (carrots, green beans, corn, and French fries) were included among their list of 19 favorite foods given by both mothers and children. Macaroni and cheese, pizza, chicken, and cereal were their four top foods, and fruit drinks, carbonated beverages, milk, and apple juice were the most commonly used beverages.

PRESCHOOLER (3 TO 6 YEARS)

Physical Characteristics and Growth

As shown in normal childhood growth charts (see Appendix I), each child tends to settle into a regular genetic growth channel as physical growth continues in spurts. On occasion the child bounds with energy. Play is hard play—running, jumping, and testing new physical resources. At other times the child will sit for increasing periods of time engrossed in passive types of activities. Mental capacities are developing, and there is more thinking and exploring of the environment. Energy needs and specific nutrients are shown in Tables 12-2 to 12-4. Protein requirements continue to increase as the child grows older. Preschool children need about 13 to 19 g/day of good-quality protein,[4] as found in milk, egg, meat, cheese, legumes, and soy. They continue to need calcium and iron to support growth and to build body stores. Because vitamins A and C and folate are often lacking in the diets of preschool children, a variety of fruits and vegetables should be provided. Vitamin D, important for calcium absorption, can be obtained in fortified milk or soy products or by spending time playing outdoors in the sun.

Psychosocial Development

Each stage of development builds on the previous one. The psychosocial developmental stage for preschool children involves increased socialization and initiative. They are beginning to develop their superego—the conscience. As powers of active movement increase, they have a growing imagination and curiosity. This is a period of increasing imitation and of sex identification. The little boy imitates his father or other male role models. The little girl copies the behavior of her mother or other female role models. Much of this becomes evident in their play by the use of grown-up clothes and role-playing in domestic or job situations. Self-feeding skills increase and eating takes on greater social aspects. The family mealtime is an important event for socialization and sex identification, as the children imitate their parents and others at the table.[33] This pattern of sex identification may have long-term implications in respect to calcium intake and health. In nearly 200 girls of kindergarten age, the best predictor of their milk intakes was the milk intakes of their mothers. If the mother drank soft drinks rather than milk, so did her daughter.[34]

Food and Feeding

The preschool child is beginning to form definite responses to various types of foods.

1. *Vegetables and fruits.* Fruits are usually well liked. However, of all the food groups, vegetables usually are the least well liked by children, yet these foods contain many vitamins and minerals needed for growth. Where there is space or opportunity, involving the young child in planting and growing vegetables in a small garden or in containers is an excellent way to draw the child's interest to vegetables to be tasted. Trips to the market or learning activities in the day care setting can help a child see a variety of shapes and colors in vegetables and discover new ones that can be prepared in a variety of ways. It is important to remember that children have a keen sense of taste; therefore flavor and texture are important. Children usually dislike strong vegetables such as cabbage and onions but do like crisp raw vegetables or fruits cut in small pieces to eat as finger foods. Tough strings and hard pieces are difficult to chew and swallow and should be

growth channel The progressive regular growth pattern of children, guided along individual genetically controlled channels, influenced by nutritional and health status.

removed. For example, it is easy to break a crisp piece of celery and remove the strings before giving it to a child. Children also react to consistency of vegetables, disliking them overcooked.

2. *Milk, cheese, egg, meat, and legumes.* It is helpful if children can set their own goals of quantities of food. Portions need to be relatively small (see *Practical Application* box). If children can pour their own milk from a small pitcher into a small glass, they will drink more. The quantity of milk needed usually declines during these years. The child will drink 2 or 3, and rarely 4, cups of milk during the day. Smaller children like their milk more at room temperature, not icy cold. Also, they prefer it in small glasses that hold about 4 oz to 6 oz rather than in large, adult-sized glasses. Cheese is a favorite finger food or snack; however, the major source of calcium in this age group is milk. Egg is usually well liked if hard-cooked or scrambled. Meat should be tender and easy to cut and chew; hence ground meat is popular, but ground meat also must be well cooked to make it safe. (To avoid the risk of foodborne illness that can be fatal in the young child, ground meat should be cooked to a temperature of 160° F, the meat should have a gray white color, and juices should be clear.)
3. *Grains.* The wide variety in which grains can be eaten adds to their appeal to children who enjoy breads, cereals, and crackers. To avoid unwanted kcalories, presweetened cereals should be used infrequently if at all.
4. *Temperature.* Because children prefer their foods lukewarm and not hot, some foods may remain on their plates and become dry and gummy such that the child refuses to eat it. Thus very small portions should be served at a time.
5. *Single foods.* Children usually prefer single foods to combination dishes such as casseroles or stews. This is a period of language learning for children. They like to learn names of foods and to be able to recognize and name them on the basis of their shape, color, texture, and taste; these identifiable characteristics need to be retained as much as possible.
6. *Finger foods.* Children like to eat food they can pick up with their fingers. When appetites lag, fruits might be substituted for vegetables. Often a variety of raw fruits and vegetables cut into finger-sized pieces and offered to children for their own selection provide a source of needed nutrition.
7. *Food jags.* Because of developing social and emotional needs, preschool children commonly follow "food jags," refusing to eat all except one particular food such as peanut butter. This may last for several days, but it is usually short lived and of no major consequence.

The preschool period is one of important growth for the young child. Lifetime food habits are forming. Food continues to play an important part in the developing personality, and group eating becomes significant as a means of socialization. The social and emotional environment and companionship at mealtime with family, other caregivers, or other children greatly influence the young child's food intake and diet quality. The child learns food patterns at the family table and follows the examples of food eaten by parents or older siblings.[35] The child may attend a day care or preschool in which group eating occurs. Food habits of preschoolers are greatly affected by peer modeling, and food preferences develop according to what the group is eating. Children in this stage of development may begin to respond to environmental cues encouraging them to consume more food than they need. In a day care setting it was found that 5-year-old children ate more food when presented with larger portions, whereas 3½-year-old children were not affected by portion size.[36] In light of the growing numbers of overweight children, we need to encourage parents to be alert to portion size when serving their children's food.

This stage of growth is also a time for the young child to develop appropriate patterns of physical exercise, and games including activities such as skipping or jumping should be encouraged in a safe environment. Physical fitness established at an early age can lower the risk of obesity in both childhood and adulthood.[37] Encouraging young children to participate in active games rather than sedentary pastimes such as watching videos or television may support appropriate food patterns as well. Even a 30-second commercial for a snack food has been shown to influence the food choices of preschool-age children.[38]

THE SCHOOL-AGE CHILD (6 TO 12 YEARS)

Physical Characteristics and Growth

The school-age period preceding adolescence has been called the latent time of growth. During this stage the rate of growth slows, and body changes occur very gradually. However, resources are being laid down for the rapid adolescent growth that lies ahead; sometimes this has been called the lull before the storm. By now the body type has been established, and growth rates vary widely. Girls usually outdistance boys in the latter part of this period.

Psychosocial Development

Psychosocial development during these early school years centers on the formal learning environment and its expectations. Children have widening horizons, new school experiences, and challenging learning opportunities. They develop increased mental powers and the ability to work out problems and face competitive activities. They learn to cooperate in group activities and begin to experience a sense of adequacy and accomplishment and sometimes the frustration of not winning. The child begins to move from a dependence on parental standards to those of peers, first steps in preparing for coming maturity and self-growth. Pressures are generated for self-control of a growing body, and inappropriate concepts of body image that lead to chronic dieting or eating disorders likely take root during this period. Negative attitudes sometimes expressed and changes in temperament are evidence of these struggles for growing independence. It is a diffuse period of gangs, cliques, hero worship, pensive daydreaming, emotional stress, and learning to get along with other children.

Food and Feeding

The slowed rate of growth during this period results in a gradual decline in the food requirement per unit of body weight. This decline continues up to the period just before approaching adolescence. Likes and dislikes are a product of earlier years. Family food attitudes are imitated, but increasing outside activities compete with family mealtimes, and family conflicts may arise.

School and the Learning Environment

Research has firmly established the close relationship between sound nutrition and childhood learning.[37] Breakfast is particularly important for the school-age child. It breaks the fast of the sleep hours and prepares the child for problem-solving and memory in the learning hours at school. The School Breakfast and Lunch Programs provide nourishing school meals that many children would not otherwise have (see Chapter 10). School programs implemented by the U.S. Department of Agriculture help to maintain sound nutrition by implementing the *Dietary Guidelines for Americans* into child breakfast and lunch programs,[39,40] developing recipes that lower the fat in school lunch entrees and desserts,[41] and preventing the initiation of snack bars that sell soft drinks and snack foods as an alternative to the cafeteria school lunch[42] (see *Issues & Answers*). Schools should also take a leadership role in promoting lifelong physical activity patterns in children. Health professionals must take a leadership role in their communities to ensure that school meal programs provide positive examples of nutritionally appropriate meal patterns and introduce children to new foods that he or she may not have tasted previously.

The school-age child has increasing exposure to both positive and negative influences on food habits. Television becomes a powerful source of food information. At the same time positive learning opportunities can occur in the classroom when nutrition education is integrated with other activities, and parents provide support and reinforcement at home. An important learning experience can be the preparation of simple meals; in an urban community, 35% of the children in third grade ate at least one meal a day that they prepared themselves or was prepared by a brother or sister.[43]

Although changes in physical activity no doubt have contributed to the growing number of overweight children, some researchers have also pointed to changes in snacking habits. A comparison of diet surveys during the past 25 years indicated that today's children do not select snacks that are higher in kcalories than children in past years but that they eat more snacks more often, which has added to their energy intakes.[44] An important message to children should be to snack only when they are hungry; snacking should not be a pastime, and the best snacks are those that are relatively low in kcalories but rich in protein, vitamins, and minerals.

Sound nutrition is especially critical for the child athlete. Children aged 6 to 12 years engaged in athletic competition need appropriate nutritional advice from parents, coaches, and trained professionals to meet their energy, protein, and fluid needs for training and competition.[45]

THE ADOLESCENT

Physical Characteristics and Growth

During the adolescent period, with the onset of puberty, the final growth spurt of childhood occurs. Maturation during this time varies so widely that chronologic age as a reference point for discussing growth ceases to be useful. Physiologic age becomes more important in dealing with individual boys and girls. Adolescent growth accounts for wide fluctuations in physical size, metabolic rate, food needs, and even illness. These capacities can be more realistically viewed only in terms of physiologic growth.

The profound body changes occurring in the adolescent result from the release of estrogen and testosterone, the sex steroid hormones that regulate the development of the sex characteristics. The rate at which these body changes occur varies widely and is particularly distinct in the growth patterns that emerge between the sexes. In girls the amount of subcutaneous fat increases, particularly in the abdominal area. The hip breadth widens in preparation for childbearing. This fat accumulation and change in body shape are often sources of anxiety to many figure-conscious young girls. In adolescent boys physical growth is manifested by an increased muscle mass and long-bone growth. The growth spurt in boys is slower than that in girls, but he soon passes her in weight and height.

Psychosocial Development

Adolescence is an ambivalent period marked by stresses and strains. On the one hand, teenagers look back to the securities of childhood; on the other hand, they reach for the maturity of adulthood. Emergence of a self-identity is the major psychosocial developmental task of the adolescent years. The search for self, begun in early childhood,

---

physiologic age Rate of biologic maturation in individual adolescents that varies widely and accounts more for wide and changing differences in their metabolic rates, nutritional needs, and food requirements than does chronologic age.

reaches its climax in the identity crisis of the teen years. The profound body changes associated with sexual development and the capability of reproduction also result in changes in body image and resulting tensions in maturing girls and boys.

The identity crisis of the adolescent years, largely revolving around sexual development and preparation for an adult role in a complex society, produces many psychologic, emotional, and social pressures. Although the period of most rapid physical growth is relatively short, only 2 or 3 years, the attendant psychosocial development continues over a much longer period. The pressure for peer group acceptance is strong, and fads in dress and food habits play out this theme. Also, in a technologically developed society such as the United States, high values are placed on education and achievement. Social tensions and family conflicts are created. These conflicts may have nutritional consequences as teenagers eat away from home more often and develop a snacking pattern of personal and peer-group food choices.

Food and Feeding

With the rapid growth of adolescence comes increased demands for energy, protein, vitamins, and minerals.

1. *Energy.* The kcalorie needs increase with the metabolic demands of growth and energy expenditure. Although individual needs may vary, girls require fewer kcalories than boys, based on their smaller body size and body composition.[4] Sometimes the large appetite, characteristic of this rapid growth period, leads adolescents to satisfy their hunger with snack foods that are high in sugar and fat and low in essential protein, vitamins, and minerals.
2. *Protein.* Adolescent growth needs for protein increase to support the pubertal changes in both sexes and the developing muscle mass in boys. Girls require 46 g/day and boys require 52 g/day to sustain daily needs and to maintain nitrogen reserves.[4]
3. *Minerals.* The calcium requirement for all adolescents rises to 1300 mg/day to meet the demands of bone growth. In fact, adolescence is a critical time for the development of bone mass under the influence of the increasing levels of the sex hormones, especially estrogen. Poor bone mineralization in adolescence increases vulnerability to bone fracture at later ages.[46] The beginning of the menses and consequent iron losses in the adolescent girl predispose her to simple iron deficiency anemia. Young female athletes such as gymnasts and runners, who begin their training before menarche, can develop secondary amenorrhea and in turn reduced bone mineral density resulting from low estrogen levels.[47] For all young athletes, fluid replacement in any exercise or performance period is essential.[45]
4. *Vitamins.* The B vitamins are needed in increased amounts to meet the extra demands of energy metabolism and tissue development. Intakes of vitamins C and A may be low because of erratic food intake and low intake of vegetables and fruits. A high prevalence of folate deficiency exists among adolescent girls, increasing the risk of neural tube defects in babies born to teenage mothers. (For a review of neural tube defects see Chapter 7.)

In the development of nutrition intervention programs for teens, it is also important to consider their cultural and ethnic backgrounds, recognizing that food habits and food problems may differ. A study of more than 2800 adolescents that included Vietnamese, Hispanic, African American, and Caucasian students showed clearly that intakes of fruits, vegetables, and dairy products differed according to group.[48] The Vietnamese adolescents were the least likely to meet the recommended three servings of dairy products each day compared with the African American, Hispanic, or Caucasian adolescents. Conversely, the Vietnamese students were the most likely to meet the goal of five fruits and vegetables a day. We also need to consider cost when making nutritional recommendations to students or mothers. Among limited-resource mothers, fruits and some vegetables were perceived as being less filling, and one mother noted it was more important to have her son's hunger satisfied than to provide particular fruits or vegetables.[49] Nutrition counseling must be individualized, taking into consideration both cultural food preferences and other circumstances existing within the family.

Eating Habits

Physical and psychosocial pressures influence adolescent eating behavior (see *To Probe Further* box). By and large, boys fare better than girls. Their large appetites and the sheer volumes of food they consume usually ensure generally adequate nutrient intakes, but the adolescent girl may be less fortunate. Two factors combine to increase her anxiety surrounding her body weight.

1. *Physiologic sex differences.* Because sexual maturation in girls brings about increased fat deposition during the adolescent growth period and because many teenage girls are relatively inactive, it is easy for them to gain weight.
2. *Social and personal tensions.* Social pressures dictating thinness sometimes cause adolescent girls to follow unwise and self-imposed crash diets for weight loss. In some cases actual self-starvation regimens lead to complex and far-reaching eating disorders such as anorexia nervosa and bulimia nervosa (see Chapter 6). These problems, which can assume severe proportions, usually involve a distorted self-image and a morbid, irrational pursuit of thinness, even when actual body weight is normal or even below age norms. In the absence of described eating disorders, constant dieting can still result in varying degrees of poor nutrition in the teenage girl at the very time in life when her body needs to be building reserves for potential reproduction. The harmful effects that bad

TO PROBE FURTHER

Food Habits of Adolescents: Where Do We Begin?

Adolescents who have entered their growth spurt seem to eat all the time. The questions for health professionals are *What are they eating?* and *How do we go about making it better?* Both quantity and quality of food are important during this period of rapid growth. Lean body mass increases by about 35 kg in boys and 19 kg in girls over these years, and 45% of total bone mass is accrued. Generous supplies of iron, zinc, calcium, and essential vitamins are needed to support these changes in body size and development.

FOOD INTAKE IN THE TEEN YEARS

Despite the critical nutrient needs in this life stage, national dietary surveys indicate that of all age groups, teens have the poorest diets. Their intakes of calcium, iron, zinc, vitamin A, and folate often fall below recommended levels. Although on the average teens eat 3 or 4 servings of vegetables each day, 1 or 2 of these servings are potatoes, most likely French fries; dark green and deep yellow vegetables are eaten infrequently. Boys and girls between the ages of 12 and 19 years eat about 1½ servings of fruit each day and about half comes from citrus sources. From the dairy group boys have only 2½ servings and girls only 1½ servings each day, which will not meet a teen's need for calcium (one dairy serving = 300 mg calcium). At the same time most adolescents are exceeding their RDA for protein. Foods such as hamburgers, pizza with cheese, tacos, and milkshakes, popular among teens, are good sources of protein. Foods high in sugar such as soft drinks and candy and items high in fat, including pastries, fatty meats, and fried foods, are eaten regularly by many teens. Both boys and girls obtain 20% of their kcalories from added sugars, 33% from fat, and 13% from saturated fat. Twenty-one percent of adolescents use vitamin-mineral supplements, but the supplement users have better diets and obtain higher intakes of nutrients from food. Teens also indulge in risk-taking behaviors: about one third smoke, and 28% of girls and 35% of boys report at least one episode of binge drinking per month.

LIFESTYLE AND NUTRITIONAL BEHAVIOR

Lifestyle choices in the teen years are influenced by peer pressure and teens' growing need to express their independence and make their own decisions. Teens also lead busy lives with school, sports, and jobs. Focus group interviews with teens in Minnesota indicated that (1) food taste and appeal, (2) time, and (3) convenience were the three most important factors influencing their food choices. They liked foods that looked good and choose the same foods over and over because they knew how they were going to taste. Foods such as pastries and other high-sugar or high-fat items were perceived as tasting better than more healthy foods such as fruits, vegetables, or dairy products. Fast food restaurants are popular because the food is served quickly. Teens often skip breakfast so they can stay in bed a little longer. Individuals in this age group do not want to spend time preparing food or cleaning up afterward. Food items must be easy to prepare or ready-to-eat, easy to eat on the bus or carry in a backpack, or delivered to the house.

Unfortunately, health is not an important personal issue at this life stage. A feeling of invulnerability and the idea that they have plenty of time in future years to worry about their health are common in teens. At the same time body weight and appearance are major concerns for 49% of girls and 43% of boys. The need to be thin causes some adolescent girls to adopt nutritionally inadequate diets or, worse, develop anorexia or bulimia nervosa (see Chapter 6). Adolescent boys trying to increase their muscle mass or "bulk up" may resort to unproven and potentially dangerous supplements or eat high-fat foods in an effort to obtain more kcalories. When working with teens who claim to be dieting, it is necessary to talk with them individually about what kind of diet they are following. For some teens dieting means drastically reducing their food intake or choosing foods erroneously believed to have special effects on appearance; for others, dieting refers to healthful practices like increasing their intakes of fruits and vegetables or cutting down on fats and sweets.

HOW DO WE HELP TEENS IMPROVE THEIR FOOD CHOICES?

Improving the food choices of this age group will require the combined efforts of parents, health professionals, food manufacturers, restaurant personnel, and food retailers. An important message to teens is that appropriate food choices along with regular physical activity can help to achieve and maintain (1) a healthy weight and positive level of fitness, (2) a high-energy level for school and work, and (3) an overall sense of well-being. Physical education and health teachers, nutrition educators, athletic coaches, school nurses, and parents must work together to develop programs that will reach teens at school and on the playing field.

Continued

TO PROBE FURTHER
Food Habits of Adolescents: Where Do We Begin?—cont'd

Teens want information that they can use now, not 10 years from now. One topic of immediate use would be selecting a lower-fat or lower-kcalorie meal at a fast food restaurant or choosing a more healthy pizza for home delivery. Snacks such as bananas, oranges, or apples; plastic containers of juice; or individual packages of ready-to-eat cereal travel well in a backpack, as do new ultrapasteurized milk drinks that do not require refrigeration. Simple to prepare or carry along breakfasts such as ready-to-eat cereal or bread or a bagel with peanut butter could be encouraged. Among junior high school students, ready-to-eat cereals provided a breakfast that was lower in cost, lower in fat, and higher in important nutrients including calcium, iron, vitamins A and D, and folate than fast food breakfast meals, granola, or toaster pastries.

Because taste is the most important factor in food selection for teens, it is important that we make healthy foods taste good. School cafeteria managers need to produce good-tasting and satisfying food that is attractively served. This means that the school meal must be viewed as an extension of the school's educational mission and supported by both teachers and parents. Salad bars have become popular among some teens, and salads to go might meet the need of both taste and convenience. Recipes that are reduced in fat and sugar but pleasing in taste and texture need to be developed for quantity food programs.

Food manufacturers must be urged to improve the nutrient quality of ready-to-eat main dishes as well as snack foods. Taste-testing parties with teens that compare lower-fat or reduced-sugar items with the less-nutritious product may help to dispel the myth that healthy foods do not taste good. Many popular foods among teens such as pizza or tacos can be exceedingly healthy foods with attention to reducing the levels of ingredients high in fat and saturated fat.

Finally, food retailers who cater to the teen audience must be urged to both sell and advertise healthy foods. Most fast food restaurants sell both orange juice and low-fat milk, but a soft drink is usually included in the combination meals and highly promoted. Salads are an option at many fast food outlets, and baked potatoes may be available as an alternative to French fried potatoes. Advertisements for soft drinks or less-healthy food items often carry the endorsements of popular sports stars. Such endorsements need to be applied to foods such as milk that are important to health and well-being. Community coalitions involving health professionals, educators, and parents concerned about adolescents and their future health will be necessary to bring about needed changes.

References

Dixon LB, Cronin FJ, Krebs-Smith SM: Let the pyramid guide your food choices: capturing the total diet concept, *J Nutr* 131:461S, 2001.

Dwyer JT et al: Do adolescent vitamin-mineral supplement users have better nutrient intakes than nonusers? Observations from the CATCH tracking study, *J Am Diet Assoc* 101(11):1340, 2001.

Hampl JS, Betts NM: Cigarette use during adolescence: effects on nutritional status, *Nutr Rev* 57:215, 1999.

Kleinman RE, ed: *Pediatric nutrition handbook,* ed 4, Elk Grove Village, Ill, 1998, American Academy of Pediatrics.

Neumark-Sztainer D et al: Factors influencing food choices of adolescents: findings from focus-group discussions with adolescents, *J Am Diet Assoc* 99:929, 1999.

Neumark-Sztainer D, Story M: Dieting and binge eating among adolescents: what do they really mean? *J Am Diet Assoc* 98:446, 1998.

Nicklas TA et al: Efficiency of breakfast consumption patterns of ninth graders: nutrient-to-cost comparisons, *J Am Diet Assoc* 102(2):226, 2002.

O'Dea JA: Children and adolescents identify food concerns, forbidden foods, and food-related beliefs, *J Am Diet Assoc* 99:970, 1999.

eating habits can have on the future course of a pregnancy are clearly indicated in many studies relating preconception nutritional status to the outcome of gestation (see Chapter 11).

TO SUM UP

Normal growth and development depend on nutrition to support heightened physiologic and metabolic processes. Nutrition in turn depends on a multitude of social, psychosocial, cultural, and environmental influences that affect individual growth potential throughout the life cycle.

Four types of growth interact during each phase of development: physical, mental, emotional, and sociocultural. Each type of growth must be evaluated when assessing the child's nutritional status and planning an effective counseling approach. Nutritional needs change with each growth period and must be individualized according to the unique growth pattern of every child.

Infants experience rapid growth. They have immature digestive systems and limited ability to absorb and excrete metabolites efficiently. Breastfeeding is preferred during the first year of life. Solid foods are not needed, nor can they be adequately tolerated, until 4 to 6 months of age.

Toddlers (aged 1 to 3 years), preschoolers (aged 3 to 6 years), and school-age children (aged 6 to 12 years) experience the slowed and erratic latent growth of childhood. Their energy requirements per unit of body weight are not as great as those of infants. Their nutritional needs center on protein for growth with attendant minerals and vitamins. Social and cultural factors influence the development of food habits in these age groups. Appropriate food behavior by parents and caregivers that can be modeled by children of these ages strongly influences the adoption of good eating habits during these periods of development.

Adolescents (aged 12 to 18 years) experience the second large growth spurt before reaching adulthood. This rapid growth involves both sexual maturation and physical growth. During this period girls increase their body proportion of fat, whereas boys increase their body proportion of muscle. Reaching peak bone mass is an important milestone for both sexes during this period of development. In general the increased kcaloric and nutrient needs of adolescence are more easily achieved by boys who consume larger amounts of food. In contrast, girls who may feel social and peer pressure to restrict food intake to avoid weight gain are less likely to meet their optimal nutrient requirements for growth. This pressure may also inhibit their ability to acquire the nutritional reserves necessary for later reproduction.

■ Questions for Review

1. How is physical growth measured? What are the NCHS Physical Growth Charts, and how are they used? What are the limitations of these charts? What are some clinical, biochemical, and dietary measures that are helpful in assessing the nutritional status of infants and children?
2. Describe the physical and psychosocial characteristics of the newborn. What are the capabilities of the newborn's digestive and renal systems and how do they relate to infant feeding?
3. Why is breastfeeding the preferred method for feeding infants (discuss both nutritional and psychosocial factors)? Describe the anatomic and hormonal components that participate in the delivery of breast milk to the nursing infant.
4. You are planning a nutrition education class to prepare pregnant mothers for breastfeeding. Outline the material that you would present, including (a) dietary needs for the new breastfeeding mother, (b) techniques for holding and feeding the baby, and (c) nipple care.
5. You are counseling a pregnant mother who has decided not to breastfeed. Describe some types of commercial formulas that would provide an appropriate alternative feeding for her infant. Describe the feeding techniques that will be important in meeting the psychosocial needs of her infant.
6. You are working with a mother whose newborn has been found to be allergic to milk proteins. What might be an available food source for this infant?
7. You are working with a low-income mother who has chosen not to breastfeed. She is concerned about the high cost of infant formula and would like to feed her infant cow's milk because it is so much cheaper. What would you tell her?
8. Outline a general schedule for a new mother to use as a guide for adding solid foods to her infant's diet during the first year of life; indicate both the time of addition and the items to be offered.
9. What changes in physical growth and psychosocial development influence eating habits in the (a) toddler, (b) preschool child, and (c) school-age child? How do these factors influence the nutritional needs of each age group?
10. What factors influence the changing nutritional needs of adolescents? Who is usually at greater nutritional risk during this stage—boys or girls? Why? What nutritional deficiencies may be associated with this vulnerable age?
11. You are the director of a school food service program in an elementary school and want to start a nutrition education program. You are working with a science teacher, a social studies teacher, and the school nurse to develop lessons that will connect learning in the classroom with good nutrition in the lunchroom. Visit the U.S. Department of Agriculture's Food and Nutrition Information Center website for Team Nutrition at *http://www.schoolmeals.nal.usda.gov:8001/* to find some ideas and materials that will assist you in this project. Develop a lesson plan for presentation in the science or social studies class that focuses on nutrition or food patterns and indicate how you will connect this lesson with the lunch program.

■ References

1. Chumlea WC, Guo SS: Physical growth and development. In Samour PQ, Helm KK, Lang CE, eds: *Handbook of pediatric nutrition,* ed 2, Gaithersburg, Md, 1999, Aspen Publishers.
2. Kuczmarski RJ et al: *CDC growth charts: United States, advance data, vital and health statistics,* No 314, Hyattsville, Md, Dec 4, 2000 (revised), CDC.
3. Strauss RS, Pollack HA: Epidemic increase in childhood overweight, 1986-1998, *JAMA* 286:2845, 2001.
4. Panel on Macronutrients, Panel on the Definition of Dietary Fiber, Subcommittee on Upper Reference Levels of Nutrients, Subcommittee on Interpretation and Uses of Dietary Reference Intakes, and the Standing Committee on the Scientific Evaluation of Dietary Reference Intakes: *Dietary reference intakes for energy, carbohydrate, fiber, fat, fatty acids, cholesterol, protein, and amino acids, parts 1 and 2,* Washington, DC, 2002, National Academy Press.

5. Kleinman RE, ed: *Pediatric nutrition handbook,* ed 4, Elk Grove Village, Ill, 1998, American Academy of Pediatrics.
6. Holst M-C: Developmental and behavioral effects of iron deficiency anemia in infants, *Nutr Today* 33(1):27, 1998.
7. Hurtado EK, Hartl Claussen A, Scott KG: Early childhood anemia and mild or moderate mental retardation, *Am J Clin Nutr* 69:115, 1999.
8. Partington S, Nitzke S, Csete J: The prevalence of anemia in a WIC population: a comparison by homeless experience, *J Am Diet Assoc* 100:469, 2000.
9. Fomon SJ: Infant feeding in the 20th century: formula and beikost, *J Nutr* 131:409S, 2001.
10. Erikson E: *Childhood and society,* New York, 1963, WW Norton.
11. Klawitter BM: Nutrition counseling. In Samour PQ, Helm KK, Lang CE, eds: *Handbook of pediatric nutrition,* ed 2, Gaithersburg, Md, 1999, Aspen Publishers.
12. McCaffree J: Rickets on the rise, *J Am Diet Assoc* 101:16, 2001.
13. Fomon SJ: Feeding normal infants: rationale for recommendations, *J Am Diet Assoc* 101(9):1002, 2001.
14. Akers SM, Groh-Wargo SL: Normal nutrition during infancy. In Samour PQ, Helm KK, Lang CE, eds: *Handbook of pediatric nutrition,* ed 2, Gaithersburg, Md, 1999, Aspen.
15. Merritt RJ, Tougas J: DHA and AA: are they essential ingredients in infant formula? Special Supplement on Infant Nutrition, *Nutr MD* 27(12), 2001.
16. Williams C et al: Stereoacuity at age 3.5 y in children born full-term is associated with prenatal and postnatal dietary factors: a report from a population-based cohort study, *Am J Clin Nutr* 73:316, 2001.
17. McCrory MA: Does dieting during lactation put infant growth at risk? *Nutr Rev* 59(1):8, 2001.
18. Fisher JO et al: Breastfeeding through the first year predicts maternal control in feeding and subsequent energy intakes, *J Am Diet Assoc* 100:641, 2000.
19. Hediger ML et al: Early infant feeding and growth status of US-born infants and children aged 4-71 mo: analyses from the third National Health and Nutrition Examination Survey 1988-1994, *Am J Clin Nutr* 72:159, 2000.
20. Hediger ML et al: Association between infant breastfeeding and overweight in young children, *JAMA* 285:2453, 2001.
21. Stettler N et al: Infant weight gain and childhood overweight status in a multicenter, cohort study, *Pediatrics* 109:194, 2002.
22. Butte NF et al: Infant feeding mode affects early growth and body composition, *Pediatrics* 106:1355, 2000.
23. Humphrey J, Iliff P: Is breast not best? Feeding babies born to HIV-positive mothers: bringing balance to a complex issue, *Nutr Rev* 59(4):119, 2001.
24. American Academy of Pediatrics, Committee on Nutrition: Hypoallergenic infant formulas, *Pediatrics* 106 (2, Pt 1): 346, 2000.
25. Merritt RJ, Tougas J: Soy protein-based infant formula: a proven record of success, Special Supplement on Infant Nutrition, *Nutr MD* 27(12), 2001.
26. Fewtrell MS et al: Catch-up growth in small-for-gestational-age term infants: a randomized trial, *Am J Clin Nutr* 74: 516, 2001.
27. Kannan S, Carruth BR, Skinner J: Cultural influences on infant feeding beliefs of mothers, *J Am Diet Assoc* 99:88, 1999.
28. Bronner YL et al: Early introduction of solid foods among urban African-American participants in WIC, *J Am Diet Assoc* 99:457, 1999.
29. Birch LL: Development of food preferences, *Ann Rev Nutr* 19:41, 1999.
30. Gerrish CJ, Mennella JA: Flavor variety enhances food acceptance in formula-fed infants, *Am J Clin Nutr* 73:1080, 2001.
31. Briley ME et al: Dietary intake at child-care centers and away: are parents and care providers working as partners or at cross-purposes? *J Am Diet Assoc* 99:950, 1999.
32. Skinner JD et al: Longitudinal study of nutrient and food intakes of white preschool children aged 24 to 60 months, *J Am Diet Assoc* 99:1514, 1999.
33. Nicklas TA et al: Family and child-care provider influences on preschool children's fruit, juice, and vegetable consumption, *Nutr Rev* 59(7):224, 2001.
34. Fisher JO et al: Maternal milk consumption predicts the tradeoff between milk and soft drink in young girls' diets, *J Nutr* 131:246, 2000.
35. Tibbs T et al: The relationship between parental modeling, eating patterns, and dietary intake among African-American parents, *J Am Diet Assoc* 101:535, 2001.
36. Rolls BJ, Engell D, Birch LL: Serving portion size influences 5-year-old but not 3-year-old children's food intakes, *J Am Diet Assoc* 100:232, 2000.
37. Johnson RK, Nicklas TA: Position of the American Dietetic Association: dietary guidance for healthy children aged 2 to 11 years, *J Am Diet Assoc* 99:93, 1999.
38. Borzekowski DLG, Robinson TN: The 30-second effect: an experiment revealing the impact of television commercials on food preferences of preschoolers, *J Am Diet Assoc* 101:42, 2001.
39. Friedman BJ, Hurd-Crixell SL, Ferris B: Texas school menu compliance with US Dietary Guidelines for Americans, *J Am Diet Assoc* 98:1325, 1998.
40. Friedman BJ, Hurd-Crixell SL: Nutrient intake of children eating school breakfast, *J Am Diet Assoc* 99:219, 1999.
41. Rankin LL, Bingham M: Acceptability of oatmeal chocolate chip cookies prepared using pureed white beans as a fat ingredient substitute, *J Am Diet Assoc* 100: 831, 2000.
42. Cullen KW et al: Effect of a la carte and snack bar foods at school on children's lunchtime intake of fruits and vegetables, *J Am Diet Assoc* 100:1482, 2000.
43. Melnick TA et al: Food consumption patterns of elementary school children in New York City, *J Am Diet Assoc* 98:159, 1998.
44. Jahns L, Siega-Riz AM, Popkin BM: The increasing prevalence of snacking among US children from 1977 to 1996, *J Pediatr* 138(4):493, 2001.
45. Manore MM, Barr SI, Butterfield GE: Nutrition and athletic performance: position of the American Dietetic Association, Dietitians of Canada, and the American College of Sports Medicine, *J Am Diet Assoc* 100:1543, 2000.
46. Wosje KS, Specker BL: Role of calcium in bone health during childhood, *Nutr Rev* 58:253, 2000.

47. Beals KA, Manore MM: Nutritional status of female athletes with subclinical eating disorders, *J Am Diet Assoc* 98:419, 1998.
48. Wiecha JM et al: Differences in dietary patterns of Vietnamese, white, African-American, and Hispanic adolescents in Worcester, Mass, *J Am Diet Assoc* 101(2):248, 2001.
49. Hampl JS, Sass S: Focus groups indicate that vegetable and fruit consumption by food stamp-eligible Hispanics is affected by children and unfamiliarity with non-traditional foods, *J Am Diet Assoc* 101(6):685, 2001.

■ Further Reading

Dwyer J: Should dietary fat recommendations for children be changed? *J Am Diet Assoc* 100:36, 2000.

Krebs NK, Johnson SL: Guidelines for healthy children, *J Am Diet Assoc* 100:37, 2000.

Satter E: A moderate view on fat restriction for young children, *J Am Diet Assoc* 100:32, 2000.

The increasing incidence of obesity in children and concern for the prevention of chronic diseases later in life have led to a discussion about the optimum level of dietary fat for children. These articles discuss this controversy.

Briley ME et al: Dietary intake at child-care centers and away: are parents and care providers working as partners or at cross-purposes? *J Am Diet Assoc* 99:950, 1999.

Cline T, White G: Local support for nutrition integrity in schools: position of the American Dietetic Association, *J Am Diet Assoc* 100:108, 2000.

Florencio CA: Developments and variations in school-based feeding programs around the world, *Nutr Today* 36(1):29, 2001.

Gable S, Lutz S: Nutrition socialization experiences of children in the Head Start program, *J Am Diet Assoc* 101:572, 2001.

Children attending day care or Head Start or schools with a breakfast and lunch program receive a major proportion of their meals for the day at that location. These articles provide some insight into the role of day care centers and schools in supporting the development of good food habits in children and the role of community health professionals in supporting school food programs, both in the United States and in developing countries.

Bronner YL et al: Early introduction of solid foods among urban African-American participants in WIC, *J Am Diet Assoc* 99:457, 1999.

Dobson B, Murtaugh MA: Position of the American Dietetic Association: breaking the barriers to breastfeeding, *J Am Diet Assoc* 101(10):1213, 2001.

Fomon SJ: Feeding normal infants: rationale for recommendations, *J Am Diet Assoc* 101(9):1002, 2001.

Mennella JA, Beauchamp GK: Early flavor experiences: research update, *Nutr Rev* 56:205, 1998.

Sills IN: Nutritional rickets: a preventable disease, *Topics Clin Nutr* 17(1):36, 2001.

These articles provide some insight into early feeding experiences and nutrition issues in feeding infants.

O'Dea J: Body basics: a nutrition education program for adolescents about food, nutrition, growth, body image, and weight control, *J Am Diet Assoc* 102(3 suppl):S68, 2002.

Reed DB et al: Clueless in the mall: a web site on calcium for teens, *J Am Diet Assoc* 102(3 suppl):S73, 2002.

Sigman-Grant M: Strategies for counseling adolescents, *J Am Diet Assoc* 102(3 suppl):S32, 2002.

Story M, Neumark-Sztainer D, French S: Individual and environmental influences on adolescent eating behaviors, *J Am Diet Assoc* 102(3 suppl):S40, 2002.

Adolescents are an important target group for nutrition education. We need to learn more about the food-related beliefs and practices of this group and strategies to improve their nutrition and health behaviors. A supplement entitled *Adolescent Nutrition: A Springboard to Health,* Volume 102, March 2002, *Journal of the American Dietetic Association* is devoted to issues and programs relevant to adolescent nutrition. The articles listed here offer practical ideas for intervention.

CASE STUDY Nutrition program for adolescents

Amanda is a graduate student of clinical nutrition assigned to the "Save Our Senior High" project in a metropolitan community of 300,000 located in northwestern United States. A representative of the city's educational advisory board approached her institution for assistance in developing a program that addresses three major problems faced by the majority of high school students: (1) popularity of fad diets among athletes, (2) obesity, and (3) iron deficiency anemia.

Amanda and other members of her class met with students who were learning other health professions (medicine, dentistry, nutrition, nursing, social work), as well as several student representatives from the high school, to plan the program. After they developed goals and objectives, they decided that the nutrition topics would be addressed in a series of workshops entitled "Nutrition and Physical Fitness," "Food for the Teen Years," and "Snack Facts."

The program was introduced to the students through an advanced bulletin distributed at the largest high school in the city, where the project was to begin. The bulletin included an article written by Amanda: "Teenage Nutrition: A Seeming Paradox." This article responded to a common concern expressed by adolescents: the apparent preoccupation of school officials with the students' food habits when they, as a group, looked and usually felt very healthy.

Amanda's article stirred a tremendous interest in the student population. Attendance at each session was high, and the discussions were lively. The evaluation results were positive. In reviewing the evaluative data and low cost of the project, the city council asked Amanda and her classmates to repeat the program at two other high schools where these problems were also prevalent. The council approached the school board about the possibility of including the project in the citywide high school curriculum for the coming year.

QUESTIONS FOR ANALYSIS

1. Outline the content of Amanda's article to reflect major points that you would have included.
2. Write a class outline for each workshop, including objectives, major topics, and questions you would expect from the students. What teaching methods and materials would you expect to be most effective in each workshop?
3. What outside influences on eating habits would you expect in this student population? How effective would you expect this educational program to be in influencing a change of behavior in eating habits?
4. Aside from in-school nutrition education programs, describe possible tactics for influencing the eating habits of teenagers.

Issues & ANSWERS

Children and Adolescents: Aim for Fitness

The *Dietary Guidelines for Americans* provide direction for the development of a healthy diet and lifestyle for all persons aged 2 years and older. The 2000 edition set goals for not only food patterns in all age groups but also appropriate physical activity (see Chapter 1, p. 26). Many chronic diseases that influence well-being in later life actually begin in childhood. Thus preventive lifestyle practices related to diet and physical activity must be introduced at an early age when patterns are being developed that will continue for a lifetime.

Aim for a healthy weight

Body weight and physical activity are intrinsically related. A regular pattern of exercise beginning in childhood will promote lifelong heart health and prevent the accumulation of excess body fat. Large numbers of U.S. children are overweight, and the numbers continue to climb. Among 5000 children between the ages of 9 and 11, the proportion classified as overweight increased by 11% during a 2-year period. There also appear to be racial, ethnic, and regional differences in overweight among children. Boys, African Americans, Hispanics, and those living in the southern states are more likely to be overweight. High-kcaloric diets coupled with inactivity patterns leading to increased body fat are associated with the growing incidence of type 2 diabetes in children of school age.

Body fat increases rapidly during the first year of life and then slows until about age 6, when again there is a normal increase in both the size and number of body fat cells. For some children, an inappropriate accumulation of body fat begins about this time or even earlier. This addition of body fat can be accelerated by a high energy intake in relation to energy needs or a sedentary life pattern with a low energy expenditure. Although there are differences in opinion on this matter, several experts suggest that children who are overweight do not consume more kcalories than normal weight children but are less physically active. The best insurance to prevent inappropriate accumulation of body fat in a child of any age is regular physical activity.

Be physically active each day

Although children and adolescents are more active than most adults, many of our youth appear to be settling into a sedentary lifestyle that is common among adults. We know that 48% of girls and 26% of boys do not exercise vigorously on a regular basis. Schools now offer fewer physical education opportunities to students, and over the past decade, daily participation in physical education dropped to 29%, although about half of all youth have such classes at least once each week. Television, computer games, the Internet, and similar sedentary pastimes are growing in popularity. About one fourth of U.S. children watch television 4 or more hours a day, and the greater the number of hours, the greater is the likelihood of overweight and increased skinfold thicknesses.

Helping children develop an active lifestyle

Parents and caregivers, schools, and communities need to work together to increase physical activity among children. Children are more likely to develop an active lifestyle if parents and role models also demonstrate such behavior. Taking your teddy bear for a walk can be a meaningful activity for a preschooler who belongs to a family who walks together regularly. School games and physical education programs should focus on activities such as walking or running that allow all students to participate, rather than on games in which several students are active but the majority sit and watch. Moving away from competitive games that discourage participation by overweight or less skilled players to such activities as kick ball or dancing or aerobics that can be done alone to music or in groups after school are worthwhile objectives for physical education. Bike-riding and jumping rope are good forms of vigorous exercise. Making school facilities such as a gymnasium or walking track available to families and students after school hours might encourage a higher level of physical activity. See Figure 12-2 for guidelines regarding activity levels for children of all ages.

Intervention for the obese child or adolescent

Interventions in childhood obesity require a team approach that includes the family or caregiver, the child, and the nutritionist. Increasing physical activity is the first goal to increase energy expenditure and support a healthy weight. The child should be encouraged to achieve 30 minutes of continuous movement every day in an activity in which he or she feels comfortable. It is important to consider the child's interests and preferences; some children enjoy group activities and others would rather exercise alone. Setting up a buddy system

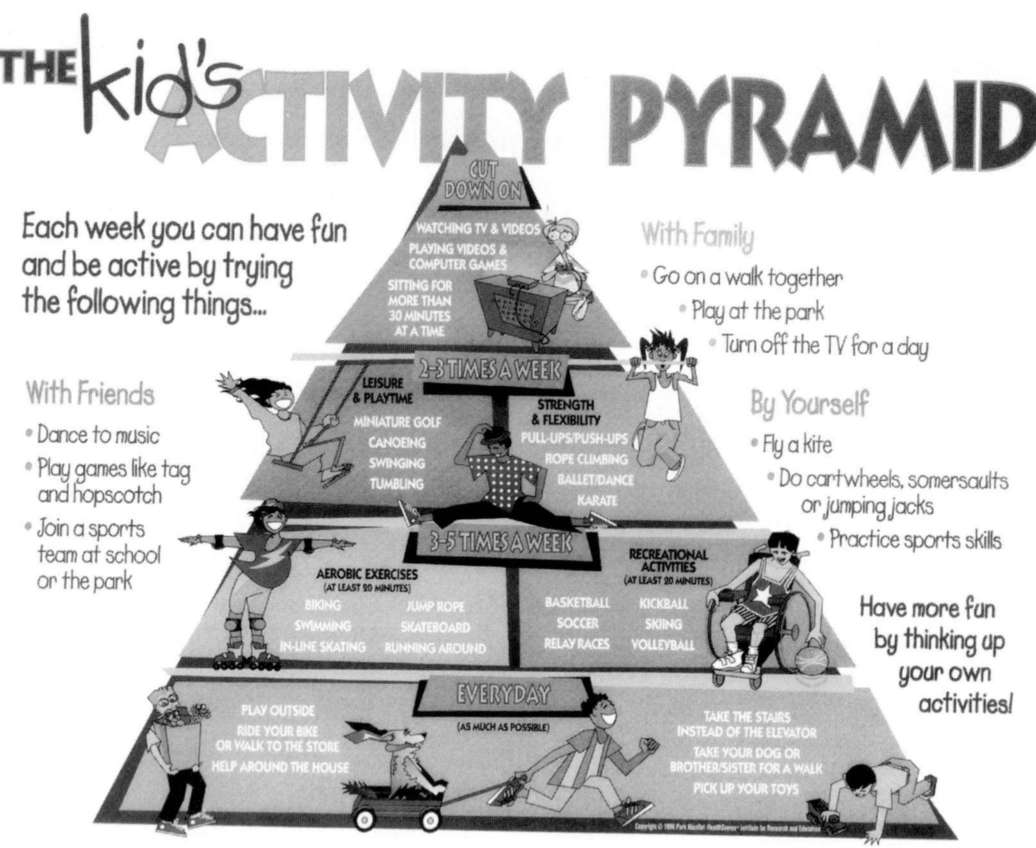

FIGURE 12-2 Fitness Pyramid for Kids. (*Copyright © 1996 Park Nicollet* HealthSource® *Park Nicollet Institute. Reprinted by permission.*)

by which they can exercise with each other may reduce feelings of self-consciousness that are likely to exist in these children. For a child soon to enter a growth spurt, limiting weight gain and promoting fitness, rather than trying to bring about active weight loss, is a reasonable goal. As the child increases in height, the body weight-to-height ratio will become more appropriate. Assist the child in recognizing environmental cues that trigger inappropriate eating, and make available healthy snack foods that can help prevent additional weight gain or initiate modest weight loss. Making food less visible around the house can help a child better control eating patterns. It is important that a health professional be involved in planning a dietary intake for an obese child to ensure that excessive kcalorie restriction does not result in a lack of protein, vitamins, and minerals for growth and health. Limiting dietary fat to no more than 30% of total kcalories and including complex carbohydrates that are good sources of fiber can help to reduce kcalorie intake, improve satiety, and reduce the risk of type 2 diabetes.

The overweight adolescent needs to be encouraged to increase physical activity to the same extent as the overweight child. If the period of rapid growth has been completed, dietary intervention to prevent further weight gain or achieve a modest weight loss is an appropriate goal (see Chapter 6 to review the benefits that can result from the loss of even 10 lb). Adjusting kcaloric intake and increasing activity to bring about the loss of ½ to 1 lb a week can provide an opportunity for the adolescent to develop new lifestyle patterns to be continued into early adulthood. Individual or group exercise should be encouraged. Family members need to be supportive, and psychologic counseling may assist in working through personal problems and avoid or correct existing eating disorders. The obese adolescent needs guidance in making food choices in social situations and at the food establishments frequented by his or her peer group. Both the teen and the parents must be helped to understand the concept of a healthy weight and the need to stay away from starvation or fad diet regimens. The nutritionist needs to be certain that important nutrients such as protein, calcium, iron, and folate are not compromised, and the *Food Guide Pyramid* remains a good tool to guide food selection. Lowering fat intake to 30% of total energy is a place to start in evaluating the diet.

REFERENCES

Duyff RL: *The American Dietetic Association's complete food & nutrition guide,* Minneapolis, Minn, 1998, Chronimed Publishing.

Dwyer JT et al: Prevalence of marked overweight and obesity in a multi-ethnic pediatric population: findings from the Child and Adolescent Trial for Cardiovascular Health (CATCH) Study, *J Am Diet Assoc* 100:1149, 2000.

Flegal KM, Troiano RP, Ballard-Barbash R: Aim for a healthy weight: what is the target? *J Nutr* 131:440S, 2001.

Johnson RK, Nicklas TA: Dietary guidance for healthy children aged 2 to 11 years: position of the American Dietetic Association, *J Am Diet Assoc* 99:93, 1999.

Kleinman RE, ed: *Pediatric nutrition handbook,* ed 4, Elk Grove Village, Ill, 1998, American Academy of Pediatrics.

Robertson SM et al: Factors related to adiposity among children aged 3 to 7 years, *J Am Diet Assoc* 99:938, 1999.

Tershakovec A: The growing epidemic of childhood obesity, *Nutr MD* 28(2):1, 2002.

Troiano RP, Macera C, Ballard-Barbash R: Be physically active each day: how can we know? *J Nutr* 131:451S, 2001.

Weaver KA, Piatek A: Childhood obesity. In Samour PQ, Helm KK, Lang CE, eds: *Handbook of pediatric nutrition,* ed 2, Gaithersburg, Md, 1999, Aspen Publishers.

Chapter

13

Nutrition for Adults: Early, Middle, and Later Years

Eleanor D. Schlenker

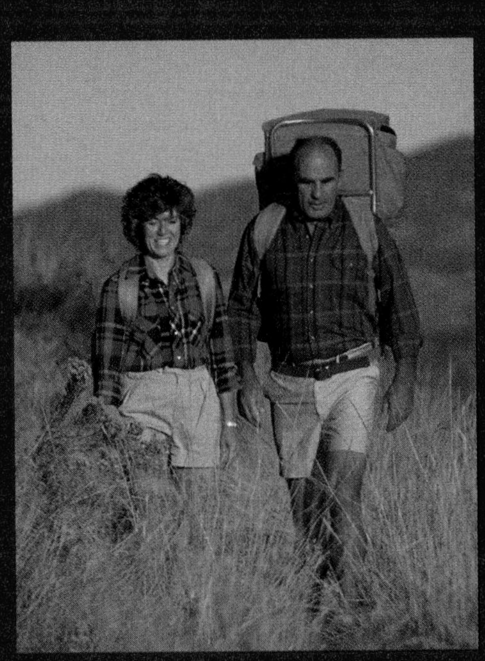

Chapter Outline

In this chapter, we complete our three-chapter sequence on nutrition through the life cycle. Following the tumultuous adolescent years come the challenges, problems, and opportunities of maturity and adulthood.

Today when adolescents come of age, they have lived only about a quarter of their potential life span. They face a changing world of accelerated pace and complexity. America reflects these changes in its aging and increasingly diverse population.

Here we review adulthood, its early, middle, and later years. We look at each stage in terms of maturing needs and the role of nutrition in maintaining optimum health and well-being.

Adulthood: Continuing Human Growth and Development

AGING THROUGHOUT THE LIFE CYCLE

Aging is a positive concept. It starts at conception and ends at death. It encompasses the whole of life, not merely its latter stages. Indeed, every stage has its unique potential and fulfillment, and the periods of adulthood—young, middle, and older—are no exception. Basic human needs continue, although in changing patterns, as persons mature and grow older.

Throughout your study, it is important to view continuing adult growth as a positive period of human life.[1] Two important concepts are significant parts of the whole process.

1. *The individual.* Although gradual aging throughout the adult years has implications for a society, this sequence of change is at its core an individual process.
2. *The total life.* Although specific changes occur at each stage of the life span, aging is a total life process.

These two basic concepts govern the needs of these years—physiologic, psychosocial, socioeconomic, and nutritional.

COMING OF AGE IN AMERICA

Young adults coming of age in America are experiencing extensive population and technology changes that affect their personal and working lives. The large population of "baby boomers" born after World War II are now in their 50s and facing a rapidly changing world of computers, high-tech medical care, and population shifts. And with our increasing life span and the growing number of older adults in our population, their personal, social, and healthcare needs are being felt in all our lives.

The Federal Interagency Forum on Aging, a coalition of nine federal agencies with special responsibilities for healthcare, housing, and other services for the aging population, compiled statistics that describe key indicators of well-being in older Americans.[2] In the next section we will summarize the changes that are occurring in the aging population and what they will mean for those of us who provide health and nutritional care for this group.

1. *Size of the aging population.* There are 35 million people in the United States who are aged 65 or older, or 1 in 8 persons. By 2030 the number of persons aged 65 or older will have increased to 1:5. The fastest growing age group among all age categories is the oldest-old, those aged 85 and older. This group tends to be in poorer health and requires more health and community services.[2]
2. *Ethnic and racial diversity.* Currently the overwhelming majority of persons aged 65 and older is white. By the year 2050 whites will represent only 64% of the older age group, 16% will be Hispanic, 12% will be black, and 7% will be Asian and Pacific Islander.[2] It will be important for health professionals to recognize the cultural differences that exist among groups in their attitudes toward health, food habits, and family roles.
3. *Education.* In 1950 only 18% of the older population had completed high school compared with 67% in 2000. About 15% of today's older generation have completed college.[2] Individuals with more education usually are able to take more responsibility for their own health and place a greater emphasis on self-care. Unfortunately, substantial educational differences exist among older racial and ethnic groups in the United States. Only 44% of Hispanic older adults and 29% of black older adults have high school diplomas compared with 72% of white older adults.[2] The older person who cannot read food labels or the directions for taking prescription or over-the-counter (OTC) drugs is less able to implement sound health practices.
4. *Income.* The number of older individuals with incomes below the poverty line declined from 13% to 8% during the past 25 years; however, certain age and sex groups are more likely to be poor. Elderly blacks and Hispanics have lower incomes than do elderly whites. Those above age 85 are more likely to be poor than are those aged 65 to 74. Single persons above age 85, particularly single women above age 85, have the highest poverty rates of all groups.[3]
5. *Living arrangements.* Because women live longer than men, older women are more likely to be widowed and older men are more likely to live with their spouse. At age 65 about half of all women are married compared with about three fourths of all men. By age 75, 72% of women live alone. Older women living alone are more likely to be poor than are older women who are married. Widowed black and Hispanic women usually live with other family members, whereas widowed white women often live alone.[3]

SHAPING INFLUENCES ON ADULT GROWTH AND DEVELOPMENT

Within our rapidly changing world, today's adults are growing and developing in many divergent ways. In terms of our interest in nutrition and health at each life stage, four areas of adult life shape the general path of development: physical, psychosocial, socioeconomic, and nutritional.

Physical Characteristics

Overall physical growth of the human body, governed by its genetic potential, levels off in the late teens and early adult years as we reach physical maturity. Physical growth is no longer marked by increasing numbers of cells and body size; rather, it is the vital process of replication, constantly growing new cells to replace old ones to maintain body structure and function, increase learning, and

TABLE 13-1 Recommended Dietary Allowances for Energy and Protein (2002*†)

Age (yr)	Weight (kg)	Weight (lb)	Height (cm)	Height (in)	Energy (kcalories)	Protein (g)
Males						
19-30	70	154	177	70	3000	56
31-50	70	154	177	70	2900	56
51-70	70	154	177	70	2700	56
≥71	70	154	177	70	2500	56
Females						
19-30	57	126	163	64	2400	46
31-50	57	126	163	64	2300	46
51-70	57	126	163	64	2100	46
≥70	57	126	163	64	2000	46

Data calculated from standards found in Panel on Macronutrients, Panel on the Definition of Dietary Fiber, Subcommittee on Upper Reference Levels of Nutrients, Subcommittee on Interpretation and Uses of Dietary Reference Intakes, and the Standing Committee on the Scientific Evaluation of Dietary Reference Intakes: *Dietary reference intakes for energy, carbohydrate, fiber, fat, fatty acids, cholesterol, protein, and amino acids, parts 1 and 2,* Washington, DC, 2002, National Academy Press.

* Because adults are urged to remain physically active throughout their lives, there is no evidence that body weight should change as adults continue to age; thus the Expert Panel has indicated that reference weights remain the same for all adult age categories.

†These energy recommendations are based on the midpoint of each age range: age 25, age 40, age 60, and age 80. Calculated values were rounded to the nearest 100. Energy needs in men decline by 10 kcalories per year after the age of 19; energy needs in women decline by 7 kcalories per year after the age of 19.

strengthen mental capacities. Then at older ages, physical growth gradually declines. Individual vigor reflects the health status of preceding years.

Psychosocial Development

Here we pick up the stages of human personality development introduced in Chapter 12. Three remaining developmental tasks of personal psychosocial growth characterize the adult years: (1) young adults—develop intimacy and expand relationships outside of parents and siblings; (2) middle adults—pursue creative expression and development of new directions; and (3) older adults—seek fulfillment and strength of purpose. Individual adults at each age experience these stages in some way, including their influence on lifestyle and health.

Socioeconomic Status

We all grow up and live our lives in a social and cultural context. Our world is rapidly changing; we are experiencing major social and economic shifts, and most adults experience some change in resources as they move through early, middle, and later adulthood. These financial pressures directly influence food security and health.

Nutritional Needs

The energy and nutrient needs of individual adults within each age group vary according to living and working situations. However, current Recommended Dietary Allowances (RDA) and Dietary Reference Intake (DRI) standards for healthy adults, presented in Tables 13-1 through 13-3, reflect general needs and serve as a point of reference for comparing these needs in our discussion.

Adult Age Groups: Nutrient Needs for Health Promotion and Disease Prevention

EARLY ADULT: 19 TO 45 YEARS

Physical Characteristics

After the turbulent physical growth and sexual development of the preceding adolescent years, the young adult's body growth pattern levels off into a state of adult homeostasis. Finely regulated gene control of neural and hormonal activity and feedback maintains a stable internal environment of "body wisdom." The body functions are fully developed, including sexual maturation and reproductive capacity.

Psychosocial Development

In the early adult years, every person is launched, for better or worse, as a socially mature individual. The core psychosocial growth task each young adult must resolve is that of building relationships outside of the core family that he or she has been a part of (Figure 13-1). It is a time of physical

replication Making an exact copy; to repeat, duplicate, or reproduce. In genetics, replication is the process by which double-stranded DNA makes copies of itself, each separating strand synthesizing a complementary strand. Cell replication is the process by which living cells, under gene control, make exact copies of themselves a programmed number of times during the life span of the organism. The process can be reproduced in the laboratory with cultured cell lines for special studies in cell biology.

TABLE 13-2 Dietary Reference Intakes for Minerals

Age (yr)	Calcium (mg)	Phosphorus (mg)	Magnesium (mg)	Iron (mg)	Zinc (mg)	Iodine (μg)	Selenium (μg)	Fluoride (mg)
Males								
19-30	1000	700	400	8	11	150	55	4
31-50	1000	700	420	8	11	150	55	4
51-70	1200	700	420	8	11	150	55	4
≥71	1200	700	420	8	11	150	55	4
Females								
19-30	1000	700	310	18	8	150	55	3
31-50	1000	700	320	18	8	150	55	3
51-70	1200	700	320	8	8	150	55	3
≥71	1200	700	320	8	8	150	55	3

Data compiled from Food and Nutrition Board, National Research Council: *Dietary reference intakes for calcium, phosphorus, magnesium, vitamin D, and fluoride,* Washington, DC, 1997, National Academy Press; Food and Nutrition Board, National Research Council: *Dietary reference intakes for thiamin, riboflavin, niacin, vitamin B_6, folate, vitamin B_{12}, pantothenic acid, biotin, and choline,* Washington, DC, 1998, National Academy Press; Food and Nutrition Board, National Research Council: *Dietary reference intakes for vitamin C, vitamin E, selenium, and carotenoids,* Washington, DC, 2000, National Academy Press; Food and Nutrition Board, National Research Council: *Dietary reference intakes for vitamin A, vitamin K, arsenic, boron, chromium, copper, iodine, iron, manganese, molybdenum, nickel, silicon, vanadium, and zinc,* Washington, DC, 2001, National Academy Press.

TABLE 13-3 Dietary Reference Intakes for Vitamins

Age (yr)	Vitamin A (μg)	Vitamin D (μg)	Vitamin E (mg)	Vitamin C (mg)	Thiamin (mg)	Riboflavin (mg)	Niacin (mg NE)	Vitamin B_6 (mg)	Folate (μg)	Vitamin B_{12} (μg)
Males										
19-30	900	5	15	90	1.2	1.3	16	1.3	400	2.4
31-50	900	5	15	90	1.2	1.3	16	1.3	400	2.4
51-70	900	10	15	90	1.2	1.3	16	1.7	400	2.4
≥71	900	15	15	90	1.2	1.3	16	1.7	400	2.4
Females										
19-30	700	5	15	75	1.1	1.1	14	1.3	400	2.4
31-50	700	5	15	75	1.1	1.1	14	1.3	400	2.4
51-70	700	10	15	75	1.1	1.1	14	1.5	400	2.4
≥71	700	15	15	75	1.1	1.1	14	1.5	400	2.4

Data compiled from Food and Nutrition Board, National Research Council: *Dietary reference intakes for calcium, phosphorus, magnesium, vitamin D, and fluoride,* Washington, DC, 1997, National Academy Press; Food and Nutrition Board, National Research Council: *Dietary reference intakes for thiamin, riboflavin, niacin, vitamin B_6, folate, vitamin B_{12}, pantothenic acid, biotin, and choline,* Washington, DC, 1998, National Academy Press; Food and Nutrition Board, National Research Council: *Dietary reference intakes for vitamin C, vitamin E, selenium, and carotenoids,* Washington, DC, 2000, National Academy Press; Food and Nutrition Board, National Research Council: *Dietary reference intakes for vitamin A, vitamin K, arsenic, boron, chromium, copper, iodine, iron, manganese, molybdenum, nickel, silicon, vanadium, and zinc,* Washington, DC, 2001, National Academy Press.

maturity, of becoming comfortable with the physical self and increasing adult role demands. If positive development is achieved, the person can build intimate relationships leading to self-fulfillment, either in marriage or in other personal relationships. If these psychosocial strengths have not been developed in the previous growing up years, the individual may become increasingly isolated from others.

Socioeconomic Status

The early adult years reflect the social and economic pressures of continued education to prepare for adult responsibilities and career beginnings and to learn new job skills. Other life tasks of the young adult are establishing one's own home, parenthood and starting young children on their way through the same life stages, and the early struggles to make one's way in the world. Given the changing work environment in today's world, many young adults face difficulties in meeting these basic goals of education, work, and family. This is also the period during which we establish the lifestyle practices of diet and exercise that will influence health in middle age and beyond.

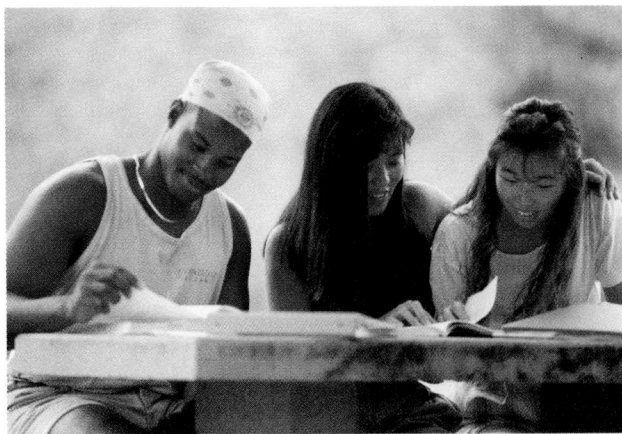

FIGURE 13-1 The early adult years center on the core problem of intimacy versus isolation. *(Credit: PhotoDisc.)*

Nutritional Needs

All of the physical, psychosocial, and socioeconomic factors just described influence nutritional needs. The distinct differences in growth patterns that emerged between males and females during adolescence are strengthened in adult bodies. The young man's larger muscle mass and long bone growth are established. The young woman's wider hip breadth and pelvic girdle of subcutaneous fat, genetically designed to support reproduction, continue to prompt concerns and sometimes unwise actions in relation to social pressures for thinness that contribute to insufficient food intake. Nutritional needs of this period center on energy, protein, and the micronutrients.

1. *Energy.* The RDA energy standard for active 19-year-old men is 3067 kilocalories (kcalories)/day, and for active 19-year-old women, 2403 kcalories/day[4] (see Table 13-1). The larger male body size and muscle mass require more energy to maintain, because lean muscle mass is metabolically active tissue. The adult resting energy expenditure (REE) per unit of body weight, a measure of metabolic rate, differs by about 10% between the genders, reflecting the female's greater proportion of body fat.[4] The remainder of the energy need is for physical activity (Figure 13-2), which makes up a smaller portion of the energy requirement than metabolic needs. The height and weight reference values in Table 13-1 are not meant to imply ideal ratios. They are actual median measurements for the designated age group reported by a large national nutrition and health survey. Women require additional energy to support pregnancy and lactation (see Chapter 11).
2. *Protein.* The RDA standard for protein during the early adult years following adolescence is 56 g/day for men and 46 g/day for women.[4] These allowances are based on a daily protein need of approximately 0.8 g/kg body weight for both genders. An additional 25 g/day of protein is needed for pregnancy; an added 25 g/day is needed for lactation. Protein intakes among most young adults in the United States are 1½ to 2 times the current RDA[5] and may over time contribute to the development of chronic kidney disease.[6]
3. *Minerals.* The DRIs for adults, as given in Table 13-2, can be met by a well-planned diet. However, two minerals, calcium and iron, need emphasis. The current DRI recommends 1000 mg of calcium each day for young adults to ensure the continued development of peak skeletal bone mass.[7] Population groups likely to consume inadequate amounts of calcium are women and older adults.[8-11] Iron is another mineral often lacking in low-kcalorie diets, resulting in iron-deficiency anemia. Women of childbearing age require more

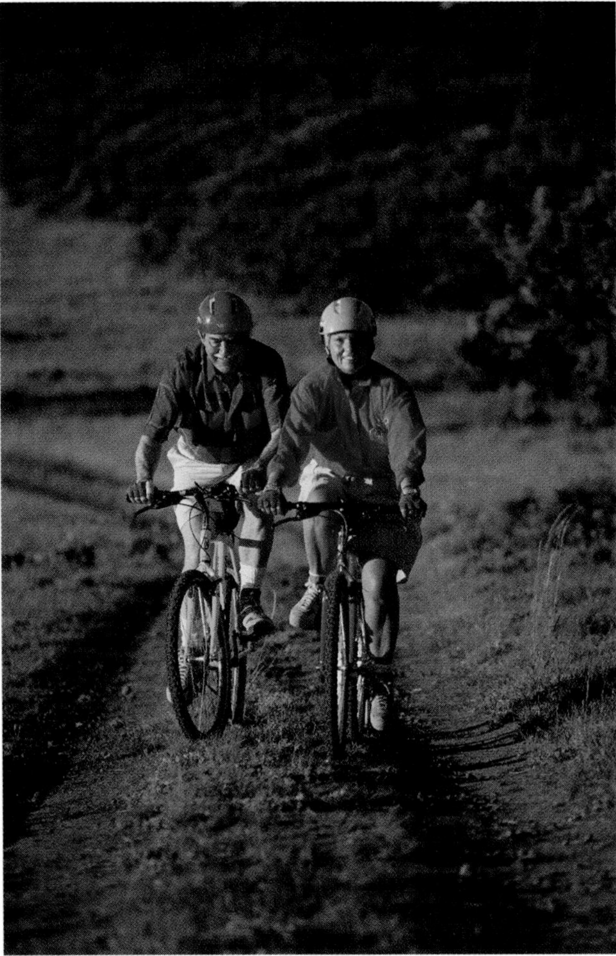

FIGURE 13-2 Energy needs vary according to degree of activity. *(Credit: PhotoDisc.)*

median In statistics, the middle number in a sequence such that half of the numbers are higher and half of the numbers are lower.

iron to offset iron loss from menstrual blood loss; therefore their RDA for iron is 18 mg/day; for men, it is 8 mg/day.[12] Iron requirements for pregnancy are 27 mg/day, which is difficult to attain by diet alone; therefore a supplement is usually prescribed. Iron needs in lactation are 9 mg daily based on the fact that the menses have not resumed.

4. *Vitamins.* The vitamin needs of young adults can be provided by food in a well-balanced diet pattern. Problems in some individuals relate more to inadequate intake than to increased need. Folate is of particular concern for young women, who may become pregnant and need good body stores of this nutrient before conception (see Chapter 7). It also appears that young adults who spend little time in the sun and do not use vitamin D–fortified dairy products or supplements containing vitamin D may be low in this vitamin and thus not able to adequately absorb the calcium present in food or supplements.[7]

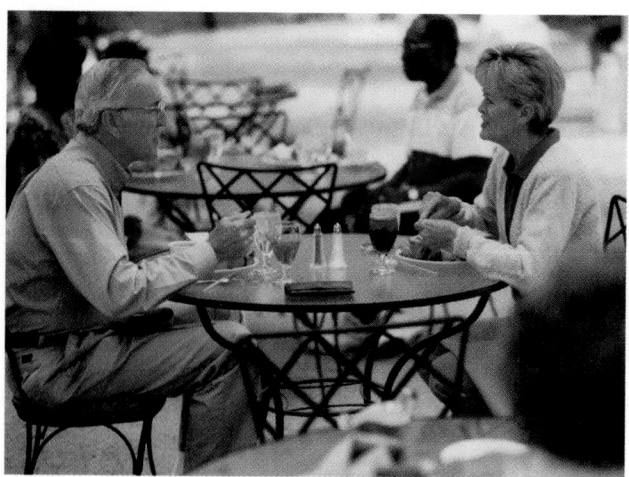

FIGURE 13-3 Middle adult years can often be a time to expand personal growth. *(Credit: PhotoDisc.)*

MIDDLE ADULT: 45 TO 65 YEARS

Physical Characteristics

Physical maintenance established during the early adult years continues into the middle adult years. However, the cell replication rate begins to slow and gradual cell loss begins. From their 30s and 40s onward, both men and women show a decline in skeletal muscle mass and muscle strength, a condition called *sarcopenia,* which means "vanishing flesh."[13] Depending on the amount of physical activity, which is often low during these years, body fat may begin to increase in both genders.[14] Regular physical examinations and laboratory tests to monitor blood lipid levels are important in this stage of life to recognize early risks of heart disease that respond to intervention.

Psychosocial Development

The middle-age adult has moved beyond the period of self-analysis and early focus on career and is now in the stage of active involvement with others—family, grandchildren, and community. Their children are now adults themselves, grown and gone to make their own lives. For some, these years have been called the "empty nest." For many, however, it is an opportunity to expand their personal horizons now that their children are independent and no longer require care on a daily basis (Figure 13-3). There is a realistic coming-to-terms with what life is all about, together with a sharing of lessons learned with younger persons. It is a regeneration of one's life in the lives of young people following in the same way. To the degree that these inner struggles are not won, there is an increasing self-absorption, a turning in on oneself, and a withering rather than a regenerating spirit of life.

Socioeconomic Status

With increasing technology in business and manufacturing, shifts in the nature of employment can bring job loss for workers at all levels of responsibility. No longer can employees expect job security with the same company all of their working lives to retirement. Women left alone as a result of divorce or others with increased time to fill now that their children are grown reenter the work force or seek new educational opportunities.

Nutritional Needs

The energy and protein needs of earlier adult years continue, and calcium takes on special importance, particularly for women. Postmenopausal women need an increased intake of calcium to reduce the loss of bone calcium when protective estrogen is no longer present.[7] The loss of estrogen in menopause and subsequent loss of bone mass increase the risk of osteoporosis and bone fracture.[15,16] Physical activity continues to decrease, adding to cardiovascular risk and possible weight gain, as well as increased vulnerability to fads that promise youth and vigor.

LATER ADULT: 65 TO 85 YEARS

Physical Characteristics

The later adult years bring a gradual waning of physical vigor, work capacity, and strength. Changes may be minimal through the years immediately after retirement but become more pronounced as individuals move through their 70s and into their 80s. Physical activity may be very limited in the later years as a result of chronic diseases such as osteoarthritis, heart disease, or pulmonary disease, adding to problems in energy balance. Increasing age brings further changes in body composition: total body water, bone mass, and muscle mass are lost while body fat mass increases. Even those elders whose body weight remains the same throughout middle and older age have more body fat at any given relative weight than do younger persons of the same weight.[14] Also, the distribution of body fat changes in later years, moving from the extremities to the body trunk, especially the abdomen, and this too has implications for health.[17] Abdominal fat contributes to a rise in serum lipids by releasing increased amounts of fatty acids into the blood and raising blood insulin levels, which raises the risk of diabetes.[18]

Psychosocial Development

Psychosocial development in the later adult years involves continuing adaptation to new challenges as physical abilities decline and emotional supports are lost. Depending on a person's resources at this point, a sense of wholeness and completeness predominates or a sense of despair prevails. If the outcomes of life's experiences have been positive, the individual arrives at older age a rich person—rich in the wisdom of the years and rewarding relationships. Building on each previous level, psychosocial growth now reaches its personal positive resolution. Nevertheless, problems associated with declining health or other circumstances over which the aging individual has no control can result in depression or failure to thrive.[19]

Socioeconomic Status

Older adults often face retirement with a limited fixed income. Others may have no stable income source and lack economic security. Lack of financial resources influences nutrient intake, and lower-income older persons have poorer diets than do higher-income older persons.[20] Living alone may influence food intake if social isolation leads to depression and the lack of incentive or ability to procure and prepare food; however, many other circumstances related to living alone contribute to food problems in the aging individual.[21] Older persons living alone are also more likely to be above age 75 and have lower incomes, which influences their ability to obtain food. Frail homebound elderly persons may have difficulty obtaining groceries on a regular basis and experience economic and social deprivation.[22] An older individual living alone with no neighbors or near relatives may go without food or adequate fluids on sick days when he or she is confined to bed.

Nutritional Needs

The new DRIs have established two age categories for persons above age 50: ages 51 to 70 and ages 71 and older (see Tables 13-1, 13-2, and 13-3). These categories were established to recognize the continuing physical changes that occur with the aging process as well as the continuing development of chronic disease. The current RDAs for energy and protein have not been updated and cover all persons above age 50. Certain prescription and over-the-counter drugs used regularly by aging individuals to manage chronic diseases influence nutrient requirements.

1. *Energy.* The current energy allowance for all adults age 19 years and over is calculated at 1.6 times the REE with adjustments for changes in body composition over the passing years. The energy need of a physically active 65-year-old man with an average weight of 77 kg is about 2600 kcalories/day, and the energy need of a physically active 65-year-old woman with an average weight of 57 kg is about 2100 kcalories/day.[4] The normal variation to account for individual needs is 20%. The kcaloric needs of older adults beyond the age of 75 years are likely to be somewhat less because of their reduced body size, REE, and physical activity. Nevertheless, physical activity to the extent possible is critical to maintain muscle mass and well-being. The sharp decline in physical activity often seen in elderly persons is not inevitable and certainly not desirable.
2. *Protein.* The daily protein allowance set in 2002 is the same for adults aged 25 to 50 and 51 and older. Currently, a level of 0.8 g/kg body weight is recommended for both genders (see Table 13-1). This makes the average allowance 56 g/day for men and 46 g/day for women.[4] This RDA is somewhat controversial. Recent research studies indicate that many older people above age 65 are not able to maintain nitrogen balance on protein intakes of 0.8 g/kg body weight per day. These older individuals continued to lose body nitrogen on a protein intake meeting the current RDA and at least some of the protein nitrogen that was lost came from muscle. In older age our bodies use protein less efficiently, and nutrition experts suggest that a protein standard of 1.0 g/kg body weight would be more appropriate for those over age 50.[23,24]
3. *Minerals.* Both calcium and iron recommendations change for persons over age 50. In older women the need for iron is decreased as menopause interrupts the monthly blood and iron loss; therefore the RDA for older women becomes the same as that for adult men (see Table 13-2). The Adequate Intake for calcium increases from 1000 to 1300 mg for both men and women after age 50 as a strategy to prevent bone loss and the development of osteoporosis.[7]
4. *Vitamins.* Daily allowances for most vitamins remain essentially the same for middle age and older age adults, with the exception of vitamin B_6 and vitamin D (see Table 13-3). Vitamin B_6 is used less efficiently by the older adult, and this may relate to the decreased amount of muscle mass that is available; muscle is the usual storage site for vitamin B_6, thus the RDA is increased.[25] To ensure an appropriate level of vitamin D to participate in calcium absorption and prevent bone loss, the Adequate Intake for vitamin D is raised from 10 μg (400 IU) to 15 μg (600 IU) for individuals aged 71 and older.[7]

OLDEST-OLD: 85 YEARS AND OLDER

U.S. Census Bureau Projections

All projections indicate that as a population we are growing older. The oldest adult group among us (those aged 85 and older) is the fastest growing age cohort within the general population, but because this is so recent a phenomenon, this "oldest-old" group is the least well understood. To distinguish the changing nature of the older adult population and to direct attention to the specific changes that continue to occur as we age, the U.S. Census Bureau now uses three classifications to distinguish persons aged 65 and older.

1. The young-old: aged 65 through 74 years
2. The old-old: aged 75 through 84 years
3. The oldest-old: aged 85 years and older

About 2 million people in the United States are now aged 85 and older. The Census Bureau projects that this number will reach 19 million by the year 2050. Looking at this increase in longevity in another way, about 65,000 persons are now age 100 or older; in the next 30 years this will increase to nearly 380,000. Given the rapid pace of biomedical research, many scientists working in this field think it is likely that life expectancy will continue to increase and the actual numbers of elderly will surpass all current projections.[2]

Nutritional Needs

Elderly persons continue to change as they age and become less efficient in nutrient absorption, overall nutrient utilization, and response to exercise, and body composition also continues to change. All of these factors influence nutritional needs. Nutrition scientists responsible for development of the DRIs gave careful attention to the research available that describes the nutritional needs and patterns of individuals aged 71 and older. Unfortunately, we know relatively little about the interactions between the aging process and chronic diseases that may affect nutrition needs and responses in the oldest-old, and research describing the nutrition and health needs of those aged 85 and older is urgently needed.

Some elderly persons—often women—with small bodies and low daily energy intakes of 1000 to 1200 kcalories or less require prudent supplementation to help meet their overall nutritional needs.[26,27] Unwanted weight loss resulting from low kcaloric intake is a major problem in caring for the oldest-old.

POSITIVE HEALTH PROMOTION: DIETARY PATTERN FOR ADULT HEALTH

Two basic tools, issued by the U.S. Department of Agriculture (USDA) and the U.S. Department of Health and Human Services (USDHHS), can serve as patterns for planning healthy diets for adults of all age groups. These are the *Food Guide Pyramid,* which provides a visual pattern for food choices from five basic food groups, and the *Dietary Guidelines for Americans,* which summarize a sound approach to reducing risks for America's leading health problems. Both of these guides, described in Chapter 1, emphasize the two basic keys to healthy diet planning and food behavior at any age: moderation and variety. The American Dietetic Association, as part of its initiative on Nutrition and Health for Older Americans, has developed a *Food Guide Pyramid for Persons Fifty Plus* that is based on the USDA *Food Guide Pyramid* and emphasizes food items that are easy to prepare and easy to chew; this *Food Guide Pyramid* is given in Figure 13-4.

The Aging Process

THE STUDY OF GERONTOLOGY

The word gerontology refers to the study of aging and can include research in the biologic, physiologic, behavioral, and sociologic aspects of aging. As the older population continues to grow, it will be important to study the role of older people in the community and how younger people can provide support for their older neighbors as well as learn from them. Researchers studying nutrition and health aspects of gerontology are trying to better understand the physical aging process as it affects both length and quality of life.

Length of Life

During the past century, the life expectancy of Americans has nearly doubled from about 49 years to almost 80 years.[3] Most of this advance resulted from reducing deaths of infants and young children, conquering the scourges of infectious diseases such as influenza, and improving sanitation standards, made possible in part through the development of antibiotics and the attention in cities to clean water and appropriate sewage and garbage systems. The harder work of increasing life expectancy lies ahead as we try to understand the normal aging process, apart from chronic disease, and how it can be influenced. The new tools of molecular biology allow us to study aging at the level of the cell and even the gene, and separate out the many factors—both genetic and environmental—that cause cells to change and grow old.

Environmental factors such as pollution or personal lifestyle habits related to diet, smoking, use of alcohol, or level of physical activity play a role in human aging. Studies thus far also support the theory that oxidative cell damage by free cell radicals influences the aging process, and this damage may affect both physiologic and mental processes. There also seems to be a critical connection between the general functional decline that occurs with advancing age and the "growing old" of human cells, which is controlled by our genes and the biologic limits to cell replication, rather than our *chronologic age* or age in years. Researchers are beginning to separate the chronic diseases of older age from the normal process of aging and lay the groundwork for a lengthened and improved end of life in humans.

Quality of Life

Demographic reports of an increasing life span and rapidly growing older population in the United States and worldwide have forced attention to the quality of this extended life. We are looking at a future of increased numbers of elderly persons and a rise in the costs of providing

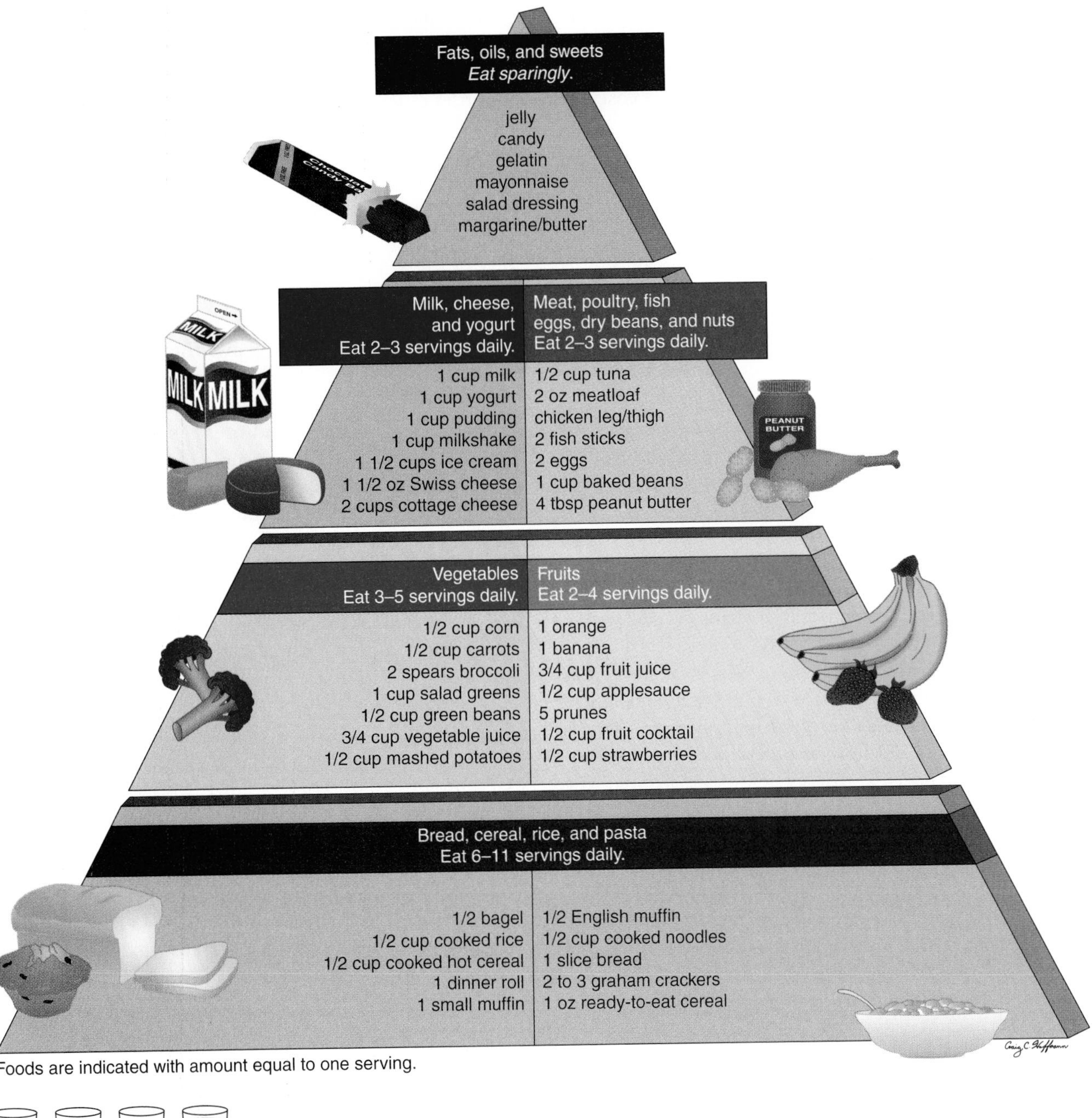

FIGURE 13-4 Food Guide Pyramid for Persons Fifty Plus. (© *2001, American Dietetic Association.* "Nutrition Management and Restorative Dining." *Used with permission.*)

for their care. In the United States, persons aged 65 and older compose only 12% of the population but incur more than one third of the nation's healthcare costs. Healthcare expenditures of persons aged 65 to 69 are $5800 per year compared with $16,500 for those aged 85 and older. Based on the rapid growth of the over-85 group, expenditures for

> demographic The statistical data of a population, especially those showing average age, income, education, births, and deaths.
>
> gerontology Study of the aging process and its remarkable progressive events.

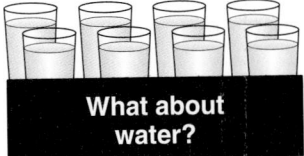

their healthcare are expected to double in the next decade. These costs will rise even more rapidly when the first of the baby boomer generation turns 85 years old in 2031.[2]

These trends and projections in healthcare costs are forcing us to consider both the nature and rate of aging changes and potential means of slowing or preventing these changes, thereby reducing chronic disease and disability. Nonfatal but highly disabling age-dependent conditions, including osteoarthritis, osteoporosis, blindness or other sensory impairments, and Alzheimer's disease, are areas of intensive study by scientists at the National Institute on Aging and universities across the country.

BIOLOGIC CHANGES IN AGING

The biologic process of growth, maturation, and gradual decline extends over the entire life span. It is conditioned by all previous life experiences and the imprint of these experiences on individual genetic heritage.

Nature of Biologic Changes

During middle and older adulthood, there is a gradual loss of cells and reduced metabolism in remaining cells, with a related gradual reduction in the performance capacity of most organ systems. These changes—both physical and mental—can occur rapidly in one organ system and slowly in another, and individuals vary widely in the rate at which these changes occur. But in general, lean body mass continues an age-related decline that accelerates in later life. For example, by the age of 70 years the kidneys lose about 28% of their weight in comparison with values in young adults, the liver loses 25% of its weight, and skeletal muscle diminishes by almost half.[13,19] Functioning units of the kidney—the nephrons—are lost as a result of the aging process and the effect of environmental factors such as our high protein intakes (see Chapter 21). Inactivity likely contributes to the loss of skeletal muscle. This gradual loss of cellular units across organ systems results in an important, overall reduction in the body's reserve capacity; therefore the older adult is less able to respond to environmental changes, physical stress, or conditions of disease and infection.

Effect of Biologic Changes on Food Intake and Utilization

Some physiologic changes that occur with age affect nutritional status. The secretion of certain digestive juices is diminished and a lack of gastric acid can lead to unwanted bacterial growth.[19] This contributes to decreased availability and absorption of important nutrients. Sensory perceptions of taste, smell, hearing, and vision may change, although these responses are highly individual.[19] These senses influence appetite and the enjoyment of food, and thus the amount of food consumed; therefore food for older adults generally needs more—not less—enhancement in seasoning. Along with these biologic changes often comes an increased concern about functional abilities and possible loss of independence, losses of loved ones and friends, financial worries, and fewer social opportunities to maintain self-esteem. All of these psychosocial and emotional responses can affect food intake.

INDIVIDUALITY OF THE AGING PROCESS

The biologic changes in aging occur in all individuals, but persons in the advancing years of life display a wide variety of individual reactions. We get old at different rates. Every person bears the imprint of individual trauma and accumulated disease experience as well as lifestyle choices, and we grow older at our own individual and unique gene-controlled rate. We can discuss aging and its nutritional needs in general terms, but individual situations and needs vary widely and must always be individually assessed. In fact all older people of a certain age are less alike than are all younger people of a certain age, because each has been exposed to a unique set of genetic and environmental influences. The greatest influence of nutrition on the aging process may occur in the early growth years, even as early as fetal life, when resources for later times are being built. Thus nutrition plays an important role in the growth and middle years in preparing us to meet the gradually declining metabolic processes of older age.

NORMAL VERSUS SUCCESSFUL AGING

Gerontologists who have studied the aging process have defined two types of human aging: normal and successful. *Normal* aging occurs as a result of both genetic and typical environmental influences. *Successful* aging occurs when individuals slow the number and rate of aging changes through positive lifestyle choices or health-related interventions.[19] A balanced diet, an active lifestyle, a positive outlook, and avoidance of addictive behaviors such as smoking and inappropriate use of alcohol all contribute to successful aging.

Individuality in Nutritional Needs of Elderly Persons

ENERGY

Reduced basal metabolic requirements caused by losses in functioning cells and reduced physical activity combine to create less energy demand as age advances. Some animal studies indicate that a diet limited in kcalories but adequate in protein, vitamins, and minerals—"undernutrition without malnutrition"—may actually lengthen life. The major difference between these animals restricted in kcalories and their counterparts consuming more kcalories is their smaller amount of body fat. We need to evaluate the influence of both the amount and the anatomical location of body fat on length of life and progression of aging changes in humans.

Individual energy needs vary with body size and physical activity, but an average estimate is about 1800 kcalories/day, more or less. However, mean energy intake is considerably lower in many older people. In a recent national survey the average daily energy intake of women aged 65 and older was about 1400 kcalories.[5] Such low-kcalorie diets are likely to be limiting in protein and important vitamins and minerals.

The kcaloric requirements of older adults vary greatly, related in part to their level of physical activity. Because living situations can be very different, a nutritional assessment must include information about daily life activities and the degree of energy they may be capable of expending. New research indicates that older adults, even relatively inactive older adults, have higher energy requirements than we previously thought and may expend more kcalories in performing a particular activity than younger persons with greater muscle coordination.[28-30] Perhaps the simplest criterion for judging adequacy of kcalorie intake is the maintenance of normal weight. However, we are currently rethinking the traditional standards for appropriate weight based on life insurance weight-for-height tables (see Chapter 6). Recent assessment of life expectancy data has raised the idea that the greatest longevity at older ages is not associated with the conventional desirable weight but with weight levels 10% to 25% greater.[31] This report has important nutritional implications for optimal energy intake of older adults. A variety of physiologic changes associated with the aging process—changes in the appetite control center in the hypothalamus, decreased taste and smell, and the use of multiple prescription medications reduce food intake in many elderly individuals. Prevention of unintentional weight loss is an important clinical responsibility in the care of older persons in both community-based and institution-based long-term care.[32,33] To meet energy needs, older adults need ample carbohydrates but limited fats.

1. *Carbohydrates.* Based on what is currently known about the optimal intake of carbohydrate, it is usually recommended that at least 50% to 55% of daily kcalories come from carbohydrate foods, and mostly complex carbohydrates such as starches. Older persons can choose freely among carbohydrate foods, according to individual needs, desires, and physical responses. In general the fasting blood glucose level does not change with advancing age in persons who do not have diabetes. Much of the observed change and increasing carbohydrate intolerance of older persons is related to factors other than biologic aging per se. Diets rich in fiber and complex carbohydrates such as legumes and a lifestyle that includes regular exercise can substantially curtail age-related changes in postmeal glucose levels and insulin resistance.[34-37]
2. *Fats.* Generally, Americans eat too much fat, and fat intake is best limited to about 30% of total kcalories. Some fat is needed as a source of energy and essential fatty acids and to support absorption of the fat-soluble vitamins. A reasonable goal is to avoid large quantities of fat, with more emphasis on the quality of the smaller amount of fat consumed, using mostly plant fats and fewer animal fats. The digestion and absorption of fats may be somewhat delayed in elderly persons, but these functions are not greatly disturbed with age. There is no need to be unduly restrictive. Sufficient fat for food palatability aids appetite and as a concentrated form of kcalories may help prevent unwanted weight loss. Increasing fat intake to 35% of total kcalories may be necessary to prevent weight loss in some very frail elderly people.
3. *Protein.* Adequate, high-quality protein is needed to preserve muscle mass, support optimum immune function, and allow normal replacement and maintenance of body proteins.
   - *Basic needs.* Although the current RDA is set at 0.8 g/kg body weight, growing evidence suggests that intakes of 1.0 to 1.2 g/kg body weight are needed to ensure the preservation of muscle mass.[23,38] Preservation of muscle mass is important for two reasons: (1) the amount of muscle present is a predictor of functional ability and the capacity for self-care, and (2) muscle serves as a store of amino acids to meet emergency needs in illness or injury. Healthy elderly with protein intakes below 1.0 g/kg body weight are more likely to have a lower immune response that improves when more protein is made available. Debilitated older people may require intakes of 1.6 g/kg body weight along with additional kcalories to adequately replace body stores.[39-40]
   - *Protein quality.* Protein needs are influenced by two basic factors: (1) the biologic value of the protein based on the quantity and ratio of its essential amino acids and (2) adequate kcalories in the diet. It is estimated that about 25% to 50% of the protein intake should come from animal sources, the only foods that are complete proteins with all the essential amino acids; the remainder of dietary protein can be from plant protein sources. In a vegetarian diet, plant proteins—with additions of milk or egg protein—ensure adequate protein intake. At this time we know very little about the ability of very elderly or frail individuals to maintain optimum protein status on a vegan diet. Protein should supply from 15% to 20% of the day's total kcalories. Healthy older adults do not need supplemental amino acid preparations because appropriate amounts and combinations are available from food. Nutritional supplements containing good-quality protein may be needed for debilitated elderly individuals but should be used only with the advice of a healthcare professional.

TO PROBE FURTHER

Thinking Processes in Older Adults: Food for Thought

Since the early studies of nutrition we have known that particular nutrients are important for the cognitive processes of thinking, reasoning, and recall. Those researchers found that certain B-complex vitamins were needed to maintain healthy tissues in the nervous system and prevent changes in personality or behavior. For example, alcohol abusers who become thiamin deficient develop dementia and experience hallucinations. The deterioration of mental status that accompanies a vitamin B_{12} deficiency is well understood. New laboratory methods that allow us to evaluate biologic changes at the subcellular level have brought about a new interest in the relationship between nutrition and brain function. Also, because some of the changes that occur in nerve tissues as a result of nutrient deficiency are similar to changes that occur with the aging process, researchers are taking a new look at the role of nutrition in preventing aging losses in the brain and nervous system.

GLUCOSE AND THE AGING BRAIN

The brain relies on glucose as the energy source to do its work; in fact, under normal circumstances, glucose is the only source of energy used by brain cells. Despite its reliance on glucose, the brain stores only enough glucose to last about 10 minutes, thus a constant supply is necessary. It also appears that more difficult tasks create an increased need for glucose compared with simple tasks, and prolonged tasks require additional glucose as work continues. Although brain glucose levels cannot be measured in humans, a glucose-containing drink has been shown to improve memory in verbal tests with older adults. Diabetes and poor glucose tolerance seem to have adverse effects on brain function in the elderly. When blood glucose levels remain high, as is the situation in uncontrolled diabetes, adaptation causes lower amounts of glucose to enter the brain and leads to poor memory performance. If insulin injections are poorly timed, and hypoglycemia ensues, mental confusion and loss of concentration will occur. Thus good glycemic control is an important goal in managing the elderly diabetic. Eating breakfast and a mid-morning snack improve mood in younger adults and replenishing brain glucose is believed to be the basis for this effect. The use of snacks by older adults to maintain stable blood glucose levels may support optimum brain function.

B-COMPLEX VITAMINS AND BRAIN FUNCTION

Vitamins can affect brain function in several different ways. Vitamin B_6 (pyridoxine) is necessary for the synthesis of various neurotransmitters, the chemicals that are needed to send nerve impulses from one nerve to another. One such transmitter is dopamine, and low levels of dopamine result in the loss of muscle control and tremors that are characteristic of Parkinson's disease. Poor intakes of vitamin B_6, resulting in lower levels of neurotransmitters, could also interfere with brain function related to memory and reasoning.

Several studies of older adults have reported a relationship between folate status and thought processes. About 10,000 persons aged 60 and older who participated in the Third National Health and Nutrition Examination Survey also completed the Mini-Mental State Examination, a brief word recall test commonly used to evaluate mental function in older adults. Years of schooling did not affect scores on this examination; however, the older persons with poorer recall had lower blood folate levels than those with higher recall. Elevated blood homocysteine levels are a sign of poor folate status. Blood homocysteine levels also were higher in the older persons having poorer recall.

Folate plays several roles in brain function. First folate participates in the formation of nucleic acids and other molecules important in the maintenance of brain tissue. Second, high blood homocysteine levels that result when folate is lacking increase atherosclerotic deposits in the lining of the blood vessels that could slow the delivery of oxygen and other nutrients to brain cells. Blood vessel changes caused by high blood homocysteine levels may be involved in the development of Alzheimer's disease.

Folate may influence mood and perceived quality of life. Liquid nutrition supplements given to a generally healthy group of older adults living in the community led to increased feelings of well-being that did not occur in older persons who were similar in age and living situation but did not receive the dietary intervention. The older adults receiving supplements had more energy and were less tired. Although the provided supplements contained many vitamins and minerals, folate was the one nutrient that appeared to contribute most to this effect.

VITAMIN E AND BRAIN FUNCTION

Vitamin E, an important antioxidant, may help prevent degenerative changes in brain and nerve tissue. Oxidation reactions that damage important brain proteins or cause structural changes in cell membranes are part of the sequence of changes that lead to the brain alterations seen in Alzheimer's disease. Vitamin E prevents the oxidation of blood cholesterol that damages

TO PROBE FURTHER

Thinking Processes in Older Adults: Food for Thought—cont'd

vessels supplying blood to the brain (see Chapter 7 to review the actions of folate, vitamin B_{12}, vitamin E, and antioxidants).

We need to learn more about how vitamin intake affects the brain. In the meantime it is important that older adults take in the recommended amounts of all vitamins that participate in memory and feelings of well-being. Remember, there is no good evidence to support the use of vitamin supplements in excess of the RDA/DRI for each of these nutrients.

References

Benton D: The impact of the supply of glucose to the brain on mood and memory, *Nutr Rev* 59:S20, 2001.

Christen Y: Oxidative stress and Alzheimer disease, *Am J Clin Nutr* 71(suppl):621S, 2000.

Houston DK et al: Age-related hearing loss, vitamin B-12, and folate in elderly women, *Am J Clin Nutr* 69:564, 1999.

Krondl M et al: Subjectively healthy elderly consuming a liquid nutrition supplement maintained body mass index and improved some nutritional parameters and perceived well-being, *J Am Diet Assoc* 99:1542, 1999.

Miller JW: Homocysteine and Alzheimer's disease, *Nutr Rev* 57:126, 1999.

Morris MS et al: Hyperhomocysteinemia associated with poor recall in the third National Health and Nutrition Examination Survey, *Am J Clin Nutr* 73:927, 2001.

Selhub J et al: B vitamins, homocysteine, and neurocognitive function in the elderly, *Am J Clin Nutr* 71(suppl):614S, 2000.

- *Strength-training needs.* Strength training or weight training has been successful in building or replacing muscle in people up to age 100. *Strength training* involves pushing against or lifting a set weight as contrasted with *endurance training,* which involves rhythmic use of the large muscles as in running or jogging. The stimulation provided by strength training leads to an increase in both size and number of muscle cells and enhances functional ability.[13] For example, older individuals who previously required assistance to rise from a chair or could not lift bags of groceries were able to accomplish these tasks without assistance after a strength training program. Both adequate protein and kcalories must be available to support these body-building exercises. Protein intakes of at least 1.2 g/kg body weight and additional kcalories to prevent loss of body weight is recommended for older people participating in strength training.[13,41]

VITAMINS

A growing concern among geriatric physicians and researchers studying nutritional needs in elderly persons is that older adults may have different nutrient needs than their younger counterparts, and these concerns led to the development of the new DRI category for adults aged 71 and older. Traditionally, it was considered unnecessary to provide additional vitamin intake in the healthy older adult, based on the idea that observed decreases in tissue vitamin stores were a normal aspect of aging. It is likely that some individual problems stem from intakes falling below the generally recommended intake rather than from an increased need. Nevertheless, particular vitamins need special attention during this period of life.

1. *Folate.* Adequate levels of this vitamin are needed to prevent the rise in blood homocysteine levels that damage the blood vessels and accelerate atherosclerosis.[25]
2. *Vitamin B_6.* As an active coenzyme in biochemical reactions involving amino acids and protein synthesis, vitamin B_6 is important to preserve or increase muscle mass.[25]
3. *Vitamin B_{12}.* The age-related decrease in gastric acid hinders the absorption of vitamin B_{12} from meat, fish, and poultry, and use of fortified breads or cereals or supplements may be needed.[42]
4. *Vitamin D.* This vitamin may be a problem for those older persons who spend most of their time indoors and do not eat vitamin D-fortified foods.[43] Moreover, sun exposure may be less effective in stimulating vitamin D synthesis in older people because of aging changes in the skin.
5. *Vitamin E.* Antioxidant vitamins and phytochemicals may reduce oxidative damage to cells and help to preserve both cognitive function and immune response.[44] (See *To Probe Further* box, which provides an overview of the role of several vitamins and other nutrients in maintaining mental function in aging.)

All of these nutrients can be obtained from a balanced diet and individual counseling should stress good food sources of these nutrients (see Chapter 7 to review food sources).

cognitive Pertaining to the mental processes of perception, memory, judgment, and reasoning, as contrasted with emotional and volitional processes.

MINERALS

In general mineral supplements are not needed for healthy elderly and current recommendations can be met on a continuing basis by a well-balanced diet. The major exception to this rule is likely calcium as it can be difficult to obtain 1200 mg daily without some modification of the usual diet, although calcium-fortified fruit and vegetable juices and cereals can complement servings of milk, cheese, yogurt, or calcium-fortified soy milk to reach the equivalent of four servings, providing 300 mg each. A particular benefit of fluid milk, fortified soy milk, or fortified yogurt is the presence of added vitamin D.

WATER

Too often the vital need for water in older adults is overlooked. Changes in the hypothalamus alter the thirst mechanism so that older persons do not get thirsty and drink as much fluid as they should, and dehydration can easily occur. Body water serves as the medium for the dilution of medications and dehydration increases the risk of adverse drug reactions. Conscious attention to adequate fluid intake, not less than 1500 ml to 2000 ml daily, is an important aspect of health maintenance and care.[24,45] Older people might be advised to develop a daily pattern in which they drink a glass of water or other noncaffeinated beverage at certain times of the day. Encouraging the use of water bottles, more typically adopted by teens and athletes, might be a way to increase regular water intake by older individuals.

NUTRIENT SUPPLEMENTATION

Healthy adults of any age regularly consuming balanced diets that include a variety of foods are unlikely to need added nutrient supplements. However, elderly persons are at greater nutritional risk, and might benefit from prudent, individually assessed supplementation. Women with a low energy intake, the oldest-old, the chronically ill or those in poor health who use multiple prescription drugs, individuals living alone or lacking social support, elderly persons with limited mobility, or those having insufficient money for food are especially at risk of low nutrient intake.[46-48] In such cases, however, it is important to remember that nutritional supplements should add to, not replace food. Also, older people must be guided as to their choice of supplements. Among 130 rural older adults nearly half used some type of supplement; however, the supplements chosen did not supply the nutrients most deficient in their diet.[49] In illness or debilitated states nutritional supplements may well be needed to replenish losses.

Preventive Health and Clinical Needs

SUCCESSFUL AGING

Many older Americans are not only living longer but also aging well. They have vigor and vitality and often participate in positive health maintenance programs. More than 80% of the oldest-old still live in the community and not in nursing homes, despite some disability or infirmity.[2] These individuals aged 85 and older, mostly women, may live alone, with friends or family in residential settings, or in adult foster care or community care homes. However, among older individuals living in nursing homes, hospitals, or the community, malnutrition is too often present and requires personal care and prevention.

MALNUTRITION

Incidence

Protein-energy malnutrition occurs in many elderly persons, especially those in hospitals or nursing homes or with serious medical problems.[33,50] Chronic disease conditions such as congestive heart failure often accentuate aging changes to produce a profound anorexia of aging.[51] Healthcare providers can and must communicate with these older adults whatever their situation may be.[10] It is not uncommon that some of these malnourished persons weigh less than 45.5 kg (100 lb) and eat fewer than 1000 kcalories daily. Wide experience has indicated that many of these older clients had no physician-recorded diagnosis of malnutrition or weight loss or any physician-prescribed nutrition supplement or nutrition assessment referral. Thus malnutrition, with or without a contributory disease, is all too common among elderly persons living in the community, and often a specific nutritional diagnosis with follow-up intervention does not occur.

Warning Signs and Preventive Care

Warning signs can alert us to early malnutrition in elderly persons. If heeded, they are crucial to preventing unnecessary and sometimes irreversible weight loss.[33,52-53]

1. *Physical signs.* Recent unintended weight loss, perhaps associated with eating problems resulting from tooth loss or poorly fitting dentures; dry mouth from decreased salivary secretions; diminished sensory perceptions such as taste, smell, or sight; or difficulty with swallowing is an obvious sign of inadequate nutrient intake (see *Practical Application* box).
2. *Multiple medications.* Long-term use of multiple medications, often termed *polypharmacy,* with actions and side effects that are often unexplained to patient and family, can interact with food and nutrients and interfere with the absorption or utilization of nutrients. Medications can also lower actual food intake by reducing appetite or producing a distorted or "bad" taste.

PRACTICAL APPLICATION

Involuntary Weight Loss: Why Does it Occur in Older Adults and What are the Consequences?

A major concern for both community caregivers and health professionals responsible for older adults in long-term care facilities is unwanted and inappropriate weight loss. Unwanted weight loss is associated with functional disability, limited nutrient reserves, and poor outcomes after surgery or serious illness.

DEFINING SERIOUS WEIGHT LOSS

Clinical care providers have taken several approaches to the characterization of serious weight loss. The standard for serious weight loss used by many long-term care facilities when monitoring body weight is the loss of 10 lb or more over a period of 6 months or the loss of 5% or more of total body weight over a period of 1 year. The Nutrition Screening Initiative (see p. 336) recommends that older adults who have lost 10 lb or more over a period of 6 months receive nutrition counseling and intervention.

FAILURE TO THRIVE AND FRAILTY

Failure to thrive is the term used to designate one weight loss condition identified in older adults. Long recognized as a syndrome in infants and children who are neglected, failure to thrive in the developing child is distinguished by a failure to grow and develop in both physical and social skills. In older persons the opposite occurs, this condition is typified as a failure to maintain, as the individual regresses in physical well-being and mental function. The first and major observation occurring in failure to thrive in older adults is weight loss, followed by increasing physical disability, loss of skills for self-care, social withdrawal, and diminished mental function and, finally, death. In failure to thrive there is no biologic or physiologic explanation for the observed weight loss and malnutrition—this downhill spiral is not the result of a terminal illness. In most cases the weight loss is related to lack of financial resources, social isolation, limited ability to obtain groceries or prepare meals, chronic disease and disability, failing eyesight, or other circumstance that limits food intake. If detected early, intervention is both possible and effective, when contributing factors are defined. Egbert referred to these older people as the "dwindles" and in most cases they are living in the community.

More recently researchers described a group of clinical symptoms associated with frailty that may have a biologic basis. In this study older adults judged to be frail had (1) unintentional weight loss of 10 lb or more in the previous year, (2) weakness as measured by low grip strength, (3) poor endurance with self-reports of chronic tiredness or exhaustion, (4) slowness based on the amount of time required to walk 15 ft, and (5) low physical activity. These symptoms were more prevalent in elderly adults who were female, African American, and older or among those with accompanying chronic conditions such as cardiovascular or pulmonary disease, arthritis, and diabetes. Cancer was not more frequent in the frail elderly compared with those who were not frail.

CONSEQUENCES OF INVOLUNTARY WEIGHT LOSS

Older adults who have experienced rapid and substantial weight loss are highly vulnerable to adverse health outcomes. These individuals are more likely to fall and, if injured, are less likely to survive or return to their own homes. The loss of muscle mass that occurs with involuntary weight loss limits the individual's ability for self-care and the downhill spiral of disability often leads to institutionalization. Frail persons have a higher risk of death within 5 years compared with older individuals who have not experienced weight loss and accompanying changes in body composition. Unwanted weight loss may actually begin with hospitalization for an unrelated condition. In nearly 500 hospitalized patients with an average age of 74, more than half received diets that provided less than 50% of their calculated energy requirements. Elderly people should be considered at high nutritional risk if their body mass index (BMI) is less than 19 and at low nutritional risk if their BMI is equal to or higher than 22.

WHY DO OLDER ADULTS EXPERIENCE UNWANTED WEIGHT LOSS?

Many situations contribute to poor food intake in elderly persons including lack of resources to obtain food, chronic disease, and depression. Chronic disease influences both energy needs and energy intake. Congestive heart failure and pulmonary disease can elevate energy requirements and lead to continuing weight loss. Certain drugs such as digoxin bring about cardiac cachexia related to both increased energy needs and low food intake. Anorexia and disordered taste are common side effects of many prescription drugs. Early satiety and aging changes in the hypothalamus appetite control center also decrease food intake (see p. 122).

Dietary restraint and eating disorders are present in some older persons. Fear of overweight or obesity and its physical consequences and perceived disease risk can reduce food intake in older individuals. Anorexia nervosa and disordered body image have been identified in the older population, although health concerns rather than social pressures to be thin are more likely to be the cause of this behavior. Loss of interest in life and depression reduce eating in some older adults. Antidepressants have been used in some skilled nursing facilities in an attempt to increase food intake. Although certain antidepressants

Continued

PRACTICAL APPLICATION

Involuntary Weight Loss: Why Does it Occur in Older Adults and What are the Consequences?—cont'd

(tricyclic antidepressants) are believed to lead to weight gain, no general trends were observed in these elderly adults. On the other hand, selective serotonin reuptake inhibitors, commonly believed to reduce food intake, do not produce this effect in the majority of older adults given these drugs. Increased social interaction, particularly at mealtime, supports increased food intake.

When studying weight loss in older persons, it is difficult to identify what factor occurred first. For example, lack of physical activity is known to heighten the loss of muscle mass as disuse leads to changes in nerve connections and muscle fibers and subsequent muscle atrophy. At the same time a loss of muscle decreases the older person's ability to move about and further limits physical activity. New studies also indicate that elderly adults are less able to regulate energy intake to maintain appropriate body weight. In younger persons a decrease in energy intake brings about a decrease in the REE as the body attempts to conserve energy and protect against unwanted weight loss. In contrast, healthy older people who were underfed for 6 weeks did not compensate for their lower kcalorie intake, lost an increased amount of weight, and failed to regain this weight over the next 6 months. Moreover, the older adults did not have increased hunger during the period of underfeeding, whereas the younger group had increased appetite. This would suggest that periods of low energy intake related to illness, emotional distress, or other circumstance can begin a sequence of weight loss in the older person that will continue uninterrupted. Researchers need to help us understand how we can prevent weight loss in the older persons in our care.

References

Egbert AM: The dwindles: failure to thrive in older patients, *Nutr Rev* 54(II):S26, 1996.

Fried LP et al: Frailty in older adults: evidence for a phenotype, *J Gerontol A Biol Sci Med Sci* 56:M146, 2001.

Moriguti JC et al: Effects of a 6-week hypocaloric diet on changes in body composition, hunger, and subsequent weight regain in healthy young and older adults, *J Gerontol A Biol Sci Med Sci* 55:B580, 2001.

Rigler SK et al: Weight outcomes among antidepressant users in nursing homes, *J Am Geriatr Soc* 49:49, 2001.

Shatenstein B, Kergoat MJ, Nadon S: Weight change, nutritional risk and its determinants among cognitively intact and demented elderly Canadians, *Can J Public Health* 92:143, 2001.

Sullivan DH, Walls RC: Protein-energy undernutrition and the risk of mortality within six years of hospital discharge, *J Am Coll Nutr* 17:571, 1998.

Wilson MM et al: Prevalence and causes of undernutrition in medical outpatients, *Am J Med* 104:56, 1998.

3. *Psychosocial signs.* Grief from loss of spouse or family and friends; depression; loneliness or living alone; being homebound with lack of sunlight; fear of physical harm from others in the home or neighborhood; or increased use or abuse of alcohol which often displaces food intake may result in lack of interest in food and reduced food intake. Distorted body image leading to self-imposed food restriction (anorexia nervosa) has been observed among older patients.
4. *Economic problems.* Low socioeconomic status, lack of sufficient money for food, inadequate housing, and homelessness place older individuals at high risk of malnutrition.
5. *Food-related difficulties.* Disability affecting food shopping or preparation can result in insufficient food stores at home, missed meals, snacks, and fluids, and a lack of fruits, vegetables, dairy foods, and grains. Poor nutrition knowledge or inappropriate food beliefs may limit the variety of foods consumed. Multiple sick days with no one available to assist with food or fluids, or an inappropriately restrictive therapeutic diet that forbids the inclusion of favorite or ethnic comfort foods can reduce food intake. About 1 in 5 elderly persons has *xerostomia,* a severe form of dry mouth caused by a greatly reduced flow of saliva. This makes swallowing difficult as food is not sufficiently moistened and can increase fear of choking. Xerostomia is associated with the use of certain medications, autoimmune diseases, or radiation therapy to the head and neck.[19]

NUTRITION SCREENING INITIATIVE

The Nutrition Screening Initiative (NSI) is a program to promote routine nutrition screening of older people in both community settings and medical facilities through a network of registered dietitians, public health and clinical nutritionists, physicians and other healthcare professionals, and community workers. This multidisciplinary project of the American Dietetic Association, the American Academy of Family Physicians, and the National Council on the Aging targets the warning signs of malnutrition in older Americans that increase the risk of chronic disease, physical disability, and institutionalization. Based on an initial comprehensive survey of research in gerontology and geriatrics and a consensus of leaders in the medical and nutrition communities, seven basic risk factors that serve as warning signs of malnutrition were identified.

The Warning Signs of poor nutritional health are often overlooked. Use this checklist to find out if you or someone you know is at nutritional risk.

DETERMINE YOUR NUTRITIONAL HEALTH

Read the statements below. Circle the number in the yes column for those that apply to you or someone you know. For each yes answer, score the number in the box. Total your nutritional score.

	YES
I have an illness or condition that made me change the kind and/or amount of food I eat.	2
I eat fewer than 2 meals per day.	3
I eat few fruits or vegetables, or milk products.	2
I have 3 or more drinks of beer, liquor or wine almost every day.	2
I have tooth or mouth problems that make it hard for me to eat.	2
I don't always have enough money to buy the food I need.	4
I eat alone most of the time.	1
I take 3 or more different prescribed or over-the-counter drugs a day.	1
Without wanting to, I have lost or gained 10 pounds in the last 6 months.	2
I am not always physically able to shop, cook and/or feed myself.	2
TOTAL	

Total Your Nutritional Score. If it's–

0-2 **Good!** Recheck your nutritional score in 6 months.

3-5 **You are at moderate nutritional risk.** See what can be done to improve your eating habits and lifestyle. Your office on aging, senior nutrition program, senior citizens center or health department can help. Recheck your nutritional score in 3 months.

6 or more **You are at high nutritional risk.** Bring this checklist the next time you see your doctor, dietitian or other qualified health or social service professional. Talk with them about any problems you may have. Ask for help to improve your nutritional health.

These materials developed and distributed by the Nutrition Screening Initiative, a project of:

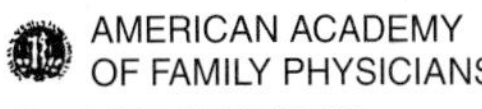
AMERICAN ACADEMY OF FAMILY PHYSICIANS

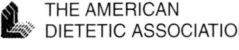

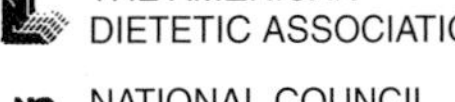
THE AMERICAN DIETETIC ASSOCIATION

NATIONAL COUNCIL ON THE AGING, INC.

Remember that warning signs suggest risk, but do not represent diagnosis of any condition. Turn the page to learn more about the Warning Signs of poor nutritional health.

FIGURE 13-5 DETERMINE Your Nutritional Health checklist. *(Reprinted with permission by the Nutrition Screening Initiative, a project of the American Academy of Family Physicians and The American Dietetic Association, funded in part by a grant from Ross Products Division, Abbott Laboratories Inc.)*

1. Inappropriate food intake
2. Poverty
3. Social isolation
4. Dependency or disability
5. Acute or chronic diseases or conditions
6. Chronic use of medications
7. Advanced age

The NSI developed a public awareness checklist for warning signs of poor nutritional health entitled Determine Your Nutritional Health (Figure 13-5). More recently the NSI has developed a checklist of warning signs for older people confined to skilled nursing facilities.

CLINICAL PROBLEMS

Diets for Chronic Disease

Physicians specializing in geriatrics and clinical nutritionists working with older adults are recommending that medically indicated diets be liberalized for elderly patients, especially those in long-term care facilities.[33,54] For patients at advanced ages, diets for lowering cholesterol

> geriatrics Branch of medicine specializing in medical problems associated with old age.

or blood pressure are of less concern than preventing inappropriate weight loss and malnutrition. Even older patients with insulin-dependent diabetes mellitus can often be managed on regular diets.[54] Highly restrictive diets leading to decreased food intake, serious weight loss, and overt malnutrition are likely to have more immediate consequences than the initial diagnosis. Instead the general practice is to follow a regular diet—well-balanced nutritionally—that offers a wide variety of food choices and some moderation in fats and sweets, as indicated for all of us (see Chapter 1).

Physical Disability

Major attention in research and clinical practice has turned to improving the functional ability of older persons to maximize their opportunities to live independently or to perform self-care to the extent possible in a supervised setting. The overall goal is to add quality of life to these extended years. Support programs for patients with osteoporosis, osteoarthritis, and other debilitating diseases and their families expand their knowledge about the disease and its management and can make a difference in the quality of life of these patients and initiate emotional support within the family. Both individual and group sessions—including nutrition assessment and counseling, physical therapy, and medical evaluation and treatment—have a positive impact on their general physical and psychologic well-being, helping them to cope with the pain and chronic nature of the condition.

COMMUNITY RESOURCES

Government Programs for Older Americans

The usual government food assistance programs for younger individuals and families also provide support for older Americans. These include the Food Stamp Program and the surplus agricultural commodities distribution programs (see Chapter 10). These programs provide needed foods and extend the food-buying resources for many older adults. However, the single greatest impact on the growing field of nutritional gerontology has been the Older Americans Act that created the national Elderly Nutrition Program.

Older Americans Act

In 1972, the Nutrition Program for Older Americans, Title VII of the Older Americans Act, was authorized by Public Law 92-258. This program was developed to meet the nutritional and social needs of persons 60 years of age and older who (1) could not afford adequate diets, (2) were unable to prepare adequate meals at home, (3) had limited mobility, or (4) were isolated and lacked incentive to prepare and eat food alone. This legislation also provided services such as outreach, escort and transportation, information and referral, health and welfare counseling, and nutrition and consumer education. Amendments authorized in 1978 provided for the coordination of nutrition services with other required services such as transportation and nutrition education, and established specific funding for both congregate and home-delivered meals. These nutrition services and education were consolidated under Title III-C of the Older Americans Act and are sometimes referred to as the Title III Nutrition Program.

1. *Congregate meals.* This program provides older Americans, particularly those with low incomes, nutritionally sound meals at little or no cost at senior centers and other public or private community facilities. Older adults can gather for a hot meal at noon and receive not only food but also social support. Food and nutrition education to help dispel nutrition myths and misleading information, to which elderly persons are often vulnerable, is also provided at meal sites.
2. *Home-delivered meals.* For those persons who are homebound by illness or disability, meals are delivered directly to the home. This service not only helps meet nutritional needs but also provides human contact and support for those who may otherwise be socially isolated. Often, the person delivering the meal is the only person the homebound individual may see that day. For some urban and rural homebound elderly persons, many of whom have poor diets, this single hot meal 5 days a week is their main source of food. As the number of homebound elderly continues to grow, programs are being forced to adopt more efficient and cost-effective ways of meal delivery. In some localities, couriers make one delivery a week of several frozen meals that can be reheated on a daily basis. It is important that alternative means of contact be established by telephone or neighbor visits to provide the social support associated with daily meal delivery. (Learn more about these programs in *Issues & Answers.*)

Research Centers of the United States Department of Agriculture

The USDA, in collaboration with universities, has established human nutrition research centers on aging, which are authorized by Congress to study the role of nutrition in the aging process. Current studies include such areas as protein needs in aged persons, the nutritional status of elderly men and women, and the influence of vitamin supplements in preventing age-related changes in immune function.

Extension Services of the United States Department of Agriculture

The USDA operates extension services in state universities and county offices in all states. Through these agencies food and nutrition educators provide counseling and practical nutrition materials for older adults and community workers.

Public Health Departments

Skilled health professionals work in the community through local and state public health departments. Health guidance for elderly persons is available through their resources. The public health nutritionist is a significant member of the healthcare team providing counseling and nutrition education services, overseeing nutrition and health screening services, and monitoring food service facilities in nursing homes licensed by the state.

State Departments for the Aging

All states receive funds under the Older Americans Act to provide nutrition and related services for older citizens and a department on aging within their state government administers the program. This state unit on aging is a source of information and technical assistance for meals programs. Area agencies on aging manage congregate and home-delivered meals programs on the local level under the supervision of the state unit on aging.

PROFESSIONAL ORGANIZATIONS AND RESOURCES

National Council on the Aging

The National Council on the Aging, established in 1950, is located in Washington, DC. It is an organization for professionals and volunteers that work on many fronts to improve the quality of life for older Americans. It serves as a nonprofit national resource for research, planning, training, technical assistance, advocacy and public policy, program and standards development, and publications that relate to all aspects of aging. This organization works with the American Dietetic Association and the American Academy of Family Physicians to identify and assist older Americans at risk for malnutrition (NSI).

American Geriatrics Society

This professional organization of physicians engaged in medical care of elderly patients promotes research in geriatrics to advance scientific knowledge of the aging process and the treatment of its diseases. A number of nurses and other health professionals are associate members. The society publishes the *Journal of the American Geriatrics Society.*

The Gerontological Society

This society's membership includes a wide range of interested health and social service professionals. This organization has stimulated increased interest in gerontology and aging problems among other professional organizations and joins with community and government agencies to advocate for the elderly. This group sponsors two publications, the *Journal of Gerontology* and *The Gerontologist.*

Community Groups

Local community groups representing health professions—such as medical societies, nursing organizations, and dietetic associations—sponsor a variety of programs to help meet the needs of elderly persons in their communities. In addition, qualified nutritionists and registered dietitians in private practice are available in most communities for individual counseling and community program support. Senior citizens centers also provide a broad range of services, including nutrition education.

Volunteer Health Organizations

Many activities of volunteer health organizations, such as the American Heart Association and the American Diabetes Association, relate to the health and nutrition needs of older persons. These organizations include professional and public members. They operate at national and community levels to fund and conduct research and education.

TO SUM UP

The challenge of meeting the nutritional needs of the older population is compounded by the lack of needed research describing the interaction of current and past social, economic, physiologic, and psychologic factors within an aging individual, and the wide range of individual differences in the biologic process of aging and chronic disease.

Nutritional requirements are influenced by the biologic changes of aging that affect organ function and body composition. Current nutrient and energy standards, however, are limited by the paucity of specific research on older adults and thus are based to a great extent on extrapolations of data gathered on younger adults. Nutrients of particular concern to the nutrition and well being of the older population include protein, folate, calcium, and vitamins B_6, B_{12}, D, and E.

Chronic illness in elderly persons is often associated with malnutrition and weight loss. Malnutrition is influenced by a number of factors, including underlying disease, disability, poverty, or various conditions affecting food intake, such as oral problems (dry mouth, lack of teeth or poorly fitting dentures, and swallowing difficulty), psychosocial problems resulting from isolation, and other personal factors contributing to boredom or apathy. The NSI, a national project sponsored by the American Dietetic Association, the American Academy of Family Physicians, and the American Council on the Aging, works in many communities to identify those elderly persons at risk for malnutrition and helps educate individuals and communities in preventive care.

■ Questions for Review

1. Briefly describe the age-related population shifts now occurring in the United States. Why have these shifts occurred? What are the implications for healthcare and associated social services?

2. Discuss the economic status, ethnic and racial composition, and living arrangements of the aging population. Illustrate how these factors have touched your own life or the life of someone you know. How might these factors influence an older person's diet or health status?
3. Select one of the adult age groups and describe their basic needs in terms of physical growth, psychosocial development, socioeconomic status, and related nutritional needs.
4. Describe some of the general biologic changes that occur with aging. How may these changes affect eating, food choices, and nutritional status?
5. You are helping a couple over age 55 with a limited income improve their food intake pattern. Plan a 1-day menu for them using the appropriate *Food Guide Pyramid.*
6. Distinguish between the terms *gerontology* and *geriatrics.* Go to your school library and find the *Journal of Gerontology* and the *Journal of the American Geriatrics Society.* Look for an article in each journal that describes food or nutrient intake or nutritional problems in older people. Compare the articles as to the type of information presented and the intended audience.
7. Identify five warning signs of malnutrition in older adults. Give an example of how each of these situations leads to poor nutrition. Suggest some ways that each situation might be improved to prevent malnutrition.
8. Visit the website of the Administration on Aging, the unit within the United States Department of Health and Human Services that has responsibility for all programs mandated by the Older Americans Act (see p. 342). Review the available information describing the most recent evaluation of the Nutrition Program for the Elderly. Does this program make a difference in the lives of the older people it serves?
9. Visit your local drug store and review the liquid supplements being marketed to the older population. Make a table describing four different supplements listing the cost and nutritional content of kcalories, protein, calcium, vitamin A, vitamin D, vitamin E, vitamin B_{12}, and folate per 1-cup serving. Using Appendix A, select a fortified cereal that would be eaten with 1 cup of milk. Compare the cost, kcalories, and leader nutrients listed above in a 1-cup serving of supplement with a usual serving size of the cereal with 1 cup of milk. Based on your findings, would you recommend the cereal serving or the liquid supplement as an evening snack? Explain.

■ References

1. Kerschner H, Pegues JAM: Productive aging: a quality of life agenda, *J Am Diet Assoc* 98:1445, 1998.
2. Federal Interagency Forum on Aging Related Statistics: *Older Americans 2000: key indicators of well-being,* Hyattsville, Md, 2000, National Institute on Aging, National Institutes of Health, available at *http://www.agingstats.gov* (accessed 8/30/02).
3. United States Department of Health and Human Services: *Health. United States, 1999 with chartbook on aging,* Rockville, Md, 1999, U.S. Government Printing Office.
4. Panel on Macronutrients, Panel on the Definition of Dietary Fiber, Subcommittee on Upper Reference Levels of Nutrients, Subcommittee on Interpretation and Uses of Dietary Reference Intakes, and the Standing Committee on the Scientific Evaluation of Dietary Reference Intakes: *Dietary reference intakes for energy, carbohydrate, fiber, fat, fatty acids, cholesterol, protein, and amino acids, parts 1 and 2,* Washington, DC, 2002, National Academy Press.
5. United States Department of Agriculture: *Continuing survey of food intake by individuals, 1994-1996,* Beltsville, Md, available at *http://www.barc.usda.gov/bhnrc/foodsurvey/Products 9496.html#table* (accessed 8/30/02).
6. Lindeman RD: The aging renal system. In Chernoff R, ed: *Geriatric nutrition: the health professional's handbook,* ed 2, Gaithersburg, Md, 1999, Aspen.
7. Food and Nutrition Board: *Dietary reference intakes for calcium, phosphorus, magnesium, vitamin D, and fluoride,* Washington, DC, 1997, National Academy Press.
8. Klesges RC et al: Predictors of milk consumption in a population of 17- to 35-year-old military personnel, *J Am Diet Assoc* 99:821, 1999.
9. Lee LT, Drake WM, Kendler DL: Intake of calcium and vitamin D in 3 Canadian long-term care facilities, *J Am Diet Assoc* 102(2):244, 2002.
10. Foote JA, Giuliano AR, Harris RB: Older adults need guidance to meet nutritional recommendations, *J Am Coll Nutr* 19:628, 2000.
11. NIH Consensus Development Panel on Osteoporosis Prevention, Diagnosis, and Therapy: Osteoporosis prevention, diagnosis, and therapy, *JAMA* 285:785, 2001.
12. Food and Nutrition Board: *Dietary reference intakes for vitamin A, vitamin K, arsenic, boron, chromium, copper, iodine, iron, manganese, molybdenum, nickel, silicon, vanadium, and zinc,* Washington, DC, 2001, National Academy Press.
13. Roubenoff R, Hughes V: Sarcopenia: current concepts, *J Gerontol A Biol Sci Med Sci* 55:716, 2000.
14. Guo SS et al: Aging, body composition, and lifestyle: the Fels Longitudinal Study, *Am J Clin Nutr* 70:405, 1999.
15. Heaney RP et al: Dietary changes favorably effect bone remodeling in older adults, *J Am Diet Assoc* 99:1228, 1999.
16. Ensrud KE et al: Low fractional calcium absorption increases the risk for hip fracture in women with low calcium intake, *Ann Intern Med* 132:345, 2000.
17. Van Itallie TB: Waist circumference: a useful index in clinical care and health promotion, *Nutr Rev* 56:300, 1998.
18. Kohrt WM: Contributing factors to insulin resistance: effect of aging, *Nutr Rev* 58(II):S19, 2000.
19. Beers MH, Berkow R, eds: *The Merck manual of geriatrics,* ed 3, Whitehouse Station, NJ, 2000, Merck Research Laboratories.
20. Dixon LB, Winkleby MA, Radimer KL: Dietary intakes and serum nutrients differ between adults from food-insufficient and food-sufficient families: Third National Health and Nutrition Examination Survey, 1988-1994, *J Nutr* 131:1232, 2001.

21. Davis MA et al: Living arrangements affect dietary quality for U.S. adults aged 50 years and older: NHANES III 1988-1994, *J Nutr* 130:2256, 2000.
22. Pierce MB, Sheehan NW, Ferris A: Older women living in subsidized housing report low levels of nutrition support, *J Am Diet Assoc* 101:251, 2001.
23. Pannemans D et al: Effect of protein source and quantity on protein metabolism in elderly women, *Am J Clin Nutr* 68:1228, 1998.
24. Weddle DO, Fanelli-Kuczmarski, M: Position of the American Dietetic Association: nutrition, aging, and the continuum of care, *J Am Diet Assoc* 100:580, 2000.
25. Food and Nutrition Board: *Dietary reference intakes for thiamin, riboflavin, niacin, vitamin B-6, folate, vitamin B-12, pantothenic acid, biotin, and choline,* Washington, DC, 1998, National Academy Press.
26. Marcus E-L, Berry EM: Refusal to eat in the elderly, *Nutr Rev* 56:163, 1998.
27. Krondl M et al: Subjectively healthy elderly consuming a liquid nutrition supplement maintained body mass index and improved some nutritional parameters and perceived well-being, *J Am Diet Assoc* 99:1542, 1999.
28. Roberts SB, Dallal GE: Effects of age on energy balance, *Am J Clin Nutr* 68(suppl):975S, 1998.
29. Roberts SB: Energy regulation and aging: recent findings and their implications, *Nutr Rev* 58:91, 2000.
30. Toth MJ, Poehlman ET: Energetic adaptation to chronic disease in the elderly, *Nutr Rev* 58:61, 2000.
31. Stevens J: Impact of age on associations between weight and mortality, *Nutr Rev* 58:129, 2000.
32. Fried LP et al: Frailty in older adults: evidence for a phenotype, *J Gerontol A Biol Sci Med Sci* 56:M146, 2001.
33. Womack P, Breeding C: Position of the American Dietetic Association: liberalized diets for older adults in long-term care, *J Am Diet Assoc* 98:201, 1998.
34. Tessari P: Changes in protein, carbohydrate, and fat metabolism with aging: possible role of insulin, *Nutr Rev* 58:11, 2000.
35. Albright A et al: American College of Sports Medicine position stand: exercise and type 2 diabetes, *Med Sci Sports Exerc* 32:1345, 2000.
36. Liu S et al: A prospective study of whole-grain intake and risk of type 2 diabetes mellitus in United States women, *Am J Public Health* 90:1409, 2000.
37. Hallfrisch J, Behall KM: Mechanisms of the effects of grains on insulin and glucose responses, *J Am Coll Nutr* 19(3 suppl):320S, 2000.
38. Campbell WW et al: The Recommended Dietary Allowance for protein may not be adequate for older people to maintain skeletal muscle, *J Gerontol A Biol Sci Med Sci* 56:M373, 2001.
39. Bourdel-Marchasson I et al: Functional and metabolic early changes in calf muscle occurring during nutritional repletion in malnourished elderly patients, *Am J Clin Nutr* 73:832, 2001.
40. Bos C et al: Short-term protein and energy supplementation activates nitrogen kinetics and accretion in poorly nourished elderly subjects, *Am J Clin Nutr* 71:1129, 2000.
41. Campbell WW et al: Effects of an omnivorous diet compared with a lacto-ovo-vegetarian diet on resistance-training-induced changes in body composition and skeletal muscle in older men, *Am J Clin Nutr* 70:1032, 1999.
42. Russell RM, Baik H, Kehayias JJ: Older men and women efficiently absorb vitamin B-12 from milk and fortified bread, *J Nutr* 131:291, 2001.
43. Semba RD et al: Vitamin D deficiency among older women with and without disability, *Am J Clin Nutr* 72:1529, 2000.
44. Food and Nutrition Board: *Dietary reference intakes for vitamin C, vitamin E, selenium, and carotenoids,* Washington, DC, 2000, National Academy Press.
45. Holben DH et al: Fluid intake compared with established standards and symptoms of dehydration among elderly residents of a long-term-care facility, *J Am Diet Assoc* 99:1447, 1999.
46. Lee JS, Frongillo EA: Nutritional and health consequences are associated with food insecurity among U.S. elderly persons, *J Nutr* 131:1503, 2001.
47. Bermudez OI, Falcon LM, Tucker KL: Intake and food sources of macronutrients among older Hispanic adults: association with ethnicity, acculturation and length of residence in the United States, *J Am Diet Assoc* 100:665, 2000.
48. Marshall TA et al: Inadequate nutrient intakes are common and are associated with low diet variety in rural, community-dwelling elderly, *J Nutr* 131:2192, 2001.
49. Vitolins MZ et al: Vitamin and mineral supplement use by older rural adults, *J Gerontol A Biol Sci Med Sci* 55:M613, 2001.
50. Hall K, Whiting SJ, Comfort B: Low nutrient intake contributes to adverse clinical outcomes in hospitalized elderly patients, *Nutr Rev* 58:214, 2000.
51. Newman AB et al: Associations of subclinical cardiovascular disease with frailty, *J Gerontol A Biol Sci Med Sci* 56: M158, 2001.
52. Jensen GL et al: Screening for hospitalization and nutritional risks among community-dwelling older persons, *Am J Clin Nutr* 74:201, 2001.
53. Klesges LM et al: Financial difficulty in acquiring food among elderly disabled women: results from the Women's Health and Aging Study, *Am J Public Health* 91:68, 2001.
54. Tariq SH et al: The use of a no-concentrated-sweets diet in the management of type 2 diabetes in nursing homes, *J Am Diet Assoc* 101(12):1463, 2001.

■ Further Reading

Bermudez OI, Falcon LM, Tucker KL: Intake and food sources of macronutrients among older Hispanic adults: association with ethnicity, acculturation and length of residence in the United States, *J Am Diet Assoc* 100:665, 2000.

Jensen GL et al: Screening for hospitalization and nutritional risks among community-dwelling older persons, *Am J Clin Nutr* 74:201, 2001.

Klesges LM et al: Financial difficulty in acquiring food among elderly disabled women: results from the Women's Health and Aging Study, *Am J Public Health* 91:68, 2001.

Mattes RD: The chemical senses and nutrition in aging: challenging old assumptions, *J Am Diet Assoc* 102(2):192, 2002.

These articles discuss some of the physical, financial, social, and ethnic influences on food habits of older persons and help us understand how we can assist our clients in selecting and obtaining nutrient-dense foods.

Minkler M, Schauffler H, Clements-Nolle K: Health promotion for older Americans in the 21st century, *Am J Health Promotion* 14:371, 2000.

This article by Minkler and her colleagues gives us some good ideas for developing health promotion programs for older adults.

Fey-Yensan N et al: Food safety risk identified in a population of elderly home-delivered meal participants, *J Am Diet Assoc* 101(9):1055, 2001.

Millen BE et al: The Elderly Nutrition Program: an effective national framework for preventive nutrition interventions, *J Am Diet Assoc* 102(2):234, 2002.

Wellman NS, Rosenzweig LY, Lloyd JL: Thirty years of the older Americans nutrition program, *J Am Diet Assoc* 102(3):348, 2002.

The website of the Administration on Aging describes many activities and materials available to serve older Americans: *http://www.aoa.dhhs.gov/* (accessed 8/30/02).

You can learn more about the Nutrition Program for the Elderly by visiting their website at *http://www.aoa.dhhs.gov/nutrition/default.htm* (accessed 8/30/02).

These articles and websites provide an overview of the Elderly Nutrition Program and other U.S. government services that are available to older persons.

Issues & ANSWERS

Community-Based Long-Term Care: Food and Nutrition Services

Evaluating the need for services

As the number of persons aged 65 and older continues to grow, government and health leaders are beginning to study the types of services that will be needed and the costs of providing those services to older adults who will no longer be able to care for themselves. Only 5% of the total population aged 65 and older currently reside in skilled nursing homes or long-term care facilities, but this rises to 19% among those aged 85 and older. As people continue to age, increasing chronic disease and frailty can lead to increasing physical disability, and they are more likely to need help with personal care and household chores.

An older person's ability to care for himself or herself is usually evaluated using the activities of daily living (ADLs) and the instrumental activities of daily living (IADLs). The ADLs listed here evaluate a person's ability to perform personal care, either independently, with some amount of help, or not at all.

- Bathing oneself
- Dressing oneself
- Feeding oneself
- Using the toilet
- Transferring between bed and chair

The IADLs relate to a person's ability to perform housekeeping chores and other activities that are required to remain independent. The IADLs are listed here.

- Prepare meals
- Perform housecleaning chores
- Handle money and balance a checkbook
- Shop without help
- Use the telephone
- Leave the house without help

Community-based long-term care

Long-term care is the term we use to refer to providing medical, social, and personal services on a continuing basis to an older person. At one time older persons who needed help with the ADLs or IADLs were likely to move to an institutional setting such as a nursing home that provided long-term care. Today we are placing more emphasis on community-based long-term care, providing services that will enable older persons to remain in the community in their own home or in the home of a family member. Most older persons who need help with the ADLs or IADLs receive help from family members; however, increasing numbers of older persons live at some distance from their children and others do not have children or other family. To fill this need, services are now being provided by home health agencies, area agencies on aging that receive state and federal funds, and private home care companies.

Nutrition is an important component of community-based long-term care services. It is important that older people maintain optimum nutritional status to help prevent or delay biologic aging and the effects of existing chronic disease. Notice that several of the ADLs and IADLs relate to food and nutritional needs. Most older people living in the community are able to feed themselves; however, obtaining groceries and preparing adequate meals can be very difficult or impossible, especially for the oldest-old. Community-based long-term care includes both in-home care services as well as community support programs for which individuals must leave their homes. Below we explore several community-based long-term care services that provide help with food and nutrition.

Nutrition services for older adults

The Older Americans Act (OAA) (see p. 338) provides funding to state departments on aging who are responsible for providing food and nutrition services to persons aged 60 and older in that state. Programs are managed locally by agencies on aging that serve a particular geographic area and offer a wide range of services. These services may include: congregate or group meals, home delivered meals (meals on wheels), transportation to congregate meals, transportation and assistance with grocery shopping, nutrition education, nutrition screening (see p. 337 for the Determine Your Health Checklist), transportation to the doctor or physical therapy, in-home nursing services, referral services, and legal aid, depending on the needs of older persons in the area and available funds.

The funding for food and nutrition services is provided under Title III of the OAA but special funding under Title VI is designated for Native Americans, Native Hawaiians, and Alaska natives. The common name given to this program across all 50 states is the Elderly Nutrition Program. The Administration on Aging of the United States Department of Health and Human Services is the agency with responsibility for setting guidelines and procedures for all programs using OAA funds. The impact of this program on the elderly population is evident from the fact that 250 million meals a year are served to 2.6 million participants. More than half of these meals are home delivered.

Congregate (group) meals

Congregate meals have been established in senior centers, churches, municipal buildings, and high rise apartment complexes, any facility that is within easy access to local older people. Most programs provide 5 meals a week served at noon. In rural areas 2 to 3 meals may be served each week. Each meal is by government regulation expected to contain at least one third of the RDAs or DRIs for persons aged 60 and older. For kcalories and those vitamins and minerals with higher recommended levels for men, the meals are expected to meet the level suggested for men. When funding is available, meal sites also provide transportation for those who may not have a car or no longer drive. For many congregate meal participants, particularly those living alone, the meal site also serves an important role in providing social support. Congregate meals promote continued health and well-being through the meal provided as well as nutrition education and screening services.

Home-delivered meals (Meals on Wheels)

Eligibility for home delivered meals requires that an individual not be physically able to leave home or be homebound as a result of caring for a disabled spouse. Traditional home delivered meal programs delivered a hot meal once a day at noon, 5 days a week. Volunteers donating their time and vehicles provided delivery services for home delivered meal programs over the years. However, with more women working outside the home and more older persons remaining in the work force beyond retirement age, it has become increasingly difficult to find volunteers. The cost of paying persons to deliver meals has forced many agencies to turn from daily delivery of a hot meal to frozen meals that can be delivered on a weekly basis.

Another problem for programs is the growing need for meals fueled by the increasing numbers of homebound older people. Based on client needs, some programs deliver extra cold or frozen meals for use on weekends or as second meals for certain days. When the Elderly Nutrition Program first began providing meals to the homebound, they were intended to supplement the food resources of the recipients. Instead, it has become apparent that for almost half of home-delivered meal recipients, the meals that are delivered are their major source of food, and these meals are divided across the day and the week.

Program evaluation

Frail and low income older people are target populations for congregate and home delivered meals programs. A national evaluation indicated that meal participants had more adequate diets than nonparticipants who were similar in age and socioeconomic status. Home delivered meal participants are a bit older and have an average age of 76, compared with congregate meal participants who have an average age of 72. Both programs contribute to the intake of important nutrients such as calcium. More than 60% of congregate and home delivered meal participants met the Adequate Intake of 1200 mg of calcium as compared with only 49% of nonparticipants. We need to continue to find ways to assist older persons in meeting their calcium needs.

Future directions for the Elderly Nutrition Program

Both congregate and home delivered meals fill important roles for older adults in the community. Unfortunately, the sharp rise in the number of requests as the older population continues to age, along with earlier hospital discharge practices brought about by the Diagnostic Related Groups (DRGs), has led to an unprecedented need for home delivered meals that is still unmet. A national survey indicated that 41% of home meal programs have waiting lists. To try to meet current needs, resources have been diverted from congregate meal programs to home delivered meals programs. Nine percent of congregate meal programs now have waiting lists and thus are less effective in preventing nutritional and physical decline in community-living older adults. It is important that health professionals support the expansion of both programs.

Both types of meal programs must also address the growing need for ethnic meals. As noted in this chapter, the older adult population is becoming more diverse, and the traditional food patterns of these groups must be respected if their nutritional needs are to be met. Health and social service professionals working with older adults need to become familiar with the Elderly Nutrition Program meals and services available in their communities.

REFERENCES

Marshall JA et al: Indicators of nutritional risk in a rural elderly Hispanic and non-Hispanic white population. San Luis Health and Aging Study, *J Am Diet Assoc* 99:315, 1999.

Millen BE et al: The Elderly Nutrition Program: an effective national framework for preventive nutrition interventions, *J Am Diet Assoc* 102(2):234, 2002.

Ponza M et al: Serving elders at risk. The Older Americans Act Nutrition Programs. National Evaluation of the Elderly Nutrition Program, 1993-1995, vol I, Princeton, NJ, 1996, Mathematica Policy Research. Can be accessed on the website of the National Policy and Resource Center on Nutrition and Aging, Florida International University at *http://www.aoa.dhhs.gov/aoa/pages/nutreval.html.*

Schlenker ED: *Nutrition in aging,* ed 3, Dubuque, Iowa, 1998, McGraw/Hill Publishers.

Vailas LI et al: Risk indicators for malnutrition are associated inversely with quality of life for participants in meal programs for older adults, *J Am Diet Assoc* 98:548, 1998.

Weddle DO, Fanelli-Kuczmarski M: Position of the American Dietetic Association: Nutrition, aging and the continuum of care, *J Am Diet Assoc* 100:580, 2000.

Wellman NS, Rosenzweig LY, Lloyd JL: Thirty years of the older Americans nutrition program, *J Am Diet Assoc* 102(3):348, 2002.

Chapter 14

Nutrition, Physical Fitness, and Stress

Sue Rodwell Williams

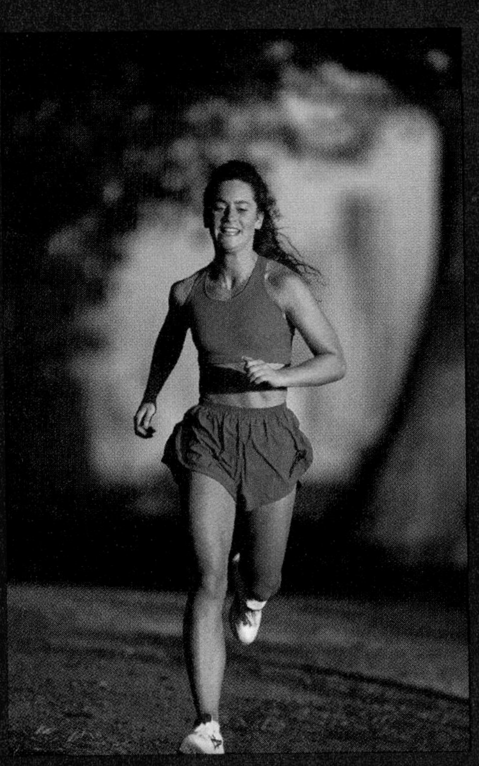

Chapter Outline

This chapter relates the three basic factors of nutrition, physical fitness, and stress to health maintenance throughout the life cycle. In an increasingly fast-paced and technologic society, building regular physical activity into our busy lives, as well as dealing with stress, requires commitment and effort. However, physical fitness is a vital cornerstone in the preventive approach to controlling the chronic diseases of modern civilization.

We examine first how nutrition works to provide energy fuels for muscle action. Then we apply these principles to enhancing athletic performance and to building a reasonable and appropriate personal exercise program. Finally, we relate how the human body manages stress in relation to our overall health goals.

Modern Civilization, Chronic Disease, and Physical Activity

MODERN DEVELOPED NATIONS AND DISEASES OF CIVILIZATION

Over thousands of years our marvelous human bodies have developed from earlier ages of human history when survival in agriculture-based societies required constant physical exertion and energy expenditure. Now, over only a few past generations, the developed nations of the world have come to live in very different circumstances. Our knowledge-based societies demand little, if any, physical activity in our work and in our lifestyles. As a result, although we live longer, our health has been paying a price. Our inactivity contributes to a host of modern ills, the so-called diseases of civilization, including coronary heart disease, diabetes, hypertension, osteoporosis, and obesity.[1]

THE PHYSICAL FITNESS MOVEMENT AND HEALTH

Americans are generally an active people—and even inactive people desire to be more active—and are increasingly aware of the benefits of physical fitness.[2,3] Physical fitness is no longer just a fad or a trend; increased participation in regular physical activity as a part of everyday life remains a national health goal, especially with healthy weight being of national concern. An estimated 60% of American adults engage in some form of leisure-time physical activity, whereas about 65% of adolescents engage in vigorous physical activity 3 or more times a week.[4] The U.S. Department of Health and Human Services, in its report *Healthy People 2010: Understanding and Improving Health,* has set health-related goals for Americans in nutrition and physical fitness to be reached by 2010. The 2010 target for participation in regular moderate-to-vigorous physical activity is for 30% of adults and 85% of adolescents.[4] Walking and swimming are our most popular outdoor activities, with bicycling and jogging close behind. Athletics, both amateur and professional, have become big business, and the health specialty of sports medicine has grown dramatically.

The health benefits of physical activity are not reserved just for athletes.[2] In everyday life, the need for exercise is serious. The modern healthcare approach of preventive medicine, as well as the necessity of dealing with chronic disease, demands positive attention to the related roles of nutrition and physical fitness in healthcare. The U.S. Department of Agriculture has published national dietary guidelines every 5 years since 1980. The latest edition, *Dietary Guidelines for Americans 2000,*[5] adds a new "Aim for Fitness" category to the well-established guidelines for what we eat. These guidelines encourage all people to, in addition to practicing healthy eating choices, be physically active each day and to aim for a healthy weight. Fitness has definite health benefits. Aerobic exercise, combined with weight training, increases fitness for all aspects of life. Exercise also has emerged as an effective therapy, along with nutritional care and weight management, in the control of hypertension, diabetes, cancer risk, and elevated blood lipids.[6] Moderate exercise helps control the health problems of many older adults.[3] Regardless of the level of exercise or active pursuits that a person can achieve, even a limited beginning builds into consistent habits. The longer people follow some form of regular exercise, the more committed they become.[7] For many, it is a matter of life and health.

Energy Sources for Physical Activity

THE NATURE OF ENERGY

The term *energy* refers to the body's ability, or power, to do work. The energy required to do body work takes several different forms: mechanical, chemical, electrical, light, radiant, and heat. Energy, like matter, can neither be created nor destroyed. It can only be changed into another form; therefore energy is constantly cycled in the body and environment. We also speak of energy as being potential (stored) or kinetic (active). Potential energy is stored energy, ready to be used. Kinetic energy is active energy, being used to do work. Energy balance in physical activity requires a base of sound nutrition to supply the substrate fuels, which along with oxygen and water meet widely varying levels of energy demand for body action.

MUSCLE ACTION: FUELS, FLUIDS, AND NUTRIENTS

Muscle Structures

The synchronized action of millions of specialized cells and structures that make up our skeletal muscle mass make possible all forms of physical activity. A finely coordinated series of small bundles within the muscle fibers (Figure 14-1), triggered by nerve endings, produce a smooth symphony of action through simultaneous and alternating contraction and relaxation. These successively smaller muscle structures include the following.

1. *Skeletal muscle.* The largest bundle in the series is the complete muscle. Each particular muscle is composed of muscle fibers called fasciculi.
2. *Muscle fiber.* Each muscle fiber is composed of bundles of still smaller strands called myofibrils.
3. *Myofibril.* Each single myofibril strand of the muscle fiber is made up of the smallest of all the fiber bundles, called myofilaments. Contraction occurs here.
4. *Myosin and actin.* Within each myofilament are the contractile proteins, myosin and actin, which are the smallest moving parts of every muscle.

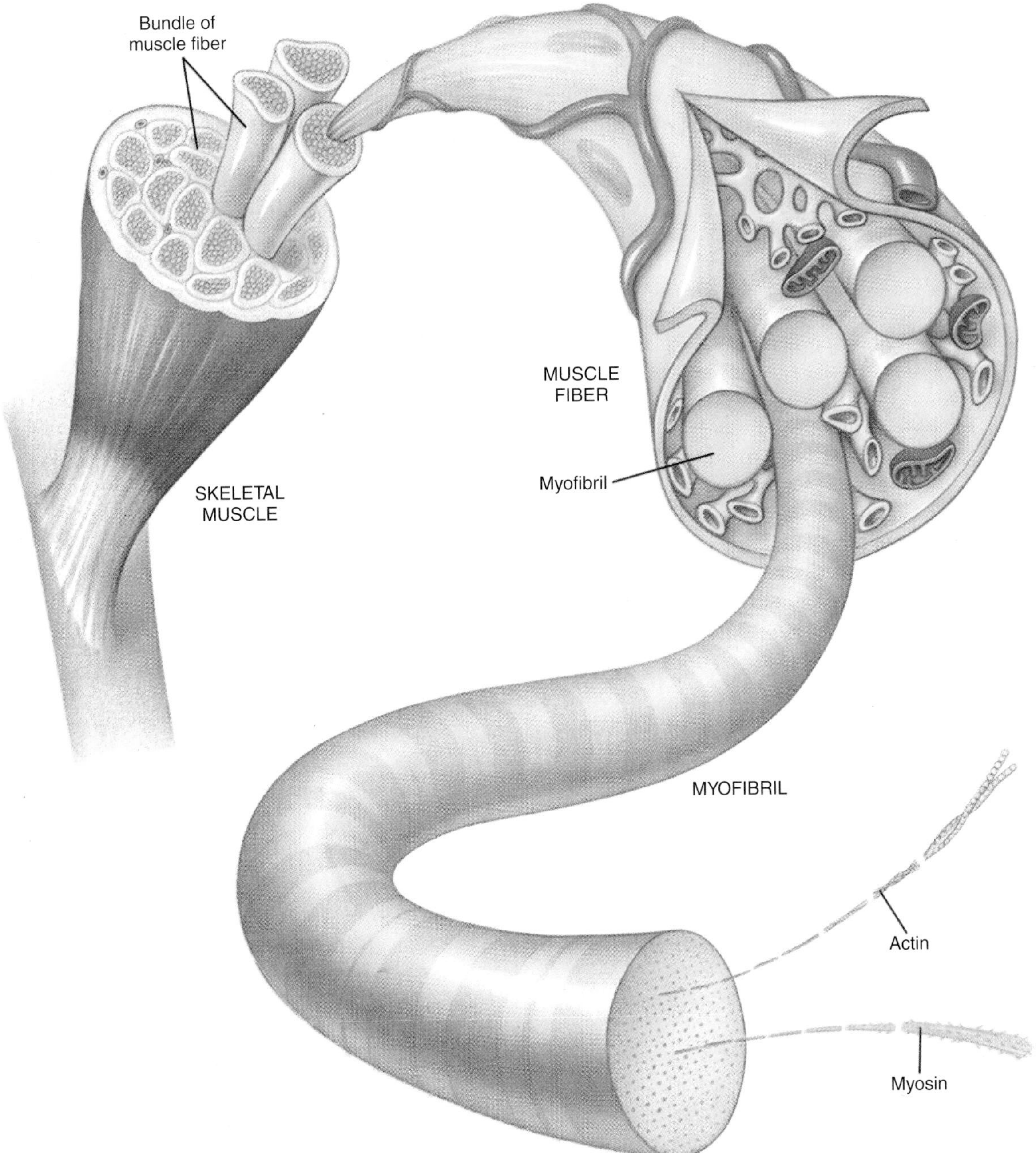

FIGURE 14-1 Skeletal muscle, showing the progressively smaller bundles within bundles. (*Modified from Barbara Cousins, from Seeley RR, Stephens TD, Tate P:* Anatomy and physiology, *ed 2, New York, 1992, McGraw-Hill. Reproduced with permission of The McGraw-Hill Companies.*)

actin Myofibril protein whose synchronized meshing action in conjunction with myosin causes muscles to contract and relax.

fasciculi A general term for a small bundle or cluster of muscle, tendon, or nerve fibers.

kinetic Energy released from body fuels by cell metabolism and now active in moving muscles and energizing all body activities.

myofibril Slender thread of muscle; runs parallel to the long axis of the muscle fiber.

myofilaments Threadlike filaments of actin or myosin, which are components of myofibrils.

myosin Myofibril protein whose synchronized meshing action in conjunction with actin causes muscles to contract and relax.

potential Energy existing in stored fuels and ready for action but not yet released and active.

substrate The specific organic substance on which a particular enzyme acts to produce new metabolic products.

Muscle Action

Inside the cell membrane, these contractile proteins, myosin and actin, are arranged in long parallel rows. These parallel rows slide together and mesh tightly when the muscle contracts and then pull apart when the muscle relaxes, allowing the muscle to shorten or lengthen as needed. When a specific motor nerve impulse excites these molecules of myosin and actin in a myofilament, they mesh together and thereby shorten the muscle. This contraction of the muscle bundles occurs instantly and simultaneously. Periods of relaxation occur between contractions. This alternating process continues until muscle fatigue builds up and the muscle can no longer respond. Muscle fatigue occurs for two reasons: (1) the supply of *glycogen,* the immediate muscle fuel, is exhausted and thus insufficient to sustain the required chemical reaction, and (2) *lactic acid,* the metabolic product of this chemical muscle reaction, accumulates during sustained high levels of exercise and cannot be removed fast enough.

Fuel Sources

Fuel sources are the basic energy nutrients in the diet, primarily carbohydrate and some fat. Their metabolic products—glucose, glycogen, and fatty acids—provide ready fuel sources for the chemical energy reactions within cells. Phosphate bonds form high-energy chemical compounds in body metabolism (see Chapter 6). The main high-energy compound of the body cells is *adenosine triphosphate (ATP).* It has rightly been called the "energy currency" of the cell. Various forms of energy are called on for successive energy needs.

1. *Immediate energy.* High-power or immediate energy demands over a short time depend on ATP being readily available within the muscle tissue. This amount is used up rapidly, and a backup compound, *creatine phosphate (CP),* is made available. These high-energy phosphate compounds, however, will sustain exercise for only about 5 to 8 seconds.
2. *Short-term energy.* If an activity lasts longer, between 30 seconds and 2 minutes, *muscle glycogen* supplies the continuing need. Although the amount of available glycogen is small, it is an important rapid source of energy for brief muscular effort.
3. *Long-term energy.* Exercise continuing more than 2 minutes requires an oxygen-dependent, or *aerobic,* energy system. A constant supply of oxygen in the blood is necessary for continued exercise. Special cell organelles, the *mitochondria,* located within each cell, produce large amounts of ATP. The ATP is produced mainly from glucose and fatty acids and supplies the continued energy needs of the body.

Fluids

Water is essential during physical activity and especially during exercise. A water deficiency can be dangerous and limits exercise capacity greatly.[8] As exercise continues, the body's temperature increases because a major part of the energy produced during muscular exertion becomes heat energy. To control this temperature increase, the body shunts as much heat as possible to the skin, where it is released in sweat, which should be replaced with 4 ounces of water every 15 minutes. Over time, and especially in hot weather, excessive sweating can lead to *dehydration.* This is a serious complication.

Nutrients

The fuel nutrients also become depleted during continued exercise. As energy demands increase, the body burns blood glucose and muscle glycogen, as well as reserves from fatty acids, to provide energy. With prolonged exercise, levels of these nutrients fall too low to sustain the body's continued demands. Fatigue follows and exhaustion threatens.

OXYGEN USE AND PHYSICAL CAPACITY

Oxygen Consumption

The most profound limit to exercise is the person's ability to deliver oxygen to the tissues and use it for the production of energy. This vital ability depends on the fitness of the pulmonary and cardiovascular systems. Because the heart is a muscle, exercise strengthens and enlarges it, enabling it to pump more blood per beat, a capacity called stroke volume. The cardiac output, how much the heart pumps out in a given period, depends on the amount of blood per contraction and on the cardiac rate, the number of contractions in a given time. In general, then, a person's aerobic capacity depends on the degree of fitness and body composition.

1. *Body fitness.* Physical fitness is defined in terms of aerobic capacity, which depends on the body's ability to deliver and use oxygen in sufficient quantities to meet the demands of increasing levels of exercise. Oxygen uptake increases with exercise intensity until either the demand is met or the ability to supply it is exceeded. This maximum rate that the body can take in oxygen (O_2), or aerobic capacity, is called the VO_2max—the maximum uptake volume of oxygen.[9] This capacity determines the intensity and duration of exercise that a person can perform. From the resting level, there is a steep rise in oxygen consumption during the first 3 minutes of exercise. After about 6 minutes the rate levels off into a steady state, indicating an equilibrium between the energy required by the exercising muscles and the aerobic energy-producing system. This aerobic capacity of an individual is measured in terms of milliliters of oxygen consumed per kilogram of body weight per minute. Thus persons of differing sizes can be compared equally.
2. *Recovery period.* During exercise, to accommodate the body's increased energy demands, the heart rate increases and breathing becomes deeper and more rapid.

After exercise stops these functions do not immediately return to their preexercise levels, especially if the exercise has been strenuous. This recovery takes time because the body must replenish its "oxygen debt."

3. *Body composition.* Gender differences in aerobic capacity reflect differences in body composition. In general, men have a higher aerobic capacity because of their larger lean body mass, the active metabolic body tissue. These highly metabolic tissues of the body thus use more oxygen than other tissues such as fat. When oxygen consumption is expressed only in terms of lean body mass instead of body weight, however, men and women have the same aerobic capacity. Women carry more body fat, a gender difference in body composition that serves critical biologic functions. Apart from stored adipose tissue fuel, essential structural and functional body fat in women is about 12% of their body weight; in men it is only 3%. And because women must, of course, carry their entire body weight as part of their total workload, their performance will be affected accordingly.
4. *Genetic influence.* A person's aerobic capacity is mainly genetically determined. But the genetic heritage is influenced, as indicated, by body composition, which is associated with sex, and by aerobic training and age. Before puberty, lean body mass is about equal in boys and girls of comparable body size, but it increases rapidly in boys at puberty under the anabolic effect of testosterone. Maximal aerobic capacity then peaks at 18 to 20 years of age and declines gradually thereafter, largely as a result of age-related losses in lean body mass.

Diet and Exercise: Fluids and Nutrients

ROLE OF WATER AND NUTRIENTS IN EXERCISE

Along with oxygen, an increased intake of water and nutrients is necessary in the course of exercise. Water is essential in any exercise but especially in prolonged exercise. A deficiency of water is dangerous and greatly limits exercise capacity. As exercise continues, the body's internal temperature increases dramatically because most of the energy produced by the processes of glycolysis is released as heat. To dissipate this increased heat, the body directs as much water as possible to the skin, where the excess heat escapes in perspiration. Excessive water loss from perspiration leads to dehydration, which is dangerous to health if it becomes severe.

Nutrients also become depleted during continued exercise as the body draws on its stored energy. As demands for cell ATP increase, the body metabolizes blood glucose and muscle glycogen to provide energy via anaerobic glycolysis. With prolonged exercise of greater intensity, however, the levels of these nutrients fall too low to sustain the body's demands. Fatigue follows, muscle failure occurs because of lactic acid buildup, and exercise cannot continue.

ENERGY-YIELDING MACRONUTRIENTS

Carbohydrate and fat in the diet are the basic fuels the body uses to maintain energy reserves, with very little energy drawn from protein. Our diet thus supplies the necessary fuel substrate from energy-yielding macronutrients. General needs apply to all individuals, although children have special needs during growth.

PROTEIN

Protein as a Fuel Substrate

Protein has only a small role as a fuel substrate in energy production during exercise. Although some amino acids can feed into the cell's basic energy cycle, the extent of this input during exercise is minimal. There is evidence that some amino acid breakdown occurs during exercise, and there is some nitrogen loss in sweat. But authorities agree that under normal circumstances protein makes a relatively insignificant contribution to energy during exercise. In endurance events, however, somewhat more protein may be used, especially when carbohydrate resources are exhausted.[9]

Protein in the Diet

Only 0.8 to 1 g of protein/kg of body weight is sufficient as a daily intake to meet the general needs of the physically active person. This amounts to the general recommended daily dietary intake standard for adults, with about 10% to 15% of the kilocalories (kcalories) in the diet coming from protein. However, most Americans actually eat about twice this amount of protein per day, putting a taxing metabolic load on the kidneys and the liver. Ill-informed athletes who purchase and use excess

aerobic capacity Milliliters of oxygen consumed per kilogram of body weight per minute; influenced by body composition.
cardiac output Total volume of blood propelled from the heart with each contraction; equal to the stroke output multiplied by the number of beats per the time unit used in the calculation.
stroke volume The amount of blood pumped from a ventricle (chamber of the heart releasing blood to body circulations) with each beat of the heart.
VO_2max Maximal uptake volume of oxygen during exercise; used to measure the intensity and duration of exercise a person can perform.

protein supplements in various forms are subjecting their bodies to an even greater taxing load and the dangers of abnormal metabolic stress. Nitrogen consumed in excess of need must be excreted. This puts a burden on the kidneys to excrete the increased urea coming from the liver, which contributes to dehydration, a serious factor during strenuous exercise. High-protein diets and supplements can also lead to increased excretion of calcium in the urine.

FAT

Fat as Fuel Substrate

Fatty acids serve as a fuel source from stored fat tissue. In the presence of oxygen, fatty acids are oxidized to provide energy. The rate at which this can occur is determined in part by the rate of mobilization of fatty acids from storage, but not all stored fat is alike. Actually, the body stores fat in two ways: (1) *depot* fat in adipose tissue, which is destined for transport back and forth to other tissues as needed for energy; and (2) *essential* fat in metabolically active tissue, such as bone marrow, heart, lungs, liver, spleen, kidneys, intestines, muscles, and nervous system, which is reserved in these places for necessary structural and functional use only. Although storage depot fat in men and women is roughly comparable, essential fat reserves make the big difference—they are about 4 times greater in women.

Free fatty acids, the fat fuel, are stored with glycerol as triglycerides in the body's adipose tissue. The enzyme *lipoprotein lipase* mobilizes these stores of fatty acids. This lipase is stimulated by exercise. Its activity is affected by levels of hormones also involved in exercise, especially growth hormone and epinephrine.

Fat in the Diet

It is important to recognize that fat as a fuel substrate is not drawn from the diet directly but rather from the body's stored adipose fat. It is not necessary to consume fat directly in food to maintain the body's adipose tissue depot fat stores because excess kcalories in the diet will be converted to fat and stored on the body regardless of the dietary source. We do not need to eat in excess of our dietary needs to burn fat, and there is no danger of depleting our fat stores before exercise has proceeded to exhaustion. Thus there is no basis for increased levels of fat in the diet. On the other hand, a moderate level of fat in the diet is needed for essential fat purposes, especially as a source of the essential fatty acid, linoleic acid. An extremely low fat intake can be medically dangerous. There are cases involving very compulsive runners who virtually eliminated fat from their diets in a desire to imitate the low-fat diet of famous runners from the Tarahumara Indians of the mountains of Mexico. Unfortunately, extreme fat elimination can create a dangerous linoleic acid deficiency. Because the heart muscle prefers fatty acids, especially linoleic acid, as an energy source, there have been reports of deaths from cardiac arrest in some of these cases. The standard recommendation that dietary fat should not exceed 25% to 30% of the total daily kcaloric intake is ample for most healthy individuals.

CARBOHYDRATES

Carbohydrates as Fuel Substrate

Although fat and protein have their special roles to play in maintaining general health, the major nutrient for energy support in exercise is carbohydrate. Carbohydrate fuels come from two sources: the circulating blood glucose and glycogen stored in muscle and the liver.

Carbohydrates in the Diet

Carbohydrates are the major energy nutrient. For active persons, carbohydrate energy should contribute about 55% to 60% of the kcalories of the daily diet. Athletes competing in prolonged endurance events should increase their energy from carbohydrates to 65% to 70% of their daily total. Complex carbohydrates (starches) are preferable to simple carbohydrates (sugars). Starches break down more slowly and help maintain blood glucose levels more evenly, avoiding low blood sugar drops, as well as maintain glycogen storage as a constant primary fuel. Simple sugars supply important daily energy and contribute to glycogen storage. Simple sugars also trigger a sharper insulin response, which in some persons may contribute to the dangers of follow-up hypoglycemia. Simple sugars, however, can supply important energy, especially for athletes in endurance events who may require as much as 5000 kcalories/day.

Many studies have shown that low-carbohydrate diets hinder exercise performance. In repeated bouts of intense exercise, diets low in carbohydrate have proved to be incapable of restoring tissue glycogen levels.[9,10] A low-carbohydrate diet decreases the body's capacity for work, which intensifies over time. Conversely, a high-carbohydrate diet restores glycogen concentrations to their regular levels. Athletes on a low-carbohydrate diet experience fatigue, ketoacidosis, dehydration, and hypoglycemia. However, athletes given carbohydrate feedings before and during exercise maintain glucose concentrations and rates of glucose oxidation necessary to exercise strenuously and thus are able to delay fatigue.[10]

Sometimes athletes try a glycogen-loading food plan to build up glycogen reserves for endurance events, but this diet manipulation carries potential side effects such as extra water storage in the muscles. A more popular modern approach consists of a depletion-tapering sequence, such as the general pattern shown in Table 14-1. This modern depletion-tapering plan extends fuel reserves and avoids the potential negative side effects of the old-style glycogen-loading program. In general, during the 3 days before the competition, athletes need to consume about 65% of their energy intake as complex carbohy-

TABLE 14-1 Modified Depletion-Taper Precompetition Program for Glycogen Loading

Day	Exercise	Diet
1	90-Minute period at 70% to 75% VO_2max	Mixed diet, 50% carbohydrate (350 g)
2-3	Gradual tapering of time and intensity	Diet above continued
4-5	Tapering of exercise time and intensity continues	Mixed diet, 70% carbohydrate (550 g)
6	Complete rest	Diet above continued
7	Day of competition	High-carbohydrate pre-event diet

From Wright ED: Carbohydrate nutrition and exercise, *Clin Nutr* 7(1):18, 1988, by permission of the publisher, Churchill Livingstone.

TABLE 14-2 Approximate Energy Expenditure per Hour for an Adult Weighing 70 kg (154 lb) and Performing Different Activities

Activity	Kcalories/hr
Sleeping	65
Lying still, awake	75
Sitting at rest	100
Standing relaxed	105
Dressing and undressing	120
Rapid typing	140
Light exercise	170
Walking slowly (2.5 mph)	200
Active exercise	290
Intensive exercise	450
Swimming	500
Running (5.5 mph)	580
Very intense exercise	600
Walking very fast (5.2 mph)	640
Walking up stairs	1110

drates or 550 g/day of carbohydrates, whichever is greater.[10]

REGULATING MICRONUTRIENTS

Vitamins and Minerals as Fuel Substrate

Vitamins and minerals cannot be used as fuel substrates. They are not oxidized or used up in the process of energy production. They are essential in the cellular energy production process but only as catalytic cofactors in enzyme reactions.

Vitamins and Minerals in the Diet

Increased physical exertion because of personal exercise or athletic training does not require a greater intake of vitamins and minerals beyond currently recommended intakes. A well-balanced diet will supply adequate amounts of vitamins and minerals, and exercise may well improve the body's efficient use of them. Because athletes, for example, have a dietary need for energy, their larger kcaloric intake from good food sources would automatically increase their general intake of vitamins and minerals. Multivitamin and mineral supplementation do not improve physical performance in healthy athletes eating a well-balanced diet; and the potential side effects from megavitamin supplements are well known (see Chapters 7 and 8). However, *therapeutic* iron supplements may be necessary for some athletes who experience the problem of sports anemia. Also, special assessment of nutrient-energy status is needed for young adolescent amenorrheic female athletes such as gymnasts and ballet dancers, who may be experiencing eating disorders such as anorexia nervosa.[11] Such disordered eating patterns may involve low calcium intake, which can have serious consequences for bone development (see *Practical Application* box).[12]

EXERCISE AND ENERGY

Physical activity requires kcalories. Table 14-2 gives some examples of the amount of kcalories expended in various activities. Physically active persons, especially athletes, need more fuel. The building of glycogen reserves in particular is important for athletes such as long distance runners who compete in endurance events. Exercise raises the body's kcaloric need and has the additional benefit of helping to regulate appetite to meet these needs. Persons at moderate exercise levels have actually been shown to eat less than inactive persons. This may relate to an internal "set point" regulating the amount of body fat the person will carry. According to this theory, the set point is raised—that is, more body fat is stored—when the individual becomes inactive. In any case, when exercise levels rise from mild or moderate amounts up to strenuous levels, kcaloric needs also rise to supply needed fuel.

Active persons, even athletes, require no more protein or fat than inactive persons. Carbohydrate is the preferred fuel and is the critical food for the active person—not only before an exercise period but also during the recovery period afterward. The complex carbohydrate forms (i.e., starches) not only sustain energy needs but also supply added fiber, vitamins, and minerals. Thus the recommended composition of energy nutrients to support physical activity is approximately the following.

- *Protein:* 10% to 15% of total kcalories (1 to 1.5 g/kg of body weight)
- *Fat:* less than 30% of total kcalories
- *Carbohydrate:* 55% to 60% of total kcalories

PRACTICAL APPLICATION

The Female Athlete Triad: How Performance and Social Pressure Can Lead to Low Bone Mass

Meredith Catherine Williams

The female athlete triad consists of three health afflictions faced by women who are extremely physically active: eating disorders, menstrual disturbances and irregularity, and osteopenia (low bone mass) or even osteoporosis. Low bone mineral density (BMD) is often the final result of the triad that affects women, and it is the leading cause of stress fractures and injuries throughout the body, some of which may be irreversible. Many women who are in top physical from are ironically the most likely to develop these three linked complications and health problems because social and performance pressure may lead women to extreme eating habits and exercise regimens. The dilemma facing women athletes today is how to maintain optimal physical performance while not increasing health risks.

Women who participate in competitive sports that require endurance, such as rowing or long distance running, or who are judged partially on physical appearance, such as in ice skating or diving, are more likely to be preoccupied with their weight and to have a negative self-image. Dancers also are affected by this pressure, especially ballerinas. Social and competitive pressure for a woman to be thin can contribute to her sense of imperfection. These demands and pressures can lead some women to develop eating disorders, which in combination with strenuous exercise will lead to low energy levels. This drop in energy will be followed by a drop in performance as the athlete loses focus and concentration and is fatigued. Some women develop extreme dietary conditions, such as bulimia, which is characterized by binge eating followed by forced vomiting, purging, or excessive laxative intakes, or anorexia, which is characterized by the refusal or inability to consume sufficient calories for daily requirements. These more serious disorders can lead to psychologic problems (depression or low self-esteem), seizures, cardiac arrhythmia, myocardial infarction, or other health complications. The seriousness of the eating disorder is linked to the amount of stress and concern the woman feels over her body image combined with the amount of emphasis put on weight by trainers, coaches, and instructors. Often women are led to believe that leanness enhances performance, and some are willing to take health risks to satisfy perfectionist needs and habits.

Poor caloric intake and eating disorders can lead to menstrual irregularity. Amenorrhea is the suppression of menstrual cycles to a level of zero to three menses a year, and primary amenorrhea is the repression of all menstrual cycles until the age of 16 years. This condition is found in young female gymnasts who, in the most competitive circles, may actually strive to delay the onset of puberty to maintain small, childlike physiques. Some women may experience oligomenorrhea instead, which are sporadic cycles that occur 3 to 9 times a year. The levels of estrogen and progesterone that regulate menses can be affected by metabolism, intensive exercise, dieting, or stress.

There are several treatments available for female athletes: sex steroid replacement, increased caloric intake, decreased exercise, weight gain, or vitamin supplements. Evidence suggests that raising estrogen and progesterone levels and increasing calcium intake are the most effective measures, yet there is a wide range of treatment prescribed. Education and further research are needed to find the optimal course.

Menstrual irregularities are related to low bone density. Before the age of 30, bone density reaches its peak, and it is vital for young women to strive for dense bones in early adulthood so as to have healthy bone density later in life. If the density of bones is diminished early on, osteopenia occurs, and if severe enough, it can be a signal of future osteoporosis. The bone loss in all areas is not permanent, but bone loss in the vertebra of the spine seems to be irreversible. Although women who were once athletes seem to recover some of their bone density loss, vertebral bone normalization is uncommon. In active young females with tightly regulated diets and menstrual inconsistency, there can be bone density as low as that of a 70-year-old woman. These thin bones increase the likelihood of stress fractures and injuries, and women are far more likely to incur such injuries than men.

Some studies, however, indicate that weight-bearing activities, such as gymnastics, seem to actually improve bone density, even perhaps in vertebra, and may help prevent density decreases later in life. Yet the problem facing women athletes who are eating improperly is that the rate of decrease in BMD increases as menstrual cycles continue to be erratic. The longer the menstrual cycles are inconsistent, the sooner bone density is lost. Weight-bearing sports will not overcome the tendency toward low BMD if diet and exercise levels are not carefully monitored.

The best course of action is to have women athletes monitor their diet to include substantial caloric intake and sufficient vitamin consumption. The prevention of osteoporosis later in life lies in the habits of the individual and the modification of factors that can lead to the triad of eating disturbances, menstrual irregularity, and low bone density. Body weight must be different for each individual depending on height and skeletal structure, and there should not be one specific weight goal for all female athletes.

PRACTICAL APPLICATION
The Female Athlete Triad: How Performance and Social Pressure Can Lead to Low Bone Mass—cont'd

However, the societal and competitive pressures that cause the initial step in this three step process must also be addressed. We cannot ask our female athletes to sacrifice their health for an image we project on them. Our need for vicarious victory must not dominate our standards of what are acceptable eating habits. In today's weight conscious society, the emphasis must not be on a perfect image, size, or body but rather on the perfect balance of health and training.

The female athlete's skeletal integrity suffers as she resorts to drastic measures in her aspiration for a perfect lean physical image, but her male athlete counterpart has no such risk because his bone density is not dependent on menstrual regularity. We as society cannot demand that our female athletes endanger their health simply because women are naturally fatter than men and are dependent on regular menstruation for proper hormone levels and thereby healthy bone density. We must draw the line and recognize the biologic differences between male and female athletes.

Everyone involved in sport must be vigilant in spotting and stopping eating disorders that women impose on themselves. The need now is to educate trainers, athletes, and health professionals about the consequences of neglected nutrition. There should be no one image of the perfect female body, and young female athletes must understand that deprivation of life's essential nutrients ultimately only does more harm than good.

References

American College of Sports Medicine: The female athlete triad position stand, *Med Sci Sports Exerc* 29:1, 1997.

Anderson JJB et al: Nutrition and bone in physical activity and sport. In Anderson JJB et al, eds: *Nutrition in exercise and sports,* ed 3, Boca Raton, Fla, 1998, CRC Press.

Brukner P, Bennell K: Stress fractures in female athletes, *Sports Med* 24:419, 1997.

Dook JE et al: Exercise and bone mineral density in mature female athletes, *Med Sci Sports Exerc* 29:291, 1997.

Keen AD, Drinkwater BL: Irreversible bone loss in former amenorrheic athletes, *Osteoporosis Int* 7:311, 1997.

Nickols-Richardson SM et al: Body composition, energy intake and expenditure, and body weight dissatisfaction in female child gymnasts and controls, *J Am Diet Assoc* 97(9):14A, 1997.

Ogawa A et al: Weight bearing exercise predicts total bone mineral content in female midshipmen, *J Am Diet Assoc* 97(9):19A, 1997.

Talbort S: The female triad, *Strength Conditioning* 4:128, 1996.

Thrash LE, Anderson JJB: The female athlete triad: nutrition, menstrual disturbances, and low bone mass, *Nutr Today* 35(5):168, 2000.

Nutrition and Athletic Performance

ATHLETES, COACHES, AND NUTRITIONAL PRACTICES

Misinformation

Athletes and their coaches are particularly susceptible to myths and claims about foods and dietary supplements. They search relentlessly for the competitive edge (see *Issues & Answers*). Knowing this, marketers unremittingly exploit this search, making this group particularly vulnerable. Manufacturers sometimes make distorted and false claims for products. For example, pangamic acid, marketed a few years ago as "vitamin B_{15}" although it is not a vitamin at all, carried claims about its ability to enhance oxygen transport during exercise. Naturally, if there were such a compound, it would be of interest to athletes and their trainers. However, scientific research has exposed these claims as unfounded.

Myths

In addition to specific fraud, the world of athletics is beset with superstitions and misconceptions. Some of these myths include the following.

- Athletes need protein for energy.
- Extra protein is needed to build bigger and stronger muscles.
- Muscle tissue is broken down during exercise, and protein supplements are needed to replace this breakdown.
- Vitamin supplements are needed to enable athletes to use more energy.
- Vitamins and minerals are burned up in workouts and training sessions.
- Electrolyte solutions are needed during exercise to replace sweat losses.
- A pregame meal of steak and eggs ensures maximal performance.
- Sugar is needed before and during performance to enhance energy levels.
- Drinking water during exercise will cause cramps.

BOX 14-1 Sample Pregame Meal

1 cup spaghetti, tomato sauce 1 slice French bread 1 cup apple juice	This sample pregame meal includes approximately 300 kcalories; high complex carbohydrate; and low protein, fat, and fiber.

Pregame and Training Meals

Traditionally, steak and eggs have been the ritual foods for the precompetition meal. However, if such a meal is eaten less than a few hours before the athletic event, it will still be in the stomach during the event. Protein and fat delay the emptying of the stomach, and neither contributes to the glycogen stores needed during exercise. On the contrary, the ideal pregame meal is now known to be a light one of approximately 300 kcalories that is eaten about 2 to 4 hours before the event, such as the meal illustrated in Box 14-1. This meal should be high is complex carbohydrates and relatively low in protein, with little fat or fiber.[3] This schedule for the meal gives the body time to digest, absorb, and transform it into stored glycogen. Good food choices include pasta, bread, bagels, muffins, and cereal with nonfat milk. Throughout the period of vigorous training, a high-carbohydrate diet with 500 to 600 g/day is recommended, such as that illustrated in Table 14-3. In addition, nutrient information may be used to calculate such diets. Small amounts of carbohydrate-containing foods or drinks may be taken up to a brief time before the event without affecting the performance. A total carbohydrate intake of 1 to 5 g/kg body weight taken from 5 minutes to 4 hours before the exercise is sufficient to enhance performance.[13,14]

TABLE 14-3 A 600-g Carbohydrate Diet*

Menu	Carbohydrates (g)
Breakfast	
1 orange	14
2 cups oatmeal	50
1 cup skim milk	12
2 bran muffins	48
Snack	
¾ cup chopped dates	98
Lunch	
Lettuce salad	
1 cup romaine lettuce	2
1 cup garbanzo beans	45
½ cup alfalfa sprouts	5.5
2 tbsp French dressing	2
3 cups macaroni and cheese	80
1 cup apple juice	28
Snack	
2 slices whole wheat toast	26
1 tsp margarine	—
2 tbsp jam	14
Dinner	
2 oz turkey breast (no skin)	—
2 cups mashed potatoes	74
1 cup peas and onions	23
1 banana	27
1 cup skim milk	12
Snack	
1 cup pasta	33
2 tsp margarine	—
2 tbsp Parmesan cheese	—
1 cup cranberry juice	36
TOTAL	628

*This diet provides 4000 kcalories, of which 61% are from carbohydrates (628 g), 14% are from protein (139 g), and 26% are from fat (118 g). A carbohydrate/protein/fat ratio of 60:15:25 is a good goal when planning a diet to aid athletic performance.

HYDRATION: WATER AND ELECTROLYTES

Water and Dehydration

Dehydration can be a serious problem for athletes. Its extent depends on the intensity and duration of the exercise, the surrounding temperature, the level of fitness, and the preexercise or pregame state of hydration. It is especially severe in endurance events. For example, marathon runners sometimes collapse from dehydration. Athletes may also have other problems such as cramps, delirium, vomiting, hypothermia, or hyperthermia—all caused by dehydration. With careful planning ahead of athletic events and providing fluid replacement throughout, many of these problems can be prevented.[15] Regular fluid intake should be planned for all types of athletes, not just runners. Sports coaches are increasingly aware of the importance of avoiding dehydration. Some strategies to increase fluid intake by players on a sports team are given in Box 14-2. A useful tool that many coaches use is mandatory weighing before and after the athletic event; then each pound (2.2 kg) of weight lost by a player during the event should be replaced by 16 oz (480 to 500 ml) of fluid.

1. *Cause of dehydration.* About 60% of the energy from the breakdown of glucose is released as heat. In minimal physical exercise this heat production maintains desirable body temperature. During heavier exercise it exceeds the body's needs and sometimes even exceeds the body's heat tolerance capacity. Sweating is our main mechanism for dissipating body heat. The major source of fluid loss in sweat is plasma fluid. Endurance events can cause the loss of several liters of water as

BOX 14-2 Strategies to Increase Fluid Intake by Sports Team Members

- Establish a regular schedule—drink during warm-up exercises and between period of play.
- Give each player a sports squeeze bottle.
- Supply players with a sports drink that tastes good while exercising.
- Make available a choice of fluids to drink.
- Offer cool fluids, which are preferred over warm fluids.
- Avoid carbonated beverages because athletes tend to drink less when the beverage is carbonated.

From Palumbo CM: Nutrition concerns related to the performance of a baseball team. Copyright by the American Dietetic Association. Adapted with permission from the *Journal of the American Dietetic Association,* vol. 100(6):704, 2000.

sweat, which is pulled from the plasma fluid to control body heat. Unless this amount is replaced, serious consequences can follow.

2. *Prevention of dehydration.* The thirst mechanism fails to keep pace with the body's increased need for fluid during exercise. The dehydrated person therefore must consciously drink more fluids. To prevent dehydration, athletes are advised to drink more water than they think is needed, in frequent small amounts, without dependence on the normal thirst mechanism (Figure 14-2). Cold water, about the temperature inside a refrigerator, is absorbed more quickly from the stomach. It is important to speed rehydration and to minimize the discomfort that a full stomach gives the athlete. During longer ultraevents such as 50-mile runs, 100-mile cycling, or triathlons, small cups of cold water, or sports drinks with mild solutions of saline and glucose, should be drunk frequently. Until quite recently it was thought that drinking water immediately before or during an athletic event would cause cramps; there is no basis for this claim.

Electrolytes

A number of special "sports drinks" are now being marketed with the indication that the electrolytes lost in sweat must be replaced (see *To Probe Further* box). This is true, but how? Sweat is more dilute than our internal fluids, and thus we lose proportionately, not just absolutely, much more water than anything else. In most instances, water is the rehydration fluid of choice; electrolytes are replaced with the athlete's next meal. However, during longer and more demanding endurance events, especially in a warm environment, a mild saline and glucose (6% solution) sports drinks that has rapid gastric emptying and intestinal absorption times may be used. A carbohydrate/electrolyte beverage may improve athletic performance in intermittent moderate- to high-intensity exercise that lasts about 60 minutes.[16,17]

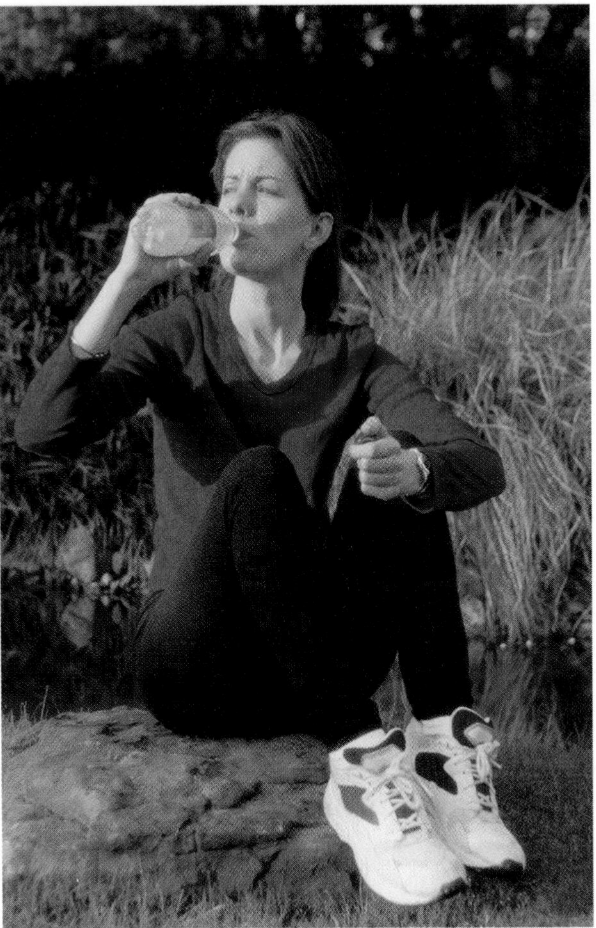

FIGURE 14-2 Frequent small drinks of cold water during extended exercise prevent dehydration. *(Credit: PhotoDisc.)*

TRAINING AND PRECOMPETITION ABUSES AMONG ATHLETES

Weight Control Measures

The sport of wrestling has a long history of widely fluctuating weight patterns among its athletes. Wrestlers often restrict food and fluid intake to certify for a weight classification that is below their off-season weight, seeking to gain advantages in strength, speed, and leverage over a smaller opponent. This practice of "making weight" still seems to be an ingrained tradition that produces large, frequent, and rapid weight loss/regain cycles, with methods such as dehydration, severe food restriction, and loss of food and fluid through induced vomiting and use of laxatives and diuretic drugs. Such disordered eating affects normal growth, and progressive dehydration impairs regulation of body temperature and cardiovascular function. Other sports such as bodybuilding and gymnastics often follow similar routines, especially before competition. In gymnastics, for example, young preadolescent girls who must maintain a small body size in the face of advancing age increasingly reduce food

TO PROBE FURTHER
Sort Out the Sports Drinks Saga

The first of the so-called sports drinks hit the market about 25 years ago, and now, with all its followers, these beverages have spawned a multimillion-dollar industry. Their claims abound, and sorting them out is not always easy for athletes and their coaches, who forever seek that prize of the competitive edge.

The current saga of the sports drinks began with a solution called Gatorade, a beverage its developers named for their university's football team. They reasoned that if they analyzed the sweat of their players, they could replace the lost minerals and water in a drink containing some flavoring, coloring, and sugars to make it acceptable, and it would taste better and do a better job than plain water. Although it has been highly profitable for the university and for the manufacturer, most athletes do not need it. Physically fit athletes engaged in regular nonendurance exercise generally do as well on plain water as on a solution such as this product and obtain their minerals from their regular diets.

However, what long-term endurance athletes do need, especially in hot weather, is water and fuel, that is, carbohydrates. For example, so much water is lost by a runner in a long-distance marathon, when the body sweats 2% to 6% of its weight, that it cannot keep cool enough and the overall system overheats, leading to heat stroke and collapse. Also, without adequate carbohydrate replacement, the muscles soon run out of glycogen stores and slow down. But simply adding sugar to water holds it in the stomach longer, where it does the body tissues no good for immediate needs.

To meet the body's dual need during such marathon events, a second category of sports drinks has now developed, using glucose polymers instead of sugar and adding less sodium. These short chains of about five glucose molecules—maltodextrins—are produced in the breakdown of starch. These drinks are less concentrated and are only slightly sweetened and flavored, and they leave the stomach rapidly, thus making them ideal as a continuing fuel source for the endurance athlete. Two such products in this category, marketed in powdered mix form, are Ross Laboratory's Exceed and Coca-Cola's Max. However, these products cannot be found in supermarkets. They are provided mainly through pharmacies to professionals working with serious athletes.

Other sports drinks to enter the market have been Gatorade clones such as the product Recharge, which claims to add no sugar yet supplies an ample amount of it as fructose and glucose in its fruit juice base. And still another category has emerged in products such as Gear Up, which adds to its base of 10 fruit juices 10 vitamins in amounts yielding 137% of the RDAs in a single 10-ounce bottle but contains no minerals. All of these extra vitamins do not help an athlete's performance, and on a hot day a perspiring athlete could easily down a megadose in four or five bottles. However, recent studies indicate that controlled use in intermittent moderate- to high-intensity exercise improves the athlete's performance.

So sort out the costs and claims of sports drinks. They are not for everyone. For the long run, special ones may meet the needs of the athlete in endurance events. But for nonendurance activities most persons do not need them. After all, water is the best solution for regular needs—and it costs far less.

References

Ball TC et al: Periodic carbohydrate replacement during 50 minutes of high-intensity cycling improves subsequent sprint performance, *Int J Sport Nutr* 5:151, 1995.

Below PR et al: Fluid and carbohydrate ingestion independently improve performance during 1 hour of intense exercise, *Med Sci Sports Exerc* 27:200, 1995.

Jackson DA et al: Effects of carbohydrate feedings on fatigue during intermittent high-intensity exercise in males and females, *Med Sci Sports Exerc* 27:S223, 1995.

Ryan M: Sports drinks: research asks for reevaluation of current recommendations, *J Am Diet Assoc* 97(suppl 2):S197, 1997.

intake and body fat, sometimes developing eating disorders. As a result, a cascade of events may follow—impaired growth, delayed puberty, induced amenorrhea from low estrogen levels, disruption or delay in bone density development, and even later osteoporosis. A similar pattern has been observed among young runners.

DRUG ABUSE

From ancient Greek runners and discus throwers in the first Olympian contests to top competitors from around the world in current Olympic events, athletes have experimented with various ergogenic aids in their eternal search for the competitive edge or the perfect body. Modern athletes—from professional football players to their aspiring high school counterparts—are doing the same thing, trying to find the magic potion in everything from bee pollen and seaweed to freeze-dried liver flakes, gelatin, amino acid supplements, and ginseng. Such efforts have been worthless in most cases but fortunately not particularly harmful. However, in the case of the group of drugs called anabolic-androgenic steroids, which are now epidemic in the sporting world, great danger and even death lie ahead for the user.[18,19] These illegal drugs must be obtained through a black market network, which adds legal jeopardy and street preparation impurities to the drug's inherent dangers to personal health. These dangers have included reported death from fatal cardiac arrest, acute heart attack, and cancer of the liver and prostate. Abuse of steroids in the United States has moved from its early use among bodybuilders to invade almost all areas of athletics, becoming epidemic among football players, significantly young junior and senior high school boys.[19] In addition, other abuses amplify the dangers of steroids. For example, a large dose of a diuretic such as furosemide (Lasix, 80 to 120 mg) is taken on the day of drug testing to dilute the urine and decrease the risk of detection. Also, large megadoses of vitamins and minerals become abused drugs and as such are used as ergogenic aids in all areas and levels of sports. Such megadoses of nutrients alter normal metabolic processes and cause severe disturbances.

RISKS FOR FEMALE ATHLETES

Some women athletes who enter highly competitive and demanding sports beginning in their preadolescent and young adolescent years face significant health risks related to anemia and low bone mineral density. These risks are especially prevalent for women athletes in sports with intensive training and with endurance events, such as gymnastics and running. Highly skilled dancers in the performing arts world often face similar risks.[11]

Sports Anemia

Reduced hemoglobin in an athlete's blood means reduced oxygen-carrying capacity, with obvious implications for aerobic capacity and the ability to sustain an exercise workload. The definition of anemia for women has been set at an hemoglobin (Hb) value of less than 12 g/dl compared with the normal value of 14 g/dl. (For men, anemia is indicated by a value of less than 14 g/dl and is normal at 16 g/dl.) Although absolute anemia is rare among competitive athletes, low normal values are typical. Heavy exercise may produce transient anemia during the initial weeks of training, with the Hb level stabilizing in the long run at the low end of normal. Strenuous continued exercise is also associated with low iron stores in athletes, which pose long-term problems. Possible causes of this sports anemia include inadequate iron in the diet, decreased iron absorption, and increased iron losses. Studies have revealed that some athlete diets are low in bioavailable iron. Women athletes have cyclic menstrual loss of iron unless they experience amenorrhea. Significant amounts of iron are lost in profuse sweating and occasionally because of *intravascular hemolysis,* which is the rupture of red blood cells caused by the stresses of heavy exercise.

Low Bone Mineral Density

Many young women athletes, as they strive for the perfect body shape and the perfect performance routine, do not realize the great danger they face of creating long-term irreversible damage to their bones. An inadequate diet, because of weight control efforts or eating disorders, combined with an interrupted menstrual and estrogen cycle can lead to lower than normal bone mineral density (osteopenia) and even in some cases to a state of osteoporosis at an abnormally young age (Figure 14-3). Because this pattern affects primarily athletes, it has been called the "female athlete triad" (see *Practical Application* box).[20-22] An estimated 40% to 60% of a woman's normal bone mineral density for her lifetime is created during adolescence when her sex hormone estrogen becomes active. The diet and hormones must work together. There must be an adequate amount of calcium in the diet, as

amenorrhea The absence of menses (menstrual cycle) entirely, or no more than three periods in a year; associated with lower than normal estrogen levels in women.

ergogenic Tendency to increase work output; various substances that increase work or exercise capacity and output.

osteopenia Below-normal level of bone mineral density, which increases the risk of stress fractures; the bone thinning is not as severe as that found in osteoporosis.

osteoporosis Abnormal thinning of bone, producing a porous, fragile, lattice-like bone tissue of enlarged spaces that is prone to fracture or deformity.

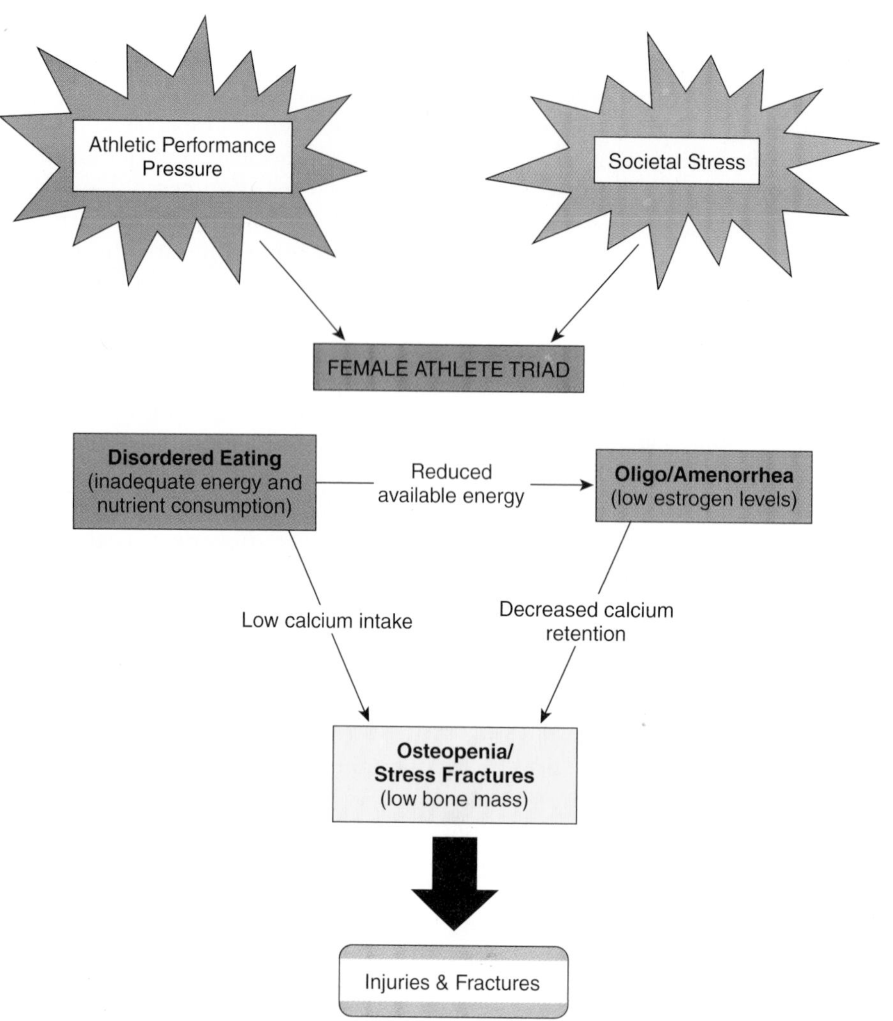

FIGURE 14-3 The female athlete triad. (*From Thrash LE, Anderson JJB: The female athlete triad: nutrition, menstrual disturbances, and low bone mass,* Nutr Today *35(5):168, 2000, Lippincott Williams & Wilkins©.*)

well as normal functioning of the female estrogen cycle that stimulates osteoblastic activity (bone growth). Unfortunately, many young female athletes and dancers restrict their diets in an effort to control their weight, growth, and optimal body fat, with resulting inadequate dietary calcium and iron.[23] Some may have more profound eating disorders, such as anorexia nervosa. At the same time, intense athletic training in young women can lead to amenorrhea, which is defined as the absence of menses entirely or no more than three periods in a year. Amenorrhea or missed periods are much more common in athletes than in nonathletes and are especially prevalent among endurance athletes such as runners. When athletic training begins at an early age before normal menarche, that onset of puberty with its normal growth and development pattern is delayed, along with the secondary sex characteristics shaping the female figure, as evidenced in the small, flat bodies of young gymnasts. Older amenorrheic adolescent runners have usually entered training after menarche and then stopped menstruating after beginning their running program. When the menstrual cycle is delayed or interrupted, normal estrogen levels are depressed. As a result, these young women athletes are at a high risk for low bone mineral density and for stress fractures.[24] Injuries and fractures can interrupt or permanently end an athletic career, and bone mineral loss may be irreversible and become a lifelong risk.[25,26]

Building a Personal Exercise Program

HEALTH BENEFITS

Exercise brings benefits to our overall health. A sense of fitness helps one to "feel good." In addition to this general sense of well-being, however, exercise—especially when it includes aerobic exercise—has special benefits for persons with certain health problems.

Coronary Heart Disease

Exercise reduces risks for heart disease in several ways related to heart function, blood cholesterol levels, and oxygen transport.

1. *Heart muscle function.* The heart is a four-chambered organ of muscle that is about the size of a fist in adults. Exercise, especially aerobic conditioning, strengthens and enlarges the heart, thereby enabling the heart to pump more blood per beat (stroke volume). A heart strengthened by exercise has an increased aerobic capacity; that is, the heart can pump more blood per minute without an undue increase in the heart rate.
2. *Blood cholesterol levels.* Exercise raises blood levels of high-density lipoprotein (HDL), which is called "good cholesterol" because it carries surplus cholesterol from the tissues to the liver for breakdown and removal from the body. Exercise also lowers blood levels of low-density lipoprotein (LDL), which is called "bad cholesterol" because it carries at least two thirds of the total blood cholesterol to body tissues, raising the potential of cholesterol deposits in major arteries of the heart. Both of these exercise effects lower the risks for diseased arteries.
3. *Oxygen-carrying capacity.* Exercise also enhances the circulatory system by increasing the oxygen-carrying capacity of the blood. The strengthened heart muscle can pump out more blood per beat, thus resulting in a healthy circulating blood volume without an increased heartbeat rate.

Hypertension

The risk for cardiovascular complications increases continuously with increasing levels of blood pressure.[27,28] When blood pressure is measured, persons with mild essential hypertension show a systolic blood pressure (i.e., the upper notation) of 140 to 159 mm Hg or a diastolic blood pressure (i.e., the lower notation) of 90 to 104 mm Hg or both. Persons with mild hypertension represent the overwhelming majority of hypertensive individuals in the general population, and exercise has become one of the most effective nondrug treatments for them. Even for persons with higher levels of blood pressure, exercise has proved to be an important adjunct to drug therapy, offsetting adverse drug effects and lowering drug needs.

Diabetes

Exercise helps control diabetes, especially type 2 non–insulin-dependent diabetes (NIDDM) in obese adults. Exercise improves the action of a person's naturally produced insulin by increasing the number of insulin receptor sites (i.e., areas where insulin may be carried into cells). In managing type 1 insulin-dependent diabetes mellitus (IDDM), the type of exercise and when it is done must be balanced with food and insulin to prevent reactions caused by drops in blood sugar.

Weight Management

Exercise is extremely beneficial in weight management because it (1) helps to regulate appetite, (2) increases the basal metabolic rate, and (3) reduces the genetic fat deposit set-point level. Together with a well-planned diet, physical exercise corrects the energy balance in favor of increased energy output and decreased energy intake (see Chapter 6). Exercise by itself has a significant effect on reducing fat and increasing lean body content.[8]

Stress Management

Exercise helps reduce stress-related eating. It also provides a physical outlet for working off the hormonal physiologic effects of adrenaline (epinephrine) produced in the body by stress, thus helping to reduce a major risk factor in the development of chronic disease.

Bone Disease

Exercise helps increase calcium deposits in bone (bone mineralization), thus reducing the risk of bone weakness and of potential osteoporosis.[29]

Mental Health

Exercise stimulates the production of brain opiates, which are substances called *endorphins.* These natural substances decrease pain (this is how aspirin works, by stimulating production of endorphins) and improve the mood, including an exhilarating kind of "high."

ASSESSMENT OF PERSONAL HEALTH AND EXERCISE NEEDS

There are many kinds of exercise. Choosing those kinds that are best depends on individual health and personal needs, the aerobic benefits involved, and personal enjoyment. Table 14-2 shows the approximate energy expenditure per hour for an adult performing different activities.

Health and Personal Needs

In planning an exercise program, it is important to assess individual health status, personal needs, present level of fitness, and resources required. Discussing an exercise program with a medical practitioner is always recommended, and getting a medical clearance before beginning an exercise program is especially important for older persons. What do you want to gain from your exercise? How much time can you commit to it? How much, if anything, does it cost? Perhaps it is even more important to ask yourself what you like to do. If the exercise you choose is not fun, you will soon stop doing it, and it will be of no benefit. It is wise to start slowly and build gradually rather than risk injury and discouragement. Moderation and regularity are the key guides.

Aerobic Benefits

To build aerobic capacity, the level of exercise must raise the pulse rate to within 70% of maximal heart

TABLE 14-4 Target Zone Heart Rate According to Age to Achieve Aerobic Physical Effect of Exercise

Age (yr)	Maximal Attainable Heart Rate (Pulse: 220 Minus Age)	Target Zone	
		70% Maximal Rate	85% Maximal Rate
20	200	140	170
25	195	136	166
30	190	133	161
35	185	129	157
40	180	126	153
45	175	122	149
50	170	119	144
55	165	115	140
60	160	112	136
65	155	108	132
70	150	105	127
75	145	101	124

TABLE 14-5 Aerobic Exercises for Physical Fitness (Maintained at Aerobic Level for at Least 20 Minutes)

Type of Exercise	Aerobic Forms
Ball playing	Handball
	Racquetball
	Squash
Bicycling	Stationary
	Touring
Dancing	Aerobic routines
	Ballet
	Disco
Jumping rope	Brisk pace
Running or jogging	Brisk pace
Skating	Ice-skating
	Roller-skating
Skiing	Cross-country
Swimming	Steady pace
Walking	Brisk pace

rate. Unless you have had an exercise tolerance or stress test and know precisely what your maximal exercising heart rate is, a good rule of thumb to determine your maximum cardiac rate is to subtract your age from 220. This calculation gives an estimate of your maximal heart rate. About 70% of this figure is your target pulse rate—the level to which you want to raise your pulse during exercise (Table 14-4). For aerobic benefits, this rate should then be maintained for approximately 20 minutes about 3 times per week. Check your resting pulse before starting the exercise period, then again during and immediately afterward, to monitor your progress in developing your target exercising heart rate and aerobic capacity.

TYPES OF PHYSICAL ACTIVITY

General Exercise

There are many exercises from which you may choose. Many of them are enjoyable and healthful but do not reach aerobic levels. For example, golf is a passion for many and gets them outdoors, but it is far too slow and sporadic to be aerobic. Also, most sports in the hands of amateurs, rather than those with fast-paced extraordinary skill to provide sustained exercise, are too slow paced to be aerobic; these include tennis, football, baseball, and basketball. Weight-lifting develops and strengthens muscles but is not an aerobic exercise. It is best to have a variety of exercises in your plan. Even though many sports do not reach aerobic levels, if they are enjoyable they should be included. If whatever you do is not fun, you will soon stop, reaping no benefits.

Aerobic Exercise

Forms of exercise that can be sustained at a necessary level of intensity to provide aerobic benefits include such activities as swimming, running, jogging, bicycling, and the popular aerobic dancing routines and workouts (Table 14-5). Perhaps the simplest and most popular form of stimulating exercise is *walking*. Figure 14-4 illustrates that aerobic walking can fit into almost anyone's lifestyle. If the pace is fast enough to elevate your pulse and it is maintained for at least the required 20 minutes, walking can be an excellent form of aerobic exercise. It is convenient and requires no equipment

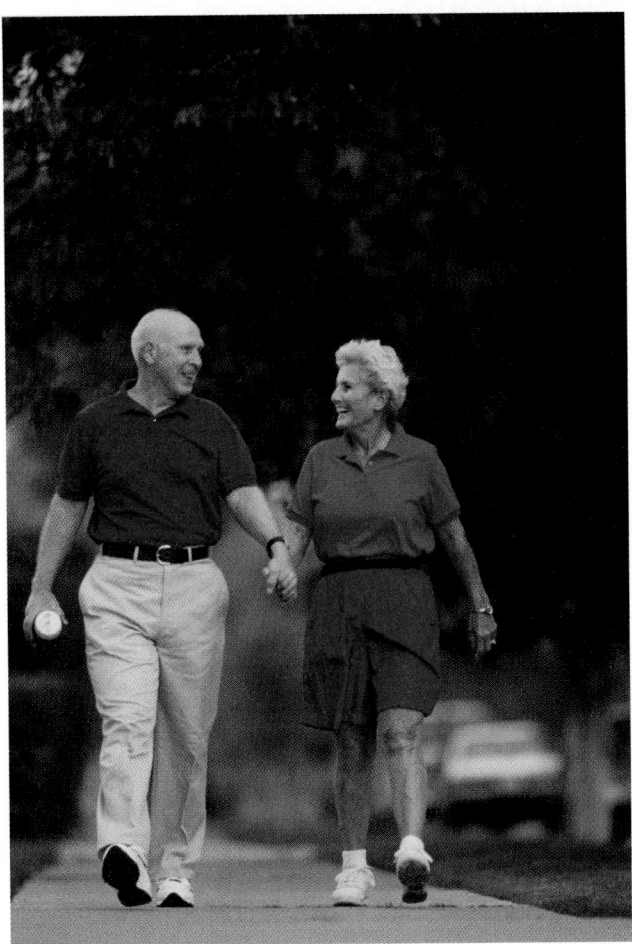

FIGURE 14-4 Aerobic walking is an enjoyable exercise that can fit into almost anyone's lifestyle. *(Credit: PhotoDisc.)*

other than good walking shoes. It is appropriate for and available to many persons.

Stress Management in Physical Fitness

Beyond planning a manageable program of physical activity, the search for physical fitness means that persons in our fast-paced society must learn to deal with physiologic responses to stress triggered through the neuroendocrine system. Successful management of stress is based in part on an awareness of the relationship among stress, disease, and nutrition.

STRESS AS A HEALTH-DISEASE RISK FACTOR

Automatic physiologic responses sweep through the body as adaptations to stress. Throughout human history these physiologic reactions have readied the body to confront or escape danger—the familiar "fight or flight" response. But this response is not well adapted to today's high-pressured and sedentary modern society and lifestyle. Often we can neither fight nor flee. These simple options are usually not appropriate in our relatively high-pressure but unphysical modern lifestyle. These repeated physiologic reactions have been linked to reduced immune function and the emergence of many of the "diseases of civilization"—coronary heart disease, hypertension, diabetes, and cancer.

STRESS AND NUTRITIONAL CARE PLANNING

The classic work of Canadian physician Hans Selye shows the close relationship of stress to the risk and incidence of disease. Selye called stress "the rate of wear and tear in the human machinery that accompanies any vital activity."[30,31]

Over the years of his monumental work, Selye established the pattern of individual physiologic response to a given stress agent. Different reactions in different persons depend on *conditioning factors,* which can inhibit or enhance one or more stress effects. These factors may be internal, such as genetic predisposition, age, or sex. Or they may be external, such as poor diet or alcohol or other drug abuse. Other investigators have validated Selye's early foundation work with applications in many areas of health and disease. Stress management has thus become a necessary part of nutrition assessment and care planning as well as an essential component of health promotion programs.

HUMAN NEEDS AND LIFE CHANGES

Change and balance are essential to continued life. The dynamic interior metabolism of the human body must interface with a changing exterior environment. Normal physiologic stress is an integral part of this interface. For example, the physiologic stress of pregnancy adapts the maternal body to sustain fetal growth and prepare for birth. Also, the normal stress of skeletal muscles pulling on bones helps maintain calcium balance between bone and blood calcium levels. And the general stress of pain warns of injury or illness.

However, severe, prolonged, uncontrolled stress, whether physical and psychosocial hunger or pain, exhausts resources and can lead to illness or death. Healthcare team members in any situation must seek to provide care based on identified human needs in the basic areas of (1) growth and development, (2) health or disease status, and (3) stress and coping balance. All of these areas include nutritional concerns.

THE NATURE OF STRESS

Perception of Stress

Individual response to stress varies according to how it is perceived. Our perception of each life experience is influenced by three factors: (1) the stimulus of external reality, (2) the message of that stimulus conveyed by the nervous system to the brain's integrative centers, where stimuli are evaluated, and (3) the interpretation we put on each experience. Subjective elements—hunger, thirst, love, fear, self-interest, personal value—influence our responses.

Common Life Stressors

Three characteristics of stress influence its effect: (1) its strength, whether it is relatively mild or severe, (2) its duration, whether it is fairly transient or long term, and (3) the strength of personal coping resources. Life stressors are (1) physical or physiologic and (2) psychologic, social, or economic. Emotional tension from multiple causes is the most common agent of human stress. It contributes to serious conditions such as cardiac and gastrointestinal diseases, especially if the body is already stressed by faulty diet or poor housing, as is often the case for high-risk families in the grip of poverty.

Physiologic-Metabolic Response to Stress

The body automatically responds to defend itself from harm. Selye called this common physiologic response to stress the *general adaptive syndrome.*[30] An understanding of this automatic cascade of physiologic events is essential for (1) identifying needs and resources, (2) planning nutritional support, both immediate and long term, and (3) rebuilding metabolic reserves. This immediate reaction of the body to stress involves actions of the combined neuroendocrine systems through three progressive stages of physiologic response (Figure 14-5).

COMBINED ACTIONS OF THE NEUROENDOCRINE SYSTEM

Both parts of the nervous system—the central nervous system and the automatic or sympathetic nervous system—constantly control and modulate reactions of the body to

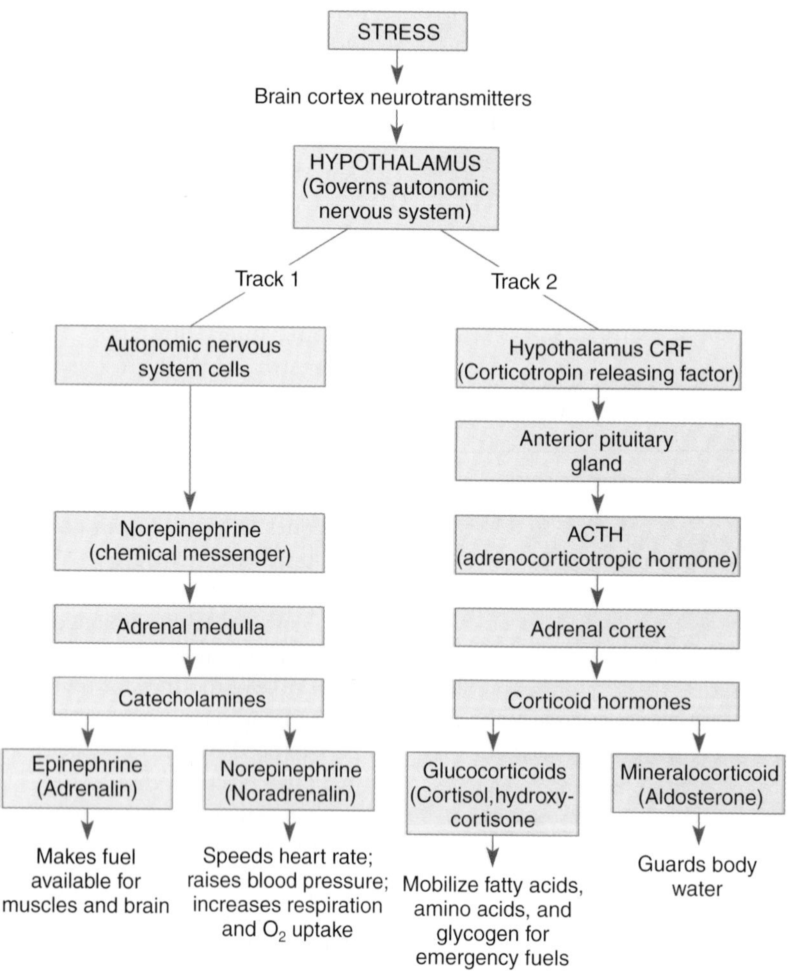

FIGURE 14-5 Progressive sequence of physiologic events in response to stress.

sensory stimuli and stress. Together with a large array of hormones and other chemical messengers, the overall neuroendocrine system provides a vast network of conscious and unconscious reactions to protect the body.[9]

Conscious Response: Central Nervous System

Certain processes in the body are under conscious direction. In response to conscious direction, the brain and central nervous system send messages to the muscles, which in turn carry out the specific actions involved, such as studying, eating, taking a walk, reading a book, or calling a friend.

Unconscious Response: Autonomic Nervous System

Other processes, such as breathing or contraction of the heart muscle, are essential to life and thus are automatically programmed and regulated. This essential control is managed by the autonomic, or sympathetic, nervous system.

Combined Neuroendocrine Response

In response to stress, the autonomic nervous system and its hormones and other chemical messengers mobilize the body's reserves for protection. From his research, Selye identified three stages of the generalized response process: (1) the initial alarm reaction, in which the body's forces are mobilized for action; (2) the adaptation-resistance stage, in which energy reserves are adjusted or rebuilt; and (3) the exhaustion stage, in which resources give out if severe stress continues. In the body's response to daily life stresses these stages overlap, reflecting the intensity of the person's life situation. The automatic physiologic response to stress increases during nervous tension, physical injury, infections, muscular work, or any other strenuous activity.

STAGE I: INITIAL ALARM REACTION

Brain Signals

In this first stage, the body's forces are mobilized for action. In response to a perceived threat, the brain instantly triggers the release of chemical messengers, *neurotransmitters,* in the brain cortex. These messengers then relay impulses along neuron tracks in the brain's outer edge to the *hypothalamus,* the "primitive" brain at the head of the brain stem that governs autonomic body functions, such as breathing, heart rate, blood pressure, digestion, hormonal balance, and many other vital activities. This part of the brain, the hypothalamus, has been called the "automatic pilot" or the "brain's brain." On receipt of the stress message, the hypothalamus instantly triggers other chemical messengers and hormones along two separate, yet integrated, tracks to adapt the body's normal physiology to changes needed to combat the danger. In Figure 14-5, you can trace these brain signals and message relays along their two tracks and note the body's important protective physiologic effects. Some liken this chain of events to a train switching freight at different stations. Others compare it to a symphony. No human creation is sufficiently well orchestrated, complex, and efficient to compare with this remarkable system of control as the body readies for crisis.

STAGE II: ADAPTATION-RESISTANCE

After the initial alarm reaction, if the particular stress does not overwhelm the person's coping resources, a second stage of resistance and adaptation follows. Here energy reserves are adjusted and rebuilt, allowing a certain tolerance to build up.

Hormonal Feedback

The body's normal hormonal feedback mechanism now comes into play to shut off continued output of the initiating hormonal agent and thus return blood levels of hormones from various target glands back to their normal levels. For example, during the initial alarm reaction, thyroid hormone and adrenal cortex corticoids—which manage massive immediate metabolic needs—flood the circulation and raise blood levels of these substances. Then, in this second stage of response, these high levels in turn feed back to the controlling master gland, the pituitary, to now shut off or lower its triggering hormones—thyroid stimulating hormone (TSH) to the thyroid and adrenocorticotropic hormone (ACTH) to the adrenal gland—for a period of automatic adjustment back to normal balance.

Rebuilding Reserves

As a result of the massive alarm reaction, normal body reserves are rapidly depleted. The blood becomes concentrated with metabolic materials, and there is marked loss of body weight. A period of restoration must eventually follow. This period allows the glands and other body tissue reserves to rebuild, the blood dilution to resume normal levels, and the body weight to return toward normal. This vital rebuilding process obviously requires positive nutrition support.

Adaptive Homeostasis

The level of this adaptation to the initial or chronic stress depends on the extent of the stress and the person's coping powers. The stress reaction is generalized throughout the body, always resulting in this general adaptive syndrome identified by Selye. When stress is superimposed on persons made vulnerable by nutritional deficiency, disorder, or disease, the effect is to make a bad situation worse. Often this is the case—for example, in high-risk populations experiencing chronic stress of poverty and malnutrition or the malnutrition seen in some hospitalized patients.

STAGE III: EXHAUSTION

After prolonged exposure to stress, the body's adaptive powers weaken and a final stage of exhaustion follows. Under severe, prolonged stress, particularly when weakened immune capacity and disease compound it, the body's adaptive energy must be restored if the person is to survive.

Immunity

Persons under stress of life events experience depressed immune function and increased vulnerability to disease. This is true of both physiologic disease and psychosocial pressure, which can bring crises both large and small. Renewed research activity in nutritional immunology has resulted.[32] The stress of protein-energy malnutrition brings atrophy to lymphoid tissue, especially the thymus gland. The stress of malnutrition particularly depresses one of the immune functions, that of the activity of the "natural killer cells." These important cells are members of the T-cell population of lymphoid cells, the lymphocytes, a type of white cell making up a major component of the body's remarkable defense system.[9] Together with a companion B-cell population of lymphoid cells, which produce antibodies for defense against disease agents, these lymphocytes come from precursor cells in the bone marrow (Figure 14-6).

The T cells make up the majority of the circulating pool of small lymphocytes in blood and lymph and in certain areas of the lymph nodes and spleen. T cells recognize invading foreign substances such as viruses by means of specific special receptors on its surface. On contact with an antigen—any foreign intruder or "non-self," an alien substance such as a virus—the T cells immediately multiply and initiate specific cellular immune responses: (1) they activate the phagocytes, special cells that have intracellular killing and degrading mechanisms for destroying invaders, and (2) they release chemical mediators that start the inflammatory process. Some T cells can do even more by becoming "killer cells" themselves and attacking antigens directly.

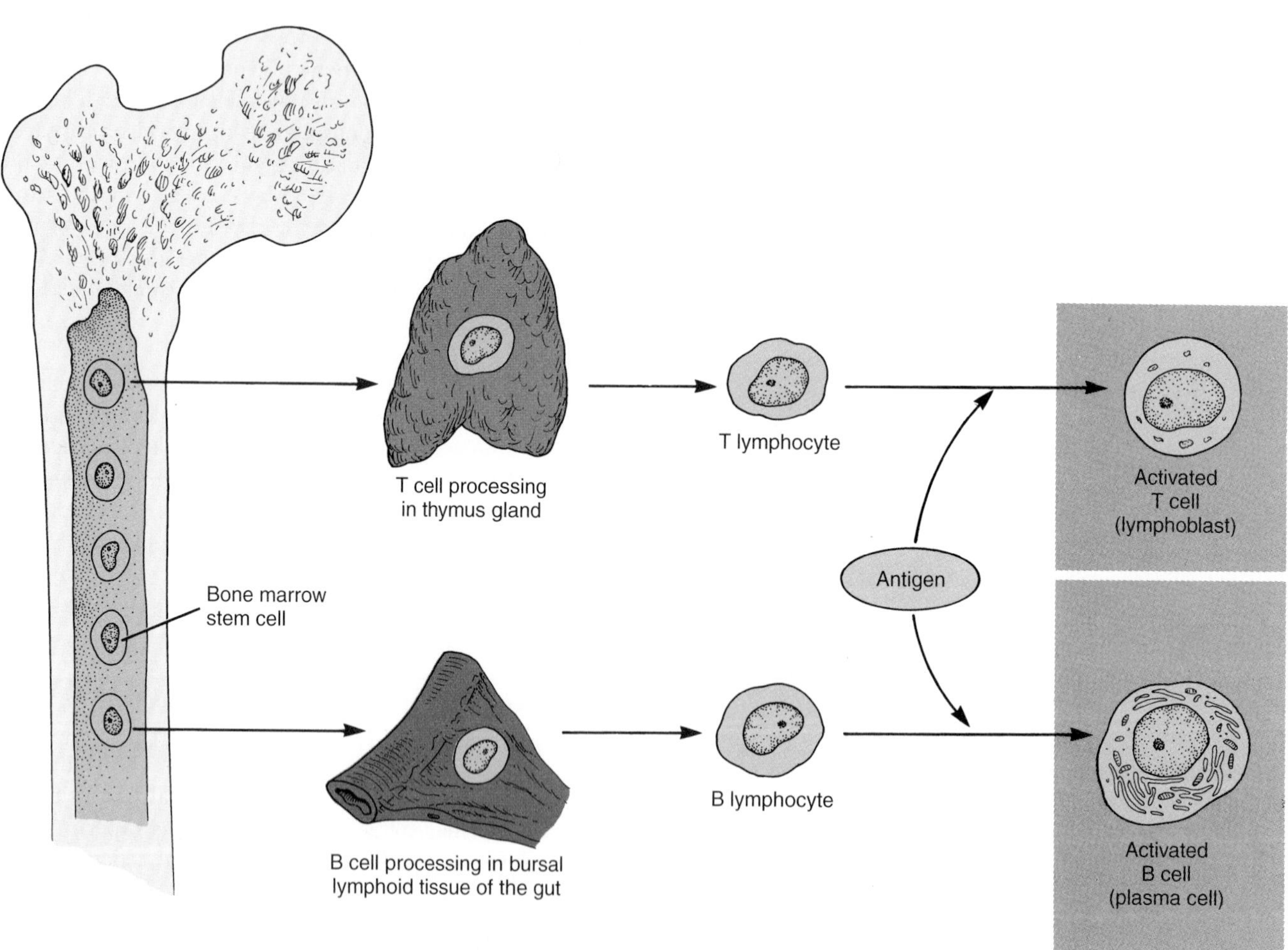

FIGURE 14-6 Development of the T and B cells, lymphocyte components of the body's immune system.

These special double-duty cells have been called "helper cell independent cytotoxic T lymphocytes," abbreviated more graphically to the name HIT cells. Also, during emergencies, cells in general produce stress proteins that repair cell damage.

Disease

Researchers studying crisis-related immunity have concluded that heightened and sustained stress can suppress immune function. But whether this condition leads to disease depends on individual conditioning factors, such as poor health and nutrition, exposure to infectious disease, and general physiologic and psychologic resources. Stress-related immunosuppression has its most significant consequences in elderly persons and others who have preexisting deficiencies in the immune system.[32]

Death

The exhaustion stage of response to stress cannot be maintained for long periods because body systems begin to wear out in their ability to cope. If resources are not restored and the stress is relentless and prolonged, finally the body's energy sources are depleted and death follows. Intervention must occur earlier to reduce stress, prevent disease, and promote health. A vital part of such intervention is nutrition support.

TO SUM UP

The energy molecule of the body is ATP, and the powerhouse of the cell is the mitochondrion. The cell's storehouse of energy is CP. These two high-energy phosphate compounds are in limited supply. They can produce energy for only a brief initial period and need to be replenished for exercise to continue. This added supply is made available by anaerobic glycolysis, with added energy made available for continued exercise by the body's aerobic system of energy production. The process of glycolysis metabolizes only carbohydrate substrate, furnished by either blood glucose or stored glycogen. Dietary carbohydrate is necessary to replenish these fuel sources. Protein contributes little to total energy production for exercise, whereas the body's ability to burn fat as fuel depends on the level of fitness. The higher the body's efficiency in using oxygen, the more fatty acids will contribute to the energy supply. Even in the best-trained athletes, fatty acid oxidation must be accompanied by glucose metabolism.

Contrary to popular belief, exercise does not require an increased intake of protein, vitamins, and minerals. The body's increased needs are well supplied by a normal healthy diet. Exercise increases the body's need for kcalories and water. Cold water taken in small, frequent amounts is the best way to prevent dehydration in most athletic events and exercise. Electrolytes lost in sweat are replaced by a continuing diet of adequate quality and quantity. Depending on the amount added, electrolytes or sugar in water may delay its emptying from the stomach and thus delay rehydration. A mild saline and glucose solution (6%) may supply fluid and fuel to sustain energy during longer endurance events. Some highly competitive athletes use harmful practices such as food and fluid deprivation for controlling weight and such ergogenic aids as illegal steroid drugs for bulking muscles.

The optimal diet for the athlete is 10% to 15% of the kcalories from protein, 30% or less from fat, and 55% to 60% from carbohydrates. The pregame meal should be small, having little or no protein and relying mainly on complex carbohydrates (starches).

The health benefits of general and aerobic exercise are many and increase with practice up to the point of overdoing. Excellent aerobic exercises include sustained fast walking, swimming, jogging, running, and aerobic dancing or workouts. Approach any exercise sensibly and choose those activities that are enjoyable.

Stress is a major risk factor for health. It triggers a physiologic "fight-or-flight" mechanism to protect the body, but in a modern stress-filled world this can only compound problems and contribute to illness. At any age, additional stress factors may increase health risks for vulnerable persons. These stress factors include physical trauma and disease, disability, and the multiple problems of poverty and general economic stress. High-stress management involves personal and social approaches based on identified individual and family needs, goals, and expectations. Methods of reducing stress and managing health risks focus on positive health and nutrition promotion, helping to build greater effective coping capacity through sound diet, relaxation, and physical activity, with a strengthened personal support system.

antibody Any of numerous protein molecules produced by B cells as a primary immune defense for attaching to specific related antigens; animal protein made up of a specific sequence of amino acids that is designed to interact with its specific antigen during an allergic response or to prevent infection.

antigen Any foreign or "non-self" substances—such as toxins, viruses, bacteria, and foreign proteins—that stimulate the production of antibodies specifically designed to interact with them.

lymphocytes Special white cells from lymphoid tissue that participate in humeral and cell-mediated immunity.

phagocytes Cells that ingest microorganisms, other cells, or foreign particles; macrophages.

Questions for Review

1. What are the component muscle structures, and how do they produce muscle action?
2. What type of substrate fuel does the body use for immediate energy needs? For short-term needs? For long-term needs?
3. How does oxygen relate to physical activity capacity and aerobic effect?
4. Outline the nutrition and physical fitness principles you would discuss with a client who is an athlete. Plan a diet for this client that would meet nutrient and energy needs.
5. Why is fluid balance vital during exercise periods? How is water and electrolyte balance achieved?
6. Describe the dangers of anabolic steroids used by some athletes for bulking muscles and gaining an edge in strength over an opponent.
7. Describe the general adaptive syndrome identified by Selye, which the body activates in response to stress, in terms of the physiologic events in each of its three stages. Why does this response create problems in today's modern society?

References

1. Lee I-M et al: Exercise intensity and longevity in men: the Harvard Alumni Health Study, *JAMA* 273(15):1179, 1995.
2. American Dietetic Association: Translating research into practice: physical activity—it's not reserved for athletes, *J Am Diet Assoc* 99(2):212, 1999.
3. American Dietetic Association: Position paper: nutrition, aging, and continuum of care, *J Am Diet Assoc* 96(10):1048, 1996.
4. U.S. Department of Health and Human Services: *Healthy people 2010: understanding and improving health,* Washington, DC, 2000, U.S. Department of Health and Human Services, Government Printing Office.
5. U.S. Department of Agriculture: *Dietary guidelines for Americans 2000,* ed 5, Washington, DC, 2000, U.S. Department of Agriculture, Government Printing Office.
6. Williams PT: High-density lipoprotein cholesterol and other risk factors for coronary heart disease in female runners, *N Engl J Med* 334(6):1298, 1996.
7. American Dietetic Association: Position paper: nutrition, aging, and continuum of care: update for 1999, *J Am Diet Assoc* 99(2):234, 1999.
8. Wilmore JH: Increasing physical activity: alterations in body mass and composition, *Am J Clin Nutr* 63(suppl): 456S, 1996.
9. Guyton AC, Hall JE: *Textbook of medical physiology,* ed 9, Philadelphia, 1996, WB Saunders.
10. Butterfield GE: Dietary requirements of the athlete. In Shephard R ed: *Current therapy in sports medicine,* ed 3, St Louis, 1994, Mosby.
11. Dox LW, Dwyer J: Lifestyle and nutrition in musical performing arts, *Nutr Today* 31(5):203, 1996.
12. Anderson JJB et al: Nutrition and bone in physical activity and sport. In Anderson JJB et al, eds: *Nutrition in exercise and sports,* ed 3, Boca Raton, FL, 1998, CRC Press.
13. American Dietetic Association Sports Cardiovascular and Wellness Nutritionists Dietetic Practice Group: *Sports nutrition: a guide for the professional working with active people,* ed 3, Chicago, 2000, American Dietetic Association.
14. McArdle WD et al: *Sports and exercise nutrition,* Philadelphia, 1999, Lippincott Williams & Wilkins.
15. Palumbo CM: Nutrition concerns related to the performance of a baseball team, *J Am Diet Assoc* 100(6):704, 2000.
16. Ryan M: Sports drinks: research asks for reevaluation of current recommendations, *J Am Diet Assoc* 16(1):S197, 1997.
17. Jackson DA et al: Effects of carbohydrate feedings on fatigue during intermittent high-intensity exercise in males and females, *Med Sci Sports Exerc* 27:S223, 1995.
18. Nnakwe N: Anabolic steroids and cardiovascular risk in athletes, *Nutr Today* 31(5):206, 1996.
19. Yesalis CE, Michael SB: Anabolic—androgenic steroids: current issues, *Sports Med* 19:326, 1995.
20. Thrash LE, Anderson JJB: The female athlete triad: nutrition, menstrual disturbances, and low bone mass, *Nutr Today* 35(5):168, 2000.
21. American College of Sports Medicine: The female athlete triad position stand, *Med Sci Sports Exerc* 29:1, 1997.
22. Talbort S: The female triad, *Strength Conditioning* 4:128, 1996.
23. Nickols-Richardson SM et al: Body composition, energy intake and expenditure, and body weight dissatisfaction in female child gymnasts and controls, *J Am Diet Assoc* 97(9): 14A, 1997.
24. Brukner P, Bennell K: Stress fractures in female athletes, *Sports Med* 24:419, 1997.
25. Keen AD, Drinkwater BL: Irreversible bone loss in former amenorrheic athletes, *Osteoporosis Int* 7:311, 1997.
26. Dook JE et al: Exercise and bone mineral density in mature female athletes, *Med Sci Sports Exerc* 29:291, 1997.
27. Franz MJ: Managing obesity in patients with comorbidities, *J Am Diet Assoc* 98(2 suppl):S39, 1998.
28. Rippe JM: Obesity as a chronic disease: modern medical and lifestyle management, *J Am Diet Assoc* 98(2 suppl):S9, 1998.
29. Ogawa A et al: Weight bearing exercise predicts total bone mineral content in female midshipmen, *J Am Diet Assoc* 97(9):19A, 1997.
30. Selye H: *The stress of life,* New York, 1956, McGraw-Hill.
31. Selye H: Hunger and stress, *Nutr Today* 5(1):2, 1970.
32. Abbas A et al: *Cellular and molecular immunology,* ed 2, Philadelphia, 1994, WB Saunders.

Further Reading

Hill JO et al: Orlistat, a lipase inhibitor, for weight maintenance after conventional dieting: a 1-year study, *Am J Clin Nutr* 69:1108, 1999.

Orlistat is a gastrointestinal lipase inhibitor that helps minimize weight regain after a successful program of needed weight loss. In this study, such regain was controlled significantly with various results according to dose level.

Schuster K: The dark side of nutrition, *Food Mgmt* 34(6):34, 1999.

Obsession with anything is usually unhealthy behavior, including unwise approaches to weight control, especially if used with children. This author discusses wise approaches to avoid obsession with weight control, especially with children, that can easily lead to eating disorders, inadequate nutrient intake for normal growth, and negative ideas about food. Instead, wise positive nutrition messages must promote variety, balance, moderation, enjoyment, and a wider healthy ideal weight range.

Steen SN: Statement of the American Dietetic Association: nutrition guidance for child athletes in organized sports, *J Am Diet Assoc* 96(6):610, 1996.

Steen SN: Statement of the American Dietetic Association: nutrition guidance for adolescent athletes in organized sports, *J Am Diet Assoc* 96(6):611, 1996.

These brief professional statements provide excellent guidelines for coaches, parents, and others involved with young growing athletes.

Issues & ANSWERS

The Winning Edge—Or Over the Edge?

Athletes, their coaches, and our entire culture have become increasingly aware that the percentage of body fat versus the percentage of lean body mass is a major influence on athletic performance. Each extra pound of body fat an athlete carries into competition is nonproductive weight. It is the muscles, the lean body mass, that provide the strength, agility, and endurance required to win.

Because of this, athletes strive to achieve as low a percentage of body fat as possible while still maintaining good health. In reaching for such a goal, however, many young athletes develop an abhorrence of body fat, resulting in food aversion and the undertaking of excessive weight-loss regimens. These self-generated excesses are commonly reinforced by those surrounding the young athletes: coaches, teammates, and perhaps the most demanding of all, parents.

Such an all-consuming focus results in compulsive behaviors, leading the young person to set unrealistic goals and resulting in abusive weight losses. The fear of failure—failure to make the team, failure in competition, and failure to live up to others' expectations—pushes young athletes in their campaign to beat the opponent, have a low level of body fat, and to win a particular contest by a large, decisive amount.

Fortunately, such excessive voluntary weight losses in young athletes are not usually caused by chronic emotional problems. The reasons typically are more superficial, resulting from an accumulation of immediate and short-term goals and concerns. These athletes usually respond well to counseling and can reverse the excessive behavior with the support of concerned friends and teammates.

Yet for a few individuals, excessive, compulsive fixation on lean body mass and the loss of body fat becomes obsessive and enduring. For example, a compulsive runner's ideal of 5% body fat is regularly found only in ballet dancers, gymnasts, fashion models, and victims of anorexia nervosa. Our mass media culture unfortunately reinforces the view that the most desirable attributes of beauty are slimness in women and physical prowess in men. When a susceptible individual enters a time of stress in search for a firm identity, he or she may turn toward cultural and media stereotypes to provide a positive self-concept. For women this stress is usually encountered during adolescence, when being physically attractive is thought by some women to be the key to social acceptance. For men the sense of self is more closely tied to their vocational and sexual effectiveness, both of which some men relate to their physical abilities. Thus the test of a man's abilities tends to occur more often in adulthood, which may result in his preoccupation with physical fitness as a way to deny any decline in strength or ability. This may be why the majority of compulsive runners, those who feel they must run despite everything, including injury or ill health, are men. Such compulsive fixation on body image in susceptible individuals often results in eating disorders that may require extensive counseling.

Our culture views compulsive dieting, as in anorexia nervosa, as a serious emotional disorder; compulsive training, on the other hand, is seen as a positive personality trait showing dedication. In reality, both may be symptomatic of unstable self-concepts and attempts to establish a firm sense of identity. They are perceptual disorders: the anorexia victim always sees herself as fat; the compulsive runner always sees himself as out of shape. Such compulsive training becomes the whole life, although it is unnatural to be pushed by whatever means possible, legal or sometimes illegal and dangerous, as in the case of anabolic steroids and cardiovascular risk. For these individuals, no goal, once attained, is sufficiently satisfying. If 5% body fat is achieved, the person strives for 4%. Such striving, often despite physical indications against it, has resulted in permanent disabilities and even death, sometimes from cardiac arrest caused by a linoleic acid deficiency.

The danger of athletic compulsion leading to eating disorders was highlighted by the 1994 death from anorexia of 22-year-old Christy Henrich, a world class American gymnast. At 4 ft 10 in (145 cm) and 95 pounds (43 kg), Christy won a silver medal at the 1989 U.S. national championships. She was known as a perfectionist who pushed herself hard, a characteristic that, when extreme, is often associated with eating disorders in athletes. She felt compelled to lose more weight and at times limited herself to only an apple a day even while continuing to train. Because of her eating disorder she eventually lost the strength to perform her routines and was forced to retire from competition. She weighed only 60 pounds (27 kg) when she died. Although her death marked the first time an American gymnast had died from an eating disorder, such problems are widely known in competitive women's gymnastics, especially at the national and international levels. In a 1992 survey of

American college women's gymnastics programs by the National Collegiate Athletics Association (NCAA), 51% of respondents reported eating disorders among their team members.

Although physical fitness and athletic accomplishments may be admirable goals, the thrill of victory for a small percentage of participants may be a hollow one if the victory is at the expense of their health and peace of mind. These driven individuals have a strict sense of self-denial and are unable to enjoy life's more receptive pleasures. The ability to slow down, stop, and enjoy smelling the roses may mean more in the long run to the quality and quantity of a person's life span than the color of a coveted ribbon or medal that may be won.

REFERENCES

Clark N: How to approach eating disorders among athletes, *Top Clin Nutr* 5(3):41, 1990.

Clark N: Counseling the athlete with an eating disorder: a case study, *J Am Diet Assoc* 94(6):656, 1994.

Kantrowitz B et al: Living with training, *Newsweek* CXX(6):24, 1992.

Nnakwe N: Anabolic steroids and cardiovascular risk in athletes, *Nutr Today* 31(5):206, 1996.

Obituary: Christy Henrich 1972-1994, *Int Gymnast* 36(10):1, 1994.

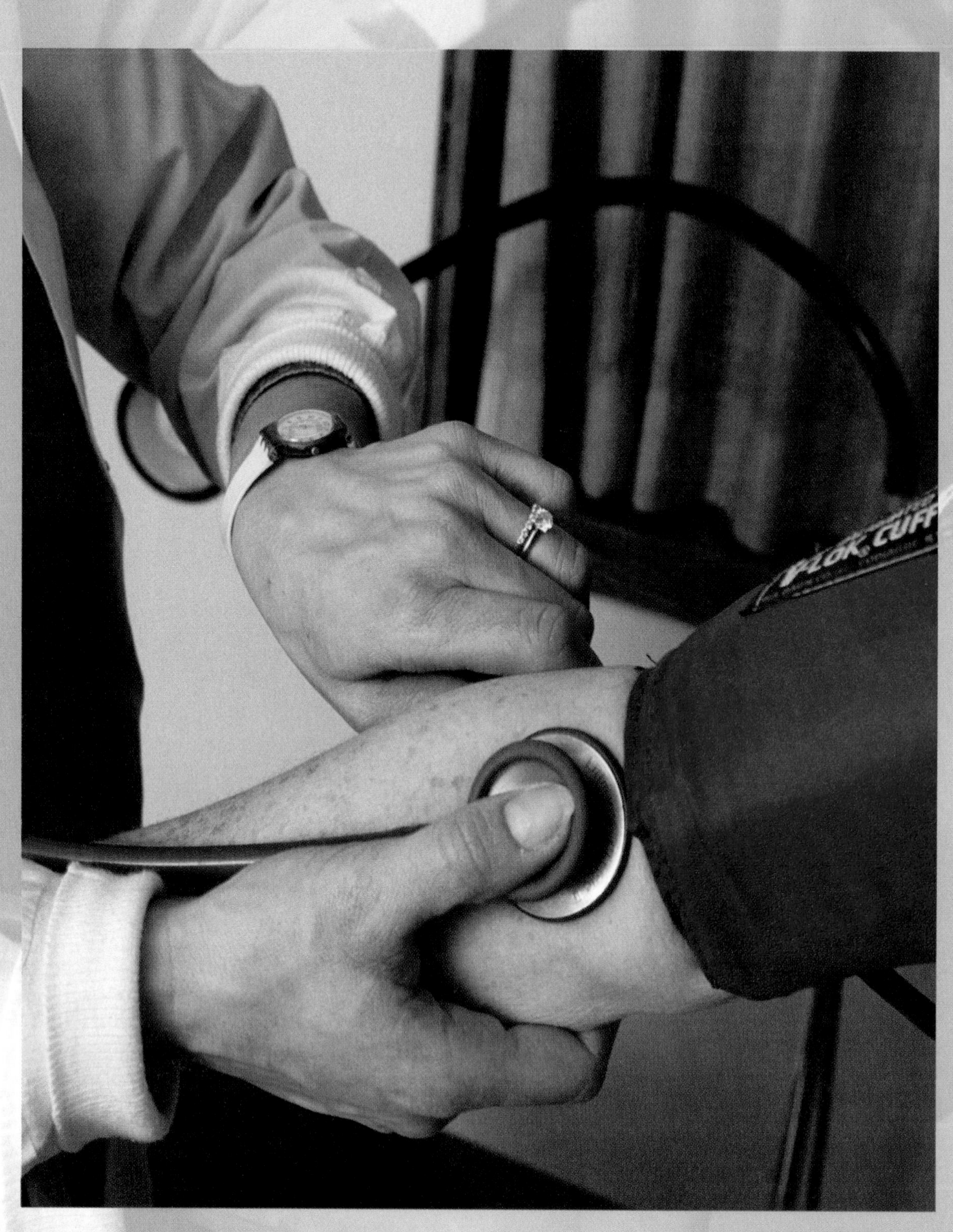

Part 3

INTRODUCTION TO CLINICAL NUTRITION

Chapter

15

Nutrition Assessment and Medical Nutrition Therapy in Patient Care

Sue Rodwell Williams

Chapter Outline

With this chapter we begin our final study sequence on clinical nutrition. In this concluding section we apply the principles of nutritional science and community nutrition that were previously discussed to nutritional needs in disease.

Here we focus on the essential first step in comprehensive nutritional care—assessing nutritional needs and developing goals as the first step in planning sensitive and valid patient care. Regardless of the place of care and the need, the healthcare team of practitioners, patient, and family work together to support the healing process and promote health.

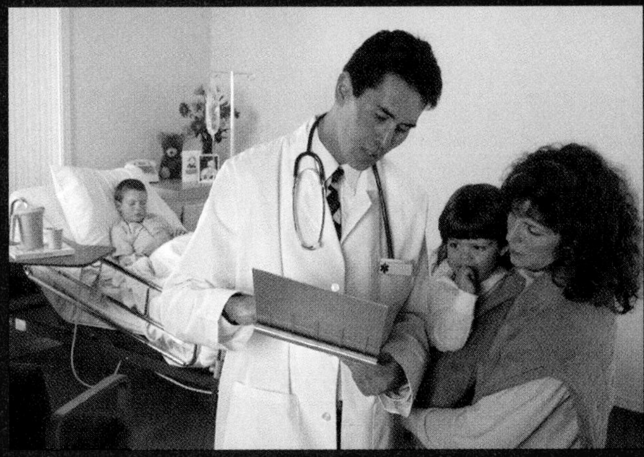

The Therapeutic Process

ROLE OF NUTRITION IN CLINICAL CARE

Persons face acute illness or chronic disease and its treatment in a variety of settings: the acute care hospital, the long-term rehabilitation center, the extended care facility, the clinic, the private office, and the home. In all instances nutritional care is fundamental. It can frequently be therapy itself. About 2500 years have passed since Hippocrates admonished us to pay closer attention to this significant connection between nutrition and disease, but we are only now, in more modern scientific times, beginning to catch a glimmer of the real depth of his valuable instruction.

Comprehensive nutritional assessment provides the necessary basis for appropriate nutritional therapy based on identified needs. Nutritional assessment and medical nutrition therapy promote multiple goals: assisting patients in recovery from illness or injury, helping persons maintain follow-up care to promote health, and helping to control healthcare costs.[1] Clinical nutritionists, all registered dietitians (RDs) and many with advanced degrees in nutritional science, use their expertise and skills to make sound clinical judgments and to work effectively with the clinical care team. These professionals provide an essential component for the successful management of the patient's plan of care.

STRESS OF THE THERAPEUTIC ENCOUNTER

In the modern hospital setting, the patient experiences a great deal of stress because he or she is sick, upset, or scared. Even the most ideal hospital stay is a very emotional experience.[2] The therapeutic encounter between healthcare providers and their patients occurs unavoidably under stressful conditions. Several factors can contribute to added nutritional toll.

Bedrest

Even though the reason for the hospitalization may indicate the need for bedrest, at the same time it has long been known that bedrest itself can result in detrimental effects on the human body.[3] For example, after just 3 days of lying supine in bed, the body begins to lose its resistance to the pull of gravity and continuing inactivity diminishes muscle tone, bone calcium, plasma volume, and gastric secretions, bringing some impairment in glucose tolerance and shifts in body fluids and electrolytes.

Hospital Malnutrition

Hospital, or iatrogenic, malnutrition has been widely documented. Hospitalized patients with hypermetabolic and physiologic stress of illness or injury can be at risk for malnutrition from their increased needs for nutritional support. Hospital operating guidelines that provide for nutrition screening on admission combined with follow-up monitoring will identify patients at malnutrition risk and provide essential medical nutrition therapy.[4] However, potential problems arising from hospital routines may contribute to a lack of adequate nourishment in some cases; these include (1) highly restricted diets remaining on order and unsupplemented too long; (2) unserved meals because of interference of medical procedures and clinical tests, and (3) unmonitored patient appetite.

Hospital Setting and System

Each injured or ill patient is a unique person and requires special treatment and care. A formidable array of staff persons seek to determine needs and implement what each patient needs as appropriate care. When individual human needs are met with personal care, within the context of carefully developed care protocols, patients will not feel intimidated and powerless.

Constant open and validating communication is essential, both among the healthcare team members and between the healthcare provider and the patient and family. It is at such times we need to remind ourselves of the time-tested fundamental ethical principles guiding all our patient care.[5,6] These principles should ensure that all we do must

- *Benefit* the patient.
- Do no *harm.*
- Preserve the patient's *autonomy.*
- *Disclose* full and truthful information for patient decisions concerning personal care.
- Provide *social justice.*

Such ethical behavior is based on the overriding fundamental principles of right action found within Anglo-American common law, which emphasizes the basic rights of privacy and free choice.[6] Continuing open communication provides the basis for such ethical practices among the healthcare team members and between the healthcare providers and the patient and family. It is especially important for many stressed elderly patients who fail to thrive. In this team effort for quality nutritional care, the RD, along with the physician, carries the primary responsibility. The nurse and other primary care practitioners provide essential support.

FOCUS OF CARE: THE PATIENT

Patient-Centered Care

The primary principle of nutritional practice, too often overlooked in the many routine procedures of the hospital setting, is evident: to be valid, nutritional care must be person centered. In this renewed partnership paradigm for patient-centered healthcare, the patient must always be a senior partner. It must be based on initial identified needs, updated constantly with the patient, with results monitored continuously in relation to therapy goals. This is necessary, of course, to provide essential physical care. But it is also necessary to support the patient's personal need to maintain self-esteem and control as much as pos-

TO PROBE FURTHER

Nutritional Assessment: When Being Objective Does Not Always Mean Being Objective

Nutritionists and other health professionals like numbers. To identify malnutrition, they monitor serum levels of liver-secreted plasma proteins, such as albumin and transferrin; take anthropometric measurements; and determine creatinine-height indexes and cell-mediated immunity response. One study now suggests that these numbers do not add up to the accuracy of the clinical examination in determining a patient's nutritional status.

Researchers from the University of Toronto and Toronto General Hospital suggest that objective measurements may sometimes be inaccurate because they are influenced by several factors: (1) the effects of the disease process itself (rather than the distinct issue of malnutrition) on changes in nutrient levels, (2) delayed response to nutritional depletion (or repletion) because of the relatively long half-lives of such indexes as serum albumin and transferrin, and (3) the wide range of confidence limits in nutritional measurements.

These workers found that two physician clinical evaluators were able to agree on the nutritional status of 81% of 59 surgical patients examined independently. The history—emphasizing weight loss, edema, anorexia, unusual food intakes, and so on—and physical examination—stressing jaundice, muscle wasting, edema, conditions of oral structures, and similar findings—provided sufficient information for them to come to conclusions that agreed with objective evaluations.

Does this mean that laboratory tests should be placed in "semiretirement," limited to use in epidemiologic surveys instead of evaluating individuals? These researchers think they should, but they acknowledge that accurate assessment tests do exist, such as total body nitrogen and total body potassium, although these are not generally available. They also suggest the possibility of combining several known indices to make a more sensitive one, even though this lends itself to the possibility of leaving out one measurement that could have an important effect on the calculations.

However, they do emphasize an important point: nutritional status is as dependent on what you see as on what you read on a laboratory sheet.

References

Baker JP et al: Nutritional assessment: a comparison of clinical judgment and objective measurements, *N Engl J Med* 306(16): 969, 1982.

Detsky AS et al: What is subjective global assessment of nutritional status? *J Parenter Enteral Nutr* 11:8, 1987.

sible. In addition, a second fundamental fact needs emphasis: despite all methods, tools, and technologies described here or elsewhere, the most therapeutic instrument of such person-centered care is yourself. It is to this seemingly simple yet profoundly personal healing encounter that you bring your skills and your dedication.

Communication with the patient at its best is an interactive, two-way process. This ideal is not always easy to achieve, however, and means much more than simply having the patient answer a few questions. All medical communication, including clinical nutritional therapies, is a form of teaching. The patient in almost all cases needs to learn new information and make the attitudinal and lifestyle changes necessary to put new knowledge to effective therapeutic use. Such teaching can take different forms, from a simple prescription concerning diet, to a persuasive appeal to emotions and attitudes, to a two-sided personal interaction (see *To Probe Further* box on p. 256). Patients today are more interested in nutrition than ever before and have more sources of information, from the media to the Internet. The websites on the Internet sponsored by Tufts University[7] and by the Hardin Library of the University of Iowa[8] are excellent sources of medically accurate nutrition information. For finding broader medical information, trustworthy advice on safe Internet searching exists for interested patients, such as the guide from Yale-New Haven Hospital.[9] The patient's personal knowledge may be accurate or erroneous, but either way will influence the patient's behavior and receptivity. Clinical practitioners often have severe time constraints in the contemporary medical environment. They nonetheless need to strive to interact with patients as sensitively and respectfully as possible.[10]

Healthcare Team

In the setting of the individual medical center, and within the essential team care provided in a managed care system, the clinical dietitian must care for the

iatrogenic Describes a medical disorder caused by physician diagnosis, manner, or treatment.

paradigm A pattern or model serving as an example; a standard or ideal for practice or behavior based on a fundamental value or theme.

patient's fundamental nutritional needs in close relationship with the medical and nursing care.[11] Sensitive communication skills are essential for all ages and degrees of health problems. Determining the patient's initial nutritional status and ongoing medical nutrition therapy needs is a primary responsibility to support healing and avoid malnutrition.[4]

PHASES OF THE CARE PROCESS

Five distinct yet constantly interacting phases are essential in the therapeutic care process.

1. *Assessment: database.* A broad base of relevant information about the patient's nutritional status, food habits, cultural context, and life situation is necessary for making accurate initial assessments. Useful background information may come from a variety of sources, such as the patient, the patient's chart, family or other relatives and friends, oral and written communication with other hospital personnel or staff, and related research. A number of valuable assessment tools have been developed, some of which are described in this chapter.
2. *Analysis: problem list.* A careful analysis of all data collected determines specific patient needs. Some needs will be immediately evident. Others will develop as the situation unfolds. On the basis of this analysis, a list of problems may be formed to guide the plan of care activities.
3. *Planning care: needs and goals.* Valid care is based on identified problems. The plan and its outcomes must always be based on personal needs and goals of the individual patient, as well as the identified medical care requirements or options discussed with the patient and family.
4. *Implementing care: actions.* The patient care plan is put into action according to realistic and appropriate activities within each situation. For example, nutritional care and education will involve decisions and actions concerning an appropriate food plan and mode of feeding, as well as the training and education needs of the patient, staff, and family who will carry it out.
5. *Evaluating and recording care: actions.* As every care activity is carried out, results are carefully evaluated to determine if the identified needs have been met. Appropriate revisions of the care plan can be made as needed for continuing care. These results are carefully recorded in the patient's medical record. Clear documentation of all activities is essential.

In our discussion here, we look at each of these phases in terms of quality nutritional care. We focus on methods and tools of nutrition assessment, practical management of nutritional therapy and care, maintenance of effective medical records, and ways of ensuring quality standards of nutritional care.

Nutritional Assessment and Analysis

THE PURPOSE AND PROCESS OF COLLECTING NUTRITIONAL DATA

The fundamental purpose of nutritional assessment in general clinical practice is to determine (1) the overall nutritional status of the patient; (2) current healthcare needs, both physical and psychosocial as well as personal; and (3) related factors influencing these needs in the person's current life situation. The first step in nutritional assessment, as with assessing any situation to determine needs and actions, is to collect pertinent information—a database—for use in identifying needs. The clinical dietitian, assisted by other healthcare team members as needed, uses several basic types of activities for nutritional assessment of patients' needs.

1. Diet evaluation and personal histories (medical, social, medications)
2. Clinical observations
3. Biochemical tests
4. Anthropometrics

Each part of this approach is important because no single parameter alone directly measures individual nutritional status or determines problems or needs (see *To Probe Further* box). Further, the overall resulting picture must be interpreted within the context of personal social and health factors that may alter nutritional requirements. Only with this type of comprehensive evaluation can nutrition assessment become the real index to the quality of life that it should be. Because such a comprehensive history is a fundamental tool for planning healthcare, history-taking is a primary skill for all health professionals. A broad number of tests may be used for research purposes in a large facility with access to highly sophisticated equipment. However, the procedures outlined here provide a good base in general practice.

DIET EVALUATION AND PERSONAL HISTORIES

A careful nutrition history, including nutritional information related to living situation and other personal, psychosocial, and economic problems, is a fundamental part of nutrition assessment. Obtaining accurate information about basic food patterns and actual dietary intake is not a simple matter because some individuals misreport or underreport what they eat. Each method of diet evaluation has particular strengths and weaknesses.[12] However, a sensitive practitioner may obtain useful information by using one or more of the basic tools described here.

Specific 24-Hour Food Record

For hospitalized patients, a record of food intake over a specific 24-hour period may be needed for tests such as a nitrogen balance study or for monitoring energy and nutrient intake. A careful explanation of purpose and procedure for the patient and staff is needed. However, such a brief recall or record in general practice has limited value in determining overall basic food habits.

Diet History

General knowledge of the patient's basic eating habits is needed to determine any possible nutritional deficiencies. In conjunction with the patient's usual living situation and related food attitudes and behaviors, social and family history, and medical history with current status and treatment, the nutrition interview provides an essential base for further personal nutrition counseling and planning of care (Figure 15-1). For example, an activity-associated day's food intake pattern, using guides discussed in Chapter 10, can provide a useful tool for obtaining a fairly valid picture of food habits and eating behaviors. In addition to food and nutrition information, drug therapy data from the medical record or the patient and family are important to determine any possible drug-nutrient interaction involved or any teaching needed by the patient (see Chapter 16). Research carefully all prescriptions and over-the-counter drugs the patient is using.

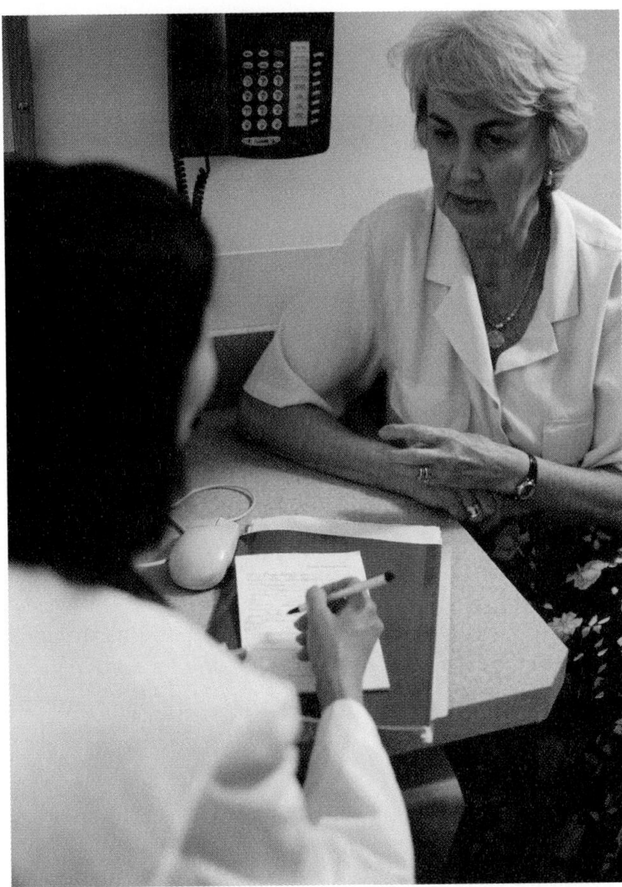

FIGURE 15-1 Interviewing patient to plan personal care. *(Credit: PhotoDisc.)*

Periodic Food Records

At various times, a 3- to 7-day food record is a helpful tool for assessing food patterns, especially when used to follow up a comprehensive initial diet history or counseling instructions for a special therapeutic diet required. A 3-day record is generally sufficient for determining overall food, energy, and nutrient intake. The 3- to 7-day periodic record can usefully be compared with the diet history to look for patterns and as a basis of interviewing to determine the prevalence of underreporting.[13] A number of appropriate software programs are available that make final computer analysis a simple matter (see *Issues & Answers*). But, of course, the accuracy of the computer analysis depends entirely on the accuracy of the food record. Sometimes a food frequency questionnaire is helpful to determine food use over an extended period, and it can provide useful data for careful interpretation, especially in combination with specific food records.[14] Food frequency questionnaires should be viewed carefully, however, as an indication of trends and relative quantities rather than as a record of absolute intakes. Research indicates a tendency among many people to underreport with this assessment tool, especially relating to their intake of dietary fat and cholesterol.[15,16]

THE PROBLEM OF UNDERREPORTING

Eating is one of life's most fundamental and universal pleasures. Is it any wonder then that many people are reluctant to divulge to others the true intimate details of what and how much they consume? Nutrition research scientists and clinical practitioners alike have long had to grapple with the psychology of eating and the emotions aroused by food.[17] Underreporting of what is actually eaten is a recurring problem in nutrition assessment.[15,18-20] The degree and type of underreporting vary. Influences on eating habits and the reporting of dietary intakes include educational level, sex, race, age, and weight.[21-23] Obese individuals (those with a high body mass index) are much more likely to underreport their food intake than are persons of normal weight.[19] Also, women are more likely to underreport than are men.[20]

The type of underreporting typically varies with the assessment instrument. Recall techniques are most likely to have simply underrecording, which in many cases can be as high as 25% of total dietary intake. Food diary methods, by contrast, can have the dual problems of both underrecording what is eaten and undereating during the period of recording in the food diary. One study found that during a period of using food diaries, obese men reduced their usual food intake by 26% (undereating) and did not record 12% of what they actually ate (underrecording).[16] A similar pattern was observed in a study of postmenopausal women; all of the women tended to undereat during the record-keeping period, whereas underrecording was most common among those who reported they were controlling their food intake to lose or maintain weight.[24]

Because underreporting of food intake is a common problem, and one intimately connected with human psychology, what measures can a dietitian or other health practitioner take to compensate? Being a careful observer is important, from the initial contact with a patient on. It is often possible in reality to identify individuals who are likely to underreport. When follow-up interviews are done, these individuals will usually admit their underreporting voluntarily to the practitioner and frequently will even provide information about both undereating and underrecording and what foods are involved.[17] The dietitian can then make reasonably informed adjustments to food records on a case-by-case basis.

CLINICAL OBSERVATIONS

For patients who are hospitalized, all clinical practitioners make use of detailed observations looking for signs of possible malnutrition. These observations are combined with the indications gained from measured vital signs and physical examination.

Clinical Signs of Malnutrition

Careful attention to physical signs of possible malnutrition provides an added dimension to the overall assessment of general nutritional status. A guide for a general examination of such signs is given in Table 15-1. A careful description of any such observations is documented in the patient's medical record.

Vital Signs and Physical Examination

Other physical data may include pulse rate, respiration, temperature, and blood pressure. A study of the common procedures of a normal physical examination will provide useful background orientation.[25]

BIOCHEMICAL TESTS

A number of laboratory tests are available for studying nutritional status. The most commonly used ones for assessing and monitoring nutritional status and planning nutritional care in clinical practice are listed here. General ranges for normal values are given in standard texts.

Measures of Plasma Protein

Basic measures include serum albumin, hemoglobin, and hematocrit. Additional ones may include prealbumin (PAB), a thyroxin-binding protein, serum transferrin, or total iron-binding capacity (TIBC) and ferritin.

Measures of Protein Metabolism

Basic 24-hour urine tests are used to measure urinary creatinine and urea nitrogen levels; these materials are products of protein metabolism. The patient's 24-hour excretion of creatinine is interpreted in terms of ideal creatinine excretion for height—the creatinine-height index (CHI) (Table 15-2). Comparison is made with standard values for this index. The patient's 24-hour urea nitrogen excretion is used with the calculated dietary nitrogen intake over the same 24-hour period to calculate nitrogen balance.

$$\text{N balance} = (\text{protein intake} \div 6.25) - (\text{urinary urea nitrogen} + 4)$$

The formula factor of 4 represents additional nitrogen loss through the feces and skin. Urinary urea nitrogen excretion reflects metabolism of dietary nitrogen, as the nitrogen balance formula indicates, and is a measure of the adequacy of protein nutrition.

Measures of Immune System Integrity: Anergy

Basic measures are made of the lymphocyte count. Additional measures may be made by skin testing, observing delayed sensitivity to common recall antigens such as mumps or purified protein derivative of tuberculin (PPD). Skin tests are read at 24 and 48 hours, with greater than 5 mm considered positive and the presence of one positive test indicating intact immunity. For hospitalized patients, this test is used with caution because there are often confounding factors that may offset the results.

ANTHROPOMETRICS

Skill gained through careful practice is necessary to minimize the margin of error in making body measurements. Selection and maintenance of proper procedures and equipment, as well as attention to careful technique, are essential in securing accurate data.

Weight

Hospitalized patients should be weighed at consistent times—for example, before breakfast after the bladder has been emptied. Clinic patients should be weighed without shoes in light, indoor clothing or an examining gown. For accuracy, use regular clinic beam scales with nondetachable weights. An additional weight attachment is available for use with very obese persons. Metric scales with readings to the nearest 20 g provide specific data; however, the standard clinic scale is satisfactory. Check all scales frequently and have them calibrated every 3 or 4 months for continued accuracy.

After careful reading and recording of the patient's weight, ask about the usual body weight and compare it with standard height-weight tables (see Chapter 6), remembering that these tables are general guidelines. It is useful to remember that research shows that underweight persons in general face greater health risks than do moderately overweight persons.[14,26,27] Interpret present weight in terms of percentage of usual and standard body weight for

TABLE 15-1 Clinical Signs of Nutritional Status

Body Area	Signs of Good Nutrition	Signs of Poor Nutrition
General appearance	Alert, responsive	Listless, apathetic, cachectic
Weight	Normal for height, age, body build	Overweight or underweight (special concern for underweight)
Posture	Erect, arms and legs straight	Sagging shoulders, sunken chest, humped back
Muscles	Well-developed, firm, good tone, some fat under skin	Flaccid, poor tone, undeveloped, tender, "wasted" appearance, cannot walk properly
Nervous control	Good attention span, not irritable or restless, normal reflexes, psychologic stability	Inattentive, irritable, confused, burning and tingling of hands and feet (paresthesia), loss of position and vibratory sense, weakness and tenderness of muscles (may result in inability to walk), decrease or loss of ankle and knee reflexes
Gastrointestinal function	Good appetite and digestion, normal regular elimination, no palpable (perceptible to touch) organs or masses	Anorexia, indigestion, constipation or diarrhea, liver or spleen enlargement
Cardiovascular function	Normal heart rate and rhythm, no murmurs, normal blood pressure for age	Rapid heart rate (above 100 beats/min tachycardia), enlarged heart, abnormal rhythm, elevated blood pressure
General vitality	Endurance, energetic, sleeps well, vigorous	Easily fatigued, no energy, falls asleep easily, looks tired, apathetic
Hair	Shiny, lustrous, firm, not easily plucked, healthy scalp	Stringy, dull, brittle, dry, thin and sparse, depigmented, easily plucked
Skin (general)	Smooth, slightly moist, good color	Rough, dry, scaly, pale, pigmented, irritated, bruises, petechiae
Face and neck	Skin color uniform, smooth, healthy appearance, not swollen	Greasy, discolored, scaly, swollen, skin dark over cheeks and under eyes, lumpiness or flakiness of skin around nose and mouth
Lips	Smooth, good color, moist, not chapped or swollen	Dry, scaly, swollen, redness and swelling (cheilosis), or angular lesions at corners of the mouth or fissures or scars (stomatitis)
Mouth, oral membranes	Reddish pink mucous membranes in oral cavity	Swollen, boggy oral mucous membranes
Gums	Good pink color, healthy, red, no swelling or bleeding	Spongy, bleed easily, marginal redness, inflamed, gums receding
Tongue	Good pink color or deep reddish in appearance, not swollen or smooth, surface papillae present, no lesions	Swelling, scarlet and raw, magenta color, beefy (glossitis), hyperemic and hypertrophic papillae, atrophic papillae
Teeth	No cavities, no pain, bright, straight, no crowding, well-shaped jaw, clean, no discoloration	Unfilled caries, absent teeth, worn surfaces, mottled (fluorosis), malpositioned
Eyes	Bright, clear, shiny, no sores at corner of eyelids, membranes moist and healthy pink color, no prominent blood vessels or mound of tissue or sclera, no fatigue circles beneath	Eye membranes pale (pale conjunctivae), redness of membrane (conjunctivae), redness of membrane (conjunctival infection), dryness, signs of infection, Bitot's spots, redness and fissuring of eyelid corners (angular palpebritis), dryness of eye membrane (conjunctival xerosis), dull appearance of cornea (corneal xerosis), soft cornea (keratomalacia)
Neck (glands)	No enlargement	Thyroid enlarged
Nails	Firm, pink	Spoon-shaped (koilonychia), brittle, ridged
Legs, feet	No tenderness, weakness, or swelling; good color	Edema, tender calf, tingling, weakness
Skeleton	No malformations	Bowlegs, knock-knees, chest deformity at diaphragm, beaded ribs, prominent scapulas

Modified from Williams SR: Nutrition assessment and guidance in prenatal care. In Worthington-Roberts BS, Williams SR: *Nutrition in pregnancy and lactation,* ed 5, New York, 1993, McGraw-Hill. Reproduced with permission of the McGraw-Hill Companies.

TABLE 15-2 Ideal Weight and Urinary Creatinine Values for Height (Adults)*

	Females		Males	
Height (cm)	Weight (kg)	Creatinine (mg)	Weight (kg)	Creatinine (mg)
140	44.9			
141	45.4			
142	45.9			
143	46.4			
144	47.0			
145	47.5		51.9	
146	48.0		52.4	
147	48.6	828	52.9	
148	49.2		53.5	
149	49.8		54.0	
150	50.4	852	54.5	
151	51.0		55.0	
152	51.5		55.6	
153	52.0	878	56.1	
154	52.5		56.6	
155	53.1	901	57.2	
156	53.7		57.9	
157	54.3	922	58.6	1284
158	54.9		59.3	
159	55.5		59.9	
160	56.2	949	60.5	1325
161	56.9		61.1	
162	57.6		61.7	
163	58.3	979	62.3	1362
164	58.9		62.9	
165	59.5	1005	63.5	1387
166	60.1		64.0	
167	60.7	1040	64.6	1421
168	61.4		65.2	
169	62.1		65.9	
170		1075	66.6	1465
171			67.3	
172			68.0	
173		1111	68.7	1516
174			69.4	
175		1139	70.1	1552
176			70.8	
177		1169	71.6	1589
178			72.4	
179			73.3	
180		1204	74.2	1639
181			75.0	
182			75.8	
183		1241	76.5	1692
184			77.3	
185			78.1	1735
186			78.9	
187				1776
188				
189				
190				1826

Data from Jeffe DB: *The assessment of the nutritional status of the community,* Geneva, 1966, World Health Organization.
*1959 Metropolitan Life Insurance Company Standards corrected for nude weight without shoe heels.

height. Check for any recent weight loss: 1% to 2% in the past week, 5% over the past month, 7.5% during the previous 3 months, or 10% in the past 6 months is significant. More than this rate can be severe. Unexplained weight loss is a problem with persons of any age. It is particularly important in elderly persons because it may be a clue to depression or a wasting disease such as cancer and needs to be on record and followed up. Values charted in the patient's record should indicate percentage of weight change.

Height

If possible, use a fixed measuring stick or tape on a true vertical flat surface. Have the patient stand as straight as possible, without shoes or cap, heels together, and looking straight ahead. The heels, buttocks, shoulders, and head should be touching the wall or vertical surface of the measuring rod. Read the measure carefully and compare it with previous recordings. Note the growth of children or the diminishing height of adults. Metric measures of height in centimeters provide a smaller unit of measure than inches.

Body Mass Index

The weight and height measures are used to calculate the patient's body mass index (BMI): weight (kilograms) divided by height $(\text{meters})^2$. This ratio is commonly used in evaluating obesity states in relation to risk factors. Details of this calculation, conversion factors, and reference values are described in Chapter 6.

Body Frame

The Metropolitan Life Insurance Company's widely used tables for height and weight of men and women use very general arbitrary categories of body frame size. Two more precise methods of establishing body frame size have been developed based on specific body joint measurements.[28]

1. *Elbow breadth.* Standards of weight and body composition by frame size and height have been developed with frame size based on measurement of elbow breadth. With the patient's arm extended and forearm bent upward to form a 90-degree angle, elbow breadth is measured with a specially developed instrument such as the Frameter, which measures the distance in centimeters between the two outer bony landmarks (medial and lateral epicondyles of the humerus).
2. *Wrist circumference.* This is a measure of height divided by wrist circumference (in centimeters). With the patient's right hand extended and using a nonstretchable metric tape, measure the wrist circumference at the joint just distal (toward the fingers) to the bony wrist bone protrusion (the styloid process). Interpret results by the following standard.

Frame Size	Male Ratio Values	Female Ratio Values
Small	10.4	11
Medium	9.6-10.4	10.1-11
Large	9.6	10.1

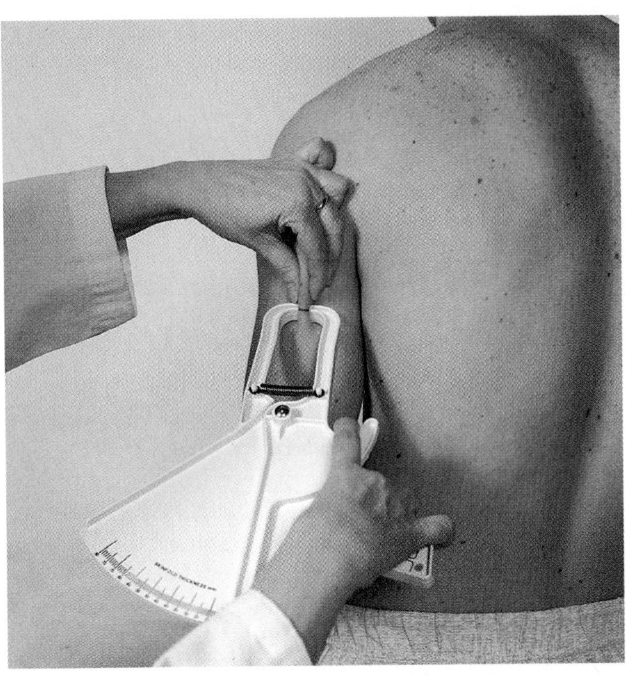

FIGURE 15-2 Assessment tools include skinfold calipers, shown here, which measure the relative amount of subcutaneous fat tissues at various body sites. (*From Jarvis C:* Physical examination and health assessment, *ed 3, Philadelphia, 2000, WB Saunders.*)

Body Measures

In general clinical practice, the clinician uses two basic body measurements—the mid-upper-arm circumference and the triceps skinfold thickness—and from these calculates a third measure, the mid-upper-arm muscle circumference. First, using a nonstretchable centimeter tape, locate the midpoint of the upper arm on the nondominant arm, unless it is affected by edema. The midarm circumference (MAC) is measured at this midpoint and read accurately to the nearest tenth of a centimeter and recorded. The resulting measure is compared with previous measurements to note possible changes. Second, using a standard millimeter skinfold caliper, take a measure of the triceps skinfold thickness (TSF) at this same midpoint of the upper arm (Figure 15-2). This measure provides an estimate of the subcutaneous fat reserves. Then, together with the midpoint circumference value at this same point, the midarm muscle circumference (MAMC) is calculated by the following formula.

$$\text{MAMC (cm)} = \text{MAC (cm)} - [3.14 \times \text{TSF (cm)}]$$

In this equation, the calculation constant 3.14 represents the value of pi (π). Because the calipers measure in millimeters, for ease of using the equation the TSF may be left in mm, with the other units remaining in cm; the calculation constant in this case is changed to 0.314.

This final derived value gives an indirect measure of the body's skeletal muscle mass, a good indicator of body composition. Finally, to interpret the patient's measurements for monitoring nutritional status, these values are compared as percentages of standards in reference tables (see Appendix J, Assessment of Nutritional Status: Percentiles).

Alternative Measures for Nonambulatory Patients

Several alternative measures can provide values for estimating height and weight of persons confined to bed.

1. *Total arm length.* With the patient holding the arm straight down by the side of the body and using a nonstretchable metric tape, measure the arm length from attachment at the shoulder to the end of the arm at the wrist. Reference standards indicate relation of this measure to height equivalents.[29] This is also a useful alternative to standing body height when body conditions distort usual standing height of ambulatory patients. For example, this measure is helpful with older persons, in whom a general thinning of weight-bearing cartilage, the bent-knee gait, and a possible kyphosis of the spine may make standing height measurement inaccurate.
2. *Arm span.* The full arm span measure is an alternate to height in adults; it is especially practical for elderly persons. Tests indicate that it may give a more accurate result than height in calculating BMI in elderly patients. Using a flexible metric tape, measure the full arm span from fingertip to fingertip in centimeters, passing the tape in front of the clavicles. A recumbent half-span measure from fingertip to body midline at the sternal notch may be used for patients with limited movement in one arm and then doubled to achieve the same result.
3. *Knee height.* With the patient lying in the supine position and the left knee and ankle each bent at a 90-degree angle, the knee height is measured with a special caliper. A simple comparative measure of knee-to-floor height in the sitting position, from the outside bony point just under the kneecap, indicating the head of the tibia, down to the floor surface, may also be used. The knee height (KH) measurement is then used to calculate the value for deriving body height equivalent:

   $$\text{Height (women)} = [(1.833 \times \text{KH}) - (0.24 \times \text{age})] + 84.88$$

   $$\text{Height (men)} = [(2.02 \times \text{KH}) - (0.04 \times \text{age})] + 64.19$$
4. *Calf circumference.* With the patient in the same supine position and the left knee bent at a 90-degree angle, and using nonstretchable metric tape, measure the calf circumference (CC) at the largest point. This measurement is then used with three other values—KH, MAC, and subscapular skinfold (SSF)—to derive body weight value.

$$\text{Weight (women)} = (1.27 \times \text{CC}) + (0.87 \times \text{KH}) + (0.98 \times \text{MAC}) + (0.4 \times \text{SSF}) - 62.35$$

$$\text{Weight (men)} = (0.98 \times \text{CC}) + (1.16 \times \text{KH}) + (1.73 \times \text{MAC}) + (0.37 \times \text{SSF}) - 81.69$$

ANALYZING NUTRITIONAL DATA

Valid patient care planning requires analysis of all nutritional data collected. On this basis problems requiring solutions can be identified. A detailed analysis of all available nutrition information helps determine nutritional diagnosis, any primary or secondary nutritional disease, and any underlying nutrition-related conditions.

The medical tests used for nutrition assessment are generally reliable in persons of any age, but conditions in elderly patients may interfere and need to be considered in evaluating test results.[30,31] For example, laboratory values are affected by hydration status, presence of chronic diseases, changes in organ function, and drugs. Nutritional assessment is an important part of the general healthcare of everyone, especially of the elderly. Health outreach programs for older persons, such as in rural areas, can use brief, easily administered tools for screening and assessing nutritional status and risk of malnutrition as part of geriatric care.[32,33]

Nutritional Diagnosis

All of the various nutritional data for each patient, collected by the Registered Dietitian and other team members through the broad assessment activities described, must be carefully analyzed to reach a valid nutritional diagnosis and plan of care. Every healthcare team member participates in this analysis through various communications, discussions, case conferences, records, and reports. The nutritional diagnosis requires information about all aspects related to the patient's needs: nutrient deficiencies, underlying disease requiring a modified nutrient or food plan, any personal cultural and ethnic needs, or economic needs, as well as the mode of feeding and dietary management.

Information about all drugs—including over-the-counter self-medications and "street drugs," as well as alcohol and prescribed drugs—is essential. Research about each drug is vital to determine any possible problems from the interaction of each drug with foods and nutrients. Many such reactions exist and are encountered with multiple drug use, especially in elderly patients with chronic diseases.

Primary and Secondary Nutritional Disease

The clinical dietitian coordinates these nutrition activities and carries a major responsibility on the healthcare team for interpreting nutrition-related data and making decisions and recommendations concerning any primary or secondary nutritional states. *Primary deficiency* disease results from a lack of essential nutrient in the diet, for whatever reason. *Secondary deficiency* disease results from one or more barriers to the use of the nutrients after they are consumed in food. This inability to use a given nutrient may stem from digestive or malabsorption problems or from lack of specific cell enzymes. Such problems may be caused by conditions such as lactose intolerance, celiac disease, inflammatory bowel disease, cell metabolism defects in genetic disease, chemotherapy, or radiation treatments.

Nutrition-Related Conditions

Related chronic disease problems with nutrition involvement are also considered; these include such conditions as heart disease, hypertension, cancer, diabetes, and liver and renal disease. Surgery also imposes nutrition demands and modifications. Any quantifiable data that are collected can be analyzed by computer. Two major nutritional tasks in which the computer excels are (1) baseline screening to identify persons at risk of malnutrition because of their disease, injury, or lifestyle and (2) analysis of intake to monitor effectiveness of ongoing treatment. Laboratory data may be handled in a similar manner, with general patterns of change monitored over time. Careful appraisal of medical and personal data from histories, records, reports, and interviews will help focus on various needs and problems and provide a realistic picture of nutritional and eating difficulties.

Problem List

On the basis of this careful analysis, a problem list is usually developed. Around such a list, realistic and relevant individualized care may be planned. Every aspect of the patient's needs is considered. In ongoing conferences with the healthcare team, the patient, family, and any other significant persons, individual goals are determined for care. These goals help establish priorities for immediate as well as long-term care.

Nutrition Intervention: Food Plan and Management

BASIC CONCEPTS OF DIET THERAPY

Normal Nutrition

A therapeutic diet is always based on the normal nutritional requirements and personal needs for each particular patient. It is modified only as the specific disease in the specific individual necessitates. In planning and counseling for nutritional care this is an important initial fact to grasp and impart to patients and clients. For example, it is a great source of encouragement to the parents of a newly diagnosed diabetic child to know that the food plan will be based on individual growth and development needs and will make use of regular foods.

Disease Application

The principles of a special therapeutic diet will be based on modifications of the nutritional components of the normal diet as a particular disease condition may require. These changes may include the following types of modifications: (1) *nutrients:* modification of one or more of the basic nutrients—protein, carbohydrate, fat, minerals, and vitamins; (2) *energy:* modification in energy value as expressed in kilocalories (kcalories); and (3) *texture:* modification in texture or seasoning, such as liquid or low residue.

Individual Adaptation

A therapeutic diet may be theoretically correct and have well-balanced food plans, but if these plans are unacceptable to the patient, they will not be followed. A workable plan for a specific person must be based on individual food habits within the specific personal life situation. This can be achieved only through careful planning with the patient, or with the parents of a child requiring a special diet, based on an initial interview to obtain a diet history, knowledge of personal food habits, living conditions, and related factors. In this way, diet principles can be understood and motivation secured to follow through. Regardless of the problems, nutritional care is valid only to the extent that it involves this kind of knowledge, skills, and insights. Individual adaptations of the diet to meet individual needs are imperative for successful therapy.

Practitioner Awareness

Within today's patient-centered care plans, all medical practitioners have a increasing awareness of the vital role of nutritional therapy and of the importance of nutrition in treatment. Medical and clinical consultations include a nutritional component today much more often than in the past. Barriers to effective therapies can exist, however. In particular, family physicians, who are the trusted primary source of information for many individuals, often face difficulties in discussing nutrition with patients.[10] The barriers include short visit times with patients both in and out of hospital, the frequently small amount of nutrition taught in medical schools, and the problem of nonhospitalized patients who fail to follow prescribed dietary changes.[34] Many efforts are under way to improve the delivery of nutrition therapy and nutrition-based patient education[35] and to expand nutrition within medical education and practice,[36,37] including the initiative of the American Society for Clinical Nutrition to fund a nutrition specialist faculty member at every U.S. medical school[38] and the publication of a variety of nutrition resources for general practitioners.[39-42] The team approach, which uses the specialized knowledge and experience of the clinical dietitian in concert with all practitioners, can lead to effective individualized care plans.

kyphosis Increased, abnormal convexity of the upper part of the spine; hunchback.

ROUTINE HOUSE DIETS

A schedule of routine "house" diets, based on some type of cycle menu plan, is usually followed in hospitals for patients who do not require a special diet modification. According to general patient need and tolerance, the diet order may be liquid (clear liquid or full liquid, with milk used on the full liquid diet), soft (no raw foods, generally somewhat bland in seasoning), and regular (a full, normal-for-age diet) (Table 15-3). Occasionally an interval step between soft and regular may be used (a light diet).

MANAGING THE MODE OF FEEDING

Depending on the patient's condition, the clinical dietitian may manage the diet by using any one of the following four feeding modes.

Oral Diet

As long as possible, of course, regular oral feeding is preferred. Supplements are added if needed. According to the patient's condition, there may also be need for assistance in eating.

Tube Feeding

If a patient is unable to eat but the gastrointestinal tract can be used, enteral delivery, or tube feeding, may provide needed nutritional support. A number of commercial formulas are available, or a blended formula may be calculated and prepared.

Peripheral Vein Feeding

If the patient cannot take in food or formula via the gastrointestinal tract, intravenous feeding is used. Solutions of dextrose, amino acids, vitamins, and minerals, with lipids as appropriate, can be fed through peripheral veins when the need is not extensive or long term.

Total Parenteral Nutrition (TPN)

If the patient's nutritional need is great and support therapy may be required for a longer time, parenteral feeding through a large central vein is needed. Placement of this

TABLE 15-3 Routine Hospital Diets

Food	Clear Liquid	Full Liquid	Soft	Regular
Soup	Clear fat-free broth, bouillon	Same, plus strained or blended cream soups	Same, plus all cream soups	All
Cereal		Cooked refined cereal	Cooked cereal, cornflakes, rice, noodles, macaroni, spaghetti	
Bread			White bread, crackers, melba toast, zwieback	All
Protein foods		Milk, cream, milk drinks, yogurt	Same, plus eggs (not fried), mild cheese, cottage and cream cheese, fowl, fish, sweetbreads, tender beef, veal, lamb, liver, bacon, gravy	All
Vegetables			Potatoes: baked, mashed, creamed, steamed, scalloped; tender cooked whole bland vegetables; fresh lettuce, tomatoes	All
Fruit and fruit juices	Fruit juices (as tolerated), flavored fruit drinks	All	Same, plus cooked fruit: peaches, pears, applesauce, peeled apricots, white cherries; ripe peaches, pears, banana, orange and grapefruit sections without membrane	
Desserts and gelatin	Fruit-flavored gelatin, fruit ices, and Popsicles	Same, plus sherbet, ice cream, puddings, custard, frozen yogurt	Same, plus plain sponge cakes, plain cookies, plain cake, puddings, pie made with allowed foods	All
Miscellaneous	Soft drinks (as tolerated), coffee and tea, decaffeinated coffee and tea, cereal beverages such as Postum, sugar, honey, salt, hard candy, Poly cose (Ross), residue-free supplements	Same, plus margarine, pepper, all supplements	Same, plus mild salad dressings	

catheter is a special surgical procedure. More concentrated special solutions can be used and monitored by a nutrition support team. The formulas are determined by the dietitian and the physician and prepared by trained pharmacists. This specialized nutrition support method was originally used only in hospitals, but advances in TPN administration now allow its use in many healthcare settings and even at home with some patients.

Evaluation: Quality Patient Care

GENERAL CONSIDERATIONS

When the nutritional care plan is carried out, patient care activities need to be considered in terms of the nutritional diagnosis and treatment objectives and the extent to which each of the care activities helps to meet the particular goals of the patient and the family. This evaluation is both continuous and thorough and requires careful, objective documentation (see *Case Study*). It seeks to validate care while it is being given as well as to determine the effectiveness of a particular course of care. Various areas need to be investigated.

1. *Estimate the achievement of nutritional therapy goals.* What is the effect of the diet or mode of feeding on the illness or the patient's situation? Is there need for any change in the nutrient ratios of the diet or formula as originally calculated, in the meal-distribution pattern, or in the feeding mode?
2. *Judge the accuracy of intervention actions.* Is there need to change any of the nutritional care plan components? For example, is there need for a change in the type of food or feeding equipment, environment for meals, procedures for counseling, or types of learning activities for nutrition education and self-care procedures?
3. *Determine patient's ability to follow the prescribed nutrition therapy.* Are there any hindrances or disabilities that prevent the patient from following the treatment plan? What is the impact of the nutrition therapy on the patient, the family, or the staff? Were the necessary nutrition assessment procedures for collecting nutrition data carried out correctly? Do the patient and family understand the information given for self-care? Have the community resources required by the patient and family been available and convenient for use? Has any needed food assistance program been sufficient to meet needs for the patient's ongoing care?

QUALITY PATIENT CARE

The current increased focus on cost control in managed healthcare reforms is leading to mechanisms for effectively evaluating patient care programs on the basis of (1) cost effectiveness and (2) provision of nutritional services by the most qualified personnel. Also, healthcare legislation concerning quality care assessment and assurance monitoring, as well as healthcare accreditation agencies such as the Joint Commission on Accreditation of Healthcare Organizations (JCAHO) to add the high standards professional seal of approval, are all increasingly mandating that such care be accurately recorded in an organized manner.

COLLABORATIVE ROLES OF THE DIETITIAN AND NURSE

The clinical dietitian works closely with the nurse in managing the nutritional care of patients. At varying times, depending on need, the nurse may provide valuable nutrition assistance as coordinator, interpreter, or teacher. Skills in consultation and referral are therefore essential.

Coordinator

Nurses coordinate special services or treatment required because of their close relationship to patients and their constant attendance. The nurse may help schedule activities to prevent conflicts or secure needed consultation for the patient with the dietitian, social worker, or other healthcare team member. Sometimes in-hospital malnutrition can develop simply because meals are constantly being interrupted by various procedures, staff interviews, or medical rounds.

Interpreter

Because of a close relationship with the patient, the nurse may often reduce tension by helping the patient understand explanations concerning various treatments and plans of care. This will include basic interpretation of the therapeutic diet from the RD and of the resulting food selections on the tray. The nurse may sometimes assist the patient in making appropriate selections from the menus provided.

Teacher or Counselor

One of the nurse's most significant roles is that of healthcare educator and counselor. There will be innumerable informal opportunities during daily nursing care for planned conversation about sound nutrition principles, reinforcing the counseling of the clinical dietitian. In addition, according to patient situations, the nurse may work with the clinical dietitian during periods of instruction about principles of the patient's diet therapy in relation

---

enteral A mode of feeding that uses the gastrointestinal tract; oral or tube feeding.

parenteral A mode of feeding that does not use the gastrointestinal tract, but instead provides nutrition by intravenous delivery of nutrient solutions.

to the disease process. The nurse will work in close cooperation with the clinical dietitian and the physician to coordinate nutritional and medical management of the patient's illness into overall nursing care. At all times the nurse will work closely with the hospital's clinical nutrition staff to support and reinforce primary nutrition education, as well as discharge planning for follow-up care. These clinical staff nutrition experts will always be excellent resources for needed nutrition consultation and referral.

Clearly, learning about the hospitalized patient's nutritional needs is a continuing activity beginning with admission. It should follow through and include plans for continuing application in the home environment. Follow-up care may be provided by the hospital's clinic dietitian, by consultation with clinical dietitians in community private practice, by public health dietitians and nurses, or by referrals to community agencies and resources.

TO SUM UP

The basis for an accurate assessment of the patient's nutritional needs begins with the individual patient and family. Physical as well as psychologic, social, economic, and cultural factors in and out of the clinical setting all play a role in evaluating the patient's health status and any possible problems with the nutritional care plan.

Nutritional assessment is based on a broad foundation of pertinent data, including food and drug uses and values. The effectiveness of an assessment based on analysis of these data depends in turn on effective communication with the patient, family members, and significant others in the development of an appropriate care plan, as well as with other members of the healthcare team. The patient's medical record is a basic means of communication among healthcare team members.

Nutritional therapy, based on a combination of the personal and physiologic needs of the patient, requires a close working relationship among nutrition, medical, and nursing staff in the healthcare facility. The nurse's schedule offers many opportunities to reinforce nutritional principles of the diet. Nutritional therapy does not end with the patient's discharge. Outpatient nutrition services, appropriate social services, and food resources in the community help meet continuing needs of patients and their families.

■ Questions for Review

1. Identify and discuss the possible effects of various psychologic factors on the outcome of nutritional therapy.
2. Outline a general procedure for assessing nutritional needs and building a care plan for a 65-year-old widower hospitalized with coronary heart disease. Include appropriate community agencies to refer the patient for follow-up care, services, and information.
3. Describe commonly used anthropometric procedures, blood tests, and urine tests for nutritional status information in terms of significance of the measure or test—what is being measured and what the results tell you.
4. Select several clinical signs used to assess nutritional status and describe what each sign shows in a malnourished person and why.
5. Describe the nature and purpose of quality assurance plans for standards of nutritional care.

■ References

1. Tucker HN, Miguel SG: Cost containment through nutrition intervention, *Nutr Rev* 54(4):111, 1996.
2. Belanger M-C, Dube L: The emotional experience of hospitalization: its moderators and its role in patient satisfaction with food services, *J Am Diet Assoc* 96(4):354, 1996.
3. Rubin M: The physiology of bed rest, *Am J Nurs* 88(1):50, 1988.
4. Gallacher-Allred CR et al: Malnutrition and clinical outcomes: the case for medical nutrition therapy, *J Am Diet Assoc* 96(4):361, 1996.
5. Bone RC: Ethical principles in critical care, *JAMA* 263(5):696, 1990.
6. Monsen ER et al: Ethics: responsible scientific conduct, *Am J Clin Nutr* 54:1, 1991.
7. Tufts University, School of Nutrition Science and Policy: *Tufts nutrition navigator,* available at *http://www.navigator.tufts.edu.*
8. University of Iowa, Hardin Library for the Health Sciences: *Hardin MD: nutrition,* available at *http://www.lib.uiowa.edu/hardin/md/nutr.html.*
9. Yale-New Haven Hospital: *Making the right choice on the web: safe surfing for health care information,* New Haven, Conn, 2001, Yale-New Haven Hospital. Also available at *http://www.ynhh.org.*
10. Truswell AS: Family physicians and patients: is effective nutrition interaction possible? *Am J Clin Nutr* 71:6, 2000.
11. Laramee SH: Position of the American Dietetic Association: nutrition services in managed care, *J Am Diet Assoc* 96(4):391, 1996.
12. Dwyer JT: Dietary assessment. In Shils ME et al, eds: *Modern nutrition in health and disease,* Baltimore, 1999, Williams & Wilkins.
13. Jain M et al: Dietary assessment in epidemiology: comparison of a food frequency and a diet history with a 7-day food record, *Am J Epidemiol* 143:953, 1996.
14. Dwyer JT: Policy and healthy weight, *Am J Clin Nutr* 63(suppl):415S, 1996.
15. Schaefer EJ et al: Lack of efficacy of a food-frequency questionnaire in assessing dietary macronutrient intakes in subjects consuming diets of known composition, *Am J Clin Nutr* 71:746, 2000.
16. Goris AHC et al: Undereating and underrecording of habitual food intake in obese men: selective underreporting of fat intake, *Am J Clin Nutr* 71:130, 2000.
17. Blundell JE: What foods do people eat? A dilemma for nutrition, an enigma for psychology, *Am J Clin Nutr* 71:3, 2000.

18. Mela DJ, Aaron JI: Honest but invalid: what subjects say about recording their food habits, *J Am Diet Assoc* 97:791, 1997.
19. Klesges RC et al: Who underreports dietary intake in a dietary recall? Evidence from the second National Health and Nutrition Survey, *J Consult Clin Psychol* 63:438, 1995.
20. Macdiarmid JI, Blundell JE: Assessing dietary intake: who, what, and why of under-reporting, *Nutr Res Rev* 11:231, 1998.
21. Kristal AR et al: Associations of race/ethnicity, education, and dietary intervention with the validity and reliability of a food frequency questionnaire, *Am J Epidemiol* 146:856, 1997.
22. Sawaya AL et al: Evaluation of four methods for determining energy intake in young and older women: comparison with doubly labeled water measurements of total energy expenditure, *Am J Clin Nutr* 63:491, 1996.
23. Weber JL et al: Validity of self-reported energy intake in lean and obese young women, using two nutrient databases, compared with total energy expenditure assessed by doubly labeled water, *Eur J Clin Nutr* 55(11):940, 2001.
24. Bathalon GP et al: Psychological measures of eating behavior and the accuracy of 3 common dietary assessment methods in healthy postmenopausal women, *Am J Clin Nutr* 71:739, 2000.
25. Seidel H et al: *Mosby's guide to physical examination,* ed 4, St Louis, 1999, Mosby, Inc.
26. Abernathy RP, Black DR: Healthy body weights: an alternative perspective, *Am J Clin Nutr* 63(suppl):448S, 1996.
27. Meisler J, St Joer S: Summary and recommendations from the American Health Foundation's Expert Panel on Healthy Weights, *Am J Clin Nutr* 63(suppl):474S, 1996.
28. Nowak RK, Schultz LO: A comparison of two methods for the determination of body frame size, *J Am Diet Assoc* 87(3):339, 1987.
29. Mitchell CO, Lipschitz DA: Arm length measurement as an alternative to height in the nutritional assessment of the elderly, *J Am Geriatr Soc* 39:492, 1991.
30. Egbert AM: The dwindles: failure to thrive in older patients, *Nutr Rev* 54(1):S25, 1996.
31. Roubenoff R et al: Nutrition assessment in long-term care facilities, *Nutr Rev* 54(1):S40, 1996.
32. Beyer K et al: Nutrition screening among rural older persons, *Nutr Today* 31(1):24, 1996.
33. Guigoz Y et al: Assessing the nutritional status of the elderly: the Mini Nutritional Assessment as part of the geriatric evaluation, *Nutr Rev* 54(1):59, 1996.
34. Mant D: Effectiveness of dietary intervention in general practice, *Am J Clin Nutr* 65(suppl):1933S, 1997.
35. American Dietetic Association: *Physician nutrition education project,* Chicago, 1998, The Association.
36. American Academy of Family Physicians: *Recommended core educational guidelines on nutrition for family practice residents,* Kansas City, Mo, 1995, American Academy of Family Physicians.
37. Society for Teachers of Family Medicine, Working Group on Nutrition Education: *Physicians' curriculum in clinical nutrition,* Kansas City, Mo, 1995, Society for Teachers of Family Medicine.
38. Jensen GL et al: Clinical nutrition: opportunity in a changing health care environment, *Am J Clin Nutr* 68:983, 1998.
39. Truswell AS: *ABC of nutrition,* ed 3, London, 1999, BMJ Books.
40. Thomas B: *Nutrition in primary care: a handbook for GPs, nurses, and primary health care professionals,* Oxford, 1996, Blackwell Science.
41. Buttriss J: *Nutrition in general practice, vol 1: basic principles,* London, 1994, Royal College of General Practitioners.
42. Buttriss J: *Nutrition in general practice, vol 2: promoting health and preventing disease,* London, 1995, Royal College of General Practitioners.

■ Further Reading

American Dietetic Association: Practice report of the American Dietetic Association: home care—an emerging practice area for dietetics, *J Am Diet Assoc* 99(11):1453, 1999.

Home care, especially for the growing numbers of older persons in our population, is increasing and the accompanying need for nutritional and nursing care reflects this pressing situation. This excellent report identifies these needs and discusses possible ways of meeting them.

Porter C et al: Dynamics of nutrition care among nursing home residents who are eating poorly, *J Am Diet Assoc* 99(11):1444, 1999.

This article provides insight into the common problem of malnutrition among nursing home residents and the apparently haphazard ways some staff members may respond, such as using liquid supplements for vitamins but not for minerals, replacing regular meals with liquid supplement drinks, or resorting to unpleasant and unethical measures such as force feeding.

CASE STUDY Nutritional assessment and therapy for a patient with cancer

Esther is a 160-cm (5 ft 4 in)-tall, medium-frame, 43-year-old patient recovering from a *gastrectomy* performed 8 days ago to treat gastric cancer. Her weight has dropped gradually for the past 4 months from an average of 59 kg (130 lb) before her illness began. She continues to follow a full-liquid diet, consuming 60 to 120 ml (2 to 4 oz) of milk every few hours, plus 1 or 2 soft-boiled eggs each day. Today she informed the nutritionist that she consumed a total of 721 ml (24 oz) of milk and 2 eggs.

In reviewing Esther's records, the nutritionist found the following nutritional assessment data: weight, 47.3 kg (103 lb); triceps skinfold, 10 mm; and midarm circumference, 17 cm. Laboratory values include serum albumin, 3 g/dl; total iron-binding capacity (TIBC), 230 μg/dl; lymphocytes, 1200 cells/m^3 (23%); hematocrit, 35%; and hemoglobin, 10.5 g/dl. Urinalysis (24 hours) included urea nitrogen, 16 g; and creatinine, 1.75 g. Skin tests were pending.

After reviewing the data, the nutritionist calculated nitrogen balance, transferrin, and creatinine-height index, which were recorded on the patient chart. Basal energy expenditure needs and kcalories and protein needed to overcome catabolism were also calculated, along with estimates for additional vitamin and mineral requirements.

The clinical nutritionist noted that the physician had ordered chemotherapy for the patient, continuing after discharge, and recommended the use of TPN, also to be continued after discharge, as a means of meeting Esther's nutritional needs. In addition, the nutritionist planned ways of meeting any feeding problems that often accompany chemotherapy, such as sore mouth, nausea, and food intolerances. Following a carefully prepared protocol developed by the hospital nutritional support team, both Esther and her husband were instructed in procuring and using the home TPN treatment. The nutritionist also provided follow-up counseling for Esther and her husband at the office and in the group sessions for cancer patients and their families.

QUESTIONS FOR ANALYSIS

1. Use a nutritional assessment data summary sheet from your hospital (or design your own) to record pertinent data given in this case study. What additional data would you collect? How would it be obtained?
2. For each test listed on your data sheet, explain what it measures and how that information contributes to an understanding of Esther's status.
3. What specific nutritional needs can you identify in this case? List them in order of priority.
4. Calculate Esther's nitrogen balance and transferrin for day 8. Why are these indices important to assessing her nutritional status?
5. What is Esther's creatinine-height index? How does it reflect her nutritional status?
6. Interpret Esther's anthropometric data, including your calculations of her midarm muscle circumference.
7. What skin tests were probably ordered? How would the results contribute to the assessment of her nutritional status?
8. What nutritional problems do you expect Esther to encounter after discharge? How could they be resolved? What community agencies might contribute to her sense of well-being after discharge?

Issues & ANSWERS

Selecting Computer Nutrient-Calculation Software

In our modern age of electronics, the computer has become a standard tool for rapid calculation procedures. In clinical and community nutrition practices as well as in population studies, it saves valuable time and provides a precise nutrient analysis of an individual's reported food intake.

Certainly computerized nutrient analyses are time-savers compared with the previous tedious manual calculations using published food value tables. But just how precise are the results? This depends on the heart of any nutrient-analysis software program—its nutrient database.

During the past few years of computer use by clinicians, researchers, and educators, it has become increasingly evident that the quality of the nutrient database on which all calculations are based determines the quality of the resulting output. Important questions that should be asked when evaluating the nutrient database in any software package being considered for purchase include the following from the University of Minnesota School of Public Health.

Does the database contain all foods and nutrients of interest?

Most databases contain the most common foods, but you may require particular foods such as ethnic, vegetarian, or fast-food items; brand-name products; and infant or nontraditional foods. The number of food items in a database does not necessarily indicate how comprehensive the system is. And adding your own foods to the database requires considerable effort.

Is the database complete for nutrients of interest?

Missing or not available values exist in available software packages and often are not flagged; therefore you may be unaware of this source of error. Inappropriate patient counseling may result. Such missing value errors in small items such as spices or other condiments may not matter, but value that is missing for total saturated fatty acids in a fast-food hamburger because the food manufacturers have not supplied it is not acceptable.

Do foods included in the database provide sufficient specific data to accurately assess nutrients of interest?

For example, if total fat and fatty acids are of concern, separate database entries must be included for such items as regular, low-fat, and nonfat dairy products and brand-name high-fat items such as margarines and salad dressings. In other cases, inclusion of food items according to preparation method, or of any dietary supplements for vitamin-mineral calculations, may be required.

Is the nutrient database current with the changing marketplace and availability of new nutrient data?

The U.S. Department of Agriculture routinely releases updates of the USDA Nutrient Data Base, the common source of data for nutrient-calculation systems, as new information becomes available. Information from food manufacturers is also available. A well-maintained software product's database should include all such data updates, and the vendor should supply information about frequency of updating and sources of data.

Are manufacturers contacted routinely for new information or reformulations of existing products?

This question extends the previous question to emphasize the still too frequent neglect of brand-name product-updating practices of software developers. Routine contact with food manufacturers is essential to maintaining an acceptable quality standard.

What quality control procedures are used to ensure database accuracy?

Because there are thousands of values for nutrients and nonnutrient information, such as food-specific serving sizes, the margin for error is great and built-in maintenance procedures for checking such errors should be present.

Vendors of nutrient-calculation software packages should be able to give answers to these important questions. Ask before you buy!

REFERENCES

Buzzard IM et al: Considerations for selecting nutrient-calculation software: evaluation of the nutrient database, *Am J Clin Nutr* 54:7, 1991.

Byrd-Bredbenner C, Juni RP: How should nutrient databases be evaluated? *J Am Diet Assoc* 96(2):120, 1996.

Haytowitz DB: Information from USDA's Nutrient Data Bank, *J Nutr* 125(7):1952, 1995.

Lee RD et al: Comparison of eight microcomputer dietary analysis programs with the USDA Nutrient Data Base for Standard Reference, *J Am Diet Assoc* 95(8):858, 1995.

Chapter

16

Drug-Nutrient Interactions

Sara Long Anderson

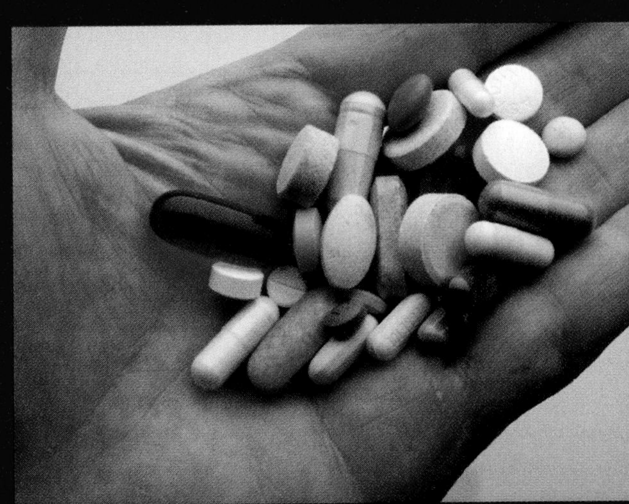

Chapter Outline

In this chapter, continuing our clinical nutrition sequence, we look briefly at some main effects of combining food and nutrients with drugs. We will see how these interactions affect nutrition therapy.

Today consumers are generally better informed about drug misuse. However, many are dangerously uninformed or misinformed about the specific drugs they may be taking, especially in relation to the food they eat.

All members of the healthcare team must have a basic knowledge of drug actions and nutrition to make the wisest and most effective use of drugs and nutritional therapy. Here we examine some of these drug-nutrient effects and how these interactions affect our nutritional therapy and education.

Drug-Nutrient Problems in Modern Medicine

PROBLEM SIGNIFICANCE: CAUSES, EXTENT, AND EFFECTS

During this century, unprecedented medical progress has resulted in decreased childhood mortality rates, which has helped to increase life expectancy. As we live longer, incidence of chronic diseases such as cardiovascular disease, type 2 diabetes mellitus, hypertension, and arthritis will continue to increase, often in comorbid manner. Furthermore, treatment of these and other chronic diseases often involves long-term use of medications, often resulting in polypharmacy.

Every year 25 to 30 new medications are introduced.[1-3] American physicians prescribe and pharmacists dispense a total amount of drugs sufficient to provide seven individual medications for each woman, man, and child in the United States. To this amount we can then add the large volume of nonprescription drugs Americans purchase over the counter.

Some concerned persons have come to view the proliferation of pills in our society with alarm. For example, epidemiologic studies in America and Europe indicate that cycles of repeated antibiotic prescriptions may increase the patient's risk of contracting an antibiotic-resistant disease organism.[4] Knowledgeable and concerned pharmacologists indicate that outside of extremely serious illness, most general medical problems can be treated with fewer than 25 drugs. The World Health Organization (WHO) has estimated only some 150 to 200 drugs are actually needed to take care of almost all ordinary illnesses around the world. Yet on our American market there are about 54,000 drugs, many of them only slight variations of other drugs, the "me, too" drugs.

DRUG USE AND NUTRITIONAL STATUS

Elderly Persons at Risk

All of us, at any age, risk harmful drug-drug or drug-nutrient interactions. However, elderly persons are particularly vulnerable,[5] and this will only become more serious. Today, adults over 65 represent approximately 12% of the U.S. population. It is projected this number will increase to 20% to 22% by 2050.[5,6] Elderly persons take a much larger percentage of prescription and nonprescription medications than their younger counterparts.[7] Twenty-three percent of women and 19% of older men over 65 years of age take five or more prescription medications a week.[8]

Several things contribute to this increased risk among the elderly.

1. They are likely to be taking more drugs for longer periods to control chronic diseases.
2. Their drugs are likely to be more toxic.
3. They respond to drugs with greater variability.
4. They have less capability to handle drugs efficiently.
5. Their nutritional status is more likely to be deficient.
6. They are more likely to make increased errors in self-care because of illness, mental confusion, or lack of drug information.

As a result of these problems, concerned physicians, nutritionists, pharmacists, and nurses are increasingly working together as a team to provide drug and nutritional education and therapy on a sounder basis. A number of drug-nutrient interactions demand this type of team work in patient care.

Nutritional Status

Well-nourished individuals are less likely to acquire diseases necessitating treatment with medication, and when they encounter specific diseases, the illness is usually less severe and responds to medication more favorably.[9] Thus poor nutritional status can have a major impact on risk for complications of drug-nutrient reactions. Nutrient-drug mechanisms that influence nutritional status include those effecting the following.

- Stimulated or suppressed appetite
- Decreased intestinal absorption
- Increased renal excretion
- Competition or displacement of nutrients for carrier protein sites
- Interference with synthesis of necessary enzyme, coenzyme, or carrier
- Hormonal effects on genetic systems
- The drug delivery system
- Components in drug formulation

In general, drugs are grouped according to primary action. Here we review briefly various effects of drugs on food and nutrients and effects of food and nutrients on drugs. In each case we give some examples for your reference in patient care.

Drug Effects on Food and Nutrients

DRUG EFFECTS ON FOOD INTAKE

Appetite Changes

The following drugs have an effect of stimulating appetite and weight gain.[10]

1. *Antihistamines.* These drugs can lead to marked increase in appetite and subsequent weight gain. One of these agents, both an antihistamine and a serotonin antagonist, is cyproheptadine hydrochloride (Periactin).
2. *Antianxiety drugs.* Some drugs in this classification may lead to hyperphagia, or excessive eating (see *Issues & Answers*). Some of these drugs include chlordiazepoxide hydrochloride (Librium), diazepam (Valium), and alprazolam (Xanax).
3. *Tricyclic antidepressants.* Tricyclic antidepressants and most antipsychotic drugs such as amitriptyline hydrochloride (Elavil), olanzapine (Zyprexa), chlorpromazine hy-

drochloride (Thorazine), and clozapine (Clozaril) may promote appetite and lead to significant weight gain.

4. *Steroids.* Anabolic steroids, including testosterone, promote nitrogen retention, increased lean body mass, and subsequent weight gain.

The following drugs have the effect of depressing the appetite.[10]

1. *Selective serotonin reuptake inhibitor (SSRI):* This class of antidepressants may cause anorexia and weight loss; an example is fluoxetine (Prozac).
2. *Amphetamines.* These drugs act as stimulants to the central nervous system and have the effect of depressing desire for food, thus leading to marked loss of weight. For this reason they have been used in the past as appetite-depressant drugs in the treatment of obesity. However, long-term use of these drugs in such treatment has caused problems, including addiction, because in most cases appetite itself is not the primary cause of the excess weight. For this reason, amphetamines are rarely used now for this purpose. Children taking amphetamines show dose-dependent growth retardation.
3. *Insulin.* Hypoglycemia can occur in persons with type 1 diabetes if food is not taken immediately after their insulin injection to balance with the rapid effect of the insulin (see Chapter 20). If some food is not readily available to counteract the rapid progression of the unrelieved severe hypoglycemia, coma and death occur.
4. *Alcohol.* Abuse of alcohol can lead to loss of appetite, reduced food intake, and malnutrition. The anorexia, or loss of appetite, can stem from various effects of alcoholism such as gastritis, lactose intolerance, hepatitis, cirrhosis, ketosis, pancreatitis, alcoholic brain syndrome, drunkenness, and withdrawal symptoms. The resulting reduced food intake can then lead to malnutrition, which further complicates the anorexia.

Taste and Smell Changes

Drugs such as the tricyclic antidepressant amitriptyline (Elavil) may impair salivary flow, causing dry mouth along with a sour or metallic taste.[10] The antibiotic clarithromycin (Biaxin) is secreted into saliva, causing a bitter taste.[10] Antibiotics such as tetracycline may suppress natural oral bacteria, resulting in oral yeast overgrowth or candidiasis. Metronidazole (Flagyl), an antibiotic, may cause *dysgeusia* (abnormal or impaired sense of taste) by causing a metallic taste in the mouth.[10] Antineoplastic medications (cisplatin or methotrexate may damage rapidly growing cells, causing stomatitis, glossitis, and/or esophagitis[10] (see *Practical Application* box).

Gastrointestinal Effects

Many drugs can affect the stomach and cause nausea, vomiting, bleeding, or ulceration; intestinal peristalsis; or intestinal flora. Nonsteroidal anti-inflammatory drugs (NSAIDs) such as acetylsalicylic acid (aspirin), ibuprofen (Advil, Motrin), and naproxen (Aleve, Anaprox) cause stomach irritation.[10] Sometimes the irritation is so severe as to cause sudden and serious gastric bleeding.[10] Anticholinergic medications (antipsychotics, antidepressants, antihistamines) slow peristalsis resulting in constipation. Ciprofloxacin (Cipro) is an antibiotic that can allow for the overgrowth of *Clostridium difficile,* resulting in pseudomembranous colitis.[10]

PRACTICAL APPLICATION
The Proof of the Pudding

The senses of taste and smell greatly affect our responses to various foods. Loss of these senses may drive persons to constantly seek elusive satisfaction by overeating, or it may stop them from eating entirely. In either case the pleasure of eating is gone, and nutritional status suffers. Patients taking drugs that affect taste and smell need counseling concerning food choices, combinations, and seasonings that can help overcome this difficulty.

Some drugs affecting taste and smell include the following.

Anesthetics, local—benzocaine, cocaine, procaine
Antibiotics—amphotericin B, ampicillin, griseofulvin, lincomycin, streptomycin, tetracyclines
Anticoagulant—phenindione
Antihistamine—chlorpheniramine maleate
Antihypertensive agents—captopril, diazoxide, ethacrynic acid
Anti-infectious agent—metronidazole
Cholesterol-lowering agent—clofibrate
Hypoglycemic agent—glipizide
Psychoactive agents—carbamazepine, lithium carbonate, phenytoin, amphetamines
Toothpaste ingredient—sodium lauryl sulfate

The proof of the pudding—our food—is in the tasting, which is easily affected by a variety of drugs, resulting in diminished appetite and necessary food intake. Patients on these drugs benefit from counseling about these taste effects, along with other effects, and ways of counteracting them in food selection, seasoning, and serving.

References

Powers D, Moore A: *Food medication interactions,* ed 6, Phoenix, Ariz, 1988, Food Medication Interactions.
Roe DA: *Diet and drug interactions,* ed 2, New York, 1989, AVI Books.
Thomas JA: Drug-nutrient interactions, *Nutr Rev* 53(10):271, 1995.
Trovato A et al: Drug-nutrient interactions, *Am Fam Physician* 44(5):1651, 1991.

DRUG EFFECTS ON NUTRIENT ABSORPTION AND METABOLISM

Nutrient Absorption

A number of drugs can increase nutrient absorption and thus benefit nutritional status. For example, cimetidine (Tagamet), a gastric antisecretory agent, helps patients with bowel resection in several ways.[10] The drug reduces gastric acid and volume output; it also lowers duodenal acid load and volume and reduces jejunal flow.[10] It maintains pH of secretions and decreases fecal fat, nitrogen, and volume, thus improving absorption of protein and carbohydrates.[10] This drug is therefore helpful in the treatment of various gastrointestinal disorders, including peptic ulcer disease (see Chapter 18).[10] On the other hand, prolonged use of cimetidine may cause decreased absorption of vitamin B_{12}, thiamin, and iron.[10]

A number of drugs can contribute to primary malabsorption. Questran (antihyperlipidemic, bile acid sequestrant [cholestyramine]) absorbs vitamins A, D, E, and K, preventing absorption of these nutrients.[10] Colchicine, a drug used in the treatment of gout, leads to vitamin B_{12} deficiency, causing megaloblastic anemia.[10] Alcohol abuse can provoke malabsorption of thiamin and folic acid, causing peripheral neuritis and anemia.[10] Laxatives can produce severe malabsorption, leading to conditions such as osteomalacia.[10]

Secondary malabsorption may also be drug induced. Some drugs can inhibit vitamin D absorption, leading to malabsorption and consequent deficiency of calcium. For example, the antibiotic neomycin causes tissue changes in the intestinal villi, precipitates bile salts, prevents fat breakdown by inhibiting pancreatic lipase, and decreases bile acid absorption.[10] These effects can lead to steatorrhea and failure to absorb the fat-soluble vitamins A, D, E, and K.[10] Malabsorption of vitamin D in turn leads to a calcium deficiency. Other drugs cause malabsorption of folic acid or impair its utilization, causing malabsorption of still other nutrients. Methotrexate, for example, used in cancer chemotherapy, is a folic acid antagonist that impairs the intestinal absorption of calcium.[10]

Summaries of medications affecting food and/or nutrients can be found in Table 16-1.

Mineral Depletion

Certain drugs can lead to mineral depletion through induced gastrointestinal losses or renal excretion.[11]

TABLE 16-1 Medications Affecting Food and/or Nutrients

Drug Class	Examples	Use	Action	Nutrients Affected	How to Avoid
Alcohol, particularly excessive use	Beer, wine, spirits		Increases turnover of some vitamins; food intake decreases	Vitamin B_{12}, folate, and magnesium	
Analgesics and NSAIDs	Salicylates (aspirin)	Pain and fever		Increases loss of vitamin C and competes with folate and vitamin K	Increase intake of foods high in vitamin C, folate, and vitamin K; take with 8 oz water
Antacids		Stomach upset	Inactivates thiamin; decreased absorption of some nutrients	Foods containing thiamin (B_1) should be consumed at a different time Depending on antacid, possibly magnesium, phosphorus, iron, vitamin A, and folate	

References: Anderson J, Hart H: *Nutrient-drug interactions and food,* Colorado State University Cooperative Extension, available at *http://www.ext.colostate.edu/pubs/foodnut/09361.html* (accessed June 3, 2002); Bland SE: Drug-food interactions, *J Pharmacy Society of Wisconsin* Nov/Dec:28, 1998; Bobroff LB, Lentz A, Turner RE: *Food/drug and drug/nutrient interactions: what you should know about your medications,* University of Florida Cooperative Extension Service, Institute of Food and Agricultural Science, available at *http://edis.ifas.ufl.edu/BODY_HE776* (accessed June 3, 2002); Brown CH: Overview of drug interactions, *US Pharmacist* 25(5), 2000, available at *http://www.uspharmacist.com/index.asp?show=archive&issue=5_2000;* Crownsville Hospital Center Pharmacy Dept: *Food/drug interactions,* 2001, available at *http://www.dhmh.state.md.us/crownsville/pharmacy/Interactions.htm;* Kuhn MA: Drug interactions with medications and food, *Nurs Spectrum,* available at *http://nsweb.nursingspectrum.com/ce/ce174.htm;* Food and Drug Administration/National Consumers League: *Food and drug interactions,* available at *http://www.nclnet.org/Food%20&%20Drug.pdf.*

TABLE 16-1 Medications Affecting Food and/or Nutrients—cont'd

Drug Class	Examples	Use	Action	Nutrients Affected	How to Avoid
Antiulcer agents (histamine blockers)	Ranitidine (Zantac), cimetidine (Tagamet), famotidine (Pepcid)	Ulcers	Decreases vitamin absorption	Vitamin B_{12}	Consult physician or registered dietitian regarding vitamin B_{12} supplementation
Antibiotics	Tetracycline, ciprofloxacin (Cipro)	Infection	Chelation of minerals; ingestion with caffeine may increase excitability and nervousness	Calcium, magnesium, iron, and zinc; caffeine	Take tetracycline at least 1 hr before or 2 hr after a meal; do not take with caffeine-containing products
Antineoplastic drugs	Methotrexate	Cancer	Causes mucosal damage, which may cause decreased nutrient absorption	Folate and vitamin B_{12}, also see Antibiotics	Consult physician or registered dietitian regarding supplementation
Anticholinergics	Elavil, Thorazine		Saliva thickens and loses ability to prevent tooth decay	Fluids	
Anticonvulsants	Phenobarbital, phenytoin (Dilantin)	Seizures, epilepsy	Increases metabolism of folate (possibly leading to megaloblastic anemia), vitamin D (especially in children), and vitamin K	Folate, vitamin D, and vitamin K	
Antidepressants	Lithium carbonate, Lithane, Lithobid, Lithonate, Lithotabs, Eskalith	Depression, anxiety	May cause metallic taste, nausea, vomiting, dry mouth, anorexia, weight gain, and increased thirst		Drink 2-3 quarts of water per day and take with food
Anti-inflammatory agents		Fever, infection	Decreases absorption	Folate	
Antihyperlipemics	Cholestyramine (Questran), colestipol (Colestid)	High serum cholesterol	Binds bile salts and nutrients	Fat-soluble vitamins (A, D, E, K), folate, vitamin B_{12}, and iron	Include rich sources of these vitamins and minerals in diet
Antituberculosis	Isoniazid (INH)	Tuberculosis	Inhibits conversion of vitamin B_6 to active form	Vitamin B_6	Vitamin B_6 supplementation is necessary to prevent deficiency and peripheral neuropathy
Corticosteroids	Prednisone, Solu-Medrol, hydrocortisone		Increases excretion	Protein, potassium, calcium, magnesium, zinc, vitamin C, and vitamin B_6	

Continued

TABLE 16-1 Medications Affecting Food and/or Nutrients—cont'd

Drug Class	Examples	Use	Action	Nutrients Affected	How to Avoid
Loop diuretics	Furosemide (Lasix)	Water retention, hypertension	Increases mineral excretion in urine	Potassium, calcium, magnesium, zinc, sodium, and chloride	Include fresh fruits and vegetables in diet
Thiazide diuretics	Hydrochlorothiazide (HCTZ)	Water retention, hypertension	Increases excretion of most electrolytes, but enhances reabsorption of calcium	Potassium, calcium, magnesium, zinc, sodium, chloride, and calcium	
Potassium-sparing diuretics	Triamterene (Dyrenium)	Water retention, hypertension	Hyperkalemia	Potassium	Avoid potassium-based salt substitutes
Laxatives	Fibercon, Mitrolan	Constipation	Decreases nutrient absorption	Vitamins and minerals	Consult physician or registered dietitian regarding supplementation
Sedatives	Barbiturates		Increases metabolism of vitamins	Folate, vitamin D, vitamin B_{12}, thiamin, and vitamin C	
Mineral oil		Laxative	Decreases absorption	Fat-soluble vitamins (A, D, E, K), beta-carotene, calcium, phosphorus, and potassium	
Oral contraceptives		Birth control	May cause selective malabsorption, or increased metabolism and turnover	Vitamin B_6 and folate	

References: Anderson J, Hart H: *Nutrient-drug interactions and food,* Colorado State University Cooperative Extension, available at *http://www.ext.colostate.edu/pubs/foodnut/09361.html* (accessed June 3, 2002); Bland SE: Drug-food interactions, *J Pharmacy Society of Wisconsin* Nov/Dec:28, 1998; Bobroff LB, Lentz A, Turner RE: *Food/drug and drug/nutrient interactions: what you should know about your medications,* University of Florida Cooperative Extension Service, Institute of Food and Agricultural Science, available at *http://edis.ifas.ufl.edu/BODY_HE776* (accessed June 3, 2002); Brown CH: Overview of drug interactions, *US Pharmacist* 25(5), 2000, available at *http://www.uspharmacist.com/index.asp?show=archive&issue=5_2000*; Crownsville Hospital Center Pharmacy Dept: *Food/drug interactions,* 2001, available at *http://www.dhmh.state.md.us/crownsville/pharmacy/Interactions.htm*; Kuhn MA: Drug interactions with medications and food, *Nurs Spectrum,* available at *http://nsweb.nursingspectrum.com/ce/ce174.htm*; Food and Drug Administration/National Consumers League: *Food and drug interactions,* available at *http://www.nclnet.org/Food%20&%20Drug.pdf.*

1. *Diuretics.* Diuretic drugs are intentionally used to reduce levels of excess tissue water and sodium, but they may also result in loss of other minerals, such as potassium, magnesium, and zinc. Potassium deficiency brings weakness, anorexia, nausea, vomiting, listlessness, apprehension, and sometimes diffuse pain, drowsiness, stupor, and irrational behavior. On the contrary, potassium-retaining diuretics such as spironolactone, as well as overuse of potassium supplementation, may cause the opposite effect of hyperkalemia.
2. *Chelating agents.* Penicillamine attaches to metals and can lead to the deficiency of such key trace elements as zinc and copper.
3. *Alcohol.* Abuse of alcohol can lead to diminished levels of potassium, magnesium, and zinc.
4. *Antacids.* These commonly used over-the-counter medications are of concern because they can produce phosphate deficiency, with symptoms of anorexia, malaise, paresthesia, profound muscle weakness, and convulsions as well as calcification of soft tissues from the prolonged hypercalcemia.
5. *Aspirin.* Salicylates such as aspirin (acetylsalicylic acid [ASA]) can induce iron deficiency by causing low-level blood loss from erosions in the stomach or intestinal tissue when taken incorrectly (see *To Probe Further* box).

TO PROBE FURTHER
The Pain Reliever Doctors Recommend Most

Aspirin has a venerable history. Being a buffered form of salicylic acid, it is a modified version of an ancient folk remedy of willow bark that had been used for many hundreds of years for fever, aches, and pain. The acetyl group in acetylsalicylic acid makes aspirin easier on the stomach than willow bark.

Aspirin is an analgesic agent, an effect enhanced in combination with caffeine, that is used for the relief of minor aches and pains. Its mechanism of action is through inhibition of certain prostaglandins (see Chapter 4), which have a profound influence on a spectrum of physiologic functions, including blood clotting, blood pressure, inflammatory process, contraction of voluntary muscles, and transmission of nerve impulses.

Studies implicate aspirin in alleviating many disorders, dangers, and discomforts, including the following.

- Risk of repeated transient ischemic attacks (TIAs), or little strokes, is reduced by 50% in men (but not in women) who have already had one.
- Many studies indicate aspirin is effective in reducing risk for myocardial infarction.
- Aspirin is one of the most effective anti-inflammatory drugs and is effective in long-term treatment of arthritis.
- Aspirin may play a role in inhibiting spread of some cancers through its action of inhibiting production of prostaglandin E_2.
- Aspirin's effect as an anticoagulant is important in treatment of phlebitis and other clot-related disorders.
- Aspirin may be effective in promoting sleep. Many scientists now believe aspirin is as effective as most prescription sedatives, and it has far fewer and less serious side effects.

It is important to remember aspirin is a drug. Many of the benefits of aspirin stem from its systemic, wide-reaching effects on metabolism, which may have unforeseen short- and long-term detrimental results. We do know aspirin is to be strictly avoided by persons with hemophilia. Also, allergic reactions to aspirin can be severe. Aspirin seems to be implicated in asthma. Children are especially vulnerable to side effects and should not be given aspirin without a physician's instructions.

Aspirin is an irritant to the stomach and intestine. Its continuous use is associated with low-level chronic loss of iron caused by mucosal erosion. This can lead to iron-deficiency anemia.

Aspirin has been linked to birth defects, especially when it is taken later in the course of pregnancy. It increases risk of infant and neonatal mortality, low birth weight, and intracranial hemorrhage.

The best way to take aspirin is on an empty stomach with a full glass of water. This is important: absorption of aspirin is facilitated by a large volume of liquid and inhibited by the presence of food. In addition, taking aspirin—especially on an empty stomach—without a large fluid intake invites erosion of the stomach lining. But aspirin should never be taken when using alcohol because it increases the bioavailability of alcohol, raising the blood concentration and thus the effect of alcohol on brain centers.

References

Koch PA et al: Influence of food and fluid ingestion on aspirin bioavailability, *J Pharm Sci* 67(11):1533, 1978.

Roine R et al: Aspirin increases blood alcohol concentrations in humans after ingestion of ethanol, *JAMA* 264(18):2406, 1990.

Schachtel BP et al: Caffeine as an aspirin adjuvant, *Arch Intern Med* 151:733, 1991.

Vitamin Depletion

Certain drugs act as metabolic antagonists and can cause deficiencies of the vitamins involved.

1. *Vitamin antagonists.* Various drugs have been used successfully to treat disease because they are antagonists of certain vitamins and thus can control key metabolic reactions in which that vitamin is involved. For example, warfarin (Coumadin) anticoagulants inhibit regeneration of vitamin K, which is necessary for blood clotting. Also, some cancer chemotherapy drugs such as methotrexate have multiple antagonist effects on folate metabolism, thus inhibiting the synthesis of cell reproduction substances—deoxyribonucleic acid and ribonucleic acid (DNA and RNA)—and protein. In a similar manner, the antimalaria drug pyrimethamine inhibits the action of folate in protein synthesis.
2. *Hypovitaminosis from use of oral contraceptives.* Some women using oral contraceptive agents (OCAs) have developed subclinical deficiencies of the vitamins folate, riboflavin, pyridoxine (B_6), cobalamin (B_{12}), and ascorbic acid (C). Apparently OCAs induce a greater demand for these vitamins.[12] However, a Canadian/U.S. study has shown that this effect does not hold true with folate.[13]

Special Adverse Reactions

Several reactions are related to specific drug interactions with particular nutrients.

paresthesia Abnormal sensations such as prickling, burning, and crawling of skin.

1. *Monoamine oxidase inhibitors (MAOIs).* These antidepressant drugs can increase the vascular effect of simple vasoactive amines, such as tyramine and dopamine, from food.[14] The resulting tyramine syndrome is marked by headache, pallor, nausea, and restlessness. With increased absorption, symptoms may escalate to apprehension, sweating, palpitations, chest pain, fever, and increased blood pressure, at times, although rarely, to the extent of hypertensive crisis and stroke. A low-tyramine food list (see Table 24-3) is provided for use by any patient taking one of these antidepressant drugs.
2. *Flushing reaction.* A number of drugs react with alcohol to produce a flushing reaction along with dyspnea and headache (Table 16-2). Central nervous system depressants, including hypnotic sedatives, antihistamines, phenothiazines, and narcotic analgesics, may cause a loss of consciousness if taken in combination with alcohol. Extreme caution must be exercised with these medications, and patients should be alerted to the dangers of mixing them with alcohol.
3. *Hypoglycemia.* Drugs such as chlorpropamide (Diabinese) and similar oral medications used to control type 2 diabetes mellitus are hypoglycemic agents. They precipitate a rapid release of insulin, which may provoke a hypoglycemic reaction. This response of a rapidly reduced blood glucose level is especially strong when the drugs are used with alcohol. Symptoms of hypoglycemia include weakness, mental confusion, and irrational behavior. If not treated, loss of consciousness can follow.
4. *Disulfiram reaction.* The drug disulfiram, commonly called Antabuse, is used in the treatment of alcoholism. It combats alcohol consumption by producing extremely unpleasant side effects when taken with alcohol. Within 15 minutes flushing ensues, followed by headache, nausea, vomiting, and chest or abdominal pain. Other drugs, including aldehyde dehydrogenase inhibitors, may have this similar disulfiram effect.

Food and Nutrient Effects on Drugs

PHYSIOLOGIC FACTORS IN DRUG ABSORPTION

Absorption of drugs is a complex matter. Physiologic events are important in a number of ways.

Solution

Before an orally administered tablet or capsule can dissolve, it must first disintegrate. The absorption of the

TABLE 16-2 Adverse Drug Reactions Caused by Alcohol and Specific Foods

Type of Reaction	Drugs	Alcohol/Foods	Effects
Flushing	Chlorpropamide (diabetes) Griseofulvin Tetrachloroethylene	Alcohol	Dyspnea, headache, flushing
Disulfiram reaction	Aldehyde dehydrogenase inhibitors: Disulfiram (Antabuse) Calcium carbamide Metronidazole Nitrofurantoin Sulfonylureas	Alcohol Foods containing alcohol	Abdominal and chest pain, flushing, headache, nausea and vomiting
Hypoglycemia	Insulin-releasing agents: Oral hypoglycemic drugs	Alcohol Sugar, sweets	Mental confusion, weakness, irrational behavior, unconsciousness
Tyramine reaction	Monoamine oxidase inhibitors (MAOIs): Antidepressants such as phenelzine Procarbazine Isoniazid (isonicotinic acid hydrazide)	Food containing large amounts of tyramine: Cheese Red wines Chicken liver Broad beans Yeast	Cerebrovascular accident, flushing, hypertension

Modified from Roe DA: Interactions between drugs and nutrients, *Med Clin North Am* 63:985, 1979; and Roe DA: *Diet and drug interactions,* ed 2, New York, 1979, AVI Books.

drug, either from solution in acid gastric secretions or in the more alkaline medium of the intestine, may be more or less complete depending on its degree of solubility. The drug then passes through the intestinal mucosa and liver circulation before entering systemic circulation. In the systemic blood circulation system, it may be subject to metabolism, deactivation, and elimination through the so-called first-pass mechanism. Food may affect eventual drug absorption at any of these points.

Stomach-Emptying Rate

Composition of the diet affects the rate at which food enters the small intestine from the stomach. Slow emptying of food from the stomach has the effect of doling out small portions of a drug, creating more optimal saturation rates on the absorptive sites in the small intestine. Fats, high temperatures, and solid meals prolong the time the food stays in the stomach. Food usually increases secretion of bile, acid, and gut enzymes. It also enhances intestinal motility and splanchnic blood flow. Drugs may adsorb to certain food particles.

Clinical Significance

Whether these physiologic events have clinical significance depends on the extent of the effect and nature of the drug. A small change in absorption is critical for a drug with a steep dose-response curve but perhaps unnoticeable for a drug with a wide range of effective concentrations. In general, the amount of absorption is clinically more important than the rate because it has greater impact on the steady-state plasma concentration of the drug after multiple doses. Table 16-3 gives some examples of drugs that

disulfiram White to off-white crystalline antioxidant; inhibits oxidation of the acetaldehyde metabolized from alcohol. It is used in the treatment of alcoholism, producing extremely uncomfortable symptoms when alcohol is ingested after oral administration of the drug.
dyspnea Labored, difficult breathing.
flushing reaction Short-term reaction resulting in redness of neck and face.
vasoactive Having an effect on the diameter of blood vessels.

TABLE 16-3 Foods and/or Nutrients Affecting Medications

Drug Class	Examples	Use	Action	Food/Nutrients	How to Avoid
Alcohol, particularly excessive use	Beer, wine, spirits		Slows absorption	Food	Consume alcohol with food or meals
Analgesics and NSAIDs	Salicylates (aspirin), ibuprofen (Motrin, Advil), naproxen (Anaprox, Aleve, Naprosyn)	Pain and fever	Alcohol ingestion increases hepatotoxicity	Alcohol	Limit alcohol intake to ≤3 drinks/day
Analgesics	Acetaminophen (Tylenol)	Pain and fever	Liver damage or stomach bleeding	Alcohol	Limit alcohol intake to ≤3 drinks/day
Antacids		Stomach upset			
Antiulcer agents (histamine blockers)	Cimetidine (Tagamet)	Ulcers	Increased blood alcohol levels; reduced caffeine clearance	Alcohol; caffeine-containing foods and beverages	
Antibiotics	Ciprofloxacin (Cipro)	Infection	Decreases absorption	Dairy products	Avoid dairy products

References: Anderson J, Hart H: *Nutrient-drug interactions and food,* Colorado State University Cooperative Extension, available at *http://www.ext.colostate.edu/pubs/foodnut/09361.html* (accessed June 3, 2002); Bland SE: Drug-food interactions, *J Pharmacy Society of Wisconsin* Nov/Dec:28, 1998; Bobrof LB, Lentz A, Turner RE: *Food/drug and drug/nutrient interactions: what you should know about your medications,* University of Florida Cooperative Extension Service, Institute of Food and Agricultural Science, available at *http://edis.ufl.edu/BODY_HE776* (accessed June 3, 2002); Brown CH: Overview of drug interactions, *US Pharmacist* 25(5), available at *http://www.uspharmacist.com/NewLook/DisplayArticle.cfm?item_num=522* (accessed June 3, 2002); Crownsville Hospital Center Pharmacy Dept: *Food/drug interactions,* 2001, available at *http://www.dhmh.state.md.us/crownsville/Pharmacy/Interactions.htm* (accessed June 9, 2002); Kuhn MA: Drug interactions with medications and food, *Nurs Spectrum,* available at *http://www.nsweb.nursingspectrum.com/ce/ce174.htm* (accessed June 9, 2002); Food and Drug Administration/National Consumers League: *Food and drug interactions,* available at *http://www.nclnet.org/Food%20&%20Drug.pdf* (accessed June 9, 2002).

Continued

TABLE 16-3 Foods and/or Nutrients Affecting Medications—cont'd

Drug Class	Examples	Use	Action	Food/Nutrients	How to Avoid
Anticoagulant	Warfarin (Coumadin)	Blood clots	Reduced efficacy; increased anticoagulation	Vitamins K and E (supplements) may reduce efficacy; alcohol and garlic may increase anticoagulation	Limit foods high in vitamin K: broccoli, spinach, kale, turnip greens, cauliflower, Brussels sprouts; avoid high dose of vitamin E (400 IU or more)
Antineoplastic drugs	Methotrexate	Cancer	Increased hepatotoxicity with chronic alcohol use	Alcohol	
Antiemetic	Amitriptyline HCl (Elavil), chlorpromazine HCl (Thorazine)	Antidepressant; antipsychotic/antiemetic	Increased sedation	Alcohol	
Anticonvulsants	Phenobarbital	Seizures, epilepsy	Increased sedation	Alcohol	
Antidepressants: Monoamine oxidase inhibitors (MAOIs)	Phenelzine (Nardil), tranylcypromine (Parnate)	Depression, anxiety	Rapid, potentially fatal increase in blood pressure	Foods or alcoholic beverages containing tyramine (beer; red wine; American processed, cheddar, bleu, brie, mozzarella, and parmesan cheeses; yogurt; sour cream; beef or chicken liver; cured meats such as sausage and salami; game meats; caviar; dried fish; avocados, bananas, yeast extracts, raisins, sauerkraut, soy sauce, miso soup; broad [fava] beans, ginseng, caffeine-containing products [colas, chocolate, coffee, tea])	
Antihistamine	Fexofenadine (Allegra), loratadine (Claritin), cetirizine (Zyrtec), astemizole (Hismanal)	Allergies	Increase drowsiness and slow mental and motor performance	Alcohol	Use caution when operating machinery or driving

References: Anderson J, Hart H: *Nutrient-drug interactions and food,* Colorado State University Cooperative Extension, available at *http://www.ext.colostate.edu/pubs/foodnut/09361.html* (accessed June 3, 2002); Bland SE: Drug-food interactions, *J Pharmacy Society of Wisconsin* Nov/Dec:28, 1998; Bobrof LB, Lentz A, Turner RE: *Food/drug and drug/nutrient interactions: what you should know about your medications,* University of Florida Cooperative Extension Service, Institute of Food and Agricultural Science, available at *http://edis.ufl.edu/BODY_HE776* (accessed June 3, 2002); Brown CH: Overview of drug interactions, *US Pharmacist* 25(5), available at *http://www.uspharmacist.com/NewLook/DisplayArticle.cfm?item_num=522* (accessed June 3, 2002); Crownsville Hospital Center Pharmacy Dept: *Food/drug interactions,* 2001, available at *http://www.dhmh.state.md.us/crownsville/Pharmacy/Interactions.htm* (accessed June 9, 2002); Kuhn MA: Drug interactions with medications and food, *Nurs Spectrum,* available at *http://www.nsweb.nursingspectrum.com/ce/ce174.htm* (accessed June 9, 2002); Food and Drug Administration/National Consumers League: *Food and drug interactions,* available at *http://www.nclnet.org/Food%20&%20Drug.pdf* (accessed June 9, 2002).

TABLE 16-3 Foods and/or Nutrients Affecting Medications—cont'd

Drug Class	Examples	Use	Action	Food/Nutrients	How to Avoid
Antihypertensives		Hypertension	Reduced effectiveness	Natural licorice and tyramine-rich foods	Avoid these foods
Antihyperlipemics (HMG-CoA reductase inhibitors) or statins	Atorvastatin (Lipitor), lovastatin (Mevacor), pravastatin (Pravachol), simvastatin (Zocor)	High serum LDL cholesterol	Enhance absorption; increase risk of liver damage	Food/meals; alcohol	Lovastatin should be taken with evening meal to enhance absorption; avoid large amounts of alcohol
Antiparkinson	Levodopa (Dopar, Larodopa)	Parkinson's disease	Decreased absorption	High-protein foods (eggs, meat, protein supplements); B_6	Spread protein intake equally in 3-6 meals/day to minimize reaction; avoid B_6 supplements or multivitamin supplement in doses >10 mg
Antituberculosis	Isoniazid (INH)	Tuberculosis	Reduced absorption with foods; increased hepatotoxicity and reduced INH levels with alcohol	Alcohol	Take on empty stomach; avoid alcohol
Bronchodilators	Theophylline (Slo-Bid, Theo-Dur)	Asthma, chronic bronchitis, and emphysema	Increased stimulation of CNS; alcohol can increase nausea, vomiting, headache, and irritability	Caffeine, alcohol	Avoid caffeine-containing foods/beverages (chocolate, colas, teas, coffee); avoid alcohol if taking theophylline medications
Corticosteroids	Prednisone (Pediapred, Preline, Solu-Medrol), hydrocortisone	Inflammation and itching	Stomach irritation	Food	Take with food or milk to decrease stomach upset
Hypoglycemic agents	Sulfonylurea (Diabinese); metformin (Glucophage)	Diabetes	Severe nausea and vomiting	Alcohol	Avoid alcohol

are better utilized when taken without food and those that should be taken with food.

EFFECTS OF FOOD ON DRUG ABSORPTION

Increased Drug Absorption

In summary, five basic circumstances contribute to increased absorption of a drug (see *Issues & Answers*).

1. *Dissolving characteristics.* When a drug does not dissolve rapidly after it has been taken, the time it remains in the stomach with food is prolonged. This increased time in the stomach may increase its effective dissolution and consequent absorption. In some instances the drug may not dissolve properly because of either the drug or gastric pH and is excreted.
2. *Gastric-emptying time.* Delayed emptying of food from the stomach can have the effect of doling out small portions of a drug, creating more optimal saturation rates on the absorption sites in the small intestine.
3. *Nutrients.* Some nutrients can promote absorption of certain drugs. For example, high-fat diets increase absorption of the antifungal drug griseofulvin. This drug is fat soluble, and high-fat diets stimulate the secretion of bile acids, which aid in absorption of the drug. Vitamin C, as well as gastric acid, enhances iron absorption. Recent studies indicate that citrus fruit

reduced lipoprotein oxidation in persons consuming a high-saturated fat diet.[15] Anticoagulant drugs interact with dietary factors, and a consistent dietary intake of vitamin K is important.[16,17] Folic acid supplementation is needed when phenytoin is used for seizure control in epileptic patients.[18]

4. *Blood flow.* Food intake increases splanchnic blood flow carrying any ingested drugs. This direct circulation to abdominal visceral organs stimulates absorption and results in an increased availability of the accompanying drugs.
5. *Nutritional status.* In addition to the presence of specific nutrients, nutritional status may also affect the bioavailability of certain drugs in different ways. For example, the antibiotic chloramphenicol is absorbed more slowly in children with protein-energy malnutrition, but elimination of the drug is slower in well-nourished children. In both cases the effect is a net increased bioavailability of the drug.

Decreased Drug Absorption

Absorption of some drugs is delayed or reduced by the presence of food.

1. *Aspirin.* Absorption of aspirin is reduced or delayed by food. It should be taken on an empty stomach with ample water, preferably cold (see *To Probe Further* box). Because aspirin increases the effect of alcohol, however, it should not be taken with alcohol.[19] In addition, caffeine enhances the analgesic effect of aspirin.[20]
2. *Tetracycline.* Nutritional status may also have an impact on drug absorption. For example, tetracycline absorption is impaired in malnourished individuals. Absorption of this commonly used antibiotic is also hindered when it is taken with milk, as well as with antacids or iron supplements. The drug combines with these materials to form new insoluble compounds that the body cannot absorb, causing loss of the minerals involved, that is, calcium or iron.[15]
3. *Phenytoin.* The presence of protein inhibits absorption of phenytoin. Carbohydrate increases its absorption, but fat has no impact.

FOOD EFFECTS ON DRUG DISTRIBUTION AND METABOLISM

Carbohydrate and Fat

Dietary carbohydrate and fat, especially their relative quantities, influence liver enzymes that metabolize drugs. For example, presence of fat increases the activity of diazepam (Valium). Fat increases the concentration of the unbound active drug by displacing it from binding sites in plasma and tissue protein.

Licorice

Licorice, a sweet-tasting plant extract used in making chewing tobacco, candy, and certain drugs, causes sodium retention and increased hypertension.[21] A person being treated for hypertension needs to avoid any natural licorice-containing product. The active ingredient in licorice is glycyrrhizic acid, which is named for its natural plant source, *Glycyrrhiza glabra,* meaning "sweet root," a member of the legume family. An analog of this active part of licorice is marketed under the trade names Biogastrone and Duogastrone, which are widely used, especially in Europe, for healing gastric ulcers, but hypertension is a side effect.

Indoles

Indoles in cruciferous vegetables (e.g., cabbage, brussels sprouts, broccoli, cauliflower) can speed up rate of drug metabolism. They apparently induce mixed-function oxidase enzyme systems in the liver.

Cooking Methods

The method of cooking foods may alter rate of drug metabolism. Charcoal broiling, for example, increases hepatic drug metabolism through enzyme induction.

Changes in Intestinal Microflora

Changes in intestinal microflora related to amount of dietary protein or fiber, for example, may influence intestinal drug metabolism.

VITAMIN EFFECTS ON DRUG ACTION

Vitamin Effects on Drug Effectiveness

Pharmacologic doses, or large megadoses beyond nutritional need, of vitamins decrease blood levels of drugs when vitamins interact with the drugs. For example, large doses of folate or pyridoxine can reduce the blood level and effectiveness of such anticonvulsive drugs as phenytoin (Dilantin) or phenobarbital that are used for seizure control. Unwise self-medication with large drug-level doses of vitamins can cause severe toxic complications. On the other hand, vitamins themselves may become important medications when used as part of the medical treatment for a secondary deficiency induced by a childhood genetic or metabolic disease. Such is the case with biotin in treating certain organic acidemias or with riboflavin in treating certain defects in fatty acid metabolism.

Control of Drug Intoxication

Riboflavin is useful in treating boric acid poisoning. Boric acid combines with the ribityl side chain of riboflavin and is excreted in the urine. Also, vitamin E combats pulmonary oxygen toxicity. Premature human infants at risk for development of bronchopulmonary dysplasia by oxygen treatment have been protected by vitamin E administration during the acute phase of respiratory distress requiring oxygen treatment.

Nutrition-Pharmacy Team

DECADES OF CHANGE

A decade or so ago hospitalized patients as a whole were less severely ill than they are today. Now, however, as a reflection of our more complex medical system and economic reform efforts, patients who are hospitalized are more acutely ill. They are more at risk for nutritional deficits and more likely to develop malnutrition, which leads to increased lengths of stay and higher costs. The task of monitoring food and drug interactions is complex and requires team responsibilities. Coordinating the pharmacy, food service, and clinical nutrition minimizes adverse drug-nutrient interactions.

CURRENT TRENDS

The movement in hospitals and other healthcare facilities today is a shift in focus toward key processes and functions, such as drug-nutrient interactions in this case, rather than the traditional strictly compartmentalized tasks of departments. Current standards focus still on departmental or service roles, but this is changing because of economic necessity as well as philosophy of care. This changing focus is being shaped, for example, in the work of the Joint Commission on the Accreditation of Healthcare Organizations (JCAHO).[22]

In the mid-1990s, JCAHO's accreditation manual reflected the philosophy that key functions often involve different disciplines coming together, partners with clearly defined responsibilities. The team of clinical nutritionist and clinical pharmacologist is clearly one of these partnerships. Current JCAHO guideline mandates monitoring of drug therapy and counseling with patients about adverse drug-nutrient interactions.[23]

TO SUM UP

Drugs can have multiple effects on the body's absorption, metabolism, retention, and nutrient status. They can provoke adverse reactions in combination with certain foods and can influence appetite, either repressing it or artificially stimulating it. Drugs can either increase an individual's absorption of nutrients or, more commonly, decrease absorption, sometimes leading to clinical deficiencies. Drugs can also induce mineral and vitamin deficiencies by their mode of action.

Just as drugs affect our use of food, food affects our use of drugs. Food can affect the absorption of drugs in a variety of ways. Foods also have an effect on subsequent distribution and metabolism of drugs. Vitamins may interfere with drug effectiveness, especially if they are taken in large doses. On the other hand, large doses of specific vitamins can be effective in countering certain toxicity conditions or a specific secondary deficiency induced by a genetic disease.

cruciferous Bearing a cross; botanical term for plants belonging to the botanical family Cruciferae or Brassicaceae, the mustard family, so-called because of cross-like four-petaled flowers; name given to certain vegetables of this family, such as broccoli, cabbage, brussels sprouts, and cauliflower.

indole A compound produced in the intestines by the decomposition of tryptophan; also found in the oil of jasmine and clove.

■ Questions for Review

1. Name four ways food may affect drug use and give examples of each.
2. If your patient were using a prescribed MAOI such as tranylcypromine sulfate (Parnate), what foods would you instruct her to avoid?
3. What is the most effective way to take aspirin? With what type of liquid? With or without food? Why?
4. What foods would you suggest to a hypertensive patient on the diuretic drug hydrochlorothiazide (HCTZ) as good sources of potassium replacement?
5. Outline suggestions you would discuss with a patient experiencing a drug-induced taste loss. How would you explain the cause of the taste loss?

■ References

1. Ament PW, Bertolino JG, Liszewski JL: Clinically significant drug interactions, *Am Fam Physician* 61(6):1745, 2000.
2. Brown CH: Overview of drug interactions, *US Pharmacist* 25(5), 2000. Available at *http://www.uspharmacist.com/index.asp?show=archive&issue=5_2000.*
3. Gnerali J: Avoiding drug interactions, *Am Fam Physician* 61(6):1628, 2000.
4. Smaglik P: Proliferation of pills, *Sci News* 151(20):310, 1997.
5. Woodard KW, Franklin RM: Treating elderly patients, *US Pharmacist* 24(8), 1999. Available at *http://www.uspharmacist.com/index.asp?show=archive&issue=8_1999.*
6. U.S. Census Bureau: *Profiles of general demographic characteristics 2000,* Washington, DC, 2001, U.S. Dept of Commerce.
7. Scheitel SM et al: Geriatric health maintenance, *Mayo Clin Proc* 71(3):289, 1996.
8. Kaufman DW et al: Recent patterns of medication use in the ambulatory adult population of the United States: the Slone survey, *JAMA* 287(3):337, 2002.
9. Albion Research: Drug-nutrient interactions: this clinical consideration will continue to grow, *Albion Res Notes* 5(4):1, 1996.
10. Pronsky ZM: *Food medication interactions,* ed 12, Birchrunville, Pa, 2002, Food Medication Interactions.

11. Murray JJ, Healy MD: Drug-mineral interactions: a new responsibility for the hospital dietitian, *J Am Diet Assoc* 91(1):66, 1991.
12. Masse PG: Nutrient intakes of women who use oral contraceptives, *J Am Diet Assoc* 91(9):1118, 1991.
13. Green TJ et al: Oral contraceptives did not affect biochemical folate indexes and homocysteine concentrations in adolescent females, *J Am Diet Assoc* 98(1):50, 1998.
14. Merriman SH: Monoamine oxidase drugs and diet, *Hum Nutr Diet* 12:21, 1999.
15. Harats D et al: Citrus fruit supplementation reduces lipoprotein oxidation in young men ingesting a diet high in saturated fat: vitamin E presumptive evidence for an interaction between vitamins C and E in vivo, *Am J Clin Nutr* 67(2):240, 1998.
16. Harris JE: Interaction of dietary factors with oral anticoagulants: review and applications, *J Am Diet Assoc* 95(5):580-584, 1995.
17. Booth SL et al: Dietary vitamin K and stability of oral anticoagulation: proposal of a diet with constant vitamin K content, *Thromb Haemost* 77(3):408, 1997.
18. Lewis DP et al: Phenytoin–folic acid interaction, *Ann Pharmacother* 29(7/8):726, 1995.
19. Roine R et al: Aspirin increases blood alcohol concentration in humans after ingestion of ethanol, *JAMA* 264(18): 2406, 1990.
20. Schachtel BP et al: Caffeine as an analgesic adjuvant, *Arch Intern Med* 151:733, 1991.
21. Morris DJ et al: Licorice, chewing tobacco, and hypertension, *N Engl J Med* 151:733, 1991.
22. Kessler DA: Communicating with patients about their medications, *N Engl J Med* 325(23):1650, 1991.
23. Joint Commission on the Accreditation of Healthcare Organizations: *Comprehensive accreditation manual for hospitals: the official handbook (CAMH),* Oakbrook, Ill, 2002, JCAHO.

■ Further Reading

Ahmed FE: Effects of nutrition on the health of the elderly, *J Am Diet Assoc* 92(9):1102, 1992.

Kerstetter JE et al: Malnutrition in the institutionalized adult, *J Am Diet Assoc* 92(9):1109, 1992.

These excellent companion articles speak to the twin problems of malnutrition and polypharmacy—multiple drug use—among elderly persons.

Clayman CB, ed: *The American Medical Association guide to prescription and over-the-counter drugs,* New York, 1988, Random House.

Clayman CB, ed: *Know your drugs and medications: the American Medical Association home medical library series,* Pleasantville, NY, 1991, Dorling Kindersley and Reader's Digest.

These two resources, prepared for public education and patient-professional reference, provide useful information about effects and interactions of drugs in common use.

Thomas JA: Drug-nutrient interactions, *Nutr Rev* 53(10):271, 1995.

This is an excellent review with numerous tables. It is a "must read" for all persons taking care of patients and clients.

Issues & ANSWERS

Grapefruit "Juices" Certain Medications

Almost all oral drugs are subject to first-pass metabolism. That is, any substance the body views as a toxin (e.g., drugs, alcohol) goes through the liver via hepatic portal circulation, thus removing some of the active substance from blood before it enters general circulation. This means a fraction of the original dose of the drug will not be "available" to systemic circulation because it has undergone biotransformation. In other words, bioavailability of the drug has been altered, or lowered. One mechanism responsible for this is an enzyme system found in the intestinal wall and liver. The cytochrome P450 3A4 system (specifically CYP3A4-mediated drug metabolism) is responsible for first-pass metabolism of many medications. Most medications are lipid soluble and readily absorbed. To eliminate toxins (i.e., drugs) from the body, however, the cytochrome P450 system either breaks them down in the gut or changes the drug in to a more water-soluble version in the liver, allowing it to be eliminated via urine.

Where does grapefruit juice come into play? Grapefruit juice blocks CYP3A4 enzyme in the wall of the small intestine, thus increasing bioavailability of the drug. This means a higher serum drug level, which may cause unpleasant consequences, including side effects and/or toxicity.

What is it in grapefruit juice that does this? The precise chemical nature of the substance responsible for inhibiting gut wall CYP3A4 enzyme is unknown, but it is believed that more than one component present in grapefruit juice may contribute to the inhibitory effect on CYP3A4.

A single glass (8 oz) of grapefruit juice has the potential to increase bioavailability and enhance beneficial or adverse effects of a broad range of medications. These effects can persist up to 72 hours after grapefruit consumption, until more CYP3A4 has been metabolized. Interactions have been found between grapefruit juice and drugs (Table 16-4).

TABLE 16-4 Interactions Between Grapefruit Juice and Medications

Category	Generic Name	Brand Name	Effect
Antihypertensive (calcium channel blockers)	Felodipine	Plendil	Flushing, headache, tachycardia, decreased blood pressure
	Nifedipine	Procardia, Adalat	
	Nimodipine	Nimotop	
	Nisoldipine	Sular	
	Nicardipine	Cardene	
	Isradipine	DynaCirc	
	Verapamil	Calan, Isoptin	Same as above plus bradycardia and atrioventricular (AV) block
Nonsedating antihistamines	Astemizole	Hismanal	
Immunosuppressant	Cyclosporine	Neoral, Sandimmune, SangCya	Kidney toxicity, increased susceptibility to infections
	Tacrolimus	Prograf	
Statin (HMG-CoA reductase inhibitors)	Atorvastatin	Lipitor	Headache, gastrointestinal complaints, muscle pain, increased risk of myopathy
	Lovastatin	Mevacor	
	Simvastatin	Zocor	
Caffeine			Nervousness, over stimulation

References: Bailey DG et al: Grapefruit juice-drug interactions, *Br J Pharmacol* 46(2):101, 1998; Kane GC and Lipsky JJ: Drug-grapefruit juice interactions, *Mayo Clin Proc* 75:933, 2000; Guo L et al: Role of furanocoumarin derivatives on grapefruit juice-mediated inhibition of human CYP3A activity, *Drug Metab Dispos* 28:766, 2000; Ho P et al: Inhibition of human CYP3A4 activity by grapefruit flavonoids, furanocoumarins and related compounds, *J Pharm Pharm Sci* 4(3):217, 2001; Hyland R et al: Identification of the cytochrome P450 enzymes involved in the N-demethylation of sildenafil, *Clin Pharmacol* 51:239, 2000; Jetter A et al: Effects of grapefruit juice on the pharmacokinetics of sildenafil; *Clin Pharmacol Ther* 71(1):21, 2002; Muirhead GJ et al: Pharmacokinetic interactions between sildenafil and saqinavir/ritonavir, *Br J Clin Pharmacol* 50:99, 2000; Pronsky ZM: *Food medication interactions,* ed 12, Birchrunville, Pa, 2002, FOOD-MEDICATION INTERACTIONS; Schmiedlin-Ren P et al: Mechanisms of enhanced oral availability of CYP3A4 substrates by grapefruit constituents, *Drug Metab Dispos* 25(1):1228, 1997; University of Illinois Chicago College of Pharmacy, Drug Information Center: *Grapefruit juice interactions,* available at *http://www.uic.edu/pharmacy/services/di/grapefru.htm* (accessed June 10, 2002); University of Michigan Health System Drug Information Service: *Selected drugs interacting with grapefruit juice,* 1999.

Continued

TABLE 16-4 Interactions Between Grapefruit Juice and Medications—cont'd

Category	Generic Name	Brand Name	Effect
Antianxiety, insomnia, or depression	Buspirone	BuSpar	Increased sedation
	Diazepam	Valium	
	Alprazolam	Xanax	
	Midazolam	Versed	
	Triazolam	Halcion	
	Zaleplon	Sonata	
	Carbamazepine	Tegretol	
	Clomipramine	Anafranil	
	Trazodone	Desyrel	
Protease inhibitors	Saquinavir	Fortovase, Invirase	Doubles bioavailability resulting in increased efficacy or toxicity depending on dose and patient variability
Sexual dysfunction	Sildenafil	Viagra	Delayed absorption (takes longer to become effective)
Medications Considered Safe for Use With Grapefruit			
	Cetirizine	Zyrtec, Reactine	
	Fexofenadine	Allegra	
	Fluvastatin	Lescol	
	Loratadine	Claritin	
	Pravastatin	Pravachol	

References: Bailey DG et al: Grapefruit juice-drug interactions, *Br J Pharmacol* 46(2):101, 1998; Kane GC and Lipsky JJ: Drug-grapefruit juice interactions, *Mayo Clin Proc* 75:933, 2000; Guo L et al: Role of furanocoumarin derivatives on grapefruit juice-mediated inhibition of human CYP3A activity, *Drug Metab Dispos* 28:766, 2000; Ho P et al: Inhibition of human CYP3A4 activity by grapefruit flavonoids, furanocoumarins and related compounds, *J Pharm Pharm Sci* 4(3):217, 2001; Hyland R et al: Identification of the cytochrome P450 enzymes involved in the N-demethylation of sildenafil, *Clin Pharmacol* 51:239, 2000; Jetter A et al: Effects of grapefruit juice on the pharmacokinetics of sildenafil; *Clin Pharmacol Ther* 71(1):21, 2002; Muirhead GJ et al: Pharmacokinetic interactions between sildenafil and saqinavir/ritonavir, *Br J Clin Pharmacol* 50:99, 2000; Pronsky ZM: *Food medication interactions,* ed 12, Birchrunville, Pa, 2002, FOOD-MEDICATION INTERACTIONS; Schmiedlin-Ren P et al: Mechanisms of enhanced oral availability of CYP3A4 substrates by grapefruit constituents, *Drug Metab Dispos* 25(1):1228, 1997; University of Illinois Chicago College of Pharmacy, Drug Information Center: *Grapefruit juice interactions,* available at *http://www.uic.edu/pharmacy/services/di/grapefru.htm* (accessed June 10, 2002); University of Michigan Health System Drug Information Service: *Selected drugs interacting with grapefruit juice,* 1999.

REFERENCES

Bailey DG et al: Grapefruit juice-drug interactions, *Br J Clin Pharmacol* 46(2):101, 1998.

Kane GC, Lipsky JJ: Drug-grapefruit juice interactions, *Mayo Clin Proc* 75:933, 2000.

Guo L et al: Role of furanocoumarin derivatives on grapefruit juice-mediated inhibition of human CYP3A activity, *Drug Metab Dispos* 28:766, 2000.

Ho P et al: Inhibition of human CYP3A4 activity by grapefruit flavonoids, furanocoumarins and related compounds, *J Pharm Pharm Sci* 4(3):217, 2001.

Hyland R et al: Identification of the cytochrome P450 enzymes involved in the N-demethylation of sildenafil, *Clin Pharmacol* 51:239, 2000.

Jetter A et al: Effects of grapefruit juice on the pharmacokinetics of sildenafil, *Clin Pharmacol Ther* 71(1):21, 2002.

Muirhead GJ et al: Pharmacokinetic interactions between sildenafil and saquinavir/ritonavir, *Br J Clin Pharmacol* 50:99, 2000.

Pronsky ZM: *Food medication interactions,* ed 12, Birchrunville, Pa, 2002, Food Medication Interactions.

Schmiedlin-Ren P et al: Mechanisms of enhanced oral availability of CYP3A4 substrates by grapefruit constituents, *Drug Metab Dispos* 25(1):1228, 1997.

University of Illinois Chicago College of Pharmacy Drug Information Center: *Grapefruit juice interactions.* Available at *http://www.uic.edu/pharmacy/services/di/grapefru.htm.*

University of Michigan Health System Drug Information Service: *Selected drugs interacting with grapefruit juice,* 1999. Available at *http://www-personal.umich.edu/~mshlafer/Lectures/grapefruit.pdf.*

Chapter 17

Nutrition Support: Enteral and Parenteral Nutrition

M. Patricia Fuhrman

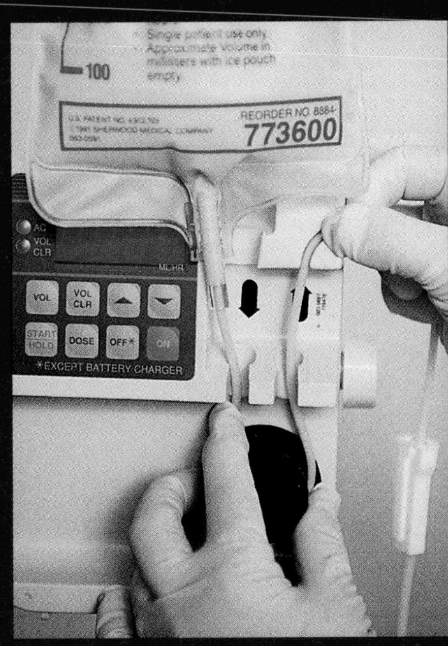

From Potter PA, Perry AG: Fundamentals of nursing: concepts, process, and practice, *ed 4, St Louis, 1997, Mosby.*

Chapter Outline

In this chapter we look at alternate modes of feeding to provide nutrition support for patients with special needs. We examine ways of feeding when the gastrointestinal tract can still be used—enteral nutrition. Then we review nutrient feeding directly into a vein when the gastrointestinal tract cannot be used—parenteral nutrition (PN).

Malnutrition, preexisting and iatrogenic, is a serious concern in hospitalized patients, especially those with critical illness or injury. Nutrition care provided by a skilled nutrition support team or clinician can have a positive affect on patient survival and recovery. This chapter will examine enteral and PN support formulas, solutions, and delivery systems for use in hospital and home.

Nutrition Assessment

NUTRITION SUPPORT AND DEGREE OF MALNUTRITION

It is an easier task to maintain positive nutrition than to replenish body stores from malnutrition. The effect of starvation on the body, even during relatively brief periods, is well documented.[1] The small amount of glycogen stored in the liver is a crucial immediate energy source. Glycogenolysis begins 2 to 3 hours after a meal and stores are depleted after 30 hours of fasting in the absence of metabolic stress. Deamination of amino acids from body tissue proteins begins after 4 to 6 hours of fasting to provide a source of blood glucose (gluconeogenesis). Also, fatty acids are mobilized from the body's adipose tissues to provide keto acids as a principal fuel for the heart, brain, and other vital organs. As adaptation to starvation occurs, the body relies less on gluconeogenesis for fuel and uses more ketones to meet metabolic needs. This reduces nitrogen losses and preserves lean body mass. During critical illness adaptation does not occur. Severely ill patients rely heavily on large amounts of glucose and protein for fuel. They often have elevated insulin levels which inhibit the mobilization of fat for energy production and thus increase the reliance on gluconeogenesis with a urinary nitrogen loss of 10 to 15 g/day or greater that continues unchecked. Critical illness can lead to severe depletion of lean body mass. Nutrition support reduces but does not reverse the process.

Any medical treatment has less chance of success if the patient is malnourished. The malnourished hospitalized patient has been referred to as "the skeleton in the hospital closet" with several reports of general malnutrition among hospitalized patients.[2-6] The lack of adequate nutrition to meet metabolic demands is increasingly recognized as a serious concern in medical and surgical patients. Adult malnutrition can be defined as inadequate nutrient intake, digestion, absorption, or metabolism that results in a significant weight change from usual body or ideal body weigh over a defined period.[7] Braunschweig et al[6] reported that as many as 54% of patients admitted to the hospital were malnourished and 31% of these patients declined nutritionally during hospitalization.

In addition, the disease process itself imposes a nutritional risk and affects nutrient requirements. The deterioration of a patient's nutritional status during hospitalization contributes to increased length of hospital stay, development of comorbidities, and cost.[6] Persons with underlying chronic disease, traumatic injury, and the elderly are particularly at risk. Thus the assessment, monitoring, and reassessment of nutritional status becomes an important part of overall care, especially for hospitalized patients (see Chapter 15). For the severely malnourished patient, especially those facing problems such as organ failure or extensive surgery, adequate and consistent provision of nutrition support is indicated. Unless the patient cannot tolerate enteral nutrition, the guiding principle for provision of nutrition support is, "If the gut works, use it." Studies have shown that patients experience fewer infectious complications and shorter length of stay and recover more rapidly when fed enterally rather than parenterally.[8,9]

A general screening and assessment program at hospital admission should be a routine procedure to identify those already in states of malnutrition as well as those at risk of potential malnutrition because of their underlying disease or injury.[6] In the hospital the attending nurse or another healthcare professional may discover eating problems or disorders in a patient and confer with the dietetics professional, who can evaluate any malnutrition risks associated with the current hospitalization and perform a full nutrition assessment.

The registered dietitian conducts the initial nutrition assessment and performs ongoing monitoring of nutritional status. Initial assessment data supply the necessary basis for (1) identifying patients requiring nutrition intervention, (2) determining the appropriate nutrition support route: enteral or parenteral; (3) calculating the patient's nutrient requirements, and (4) determining the specific formulations to meet the requirements. Once therapy begins, careful monitoring maintains optimal therapy and avoids metabolic, septic, and gastrointestinal complications.

GUIDELINES FOR NUTRITION ASSESSMENT

Nutrition assessment is done through a standard approach and includes several key parameters: (1) evaluation of nutrient intake and adequacy, (2) nutrition-focused physical assessment, (3) biochemical laboratory data, (4) anthropometrics, and (5) comprehensive review of medical and surgical histories.[10] Nutrition assessment techniques and parameters are described in detail in Chapter 15. However, the standard nutrition assessment parameters are skewed by the effects of critical illness and the inflammatory response. Adequacy of nutrients is affected by requirements which change with different disease states and metabolic conditions. Weight is often affected by fluid status and may no longer be indicative of usual or current body weight. Laboratory values are often not reflective of nutrition, particularly if patients have inadequate liver or renal function, acid-base imbalance, or abnormal hydration status. Constitutive hepatic proteins such as serum albumin, transferrin, and prealbumin are decreased as a result of inflammation and no longer reflect nutritional status; therefore the clinician must rely primarily on subjective global assessment (Box 17-1) and astute clinical judgment to perform and interpret the assessment of nutri-

BOX 17-1 Subjective Global Assessment Components

History
Change in weight
Change in dietary intake
Gastrointestinal symptoms
Functional capacity
Nutritional requirements of disease

Physical Assessment
Loss of subcutaneous fat
Muscle loss
Fluid retention
- Ankle and sacral edema
- Ascites

From Detsky AS et al: What is subjective global assessment of nutritional status? *J Parenter Enteral Nutr* 11(1):8-13, 1987.

TABLE 17-1 Categorization of Severity of Weight Loss by Percentage of Weight Lost Over Time

Time Period	Significant Weight Loss (%)	Severe Weight Loss (%)
1 wk	1-2	>2
1 mo	5	>5
3 mo	7.5	>7.5
6 mo	10	>10

Adapted from the American Society for Parenteral and Enteral Nutrition (A.S.P.E.N.): Nutritional and metabolic assessment of the hospitalized patient, *J Parenter Enteral Nutr* 1(1):11-22, 1977. NOTE: A.S.P.E.N. does not endorse the use of this material in any other form than its entirety.

tional status.[5] Subjective global assessment focuses on two features: history and physical examination.[5] This technique eliminates the ambiguity and nonspecific, nonsensitive nature of laboratory values during critical illness and inflammation.

History

The history includes all aspects of the patient's health: weight change, nutrient intake, gastrointestinal function and symptoms, functional capacity, and the diagnosis and its nutritional impact. The clinician should identify whether the patient has experienced a weight change from normal or usual weight and the time frame during which the weight loss occurred. The extent of weight loss is not always clear, particularly if the patient has lost lean body mass but is retaining fluid as occurs with end-stage liver, heart, and kidney diseases. Current or actual body weight (ABW) and height are interpreted according to changes from usual body weight (UBW) and the percent of recent weight change:

$$\text{Percent usual body weight} = \text{ABW} \div \text{UBW} \times 100$$

$$\text{Percent weight change} = [(\text{UBW} - \text{ABW}) \div \text{UBW}] \times 100$$

The amount of recent weight change is compared with values associated with malnutrition (Table 17-1). However, weight can be misleading if the patient has fluid retention with edema and anasarca or if the patient has undergone an amputation.

Changes in appetite and dietary intake must be assessed to identify overall nutrient adequacy of the diet and potential contributing factors for reported weight loss. It is important to identify diet modifications followed and nutritional supplements consumed by the patient. Gastrointestinal function determines the ability to assimilate nutrients. The presence of nausea, vomiting, diarrhea, and anorexia inhibits nutrient intake and availability. Assessment of the functional capacity of the patient determines whether the patient can perform the activities of daily living completely or in part or if the patient is bedridden and totally dependent on others for care. Medical and surgical history entails examination of what the past and current medical problems have been and enables the clinician to identify potential risks for nutrient inadequacies and deficiencies.

Physical Examination

During the physical assessment, the clinician looks for the signs of muscle and fat wasting. Inspection of the upper body can identify temporal, clavicular, and torso wasting of skeletal muscle mass and subcutaneous fat. Signs of edema and ascites indicate inability to keep fluid in the vascular space with subsequent interstitial fluid accumulation. The physical manifestations are then correlated to the patient's disease process and current medical condition.

Basal Energy Expenditure

An estimate of an adult patient's energy needs can be performed using more than 200 different calculations. The Harris-Benedict equations (HBE) are the most commonly used formulas for estimating basal energy expenditure. Energy requirements are estimated by determining basal energy expenditures (BEE), disease/injury energy needs, and physical activity (see Chapter 6). The energy needs of critically ill patients are not as great as originally thought. In hospitalized patients, the increased energy requirements of the disease are often offset by decreased levels of activity.

enteral A feeding modality that provides nutrients, either orally or by tube feeding through the gastrointestinal tract.

The HBE involve measures of weight in kilograms, height in centimeters, and age in years.[11]

$$\text{Women: BEE} = 655\ [9.6 \times \text{weight (kg)}] + [1.8 \times \text{height (cm)}] - [4.7 \times \text{age (yr)}]$$

$$\text{Men: BEE} = 66.5\ [13.8 \times \text{weight (kg)}] + [5.0 \times \text{height (cm)}] - [6.8 \times \text{age (yr)}]$$

The term resting energy expenditure (REE) is often used interchangeably with BEE in discussing basal energy needs. In general, caloric provision to critically ill patients should not exceed 20% above BEE/REE. However, there are metabolic conditions such as severe burns or head injury that create energy needs up to 50% to 100% above BEE. The more malnourished a patient is, the more carefully resumption of nutrition should be done. Refeeding syndrome is a life-threatening response to overaggressive provision of kilocalories (kcalories) to a patient who has been chronically starved. The hallmark symptoms of refeeding are an intracellular shift of electrolytes with resulting hypokalemia, hypophosphatemia, and hypomagnesemia along with hyperglycemia and fluid retention.[12] The end result can be congestive heart failure and death.

Critically ill patients with major trauma, sepsis, and systemic inflammatory response syndrome (SIRS) demonstrate catabolism resulting in a net loss of body mass. Nitrogen lost in the urine can be as high as 15 to 30 g over 24 hours. This results in a negative nitrogen balance because the patient is losing more nitrogen than is provided from nitrogen/protein sources. Catabolic periods with losses of body resources are inevitable after trauma and extensive surgery. The catabolic process increases nutrient demand and requirements. Initiating nutrition support in these patients reduces, but does not eliminate, the negative nitrogen balance that occurs after traumatic injury or critical illness.

Nitrogen Balance

Nitrogen balance studies are calculations that estimate of the degree of catabolism. The patient's intake of protein (nitrogen) is subtracted from nitrogen output through urinary and insensible losses:

$$N_2 \text{ balance} = N_2 \text{ intake} - N_2 \text{ loss}$$

N_2 intake = protein intake ÷ 6.25* $\quad$ N_2 loss = urinary urea nitrogen + 4**

*6.25 g of protein yields 1 g N_2 $\quad$ **Estimated insensible losses of N_2

However, nitrogen balance calculation is not accurate with renal failure or retained nitrogen such as elevated blood urea nitrogen. Other sources of nitrogen such as blood products as well as losses of nitrogen from wounds, stool, nasogastric suction, and bleeding must also be taken into account when calculating nitrogen balance. The 4 g of insensible nitrogen loss may not be an accurate estimate and could affect accuracy of the results. Measurement of urinary urea nitrogen requires an accurate 24-hour urine collection. Nitrogen balance should be performed serially to monitor changes in status because the patient's condition does not remain constant.

Hepatic Proteins as Nutrition Indicators

Hepatic proteins, albumin, transferrin, and prealbumin are often used as indicators of nutrition status. During critical illness, the hepatic production of constitutive proteins—albumin, transferrin, and prealbumin—is decreased in favor of increased production of acute phase reactants required for survival.[13] A decreased serum value of the plasma constitutive proteins therefore signifies an inflammatory process and not nutritional status. Serum albumin (half-life, 21 days) is neither sensitive nor specific for nutrition in critically ill patients. The half-live of transferrin is 8 to 10 days. However, when evaluating transferrin it is important to evaluate serum iron and ferritin to determine other factors that could be affecting serum transferrin levels. Prealbumin (half-life, 2 to 3 days) is a more sensitive marker of current status but is also affected by inflammation and therefore requires interpretation with consideration for the patient's condition. Serum levels of albumin, transferrin, and prealbumin can be followed serially over time, and trends in improvement can be monitored for abatement of the inflammatory process.

MANAGEMENT OF NUTRITION SUPPORT PATIENTS

The management of nutrition support is ideally performed by an official interdisciplinary nutrition support committee or team composed of designated members from the departments of medicine, surgery, nutrition, nursing, and pharmacy.[14] Each team member should be certified in nutrition support by an accrediting body such as the National Board of Nutrition Support Certification and the Board of Pharmaceutical Specialties. The American Society for Parenteral and Enteral Nutrition has developed standards of practice for nutrition support professionals and interdisciplinary nutrition support competencies.[15-19] However, in many facilities, nutrition support management is overseen by an informal collection of interested clinicians, a sole nutrition support practitioner, or no one person in particular. The new standards of the Joint Commission on Accreditation of Healthcare Organizations (JCAHO) and the Accreditation Manual for Hospitals (AMH) have focused on key multidisciplinary processes that ensure performance of nutrition screening and assessment to promote quality patient outcomes.[20]

Baseline nutritional data obtained before starting nutrition support provide a means of measuring effectiveness of treatment. At designated periods during therapy, certain tests are repeated to monitor the patient's course and reduce metabolic complications. Specific protocols vary in different medical centers. However, a general guide for standard monitoring data is summarized in Box 17-2.[21]

Generally, clinicians give primary importance to three major monitoring procedures: (1) serial weights to determine adequacy of total kcal provision and monitor fluid status, (2) physical examination for micronutrient adequacy and changes in body fat and muscle mass, and, ultimately, (3) improvement in functional status. All baseline and monitoring data are recorded in the patient's chart, along with all enteral and parenteral solution orders.

There are no evidence-based "rules" for when patients should begin specialized nutrition support. The determination of when to initiate nutrition support depends on the patient's nutritional status and the anticipated time period before oral diet can be resumed and tolerated. The American Society for Parenteral and Enteral Nutrition (A.S.P.E.N.) guidelines recommend that nutrition support should be considered when patients have had an inadequate oral intake for 7 to 14 days or the patient's oral intake is anticipated to remain inadequate for 7 to 14 days.[7] Other guidelines available to identify when to feed are the "rule of five" and degree of weight loss. The "rule of five" states that if a patient has had no food for 5 days and is unable to tolerate an oral diet for an additional 5 days, nutrition support should be considered to reduce the risk of developing iatrogenic malnutrition. The weight loss rule stratifies patients according to the percentage of weight loss of their usual body weight over a designated period (see Table 17-1). Patients who have undergone severe the weight loss and are unable to tolerate oral nutrition for 5 to 7 days or longer are potential candidates for nutrition support.

BOX 17-2 Clinical Parameters to Monitor During Nutrition Support

Daily input and output (I/O)
Daily weights
Physical examination
Temperature, pulse, respirations
Laboratory parameters

- Acid-base status
- Blood urea nitrogen (BUN)
- Complete blood cell count (CBC)
- Creatinine
- Electrolytes
- Glucose
- Hepatic proteins
- International normalized ratio (INR)
- Liver function tests
- Osmolarity, serum and urine
- Platelet Count
- Prothrombin time (PT)
- Triglyceride level
- Urinary urea nitrogen
- Urine specific gravity
- Vitamins and minerals

Enteral Nutrition Versus Parenteral Nutrition

There is ongoing debate concerning evidence-based effectiveness of parenteral and enteral nutrition support. Questions focus on what constitutes early enteral nutrition, how to select the most appropriate enteral feeding formula according to each patient's specific disease state, what is the preferred method of formula delivery, and which factors contribute to tube feeding-related complications, such as diarrhea or respiratory problems.[22] In all cases when the gastrointestinal tract is functioning, enteral nutrition support should be used to restore or maintain an optimal state of nutrition. PN should be reserved for patients without a functional gastrointestinal tract. In some cases the patient can take some enteral feeding but impairment in either digestive or absorptive capacity requires supplementation with parenteral therapy. The VA Cooperative Study showed that perioperative nutrition support was beneficial for severely malnourished patients but contributed to increased complications in mild to moderately malnourished patients.[23] The gastrointestinal tract should always be the first choice for nutrition support. Figure 17-1 provides an algorithm for determining the route of nutrition support.[24]

PN is associated with serious complications, as shown in Box 17-3. Reliance on PN when the gastrointestinal tract is functional can contribute to disuse of the alimentary tract with subsequent bacterial overgrowth, hepatic abnormalities, deterioration of gastrointestinal integrity with subsequent migration of intestinal bacteria into the systemic circulation, and sepsis. Patients reliant solely on PN are at risk for septic and hepatic complications that can contribute to morbidity and mortality. Some of the adverse effects of PN may be related to the inability to provide all the necessary nutrients parenterally. Parenteral solutions are not as "complete" (i.e., do not contain the variety of nutrients) as enteral formulas or oral diet. Certain nutrients, such as glutamine, choline, and short-chain fatty acids, are not standard components of commercially available parenteral formulas. Nutrients that are considered nonessential, such as phytochemicals,

constitutive proteins Albumin, prealbumin, transferrin. Plasma proteins often used to assess the response to nutrition support. Serum levels are nonspecific and nonsensitive to the nutritional care or requirements of critically ill patients.

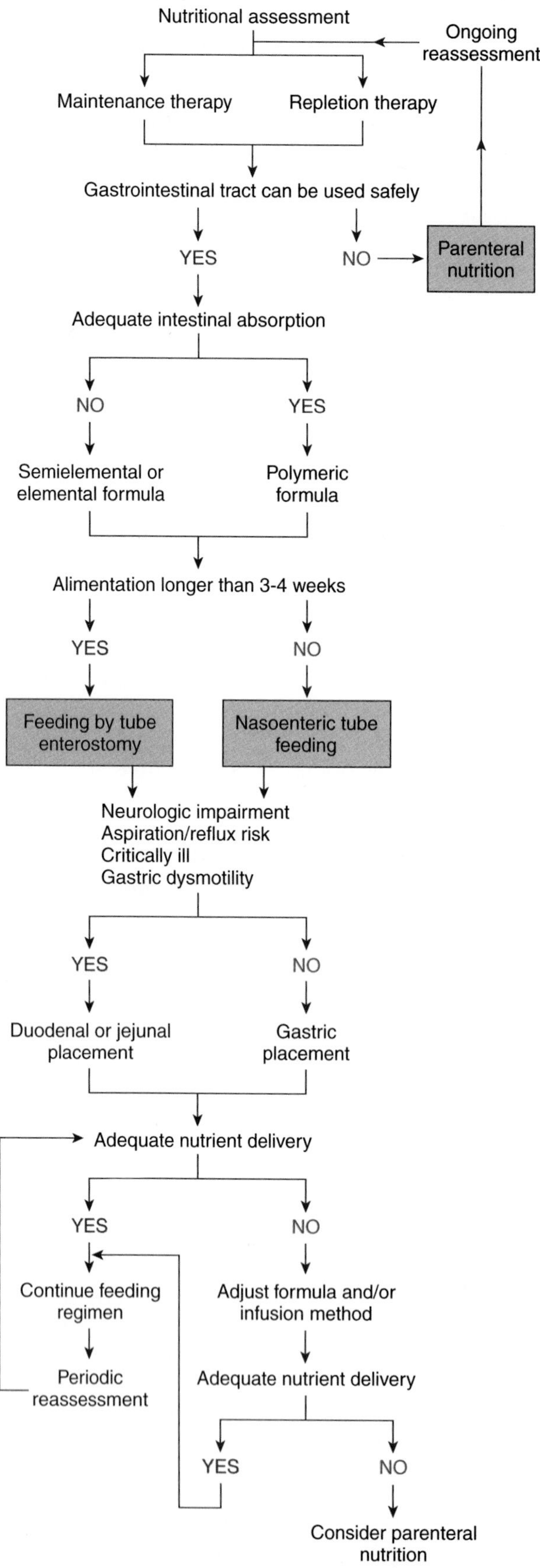

FIGURE 17-1 Algorithm for providing nutrition support. (*Adapted from Guenter P et al: Delivery systems and administration of enteral feeding. In Rombeau JL, Rolandelli RH, eds:* Clinical nutrition: enteral and tube feeding, *ed 3, Philadelphia, 1997, WB Saunders.*)

BOX 17-3 Complications Associated With Parenteral Nutrition

Catheter related	Gastrointestinal	Metabolic
Air embolism	Fatty liver	Acid-base imbalance
Catheter embolization	Gastric hyperacidity	Electrolyte abnormalities
Catheter occlusion	Gastrointestinal atrophy	Essential fatty acid deficiency
Improper tip location	Hepatic cholestasis	Fluid imbalance
Phlebitis		Glucose intolerance
Pneumothorax		Mineral abnormalities
Sepsis		Overfeeding
Venous thrombosis		Refeeding syndrome
		Triglyceride elevation

carotenoids, and fiber, are not contained in PN formulas. Nutrients such as manganese may be provided in excess of needs, whereas other nutrients such as antioxidants may not be given in adequate amounts for specific disease requirements.

Enteral Feeding in Clinical Nutrition

MODES OF ENTERAL NUTRITION SUPPORT

Many patients with a functioning gastrointestinal tract do not or cannot eat a sufficient amount of nutrients by mouth to restore, repair, or maintain physiologic systems or body tissues. The first option for providing adequate nutrition should be to deliver nutrients orally. The patient can be given small, frequent nutrient-dense meals with an oral defined formula supplement. If oral intake remains suboptimal despite attempts to augment kcal with supplements and diet modulation, enteral tube feeding can be initiated to meet nutrient requirements for restoration of health. If it is not feasible to use the gastrointestinal tract for feeding or if the gastrointestinal tract cannot effectively provide consistent and adequate nutrition, PN may be an appropriate feeding modality. Therefore the questions that must be answered are as follows.

1. Does the patient require nutrition support?
2. What is the optimal route of feeding?
3. What formulation is needed, and how should it be provided?
4. Does the patient require long-term nutrition support?

Oral Diet

When a patient does not consume a nutritionally complete diet, the energy value of foods in the oral diet can be increased according to patient tolerance and preference with added sauces, seasonings, and dressings. Frequent, less bulky, concentrated small meals may be helpful so that the patient is not overwhelmed or discouraged by a tray full of food. If a patient is on a modified diet, liberalization of the diet as much as feasible can help improve oral intake. For example, changing from a regimented 1800-kcalorie diabetic diet to a no-concentrated-sweets diet allows the patient more flexibility in food selection. It may be necessary to liberalize to a nonrestricted diet. Depending on the patient's condition and food preferences, an oral liquid nutritional supplement, commercially available or made in-house, can be provided with or between meals. However, taste fatigue can happen fairly rapidly when patients are receiving two to six cans of an oral supplement per day. It is important to offer supplements in a variety of flavors and textures to maintain adequate consumption. Some facilities, particularly long-term care providers, have found that dispensing oral supplements in small amounts of 30 to 60 ml during times when medications are administered improved oral nutritional supplement intake and nutrient delivery.[25,26]

Tube Feeding

If a sufficient oral intake of nutrients is not possible, then the next option is enteral nutrition by tube feeding, either as a supplement to oral dietary intake or as the sole source of nutrition.

INDICATIONS FOR ENTERAL NUTRITION

The American Society for Parenteral and Enteral Nutrition has published guidelines for indications for nutrition support.[7] Enteral nutrition support is indicated for patients who are or who are likely to become malnourished and unable or unwilling to consume adequate nutrition. Factors that affect the decision to provide enteral nutrition include the patient's preadmission nutritional state, risk for malnutrition based on current disease/condition, ability to consume a nutritionally complete oral diet, and functional status of the gastrointestinal tract. An indication for nutrition support for a previously well-nourished medical-surgical patient is the inability to eat for more than 7 to 14 days. Research finds no benefit of aggressive early enteral nutrition support for patients who were not malnourished versus those who waited 6 days to begin an

TABLE 17-2 Categories and Macronutrient Sources for Various Types of Enteral Formulas

Type of Formula	Protein Sources	Carbohydrate Sources	Fat Sources	Kcalories/ml	Protein Content	Nonprotein Calorie-to-Nitrogen Ratio	Examples
Intact (Polymeric)							
	Calcium and magnesium caseinates Sodium and calcium caseinates Soy protein isolate Calcium-potassium caseinate Delactosed lactalbumin Egg white solids Beef Nonfat milk	Maltodextrin Corn syrup solids Sucrose Cornstarch Glucose polymers Sugar Vegetables Fruits Nonfat milk	Medium-chain triglycerides Canola oil Corn oil Lecithin Soybean oil Partially hydrogenated soybean oil High-oleic safflower oil Beef fat	1-2	30-84 g/L	75-177:1	Boost (MJ) Compleat (No) Compleat Modified (No) Fibersource Standard (No) Isocal (MJ) Isosource Standard (No) Jevity (R) Magnacal Renal (MJ) Nepro (R) Nutren 1.0 (Ne) Osmolite (R) Resource Plus (No) Suplena (R) TwoCal HN (R) Ultracal (MJ)
Hydrolyzed (Oligomeric or Monomeric)							
	Enzymatically hydrolyzed whey or casein Soybean or lactalbumin hydrolysate Whey protein Free amino acids Soy protein hydrolysate	Hydrolyzed cornstarch Sucrose Fructose Maltodextrin Tapioca starch Glucose oligosaccharides	Medium-chain triglycerides Sunflower oil Lecithin Soybean oil Safflower oil Corn oil Coconut oil Canola oil Sardine oil	1-1.33	21-52.5 g/L	67-282:1	Advera (R) AlitraQ (R) Criticare HN (MJ) Crucial (Ne) Peptamen (Ne) Perative (R) Reabilan (Ne) Tolerex (No) Vital HN (R) Vivonex Plus (No)
Modular							
Protein	Low-lactose whey and casein Calcium caseinate Free amino acids	—	—	**Per 100 g** 370-424	**Per 100 g** 75-88.5	—	Casec (MJ) ProMod (R) Resource Protein Powder (No)
Carbohydrate	—	Maltodextrin Hydrolyzed cornstarch	—	**Per 100 g** 380-386	—	—	Moducal (MJ) Polycose (R)
Fat	—	—	Safflower oil Polyglycerol esters of fatty acids Soybean oil Lecithin Medium-chain triglycerides Fish oil	**Per 1 tbsp** 67.5-115	—	—	MCT Oil (MJ) Microlipid (MJ)

Adapted from Gottschlich MM, Shronts EP, Hutchins AM: Defined formula diets. In Rombeau JL, Rolandelli RH, eds: *Clinical nutrition: enteral and tube feeding,* ed 3, Philadelphia, 1997, WB Saunders.
MJ, Mead Johnson; *No,* Novartis; *R,* Ross; *Ne,* Nestle.

oral diet.[27] Patients who are malnourished before hospitalization should be fed sooner, within 5 to 7 days.

Enteral Formulas

COMPLETE ENTERAL FORMULAS

Blenderized or Commercial

Our current age of advanced nutrition science and technology has brought a variety of commercial formulas and smaller, safer, more comfortable feeding tubes. The majority of tube feedings in healthcare facilities are given with a defined, commercially prepared enteral formula. However, financial or personal reasons may motivate a patient or family to use blenderized formulas for home enteral feeding. Although there may be emotional comfort in the use of home-prepared food, there are problems involved. These problems involve its physical form, safety, digestion and absorption, and nutrient adequacy.

Physical form. Foods broken down and mixed in a blender generally yield a viscous solution that is difficult to infuse through a feeding tube. Thus because of particle size and tendency to stick to the tube, a large-bore feeding tube that is more uncomfortable is required. The tube must be aggressively flushed with water after each feeding to prevent tube clogging.

Safety. Blenderized formulas are associated with a risk of bacterial growth and inconsistent nutrient composition from settling out of solid components. Preparation and storage methods affect the safety and contamination risk of blenderized formulas. Good hand-washing and thorough washing of the blender and equipment are imperative to reducing bacterial contamination of the enteral formula. The formula must be infused into the stomach and cannot be used for small bowel feedings. The hydrochloric acid and low pH of the stomach are necessary to kill bacteria present in the foods used for formula preparation.

Digestion and absorption. The blended food formula requires a fully functioning digestive and absorptive system to assimilate the nutrients contained in the formula. Patients with gastrointestinal deficits that require nutrients with varying degrees of predigestion (hydrolysis) cannot tolerate the larger molecules contained in a blenderized food formula.

Nutrient adequacy. Food preparation techniques and the variety of foods used to prepare a blenderized food formula will determine the nutrient content, which will vary with different preparation methods and types of foods used. Patients may need to take a micronutrient supplement to meet requirements for all vitamins and minerals.

• • •

In contrast, commercial formulas provide sterile, nutritionally complete, homogenized solutions suitable for small-bore feeding tubes. Enteral formulas are available as polymeric, semielemental or oligomeric, and elemental or monomeric[28] (Table 17-2). It is important to keep abreast of what products are currently available because new formulations and enteral products are constantly being developed. Polymeric enteral formulas require digestion and are available with and without fiber. The macronutrients and micronutrients of a polymeric formula can be modified for the specific needs of patients with various disease states. Semielemental or oligomeric are partially digested or hydrolyzed. The smaller molecules increase the osmolality of the formula. Elemental or monomeric formulas are completely predigested and require only absorption for assimilation into the body. These formulas have the highest osmolality, lowest viscosity, and worst taste of all the enteral formulas. Formulas will also vary according to nutrient density from 1 to 2 kcalories/ml. More concentrated formulas are designed for patients with fluid intolerance, such as those with renal, hepatic, or cardiac failure, as well as for patients who desire less volume or fewer feedings per day. However, it is imperative to provide adequate hydration for patients without a fluid restriction receiving a concentrated enteral formula. A new development in enteral formulas is the addition of microbial inhibitors to protect against bacterial contamination.

NUTRIENT COMPONENTS

Carbohydrates

From 50% to 60% of the kcalories in the American diet come from carbohydrates, starches, and sugars. Carbohydrates are the body's primary energy source. Although the large starch molecules are well tolerated and easily digested by most patients, their relative insolubility creates problems in enteral formulas. Thus the smaller saccharides formed by partial or complete hydrolysis of corn starch are common formula components[28] (see Table 17-2). In addition to the simple sugars glucose and sucrose, the carbohydrate components include intermediate glucose polymers of

osmolality The ability of a solution to create osmotic pressure and determine the movement of water between fluid compartments; determined by the number of osmotically active particles per kilogram of solvent; serum osmolality is 280 to 300 mOsm/kg.

viscous Physical property of a substance dependent on the friction of its component molecules as they slide by one another; viscosity.

varying chain lengths. Very few enteral nutrition formulas contain the disaccharide lactose because lactose intolerance is common among hospitalized patients. Formulas can also contain soluble and insoluble fiber. There is considerable controversy as to the benefit of providing fiber in enteral formulations.[22,28] Insoluble fiber increases stool volume and thus is used to treat problems with gastric motility: constipation and diarrhea. Soluble fiber has been promoted to improve glycemic control, reduce serum cholesterol levels, and maintain colonic mucosal integrity. The focus on maintaining intestinal flora has resulted in increased research and availability of prebiotics and probiotics given with or in enteral feeding formulas. Prebiotics, nondigestible food components, provide the fuels to enhance repletion of the normal bacterial milieu of the gastrointestinal tract, whereas probiotics, live microbes, are designed to repopulate by providing the "good" bacteria directly to the gastrointestinal tract.[29]

Protein

The protein content of standard enteral formulas maintains the body cell mass and promotes tissue synthesis and repair (see Chapter 5). The biologic quality of dietary protein depends on its amino acid profile, especially its relative proportions of essential amino acids. To supply these needs, three major forms of protein are used in nutrition support enteral formulas: intact proteins, hydrolyzed proteins, and crystalline amino acids[28] (see Table 17-2).

1. *Intact proteins.* Intact proteins are the complete and original forms as found in foods, although protein isolates such as lactalbumin and casein from milk are intact proteins that have been separated from their original food source.
2. *Hydrolyzed proteins.* Hydrolyzed proteins are protein sources that have been broken down by enzymes into smaller protein fragments and amino acids. These smaller products—tripeptides, dipeptides, and free amino acids—are absorbed more readily into the blood circulation. The larger peptides must be broken down further before they can be absorbed.
3. *Crystalline amino acids.* Pure crystalline amino acids are easily absorbed. The small size of the amino acid results in an increase in the osmolality of the formula. Amino acids result in a bitter-tasting formula. If an elemental formula is used as an oral supplement, it requires flavoring aids or special preparation methods to improve palatability, for example, pudding, frozen slush, or Popsicle. However, despite flavorings, the taste can still be unacceptable to a sick patient or can quickly lead to taste fatigue and refusal by the patient.

Fat

The major roles of fat in an enteral nutrition formula are to supply a concentrated energy source, essential fatty acids, and a transport mechanism for fat-soluble vitamins. The major forms of fat used in standard formulas are butterfat in milk-based mixtures; vegetable oils from corn, soy, safflower, or sunflower; medium-chain triglycerides (MCT); and lecithin[28] (see Table 17-2). Vegetable oils supply a rich source of the essential fatty acids—linoleic and linolenic acids. Current research is examining outcomes related to enteral formulas containing various combinations of short-chain fatty acids, medium-chain fatty acids, and omega-3 fatty acids (see Chapter 4).[30,31]

Vitamins and Minerals

Standard whole diet commercial formulas provide 100% of the Recommended Dietary Allowance (RDA) and Dietary Reference Intake (DRI) for vitamins and minerals when the formula is provided at a specific volume per day. The volume required to provide the RDA/DRI varies with each formula and the nutrient requirements of the patient. Delivery of reduced kcalories and use of diluted formulas may require supplementation with vitamin and mineral preparations. Patients with nutrient deficiencies may require supplementation of some micronutrients in addition to the standard vitamin and mineral composition of the enteral formula. Several enteral formulas are designed for specific patient populations and contain micronutrients designed to meet the requirements of the particular disease state or condition.

PHYSICAL PROPERTIES

After selecting a formula according to the patient's nutritional requirements and gastrointestinal function, the clinician must consider the physical properties of the formula that can affect tolerance. Individual intolerance is reflected in gastric retention, abdominal distention and pain, diarrhea, or constipation. A factor often evaluated when a patient demonstrates intolerance is the osmolality of the enteral formula. Osmolality is based on the concentration of the formula and defined as the number of osmotic particles per kilogram of solvent (water), the kcalorie-nutrient density, and residue content. However, there is no evidence that enteral formula osmolality is the primary contributor to formula intolerance. Manifestations of enteral feeding intolerance, of which diarrhea is the most common, are more often related to inappropriate tube-feeding techniques or drug interactions (see *Issues & Answers*).

MEDICAL FOODS FOR SPECIAL NEEDS

Certain formulas designed for special nutrition therapy are called medical foods. The U.S. Food and Drug Administration (FDA) first recognized the concept of medical foods as distinct from drugs in 1972, when the first special formula was developed for treatment of the genetic disease phenylketonuria (PKU) in newborns (see Chapter 18). The definition of "medical foods" remained rather murky as medical research developed an increasing number of special formulas. In 1988 Congress amended the Orphan Drug Act to include medical foods, defining them as food specifically formulated for use under medical supervision for primary treatment of metabolic-genetic diseases having distinctive nutritional requirements based on recognized scientific principles.[32] The Orphan Drug Act Amendment was subsequently incorporated into the reformed Nutrition Labeling and Education Act of 1990.

There has been an explosion of specialty enteral formulas developed over the past 10 years. There are several products available in each category of disease- or condition-specific formulation: (1) end-stage renal disease, (2) hepatic disease, (3) pulmonary disease, (4) diabetes mellitus, (5) malabsorption syndromes, (6) immunoincompetence, and (7) metabolic stress. Indications for specialty enteral formulas are limited to a small subset of patients within each disease state classification for which a specialty formula is designed. There is considerable discussion on the treatment- and cost-effectiveness of specialty enteral formulas with continued need for scientific evidence to support their use.[22]

MODULAR ENTERAL FORMULAS

The commercial complete enteral formula products for tube feeding are designed with a fixed ratio of nutrients to meet general standards for nutritional needs. However, some patients' particular needs are not met by these standard fixed-ratio formulas, and they require an individualized modular formula. An individual formula, composed completely of modular components, is planned, calculated, prepared, and administered with the expertise of the registered dietitian. Modular enteral components are listed in Table 17-2. However, the more common use of modular components is the addition of either carbohydrate, fat, or protein to a commercial formula to individualize the calorie and protein content of the formula for the patient. Other modular nutrients such as fiber and probiotics or prebiotics can also be added to the feeding regimen but should be given separately through the feeding tube and not added directly to the commercial enteral formulation. Every component added to an enteral formula can increase the osmolality and viscosity of the formula and contribute to feeding intolerance, bacterial contamination, or occlusion of the feeding tube.

Blue food dye is often added to enteral formulas to detect aspiration of the formula into the trachea and lungs. There is considerable debate as to the safety, specificity, and sensitivity of blue dye in identifying aspiration in tube fed patients. The addition of blue food dye increases the risk of bacterial contamination, false-positive occult stool test, discoloration of the skin and body fluids, and death.[33,34] There also is no standardization for how much food dye to add per liter of enteral formula, with formula hues ranging from pale to cobalt blue. In general, about 1 ml of blue food dye for each liter of enteral formula is sufficient.[35] Blue food dye should only be added if aspiration is suspected and should not be added for a prolonged period or to septic patients. Methylene blue should not be added to enteral feeding formulas because it can adversely affect cellular function.[36] Development of a completely modular formula or the addition of a modular component to a commercial formula increases the risk of bacterial contamination of the formula.

Enteral Nutrition Delivery Systems

FEEDING EQUIPMENT

Nasoenteric Feeding Tubes

Small-bore nasoenteric feeding tubes, generally from 8 to 12 French, made of softer, more flexible polyurethane and silicone materials have replaced former large-bore stiff tubing. Small-bore feeding tubes are more comfortable for patients and permit the infusion of commercially available enteral nutrition formulas. Nasoenteric tubes can be inserted into either the stomach or beyond the pyloric valve into the small intestine: duodenum or jejunum[37] (Figure 17-2). Distal placement of a feeding tube beyond the ligament of Treitz is often preferred for patients with a history or risk of aspiration, gastric dysmotility, depressed gag reflex, neurologic impairment, and critical illness.[24] Insertion can be done blindly at the bedside or using radiographic visualization. Placement of a feeding tube should be performed by experienced, trained personnel. Feeding tube placement is an invasive procedure and carries the risk of misplacement into the lungs or brain, as well as perforation of the gastrointestinal tract. During placement, aspirates of gastrointestinal contents can be checked for pH and enzyme concentration, as well as visually inspected to reduce the number of radiographs required to determine when the desired location has been reached.[38] However, no enteral infusion of nutrients should be started until feeding tube placement is confirmed by radiography.

Feeding Enterostomies

Nasoenteric tube placement is usually indicated for short-term therapy. However, for enteral feeding anticipated to exceed more than 3 to 4 weeks, surgically or endoscopically placed enterostomies at progressive points along the gastrointestinal tract are preferred[37] (see Figure 17-2).

medical foods Specially formulated nutrient mixtures for use under medical supervision to treat various metabolic diseases.

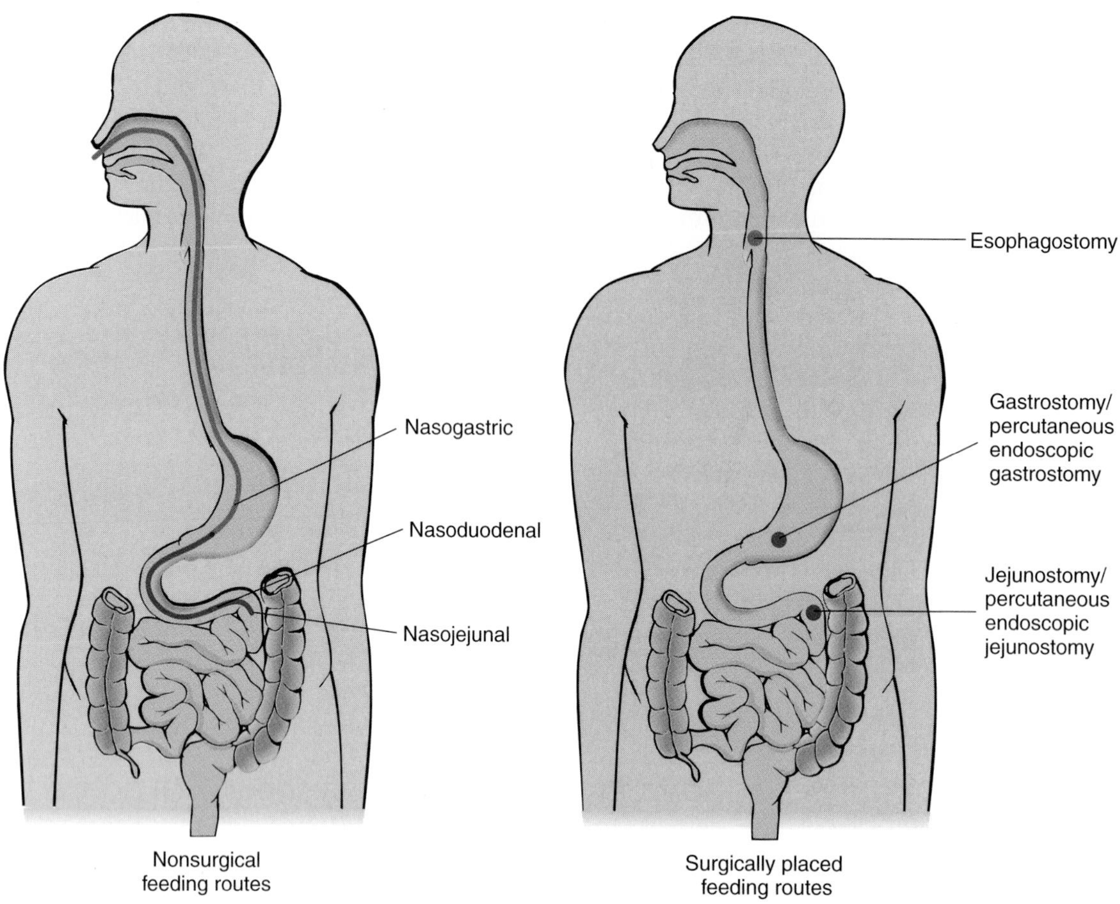

FIGURE 17-2 Types of enteral feeding routes. (*From Rolin Graphics in Grodner M, Anderson SL, DeYoung S:* Foundations and clinical applications of nutrition: a nursing approach, *ed 2, St Louis, 2000, Mosby.*)

General Comfort Tips for Patients on Nasoenteric Tube Feedings

- *Thirst, oral dryness.* Lubricate lips, chew sugarless gum, brush teeth, rinse mouth frequently with water, suck lemon drops occasionally. If small amounts of water by mouth is permitted, let ice cubes melt in mouth to soothe mouth and esophagus.
- *Tube discomfort.* Gargle with a mixture of warm water and mouthwash, gently blow nose, and clean tube regularly with water-soluble lubricant. If persistent, pull tube out gently, clean it, and reinsert a new tube. (Many long-term users of tube feeding have learned to pass their own nasogastric tubes.)
- *Tension, fullness.* Relax and breathe deeply after each feeding.
- *Loud stomach noises.* Take feedings in private.
- *Limited mobility.* Change positions in bed or chair, and walk around the house or hospital corridor. Perform range-of-motion exercises while confined to bed.
- *General gustatory distress with feeding.* Warm or chill feedings, but avoid having formula too cold because that increases risk of diarrhea. Consider occasional use of blender-mixed "regular" foods—only if patient is fed into the stomach.
- *Persistent hunger.* Chew a favorite food, then spit it out; chew gum, or suck lemon drops.
- *Inability to drink.* Rinse mouth frequently with water or other liquids.

- *Esophagostomy.* A cervical esophagostomy can be placed at the level of the cervical spine to the side of the neck after head and neck surgeries for cancer or traumatic injury. This removes the discomfort of a nasoenteric tube, and the entry point can be concealed under clothing.
- *Gastrostomy.* A gastrostomy tube is surgically or endoscopically placed in the stomach if the patient is not at risk for aspiration and has normal gastric motility.
- *Jejunostomy.* A jejunostomy tube is surgically or endoscopically placed in the jejunum or distal duodenum, the middle section of the small intestine. This proce-

dure is indicated for patients with neurologic impairment, a risk or history of aspiration, an incompetent gag reflex or gastric dysfunction. Gastric dysfunction can be related to gastric atony, gastroparesis, gastric cancer, gastric outlet obstruction, or gastric ulcerative disease.

Care and Maintenance of Enteral Feeding Tubes

Enteral feeding tubes should be flushed routinely with water to maintain patency and prevent clogging. Tap water is generally sufficient. If there is concern about the safety of the water source or if the patient is immunosuppressed, sterile water should be used to flush the feeding tube. Standard flushing volumes are 30 ml of water every 4 hours during continuous feedings. Water flushes for intermittent and bolus enteral feedings are a minimum of 30 ml immediately after each feeding. The amount of water flushed through the tube is adjusted according to the patient's fluid requirements and tolerance. Larger fluid volumes will be needed for patients who cannot drink water for hydration; smaller fluid volumes are needed for patients on fluid restrictions.

Ideally no medications should be put down small-bore feeding tubes because medications are a primary contributor to feeding tube clogs. However, the reality of life often requires the administration of medications via feeding tubes. Flush with 30 ml water before and after medication administration. Each medication should be administered separately with 5 ml water flushed through the tube between each medication. Check with a pharmacist when determining which medications are compatible with administration through a feeding tube. Medications should never be added directly to the enteral formula because of the risk of drug-nutrient interactions. Warm water, a 30- to 60-ml syringe, and a pumping action can be used to dislodge a clog within the feeding tube. No evidence supports the use of other liquids such as soft drinks or juices to declog feeding tubes.[39] A pancreatic enzyme and bicarbonate mixture may be effective against formula clogs but will not affect medication clogs.[40]

Containers and Pumps

The enteric tube feeding system includes the formula container, connection tubing, and often an infusion pump. A variety of containers and feeding sets are available. Formulas can be administered by syringe, gravity drip, or a volumetric pump. A pump may be needed for more accurate control, which is essential for feedings given directly into the small intestine or for more viscous formulas. Critically ill patients should also be enterally fed by volumetric pump to increase tolerance to enteral nutrition support.

Delivery systems are categorized as either open or closed. An open delivery system involves pouring a volume of formula from a can or mixing bowl/container into an empty bag, syringe, or infusion container. The infusion bag/container is reopened and refilled periodically with more formula. Clean technique is required when decanting the formula into the bag and when handling the tubing connections. Formula hang time is limited to 8 hours or less.[20,41] The hang time is further reduced if additives such as protein powder or food dye are placed into the formula. The infusion bag should be rinsed with sterile water before the initial filling and subsequent refilling with formula.[20] The administration set, tubing and infusion bag, should be changed every 24 hours. The primary benefit of the open system is the ability to modulate the enteral formula.

The closed system is composed of a sterile vessel that is purchased prefilled with enteral formula. The container is spiked and connected to an infusion pump. There is less manipulation of the formula and tubing and hence less risk of bacterial contamination.[42,43] The hang time is expanded to 24 to 48 hours (refer to manufacturer's guidelines for hang time of product being used). The benefits of the closed system are a reduction of time, labor, and contamination risk. Caveats of the closed system are its higher cost and the inability to modulate the formula. Regardless of the system used, good hand-washing is essential for reduction in bacterial contamination. In the final analysis, regardless of the type of formula and equipment that are used, microbiologic quality control programs maintained by healthcare personnel are essential.[42,43] Clinicians working with patients on tube feedings need to be familiar with the different delivery systems, types of enteral feeding tubes, and features of enteral feeding pumps to determine which products are preferable for their facility and patient population.

Infusion of Enteral Tube Feeding

Tube feedings can be provided via bolus, intermittent, or continuous infusion through a feeding tube. Patients can progress from one infusion modality to another as their medical condition changes. All enteral feedings should be initiated at full strength. Tolerance to tube feeding has not been shown to be improved with dilution of the formula.[44] Enteral feedings should be introduced gradually and progressed per patient tolerance. Gastric feedings can be given as bolus, intermittent, or continuous feedings. Small bowel feedings are given as continuous feedings.

Bolus feeding is generally initiated with 120 to 240 ml of formula every 3 to 4 hours and increased by 60 to 240 ml every 8 to 12 hours depending on degree of illness and tolerance. The infusion period is relatively short, 10 to 20 minutes, and is infused through a syringe or from a bag by the flow of gravity.[45] The infusion should not exceed 40 to 60 ml/min. Gravity infusion is controlled by a roller clamp, raising or lowering the formula container, or advancing the plunger into the syringe.

Intermittent feedings are similar to bolus feedings but are given over a longer time period of 30 to 60 minutes every 3 to 6 hours. The enteral formula is placed in a bag with the rate controlled by a roller clamp. This method is used to provide periodic gastric feedings to patients who do not tolerate the more rapid infusion of a bolus feeding. The maximum amount of formula given by bolus or intermittent feedings varies from 300 to 500 ml per feeding and is based on patient tolerance and requirements.

Continuous feedings are provided over a defined period with the formula infused by gravity or pump. Continuous feedings can be given over 24 hours or cycled over a shorter period, such as 8 to 20 hours per day. Enteral feeding tolerance is generally better in critically ill patients who are fed continuously regardless of whether fed into the stomach or small bowel.

All patients fed through a feeding tube should have the head of the bed elevated 30° to 45° to reduce the risk of aspiration of gastric contents.[46] Patients fed with a tube into the small bowel can still aspirate gastric contents and may require concomitant gastric decompression during small bowel feeding.[47] In addition, feeding tubes, particularly nasoenteric feeding tubes, can migrate from the small bowel into the stomach. Patients who must lie flat or in Trendelenburg's position should have enteral feedings stopped.

Monitoring the Tube-Fed Patient

Monitoring of the tube-fed patient should focus on transitioning to an oral diet and reducing or eliminating dependency on tube feeding. All patients who are being nourished by tube feeding should be carefully monitored for signs and symptoms of enteral feeding intolerance. Tolerance to enteral nutrition is determined by gastrointestinal signs of vomiting, abdominal distention or bloating, and frequency and consistency of bowel movements. If problems occur, the feeding may need to be changed to a different formula or the infusion adjusted to be given more slowly with continuous rather than intermittent or bolus feeding until tolerance improves and symptoms subside. However, in most instances, the enteral formula itself is not the causative agent for the intolerance. Two parameters—residual volume and diarrhea—are often used to determine tolerance to tube feeding. Both are nebulous terms often used with no standardized meaning within each institution, much less nationwide standard definitions.

Diarrhea is generally defined by the person cleaning it up and can be based on volume, frequency, or consistency of the stools. There are 14 definitions of diarrhea in the literature.[48] Commonly used definitions are greater than three stools per day or more than 500 ml of stool/day for 2 consecutive days.[49] Each healthcare facility should define diarrhea and then create an algorithm or protocol for treatment to reduce unnecessary interruptions of enteral feeding.[49] The most common etiology of diarrhea in the tube-fed patient is medications, primarily antibiotics and medications containing sorbitol (see *Issues & Answers*).

Residual volume interpretation is also often determined by caregiver experience and not evidence-based guidelines. A research study defined acceptable residual volume as less than 200 ml with an nasogastric tube and less than 100 ml with a gastrostomy tube.[50] The authors suggested that high residual volumes be correlated with the presence of physical signs of intolerance before stopping enteral feeding. Another study found that if patients were given a prophylactic prokinetic agent, a residual volume of 250 ml was tolerated.[51] Residual volume can vary based on the position of the patient, for example, a patient who is lying on his or her right side could have a greater residual volume than if the patient were lying flat or sitting upright. It is best to measure the residual volume when the patient is in a semirecumbent or upright sitting position. There should be no residual volume with small bowel feeding. If residual volumes occur with small bowel feedings, verify tube placement because small-bore tubes often migrate back into the proximal small bowel, stomach, and esophagus, particularly in critically ill patients with nasoenteric feeding tubes.

It is imperative that the staff nurse or clinician administering the formula to the patient checks for gastric residuals or gastric emptying rate, noting any signs of abdominal distention or bloating, and monitors vital signs—temperature, pulse, and respiration. Because gastrointestinal aspirates contain gastric enzymes and hydrochloric acid required for digestion, electrolytes, enteral formula, and fluid, the aspirates should be returned to the patient after determining the volume. However, if doing so would make the patient uncomfortable or if the volume removed exceeds 300 ml, discard the residuals and recheck in 1 to 2 hours. The feeding tube should be flushed with 30 ml water after checking and returning residuals to be sure the gastric contents with digestive enzymes are no longer within the lumen of the feeding tube. Attending nurses also monitor the flow rate and record the intake of formula, water flushes, and other fluids, as well as observe and report all outputs in addition to all patient responses to the enteral feeding regimen. The clinical dietitian monitors tolerance of the formula, state of hydration, and nutritional response using data collected from a variety of sources, including laboratory, anthropometric, physical and clinical assessment, and nursing records. Protocols for enteral nutrition can provide guidelines for troubleshooting problems and improve nutrient delivery.[52]

CLINICAL AND LABORATORY PARAMETERS TO MONITOR

Daily blood and urine tests for glucose and acetone during the first week or so, according to protocol, reflect carbohydrate tolerance. Patients who are diabetic or those who are severely stressed or septic may have difficulty metabolizing carbohydrate and are monitored closely. It is important not to overfeed patients on nutrition support. Insulin should be provided as needed to maintain serum glucose level at less than 200 mg/dl.

Daily weights, compared with a baseline weight before start of the formula, along with daily input and output measures are essential for an accurate assessment of patient tolerance and nutrient adequacy. Routine monitoring includes serum tests for glucose, potassium, sodium, chloride, carbon dioxide, creatinine, and blood urea nitrogen and complete blood cell counts along with periodic tests for urine specific gravity. Sudden weight changes can indicate hydration imbalance and need to be investigated. Box 17-2 provides a list of nutrition support monitoring parameters.

HYDRATION STATUS

Signs of volume deficit or dehydration include weight loss, poor skin turgor, dry mucous membranes, and low blood pressure from decreased blood volume. Patients also demonstrate increased serum levels of sodium, albumin, hematocrit, and blood urea nitrogen, as well as elevated urine specific gravity levels. Severe dehydration is critical and life threatening. It can be prevented by careful monitoring and supplying the patient's daily fluid requirements with water or other hydration fluids given through the tube. Fluid requirements can be estimated by several available formulas, such as 1 ml water/kcalorie or 30 to 35 ml/kg. The water content of the enteral formula and the amount of water given with medications and routine flushing are taken into consideration when determining the patient's hydration status and fluid requirements. Fluids must be monitored for adequacy and adjusted as necessary to attain and maintain euvolemia. Patients with excessive fluid losses, such as fistulas and drains, may require intravenous hydration in conjunction with enteral nutrition.

Signs of volume excess or overhydration include weight gain, edema, jugular vein distension, elevated blood pressure, and decreased serum levels of sodium, albumin, blood urea nitrogen, and hematocrit. Patients with renal, cardiac, and hepatic impairment may require less hydration than do other patients. The clinical dietitian monitors the patient's fluid requirement and response with routine nutrition assessments and follow-up according to the hospital's established protocol.

DOCUMENTATION OF THE ENTERAL NUTRITION TUBE FEEDING

The patient's medical record is an essential means of communication among the members of the healthcare team. The clinical dietitian is involved in actions and documentation related to (1) all ongoing nutrition analyses of actual formula intake, (2) tolerance of the formula and any complications, (3) recommendations for adjustments in enteral formula, routine flushing, and method and rate of delivery, and (4) education of patient and family.

Parenteral Feeding in Clinical Nutrition

Parenteral nutrition should be reserved for patients unable to receive adequate nutrition via the enteral route. The A.S.P.E.N. has published general guidelines to determine when PN support is appropriate.[7] Indications and contraindications for PN are listed in Box 17-4.

BOX 17-4 Indications and Contraindications for Parenteral Nutrition

Indications

1. Nonfunctional gastrointestinal (GI) tract
   a. Obstruction
   b. Intractable vomiting or diarrhea
   c. Short bowel syndrome
   d. Paralytic ileus
2. Inability to adequately utilize GI tract
   a. Slow progression of enteral nutrition
   b. Limited tolerance of enteral nutrition
   c. Enteric fistula
3. Preoperative
   a. Severely malnourished and NPO for at least 1 week before surgery

Contraindications

1. No central venous access
2. Grim prognosis when PN will be of no benefit
3. Enteral nutrition is an alternative means of support

Conditions Previously Treated With PN That Benefit From Enteral Feeding

1. Inflammatory bowel disease
2. Pancreatitis

Modified from Fuhrman MP: Parenteral nutrition, *Dietitian's Edge* 2(1):53-57, 2001.

parenteral A feeding modality that provides nutrient solutions intravenously rather than through the gastrointestinal tract.

BASIC TECHNIQUE

Guidelines for ordering PN are given in Box 17-5, and an example of a basic PN solution is given in Box 17-6. PN refers to any intravenous feeding method. Nutrients are infused directly into the blood circulation when the gastrointestinal tract cannot or should not be used. Two parenteral routes are available[53] (Figure 17-3).

1. *Central parenteral nutrition (CPN).* A large central vein is used to deliver concentrated solutions for nutrition support. The osmolarity of central vein parenteral formulas can be as high as 1700 to 1900 mOsm. The high formula osmolarity requires infusion of the formula into a large vessel with rapid blood flow. A central line generally originates from the subclavian, internal jugular, or femoral vein with the tip in the superior vena cava, right atrium of the heart, or inferior vena cava. Central line access can also be achieved with a peripherally inserted central catheter (PICC) that is inserted in the basilic vein with the tip in the superior vena cava or right atrium.
2. *Peripheral parenteral nutrition (PPN).* A smaller peripheral vein, usually in the distal arm or hand, is used to deliver less-concentrated solutions for periods less than 14 days. The osmolarity of PPN is limited to 900 mOsm or less to reduce the risk of thrombophlebitis in the smaller vessels of the upper distal extremities.[54]

BOX 17-5 Guidelines for Ordering Parenteral Nutrition

1. Determine that the patient has central IV access.
2. Identify the amount of calories, protein, and fluid desired.
3. Determine the desired distribution of dextrose and lipids.
4. Indicate additives desired
   a. Vitamins
   b. Minerals
   c. Electrolytes
   d. Medications

PARENTERAL NUTRITION DEVELOPMENT

The pioneering work of American surgeons such as Jonathan Rhodes and Stanley Dudrick in the late 1960s propelled PN from theory into reality.[55] In the following years, the development of the surgical technique, equip-

BOX 17-6 Example of a Basic PN Formula for a 55-kg Patient

Base Solution			
70% Dextrose	350 ml	245 g	833 kcalories
10% Amino acids	800 ml	80 g	320 kcalories
20% Lipid	250 ml	50 g	500 kcalories
Total	1400 ml		1653 kcalories
Additives			
Standard Electrolytes			
Sodium		55 mEq	
Potassium		40 mEq	
Phosphate		13 mmol	
Calcium		11 mEq	
Magnesium		14 mEq	
Chloride and acetate balanced with salts			
Multivitamin Preparation		10 ml	
Trace Element Preparation		5 ml	
Chromium			
Copper			
Manganese			
Selenium			
Zinc			
Medications			
Regular insulin		Only add if hyperglycemia occurs	
H_2 antagonists		Dose depends on H_2 antagonist and renal function	

ment, and solutions to meet the nutritional requirements of catabolic illness and injury and the development of antibiotics and diuretics led to its current widespread use and future directions.[22,56] PN was preferentially used to treat critically ill patients until a resurgence in enteral nutrition in the 1990s as more was learned about the importance of maintaining gastrointestinal integrity. PN is associated with potentially serious mechanical, metabolic, and gastrointestinal complications (see Box 17-1). PN should be used judiciously to minimize the risks involved. PPN can be used in many cases as a viable alternative for brief periods for patients without central vein access.[57]

Basic factors govern decisions about the use of PN: availability and functional capacity of the gastrointestinal tract, prognosis, and availability of central intravenous access.[7] The cost of PN is generally greater than that of enteral feeding, and institutions have demonstrated cost savings when inappropriate use of PN has been decreased.[58,59] PN should not be given to patients with a grim prognosis because nutrition will not change the disease course or survival. Patients must have a central intravenous access line to receive PN with one port designated exclusively for PN. Thus careful assessment of each of situation should weigh the benefits and burdens of providing PN for nutrition support.

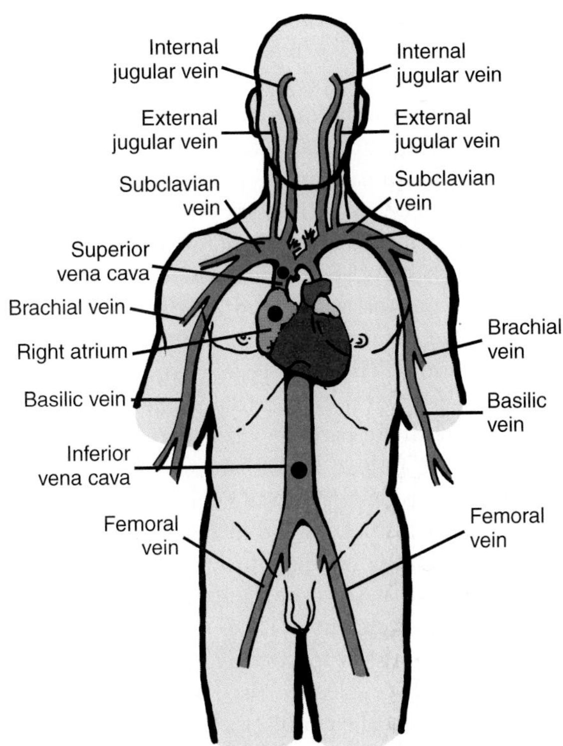

FIGURE 17-3 Sites of central venous access for parenteral nutrition. (*From Fuhrman MP: Management of complications of parenteral nutrition. In Matarese LE, Gottschlich MM, eds:* Contemporary nutrition support practice: a clinical guide, *Philadelphia, 1998, WB Saunders.*)

Indications for PN include inaccessibility to or nonfunctioning of the gastrointestinal tract. Patients may also have inadequate absorption of nutrients in the gastrointestinal tract because of reduced bowel length or inflammation. Examples of indications for PN are obstruction, fistula, severe inflammation, intractable vomiting or diarrhea, or gastrointestinal bleeding (see Box 17-4). If the gastrointestinal tract is functional but the patient cannot or will not consume sufficient nutrients orally, enteral tube feeding should be considered. Many conditions that had been previously thought to be an indication for PN are treated with enteral nutrition, such as pancreatitis, severe malnutrition, ileus, and coma.

CANDIDATES FOR PARENTERAL NUTRITION

Specialized nutrition support should be reserved for patients unable to receive or tolerate adequate nutrients via the enteral route. On the basis of these general considerations, a number of clinical situations suggest a need for aggressive PN support.

1. *Preoperative nutrition intervention* may benefit moderately to severely malnourished patients who can receive nutrition support for 7 to 14 days preoperatively.[7] PN should only be given if enteral nutrition support is not feasible or tolerated. The VA Cooperative Study demonstrated that the greatest benefit of perioperative PN was experienced by severely malnourished patients.[23]
2. *Postoperative surgical complications.* Complications that often result in initiation of PN are prolonged paralytic ileus and obstruction; stomal dysfunction; short bowel syndrome; enterocutaneous, biliary, or pancreatic fistula; chylothorax; chylous ascites; and peritonitis. However, there are reports of successful enteral feeding with short bowel syndrome, fistula, and chylous leaks when patients are given an elemental or semielemental, low-fat enteral formula.[60-62] PN is not indicated in patients who can resume enteral nutrition within 7 to 10 days postoperatively.[7]
3. *Inflammatory bowel disease.* Intractable gastroenteritis, regional enteritis, ulcerative colitis, extensive diverticulitis, and radiation enteritis may require PN if the gastrointestinal inflammation is severe and prolonged.[7] Studies have shown that in some cases enteral feeding

fistula Abnormal connection between two internal organs, an internal organ and the skin, or an internal organ and a body cavity.

osmolarity The number of millimoles of liquid or solid in a liter of solution; parenteral nutrition solutions given by central vein have an osmolarity around 1800 mOsm/L; peripheral parenteral solutions are limited to 600 to 900 mOsm/L (dextrose and amino acids have the greatest impact on a solution's osmolarity).

can be feasible and beneficial in inflammatory bowel disease.[63]

4. *Malabsorption.* Nutrient losses and interference with nutrient absorption occur with chemotherapy and radiation therapy. The malabsorption that is associated with severe gastrointestinal inflammation, acute severe pancreatitis, and massive burns can exceed the ability to meet nutrient requirements enterally.

Peripheral Parenteral Nutrition

Generally, decisions to use PPN instead of CPN are based on energy demands, anticipated time of use, and availability of intravenous access. PPN cannot be used when the patient has problems with fluid retention or hyperlipidemia. Characteristics of PPN include caloric value generally less than 2000 kcalories/day, of which 50% to 60% is provided by lipids; infusion volume of 2 to 3 L (dilution of the formula is required for peripheral vein tolerance); and use of infusion for less than 14 days.[57]

Parenteral Solutions

THE PARENTERAL NUTRITION PRESCRIPTION

The PN prescription and plan of care are based on the calculation of basic nutritional requirements plus additional needs resulting from the patient's degree of catabolism, malnutrition, and any activity. An example of a basic PN formula plan is shown in Box 17-6. The same principles of nutrition therapy are applied whether the patient is fed enterally or parenterally. Nutrition needs are fundamental—energy, protein, electrolytes, minerals, and vitamins. Guidelines are available that address PN labeling, compounding, formulations, stability, and filtering.[64] The guidelines are designed to reduce errors and complications in preparing and infusing parenteral solutions.

ENERGY REQUIREMENTS

The energy requirements for hospitalized patients on PN support vary with the degree of metabolic stress but generally range from 20 to 35 kcalories/kg. Regardless of the calculation used to estimate energy expenditure, it is important to monitor the impact of the nutrients provided to determine changes that are needed to maintain or replete the patient. The kcalories are adjusted based on patient tolerance and desired versus actual response to nutrient provision.

PREPARATION OF THE PARENTERAL NUTRITION SOLUTION

There are a variety of PN component solutions with varying concentrations and nutrient compositions. Standard components of PN can include dextrose, lipids, amino acids, electrolytes, vitamins, minerals, and medications.

TABLE 17-3 Caloric Value per Milliliter of Parenteral Components

Nutrient	Concentration (%)	Kcalories/ml
Dextrose	70	2.38
	50	1.85
Lipids	30	3.0
	20	2.0
	10	1.1
Amino acids	15	0.6
	10	0.4
	8.5	0.34

Although PN is compounded with modular components and hence an ability to adjust kcalorie and protein independent of each other, the kcalories provided to meet estimated or measured energy needs should include total kcalories from carbohydrate, fat, and protein (Table 17-3).

Protein-Nitrogen Source

Nitrogen is supplied by essential and nonessential crystalline amino acids in the PN solution. Standard commercial amino acid solutions produced by various manufacturers range in concentration from 3% to 20%. Standard amino acid solutions are appropriate for almost all adult patients receiving PN. Protein has a caloric value of 4 kcalories/g (see Table 17-3) and usually provides 10% to 20% of the total kcalories provided in PN.

In addition to standard amino acid solutions, three types of specialized amino acid solutions have been formulated for specific disease states. The disease-specific formulas are more expensive than standard solutions and their effectiveness has not been demonstrated. Two types are enriched with branched-chain amino acids (BCAAs) isoleucine, leucine, and valine and are designed for patients with either extensive trauma and severe catabolic stress or liver failure. The other type is enriched with essential amino acids and designed to prevent the development of hyperuremia in patients with acute renal failure. Neither the renal failure formula with only essential amino acids nor the BCAA formula designed for trauma and critical illness has been found to improve outcome in these patient populations.[7] The infusion of BCAA may be beneficial in patients with chronic encephalopathy that is unresponsive to drug therapy.[7] There also are amino acid formulas that are designed specifically for the needs of pediatric patients and are selected based on the age and nutrient requirements of the child.

Carbohydrate—Dextrose

Dextrose is the most common and least expensive source of kcalories used for PN support. Dextrose is available in concentrations ranging from 2.5% to 70%. Hypertonic solutions of 50% to 70% dextrose are often used in PN formulations and provide 50 or 70 g of dextrose/100 ml, respectively. Glucose used in PN support is commercially available as dextrose monohydrate ($C_6H_{12}O_6H_2O$), which has an energy value of 3.4 kcalories/g, versus the energy value of 4 kcalories/g of dietary glucose ($C_6H_{12}O_6$). The caloric value of dextrose solutions is given in Table 17-3. The initial dextrose content of PN should not exceed 200 g. The gradual introduction of dextrose enables the clinician to evaluate glycemic response and, if necessary, institute insulin therapy. The amount of dextrose provided is increased to goal according to patient tolerance and should not exceed 5 mg/kg/min.

Glycerol is another form of carbohydrate used in parenteral solutions. It provides 4.3 kcalories/g and is available as a component along with amino acids in a commercially available PPN solution.

Fat—Lipids

Lipid emulsions provide a concentrated energy source, 9 kcalories/g, as well as the essential fatty acids linoleic and linolenic acid. A minimum of 4% to 10% of the daily kcalorie intake should consist of fat to prevent essential fatty acid deficiency. Lipids are available in 10% (1.1 kcalories/ml), 20% (2 kcalories/ml), and 30% (3 kcalories/ml) products (see Table 17-3). A 500-ml bottle of 10%, 20%, or 30% fat emulsion provides 555, 1000, and 1500 kcalories, respectively. Commercial lipid emulsion products consist of soybean and safflower oils combined or soybean oil alone. The content of lipid in a parenteral solution is usually limited to 20% to 30% of total kcalories because lipids have been reported to adversely affect the immune system.[65] However, the infusion of lipids over 24 hours may limit this adverse effect. Research on alternative lipid sources includes forms such as short-chain fatty acids, medium-chain fatty acids, omega-3 fatty acids, and blended or structured lipids. Lipid emulsions can be infused separately through the Y-port of the intravenous catheter (piggybacked) or combined with the dextrose and amino acid base in what is called a total nutrient admixture (TNA) or 3-in-1.[64]

Electrolytes

The body maintains a balance of fluid and electrolytes in intracellular and extracellular spaces of all tissues to maintain homeostasis (see Chapter 8). Electrolyte status is affected by the disease state and metabolic condition of the patient. Electrolytes in PN formulas are based on normal electrolyte balance with adjustments according to individual patient requirements. Electrolytes should be routinely monitored to determine electrolyte requirements in PN.

In general, the basic electrolyte needs are as shown in Table 17-4, with chloride and acetate balanced among the salts. Commercial amino acid formulations are available with or without added electrolytes. The amounts of electrolytes present in the amino acid solution must be taken into account when calculating additions for a specific patient. Guidelines for electrolyte management include (1) identify and correct any preexisting deficits before initiating PN, (2) determine the etiology of electrolyte abnormalities, (3) replace excessive fluid and electrolyte losses, and (4) monitor and assess electrolyte status daily. Depending on the requirements for electrolyte replacement, it may be necessary to replete electrolytes outside the PN because there are limitations on what can be added to a parenteral solution based on stability and compatibility.[61] Selected electrolytes can be omitted from the parenteral solution when serum levels exceed normal values, such as potassium and phosphorus with renal failure. Electrolyte levels should be checked in all patients before starting PN.

TABLE 17-4 Electrolytes and Parenteral Nutrition

Standard Electrolytes		General Guidelines
Potassium (K)	80 mEq/day	0.7-1.5 mEq/kg/day
Sodium (Na)	80 mEq/day	1.0-1.5 mEq/kg/day
Phosphate (HPO_4)	30 mmol/day	7-9 mmol/1000 kcalories
Magnesium (Mg)	10 mEq/day	0.25-0.45 mEq/kg/day
Calcium (Ca)	9.4 mEq/day	0.2-0.3 mEq/kg/day

From Furman MP: Parenteral nutrition, *Dietitian's Edge* 2(1):55, 2001.

Vitamins

Vitamin requirements are based on normal standards (see current RDA/DRI listed inside front cover of this book), with adjustments made according to metabolic states. Individual nutrients may be added as needed to cover increased metabolic and depletion states. All patients on PN should receive daily provision of vitamins. Serum levels of vitamins should be monitored in patients requiring chronic PN or when deficiencies or excesses are suspected.

The Nutrition Advisory Group of the American Medical Association has established guidelines for parenteral administration of 12 vitamins: A, D, E, thiamin, riboflavin, niacin, pantothenic acid, pyridoxine, folate, biotin, cobalamin, and ascorbic acid.[66] Multivitamin preparations based on these guidelines are available. However, during a recent injectable multivitamin shortage, vitamin products without all 12 vitamins were more widely used. It is important to know the content of the vitamin preparation used in your facility and to replace "missing" vitamins separately. Vitamin K has not been a component of any injectable vitamin formulation for adults. If needed for individual maintenance as evidenced by the international normalized ratio (INR), it was added to the solution or given as an intramuscular

admixture A mixture of ingredients that each retain their own physical properties; a combination of two or more substances that are not chemically united or that exist in no fixed proportion to each other.

injection. The Food and Drug Administration has mandated changes in parenteral vitamin formulations that include the addition of 150 μg of vitamin K to injectable multivitamin preparations.[67] It will be important to monitor INR levels, particularly for patients started or stopped on PN who are also on anticoagulation therapy.

Trace Elements

The American Medical Association has set guidelines for the addition of four trace elements in PN solutions: zinc, copper, manganese, and chromium.[68] Trace element preparations are available with combinations of the aforementioned four trace elements only, the standard four plus selenium, or the standard four plus selenium, molybdenum, and iodine. Each trace element is also available as a single injectable mineral product. There is a growing amount of literature as to the importance of providing selenium to PN patients who are critically ill[69,70] and those who require long-term PN.[71] Iron is not routinely added to PN because of incompatibility issues. If it is needed by an individual patient, it is administered apart from the PN admixture.

Patients on long-term PN without trace element supplementation are at risk for micronutrient deficiencies.[71,72] There have also been reports of excess trace element levels with current levels of supplementation.[73] Caution is needed when adding minerals to the PN solution. Incompatibilities of certain electrolytes and other components may form insoluble substances that precipitate from the solution, depending on ion concentration, mixing sequence, temperature, and solution pH.

Medications

Medication that are often added to PN include insulin, H_2-antagonists, heparin, metoclopramide, and octreotide. The inclusion of these medications and others will depend on each institution's guidelines for addition of medications to PN solutions. There are a plethora of issues concerning compatibility, bioavailability, efficacy, interactions, and safety when including medications in PN solutions. Consult a pharmacist whenever considering the addition of a medication to PN solutions.

Parenteral Nutrition Delivery System

EQUIPMENT

Strict aseptic technique throughout PN administration by all healthcare personnel is absolutely essential. This includes (1) the solution preparation by the pharmacist, (2) the surgical placement of the venous catheter by the physician, and (3) the care of the catheter site and all external equipment and administration of the solution by the nurse. At every step of the PN process, strict infection control is a primary responsibility of all healthcare professionals.

Venous Catheter

Surgical placement of the venous catheter is done by the physician at the bedside or in a surgical suite, using local or general anesthesia. Commercially prepared sterile kits contain all the necessary equipment items for gaining access to a large central vein for infusion of the nutrition support solution directly into the central blood circulation. Intravenous catheters are available with single, double, triple, or quadruple lumens. There is inconsistent data as to whether the number of lumens contributes to the risk of catheter-related infection.[74-76] Catheters are also categorized as either temporary or permanent. Temporary catheters involve a direct percutaneous puncture into a major vessel and are used in the short term during hospitalization. Permanent catheters are designed for long-term use and are available as implanted ports, tunneled, and PICCs. The tip of a central venous catheter is located in the inferior or superior vena cava, which leads directly into the heart[53] (see Figure 17-3). Placement of the catheter tip in the vena cava allows the infusion of concentrated solutions, 5 times the concentration of blood plasma, to be infused at a rate of 2 to 3 ml/min. The hypertonic solutions are immediately diluted by the large blood flow of 2 to 5 L/min in the vena cava.

Catheter-related sepsis is a serious complication, particularly with the increase in colonization with resistant strains of microorganisms that limit the available treatment options. Antibiotic-impregnated catheters and dressings are available and are associated with reduced catheter-related septic complications.[77-79] Filters on intravenous catheter tubing prevent infusion of not only particulate matter but also certain microorganisms.[64] Clinicians must use aseptic technique when inserting and caring for intravenous catheters.

Solution Infusion and Administration

Volumetric infusion pumps should be used to deliver the parenteral solution at a constant rate to prevent metabolic complications. Protocols for external delivery system tubing changes are provided by infection control guidelines. Routine flushing of intravenous catheters is recommended to maintain catheter patency. Needleless intravenous access devices reduce the risk of needlestick injuries but can increase the risk of catheter-related infections. According to the Intravenous Nurses Society standards of practice needleless devices should be changed every 24 hours, the injection port should be disinfected with alcohol before accessing, and all junctions should be secured with Luer-locks, clasps, or threaded devices.[80]

Infusion of PN is generally over 24 hours, particularly in the critically ill. PN can be cycled over 10 to 12 hours if desired and if the patient can tolerate the larger volume over a shorter period. The rate of infusion is based on the final compounded volume and the length of time the infusion is to be given. The administration of PN should be adjusted based on the patient's response and tolerance to the regimen (see *Practical Application* box).

PRACTICAL APPLICATION
Parenteral Nutrition Administration

Of all the various ways of nourishing the human body—normal eating, liquid diets, enteral nutrition, and parenteral nutrition (PN)—PN requires the highest degree of skilled and precise administration. There is always a risk of potentially life-threatening complication and infection. The roles of trained nutrition support clinicians are central to the success of PN. The nutrition support nurse administers the PN solution according to the nutrition support team protocol, monitoring the entire PN system frequently to see that it is operating accurately.

Specific clinical protocols will vary somewhat, but they usually include the following points.

- *Start slowly.* Give the patient time to adapt to the glucose and electrolyte concentration of the solution.
- *Schedule carefully.* PN volume can vary from 1 to 3 L and should be infused by continuous drip. The rate should be regulated by an infusion pump and is based on the total volume of the compounded solution.
- *Monitor closely.* Note metabolic effects of glucose (blood glucose levels not to exceed 200 mg/dl) and electrolytes. First-day formulas generally contain only 200 g dextrose. Monitor glycemic tolerance closely particularly the first couple of days as the feeding is advanced. Electrolyte status and glucose levels should be determined before and throughout PN administration. Increase kcalories only as patient tolerates macronutrient content.
- *Make changes cautiously.* Monitor and report the effect of all changes and proceed slowly.
- *Maintain a constant rate.* Keep to the correct hourly infusion rate, with no "catch-up" or "slow-down" effort to meet the original volume order.
- *Discontinue PN.* Reduce the rate by one half for 1 hour before discontinuing. If patient has had insulin added to PN and is not receiving enteral feeding, monitor for rebound hypoglycemia (check serum glucose 2 hours after stopping PN infusion).

MONITORING

The complications of PN include catheter, gastrointestinal, and metabolic problems (see Box 17-3). In the hands of well-trained PN clinicians, risks can be minimized and complications controlled.[81] Specific protocols, updated periodically as needed, guide continuing assessment and monitoring.[82] Every patient on PN should undergo a routine reassessment with adjustments made in the feeding regimen according to the patient's metabolic and nutritional needs. Every effort should be made to transition the patient from PN to enteral tube feeding or oral diet whenever feasible or appropriate. Providing at least a portion of kcalories enterally may help reduce the adverse effects associated with PN.[53]

Home Nutrition Support

HOME ENTERAL NUTRITION

Patient Selection

Patients being considered for home tube-feeding should be screened for an adequate support system and safe environment for administration of the feeding. Developments in enteral formulas and portable, lightweight, infusion equipment have simplified home enteral feeding and made it easier to manage. As a result, the number of patients using home enteral nutrition continues to grow as a means of cutting hospital costs and allowing earlier family support at home. Home care requires education and training of both patient and family.[83]

BOX 17-7 Home Enteral Nutrition Topics and Tasks

- What enteral formulation is used and why
- How to prepare the formula for infusion
- How to infuse the formula through the feeding tube
- How to correctly use and troubleshoot problems with the equipment
- How much water and how often to flush the feeding tube
- How to care for the tube site
- How to recognize formula intolerance
- How to avoid and treat complications
- How to give medications and other separate nutrients through the feeding tube
- When to call the physician or home care provider

Teaching Plan

Educating the patient and family or caregiver for home care is a team responsibility. This team may be hospital based or affiliated with the home care agency that will manage the patient's care after discharge. The dietitian, nurse, and pharmacist develop and carry out a teaching plan, which includes topics and related tasks in preparing patients and families for discharge on home enteral feeding[78] (Box 17-7).

The hospital or home care agency should provide a teaching manual with illustrations to guide the teaching-learning process and to be used as a reference at home. The teaching plan should start as soon as the decision for home tube feeding is made. A social worker identifies and if possible resolves any personal, psychosocial, safety, or economic issues with home care.

Finally, the teaching plan should allow sufficient time before discharge for the patient and family to demonstrate competency in (1) administering the formula and (2) recording all necessary information about formula and fluid intake, formula tolerance, and complications. Directions for recording information are included in the home care manual. Records are reviewed regularly by nutrition support specialists providing follow-up care at home and in the outpatient clinic.

Follow-Up Monitoring

The plan for follow-up monitoring should be guided by the specific protocol schedule developed by the institution for laboratory, clinical, and nutrition assessments. The interdisciplinary team checks the patient's progress and works with the patient and family to troubleshoot any problems that arise and make required adjustments in the formula or feeding plan. As mentioned previously, whenever feasible and appropriate the patient is transitioned to oral intake.

HOME PARENTERAL NUTRITION

The patient sent home with PN requires education and training on the provision of PN in the outpatient setting. In the hands of knowledgeable and capable patients and their families, home PN allows mobility and independence. The patient and family must be trained to use aseptic technique for adding micronutrients and medications to the solution and for accessing the intravenous catheter or port. Special equipment, solutions, and guidelines for training and supervising patients and families have been developed and are successfully used by hundreds of patients. The Oley Foundation provides a network of support for patients on chronic, long-term home PN. (Refer to Internet resources for the website of the Oley Foundation.) Ongoing assessment of gastrointestinal function must be performed to determine if the patient is able to transition to enteral feedings either orally or via feeding tube. Patients are also monitored closely for the development of complications associated with long-term PN infusion.

TO SUM UP

For patients with functioning gastrointestinal tracts, enteral nutrition support has proved to be a potent tool against present or potential malnutrition. Enteral nutrition support is achieved by an oral diet with nutrient-dense supplementation or alternately by tube feeding when the patient cannot, will not, or should not eat. Commercial products with or without modular enhancement provide complete nutrition when provided in adequate amounts. It is also possible to prepare blenderized formulas from common foodstuffs. Enteral nutrition can be provided through nasoenteric or enterostomy feeding tubes with an open versus closed delivery system. Tubing and container adaptations and the development of small, mobile infusion pumps, together with a comprehensive teaching plan for patient and family and follow-up monitoring by a clinical team, allow many patients the option of home enteral feeding.

For patients with a dysfunctional gastrointestinal tract, PN support allows the provision of required nutrients. This feeding method depends heavily on biomedical technology for the development of tubes, bags, pumps, and other equipment for feeding nutrients directly into veins for circulation through the blood to the cells. The route of entry may be a large central vein for intravenous feeding over a long period or a smaller peripheral vein for feeding less-concentrated solutions for a shorter period. Home PN is successfully used by many patients, with the support of families, friends, and nutrition support specialists.

■ Questions for Review

1. Describe several types of patient situations in which enteral nutrition support may be indicated. What nutrition assessment procedures may help to identify these individuals?
2. Describe the nutrient components of a typical complete polymeric enteral formula. How does it differ from a modular formula? How does it differ from a semielemental and an elemental formula?
3. Define PN and identify examples of conditions in which it would be used.

The following questions apply to the case of a man referred to nutrition support services. Imagine you are caring for this patient.

A previously healthy 45-year-old man, while on a long transport haul as a truck driver, was in an accident in which he sustained a severe abdominal injury requiring extensive surgical repair and leaving the gastrointestinal tract unavailable for use for an undetermined period. He is referred to the nutrition support team for PN. Early in this care he asks you how this feeding works.

1. How would you describe and explain the PN feeding process?
2. What nutrition assessment parameters would be beneficial in identifying his risk of developing malnutrition and his tolerance to parenteral therapy?
3. List the typical components of a basic PN formula that he may require, and describe the purpose of each to help reassure him of its adequacy and importance.
4. Sufficient energy (kcalorie) intake is essential to immediately meet his metabolic needs after surgery. Assume a normal preinjury weight (175 lb) and height (70

inches) and an added stress factor of 1.2 times his basal energy expenditure (BEE). Calculate his total kcalorie requirement, using the Harris-Benedict equation.

5. Define hepatic proteins and describe why they are not appropriate static indicators of nutritional status in critically ill patients. How can you monitor the effectiveness of the PN formula in meeting his nutrition support needs for recovery?

References

1. Borum PR: Nutrient metabolism. In Gottschlich MM et al, eds: *The science and practice of nutrition support: a case-based core curriculum,* Dubuque, Iowa, 2001, Kendall/Hunt Publishing.
2. Butterworth CE: The skeleton in the hospital closet, *Nutr Today* 9:4, 1974.
3. Bistrian BR et al: Protein status of general surgical patients, *JAMA* 230:858, 1974.
4. Naber T et al: Prevalence of malnutrition in nonsurgical hospitalized patients and its association with disease complications, *Am J Clin Nutr* 66:1232, 1997.
5. Detsky AS et al: What is subjective global assessment of nutritional status? *J Parenter Enteral Nutr* 11(1):8, 1987.
6. Braunschweig C et al: Impact of declines in nutritional status on outcomes in adult patients hospitalized for more than seven days, *J Am Diet Assoc* 100:1316, 2000.
7. A.S.P.E.N. Board of Directors and The Clinical Guidelines Task Force: Guidelines for the use of parenteral and enteral nutrition in adult and pediatric patients, *J Parenter Enteral Nutr* 26:1SA, 2002.
8. Moore FA et al: Early enteral feeding, compared with parenteral, reduces postoperative septic complications: the results of a meta-analysis, *Ann Surg* 216:172, 1992.
9. Lipman TO: Grains or veins: is enteral nutrition really better than parenteral nutrition? a look at the evidence, *J Parenter Enteral Nutr* 22:167, 1998.
10. Shopbell JM et al: Nutrition screening and assessment. In Gottschlich MM et al, eds: *The science and practice of nutrition support: a case-based core curriculum,* Dubuque, Iowa, 2001, Kendall/Hunt Publishing.
11. Harris JA, Benedict FG: *A biometric study of basal metabolism,* Washington, DC, 1919, Carnegie Institution of Washington.
12. Solomon SM, Kirby DF: The refeeding syndrome: a review, *J Parenter Enteral Nutr* 14:90, 1990.
13. Vanek VW: The use of serum albumin as a prognostic or nutritional marker and the pros and cons of IV albumin therapy, *Nutr Clin Pract* 13:110, 1998.
14. Meyer J et al: Benefits of a nutrition support service in an HMO setting, *Nutr Clin Pract* 16:25, 2001.
15. American Society for Parenteral and Enteral Nutrition Board of Directors: Standards of practice for nutrition support nurses, *Nutr Clin Pract* 16:56, 2001.
16. American Society for Parenteral and Enteral Nutrition Board of Directors: Standards of practice for nutrition support pharmacists, *Nutr Clin Pract* 14:275, 1999.
17. American Society for Parenteral and Enteral Nutrition Board of Directors: Standards of practice for nutrition support physicians, *Nutr Clin Pract* 11:235, 1996.
18. American Society for Parenteral and Enteral Nutrition Board of Directors: Standards of practice for nutrition support dietitians, *Nutr Clin Pract* 15:53, 2000.
19. Board of Directors, American Society for Parenteral and Enteral Nutrition: Interdisciplinary nutrition support core competencies, *Nutr Clin Pract* 14:331, 1999.
20. JCAHO Board of Directors: *Comprehensive accreditation manual for hospitals,* Oakbrook Terrace, Ill, 2000, Joint Commission on Accreditation of Healthcare Organizations.
21. Fuhrman MP: Parenteral nutrition: a clinician's perspective, *Dietitians Edge* 2(1):53, 2001.
22. Charney P: Enteral nutrition: indications, options and formulations. In Gottschlich MM et al, eds: *The science and practice of nutrition support: a case-based core curriculum,* Dubuque, Iowa, 2001, Kendall/Hunt Publishing.
23. Veterans Affairs Total Parenteral Nutrition Cooperative Study Group: Perioperative total parenteral nutrition in surgical patients, *N Engl J Med* 325:525, 1992.
24. Guenter P et al: Delivery systems and administration of enteral feeding. In Rombeau JL, Rolandelli RH, eds: *Clinical nutrition: enteral and tube feeding,* ed 3, Philadelphia, 1997, WB Saunders.
25. Lewis DA, Boyle K: Nutritional supplement use during medication administration: selected case studies, *J Nutr Elderly* 17(4):53, 1998.
26. Turic A et al: Nutrition supplementation enables elderly residents in long-term care facilities to meet or exceed RDAs without displacing energy or nutrient intakes from meals, *J Am Diet Assoc* 98:1457, 1998.
27. Watters JM et al: Immediate postoperative enteral feeding results in impaired respiratory mechanics and decreased mobility, *Ann Surg* 266:369, 1997.
28. Gottschlich MM et al: Defined formula diets. In Rombeau JL, Rolandelli RH, eds: *Clinical nutrition: enteral and tube feeding,* ed 3, Philadelphia, 1997, WB Saunders.
29. Kopp-Hoolihan L: Prophylactic and therapeutic uses of probiotics: a review, *J Am Diet Assoc* 101:229, 2001.
30. Gadek JE et al: Effect of enteral feeding with eicosapentaenoic acid, γ-linolenic acid, and antioxidants in patients with acute respiratory distress syndrome, *Crit Care Med* 27:1409, 1999.
31. Consensus recommendations form the U.S. Summit on Immune-Enhancing Enteral Therapy, *J Parenter Enteral Nutr* 25:S61, 2001.
32. Talbot JM: Guidelines for the scientific review of enteral food products for special medical purposes, *J Parenter Enter Nutr* 15(suppl 3):100S, 1991.
33. Metheny NA, Clouse RE: Bedside methods for detecting aspiration in tube-fed patients, *Chest* 111:724, 1997.
34. Maloney JP et al: Systemic absorption of food dye in patients with sepsis [letter], *NEJM* 343:1047, 2000.
35. Metheny NA et al: A survey of bedside methods to detect pulmonary aspiration of enteral formula in intubated tube-fed patients, *Am J Crit Care* 8(3):160, 1999.
36. Cannon R et al: *Methods and tubes for establishing enteral access: discussion. Enteral nutrition support for the 1990s: innovations in nutrition, technology, and techniques.* Report of the 12th Ross Roundtable on Medical Issues. Columbus, Ohio, 1992, Ross Products Division, Abbott Laboratories.
37. Moore MC, ed: Enteral nutrition. In *Mosby's pocket guide series: nutritional care,* ed 4, St Louis, 2001, Mosby.

38. Metheny NA et al: pH and concentration of bilirubin in feeding tube aspirates as predictors of tube placement, *Nurs Res* 48(4):189, 1999.
39. Metheny N et al: Effect of feeding tube properties and three irrigants on clogging rates, *Nurs Res* 37:165, 1988.
40. Sriram K et al: Prophylactic locking of enteral feeding tubes with pancreatic enzymes, *J Parenter Enteral Nutr* 21(6):353, 1997.
41. Orlee K et al: Enteral formulations. In A.S.P.E.N. Board of Directors, ed: *A.S.P.E.N. nutrition support practice manual,* Silver Spring, Md, 1998, American Society for Parenteral and Enteral Nutrition.
42. Vanek VW: Closed versus open enteral delivery systems: a quality improvement study, *Nutr Clin Pract* 15:234, 2000.
43. Herlick SJ et al: Comparison of open versus closed systems of intermittent enteral feeding in two long-term care facilities, *Nutr Clin Pract* 15:287, 2000.
44. Keohane PP et al: Relation between osmolarity of the diet and gastrointestinal side effects in enteral nutrition in enteral nutrition. *BJM* 288:678, 1984.
45. Lysen LK, Samour PQ: Enteral equipment. In Matarese LE, Gottschlich MM, eds: *Contemporary nutrition support practice: a clinical guide,* Philadelphia, 1998, WB Saunders.
46. Ibanaez J et al: Gastroesophageal reflux in intubated patients receiving enteral nutrition: effect of supine and semirecumbent positions, *J Parenter Enteral Nutr* 16:419, 1992.
47. Cogen R et al: Complications of jejunostomy tube feeding in nursing facility patients, *Am J Gastroenterol* 86:1610, 1991.
48. Mobarhan S, Demeo M: Diarrhea induced by enteral feeding, *Nutr Rev* 53:67, 1995.
49. Fuhrman MP: Diarrhea and tube feeding, *Nutr Clin Pract* 14:83, 1999.
50. McClave SA et al: Use of residual volume as a marker for enteral feeding tolerance: prospective, blinded comparison with physical examination and radiographic findings, *J Parenter Enteral Nutr* 16(2):99, 1992.
51. Pinilla JC et al: Comparison of gastrointestinal tolerance to two enteral feeding protocols in critically ill patients: a prospective, randomized trial, *J Parenter Enteral Nutr* 25:81, 2001.
52. Spain DA et al: Infusion protocol improves delivery of enteral tube feeding in the critical care unit, *J Parenter Enteral Nutr* 23:288, 1999,
53. Fuhrman MP: Management of complications of parenteral nutrition. In Matarese LE, Gottschlich MM, eds: *Contemporary nutrition support practice: a clinical guide,* Philadelphia, 1998, WB Saunders.
54. Mirtallo JM: Introduction to parenteral nutrition. In: Gottschlich MM et al, eds: *The science and practice of nutrition support: a case-based core curriculum,* Dubuque, Iowa, 2001, Kendall/Hunt Publishing.
55. Dudrick SJ et al: Can intravenous feeding as the sole means of nutrition support growth in the child and restore weight loss in an adult? *Ann Surg* 169:974, 1969.
56. Klein S et al: Nutrition support in clinical practice: review of published date on recommendations for future directions, *J Parenter Enter Nutr* 21(3):133, 1997.
57. Stokes MA, Hill GL: Peripheral parenteral nutrition: a preliminary report on its efficacy and safety, *J Parenter Enteral Nutr* 17(2):145, 1993.
58. Trujillo ED et al: Metabolic and monetary costs of avoidable parenteral nutrition use, *J Parenter Enteral Nutr* 23:109, 1999.
59. Speerhas RA et al: Five year follow-up of a program to minimize inappropriate use of parenteral nutrition [abstract], *J Parenter Enteral Nutr* 25:S4, 2001.
60. Tulsyan N et al: Enterocutaneous fistulas, *Nutr Clin Pract* 16:74, 2001.
61. Byrne TA et al: Beyond the prescription: optimizing the diet of patients with short bowel syndrome, *Nutr Clin Pract* 15:306, 2000.
62. Spain DA, McClave SA: Chylothorax and chylous ascites. In Gottschlich MM et al, eds: *The science and practice of nutrition support: a case-based core curriculum,* Dubuque, Iowa, 2001, Kendall/Hunt Publishing.
63. Kelly DG, Nehra V: Gastrointestinal disease. In Gottschlich MM et al, eds: *The science and practice of nutrition support: a case-based core curriculum,* Dubuque, Iowa, 2001, Kendall/Hunt Publishing.
64. National Advisory Group on Standards and Practice Guidelines for Parenteral Nutrition: Safe practices for parenteral nutrition formulations, *J Parenter Enteral Nutr* 22:49, 1998.
65. Seidner DL et al: Effect of long-chain triglyceride emulsions on reticuloendothelial system function in humans, *J Parenter Enteral Nutr* 13:614, 1989.
66. American Medical Association, AMA Department of Foods and Nutrition: Multivitamin preparations for parenteral use: a statement by the Nutrition Advisory Group, *J Parenter Enteral Nutr* 3:258, 1979.
67. Parenteral multivitamin products; drugs for human use; drug efficacy study implementation; amendment (21 CFR 5.70), *Federal Register* 65:21200, 2000.
68. Expert Panel for Nutrition Advisory Group, AMA Department of Foods and Nutrition: Guidelines for essential trace element preparations for parenteral use, *JAMA* 241:2051, 1979.
69. Forceville F et al: Selenium, systemic immune response syndrome, sepsis, and outcome in critically ill patients, *Crit Care Med* 26:1536, 1998.
70. Angstwurm MAW et al: Selenium replacement in patients with severe systemic inflammatory response syndrome improves clinical outcome, *Crit Care Med* 27:1807, 1999.
71. Cohen HJ et al: Glutathione peroxidase and selenium deficiency in patients receiving home parenteral nutrition: time course for development of deficiency and repletion of the enzyme activity in plasma and blood cells, *Am J Clin Nutr* 49:132, 1989.
72. Fuhrman MP et al: Pancytopenia following removal of copper from TPN, *J Parenter Enteral Nutr* 24:361, 2000.
73. Masumoto K et al: Manganese intoxication during intermittent parenteral nutrition: report of two cases, *J Parenter Enteral Nutr* 25:95, 2001.
74. Pemberton L et al: Sepsis from triple- vs single-lumen catheters during total parenteral nutrition in surgical or critically ill patients, *Arch Surg* 121:591, 1986.
75. Farkas J et al: Single- versus triple-lumen central catheter-related sepsis: a prospective randomized study in a critically ill population, *Am J Med* 93:277, 1992.
76. Savage AP et al: Complications and survival of multilumen central venous catheters used for total parenteral nutrition, *Br J Surg* 80:1287, 1993.

77. Maki DG et al: Prevention of central venous catheter-related bloodstream infection by use of an antiseptic-impregnated catheter: a randomized, controlled trial, *Ann Intern Med* 127:257, 1997.
78. Veenstra DL et al: Cost-effectiveness of antiseptic-impregnated central venous catheters for the prevention of catheter-related bloodstream infection, *J Am Med Assoc* 282:554, 1999.
79. Hanazaki K et al: Chlorhexidine dressing for reduction in microbial colonization of the skin with central venous catheters: a prospective randomized controlled trial [letter], *J Hosp Infect* 42:165, 1999.
80. Intravenous Nurses Society: Infusion nursing standards of practice, *J Intravenous Nurs* 23(6S):S1-S85, 2000.
81. Dodds ES et al: Metabolic occurrences in total parenteral nutrition patients managed by a nutrition support team, *Nutr Clin Pract* 16:78, 2001.
82. Klein CJ et al: Nutrition support care map targets monitoring and reassessment to improve outcomes in trauma patients, *Nutr Clin Pract* 16:85, 2001.
83. American Society for Parenteral and Enteral Nutrition Board of Directors: Standards for home nutrition support, *Nutr Clin Pract* 14:151, 1998.

■ Further Reading

American Dietetic Association and Morrison Health Care: *Medical nutrition therapy across the continuum of care,* ed 2, and *Medical nutrition therapy across the continuum of care: supplement 1,* Chicago, Ill, 1998 and 1997, American Dietetic Association.

Fisher GG, Opper FH: An interdisciplinary nutrition support team improves quality of care in a teaching hospital, *J Am Diet Assoc* 96(2):176, 1996.

Fuhrman MP: Antioxidant supplementation in critical illness: what do we know? *Nutrition* 16:470, 2000.

Herrmann VM: Nutrition support: ethical or expedient, and who will choose? *J Parenter Enteral Nutr* 23:195, 1999.

Hester DD et al: Evaluation of the appropriate use of parenteral nutrition in an acute care setting, *J Am Diet Assoc* 96(6):602, 1996.

Klein CJ et al: Overfeeding macronutrient to critically ill adults: metabolic complications, *J Am Diet Assoc* 98:795, 1998.

Krzywda EA et al: Catheter infections: diagnosis, etiology, treatment, and prevention, *Nutr Clin Pract* 14:178, 1999.

Miles JM, Klein JA: Should protein be included in calorie calculations for a TPN prescription? *Nutr Clin Pract* 11:204, 1996.

Misra S, Kirby DF: Micronutrient and trace element monitoring in adult nutrition support, *Nutr Clin Pract* 15:120, 2000.

Proceedings of the second annual Ross medical nutrition and device roundtable: enteral nutrition and device use in alternative care settings, *Nutr Clin Pract* 15(suppl):S1-S80, 2000.

Ryder M: The future of vascular access: will the benefits be worth the risk? *Nutr Clin Pract* 14:165, 1999.

Schauster H, Dwyer J: Transition from tube feedings to feedings by mouth in children: preventing eating dysfunction, *J Am Diet Assoc* 96(3):277, 1996.

Schwartz DB: Enhanced enteral and parenteral nutrition practice and outcomes in an intensive care unit with a hospital-wide performance improvement process, *J Am Diet Assoc* 96(5):484, 1996.

Seidner DL, Licata A: Parenteral nutrition-associated metabolic bone disease: pathophysiology, evaluation, and treatment, *Nutr Clin Pract* 15:163, 2000.

Shatsky F, Borum P: Should carnitine be added to parenteral nutrition solutions? *Nutr Clin Pract* 15:152, 2000.

Shronts EP: Essential nature of choline with implications for total parenteral nutrition, *J Am Diet Assoc* 97(6):639, 1997.

■ Websites of Interest

http://www.nutritioncare.org American Society for Parenteral and Enteral Nutrition

http://www.eatright.org American Dietetic Association

http://www.dnsdpg.org Dietitians in Nutrition Support

http://www.tpnpro.com Tutorial on parenteral nutrition

http://www.oley.org Oley Foundation

Issues & ANSWERS

Troubleshooting Diarrhea in Tube-Fed Patients: A Costly Chase

Diarrhea is one of the most common complications associated with tube feeding, yet the reported incidence ranges widely from as little as 2% to as much as 70% in general patient populations and as high as 80% in intensive care patients. Questions that relate to this wide variance and that plague investigators apparently center on definition and cause. But the ultimate bottom line for patient and family and their health insurers is the price of the clinical search for the etiology and appropriate method of treatment. Although clinicians search for an effective treatment, diarrhea results in reduced kcalorie intake, dehydration, electrolyte abnormalities, and skin breakdown. Diarrhea also causes the patient discomfort, embarrassment, and frustration.

Problem of definition

If we are ever going to determine an accurate occurrence rate, etiology, and treatment of diarrhea, there must be a precise operational definition on which to establish a research design and evaluate results. There are at least 14 definitions for diarrhea in the literature. However, there is little agreement on which definition most accurately reflects diarrhea that requires intervention. Common definitions include output of more than 500 ml on 2 consecutive days or more than three stools per day. From a nursing standpoint, the collection and measurement of stool outputs are much less desirable than tracking the number of occurrences. However, the true definition of diarrhea may need to reflect consistency, frequency, and volume and not just number of stools per 24 hours. In most cases, diarrhea is defined by the person cleaning it up. The diagnosis of the etiology of diarrhea and the subsequent treatment consume time and healthcare resources. Meanwhile the patient is losing fluid, electrolytes, and nutrients through uncontrolled stool output. This can further exacerbate impaired nutritional status. Diarrhea not only takes a physical and nutritional toll on the patient but also has a psychologic effect of embarrassment and humiliation from an inability to control bodily functions and the loss of privacy.

Factors contributing to diarrhea

Reported causes of diarrhea in tube-fed patients also vary. The finger of blame for diarrhea usually is aimed at the formula itself. This results in manipulation of the formula—selection and concentration and infusion methods—usually to no avail because feeding intolerance is generally a manifestation, not the etiology, of diarrhea. A variety of causes for diarrhea have been reported. The most common contributors to diarrhea in tube fed patients are medications or some aspect of the patient's condition. However, many times there is not one single contributor but rather a combination of events or therapies that result in diarrhea.

Formula. The formula osmolality or concentration and rate of delivery are often blamed for instigating diarrhea. However, conflicting reports have shown no increase in the incidence of diarrhea when the formula concentration varied widely from 145 to 430 mOsm, and no significant association has been made between malabsorption and formula osmolality or rate of delivery. Formulas providing more than 30% of total kcalories as fat have been associated with a higher incidence of diarrhea, whereas those providing 20% fat rarely were involved. Further study of fat composition is needed, specifically comparing medium-chain versus long-chain triglycerides and omega-3 versus omega-6 fatty acids. Studies of the role of fiber in tube feedings have also been conflicting. There is no consistency in the types and amount of fiber in enteral formulas. Soluble fiber can increase colonic absorption of water. However, when the fiber given to a patient is increased rapidly, the patient will experience flatulence, abdominal distention, and constipation. Reviewers have found that the studies thus far have been few, the models used variable, the limitations substantial, and the conclusions of the investigators mixed. In general the amount and type of fiber in enteral formulas are not significant enough to prevent or contribute to diarrhea.

Bacterial contamination. There are studies that have shown that the more manipulation and additives, such as modular components, that are added to an enteral formula, the more likely the formula will become contaminated. Formula hang time, open versus closed delivery systems, and preparation technique can affect the risk of bacterial contamination of the enteral formula. Formula added to open delivery systems should hang no longer than 8 hours (even shorter periods of time if additives are combined with the formula). Closed systems that use containers prefilled with formula can hang 24 to 48 hours. The fewer times any system is handled and opened, the less chance there is for contamination. Commercial formula manufacturers are making formulas now that contain microbial inhibitors to reduce the risk of bacterial contamination of the enteral formula itself.

Infusion method. Intragastric feedings are associated with an increased incidence of diarrhea. The infusion of a large amount of kcalories into the stomach stimulates the colon to secret water, sodium, and chloride with resulting inability of the colon to absorb nutrients.

Patient's condition. Malnourished or critically ill patients are more susceptible to mucosal tissue breakdown and malabsorption leading to diarrhea. Hypoalbuminemia has also been reported to be a potential cause of diarrhea because of its effect on reducing colloidal osmotic pressure within blood vessels, which could lead to edema of the intestinal mucosa, malabsorption, and diarrhea. However, there has been no correlation between patients with hypoalbuminemia and incidence of diarrhea. Patients with pancreatic insufficiency, celiac disease, small bowel syndrome, fecal impaction, diabetes mellitus, or gastrointestinal inflammation are at greater risk for diarrhea.

Medications. Multiple medications routinely given to hospitalized patients have been related to diarrhea. Antibiotics are most often associated with gastrointestinal side effects. However, the patients more susceptible to developing diarrhea are those who are critically ill and on multiple medications. Extensive treatment with antibiotics and disuse of the gastrointestinal tract contribute to a change in the bacterial milieu of the intestine with proliferation of the enteric pathogen *Clostridium difficile.* Other medications associated with the development of diarrhea are H_2-blockers, lactulose or laxatives, magnesium-containing antacids, potassium and phosphorus supplements, antineoplastic agents, and quinidine. Medications are often hyperosmolar and require dilution before infusion through a feeding tube. In general, drug reactions may relate to the metabolically active agent or to another ingredient added for its physical properties in the form of the drug, such as tablet or liquid, as the following case illustrates.

The case of the costly chase

A recently reported case of unexplained diarrhea in a tube-fed patient illustrates the difficult, and often costly, search for the cause. Max was a 55-year-old man who had had an aortic aneurysm and underwent emergency surgery to repair it. In the intensive care unit, the postoperative course was complicated by respiratory problems requiring ventilator assistance. He was administered a bronchodilator drug, theophylline, in tablet form, crushed and administered by nasogastric tube with water. When Max was able to take nourishment, an isotonic formula given by enteral tube feeding was started, and the crushed theophylline tablets were changed to a sugar-free theophylline solution. Within a day, Max began to have progressive abdominal distention and continuous liquid diarrhea. To rule out an abdominal catastrophe related to the aneurysm or surgery, a computed abdominal tomography scan, an aortogram, and colonoscopy were performed, but all of these studies were normal.

Despite stopping the enteral feeding, the distention and diarrhea continued. Stool specimens were tested for fecal leukocytes, parasites, and *C. difficile* toxin, and an enteric pathogen culture was prepared. All were nondiagnostic. Extensive additional serum and urine tests, as well as a sigmoidoscopy with rectal biopsy, gave no clue. Then stool electrolytes and osmolality measures suggested an osmotic diarrhea. Because Max was not receiving enteral feedings, his physicians thought a secretory bacterial toxin was probably causing the continuing diarrhea, so the previous studies were repeated to confirm the osmotic nature of the diarrhea. In addition, all of the medications were reviewed, but none appeared to be the cause.

Because the continued diarrhea prohibited enteral feeding and Max needed nourishment, parenteral nutrition was ordered. This move immediately brought an automatic Nutrition Support Service consultation, which included further assessment of medications. This evaluation revealed that the sugar-free theophylline solution was 65% sorbitol.

Sorbitol is a polyhydric alcohol used as a sweetener in many sugar-free products such as dietetic foods and chewing gum. There was no information about sorbitol on the label or package insert of the drug because sorbitol is considered an "inactive" ingredient. The sorbitol content was obtained by contacting the manufacturer.

Fortunately for Max, however, the nutrition support team did know the components of the medication and found the hidden culprit. The registered dietitian knew that sorbitol in larger doses is a laxative! Calculations of the regular daily amount of the theophylline Max was taking showed that he was receiving nearly 300 g of sorbitol daily when the usual laxative dose was only 20 to 50 g. The nutrition support team immediately recommended that this sorbitol-sweetened solution of theophylline be discontinued and that a sorbitol-free form of the medication be used instead. Almost immediately the diarrhea began to decrease, and in 3 days it was gone.

The extent of this costly chase was revealed in Max's hospital bill. He had continued to receive the faulty drug for almost half of his 3-month hospital stay, during which time the diarrhea prevented enteral feeding and he had to have the more expensive parenteral nutrition. The parenteral nutrition cost $4860 more than the enteral feedings would have cost for the same period. In addition, all the extensive investigations to find the cause of the diarrhea cost $4250, which together with the indirect costs for extra days of care and supplies made a total hospital bill of about $170,000.

The causes of diarrhea in tube-fed patients are many, but in the hands of a skilled nutrition support team, the formula is seldom one of them. It is often found in the medications. Just remember what this medication's hidden ingredient—sorbitol—cost Max.

REFERENCES

Bowling TE: Enteral-feeding-related diarrhea: proposed causes and possible solutions, *Proc Nutr Soc* 54:579, 1995.

Fuhrman MP: Diarrhea and tube feeding, *Nutr Clin Pract* 14:83, 1999.

Hill DB et al: Osmotic diarrhea induced by sugar-free theophylline solution in critically ill patients, *J Parenter Enteral Nutr* 15(3):332, 1991.

Mobarham S, DeMeo M: Diarrhea induced by enteral feeding, *Nutr Rev* 53(3):67, 1995.

Ringel AF, Jameson GL, Foster ES: Diarrhea in the intensive care patient, *Crit Care Clin North Am* 11:465, 1995.

Williams MS et al: Diarrhea management in enterally fed patient, *Nutr Clin Pract* 13:225, 1998.

Wong K: The role of fiber in diarrhea management, *Support Line* 20:16, 1998.

Chapter

18

Gastrointestinal Diseases

Georgia Clark-Albert

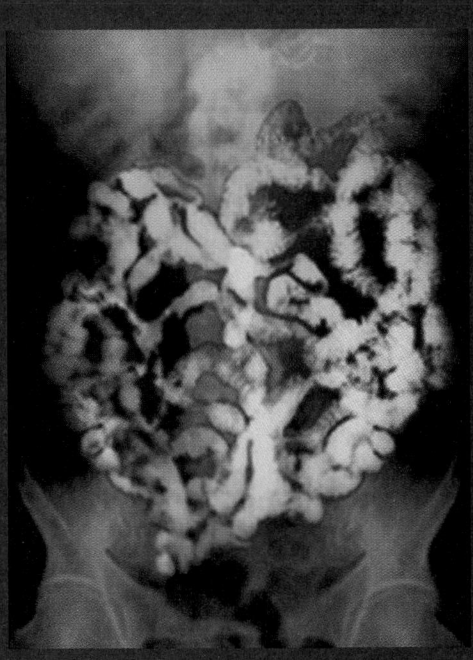

Chapter Outline

In this chapter, we consider diseases of the gastrointestinal tract and its surrounding accessory organs—the liver, gallbladder, and pancreas. In health, the digestion and absorption of our food are accomplished through a series of intimately interrelated actions among these organ systems. To the extent that disease or malfunction at any point interferes with this finely interwoven process, nutrition therapy must be used to modify food intake.

The gastrointestinal tract is a sensitive mirror of the individual human condition. It often reflects both physical and emotional conditioning. Its physiologic function reflects physical and psychologic conditioning. In this chapter we relate these basic functions and the healing process not only to the nutrition therapy indicated but also to the individual's personal needs.

Digestive Process

When food is taken into the mouth, the act of eating stimulates the gastrointestinal tract into accelerated action. Throughout the digestive process, highly coordinated systems and interactive functions respond (see Figure 2-1). Secretory functions provide the necessary environment and agents for chemical digestion, and peristalsis and gravity move the food mass along. Nutrients are absorbed into the blood circulation and carried to the cells, which take up what is needed to nourish the body. Emotional factors influence the overall individual response pattern. This highly individual and interrelated functional network forms the basis for medical nutrition therapy in disease. After food is taken into the mouth and masticated, *swallowing* (the act of the sphincter relaxing) occurs, allowing the bolus to pass from the laryngopharynx into the esophagus entrance at the upper esophageal sphincter. Food is pushed through the esophagus by gravity and involuntary muscular movements called *peristalsis,* controlled by the medulla oblongata. Circular muscle fibers contract, constricting the esophageal wall and squeezing the bolus toward the stomach. The lower esophageal sphincter muscle at the entry to the stomach forms a controlling valve, relaxing to receive the bolus and then closing to hold each bolus for some initial digestive action of enzymes. The stomach cells produce enzymes to break down food particles and to protect themselves from being broken down. The passage of food from the mouth to the stomach takes about 4 to 8 seconds.

The *chyme* (semiliquid mass) is released by the stomach through the pyloric sphincter into the duodenum, the first section of the small intestine. Most digestion occurs in the small intestine. A number of small intestine and accessory organ conditions may interfere with normal food passage and create malabsorption problems. These overall conditions vary widely from brief periods of functional discomfort to serious disease and complete obstruction. In making medical nutrition therapy recommendations for food choices and feeding mode, the nutrition practitioner will take into account the degree of dysfunction.

Problems of the Mouth and Esophagus

MOUTH PROBLEMS

The teeth and jaw muscles in the mouth work together to break down food into a form that can be easily swallowed. Conditions that interfere with this process interfere with nutrition.

Tissue Inflammation

The tissues of the mouth often reflect a person's basic nutritional status. In malnutrition the tissues of the mouth deteriorate and become inflamed and are more vulnerable to local infection or injury, causing pain and difficulty with eating. These conditions in the oral cavity include (1) *gingivitis,* inflammation of the gums, involving the mucous membrane with its supporting fibrous tissue circling the base of the teeth; (2) *stomatitis,* inflammation of the oral mucosa lining the mouth; (3) *glossitis,* inflammation of the tongue; and (4) *cheilosis,* a cracking and dry scaling process at the corners of the mouth affecting the lips and corner angles, making opening the mouth to receive food difficult.

These oral tissue problems may also be nonspecific and unrelated to nutritional factors. In some cases, gingivitis and stomatitis occur in mild form in relation to another disease or stress. Occasionally a severe form of acute necrotizing ulcerative gingivitis occurs. It is caused by a specific infectious bacterium, *Fusobacterium nucleatum,* often in conjunction with the spirochete *Treponema vincentii;* it is also known as Vincent's disease, from the Paris physician Henri Vincent (1862-1950), who first identified the disease process. The gums around the bases of the teeth become puffy, shiny, and tender overlapping the teeth margins. Affected gums often bleed, especially during toothbrushing. This serious condition destroys gum tissue and the supporting tissues of the teeth and requires a course of antibiotic treatment.

Mouth pain in these conditions often causes decreased food intake. Maintaining adequate nutritional intake then becomes a major problem. Generally, patients are given high-protein, high-kilocaloric (kcaloric) liquids and then soft foods, usually nonacidic and without strong spices to avoid irritation. Temperature extremes may also be avoided if they cause pain. Gradually foods are increased according to toleration, and foods are often supplemented with vitamins and minerals. In severe disease, the use of a mouthwash containing a mild topical local anesthetic before meals helps relieve the pain of eating.

Dental Problems

The incidence of dental caries has recently been reduced in children and young adults. However, it is still present in many older adults, especially those unable to afford regular dental care, and causes tooth loss and chewing problems. In older adults, some 65 million in the United States alone, periodontal disease is a major cause of tooth loss. Especially if dental caries is untreated or if dental hygiene is poor, gum tissue at the base of the teeth becomes damaged and pockets form between the gums and the teeth. Dental plaque forms from a sticky deposit of mucus, food particles, and bacteria. The plaque hardens into *calculus,* a mineralized coating developed from the plaque and saliva. These hardened particles then collect in the pocket openings at the base of the teeth, where the bacte-

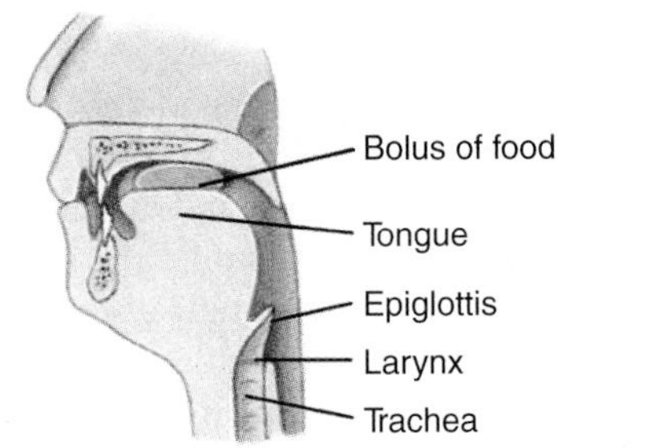

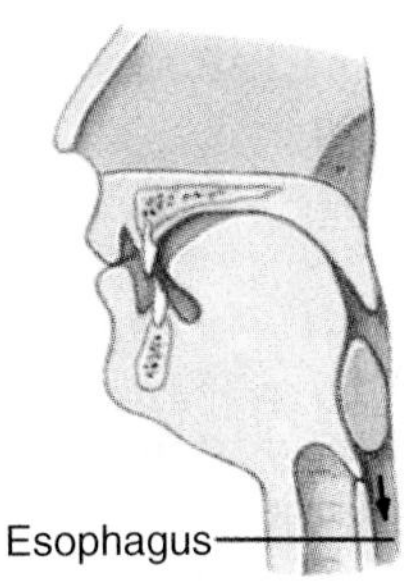

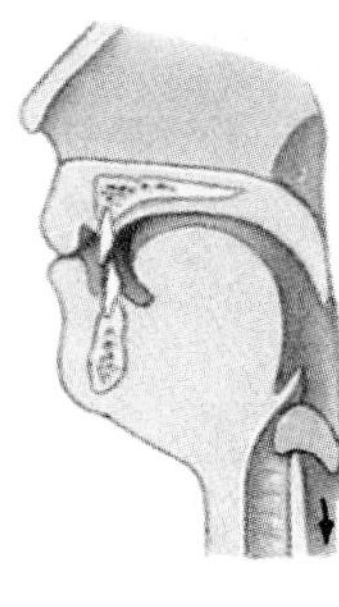

FIGURE 18-1 Parts of mouth, pharynx, and esophagus involved in the swallowing process. (*From Wardlaw GM, Insel PM:* Perspectives in nutrition, *ed 2, New York, 1993, McGraw-Hill. Reproduced with permission of the McGraw-Hill Companies.*)

ria attack the periodontal tissue. The result is bacterial erosion of bone tissue surrounding affected teeth and subsequent tooth loss. Preventive care through daily dental care with fluoridated toothpaste, careful flossing, and periodic plaque removal by the dental hygienist form the best approach. Extensive tooth loss leads to the need for tooth replacement with dentures. In many elderly people these dentures become ill fitting, especially when weight loss occurs, and hinder adequate chewing. All of these dental problems need to be reviewed as part of the physical assessment in any patient's nutritional history so that food textures and forms can be adjusted to individual needs.

Salivary Glands and Salivation

Disorders of the salivary glands affect eating because saliva carries an *amylase* that begins starch breakdown and is vital in moistening the food to facilitate chewing. Problems may arise from infection, such as infection with the mumps virus, which attacks the parotid gland. Other problems come from excessive salivation, which occurs in numerous disorders affecting the nervous system, such as Parkinson's disease, and from local disorders such as mouth infections or injury. Problems may arise from any disease or drug that causes overactivity of the parasympathetic division of the autonomic nervous system, which controls the salivary glands.

Conversely, lack of salivation, which causes *xerostomia* (dry mouth), may be a temporary condition caused by fear, salivary gland infection, or action of anticholinergic drugs that hinder the normal action of neurotransmitters. Clients with dry mouth best tolerate moist, soft foods with added gravies and sauces. Permanent xerostomia is rare but does occur in Sjögren's syndrome, a symptom complex of unknown cause that is thought to be an abnormal immune response. It occurs in middle-aged or older women and is marked by dry mouth and enlargement of the parotid glands; it is often associated with rheumatoid arthritis. It may also result from radiation therapy. There is difficulty in swallowing and speaking, interference with taste, and tooth decay. Salty foods dry the mouth and should be avoided. Chewing gum or sucking on sugarless candy can increase salivary secretions. The extreme mouth dryness may be partially relieved by spraying the inside of the mouth with an artificial saliva solution.

Swallowing Disorders

Most people take swallowing for granted. Each day we eat, chew, and swallow without giving it a second thought. However, the process of swallowing involves highly integrated actions of the mouth, pharynx, and esophagus (Figure 18-1). Swallowing difficulty, known medically as *dysphagia,* is a fairly common problem arising from many causes including stroke, aging, developmental disabilities, and nervous system diseases. It may be only temporary, such as a piece of food lodged in the back of the throat, for which the Heimlich maneuver is appropriate first aid, or it may be involved with insufficient production of saliva and xerostomia. Such dysfunctional swallowing often causes children and adults alike to aspirate food particles, in turn causing coughing and choking episodes. Dysphagia is of concern for many reasons. Foods may enter the trachea and aspirate into the lungs, allowing bacteria to multiply, leading to pneumonia. Clients with dysphagia are usually referred to a special interdisciplinary team that includes a physician, speech pathologist, nurse, clinical dietitian, physical therapist, and an occupational therapist, with special training in swallowing problems. Thin liquids are the most difficult food form to swallow. Depending on the level of dysphagia, liquids may need to be thickened. Thickening agents include baby rice, commercially

---

Heimlich maneuver — A first-aid maneuver to relieve a person who is choking from blockage of the breathing passageway by a swallowed foreign object or food particle. Standing behind the person, clasp the victim around the waist, placing one fist under the sternum (breastbone) and grasping the fist with the other hand. Then make a quick, hard, thrusting movement inward and upward.

---

prepared thickeners, potato flakes, or mashed potatoes. Levels of thickness include thick (yogurt or pudding consistency) and medium thick (nectar consistency).

ESOPHAGEAL PROBLEMS

Central Problems

The esophagus is a long, muscular tube lined with mucous membranes that extends from the pharynx, or throat, to the stomach (see Figure 18-1). It is bounded on both ends by circular muscles, or sphincters, that act as valves to control food passage. The upper sphincter remains closed except during swallowing, thus preventing airflow into the esophagus and stomach. Disorders along the tube that may disrupt normal swallowing and food passage include esophageal spasm (uncoordinated contractions of the esophagus), esophageal stricture (a narrowing caused by a scar from previous inflammation, ingestion of caustic chemicals, or a tumor), and esophagitis (an inflammation). These problems hinder eating and require medical attention through dilation, stretching procedures, or surgery to widen the tube or drug therapy.

Lower Esophageal Sphincter Problems

Defects in the operation of the lower esophageal sphincter (LES) muscles may come from changes in the smooth muscle itself or from the nerve-muscle hormonal control. In general, these LES problems arise from spasm, stricture, or incompetence.

Achalasia

If the LES does not relax normally when presented with food during swallowing, the condition is call achalasia (*a* = "without," *chalasia* = "relaxation"). Spasms occur when the LES muscles maintain an excessively high muscle tone, even while resting, and thus fail to open normally when the person swallows. Achalasia is also known as *cardiospasm,* from the proximity of the heart, although it has no relation to heart action. Peristalsis in the upper esophagus is often found, resulting in the esophagus becoming shaped like a funnel or bag. Patient symptoms include swallowing problems, frequent vomiting, feelings of chest fullness, and weight loss. Protein-calorie malnutrition and pulmonary infections secondary to reduced oral intake and aspiration of food and saliva may occur in severe cases.[1]

Medical treatment includes endoscopic dilation of the LES or surgical release of the muscle.[1] The stricture improves but the peristalsis does not. Nutrition requirements of patients with achalasia vary with the severity of the disease and the approach to treatment. Generally, nutrient-dense liquids and semisolid foods, taken at moderate temperatures, in small quantities, and at frequent intervals are usually tolerated by patients with achalasia.[1] General guidelines for nutritional management are given in Table 18-1.

Gastroesophageal Reflux Disease

Gastroesophageal reflux disease (GERD), the backflow or regurgitation of gastric contents from the stomach into the esophagus, is a very common disease that affects at least 44% of adults in the United States.[2] Regurgitation of the acid gastric contents into the lower part of the esophagus creates constant tissue irritation because the wall of the esophagus is not protected from the acid of the stomach and, during reflux, many patients feel a burning sensation behind the sternum that radiates toward the mouth. This common symptom of GERD, heartburn (pyrosis), is unrelated to disease of the heart. Additional symptoms include acid indigestion and/or regurgitation, which often occurs after meals, especially if the meal is large or of a high fat content.[3] Other less common symptoms include iron deficiency anemia with chronic bleeding and aspiration, which may cause cough, dyspnea, or pneumonitis. Sometimes substernal pain radiates into the neck and jaw or down the arms. Acid reflux may be caused by a hiatal hernia, pregnancy (estrogen and progesterone have been shown to reduce LES pressure), obesity, pernicious vomiting, or nasogastric tubes. A number of drugs also lower LES pressure, causing GERD and heartburn to be a side effect of drugs used in the treatment of other conditions.

The acid and pepsin cause tissue erosion with symptoms of substernal burning, cramping, pressure sensation, or severe pain. Symptoms are aggravated by lying down or by any increase of abdominal pressure, such as that caused by tight clothing. The condition is related to (1) a nonfunctioning gastroesophageal sphincter, (2) frequency and duration of the acid reflux, and (3) inability of the esophagus to produce normal secondary peristaltic waves to pre-

TABLE 18-1 Dietary Principles for Care of Achalasia

Principles	Foods Included
Energy nutrients	Modified protein and carbohydrates and increased fat to help reduce lower esophageal sphincter pressure and gastric section
Texture	Liquid or semisolid food as tolerated
	Moderate to low fiber if it aids swallowing
Temperature	No very hot or very cold foods
Irritants	No citrus juices to injure mucosa if retained
	No highly spiced foods to irritate if retained
Meal pattern	Frequent, small meals as tolerated
Eating pace	Eat slowly in small bites and swallows

Modified from Zeman FJ: *Clinical nutrition and dietetics,* ed 2, Englewood Cliffs, NJ, 1991, Prentice Hall.

vent prolonged contact of the mucosa with the acid pepsin. A hiatal hernia may or may not be present. The most common complications of GERD are stenosis and esophageal ulcer. In long-term studies a significant number of patients with reflux esophagitis and *Helicobacter pylori* infection, treated with the antacid omeprazole, showed increased risk of atrophic gastritis and the cascading events that can lead to gastric cancer.[4]

From 85% to 90% of patients with GERD respond to weight reduction and conservative measures. Lifestyle modifications that decrease distal esophageal acid exposure include cessation of smoking, avoiding lying down 2 to 3 hours postprandially, decreasing fat intake, and raising of the head of the bed.[5] Foods found to increase LES, and therefore should be avoided, include chocolate, alcohol, peppermint, spearmint, strong tea, and coffee. Antacids and over-the-counter acid suppressants are helpful in relieving symptoms in milder forms of GERD. Table 18-2 summarizes these management principles.

TABLE 18-2 Dietary Care of Gastroesophageal Reflux

Outcome	Action
Decrease esophageal irritation	Avoid common irritants such as coffee, carbonated beverages, tomato and citrus juices, and spicy foods
Increase lower esophageal sphincter pressure	Increase protein foods
	Decrease fat to about 45 g/day or less; use nonfat milk
	Avoid strong tea, coffee, and chocolate if poorly treated
	Avoid peppermint and spearmint
Decrease reflux frequency and volume	Eat small, frequent meals
	Sip only a small amount of liquid with meal; drink mostly between meals
	Avoid constipation; straining increases abdominal pressure reflux
Clear food materials from the esophagus	Sit upright at the table or elevate the head of bed
	Do not recline for 2 hours or more after eating

Modified from Zeman FJ: *Clinical nutrition and dietetics,* ed 2, Englewood Cliffs, NJ, 1991, Prentice-Hall.

Hiatal Hernia

The esophagus normally enters the chest cavity at the *hiatus,* an opening in the diaphragm membrane, and immediately joins the upper portion of the stomach. A hiatal hernia occurs when a portion of the upper part of the stomach at this entry point of the esophagus protrudes through the hiatus alongside the lower portion of the esophagus (Figure 18-2). Food is easily held in this

achalasia Failure to relax the smooth muscle fibers of the gastrointestinal tract at any point of juncture of its parts; especially failure of the esophagogastric sphincter to relax when swallowing, as a result of degeneration of ganglion cells in the wall of the organ. The lower esophagus also loses its normal peristaltic activity. Also called cardiospasm.

gastritis Inflammation of the stomach.

pyrosis Heartburn.

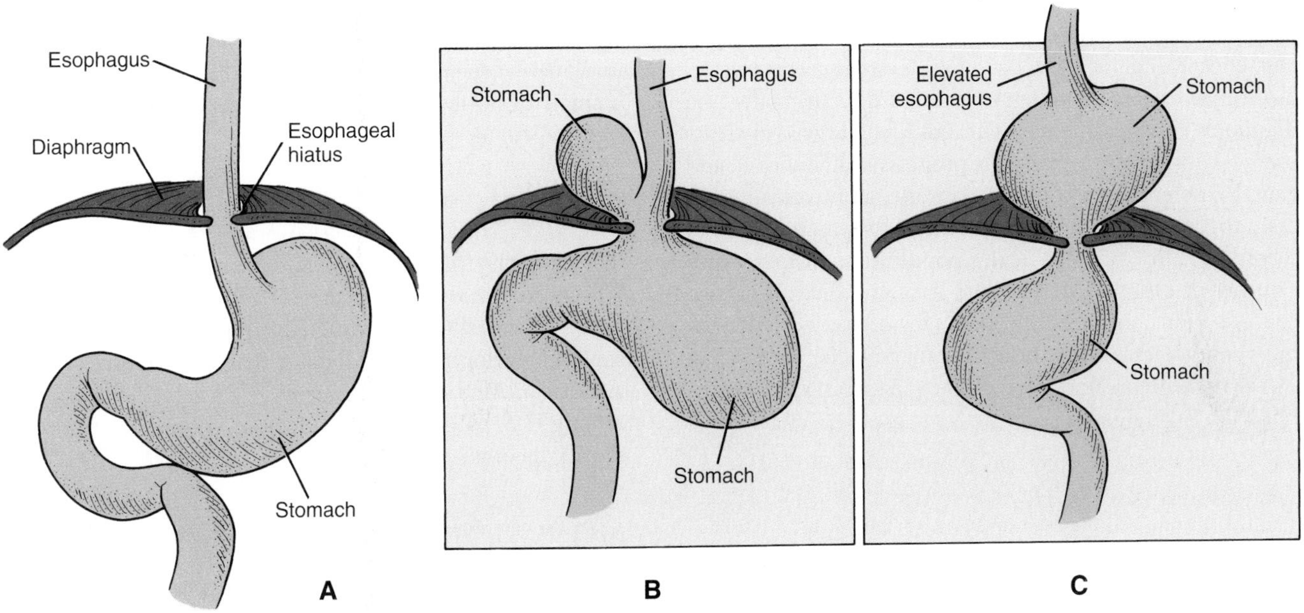

FIGURE 18-2 Hiatal hernia compared with normal stomach placement. **A,** Normal stomach. **B,** Paraesophageal hernia (esophagus in normal position). **C,** Esophageal hiatal hernia (elevated esophagus).

herniated area of the stomach and mixed with acid and pepsin; then it is regurgitated back up into the lower part of the esophagus. Gastritis can occur in this herniated portion of the stomach and cause bleeding and anemia. The reflux of gastric acid contents causes symptoms similar to those described earlier.

A regular diet of choice using frequent small feedings for comfort is usually tolerated. Also, because obesity is often associated with hiatal hernia, weight reduction is a primary goal. Avoiding tight clothing helps relieve discomfort. Patients will need to avoid leaning over or lying down immediately after meals and should sleep with the head of the bed elevated. Antacids help relieve the burning sensation. Large hiatal hernias or smaller sliding hernias may require surgical repair.

Problems of the Stomach and Duodenum: Peptic Ulcer Disease

INCIDENCE

Peptic ulcer disease (PUD) was uncommon in the 1800s, but it began to increase greatly during the early part of the 1900s. The increase seems to have peaked about the mid-1950s, as a result of increased knowledge of the disease process and rapid progress in its medical management. The Centers for Disease Control and Prevention (CDC) reports that close to 10% of the U.S. population will be affected by peptic ulcers sometime during their lives, with peptic ulcers accounting for some 1 million hospitalizations and 6500 deaths each year, with direct and indirect costs of nearly $6 billion annually.[6] The development of simple, cost-effective, highly exact serologic tests and effective *H. pylori* eradication therapies have had a dramatic effect on diagnoses and treatment, quality of life, and cost of treatment.[6] Despite the remarkable progress in knowledge and care, PUD remains a common, chronic, and recurring disease, still one of the most prevalent of the gastrointestinal disorders. Now with an aging population, an increasing number of older adult patients have the disease. Major complications are bleeding, perforation, and obstruction, but these are rare with modern management. Fewer than 2% of the patients under treatment experience such a complication in any given year.[7]

GENERAL NATURE

An *ulcer* is the loss of tissue on the surface of the mucosa. In the gastrointestinal tract, an ulcer extends through the mucosa, submucosa, and often into the muscle layer. *Peptic ulcer* is the general term for an eroded mucosal lesion in the central portion of the gastrointestinal tract. A peptic ulcer can occur in any area of the stomach that is exposed to pepsin. The areas affected include the lower portion of the esophagus, the stomach, and the first portion of the duodenum, called the *duodenal bulb.* Esophageal and gastric ulcers are less common. Most ulcers occur in the duodenal bulb, where gastric contents emptying into the duodenum through the pyloric valve are most concentrated. Gastric ulcers occur usually along the lesser curvature of the stomach. PUD itself is a benign disease, but ulcers do tend to recur. Gastric ulcers are more prone to develop into malignant disease. Weight loss is common in patients with gastric ulcers. Patients with duodenal ulcers may gain weight from frequent eating to counteract pain.

DISCOVERY OF THE CAUSATIVE MICROBE

An Australian team of pathologists working at the Royal Perth Hospital discovered the causative microbe, a corkscrew-shaped bacterium, later named *Helicobacter pylori* because of its coiled helix structure ("helico") and its major infection site surrounding the pyloric valve area between the lower stomach and the first section of the small intestine, the duodenal bulb ("pylori").[8-10] They published their first report early in 1983 and followed with a more definitive study in 1984.[8]

INCIDENCE

As with other infectious processes, *H. pylori* grows vigorously in areas where people are poor and living in crowded conditions. For example, in developing countries the infection occurs early in life, usually at 6 to 8 months of age, and persists as a chronic condition infecting 80% of the population by the age of 20 years.[10] In contrast, in developed countries the infection rate increases slowly with age and 50% of the persons 60 years old are infected, but only a small minority of these people develop gastric pathology, peptic ulcers, or gastric cancer.[10,11]

ETIOLOGY

The causative role of *H. pylori* is now clearly established. The U.S. National Institutes of Health (NIH) has officially approved these findings in a report by an NIH Consensus Development Conference that was endorsed by the American Medical Association.[12] Reported risk factors among U.S. adults include older age, short education, low family income, and smoking.[13]

MEDICAL MANAGEMENT

In the past few years, with the discovery and knowledge of *H. pylori* infection as the direct cause of PUD and gastric acidity as the indirect supporting factor, we have seen a revolution in our understanding of the pathophysiology of PUD. Three components of the disease and its medical management form the basis of clinical therapy.[14]

Gastric Acid and Pepsin

There is hypersecretion of gastric hydrochloric acid and pepsinogen, which the acid quickly converts to the strong active protein enzyme pepsin. The amount of acid varies, but the classic medical dictum—"no acid, no ulcer"—still holds.

Nonsteroidal Anti-inflammatory Drugs

Widely used nonsteroidal anti-inflammatory drugs (NSAIDs), the most commonly known of which is ibuprofen (Advil, Motrin), as well as the common analgesic aspirin (acetylsalicylic acid [ASA]), irritate the gastric mucosa and cause bleeding, erosion, and ulceration, especially with prolonged or excessive use. The NSAID group of drugs are so named to distinguish them from the corticosteroids, synthetic variants of the natural adrenal hormones. The NSAIDs include a dozen anti-inflammatory drugs.

Clinical Symptoms

Basic symptoms of peptic ulcer are increased gastric tone and painful hunger contractions when the stomach is empty. In duodenal ulcer, the amount and concentration of hydrochloric acid are increased. In gastric ulcer it may be normal. Nutritional deficiencies are evident in low plasma protein levels, anemia, and loss of weight. Hemorrhage may be the first sign in some patients. Diagnosis is based on clinical findings, radiographs, or visualization by fiberoptic gastroscopy.

MEDICAL MANAGEMENT

The primary goal of medical management for PUD is the control of *H. pylori.* Additional supportive goals are to (1) alleviate the symptoms, (2) promote healing, (3) prevent recurrences, and (4) prevent complications. In addition to general traditional measures, the rapidly expanding knowledge base and development of a number of new drugs have increased the physician's available management tools.

General Therapeutic Measures

Adequate rest, relaxation, and sleep have long been a foundation for general care of PUD to enhance the body's natural healing process. Positive stress coping and relaxation skills, which help patients deal with personal psychosocial stressors, can be learned and practiced. Simple encouragement to talk about anxieties, anger, and frustrations helps to make patients feel better, and as soon as they are able, appropriate physical activity helps work out tensions. Habits that contribute to ulcer development, such as smoking and alcohol use, should be eliminated. Common drugs such as aspirin and NSAIDs should be avoided.

Medical Management

Current medical management of PUD has a wider choice of drugs to control underlying physiologic causes and clinical symptoms and to support healing. In various ways, five types of drugs now suppress gastric acid and pepsin secretion, protect mucosal tissue, buffer acid, and eliminate infection.

1. *Histamine H_2-receptor antagonists.* These agents, commonly called H_2-blockers, are popular drugs for controlling gastric acid secretion. They decrease hydrochloric acid production by competing with histamine for receptor sites on parietal cells. Normally, histamine attached to its specific cellular receptors (type H_2) on the acid-producing parietal cells of the gastric mucosa and mediate their secretion of hydrochloric acid. Thus their blocking action effectively controls acid and pepsin because the inactive pepsinogen requires the acid for activation. Four of these drugs have now been reclassified for over-the-counter purchase: (1) cimetidine (Tagamet), (2) ranitidine (Zantac), (3) famotidine (Pepcid), and (4) nizatidine (Axid).
2. *Proton pump inhibitors.* This newer class of drugs, more potent than the H_2-blockers, also suppresses gastric acid, but by a different action. Without competition, in the parietal cells they irreversibly prevent action of a key enzyme that actively secretes hydrogen ions needed for hydrochloric acid (HCI) production. Without available H+ ions, the HCI cannot be made. Then without the acid, ulcers heal rapidly. An example of this type drug is omeprazole (Prilosec). Proton pump inhibitors may interfere with liver metabolism of anticoagulants, diazepam (Valium), or phenytoin (Dilantin). Serum levels of these drugs should be monitored during concurrent therapy.
3. *Mucosal protectors.* Drugs of this type act as cytoprotective agents by helping the stomach heal itself. They produce a gel-like suspension that binds to the ulcer base and covers it and the surrounding normal mucosal tissue to protect the involved tissue from harm while it heals. This drug also forms complexes with pepsin that inactivates the pepsin. An example of this type of drug is sucralfate.
4. *Antacids.* These well-known substances counteract or neutralize acidity. The two main types are (1) magnesium-aluminum compounds (Maalox TC, Mylanta II, or Riopan) and (2) aluminum hydroxide (Basaljel, Amphojel). Aluminum-based preparations may cause constipation; magnesium-based preparations may cause diarrhea.
5. *Antibiotics.* Drugs of this type are used to control the *H. pylori* infection associated with PUD. Although the organism is easily suppressed, it seems to be more difficult to eradicate. However, combinations being used by investigators and clinicians include the following bacterial or suppressant agents.

- Bismuth (Pepto-Bismol), bismuth subsalicylate, or colloid bismuth subcitrate
- Metronidazole (Flagyl), a bacterial and protozoan killer
- Amoxicillin (Amoxil, Polymox), a penicillin derivative, or tetracycline (Achromycin-V, Panmycin) a frequently used wide-spectrum antibody

Other drugs for general needs include acetaminophen (Tylenol) to replace aspirin or NSAIDs. Also, if needed briefly for mild sedation to aid the initial need for relaxation and sleep, a tricyclic antidepressant such as amitriptyline (Elavil) may be prescribed.

Many regimens have been devised for eradicating *H. pylori,* and debate continues over the best treatment.[7] Bismuth triple therapy was the first regimen to show eradication rates above 80%. Since then many studies have shown eradication rates consistently of 87% to 89% in populations with unknown prevalence of imidazole resistance. In patients infected with metronidazole resistant strains, however, efficacy drops to 48%. The main challenge now is to develop a maintenance therapy that prevents recurrence of the disease.[15,16] Currently the best approach seems to include continuous low-dose drug therapy, intermittent full-dose treatment, or symptomatic self-care with the same agents used to heal the ulcer. Success rates hinge on the relative strengths of risk factors that influence recurrence (Table 18-3). Acid-independent mechanisms used include the use of sucralfate (Carafate) to coat the stomach and adhere to the ulcer surface, reinforcing the mucous barrier. Misoprostol (Cytotec) aids in mucus production and inhibits acid secretion by parietal cells. It is useful in maintenance therapy to prevent ulcers in patients who use NSAIDs. Metoclopramide (Reglan) prompts the LES to tighten preventing reflux in GERD.

TABLE 18-3 Recurrent Peptic Ulcer Risk Factors

Chance of Recurrence	Risk Factors
Possible	Positive family history
	Emotional stress
	Continued use of concentrated alcohol
Good	History of recurrences and complications
	Continued use of aspirin and other NSAIDs
	Increased *Helicobacter pylori* infection
Strong	Poor compliance with maintenance diet or drug plan
	Continued smoking (≥10 cigarettes/day)
	Gastric acid hypersecretion

Modified from Earnest DL: Maintenance therapy in peptic ulcer disease, *Med Clin North Am* 75(4):1013, 1991.

Nutritional Management

The revolutionary advance in knowledge of PUD and development of drugs for its medical management have also brought welcome reevaluation of the role of nutrition in its basic care. There is now both medical and nutritional agreement that the old restrictive bland milk-based diet routines of the past, long since known to be ineffective and potentially harmful, have no role in the modern management of PUD.[11,12,16-18] Instead, a positive nutrition approach and basic dietary principles guide our current practice.

1. *Current positive nutrition approach.* The current medical nutrition therapy is that of basic health maintenance or preventive approach in overall healthcare today.[15] As with any disease process involving tissue injury, the prime nutritional requirement is clear: sufficient energy-nutrient intake supplied by a regular well-balanced diet to support the primary medical management of (1) tissue healing and (2) tissue maintenance of structural and functional integrity. Initial and periodic reassessment of nutritional needs is necessary to determine energy-nutrient status and any area of individual deficiencies.
2. *Nutrition principles.* The basic nutrition principles of a well-balanced diet are found in the regular guidelines of the Recommended Dietary Allowance (RDA) energy-nutrient standards and the *Dietary Guidelines for Americans* for health promotion (see Chapter 1). In addition to the major goal of optimal nutritional support, a second dietary goal is to avoid stimulating excess acid secretion and directly irritating the gastric mucosa. Only a few related food factors or habits have been shown to cause excess acid secretion and irritation.
   - *Meal pattern.* Eat three regular meals a day without frequent snacks, especially at bedtime. Any food intake stimulates more acid output.
   - *Food quantity.* Avoid stomach distention with large quantities of food at a meal.
   - *Milk intake.* Avoid drinking milk frequently. It stimulates significant gastric acid secretion and has only a transient buffering effect. Also, the milk sugar lactose creates problems of abdominal cramping, gas, and diarrhea for many persons with lactose intolerance caused by a deficiency of the enzyme lactase.
   - *Seasonings.* Individual tolerance is the rule. However, several agents have caused variable results and may need to be watched: hot chili peppers, black pepper, and chili powder.
   - *Dietary fiber.* There is no evidence for restricting dietary fiber. Some fibers, especially soluble forms, are beneficial. Adequate fiber will counteract the constipating effects of drug therapy.

- *Coffee.* Avoid regular and decaffeinated coffee. Coffee stimulates acid secretion and may cause dyspepsia. The comparative effect of regular tea and colas may be milder with some persons, but these beverages also stimulate acid secretion.
- *Citric acid juices.* These juices may induce gastric reflux and discomfort in some persons.
- *Alcohol.* Avoid alcohol in concentrated forms, such as 40% (80 proof) alcohol. Other less concentrated forms, such as wine, taken with food in moderate amounts, are tolerated well by some patients. Avoid beer; it has been shown to be a potent stimulant of gastric acid. For patients who find it particularly difficult to avoid alcohol and coffee completely, some physicians have suggested they may try a small serving of wine with dinner occasionally or a small cup (demitasse) of coffee at the close of the meal to minimize the acid secretion.
- *Smoking.* The habit of smoking is often associated with food intake. It is best eliminated completely at any time. It not only affects gastric acid secretion but also influences the effectiveness of drug therapy.
- *Food environment.* Finally, consider the food environment. Eat slowly and savor the food in a calm environment. Respect individual responses or tolerances to specific foods experienced at any time. Remember that the same food may evoke different responses at different times depending on the stress factor.

Personal Focus

Sound nutritional management plays an important supportive role in the total medical care of persons with PUD. The individual must be the focus of treatment. The patient is not "an ulcer," but a person with an ulcer. The course of the disease is conditioned by the individuality of the patient and his or her life situation. The presence of the ulcer affects the patient's life. In the long run, a wide range of foods, attractive to the eye and the taste, and regular, unhurried eating habits provide the best course of action.

Small Intestine Diseases

CONDITIONS OF MALABSORPTION AND DIARRHEA

Diarrhea

Diarrhea is not a disease but a symptom that can be attributed to many medical conditions. *Diarrhea* is defined as an increase in the frequency of bowel moments compared with the usual pattern or the excess water content of the stools affecting consistency or volume or both. Diarrhea most directly involves the large intestine but may be caused by disease of the small intestine, pancreas, or gallbladder. General diarrhea may result from basic dietary excesses. There may be fermentation of sugars involved or excess fiber stimulation of intestinal muscle function.

Chronic diarrhea may occur as a result of gastrointestinal tract motility dysfunction such as irritable bowel syndrome, malabsorption, metabolic disorders, food intolerances (i.e., lactose intolerance), food poisoning, infections, and human immunodeficiency virus (HIV) infection. In the case of lactose intolerance, the accumulated concentration of undigested lactose in the intestine, resulting from the lack of the enzyme lactase, creates increased osmotic pressure. This pressure effectively draws water into the gut and stimulates hypermotility, abdominal cramping, and diarrhea. Milk treated with lactase enzyme is tolerated by these persons without the difficulty encountered with regular milk. Secretory, osmotic, and inflammatory processes in the intestine result in increased losses of fluid and electrolytes from diarrhea[19] (see *Issues & Answers*).

Malabsorption

In a normally functioning body, foods are digested and then nutrients are absorbed into the bloodstream, mostly from the small intestine. Malabsorption occurs either because a disorder interferes with how food is digested or because a disorder interferes with how nutrients are absorbed There are multiple causes of a malabsorption condition.[19] Symptoms of malabsorption include a change in bowel habits, apathy, fatigue, and a smooth surface on the lateral tongue. Some of these causes include the following.

- *Maldigestion problems:* pancreatic disorders, biliary disease, bacterial overgrowth, ileal disease (inflammatory bowel disease [IBD])
- *Intestinal mucosal changes:* mucosal surface alterations, intestinal surgery such as resections that shorten the bowel, lymphatic obstruction, intestinal stasis
- *Genetic disease:* cystic fibrosis with its complications of pancreatic insufficiency and lack of the pancreatic enzymes lipase, trypsin, and amylase
- *Intestinal enzyme deficiency:* lactose intolerance caused by lactase deficiency
- *Cancer and its treatment:* absorbing surface effect of radiation and chemotherapy
- *Metabolic biochemical defects:* absorbing surface effects of pernicious anemia or gluten-induced enteropathy (celiac sprue)

Here we briefly review four of these malabsorptive conditions—celiac sprue, cystic fibrosis, IBD, and short-bowel syndrome (SBS).

CELIAC SPRUE

Metabolic Defect

In 1889 a London physician named Gee observed a number of malnourished children having extensive fatty diarrhea, steatorrhea, and distended abdomens. He gave the name "celiac" to the general clinical condition from the

Greek word *kolia,* meaning "belly" or "abdomen." It was not until the mid-1950s that the Dutch pediatrician Willem-Karel Dicke and his associates discovered the causative agent. Their tissue studies confirmed that the gliadin fraction of the protein gluten in wheat produced the fat malabsorption and further that what had been called celiac disease in children and nontropical sprue in adults was a single disease, which came to be called *celiac sprue.*[20] As currently used, the alternate terms *celiac disease* and *gluten-sensitive enteropathy* are synonymous with celiac sprue. In all cases, such diseased tissues consistently show an eroded mucosal surface lacking the number and form of normal villi and having few microvilli. This erosion effectively reduces the absorbing surface by as much as 95%.

Clearly, gluten molecules combine with antibodies in the small intestine, causing the usually brushlike lining of the intestine to flatten, thereby being much less able to digest and absorb foods. When foods containing gluten are avoided, the lining of the intestine is restored and functions efficiently. Studies indicate a biochemical metabolic defect probably involving an enzyme deficiency and a genetic base. It is now apparent that the steatorrhea (about 80% of the ingested fat appears in the stools) and the progressive malnutrition are secondary effects caused by the primary biochemical reaction to gliadin in sensitive persons.

Nutritional Management

The goal of nutritional management is to control the intake of dietary gluten and prevent malnutrition. The diet is better defined as low gluten rather than gluten free because it is impossible to completely remove all gluten. Usually a small amount is tolerated by most patients, except in the prolonged use of newer products labeled "gluten free" but containing wheat starch as a thickening agent, which cannot be recommended.[21] Wheat and rye are the main sources of gluten; it is also present in oats and barley. Thus these four grains have always been eliminated from the diet. However, a growing body of evidence now suggests that moderate amounts of oats may be safely used in the diets of most adults with celiac disease.[22] Corn and rice are usually the substitute grains used. Parents of children with celiac sprue need special instructions about food products to avoid, what constitutes a basic meal pattern, and recipes for food preparation. Careful label reading must be discussed because many commercial products use the offending grains as thickeners or fillers, and parents' knowledge of gluten-containing food products is highly variable and influences the child's attitudes toward dietary compliance. With an increasing number of processed foods being marketed, as well as increasing use of ethnic foods in Western society, it is difficult to detect all foods containing gluten; therefore a home test kit for gluten has been developed.[23] Good dietary management varies according to the child's age, pathologic conditions, and clinical status. Generally, a dietary program based on the low-gluten diet given in Table 18-4 may be followed. In a small subgroup of patients, the symptoms persist despite strict adherence to the diet. In rare instances, persons with such a refractory form of the disease respond only to parenteral nutrition support.[20]

CYSTIC FIBROSIS

Genetic-Metabolic Defect

Cystic fibrosis is inherited as an autosomal recessive trait mainly in white populations in which 1:20 is a carrier and now 1:2500 newborns is affected.[24] It occurs rarely in other populations—for example, 1:17,000 black live births and 1:90,000 Oriental live births. It is the most common fatal genetic disease in North America. In past years, children carrying the disease have generally lived to about the age of 10 years, dying from complications such as chronic obstructive pulmonary disease (COPD) with progressive damage to airway epithelial cells and pancreatic insufficiency from fibrosis and resulting lack of pancreatic enzymes. Improved management of the disease based on increasing scientific knowledge has the outlook is much brighter, with some surviving into their 40s and even 50s. Currently, a screening test for newborns helps detect the disease early. Then early intervention and support of a skilled cystic fibrosis team of healthcare specialists can accurately assess individual needs, help families cope, and develop an appropriate therapeutic plan.[24]

In the summer of 1989, the cystic fibrosis gene was discovered; shortly after that, continuing studies disclosed the underlying biochemical defect.[25] The normal gene's large protein product, composed of 1480 amino acids in five domains (see Chapter 5), controls the opening and closing of ion channels that actively transports chloride ions across epithelial cell membranes. Scientists have named this large protein for its function: cystic fibrosis transmembrane conductance regulator (CFTR).[25] The mutant cystic fibrosis gene cannot produce this controlling protein product called CFTR. Thus because of the resulting defective epithelial iron transport, chloride is trapped in the cells and excess sodium is also absorbed, causing abnormally high electrolyte concentrations in the sweat. This imbalance leads to the thickened mucus formation and clinical effects in the various organ systems involved.

Clinical Symptoms

The classic clinical symptoms of cystic fibrosis include the following effects in body organ systems.[26,27]

1. Thick mucus in the lungs that accumulates and clogs air passages, damages the epithelial tissue of these airways, and leads to COPD and frequent respiratory infections, both contributing to increased metabolism and increased energy-nutrient needs
2. Pancreatic insufficiency caused by progressive clogging of pancreatic ducts and functional tissue degeneration, resulting in lack of normal pancreatic enzymes: protein-splitting trypsin, chymotrypsin, carboxypeptidase; fat-splitting lipase; and starch-splitting amylase; progres-

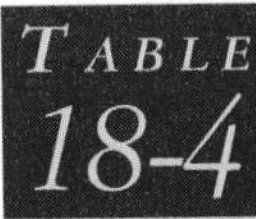

TABLE 18-4 Low-Gluten Diet for Children With Celiac Disease

Dietary Principles

Kilocalories—high, usually about 20% above normal requirement to compensate for fecal loss
Protein—high, usually 6-8 g/kg weight
Fat—low, but not fat free, because of impaired absorption
Carbohydrates—simple, easily digested sugars (fruits, vegetables) should provide about one half of the kcalories
Feedings—small, frequent feedings during ill periods; afternoon snack for older children
Texture—smooth, soft, avoiding irritating roughage initially, using strained foods longer than usual for age, adding whole foods as tolerated and according to age of child
Vitamins—supplements of B vitamins, vitamins A and B in water-miscible forms, and vitamin C
Minerals—iron supplements if anemia is present

Food Groups	Foods Included	Foods Excluded
Milk	Milk (plain or flavored with chocolate or cocoa) Buttermilk	Malted milk; preparations such as Cocomalt, Hemo, Postum, Nestle's chocolate
Meat or substitute	Lean meat, trimmed well of fat Eggs, cheese Poultry, fish Creamy peanut butter (if tolerated)	Fat meats (sausage, pork) Luncheon meats, corned beef frankfurters, all common prepared meat products with any possible wheat filler Duck, goose Smoked salmon Meat prepared with bread, crackers, or flour
Fruits and juices	All cooked and canned fruits and juices Frozen or fresh fruits as tolerated, avoiding skins and seeds	Prunes, plums (unless tolerated)
Vegetables	All cooked, frozen, canned as tolerated (prepared *without* wheat, rye, oat, or barley products); raw as tolerated	Any causing individual discomfort All prepared with wheat, rye, oat, or barley products
Cereals	Corn or rice	Wheat, rye, oat, barley; any product containing these cereals
Breads, flours, cereal products	Breads, pancakes, or waffles made with suggested flours (cornmeal, cornstarch; rice, soybean, lima bean, potato, buckwheat)	All bread or cracker products made with gluten; wheat, rye, oat, barley, macaroni, noodles, spaghetti; any sauces, soups, or gravies prepared with gluten flour, wheat, rye, oat, or barley
Soups	Broth, bouillon (no fat or cream; no thickening with wheat, rye, oat, or barley products); soups and sauces may be thickened with cornstarch	All soups containing wheat, rye, oat, or barley products

sive loss of functional insulin-producing beta cells in the Islets of Langerhans, resulting in insulin-dependent diabetes mellitus (IDDM)

3. Malabsorption of undigested food nutrients and extensive malnutrition and stunted growth
4. Biliary cirrhosis caused by progressive clogging of bile ducts producing biliary obstruction and functional liver tissue degeneration
5. An elevation of sodium and/or chloride concentration in sweat found by using the only reliable test—the quantitative pilocarpine iontophoresis sweat test.

Nutritional Management

Current nutritional management of cystic fibrosis follows guidelines developed by a consensus committee of the U.S. Cystic Fibrosis Foundation (CFF).[26] This more aggressive nutritional management program, used in all of the CFF centers throughout the United States, results from three factors: (1) increased knowledge of the disease process, (2) early diagnosis and intervention, and (3) improved therapeutic products such as replacement pancreatic enzymes in the form of capsule-encased enteric-coated microspheres—"beads"—that correct the maldigestion and help support energy-nutrient growth needs.[28] With this pancreatic enzyme replacement therapy, commonly called "PERT," it is now recommended that persons with cystic fibrosis consume a high-energy, high-protein diet with no fat restriction.

cirrhosis Chronic liver disease, characterized by loss of functional cells, with fibrous and nodular regeneration.

However, some persons continue to follow the low-fat advice given to them before the development of the enteric-coated enzyme preparations.[29] Treatment with PERT is very individualized. Even with maximum use, 10% to 20% of the ingested energy will usually be malabsorbed. The overall goal is to support normal nutrition and growth for all ages.

This PERT management program is based on an initial and ongoing schedule for assessment, including anthropometrics, laboratory studies, and nutrition evaluation (Table 18-5). Related therapy is then outlined in five levels according to individual assessment results and nutritional care needs and actions (Table 18-6).

TABLE 18-5 Basic Nutritional Assessment for Nutritional Management of Cystic Fibrosis

Key Assessments	Monitoring Schedule and Indications		
Anthropometry		***Biochemical Data***	
Weight	Every 3 months or as needed for growth evaluation and routine	CBC†	Yearly routine care, interim as needed to detect deficiencies, iron status
Height (length)		TIBC,† serum iron, ferritin	
Head circumference (until age 2 yr)		Plasma/serum retinol, alpha-tocopherol	As indicated, weight loss, growth failure, clinical deterioration
Midarm circumference		Albumin, prealbumin	
Triceps skin fold		Electrolytes, acid-base balance	Summer heat, prolonged fever
Midarm muscle circumference (derived)*			
		Dietary evaluation	
		Dietary intake	As indicated, history and food records, full energy-nutrient analysis
		3-day fat balance study‡	As indicated, weight loss, growth failure, clinical deterioration
		Anticipatory guidance	Yearly, interim as needed according to growth or situational needs

*See Chapter 15 for equations.
†*CBC,* Complete blood count; *TIBC,* total iron-binding capacity.
‡Three-day food records for analysis of fat intake; stool collections for analysis of fat content and degree of malabsorption.
Modified from CFF Consensus Report; Ramsey B et al: Nutrition assessment and management in cystic fibrosis: a consensus report, *Am J Clin Nutr* 55:108, 1992.

TABLE 18-6 Levels of Nutritional Care for Management of Cystic Fibrosis

Levels of Care	Patient Groups	Nutrition Actions
Level I—Routine care	All	Diet counseling, food plans, enzyme replacement, vitamin supplements, nutrition education, exploration of problems
Level II—Anticipatory guidance	Above 90% ideal weight-height index, but at risk of energy imbalance; severe pancreatic insufficiency, frequent pulmonary infections, normal periods of rapid growth	Increased monitoring of dietary intake, complete energy-nutrient analysis, increased kcaloric density as needed; assess behavioral needs; provide counseling, nutrition education
Level III—Supportive intervention	85%-90% ideal weight-height index, decreased weight-growth velocity	Reinforce all the above actions, add energy-nutrient–dense oral supplements
Level IV—Rehabilitative care	Consistently below 85% ideal weight-height index, nutritional and growth failure	All of the above plus enteral nutrition support by nasoenteric or enterostomy tube feeding (see Chapter 17)
Level V—Resuscitative or palliative care	Below 75% ideal weight-height index, progressive nutritional failure	All of the above plus continuous enteral tube feedings or TPN (see Chapter 17)

Modified from CFF Consensus Report; Ramsey B et al: Nutrition assessment and management in cystic fibrosis: a consensus report, *Am J Clin Nutr* 55:108, 1992.

Directions for calculating energy needs for cystic fibrosis patients, basal metabolic rate (BMR) and daily energy requirements (DER), physical activity, and disease status, are included in Appendix N, Guidelines for Nutritional Assessment and Care of Cystic Fibrosis.

INFLAMMATORY BOWEL DISEASES

Nature and Incidence

Irritable bowel syndrome, first described by the British physician Frederick Osler in 1892, has confounded physicians for more than a century.[30] The general term *inflammatory bowel disease (IBD)* is now used to apply to two intestinal conditions with similar symptoms but different underlying clinical problems—Crohn's disease and ulcerative colitis.[31,32] Both of these conditions produce extended mucosal tissue lesions, although these lesions differ in extent and nature. However, they have been classified medically in a single group because they are similar in their clinical symptoms and management. Their causes remain unknown, although heredity, environment, and immune functions are thought to be contributing factors.[33] The incidence of these diseases, especially Crohn's disease, has increased worldwide. Crohn's disease is particularly prevalent in industrialized areas of the world. It also appears among otherwise low-risk persons who move from rural to urban centers, with incidence being highest among people from 20 to 40 years of age and in Jews. Although epidemiologic and clinical studies continue to increase knowledge of the disease processes involved, the causes of these two IBDs remain unknown. Sensitive or specific serologic or genetic markers have yet to be identified.[34,35]

Ulcerative colitis and Crohn's disease have severe, often devastating tissue effects and nutritional consequences. They can be distinguished by two main differences: (1) anatomic distribution of the inflammatory process and (2) the nature of tissue changes involved. Crohn's disease occurs in any part of the intestinal tract; in contrast, ulcerative colitis is confined to the colon and rectum. In Crohn's disease, the inflammatory tissue changes become chronic and can involve any part of the intestinal wall and may penetrate the entire wall. Often this extensive tissue involvement leads to partial or complete obstruction and to fistula formation.[35] Fistulas can develop in an inflamed loop of intestine sticks to another loop or to another organ or to the skin. A fistula may form between the stomach or the upper port of the small intestine and the colon, causing food to be shunted directly into the colon, leading to further malabsorption. In contrast, the tissue changes in ulcerative colitis are usually acute, last for brief periods, and are limited to the mucosal and submucosal tissue layers of the intestinal wall.

Clinical Symptoms

A chronic bloody diarrhea is the most common clinical symptom, occurring at night as well as during the day. Ulceration of the mucous membrane of the intestine leads to various associated nutritional problems such as anorexia, nutritional edema, anemia, avitaminosis, protein losses, negative nitrogen balance, dehydration, and electrolyte disturbances. Clinicians have observed evidence of specific deficiencies of zinc and vitamin E, with improvement occurring when supplements of the particular nutrients involved are taken. There is generally weight loss, fever, diarrhea, malabsorption, cramping abdominal pain, skin lesions, and arthritic joint involvement. In Crohn's disease, the overall malnutrition resembles kwashiorkor and is an important cause of abnormal immunologic function.

Medical Management

Over the years, the precise nature and cause of IBD have continued to puzzle practitioners. Gastroenterologists have aptly called it "a dilemma within a dilemma surrounded by dilemmas."[36] Medical management of IBD has centered on drug therapy to control the inflammatory process and promote healing, as well as the moderate use of antidepressants for reactions to situational stress factors. Ongoing development of new agents in addition to mainstays of the past hold promise for future therapy.[35-37] The physician has available three types of drugs to use in developing individual therapy for IBD: (1) a corticosteroid—prednisone; (2) an anti-inflammatory agent—sulfasalazine, which is a combination of sulfapyridine and 5-aminosalicylic acid; and (3) an immunosuppressant agent especially for Crohn's disease—mercaptopurine.[35,37]

In general, after comprehensive tests and examinations to rule out organic disease, drug therapy consists largely of (1) moderate use of antidepressant agents for transient reactions to situational stress factors seen in the larger patient group in general medical care, with referrals as needed to counseling or psychiatric services, and (2) frequent use of anticholinergic agents to reduce the impact of neurotransmitters of the enteric nervous system on smooth muscles of the intestine causing spastic contractions.[36] Other drugs used include stool bulk formers and antidiarrheal agents. Effects of these drugs become important aspects of planning supportive nutritional care. Optimal treatment of patients with IBD focuses on symptom severity and degree of disability.[31]

Medical Nutrition Therapy

Nutrition therapy centers on supporting the healing process and avoiding nutritional deficiency states. In general, a high-fiber, low-fat diet is used, with individual adjustments as needed. In serious conditions, enteral nutrition support includes elemental formulas of absorbable isotonic preparations of amino acids, glucose, fat, minerals, and vitamins. When patients tolerate these feedings, there is diminished gastrointestinal protein loss and improved nutrition, accompanied by clinical remission. In cases where the small bowel has been shortened or the disease process is extensive, as in Crohn's disease, total parenteral nutrition (TPN) support is most effective.[38] Such vigorous nutritional therapy is particularly important in childhood to prevent severe growth retardation. Nutritional repletion improves symptoms dramatically. There is diminished gastrointestinal secretion and motility, decreased disease activity, relief of partial intestinal obstruction, occasional closure of enteric fistulas, and renewed immunocompetence. Nutritional supplements are usually necessary to avoid deficiencies in agents such as zinc, copper, chromium, selenium, and other nutrients.

General Continuing Nutrition Therapy

With a careful history as a base, a reasonable and appropriate food plan may be developed with the patient and family. Periodic food records and related symptoms provide the basis for continued counseling and adjustments. In general, the food plan gives attention to the following basic principles.

1. *Increase dietary fiber.* Increased dietary fiber aids functions of the large intestine mainly by (1) increasing and softening the fecal output, (2) regulating transit time of the final food mass through the colon, and (3) lowering segmental pressures in the final section of the colon, especially the sigmoid area. A regular diet with optimal energy-nutrient composition and dietary fiber food sources, such as whole grains, fruits, and vegetables, should provide the basic therapy (Table 18-7). Moderate supplemental dietary fiber may be used if needed, with controlled additions of bran, often better tolerated in cooked forms, or more soluble forms of bulking agents such as psyllium seed products (Metamucil).
2. *Recognize gas formers.* Some foods are recognized gas formers for many people because of known constituents such as certain oligosaccharides, as in the case of legumes (see Chapter 3). Others provide gaseous discomfort on an individual basis, such as the cruciferous family of vegetables, including cabbage, Brussels sprouts, broccoli, turnips, and radishes. The use of a few drops of a product such as Beano (appropriately called "beanase" enzyme by the manufacturer) can be mixed with the first few bites of a food to reduce breath hydrogen.
3. *Respect food intolerances.* Lactose intolerance, caused by a deficiency of the digestive enzyme, is a well known disorder resulting in intestinal cramping, bloating, and diarrhea after drinking milk or consuming other dairy products. However, preparations of lactase enzyme such as Lactaid allow lactose-intolerant persons to successfully consume dairy products.
4. *Reduce total fat intake.* Excess fat delays gastric emptying and contributes to malabsorption problems in the intestine and subsequent diarrhea. Additionally, moderation in total dietary fat intake helps reduce risks of fatty buildup in major blood vessels that leads to heart disease problems.
5. *Avoid large meals.* Large amounts of food in one meal create discomfort from gastric distention and gas generated in the stomach, especially when the meals are of high caloric content. Smaller, more frequent meals may reduce these symptoms.
6. *Decrease air-swallowing habits.* Certain habits of eating contribute to gas swallowed or generated in the stomach; these include eating rapidly, eating large amounts, and consuming excessive fluids, especially carbonated beverages. Habits of chewing gum and smoking also contribute to gas formation.

SHORT-BOWEL SYNDROME

Etiology

SBS is a pattern of varying metabolic and physiologic consequences of surgical removal of parts of the intestine with extensive dysfunction of the remaining portion of the organ.[37] Typically in an adult the small intestine is 20 feet long and the large intestine is 7 feet long. A general definition for SBS is a shortening (resecting) of the small intestine by about 50%. Resections result from inherent conditions such as Crohn's disease or radiation enteritis, surgical bypass, or massive abdominal injury and trauma. They may also be required for vascular problems such as blood clots causing death of involved tissue or for extensive fistula formation, radiation injury, congenital abnormalities, or cancer.

Nutritional Management

Degrees of surgical resection create different problems and nutrition therapy must be tailored to individual functional capacity remaining. Early enteral or parenteral nutrition support usually supplies initial needs. Frequent monitoring of nutritional responses, especially fluid and electrolyte balances and malnutrition signs, is essential. The patient is weaned from nutrition support to an oral diet as tolerated, accompanied by vitamin and mineral supplementation. Nutritional status should continue to be monitored. As adaptation progresses, the early restriction of fat may be liberalized somewhat with moderate use of the more easily absorbed medium-chain triglycerides (MCT oil) to obtain needed kcalories.

Large Intestine Diseases

DIVERTICULAR DISEASE

Nature and Etiology

A *diverticulum* is a small tubular sac that protruded from a main canal or cavity in the body. The formation and presence of small diverticula protruding from the intestinal lumen, usually the colon, produce the condition diverticulosis. More often diverticulosis occurs in older adults. It develops at points of weakened musculature in the bowel wall, along the track of blood vessels entering the bowel from within. The direct cause is a progressive increase in

TABLE 18-7 Dietary Fiber and Kilocalorie Values for Selected Foods

Foods	Serving	Dietary Fiber (g)	Kilocalories
Breads and Cereals			
All Bran	⅓ cup	8.5	70
Bran (100%)	½ cup	8.4	75
Bran Buds	⅓ cup	7.9	75
Corn Bran	⅔ cup	5.4	100
Bran Chex	⅔ cup	4.6	90
Cracklin' Oat Bran	⅓ cup	4.3	110
Bran Flakes	¾ cup	4.0	90
Air-popped popcorn	1 cup	2.5	25
Oatmeal	1 cup	2.2	144
Grapenuts	¼ cup	1.4	100
Whole-wheat bread	1 slice	1.4	60
Legumes, Cooked			
Kidney beans	½ cup	7.3	110
Lima beans	½ cup	4.5	130
Vegetables, Cooked			
Green peas	½ cup	3.6	55
Corn	½ cup	2.9	70
Parsnip	½ cup	2.7	50
Potato, with skin	1 medium	2.5	95
Brussels sprouts	½ cup	2.3	30
Carrots	½ cup	2.3	25
Broccoli	½ cup	2.2	20
Beans, green	½ cup	1.6	15
Tomato, chopped	½ cup	1.5	17
Cabbage, red and white	½ cup	1.4	15
Kale	½ cup	1.4	20
Cauliflower	½ cup	1.1	15
Lettuce (fresh)	1 cup	0.8	7
Fruits			
Apple	1 medium	3.5	80
Raisins	¼ cup	3.1	110
Prunes, dried	3	3.0	60
Strawberries	1 cup	3.0	45
Orange	1 medium	2.6	60
Banana	1 medium	2.4	105
Blueberries	½ cup	2.0	40
Dates, dried	3	1.9	70
Peach	1 medium	1.9	35
Apricot, fresh	3 medium	1.8	50
Grapefruit	½ cup	1.6	40
Apricot, dried	5 halves	1.4	40
Cherries	10	1.2	50
Pineapple	½ cup	1.1	40

Modified from Lanza E, Butrum RR: A critical review of food fiber analysis and data, *J Am Diet Assoc* 86:732, 1986.

pressure within the bowel from segmental circular muscle contractions that normally move the remaining food mass along and form the feces for elimination. When pressures become sufficiently high in one of these segments and dietary fiber is insufficient to maintain the necessary bulk for preventing high internal pressures within the colon,

immunocompetence The ability or capacity to develop an immune response, that is, antibody production and/or cell-mediated immunity, after exposure to antigen.

diverticula, small protrusions of the muscle layer, develop at that point. The condition causes no problem unless the small diverticula become infected and inflamed from fecal irritation and colon bacteria. This diseased state is called *diverticulitis.* The commonly used collective term covering diverticulosis and diverticulitis is *diverticular disease.*

Clinical Symptoms

As the inflammatory process grows, increased hypermotility and pressures from luminal segmentation cause pain. The pain and tenderness are usually localized in the lower left side of the abdomen and are accompanied by nausea, vomiting, distention, diarrhea, intestinal spasm, and fever. If the process continues, intestinal obstruction or perforation may necessitate surgical intervention.

Nutritional Management

Diverticular disease is a common gastrointestinal disorder among middle-aged and elderly persons. It may often be accompanied by malnutrition. Aggressive nutritional therapy hastens recovery from an attack, shortens the hospital stay, and reduces costs. Numerous studies and extensive clinical practice have demonstrated better management of chronic diverticular disease with an increased amount of dietary fiber than with old practices of restricting fiber. In acute episodes of active disease, however, the amount of dietary fiber should be reduced. The relationship of dietary fiber and diverticular disease has been further reinforced by studies of populations, such as those in Japan, that have recently experienced the westernization of their culture. Chapter 2 provides an extended discussion of dietary fiber and its relation to health and disease.

CONSTIPATION

A common disorder, usually of short duration, constipation is characterized by retention of feces in the colon beyond the normal emptying time. It is a problem for which Americans spend a quarter of a billion dollars each year for laxatives. However, the "regularity" of elimination is highly individual, and it is not necessary to have a bowel movement every day to be healthy. Usually, this common short-term problem results from various sources of nervous tension, worry, and changes in social setting. Such situations include vacations and travel, with alterations in usual routines. Also, it may be caused by prolonged use of laxatives or cathartics, low-fiber diets, inadequate fluid intake, or lack of exercise, all of which can contribute to a decreased intestinal muscle tone. Increasing activity and improving dietary intake to include adequate fiber (goal of 25 to 35 g/day) and fluid are usually sufficient strategies to remedy the situation. If chronic constipation persists, however, agents that increase stool bulk may be necessary. These bulking agents include bran or more soluble forms of fiber. Taking laxatives or enemas on a regular basis should be avoided. The problem of constipation occurs in all age groups but is almost epidemic in elderly people. In all cases a personalized approach to management of constipation is fundamental.

Food Allergies and Sensitivities

UNDERLYING ETIOLOGY

Hippocrates was among the first to record an adverse reaction to food more than 2000 years ago. The word *allergy* comes from the Greek words *allos* ("other") and *ergon* ("work"). The American Academy of Allergy, Asthma & Immunology and the National Institute of Allergy and Infectious Disease, NIH, developed standardized nomenclature to use in discussing food-related reactions. An *adverse food reaction* is a generic term referring to any unfavorable reaction after the ingestion of a food. Adverse food reactions are further categorized into food allergy (food hypersensitivity) or food intolerance. A food allergic reaction is an abnormal immunologic response. Immunoglobulin E (IgE) is found in low concentration in normal serum but in high concentration in the serum of patients with allergies. The term *food allergy* should be used only for hypersensitivity that is caused by IgE, the immunoglobulin class responsible for allergic antibodies.[39]

Food intolerances, which constitute the majority of adverse reactions to foods, are the result of nonimmunologic mechanisms. Milk, eggs, or peanuts cause almost 75% of adverse reactions to food.[40] Adverse reactions to single foods is common; adverse reactions to multiple foods is very rare.

In general, the process of diagnosis and treatment of adverse reactions to foods includes clinical assessment, dietary manipulation, and laboratory tests. Appropriate medical nutrition therapy is essential.

COMMON FOOD ALLERGENS

The care of a child who has had an allergic reaction presents many problems. A wide variety of environmental, emotional, and physical factors influence reaction, and a suitable regimen is sometimes difficult to find. Because sensitivity to protein substances is a common basis for food allergy, the early foods of infants and children are frequent offenders. Fortunately, however, children tend to become less allergic to food sources as they become older.

Milk

Cow's milk has long been a common cause of allergic response in infants.[41,42] In sensitive children it causes gastrointestinal difficulties such as vomiting, diarrhea, and colic, or it may cause respiratory and skin problems. The problem is generally identified by clinical symptoms, family history, and a trial on a milk-free diet, using an appropriate substitute hypoallergenic formula such as the casein hydrolysate formulas Nutramigen and Pregestimil (both from Mead Johnson) or the special hydrolysate formula Alimentum (Ross).[43] Freedom from symptoms on a milk-free diet is then followed by a retrial on milk to determine if it causes the symptoms to reappear; only then is the diagnosis of milk allergy established. Often symptoms appear and disappear spontaneously, regardless of dietary changes; however, they tend to be more often caused by food if gastrointestinal problems are present.

Eggs, Wheat, and Other Foods

Among the dominant food allergens noted in infants are chicken eggs, cow's milk, and wheat. The specific biochemical sensitivity to gluten (a protein found in wheat) in the child with gluten-induced celiac sprue is caused by a specific biochemical defect in the mucosal cells in celiac disease and represents a different sensitivity mechanism from the immunophysiology causing a true food allergy. Other true food allergens among children, some continuing through adulthood, include peanuts, soy, tree nuts, other cereal grains, and shellfish.[44]

NUTRITIONAL MANAGEMENT

In the diet of a child with an allergy, solid foods are usually added slowly to the original formula, with common offenders excluded in early feedings. The following basic list of most frequently offending food allergens must be avoided.[44,45]

- Chicken eggs
- Cow's milk
- Wheat
- Peanuts
- Tree nuts
- Soy products
- Shellfish, fish

Citrus fruits, berries, and tomatoes may cause skin rash, but this is a local reaction; it is not the immunologic response that identifies a true allergy.[44]

The initial nutrition evaluation of a patient suspected of having a food allergy should focus on a careful food history that includes intake of suspected foods, approximate quantity ingested, and time between the ingestion and development of symptoms. In some cases a series of diagnostic food elimination diets may be used to identify offending food allergens. A core of less-often offending foods is used initially, with gradual addition of other single foods one at a time to test the response. If a given food causes return of the allergy, the food is then identified as an allergen and eliminated from use. It may be retested later to determine if it is still an allergen. Guidance in the substitution of special food products and in the use of special recipes can be provided for the child's parents. Most food allergies tend to lessen as the child grows older. However, serious allergy to a few key foods, especially peanuts, may continue into adulthood and requires constant monitoring of food products and dishes to avoid severe attacks.[45] These attacks of severe anaphylactic shock are marked by sudden bronchial spasms, vomiting, dropping blood pressure, and irregular heart rhythm.

FAMILY EDUCATION AND COUNSELING

The education of the parents and family of a child with an allergy must include knowledge and understanding of the allergic state and the many factors that may influence it. If specific foods have been definitely identified as offenders, careful guidance to eliminate these from the diet is needed. Common uses of the offending food in daily meal patterns and its occurrence in a number of commercial products and other hidden sources should be discussed. Label reading and recipe adaptation are important. As a child with an allergy grows older, reaction to a given food may wane, and it can gradually be added to the diet.

Food Intolerances From Genetic-Metabolic Disease

Certain food intolerances may stem from underlying genetic disease that affects the metabolism of one or more specific nutrients. Genetic disease results from the individual's specific gene inheritance. Genes in each cell control the metabolic functions of the cell. They regulate the synthesis of some 1000 or more specific cell enzymes that control metabolism within the cell. When a specific gene is abnormal *(mutant)*, the enzyme whose synthesis that gene controls cannot be made. In turn, the specific metabolic reaction controlled by that specific missing enzyme cannot take place. The specific genetic disease caused by this metabolic block then manifests clinical symptoms connected with resulting abnormal metabolic products. As primary examples here, we look briefly at two such genetic diseases affecting food-nutrient intolerances: (1) phenylketonuria (PKU), which affects amino acid metabolism and hence protein foods; (2) galactosemia, which affects carbohydrate metabolism, specifically food sources of lactose. Both are detected by newborn screening procedures that are mandatory by law.

PHENYLKETONURIA

Metabolic Defect and Clinical Symptoms

PKU results from the missing cell enzyme, phenylalanine hydroxylase, which metabolizes one of the essential amino acids, phenylalanine, to tyrosine, another nonessential amino acid. Phenylalanine then accumulates in the blood, and its alternate metabolites, the phenyl acids, are excreted in the urine. One of these urinary acids, phenylpyruvic acid, is a phenylketone; hence the name of the disease. Untreated PKU can produce devastating effects, but present medical nutritional therapy can avoid these results.[46] In past years, before current newborn screening laws and dietary treatment practices from birth, the most profound effect observed in persons with untreated PKU was severe mental retardation. The IQ of affected persons was usually below 50 and often less than 20. Central nervous system damage caused irritability, hyperactivity, convulsive seizures, and bizarre behavior.

Medical Nutrition Therapy

PKU can now be well controlled by special nutrition therapy. After screening at birth a special low-phenylalanine diet effectively controls the serum phenylalanine levels so they are maintained at appropriate amounts to prevent clinical symptoms and promote normal growth and development.[46] Because phenylalanine is an essential amino acid necessary for growth, it cannot be totally removed from the diet. Blood levels of phenylalanine are constantly monitored, and the metabolic team nutritionist calculates the special diet for each infant and child to allow only the limited amount of phenylalanine tolerated. Based on extensive studies, guidelines for nutrition management of PKU are currently being used effectively to build lifetime habits; research now indicates that there is no safe age at which a child may discontinue the diet.[46] This dietary management is built on two basic components: (1) a substitute for milk, a special medical food continued past infancy and childhood into adolescence and adulthood; and (2) guidelines for adding solid foods, both regular and special low-protein products, and then building continuing food habits.

Family Education and Counseling

Initial education and continuing support of parents is essential because dietary management of PKU is the only known effective method of treatment and because maintaining the diet becomes more difficult as the child grows older. Parents must understand and accept the necessity of the diet, and this requires patience, understanding, and continued reinforcement. The PKU team, together with parents, provides initial and continuing care so that the child with PKU will grow and develop normally. When PKU is diagnosed at birth, as a result of widespread screening programs, a child can have a healthy and happy life, instead of the profound disease consequences experienced in the past. The current practice of long-term nutrition management is especially critical for young women with PKU who are considering pregnancy. At least 6 months before becoming pregnant, women with PKU should meet with a metabolic team to discuss treatment and follow-up. It is possible for women with PKU to have normal children. However, maternal PKU presents the possibility of a potentially high-risk pregnancy if a low-phenylalanine diet is not strictly followed.

GALACTOSEMIA

Metabolic Defect and Clinical Symptoms

This genetic disease affects carbohydrate metabolism so that the body cannot use the monosaccharide galactose. Three enzymes are responsibly for the conversion of galactose to glucose, and in galactosemia at least one of the enzymes is defective or missing. Milk, the infant's first food, contains a large amount of the precursor lactose (milk sugar). When infants with galactosemia are given breast milk or regular infant formula, they vomit and have diarrhea. After galactose is initially combined with phosphate to begin the metabolic conversion to glucose, it cannot proceed further in the infant with galactosemia. Galactose rapidly accumulates in the blood and in various body tissues. In the past the excess tissue accumulations of galactose caused rapid damage in the untreated infant. Clinical symptoms appeared soon after birth and the child failed to thrive. Continued liver damage brought jaundice, an enlarged liver with cirrhosis, enlarged spleen, and ascites. Without treatment, death usually resulted from liver failure. If the infant survived, continuing tissue damage and hypoglycemia in the optic lens and the brain caused cataracts and mental retardation. Now, however, with newborn screening programs, infants with galactosemia are diagnosed at birth and started on special dietary management. With this vital nutrition therapy, children can grow and develop normally.

Medical Nutrition Therapy

The main indirect source of dietary galactose is the lactose in milk. A galactose-free diet (free of all forms of milk and lactose) is followed and the infant is fed a soy-based formula. Breastfeeding is not an option when this genetic condition is present. The body synthesizes the amount of galactose needed for body structures. As solid foods are added to the infant's diet at about 6 months of age, careful attention must be given to avoiding lactose from other food sources. Parents quickly learn to check labels carefully on all commercial products to detect any lactose or lactose-containing substances.

Diseases of the Gastrointestinal Accessory Organs

Three major accessory organs (liver, gallbladder, and pancreas) lie adjacent to the gastrointestinal tract and produce important digestive agents that enter the intestine and aid in the processing of food substances. Specific enzymes are produced for each of the major nutrients, and bile is added to assist in the enzymatic digestion of fats. Diseases of these organs can easily affect gastrointestinal function and cause problems in the normal handling of specific types of food.

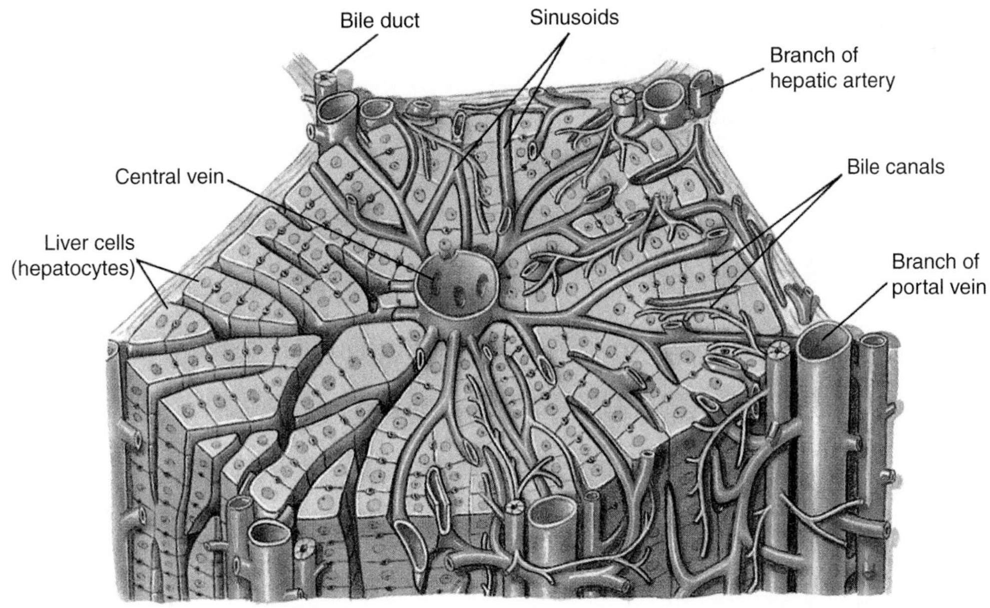

FIGURE 18-3 Liver structure showing hepatic lobule and hepatic cell.

VIRAL HEPATITIS

Structural Scheme of the Liver Lobules

The unique structural design of these basic functional units of the liver enables this vital organ to do its life-sustaining work. Each liver lobule is constructed around a central vein that empties into the hepatic veins that flow into the vena cava. From this central vein many hepatic cellular plates radiate outward like spokes in a wheel (Figure 18-3).

Etiology

Viral hepatitis (inflammation of the liver) is a major public health problem throughout the world, affecting hundreds of millions of people. It causes considerable illness and death in human populations from the acute infection or its effects, which may include chronic active hepatitis, cirrhosis, and primary liver cancer.[47] During the past few years, knowledge of the viruses causing different types of hepatitis has grown rapidly. Currently, six unrelated human hepatitis viruses, A, B, C, D, E, and the newly discovered hepatitis virus G, have been isolated and described.[48-50] The two most common and well known are A and B, which serve as examples.

- *Hepatitis A virus (HAV).* HAV, the infectious agent of hepatitis type A, was formerly called infectious hepatitis. It was discovered in the early 1970s in the feces of infected patients and is transmitted via the classic oral-fecal route through contaminated food and water. It is a prevalent infection worldwide, especially where there is overcrowding and poor hygiene or sanitation. An HAV vaccine has been developed that is far more effective than the former large and painful injection of gamma globulins, antibodies isolated from the blood. This vaccine protects travelers to developing countries, where the virus is endemic and may easily contaminate water and food.[51]
- *Hepatitis B virus (HBV).* HBV, the infectious agent of hepatitis type B, was formerly called serum hepatitis. It was discovered in the late 1960s, mainly spread sexually and by sharing of contaminated needles among drug abusers. It has now been implicated worldwide as the major causative factor in chronic liver disease and associated liver cancer. The HBV infection is closely related to the body's immune system. The estimate of carriers is about 300 million worldwide, of whom 75% are Asians. The World Health Organization (WHO) indicates that about 40% of these infected persons will die of chronic active hepatitis or liver cancer.[52] An improved vaccine was developed in 1986 and is now being used with high-risk groups such as healthcare personnel and babies of antibody-carrier mothers in most developed countries.[53] In some endemic areas, all newborns are routinely vaccinated.

endemic Characterizing a disease of low morbidity that remains constantly in a human community but is clinically recognizable in only a few.
jaundice A syndrome characterized by hyperbilirubinemia and deposits of bile pigment in the skin, mucous membranes, and sclera, giving a yellow appearance to the patient.

Clinical Symptoms

The viral agents of hepatitis produce diffuse injury to liver cells, especially the parenchymal cells. In milder cases the liver injury is largely reversible, but with increasing severity, more extensive necrosis occurs. In some cases massive necrosis may lead to liver failure and death. A cardinal symptom of hepatitis is anorexia, contributing to the risk of malnutrition. Varying clinical symptoms appear depending on the degree of liver injury. Jaundice, a major symptom, may or may not be obvious, depending on the severity of the disease and can have both nutritional and psychologic effects (see *Practical Application* box). In an

PRACTICAL APPLICATION

Jaundice: When to Expect It and What to do About It

Because jaundice is not usually a life-threatening condition, it is easy for the healthcare professional to take it lightly. The resulting yellow-to-orange skin color seems harmless, only reflecting an accumulation of excessive bile pigments in the blood that results from a rise in bilirubin, a product of heme released when red blood cells are destroyed. The underlying condition resulting in hemolysis, not the jaundice itself, is the major issue.

This may be true in a biologic sense. However, in a psychologic sense, jaundice can be devastating. The embarrassment of an altered body image, with accompanying depression and withdrawal, can affect the appetite and willingness to comply with the therapy that is recommended for the illness. To promote a healthy recovery, health workers must treat jaundice as seriously as these effects dictate. Several actions would be helpful.

1. *Explain to the patient the reason for jaundice.*
   - *Prehepatic jaundice.* Prehepatic jaundice most often is caused by a massive breakdown in red blood cells. It is seen most often in Rh factor sensitization, hemolytic anemias, sickle cell anemia, massive lung infarctions, transfusion reactions, and septicemia. The result is an excessive amount of bilirubin in a form that cannot be excreted—that is, fat soluble. The body's bilirubin transport system, based on albumin, then deposits the excess in the patient's skin and in a few other tissues.
   - *Hepatic jaundice.* In hepatic jaundice the liver cannot convert fat-soluble bilirubin into the water-soluble form required for its removal from the blood. This condition is seen in hepatitis, cirrhosis, metastatic cancer, and prolonged drug use, especially of drugs broken down by the liver.
   - *Posthepatic jaundice.* Posthepatic jaundice occurs when the flow of bile into the duodenum is blocked. Because bile carries water-soluble excretable bilirubin, this blockage backs up the bile, resulting in a backlog of bilirubin in the blood. Blockage often occurs with inflation, scar tissue, stones, or tumors in the liver, bile, or pancreatic systems.
2. *Explain to the patient assessment procedures and tests.* A careful and comprehensive assessment process involving members of the healthcare team provides vital information for medical, nutritional, and nursing care plans.
   - *Include a careful history and anthropometry.* A full personal, family, psychosocial, medical, and nutritional history will help detect any possible hepatic virus sources and current nutritional status and needs.
   - *Check anthropometric data.* Routine body measures including skinfold thicknesses help determine nutritional status.
   - *Evaluate results of routine biochemical tests.* Relate these tests to medical diagnosis and nutritional status and needs.
   - *Explain each procedure.* A clear explanation of each procedure will help the patient participate more meaningfully in diagnostic and care-planning processes and will allay anxieties about the jaundice.
3. *Identify nutrition-related problems.* Jaundice is often associated with anorexia, indigestion, nausea, and vomiting.
   - *Help resolve nutrition-related problems.* To overcome indigestion or anorexia, recommend small meals that offer some of the patient's favorite foods. To overcome nausea or vomiting, simple foods may be necessary. Also, foods rich in fat and caffeine should also be avoided.
   - *Encourage the patient to discuss personal feelings and concerns.* Such information is essential for the nurse and nutritionist to develop a treatment plan. Also, this counseling may help the patient feel psychologically stronger and ready to contribute to the healthcare process.
   - *Discuss pertinent needs with the patient's family and friends.* Often other significant persons avoid the patient out of embarrassment or lack of understanding. A discussion of the patient's need for support may help other persons accept the patient socially and support any other efforts made to resolve the underlying health problem.
   - *Make appropriate referrals as needed.* If jaundice was the result of alcohol or drug abuse, the patient and possibly the patient's family may require special counseling. Referral to community programs after hospital discharge may help provide needed follow-up therapy.

References

Sherlock S: *Diseases of the liver and biliary system,* ed 8, Cambridge, Mass, 1989, Blackwell Scientific Publications.

Vail BA: Management of chronic viral hepatitis, *Am Fam Physician* 55(8):2749, 1997.

outbreak of hepatitis, many infected persons may be non-icteric and thus go undiagnosed and untreated because jaundice has not developed sufficiently to be seen. Malnutrition and impaired immunocompetence contribute to spontaneous infections and continuing liver disease. General symptoms, in addition to the main sign of anorexia, include malaise, weakness, nausea and vomiting, diarrhea, headache, fever, enlarged and tender liver, and enlarged spleen. When jaundice develops, it usually occurs for a preicteric period of 5 to 10 days, deepens for 1 to 2 weeks, then levels off and decreases. After this crisis point there is a sufficient recovery of injured cells and a convalescence of 3 weeks to 3 months follows. Optimal care during this time is essential to avoid relapse.

General Treatment

Bedrest is essential. Physical exercise increases both severity and duration of the disease. A daily intake of 3000 to 3500 ml of fluid guards against dehydration and gives a general sense of well-being and improved appetite. However, optimal nutrition is the major therapy. It provides the essential foundation for recovery of the injured liver cells and overall return of strength.

Medical Nutrition Therapy

A complete nutrition assessment and initial personal history provide the basis for planning care. Nutritional therapy principles relate to the liver's function in metabolizing each of the nutrients.

1. *Adequate protein.* Protein is essential for liver cell regeneration, as well as for maintaining all of the body's essential functions. It also provides lipotropic agents such as methionine and choline for the conversion of fats to lipoproteins and removal from the liver, thus preventing fatty infiltration. The daily diet should supply 1.5 to 2 g/kg of actual body weight, or about 100 to 150 g, of high-quality protein. This amount is usually enough to achieve a positive nitrogen balance.
2. *High carbohydrate.* Sufficient available glucose must be provided to restore protective glycogen reserves and meet the energy demands of the disease process. Also, adequate glucose for energy ensures the use of protein for vital tissue regeneration. The diet should supply about 50% to 55% of the total kcalories as carbohydrates, or about 300 to 400 g/day.
3. *Moderate fat.* A moderate amount of fat makes the food more palatable and therefore encourages the anorexic patient to eat. If steatorrhea is present, a more easily absorbed medium-chain triglyceride product such as MCT oil may be used for a brief time. Then regular vegetable oil products and small amounts of butterfat may be resumed to ensure adequate amounts of essential linoleic acid. The diet should supply about 30% to 35% of the total kcalories as fat, or about 80 to 100 g/day.
4. *Increased energy.* The classic Harris-Benedict equations are used to estimate basal energy expenditure (BEE) (see Chapter 17). For total energy needs, a malnourished patient should receive 150% of the BEE value. Ambulatory patients require more energy intake, about 2500 to 3000 kcalories/day, to cover physical activity. This increased energy requirement is needed to furnish demands of the tissue regeneration process, to compensate for losses from fever and general debilitation, and to renew strength and recuperative powers.
5. *Micronutrients.* Fat-soluble vitamins in water-soluble form should be provided in amounts twice the normal Reference Daily Intakes (RDIs). Other water-soluble vitamins also require supplementation.

Meals and Feedings

The problem of supplying a diet adequate to meet the increased nutritional demands of a patient, with an illness that makes food almost repellent, calls for creativity and supportive encouragement. Food may need to be in liquid form at first, using concentrated commercial or blended formulas for frequent feedings (Table 18-8). As the patient improves, appetizing and attractive food is needed. Because nutrition therapy is the key to recovery, a major nutrition and nursing responsibility requires devising ways to encourage the increased amounts of food

TABLE 18-8 High-Protein, High-Kilocalorie Formula for Patient With Hepatitis

Ingredients	Amount	Approximate Food Value	
Milk	1 cup	Protein	40 g
Egg substitute	Equivalent of 2 eggs	Fat	30 g
Skimmed milk powder or	6 to 8 tbsp	Carbohydrates	70 g
Casec	2 tbsp	Kilocalories	710
Sugar	2 tbsp		
Ice cream	2.5 cm (1 in) slice or 1 scoop		
Cocoa or other flavoring	2 tbsp		
Vanilla	Few drops, as desired		

icteric Alternate term for jaundice: nonicteric indicates absence of jaundice; preicteric indicates a state before development of icterus, or jaundice.

necrosis Cell death caused by progressive enzyme breakdown.

parenchymal cells Functional cells of an organ, as distinguished from the cells comprising its structure or framework.

TABLE 18-9 High-Protein, High-Carbohydrate, Moderate-Fat Daily Diet

Food	Amount
Milk	1 L (1 qt)
Egg substitute	Equal to 1-2 eggs
Lean meat, fish, or poultry	224 g (8 oz)
Vegetables (4 servings)	
Potato or substitute	2 servings
Green leafy or yellow	1 serving
Other vegetables (including 1 raw)	1-2 servings
Fruit (3-4 servings, includes juices often)	
Citrus (or other good source of ascorbic acid)	1-2 servings
Other fruit	2 servings
Bread and cereal (whole grain or enriched)	6-8 servings
Cereal	1 serving
Sliced bread or crackers	5-6 servings
Butter or fortified margarine	2-4 tbsp
Jam, jelly, honey, and other carbohydrates	As patient desires and is able to eat them
Sweetened fruit juices	To increase carbohydrates and fluids

intake needed, as suggested in Table 18-9. The clinical dietitian and the nursing staff should work together to achieve mutual goals planned for the patient. All staff attendants must follow appropriate precautions in handling patient trays to prevent spread of the infection.

CIRRHOSIS

Cirrhosis is the general term used for advanced stages of liver disease, regardless of the initial cause of the disease. Among all digestive diseases, cirrhosis of the liver, caused by chronic alcohol abuse, is the leading nonmalignant cause of death in the United States and most of the developed world. The majority of deaths occur among young and middle-aged adults. The French physician René Laënnec (1781-1826) first used the term *cirrhosis* (from the Greek work *kirrhos,* meaning "orange yellow") to describe the abnormal color and rough surface of the diseased liver. The cirrhotic liver is a firm, fibrous, dull yellowish mass with orange nodules projecting from its surface (Figure 18-4).

Etiology

Some forms of cirrhosis result from biliary obstruction, with blockage of the biliary ducts and accumulation of bile in the liver.[54] Other cases may result from liver necrosis from undetermined causes or, in some cases, from previous viral hepatitis. A common problem is fatty cirrhosis, associated with the complicating factor of malnutrition. Continuing fatty infiltration causes cellular destruction and fibrotic tissue changes.

Clinical Symptoms

Early signs of cirrhosis include gastrointestinal disturbances such as nausea, vomiting, loss of appetite, distention, and epigastric pain. In time, jaundice may appear, with increasing weakness, edema, ascites, and anemia from gastrointestinal bleeding, iron deficiency, or hemorrhage. A specific macrocytic anemia from folic acid deficiency is also frequently observed. Steatorrhea is a common symptom. Major symptoms are caused by a basic protein deficiency and its multiple metabolic problems: (1) plasma protein levels fall leading to failure of the capillary fluid shift mechanism (see Chapter 8), causing ascites, (2) lipotropic agents are not supplied for fat conversion to lipoproteins and damaging fat accumulates in the liver tissue, (3) blood-clotting mechanisms are impaired because factors such as prothrombin and fibrinogen are not adequately produced, and (4) general tissue catabolism and negative nitrogen balance continue the overall degenerative process.

As the disease progresses, the increasing fibrotic scar tissue impairs blood circulation through the liver, and portal hypertension follows.[55] Contributing further to the problem is the continuing ascites. The impaired portal circulation with increasing venous pressure may lead to esophageal varices, with danger of rupture and fatal massive hemorrhage.

Drug therapy includes the use of broad-spectrum antibiotics to limit the growth of intestinal bacteria and laxatives to speed intestinal transit time, limiting the amount of time available for bacteria to produce ammonia in the gastrointestinal tract. Lactulose, a synthetic derivative of lactose consisting of one molecule of galactose and one molecule of fructose, is a laxative that is used in the treatment of hepatic encephalopathy. Lactulose is ionized, cannot diffuse across the colon membrane, and is excreted in the stool. Lactulose can reduce blood ammonia levels by 25% to 50%. Diuretics may be given to reduce fluid retention and prevent ascites.

Medical Nutrition Therapy

When alcoholism is an added underlying problem, treatment is difficult. Each patient requires supportive care. Therapy is usually aimed at correcting fluid and electrolyte problems and providing as much nutrition support as possible for hepatic repair. In any case, guidelines for nutrition therapy for cirrhosis of the liver should include the following principles.

1. *Protein intake.* Intake should be adequate to regenerate liver cells and prevent infections but not excessive to the point of aggravating ammonia buildup and inducing hepatic coma.
   - *Protein in cirrhosis.* From 1.0 to 1.5 g of protein per kilogram of body weight per day

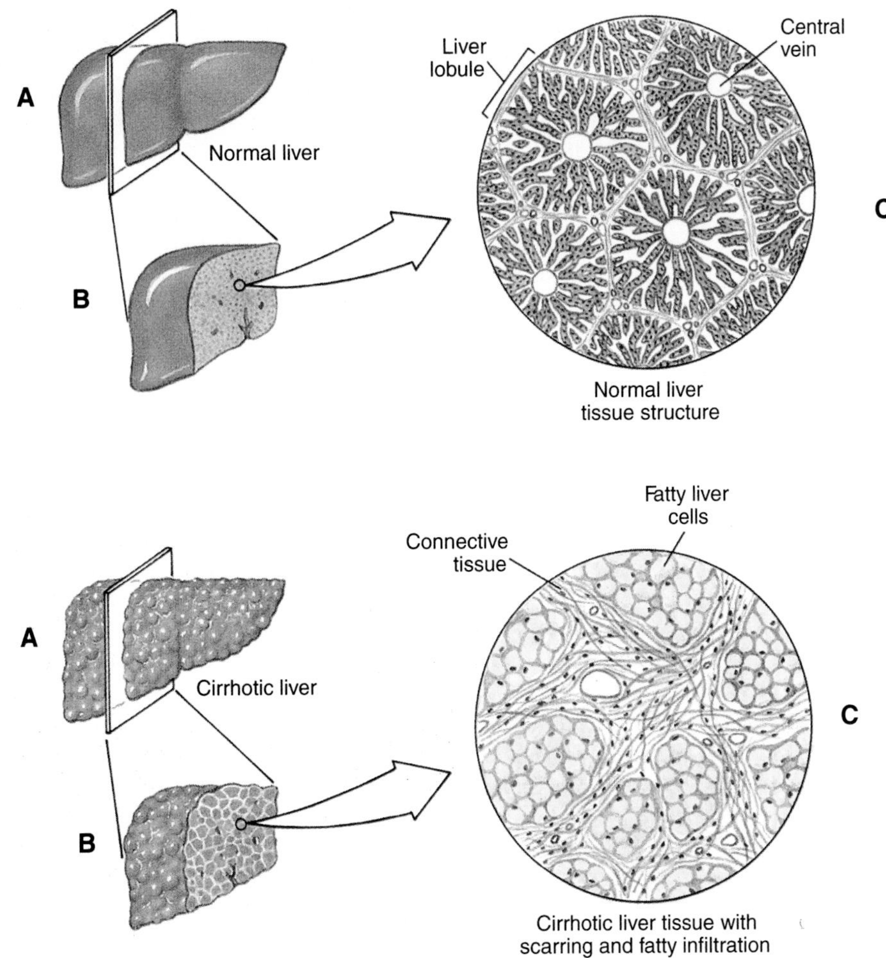

FIGURE 18-4 Comparison of normal liver and liver with cirrhotic tissue changes. **A**, Anterior view of organ. **B**, Cross-section. **C**, Tissue structure.

- *Protein in impending coma.* From 40 to 60 g/day from foods; additional protein to meet needs supplied from special formulas
- *Protein in hepatic coma.* Protein from all sources may need to be restricted. Tolerance is determined on an individual basis, and protein intake can be increased as the condition of the patient improves.

2. *Sodium.* Intake is usually restricted to about 1000 to 2000 mg/day to help reduce fluid retention. A sodium intake level of less than 2000 mg/day is considered quite restrictive, and palatability of food is usually a problem. It may be necessary to liberalize the sodium restrictions to improve intake.
3. *Texture.* If esophageal varices develop, it may be necessary to give soft foods that are smooth in texture to prevent the danger of rupture and hemorrhage.
4. *Carbohydrate.* Adequate intake is needed to prevent catabolism of body protein for energy, which would further increase blood ammonia. Intestinal bacteria make ammonia from undigested proteins (proteins from shed mucosal cells, protein from gastrointestinal tract bleed, and dietary proteins).
5. *Fat.* Fat helps make food more appealing and increases kcalorie content, making it important in the diet of a person with cirrhosis. Fat intake only needs to be restricted when there is steatorrhea, and even then MCT oil can be used.
6. *Vitamins and minerals.* The central role of the liver is to metabolize and store vitamins and minerals. Usually all people with advanced liver disease require supplementation of some vitamins, minerals, and trace elements. Nutrient supplementation is determined by monitoring serum levels and checking for clinical signs of deficiencies.
7. *Alcohol.* To protect the liver from further injury abstinence from alcohol is mandatory.

HEPATIC ENCEPHALOPATHY

The term *encephalopathy* refers to any disease or disorder that affects the brain, especially chronic degenerative conditions.

The effect on the brain in hepatic encephalopathy is a major serious complication of end-stage liver disease. The accumulation of toxic substances in the blood as a result of liver failure impairs consciousness and contributes to memory loss, personality change, tremors, seizures, stupor, and coma.

Etiology

As cirrhotic changes continue in the liver, the portal blood circulation diminishes and liver functions begin to fail. The normal liver has a major function of removing ammonia from the blood by converting it to urea for excretion. The failing liver can no longer inactivate or detoxify substances or metabolize others. A key factor involved in the progressive disease process is an elevated blood level of ammonia, although it is by no means the sole agent. The resulting hepatic encephalopathy brings changes in consciousness, behavior, and neurologic status.

Clinical Symptoms

Typical response involves disorders of consciousness and alterations in motor function. There is apathy, confusion, inappropriate behavior, and drowsiness, progressing to coma. The speech may be slurred or monotonous. A coarse, flapping tremor known as *asterixis* is observed in the outstretched hands, caused by a sustained contraction of a group of muscles. The breath may have a fecal odor, *fetor hepaticus.*

Basic Treatment Objectives

The fundamental objective of treatment is twofold: (1) removal of the sources of excess ammonia and (2) provision of nutritional support. Parenteral fluid and electrolytes are used to restore normal balances. Lactulose and neomycin may be used to control ammonia levels. Neomycin is an antibiotic that reduces the population of urea-splitting organisms within the bowel that produce ammonia. To stop bleeding into the intestine thereby reducing the amount of intestinal ammonia, a Sengstaken-Blakemore tube may be used.

Medical Nutrition Therapy

General nutrition support for hepatic encephalopathy is based on the following principles of dietary management.

1. *Low protein.* General protein intake is reduced individually as necessary to restrict the dietary sources of nitrogen in amino acids. The amount of restriction varies with the circumstances, but the usual amount ranges from 30 to 50 g/day, depending on whether symptoms are severe or mild. A simple method for controlling dietary protein uses a base meal pattern containing approximately 15 g protein and then adds small items of protein foods according to the level of protein desired (Table 18-10).
2. *Branched-chain amino acids.* The three branched-chain amino acids (BCAAs)—leucine, isoleucine, and valine—are not catabolized by the liver but are taken up by other tissues. Thus they can be metabolized without depending on healthy liver tissue, as is the case with the other amino acids. They provide a useful energy source, as well as a better-tolerated source of needed protein that may be used directly by the muscles, heart, liver, and brain. Oral BCAA formula has been used, with the patients becoming neurologically normal. The clinical use of BCAA supplementation in enteral and parenteral nutrition support formulas is an important part of standard therapy in liver failure and may improve the chance of survival.
3. *Kilocalories and vitamins.* Adequate energy intake is crucial to the patient's recovery, especially through the impact of kcaloric intake on liver glycogen reserves and their protective role in the healing process. The amounts of kcalories and vitamins are prescribed according to need. About 2000 kcalories/day is needed to prevent tissue catabolism, with sufficient carbohydrate as the primary energy source and some fat as tolerated. Vitamin K is usually given parenterally, along with other vitamins and minerals, especially zinc, in which the patient may be deficient.
4. *Fluid intake.* Fluid intake-output balance is carefully controlled.

LIVER TRANSPLANTATION

The development of liver transplantation as an acceptable therapy for end-stage liver disease has been an important medical advance. Candidates for transplant include patients with end-stage chronic liver disease or acute liver failure, progressive liver disease for which conventional treatment has failed, and a prognosis that indicates a survival of less than 10%.[56] In such cases, orthotopic (normal placement) liver transplantation remains the best chance of prolonged survival, especially with end-stage disease in children.[57] Liver transplantation is indicated for patients, mostly women, with intractable symptoms of primary biliary cirrhosis.[58] Less suitable cases include problems such as alcoholic cirrhosis and malignant tumors and those complicated by sepsis or advanced lung and kidney disease. As with all major surgery, aggressive nutritional support reduces risks. Careful pretransplantation nutrition assessment and support helps prepare the patient for the surgery. Enteral or parenteral nutrition support may be required for optimal postoperative nutritional status. A number of posttransplantation young women, with new healthier livers and good nutrition support, have experienced the return of fertility and been able to conceive and maintain the high-risk pregnancy to a successful conclusion with closely monitored medical and nutritional management.[59] In such cases, immediate follow-up contraception with a barrier method is recommended because birth control pills may interfere with accurate cyclosporine dosing for maintaining the transplant.

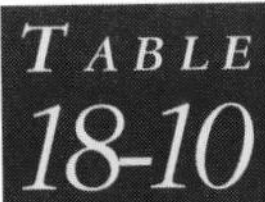

Low-Protein Diets (15, 30, 40, and 50 g Protein)

General Description

The following diets are used when dietary protein is to be restricted.

The patterns limit foods containing a large percentage of protein, such as milk, eggs, cheese, meat, fish, fowl, and legumes.

Avoid meat extractives, soups, broth, bouillon, gravies, and gelatin desserts.

Basic Meal Patterns

Breakfast (Approximately 15 g of Protein)	Lunch (Approximately 15 g of Protein)	Dinner (Approximately 15 g of Protein)
½ cup fruit or fruit juice	1 small potato	1 small potato
½ cup cereal	½ cup vegetable	½ cup vegetable
1 slice toast	Salad (vegetable or fruit)	Salad (vegetable or fruit)
Butter	1 slice bread	1 slice bread
Jelly	Butter	Butter
Sugar	1 serving fruit	1 serving fruit
2 tbsp cream	Sugar	Sugar
Coffee	Coffee or tea	Coffee or tea

	Examples of Meat Portions
For 30 g of Protein Add: 1 cup milk plus: 28 g (1 oz) meat, 1 egg, or equivalent	28 g (1 oz) meat = 1 thin slice roast, 4 × 5 cm (1½ × 2 in) 1 rounded tbsp cottage cheese 1 slice American cheese
For 40 g of Protein Add: 1 cup milk plus: 70 g (2½ oz) meat, or 1 egg + 42 g (1½ oz) meat	70 g (2½ oz) meat = Ground beef patty (5 can be made from 448g [1 lb]) 1 slice roast
For 50 g of Protein Add: 1 cup milk plus: 112 g (4 oz) meat, or 2 eggs + 56 g (2 oz) meat	112 g (4 oz) meat = 2 lamb chops 1 average steak

The use of a HemoTherapies Unit as new treatment for liver disease patients has been cleared for use by the U.S. Food and Drug Administration (FDA). The device is used with acute hepatic encephalopathy and severe drug overdoses from aggressive drug therapies and certain types of toxic exposures.

GALLBLADDER DISEASE

Metabolic Function

The basic function of the gallbladder is to concentrate and store the bile produced in its initial watery solution by the liver. The liver secretes about 600 to 800 ml of bile/day, which the gallbladder normally concentrates fivefold to tenfold to accommodate this daily bile production in its small capacity of 40 to 70 ml. Through the cholecystokinin (CCK) mechanism, the presence of fat in the duodenum stimulates contraction of the gallbladder with the release of concentrated bile into the common duct and then into the small intestine.

Cholecystitis and Cholelithiasis

The prefix *chole-* of the two terms *cholecystitis* and *cholelithiasis* comes from the Greek word *chole,* which means "bile." Thus cholecystitis is an inflammation of the gallbladder, and cholelithiasis is the formation of gallstones.

Inflammation of the gallbladder usually results from a low-grade chronic infection and may occur with or without gallstones. However, in 90% to 95% of patients, acute cholecystitis is associated with gallstones and is caused by the obstruction of the cystic duct by stones, resulting in acute inflammation of the organ. Gallstones can be classified into two main groups: cholesterol and pigment stones.

1. *Cholesterol stones.* In the United States and most Western countries, more than 75% of the gallstones are cholesterol stones. The infectious process produces changes in the gallbladder mucosa, which affects its absorptive powers. The main ingredient of bile is cholesterol, which is insoluble in water. Normally, cholesterol is kept in solution by the other ingredients in bile. However, when the absorbing mucosal tissue of the gallbladder is inflamed or infected, changes occur in the tissue. The absorptive powers of the gallbladder may be altered, affecting the solubility of the bile ingredients. Excess water or excess bile acid may be absorbed. Under these abnormal absorptive conditions cholesterol may precipitate, forming gallstones of almost pure cholesterol. Excessive use of dietary fat over a long

period of time predisposes persons to gallstone formation because of the constant stimulus to produce more cholesterol as a necessary bile ingredient to metabolize fat.[60]

2. *Pigment stones.* Both black and brown pigment gallstones, although they differ in chemical composition and clinical features, are colored by the presence of *bilirubin,* the pigment in red blood cells. They are associated with chronic hemolysis in conditions such as sickle cell disease, thalassemia, cirrhosis, long-term TPN, and advancing age. Pigment stones are often found in the bile ducts and may be related to a bacterial infection with *Escherichia coli.*

Clinical Symptoms

When inflammation, stones, or both are present in the gallbladder, contraction from the cholecystokinin-pancreozymin (CCK-PZ) mechanism causes pain. Sometimes the pain is severe. There is fullness and distention after eating and particular difficulty with fatty foods.

General Treatment

Surgical removal of the gallbladder, a cholecystectomy, is usually indicated. If the patient is obese, some weight loss before surgery is advisable if surgery can be delayed. Supportive therapy is largely nutritional. Several new nonsurgical treatments for removing the stones, using chemical dissolution or mechanical stone fragmentation, have been developed (see *To Probe Further* box). These methods provide effective alternatives to surgery in some cases.

Medical Nutrition Therapy

Basic principles of nutritional therapy for gallbladder disease include the following.

1. *Fat.* Because dietary fat is the principal cause of contraction of the diseased organ and subsequent pain, it is poorly tolerated. Energy should come primarily from carbohydrate foods, especially during acute phases. Control of fat will also contribute to weight control, a primary goal because obesity and excess food intake have been repeatedly associated with the development of gallstones.

TO PROBE FURTHER

Dissolution and Fragmentation: Alternate Solutions to the Problem of Gallstones

The 25 million Americans with gallstones may be able to have relief without surgery. Chemical dissolution by use of a drug, alone or combined with mechanical fragmentation by ultrasound waves, offers possible alternatives.

Chenodiol (chenodeoxycholic acid [CDCA]) and its companion, ursodiol (ursodeoxycholic acid [UDCA]), are two natural bile acids that reduce the concentration of cholesterol in bile and dissolve cholesterol stones harmlessly, thus sparing many persons the discomfort, risk, and cost of major surgery. Their biologic activity prevents excessive cholesterol from separating out of bile to form the most common type of gallstone. Other stones consisting of combinations of calcium carbonate, bilirubin, and other compounds make up only 15% to 20% of all gallstones.

These two naturally occurring bile acids, CDCA and UDCA, have been studied for a number of years and are now used to treat gallstones in more than 40 countries. Clinically, they appear to be effective at dissolving "floating" gallstones less than 1.25 cm (½ in) in diameter with few side effects (such as diarrhea) and only temporary reversible changes in some liver enzymes. This makes it potentially beneficial to patients who are surgical risks because of other medical problems.

Other nonsurgical methods of removing gallstones are also now in experimental stages of development and may expand these alternatives still further. An additional chemical dissolution method is the instillation of liquid solvents such as methyl tert-butyl ether (MTBE) directly into the gallbladder or the common bile duct. Additional mechanical fragmentation by pulsed lasers is being studied.

These alternate means may help patients avoid gallbladder surgery, but they do not eliminate the need for a diet emphasizing carbohydrates and fiber and controlling fat as a method of weight management. Most of these alternatives work mainly on small stones rather than on larger clumps of cholesterol. Also, they are not recommended for everyone. Chronic liver disease or a bile duct obstruction may rule them out, as does pregnancy. For many persons, however, these alternatives may provide successful treatments. Those who have gallstones may be able to say good-bye to pain, indigestion, nausea, and jaundice without fear of surgery.

References

Albert MB, Fromm H: Nonsurgical alternatives in the management of gallstones, *J Intensive Care Med* 4(1):3, 1989.

Editorial: Bile acid therapy in the 1990s, *Lancet* 340:1260, 1992.

Hochberger J et al: Lithotripsy of gallstones by means of a quality-switched giant-pulse neodymium:yttrium-aluminum-garnet laser: basic in vitro studies using a highly flexible fiber system, *Gastroenterology* 101(5):1391, 1991.

2. *Kilocalories.* If weight loss is indicated, kcalories will be reduced according to need. Principles of weight management are discussed in Chapter 6. Usually such a diet will have a relatively low percentage of calories from fat, meeting the needs of the patient for fat moderation.
3. *Cholesterol and "gas formers."* Two additional modifications usually found in traditional diets for gallbladder disease concern restriction of foods containing cholesterol and foods labeled "gas formers." Neither modification has a valid rationale. The body daily synthesizes more cholesterol than is present in an average diet. Thus restriction of dietary cholesterol has little effect in reducing gallstone formation. Total dietary fat reduction is more important. As for the use of "gas formers," such as legumes, cabbage, or fiber, blanket restriction seems unwarranted because food tolerances in any circumstances are highly individual.

DISEASES OF THE PANCREAS

Pancreatitis

Acute inflammation of the pancreas (pancreatitis) is caused by the digestion of the organ tissues by the enzymes it produces, principally *trypsin.* Normally, enzymes remain in the inactive form until the pancreatic secretions reach the duodenum through the common duct. However, gallbladder disease may cause a gallstone to enter the common bile duct and obstruct the flow from the pancreas or cause a reflux of these secretions and bile from the common duct back into the pancreatic duct. This mixing of digestive materials activates the powerful pancreatic enzymes within the gland. In such activated form, they begin their damaging effects on the pancreatic tissue itself, causing acute pain. Sometimes infectious pancreatitis may occur as a complication of mumps or a bacterial disease. Mild or moderate pancreatitis may subside completely, but it has a tendency to recur.

General Treatment

Initial care consists of measures recommended for acute disease involving shock. These measures include intravenous feeding at first, replacement therapy of fluid and electrolytes, blood transfusions, antibiotics and pain medications, and gastric suction.

Medical Nutrition Therapy

In early stages, nutritional status is maintained by parenteral nutrition support. Oral feedings are withheld because entry of food into the intestines stimulates pancreatic secretions. As healing progresses and oral feedings are resumed, a light diet is used to avoid excessive stimulation of pancreatic secretions. Alcohol and caffeine should be avoided to decrease pancreatic stimulation. Alcohol in Western societies and malnutrition worldwide are the major causes of chronic pancreatitis. Persons with this disease are usually thin and have low serum lipid concentrations, suggesting that they have latent digestion disorders or malabsorption.[61]

TO SUM UP

Nutrition therapy for gastrointestinal disease is based on careful consideration of four major factors: (1) secretory functions, providing the chemical agents and environment necessary for digestion to occur; (2) neuromuscular functions, required for motility and mechanical digestion; (3) absorptive functions, enhancing the entry of nutrients into the circulatory system; and (4) psychologic factors, reflected by changes in gastrointestinal function.

Esophageal problems vary widely from simple dysphagia to serious diseases or obstruction. Nutritional therapy and mode of intake vary according to degree of dysfunction.

PUD is a common gastrointestinal problem affecting millions of Americans. It is an erosion of the mucosal lining, mainly in the duodenal bulb and less commonly in the lower antrum portion of the stomach. It results in increased gastric tone and painful hunger contractions on an empty stomach, as well as nutritional problems such as low plasma protein levels, anemia, and weight loss. Current medical management consists of acid and infection control with a coordinated system of drugs, rest, and a regular diet with few food and drink considerations to supply the essential nutritional support for tissue healing.

Intestinal diseases are classified as (1) anatomic changes, such as the development of small tubular sacs branching off the main alimentary canal in diverticular disease; (2) malabsorption, from multiple maldigestive and malabsorptive conditions; and (3) IBD, resulting from mucosal changes and infectious processes, as seen in ulcerative colitis and Crohn's disease, or (4) SBS, resulting from surgical resection of parts of the intestine. Nutritional therapy involves fluid and electrolyte replacement, modifications in the diet's protein and energy content and food texture, and increased vitamins and minerals, with continuous adjustment of the diet according to changes in toleration for specific foods. Allergic responses to common food allergens, as well as missing cell enzymes in genetic disease, may also contribute to gastrointestinal and metabolic problems from related food intolerances.

Accessory organs to the gastrointestinal tract—liver, gallbladder, and pancreas—have important functions related to nutrient digestion, absorption, and metabolism, and their diseases interfere with these normal functions. Common liver disorders include hepatitis, usually caused by viral infection, and cirrhosis, an advanced liver disease leading to hepatic encephalopathy and progressive liver failure. Nutrient and energy levels required vary with each condition.

Diseases of the gallbladder include cholecystitis, inflammation that interferes with the absorption of water and bile acids, and cholelithiasis, or gallstone formation. Treatment involves a generally reduced-fat diet and surgical removal of the gallbladder. Diseases of the pancreas include acute and chronic forms of pancreatitis, in which alcohol abuse can be a primary cause. Other causes include biliary disease, malnutrition, drug reactions, abdominal injury, and genetic predisposition. In acute pancreatitis, pain is severe because of pancreatic enzyme reflux with self-digestion of pancreatic tissue by its own enzymes. Parenteral nutrition support is used to avoid enzyme stimulus, with gradual return to small, frequent meals as the attack subsides. In chronic pancreatitis, which is caused by alcoholism in Western societies and malnutrition worldwide, maldigestion from lack of enzymes because of pancreatic insufficiency creates nutritional problems. Nutritional care focuses on a nourishing diet with enzyme replacement and vitamin-mineral supplementation.

Questions for Review

1. What is the basic principle of diet planning for patients with esophageal problems? Outline a general nutritional care plan for a patient with GERD complicated by a hiatal hernia.
2. In current practice, what are the basic principles of diet planning for patients with PUD? How do these principles differ from former traditional therapy?
3. Outline a course of nutritional management for a person with PUD, based on the current approaches to medical management. How would you plan nutrition education for continuing self-care and avoidance of recurrence?
4. Describe the etiology, clinical signs, and treatment of each of the following intestinal diseases: malabsorption and diarrhea, IBD, diverticular disease, irritable bowel syndrome, and constipation.
5. Compare the basis of food intolerances resulting from food allergy and a specific genetic disease such as PKU.
6. How are the major metabolic functions of the liver affected in liver disease? Give some examples.
7. What is the rationale for treatment in the spectrum of liver disease—hepatitis, cirrhosis, and hepatic encephalopathy?
8. Develop a 1-day food plan for a 45-year-old man, 183 cm (6 ft 1 in) tall, weighing 90 kg (200 lb), with infectious hepatitis; develop another plan for a similar patient with cirrhosis of the liver and another for a patient with hepatic encephalopathy. What principles of diet therapy apply for each?
9. What are the principles of nutrition therapy for gallbladder disease? Write a 1-day meal plan for a 30-year-old woman, 165 cm (5 ft 6 in) tall, weighing 81 kg (180 lb), who has an inflamed gallbladder with stones and is awaiting a cholecystectomy.
10. Compare acute and chronic forms of pancreatitis in terms of etiology, symptoms, and nutritional therapy. What role does special enteral and parenteral nutrition support play in this therapy?

References

1. Williams S: Gastrointestinal diseases. In Smith, ed: *Diet therapy,* St Louis, 1995, Mosby.
2. Sontag S: The medical management of reflux esophagitis, role of antacids and acid inhibition, *Gastroenterol Clin North Am* 19:683, 1990.
3. Grant JC, Quinn Jr B: *Gastroesophageal reflux disease and the otolaryngologic manifestations,* Galveston, Tex, 1999, Department of Otolaryngology, University of Texas Medical Branch, Grand Rounds.
4. Kuipers EJ et al: Atrophic gastritis and *Helicobacter pylori* infection in patients with reflux esophagitis treated with omeprazole or fundoplication, *N Engl J Med* 334(16):1018, 1996.
5. Devault KR, Castell DO: Updated guidelines for the diagnosis and treatment of gastroesophageal reflux disease, *Am J Gastroenterol* 94(6):1434, 1999.
6. CDC, Division of Bacterial and Mycotic Diseases: *Economics of peptic ulcer disease and* H. pylori *infection,* 1998, accessible at *http://www.cdc.gov/ulcer/economic.htm.*
7. Katz J: The course of peptic ulcer disease, *Med Clin North Am* 75(4):1013, 1991.
8. Marshall BJ, Warren JR: Unidentified curved bacilli in the stomach of patients with gastritis and peptic ulceration, *Lancet* 8390:1311, 1984.
9. Blaser MJ: The bacteria behind ulcers, *Sci Am* 274(2):104, 1996.
10. Marchetti M et al: Development of a mouse model of *Helicobacter pylori* infection that mimics human disease, *Science* 267(5204):1655, 1995.
11. Megraud F: Epidemiology of *Helicobacter pylori* infection, *Gasteroenterol Clin North Am* 22(1):73, 1993.
12. NIH Consensus Development Panel on *Helicobacter pylori* in peptic ulcer disease, *JAMA* 65:272, 1994.
13. Sonnenberg A, Everhart JE: The prevalence of self-reported peptic ulcer in the United States, *Am J Pub Health* 86(2): 200, 1996.
14. Walsh JH, Peterson WL: The treatment of *H. pylori* in the management of peptic ulcer disease, *N Engl J Med* 333(15): 984, 1995.
15. Hentschel E et al: Effect of ranitidine and amoxicillin plus metronidazole on the eradication of *Helicobacter pylori* and the recurrence of duodenal ulcer, *N Engl J Med* 328(5):308, 1993.
16. Damianos AJ, McGarrity TJ: Treatment strategies for *Helicobacter pylori* infection, *Am Fam Physician* 55(8):2765, 1997.
17. Tompkins LS, Falkow S: The new path to preventing ulcers, *Science* 267(5204):1621, 1995.
18. Nowak R: The gold bug: *Helicobacter pylori, Science* 267 (5195):173, 1995.
19. Caspary WF: Physiology and pathophysiology of intestinal absorption, *Am J Clin Nutr* 55(suppl):299S, 1995.
20. Trier JS: Celiac sprue, *N Engl J Med* 325(24):1709, 1991.
21. Chartrand LJ et al: Wheat starch intolerance in patients with celiac disease, *JAMA* 97(6):612, 1997.

22. Thompson T: Do oats belong in a gluten-free diet? *J Am Diet Assoc* 97(12):1413, 1997.
23. Skerritt JH, Hill AS: Self-management of dietary compliance in celiac disease by means of ELISA "home test" to detect gluten, *Lancet* 337:379, 1991.
24. Marcus MS et al: Nutritional status of infants with cystic fibrosis associated with early diagnosis and intervention, *Am J Clin Nutr* 54:578, 1991.
25. Thomas PJ et al: Cystic fibrosis transmembrane conductance regulator: nucleotide binding to a synthetic peptide, *Science* 251:553, 1991.
26. Cystic Fibrosis Foundation: Guidelines for patient services, evaluation, and monitoring in cystic fibrosis centers, *Am J Dis Child* 144:1311, 1990.
27. Moran A et al: Pancreatic endocrine function in cystic fibrosis, *J Pediatr* 118:715, 1991.
28. Brady MS et al: Effectiveness of enteric coated pancreatic enzymes given before meals in reducing steatorrhea in children with cystic fibrosis, *J Am Diet Assoc* 92(7):813, 1992.
29. Dowsett J: Nutrition in the management of cystic fibrosis, *Nutr Rev* 54(1):31, 1996.
30. Maxwell PR et al: Irritable bowel syndrome, *Lancet* 350: 1691, 1997.
31. Dalton CB, Drossman DA: Diagnosis and treatment of irritable bowel syndrome, *Am Fam Physician* 55(3):875, 1997.
32. Fackelman K: Gastrointestinal blues, *Sci News* 150(19): 302, 1996.
33. Kim Y: Can fish oil maintain Crohn's disease in remission? *Nutr Rev* 54:248-257, 1996.
34. Hoffenberg EF et al: Circulating antioxidant concentrations in children with inflammatory bowel disease, *Am J Clin Nutr* 65:1482, 1997.
35. Hanauer SB: Inflammatory bowel disease, *N Engl J Med* 334(13):841, 1996.
36. Friedman G: Treatment of the irritable bowel syndrome, *Gastroenterol Clin North Am* 20(2):325, 1991.
37. Rosenberg IH, Mason JB: Intestinal disorders: inflammatory bowel disease. In Shils ME, Olson JA, Shike M, eds: *Modern nutrition in health and disease,* ed 8, vol 2, Philadelphia, 1994, Lea & Febiger.
38. Jeejeebhoy KN: Intestinal disorders: short-bowel syndrome. In Shils ME, Olson JA, Shike M, eds: *Modern nutrition in health and disease,* ed 8, vol 2, Philadelphia, 1994, Lea & Febiger.
39. Anderson JA: Milk, eggs, and peanuts: food allergies in children, *Am Fam Physician* 56(5):1365, 1997.
40. Bock SA, Atkins FM: Patterns of food hypersensitivity during sixteen years of double-blind, placebo-controlled food challenges, *J Pediatr* 117:561-567, 1990.
41. Parker SL et al: Foods perceived by adults as causing adverse reactions, *J Am Diet Assoc* 93(1):40, 1993.
42. Bishop JM et al: Natural history of cow milk allergy: clinical outcome, *J Pediatr* 116:862, 1990.
43. Sampson HA et al: Safety of casein hydrolysate formula in children with cow milk allergy, *J Pediatr* 118:520, 1991.
44. Björkstén B: Dietary management of food allergy, *Semin Pediatr Gastroenteral Nutr* 3(2):13, 1992.
45. Nash JM et al: Allergies, *Time* 139(25):54, 1992.
46. Elsas II LJ, Acosta PB: Nutritional support of inherited metabolic disease. In Shils ME, Olson JA, Shike M, eds: *Modern nutrition in health and disease,* ed 8, vol 2, Philadelphia, 1994, Lea & Febiger.
47. Lau JYN et al: Viral hepatitis, *Gut* 32(suppl 9):47, 1991.
48. Vail BA: Management of chronic viral hepatitis, *Am Fam Physician* 55(8):2749, 1997.
49. Martinot M et al: Influence of hepatitis G virus infection on the severity of liver disease and response to interferon-α in patients with chronic hepatitis C, *Ann Intern Med* 126(11): 874, 1997.
50. Koff RS: Interferon-α for chronic hepatitis C: reducing the uncertainties, *Ann Intern Med* 127(10):1997.
51. Hoffman M: Hepatitis A vaccine shows promise, *Science* 254:1581, 1991.
52. *Bull World Health Organ* 66:443, 1988.
53. Lee WM: Hepatitis B virus infection, *N Engl J Med* 337(24):1733, 1997.
54. Silk DBA et al: Nutritional support in liver disease, *Gut* 32(suppl 9):29, 1991.
55. Everhart JE, Hoofnagle JH: Hepatitis B-related end-stage liver disease, *Gastroenterology* 103(5):1692, 1992.
56. Poterucha JJ, Wiesner RH: Liver transplantation and hepatitis B, *Ann Intern Med* 126(8):805, 1997.
57. Holt RIG et al: Orthotopic liver transplantation reverses the adverse nutritional changes of end-stage liver disease in children, *Am J Clin Nutr* 65:534, 1997.
58. Neuberger J: Primary biliary cirrhosis, *Lancet* 350(Sept 20):875, 1997.
59. Laifer SA et al: Pregnancy in liver transplant patients—and vice versa, *Gastroenterology* 10(5):1443, 1991.
60. Ortega RM et al: Differences in diet and food habits between patients with gallstones and controls, *J Am Coll Nutr* 16(1):88, 1997.
61. Vaona B et al: Food intake of patients with chronic pancreatitis after onset of the disease, *Am J Clin Nutr* 65:851, 1997.

■ Further Reading

Anderson JA: Milk, eggs, and peanuts: food allergies in children, *Am Fam Physician* 56(5):1365, 1997.

Lallè JP, Peltre G: Biochemical features of grain-legume allergens in humans and animals, *Nutr Rev* 54(4):101, 1996.

These two articles will aid in counseling with patients who have allergies to commonly used foods.

Chartrand LJ et al: Wheat starch intolerance in patients with celiac disease, *J Am Diet Assoc* 97(6):612, 1997.

Thompson T: Do oats belong in a gluten-free diet? *J Am Diet Assoc* 97(12):1413, 1997.

These two articles provide a helpful resource for practical ways of providing food for special diets.

Dalton CB, Drossman DA: Diagnosis and treatment of irritable bowel syndrome, *Am Fam Physician* 55(3):875, 1997.

The authors present a sensitive article about this common but frustrating condition in elderly persons, providing helpful background for all those who care for these patients.

Mann LL, Wong K: Development of an objective method for assessing viscosity of formulated foods and beverages for the dysphagic diet, *J Am Diet Assoc* 96(6):585, 1996.

Here are practical ways of providing soft foods for persons with a range of swallowing disorders, a real need especially when the disorder is long term or permanent and economy is a problem.

■ Websites of Interest

Celiac Sprue

http://www.csaceliacs.org Celiac Sprue Association

http://www.celiac.com Celiac Disease and Gluten-Free Diet Support Page

http://www.gastromd.com Front Range Gastroenterology Associates

http://www.dietitian.com/gluten.html Ask the Dietitian: Gluten and Celiac Sprue

Cirrhosis

http://www.niddk.nih.gov National Institute of Diabetes & Digestive & Kidney Diseases

http://www.gastro.org/public/cirrhosis.html The American Gastroenterological Association: Cirrhosis of the Liver

http://www.liverfoundation.org American Liver Foundation

Dysphagia

http://www.dysphagia.com Dysphagia Resource Center

http://www.dysphagia-diet.com Dysphagia Diet

http://www.dysphagiaonline.com Dysphagiaonline.com

Food Allergies

http://www.aafa.org Asthma and Allergy Foundation of America

http://www.aaamc.org Monterey County Area Agency on Aging

http://www.foodallergy.org The Food Allergy and Anaphylaxis Network

http://www.peanutallergy.com PeanutAllergy.com

http://www.aaaai.org American Academy of Allergy, Asthma and Immunology

Gastroesophageal Reflux Disease (GERD)

http://www.gerd.com GERD Information Resource Center

http://www.aboutgerd.org About GERD

http://www.gastro.org The American Gastroenterological Association

Irritable Bowel Syndrome (IBS)

http://www.aboutibs.org About IBS

Lactose Intolerance

http://www.niddk.nih.gov National Institute of Diabetes & Digestive & Kidney Diseases

http://www.lactose.net Lactose.net

http://www.lactose.co.uk Lactose.co.uk

http://www.gastro.org The American Gastroenterological Association

Pancreatitis

http://www.niddk.nih.gov National Institute of Diabetes & Digestive & Kidney Diseases

http://www.emedicine.com emedicine

http://www.tummyhealth.com Tummyhealth.com

Peptic Ulcer Disease

http://www.nlm.nih.gov/pubs/cbm/pepulcer.html National Library of Medicine: *Helicobacter pylori* in Peptic Ulcer Disease

http://www.niddk.nih.gov National Institute of Diabetes & Digestive & Kidney Diseases

Phenylketonuria (PKU)

http://www.pkunews.org National PKU News

http://www.thearc.org/faqs/pku.html The Arc: Phenylketonuria (PKU)

http://www.pku-allieddisorders.org National Coalition for PKU and Allied Disorders

http://www.pkunetwork.org Children's PKU Network

CASE STUDY The patient with peptic ulcer disease

Lowell is a 40-year-old businessman who was admitted to the city hospital 3 weeks ago after an incidence of vomiting bright-red blood. A medical history revealed that a dull, gnawing pain in the upper abdomen began several months ago and has increased in severity during that time. It became more severe after his most recent out-of-state trip to one of his stores. Because the pain was usually accompanied by headaches, he took aspirin to help relieve it.

Initial hospital treatment consisted of blood transfusions, intravenous fluids and electrolytes, and vitamin C. Lowell continued to feel nauseous and weak, but he stopped vomiting. However, he passed several large, tarry stools during the first 24 hours. His initial nutritional assessment results included weight 68 kg (150 lb), height 175 cm (70 in), albumin 2.8 g/dl, prealbumin 14 mg/dl, transferrin 18% saturation value, hemoglobin 11 g/dl, and hematocrit 35%. His medications included cimetidine, sucralfate, magnesium-aluminum hydroxide; and triple antibiotic therapy.

The patient began slowly to tolerate sips of clear liquids and then advanced to a regular diet as tolerated, showing continued improvement. Before he was discharged at the end of the second week, the nutritionist and the nurse discussed general nutritional needs with Lowell and his wife. They advised him to eat his meals regularly in as relaxed a setting and manner as possible, eliminate his frequent between-meal snacks, and take his multivitamin supplement daily with his meals. Also, they reviewed his general guidelines sheet, listing a few food-related items or habits to avoid. They also advised him to stop smoking and to rest as much as possible before returning to work. His physician had also advised him to reduce his workload and scheduled a follow-up appointment in 1 week.

Lowell's wife accompanied him to the next appointment and reported that she was pleased with his ability to put aside business duties and take more time to enjoy his family. Lowell stated that his two teenage sons had been surprisingly supportive in assisting him in following the prescribed regimen and that he plans to make it his general habit.

QUESTIONS FOR ANALYSIS

1. The radiographic diagnosis of Lowell illness was a gastric ulcer in the antrum lesser curvature. What does this mean? Where do most ulcers occur? Why?
2. What factors contributed to Lowell's ulcer? What effect did each of them have?
3. Evaluate the results of Lowell's initial nutritional assessment date. How would you use this information in nutrition counseling?
4. Identify Lowell's basic nutritional needs. Outline a teaching plan based on these needs that you would use to help him with his new diet plan. How would you include his wife in formulating and implementing his nutritional care plan?
5. What role does vitamin C play in Lowell's therapy? What other vitamins and minerals play a significant role in his care? Describe each role.
6. Why should Lowell give up coffee, cigarettes, and alcohol? What problems do you think he may encounter in trying to change these habits?

Issues & ANSWERS

Nutritional Aspects of Diarrhea

Gastrointestinal disease so often presents barriers to efficient nutrient absorption that nutritional deficiencies are planned for automatically. Ironically many of these conditions also frequently lead to diarrhea, which results in further loss of fluids and electrolytes. As expected, their replacement is the initial and primary concern of therapy. However, different types of diarrhea also present other differences; the control of type-specific problems requires different modes of treatment coordinated with the treatment of the disease it accompanies. Before looking into possible treatment modes, examine first three of the most common types of diarrhea: watery, fatty, and small volume.

Watery diarrhea occurs when the amount of water and electrolytes moving into the intestinal mucosa exceeds that amount absorbed into the bloodstream. This movement of water and electrolytes into the mucosa may be secretive or osmotic.

If this movement of water and electrolytes into the mucosa is secretive, it may be active or passive. Active movement occurs with excessive gastric hydrochloric acid secretion or enterotoxin-induced infections such as cholera. Passive movement occurs with a rise in hydrostatic pressure that accompanies such infectious diseases as salmonellosis or tuberculosis, nonbacterial infections, fungal infections, renal failure, irradiation enteritis, and IBD. Other conditions associated with watery diarrhea include hyperthyroidism, thyroid carcinoma, and hypermotility of the gastrointestinal tract.

If this movement of water and electrolytes into the mucosa is osmotic, it will occur when these nutrients are not absorbed because of intolerable levels of nonabsorbable particles present in the intestinal chyme. Such particles include lactose (milk sugar) in individuals with lactase deficiency or gluten (a cereal protein found in wheat and rye, and to a lesser degree in barley and oats) in persons with a reduced gastrointestinal transit time caused by the removal of part of the intestinal tract.

Fatty diarrhea, or *steatorrhea,* occurs with maldigestion or malabsorption. Maldigestion involves a lack of enzymatic activity required to completely digest food, such as reduced pancreatic exocrine activity (release of intestinal enzymes from the pancreas) caused by pancreatic insufficiency.

Malabsorption means that digested materials do not make it across the intestinal mucosa to enter the bloodstream. This failure occurs in conditions in which the intestinal villi are destroyed, such as celiac disease.

Small-volume diarrhea occurs mainly when the rectosigmoid area of the colon is irritated, such as in IBD (Crohn's disease or ulcerative colitis). It also occurs when inflammatory conditions affect areas adjacent to the colon, as in pelvic inflammatory disease, diverticulitis, appendicitis, or hemorrhagic ovarian cysts.

The metabolic consequences of each type of diarrhea are similar. Uncontrolled, they result in syncope, hypokalemia, acid-base imbalances, and hypovolemia, with resulting renal failure. They may also be accompanied by low levels of fat-soluble vitamins, vitamin B_{12}, or folic acid or eventually lead to protein-energy malnutrition. In addition to these conditions, each type also manifests problems associated with the disorder they accompany. Workers with the Memorial Sloan-Kettering Cancer Center in New York and the Department of Medicine at Brooke Army Medical Center in Texas have developed recommendations for treating gastrointestinal diseases associated with each type of diarrhea. These are summarized here, with the focus on the diarrheal aspects of disease.

- Watery diarrhea often accompanies inflammatory bowel conditions, such as Crohn's disease, for which diet therapy involves (1) increased protein and kcalories, (2) low fats and lactose, and (3) avoidance of foods that stimulate peristalsis. Thus secretive diarrhea is reduced by eliminating foods that may stimulate gastric acid secretion, and all types of watery diarrhea are avoided by reducing the motility of the gastrointestinal tract. In other conditions in which osmotic diarrhea occurs, such as dumping syndrome, this problem is avoided by giving fluids between meals to avoid any extreme difference in osmotic pressures on either side of the intestinal wall. Small, frequent meals also help prevent this problem, as well as painful distention.
- Fatty diarrhea frequently accompanies conditions associated with maldigestion, such as chronic pancreatitis. The nutrition management of this disease involves (1) frequent meals that are high in protein and carbohydrates and low in fat; (2) use of medium-chain triglycerides, which are more easily absorbed under adverse conditions; and (3) avoiding gastric stimulants, especially caffeine and alcohol. Fatty diarrhea also accompanies conditions of malabsorption, such as gluten-sensitive enteropathy. In addition to nutrition management strategies listed, treating this type of diarrhea

requires the removal of products that damage the mucosal villi, including lactose and gluten, which is found in wheat, rye, barley, and oats, and food products and fillers such as hydrolyzed vegetable protein products. It sometimes requires restricting fat as well. In both cases the primary concern is to monitor fats that would otherwise appear in the feces. As the therapy progresses, the fat content of the meal can be increased as tolerated to normal levels to improve palatability.

- Small-volume diarrhea may accompany diverticulosis of the colon. A high-residue diet is recommended to increase fecal bulk, thereby preventing diarrhea. To prevent flatulence and distention, fiber should be added to the diet gradually.

All types of diarrhea can result in malnutrition, primarily because of electrolyte and fluid losses. It is important to identify the type of diarrhea occurring with each patient; only then can an effective nutritional management strategy be designed to replace those losses, as well as to eliminate or prevent other nutrition-related problems that are possible for each case.

REFERENCES

Banwell JG: Pathophysiology of diarrheal disorders, *Rev Infect Dis* 12(suppl 1):30, 1990.

Barrett KE, Dharmsathaphorn K: Secretion and absorption: small intestine and colon. In Yamada T, ed: *Textbook of gastroenterology,* Philadelphia, 1991, JB Lippincott.

Gorbach SL: Efficacy of lactobacillus in treatment of acute diarrhea, *Nutr Today* 31(suppl 6):19S, 1996.

Kaaila M, Isolauri E: Nutritional management of acute diarrhea, *Nutr Today* 31(suppl 6):16S, 1996.

Chapter

19

Diseases of the Heart, Blood Vessels, and Lungs

Sara Long Anderson

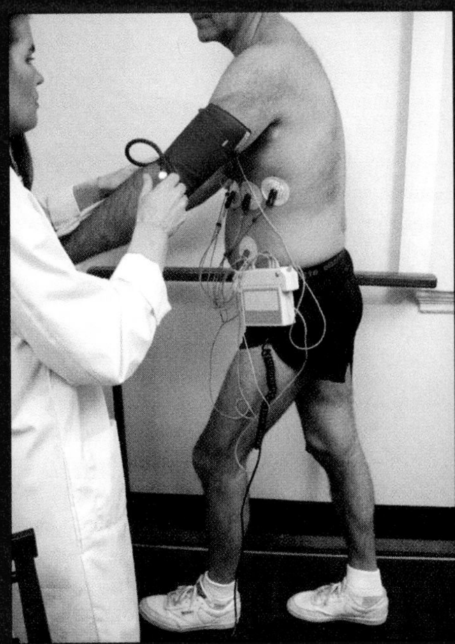

Chapter Outline

In this chapter, we consider interrelated diseases of the circulatory system—heart, blood vessels, and lungs. In recent decades these diseases of modern civilization have become the major causes of death in the United States and most other Western societies. The magnitude of this overall healthcare problem is enormous.

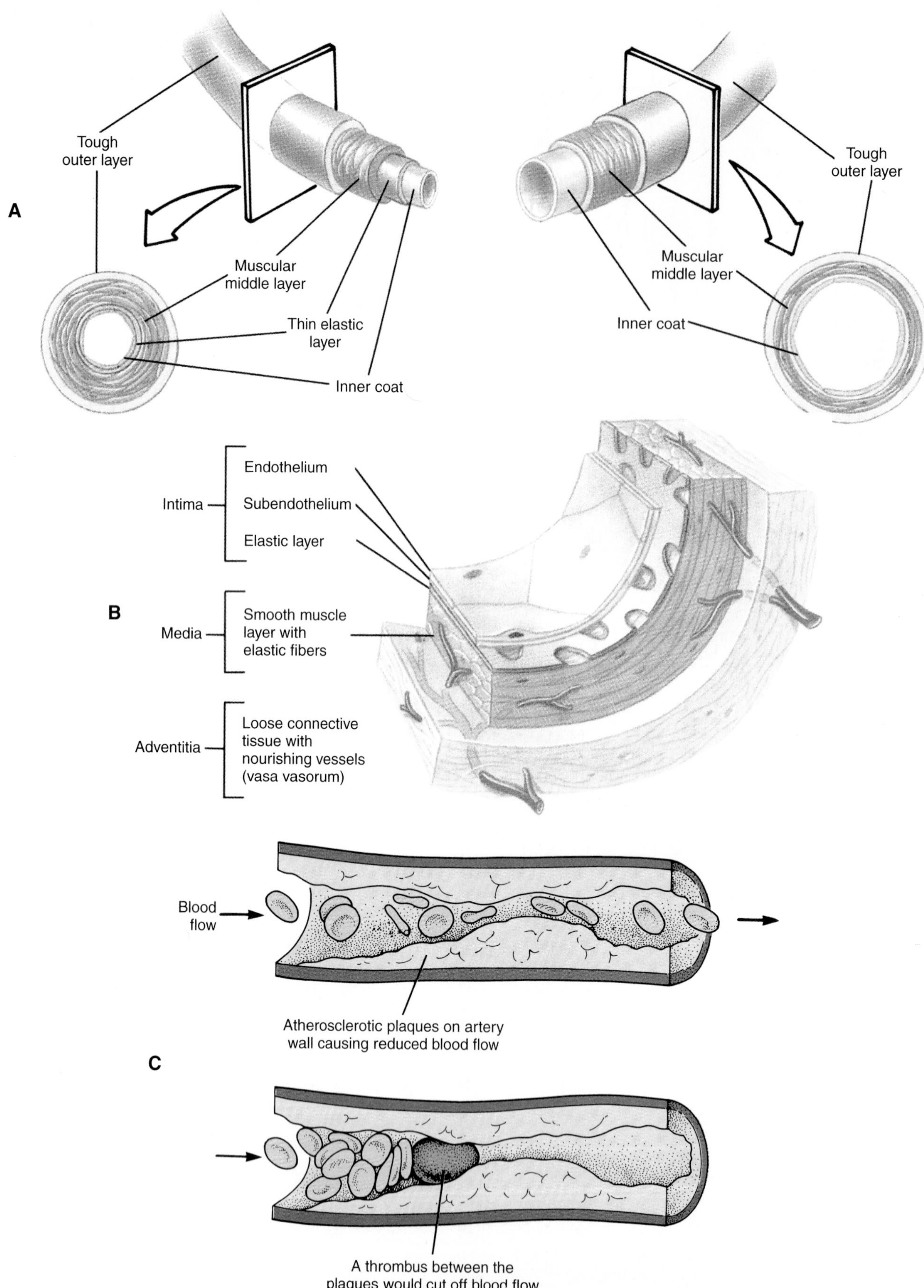

FIGURE 19-1 Blood vessel structure and diseased arteries. **A,** Comparative wall thicknesses and inner lumen size of arteries *(left)* and veins *(right)*. **B,** Cutout of vessel wall showing three basic layers of tissue involved: intima, media, and adventitia. **C,** Atherosclerotic plaque in artery.

Coronary Heart Disease: The Problem of Atherosclerosis

THE UNDERLYING DISEASE PROCESS

Atherosclerosis, the major arteriosclerosis disease and underlying pathologic process in coronary heart disease (CHD), is paramount in ongoing study in modern medicine. The characteristic lesions involved are raised fibrous plaques (Figure 19-1). They appear on the interior surface, the intima, of blood vessel as discrete lumps elevated above unaffected surrounding tissue and ranging in color from pearly gray to yellowish gray. The main cellular component of plaque is a smooth muscle cell similar to the major cell of the normal artery wall. Plaque usually contains fatty material, such as lipoproteins, that carry cholesterol in the blood. Deep in the lesions are debris from dead and dying cells and varying amounts of lipids. Crystals of cholesterol can be seen with the unaided eye in the softened cheesy debris of advanced lesions.

It is this fatty debris that suggested the original name *atherosclerosis,* from the Greek words *athera* ("gruel") and *sclerosis* ("hardening"). This fatty degeneration and thickening narrow the vessel lumen and may allow a blood clot, an embolus, to develop from its irritating presence. Eventually the clot may cut off blood flow in the involved artery. If the artery is a critical one, such as a major coronary vessel, a heart attack occurs. Tissue area serviced by the involved artery is deprived of its vital O_2 and nutrient supply, a condition called ischemia, and the cells die. The localized area of dying or dead tissue is called an infarct. Because the artery involved supplies cardiac muscle, the *myocardium,* the result is called an *acute myocardial infarction (AMI).* The two major coronary arteries, with their many branches, are so named because they lie across the brow of the heart muscle and resemble a crown (Figure 19-2). Figure 19-3 shows the anterior internal view of the normal human heart.

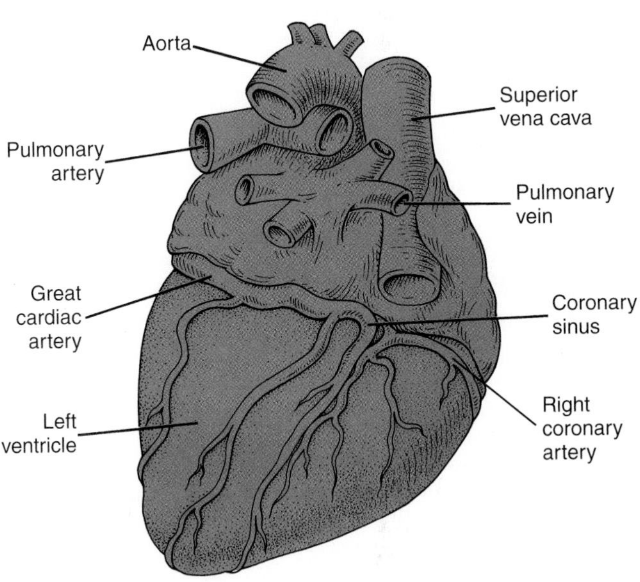

FIGURE 19-2 Coronary blood circulation. Posterior external view showing coronary arteries.

Thus the focus of the problem in CHD is development of these characteristic fatty plaques called atheromas. Injury to the important inner endothelial lining of the blood vessel wall leads to a thickening thrombosis and lipid deposits, with the development of atherosclerosis. According to the American Heart Association, three proven causes of damage to arterial walls are (1) elevated levels of serum cholesterol and triglycerides, (2) high blood pressure, and (3) tobacco smoke.[1] The major role-player in plaque development is a lipoprotein, low-density lipoprotein (LDL) cholesterol, that carries cholesterol in the blood.[2,3] Additional risk factors are shown in Box 19-1.

CHOLESTEROL, LIPOPROTEINS, AND LIPIDS

Cholesterol is a soft, fat-like substance found in all cell membranes and blood and is a precursor of bile acids and steroid hormones. Cholesterol and triglycerides (TG) cannot dissolve in blood and must be transported to and from cells by individual components containing both lipid and proteins (lipoproteins).[1-3] The five types of lipoproteins are classified according to fat content and thus their density, with those having the highest fat content possessing the lowest density.

1. *Chylomicrons* have the highest lipid content and lowest density and are composed mostly of dietary TG, with a

---

arteriosclerosis Blood vessel disease characterized by thickening and hardening of artery walls, with loss of functional elasticity, mainly affecting the intima (inner lining) of the arteries.

atheroma A mass of fatty plaque formed in inner arterial walls in atherosclerosis.

atherosclerosis Common form of arteriosclerosis, characterized by the gradual formation—beginning in childhood in genetically predisposed individuals—of yellow cheeselike streaks of cholesterol and fatty material that develop into hardened plaques in the intima or inner lining of major blood vessels, such as coronary arteries, eventually in adulthood cutting off blood supply to the tissue served by the vessels; the underlying pathology of coronary heart disease.

infarct An area of tissue necrosis caused by local ischemia, resulting from obstruction of blood circulation to that area.

ischemia Deficiency of blood to a particular tissue, resulting from functional blood vessel constriction or actual obstruction walls in atherosclerosis.

intima General term indicating an innermost part of a structure or vessel; inner layer of the blood vessel wall.

plaque Thickened deposits of fatty material, largely cholesterol, within the arterial wall that eventually may fill the lumen and cut off blood supply to the tissue served by the damaged vessel.

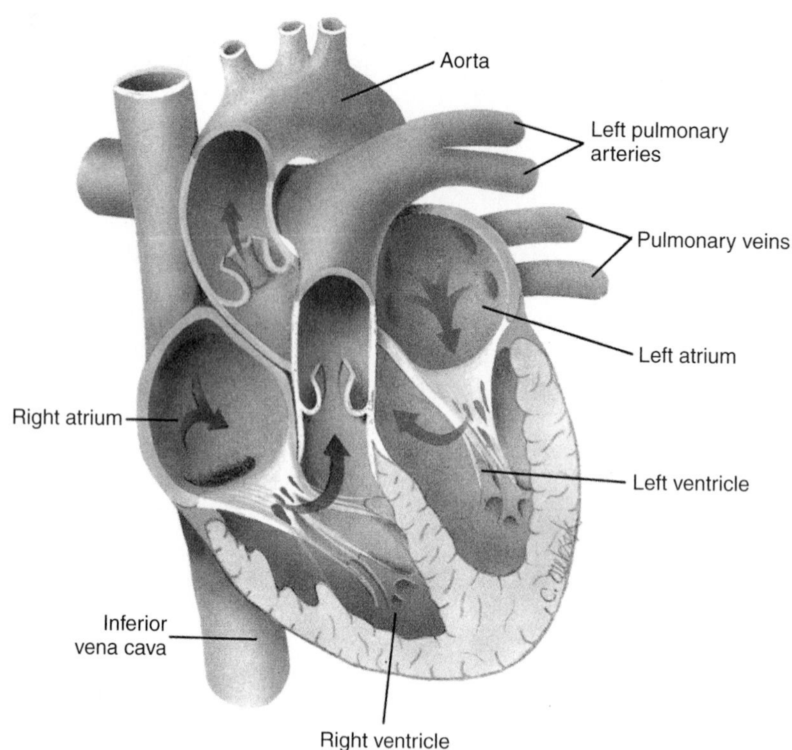

FIGURE 19-3 The normal human heart. Anterior internal view showing cardiac circulation. (*From Seeley RR, Stephens TD, Tate P:* Anatomy and physiology, *ed 2, New York, 1992, McGraw-Hill. Reproduced with permission of the McGraw-Hill Companies.*)

BOX 19-1 Major Risk Factors in Cardiovascular Disease

Lipid Risk Factors

- ↑ LDL cholesterol (>100 mg/dl)
- ↓ HDL cholesterol (<40 mg/dl)
- ↑ Triglycerides (>150 mg/dl)

Nonlipid Risk Factors

Modifiable

- Tobacco smoke and exposure to tobacco smoke
- High serum cholesterol (>200 mg/dl)
- Hypertension (>140/90 mm Hg)
- Physical inactivity
- Obesity (BMI >30 kg/m^2) and overweight (BMI 25-29.9 kg/m^2)
- Diabetes mellitus
- Atherogenic diet (↑ intakes of saturated fats and cholesterol)
- Stress and coping
- Excessive alcohol consumption (>1 drink/day for women and >2 drinks/day for men)
- Individual response to stress and coping
- Some illegal drugs (cocaine and IV drug abuse)

Nonmodifiable

- Male gender
- Increasing age (males >45 years, females >55 years)
- Heredity (including race)
- Family history of premature CHD (MI or sudden death <55 years of age in father or other male first-degree relative, or <65 years of age in mother or other female first-degree relatives)

References: American Heart Association, Heart and stroke facts, 1992-2001; Grundy SM et al: Primary prevention of coronary heart disease: guidance from Framingham, *Circulation*: 97:1876, 1998; National Cholesterol Education Program (NCEP): *Third report of the NCEP Expert Panel on Detection, Evaluation, and Treatment of High Blood Cholesterol in Adults (Adult Treatment Panel III) Executive Summary,* NIH Publication No 01-3670, Washington, DC, 2001, National Institutes of Health, National Heart, Lung, and Blood Institute, available at *http://www.nhlbi.nih.gov/guidelines/cholesterol/atp3xsum.pdf*; National Cholesterol Education Program (NCEP): *Third report of the NCEP Expert Panel on Detection, Evaluation, and Treatment of High Blood Cholesterol in Adults (Adult Treatment Panel III), Full Report,* Washington, DC, 2001, National Institutes of Health, National Heart, Lung, and Blood Institute, available at *http://www.nhlbi.nih.gov/guidelines/cholesterol/atp3_rpt.pdf*.

TABLE 19-1 Characteristics of the Classes of Lipoproteins

Characteristic	Chylomicrons	Very Low-Density (VLDL)	Intermediate-Density (IDL)	Low-Density (LDL)	High-Density (HDL)
Composition					
Triglycerides (TG)	80%-95%; diet, exogenous	60%-80%; endogenous	40%; endogenous	10%-30%; endogenous	5%-10%; endogenous
Cholesterol	2%-7%	10%-15%	30%	45%-50%	20%
Phospholipid	3%-6%	15%-20%	20%	15%-22%	25%-30%
Protein	1%-2%	5%-10%	10%	20%-25%	45%-50%
Function	Transport dietary TG to plasma and tissues, cells	Transport endogenous TG to cells	Continue transport of endogenous TG to cells	Transport cholesterol to peripheral cells	Transport free cholesterol from membranes to liver for catabolism
Place of synthesis	Intestinal wall	Liver	Liver	Liver	Liver
Size, density					
Description	Largest, lightest	Next largest, next lightest	Intermediate size, lighter	Smaller, heavier	Smaller, densest, heaviest
Density	0.095	0.095-1.006	1.00-1.03	1.019-1.063	1.063-1.210
Size in nanometers (nm)	75-100	30-80	25-40	10-20	7.5-10

small amount of carrier protein. They accumulate in portal blood after a meal and are efficiently cleared from the blood by the specific enzyme lipoprotein lipase.

2. *Very low-density lipoproteins (VLDL)* still carry a large lipid (TG) content but include about 10% to 15% cholesterol. These lipoproteins are formed in the liver from endogenous fat sources.
3. *Intermediate-density lipoproteins (IDL)* continue the delivery of endogenous TG to cells and carry about 30% cholesterol.
4. *LDL* carries, in addition to other lipids, about two thirds or more of total plasma cholesterol formed in blood serum from catabolism of VLDL. Because LDL carries cholesterol to cells for deposit in tissues, it is considered the main agent in elevated serum cholesterol levels, or the "bad" cholesterol.
5. *High-density lipoproteins (HDL)* carry less total lipid and more carrier protein. They are formed in the liver from endogenous fat sources. Because HDL carries cholesterol from tissues to the liver for catabolism and excretion, higher serum levels of this "good" cholesterol form are considered protective against cardiovascular disease. A value of 60 mg/dl or above contributes definite protection and decreased risk.

Characteristics of these classes of lipoproteins are summarized in Table 19-1.

FUNCTIONAL CLASSIFICATION OF LIPID DISORDERS

Current clinical practice is based on a useful functional classification that reveals two important factors: (1) recognition of genetic factors involved and (2) focus on the role of apolipoproteins in the course of lipoprotein formation, transport, or destruction. Both factors will be encountered in readings and in clinical work with patients. Thus the outline provided in this discussion and summaries in Table 19-2 of apolipoproteins and in Table 19-3 of the functional classification of lipid disorders are useful in understanding clinical problems involved and in counseling patients.

Apolipoproteins

The term *apolipoprotein* refers to a major protein part of a combined metabolic product, in this case a specific protein part of a combined lipid-protein molecule. These apolipoproteins are increasingly recognized as important parts of the lipoprotein molecule as more of them are identified, analyzed, and classified by letter and number. For example, apolipoprotein B is a common attachment to LDL and serves two basic functions: (1) aids transport of lipids in a water medium, blood, and (2) transports lipids into cells for metabolic purposes. When apolipoprotein B-100, a single large protein molecule, attaches to one pole of the LDL, it provides a recognition site for LDL receptors on the cell, causing the entire LDL to be transported by pinocytosis into the cell for use in cell metabolism.[4] Various types of LDL have specific receptor sites for

apolipoprotein A separate protein compound that attaches to its specific receptor site on a particular lipoprotein and activates certain functions, such as protein synthesis of a related enzyme. For example, apolipoprotein C-II is an apolipoprotein of HDL and VLDL that functions to activate the enzyme lipoprotein lipase.

TABLE 19-2 Apolipoproteins in the Structure of Human Plasma Lipoproteins

Apolipoprotein	Related Lipoprotein	Tissue Origin	Function
A-I	CM, VLDL, HDL	Intestine, liver	Activates LCAT
A-II	CM, VLDL, HDL	Intestine, liver	Unclear
A-III	Subfraction of HDL		Catalyzes transfer of cholesterol esters among lipoproteins
A-IV	CM, VLDL, HDL, free in plasma	Intestine, liver	May activate LCAT
B-48	CM	Intestine	Secretes CM; transports cholesterol and TGs
B-100	VLDL, IDL, LDL	Liver	Secretes VLDL; recognizes LDL receptor
C-I	CM, VLDL, HDL	Liver	Inhibits hepatic uptake of lipoproteins
C-II	CM, VLDL, HDL	Liver	Activates lipoprotein lipase
C-III	CM, VLDL, HDL	Liver	Inhibits lipoprotein lipase and premature remnant clearance
D	HDL	Spleen, liver, intestine, and adrenal glands	Functions in cholesterol ester transfer complex
E	CM, VLDL, IDL, trace amounts in LDL and HDL	Liver, macrophages, and body tissues except the intestine	Recognizes remnant and LDL receptor; acts as regulator in immune system; modulates cell growth

CM, Chylomicron; *HDL,* high-density lipoprotein; *IDL,* intermediate-density lipoprotein; *LDL,* low-density lipoprotein; *VLDL,* very low–density lipoprotein; *LCAT,* lecithin-cholesterol acyltransferase; *TG,* triglyceride.

TABLE 19-3 Functional Classification of Lipid Disorders

Type of Defect or Lipid Disorder	Abnormal Lipid Pattern	Clinical Characteristics	Nutritional Therapy
Defective Synthesis of Apolipoproteins			
Apolipoprotein A deficiency	Decreased HDL level Increased tissue cholesterol level Decreased serum cholesterol level Increased serum TG level	Rare Genetic Tangier disease	Low cholesterol Low fat
Apolipoprotein B deficiency	High mucosal tissue fat No lipoprotein synthesis possible	Rare Genetic Serious prognosis for child Malabsorption Steatorrhea	Very low fat
Apolipoprotein C deficiency	Increased TG level Increased chylomicron level	Rare Genetic Early childhood Abdominal pain (pancreatitis) Lipidemia, retinalis Xanthomas	Very low fat (20 g) High carbohydrate Medium-chain triglycerides (MCTs)
Apolipoprotein E deficiency	Increased chylomicron remnants Decreased serum LDL level Increased cholesterol level	Relatively uncommon Genetic Xanthomas Premature atherosclerosis	Low cholesterol (<300 mg) Low saturated fat Increased substitution of polyunsaturated fat Weight reduction
Enzyme Deficiency			
Lipoprotein lipase deficiency	Increased chylomicron level	Rare Genetic Early childhood Abdominal pain (pancreatitis) Lipidemia, retinalis Xanthomas Hepatosplenomegaly	Very low fat (20 g) High carbohydrate MCTs

TABLE 19-3 Functional Classification of Lipid Disorders—cont'd

Type of Defect or Lipid Disorder	Abnormal Lipid Pattern	Clinical Characteristics	Nutritional Therapy
Enzyme Deficiency—cont'd			
Lecithin-cholesterol acyltransferase deficiency	Overall abnormal lipid pattern: all lipoproteins have low amounts of cholesterol esters and high concentrations of free cholesterol and lecithin Accumulation of large LDL particles rich in unesterified cholesterol	Rare Genetic Abnormal cornea Anemia Kidney damage	Low cholesterol Low fat
LDL Receptor Deficiency			
Familial hypercholesterolemia	Increased LDL level Increased total cholesterol level Increased VLDL level	Common Genetic Increased atherosclerosis All ages Xanthomas	Low cholesterol (<300 mg) Low saturated fat Substitution of polyunsaturated fat
Other Inherited Hyperlipidemias			
Familial hypertriglyceridemia	Increased VLDL level Increased TG level Increased cholesterol level Sometimes increased blood sugar level	Common Genetic Glucose intolerance Possible type II (non–insulin-dependent) diabetes mellitus Obesity Accelerated atherosclerosis	Weight reduction Low simple carbohydrates Low saturated fat Low cholesterol
Familial multiple hyperlipoproteinemia	Increased VLDL level Increased LDL level	Fairly common Genetic Adult Xanthomas; vascular disease	Low cholesterol (<300 mg) Low saturated fat Substitution of polyunsaturated fat Weight reduction
Familial type V hyperlipoproteinemia	Increased chylomicron level Increased VLDL level Increased cholesterol level Increased TG level	Rare Glucose intolerance Obesity Abdominal pain (pancreatitis) Hepatosplenomegaly	Weight reduction Controlled carbohydrate and fat intake High protein

particular apolipoproteins to which the apolipoprotein is attracted and which in large measure determine function.

Function

When lipoproteins are synthesized in the intestinal wall, liver, and blood serum, the protein component is made up of varying kinds of apolipoprotein parts. These genetically determined components influence the structure, receptor binding, and metabolism of lipoproteins. It is an apolipoprotein component that helps form special spherical droplets of lipid material for transport in the bloodstream (see Chapter 3). Apolipoprotein determination is currently a useful laboratory tool for identifying persons at high risk for CHD.[5,6]

Classes

A number of apolipoproteins and their corresponding apolipoproteins have been identified. Class designations in common use are apolipoprotein A, B, C, D, and E. In turn, each class consists of several different proteins, for example, A-I, A-II, A-III, and A-IV and C-I, C-II, and C-III. All of these classes of apolipoproteins are made by the liver, and the intestinal mucosa makes apolipo-proteins A and B. Table 19-2 lists these various classes of apolipoproteins with their related lipoproteins and functions.

Defects in Synthesis of Apolipoproteins

Current functional approach classifies lipid disorders into four major groups based on the underlying functional problem: (1) defects in apolipoprotein synthesis, (2) enzyme deficiencies, (3) LDL-receptor deficiency, and (4) other inherited hyperlipidemias. The summary of these lipid disorders in Table 19-3 provides a review of these basic related conditions and nutritional therapies.

TABLE 19-4 Essential Components of Therapeutic Lifestyle Changes (TLC)

Component	Recommendation
LDL-raising nutrients	
Saturated fats	<7% of total energy intake
Dietary cholesterol	<200 mg/d
Therapeutic options for LDL lowering	
Plant stanols/sterols	2 g/day
Soluble fiber	10-25 g/day
Total energy (kcals)	Adjust total energy intake to maintain desirable body weight/prevent weight gain
Physical activity	Include enough moderate exercise to expend at least 200 kcal/day

Reference: National Cholesterol Education Program (NCEP): *Third report of the NCEP expert panel on detection, evaluation, and treatment of high blood cholesterol in adults (Adult Treatment Panel III), Full Report,* Washington, DC, 2001, National Institutes of Health, National Heart, Lung, and Blood Institute, available at *http://www.nhlbi.nih.gov/guidelines/cholesterol/atp3_rpt.pdf.*

TABLE 19-5 Nutrient Composition of the Therapeutic Lifestyle Changes (TLC) Diet

Component	Recommendation
Polyunsaturated fat	Up to 10% total energy intake
Monounsaturated fat	Up to 20% total energy intake
Total fat	25%-35% total energy intake*
Carbohydrate†	50%-60% total energy intake
Dietary fiber	20-30 g/day
Protein	Approximately 15% total energy intake

References: National Cholesterol Education Program (NCEP): *Third report of the NCEP Expert Panel on Detection, Evaluation, and Treatment of High Blood Cholesterol in Adults (Adult Treatment Panel III) Executive Summary,* NIH Publication No 01-3670, Washington, DC, 2001, National Institutes of Health, National Heart, Lung, and Blood Institute, available at *http://www.nhlbi.nih.gov/guidelines/cholesterol/atp3xsum.pdf*; National Cholesterol Education Program (NCEP): *Third report of the NCEP Expert Panel on Detection, Evaluation, and Treatment of High Blood Cholesterol in Adults (Adult Treatment Panel III),* Washington, DC, 2001, National Institutes of Health, National Heart, Lung, and Blood Institute, available at *http://www.nhlbi.nih.gov/guidelines/cholesterol/atp3_rpt.pdf.*

*ATP III allows for increase of total fat to 35% total energy intake and reduction in carbohydrate to 50% for persons with the metabolic syndrome. Any increase in fat intake should be in the form of either polyunsaturated or monounsaturated fat.

†Carbohydrates should come primarily from foods rich in complex carbohydrates including grains—especially whole grains—fruits and vegetables.

GENERAL PRINCIPLES OF NUTRITIONAL THERAPY

Basic Guidelines

The National Cholesterol Education Program (NCEP) periodically publishes revised guidelines for clinical management of high serum cholesterol. ATP I delineated strategy for primary prevention of CHD in persons with high levels of LDL cholesterol (160 mg/dl), or those with borderline-high LDL cholesterol (130-159 mg/dl) and two or more risk factors. ATP II substantiated these strategies and made further recommendations for intensive management of LDL cholesterol in persons with established CHD. A new, lower LDL cholesterol of 100 mg/dl was established. The third Adult Treatment Panel (ATP III) report identifies more intensive LDL-lowering therapy. The Adult Treatment Panel III (ATP III)[2,3] suggests a comprehensive lifestyle approach to reducing risk for CHD called therapeutic lifestyle changes (TLC) and incorporates the following components.[2,3]

- Reduced intake of saturated fats and cholesterol
- Therapeutic dietary options for enhancing LDL lowering (plant stanols/sterols and increased soluble fiber)
- Weight reduction
- Increased regular physical activity

Components of TLC are outlined in Table 19-4. ATP III also suggests ranges for other macronutrients in the TLC Diet (Table 19-5). Overall composition of the TLC Diet is consistent with recommendations of the *Dietary Guidelines for Americans 2000* (see Appendix M).[7]

Components of the TLC Diet

Saturated fat and cholesterol. In view of the fact that the major LDL-raising nutrient components are saturated fat and cholesterol, reducing saturated fat (<7% of total energy intake) and cholesterol (<200 mg/d) in the diet is the foundation of the TLC Diet.[2,3] The strongest nutritional influence on serum LDL cholesterol levels is saturated fats.[8] In fact, there is a "dose-response relationship" between saturated fats and LDL cholesterol levels.[3] For every 1% increase in kilocalories (kcalories) from saturated fats as a percent of total energy, serum LDL cholesterol increases approximately 2%. On the other hand, a 1% decrease in saturated fats will lower serum cholesterol by about 2%.[9,10] Although weight reduction by itself, even of a few pounds, will reduce LDL cholesterol levels,[3,11,12] weight reduction attained using a kcalorie-controlled diet low in saturated fats and cholesterol will improve and maintain LDL cholesterol lowering.[3,13,14] Although dietary cholesterol does not have the same influence of saturated fat on serum LDL cholesterol levels,[3] high cholesterol intakes raise LDL cholesterol levels.[3,15,16] Therefore reducing dietary cholesterol to less than 200 mg/day decreases serum LDL cholesterol in most persons.[3]

Monounsaturated fat. The TLC Diet recommends the substitution of monounsaturated fat for saturated fats at an intake level of up to 20% of total energy intake[2,3] because monounsaturated fats lower LDL cholesterol levels relative to saturated fats[3,9] without decreasing HDL cholesterol or TG levels.[3,9,17,18] It is recommended that plant oils and nuts be used because they are the best sources of monounsaturated fats.[3]

Polyunsaturated fats. Polyunsaturated fats, in particular linoleic acid, reduces LDL cholesterol levels when used instead of saturated fats. However, they can also bring about small reductions in HDL cholesterol when compared side by side with monounsaturated fats.[3,9] The TLC Diet recommends liquid vegetables oils, semiliquid margarines, and other margarines low in *trans* fatty acids be used because they are the best sources of polyunsaturated fats; intakes can range up to 10% of total energy intake.[2,3]

Total fat. In view of the fact that only saturated fats and *trans* fatty acids increase LDL cholesterol levels,[19] serum levels of LDL cholesterol are unrelated to total fat intake per se.[3] For that reason, the ATP III suggests it is not crucial to limit total fat intake for the specific goal of reducing LDL cholesterol levels, provided saturated fats are decreased to goal levels.[2,3]

Carbohydrate. When saturated fats are replaced with carbohydrates, LDL cholesterol levels are reduced. On the other hand, very high intakes of carbohydrates (>60% total energy intake) are associated with a reduction in HDL cholesterol and a increase in serum TG.[3,9,17,20,21] Increasing soluble fiber intake can sometimes reduce these responses.[3,21-23] On average, increasing soluble fiber to 5 to 10 g/day is accompanied by an approximately 5% reduction in LDL cholesterol.[24,25]

Protein. Despite the fact that dietary protein as a rule has an insignificant effect on serum LDL cholesterol level, replacing animal protein with plant-based protein has been reported to decrease LDL cholesterol.[3,26] This may be due to plant-based proteins (legumes, dry beans, nuts, whole grains, and vegetables) containing less saturated fat than many animal proteins and no cholesterol. This is not to say animal proteins cannot be low in saturated fat and cholesterol. Fat-free and low-fat dairy products, egg whites, fish, skinless poultry, and lean cuts of beef and pork are also low in saturated fat and cholesterol. All foods of animal origin will contain cholesterol.

Further dietary options for reducing LDL cholesterol. Adding 5 to 10 g of soluble fiber (oats, barley, psyllium, pectin-rich fruit, and beans)/day is associated with approximately a 5% reduction in LDL cholesterol[24,25] and is regarded as a therapeutic option to enhance reduction of LDL cholesterol[3] (see *To Probe Further* box). Plant sterols present an additional therapeutic option.[3] Daily intakes of 2 to 3 g plant stanol/sterol esters (isolated from soybean and tall pine-tree oils) have been shown to lower LDL cholesterol by 6% to 15%.[27-33]

General Approach to Therapeutic Lifestyle Changes (TLC)

The ATP III[2,3] suggests patients at risk for CHD or with CHD be referred to registered dietitians or other qualified nutritionists for the duration of all stages of medical nutrition therapy (MNT). After 6 weeks of TLCs, LDL cholesterol should be measured to evaluate response to TLC. If the LDL cholesterol target has been realized or an improvement in LDL lowering has occurred, MNT should be uninterrupted. If the goal has not been attained, there are a number of alternatives from which the physician can select. First, MNT can be re-explained and reinforced. Next, therapeutic dietary options can be integrated into TLC. Response to MNT should be assessed in an additional 6 weeks. If the LDL cholesterol target is achieved, the current intensity of MNT should be continued indefinitely. If there is downward movement in LDL cholesterol measures, thought should be given to continuing MNT before adding LDL-lowering medications. If it looks unlikely the LDL target will be realized with MNT, medications should be considered.[2,3] The Guide to Therapeutic Lifestyle Changes (TLC) Healthy Lifestyle Recommendations for a Healthy Heart is shown in Box 19-2.

DRUG THERAPY

Although the use of TLC will attain the LDL cholesterol target goal for many, a segment of the population will have need of LDL-lowering medications to achieve the prescribed goal for LDL cholesterol.[2,3] If treatment with TLC alone is unsuccessful after 3 months, the ATP III recommends the initiation of drug treatment. When drugs are used, however, TLC also should continue to be used concomitantly. MNT affords further CHD risk reduction beyond drug efficacy.[3] Actions of the combined use of TLC and LDL cholesterol-lowering medications may include the following.[3]

1. Intensive LDL lowering with TLC, including therapeutic dietary options
    - May prevent need for drugs
    - Can augment LDL-lowering medications
    - May allow for lower doses of medications
2. Weight control plus increased physical activity
    - Reduces risk beyond LDL cholesterol lowering
    - Constitutes principal management of metabolic syndrome
    - Raises HDL cholesterol
3. Initiating TLC before medication consideration
    - For most people, a trial of MNT of about 3 months is advised before initiating drug therapy
    - Ineffective trials of MNT exclusive of medications should not be protracted for an indefinite period if goals of therapy are not approached in a reasonable period; medications should not be withheld if it is needed to reach targets in persons with a short-term and/or long-term CHD risk that is high
4. Initiating drug therapy simultaneously with TLC
    - For severe hypercholesterolemia in which MNT alone cannot attain LDL cholesterol targets

---

metabolic syndrome Multiple metabolic risk factors in one individual: overweight/obesity, physical inactivity, and genetic factors.

trans fatty acids Fatty acids that have been hydrogenated to be used in margarine and in the food industry; have been shown to increase LDL cholesterol and lower HDL cholesterol

TO PROBE FURTHER
Added Food Factors in Coronary Heart Disease Therapy

The primary focus of medical nutritional therapy for CHD focuses on control of lipid factors, including cholesterol and saturated fats. Two other food factors, however, play a different role. In varying ways they help to protect us from the development of CHD.

DIETARY FIBER

Studies indicate water-soluble types of dietary fiber have significant cholesterol-lowering effect. Soluble fiber includes gums, pectin, certain hemicelluloses, and the body's storage polysaccharide, glycogen. Foods rich in soluble fiber include oat bran and dried beans, with additional amounts in barley and fruits. Oat bran, for example, contains a primary water-soluble gum, beta-glucan, which is a lipid-lowering agent. Soluble dietary fiber has the following properties.

- Delays gastric emptying
- Slows intestinal transit time
- Slows glucose absorption
- Is fermented in colon into short-chain fatty acids that may inhibit liver cholesterol synthesis and help clear LDL cholesterol

On the other hand, insoluble dietary fiber—cellulose, lignin, and many hemicelluloses—found in vegetables, wheat, and most other grains does not have these lipid-lowering effects. Thus an increased use of soluble fiber food sources, especially oat bran and legumes, would have beneficial effects.

OMEGA-3 FATTY ACIDS

Studies indicate omega-3 fatty acids, eicosapentaenoic acid (EPA), and docosahexaenoic acid (DHA) (see Chapter 4), found mostly in seafood and marine oils, also have protective functions. They can do the following.

- Change pattern of plasma fatty acids to alter platelet activity and reduce platelet aggregation that causes blood clotting, thus lowering the risk of coronary thrombosis
- Decrease the synthesis of VLDL
- Increase anti-inflammatory effects

It would seem, then, that factors in foods such as oats, dried beans, and fatty fish would provide valuable lipid-lowering additions to our diets.

References

Anderson JW, Gustafson NJ: Dietary fiber and heart disease: current management concepts and recommendations, *Top Clin Nutr* 3:21, 1988.

National Cholesterol Education Program (NCEP): *Third report of the NCEP Expert Panel on Detection, Evaluation, and Treatment of High Blood Cholesterol in Adults (Adult Treatment Panel III), Full Report,* Washington, DC, 2001, National Institutes of Health, National Heart, Lung, and Blood Institute, available at *http://www.nhlbi.nih.gov/guidelines/cholesterol/atp3_rpt.pdf.*

National Cholesterol Education Program (NCEP): *Third report of the NCEP Expert Panel on Detection, Evaluation, and Treatment of High Blood Cholesterol in Adults (Adult Treatment Panel III) Executive Summary,* NIH Publication No. 01-3670, May 2001, Washington, DC, 2001, National Institutes of Health, National Heart, Lung, and Blood Institute, available at *http://www.nhlbi.nih.gov/guidelines/cholesterol/atp3xsum.pdf.*

Simopoulos AP: Omega-3 fatty acids in growth and development, part II: the role of omega-3 fatty acids in health and disease—dietary implications, *Nutr Today* 23:12, 1988.

- For those with CHD or CHD risk equivalents in whom MNT alone will not attain LDL cholesterol targets

The general strategy for initiation and progression of drug therapy is outlined in Figure 19-4. Major drugs used to treat hypercholesterolemia are outlined in Table 19-6.

ACUTE CARDIOVASCULAR DISEASE: MYOCARDIAL INFARCTION

Medical Management

Initial medical treatment of MI, or heart attack, usually includes strong analgesics for the severe unremitting pain, O_2 therapy, and intravenous fluids for shock. Drugs may include (1) lidocaine, an antiarrhythmic drug to reduce the risk of ventricular fibrillation (irregular heartbeat); (2) diuretics for heart failure to avoid accumulation of fluid in the lungs; and (3) beta-blockers that occupy the beta-receptors and prevent stimuli of norepinephrine to the muscles. In some hospitals patients who arrive shortly after the heart attack are treated with a fast-acting thrombolytic drug, streptokinase, an enzyme that dissolves blood clots, followed by angioplasty, a procedure used to widen the narrowed coronary arteries. In this procedure, which is performed under local anesthesia and guided by x-ray imaging, a balloon at the tip of a catheter is inserted into the artery and positioned at the narrowed point. The balloon is then inflated and deflated a few times to widen the vessel and then withdrawn. Follow-up use of the cholesterol-lowering drug pravastatin has proved to be successful in maintaining a blood cholesterol level lower than the average of 210 mg/dl, which is too high.[34]

Nutritional Management

In the initial acute phase of cardiovascular disease, a MI requires close attention to dietary modifications. The basic clinical objective is cardiac rest to allow the healing process

BOX 19-2 Guide to Therapeutic Lifestyle Changes (TLC): Healthy Lifestyle Recommendations for a Healthy Heart

Food Items to Choose More Often

Breads and Cereals

≥6 servings per day, adjusted to caloric needs

Breads, cereals, especially whole grains; pasta; rice; potatoes; dry beans and peas; low-fat crackers and cookies

Vegetables

3-5 servings per day fresh, frozen, or canned without added fat, sauce, or salt

Fruits

2-4 servings per day fresh, frozen, canned, dried

Dairy Products

2-3 servings per day fat-free, ½%, 1% milk, buttermilk, yogurt, cottage cheese, fat-free and low-fat cheese

Eggs

<2 egg yolks per week; egg whites or egg substitute

Meat, Poultry, Fish

≤5 oz per day

Lean cuts loin, leg, round, extra lean hamburger; cold cuts made with lean meat or soy protein; skinless poultry; fish

Fats and Oils

Amount adjusted to caloric level: unsaturated oils; soft or liquid margarines and vegetable oil spreads; salad dressings, seeds, and nuts

TLC Diet Options

Stanol/sterol-containing margarines; soluble fiber food sources: barley, oats, psyllium, apples, bananas, berries, citrus fruits, nectarines, peaches, pears, plums, prunes, broccoli, Brussels sprouts, carrots, dry beans, soy products (tofu, miso)

Food Items to Choose Less Often

Breads and Cereals

Many baked products, including doughnuts, biscuits, butter rolls, muffins, croissants, sweet rolls, Danish, cakes, pies, coffee cakes, cookies

Many grain-based snacks, including chips, cheese puffs, snack mix, regular crackers, buttered popcorn

Vegetables

Vegetables fried or prepared with butter, cheese, or cream sauce

Fruits

Fruits fried or served with butter or cream

Dairy Products

Whole milk, 2% milk, whole-milk yogurt, ice cream, cream, cheese

Eggs

Egg yolk, whole eggs

Meat, Poultry, Fish

Higher-fat meat cuts: ribs, t-bone steak, regular hamburger, bacon, sausage; cold cuts: salami, bologna, hot dogs; organ meats: liver, brains, sweetbreads; poultry with skin fried meat; fried poultry, fried fish

Fats and Oils

Butter, shortening, stick margarine, chocolate, coconut

Recommendations for Weight Reduction

Weigh Regularly

Record weight, body mass index, and waist circumferences

Lose Weight Gradually

Goal: lose 10% of body weight in 6 months. Lose ½-1 lb per week

Develop Healthy Eating Patterns

Choose healthy foods (see Column 1)

Reduce intake of foods in Column 2

Limit number of eating occasions

Avoid second helpings

Identify and reduce hidden fat by reading food labels to choose products lower in saturated fat and calories, and ask about ingredients in ready-to-eat foods prepared away from home

Identify and reduce sources of excess carbohydrates such as fat-free and regular crackers; cookies and other desserts; snacks; and sugar-containing beverages

Recommendations for Increased Physical Activity

Make Physical Activity Part of Daily Routines

Reduce sedentary time

Walk, wheel, or bike ride more, drive less; take the stairs instead of an elevator; get off the bus a few stops early and walk the remaining distance; mow the lawn with a push mower; rake leaves; garden; push a stroller; clean the house; do exercises or pedal a stationary bike while watching television; play actively with children; take a brisk 10-minute walk or wheel before work, during your work break, and after dinner

Make Physical Activity Part of Exercise or Recreational Activities

Walk, wheel, or jog; bicycle or use an arm pedal bicycle; swim or do water aerobics; play basketball; join a sport team; play wheelchair sports; golf (pull cart or carry clubs); canoe; cross-country ski; dance; take part in an exercise program at work, home, school, or gym

From the National Cholesterol Education Program (NCEP): *Third report of the NCEP Expert Panel on Detection, Evaluation, and Treatment of High Blood Cholesterol in Adults (Adult Treatment Panel III), Full Report,* Washington, DC, 2001, National Institutes of Health, National Heart, Lung, and Blood Institute.

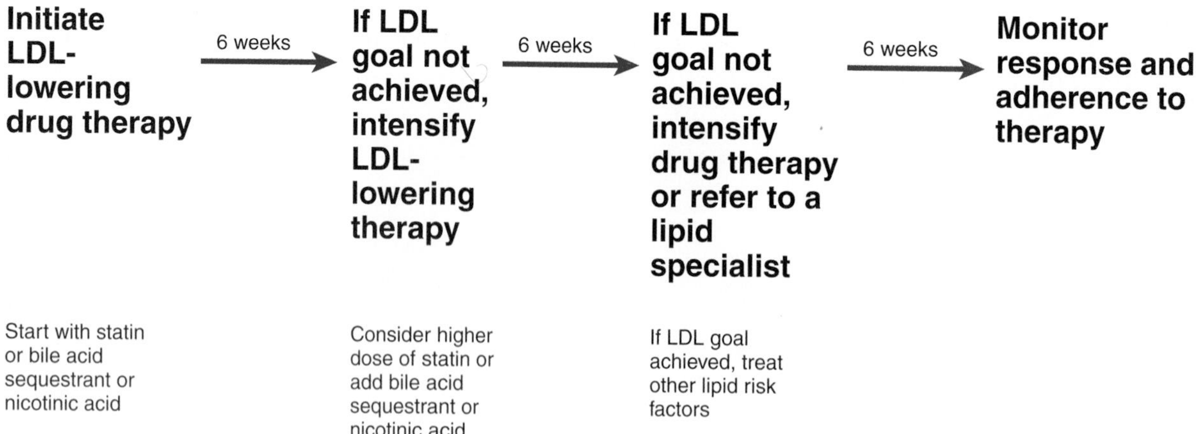

FIGURE 19-4 Progression of drug therapy. (*From the National Cholesterol Education Program {NCEP}:* Third report of the NCEP Expert Panel on Detection, Evaluation, and Treatment of High Blood Cholesterol in Adults [Adult Treatment Panel III], Full Report, *Washington, DC, 2001, National Institutes of Health, National Heart, Lung, and Blood Institute.*)

TABLE 19-6 Major Drugs Used to Treat Hypercholesterolemia

Drug Class	Available Drugs	Lipid/Lipoprotein Effects	Major Side Effects	ATP III Recommendation
HMG CoA reductase inhibitors (statins)	Lovastatin, Pravastatin, Simvastatin, Fluvastatin, Atorvastatin	↓ LDL cholesterol 18%-55% ↑ HDL cholesterol 5%-15% ↓ Triglycerides 7%-30%	Myopathy, increased liver transaminases	Should be considered as the drug of choice when LDL-lowering medications are indicated to achieve LDL treatment goals
Bile acid sequestrants	Cholestyramine, colestipol, colesevelam	↓ LDL cholesterol 15%-30% ↑ HDL cholesterol 3%-5% Triglycerides no effect or ↑	Upper and lower GI complaints common Decrease absorption of other drugs	Should be considered as LDL-lowering therapy for persons with moderate elevations in LDL cholesterol, younger persons with elevated LDL cholesterol, women with elevated LDL cholesterol who are considering pregnancy, persons needing only modest reductions in LDL cholesterol, and combination therapy with statins in persons with very high LDL cholesterol
Nicotinic acid (niacin)	Crystalline nicotinic acid Sustained-release (or timed release) nicotinic acid Extended-release nicotinic acid (Niaspan)	↓ LDL cholesterol 5%-25% ↑ HDL cholesterol 15%-35% ↓ Triglycerides 20%-50%	Flushing, hyperglycemia, hyperuricemia or gout, upper GI distress, hepatotoxicity, especially for sustained-release form	Should be considered as a single agent in higher-risk person's atherogenic dyslipidemia who do not have a substantial increase in LDL cholesterol levels, and in combination therapy with other cholesterol-lowering medications in higher-risk persons with atherogenic dyslipidemia combined with elevated LDL cholesterol levels. Should be used with caution in those with active liver disease, recent peptic ulcer, hyperuricemia and gout, and type 2 diabetes. High doses (>3 g/day) generally should be avoided in persons with type 2 diabetes, although lower doses may effectively treat diabetic dyslipidemia without significantly worsening hyperglycemia.

Reference: National Cholesterol Education Program (NCEP): *Third report of the NCEP Expert Panel on Detection, Evaluation, and Treatment of High Blood Cholesterol in Adults (Adult Treatment Panel III), Full Report,* Washington, DC, 2001, National Institutes of Health, National Heart, Lung, and Blood Institute.

TABLE 19-6 Major Drugs Used to Treat Hypercholesterolemia—cont'd

Drug Class	Available Drugs	Lipid/Lipoprotein Effects	Major Side Effects	ATP III Recommendation
Fibric acid derivatives (fibrates)	Gemfibrozil, fenofibrated, clofibrate	↓ LDL cholesterol 5%-20% (in non-hypertriglyceridemic persons; may be increased in hypertriglyceridemic persons) ↑ HDL cholesterol 10%-35% (more in severe hypertriglyceridemia) ↓ Triglycerides 20%-50%	Dyspepsia, various upper GI complaints, cholesterol gallstones, myopathy	Can be recommended for persons with very high triglycerides to reduce risk for acute pancreatitis. Can also be recommended for persons with elevated beta-VLDL. Should be considered an option for treatment of those with established CHD who have low levels of LDL cholesterol and atherogenic dyslipidemia. Also should be considered in combination with statin therapy in those with elevated LDL cholesterol and atherogenic dyslipidemia

to begin. All care is directed toward this basic need for cardiac rest so the damaged heart can be restored to normal functioning. The diet is therefore modified in energy value and texture, as well as in fat and sodium.

1. *Energy (kcalories).* A brief period of undernutrition during the first few days after the attack is advisable. Metabolic demands for digestion, absorption, and metabolism of food require a generous cardiac output volume. Small intakes of food at a time, spread over the day, decrease the metabolic workload to a level the weakened heart can accommodate. The patient progresses to consume more food as healing occurs. During initial recovery stages, the diet may be limited to about 1200 to 1500 kcalories to continue cardiac rest from metabolic workloads. If the patient is obese, this kcalorie level may be continued for a longer period to help the patient begin very gradually to lose some of the excess weight.
2. *Texture.* Early feedings generally include foods soft in texture or easily digested to avoid excess effort in eating. Smaller meals served more frequently may give needed nutrition without undue strain or pressure. Avoid temperature extremes in solid and liquid foods, and avoid foods that may constipate and cause straining.
3. *Lipids.* The general prudent diet controls the amount and kind of fat, as well as cholesterol, for most patient needs. Individual modifications may be used to meet any additional needs.
4. *Sodium.* A moderately reduced sodium content in foods selected is also emphasized. This will help control any tendency to fluid accumulation in body tissues. Added tissue fluid causes more work for the heart to maintain an increased blood volume circulation.

Additional Risk Factors

Heavy coffee drinking has an effect on blood cholesterol levels and disrupts heart rhythms. An abnormal heart rhythm is seen after only one or two cups of coffee in patients with a history of irregular heart rate. The best practice is to avoid caffeine or to limit regular coffee to two cups per day.[35,36] Heavy use of alcohol also increases TG levels and atherosclerotic risk. If alcohol is used, the amount should be moderate. In addition, stress and anxiety have been shown to increase risk of heart disease complications and management.[37,38] This is particularly true, for example, for persons who have long-term exposure to little or no control in their working situation.[39]

CHRONIC CORONARY HEART DISEASE: CONGESTIVE HEART FAILURE

In chronic CHD, a condition of congestive heart failure may develop over time. Each year in the United States, this is responsible for more than 700,000 hospitalizations.[40] The progressively weakened heart muscle, the *myocardium,* is unable to maintain an adequate cardiac output to sustain normal blood circulation. Resulting fluid imbalances cause edema, especially pulmonary edema, to develop. This condition brings added problems in breathing called respiratory distress or dyspnea, which places added stress on the laboring heart. Thus heart failure is now considered a disorder of circulation, not merely a disease of the heart.[41]

Etiology: Relationship to Sodium and Water

Fluid congestion of chronic heart disease relates to imbalances in the body's capillary fluid shift mechanism and its resulting hormonal effects.

1. *Imbalance in capillary fluid shift mechanism.* As the heart fails to pump out returning blood fast enough, the venous return is retarded. This causes a disproportionate amount of

pulmonary edema Accumulation of fluid in tissues of the lung.

blood to accumulate in the vascular system working with the right side of the heart. Venous pressure rises, a sort of "backup" pressure effect, and overcomes the balance of filtration pressures necessary to maintain the normal capillary fluid shift mechanism (see Chapter 8). Fluid that would normally flow between interstitial spaces and blood vessels is held in the tissue spaces rather than recirculated.

2. *Hormonal mechanisms.* Two hormonal mechanisms are involved in fluid balance in normal circulation. In this instance, both contribute to cardiac edema.
   - *Aldosterone mechanism.* This mechanism, described more completely by its full name of the renin-angiotensin-aldosterone mechanism, is normally a lifesaving sodium- and water-conserving mechanism to ensure essential fluid balances. In this case, however, it only compounds the edema problem. As the heart fails to propel blood circulation forward, deficient cardiac output effectively reduces blood flow through kidney nephrons. Decreased renal blood pressure triggers the renin-angiotensin system. Renin is an enzyme from the renal cortex that combines in blood with its substrate, angiotensinogen, which is produced in the liver, to produce in turn angiotensin I and II. Angiotensin II acts as a stimulant to the adrenal glands to produce aldosterone. This hormone in turn effects a reabsorption of sodium in an ion exchange with potassium in the distal tubules of the nephrons, and water reabsorption follows. Ordinarily this is a lifesaving mechanism to protect the body's vital water supply. In congestive heart failure, however, it only adds to the edema problem. The mechanism reacts as if the body's total fluid volume is reduced, when in truth the fluid is excessive; it is just that it is not in normal circulation but is being retained in the body's tissues.
   - *Antidiuretic hormone mechanism.* This water-conserving hormonal mechanism also adds to edema. Cardiac stress and reduced renal flow cause the release of antidiuretic hormone (ADH), also known as vasopressin, from the pituitary gland. ADH then stimulates still more water reabsorption in nephrons of the kidney, further increasing the problem of edema.

Increased Cellular Free Potassium

As reduced blood circulation depresses cell metabolism, cell protein is broken down and releases its bound potassium in the cell. As a result, the amount of free potassium inside the cell is increased, which increases intracellular osmotic pressure. Sodium ions in fluid surrounding the cell then also increase in number to balance increased osmotic pressure within the cell and to prevent cell dehydration. In time, the increased sodium outside the cell causes still more water retention.

Nutritional Management

The basis for all care of the person with congestive heart disease is reduction of the work load of the heart. Medical treatment involves O_2 therapy, decreased physical activity, and drug therapy with (1) diuretic agents to control fluid congestion in the lungs, and (2) digitalis drugs to strengthen contractions of the heart muscle. Nutritional support involves the following.

- *Low sodium.* Sodium is usually restricted to 500 to 1000 mg/day. Additionally, individual fluid restriction may be needed to help reduce fluid retention. Amounts may vary depending on severity of the heart failure and tissue fluid accumulation.
- *Food texture and meal pattern.* Food should have a relatively soft texture, require little physical effort to eat, and be divided into small feedings that are eaten slowly.
- *The kcalories.* The kcalories should be decreased to reduce obesity, as well as to decrease the work of the heart to meet circulatory demands for digestion and absorption.
- *Vitamins and minerals.* The person with CHD should receive a full allowance of vitamins and minerals, with special attention to any drug-nutrient interactions causing losses. For example, potassium replacement is needed when potassium-depleting diuretics are used, and added vitamin B_6 may be needed when the vasodilator hydralazine is used for hypertension control; this drug binds vitamin B_6 and increases its excretion.

CARDIAC CACHEXIA

Etiology

Sometimes with prolonged myocardial insufficiency and heart failure an extreme clinical condition of cardiac cachexia develops. Progressive, profound malnutrition results from an insufficient O_2 supply that cannot meet demands of red blood cell formation by the bone marrow or energy needs for basic breathing. The enlarged, laboring heart is unable to maintain a sufficient blood supply to the body tissues, and nutrient delivery to cells is impaired. Edema, unpalatable sodium-restricted diets, drug reactions, and postoperative complications of cardiac surgery all worsen the anorexia and reduce food intake. In addition, the individual has probably become hypermetabolic and hypercatabolic. It should be no surprise the incidence of nosocomial (hospital-induced) cardiac cachexia is a common occurrence.

Nutritional Therapy

The goal is to help restore heart-lung function as much as possible and to rebuild body tissue. Team care involving the physician, clinical dietitian, nurse, patient, and family is essential. Nutrition support focuses on energy, nutrients, supplements, and feeding plan.

- *Energy.* Sufficient kcalories are needed to cover basal energy needs, as well as energy for minimal activity and the hypermetabolism of severe congestive heart failure; more kcalories may be needed if major surgery is planned. Depending on the extent of malnutrition indicated by nutritional assessment, an increase of 30% to 50% of basal needs may be indicated.
- *Fluids.* Sufficient but not excessive fluid intake is needed, at a rate of about 0.5 ml/kcalorie/day or 1000 to 1500 ml/day.

- *Protein.* Approximately 0.8 to 1 g/kg body weight is needed to replace tissue losses and cover malabsorption.
- *Fat.* Using a medium-chain triglyceride (MCT) oil for part of the fat allowance modifies losses from malabsorption.
- *Sodium.* Sodium restriction varies with individual status, usually in a range of 500 to 2000 mg/day, with attention to multiple alternate seasonings to enhance palatability of food (see Appendix H).
- *Mineral-vitamin supplementation.* General supplementation at 1½ to 2 times the Dietary Reference Intakes (DRIs)/Recommended Dietary Allowances (RDAs), with follow-up monitoring of blood concentrations, is usually provided to meet needs for tissue rebuilding, malabsorption losses, and hypermetabolic state.
- *Feeding plan.* Small, frequent feedings are better tolerated. Large meals add to the risk of CO_2 accumulation and respiratory failure.
- *Enteral and parenteral nutrition support.* Tube feedings or parenteral nutrition may be appropriate. Several enteral feeding formulas that have a low volume with a high density of kcalories are available. These are suitable for patients requiring fluid restriction.

Essential Hypertension and Vascular Disease

BLOOD PRESSURE CONTROLS

Arterial Pressure

As commonly measured, blood pressure is an indication of arterial pressure in vessels of the upper arm. This measure is obtained by an instrument for determining the force of the pulse (Figure 19-5). This instrument is called a *sphygmomanometer,* from the Greek words *sphygmos* ("pulse"), *manos* ("thin"), and *metron* ("measure"). Pulse pressure is measured in millimeters of mercury (mm Hg) rise in thin contained tubes, or in equivalent values read on gauges or digital indicators. The higher, or upper, value recorded is systolic pressure from contraction of the heart muscle. The lower value recorded is diastolic pressure, produced during the relaxation phase of the cardiac cycle.

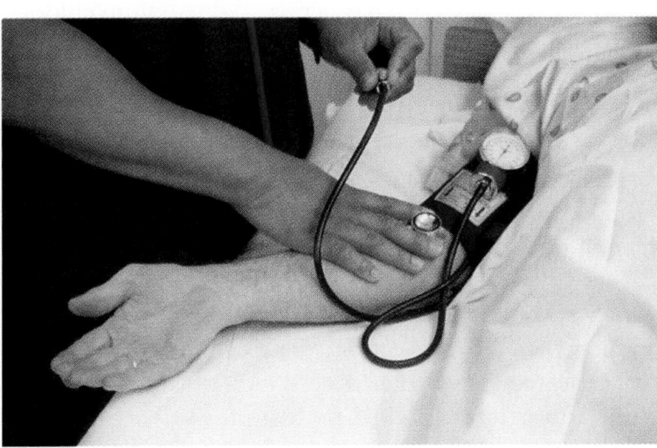

FIGURE 19-5 Monitoring blood pressure. (*From Potter PA, Perry AG:* Basic nursing: essentials for practice, *ed 5, St Louis, 2003, Mosby.*)

Several factors contribute to maintaining fluid dynamics of normal blood pressure: (1) increased pressure on forward blood flow; (2) increased resistance from containing blood vessels; and (3) increased viscosity of blood itself, making movement through vessels more difficult. Of these factors, increased viscosity is a rare event. Thus in discussing high blood pressure in general terms, we are dealing with the first two factors, pumping pressure of the heart muscle propelling blood forward and resistance to this forward flow presented by blood vessel walls normally or by any abnormal added constriction or thickening.

Muscle Tone of Blood Vessel Walls

In hypertension, the body's finely tuned mechanisms designed to maintain fluid dynamics are not operating effectively. Normally, these systems include several agents that act to variously dilate and constrict blood vessels to meet whatever need is present at a given time. In a person with hypertension, however, dilation or constriction of blood vessels does not occur in the normal manner. If not effectively treated, uncontrolled elevated blood pressure results. Body systems that operate to help maintain normal blood pressure include (1) neuroendocrine functions of the sympathetic nervous system, mainly mediated by chemical neurotransmitters, such as norepinephrine; (2) hormonal systems such as the renin-angiotensin-aldosterone mechanism and its vasopressor effect; and (3) enzyme systems such as the kallikrein-kinin mechanism (sometimes operating with prostaglandins), which controls substances that act to dilate or constrict smooth muscle as needed.

THE PROBLEM OF HYPERTENSION

High blood pressure is one of the most prevalent vascular diseases worldwide.[42] It is a common problem in the United States affecting the lives of approximately 43 million people.[43,44] It is a major factor in the approximately 500,000 strokes and 1.25 million heart attacks that occur each year. At least 95% of these persons have essential hypertension, meaning that its cause is unknown, although there is apparently a strong familial predisposition with its onset in young teenaged years. It has become the fourth largest public health problem in America. It has often been called the "silent disease" because it carries no overt signs, but it can

antidiuretic hormone (ADH) Water-conserving hormone from posterior lobe of pituitary gland; causes resorption of water by kidney nephrons according to body need.
essential hypertension An inherent form of hypertension with no specific discoverable cause and considered to be familial; also called primary hypertension.
vasopressin Alternate name of ADH.

TABLE 19-7 Classification of Blood Pressure for Adults

Category	Systolic (mm Hg)		Diastolic (mm Hg)
Optimal*	<120	and	<80
Normal	<130	and	<85
High-normal	130-139	or	85-89
Hypertension†			
Stage 1	140-159	or	90-99
Stage 2	160-179	or	100-109
Stage 3	≥180	or	≥110

Reference: The Sixth Report of the Joint National Committee on Prevention, Detection, Evaluation, and Treatment of High Blood Pressure, NIH Publication No. 98-4080, Washington, DC, 1997, National Institutes of Health, National Heart, Lung, and Blood Institute.

*Optimal blood pressure with respect to cardiovascular risk is below 120/80 mm Hg. However, unusually low readings should be evaluated for clinical significance.

†Based on the average of 2 or more readings taken at each of 2 or more visits after initial screening.

BOX 19-3 Lifestyle Modifications for Hypertension Prevention and Management

- Lose weight if overweight.
- Limit alcohol intake to no more than 1 oz (30 ml) ethanol (e.g., 24 oz [720 ml] beer, 10 oz [300 ml] wine, or 2 oz [60 ml] 100-proof whiskey) per day or 0.5 oz (15 ml) ethanol per day for women and lighter weight people.
- Increase aerobic physical activity (30-45 min most days of the week).
- Reduce sodium intake to no more than 100 mmol/day (2.4 g sodium or 6 g sodium chloride).
- Maintain adequate intake of dietary potassium (approximately 90 mmol/day).
- Maintain adequate intake of dietary calcium and magnesium for general health.
- Stop smoking and reduce intake of dietary saturated fat and cholesterol for overall cardiovascular health.

Reference: The Sixth Report of the Joint National Committee on Prevention, Detection, Evaluation, and Treatment of High Blood Pressure, NIH Publication No. 98-4080, Washington, DC, 1997, National Institutes of Health, National Heart, Lung, and Blood Institute.

have serious implications if not treated and controlled. The large United States study—DASH (Dietary Approaches to Stop Hypertension)—has clearly indicated that a diet rich in fruits, vegetables, and low-fat dairy foods and with reduced saturated and total fat can substantially lower blood pressure.[43,44] Individual treatment uses current antihypertensive drugs as needed. However, other sociocultural factors—such as stressors related to racial discrimination and environmental factors, access to medical care, health education, and lifestyle—influence mass population hypertension and stroke risk in the "high normal blood pressure and mild hypertensive" groups.[45,46] During the past decade, the U.S. National Heart, Lung, and Blood Institute (NHLBI) of the National Institutes of Health (NIH) initiated a public education campaign about the serious problem of hypertension and the value of preventive care.

Classifications of Blood Pressure

Hypertension is defined as systolic blood pressure of 140 mm Hg or higher, diastolic blood pressure of 90 mm Hg or higher, or taking antihypertensive medication. The objective of identifying and treating hypertension is to reduce morbidity and mortality. For that reason, classification of adult (≥18 years of age) blood pressure (Table 19-7) provides a mechanism for identifying high-risk individuals and provides guidelines for follow-up and treatment.[47]

Prevention and Treatment

The goal of the prevention and management of hypertension is to reduce morbidity and mortality by the least intrusive means possible.[47] Lifestyle modifications (Box 19-3) offer potential for preventing hypertension, have been shown capable of lowering blood pressure, and can reduce cardiovascular risk factors at minimal cost and risk.[48]

Nutritional Management of Hypertension

Taste for a given amount of salt with food is an acquired one, not a physiologic necessity. Sufficient sodium for the body's need is provided as a natural mineral in foods consumed. Some persons salt their foods heavily and thus form high salt taste levels. Others form lighter tastes by using smaller amounts. Common daily adult intakes of sodium range widely from about 2 to 4 g with lighter tastes to as high as 10 to 12 g with heavier use. Salt (sodium chloride [NaCl]) intakes are about twice these amounts because sodium (Na) makes up about 40% of the NaCl molecule. The large amount of salt in the American diet, estimated to be about 6 to 15 g sodium/day (260 to 656 mEq), is largely a result of the increased use of many processed food products. The main source of dietary sodium is food processing (about 75%). Approximately 10% to 11% occurs naturally in foods, about 15% is discretionary (half of which is contributed by table salt and half by cooking), and less than 1% comes from water.[47,49-51]

Other nutrients that affect blood pressure are potassium and calcium. High potassium intake from food sources (see *Practical Application* box and *Issues & Answers*) such as fresh fruits and vegetables may protect against developing hypertension and improve blood pressure con-

PRACTICAL APPLICATION

DASH Diet Pattern

The DASH diet is based on 2000 kcalories/day. The following table indicates the number of recommended daily servings from each food group with examples of food choices. The number of servings may increase or decrease, depending on individual calorie needs.

Food Group	Daily Serving (Except Where Noted)	Serving Sizes	Examples and Notes	Significance to the DASH Diet Pattern
Grains and grain products	7-8	1 slice bread 1 oz dry cereal* ½ cup cooked rice, pasta, or cereal	Whole-wheat bread, English muffin, pita bread, bagel; cereals; grits; oatmeal	Major source of energy and fiber
Vegetables	4-5	1 cup raw, leafy vegetable ½ cup cooked vegetables 6 oz vegetable juice	Tomatoes, potatoes, carrots, peas, squash, broccoli, turnip greens, collard, kale, spinach, artichokes, beans, sweet potatoes	Rich sources of potassium, magnesium, and fiber
Fruits	4-5	6 oz fruit juice 1 medium fruit ¼ cup dried fruit ½ cup fresh, frozen, or canned fruit	Apricots, bananas, dates, grapes, oranges, orange juice, tangerines, strawberries, mangoes, melons, peaches, pineapple, prunes, raisins	Important sources of potassium, magnesium, and fiber
Low-fat or nonfat dairy foods	2-3	8 oz milk 1 cup yogurt 1.5 oz cheese	Fat-free or 1% milk, fat-free or low-fat buttermilk; nonfat or low-fat yogurt; part-nonfat mozzarella cheese, nonfat cheese	Major sources of calcium and protein
Meat, poultry, and fish	<2	3 oz cooked meats, poultry, or fish	Select only lean meats; trim away visible fats; broil, roast, or boil, instead of frying; remove skin from chicken	Rich sources of protein and magnesium
Nuts, seeds, and legumes	4-5/wk	1.5 oz or ½ cup nuts 0.5 oz or 2 tbsp seeds ½ cup cooked legumes	Almonds, filberts, mixed nuts, peanuts, walnuts, sunflower seeds, kidney beans, lentils	Rich sources of energy, magnesium, potassium, protein, and fiber
Fats and oils†	2-3	1 tsp soft margarine 1 tbsp low fat mayonnaise or salad dressing 2 tbsp light salad dressing 1 tsp vegetable oil	Soft margarine, lowfat mayonnaise, light salad dressing, vegetable oil (such as olive, corn, canola, or safflower)	DASH has 27% of calories as fat, including that in or added to foods
Sweets	5/wk	1 tbsp sugar 1 tbsp jelly or jam ½ oz jelly beans 8 oz lemonade	Maple syrup, sugar, jelly, jam; fruit-flavored gelatin, jelly beans, fruit punch, sorbet, ices, hard candy	Sweets should be low in fat

*Equals ½-1¼ cup depending on cereal type. Check the product's nutrition label.

†Fat content changes serving counts for fats and oils. For example: 1 tbsp of regular salad dressing equals 1 serving; 1 tbsp of low-fat dressing equals ½ serving; 1 tbsp of fat-free dressing equals 0 servings.

Reference

U.S. Dept. of Health and Human Services, Public Health Service, National Institutes of Health, National Heart, Lung, and Blood Institute: *The DASH diet,* NIH Publication No. 01-4082. Revised May 2001, available at *http://www.nhlbi.nih.gov/health/public/heart/hbp/dash/new_dash.pdf.*

trol in those who do have hypertension.[47,52] Low calcium intake is also associated with increased prevalence of hypertension.[47,53] Increased calcium intake may lower blood pressure in some, but overall effect is minimal[54]; thus there is no current recommendation for use of calcium supplementation to lower blood pressure.[47]

CEREBROVASCULAR ACCIDENT

Arteriosclerotic vascular injury and hypertension may also affect blood vessels in the brain. A cerebrovascular accident (CVA), or stroke, occurs when a blood vessels carrying O_2 and nutrients to the brain ruptures *(hemorrhagic stroke)* or is clogged by a blood clot *(ischemic stroke),* interrupting blood flow to an area of the brain. When any part of the brain does not receive blood and O_2, nerve cells in the affected area die, resulting in loss of control of abilities that area of the brain once controlled. During the past two decades, with the declining U.S. early death rate from heart disease, stroke stands in third place as a leading cause of death of adults aged 25 to 65 years.[48] Nearly 160,000 Americans die annually of stroke, meaning someone in the United States experiences a stroke every 45 seconds.[55] Among all U.S. population groups, the incident rate for first stroke among African Americans is almost double that of European Americans.[55]

There are four main types of stroke: two are caused by blood clots and two are caused by ruptured blood vessels. Cerebral thrombosis and cerebral embolism account for approximately 70% to 80% of all strokes. Cerebral thrombosis, the most common stroke, occurs when a thrombus forms and blocks blood flow in an artery bringing blood to part of the brain. They usually occur at night or first thing in the morning when blood pressure is low. They are often preceded by a transient ischemic attack (TIA), or "ministroke." Cerebral embolism occurs when an embolus forms away from the brain, usually in the heart. The clot is carried in the bloodstream until it lodges in an artery leading to or in the brain and blocks the flow of blood.[1] A *subarachnoid hemorrhage* occurs when a blood vessel on the brain's surface ruptures and bleeds into the space between the brain and skull. A *cerebral hemorrhage* occurs when a defective artery in the brain bursts, flooding the surrounding tissue with blood.[1]

PERIPHERAL VASCULAR DISEASE

Peripheral vascular disease (PVD) is characterized by narrowing of blood vessels in the legs and sometimes the arms. Blood flow is restricted and causes pain in affected area. Contributory risk factors include hypertension and diabetes mellitus. However, the greatest risk factor is cigarette smoking, which constricts blood vessels. More than 90% of patients with PVD are or were moderate to heavy smokers.

Symptoms and Complications

As arteries gradually narrow because of atherosclerosis (the most common cause), an aching, tired feeling occurs in leg muscles when walking. Resting the leg for a few minutes relieves pain, but it recurs shortly when walking is resumed. For this reason the symptom is called intermittent claudication. Sometimes, a sudden arterial blockage occurs when a blood clot develops on the top of a plaque or a clot formed in the heart is carried to a peripheral artery and blocks it. The blockage causes sudden severe pain in the affected area, which becomes cold and either pale or blue and has no pulse. Movement and sensation are lost.

Treatment

By far the most important treatment for the patient is to stop smoking. As with coronary vessels, surgery on diseased vessels is sometimes required: (1) arterial reconstructive surgery to bypass them, (2) endarterectomy to remove obstructing fatty deposits on inner linings, or (3) balloon angioplasty to widen vessels. Drug therapy may include antiplatelet or anticoagulant agents to prevent blood clotting. Nutritional therapy consists of regular fat and cholesterol modifications described for CHD. Exercise is also important. The person should walk every day with medical clearance, gradually increasing to about 1 hour—stopping whenever intermittent pain occurs and resuming when it stops. Regular inspection of feet, daily washing and stocking change, good-fitting shoes to avoid pressure, and scrupulous foot care (ideally by a podiatrist) are essential to prevent infection.

Chronic Obstructive Pulmonary Disease

CLINICAL CHARACTERISTICS

Progressive congestive heart failure, as well as other respiratory problems, contributes to lung disease and risk of respiratory failure. Malnutrition is common with the debilitating condition of chronic obstructive pulmonary disease (COPD). This term describes a group of disorders in which airflow in the lungs is limited and respiratory failure develops. Two main interrelated COPD conditions are chronic bronchitis and emphysema. Malnutrition usually accompanies COPD, and its presence increases illness and death rates associated with the disease process. Anorexia and significant weight loss reflect a growing inability to maintain adequate nutritional status, which in turn severely compromises pulmonary function. Progression of the disease process, with its increasing shortness of breath, prevents the person from living a normal life, and prognosis is poor. Eventually, in progressive respiratory failure, the patient becomes dependent on a mechanical respirator and controlled O_2 supply. A poor prognosis is associated with a compromised nutritional status in these patients.

NUTRITIONAL MANAGEMENT

Respiratory failure is actually a failure of pulmonary exchange of O_2 and CO_2. Thus its common manifestations are hypoxemia, deficient oxygenation of blood, and hypercapnia, excess CO_2 in the blood. Patients with COPD have greater energy requirements, which will vary for each individual. Requirements for carbohydrate, protein, and fat will be determined by the underlying lung disease, oxygen therapy, medications, weight status, and any acute fluid fluctuations.[56] A balanced proportion of protein (15% to 20% total kcalories) with fat (30% to 45% total kcalories and carbohydrate (40% to 55% total kcalories) is necessary to maintain a appropriate respiratory quotient (RQ) from substrate utilization.[56] It is important not to overfeed patients with COPD. Commonly, other coexisting diseases (CVD, DM, renal disease, or cancer) may well be present, thereby influencing total amount and kind of carbohydrate, protein, and fat prescribed.[56]

General guidelines for dietary modification in chronic pulmonary disease for professional use based on these nutrition support principles are available.[57] Suggestions for use in counseling COPD clinical patients in menu planning and food preparation are included.

TO SUM UP

CHD remains the leading cause of death in the United States. Atherosclerosis, its underlying pathology, involves the formation of plaque, a fatty substance that builds up along the interior surfaces of blood vessels, interfering with blood flow and damaging blood vessels. If this buildup becomes severe, it cuts off blood supplies of O_2 and nutrients to tissue cells, which in turn begin to die. When this occurs in a coronary artery, the result is an MI, or heart attack. When it occurs in a brain vessel, the result is a cerebrovascular accident, or stroke.

Risk for atherosclerosis increases with amount and type of blood lipids (lipoproteins) available. The apolipoprotein portion of lipoproteins is an important genetically determined part of the disease process. Elevated serum LDL cholesterol level is a primary factor in atherosclerosis development.

Initial dietary recommendations for acute cardiovascular disease (heart attack) include caloric restriction, soft-textured foods, and small, frequent meals to reduce the metabolic demands of digestion, absorption, and metabolism of foods and their nutrients. Maintenance of a lean body weight is important. Persons with chronic CHD (congestive heart failure) and those with essential hypertension benefit from weight management, exercise, and sodium restriction to overcome cardiac edema and to help control elevated blood pressure.

Current dietary recommendations to help prevent CHD involve maintaining a healthy weight; limiting fats to 25% to 30% of all kcalories, with the majority being unsaturated food forms; limiting sodium intake to 2 to 3 g/day; and increasing exercise.

Concerted efforts are needed to combat development of cardiac cachexia in progressive heart failure. Also, atherosclerotic plaques may occur in the extremities, usually the legs, causing PVD and the pain of intermittent claudication when walking. Progressive respiratory failure interferes with normal exchange of blood gases, O_2 and CO_2, and results in COPD, for which changed ratios of the fuel macronutrients are sometimes indicated.

Questions for Review

1. Which types of hyperlipoproteinemia occur most often? Identify lipids that are elevated in each case, as well as predisposing factors. Describe the types of diet recommended for each.
2. Identify four dietary recommendations that should be made for the person with a heart attack. Describe how each recommendation helps recovery.
3. What dietary changes can the average American make to reduce saturated fats and to substitute polyunsaturated fats?
4. What does the term *essential hypertension* mean? Why would weight management and sodium restriction contribute to its control?
5. Outline nutritional therapy for cardiac cachexia and discuss the rationale for each aspect of the feeding plan.
6. Discuss cause and treatment of peripheral vascular disease.
7. Outline nutritional therapy for COPD and discuss the rationale for the fuel macronutrient adjustments.

---

hypercapnia Excess CO_2 in the blood.

hyperlipoproteinemia Elevated level of lipoproteins in the blood.

hypoxemia Deficient oxygenation of the blood, resulting in hypoxia, reduced O_2 supply to tissue.

intermittent claudication A symptomatic pattern of peripheral vascular disease, characterized by the absence of pain or discomfort in a limb, usually the legs, when at rest, which is followed by pain and weakness when walking, intensifying until walking becomes impossible, and then disappearing again after a rest period; seen in occlusive arterial disease.

■ References

1. American Heart Association: *Heart and stroke facts, 1992-2001,* available at *http://216.185.112.5/downloadable/heart/1014833865440101319123698 5HSfacts02.pdf.*
2. National Cholesterol Education Program (NCEP): *Third report of the NCEP Expert Panel on Detection, Evaluation, and Treatment of High Blood Cholesterol in Adults (Adult Treatment Panel III) Executive Summary,* NIH Publication No. 01-3670, Washington, DC, 2001, National Institutes of Health, National Heart, Lung, and Blood Institute, available at *http://www.nhlbi.nih.gov/guidelines/cholesterol/atp3xsum.pdf.*
3. National Cholesterol Education Program (NCEP): *Third report of the NCEP Expert Panel on Detection, Evaluation, and Treatment of High Blood Cholesterol in Adults (Adult Treatment Panel III), Full Report,* Washington, DC, 2001, National Institutes of Health, National Heart, Lung, and Blood Institute, available at *http://www.nhlbi.nih.gov/guidelines/cholesterol/atp3_rpt.pdf.*
4. Guyton AC: *Textbook of medical physical physiology,* ed 9, Philadelphia, 1996, WB Saunders.
5. Anding JD et al: Blood lipids, cardiovascular fitness, obesity, and blood pressure: the presence of potential coronary heart disease risk factors in adolescents, *J Am Diet Assoc* 96:238, 1996.
6. National Cholesterol Education Program: *Report of the expert panel on blood cholesterol levels in children and adolescents,* USDHHS (PHS), National Institutes of Health, National Heart, Lung, and Blood Institute, Publication No. 91-2732, Washington, DC, 1991, U.S. Government Printing Office.
7. U.S. Department of Agriculture, U.S. Department of Health and Human Services: *Nutrition and your health: Dietary Guidelines for Americans,* ed 5, Home and Garden Bulletin No. 232, Washington, DC, 2000, U.S. Government Printing Office.
8. Grundy SM, Denke MA: Dietary influences on serum lipids and lipoproteins, *J Lipid Res* 31:1149, 1990.
9. Mensink RP, Katan MB: Effects of dietary fatty acids on serum lipids and lipoproteins: a meta-analysis of 27 trials, *Arterioscler Thromb* 12:911, 1992.
10. Kris-Etherton PM, Yu S: Individual fatty acids effects on plasma lipids and lipoproteins: human studies, *Am J Clin Nutr* 65(suppl5):1628S, 1997.
11. National Institutes of Health: *Clinical guidelines on the identification, evaluation, and treatment of overweight and obesity in adults—the evidence report,* NIH Publication No. 98-4083, Bethesda, Md, 1998, National Heart, Lung, and Blood Institute, available at *http://www.nhlbi.nih.gov/guidelines/obesity/ob_gdlns.pdf.*
12. National Institutes of Health: Clinical guidelines on the identification, evaluation, and treatment of overweight and obesity in adults—the evidence report, *Obesity Res* 6(suppl 2):51S, 1998.
13. Caggiula AW et al: The Multiple Risk Intervention Trial (MRFIT): IV—intervention on blood lipids, *Prev Med* 10: 443, 1981.
14. Stamler J et al: Relation of changes in dietary lipids and weight, trial years 1-6, to change in blood lipids in the special intervention and usual care groups in the Multiple Risk Factor Intervention Trial, *Am J Clin Nutr* 65:272S, 1997.
15. Hopkins PN: Effects of dietary cholesterol on serum cholesterol: a meta-analysis and review, *Am J Clin Nutr* 55: 1060, 1992.
16. Clarke R et al: Dietary lipids and blood cholesterol: quantitative meta-analysis of metabolic ward studies, *BMJ* 314:112, 1997.
17. Garg A: High-monounsaturated-fat diets for patients with diabetes mellitus: a meta-analysis, *Am J Clin Nutr* 67(suppl 3):577S, 1998.
18. Kris-Etherton PM et al: High-monounsaturated fatty acid diets lower both plasma cholesterol and triacylglycerol concentrations, *Am J Clin Nutr* 70:1009, 1999.
19. National Research Council: *Diet and health: implications for reducing chronic disease risk,* Washington, DC, 1989, National Academy Press.
20. Knopp RH et al: Long-term cholesterol-lowering effects of 4 fat-restricted diets in hypercholesterolemic and combined hyperlipidemic men: the Dietary Alternatives Study, *JAMA* 278:1509, 1997.
21. Turely ML et al: The effect of a low-fat, high-carbohydrate diet on serum high density lipoprotein cholesterol and triglyceride, *Eur J Clin Nutr* 52:728, 1998.
22. Jenkins DJ et al: Effect on blood lipids of very high intakes of fiber in diets low in saturated fat and cholesterol, *N Engl J Med* 329:21, 1993.
23. Vuksan V et al: Beneficial effects of viscous dietary fiber from Konjac-mannan in subjects with the insulin resistance syndrome: results of a controlled metabolic trial, *Diabetes Care* 23:9, 2000.
24. U.S. Department of Health and Human Services, Food and Drug Administration: Food labeling: health claims; soluble fiber from certain foods and coronary heart disease—final rule, *Federal Register* 28234, 1997.
25. U.S. Department of Health and Human Services, Food and Drug Administration: Food labeling: health claims; soluble fiber from certain foods and coronary heart disease—final rule, *Federal Register* 8103, 1998.
26. Anderson JW: Dietary fibre, complex carbohydrate and coronary heart disease, *Can J Cardiol* 11(suppl G):55G, 1995.
27. Vuorio AF et al: Stanol ester margarine alone and with simvastatin lowers serum cholesterol in families with familial hypercholesterolemia caused by the FH-North Karelia Mutation, *Arterioscler Thromb Vasc Biol* 20:500, 2000.
28. Gylling H, Miettinen TA: Cholesterol reduction by different plant stanol mixtures and with variable fat intake, *Metabolism* 48:575, 1999.
29. Gylling H et al: Reduction of serum cholesterol in postmenopausal women with previous myocardial infarction and cholesterol malabsorption induced by dietary sitostanol ester margarine: women and dietary sitostanol, *Circulation* 96:4226, 1997.
30. Hallikainen MA, Uusitupa MI: Effects of 2 low-fat stanol ester-containing margarines on serum cholesterol concentrations as part of a low-fat diet in hypercholesterolemic subjects, *Am J Clin Nutr* 69:403, 1999.
31. Hendricks HF et al: Spreads enriched with three different levels of vegetable oil sterols and the degree of cholesterol lowering in normocholesterolaemic and mildly hypercholesterolaemic subjects, *Eur J Clin Nutr* 53:319, 1999.

32. Miettinen TA et al: Reduction of serum cholesterol with sitostanol-ester margarine in a mildly hypercholesterolemic population, *N Engl J Med* 333:1308, 1995.
33. Vanhanen HT et al: Serum cholesterol, cholesterol, precursors, and plant sterols in hypercholesterolemic subjects with different apoE phenotypes during dietary sitostanol ester treatment, *J Lipid Res* 34:1535, 1993.
34. Sacks FM et al: The effect of pravastatin on coronary events after myocardial infarction in patients with average cholesterol levels, *N Engl J Med* 335(14), 1996.
35. Soroko S et al: Reasons for changing caffeinated coffee consumption: the Rancho Bernardo Study, *J Am Coll Nutr* 15:97, 1996.
36. Nygård O et al: Coffee consumption and plasma total homocysteine: the Hordaland Homocysteine Study, *Am J Clin Nutr* 65:136, 1997.
37. Moser D, Dracup K: Is anxiety early after myocardial infarction associated with subsequent ischemia and arrhythmic events? *Psychosom Med* 58:395, 1996.
38. Roush W: Profile: Herbert Benson: mind-body maverick pushes the envelope, *Science* 276(5311):357, 1997.
39. Johnson JV et al: Long-term psychosocial work environment and cardiovascular mortality among Swedish men, *Am J Public Health* 86:324, 1996.
40. Chin MH, Goldman L: Factors contributing to the hospitalization of patients with congestive heart failure, *Am J Public Health* 87:643, 1997.
41. Packer M: Pathophysiology of chronic heart failure, *Lancet* 340:88, 1992.
42. Kannel WB, Wolf PA: Inferences from secular trend analysis of hypertension control, *Am J Public Health* 82:1593, 1992.
43. Appel LJ et al: A clinical trial of the effects of dietary patterns on blood pressure, *N Engl J Med* 336:1117, 1997.
44. Taubes G: New study says low-fat diet can lower blood pressure, *Science* 276(5311):350, 1997.
45. Casper M et al: Antihypertensive treatment and US trends in stroke mortality, 1962 to 1980, *Am J Public Health* 82:1596, 1992.
46. Jacobs DR et al: The United States decline in stroke mortality: what does the ecological analysis tell us? *Am J Public Health* 82:1596, 1992.
47. National High Blood Pressure Program: *The Sixth Report of the Joint National Committee on Prevention, Detection, Evaluation, and Treatment of High Blood Pressure. National Institutes of Health. National Heart, Lung, and Blood Institutes,* NIH Publication No. 98-4080, Washington, DC, 1997, U.S. Government Printing Office, available at *http://www.nhlbi.nih.gov/guidelines/hypertension/jnc6.pdf.*
48. National Center for Health Statistics, Centers for Disease Control and Prevention: *Stroke,* available at *http://www.cdc.gov/nchs/fastats/stroke.htm* (accessed June 2, 2002).
49. National High Blood Pressure Education Program: *Implementing recommendations for dietary salt reduction,* National Institutes of Health, National Heart, Lung, and Blood Institute, NIH Publication No. 55-728N, Washington, DC, November 1996, U.S. Government Printing Office.
50. Kaplan NM: New evidence on the role of sodium in hypertension: the Intersalt Study, *Am J Hypertens* 3:168, 1990.
51. Law MR et al: By how much does dietary salt reduction lower blood pressure? *Br Med J* 302:811, 1991.
52. Whelton PK et al: Effects of oral potassium on blood pressure: meta-analysis of randomized controlled clinical trials, *JAMA* 277:1624, 1997.
53. Cappuccio FP et al: Epidemiologic association between dietary calcium intake and blood pressure: a meta-analysis of published data, *Am J Epidemiol* 142:935, 1995.
54. Allender PS et al: Dietary calcium and blood pressure: a meta-analysis of randomized clinical trials, *Ann Intern Med* 124:825, 1996.
55. National Stroke Association: *Brain attack statistics,* available at *http://www.stroke/org/brain-stat.cfm* (accessed June 2, 2002).
56. Mueller DH. Medical nutrition therapy for pulmonary disease. In Mahan LK, Escott-Stump S: *Krause's food, nutrition, and diet therapy,* ed 10, Philadelphia, 2000, WB Saunders.
57. *Dietary modification in chronic pulmonary disease* (monograph), Columbus, Ohio, 1986, Ross Laboratories.

■ Further Reading

Sacks FM et al.: Effects on blood pressure of reduced dietary sodium and the Dietary Approaches to Stop Hypertension (DASH) diet, *N Engl J Med* 344:3, 2001.

This article presents the research methods and data that demonstrate decreased sodium intake and increased intake of fruits, vegetables, and low-fat dairy foods lower blood pressure.

McNamara DJ: Cholesterol intake and plasma cholesterol: an update, *J Am Coll Nutr* 16(6):530, 1997.

This article is "must" reading for professionals and students in the field of nutrition and heart disease. It presents an alternate view, based on recent and ongoing studies, that dietary cholesterol itself is not related to either blood cholesterol or heart disease deaths. Consistent clinical and epidemiologic data seem to indicate increasingly that dietary cholesterol has little effect on plasma cholesterol in most individuals and raises a number of questions about the justification of population-wide restrictions on dietary cholesterol intake.

Connor WE, Connor SL: Should a low-fat, high-carbohydrate diet be recommended for everyone? The case for a low-fat, high-carbohydrate diet, *N Engl J Med* 337(Aug 21):562, 566, 1997.

Katan MB, Grundy SM, Willett WC: Should a low-fat, high-carbohydrate diet be recommended for everyone? beyond low-fat diets, *N Engl J Med* 337(Aug 21):563, 567, 1997.

These well-known researchers in the field of heart disease also emphasize the role of obesity and little physical exercise as risk factors in heart disease.

Brownson RC et al: Preventing cardiovascular disease through community-based risk reduction: the Bootheel Heart Health Project, *Am J Public Health* 86(2):206, 1996.

This interesting heart disease risk reduction project in six southeastern Missouri counties—using community-based activities such as exercise groups, healthy cooking demonstrations, blood pressure and cholesterol screenings, and cardiovascular disease education—clearly shows how such a program can achieve positive results within a relatively brief period, even with modest resources.

Oster G, Thompson D: Estimated effects of reducing dietary saturated fat intake on the incidence and costs of coronary heart disease in the United States, *J Am Diet Assoc* 96(2):127, 1996.

Rhodes KS et al: Intensive nutrition counseling enhances outcomes of National Cholesterol Education Program dietary therapy, *J Am Diet Assoc* 96(10):1003, 1996.

These two brief reports focus on the cost of heart disease. They indicate how population-based interventions that encourage persons to reduce dietary intake of saturated fat can prevent tens of thousands of cases of coronary heart disease and save billions of dollars in related costs.

CASE STUDY The patient with myocardial infarction

Edward is a 37-year-old sedentary executive who was seen for an annual physical examination 6 months ago. He had no complaints other than feeling the "everyday pressures" of his job as a corporate attorney and head of the legal division. He admitted smoking two packs of cigarettes a day as a means of relieving stress.

Edward is 175 cm (5 ft 10 in) tall and at the time of his examination weighed 83 kg (185 lb). His blood pressure was 148/90 mm Hg, and his serum cholesterol level was 285 mg/dl. He was advised to quit smoking, exercise daily at a moderate pace, and lose 9 kg (20 lb).

He arrived in the hospital emergency department 3 months later complaining of severe chest pains and difficulty breathing. His wife reported he had appeared pale that evening, had broken out into a cold sweat, and had vomited shortly after arriving home from work. Once regular breathing was restored by the emergency medical team and his pain subsided, a number of laboratory tests were ordered. These tests included serum glutamic-oxaloacetic transaminase (SGOT), lactate dehydrogenase (LDH), prothrombin time, lipid panel plus HDL cholesterol, sedimentation rate, coagulation times, fasting blood sugar (FBS), blood urea nitrogen (BUN), and complete blood count (CBC). An electrocardiogram (ECG) was also ordered. The patient was then transferred to the coronary care unit for closer monitoring.

The following tests results were elevated: SGOT, LDH, LDL and total cholesterol, TG, glucose, prothrombin time, white blood cell count, and sedimentation rate. HDL level was low. The ECG revealed an infarction of the posterior wall of the myocardium. The diagnosis was MI, with underlying familial hypercholesterolemia.

In consultation with the clinical nutritionist, the cardiologist ordered a liquid diet, increasing it to a soft diet with low saturated fats 2 days later. The nutritionist noted continued improvement in the patient's appetite accompanying recovery and recommended changing the diet order to the Therapeutic Lifestyle Changes (TLC) diet.

A week later Edward was discharged. During convalescence the nutritionist and nurse met with him and his wife several times to discuss his continuing care at home. At each follow-up clinic visit with the physician and nutritionist, Edward showed good general recovery and enjoyment of his new modified fat and cholesterol food habits.

QUESTIONS FOR ANALYSIS

1. What predisposing factors in Edward's lifestyle place him in the high-risk category for CHD?
2. Why was moderate, consistent exercise originally recommended?
3. Explain the causes for Edward's initial symptoms.
4. How does each laboratory test ordered in the emergency department relate to cell metabolism? Why were results elevated?
5. Explain the association between the final diet order and his lipid disorder.
6. Outline a 1-day menu for Edward that complies with the final hospital diet order.
7. What nondietary needs might Edward have while convalescing at home? What community agencies might be of assistance?

Issues & ANSWERS

Strategies for Adopting DASH

Dietary changes are best achieved through small changes in food selections. Use this list of tips as a way to initiate discussion and dietary compliance to reduce hypertension among your clients.

Tips on eating the DASH way

Change gradually.

- If you now eat one or two vegetables a day, add a serving at lunch and another at dinner.
- If you do not eat fruit now or have only juice at breakfast, add a serving to your meals or have it as a snack.
- Gradually increase your use of fat-free and low-fat dairy products to three servings a day. For example, drink milk with lunch or dinner instead of soda, sugar-sweetened tea, or alcohol. Choose low-fat (1%) or fat-free (skim) dairy products to reduce your intake of saturated fat, total fat, cholesterol, and kcalories.
- Read food labels on margarines and salad dressings and choose those lowest in unsaturated fat. Some margarines are now *trans* fat free.

Treat meat as one part of the whole meal instead of the focus.

- Limit meat to 6 oz a day (2 servings)—all that is needed. Three to 4 oz is about the size of a deck of cards.
- If you now eat large portions of meat, cut them back gradually—by one half or one third at each meal.
- Include two or more vegetarian-style (meatless) meals each week.
- Increase servings of vegetables, rice, pasta, and dry beans at meals. Try casseroles, pasta, and stir-fry dishes that have less meat and more vegetables, grains, and dry beans.

Use fruit or other foods low in saturated fat, cholesterol, and kcalories as desserts and snacks.

- Fruits and other low-fat foods offer great taste and variety. Use fruits canned in their own juice. Fresh fruits require little or no preparation. Dried fruits are a good choice to carry with you or to have ready in the car.
- Try these snacks ideas: unsalted pretzels or nuts mixed with raisins, graham crackers, low-fat and fat-free yogurt and frozen yogurt, popcorn with no salt or butter added, and raw vegetables.

Try these other tips.

- Choose whole grain foods to get added nutrients such as minerals and fiber. For example, choose whole wheat bread and whole grain cereals.
- If you have trouble digesting dairy products, try taking lactase enzyme pills or drops (available at drugstores and groceries) with the dairy foods, or buy lactose-free milk or milk with lactase enzyme added to it.
- Use fresh, frozen, or no-salt-added canned vegetables.

REFERENCE

U.S. Dept. of Health and Human Services, Public Health Service, National Institutes of Health, National Heart, Lung, and Blood Institute: *The DASH diet,* NIH Publication No. 01-4082. Revised May 2001, available at *http://www.nhlbi.nih.gov/health/public/heart/hbp/dash/new_dash.pdf.*

Chapter 20 Diabetes Mellitus

Sara Long Anderson

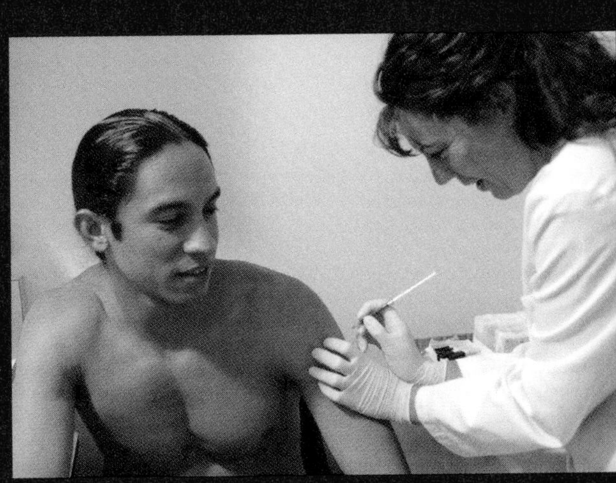

Chapter Outline

In this chapter of our continuing clinical nutrition series, we look at the problem of diabetes. We seek to understand its nature and how it can be managed to maintain good health and avoid complications.

Diabetes is a serious, costly, and increasingly common chronic disease. In the United States nearly 16 million (5.9%) of the population have diabetes. An estimated 10.3 million Americans have diagnosed diabetes and an additional 5.4 million have undiagnosed diabetes. The rate of diagnosed diabetes among American adults increased by one third between 1990 and 1998.[1] *There are approximately 800,000 newly diagnosed cases of diabetes each year. Diabetes can be diagnosed on the basis of two fasting glucose readings of 126 mg/dl or higher or a random glucose level of 200 mg/dl or higher and symptoms such as increased thirst, increased urination, and weight loss.*[2]

Although elevation of blood glucose level is the hallmark characteristic of diabetes, it is a group of metabolic disorders resulting from a defect in insulin secretion, insulin action, or both. These defects interfere with normal cellular uptake of glucose and utilization of glucose within cells. Restoring normal metabolic function is the goal in diagnosing and treating diabetes early. Restoration of normal metabolism can prevent many of the short-term complications such as hyperglycemia and hyperglycemia and the longer-term microvascular, macrovascular, and neurologic complications that affect multiple body systems.

Direct and indirect health costs of diabetes are nearly $100 billion a year in the United States.[3] *The death rate among middle-aged people with diabetes is double the death rate of those who do not have diabetes. Diabetes causes preventable complications that can be life threatening, including heart disease. Lifestyle changes can delay the progression of diabetes, as can controlling blood glucose, lipids, and blood pressure.*

Nature of Diabetes

HISTORY

The metabolic disease we know today as diabetes mellitus has been with us for a long time. Ancient records describe its devastating effects as observed by early healers. In the first century AD the Greek physician Aretaeus wrote of a malady in which the body "ate its own flesh" and gave off large quantities of urine. He gave it the name *diabetes,* from the Greek word meaning "siphon" or "to pass through." Much later, in the seventeenth century, the word *mellitus,* from the Latin word for "honey," was added because of the sweet nature of the urine. This addition also distinguished it from diabetes insipidus ("insipid," meaning tasteless, or not sweet), another disorder, although uncommon, in which the passage of copious amounts of urine had been observed. Today, use of the single name diabetes always means diabetes mellitus.

As medical knowledge began to grow, early clinicians—such as Rollo in England and Boushardat in France—observed that diabetes became less severe in overweight patients who lost weight. Later another French physician, Lancereaux, and his students described two kinds of diabetes: diabete gras—"fat diabetes," and diabete maigre—"thin diabetes."[4] All these observations preceded any knowledge about insulin or any relation to the pancreas. During these times, which have aptly been called the "diabetic dark ages," persons with diabetes had short lives and were maintained on a variety of semistarvation diets.[5]

Later, evidence began to point to the pancreas as a primary organ involved in the disease process. Paul Langerhans (1847 to 1888), a young German medical student, found special clusters—or islets—of cells scattered throughout the human pancreas that were different from the rest of the tissue. Although their function was still unknown, these special islet cells were named for their young discoverer: the *islets of Langerhans.* Research at that time focused on the pancreas. Finally, in the years of 1921 and 1922 a University of Toronto team discovered and successfully used the controlling agent from the "island cells," naming it insulin for its source (see *To Probe Further* box).[6]

CLASSIFICATION

The American Diabetes Association classifies diabetes into the following categories: (1) type 1 diabetes, formerly called insulin-dependent diabetes mellitus, (2) type 2 diabetes, formerly called non–insulin-dependent diabetes mellitus, (3) gestational diabetes mellitus (GDM), and (4) impaired glucose tolerance (IGT) and impaired fasting glucose (IFG).[2] The terms "insulin-dependent diabetes mellitus" and "non–insulin-dependent diabetes mellitus" and their acronyms, IDDM and NIDDM, should no longer be used because they are confusing and have often resulted in classifying patients based on treatment rather than etiology of their diabetes.[2]

Type 1 diabetes is characterized by sudden, severe insulin deficiency requiring insulin therapy to prevent ketoacidosis, coma, and death. Type 1 diabetes generally appears during childhood or adolescence and accounts for 5% to 10% of the cases of diabetes. However, type 1 diabetes can occur at any age, and almost half of new cases are diagnosed after 20 years of age. There are two forms of type 1 diabetes: immune-mediated diabetes and idiopathic diabetes. Immune-mediated diabetes results from a cellular-mediated autoimmune destruction of the beta cells of the pancreas.[7] Idiopathic diabetes has no known etiology.

The onset of type 1 diabetes is often rapid, accompanied by classic symptoms of weight loss and increased urination and thirst, especially if a viral infection or other stress increases the need for insulin. Onset may be less acute or there may be a "honeymoon period" of 6 to 12 months in which the diabetes may appear to be "cured" after an initial acute onset and initiation of insulin therapy. Destruction of the beta cells in the pancreas and loss of insulin production are usually gradual, accounting for the honeymoon period after insulin therapy restores normal glucose and the metabolic stress is resolved.

Type 2 diabetes is associated with insulin resistance and obesity combined with inadequate insulin produced in the pancreatic beta cells to compensate for the insulin resistance or an insulin secretory defect with insulin resistance.[2] Type 2 diabetes accounts for 90% to 95% of all cases of diabetes, and symptoms may include poor wound healing, blurred vision, or recurrent gum or bladder infections. Many individuals are not symptomatic, and the diabetes may be detected as the result of a routine blood test. Obesity and physical inactivity are strong risk factors for type 2 diabetes.[8-10] A large waist circumference is considered to be a biomarker for insulin resistance and the metabolic syndrome associated with diabetes, hypertension, and dyslipidemia (typically low high-density cholesterol and elevated triglyceride levels).[11] Although type 2 diabetes is associated with insulin resistance and is typically diagnosed after 40 years of age, it is occurring in epidemic proportions in younger populations, including children and adolescents. Called *maturity-onset diabetes of the young (MODY),* the incidence and prevalence of type 2 diabetes in children have increased 30-fold during the past 20 years.[12-18] Obesity is the most prominent clinical risk factor for type 2 diabetes in children and adolescents.[15]

GDM is defined as carbohydrate intolerance of variability severity with onset or first recognition during pregnancy. GDM develops in 2% to 5% of all pregnancies, and 30% to 40% of women with GDM are likely to develop type 2 diabetes.[19] In both type 2 diabetes and GDM, there is a relative insulin deficiency because the pancreas fails to produce the level of insulin needed to compensate for insulin resistance.

Judith Wylie-Rosett, EdD, RD, of Albert Einstein College of Medicine, Bronx, New York, provided some revisions to this chapter.

TO PROBE FURTHER
Insulin: Saga of a Success Story

Looking at numbers only, it would appear that the development of insulin was a causal factor in changing the status of diabetes mellitus from a rare disease to one that affects almost 16 million Americans. Closer inspection of the facts, however, reveals the disease was thought to be rare only because its victims died young—fewer persons were around who had the disease. Today insulin enables clients with type 1 diabetes live longer and enjoy productive lives.

The success story behind insulin lies not only in its ability to extend the life span of the person with diabetes but also in its own resilience. Insulin was discovered during the summer of 1921 at the University of Toronto by Frederick Banting, a surgeon who, according to newspaper accounts of the day, solved the mystery of insulin in his sleep, and Charles Best, a college graduate who was not yet enrolled in medical school. Their insulin was derived from the pancreas of dogs by tying off pancreatic ducts, waiting for the organ to "die," and then making an extract of the remaining tissue.

The extract worked fairly well in their tests with dogs. An extract that worked in humans was not developed for another 6 months, partly because their extract was originally given by mouth. Even when injected, their formula failed, which indicated that faulty purification methods may have been involved.

Finally, in January 1922, a successful extract was developed by a new member who joined the research team, J.B. Collip. Its effect on one patient's diabetic condition was not enough to counteract the effect of the treatment of the day—a diet that derived almost 71% of its kcalories from fat. The patient died at age 27 years with atherosclerosis and coronary heart disease. However, the team was successful with their third patient. The young girl, who was first diagnosed as having diabetes when she was 11 years old, lived to be 73 years of age. After insulin therapy was initiated, she was taken off the popular "starvation" diet of the day, gained weight, and led a normal life.

Ironically, despite Collip's successful extraction procedure, his subsequent actions almost stopped their project. Jealousies developed and, with the permission of the head of the university's physiology department, Collip refused to share his purification methods with Banting. Then, after his extraction product was a success, Collip conveniently "forgot" how to make it! As a result of this foolish battle, at least one patient died because the researchers ran out of original extract.

Fortunately, Collip miraculously "remembered" how to make his extract the next May. Soon after, insulin was being mass-produced and made available to the growing number of persons who depended on it for their survival.

References

Altman LK: The tumultuous discovery of insulin: finally, the hidden story is told, *New York Times* Sept 14, 1982.

Bliss M: *The discovery of insulin,* Chicago, 1982, University of Chicago Press.

Nestle M et al: A case of diabetes mellitus, *N Engl J Med* 81:127, 1982.

About 13.4 million, or 7% of the population, have impaired fasting glucose (IFG) or impaired glucose tolerance (IGT) depending on whether it is identified through fasting blood glucose or an oral glucose tolerance test (OGTT).[12] Formerly called "borderline diabetes," both are associated with greater risk of heart disease and subsequent development of diabetes. Research has shown that lifestyle interventions can reduce the rate of progression to type 2 diabetes.[20-22] Criteria for diagnosing diabetes are outlined in Table 20-1.

CONTRIBUTING CAUSES

Genetics

For some time, early insulin assay tests developed to measure the level of insulin activity in the blood found insulin-like activity in diabetes to be 2 or 3 times normal

diabetes insipidus A condition of the pituitary gland and insufficiency of one of its hormones, vasopressin (antidiuretic hormone); characterized by a copious output of a nonsweet urine, great thirst, and sometimes a large appetite. However, in diabetes insipidus these symptoms result from a specific injury to the pituitary gland, not a collection of metabolic disorders as in diabetes mellitus. The injured pituitary gland produces less vasopressin, a hormone that normally helps the kidneys reabsorb adequate water.

insulin Hormone formed in the beta cells of the islets of Langerhans in the pancreas. It is secreted when blood glucose and amino acid levels rise and assists their entry into body cells. It also promotes glycogenesis and conversion of glucose into fat and inhibits lipolysis and gluconeogenesis (protein breakdown). Commercial insulin is manufactured from pigs and cows; new "artificial" human insulin products have recently been made available.

TABLE 20-1 Criteria for Diagnosing Diabetes

Diabetes Type	Former Term	Etiology	Criteria
Type 1 diabetes*: immune mediated or idiopathic	Insulin-dependent diabetes mellitus (IDDM), type 1 diabetes, juvenile-onset diabetes, ketosis-prone diabetes, brittle diabetes	Beta cell destruction, usually leading to absolute insulin deficiency	Symptoms† of diabetes mellitus and casual plasma glucose ≥200 mg/dl (casual is defined as any time of day without regard to last meal) **OR** Fasting plasma glucose (FPG) ≥126 mg/dl (fasting is defined as no kcaloric intake for at least 8 hr) **OR** 2-hr postprandial plasma glucose (PPG) ≥200 mg/dl during oral glucose tolerance test (OGTT) (performed as described by the World Health Organization using glucose load containing the equivalent of 75 g anhydrous glucose dissolved in water)
Type 2 diabetes (adults)	Non–insulin-dependent diabetes mellitus (NIDDM), type 2 diabetes, adult-onset diabetes, maturity-onset diabetes, ketosis-resistant diabetes, stable diabetes	Insulin resistance with insulin secretory defect	
Type 2 diabetes (children)			Overweight (body mass index [BMI] >85th percentile for age and gender, weight for height >85th percentile, or weight >120% of ideal for height) **PLUS** Any 2 of the following: Family history of type 2 DM in first- or second-degree relative Native American, African-American, Latino, Asian-American, Pacific Islander Signs of insulin resistance or conditions associated with insulin resistance (acanthosis nigricans, hypertension [HTN], dyslipidemia, or polycystic ovary syndrome [PCOS])
Gestational diabetes (GDM)	Gestational diabetes, type 3 diabetes		*One-step approach:* Diagnostic OGTT *Two-step approach:* Initial screening to measure plasma or serum glucose concentration 1 hr after 50 g oral glucose load (glucose challenge test [GCT]) and perform diagnostic OGTT on those women exceeding glucose threshold value on GCT. Glucose threshold ≥140 mg/dl identifies ~80% of women with GDM
Impaired glucose tolerance (IGT)	Borderline diabetes, chemical diabetes		2-hr PPG ≥140 mg/dl and <200 mg/dl **OR** 2-hr PPG 140 mg/dl to 199 mg/dl

*Patients with any form of diabetes may require insulin treatment at some stage of their disease. Such use of insulin does not classify the patient as having type 1 diabetes.

†Symptoms include polyuria, polydipsia, and unexplained weight loss.

insulin levels. It is now evident that diabetes is a syndrome with multiple forms, resulting from (1) lack of insulin and/or (2) insulin resistance.[2]

Diabetes has long been associated with excess body weight, since the early observations of differences in "fat diabetes" and "thin diabetes."[4] Current research has reinforced the relation of the overweight state to the development of diabetes. Obesity can increase circulating insulin levels, which will ultimately lead to increased insulin resistance. In addition, individuals with a family history may have mutations on genes that control insulin production or may inherit insulin resistance not directly related to obesity. Thus, multiple genetic mutations may interact to increase the risk of type 2 diabetes.

Diabetes has often been defined in terms of heredity, but increasing evidence indicates that there is considerable genetic variation between the two main types of diabetes. Studies of Type 1 diabetes have shown an autoimmune attack by the body's insulin-producing cells is at fault, but its development is also associated with viruses such as coxsackievirus, mumps, and rubella. Insulin resistance is common in Western societies and sometimes termed *metabolic syndrome* or *syndrome* X. Insulin resistance is associated with a variety of conditions, including obesity, hypertension, hyperlipidemia, and hyperuricemia, as well as a sedentary lifestyle.[23]

Environmental Role: "Thrifty Gene"

Environmental factors apparently play a role in unmasking the underlying genetic susceptibility, a "thrifty" diabetic genotype that probably developed from primitive times for survival. This theory indicates diabetes may be associated with past genetic modifications for survival during varying periods of food availability. Gene mutations and the "thrifty" trait associated with type 2 diabetes facilitated more efficient use of limited food during times under difficult survival conditions. As food supplies became more plentiful, negative aspects of the "thrifty" trait began to appear. Such is indeed the case, for example, with the experience of Pima Indians in Arizona, as earlier studies and recent archaeological excavations there have indicated.[23-25] In earlier times, this group ate a limited diet mainly of carbohydrate foods harvested through heavy physical labor in a primitive agriculture. Now, however, with the "progress" of civilization, Pimas have become obese, and half of the adults have type 2 diabetes, the highest reported rate of this type of diabetes in the world. Native Americans develop diabetes at almost 3 times the rate as Caucasians. This same pattern is seen among populations of now-urbanized Pacific Islanders, South Asians, Asian Indians, and Creoles, although less is know about the exact numbers.[8,9] Other at-risk populations include Hispanic/Latino Americans, who are twice as likely develop diabetes as Caucasians, and African Americans, who develop diabetes at 1.9 times the rate of Caucasians.[3] Thus evidence suggests these groups have a genetic susceptibility to type 2 (diabetic genotype) and the disease is triggered by environmental factors, including obesity. Several specific genes involved in energy metabolism are thought to increase the risk for developing obesity and/or type 2 diabetes. As we commonly observe, lifestyle (dietary and physical activity habits) can interact with genetics in the development of type 2 diabetes.

SYMPTOMS

Symptoms of type 1 diabetes in its uncontrolled state include the following.

- Increased thirst (polydipsia)
- Increased urination (polyuria)
- Increased hunger (polyphagia)
- Weight loss (more common with type 1 diabetes)
- Fruity smell to breath (symptom of ketoacidosis)
- Fatigue or weakness

These symptoms occur because in an insulin-deficient state, glucose is filtered by the kidney into the urine rather than being used by cells for energy. Urine volume increases as the level of glucose excreted increases and the body compensates for this abnormal state by breaking down fat. Ketones are formed as the result of using fat as a primary energy source.

Type 2 diabetes may be asymptomatic or the symptoms may be more subtle and may include the following.

- Poor wound healing or recurrent infections
- Blurred vision (result of effects of hyperglycemia on shape of the cornea, which is returned to normal after glucose levels are stabilized)
- Skin irritation or infection
- Recurrent gum or bladder infections

The classic symptoms of diabetes are the result of the short-term effects of hyperglycemia. These symptoms are reversible if blood glucose levels are returned to a normal or near-normal level.

THE METABOLIC PATTERN OF DIABETES

Overall Energy Balance and the Energy Nutrients

Because initial symptoms of glycosuria and hyperglycemia are related to excess glucose, historically diabetes was called a disease of carbohydrate metabolism. However, as more becomes known about the intimate interrelationships of carbohydrate, fat, and protein metabolism, we view it in more general terms. It is a metabolic disorder resulting from lack of insulin (absolute, partial, or unavailable) affecting more or less each basic energy nutrient. It is especially related to metabolism of the two fuels, carbohydrate and fat, in the body's overall energy system.

Normal Blood Glucose Control

Control of blood glucose level within its normal range of 70 to 120 mg/dl (3.9 to 6.7 mmol/L) is vital to normal overall fuel metabolism and other metabolic functions. A knowledge of factors involved in maintaining a normal blood glucose level is essential to understanding the impairment of these factors (see Chapters 3 and 4). An overview of these normal balancing controls is given in Figure 20-1.

Sources of Blood Glucose

Two sources of blood glucose ensure a constant supply of this primary body fuel: (1) diet, the energy nutrients in our food (i.e., dietary carbohydrate, protein, and fat), and (2) glycogen, the backup source from constant turnover of "stored" liver glycogen by a process called glycogenolysis.

---

glycogenolysis Production of blood glucose from liver glycogen.

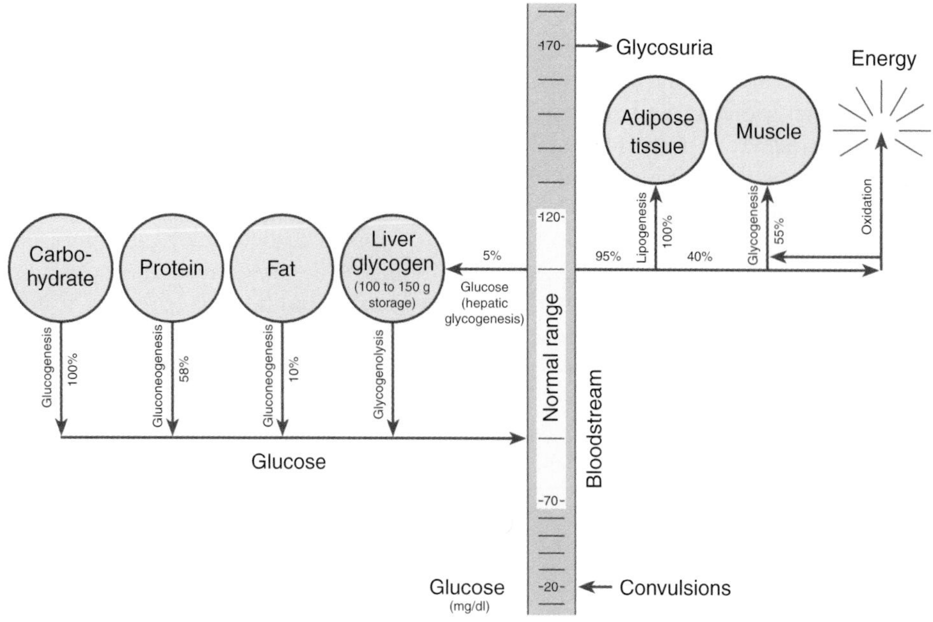

FIGURE 20-1 Sources of blood glucose (food and stored glycogen) and normal routes of control.

Uses of Blood Glucose

To prevent continued rise of blood glucose above normal limits, several basic uses for blood glucose are constantly available according to need. These include the following: (1) glycogenesis, conversion of glucose to glycogen for "storage" in liver and muscle; (2) lipogenesis, conversion of glucose to fat and storage in adipose tissue; and (3) glycolysis, cell oxidation of glucose for energy.

Pancreatic Hormonal Controls

Three types of islet cells scattered in clusters throughout the pancreas (islets of Langerhans) provide hormones closely interbalanced in the regulation of blood glucose levels. This specific arrangement of human islet cells is illustrated in Figure 20-2.

- *Alpha cells.* Arranged around the outer rim of the islets are alpha cells, one to two cells thick, making up about 30% of the total cells. These cells synthesize glucagon.
- *Beta cells.* The largest portion of islets is occupied by beta cells filling the central zone or about 60% of the gland. These primary cells synthesize insulin.
- *Delta cells.* Interspersed between alpha and beta cells—or occasionally between alpha cells alone—are delta cells, the remaining 10% of total cells. These cells synthesize somatostatin.

Interrelated Hormone Functions

Juncture points of the three types of islet cells act as sensors of blood glucose concentration and its rate of change. They constantly adjust and balance the rate of secretion of insulin, glucagon, and somatostatin to match whatever conditions prevail at any time. Each one of the three hormones has specific interbalanced functions.

1. *Insulin.* Although precise mechanisms are not entirely clear in every case, insulin has a profound effect on glucose control. It functions extensively in the metabolism of all three energy nutrients:
   - Insulin facilitates transport of glucose through cell membranes by way of special insulin receptors. These receptors are located on the membrane of insulin-sensitive cells, including those in adipose tissue, muscle tissue, and monocytes. Researchers are reaching a better understanding of these special receptors and how to treat the disease by studying insulin receptors.[26] These insulin receptors mediate all metabolic effects of insulin. Research has shown that cells of obese persons with diabetes have fewer than the normal number of insulin receptors. Weight loss in obese individuals and physical exercise increase the number of these receptors. The insulin receptor also appears to control several metabolic steps within the cell.
   - Insulin enhances conversion of glucose to glycogen and its consequent storage in the liver (glycogenesis).
   - Insulin stimulates conversion of glucose to fat (lipogenesis) for storage as adipose tissue.
   - Insulin inhibits fat breakdown (lipolysis) and the breakdown of protein.
   - Insulin promotes uptake of amino acids by skeletal muscles, thus increasing protein synthesis.
   - Insulin influences glucose oxidation through the main glycolytic pathway.
2. *Glucagon.* The hormone glucagon functions as a balancing antagonist to insulin. It rapidly causes breakdown of liver glycogen, and—to a lesser extent—

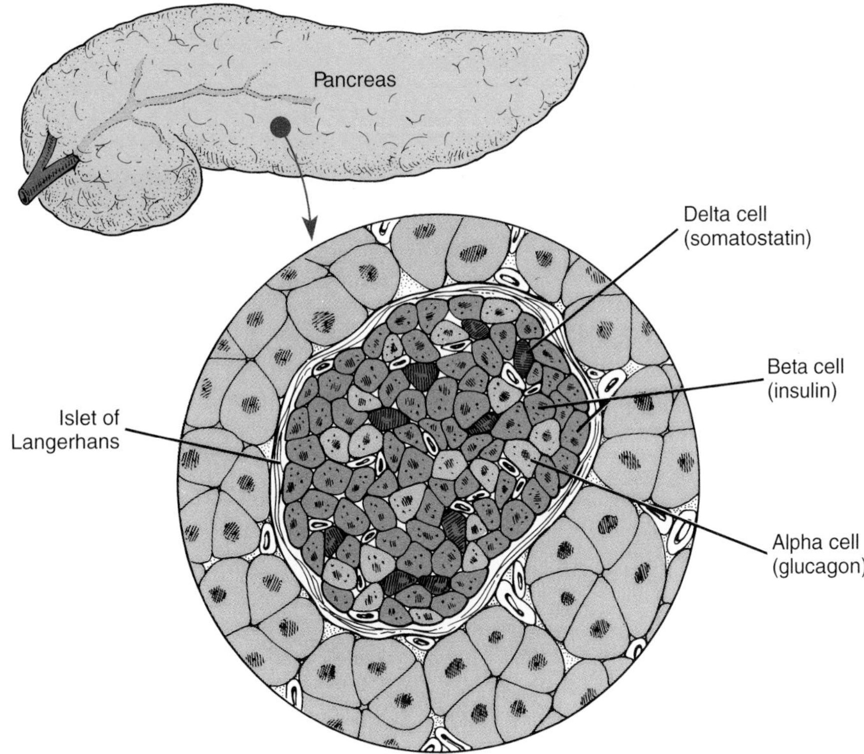

FIGURE 20-2 Islets of Langerhans, located in the pancreas.

fatty acids from adipose tissue to serve as body fuel. This action raises blood glucose levels to protect the brain and other body tissues. It helps maintain normal blood glucose levels during fasting hours of sleep. A lowering of the blood glucose concentration, increased amino acid concentrations, or sympathetic nervous system stimulation triggers glucagon secretion.

3. *Somatostatin.* Although pancreatic islet delta cells are the major source of somatostatin, this hormone is also synthesized and secreted in different regions of the body, including the hypothalamus. It acts in balance with insulin and glucose to inhibit their interactions as needed to maintain normal blood glucose levels. It also helps regulate blood glucose levels by inhibiting the release of a number of other hormones as needed.

Endocrine Function of Fat Cells

Historically, the primary role of body fat was considered to be stored energy and its role in secreting peptides was largely unknown. With the discovery of leptin in the 1990s, a growing number of peptides secreted from fat have been identified. These peptides appear to have an endocrine function and may play an important role in regulating appetite, body weight, and aspect of glucose metabolism.

METABOLIC CHANGES IN DIABETES

In uncontrolled diabetes, insulin is lacking to facilitate operation of normal blood glucose controls. Abnormal metabolic changes occur that affect glucose, fat, and protein and account for symptoms of diabetes.

Glucose

Blood glucose cannot be oxidized properly through the main glycolytic pathway in the cell to furnish energy

glycogenesis Synthesis of glycogen from blood glucose.
glycolysis Cell oxidation of glucose for energy.
glucagon A polypeptide hormone secreted by the alpha cells of the pancreatic islets of Langerhans in response to hypoglycemia; has an opposite balancing effect to that of insulin, raising the blood sugar, and thus is used as a quick-acting antidote for the hypoglycemic reaction of insulin. It stimulates the breakdown of glycogen (glycogenolysis) in the liver by activating the liver enzyme phosphorylase, and thus raises blood sugar levels during fasting states to ensure adequate levels for normal nerve and brain function.
lipogenesis Synthesis of fat from blood glucose.
somatostatin A hormone formed in the delta cells of the pancreatic islets of Langerhans and the hypothalamus. It is a balancing factor in maintaining normal blood glucose levels by inhibiting insulin and glucogen production in the pancreas as needed.

(see Chapter 6). Therefore it builds up in the blood (hyperglycemia).

Fat

Formation of fat (lipogenesis) is curtailed, and fat breakdown (lipolysis) increases. This leads to excess formation and accumulation of ketones (ketoacidosis). The appearance of the major ketone, acetone, in urine indicates development of ketoacidosis.

Protein

Tissue protein is also broken down in an effort to secure energy. This causes weight loss and nitrogen excretion in the urine.

General Management of Diabetes

TREATMENT GOALS

Basic Objectives

The diabetes healthcare team—physician, dietitian, nurse, and person with diabetes—is guided by three basic objectives in the care of each person with diabetes.

1. *Maintain optimal nutrition.* The first objective is to fulfill the basic nutritional requirement for health, growth and development, and a desirable body weight.
2. *Avoid hypoglycemia or hyperglycemia.* This second objective is designed to keep the person relatively free of hypoglycemia or insulin reaction, which requires immediate countermeasures, and hyperglycemia, which, if untreated, contributes to more serious ketoacidosis or diabetic coma.
3. *Prevent complications.* The third objective recognizes increased risk a person with diabetes faces for developing complicating problems that reflect damaging effects of chronic diabetes on tissues of small and large blood vessels and peripheral nerves.[27,28] These damages may occur in tissues such as eyes (retinopathy), nerve tissues (neuropathy), and renal tissues (nephropathy). In addition, coronary artery disease occurs in persons with diabetes about 4 times as often as in the general population. Peripheral vascular disease occurs about 40 times as often.

In all of these areas there is evidence that consistent, well-planned food habits and exercise, balanced as needed with early aggressive insulin therapy, can significantly help normalize metabolism and thereby reduce risks of these potentially serious complications.[29]

This aggressive insulin therapy consists of multiple daily injections or continuous subcutaneous infusion by pump. Self-monitoring of blood glucose levels is used to guide decisions to improve glycemic control. The added cardiovascular risk associated with diabetes is reflected in having blood pressure and lipid goals for diabetes management that are similar to those used in treating individuals who have diagnosed cardiovascular disease (Table 20-2).

Self-Care Role of the Person With Diabetes

To effectively control diabetes, the person with diabetes must play a central role. Daily self-discipline and informed self-care, supported by a skilled and sensitive healthcare team, are required for sound diabetes management. Ultimately, all persons with diabetes must treat themselves. This is especially true with the tighter nor-

TABLE 20-2 Metabolic Goals in Diabetes Management

Indicator	Normal Value	Goal	Additional Action Suggested*
Plasma values (mg/dl)			
Average preprandial glucose	<110	90-130	<90/>150
Average bedtime glucose	<120	110-150	<110/>180
Whole blood values† (mg/dl)			
Average preprandial glucose	<100	80-120	<80/>140
Average bedtime glucose	<110	100-140	<100/>160
Hb_{A1c} (%)	<6	<7	>8
LDL cholesterol		<100 mg/dl	
HDL cholesterol		Men: >55 mg/dl Women: >55 mg/dl	
Triglycerides		<150 mg/dl	
Blood pressure		<130/80	

*Depends on individual patient circumstances.

†Measurement of capillary blood glucose.

mal blood glucose control currently being used, with frequent self-monitoring of blood glucose and multiple insulin injections or an insulin infusion pump. Thus there is even greater need now for comprehensive diabetes education programs that encourage self-monitoring and self-care responsibility. Diabetes-related issues also need to be addressed as an integral component of primary care. Weight, activity, variety, and excess are themes that are relevant for assessing basic needs and providing basic recommendations. The WAVE pocket guide was developed to help primary care providers to briefly assess needs and provide guidance to clients with diabetes or at risk for developing diabetes.[30] (The WAVE pocket guide is available as a downloadable pdf file at *http://biomed.brown.edu/courses/nutrition/naa/wave.pdf*.)

Rationale for Diabetes Medical Nutrition Therapy

Medical nutrition therapy for diabetes is multifaceted. Physicians and nurses can no longer rely on preprinted diet sheets to assume they are providing nutrition care for patients.[31] There is no standard "ADA" or "diabetic" diet. The American Diabetes Association does not sanction any single meal plan or specific percentages of nutrients.[32] It is essential that persons with diabetes are assessed by a registered dietitian to determine an appropriate nutrition prescription and plan for self-management education.[12,32] Additionally, diet orders such as "no sugar added," "no concentrated sweets," "low sugar," and "liberal diabetic" are not considered suitable because they do not reflect diabetes nutrition recommendations and pointlessly restrict sucrose. Such meal plans support the erroneous concept that simply limiting sucrose-sweetened foods will enhance blood glucose control.[32]

Medical nutrition therapy should be individualized, taking usual eating habits and other lifestyle factors into consideration.[33] Consistency within an eating pattern will result in better glycemic control than abiding by an arbitrary eating style.[34] Nutrition recommendations are the same for individuals with diabetes as for the general population in regard to total fat, saturated fat, cholesterol, fiber, vitamins, and minerals. Recommendations for protein, carbohydrates, sucrose, and alcohol are modified depending on the nature of diabetes in relation to carbohydrate metabolism or effects of complications.[31]

TYPE 1 DIABETES MELLITUS (TYPE 1)

Recognizing the need for a more comprehensive program of care of diabetes, based on the individual metabolic balance concept and designed to help delay or avoid life-threatening complications of this chronic disease, a national U.S. clinical research study supported by the National Institutes of Health was organized. The Diabetes Control and Complications Trial (DCCT)[29] involved 1441 subjects in 29 clinical centers across the country for approximately 10 years. The study was designed to compare the effects of intensive insulin therapy aimed at achieving blood glucose levels as close as possible to the normal nondiabetic range with effects of conventional therapy on early microvascular complications of type 1 diabetes. The DCCT demonstrated that lowering Hb_{A1c} from 9% to 7% in the intensively treated group reduced the risk of the development or progression of eye, kidney, and neurologic complications by 50% to 75%.[12,35] Dietary strategies played an important role in achieving control in the intensively treated group.[36] The reduction in complications was linearly related to improvement in glycemic control, indicating risk reduction can be achieved even if intensification of treatment fails to achieve a near-normal Hb_{A1c}.[31,37] Adverse affects of intensive therapy included a two- to three-fold increase in severe hypoglycemia and a weight gain of 10 lb (4.5 kg).[29] Initial weight was considerably higher, but providing consultation about overeating to prevent or treat hypoglycemia appears to attenuate the weight gain. The DCCT results indicated the strength of the expanded role of the registered dietitian, assisted as needed by the diabetes team nurse, in individualizing medical nutrition therapy with various diet management tools and insulin balance.[38,39]

TYPE 2 DIABETES MELLITUS (TYPE 2)

The United Kingdom Prospective Diabetes Study (UKPDS) evaluated the effects of treatments to improve glycemic control and cardiovascular risk factors in individuals with newly diagnosed diabetes. Glycemic control and cardiovascular risk reduction therapies reduced rates of both macrovascular and microvascular complications.

nephropathy Disease of the kidneys; in diabetes, renal damage associated with functional and pathologic changes in the nephrons, which can lead to glomerulosclerosis and chronic renal failure.
neuropathy General term for functional and pathologic changes in the peripheral nervous system; in diabetes, a chronic sensory condition affecting mainly the nerves of the legs, marked by numbness from sensory impairment, loss of tendon reflexes, severe pain, weakness, and wasting of muscles involved.
retinopathy Noninflammatory disease of the retina—the visual tissue of the eye—characterized by microaneurysms, intraretinal hemorrhages, waxy yellow exudates, "cotton wool" patches, and macular edema; a complication of diabetes that may lead to proliferation of fibrous tissue, retinal detachment, and blindness.

The UKPDS confirmed the DCCT finding with respect to preventing microvascular complications of diabetes and provided evidence that a comprehensive risk reduction approach could also reduce macrovascular complications.[40-43] The major cause of morbidity and mortality in persons with diabetes is cardiovascular disease. Type 2 diabetes and its common coexisting conditions (e.g., hypertension and dyslipidemia) are considered to be independent risk factors for macrovascular disease.[12]

GESTATIONAL DIABETES MELLITUS

For women with preexisting diabetes or GDM, risks of fetal abnormalities and mortality are increased in the presence of hyperglycemia. Maternal insulin does not cross the placenta, but glucose does, causing the fetus's pancreas to increase insulin production if the mother becomes hyperglycemic. This increased production of insulin causes macrosomia—the most typical characteristic of babies born to women with diabetes. Other problems such as respiratory difficulties, hypocalcemia, hypoglycemia, hypokalemia, and/or jaundice may occur.[44] Therefore every effort should be made to control blood glucose levels.[12] All women with GDM should receive counseling by a registered dietitian when possible.[45] Individualized medical nutrition therapy, contingent on maternal weight and height, should include provision of adequate kilocalories (kcalories) and nutrients to meet the needs of the pregnancy and be consistent with established maternal blood glucose goals.[45] At the start, self-monitoring of blood glucose should be planned 4 times a day (fasting and 1 or 2 hours postprandial).[46] Frequency can be decreased one glycemic control is established. Blood glucose goals during pregnancy are as follows.[47]

- Fasting: less than 95 mg/dl
- 1 Hour postprandial: 140 mg/dl
- 2 Hours postprandial: less than 120 mg/dl

Implementing Medical Nutrition Therapy

Nutrition intervention is governed by consideration of treatment goals and lifestyle changes the person with diabetes is ready to make, preferably to predetermined energy levels and percentages of carbohydrates, protein, and fat.[31] The objective of medical nutrition therapy (MNT) is to support and facilitate individual lifestyle and behavior changes that will lead to improved glycemic control.[31] Cultural and ethnic preferences should be taken into consideration, and persons with diabetes should be included in the decision-making process.[31]

Current nutrition principles and recommendations focus on lifestyle goals and strategies for treatment of diabetes. For the first time, the 2002 evidence-based nutrition recommendations purposely address lifestyle approaches to diabetes prevention as MNT for treating and managing diabetes may not necessarily be the same for preventing or delaying onset of diabetes.[31] Goals of MNT that apply to all persons with diabetes are as follows.[31]

1. Attain and maintain optimal metabolic outcomes including
   - Blood glucose levels in the normal (or near-normal) range
   - Lipid and lipoprotein profiles that reduce risk for macrovascular diseases
   - Blood pressure levels that reduce risk for vascular disease
2. Prevent and treat chronic complications.
3. Improve health through healthy food choices and physical activity.
4. Address individual nutritional needs taking into consideration personal and cultural preferences and lifestyle while respecting individuals' wishes and willingness to change.

Additional, more specific medical nutrition goals include the following.

1. *Youth with type 1 diabetes.* MNT goals for children and adolescents with type 1 diabetes should ensure provision of sufficient energy for normal growth and development. Insulin regimens should be integrated into usual eating and physical activity habits.[31]
2. *Youth with type 2 diabetes.* Goals for MNT for children and adolescents with type 2 diabetes should facilitate changes in eating and physical activity habits to decrease insulin resistance and enhance metabolic status.[31]
3. *Pregnant and lactating women.* MNT goals for pregnant and lactating women should provide adequate energy and nutrients necessary for optimal pregnancy outcomes.[31]
4. *Older adults.* Nutritional and psychosocial needs of an aging individual should be provided in MNT goals.[31]
5. *Individuals treated with insulin or insulin secretagogues.* Self-management education for treatment and prevention of hypoglycemia, acute illness, and exercise-related blood glucose problems should be included in MNT goals for individuals treated with insulin or insulin secretagogues.
6. *Individuals at risk for diabetes.* For those at risk for developing diabetes, physical activity should be encouraged and food choices that facilitate moderate weight loss (or at least prevent weight gain) should be promoted.

MNT recommendations for management of type 1 and type 2 diabetes are outlined in Table 20-3.

TABLE 20-3 Summary of 2002 Medical Nutrition Therapy Recommendations for Diabetes Mellitus

Nutrition principles and recommendations are classified into four categories according to levels of supporting evidence: A—those for which there is strong supporting evidence, B—some supporting evidence, C—limited supporting evidence, or D—those based on expert consensus.

Nutrition Recommendation	Grading
Carbohydrates	
Whole grains, fruits, vegetables, and low-fat milk should be included.	A
Total amount of carbohydrates in meals and snacks is more important than the source or type of carbohydrate.	A
Individuals receiving intensive insulin therapy should adjust their premeal insulin doses based on the carbohydrate content of the meal.	A
Individuals receiving fixed daily insulin doses should try to be consistent in day-to-day carbohydrate intake.	B
There is not sufficient evidence of long-term benefit to recommend or use of low-glycemic index diets as a primary strategy in food/meal planning for individuals with type 1 diabetes.	B
As for the general public, consumption of fiber should be encouraged.	B
Percentages of carbohydrates should be based on individual nutrition assessment.	B
Carbohydrate and monounsaturated fat together should provide 60%-70% of energy intake.	D
Nutrative Sweeteners	
Sucrose does not increase glycemia to a greater extent than isocaloric amounts of starch.	A
Sucrose and sucrose-containing food do not need to be restricted; however, if included in the food/meal plan, it should be substituted for other carbohydrate sources or, if added, be adequately covered with insulin or other glucose-lowering medication.	A
Fructose reduces postprandial glycemia when it replaces sucrose or starch.	B
Consumption of fructose in large amounts may have adverse effects on plasma lipids.	B
Use of sugar alcohols as sweetening agents appears to be safe.	B
Sugar alcohols may cause diarrhea, especially in children.	B
Use of added fructose as a sweetening agent is not recommended.	C
Sucrose and sucrose-containing food should be eaten in the context of a healthy diet, and the intake of other nutrients ingested with sucrose, such as fat, should be taken into account.	D
There is no reason to recommend avoidance of naturally occurring fructose in fruits, vegetables, and other food.	D
It is unlikely sugar alcohols in amounts ingested in individual food servings or meals will contribute to a significant reduction in total energy or carbohydrate intake (although no studies have been conducted to support this).	D
Resistant Starches	
Resistant starches (nondigestible) have no established benefit.	C
Nonnutritive Sweeteners	
Nonnutritive sweeteners are safe when consumed within the acceptable daily intake established by the FDA.	A
It is unknown if use of nonnutritive sweeteners improves long-term glycemic control or assists in weight loss.	D
Dietary Protein	
In those with controlled type 2 diabetes, ingested protein does not increase plasma glucose concentrations, although ingested protein is just as potent a stimulant of insulin secretion as carbohydrate.	A
There is no evidence to suggest that usual protein intake (15%-20% of total daily energy) should be modified if renal function is normal.	B
Protein requirements may be greater than the RDA, but not greater than usual intake for those with less-than-optimal glycemic control.	B
Dietary protein does not slow absorption of carbohydrate and dietary protein and carbohydrate do not raise plasma glucose later than carbohydrate alone and thus do not prevent late-onset hypoglycemia.	B
It may be prudent to avoid protein intake >20% of total daily energy.	C
Long-term effects of diets high in protein and low in carbohydrate are unknown. Although such diets may produce short-term weight loss and improved glycemia, it has not been established that weight loss is maintained. Long-term effect of such diets on plasma LDL cholesterol is also a concern.	D
Dietary Fat	
In all, <10% of energy intake should be derived from saturated fats. Some (i.e., those with LDL cholesterol ≥100 mg/dl) may benefit from lowering saturated fat intake to <7% of energy intake.	A
Dietary cholesterol intake should be <300 mg/day. Some (i.e., those with LDL cholesterol ≥100 mg/dl) may benefit from lowering dietary cholesterol to <200 mg/day.	A

Continued

TABLE 20-3 Summary of 2002 Medical Nutrition Therapy Recommendations for Diabetes Mellitus—cont'd

Nutrition Recommendation	Grading
Dietary Fat—cont'd	
Intake of transunsaturated fatty acids should be minimized.	A
Current fat replacers/substitutes approved by the FDA are safe for use in food.	A
To lower plasma LDL cholesterol, energy derived from saturated fat can be reduced if concurrent weight loss is desirable or replaced with carbohydrate or monounsaturated fat if weight loss is not a goal.	A
Polyunsaturated fat intake should be ~10% of energy intake.	B
In weight-maintaining diets, when monounsaturated fat replaces carbohydrate, it may beneficially affect postprandial glycemia and plasma triglycerides but not necessarily fasting plasma glucose of Hb_{A1c}.	B
Incorporation of 2 or 3 servings of plant stanols/sterols (~2 g) food/day, substituted for similar food, will lower total and LDL cholesterol.	B
Reduced-fat diets when maintained long term, contribute to modest loss of weight and improvement of dyslipidemia.	B
Two or more servings of fish per week provide dietary n-3 polyunsaturated fat and can be recommended.	C
Monounsaturated fat and carbohydrate together should provide 60%-70% of energy intake. However, increasing fat intake may result in increased energy intake.	D
Fat intake should be individualized and designed to fit ethnic and cultural backgrounds.	D
Use of low-fat food and fat replacers/substitutes may reduce total fat and energy intake and thereby facilitate weight loss.	D
Energy Balance and Obesity	
In insulin-resistant individuals, reduced energy intake and modest weight loss improve insulin resistance and glycemia in the short term.	A
Structured programs that emphasize lifestyle changes, including education, reduced fat (<30% daily energy) and energy intake, regular physical activity, and regular participant contact can produce long-term weight loss of 5%-7% of starting weight.	A
Exercise and behavior modification are most useful as adjuncts to other weight-loss strategies. Exercise is helpful in maintaining weight loss.	A
Nutrition interventions, such as standard weight-reduction diets, when used alone are unlikely to produce long-term weight loss. Structured, intensive lifestyle programs are necessary.	A
Optimal strategies for preventing and treating obesity long term have yet to be defined.	A
Currently available weight-loss drugs have modest beneficial effects. These drugs should be used only in people with BMI >27.0 kg/m².	B
Gastric reduction surgery can be considered for patients with BMI >35.0 kg/m². Long-term data comparing benefits and risks of gastric reduction surgery to those of medical therapy are not available.	C
Micronutrients	
There is no clear evidence of benefit from vitamin and mineral supplementation for persons who do not have underlying deficiencies. Exceptions include folate for prevention of birth defects and calcium for prevention of bone disease.	B
Although difficult to ascertain, if deficiencies of vitamins and minerals are identified, supplementation can be beneficial.	B
Routine supplementation of the diet with antioxidants is not advised because of uncertainties related to long-term efficacy and safety.	B
Select populations, such as elderly individuals, pregnant or lactating women, strict vegetarians, and people on kcalorie-restricted diets, may benefit from supplementation with a multivitamin preparation.	D
There is no evidence to suggest long-term benefit from herbal preparations.	D
Alcohol	
If individuals choose to drink alcohol, daily intake should be limited to 1 drink for adult women and 2 drinks for adult men. One drink is defined as a 12-oz beer, 5-oz glass of wine, or 1.5-oz glass of distilled spirits.	A
The type of alcoholic beverage consumed does not make a difference.	A
When moderate amounts of alcohol are consumed with food, blood glucose levels are not affected.	A
To reduce risk of hypoglycemia, alcohol should be consumed with food.	A
Ingestion of light-to-moderate amounts of alcohol does not raise blood pressure; excessive, chronic ingestion of alcohol raises blood pressure and may be a risk factor for stroke.	A
Pregnant women and people with medical problems such as pancreatitis, advanced neuropathy, severe hypertriglyceridemia, or alcohol abuse should be advised not to ingest alcohol.	A
There are potential benefits from ingestion of moderate amounts of alcohol, such as decreased risk of type 2 diabetes, coronary heart disease, and stroke.	B
Alcoholic beverages should be consumed in addition to the regular food/meal plan for all patients with diabetes. No food should be omitted.	D

Issues Related to Medical Therapy

INSULIN THERAPY

The management goal for persons with type 1 diabetes is to maintain a normal blood glucose level as closely as possible. Strong evidence from the DCCT, as well as accumulating practice experience, indicates that maintaining such a "normoglycemic" state helps prevent the chronic complications of long-term uncontrolled hyperglycemia.[28,48] To achieve this goal, more intensive insulin therapy with the different types of insulin now available is being used. Insulin is increasingly being used as adjunctive therapy in type 2 diabetes.

Types of Insulin

A number of insulin preparations are available for therapeutic use, and new ones are constantly being developed to meet medical care needs for individual patients and market changes. Individual responses to these insulins are highly variable. According to time of action, they are rapid, intermediate, and long acting.

1. *Rapid-acting insulins.* These insulins have various names, depending on the manufacturer (e.g., Humulin R, Regular, Semilente, and Velosulin R). Rapid-acting insulins have their onset of action within approximately ½ hour after injection and stay in the body for less than 5 hours. This type of insulin peaks about 2 hours after injection. A recently developed human insulin analogue, Humalog (generic name, insulin lispro), approved by the Food and Drug Administration in 1996, has the shortest time-action curve of any insulin currently available.[49,50] Short-acting insulins have their onset of action in ½ to 1 hour and have a 6- to 8-hour duration. Short-acting insulins peak around 3 hours. A number of variables influence absorption rate, such as site of injection, physical activity, skin temperature, and any circulating anti-insulin antibodies. Effect on blood glucose can be detected in about 1 hour, peaks at 4 to 6 hours, and lasts about 12 to 16 hours.
2. *Intermediate-acting insulins.* These insulins include Humulin L, Lente, NPH, Insulatard N, and Insulatard. Effect is detected in about 2 hours, peaks at about 11 hours, and lasts about 20 to 29 hours.
3. *Long-acting insulins.* These insulins include Humulin U and Ultralente. Their duration is somewhat longer than that of the intermediate-acting insulins. They can be difficult to use because basal insulin is difficult to predict or control when the insulin peaks. Insulin glargine rDNA, which was first released in 2001, is a recombinant DNA insulin analog specifically formulated to provide a long, flat response. However, insulin glargine rDNA (trade name Lantus) cannot be mixed with other insulins, and two injections are needed to combine the action with a short-acting insulin. It is a long-acting insulin that works slowly over 24 hours and may not be used in combination with another type of insulin or an oral hypoglycemic medication to keep blood glucose regulated. Treatment algorithms are developed to adjust insulin on the basis of lifestyle and self-monitoring of blood glucose.

The process of intensifying type 1 diabetes management occurs in several stages. The initial dose of insulin is usually calculated based on current body weight with 0.5 to 0.6 unit of insulin/kg/day, with approximately half being for basal needs and half being as boluses for meals. During this initial phase a consistent carbohydrate intake is needed to identify a blood glucose pattern. After mastering an understanding, the client can move on to more complex planning using monitoring results to achieve better glycemic control and a more flexible lifestyle. Bolus requirement varies widely, but the initial dose is often estimated to provide 1 unit of short-acting insulin/15 g of carbohydrate. Gradually the client learns to adjust insulin for changes in food or activity using a ratio of carbohydrate intake to insulin dosage. A similar approach is used for insulin therapy in other forms of diabetes. In the treatment of type 2 diabetes, insulin may be used alone or in conjunction with an oral agent.[51]

Sources of Insulin

Human insulin has replaced beef and pork insulins that were traditionally used to treat diabetes. These animal-derived insulins are immunogenic to humans, beef more so than pork; in time they induce anti-insulin antibodies that delay or blunt their action. Human insulin is available from two sources: (1) biosynthesis by recombinant DNA technology through rapidly reproducing bacteria that have been given the human gene and (2) chemical substitution of the terminal amino acid of the beta-chain of pork insulin. Because they carry the human insulin structure, these newer insulins are almost nonimmunogenic.

Insulin and Exercise Balance

Exercise benefits all persons with diabetes through its action in increasing the number of insulin receptors on muscle cells, thus increasing insulin efficiency.[52] However, physical activity must be regular to be effective.[53] A detailed history of personal activity and exercise habits provides information that is needed to help a client plan a wise program of regular moderate exercise. Guidelines for extra food to cover periods of heavier exercise, athletic practice, or competition can be included (Table 20-4). Gregory et al[54] report the experience of a college football player with diabetes and his carefully planned blood sugar control during games. In general, exercise programs make persons feel better both physically and psychologically. This improved sense of well-being should not be underestimated in persons facing a chronic disease.

TABLE 20-4 Meal-Planning Guide for Active People With Type 1 Diabetes Mellitus

Exchange Needs	Sample Menus
Moderate Activity	
30 Minutes	
1 bread *or*	1 bran muffin *or*
1 fruit	1 small orange
1 Hour	
2 bread + 1 meat *or*	Tuna sandwich *or*
2 fruit + 1 milk	½ cup fruit salad + 1 cup milk
Strenuous Activity	
30 Minutes	
2 fruit *or*	1 small banana *or*
1 bread + 1 fat	½ bagel + 1 tsp cream cheese
1 Hour	
2 bread + 1 meat + 1 milk *or*	Meat and cheese sandwich + 1 cup milk *or*
2 bread + 2 meat + 2 fruit	Hamburger + 1 cup orange juice

Insulin Delivery Systems

Intensive insulin therapy for maintaining more normal blood glucose control requires multiple injections of rapid-acting insulin, alone or in combination with basal intermediate-acting insulin. This is accomplished either by regular injection with disposal syringes or with an insulin pump. The pump is not for everyone, but for many it has made life easier to use an insulin pump to achieve a basal insulin infusion and bolus insulin for meals. It is a small device that is easily worn on the belt with a subcutaneous needle in the abdomen and buttons the wearer pushes to obtain a fixed programmed flow of insulin in balance with food intake. Frequent monitoring is needed to adjust insulin dosage with either multiple injections or the insulin pump.

Oral Antidiabetic Drugs

There are five classes of oral antidiabetic drugs used to treat hyperglycemia in type 2 diabetes: sulfonylurea, biguanide, thiazolidinedione, meglitidine, and alpha-glucosidase inhibitor. When lifestyle changes alone cannot normalize metabolism, MNT should help optimize metabolic control and reduce potential medication side effects. Table 20-5 provides a brief review of insulin and oral antidiabetic drugs.

Insulin is often used in type 2 diabetes as adjunctive therapy when oral agents are not achieving glycemic control. A nighttime dose of insulin is commonly used to help reduce fasting glucose levels, especially if fasting levels are 13.9 mmol/L (250 mg/dl) or higher. Insulin therapy is also commonly used as adjunctive therapy when glycemic control is not achieved with oral agent monotherapy or combination therapy.

Testing Methods for Monitoring Results

Frequent testing of blood glucose levels is necessary for successful "tight" control of type 1 diabetes and to reduce the risk of complications.

Self-monitoring of blood glucose. For insulin doses to be administered in sufficient time intervals and amounts to maintain normal blood glucose, close monitoring of immediate blood glucose levels is mandatory.[50] Small, lightweight, easy-to-use, hand-size meters, easily carried in pockets and handbags, are available for convenient use. A reagent test strip is inserted into the blood glucose meter, a drop of capillary blood from the finger obtained with an automatic lancer is placed on the reagent test strip, and a digital reading of the blood glucose level appears on the meter. Frequency of monitoring varies according to need for control and goal of care. More frequent self-monitoring is indicated for unstable forms of diabetes, persons using insulin pumps, and those who want close control and freedom of movement. Usually two to eight before- and after-meal tests are performed daily. During pregnancy postprandial monitoring is performed at 1 hour after meals. Glucose goals are lower during pregnancy because of the dilution effect of having a greater blood volume.

Glycated hemoglobin. The most common glycated hemoglobin test is the Hb_{A1c}. Glycated hemoglobins are relatively stable molecules within the red blood cell. During the 120-day life of the red blood cell, glucose molecules attach themselves to hemoglobin. This irreversible glycosylation of hemoglobin depends on the concentration of blood glucose. Glycosylation of proteins in various body systems appears to play a role in the development of diabetic complications. The higher the level of circulating glucose over the life of the red blood cells, the higher the concentration of glycohemoglobin. Thus measurement of hemoglobin A1c (Hb_{A1c}) relates to the level of blood glucose over a longer period. It provides an effective tool for evaluating the long-term management of diabetes and degree of control.[12] Because glucose attaches to hemoglobin over the life of the red blood cell, the test gives an accumulated history of glucose levels over time, providing an effective management tool for evaluating progress and making decisions about treatment changes. Obtaining a Hb_{A1c} level every 6 to 8 weeks can be used to monitor the overall glucose control.

Physical Activity Habits

In counseling clients with diabetes, a detailed history of personal activity and physical exercise habits should be discussed. This information is then used as a basis for planning together a wise program of regular moderate exercise. Guidelines for extra food to cover periods of

TABLE 20-5 Medications Used to Treat Diabetes

Drug Class	Drug Name(s)	Action	Target Organ(s)	Side Effects	How Taken
Alpha-glucosidase inhibitor	*Acarbose:* Precose, Glucobay, Prandese, Glucor *Miglitol:* Glyset, Miglibay, Bayglitol	Delays absorption of glucose from GI tract	Small intestine	Excess flatulence, diarrhea (particularly after high-carbohydrate meal), abdominal pain, may interfere with iron absorption	Must be taken with meals
Biguanides	*Metformin:* Glucophage *Metformin + glibenclamide:* Glucovance, Glucophage + Glyburide	Decrease hepatic glucose production and intestinal glucose absorption; improves insulin sensitivity	Liver, small intestine, and peripheral tissues	Less likely to gain weight; may lose weight; anorexia, nausea, diarrhea, metallic taste, may reduce absorption of vitamin B_{12} and folic acid, rarely suitable for adults >80 yr of age	Take with first main meal
Insulin and related agents	*Insulin mixtures:* Humulin 50/50, Humulin 70/30, Novolin 70/30	Exogenous insulin preparations		Hypoglycemia, fatigue, hunger, nausea, muscular weakness or trembling, headache, sweating, blurred vision, fainting, weight gain, skin irritation	Subcutaneous injection
	Intermediate acting: Humulin L, Humulin N, Iletin II Lente, Iletin II NPH, Novolin L, Novolin N	Exogenous insulin preparations		Hypoglycemia, fatigue, hunger, nausea, muscular weakness or trembling, headache, sweating, blurred vision, fainting, weight gain, skin irritation	Subcutaneous injection
	Long-acting: Humulin U, Lantus (insulin glargine)	Exogenous insulin preparations		Hypoglycemia, fatigue, hunger, nausea, muscular weakness or trembling, headache, sweating, blurred vision, fainting, weight gain, skin irritation	Subcutaneous injection
	Rapid-acting: Humalog, Insulin Lispro, Insulin Aspart	Exogenous insulin preparations		Hypoglycemia, fatigue, hunger, nausea, muscular weakness or trembling, headache, sweating, blurred vision, fainting, weight gain, skin irritation	Subcutaneous injection, intramuscular or intravenous in special situations
	Short-acting: Humulin R, Iletin II Regular, Novolin R, Novolin BR	Exogenous insulin preparations		Hypoglycemia, fatigue, hunger, nausea, muscular weakness or trembling, headache, sweating, blurred vision, fainting, weight gain, skin irritation	Subcutaneous injection, intramuscular or intravenous in special situations

Compiled from: Setter SM: New drug therapies for treatment of diabetes, *On the Cutting Edge Diabetes Care and Education Newsletter* 19(2):3-7, 1998; Sharp AR: Nutritional implications of new medications to treat diabetes, *On the Cutting Edge Diabetes Care and Education Newsletter* 19(2):1998; White JR, Campbell RK: Recent developments in the pharmacological reduction of blood glucose in patients with Type 2 diabetes, *Clin Diabetes* 19:153-159, 2001, available at *http://clinical.diabetesjournals.org/cgi/content/full/19/4/153*; Rosen ED: Drug classes for diabetes, *Veritas Medicine for Patients,* available at *http://www.veritasmedicine.com*.

Continued

TABLE 20-5 Medications Used to Treat Diabetes—cont'd

Drug Class	Drug Name(s)	Action	Target Organ(s)	Side Effects	How Taken
Meglitinides (non-sulfonylurea insulin releasers)	*Nateglinide:* Starlix *Repaglinide:* Prandin, Aculin	Stimulates secretion of insulin	Pancreatic beta cells	Hypoglycemia and weight gain; *repaglinide* has a slightly increased risk for cardiac events	Take with meals
Sulfonylureas	*Acetohexamide:* Dymelor *Tolazamide:* Tolinase *Tolbutamide:* Orinase *Chlorpropamide:* Diabinese *Glimepiride:* Amaryl *Glyburide:* DiaBeta, Micronase, Glynase PresTabs	Stimulates secretion of insulin	Pancreatic beta cells	Hypoglycemia and weight gain; *tolbutamide* may be associated with cardiovascular complications; *chlorpropamide* can cause hyponatremia; should not be used by women who are pregnant or nursing, or by individuals allergic to sulfa drugs; sulfonylurea interact with many other drugs (prescription, OTC, and alternative); *Diabinese:* avoid alcohol	Take before or with meals
Thiazolidinediones (TZDs)	*Pioglitazone:* Actos *Rosiglitazone:* Avandia	Improves insulin sensitivity	Activates genes involved with fat synthesis and carbohydrate metabolism	Possible liver damage, weight gain, mild anemia	Once or twice daily

Compiled from: Setter SM: New drug therapies for treatment of diabetes, *On the Cutting Edge Diabetes Care and Education Newsletter* 19(2):3-7, 1998; Sharp AR: Nutritional implications of new medications to treat diabetes, *On the Cutting Edge Diabetes Care and Education Newsletter* 19(2):1998; White JR, Campbell RK: Recent developments in the pharmacological reduction of blood glucose in patients with Type 2 diabetes, *Clin Diabetes* 19:153-159, 2001, available at *http://clinical.diabetesjournals.org/cgi/content/full/19/4/153*; Rosen ED: Drug classes for diabetes, *Veritas Medicine for Patients,* available at *http://www.veritasmedicine.com.*

heavier exercise or athletic practice and competition are included[55] (see Table 20-4). Self-monitoring is a regular procedure now used by most persons with type 1 diabetes. It is a helpful means of determining the balance needed at any point in time between exercise, insulin, and food.

GESTATIONAL DIABETES

Occasionally, the stress of pregnancy may bring about GDM, which is a form of glucose intolerance that has onset during pregnancy and is resolved on parturition.[56] Risk of fetal abnormalities and mortality are increased in the presence of hyperglycemia; therefore every effort should be made to control blood glucose levels. All women with GDM should receive nutrition counseling by a registered dietitian when possible.[45]

Changes that take place during pregnancy greatly affect insulin utilization. Some hormones and enzymes produced by the placenta are antagonistic to insulin, thus reducing its effectiveness. Maternal insulin does not cross the placenta, but glucose, does causing the fetal pancreas to increase insulin production if maternal blood glucose levels get too high. Increased production of insulin causes the most predictable characteristic of infants born to women with diabetes—macrosomia, in addition to other problems such as respiratory difficulties, hypocalcemia, hypoglycemia, hypokalemia, and jaundice.[44]

Individualization of MNT based on maternal weight and height is recommended.[45] MNT should include the provision of adequate kcalories and nutrients to meet pregnancy needs and should be consistent with accepted maternal blood glucose goals.[45] Self-monitoring of blood glucose (SMBG) provides important information about the impact of food on blood glucose levels.[46] At the beginning of the pregnancy, minimal daily SMBG should be planned 4 times a day (fasting and 1 or 2 hours after each meal).[46] Blood glucose goals during pregnancy are fasting less than 95 mg/dl, 1-hour postprandial 140 mg/dl, and 2-hour postprandial less than 120 mg/dl.[32] Frequency of SMBG may be decreased once blood glucose control is established. However, some monitoring should continue throughout pregnancy.[46]

Recommended weight gains and nutrient requirements are the same as for established pregnancy guidelines.[57]

- Underweight (BMI <19.8): 28 to 40 lb
- Normal/healthy weight (BMI 19.8 to 26): 25 to 35 lb
- Overweight (BMI 26 to 29): 15 to 25 lb
- Obese (BMI >29): At least 15 lb

No kcalorie modifications are needed for the first trimester.[31,56] During the second and third trimesters, increased energy intake of approximately 100 to 300 kcalories/day is suggested.[31,56] High-quality protein should be increased by 10 g/day.[56] As with any pregnancy, 400 μg/day of folic acid is recommended for prevention of neural tube defects and other congenital abnormalities.[31] Alcohol consumption is not recommended in any amount.

The kcaloric restriction must be considered with care. A minimum of 1700 to 1800 kcalories/day of carefully selected foods has been shown to prevent ketosis.[58] Intakes below this level are not advised.[46] Weight gain goals are established using prepregnancy BMI. Weight gain should still occur even if patients have gained substantial weight before the onset of GDM.[46] Each patient with GDM should be evaluated individually by a registered dietitian, should have care plans fine-tuned, and should have patient education provided as required to realize weight goals.[46]

IMPAIRED FASTING GLUCOSE AND IMPAIRED GLUCOSE TOLERANCE

The terms *impaired fasting glucose (IFG)* and *impaired glucose tolerance (IGT)* refer to a metabolic stage somewhere between normal glucose homeostasis and overt diabetes. Although not clinical entities in their own right, these conditions are risk factors for future diabetes and cardiovascular disease.[2,12] Lifestyle interventions should be consistent with current guidelines for overweight and obesity and address cardiovascular risk factors and common concomitant conditions. The Da Quing IGT and Diabetes study provided preliminary evidence that diet and exercise intervention can lower the conversion to overt diabetes during the 6-year period.[21] The Finnish Diabetes Prevention Study demonstrated that a lifestyle change program could reduce the risk for developing diabetes by 58% during a 3-year period.[20] In the United States, the Diabetes Prevention Program (DPP) has confirmed the findings of the Finnish trial in a highly diverse American population with IGT. The DPP addressed how an intensive diet and exercise intervention compares with metformin in a three-arm randomized clinical trial that uses placebo as the third arm.[59]

Management of Diabetes Medical Nutrition Therapy

COUNSELING PROCESS IN MEDICAL NUTRITION THERAPY FOR DIABETES

MNT for diabetes is highly individualized. The American Diabetes Association recommendations clearly state that there is no one "diabetic" or "ADA" diet. Now the "recommended diet" is a dietary prescription based on individual nutritional assessment and treatment goals.[33] This new model emphasizes actions of the diabetes team clinical dietitian in an individualized, integrated four-point approach: assessment, goal setting, nutrition intervention, and evaluation.

1. *Assessment.* The first step involves a comprehensive assessment of the client's background. It includes clinical information, medical and lifestyle data such as personal self-monitoring of blood glucose, and dietary history. Interview follow-up tools such as questionnaires and food records assess general food patterns and nutrient intake.
2. *Goal setting.* The second step guides the client in setting up personal goals in the self-care of diabetes. To be valid, these goals must be reasonable and negotiable as follow-up experience may indicate.
3. *Nutrition intervention.* The third step guides the client in selecting and using the most appropriate meal-planning guide from the number that are now available, based on individual needs for knowledge and skills to change or maintain eating habits and daily living practices.
4. *Evaluation.* Together the client and dietitian evaluate goals and nutrition intervention, as well as ongoing clinical data, to help the client succeed at the established individual program. They then make any desired adjustments, and the dietitian provides continuing counseling and education as needed.

DIABETES MEAL PLANNING TOOLS

Since the DCCT there has been growing emphasis on selecting a planning approach that meets the needs of each client from a wide array of meal-planning guides. Regardless of the diabetes MNT management tool, the first vital principle in working with persons who have diabetes is to start where they are. Any food-planning process must focus first on the unique individual rather than on the "case" or disease. Numerous planning approaches are used by skilled and sensitive clinical dietitians who tailor their actions to the person's learning needs and abilities, nutritional needs, personal needs,

macrosomia Unusually large size.

and lifestyle issues. Because of the widespread use of the exchange lists as a dietary management tool, they are outlined in Appendix L.

PLANNING FOR SPECIAL NEEDS

Sick Days

When general illness occurs, food and insulin amounts must be adjusted accordingly. Texture may be modified as needed to use easily digested and absorbed liquid foods while still maintaining as much as possible glucose equivalents of the usual food plan.

Physical Activity

For any strenuous physical activity, the client with type 1 diabetes must make special plans ahead. This is particularly true of a young person with diabetes who is engaging in athletic practice or competition.[53,54] Energy demands of exercise are discussed in Chapter 14.

Travel

When a trip is planned, the clinical dietitian must confer with the client to guide food choices according to what will be available. Self-monitoring of blood glucose levels and insulin therapy equipment and making food plans are as important on vacation or a business trip as they are at home. The traveler always needs to plan ahead with the healthcare team (see *Practical Application* box).

Eating Out

Provide similar guidelines and suggestions for various situations when the client eats meals away from home. As a general rule, the plan must be made ahead of time; therefore accommodations for what is eaten at home before and after the meal eaten away from home reflect continuing balance needs of the day. Have the client get the menu ahead of time. Many restaurants are willing to fax their menus or they may be available on web sites.

Stress

Any form of emotional stress is reflected in variations of diabetes control.[60,61] These variations are caused by hormonal responses that act as antagonists to insulin. The clinical dietitian must help the client learn and practice a variety of useful stress-reduction activities.

Diabetes Education Program

GOAL: PERSON-CENTERED SELF-CARE

In past years the traditional medical model has guided diabetes education in its methods, language, and respective roles assumed. Professionals have viewed themselves as having major authoritative roles and have assigned to the person with diabetes the more passive role of "patient." With notable exceptions in certain places, this model has been followed in most cases. However, with the increasing movement toward changing roles of practitioners and consumers in the healthcare system, persons with diabetes are assuming a more active voice in planning and conducting their own care. Several barriers in our traditional system stem from three sources: (1) our culture, (2) our healthcare delivery system, and (3) our professional training habits. Essentially, much of the core problem focuses on communication. For example, a list of words we use too commonly that may be objectionable to persons with diabetes, along with the preferred language, include the following.

1. *"Diabetic"* used as a noun. The word *diabetic* is an adjective and should not be used alone as a noun. Use instead the phrase *person with diabetes.*
2. *Compliance.* The word *compliance* raises red flags in minds of persons with diabetes. It is a purely medical term and connotes an authoritative physician position. Instead, the word *adherence* should be used, which has been adopted by national committees and associations working in the field of diabetes. The word *adherence* indicates placement of more decision-making responsibility on the person with diabetes to determine courses of action in varying situations, which is, of course, the necessity.
3. *Patient.* Instead of *patient,* the phrase *person with diabetes* should be used. Persons with diabetes, like any other person, are patients only when they are in the hospital or seeing a physician for an illness.
4. *Cheating.* A particularly abusive word in the minds of many persons with diabetes, especially parents of children and young people with diabetes, is the word *cheating.* This flagrant language abuse suggests dishonesty or failure to live up to an external code. By and large, persons with diabetes do not "cheat." They may kid themselves or they may be inaccurate in their reporting, but they do not cheat. Instead phrases such as *having difficulty* or *having a problem with* should be used.

CONTENTS: TOOLS FOR SELF-CARE

A plan for diabetes education must recognize the need for building self-sufficiency and responsibility within persons with diabetes and their families. It should provide practical guidelines that build on necessary skills that a person with diabetes must have for the best possible control, as well as additional surrounding factors related to life situations and psychosocial needs. Content areas include needs in relation to the nature of diabetes, nutrition and basic meal-planning, insulin (or oral medication) effects and how to regulate them, monitoring of blood glucose, how to deal with illness, and, if relevant, urine ketones.

PRACTICAL APPLICATION
Travel and Illness: "Real-Life" Situations

People with diabetes do not stop living their lives just because they have diabetes. They still travel and they still catch colds and flu and other common illnesses. Special considerations to all areas of diabetes management will enhance safe traveling, as well as the traveler's health. What kind of information does the person with diabetes need to know when traveling or if he or she becomes too ill to eat? How did the tragic events of September 11, 2001, affect airline travel for persons with diabetes? The following are a few helpful hints you may want to offer clients for these common situations.

TRAVELING SAFELY WITH DIABETES

General Tips

1. Make sure there is sufficient medication (insulin or oral glucose-lowering medication) for the entire trip.
2. Carry some form of medical identification that includes type of diabetes, name, address, telephone number(s), emergency contact information, medications taken, physician's name and phone number, and additional relevant medical conditions. Preferably, this information should be worn on a necklace or bracelet (rather than carrying it in a wallet or purse).
3. Take extra snacks such as cereal bars, vanilla wafers, peanut butter crackers, or glucose tablets or gel.
4. Always keep insulin cool, especially if vacationing in the tropics or to the beach.
5. Keep some money available for food purchases if necessary. Change for a vending machine may be hard to come by.
6. Always carry blood glucose monitoring equipment. Blood glucose levels should be checked before beginning a trip, as well as every 2 hours. An extra check should be done anytime symptoms of hypoglycemia occur, even if recent blood glucose checks were acceptable.
7. Walking around and stretching every 2 to 4 hours helps stimulate circulation.
8. Whenever possible, travel with a companion.
9. Wear comfortable shoes.
10. Plan for time zone changes. Meal schedules may need to be revised to balance with insulin activity pattern.
11. If traveling abroad, learn to say the following in the local language: "I have diabetes. Please give me something sweet to drink."
12. If travel is frequent, contact a registered dietitian or diabetes educator for ideas for healthful, portable meals/snacks.

Driving Tips

1. If diabetes medication has potential to cause hypoglycemia, medications and meals will need to be timed during a long trip.
2. If diabetes medications have potential to cause hypoglycemia, food should be eaten before leaving home or snacks should be taken in the automobile. Traffic may not be conducive to stopping at a favorite store or restaurant for a quick meal or snack.
3. Keep nonperishable, carbohydrate-containing foods in the automobile in case of flat tires, traffic jams, or breakdowns occur. Handy, premeasured carbohydrate amounts may be beneficial to avoid over- or undereating. Replenish the food supply as needed to avoid running out an inopportune times.
4. Always carry blood glucose monitoring equipment when driving. Blood glucose levels should be checked before the trip begins, as well as every 2 hours while driving. An extra check should be done if symptoms of hypoglycemia occur (even if recent blood glucose checks have been acceptable).
5. An extra glucose meter should not be kept in automobiles. Internal automobile temperatures can get very hot and very cold. Strips and meters exposed to extreme temperatures may not be accurate or function properly.
6. High blood glucose levels may cause the following symptoms that can affect driving.
   - Fatigue related to the body's inability to use glucose for energy
   - Increased urination, causing preoccupation, repeated stops, and a delay in arriving at destination
   - Blurry vision, which may impair ability to see road signs clearly; blurry vision may be especially problematic at night or while driving in rain or snow
   - Numbness or tingling in hands or feet, which may impair perception or sensation steering or when applying pressure to gas or brake pedals
7. Prompt attention to hypoglycemia and treatment is necessary to prevent mental confusion and even losing consciousness. When blood glucose is low, the first organ affected is the brain! Keep appropriate sources of carbohydrates available in the automobile.
8. If driving hours at a time, it is important to stop the automobile, get out and stretch, and walk around every 2 to 4 hours.
9. Wear medical identification. Law enforcement officers may not be familiar with diabetes or symptoms of hypoglycemia or hyperglycemia. They can mistake impaired awareness and judgment for drunkenness.
10. Whenever possible, drive with a friend.
11. If driving over several hours, set an alarm as a reminder for blood glucose checks, meals, and even times to stretch and walk.
12. Visual disturbances can occur with either hyperglycemia or hypoglycemia.

Continued

PRACTICAL APPLICATION

Travel and Illness: "Real-Life" Situations—cont'd

13. If driving long distances, take twice as many diabetes supplies as thought to be needed. Be aware of all medicines taken (prescription and over-the-counter).
14. Always carry money for toll booths, parking, and telephone calls. Consider keeping a cell phone to call for assistance.

Flying Tips

1. Call ahead to airlines to advise them of the diabetes and supplies needed.
2. Carry a copy of physician's prescription for insulin and/or other medications.
3. Carry a letter from the physician explaining the need to carry syringes/injection devices and insulin.
4. If problems are encountered, request to speak to a manager or supervisor.
5. Carry insulin onto the aircraft. Insulin should not be packed in luggage that will be stored in the hold of an airplane. Low temperatures can damage the insulin.
6. Pack insulin and syringes/needles in a small, separate carrier bag so it can be handed to personnel aboard the plane if they request the syringes for safekeeping. The limit of one carry-on and one personal bag (e.g., purse or briefcase) for each traveler does not apply to medical supplies and/or assistive devices.

SICK DAY SURVIVAL

1. Keep taking diabetes medications even if solid foods cannot be eaten.
2. For insulin users, the physician may prescribe extra doses or increased amounts of insulin during an illness.
3. Blood glucose should be tested and recorded every 4 hours.
4. Test for ketones in urine if blood glucose level stays at or over 240 mg/dl for at least 4 hours.
5. Try to use regular meal plan/diet, but if that is not possible, soft foods or liquids can be consumed to take the place of carbohydrates usually eaten. Some easily digested foods to replace one serving (15 g) of carbohydrate include:
   - ⅓ to ½ cup fruit juice
   - ½ cup regular soft drink
   - ½ cup regular gelatin
   - ½ cup hot cereal
   - ½ cup vanilla ice cream
   - 1 cup broth-based soup
6. To prevent dehydration, sip 3 to 6 oz of noncaffeinated, sugar-free beverages or water every hour. Sugar-free fluids may be alternated with liquids containing sugar to help control blood glucose levels.
7. Keep a thermometer on hand to determine body temperature.
8. When buying over-the-counter medicines, choose one that is sugar-free. In addition to the word "sugar" on labels, "dextrose," "fructose," "lactose," "sorbitol," "mannitol," "xylitol," and "honey" indicate a product contains sugar.
9. Over-the-counter cold medications containing epinephrine-like compounds (including ephedrine, pseudoephedrine, phenylpropanolamine, phenylephrine, and epinephrine) can raise blood glucose levels and should only be used with a physician's approval.
10. *Planning ahead:* Keep the following items on hand in case of colds, flu, or other kinds of illnesses.
    - Thermometer
    - Urine test strips for ketones (check expiration date periodically)
    - Approved over-the-counter cold and flu medicines
    - Syringes or prescription for them (if insulin is not usually taken but is part of a sick day plan)
    - Short-acting insulin (keep refrigerated)
    - Extra prescriptions for all medications usually taken (or have on file at pharmacy)
    - Nonperishable foods such as noncaffeinated soft drinks (regular and diet), regular gelatin, popsicles, sport drinks, saltines, and canned fruit juices
11. Call the physician if any of the following occur.
    - Vomiting over several hours
    - Diarrhea recurring within 6 hours
    - Difficulty breathing
    - Blood glucose levels greater than 240 mg/dl for 24 hours if using oral medications; blood glucose levels greater than 240 mg/dl for 2 consecutive tests (4 hours apart) after taking supplemental insulin
    - Blood glucose levels less than 60 mg/dl
    - Moderate to large amounts of ketones in urine and no improvement after at least 12 hours
    - Signs of dehydration such as dry skin or mouth, sunken eyes, or weight loss
    - Sickness that continues from 12 to 48 hours without improvement
    - Increased fatigue
    - Stomach or chest pain
    - Temperature that stays at higher than 101° F
    - Acute loss of vision
12. When calling the physician, he or she will want to know blood glucose levels and urine ketone levels, how long the illness has lasted, what medicines have been taken, temperature, how much has been eaten or drunk, and other symptoms that have been experienced.

PRACTICAL APPLICATION
Travel and Illness: "Real-Life" Situations—cont'd

13. If necessary to go to the emergency department, staff should be informed of the diabetes.

In summary, in all cases the client must be advised to (1) maintain a steady intake of food every day, (2) replace the carbohydrate value of solid foods with that of liquid or soft foods as needed, (3) monitor blood and urine frequently for sugar and ketone levels, and (4) contact the physician if the illness lasts more than a day or so.

References

FAA Office of Public Affairs Press Releases: *FAA Advises air travelers on airport, airline security measures,* available at *http://www.faa.gov/apa/index.cfm.*

Hieronymus L, Cherolis J: On the road: driving safely with diabetes, *Diabetes Self-Manage* Nov/Dec 2001, available at *http://www.diabetesselfmanagement.com.*

Irons MJ: Fighting colds and flu, *Diabetes Self-Manage* Jan/Feb 1998, available at *http://www.diabetesself management.com.*

National Diabetes Information Clearinghouse: *What I need to know about eating and diabetes,* NIH Publication No. 02-5043, May 2002, available at *http://www.niddk.nih.gov/health/diabetes/pubs/eating/nutri.htm.*

The Diabetes Mall: FAA regulations for diabetes supplies, *Diabetes News* for Oct. 7, 2001, available at *http://www.diabetesnet.com/news/news100701.html.*

The Diabetes Pro: *Air travel with diabetes,* available at *http://www.diabetesnet.com/diabetes_information/diabetes_travel.php.*

UCL Hospitals: Traveling with your diabetes patients on insulin, *UCLH Diabetes* available at *http://www.uclh.org/services/diabetes/protocol/travel/travel_diab.shtml.*

U.S. Department of Transportation: *Fact sheet: steps taken to ensure new security requirements preserve and respect the civil rights of people with disabilities,* issued 10/29/01 by the Office of the Assistant General Counsel for Aviation Enforcement and Proceedings and its Aviation Consumer Protection Division, available at *http://www.pva.org/NEWPVASITE/newsroom/PR2001/pr01127.htm.*

EDUCATIONAL MATERIALS: PERSON-CENTERED STANDARDS

A broad, confusing array of diabetes education materials are available. Some are excellent, and some should be discarded. Whatever is used should measure up to several basic person-centered requirements by doing the following.

1. Give the intended receiver credit for having some intelligence and wanting new information.
2. Inform persons fully and completely, giving both sides when experts disagree—as they surely do on occasion.
3. Appeal to various levels of audience, ranging from basic to sophisticated.
4. Never be patronizing, dehumanizing, or childish.

Whatever methods or materials we use, one central fact remains: the person who has diabetes is the most important and a fully equal member of the diabetes care team. Interdisciplinary approaches and strategies that involve this recognition can be developed.

TO SUM UP

Diabetes mellitus is a syndrome composed of many metabolic disorders collectively characterized by hyperglycemia and other symptoms. Treatment relies heavily on a basic type of therapy—a carefully controlled diet. Diabetes is classified in four categories: type 1, type 2, GDM, and IGT.

Blood glucose levels are controlled primarily by hormones of pancreatic islet cells: insulin, which facilitates passage of glucose through cell membranes via special membrane receptors; glucagon, which ensures adequate levels of glucose to prevent hypoglycemia; and somatostatin, which controls the actions of insulin and glucagon to maintain normal blood glucose levels. Diabetes results from inadequate insulin secretion or insulin resistance from too few receptor sites. Symptoms range from polydipsia, polyuria, polyphagia, and signs of abnormal energy metabolism to fluid and electrolyte imbalances, acidosis, and coma in seriously uncontrolled conditions.

Type 1 affects about 5% to 10% of all persons with diabetes. It often develops during childhood or adolescence. Treatment involves blood glucose self-monitoring, insulin administration, and regular meals and exercise to balance insulin activity. Type 2 occurs mostly in adults, particularly those who are overweight. Acidosis is rare. Treatment consists of weight management and exercise. The food plan for both types of diabetes should be low in saturated fats and cholesterol to reduce cardiovascular risk. Moderate regular exercise increases efficiency of insulin and aids in weight management. GDM occurs in 2% to 5% of all pregnancies.

■ Questions for Review

1. Describe the major characteristics of type 1 and type 2 diabetes mellitus. Explain how these characteristics influence differences in nutrition therapy. List and describe medications used to control these conditions.
2. Identify and explain symptoms of uncontrolled chronic diabetes mellitus.
3. Describe three major complications of uncontrolled chronic diabetes and therapy used in the DCCT designed to achieve and maintain normal blood glucose levels and help avoid these complications.
4. Glenn just found out that he has diabetes mellitus. He is a sedentary, 45-year-old man who is 170 cm (5 ft 8 in) tall and weighs 94 kg (210 lb). No medications were prescribed for him. What is his BMI? If he decides to drink, how much alcohol could be allowed and how should he fit it into his diet? Defend your answer. Glenn wants to help his children reduce their chances of developing diabetes. What advice would you offer?

■ References

1. Centers for Disease Control and Prevention, Diabetes Press Release from CDC: *Diabetes rates rise another 6 percent in 1999,* available at *http://www.cdc.gov/diabetes/news/docs/010126.htm.*
2. Expert Committee: Report of the Expert Committee on the Diagnosis and Classification of Diabetes Mellitus, *Diabetes Care* 25:S5, 2002.
3. National Diabetes Information Clearinghouse: *National diabetes statistics: general information and national estimates on diabetes in the United States, 2000,* available at *http://www.niddk.nih.gov/health/diabetes/pubs/dmstats/dmstats.htm.*
4. Whitehouse FW: Classification and pathogenesis of the diabetes syndrome: a historical perspective, *J Am Diet Assoc* 81(3):243, 1982
5. Nestle et al: A case of diabetes mellitus, *N Engl J Med* 81:127, 1982.
6. Bliss M: *The discovery of insulin,* Chicago, 1982, University of Chicago Press.
7. Atkinson MA, Maclaren NK: The pathogenesis of insulin dependent diabetes, *N Engl J Med* 331:1428, 1994.
8. McKeigue PM et al: Relation of central obesity and insulin resistance with high diabetes prevalence and cardiovascular risk in South Asians, *Lancet* 337:382, 1991.
9. Dowse GK et al: Abdominal obesity and physical inactivity as risk factors for NIDDM and impaired glucose tolerance in Indian, Creole, and Chinese Mauritians, *Diabetes Care* 14(4):271, 1991.
10. Connell JE, Thomas-Doberson D: Nutritional management of children with insulin-dependent diabetes mellitus: a review by the Diabetes Care and Education Dietetic Practice Group, *J Am Diet Assoc* 91(12):1556, 1991.
11. Kissebah AH et al: Relation of body fat distribution to metabolic complications of obesity, *J Clin Endocrinol Metab* 54:254, 1982.
12. American Diabetes Association: Standards of medical care for patients with diabetes mellitus, *Diabetes Care* 25(suppl): 33S, 2002.
13. American Diabetes Association: Type 2 diabetes in children and adolescents, *Pediatrics* 105:671, 2000.
14. American Diabetes Association: Type 2 diabetes in children and adolescents, *Diabetes Care* 23:381, 2000.
15. Pinhas-Hamiel O: Type 2 diabetes: not just for grownups anymore, *Contemp Pediatr* 1:102, 2001.
16. Sinha R et al.: Prevalence of impaired glucose tolerance among children and adolescents with marked obesity, *N Engl J Med* 346:802, 2002.
17. Levetan C: Into the mouths of babes: the diabetes epidemic in children, *Clin Diabetes* 19:102, 2001.
18. Rosenbloom AL et al: Emerging epidemic of type 2 diabetes in youth, *Diabetes Care* 22:345, 1999.
19. American Diabetes Association: *The impact of diabetes,* available at *http://www.diabetes.org/main/info/facts/impact/default.jsp.*
20. Tuomilehto J et al: Prevention of type 2 diabetes mellitus by changes in lifestyle among subjects with impaired glucose tolerance, *N Engl J Med* 344:13453, 2001.
21. Pan XR et al: Effects of diet and exercise in preventing NIDDM in people with impaired glucose tolerance: the DaQing IGT and diabetes study, *Diabetes Care* 20:537, 1997.
22. National Institutes of Diabetes and Digestive and Kidney Diseases: Diet and exercise dramatically delay type 2 diabetes: diabetes medication metformin also effective, available at *http://www.niddk.nih.gov/welcome/releases/8_8_01.htm.*
23. Polonsky KS et al: Non–insulin-dependent diabetes mellitus—a genetically programmed failure of the beta cell to compensate for insulin resistance, *N Engl J Med* 334(12): 777, 1996.
24. Walston J et al: Time of onset of non–insulin-dependent diabetes mellitus and genetic variation in the β3-adrenergic receptor gene, *N Engl J Med* 333(6):343, 1995.
25. Wendorf M, Goldfine ID: Archeology of NIDDM-excavation of the thrifty genotype, *Diabetes* 40:161, 1991.
26. Bell GI: Molecular defects in diabetes mellitus, *Diabetes* 40:413, 1991.
27. Porte D Jr, Schwartz MW: Diabetes complications: why is glucose potentially toxic? *Science* 272(5262):699, 1996.
28. Clarke CM Jr, Lee DA: Prevention and treatment of the complications of diabetes mellitus, *N Engl J Med* 332(18): 1210, 1995.
29. Diabetes Control and Complications Trial Research Group: The effect of intensive treatment of diabetes on the development and progression of long-term complications in insulin-dependent diabetes mellitus, *N Engl J Med* 329:977, 1993.
30. Barner CW et al: WAVE: a pocket guide for a brief nutrition dialogue in primary care, *Diabetes Educ* 27:352, 2001.
31. Franz MJ et al: Evidence-based nutrition principles and recommendations for the treatment and prevention of diabetes and related complications, *Diabetes Care* 25:148, 2002.
32. American Diabetes Association: Translation of the diabetes nutrition recommendations for health care institutions, *Diabetes Care* 25(suppl):61S, 2002.
33. American Dietetic Association: Nutrition recommendations and principles for people with diabetes mellitus, *J Am Diet Assoc* 94(5):504, 1994.

34. Schlundt DG et al: Situational obstacles to dietary adherence for adults with diabetes, *J Am Diet Assoc* 94(8):874, 1994.
35. American Diabetes Association: Implications of the Diabetes Control and Complications Trial (position statement), *Diabetes Care* 25:S25, 2002, available at *http://care.diabetesjournals.org/cgi/content/full/25/suppl_1/s25*.
36. Delahanty LM, Halford BN: The role of diet behaviors in achieving improved glycemic control in intensively treated patients in the Diabetes Control and Complications Trial, *Diabetes Care* 16:1453, 1993.
37. Harris MI, Eastman RC: Is there a glycemic threshold for mortality risk? *Diabetes Care* 21:331, 1998.
38. Delahanty L et al: Expanded role of the dietitian in the Diabetes Control and Complications Trial: implications for clinical practice, *J Am Diet Assoc* 93(7):758, 1993.
39. Lyon RB, Vinci DM: Nutrition management of insulin-dependent diabetes mellitus in adults: review by the Diabetes Care and Education Dietetic Practice Group, *J Am Diet Assoc* 93(3):309, 1993.
40. Oxford Center for Diabetes, Endocrinology and Metabolism Diabetes Trials Unit: *UK prospective diabetes study*, available at *http://www.dtu.ox.ac.uk/ukpds/results.html*.
41. Robertson KE: What the UKPDS really says about cardiovascular disease and glycemic control, *Clin Diabetes* 17:109, 1999.
42. Ousman Y, Sharma M: The irrefutable importance of glycemic control, *Clin Diabetes* 19:71, 2001.
43. American Diabetes Association: Implications of the United Kingdom Prospective Diabetes Study, (position statement), *Diabetes Care* 25:S28, 2002.
44. Orland MJ: Diabetes mellitus. In Carey CF, Lee HH, Woeltje KF, eds: *The Washington manual of medical therapeutics,* ed 29, Philadelphia, 1998, Lippincott Williams & Wilkins.
45. American Diabetes Association: Gestational diabetes mellitus (position statement), *Diabetes Care* 25(suppl):94S, 2002.
46. Reader D, Sipe M: Key components of care for women with gestational diabetes, *Diabetes Spectrum* 14:188, 2001.
47. American Diabetes Association: Gestational diabetes mellitus (position statement), *Diabetes Care* 24:77S, 2001.
48. Anderson EJ et al: The DCCT Research Group: nutrition interventions for the intensive therapy in the Diabetes Control and Complications Trial, *J Am Diet Assoc* 93(7):768, 1993.
49. Thom S: Humalog (insulin lispro): nutritional implications and educational considerations, *On Cutting Edge* 17(4):8, 1996.
50. Trautmann ME et al: Intensive insulin therapy with insulin lispro in patients with type I diabetes reduces the frequency of hypoglycemia episodes, *Endocrinol Diabetes* 104:25, 1996.
51. Setter SM: New drug therapies for the treatment of diabetes, *On Cutting Edge* 19(2):3, 1998.
52. Hayes C: Pattern management: a tool for improving blood glucose control with exercise, *On Cutting Edge* 17(4):4, 1996.
53. Joyce M, King J: Consideration in selecting appropriate blood glucose monitoring devices, *On Cutting Edge* 17(4): 16, 1996.
54. Gregory RP et al: Nutrition management of a collegiate football player with insulin-dependent diabetes: guidelines and a case study, *J Am Diet Assoc* 94(4):775, 1994.
55. Beebe C: Implementation of the 1994 Nutrition Recommendations in Clinical Practice: NIDDM, *On Cutting Edge* 16(2):11, 1995.
56. Metzger BE, Coustan DR, eds: Proceedings of the fourth international workshop conference on gestational diabetes mellitus, *Diabetes Care* 21(suppl):1B, 1998.
57. American Dietetic Association: *Manual of clinical dietetics,* ed 6, Chicago, 2000, The Association.
58. Rizzo T et al: Correlations between antepartum maternal metabolism and intelligence of offspring, *N Engl J Med* 325:911, 1991.
59. Diabetes Prevention Program Research Group: The diabetes prevention program: recruitment methods and results, *Control Clin Trials* 23:157, 2002.
60. Holler HJ, Pastors JG: *Diabetes medical nutrition therapy: a professional guide to management and nutrition education,* Chicago, 1996, American Dietetic Association.
61. Chapman KM et al: Applying behavioral models to dietary education of elderly diabetic patients, *J Nutr Educ* 27(2):75, 1995.

■ Further Reading

Gregory RP et al: Nutrition management of a collegiate football player with insulin-dependent diabetes: guidelines and a case study, *J Am Diet Assoc* 94(7):775, 1994.

This interesting account of balancing insulin, high level of physical activity, and a daily training diet of 6200 kcalories relates a sample game day schedule of meals and interval blood tests with related amounts of a sports drink before the game, at half-time, and after the game. This college athlete had no problem finishing the 11-game season (his senior year) with excellent game performances.

Warshaw H: *Guide to healthy restaurant eating,* ed 2, Chicago, 2002, American Diabetes Association.

This useful book reviews more than 3500 menu items from over 55 major restaurant chains. Nutrition information is included for kcalories, fat, percent kcalories from fat, saturated fat, cholesterol, sodium, carbohydrate, fiber, and protein with serving sizes and/or exchanges for each item. Restaurant pitfalls and strategies for "defensive" restaurant dining are included.

■ Websites of Interest

- ***http://ndep.nih.gov*** National Diabetes Education Program (NDEP) (1-800-860-8747)

The NDEP is a federally sponsored initiative that involves public and private partnerships to improve the treatment and outcomes for people with diabetes through a variety of activities. The NDEP publications include a newsletter, materials for people with diabetes (in several languages), materials for health-care providers, materials for organization and media kits. Single copies of most materials are available free of charge or can be downloaded from the NDEP website.

- ***http://diabetes.org*** American Diabetes Association (ADA) (1-800-DIABETES)

The American Diabetes Association publishes many health professional and client material in addition to its scientific journals. In an annual supplement to *Diabetes Care,* the ADA reissues its practice guidelines that address a wide array of clinical issues including nutrition. These guidelines can be downloaded from the ADA website free of charge. Local information about ADA activities can be obtained from either the website or the 800 number. Diabetes self-management educational programs that are reviewed and receive ADA "recognition" are covered by Medicare and other third-party payers.

- ***http://eatright.org*** or ***http://www.dce.org*** Diabetes Care and Education (DCE) Practice Group of the American Dietetic Association

The DCE publishes *On the Cutting Edge,* a theme-centered newsletter on timely topics related to nutrition and diabetes. Educational materials develop by the DCEP are available for purchase from the ADA. The DCE website provides information about the Medicare MNT benefits for persons with diabetes, Health Care Financing Administration (HFCA) rules for ADA Education Recognition Programs reimbursement, and CPT codes for MNT. The website also provides information about the DCE publications and email listserv.

- ***http://www.cdc.gov/diabetes*** Division of Diabetes Translation of the Centers for Disease Control and Prevention (1-877-CDC-DIAB)

The website has information about the Diabetes Control Program in each state and diabetes-related statistics such as the rise in the prevalence and incidence of diabetes. The National Diabetes Fact Sheet *CDC Information* is available as a downloadable file.

- ***http://www.niddk.nih.gov/health/diabetes/diabetes.htm*** National Institutes of Diabetes & Digestive & Kidney Diseases (NIDDK)

The NIDDK website provides information about its diabetes-related clinical trials and other research programs, a directory of diabetes organizations, health education programs, and diabetes-related topics. Downloadable files include *Diabetes Dateline,* an NIDDK newsletter; client education materials; and information for health professionals. The NIDDK website also includes the National Diabetes Information Clearinghouse, which disseminates information about online and print materials and provides access to database searches for diabetes-related references.

- ***http://aadenet.org*** American Association of Diabetes Educators (AADE)

As a multidisciplinary organization of health professionals who teach about diabetes, the AADE and its website provide information about the scope of practice and standards related to diabetes education. The website also has information and AADE publications.

CASE STUDY: The patient with type 1 diabetes

Angela is a 35-year-old woman diagnosed 2 years ago with type 2 diabetes. She has three children whose birth weights were in the range of 4.5 to 5 kg (10 to 11 lb). The children, now teenagers, show no signs of diabetes, and their weights are reported to be within normal limits despite their mother's fondness for cooking. Her husband, an underpaid construction worker, is slightly overweight.

Six months ago, Angela was seen with a complaint of a series of infections that lasted longer than usual during the past 2 months. At that time she was measured as 165 cm (5 ft 5 in) and 71 kg (156 pounds). Her glucose tolerance test was positive. She was seen for follow-up twice during the following month, each time showing hyperglycemia and glycosuria. At the second follow-up, an oral antidiabetic medication was prescribed, and she was referred for MNT.

Angela did not keep this appointment or her subsequent medical appointment. She was not seen again until 1 month ago, when she was seen in the emergency department with ketoacidosis. She responded well to treatment and was placed on a 1200-kcalorie diet and a mixture of intermediate- and rapid-acting insulin given in two injections a day. Her discharge plan included a referral for MNT consultation session and diabetes education classes.

QUESTIONS FOR ANALYSIS

1. What factors do you think contributed to the ketoacidosis? Why?
2. What relation do these factors have to diabetes control?
3. Why did Angela first appear to have type 2 diabetes?
4. Assume that Angela administers insulin before breakfast and before the evening meal. What additional information is necessary to develop an individualized meal plan?
5. Identify any personal factors that may affect Angela's follow-through with her treatment plan. Do you anticipate any problems?
6. If so, how would you attempt to help her solve them?
7. Outline a diabetes education plan for Angela.

Issues & ANSWERS

Nutrition Questions From Persons With Diabetes

Persons with diabetes have many questions about their diets especially when they are newly diagnosed and anxieties are high. They do not want just a "Yes" or "No" answer. For any item of concern, they want to know if it can be used at all and if use is limited, why, and by how much. Questions about alcohol and various sweeteners are common.

Alcohol and diabetes: do they mix?

People with diabetes should follow the same sensible drinking guidelines as people without diabetes.

- Use alcohol only in moderation (1 drink/day for women, 2 drinks/day for men).
    - 1 drink = 12 oz regular beer, 5 oz wine, or 1.5 oz of 80-proof distilled spirits (whiskey, Scotch, rye, vodka, brandy, cognac, rum).
- Never drink alcohol on an empty stomach.
- Some medications may not mix with alcohol; check with physician or pharmacist.
- Never drink and drive.
- Never drink if pregnant or trying to become pregnant.
- Above all, use common sense.

Having diabetes should not prevent consumption of alcohol; however, some considerations must be made. Alcohol can cause hyperglycemia and hypoglycemia. Alcohol moves very quickly from the stomach into the bloodstream; it does not require digestion or metabolism. Thirty to 90 minutes after an alcoholic drink, alcohol in the bloodstream is at its highest concentration. Because the liver plays the biggest role in removing alcohol from the blood, it stops making glucose while cleansing alcohol from the body. If blood glucose levels are falling during the same time, hypoglycemia can occur very quickly. For those taking insulin or oral hypoglycemic agents, they too are lowering blood glucose levels. This is why two shots of whiskey on an empty stomach lowers blood sugar dramatically.

Alcohol is high in kcalories (and low in food value) and can raise blood glucose, especially if mixed with sweet mixers, fruit juices, or ice cream. Two ounces of 90-proof alcohol contain almost 200 kcalories. Wine coolers, liqueurs, and port wines are also high in sugar and kcalories. This can interfere with weight loss goals and practicing tight control. Alcohol also increases serum cholesterol levels, although this effect is transient. And it can lead to hyperlipoproteinemia with high triglyceride levels in susceptible persons, including persons with diabetes, when it is excessive. Alcohol can also make neuropathy and retinopathy worse.

For clients who choose to use alcohol, they should ask themselves three basic questions.

1. Is my diabetes under control?
2. Does my healthcare provider agree that I am free from health problems that alcohol can make worse (e.g., high blood pressure, neuropathy)?
3. Do I know how alcohol can affect me and my diabetes?

If "yes" is the answer to all three questions, then it is okay for him or her to have an occasional drink. In addition to the sensible drinking guidelines listed earlier, the following also need to be discussed.

- Discuss the use of alcohol with your physician or dietitian.
- Drink with caution and carry identification.
- Pick drinking buddies wisely. (Make sure at least one friend or trusted companion knows that you have diabetes and is aware of what should be done in case of hypoglycemia.)
- Have a snack before going to bed to prevent hypoglycemia during sleep.
- A person with diabetes should not drink if he or she is practicing tight control (alcohol impairs judgment); has neuropathy, hypertriglyceridemia, or hypertension; is taking Diabinese (causes nausea, flushing, headache, or dizziness when mixed with alcohol); or is taking Glucophage (can cause lactic acidosis).
- Always sip alcoholic drinks slowly.
- Male clients **taking insulin** can include two alcoholic beverages in addition to their regular meal plan. Women can include one alcoholic beverage. No food should be omitted in exchange for an alcoholic drink.
- Clients who are **not taking insulin** (and who are watching their weight) should substitute alcohol for fat choices and in some cases extra starch choices (sweet wines, sweet vermouth, and wine coolers).

Can I use fructose in my diabetic diet?

How would you answer this question from your diabetic client? Fructose has been touted as a sweetener for persons with diabetes because it is a naturally occurring sugar that is as much as 1 to 1½ times as sweet as sucrose. But can the person with diabetes use it safely?

Although fructose as a sweetener is not for all persons with diabetes, generally you can reply, "Yes, but with qualifications."

- Advertising claims promoting fructose are sometimes so misleading that many consumers mistakenly believe that it can be used as a "free" food. However, fructose has the same nutritive value as other sugars—4 kcalories/g. Persons with type 1 diabetes should especially be instructed to use fructose as carefully as they use any other food with a caloric and carbohydrate value.
- The quantity must be limited. If used, the maximum amount is 75 g/day.
- Consumption of fructose in large amounts may have adverse effects on plasma lipids.
- The sweetness of fructose varies with temperature, acidity, and dilution. It has been used satisfactorily in some cooked desserts. However, with high temperatures, a rise in pH, and increased concentration of solution, its sweetness is reduced.

REFERENCES

American Diabetes Association: *Alcohol, alcohol, everywhere: but is it safe to drink?* available at *http://www.diabetes.org*.

Detroit Medical Center: *Nutrition for diabetics: use of alcohol,* available at *http://www.sinaigrace.org/health_info/topics/nutr3311.html*.

Department of Nutrition and Dietetics, The Ohio State University: *Health for life: alcohol and diabetes,* available at *http://www.osu.edu/units/osuhosp/patedu/homedocs.pdf/nut-diet.pdf/nut-othe.pdf/alc-diab.pdf*.

Ford-Martin P: *Drinking while diabetic: a guide to safely imbibing, and knowing when to just say no,* available at *http://diabetes.about.com/library/weekly/aa031201a.htm*.

Franz MJ et al: Evidence-based nutrition principles and recommendations for the treatment and prevention of diabetes and related complications, *Diabetes Care* 25:148, 2002.

Joslin Diabetes Center: *Managing diabetes: fitting alcohol into your meal plan,* available *http://www.joslin.org/education/library/index.shtml*.

Stockwell P: Alcohol and diabetes, available at *http://www.faqs.org/faqs/diabetes/faq/part3/section-20.html*.

University of Michigan Health System: *Diabetes: the use of alcohol,* available at *http://www.med.umich.edu/1libr/topics/diabet07.htm*.

Chapter

21

Renal Disease

D. Jordi Goldstein-Fuchs

Chapter Outline

This chapter reviews basic kidney function and pathophysiology of kidney diseases. Nutrition assessment methodology and nutrition recommendations for chronic kidney disease (CKD), maintenance dialysis therapy, postrenal transplantation, acute renal failure (ARF), renal stones, and urinary tract infection (UTI) are discussed.

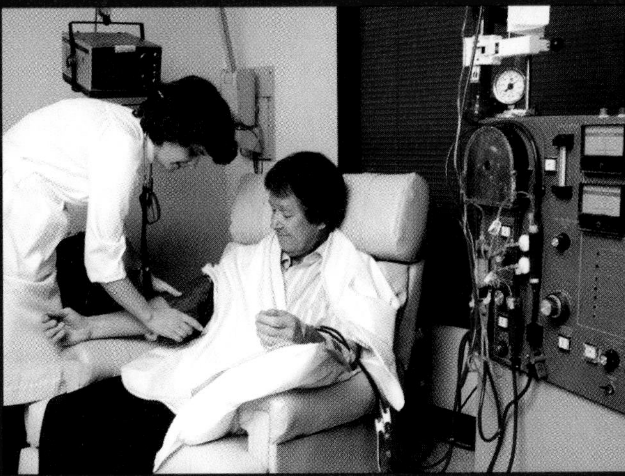

Basic Kidney Function

The main functions of the kidney are excretory, regulatory, and endocrine. The excretory function serves to remove potentially toxic metabolic waste products such as urea, the major end product of protein metabolism, from the blood. The regulatory function controls electrolyte, acid-base, and fluid balance. The result is maintenance of the proper serum concentrations of sodium, potassium, calcium, phosphorus, chloride, bicarbonate, and hydrogen ions. The endocrine functions include the conversion of the biologically inactive form of vitamin D (25-hydroxycholecaliciferol) to the biologically active vitamin D (1,25-dihydroxycholecalciferol), the synthesis of erythropoietin (needed for red blood cell production in the bone marrow), and the synthesis and release of renin, which regulates systemic blood pressure.[1-4]

These functions are accomplished by the unique architecture of the nephron, the basic functioning unit of the kidney. Each human adult kidney consists of approximately 1 million nephrons (Figure 21-1). The key structures of the nephron are the glomerulus and the tubules.[4]

GLOMERULUS

At the head of each nephron, blood enters in a single capillary and then branches into a group of collateral capillaries. This tuft of collateral capillaries is held closely together in a cup-shaped membrane. This cup-shaped capsule is named *Bowman's capsule* for the young English physician Sir William Bowman. In 1843 Bowman established the basis of plasma filtration and consequent urine secretion from the interrelationship of the blood-filled glomeruli and the enveloping membrane. The filtrate formed here is cell free and virtually protein free.

TUBULES

Continuous with the base of Bowman's capsule, the nephron tubules wind in a series of convolutions toward their terminal in the renal pelvis. Specific reabsorption functions performed by the four sections of the tubule are the following.

1. *Proximal tubule.* In the first section nearest the glomerulus, major nutrient reabsorption occurs. Essentially 100% of the glucose and amino acids and 80% to 85% of the water, sodium, potassium, chloride, and most other substances are reabsorbed. Only 15% to 30% of the filtrate remains to enter the next section.
2. *Loop of Henle.* This narrowed midsection of the renal tubule is named for the German anatomist Friedrich Henle, who in 1845 first demonstrated its unique

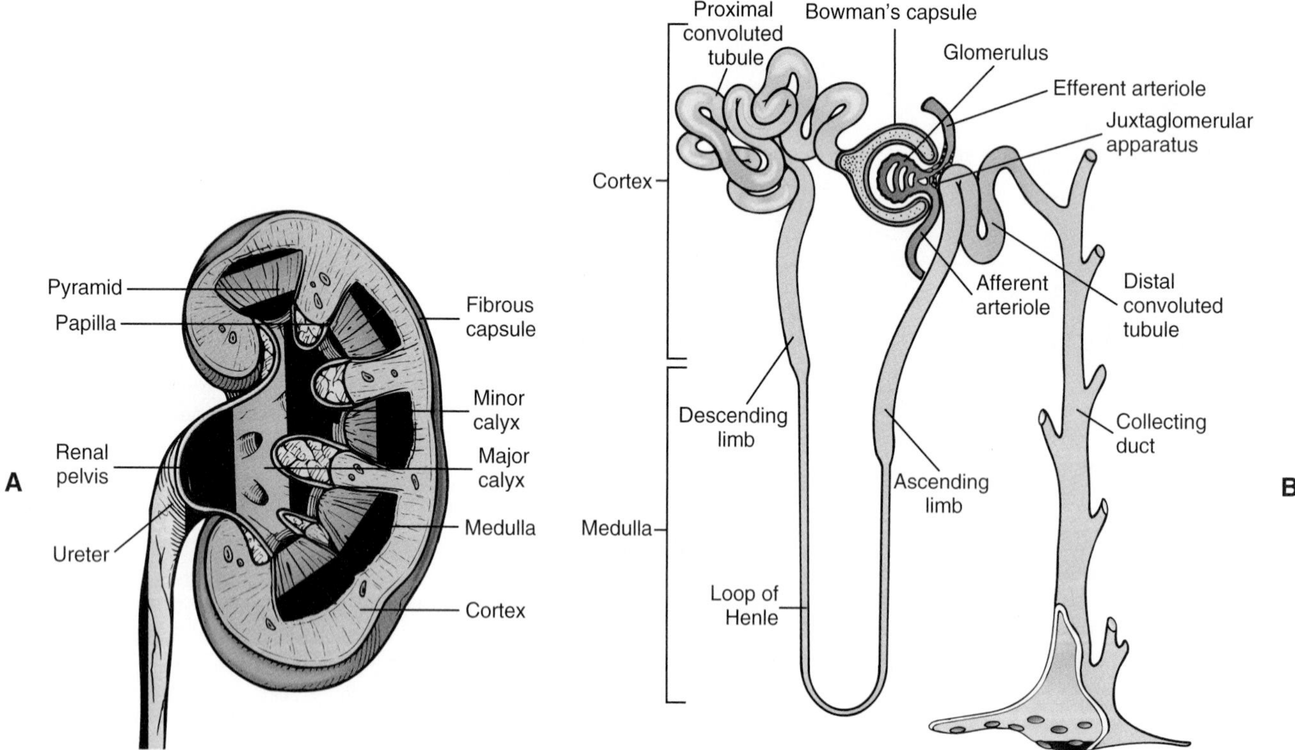

FIGURE 21-1 A, Longitudinal section of the kidney. B, Nephron of the kidney. (*From Lewis SM, Collier IC, Heitkemper MM:* Medical-surgical nursing: assessment and management of clinical problems, *ed 4, St Louis, 1996, Mosby.*)

structure and function in creating the necessary fluid pressures for ultimately forming a concentrated urine. At this narrowed midsection, the thin loop of the tubule dips into the central renal medulla. Here, through a balanced system of water and sodium exchange through sodium pumps in the limbs of the loop (the countercurrent system), important fluid density is created surrounding the loop. This area of increased density in the central part of the kidney is important to concentrate the urine through osmotic pressure as the lower collecting tubule later passes through this same area of the kidney.

3. *Distal tubule.* This latter portion of the tubule functions primarily in providing acid-base balance through secretion of ionized hydrogen. It also conserves sodium by reabsorbing it under the influence of the hormones aldosterone and vasopressin (also called antidiuretic hormone [ADH]).
4. *Collecting tubule.* In this final widened section of the tubule, the filtrate is concentrated to save water and form urine for excretion. Water is absorbed under the influence of the pituitary hormone vasopressin (ADH) and the osmotic pressure of the more dense surrounding fluid in this central part of the kidney. The resulting volume of urine, now concentrated and excreted, is only 0.5% to 1% of the original water and solutes filtered at the beginning in Bowman's capsule.

It is through these specialized anatomic components that the kidney serves to maintain homeostasis of the body's internal environment.[2,4]

Chronic Kidney Disease

Chronic renal failure is a disease syndrome in which progressive, irreversible losses of the excretory, endocrine, and metabolic capacities of the kidney occur as a result of kidney damage. Determination of renal function requires evaluation of the glomerular filtration rate (GFR), which is accomplished through clearance tests. Clearance tests measure the rate at which substances are cleared from the plasma by the glomerulus.[5] In clinical practice, the GFR is best approximated by using prediction equations and factoring in the serum creatinine concentration, age, gender, race, and body size. Recommended prediction equations for adults are the Modification of Diet in Renal Disease (MDRD) study and Cockroft-Gault equations.[6] A normal GFR is 125 ml/min/1.73 m^2.[5] As kidney disease progresses, the GFR falls. Chronic renal failure progresses slowly over time and may include periods during which kidney function remains stable. However, once the disease progresses to end stage (GFR $<$15 ml/min/1.73 m^2), continuance of life requires the initiation of maintenance dialysis therapy or subsequent kidney transplantation.[7]

CKD is a public health problem. The incidence and prevalence of end-stage renal disease (ESRD) has doubled in the United States during the past decade.[8] In 1998 the prevalence rate was 1160 per million. In 1999 the rate increased to 1217 per million.[9] The point prevalence on December 31, 1998, was more than 1160 per million population, of which 835 per million population were receiving dialysis replacement therapy. Of the group being treated by dialysis, 97 per million were over 70 years of age compared with 2.1 per million being children.[10] The total cost for the ESRD program continues to increase. In 1997 the cost was $15.64 billion; in 1998, $16.7 billion; and in 1999, $17.9 billion.[8,9]

The life expectancy for a person with ESRD is significantly below that of the general U.S. population. For example, a 40- to 44-year-old person on dialysis has a projected 6.6 to 10.9 years of additional life compared with the expected 37.4 years for a person of the same age without disease.[9] CKD is accompanied by significant comorbidities, including cardiovascular disease (CVD), malnutrition, and anemia. Lost working days and income, frequent intercurrent illness, and psychosocial adjustments all lend to a difficult life quality.

The most common causes of ESRD are diabetic nephropathy and hypertension. In 1999 43% of new cases of CKD were the result of diabetes and 26% were the result of hypertension.[9] Other common causes of kidney failure include glomerulonephritis, cystic kidney disease, and urologic disease.[9] Table 21-1 lists a classification of kidney disease.

dialysis Process of separating crystalloids and colloids in solution by the difference in their rates of diffusion through a semipermeable membrane; crystalloids pass through readily and colloids pass through only very slowly or not all.

glomerulonephritis A form of nephritis affecting the capillary loops in an acute short-term infection. It may progress to a more serious chronic condition leading to irreversible renal failure.

medulla Inner tissue substance of the kidney.

nephron Microscopic anatomic and functional unit of the kidney that selectively filters and resorbs essential blood factors, secretes hydrogen ions as needed for maintaining acid-base balance, and then resorbs water to protect body fluids and forms and excretes a concentrated urine for elimination of wastes. The nephron includes the renal corpuscle (glomerulus), the proximal convoluted tubule, the loop of Henle, the distal convoluted tubule, and the collecting tubule, which empties the urine into the renal medulla. The urine passes into the papilla and then to the pelvis of the kidney. Urine is formed by filtration of blood in the glomerulus and by the selective reabsorption and secretion of solutes by cells that comprise the walls of the renal tubes. There are approximately 1 million nephrons in each kidney.

TABLE 21-1 Simplified Classification of Chronic Kidney Disease by Diagnosis

Disease	Major Types (Examples)
Diabetic kidney disease	Type 1 and type 2 diabetes
Nondiabetic kidney disease	Glomerular diseases (autoimmune diseases, systemic infections, drugs, neoplasia) Vascular diseases (large vessel disease, hypertension, microangiopathy) Tubulointerstitial diseases (urinary tract infection, stones, obstruction, drug toxicity) Cystic diseases (polycystic kidney disease)
Diseases in the transplant	Chronic rejection Drug toxicity (cyclosporine or tacrolimus) Recurrent diseases (glomerular diseases) Transplant glomerulopathy

From National Kidney Foundation: K/DOQI clinical practice guidelines for chronic kidney disease: evaluation, classification and stratification, *Am J Kidney Dis* 39(suppl 1):s1-s266, 2002.

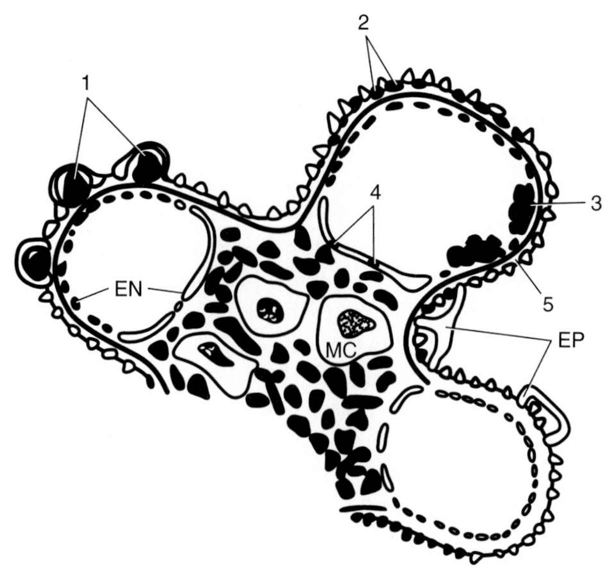

FIGURE 21-2 Schematic depiction of the anatomy of the glomerulus and possible intraglomerular sites of immune complex deposition. (*From Couser WG: Mechanisms of glomerular injury in immune-complex disease,* Kidney Int *28:569, 1985.*)

PATHOPHYSIOLOGY OF GLOMERULAR DISEASE

The majority of nondiabetic glomerular diseases are the result of immune-mediated mechanisms. Although renal injury induced by antibody alone is known to occur, the mechanisms involved in renal injury resulting from antigen-antibody complex formation are better understood. Antigen-antibody complex formation occurs as a result of antibody reacting either to circulating antigens or to native kidney antigens expressed on renal cell membranes. Immune complex deposition may occur within the glomerular basement membrane (GBM), between the GBM and epithelial cell (subepithelial), between the GBM and endothelial cell (subendothelial), or within the mesangial matrix. The pattern of immune complex deposition within the glomerulus is helpful diagnostically because different diseases have characteristic patterns.[4,11,12] For example, membranous nephropathy is characterized in part by subepithelial immune complex deposition (Figures 21-2 and 21-3).

Deposition of immune complexes leads to activation of the complement system, which mediates injury through inflammatory or noninflammatory mechanisms. Chemotactic complement components formed as products of the activated complement cascade result in the migration of inflammatory cells into glomeruli. These cells, which include platelets, macrophages, and polymorphonuclear neutrophils (leukocytes), all produce products that are either directly cytotoxic or serve as mediators for further cell or matrix injury (e.g., proteases, reactive oxygen species, lipid mediators, and cytokines). When subepithelial immune complexes activate complement, a noninflammatory mechanism is responsible for glomerular injury.[4,11,12]

TREATMENT OF KIDNEY DISEASE

The approach to the treatment of kidney disease has shifted focus from diagnosis and treatment of established kidney diseases to detection and treatment at much earlier stages.[13] Studies in patients with diabetic nephropathy have demonstrated that the clinical course of this disease can be significantly improved if specific interventions are instituted early in the development of the disease. These include annual screening for microalbuminuria ($\geq$30 mg/day or 20 μg/min of albumin in the urine); improving glycemic control; aggressive antihypertensive therapy with angiotensin-converting enzymes or angiotensin receptor blockers; and lifestyle modifications that include weight loss, reduction in salt and alcohol intake, and exercise.[14]

Less traditional interventions that have been explored for their beneficial effects on renal disease include nutrients such as amino acids and carbohydrates. A class of nutrients that continues to be investigated for potential benefits on progression of renal disease is the omega-3 fatty acids (see *To Probe Further* box.)

Through their initiative entitled "K/DOQI: Kidney Disease Outcomes Quality Initiative," The National Kidney Foundation recently published clinical practice guide-

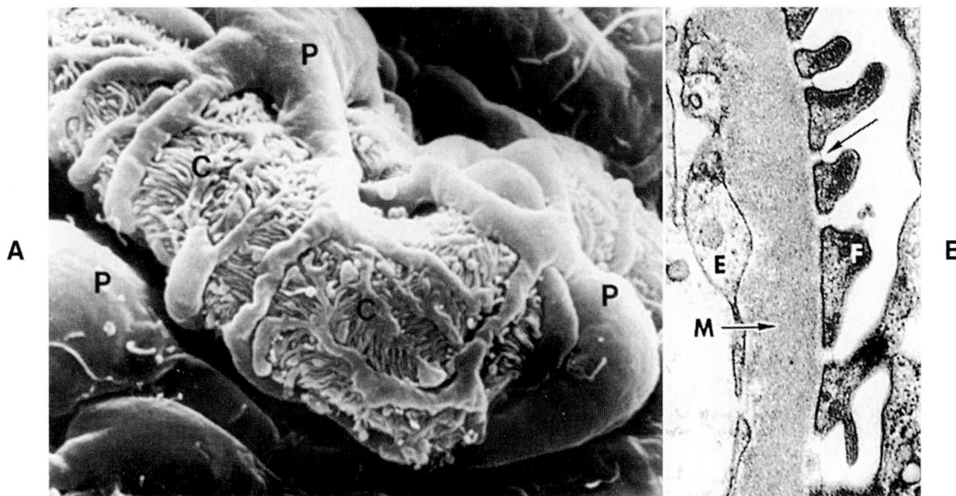

FIGURE 21-3 Glomerular capillary. **A,** Scanning electron micrograph of normal glomerular capillary *(C)* enclosed by podocytes *(P)* with primary processes and interdigitating foot processes. **B,** Glomerular capillary wall showing foot processes of endothelial podocytes *(F),* filtration slit membrane *(arrow),* basement membrane *(M),* and fenestrated endothelium *(E)* (magnification, ×40,000). *(From Kissane JM, ed:* Anderson's pathology, *ed 9, St Louis, 1990, Mosby.)*

lines for the evaluation, classification, and stratification of CKD.[15] A main rationale for the development of these clinical guidelines was the accumulation of evidence that the adverse effects of CKD including kidney failure, CVD, and premature death can be prevented or delayed by earlier testing and treatment of CKD.[13]

The K/DOQI guidelines for CKD recommend that all individuals during health evaluations be evaluated as to whether they are at increased risk of having or developing renal disease. Patients are to be considered at risk if they have diabetes, hypertension, autoimmune diseases, systemic infections, exposure to drugs or procedures associated with acute decline in kidney function, recovery from acute kidney failure, age greater than 60 years, family history of kidney disease, or reduced kidney mass.[16] Table 21-2 identifies stages of disease and associates that stage with a level of GFR and clinical manifestations. As the GFR falls below 60 ml/min/1.73 m^2, nutritional intervention becomes an important component of medical care.

MALNUTRITION, MORBIDITY, AND INFLAMMATION

Malnutrition is a significant comorbidity of chronic renal failure, including patients on hemodialysis or peritoneal dialysis therapy.[17,18] The prevalence of malnutrition and characterization of the nutritional status of the predialysis patient with chronic, progressive disease have not been definitively described. The largest set of data concerning the nutritional status of the patient with chronic kidney disease is available from the MDRD study.[19] This study reported correlations between GFRs, diet intake, and indices of nutritional status, including serum albumin, transferrin, and body weight. The earliest relationship reported was for GFRs equivalent to serum creatinine levels in the ranges of approximately 2.3 and 2.5 mg/dl for females and males, respectively (GFR = 35 ml/min/1.73 m^2). As kidney failure progressed as evidenced by worsening GFR, there was a deterioration in nutritional status. Being that the MDRD study excluded patients who presented with malnutrition, the overall prevalence of malnutrition in this patient group could not be calculated.

The nutritional status of the patient on maintenance dialysis therapy has been widely documented. Surveys report 23% to 76% of patients on hemodialysis and 18% to 50% of patients on peritoneal dialysis therapy are malnourished.[17] Life-threatening malnutrition is present in 5% to 10% of patients and moderate malnutrition is present in an

complement A complex series of enzymatic proteins occurring in normal serum that interact to combine with and augment (fill out, complete) the antigen-antibody complex of the body's immune system, producing lysis when the antigen is an intact cell; composed of 11 discrete proteins or functioning components, activated by the immunoglobulin factors IgG and IgM.
hemodialysis Removal of certain elements from the blood according to their rates of diffusion through a semipermeable membrane—e.g., by a hemodialysis machine.
peritoneal dialysis Dialysis through the peritoneum into and out of the peritoneal cavity.

TO PROBE FURTHER
Omega-3 Fatty Acids and Renal Disease

Recent statistics available report there are currently 300,000 Americans living with the diagnosis of end-stage renal disease (ESRD).[1] Despite countless research efforts, the mechanisms responsible for the progressive nature of renal disease remain elusive. Historically, nutrition science has been an inherent component of research directed toward identifying nutrient manipulations that ameliorate kidney disease, metabolic abnormalities associated with chronic renal insufficiency, and mechanisms by which nutrients modulate factors involved in promoting exacerbation of existing disease. In all of these research areas, dietary protein, phosphorus, and caloric deprivation have been more widely studied than other nutrients. However, more recently there has been a shift of research interest directed toward dietary essential fatty acids (EFAs). This shift is in response to a growing body of evidence indicating that fatty acid substitution of cell membrane phospholipids modulates biochemical pathways implicated in both the pathophysiology of progressive kidney disease and the CVD so prominent in the renal patient population.

It has been demonstrated that altering the availability of EFAs can influence the natural course of several important diseases in the mammalian organism. For example, epidemiologic studies of the Dutch, Japanese, and native Greenland Eskimo populations attribute their low incidence of heart disease to a fish diet high in omega-3 fatty acids. Several investigations exploring the effects of polyunsaturated fatty acid–supplemented diets in experimental immune and nonimmune models of renal disease have been reported.[1-7] Beneficial observations have included an improved lipid profile, prolonged survival, and improved renal function.

Dietary EFAs are the direct precursors to the biologically diverse and potent class of compounds called eicosanoids. EFAs can also modulate cellular production of interleukins. Several chronic inflammatory and renal diseases are characterized in part by an overproduction of eicosanoids and interleukins. These facts, which have been demonstrated in animal and some human studies, suggest that manipulation of dietary fatty acids might contribute a therapeutic influence by altering proinflammatory and other activated pathways in disease processes. In vitro, manipulation of fatty acids has been found to modify macrophage function, production of vasoactive substances, and membrane signal transduction.[6] Alteration of phospholipid fatty acid composition in cell membranes achieved through manipulation of cell medium fatty acid content has been observed to affect many cellular properties; examples include cell membrane fluidity, receptor binding, cell-mediated transport, ion channels, eicosanoid formation, and intracellular calcium concentration.[1-7]

Although studies in humans have been few in number, recent reports are encouraging. Kutner and colleagues[2] explored the effect of fish consumption in 216 incident dialysis patients. Patient survival was followed for 3 years. This study found that fish intake was associated with patient survival. Patients who ate fish were 50% less likely to die during the study interval. Donadio[3] demonstrated in human trials that omega-3 fatty acids have a beneficial effect on immunoglobulin A nephropathy (IgAN). IgAN is the most prominent cause of glomerulosclerosis in the world. It affects young adults of whom 20% to 40% will develop progressive renal disease and ultimately kidney failure. The rationale for interest of omega-3 fatty acids in IgAN was based on the effect of these fatty acids on altering the production of eicosanoids and inflammatory mediators. In clinical trials, Donadio and colleagues observed that patients with IgAN treated with 1.8 g of eicosapentaenoic acid (EPA) and 1.2 g of docosahexaenoic acid (DHA) had a slower loss of renal function. In a different trial, patients treated with placebo had a higher rate of developing renal failure than those treated with EPA and DHA.

Additional research is needed to elucidate the beneficial effects of omega-3 fatty acid intake in patients with chronic renal disease. However, the current body of research indicating inflammatory mechanisms responsible for the high prevalence of CVD in this patient population, and the interrelationships between markers of malnutrition and inflammation, certainly encourage continued research in the role of omega-3 fatty acids modulating these common biochemical pathways.

References

1. U.S. Renal Data System: Annual data report: executive summary, *Am J Kidney Dis* 34:s9-s19, 1999.
2. Kutner N et al: Association of fish intake and survival in a cohort of incident dialysis patients, *Am J Kidney Dis* 39(5):1018, 2002.
3. Donadio J: The emerging role of omega-3 polyunsaturated fatty acids in the management of patients with IgA nephropathy, *J Ren Nutr* 11(3):122, 2001.
4. Donadio J et al: A controlled trial of fish oil in IgA nephropathy, *N Engl J Med* 331:1194, 1994.
5. Goldstein DJ et al: Fish oil ameliorates renal injury and hyperlipidemia in the Milan normotensive rat model of focal glomerulosclerosis, *J Am Soc Nephrol* 6:1468, 1995.
6. Goldstein DJ, Wheeler DC, Salant DJ: The effects of omega-3 fatty acids on complement-mediated glomerular epithelial cell injury, *Kidney Int* 50:1863, 1996.
7. Weise W et al: Fish oil has protective and therapeutic effects on proteinuria in passive Heymann nephritis, *Kidney Int* 43:359, 1993.

TABLE 21-2 Stages of Chronic Kidney Disease: Clinical Presentations

Stage	Description	GFR Range (ml/min/1.73 m^2)	Clinical Presentations*
	At increased risk	≥90 (without markers of damage)	CKD risk factors
1	Kidney damage with normal or ↑ GFR	≥90	Markers of damage (nephrotic syndrome, nephritic syndrome, tubular syndromes, urinary tract symptoms, asymptomatic urinalysis abnormalities, asymptomatic radiologic abnormalities, hypertension due to kidney disease)
2	Kidney damage with mild ↓ GRF	60-89	Mild complications
3	Moderate ↓ GFR	30-59	Moderate complications
4	Severe ↓ GFR	15-29	Severe complications
5	Kidney failure	<15 (or dialysis)	Uremia, cardiovascular disease

From National Kidney Foundation: K/DOQI clinical practice guidelines for chronic kidney disease: evaluation, classification and stratification, *Am J Kidney Dis* 39(suppl 1):s1-s266, 2002.

*Includes presentations from preceding stages. Chronic kidney disease is defined as either kidney damage or GFR <60 ml/min/1.73 m^2 for ≥3 months. Kidney damage is defined as pathologic abnormalities or markers of damage, including abnormalities in blood or urine tests or imaging studies.

GFR, Glomerular filtration rate; *CKD,* chronic kidney disease.

additional 20% to 40%.[20] Factors contributing to malnutrition in patients with renal failure are listed in Box 21-1.

It is now recognized that malnutrition is an important risk factor for death.[21,22] In a study of more than 14,000 hemodialysis patients, Lowrie and Lew[21] found that those with a serum albumin concentration of less than 2.5 g/dl had a risk of death 20 times higher than patients with albumin levels of greater than 4.0 g/dl. Patients with albumin levels of 3.5 to 4.0 had a risk of death 2 times higher than that of patients with albumin levels greater than 4.0 g/dl. Other indices of nutritional status have since been identified to be important predictors of mortality; these include serum cholesterol, creatinine, and prealbumin. As a result, it has been hypothesized that malnutrition is a main cause of death in the dialysis patient population.

Interventions to improve serum albumin and other markers of nutritional status have had mixed results. It has been recently hypothesized that the parameters reflecting malnutrition are influenced not only by nutritional status but by an inflammatory process that may or may not be related to the presence of active CKD.[23-25] The inflammatory response is mediated by cytokines including interleukin-1, interleukin-6, and tumor necrosis factor-alpha. Cytokines induce anorexia, decreases in fat mass, loss of lean muscle mass, augmented catabolism, and decreases in serum levels of albumin, prealbumin, and transferrin. Similar changes are induced by malnutrition. Studies have demonstrated increased levels of these cytokines in surveys of hemodialysis and peritoneal dialysis patients.[26]

Several parameters used for nutrition assessment and nutritional monitoring are negative acute-phase reactant proteins (ARPs), including albumin, prealbumin, and transferrin. In response to inflammation, hepatic synthesis

BOX 21-1 Factors Contributing to the Presence of Malnutrition in Patients With Chronic Renal Failure

1. Anorexia due to
   - Nausea, emesis, medications
   - Uremia/uremic state of metabolism
   - Underdialysis
   - Accumulation of uremic toxins not completely removed by dialysis
2. Metabolic acidosis
3. Endocrine disorders (insulin resistance, hyperparathyroidism, impaired response to insulin-like growth factor I)
4. Comorbidity (infections, intercurrent illnesses)
5. Reduced nutrient intake
6. Dialysis related
   - Inadequate dose
   - Catabolism (bioincompatible membrane)
   - Loss of amino acids and protein to the dialysate
   - Reuse with bleach
7. Psychosocial
   - Depression
   - Inability to purchase or prepare food adequately
   - Loss of or poorly fitting dentures

From Wolfson M: Causes, manifestations, and assessment of malnutrition in chronic renal failure. In Kopple J, Massry S, eds: *Nutritional management of renal disease,* Philadelphia, 1997, Williams & Wilkins.

and serum levels of the above negative ARPs diminish. At the same time, the synthesis and serum levels of positive ARPs increase; these include c-reactive protein (CRP), serum amyloid A, and ferritin. In dialysis patients, the serum albumin concentration is negatively associated with positive ARPs.[27] Therefore indicators traditionally viewed to be signs of malnutrition, such as decreased serum concentrations of albumin and prealbumin, loss of muscle mass, and weight loss, may not be the result of malnutrition but may instead be the result of an inflammatory response or some combination of inflammation and malnutrition. The clinical or biologic stimuli/stimulus activating a proinflammatory response with symptoms of malnutrition is currently unknown. Hypotheses include unrecognized clinical infection, bioincompatible membranes, oxidative stress, increased production of glycosylated end products, endothelial dysfunction, or vascular disease.[23-27]

The main cause of death in patients with ESRD is CVD.[28] In dialysis patients, the death rate from CVD is 10 to 20 times higher than that in the general population.[29] Atherosclerosis is an inflammatory disease characterized by increased adhesiveness of the endothelium for platelets, leukocytes, increased vascular permeability, formation of vasoactive cytokines, and growth factors. CRP is a powerful predictor of cardiovascular events. Elevated levels are commonly observed in patients with chronic renal disease.

Elevated CRP levels in renal patients suggest a chronic state of inflammation. Stenvinkel and colleagues[23] have hypothesized that interactions exist between malnutrition, inflammation, and CVD, referred to as the Malnutrition, Inflammation, Atherosclerosis (MIA) syndrome. It is possible that some patients are malnourished as a result of (1) anorexia and hypercatabolism related specifically to renal disease, (2) inflammation and CVD, and (3) a mixed type of malnutrition (Table 21-3 and Figure 21-4). These newer hypotheses are the beginning to a different approach to the treatment of malnutrition in renal disease. As the etiology and discrimination of nutrition parameters become possible, more successful interventions can be developed.

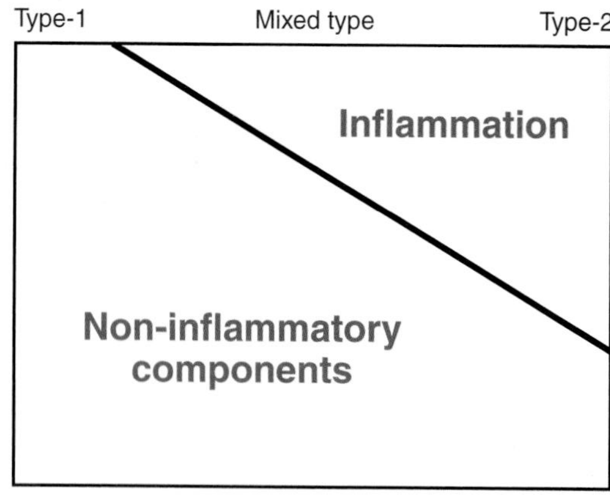

FIGURE 21-4 Proposed relative contribution of noninflammatory components (e.g., low intake of protein and energy because of uremic anorexia, underdialysis, physical activity) and the inflammatory components of malnutrition in patients with type 1 and type 2 malnutrition, respectively. *(From Stenvinkel P et al: Are there two types of malnutrition in chronic renal failure? evidence for relationships between malnutrition, inflammation and atherosclerosis {MIA syndrome},* Nephrol Dial Transplant *15{7}:953, 2000, by permission of Oxford University Press.)*

TABLE 21-3 Proposed Features of Type 1 and Type 2 Malnutrition

	Type 1	Type 2
Serum albumin	Normal/low	Low
Comorbidity	Uncommon	Common
Presence of inflammation	No	Yes
Food intake	Low	Low/normal
Resting energy expenditure	Normal	Elevated
Oxidative stress	Increased	Markedly increased
Protein catabolism	Decreased	Increased
Reversed by dialysis and nutritional support	Yes	No

From Stenvinkel P et al: Are there two types of malnutrition in chronic renal failure? evidence for relationships between malnutrition, inflammation and atherosclerosis (MIA syndrome), *Nephrol Dial Transplant* 15(7):953, 2000, by permission of Oxford University Press.

Nutrition Assessment of Patients With Kidney Disease

Evaluating and monitoring nutritional status are vital components of nutritional care of the patient with kidney disease. The high prevalence of malnutrition, the large number of aberrations in normal metabolism, and complications including anorexia and catabolism all indicate the need for consistent monitoring. Nutrition assessment is best completed by a registered dietitian who has received special training in renal nutrition care.

When completing a nutrition assessment, an array of indices, each representing a specific data category, are measured independently and then evaluated collectively to ascertain the nutritional status of the renal patient. Box 21-2 lists the data categories that encompass the nutritional assessment of the renal patient. Specific indices that have been used to evaluate each data category are listed in Box 21-3. The following is a review of the indices most commonly measured from each data category.[30-32]

Subjective global assessment (SGA) is an approach to completing a nutrition assessment that has been validated in the ESRD population. However, current efforts for identifying methods for nutrition assessment are focusing on developing objective methodologies.

BOX 21-2 Five Data Categories and Constituents Inherent to Nutritional Assessment

1. Clinical	2. Food and Diet Intake	3. Biochemical	4. Body Weight	5. Body Composition
Physical examination Nutrient physical examination (NPE) Medical history Psychosocial history Demographics Physical activity level Current medical/ surgical issues	Diet history Appetite assessment Quantitative food intake Qualitative food intake Food habits and patterns Fluid intake/ balance	Visceral protein stores Static protein reserves Other estimates of protein nutriture Immune competence Vitamins, minerals, and trace elements Fluid, electrolyte, and acid-base balance Lipid status	History Actual Compared to standards Body mass index (BMI) Weight change over time Goal weight	Adipose stores Lean body mass (skeletal muscle)

From Goldstein DJ: Assessment of nutritional status in renal disease. In Mitch WE, Klahr S, eds: *Nutrition and the kidney,* ed 4, Philadelphia, 2002, Lippincott Williams & Wilkins.

BOX 21-3 Biochemical Parameters for Assessing the Nutritional Status of the Patient With Renal Disease

A. Visceral Protein Stores

Albumin
Prealbumin (thyroxin binding prealbumin)
Retinol-binding protein
Transferrin (siderophilin)
Somatomedin C (insulin-like growth factor I)
Acute-phase proteins (ceruloplasmin, complement components, C-reactive protein, fibrinogen)
Fibronectin
Pseudocholinesterase
Ribonuclease
Total protein
Albumin/globulin ratio

B. Static (Somatic) Protein Reserves

Urinary and serum creatinine
Creatinine height index
3-Methylhistidine

C. Other Estimates of Protein Reserves

Plasma amino acid profiles
Protein turnover studies
Biochemical analysis of skeletal muscle
Nitrogen balance

D. Immune Competence

Total lymphocyte counts
Delayed cutaneous hypersensitivity responses: *Candida,* mumps, *Trichophyton,* streptokinase-streptodornase (SKSD), and purified protein derivative (PPD)
Specific immunoglobulin levels
Complement proteins

E. Vitamin, Mineral, Trace Element Nutriture

Serum levels of water-soluble vitamins, fat-soluble vitamins, and specific minerals and trace elements
Nutrition physical examination

F. Fluid, Electrolyte, and Acid-Base Status

Serum chemistries: sodium, potassium, calcium, phosphorus, bicarbonate, chloride, glucose

G. Indirect Indices of Renal Function and Dialysis Adequacy

Serum creatinine
Blood urea nitrogen

H. Anemia

Hemoglobin
Hematocrit
Mean cell corpuscular volume
Total iron-binding capacity
Serum iron
Percent transferrin saturation
Ferritin
Red blood cell count
Reticulocyte count
White blood cell count

I. Hyperlipidemia

Serum: Cholesterol
Triglycerides

J. Renal Osteodystrophy

Serum: Calcium
Vitamin D
Alkaline phosphatase

From Goldstein DJ: Assessment of nutritional status in renal disease. In Mitch WE, Klahr S, eds: *Nutrition and the kidney,* ed 4, Philadelphia, 2002, Lippincott Williams & Wilkins.

CLINICAL

Medical History

The medical history should include any information about the patient's appetite, food intake, and ability to metabolize food. This requires past medical and surgical history, current medical diagnosis and problems, prescribed medications, drug use including alcohol, bowel habits, and weight history. Record of any major organ or gastrointestinal diseases, surgeries, or previous symptoms of malabsorption or other digestive problems, including nausea, vomiting, and diarrhea, should be noted. Impairment in fluid and electrolyte balance, hypertension/hypotension, proteinuria, and any previous symptoms of uremia that affect appetite, food intake, digestion, or nutritional status should also be noted.

Psychosocial History

This evaluates the patient's mental status as well as factors regarding the economics, education level, physical home environment, food shopping and preparation capabilities, and available support systems. The goal is to create an individualized intervention that the patient or patient's support system can understand and apply. Factors that might compromise nutritional status include depression or improper food preparation and storage equipment. This component of the assessment process helps identify patients requiring social services to assist with economic needs or special services to provide regular access to food and medications.

Demographics

Information on age, marital status, gender, and ethnicity is needed to assess nutritional status. Many of the reference standards used to classify clinical indices adjust for gender and age. Knowledge of ethnicity affects the ability to individualize the diet therapy; marital status helps identify support systems.

Physical Activity

Assessment of the patient's physical capabilities is needed to maintain activities of daily living and the proper level of physical exercise for psychological and physical therapeutics. The following questionnaires have been validated for the purpose of measuring physical activity and physical functioning in the ESRD patient population: the Stanford 7-Day Physical Activity Recall, the Physical Activity Scale for the Elderly, the Human Activity Profile, and the Medical Outcomes Study Short-Form 36-item questionnaire.

Current Medical/Surgical Issues

Identification of nutritional implications of medical and surgical problems is imperative for the nutritional assessment procedure. For the patient with chronic, progressive disease, this requires acknowledgment of any newly diagnosed medical/surgical illnesses.

DIET AND FOOD INTAKE

This category relies on subjective patient reporting to evaluate qualitative and quantitative aspects of food intake. One of the most useful outputs from this category is the calculation of nutrient intake. Other outputs include information related to past and current food intake (qualitative and quantitative), eating patterns, and specific food preferences. This information allows an approximation of the diet's adequacy. It also helps to identify nutrient factors that may be contributing to medical problems. The qualitative data are essential for the formulation of individual diet therapy, including meal plans and menus.

Diet History

The diet history is usually obtained at the initial meeting. It is an all-inclusive collection of some objective but primarily subjective information concerning the patient's food, such as aversions, allergies, preferences, and intake. Information on previous and current diet intake assists in devising interventions to improve the diet or devising an acceptable therapeutic meal plan. The most commonly used tools to obtain food intake information differ in the approach to data collection, retrospective versus prospective, and whether the information is a qualitative description of intake versus a quantitative one.

Food record. A food record provides qualitative and approximate quantitative food intake information that is best collected prospectively. The minimal time recommended for data collection is 3 days; a reasonable maximum is 5 days. The patient should provide intake information for both weekends and weekdays so that variability can be determined. For the dialysis patient, it is strongly recommended that the food record include intake for dialysis as well as nondialysis days, in addition to the weekend-versus-weekday pattern. A difference in food intake between dialysis and nondialysis days has been noted in both type and amount of food selected.

The patient should be provided with instructions on how to approximate food portion sizes and servings of fluid to ensure accurate reporting. The use of food models is very helpful. The food record should include the time of day of any intake (both meals and snacks), the names of the foods eaten, the approximately amount of food ingested, the method of preparation, and special recipes or steps taken in the food preparation. The same instructions apply to fluid intake. Brand names are requested when available.

Some patients find that it is more convenient to record food intake at the end of the day. This is an inferior method because the data collection becomes retrospective and more subject to error. Calculation of the intake of total protein, protein quality, carbohydrate, fat, fatty acid classes, and other selected nutrients is best completed by a computerized nutrient analysis program.

24-Hour food recall. The 24-hour food recall is an interactive tool in which the clinician assists the patient in remembering qualitative and quantitative food intake via prompting. The clinician can sit with a patient during dialysis and slowly help the patient recall the previous day's intake of both food and fluid. Food models or drawings can be used to help the patient identify portion size. One 24-hour recall, however, does not provide sufficient information to ascertain total food intake.

A variation of the 24-hour recall for a dialysis patient is to meet with the patient during three consecutive treatments, or at least four sessions within a 2-week period, and obtain one 24-hour recall at each visit. Effort should be made to obtain a recall for a weekend day, a dialysis day, and a nondialysis day. To obtain a total food intake on a dialysis day, the practitioner can ask the patient what he or she had to eat so far that day and record it. The patient or family member can finish recording for the rest of the day, or the clinician can meet with the patient at the next session to help him or her recall what was eaten for the rest of that day. Calling the patient's home on a daily basis to obtain the needed information is an option but is not practical.

Food frequency questionnaires (FFQs). FFQs approximate nutrient intake by identifying the periodicity of intake of specific foods within food groups that are significant sources of a particular nutrient or nutrients (e.g., dairy products are a good source of calcium, vitamin D, and protein). A food frequency consists of listing foods according to group, such as vegetables, fruits, dairy, protein, and so forth. The patient is questioned as to how often he or she eats this food per day, per week, and per month. An approximation of the adequacy of intake of specific nutrients can be calculated from the results. Although FFQs have not been widely used to assess the intake of renal patients, a recent study in hemodialysis patients provides preliminary data indicating the Block (version 98) FFQ can be a useful tool for this purpose.[33]

BIOCHEMICAL VALUES

Serum biochemical values are used to assess and monitor nutritional status over time. Selected serum values pertain to visceral protein stores, static protein reserves, overall protein nutriture, immune competence, iron stores, and vitamin, mineral, and trace element status. In addition to these components, nutritional assessment involves evaluating fluid, electrolyte, and acid-base status; renal function; dialysis adequacy for the patient receiving replacement therapy; serum lipid levels; and bone health.

Visceral Protein Stores

Serum levels of albumin, transferrin, prealbumin, and retinol-binding protein (RBP) are the biochemical markers most often used to assess visceral protein stores, monitor response to nutrition intervention, and identify which patients are at risk for development of complications or are responding poorly to medical/surgical treatment. The assumption—not yet proved—is that serum concentration represents hepatic protein synthetic mass and, indirectly, the functional protein mass of the internal viscera (i.e., heart, lung, kidneys, intestines).[30]

Serum albumin. Albumin, the most abundant plasma protein, functions to maintain plasma oncotic pressure and serves as a major carrier protein for drugs, hormones, enzymes, and trace elements. Clinically significant hypoalbuminemia occurs with different types of malnutrition besides kidney disease (e.g., protein-energy kwashiorkor, uncomplicated), in both children and adults. In these conditions, hypoalbuminemia usually indicates other metabolic derangements as well as a poor prognosis. From these observations, serum albumin became a part of routine nutritional assessment of the hospitalized patient and, subsequently, the renal patient.

The causes of significant hypoalbuminemia associated with malnutrition are not known. (See earlier section on the MIA syndrome.) Although serum albumin levels have been used extensively in clinical practice, research studies, and nutritional surveys to assess the nutritional status of the chronic and end-stage renal patient population, the reliability and sensitivity of this parameter have been questioned. The concerns are independent of the conditions that change serum albumin as a marker of visceral protein stores. The use of albumin for assessment purposes has been criticized because of its long half-life, averaging 14 to 20 days, and large body pool, 4 to 5 mg/kg, making albumin slow to respond to changes in visceral protein stores. It is therefore a late marker of malnutrition.[18,27]

Prealbumin (thyroxine-binding prealbumin, transthyretin). Prealbumin is a carrier protein for RBP and thus has a major role in the transport of thyroxine. Its short half-life of 2 to 3 days and its small body pool make it more sensitive than albumin to changes in protein status. This was the first visceral protein found to be low in healthy children who were eating marginal amounts of protein. In primates, prealbumin reflects overall nitrogen balance during starvation and refeeding. Decreases in serum levels occur independently of nutritional status when there is acute metabolic stress, including trauma, minor stress, and inflammation. The serum concentration has also been observed to decrease in liver disease and with iron supplementation. Prealbumin can be useful as a nutritional marker after acute metabolic stress.

The low molecular weight of prealbumin (approximately 54,980 daltons) precludes its use as a marker of nutritional status in patients with chronic renal disease who have a decreased GFR. Prealbumin levels have been reported to be elevated in the euvolemic patient with chronic renal failure. In hemodialysis patients, high levels have been observed and are attributed to decreased renal catabolism. A decline in the proportion of circulating free

proteinuria The presence of an excess of serum proteins, such as albumin, in the urine.

prealbumin versus that complexed with RBP may explain the diminished catabolism and therefore elevated levels. A concentration of less than 30 mg/dl (normal range, 10 to 40 mg/dl) may indicate malnutrition in the hemodialysis patient and has recently been associated with an increased risk of death. These studies indicate that the prealbumin level may serve as a better nutrition assessment tool and predictor of patient outcome than the traditionally used serum albumin in the dialysis population.[20,22]

Retinol-binding protein. This protein circulates in a 1:1 molar ratio with prealbumin and transports the alcohol fraction of vitamin A. Its short half-life of 10 to 12 hours and small body pool enable it to respond quickly and specifically to changes in protein status. RBP is not an appropriate marker of nutritional status for the patient with chronic renal disease or ESRD because it is catabolized in renal proximal tubular cells. With renal disease, the half-life is reported to be prolonged, and serum levels increase. Other limitations of RBP for nutritional assessment are that serum levels become low in hyperthyroidism, vitamin A deficiency, and acute catabolic states (i.e., levels change inversely with acute-phase proteins).

Transferrin (siderophilin). The main function of transferrin is to bind ferrous iron and to transport iron to the bone marrow. The half-life of 8 to 10 days and small body pool enable it to respond more rapidly to short-term changes in protein status, compared with albumin. Studies in malnourished children as well in hospitalized patients have demonstrated a correlation between transferrin and the severity and prognosis of disease, as well as an improvement in serum levels with nutrition intervention.[30]

Before it was practical to measure transferrin levels, the total iron-binding capacity was thought to be equivalent to the amount of iron required to saturate plasma transferrin. This assumption turned out to be true only in normal and iron-deficient subjects. The most common estimate is obtained from the total iron-binding capacity (TIBC) using this formula: transferrin $= (0.8 \times \text{TIBC}) - 43$. However, this formula has not been validated as an estimate of serum transferrin in the renal patient, and a direct measure is recommended. The use of this protein in the nutritional assessment of the renal patient is confounded by many factors that influence the serum levels. Iron deficiency increases hepatic synthesis and plasma levels. Reduced transferrin concentrations are observed in association with uremia, protein-losing enteropathy, nephropathy, acute catabolic states, chronic infections, and iron loading. In chronic renal failure, transferrin is reliable for the evaluation of iron status. Most patients on renal replacement receive erythropoietin therapy and iron supplementation. The use of transferrin should be reserved for those patients who have a stable erythropoietin regimen with adequate iron replacement.

Insulin-like growth factor I (somatomedin C). Insulin-like growth factor I (IGF-I) is a serum protein with mitogen properties and insulin-like activities; it may be a sensitive biochemical indicator of nitrogen balance. With a half-life of 2 to 6 hours, IGF-I represents an acute-phase response. Studies of hospitalized, hypercatabolic patients indicate that IGF-I is a better marker of nitrogen balance than other serum proteins. In humans, IGF-I levels fall during fasting and increase with refeeding, and it has been reported to be a reliable marker of malnutrition in children. A serum concentration below 300 ng/ml indicates a poor nutritional status in hemodialysis patients.

Static Protein Reserves (Somatic Protein, Muscle Stores)

Measures of muscle mass are thought to be good indicators of static protein reserves because approximately 60% of total body protein is contained in muscle. Skeletal muscle is the predominant source of amino acid mobilization during periods of nutrition deficiency. Both anthropometric and biochemical markers are used to assess muscle mass. Anthropometric techniques are discussed in Body Composition.

Urinary and serum creatinine. Creatinine is formed at a relatively constant rate from creatine, a compound found predominantly in muscle; therefore urinary creatinine is proportional to muscle creatine content and hence to total body muscle mass. Urinary excretion of creatinine correlates with lean body mass measured by isotope dilution and ^{40}K total body counting techniques.

For the patient with renal insufficiency or deteriorating renal function, urinary creatinine cannot be used for nutritional assessment purposes. There is no role for urinary creatinine excretion in nutritional assessment for the end-stage patient who has zero or insignificant residual renal function and accumulates creatinine.

For a chronic renal patient with a stable GFR, and for the dialysis patient, changes in serum creatinine over time (about 3 months) may indicate a change in muscle mass. Verification of a change in muscle mass based on the serum creatinine must be confirmed by assessing other parameters of somatic protein stores, as well as by evaluating the patient's weight, overall food intake, and biochemical markers of visceral stores.

Immune competence. A comprehensive nutritional assessment includes tests of immune function. The total lymphocyte count and delayed cutaneous hypersensitivity responses are tests of humoral immunity and have limited use in nutritional assessment because of altered host defenses. The use of serum complement system components and serum immunoglobulins to test humoral immunity is complex because of the discrepancies concerning which proteins are altered in renal failure or improve with adequate nutrition.

BODY WEIGHT

Initial assessment of body weight and monitoring of weight change over time represent critical components of the nutritional assessment process. Weight loss in excess of 5% to 10%, depending on the patient's overall nutritional status, or substandard weight for height, should be considered a risk factor for malnutrition. Interrelationships between weight loss over time and outcome in the renal patient population have not yet been reported.

Body mass index (weight [kg]/height [m^2]), current weight, usual weight, ideal body weight, percent usual weight, percent ideal body weight, and particularly percent weight change over a defined time period are important parameters of body weight. A database or sheet in the patient's chart that is committed to record body weight is recommended for every patient.

BODY COMPOSITION

Measures of body composition to ascertain fat stores and lean body mass are included. Other than the initial investment for skinfold calipers and an accurate tape measure, anthropometry is an inexpensive technique. The measurements obtained are compared with standards that classify the patient as normal, "at risk" for malnutrition, or having a type and degree of malnutrition. In general, measurements below the 35th to 40th percentile suggest mild depletion; below the 25th to 35th percentile, moderate depletion; and below the 25th percentile, severe depletion.

Anthropometry

Fat stores. Approximately half of human fat is found in the subcutaneous layer. Therefore measurement of subcutaneous fat provides a reasonably accurate index of total body fat. The triceps skinfold thickness and subscapular skinfold are commonly used to quantify adipose tissue thickness on the limbs and trunk. Other body points that can be measured to ascertain adipose stores using skinfold thickness are biceps, abdomen, suprailiac, medial calf, and anterior thigh. Loss of fat from subcutaneous stores occurs proportionally; therefore repeat measures from a selected group of sites in an individual patient can provide reliable information on trends of adipose stores. In dialysis patients, it is recommended that arm measures be completed using the nonaccess arm. Otherwise, the right arm is recommended for use in measurements.

Skeletal muscle (somatic protein mass, static protein reserves). Anthropometric measures of muscle mass can serve as an indirect assessment of muscle stores because approximately 60% of total body protein is located in skeletal muscle. In response to poor nutrition, skeletal muscle is the primary source of amino acids. The most commonly used anthropometric measures to assess skeletal muscle are the midarm muscle circumference (MAMC) and midarm circumference (MAC). There are several limitations to these anthropometric measures: a 10% error occurs between measurements even when performed by the same clinician, and there is a poor correlation reported between visceral stores and upper arm measurements. Therefore anthropometric measures alone cannot be relied on to evaluate muscle and fat stores. Anthropometric measures are best used in conjunction with data from the other categories (see Box 21-2).

Advanced Methods of Body Composition Analysis

Methods available to determine fat-free mass are measures of body water, potassium, nitrogen, and calcium and two electrical approaches, bioelectrical impedance (BIA) and electromagnetic scanning, referred to as TOBEC and EMSCAN, respectively. Techniques to estimate total body fat other than anthropometry are inert gas absorption, infrared interactance, total body carbon using neutron activation, computed tomography, magnetic resonance imaging, and dual-energy x-ray absorptiometry (DEXA). Although several of these techniques have been used for body composition analysis in renal patients, they have not been adopted for routine use.

Altered Nutrient Requirements With Chronic Kidney Disease

The nutrition intervention for patients with CKD includes modifications for sodium, fluid, potassium, phosphorus, calcium, vitamin D, iron, calories, and protein. Although global recommendations are available, nutritional care must be individualized based on serum chemistries, fluid balance, and nutritional status. These concerns are addressed in the following discussion.

SODIUM AND POTASSIUM

As kidney function declines, the ability of the nephrons to maintain sodium balance through sodium excretion diminishes. However, an adaptive mechanism results in the undamaged nephrons to be able to excrete a higher percentage of filtered sodium with the effect being a decrease in the fractional reabsorption and an increase in the fractional excretion of sodium by the renal tubules. As the GFR falls to 10 ml/min, a 2.0- to 3.0-g sodium restriction may be required to maintain both sodium and fluid balance. Clinical symptoms of excessive sodium intake include shortness of breath, hypertension, congestive heart failure, and edema. Alternatively, a patient who continues to have a urine output of at least 1000 ml/day may be able to maintain sodium balance on an unrestricted intake.[1,3,4]

---

hyperthyroidism Abnormally increased activity of the parathyroid gland, resulting in excessive secretion of parathyroid hormone, which usually helps regulate serum calcium levels in balance with vitamin D hormone; excess secretion occurs when the serum calcium level falls below normal, as in chronic renal disease or in vitamin D deficiency.

TABLE 21-4 Recommended Dietary Nutrient Intake for Patients With Chronic Renal Failure Not Undergoing Dialysis[a,b,c]

Protein: low-protein diet (g/kg/day)	GFR <25 ml/min: 0.6 g protein/kg/day; if patient unable to maintain adequate intake of calories or will not accept this diet, 0.75 g protein/kg/day
Energy (kcalories/kg/day)	GFR <25 ml/min: 35 kcalories/kg/day if <60 years of age; 30-35 kcalories/kg/day if ≥60 years of age
Fat (percentage of total energy intake)[d,e]	30
Polyunsaturated/saturated fatty acid ratio[e]	1.0:1.0
Carbohydrate[e,f]	Remainder of nonprotein calories
Total fiber intake (g/day)[e]	20-25
Minerals (range of intake)	
Sodium (mg/day)	1000-3000[g]
Potassium (mEq/day)	40-70
Phosphorus (mg/kg/day)	5-10[h]
Calcium (mg/day)	1400-1600[i]
Magnesium (mg/day)	200-300
Iron (mg/day)	≥10-18[j]
Zinc (mg/day)	15
Water (ml/day)	Up to 3000 as tolerated[g]
Vitamins	Diet may be supplemented with these quantities
Thiamin (mg/day)	1.5
Riboflavin (mg/day)	1.8
Pantothenic acid (mg/day)	5
Niacin (mg/day)	20
Pyridoxine HCl (mg/day)	5
Vitamin B_{12} (μg/day)	3
Vitamin C (mg/day)	60
Folic acid (mg/day)	1
Vitamin A	Refer to chapter text for additional information
Vitamin D	Refer to chapter text for additional information
Vitamin E (IU/day)	15
Vitamin K	None[k]

From National Kidney Foundation: K/DOQI clinical practice guidelines for chronic kidney disease: evaluation, classification and stratification, *Am J Kidney Dis* 39(suppl 1):128, 2002; modified from Kopple J: Nutrition management of nondialyzed patients with chronic renal failure. In Kopple JD, Massey SG, eds: *Nutritional management of renal diseases,* Philadelphia, 1997, Williams & Wilkins.

GFR, Glomerular filtration rate.

[a]GFR >4-5 ml/min/1.73 m^2 and <25 ml/min/1.73 m^2.

[b]The protein intake is increased by 1.0 g/day of high-biologic-value protein for each g/day of urinary protein loss.

[c]When recommended intake is expressed per kilogram of body weight, this refers to the patient's normal weight, as determined from the NHANES data, or adjusted body weight.

[d]Refers to percentage of total energy intake (diet plus dialysate); if triglyceride levels are very high, the percentage of fat in the diet may be increased to about 40% of total calories; otherwise, 30% of total calories is preferable.

[e]These dietary recommendations are considered less crucial than the others. They are emphasized only if the patient has a specific disorder that may benefit from this modification or has expressed interest in his dietary prescription and is complying well with more important aspects of the dietary treatment.

[f]Should be primarily complex carbohydrates.

[g]Can be higher in patients who have greater urinary losses.

[h]Phosphate binders (aluminum carbonate or hydroxide, or calcium carbonate, acetate, or citrate) often are needed to maintain normal serum phosphorus levels.

[i]Dietary intake usually must be supplemented to provide these levels. Higher daily calcium intakes are commonly ingested because of the use of calcium binders of phosphate.

[j]At least 10 mg/day for males and nonmenstruating females; ≥18 mg/day for menstruating females.

[k]Vitamin K supplements may be needed for patients who are not eating and who receive antibiotics.

Kidney regulation of potassium balance is obtained by renal excretion of potassium in an amount equal to that absorbed by the gastrointestinal tract. Potassium balance is dependent on the ability of the tubules to continue to secrete potassium into the ultrafiltrate. This ability will decrease as kidney failure progresses. Once the patient becomes oliguric or GFR drops to about 10 ml/min, dietary potassium restriction to approximately 2 g/day is required to maintain the serum levels within the normal range of 3.5 to 5.0 mEq/L.[1,3,4]

PHOSPHORUS, CALCIUM, AND VITAMIN D

The consequence of the abnormalities of calcium, phosphorus, and vitamin D metabolism that are seen in chronic kidney disease is the development of bone diseases, which are referred to as renal osteodystrophy. The diagnoses include osteoporosis, osteosclerosis, osteomalacia, and osteitis fibrosa. The healthy kidney filters about 7 g of phosphorus/day, of which 80% to 90% is reabsorbed by the renal tubules and the remaining 10% is excreted into the urine. Phosphorus balance can be maintained until the GFR falls under 20 ml/min. At that point, phosphorus accumulation occurs in the serum. In addition, the conversion of vitamin D to the active form 1,25-dihydrocholecalciferol is diminished, resulting in low serum calcium levels and elevated parathyroid hormone levels. The dietary intervention for bone disease management is dietary phosphorus restriction to 5 to 10 mg phosphorus/kg body weight/day. In addition to dietary phosphate restriction, most patients require oral calcium and/or oral or intravenous vitamin D or vitamin D analogues. Serum parathyroid hormone, calcium, and phosphorus levels must be monitored closely to avoid excesses and deficiencies that can exacerbate the bone disease.[30,34]

IRON

Because of the diminished ability of the failing kidney to synthesize adequate amounts of erythropoietin, most patients with chronic renal failure develop anemia if left untreated. Recommended levels for the hematocrit are 33% to 36%; for hemoglobin, 11 to 12 g/dl. These target levels are accomplished through the administration of recombinant human erythropoietin (rHuEPO) and 10 to 18 mg oral iron. Doses are individualized. If left untreated, adverse clinical events can occur, including increased mortality rates, malnutrition, angina, cardiac enlargement, and impaired immunologic response.[35,36]

CALORIES AND PROTEIN

Historically, dietary protein was restricted in patients with chronic renal disease to levels as low as 0.3 g protein/kg body weight/day when supplemented with essential amino acids or nitrogen-free analogues called *keto-acids.* A more common protein restriction was 0.6 g/kg/day. The rationale for the restriction was based on observations in animals and human studies that, in general, high-protein diets resulted in proteinuria, mortality, and renal damage, whereas restriction of dietary protein resulted in improvements.[31] There are a large number of human studies that have demonstrated that low-protein diets initiated early in chronic renal failure improve uremic symptoms by decreasing the formation of nitrogenous compounds. These diets were to be calorically dense, in the range of 35 kilocalories (kcalories)/kg to promote protein sparing and minimize the formation of protein metabolic byproducts. However, the beneficial effects of these diets on preventing the progression of kidney disease were never demonstrated. Patients often became malnourished. Whether this was because of the inability to adhere to the diet or from some other catabolic event was not discriminated in the majority of studies.[31]

In 1990, the MDRD study was implemented to test, in a large multicenter trial, the use of low-protein diets in delaying the progression of renal disease.[19] Two groups of patients were studied. Group A patients had GFRs in the range of 25 to 55 ml/min/1.73 m^2 and were randomized to a diet of 1 or more g protein/kg/day or 0.6 g/kg/day. Mean blood pressures were maintained at 105 or 92 mm Hg. Group B patients had GFRs in the range of 13 to 24 ml/min/1.73 m^2 and were assigned diets containing 0.6 or 0.3 g protein/kg/day plus a keto-acid supplement. Blood pressure goals were the same. Renal function was monitored for 2.2 years by measuring ^{125}I-iothalamate renal clearance. The MDRD study results demonstrated that neither the low-protein diet nor the blood pressure control decreased the loss of GFR.

The K/DOQI guidelines for CKD include recommendations for protein and calories based on a comprehensive review of the literature.[15] These guidelines recommend 0.6 g protein/kg body weight/day when GFR is less than 25 ml/min and the patient is not on dialysis. For individuals who do not want to follow this diet or are unable to maintain adequate caloric intake, a diet providing 0.75 g protein/kg/day is recommended to be considered. At this same level of GFR, caloric intake for patients younger than 60 years of age is recommended to be 35 kcalories/kg/day; for those 60 years of age or older, 30 to 35 kcalories/kg/day. Other diet recommendations that integrate current data concerning protein, calories, fatty acids, vitamins, and minerals until additional data are available are listed in Table 21-4.

Medical Nutrition Therapy

As of January 2002, Medicare began to provide payment for medical nutrition therapy for patients with chronic renal insufficiency. The Institute of Medicine (IOM) defines chronic renal insufficiency as the stage of renal disease associated with a reduction in renal function not severe enough to require dialysis or transplantation (GFR = 13 to 50 ml/min/1.73 m^2).[16,37] The

osteodystrophy Defective bone formation.

Renal Practice Group of the American Dietetic Associate recently published guidelines of care for the patient with kidney disease that includes expected outcomes of medical nutrition therapy.[37] These guidelines identify outcome assessment parameters, expected outcome to therapy, and ideal/goal value of indices being monitored (Table 21-5).

MAINTENANCE HEMODIALYSIS

Since the advent of the artificial kidney machine, a number of kidney dialysis centers have been established for the treatment of progressive chronic renal insufficiency. Home units are also available, although considerable skill and expense are required to operate them. Much of the cost is paid under a provision of Medicare. A patient re-

TABLE 21-5 Expected Outcomes of Medical Nutrition Therapy for Adults With Chronic Kidney Disease Not Requiring Dialysis Replacement Therapy

	Expected Outcomes of Medical Nutrition Therapy	
Outcome Assessment Factors	Expected Outcome of Therapy	Ideal/Goal Value
Clinical Outcomes	***Measure <30 Days Before Nutrition Session***	
Biochemical Parameters		
Blood urea nitrogen, creatinine	Levels stabilized	Levels stabilized
Albumin	Level maintained within goal range (stabilized in nephrotic syndrome)	3.5-5.0 g/dl (may be lower in nephrotic syndrome)
Potassium	Level maintained within goal range	3.5-5.5 mEq/L
Phosphorus	Level progressing toward goal range	2.5-5.0 mg/dl
Calcium	Level progressing toward goal range	8.5-10.5 mg/dl
Serum glucose (premeal)	Maintained within goal range	80-120 mg/dl
Hb_{A1c} (diabetes)	Maintained within goal range	<7%
Cholesterol	Level progressing toward goal range	120-240 mg/dl
Triglycerides (fasting)	Level progressing toward goal range	<200 mg/dl
Creatinine clearance/GFR	Decline minimized	Stabilized
Hematologic Parameters		
Hematocrit/hemoglobin	Adequate erythropoiesis maintained	Hematocrit 33%-36%; hemoglobin 11.0-12.0 g/dl
Ferritin	Adequate iron stores maintained for erythropoiesis	Ferritin 100-800 ng/ml
Transferrin saturation		Transferrin saturation 20%-50%
Anthropometrics		
Weight	Reasonable weight achieved/maintained	Within reasonable body weight (body mass index, 20-25 kg/m^2)
	Adequate body mass maintained	Adequate muscle/fat stores
Clinical Signs and Symptoms		
	Level of functional ability maintained	Optimum functional ability Minimum gastrointestinal symptoms
	Good appetite maintained	Food intake >80% recommended intake
	Appropriate blood pressure control maintained	Blood pressure within appropriate limits
Patient/Caregiver Behavioral Outcomes		*MNT Goals*
Food selection/meal planning	Exhibits positive changes in food selection and amounts If diabetic, times meals and snacks appropriately	1. Makes appropriate food choices and takes medications as prescribed 2. Maintains appropriate protein intake 3. Maintains lab values within acceptable limits
Nutrient needs	Identifies foods with a significant protein content	4. If diabetic, maintains stable glucose levels through appropriate dietary practices
Potential food/drug interactions	Verbalizes potential food/drug interactions	5. If no medical limitations, maintains an exercise program
Exercise	If no medical limitations, gradually increases or continues physical activity level	

quiring maintenance hemodialysis usually requires two or three treatments per week, with each treatment lasting 2½ to 5 hours.

During treatment the patient's blood circulates through the dialysis solution in an artificial kidney (the dialyzer), maintaining normal blood levels of life-sustaining substances that the patient's own kidneys can no longer accomplish. An alternative form of peritoneal dialysis is practical for long-term ambulatory therapy at home (see *Practical Application* box).

The diet of a patient on kidney dialysis is a vital aspect of maintaining biochemical control. Several basic objectives govern each individually tailored diet, designed to (1) maintain adequate protein and calorie intake, (2) prevent dehydration or fluid overload, (3) maintain normal serum potassium and sodium blood levels, and (4) maintain acceptable phosphate and calcium levels.

Protein and Calories

The K/DOQI initiative completed a comprehensive evaluation regarding protein and energy intake for patients receiving maintenance hemodialysis and peritoneal dialysis therapy.[38] The recommendation is that patients on hemodialysis therapy maintain a protein intake of 1.2 g protein/kg body weight/day. Patients receiving peritoneal dialysis are recommended to receive 1.2 to 1.3 g protein/kg body weight/day. Calorie intake is advised to be 35 kcalories/kg body weight/day for those who are younger than 60 years and 30 to 35 kcalories/kg body weight/day for individuals 60 years or older.[38]

Fluid

Fluid intake is recommended to be equal to approximately 500 ml/day, plus an amount equal to urinary output, if any. The total intake must account for additional fluids in the foods consumed. Even with this restriction there is an expected daily weight gain between dialysis treatments. The interdialytic weight gain is ideally no greater than 2% to 5% body weight or no greater than an average of 2.5 kg.[37]

Sodium, Potassium, and Phosphorus

To control body fluid retention and hypertension, sodium should be limited to 2000 to 3000 mg of sodium/day. This restriction helps to prevent pulmonary edema or congestive heart failure from fluid overload.

Potassium restriction is imperative to prevent hyperkalemia. Potassium accumulation can induce cardiac arrhythmias or cardiac arrest. Thus a dietary allowance of 2000 to 3000 mg of potassium/day is usually followed.

To prevent serum phosphorus levels from exceeding 4.0 to 6.0 mg/dl and to prevent bone disease, dietary phosphorus is recommended to be 800 to 1200 mg/day or less than 17 mg/kg.

Vitamins

During the dialysis treatments, water-soluble vitamins from the blood are lost in the dialysate filtered out of the circulating blood. A daily supplement providing water-soluble vitamins is recommended.

Table 21-6 summarizes the dietary recommendations for patients receiving hemodialysis and peritoneal dialysis.

Peritoneal Dialysis

An alternate form of dialysis, peritoneal dialysis, allows dialysate solutions to flow directly through a catheter port established through the abdominal wall into the abdominal cavity. The solution is typically a dextrose-salt solution. The high osmolality of the solution causes the waste materials to diffuse across the saclike peritoneum lining the abdominal cavity (see *Practical Application* box). Then this dialysate collection of waste materials flows back into the dialysate bag for disposal. The peritoneal membrane serves as the filtering mechanism.[31]

There are two main types of peritoneal dialysis: (1) continuous ambulatory peritoneal dialysis (CAPD), in which a dialysis solution in a plastic pouch is infused and drained via gravity each day (24 hours), 5 times at 4-hour intervals; and (2) continuous cyclic peritoneal dialysis (CCPD), in which three or four machine-delivered exchanges are given at night, about 3 hours each, leaving about 2 L of dialysate solution in the peritoneal cavity for 12 to 15 hours during the day.

Nutrition concerns specific to peritoneal dialysis involve the calories contributed by the dialysate, which are usually 1.5%, 2.5%, or 4.25% dextrose in 1.5 to 2 L of solution, and fluid and potassium intake can be liberalized compared with hemodialysis because of the enhanced clearance of potassium.

KIDNEY TRANSPLANTATION

Incident rates for kidney transplantation have increased 6.3% annually from 1995 to 1999.[39] There are currently 101,000 patients living with a functioning kidney transplant. Patients with kidney transplants often face nutritional challenges related to posttransplantation medications. Hyperlipidemia, weight gain, and abnormal blood glucose levels can result, often because of side effects of the antirejection medications such as corticosteroids and cyclosporin A.[40] In addition, transplant recipients are at increased risk for CVD. The death rate from CVD is 40% in this patient population, and 60% of patients

peritoneum A strong smooth surface—a serous membrane—lining the abdominal/pelvic walls and the undersurface of the diaphragm, forming a sac enclosing the body's vital visceral organs within the peritoneal cavity.

PRACTICAL APPLICATION
Peritoneal Dialysis

A variety of types of peritoneal dialysis exist, with the two main types being continuous ambulatory peritoneal dialysis (CAPD) and continuous cyclic peritoneal dialysis (CCPD). Similar to the decision to choose hemodialysis or peritoneal dialysis, which type of peritoneal dialysis is performed is dependent on lifestyle and clinical considerations. CAPD is an ambulatory dialysis procedure that introduces dialysate directly into the peritoneal cavity. Solutes and water flow across the peritoneal membrane into the dialysate fluid. This is accomplished by attaching a disposable bag containing the dialysate to a catheter permanently inserted into the peritoneal cavity, waiting an individually prescribed amount of time (i.e., "dwell time") for the solution exchange, and then lowering the bag to allow the force of gravity to cause the waste-containing fluid to drain into it. When the bag is empty, it can be folded around the waist or tucked into a pocket, allowing the user mobility.

The exchange takes place via osmosis and diffusion, with the rate being determined in part by the amount of dextrose in the solution. The most common dialysate solutions are 1.5%, 2.5%, or 4.25% dextrose in 1.5 to 2 L of solution. The actual rate of solute transport, the type of number of peritoneal dialysis exchanges, and solution dwell times vary among patients. Each patient is prescribed an individualized dialysis prescription that includes the number and type of dialysate solutions to use each day and the length of dwell times. A method to determine membrane function and the optimal peritoneal dialysis method for each patient is the peritoneal equilibration test. Peritoneal solute and solvent movement rates vary among patients and over time can vary even within the same patient. Therefore clinical monitoring of dialysis adequacy is important. Patients using CAPD as a renal replacement therapy have greater mobility than those on hemodialysis and typically have a more liberal diet in regard to dietary potassium, phosphorus, and total fluid intake due in large part to the more continuous nature of the therapy. The protein requirement is higher and can be a challenge for some patients. Table 21-6 lists the nutritional recommendations for patients on peritoneal dialysis. Special nutrient considerations are as follows.

- *Protein and amino acid* losses are significant and therefore the recommendation for dietary protein intake is higher than that for hemodialysis patients (see Table 21-6). Protein losses average 5 to 15 g/24 hours. Amino acid losses average 3 g/day.
- *Potassium* requirements depend on the number of solution exchanges, whether the patient has any residual renal function, and the individual clearance characteristics of the patient's peritoneal membrane. On average, the potassium recommendation is 3 to 4 g of potassium/day. Some patients will require potassium supplementation.
- *Phosphorus-binding antacids* are not as needed because of improved control of phosphorus blood levels with CAPD use.
- The dietary *sodium* restriction is usually 2 to 4 g/day. The recommendation must be individualized in accordance to the patient's fluid status, blood pressure, and thirst.
- *Fluid* requirements depend on weight, blood pressure, and residual renal function.

CAPD poses nutrition-related problems related to weight gain from the dialysate and, on the other end of the spectrum, anorexia because of glucose absorption from the dialysate.

One method available to calculate glucose absorption in an individualized manner is the D/D_0 formula: grams of glucose absorbed.

$$\text{Glucose (g)} = (1 - D/D_0) \times G_i$$

where D_0 is initial dextrose in the dialysate at zero hours (g); D is remaining dextrose in the dialysate after an appropriate dwell time (g); D/D_0 is fraction of glucose remaining in the dialysate; and G_i is initial glucose instilled.
13 g/L for 1.5% dextrose
22 g/L for 2.5% dextrose
38 g/L for 4.25% dextrose

In addition to posing possible weight-management problems, the extra dextrose can lead to elevated triglycerides and low-density lipoprotein (LDL) levels and depressed levels of protective high-density lipoproteins (HDL), thus increasing the risk of coronary heart disease in long-term users.

Nutritionists and nurses who counsel patients being transferred from hemodialysis to the CAPD regimen may find that patients need guidance in adjusting to their new diet. The following guidelines may be helpful.

- Increase potassium intake by eating a wide variety of fruits and vegetables each day.
- Encourage liberal fluid intake to prevent dehydration.
- Encourage complex carbohydrates while avoiding overindulging in concentrated sweets to help control triglyceride and HDL levels.
- Maintain lean body weight by incorporating the kcalories provided by the dialysate into the total meal plan (to be calculated and explained to the patient by the renal dietitian).

References

National Kidney Foundation: K/DOQI clinical practice guidelines for nutrition in chronic renal failure, *Am J Kidney Dis* 35(6):s42, 2000.

National Kidney Foundation: K/DOQI clinical practice guidelines peritoneal dialysis adequacy, 2000, *Am J Kidney Dis* 37:s81, 2001.

Passadakis T, Vagemezis V, Oreopoulos D: Peritoneal dialysis: better than, equal to, or worse than hemodialysis? data worth knowing before choosing a dialysis modality, *Peritoneal Dialy Int* 21:25, 2001.

Valderrabano F, Lopez-Gomez J: Quality of life in end-stage renal disease patients, *Am J Kidney Dis* 38(3):443, 2001.

Wiggins K: *Guidelines for nutrition care of renal patients,* ed 3, Chicago, 2002, American Dietetic Association.

TABLE 21-6 Nutritional Recommendations for Patients on Hemodialysis and Peritoneal Dialysis Therapy

Nutrient	Hemodialysis	Peritoneal Dialysis
Protein (g/kg)*	1.2-1.3; at least 50% high biologic value	1.2-1.3; at least 50% high biologic value
Energy (kcal/kg or kJ/kg)* If patient <90% or >115% of median standard weight, use aBW_{ef}	30-35 (125-145) if ≥60 years of age and 35 (145) if <60 years of age	30-35 (125-145) if ≥60 years of age and 35 (145) if <60 years of age
Phosphorus	800-1200 mg/day or <17 mg/kg*	1200 mg/day or <17 mg/kg*
Sodium	2000-3000 mg/day (88-130 mmol/day)	Individualized based on blood pressure and weight; CAPD and APD: 3000-4000 mg/day (130-175 mmol/day)
Potassium	40 mg/kg* or approximately 2000-3000 mg/day (50-80 mmol/day)	Generally unrestricted with CAPD and APD (approximately 3000-4000 mg/day [80-105 mmol/day] unless serum level is increased or decreased
Fluid	500-1000 ml/day + daily urine output	CAPD and APD approximately 2000-3000 ml/day based on daily weight fluctuations, urine output, ultrafiltration, and blood pressure; unrestricted if weight and blood pressure are controlled and residual renal function = 2-3 L/day
Calcium	Approximately 1000-1800 mg/day; supplement as needed to maintain normal serum level	Approximately 1000-1800 mg/day; supplement as needed to maintain normal serum level

From Goldstein DJ, McQuiston B: Nutrition and renal disease. In Coulston A, Rock C, Monson E, eds: *Nutrition in the prevention and treatment of disease,* San Diego, 2001, Academic Press.

*For continuous ambulatory peritoneal dialysis (CAPD) and automated, or "cycler," peritoneal dialysis (APD) include dialysate calories.

develop hypercholesterolemia.[40-42] Therefore nutrition therapy for the kidney transplant recipient is designed to control blood lipids, blood glucose, and blood pressure within normal ranges; to maintain normalized electrolyte imbalances; to prevent weight gain; and to promote good nutritional health.[41,42] A low-fat diet and exercise plan are generally recommended.[39-41] A summation of nutrition guidelines for this patient group is provided in Table 21-7.

ACUTE RENAL FAILURE

The catabolic ARF patient, most frequently encountered in the intensive care setting, presents a management challenge to the entire team of physicians, nurses, dietitians, respiratory therapists, dialysis staff, pharmacy, and other technicians. These patients are in negative nitrogen balance and generate much urea resulting from the catabolic process. Infection is a major threat, and it aggravates the existing malnutrition.

Disease Process

Renal failure may occur as an acute phase with sudden shutdown of renal function following some metabolic insult or traumatic injury to normal kidneys. The situation is often life threatening, and the mortality rate associated with renal failure is high. Survival is less than 50%, especially after surgery.[43,44] In this medical emergency, the nutritionist and nurse play important supportive roles. Immediate and continuing nutritional support is essential.

ARF may have various causes, as follows: (1) severe injury such as extensive burns or crushing injuries that cause widespread tissue destruction; (2) infectious diseases such as peritonitis; (3) traumatic shock after surgery on the abdominal aorta; (4) toxic agents in the environment such as carbon tetrachloride or poisonous mushrooms; or (5) immunologic drug reactions in allergic or sensitive persons, such as penicillin reaction.[43-45]

Clinical Symptoms

The major sign of ARF is oliguria, diminished urine output, often accompanied by proteinuria or hematuria. This diminished urine output is brought on by the underlying tissue problems that characterize ARF. Usually there is blockage of the tubules caused by cellular debris from tissue trauma or urinary failure with backup retention of filtrate materials.[45]

hematuria The abnormal presence of blood in the urine.
oliguria Secretion of a very small amount of urine in relation to fluid intake.

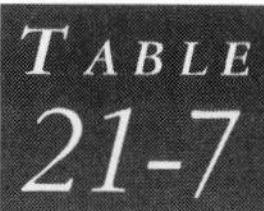

TABLE 21-7 Nutrition Guidelines for Adult Kidney Transplant Recipients

Nutrient	Prescription	Purpose
First 6-8 Weeks After Transplantation and During Treatment for Acute Rejection		
Protein	1.3-1.5 g/kg	Counteract protein catabolism; promote wound healing
Calories	30-35 kcalories (125-145 kJ)/kg	Meet postsurgery energy demands and allow protein to be used for anabolism
After 6-8 Weeks		
Protein	1.0 g/kg	Minimize muscle protein wasting
Calories	Sufficient to achieve optimal weight for height	Achieve/maintain optimal weight
At All Times		
Carbohydrates	Consistent carbohydrate intake; increase fiber content	Meet energy demands; promote bowel regularity
Fats	No more than 30% of calories; cholesterol <300 mg/day	Reduce posttransplant hyperlipidemia; help prevent progression of atherosclerosis
Potassium	Variable; restrict or supplement as necessary based on serum level	Maintain acceptable potassium level
Sodium	2-4 g (87-175 mmol) may be necessary	Maintain blood pressure control in salt-sensitive individuals; minimize edema
Calcium	1000-1500 mg	Minimize further bone demineralization; correct calcium/phosphorus imbalance
Phosphorus	1200-1500 mg; some patients may require supplements	Minimize further bone demineralization; correct calcium/phosphorus imbalance
Fluids	Ad libitum	Maintain adequate hydration

Oliguria. Diminished urinary output is a cardinal symptom, often with proteinuria or hematuria accompanying the small output. Water balance becomes a crucial factor. The course of the disease is usually divided into an oliguric phase followed by a diuretic phase. The urinary output during the oliguric phase varies from as little as 20 to 200 ml/day.

Anorexia, nausea, and lethargy. During this initial phase of ARF, the patient may be lethargic and anorectic and experience nausea and vomiting. Blood pressure elevation and signs of uremia may be present. Oral intake is usually difficult in this catabolic period.[46]

Increasing serum urea nitrogen and creatinine levels. During the initial catabolic period after injury, surgery, or some other metabolic dysfunction, the serum urea nitrogen level increases along with the creatinine level. These increases result from the tissue breakdown of muscle mass. Blood potassium, phosphate, and sulfate levels also increase, and sodium, calcium, and bicarbonate levels decrease.[2,46]

General Medical Management

Usually after initial conservative medical therapy, recovery occurs in a few days to 6 weeks. However, in more complicated cases in which the oliguria continues for 4 to 5 days, more aggressive therapy, including hemodialysis and total parenteral nutrition (TPN), is instituted.

Basic treatment goals. Treatment must be individual, adjusted according to progression of the illness, the type of treatment being used, and the patient's response. In general, however, basic therapy objectives are as follows.[2,46]

- Reduce and minimize protein breakdown
- Prevent protein catabolism and minimize uremic toxicity
- Avoid dehydration or overhydration
- Correct acidosis carefully
- Correct electrolyte depletions and avoid excesses
- Control fluid and electrolyte losses from vomiting and diarrhea
- Maintain optimal nutritional status
- Maintain appetite, general morale, and sense of well-being
- Control complications—hypertension, bone pain, nervous system problems

Nutrition Requirements for Patients With Acute Renal Failure

The ARF patient's nutrition requirements are directly influenced by the type of renal replacement therapy (if any), nutritional and metabolic status, and the degree of hypercatabolism. The current recommendations for protein and calories for this patient population are defined in the following discussion.[43-48]

Protein is expressed as grams per kilogram of ideal body weight per day. Protein sources containing both essential and nonessential amino acids should be provided. For patients whose ARF is expected to resolve in a few days and who will not need dialysis, 0.55 to 1 g of protein is recommended.[43,44] The patient's nutrition and metabolic status and the renal diagnosis determine the exact dose. For patients receiving acute hemodialysis the recommendation is 1.2 to 1.4 g of protein; for those on acute intermittent or CAPD, 1.2 to 1.5 g; and for those on chronic renal replacement therapies, 1.5 to 2.0 g.[2,43,44]

When energy requirements cannot be measured directly, calorie requirements can usually be met by providing 35 to 50 kcalories/kg ideal body weight, reserving the upper limit of the range for patients who are severely catabolic and whose nitrogen balance does not improve at lower intakes. In general, 60% of calories should be provided as carbohydrate and 20% to 35% as fat. Any patient receiving TPN for more than 5 to 7 days should receive 50 to 100 g of lipids as an emulsion, to avoid essential fatty acid deficiency.[2,43-47]

The total fluid intake for any patient depends on the amount of residual renal function (i.e., is the patient oliguric? anuric?) and fluid and sodium status. In general, fluid intake can be calculated by adding to the 24-hour urine output 500 ml for insensible losses.

Supplementation of minerals, electrolytes, and trace elements is determined by monitoring serum and urine levels, when appropriate, to prevent excess or deficiency states from arising. Although the specific vitamin requirements of ARF patients are not known, the following guidelines are available.[43-47]

- Supplementation of vitamin A is not recommended for at least 2 weeks because levels are elevated with chronic renal failure.
- Vitamin K supplements should be given particularly to patients who are taking antibiotics that suppress intestinal growth of bacteria that usually synthesize it.
- To avoid vitamin B_6 deficiency, 10 mg of pyridoxine hydrochloride/day (8.2 mg of pyridoxine/day) is recommended.
- Limiting ascorbic acid to 60 to 100 mg/day prevents increased oxalate production and serum oxalate levels.

Route of nutrition support. The criteria for deciding which route of nutrition support to use, enteral or parenteral, for critically ill patients have become increasingly complex. In addition to the increased costs associated with the parenteral route, some studies report an increased incidence of infectious complications with parenteral, compared with enteral, nutrition.[49] Parenteral nutrition has also been associated with atrophy of gut mucosa, reduced levels of secretory immunoglobulin A, enhanced bacterial and endotoxin translocation, and exaggerated hormonal and metabolic responses to septic challenge.[46] Therefore patients with catabolic ARF should be evaluated for route of nutrient delivery; enteral nutrition should be used if the gut is functional.[49]

Because uremia is a potent catabolic signal, metabolic studies in patients with ARF and CRF have traditionally limited the intake of nonessential amino acids in an attempt to reduce urea production. Proteins of high biologic value, but in quantities much smaller than are usually given (<0.5 g/kg/day), were administered along with adequate calories, usually in the form of glucose. The same approach was used with TPN. A central venous infusion of an essential amino acid solution and a hypertonic dextrose solution was frequently administered to provide calories and a small quantity of essential nitrogen. It was thought that this approach would prevent malnutrition and at the same time reduce protein catabolism and minimize the rise in blood urea nitrogen (BUN) level.[44]

This clinical approach to nutrition therapy has not reduced mortality rates.[43,48] In the mid-1990s, the aggressive use of dialysis (early intervention and large doses) and the use of parenteral solutions (for those not candidates for enteral) containing mixed amino acids, dextrose, and lipids were becoming standard practice. Dialysis therapy can be adjusted to the patient in terms of clearing catabolic products and allowing for increased administration of protein and calories. Continuous renal replacement therapy (CRRT) has made possible aggressive nutrition support for hypercatabolic patients who have failing kidney function.[43-46]

Debate continues about the optimal amino acid composition of TPN solutions.[49] Despite some question about the relative nephrotoxicity of certain amino acids, current recommendations call for formulations containing mixed amino acids, essential and nonessential. There is currently no conclusive evidence that specialized formulations such as those additionally enriched with branched-chain amino acids have a beneficial effect on outcome.

Because available data on nutrition therapy for ARF are both limited and conflicting, no treatment plan can be enthusiastically advocated for such patients. Depending on whether the dialysis is initiated or not, general recommendations for protein are 0.6 to 1.4 g/kg/d. Adequate kcalories should also be provided (30 to 35 kg/kg/d). The percentage of increases in protein and calorie needs in catabolic ARF patients is generally related to the precipitating event. Not only must protein and calorie requirements be estimated, but altering intake of vitamins and electrolytes should be considered in view of the degree of renal dysfunction. Strategies for fluid and electrolyte management include continuous renal replacement therapies such as continuous arteriovenous hemodialysis (CAVHD). These treatment modalities can allow for sufficient nutrition while avoiding fluid and electrolyte complications. Dialysis interventions require close monitoring and assessment to allow ongoing adjustment of the total treatment regimen.[2,43-48]

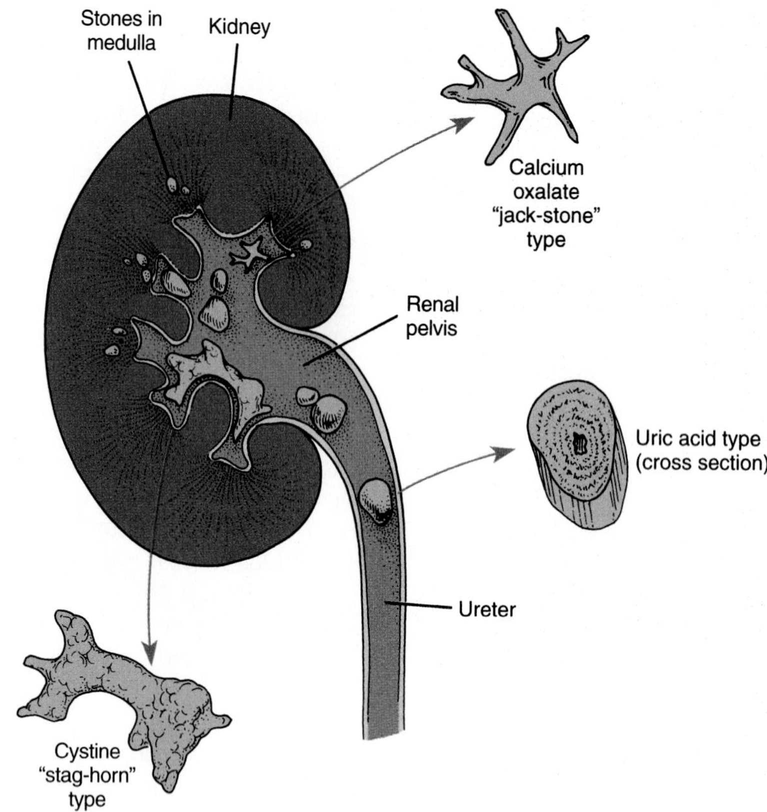

FIGURE 21-5 Renal stones in kidney, pelvis, and ureter.

Noncatabolic patients may not require dialysis therapy if normal fluid and electrolyte balance can be maintained and blood urea nitrogen (BUN) does not exceed 80 mg/dl. This group of ARF generally results from ingestion of nephrotoxic drugs or exposure to contrast dyes used for diagnostic imaging. These patients are not normally nutritionally depleted and have lower urea generation rates. Oral and enteral feedings are preferred as long as the gastrointestinal tract is functioning normally. However, catabolic ARF patients are most frequently encountered in the intensive care setting. Despite the improvements in dialysis technology and intensive care medicine, the mortality rate of critically ill patients with ARF remains over 50%.[43,44] Work is being conducted with this patient population to improve the approaches of study design so that better intervention studies can be conducted in the future.[48]

Kidney Stone Disease

DISEASE PROCESS

Kidney stone disease is an ancient medical problem. Since the days of Hippocrates, records of its incidence have appeared in medical documents. It continues to be a prevalent health problem. Multiple stone attacks affect 12% to 20% of American men and 5% to 10% of women during their lifetimes, with most of the stones today composed of calcium oxalate mixed with varying proportions of calcium phosphate.[50] Kidney stone disease appears to be chronic and recurrent. The basic cause is unknown, but many predisposing risk factors have been found to be involved with calcium, protein, and sodium, with sodium—mostly in the form of dietary salt (NaCl)—receiving the most attention.[50] Although the basic cause of kidney stones remains unknown, many factors contribute directly or indirectly to their formation. These factors relate to the nature of the urine itself or to the conditions of the urinary tract environment. According to the concentration of urinary constituents, the major stones formed are calcium stones, struvite stones, uric acid stones, and cystine stones (Figure 21-5).

Major Types of Stones

Calcium stones. Most kidney stones are composed of calcium compounds, usually calcium oxalate or calcium oxalate mixed with calcium phosphate. In persons who form stones, which is a familial tendency, the urine produced is supersaturated with these crystalloid elements, and there is a lack of normal urine substances that prevent the crystals from forming stones.[51] Theories as to how excessive urinary calcium may result include the following.

BOX 21-4 Food Sources of Oxalates

Fruits	Vegetables	Nuts	Beverages	Other
Berries, all	Baked beans	Almonds	Chocolate	Grits
Currants	Beans, green and wax	Cashews	Cocoa	Tofu
Concord grapes	Beets	Peanuts	Draft beer	Soy products
Figs	Beet greens	Peanut butter	Tea	Wheat germ
Fruit cocktail	Celery			
Plums	Chard, Swiss			
Rhubarb	Chives			
Tangerines	Collards			
	Eggplant			
	Endive			
	Kale			
	Leeks			
	Mustard greens			
	Okra			
	Peppers, green			
	Rutabagas			
	Spinach			
	Squash, summer			
	Sweet potatoes			
	Tomatoes			
	Tomato soup			
	Vegetable soup			

1. *Excess calcium intake.* This results from the prolonged use of large amounts of milk, alkali therapy for peptic ulcer, use of a hard water supply, or supplemental calcium.[52-53]
2. *Excess salt (NaCl) intake.* Recent research, both salt-loading studies and reports of free-living populations, confirms earlier observations that high intakes of NaCl result in hypercalciuria.[50]
3. *Excess vitamin D.* Hypervitaminosis D may cause increased calcium absorption from the intestine as well as increased withdrawal from bone.
4. *Prolonged immobilization.* Body casting or immobilization from illness or disability may lead to withdrawal of bone calcium and increased urinary concentration.
5. *Hyperparathyroidism.* Primary hyperparathyroidism causes excess calcium excretion. About two thirds of the persons with this endocrine disorder have kidney stones, but this disorder accounts for only about 5% of total calcium stones.
6. *Renal tubular acidosis.* Excess excretion of calcium is caused by defective ammonia formation.
7. *Idiopathic calcinuria.* Some persons, even those on a low-calcium diet, for unknown reasons may excrete as much as 500 mg of calcium/day.
8. *Oxalate.* Because of a metabolic error in handling oxalates, about half of the calcium stones are compounds with this material. Oxalates occur naturally only in a few food sources (Box 21-4), and individual absorption/excretion rates influence availability. Studies in normal volunteers consuming oxalate-rich foods have indicated that the increased urinary oxalate values were not proportional to the oxalate values of food.[51] Only eight foods caused a significant increase in urinary oxalate excretion: spinach, rhubarb, beets, nuts, chocolate, tea, wheat bran, and strawberries. Nutrition therapy for stone-forming individuals may be limited to restriction of these eight foods, with results monitored by laboratory analysis of urine composition.
9. *Animal protein.* A diet high in animal protein, such as the typical American diet, has been linked to increased excretions of calcium, oxalate, and urate. A vegetarian-type diet has been recommended by some investigators as a wise choice for stone-forming persons.
10. *Dietary fiber.* Added dietary fiber has been found to reduce risk factors for stone formation, especially calcium stones.

blood urea nitrogen (BUN) The nitrogen component of urea in the blood; a measure of kidney function; elevated levels of BUN indicate a disorder of kidney function.

Struvite stones. Next to calcium stones in frequency are struvite stones, composed of a single compound—magnesium ammonium phosphate ($MgNH_4PO_4$). These are often called "infection stones" because they are associated with UTIs. The offending organism in the infection is *Proteus mirabilis.* This is a urea-splitting bacterium that contains urease, an enzyme that hydrolyzes urea to ammonia. Thus the urinary pH becomes alkaline. In the ammonia-rich environment struvite precipitates and forms large, "staghorn" stones. Surgical removal is usually indicated.

Uric acid stones. Excess uric acid excretion may be caused by an impairment in the intermediary metabolism of purine, as occurs in gout. It may also result from a rapid tissue breakdown in wasting disease.

Cystine stones. A heredity metabolic defect in renal tubular reabsorption of the amino acid cystine causes this substance to accumulate in the urine. This condition is called *cystinuria.* Because this is a genetic disorder, it is characterized by early onset and a positive family history. This is one of the most common metabolic disorders associated with kidney stones in children before puberty.

Urinary Tract Conditions

The physical changes in the urine and the organic stone matrix provide urinary tract conditions that lead to the formation of kidney stones.

Physical changes in the urine. Susceptible persons form stones when physical changes in the urine predispose to such formation. Such physical conditions include the following.

1. *Urine concentration.* The concentration of the urine may result from a lower water intake or from excess water loss, as in prolonged sweating, fever, vomiting, or diarrhea.
2. *Urinary pH.* Changes in urinary pH from its mean 5.85 to 6 may be influenced by the diet or altered by the ingestion of acid or alkali medications.

Organic stone matrix. Formation of an organic stone matrix provides the necessary core or nucleus (nidus) around which crystals may precipitate and form a mucoprotein-carbohydrate complex. In this complex, galactose and hexosamine are the principal carbohydrates. Some possible sources of these organic materials include (1) bacteria masses from recurrent UTIs; (2) renal epithelial tissue of the urinary tract that has sloughed off, possibly because of vitamin A deficiency; and (3) calcified plaques (Randall's plaques) formed beneath the renal epithelium in hypercalciuria. Irritation and ulceration of overlying tissue cause the plaques to slough off into the collecting tubules.

Clinical Symptoms

Severe pain and numerous urinary symptoms may result, with general weakness and sometimes fever. Laboratory examination of urine and chemical analysis of any stone that is passed help determine treatment.

General Treatment

Fluid intake. Large fluid intake produces a more dilute urine and is a foundation of therapy. The dilute urine helps to prevent concentration of stone constituents.

Urinary pH. An attempt to control the solubility factor is made by changing the urinary pH to an increased acidity or alkalinity, depending on the chemical composition of the stone formed. An exception is calcium oxalate stones because the solubility of calcium oxalate in urine is not pH dependent. Conversely, however, calcium phosphate is soluble in an acid urine.

Stone composition. When possible, dietary constituents of the stone are controlled to reduce the amount of the substance available for precipitation.

Binding agents. Materials that bind the stone elements and prevent their absorption in the intestine cause fecal excretion. For example, sodium phytate is used to bind calcium, and aluminum gels are used to bind phosphate. Glycine and calcium have a similar effect on oxalates.

Nutrition Therapy

Nutrition therapy is directly related to the stone chemistry.

Calcium stones. The traditional dietary approach for calcium stones has been to limit dietary calcium intake to about 400 mg/day. This has raised concerns regarding effects on bone density when used long term.[53,54] In addition, because calcium stones have an alkaline chemistry, an acid ash diet has been thought to help create a urinary environment less conducive to the precipitation of the basic stone elements. The classification of food groups is based on the pH of the metabolic ash produced (Box 21-5). An acid ash diet increases the amount of meat, grains, eggs, and cheese. It limits the amounts of vegetables, milk, and fruits. An alkaline ash diet outlines the opposite use of

BOX 21-5 Acid and Alkaline Ash Food Groups

Acid Ash	Alkaline Ash	Neutral
Meat Whole grains Eggs Cheese Cranberries Prunes Plums	Milk Vegetables Fruits (except cranberries, prunes, and plums)	Beverages (coffee, tea)

these foods. The use of cranberry juice has been promoted to assist in the acidification of urine. However, the commercially prepared cranberry juices on the consumer market are too dilute to be effective because they contain only about 26% cranberry juice. Thus an inordinate volume would be required to achieve any consistent effectiveness as a urinary acidifying agent. Instead, to effect a sustained acidifying of urinary pH, most physicians rely on drugs.

A recent study by Borghi and colleagues[54] indicates that a calcium-rich diet low in salt and animal protein significantly reduces the recurrence of kidney stones in men. In this study, 120 men with recurrent calcium oxalate stones and hypercalciuria were randomized to receive a normal calcium diet (30 mmol/day, n = 60) with a dietary protein restriction of 52 g/day and salt restriction of 50 mmol/day. The other 60 men in the study were randomized to receive the traditional low-calcium diet, 10 mmol. At the end of 5 years, 20% of the patients on the normal-calcium, low-protein and salt diet and 38% of the men on the low-calcium diet had relapses. The relative risk for the normal-calcium diet compared with the low-calcium diet was 0.49. Urinary calcium levels dropped in both group, but urinary oxalate excretion fell in the normal calcium group and increased in the men on the low-calcium diet. Although the exact mechanisms are still being debated, the study does indicate that a low-animal protein diet and salt diet with normal-calcium intake protects against recurrence of kidney stones compared with the traditional low-calcium diet.

Uric acid stones. About 4% of the total incidence of renal calculi are uric acid stones. Because uric acid is a metabolic product of purines, dietary control of this precursor is indicated. Purines are found in active tissue such as glandular meat, other lean meat, meat extractives, and, in lesser amounts, plant sources such as whole grains and legumes. An effort to produce an alkaline ash to help increase the urinary pH is indicated.

Cystine stones. About 1% of the total stones produced are cystine; this condition is a relatively rare genetic disease. Cystine is a nonessential amino acid produced from the essential amino acid methionine; thus a diet low in methionine is used. This diet is used with high fluid intake and alkaline diet therapy.

Urinary Tract Infection

DISEASE PROCESS

The term *urinary tract infection* refers to a wide variety of clinical infections in which a significant number of microorganisms are present in any portion of the urinary tract.[56,57] A common form is cystitis, an inflammation of the bladder that is very prevalent in young women. At least 20% of women experience a UTI during their lifetime, of which the vast majority are cases of uncomplicated cystitis.[55,56] The condition is called recurrent UTI if three or more bouts are experienced in 1 year.

The majority of cases are caused by aerobic members of the fecal flora, especially *Escherichia coli.*[57] The presence of these organisms in the urine is termed *bacteriuria.* Urine produced by the normal kidney is sterile and remains so as it travels to the bladder. In UTI, however, the normal urethra has microbial flora; therefore any voided urine generally contains many bacteria. Bacteriuria is present when the quantity of organisms is more than 100,000 bacteria/ml of urine. The female anatomy is more conducive to entry of these bacteria into the urinary tract. Recurrent cystitis occurs mostly in young and otherwise healthy women who have infections that usually correspond with sexual activity and continued diaphragm use. In most cases, simply changing to another birth control method will solve the problem. Cystitis is characterized by frequent voiding and burning on urination.

TREATMENT

Currently antibiotic treatment of UTI has been cut back a great deal. General nutritional measures include acidifying the urine by taking vitamin C (because cranberry juice is not effective) and drinking plenty of fluids to produce a dilute urine. Control of UTI is an important measure because it is a risk factor in stone formation. Current medical research shows promise for the development of new vaccines to prevent UTIs.[57]

Resources

The renal diet is complex and presents a challenge to practitioners and, even more so, to patients. A basic resource, the National Renal Diet educational series, provides valuable guides. These standardized guidelines for nutrition intervention and patient education in renal disease have been developed by the collaborative work of renal dietitians from The American Dietetic Association Renal Dietitians Dietetic Practice Group and the National Kidney Foundation Council on Renal Nutrition. The Professional Guide can be used in conjunction with ADA's other guides for the care of renal disease patients. Because dietary management must be tailored to the stage of the disease and method of treatment, the series of materials contains a professional guide and six client booklets, each designed with special food lists to meet specific needs of the various renal disease requirements. These ADA resources give the practitioner a comprehensive basis for individualizing dietary instructions and provide the patient and family with a practical guide for everyday decisions and plans for food choices.

The Council on Renal Nutrition of the National Kidney Foundation is an expert resource for information. Membership includes a subscription to the *Journal of Renal Nutrition,* a quarterly publication geared toward nutritionists, scientists, and physicians interested and working in the fields of nephrology and renal nutrition. For contact information, see "Websites of Interest" at the end of this chapter.

The importance of nutritional status and care has been documented to have a role in patient outcomes; therefore the interest in renal nutrition and the number of online resources have substantially increased. See "Websites of Interest" at the end of this chapter for a listing of websites that provide excellent information and links to other sites pertaining to renal nutrition and nephrology.

TO SUM UP

Through its unique functional units, the nephrons, the kidneys act as a filtration system, reabsorbing substances the body needs, secreting additional hydrogen ions to maintain a proper pH balance in the blood, and excreting unnecessary materials in a concentrated urine.

Renal function may be impaired by a variety of conditions. These include inflammatory and degenerative diseases, infection and obstruction, chronic diseases such as hypertension and diabetes, environmental agents such as insecticides and solvents and other toxic substances, and some medications and trauma. Some clinical conditions affecting structure and function include glomerulonephritis, acute and chronic renal failure, renal calculi, and UTI.

CKD and its result, ESRD, are treated by dialysis—hemodialysis or peritoneal dialysis—and kidney transplantation. The diet for CKD needs to include ample calories and protein with restrictions for GFR of less than 25 ml/min/1.72 m^2, only if the patient is able to maintain adequate caloric intake. Dialysis patients must be monitored closely for calories, protein, fluid, and electrolyte balance. All of the diets need to be individualized to ensure overall nutritional adequacy and adherence. Monitoring of nutritional status is important for all patients.

Questions for Review

1. For each of the following conditions, outline the nutritional components of therapy, explaining the impact of each on kidney function: glomerulonephritis, ARF (renal insufficiency), and chronic renal failure.
2. Identify four clinical conditions that impair renal function. Give an example of each, describing its effect on various structures in the kidney.
3. List the nutritional factors that must be monitored in individuals undergoing renal dialysis.
4. Summarize the rationale and nutrient recommendations for patients who have received a renal transplant.
5. Outline the nutritional therapy used for patients with various types of kidney stones. Describe each type of stone and explain the rationale for each aspect of therapy.
6. For what condition is a UTI a predisposing factor? What general nutritional principles are recommended in the treatment of such infections?

References

1. Chatoth D: Elements of renal structure and function. In Carpenter G, Griggs R, Loscalzo J, eds: *Cecil essentials of medicine,* Philadelphia, 2001, WB Saunders.
2. Goldstein DJ, Beth McQuiston: Renal Nutrition. In Matarese L, Gottschlich M, eds: *Contemporary nutrition support practice,* ed 2, Philadelphia, 2002, WB Saunders.
3. Robertson GL, Berl T: Pathophysiology of water metabolism. In Brenner BM, Rector FC, eds: *The kidney,* ed 5, Philadelphia, 1996, WB Saunders.
4. Rose BD: Clinical assessment of renal function. In Rose BD, ed: *Pathophysiology of renal disease,* ed 2, New York, 1987, McGraw-Hill.
5. Gregory, MC: Renal function tests. In Jones S, ed: *Clinical laboratory pearls,* New York, 2001, Lippincott Williams & Wilkins.
6. National Kidney Foundation: K/DOQI clinical practice guidelines for chronic kidney disease: evaluation, classification and stratification, *Am J Kidney Dis* 39(suppl 1):s76, 2002.
7. Zawada E: Initiation of dialysis. In Daugirdas J, Plake P, Ing T, eds: *Handbook of dialysis,* ed 2, Philadelphia, 2001, Lippincott Williams & Wilkins.
8. U.S. Renal Data System: Annual data report II: incidence and prevalence of ESRD, *Am J Kidney Dis* 34:s40,1999.
9. U.S. Renal Data System: Excerpts from the USRDS 2001 annual data report: atlas of end-stage renal disease in the United States, *Am J Kidney Dis* 38(4):s37, 2001.
10. National Kidney Foundation: K/DOQI clinical practice guidelines for chronic kidney disease: evaluation, classification and stratification, *Am J Kidney Dis* 39(suppl 1):s62, 2002.
11. Lu CY, Salant DJ: Renal immunology and pathology, *Curr Opin Nephrol Hypertens* 7(3):27, 1998.
12. Couser W: Mediation of immune glomerular injury. *J Am Soc Nephrol* 1:13, 1990.
13. National Kidney Foundation: K/DOQI clinical practice guidelines for chronic kidney disease: evaluation, classification and stratification, *Am J Kidney Dis* 39(suppl 1):s32, 2002.
14. American Diabetes Association: Diabetic nephropathy, *Diabetes Care* 25(suppl 1):s85, 2002.
15. National Kidney Foundation: K/DOQI clinical practice guidelines for chronic kidney disease: evaluation, classification and stratification, *Am J Kidney Dis* 39(suppl 1): s1-s266, 2002.
16. National Kidney Foundation: K/DOQI clinical practice guidelines for chronic kidney disease: evaluation, classification and stratification, *Am J Kidney Dis* 39(suppl 1):s14, 2002.
17. Qureshi AR et al: Factors influencing malnutrition in hemodialysis patients: a cross-sectional study, *Kidney Int* 53:773, 1998.

18. Goldstein DJ, Callahan C: Strategies for nutritional intervention in patients with renal failure, *Miner Electrolyte Metab* 24(1):82-91, 1997.
19. Klahr S et al: The effects of dietary protein restriction and blood pressure control on the progression of chronic renal failure: modification of diet in renal disease study group, *N Engl J Med* 330:878, 1994.
20. Chertow G, Lazarus M: Malnutrition as a risk factor for morbidity and mortality in maintenance patients. In Kopple J, Massry S, eds: *Nutritional management of renal disease,* Philadelphia, 1997, Williams & Wilkins.
21. Lowrie EG, Lew NL: Death risk in hemodialysis patients: the predictive value of commonly measured variables and an evaluation of death rate between facilities, *Am J Kidney Dis* 15:458, 1990.
22. Owen WF: Nutritional status and survival in end-stage renal disease patients, *Miner Electrolyte Metab* 2:(1):72, 1997.
23. Stenvinkel P et al: Are there two types of malnutrition in chronic renal failure? evidence for relationships between malnutrition, inflammation and atherosclerosis (MIA syndrome), *Nephrol Dial Transplant* 15(7):953, 2000.
24. Kaysen G: Role of inflammation and its treatment in ESRD patients, *Blood Purif* 20:70, 2002.
25. Bistrian BR: Interaction between nutrition and inflammation in end-stage renal disease, *Blood Purif* 18(4):333, 2000.
26. Don BR, Kaysen G: Assessment of inflammation and nutrition in patients with end-stage renal disease, *J Nephrol* 13(4):249, 2000.
27. Kaysen G: Malnutrition and the acute-phase reaction in dialysis patients-how to measure and how to distinguish, *Nephrol Dial Transplant* 15(10):1521, 2000.
28. Hasselwander O: Oxidative stress in chronic renal failure, *Free Radic Res* 29(1):1-11, 1998.
29. Eikelboom J, Hankey G: Associations of homocysteine, C-reactive protein and cardiovascular disease in patients with renal disease, *Curr Opin Nephrol Hypertens* 10:377, 2001.
30. Goldstein DJ: Assessment of nutritional status in renal disease. In Mitch WE, Klahr S, eds: *Nutrition and the kidney,* ed 4, Philadelphia, 2002, Lippincott Williams & Wilkins.
31. Goldstein DJ, McQuiston B: Nutrition and renal disease. In Coulston A, Rock C, Monson E, eds: *Nutrition in the prevention and treatment of disease,* San Diego, 2001, Academic Press.
32. Wolfson M: Causes, manifestations, and assessment of malnutrition in chronic renal failure. In Kopple J, Massry S, eds: *Nutritional management of renal disease,* Philadelphia, 1997, Williams & Wilkins.
33. Kalantar-Zadeh K et al: Food intake characteristics of hemodialysis patients as obtained by food frequency questionnaire, *J Ren Nutr* 12:17, 2002.
34. Bro S, Olgaard K: Effects of excess parathyroid hormone on nonclassical target organs, *Am J Kidney Dis* 30:606, 1997.
35. Frankenfield D et al: Anemia management of adult hemodialysis patients in the U.S.: results from the 1997 Core Indicators project, *Kidney Int* 57:578, 2000.
36. Tarng D et al: Erythropoietin hyporesponsiveness: from iron deficiency to iron overload, *Kidney Int* 55:s107, 1999.
37. Renal Dietitians Dietetic Practice Group, American Dietetic Association: *Guidelines for nutrition care of renal patients,* ed 3, Chicago, 2002, American Dietetic Association (edited by K Wiggins).
38. National Kidney Foundation: K/DOQI clinical practice guidelines for nutrition in chronic renal failure, *Am J Kidney Dis* 35(6; suppl 2):s9-s140, 2000.
39. U.S. Renal Data System: Excerpts from the USRDS 2001 annual data report: atlas of end-stage renal disease in the United States, *Am J Kidney Dis* 38(4):s18, 2001.
40. Weil SE: Nutrition in the kidney transplant recipient. In Danovitch GM, ed: *Handbook of kidney transplantation,* ed 2, Boston, 1996, Little, Brown.
41. Jaggers H, Allman M, Chan M: Changes in clinical profile and dietary considerations after renal transplantation, *J Renal Nutr* 6:12, 1996.
42. Blue L: Adult kidney transplantation. In Hasse J, Blue L, eds: *Comprehensive guide to transplant nutrition,* Chicago, 2002, American Dietetic Association.
43. Weiner Feldman R: Nutrition in acute renal failure, *J Renal Nutr* 4(2):97, 1994.
44. Matarese L: Assessment and nutrition management of the patient with renal disease. In Winkler M, Lysen L, eds: *Suggested guidelines for nutrition and metabolic management of adult patients receiving nutrition support,* ed 2, Chicago, 1993, American Dietetic Association.
45. Williams S: *Essentials of nutrition and diet therapy,* ed 7, St Louis, 1999, Mosby.
46. Monson P, Mehta R: Nutrition in acute renal failure: a reappraisal for the 1990s, *J Renal Nutr* 4(2):58, 1994.
47. Druml W: Nutritional management of acute renal failure. In Jacobson H, Striker G, Skaher S, eds: *The principles and practices of nephrology,* St Louis, 1995, Mosby.
48. Mehta R et al: Refining predictive models in critically ill patients with acute renal failure, *J Sm Soc Nephrol* 13(5) 1350:2002.
49. Burtis WJ et al: Dietary hypercalciuria in patients with calcium oxalate kidney stones, *Am J Clin Nutr* 60(3): 1995.
50. Massy LK, Whiting SJ: Dietary salt, urinary calcium, and kidney stone risk, *Nutr Rev* 53(5):131, 1995.
51. Massy LK et al: Effect of dietary oxalate and calcium on urinary oxalate and risk of formation of calcium oxalate kidney stones, *J Am Diet Assoc* 93(8):901, 1993.
52. Curhan GC et al: Comparison of dietary calcium with supplemental calcium and other nutrients as factors affecting the risk for kidney stones, *Ann Intern Med* 126(7):497, 1997.
53. Coe FL et al: Diet and calcium: the end of an era? *Ann Intern Med* 126(7):553, 1997.
54. Borghi L et al: Comparison of two diets for the prevention of recurrent stones in idiopathic hypercalciuria, *N Eng J Med* 346(2):77, 2002.
55. Dranov P: Urinary tract infection, *Am Health* 14(4):66, 1995.
56. Service RE: New vaccines may ward off urinary tract infections, *Science* 276(5312):533, 1997.
57. Langermann S et al: Prevention of mucosal *Escherichia coli* infection by FimH-adhesin-based system vaccination, *Science* 276(5312):607, 1997.

Further Reading

National Kidney Foundation: Kidney disease outcomes quality initiative (K/DOQI): practice guidelines for peritoneal dialysis adequacy, *Am J Kidney Dis* 37(suppl 1):s55, 2001.

One of the publications from the K/DOQI series, this supplement addresses the main aspects of peritoneal dialysis care and offers to the clinician relevant applicable guidelines based on an extensive review and analysis of the medical literature that can be used to guide clinical management.

Ikizler T et al: Association of morbidity with markers of nutrition and inflammation in chronic hemodialysis patients: a prospective study, *Kidney Int* 55:1945-1951, 1999.

This article provides an analysis of clinical parameters reflective of malnutrition and inflammation that are associated with clinical outcomes.

National Kidney Foundation: Kidney disease outcomes quality initiative: Clinical practice guidelines for the treatment of anemia of chronic renal failure, *Am J Kidney Dis* 37(suppl 1):s182-s235, 2001.

One of the publications from the K/DOQI series, this supplement provides applicable guidelines that the clinician can use to manage the anemia associated with CKD.

Daugirdas J, Van Stone J, Boag J: Hemodialysis apparatus: In Daugirdas J, Blake P, Ing T, eds: *Handbook of dialysis*, ed 3, Philadelphia, 2001, Lippincott Williams & Wilkins.

An excellent overview of what equipment is needed for hemodialysis therapy and how it all works.

Albright RC: Acute renal failure: a practical update, *Mayo Clin Proc* 76:67-74, 2001.

An excellent update on the management of patients with ARF.

Herselman M et al: Protein-energy malnutrition as a risk factor for increased morbidity in long term hemodialysis patients, *J Ren Nutr* 10:7-15, 2000.

Interesting data demonstrating that malnutrition is associated with morbidity in dialysis patients.

Websites of Interest

http://www.jrnjournal.org *Journal of Renal Nutrition* with links to the homepage of the National Kidney Foundation and the Council on Renal Nutrition

http://www.kidney.org National Kidney Foundation

http://www.eatright.org American Dietetic Association

http://www.hdcn.com Hemodialysis, clinical nephrology

http://www.nephronline.com *Nephrology News & Issues*

http://renalsoc.ucdavis.edu/ International Society on Renal Nutrition and Metabolism

http://www.jasn.org *Journal of the American Society of Nephrology*

http://www.ajkd.org *American Journal of Kidney Diseases*

CASE STUDY The patient with chronic renal failure

Mr. Steinberg is 45 years old, married, and works as a city planner for a large municipal government. He cited a recent history of nausea, anorexia, hematuria, and swollen ankles during a physical examination. His wife reported that he had been tiring more easily than usual during the past year. A history of prior illnesses proved negative, except for a severe case of influenza with sore throat 10 years before during an epidemic when he was stationed with the Army overseas. Tests were ordered, and the patient was advised to return in a week for review of the test results and sooner if there were any changes in his symptoms.

Mr. Steinberg did return, with additional symptoms of headaches and occasionally blurred vision. At that time his blood pressure was 160/98, his temperature was 37.5° C (99.6° F), and he had lost 4 kg (8.75 lb). The laboratory tests showed albumin and red and white blood cells in the urine, with an elevated BUN; a PSP indicated a reduced filtration rate. The diagnosis was chronic renal failure.

The physician discussed the diagnosis and its serious prognosis with Mr. and Mrs. Steinberg, giving them the benefits and disadvantages of both hemodialysis and kidney transplantation. Antihypertensive medication was prescribed along with other drugs to minimize discomfort.

During the following weeks Mr. Steinberg continued to lose weight, had increasing joint pain, and became anemic. He found it increasingly difficult to maintain his hectic schedule of frequent meetings, conferences, and public speeches because of gastrointestinal bleeding, increasing nausea, and occasional muscle spasms. Small mouth sores made eating very difficult.

Finally the Steinbergs informed the physician of their decision to accept the kidney transplant as a means of controlling the disease process. They were referred to the clinical nutritionist for renal diet counseling to control protein, sodium, potassium, phosphate, and fluids, as well as to ensure adequate kcalories. After discussing these needs for nutritional maintenance before surgery, the nutritionist helped them develop a meal plan based on Mr. Steinberg's food preferences. Food selection and preparation were discussed in detail, with many ideas for building in as much variety and taste appeal as possible.

The Steinbergs' follow-up with the food plan was excellent. One month later the laboratory values were almost normal, blood pressures averaged 140/88, the headaches and blurred vision had virtually disappeared, and Mr. Steinberg had gained 3.2 kg (7 lb) of his lost weight. The nutrient supplements, including the amino acid analogues, were taken each day as instructed.

Fortunately a kidney donor was soon found, and with the aid of drug control of immune responses the transplant surgery was apparently a success. Mr. Steinberg convalesced well at home, kept all follow-up visits with the healthcare team, and has continued to be asymptomatic 1 year following surgery.

QUESTIONS FOR ANALYSIS

1. Identify a metabolic imbalance caused by renal failure that may account for each symptom presented by Mr. Steinberg.
2. What would be the objectives in care of renal failure such as Mr. Steinberg was experiencing?
3. What factors affect the amount of protein needed by persons with chronic renal failure? What amounts are usually used? Why? What are the amino acid analogues used with the low-protein diet, and why are they used?
4. What factors affect the amount of sodium needed by persons with chronic renal failure? How much is usually recommended?
5. Why is it important to control potassium levels? How much is recommended? What clinical signs presented by Mr. Steinberg may indicate that he had not been getting enough potassium?
6. Why is control of phosphate important in the diet for chronic renal failure? What additional means may be used to control it?
7. What factors affect fluid balance in chronic renal failure? How much is usually allowed?
8. What is the basic principle of the low-protein dietary regimen? List and explain each factor in the diet and potential problems in its management.
9. Outline a general teaching plan you would use to instruct the Steinbergs about the presurgical and postsurgical dietary needs.

Issues & ANSWERS

Kidney Transplantation

Approximately 273,000 Americans receive maintenance dialysis as their kidney replacement. Some patients await transplantation.[1,2] Others cannot consider a transplant because of medical and/or psychosocial issues. Overall, kidney transplantation remains the treatment of choice for the majority of patients with ESRD. Advances in solid organ transplantation and immunosuppressive therapy have resulted in improved patient survival and improved viability of transplanted kidneys.[1-4]

Nearly 50% of all kidney transplant recipients will be alive with a successful functioning transplant 10 years after transplantation.[2] One-year cadaver kidney success rates are 89%, and 5-year success rates are 65%. In comparison the success rates for recipients of living-donor kidneys are 97% at 1 year and 78% at 5 years. A patient who is trouble free for the first 3 months after the transplantation has an excellent prognosis. The most common causes of death after the first year are CVD, infection, and cancer.[2]

The patient who receives a kidney transplant has a challenging first year. Visits to the transplant team occur an average of 2 or 3 times per week during the first month and once per week for up to 3 months after the surgery. Visits then drop to once monthly during the first year if there are no problems. After the first year, it is recommended that patients have their laboratory parameters monitored every 1 to 2 months.[2-4]

Medication regimens are challenging for the transplant recipient. Immunosuppressive agents, lipid-lowering drugs, antihypertensives, and hypoglycemic agents are needed for quite some time. There can be significant side effects to these medicines, and adherence to the rigid medication schedule is critical for successful allograft survival. Medical problems that can develop during the first year include infections such as cytomegalovirus, hyperlipidemia, bone disease, diabetes, CVD, hypertension, and dental problems. Weight gain as a side effect of medications can also become a problem (see text for nutritional recommendations for the kidney transplant recipient).[1-4]

The morbidity and mortality rates for kidney transplantation are clinically significant. These statistics should improve as advances in the technology of the surgery and pharmacologic management occur over time. Not every patient will medically qualify for transplantation, and every candidate must be assessed for their ability to meet the demands of the posttransplantation period. In the future, perhaps the availability of organs for transplantation will be increased by improvements in living related surgeries, development of artificial organs, and/or, most optimistically, finding a cure for progressive kidney disease.[1-4]

REFERENCES

1. Baiardi F et al: Effects of clinical and individual variables on quality of life in chronic renal failure patients, *J Nephrol* 15(1):61, 2002.
2. Braun WE: Update on kidney transplantation: increasing clinical success, expanding waiting lists, *Cleve Clin J Med* 69(6):501, 2002.
3. Matas A et al: Life satisfaction and adverse effects in renal transplant recipients: a longitudinal analysis, *Clin Transplant* 16(2):113, 2002.
4. Centers for Medicare & Medicaid Services: 2001 Annual Report: End Stage Renal Disease Clinical Performance Measures Project, *Am J Kidney Dis* 39(suppl 2):s1, 2002.

Chapter

22

Nutritional Care of Surgery Patients

Gail A. Cresci

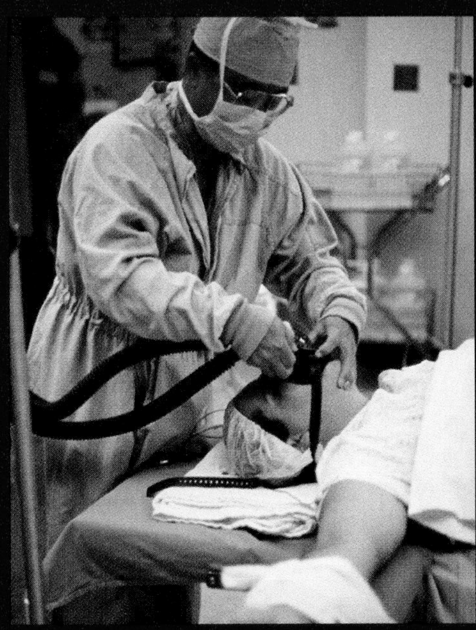

Chapter Outline

In this chapter, various surgical procedures are discussed, with a focus on surgical procedures and situations that could bear a large nutritional consequence, particularly those of the alimentary tract. Understanding the surgical procedure performed, with knowledge of the nutritional and absorptive function and capacity of the alimentary tract, is imperative to providing optimal nutritional care of surgery patients. An understanding of the body's response to metabolic stress is also important when determining the optimal timing and type of nutritional intervention for the patient.

Nutritional Needs of General Surgery Patients

PREOPERATIVE NUTRITION

The nutritional needs of surgery patients varies based on several factors, including the patient's disease process, other comorbidities, and baseline nutritional status. Many general surgery patients are adequately nourished preoperatively and therefore do not have any special nutrient requirements. The disease itself often lends to poor nutrient intake and a hypermetabolic state that places the patient at nutritional risk. Malnutrition is associated with altered immune function, poor wound healing, and increased morbidity and mortality rates.[1] It is estimated that more than 50% of hospitalized patients are malnourished on both hospital admission and hospital discharge.[2-5] Ideally, for optimal outcomes a malnourished patient should be nutritionally repleted for 7 to 10 days before surgery if time permits.[6] Unless the gastrointestinal tract is nonfunctional, nutrient provision should be provided enterally rather than parenterally[7] (see *Practical Application* box).

1. *Energy.* Adequate calories should be consumed to prevent loss of endogenous stores of carbohydrate, fat, and protein. Carbohydrates should comprise the majority of the calories (50% to 60%). A minimum of about 150 g of carbohydrates/day is needed for central nervous system function.
2. *Protein.* Most patients do not have excessive preoperative protein requirements, but body stores should be assessed. Adequate protein status is imperative to facilitate optimal wound healing.
3. *Vitamins and minerals.* Any deficiency state such as anemia should be corrected. Electrolytes and fluids should be normalized and in balance with correction of dehydration, acidosis, or alkalosis.

PRACTICAL APPLICATION

Energy and Protein Requirements in General Surgery Patients

The nutritional needs of general surgery patients vary based on several factors, including the patient's disease process, other comorbidities, surgery to be performed, and baseline nutritional status. For example, compare the following patient situations.

ADEQUATELY NOURISHED PREOPERATIVE PATIENT

For the patient with normal energy and nitrogen balance, approximately 25 kcalorie/kg/day and 0.8 to 1.0 g protein/kg/day should maintain these balances.

ADEQUATELY NOURISHED POSTOPERATIVE PATIENT

After surgery, if no complications occurred, energy requirements remain about the same—25 kcalorie/kg/day. Protein requirements increase slightly due to increased metabolism and need for wound healing in the postoperative period to 1.0 to 1.1 g/kg/day.

ADEQUATELY NOURISHED STRESSED PATIENT

This patient is assumed to have adequate nutrient stores; therefore replenishment is not the goal. The metabolic stress increases metabolic and catabolic rates, making energy and protein needs elevated. Energy needs are estimated at 25 to 30 kcalories/kg/day; protein needs, 1.2 to 1.5 g/kg/day. Postoperatively the patient should be reassessed and protein needs may increase up to 2 g/kg/day.

NUTRITIONALLY DEPLETED NONSTRESSED PATIENT

Upcoming Surgery: GI Tract Resection Resulting From Obstruction

Because of reduced dietary intake, this patient's nutrient stores (mostly glycogen and fat) may be depleted. In the nonstressed state, protein stores are spared for the most part. Energy needs are similar to those of the nourished preoperative patient at 25 kcalories/kg/day. However, protein needs are slightly elevated to 1.0 to 1.2 g/kg/day. Postoperatively this patient's energy needs will remain near the same at 25 kcalories/kg/day, but protein needs are increased to 1.2 to 1.5 g/kg/day.

NUTRITIONALLY DEPLETED STRESSED PATIENT

This patient has both elevated energy and protein requirements because of cytokine and hormonal shifts causing a hypermetabolic and hypercatabolic state. Energy needs are 25 to 30 kcalories/kg/day with caution to avoid overfeeding. Overfeeding in a hypermetabolic state can result in hyperglycemia, hypercarbia, hepatic steatosis, and overall immune suppression. Protein needs are elevated to 1.5 to 2.0 g/kg/day. Postoperatively the nutrient needs remain about the same. At this point, the goal is to minimize loss of lean body mass, not to replenish it. Once the patient is stable and anabolic, calories can be increased to 35 kcalories/kg/day as needed for rehabilitation.

References

A.S.P.E.N. Board of Directors: Guidelines for the use of parenteral and enteral nutrition in adult and pediatric patients, *J Parent Enteral Nutr* 26, 2002.

Frakenfield D: Energy and macrosubstrate requirements. In *The science and practice of nutrition support,* ed 3, Dubuque, Iowa, 2001, Kendall/Hunt.

Immediate Preoperative Period

Typical dietary preparation for surgery involves giving nothing by mouth 8 to 12 hours before surgery. The rationale is to ensure that the stomach is empty of food and liquids to prevent vomiting or aspiration during surgery or anesthesia recovery. In an emergency situation, gastric suction is used to remove stomach contents. With surgery involving the gastrointestinal (GI) tract, food and fecal matter may interfere with the procedure itself and cause contamination. Therefore before lower GI surgery, a low-residue diet may be prescribed to reduce fecal residue. Although restricting dietary intake may prevent risks of anesthesia, it can also impair the patient's ability to respond to the metabolic stress of surgery. Recent research is investigating the provision of a carbohydrate-containing drink 2 to 3 hours before surgery to prevent glycogen depletion and hence lack of body fuel when energy needs are increased.

POSTOPERATIVE NUTRITION

Nutrient provision in the postoperative period depends on several factors, including the surgical procedure performed and anticipated time to resumption of oral intake, complications of surgery and postoperative clinical status, and preoperative nutritional status. The well-nourished patient undergoing elective surgery will typically resume oral feeding by postoperative day 3 to 7, depending on the return of bowel function. In this situation, supplemental nutrition in the form of enteral and parenteral nutrition is not indicated. The malnourished patient who is undergoing elective or emergency surgery and not anticipated to be able to meet his or her nutritional needs orally for a period of 7 to 10 days should receive specialized nutrition support.[6] This nutrition support should be provided enterally rather than parenterally to minimize the incidence of complications.[6] The duration of this therapy will then depend on the patient's clinical status and transition to an adequate oral dietary consumption.

Energy Requirements

In the immediate postoperative period, especially in the critically ill, the goal of nutritional support is maintenance of current lean body mass, not repletion, and should serve as an adjunct to other critical therapies. Numerous factors are present that limit the effectiveness of exogenously administered nutritional substrates from preventing catabolism regardless of the level of support. It should not be expected to convert a catabolic septic patient into an anabolic state at this time. Many undesirable metabolic complications can occur in attempting to do so, such as hypercapnia, hyperglycemia, hypertriglyceridemia, hepatic steatosis, and azotemia.[7-11] Once the hypermetabolic process is corrected, anabolism is favored and repletion can occur.

There are multiple methods for determining energy requirements. Indirect calorimetry involves the actual measurement of energy expenditure and remains the "gold standard."[12] However, there are many disadvantages to this method, including increased cost, trained personnel, and inaccurate readings in patients with an FIO_2 of 50% or greater, malfunctioning chest tubes, endotracheal tubes, or bronchopleurofistulas. Because of these flaws, many institutions do not have the technology available and rely on predictive equations. Predicting energy needs can be difficult because of uncertainties regarding multiple factors on energy expenditure (Table 22-1).[13] Predictive equations (Box 22-1) may overestimate energy needs for those mechanically ventilated and sedated, and neuromuscular paralysis can decrease energy requirements by as much as 30%.[14] Calculated results are only as accurate as the variables used in the equation. Obesity and resuscitative water weight complicate the use of these equations and lead to a tendency for overfeeding.[15] It is unclear as to whether ideal body weight (IBW) or total body weight should be used in predictive energy equations. It has been reported that obese patients should receive 20 to 30 kilocalories (kcalories)/kg IBW/day,[16] as well as utilization of adjusted body weight, particularly in those greater than 130% IBW.[15] Predictive equations have been developed to account for obesity, using actual body weight, as well as trauma, burns, and ventilatory status.[17] Patino et al[18] reported a hypocaloric-hyperproteinic nutrition regimen provided during the first days of the flow phase of the adaptive response

TABLE 22-1 Influences on Resting Energy Expenditure

Clinical Condition	REE (%)*
Elective Uncomplicated Surgery	Normal
Major Abdominal, Thoracic, and Vascular Surgery	
ICU + mechanical ventilation	105-109 ± 20-28
Cardiac Surgery	
ICU + mechanical ventilation	119 ± 21
Multiple Injury	
ICU + mechanical ventilation	138 ± 23
Spontaneous ventilation	119 ± 7
Head and multiple injury, ICU + mechanical ventilation	150 ± 23
Head Injury	
ICU + spontaneous ventilation	126 ± 14
ICU + mechanical ventilation	104 ± 5
Infection	
Sepsis + spontaneous ventilation	121 ± 27
ICU + septic shock + mechanical ventilation	135 ± 28
Sepsis + mechanical ventilation	155 ± 14
Septic shock + mechanical ventilation	102 ± 14
Multiple injury + sepsis + mechanical ventilation + TPN	191 ± 38

*Values are percentage of reference value (±SD).

REE, Resting energy expenditure; *ICU,* intensive care unit; *TPN,* total parenteral nutrition.

Adapted from Chiolero R, Revelly JP, Tappy L: Energy metabolism in sepsis and injury, *Nutrition* 13(Suppl):45S-51S, 1997, with permission from Elsevier Science.

BOX 22-1 Selected Methods for Estimating Energy Requirements

Harris-Benedict Basal Energy Expenditure Equation (BEE)

$$\text{Male: } 13.75(W) + 5(H) - 6.76(A) + 66.47$$

$$\text{Female: } 9.56(W) + 1.85(H) - 4.68(A) + 655.1$$

Where W is weight (in kilograms); H, height (in centimeters); and A, age (in years).

NOTE: To predict total energy expenditure (TEE), add an injury/activity factor of 1.2 to 1.8 depending on the severity and nature of illness.

Ireton-Jones Energy Expenditure Equations (EEEs)

Obesity

$$EEE = (606 \times S) + (9 \times W) - (12 \times A) + (400 \times V) + 1444$$

Spontaneously Breathing Patients

$$EEE\ (s) = 629 - 11(A) + 25(W) - 609(O)$$

Ventilator-Dependent Patients

$$EEE\ (v) = 1784 - 11(A) + 5(W) + 244(S) + 239(T) + 804(B)$$

Where EEE is given in kcalories/day; *v,* ventilator dependent; *s,* spontaneously breathing; *A,* age (in years); *W,* body weight (in kilograms), *S,* sex (male = 1, female = 0); *V,* ventilator support (present = 1, absent = 0), *T,* diagnosis of trauma (present = 1, absent = 0); *B,* diagnosis of burn (present = 1, absent = 0); and *O,* obesity >30% above IBW (from 1959 Metropolitan Life Insurance tables; present = 1, absent = 0).

Curreri Burn Formula (Estimated Energy Expenditure)

$$\text{EEE for ages 18 to 59 years} = (25\ \text{kcalorie} \times W) + (40 \times \text{TBSA burn})$$

$$\text{EEE for ages} \geq 60\ \text{years} = BEE + (65 \times \text{TBSA burn})$$

Where EEE is given in kcalories/day; *W,* weight (in kilograms); *TBSA,* total body surface area (in percent).

to injury, sepsis, and critical illness. The regimen consists of a daily supply of 100 to 200 g of glucose and 1.5 to 2.0 g of protein per kg IBW. Overall, energy requirements for surgery patients range from 20 to 35 kcalories/kg usual body weight/day.[19]

Protein Requirements

Dietary protein is required to build new and maintain existing body tissue and has many functions in the body. Protein can also be oxidized directly for ATP and is critical to the body's ability to perform gluconeogenesis. Therefore protein is an important energy substrate in addition to its role in tissue building and repair.

Protein requirements in the surgical patient are typically elevated, particularly in the critically ill. Increased requirements are the result of the need for tissue synthesis and wound healing, maintenance of oncotic pressure, adequate blood volume, maintenance of immune function, and energy substrate. Stressed critically ill patients require protein in the range of 1.5 to 2.0 g/kg/day.[18] Achieving positive nitrogen balance is nearly impossible immediately after the metabolic insult, but after the primary insult is controlled or resolved, positive nitrogen balance is feasible. Protein requirements do not decrease with increasing age. Reduction in lean body mass and obligatory loss of protein during physiologic stress increase protein requirements for the critically ill older patient to that similar to that for a younger patient.[20] Protein tolerance as opposed to protein requirement often determines the amount of protein delivered. The onset of azotemia, impaired renal or hepatic function, signals the need to reduce protein delivery. Most studies that examined graded protein intakes in septic, injured, or burned patients have found no protein-sparing benefit to giving protein in excess of the above recommendations.[21]

Fluid Requirements

Water is the medium within which all systems and subsystems function. It is necessary in the digestion, absorption, transport, and utilization of nutrients as well as the elimination of toxins and waste products. Water also provides structure to cells and is a vital component of thermoregulation. Water is the most abundant substance in the human body, accounting for approximately 60% of body weight of adult males and 50% of body weight of adult females. The majority of water intake comes from ingested fluid and food; a small amount is produced as a byproduct of metabolic processes, primarily carbohydrate metabolism. The main source of water loss is in the form of urine. However, sizeable amounts are also lost insensibly through the skin and respiratory tract. Smaller amounts of water are lost in sweat and feces (Table 22-2).

Normal body water requirements can be estimated using a variety of methods. The National Research Council recommends 1 ml/kcalorie energy expenditure for adults with average energy expenditure living under average environmental conditions. Fluid requirements increase with several conditions, including fever, high altitude, low humidity, profuse sweating, watery diarrhea, vomiting, hemorrhage, diuresis, surgical drains, and loss of skin integrity (e.g., burns, open wounds).

Therefore fluid balance is of vital concern after surgery. Patients often receive large volumes of fluid intraoperatively. These volumes are normally diuresed postoperatively, but occasionally the patient may require diuretics to facilitate this. Typically surgical patients are provided with intravenous fluids until oral intake is resumed and tolerated to

TABLE 22-2 Normal Daily Fluid Gains and Losses in Adults

Fluid Gains		Fluid Losses	
Sensible		***Sensible***	
Food	1000 ml	Urine	1500 ml
Fluid	1200 ml	Feces	100 ml
		Sweat	50 ml
Insensible		***Insensible***	
Oxidative metabolism	350 ml	Skin	500 ml
		Lungs	400 ml
TOTAL	2550 ml	TOTAL	2550 ml

From The Science and Practice of Nutrition Support: A Case-Based Core Curriculum by American Society for Parenteral and Enteral Nutrition, ed 3. Copyright © 2001 by ASPEN. Reprinted by permission of Kendall/Hunt Publishing Company.

maintain fluid balance. Daily weight measurement of the patient provides a guideline for fluid balance.

Vitamins and Minerals

Adequate levels of vitamins and minerals are very important for optimal postoperative recovery. Vitamin C serves many functions in the body. In addition to being an antioxidant, it is required for the synthesis of collagen, carnitine, and neurotransmitters and for the immune-mediated and antibacterial functions of white blood cells. Iron is an essential component of hemoglobin, which is necessary for oxygen transport; of myoglobin, which is necessary for muscle iron storage; and in cytochromes, which are necessary for the oxidative production of cellular energy. Vitamin K is essential in the blood-clotting mechanism. Surgical patients with elevated enteric losses (e.g., ostomy, stool, fistula) are at risk for several trace element deficiencies (e.g., zinc, copper). If losses exceed 800 ml/day, extra supplementation of micronutrients should be considered. Various GI operations may also place a surgical patient at risk for several micronutrient deficiencies, depending on the location of bowel resected.

DIETS

Oral Diet

The preferred route of nutrient delivery is for the patient to be able to self-consume adequate nutrients. Fortunately the majority of surgical patients can accomplish this by postoperative day 7 at the latest. Routine intravenous fluids are intended to provide hydration and electrolytes, not energy and protein requirements. For example, 1 L of routine intravenous fluids of a 5% dextrose solution provides 50 g of dextrose, with an energy value of only 170 kcalories; no protein is provided. If adequate calories and protein are not consumed, then the patient's diet may be supplemented. Often the addition of between-meal feedings consisting of soft, high-protein foods is adequate. However, sometimes commercially available oral supplements may be provided because they are a concentrated source of energy, protein, and vitamins/minerals.[23] Not all patients tolerate these supplements because they tend to be very sweet and patients develop taste fatigue. Every effort should be made to maximize the patient's diet for their diet preferences to improve inadequate dietary consumption.

BOX 22-2 Typical Foods in Postoperative Diets

Clear Liquid
Broth
Clear juice (apple, grape, cranberry)
Jello
Sodas (Sprite, Ginger Ale)
Tea
Coffee

Full Liquid
Juice (any)
Milk
Milkshakes
Ice cream
Cream soups
Thinned oatmeal, corn grits
Scrambled eggs (in some institutions)
Oral liquid nutrition supplements (e.g., Ensure, Boost)

Soft/Regular
Juice
Canned fruits
Cooked vegetables
Soft meats (baked chicken, stews, roasts)
Scrambled eggs
Pancakes, biscuits, muffins
Soups
Soft sandwiches (egg, tuna, chicken salad, turkey, ham and cheese)
Soft starches (mashed potatoes, pasta, rice)
Milk, tea, coffee
Ice cream
Puddings, yogurt
Soft desserts (cake, pies, soft cookies)

Routine Postoperative Diets

A diet order is typically prescribed postoperatively once the patient exhibits adequate bowel function (e.g., flatus, bowel sounds present). Historically the first diet order is a clear liquid diet (Box 22-2). This diet contains hyperosmolar

sepsis Presence in the blood or other tissues of pathogenic microorganisms or their toxins; conditions associated with such pathogens.

BOX 22-3 Indications for Parenteral Nutrition

- Bowel obstruction
- Persistent intolerance of enteral feeding (e.g., emesis, diarrhea)
- Hemodynamic instability
- Major upper gastrointestinal bleed
- Ileus
- Unable to safely access intestinal tract

Relative Indications

- Significant bowel wall edema
- Nutrient infusion proximal to recent gastrointestinal anastomosis
- High output fistula (>800 ml/day)

BOX 22-4 Methods of Enteral Access

Short Term (<4 wk)	Long Term (>4 wk)
Nasoenteric Feeding Tube	***Percutaneous Feeding Tube***
Spontaneous passage	*Percutaneous Endoscopic*
Bedside—prokinetic agent	Gastric (PEG)
Active Passage	Gastric/jejunal (PEG/J)
Bedside—assisted	Direct jejunal (DPEJ)
Endoscopic	***Laparoscopic***
Fluoroscopic	Gastrostomy
Operative	Jejunostomy
	Surgical
	Gastrostomy
	Jejunostomy

fluids, calories from primarily simple sugars, very little protein, and a fair amount of sodium and chloride. Because this diet is an incomplete diet and very unpalatable, patients should be advanced to either a full liquid or soft/regular diet as soon as the clear liquid diet is tolerated. These diets are complete diets in that calorie, protein, and vitamin/mineral requirements can be met if adequate amounts are consumed. Recently this historical diet progression after GI surgery was challenged.[24] Patients randomized to a regular diet as their first postoperative diet after abdominal surgery had equal tolerance and improved nutrient intake compared with those receiving a clear liquid diet.

Specialized Nutrition Support

If an oral diet is not tolerated or feasible, then enteral or parenteral nutrition may be provided. Enteral nutrition is indicated for patients with an adequately functional GI tract and whose oral nutrient intake is insufficient to meet estimated needs.[6] Enteral nutrition maintains the nutritional, metabolic, immunologic, and barrier functions of the intestines; it is less expensive and safer than parenteral nutrition.[25] Although enteral nutrition is the preferred route of nutrient delivery, it is not innocuous and there are some situations where enteral feeding is not feasible (Box 22-3) and parenteral nutrition should be used. The expected length of therapy, clinical condition, risk of aspiration, and local expertise usually determine route of administration and type of access for tube feedings. There are multiple methods for obtaining enteral access (Box 22-4), all of which carry various degrees of expertise, risk, and expense. Nasoenteric or oroenteric tubes are generally used when therapy is anticipated to be of short duration (e.g., <4 weeks) or for interim access before the placement of a long-term device. Long-term access requires a percutaneous or surgically placed feeding tube. It is not always clear when enteral nutrition will be tolerated. If the individual's needs are not met enterally, then parenteral nutrition may be implemented for either full nutrient provision or concurrently with the enteral delivery to provide the balance of nutrients not tolerated.

The majority of postoperative surgical patients can tolerate a standard enteral formulation that provides their energy and protein requirements. Recently research studies have evaluated the use of "immune-enhancing" enteral formulas in postoperative gastrointestinal cancer patients, trauma patients, and patients with critical illness. These formulas are supplemented with various "immune-enhancing" nutrients, including L-arginine, L-glutamine, omega-3 fatty acids, nucleic acids, and various vitamins and minerals. When these diets were used in these surgical populations, decreases in infectious complications and hospital length of stay were noted.[6,26]

Nutritional Concerns for Patients Undergoing Alimentary Canal Surgery

The digestive tract is a metabolically active organ involved in the digestion, absorption, and metabolism of many nutrients; therefore various surgical interventions involving the GI tract can result in malabsorption and maldigestion and nutritional deficiencies.

HEAD AND NECK SURGERY

These patients often present for surgery malnourished due to their disease state. Many times surgical intervention is required due to a tumor that may be inhibiting the patient's ability to chew and swallow normally. Typically the loss of this ability is what makes the patient seek medical attention. Patients with head and neck cancer usually have a long history of alcohol and tobacco use, which may also affect optimal nutritional status.

Depending on the patient's treatment, optimization of nutrition preoperatively is ideal. This also depends on the individual's disease progression and ability to swallow. Many times preoperative treatment involves radiation and/or chemotherapy to reduce the tumor size. In these situations ability to swallow may worsen due to the negative side effects of these therapies. Ideally, placement of a percutaneous endoscopic gastrostomy (PEG) feeding tube can be performed to allow for nutrition, hydration, and medication administration to maintain and/or improve nutritional status preoperatively. The patient may also still be able to swallow soft foods or liquids, which should be maximized for caloric and protein density. If a PEG tube is not placed preoperatively, it can be placed intraoperatively or a nasoenteric tube may be placed. These feeding tubes are then used postoperatively until the patient is able to resume an oral diet.

ESOPHAGEAL SURGERY

There are several medical conditions affecting the esophagus that can prevent swallowing and thus nutrient intake. Common conditions include corrosive injuries and perforation, achalasia, gastroesophageal reflux disease (GERD), and partial or full obstruction caused by cancer, congenital abnormalities, or strictures. These conditions usually require surgical intervention involving removal of a segment or the entire esophagus. The esophageal tract is then replaced with either the stomach (gastric pull-up) or the intestine (colonic/jejunal interposition). A gastric pull-up procedure involves drawing the stomach up to the esophageal stump, causing displacement of the stomach into the thoracic cavity. This procedure results in a reduction of stomach volume capacity, with potential delayed gastric emptying and dumping syndrome (Table 22-3). The colonic/jejunal interposition procedure involves forming a new conduit by anastomosing the selected portion of bowel between the esophagus and stomach. Complications following this procedure include swallowing difficulties, strictures, and leakage at the anastomotic site.

Preoperative nutrition for these patients may be a tolerated oral diet, often liquids because of dysphasia and obstruction. If a patient is unable to consume his or her full nutrient needs orally, then a feeding tube may be placed if the esophagus is not obstructed. A PEG tube is not indicated if a gastric pull-up procedure is to be performed because the stomach is used to make the esophageal conduit and a hole resulting from a gastrostomy tube would be contraindicated. These patients may require preoperative parenteral nutrition if the esophagus is obstructed. Intraoperatively, a jejunal feeding tube may be placed to allow for postoperative enteral nutrition until the anastomosis heals and oral intake is resumed. If enteral access is not obtained intraoperatively, then parenteral nutrition is indicated because these patients may not resume oral intake for 7 to 10 days.

For patients with chronic GERD, a Nissen fundoplication procedure may be performed. This is the most commonly performed antireflux procedure operation for patients with gastroesophageal reflux refractory to medical management. This procedure involves wrapping the stomach around the base of the esophagus, near the lower esophageal sphincter; this places pressure and narrows

---

anastomosis A surgical joining of two ducts to allow flow from one to the other.

dumping syndrome Constellation of postprandial symptoms that result from rapid emptying of hyperosmolar gastric contents into the duodenum. The hypertonic load in the small intestine promotes reflux of vascular fluid into the bowel lumen, causing a rapid decrease in the circulating blood volume. Rapid symptoms of abdominal cramping, nausea, vomiting, palpitations, sweating, weakness, reduced blood pressure, tremors, and osmotic diarrhea occur. Symptoms of early dumping begin 10 to 30 minutes after eating; late dumping syndrome occurs 1 to 4 hours after a meal. Late dumping is a result of insulin hypersecretion in response to the carbohydrate load dumped into the small intestine. Once the carbohydrate is absorbed, the hyperinsulinemia causes hypoglycemia, which results in vasomotor symptoms such as diaphoresis, weakness, flushing, and palpitations. Individuals who have undergone gastrointestinal surgery resulting in a reduced or absent gastric pouch are more prone to dumping syndrome.

gastroesophageal reflux disease (GERD) Describes symptoms that result from reflux of gastric juices, and sometimes duodenal juices, into the esophagus. Symptoms include substernal burning (heartburn), epigastric pressure sensation, and severe epigastric pain. Prolonged and severe GERD can lead to esophageal bleeding, perforation, strictures, Barrett's epithelium, adenocarcinoma, and pulmonary fibrosis (from aspiration). Conservative dietary therapy involves weight reduction; restriction of carbonated beverages, caffeine, fatty foods, peppermint, chocolate, and ethanol; small frequent meals; and wearing of loose clothing to promote symptomatic relief.

malabsorption and maldigestion Malabsorption is a syndrome in which normal products of digestion do not traverse the intestinal mucosa and enter the lymphatic or portal venous branches. Maldigestion, which may be clinically similar to malabsorption, describes defects in the intraluminal phase of the digestive process caused by inadequate exposure of chyme to bile salts and pancreatic enzymes. Clinical symptoms of malabsorption include diarrhea, steatorrhea, and weight loss. Laboratory signs include depressed serum fat-soluble vitamin levels, accelerated prothrombin time, hypomagnesemia, and hypocholesterolemia. Patients with symptoms of malabsorption should have a laboratory work-up to determine the presence and degree of nutrient loss.

sphincter A circular band of muscle fibers that constricts a passage or closes a natural opening in the body (e.g., lower esophageal sphincter, pyloric sphincter).

TABLE 22-3 Common Gastrointestinal Operations and Nutritional Consequences

Location	Potential Consequences
Esophagus	
Resection/replacement	Weight loss due to inadequate intake
Gastric pull-up	↑ Protein loss due to catabolism
Colonic interposition	May require enteral/parenteral nutrition until oral intake appropriate
	Antidumping diet; may malabsorb fat/fat-soluble vitamins, simple sugars, and various vitamins/minerals
	Early satiety due to reduced storage capacity (gastric pull-up)
Stomach	
Partial gastrectomy/ vagotomy	Early satiety due to reduced storage capacity
	Delayed gastric emptying of solids due to stasis
	Rapid emptying of hypertonic fluids
Total gastrectomy	Weight loss due to dumping/malabsorption, early satiety, anorexia, inadequate intake, unavailability of bile acids and pancreatic enzymes due to anastomotic changes
	Malabsorption may lead to anemia, metabolic bone disease, protein-calorie malnutrition
	Bezoar formation
	Vitamin B_{12} deficiency due to lack of intrinsic factor
Intestine*	
Proximal	Malabsorption of vitamins/minerals (Ca^{2+}, Mg^{2+}, iron, vitamins A and D)
Gastric bypass	Protein-calorie malnutrition from malabsorption due to dumping, unavailability of bile acids and pancreatic enzymes due to anastomotic changes
	Bezoar formation
Distal	Malabsorption of vitamins/mineral (water soluble—folate, vitamins B_{12}, C, B_1, B_2, pyridoxine)
	Protein-calorie malnutrition due to dumping
	Fat malabsorption
	Bacterial overgrowth if ileocecal valve resected
Colon	Fluid and electrolyte (K^+, Na^+, Cl^-) malabsorption

*Note that consequences only may occur with extensive disease process and resection.

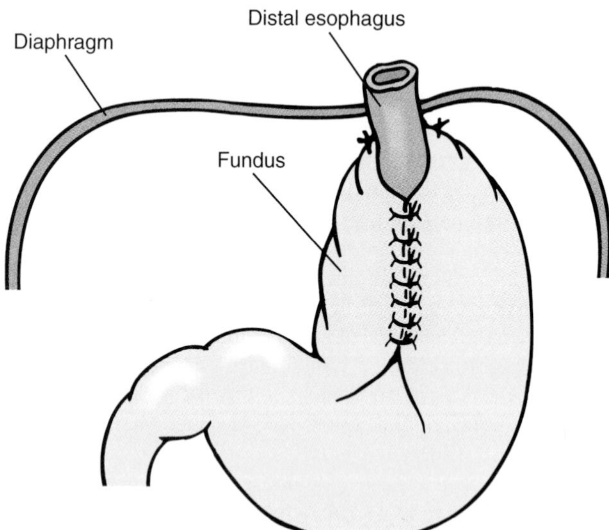

FIGURE 22-1 Nissen fundoplication. *(From Lewis SM, Heitkemper MM, Dirksen SR:* Medical-surgical nursing: assessment and management of clinical problems, *ed 5, St Louis, 2000, Mosby.)*

the lower esophageal opening to prevent reflux (Figure 22-1). Patients are typically placed on a pureed diet for 2 weeks after this procedure with small frequent meals, no gulping of liquids, and crushed or liquid medications. After this time solid foods are gradually added to the diet with future avoidance of bread products, nuts, and seeds because these can become lodged in the lower esophagus and cause an obstruction.

GASTRIC SURGERY

A number of nutrition problems may develop after gastric surgery, depending on the type of surgical procedure and the patient's response (see Table 22-3). There are several indications for gastric surgery, including tumor removal, ulcer disease, perforation, hemorrhage, Zollinger-Ellison syndrome, gastric polyposis, and Menetrier's disease. A vagotomy is often performed to eliminate gastric acid secretion. Vagotomy at certain levels can alter the normal physiologic function of the stomach, small intestine, pancreas, and biliary system. The total gastric and truncal vagotomy procedures impair proximal and distal

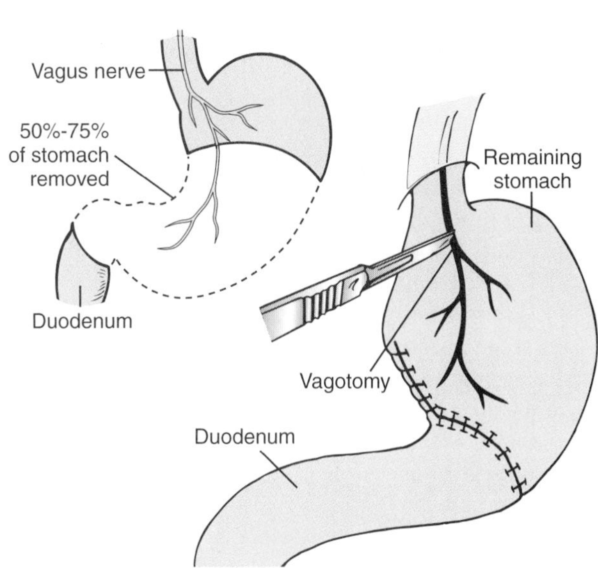

FIGURE 22-2 Billroth I (gastroduodenostomy). (*From Lewis SM, Heitkemper MM, Dirksen SR:* Medical-surgical nursing: assessment and management of clinical problems, *ed 5, St Louis, 2000, Mosby.*)

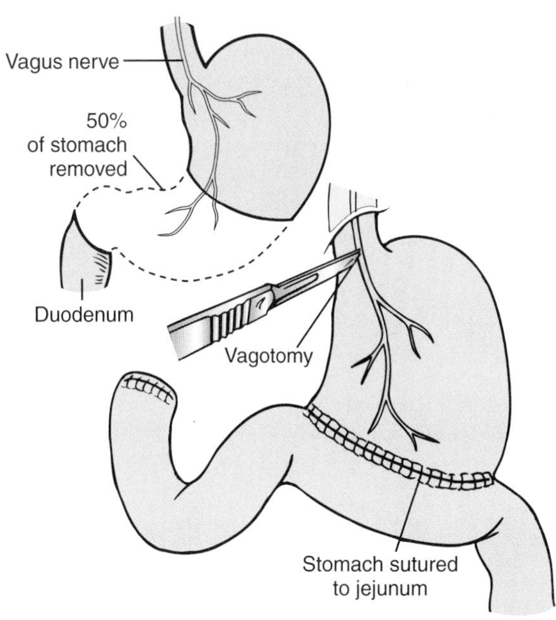

FIGURE 22-3 Billroth II (gastrojejunostomy). (*From Lewis SM, Heitkemper MM, Dirksen SR:* Medical-surgical nursing: assessment and management of clinical problems, *ed 5, St Louis, 2000, Mosby.*)

motor function of the stomach. Digestion and emptying of solids are retarded while emptying of liquids is accelerated.[27] These vagotomy procedures are commonly accompanied by a drainage procedure (antrectomy or pyloroplasty) that helps the stomach to empty. Nutrition complications associated with vagotomy and pylorplasty include dumping syndrome, steatorrhea, and bacterial overgrowth.

A total gastrectomy involves removal of the entire stomach. A storage reservoir may be created using a section of the jejunum. A subtotal or partial gastrectomy involves removal of a portion of the stomach accompanied by a reconstructive procedure. A Billroth I (gastroduodenostomy) involves an anastomosis of the proximal end of the intestine (duodenum) to the distal end of the stomach (Figure 22-2). A Billroth II (gastrojejunostomy) involves an anastomosis of the stomach to the side of the jejunum, which creates a blind loop (Figure 22-3). Any gastric surgery carries some potential for the development of malnutrition. Common consequences include weight loss, dumping syndrome, malabsorption, anemia, and metabolic bone disease. Dumping syndrome, epigastric fullness, nausea, and vomiting often occur in the early postoperative period. These symptoms are managed with dietary modifications and antiemetic medications.[27]

Generally after gastric surgery, small frequent oral feedings are resumed according to the patient's tolerance (Box 22-5). For the first 2 weeks after surgery, soft, bland foods with a low fiber content should be consumed in small portions. Simple sugars, lactose, and fried foods should be avoided; beverages should be consumed at least 30 minutes before and after meals; and foods high in complex carbohydrates and protein should be emphasized. Generally these diet modifications are necessary for only the short term because most patients can resume a regular diet. However, some individuals may need an antidumping diet indefinitely. For individuals who were malnourished preoperatively, a small bowel feeding tube may be placed intraoperatively. Low-rate enteral feedings using a standard formulation may be initiated on postoperative day 1. Tube feedings are adjusted according to the patient's clinical progress and tolerance of an oral diet. Patients may be discharged home with nocturnal tube feedings until their oral diet consumption is optimal.

gastric polyposis An abnormal condition characterized by the presence of numerous polyps in the stomach.

Menetrier's disease (giant hypertrophic gastritis) Rare disease characterized by large folds of nodular gastric rugae that may cover the wall of the stomach, causing anorexia, nausea, vomiting, and abdominal distress.

vagotomy Cutting of certain branches of the vagus nerve, performed with gastric surgery, to reduce the amount of gastric acid secreted and lessen the chance of recurrence of a gastric ulcer.

Zollinger-Ellison syndrome A condition characterized by severe peptic ulceration, gastric hypersecretion, elevated serum gastrin, and gastrinoma of the pancreas or the duodenum. Total gastrectomy may be necessary.

BOX 22-5 Postgastrectomy Antidumping Diet

Principles of Diet

After surgery, some discomfort or diarrhea may occur, therefore to reduce the likelihood of those symptoms, a healthy, nutritionally complete diet should be followed. Each person may react to food differently. Foods should be reintroduced into the diet slowly.

Steps of Diet

1. Intake of complex carbohydrates is unlimited (e.g., bread, vegetables, rice, potatoes).
2. Intake of simple sugars (e.g., sugar, candy, cake, pies, jelly, honey) should be kept to a minimum. Artificial sweeteners may be used.
3. Fat intake should be moderate (≤30% total calories).
4. Protein should be unlimited because it helps with wound healing (e.g., meats, legumes).
5. Milk contains lactose, which may be hard to digest. Introduce milk and milk products slowly several weeks after surgery.
6. Eat small, frequent meals, approximately 6 meals per day, to avoid loading the stomach.
7. Limit fluids to 4 oz (½ cup) during mealtimes. This prevents the rapid movement of food through the upper gastrointestinal tract.
8. Drink fluids 30-45 minutes before and after eating to prevent diarrhea.
9. Relatively low-roughage foods and raw foods are allowed as tolerated after postoperative day 14.
10. Eat and chew slowly.
11. Avoid extreme temperatures of foods.

Sample Menu

Breakfast	Lunch	Dinner
Scrambled egg, 1	Bread, 2 slices	Chicken breast, 3 oz
Toast, 1 slice	Ham, 2 oz	Mashed potatoes, ½ cup
Margarine, 1 tsp	Cheese, 1 oz	Green beans, ½ cup
Low-sugar jelly, 1 tsp	Mustard, 2 tsp	Margarine, 2 tsp
Banana, 1 small	Canned fruit, water packed	Yogurt, sugar-free, 4 oz
	Yogurt, sugar-free, 4 oz	
Mid-Morning Snack	**Mid-Afternoon Snack**	**Evening Snack**
Canned fruit, water packed, ½ cup	Saltine crackers, 3 squares	Sugar-free pudding, ½ cup
Graham crackers, 2 squares	Peanut butter, 1 tbsp	Vanilla Wafers, 3 pieces

Oral supplements may be provided to increase nutrient intake; however, they need to be isotonic, containing no simple sugars, to avoid dumping. Unfortunately, most oral liquid supplements are hyperosmolar, containing simple sugars, and therefore are not well tolerated after gastric surgery. Parenteral nutrition is indicated only if enteral access is not available and the patient is malnourished and not able to tolerate adequate nutrients orally.

Anemia is a common consequence of gastric surgery. Anemia can be attributed to a deficiency or malabsorption of one or more nutrients, including iron, vitamin B_{12}, and folate. Assimilation of vitamin B_{12} requires liberation of the vitamin from protein and binding of the vitamin to intrinsic factor, both of which occur in the stomach. Failure of either of these reactions to occur results in vitamin B_{12} malabsorption, which with time produces anemia.[27] Total gastrectomy patients require periodic intramuscular vitamin B_{12} injections. Metabolic bone disease can be a late complication of gastric surgery. The cause of metabolic bone disease varies with the surgical procedure. The Billroth II procedure is associated with more complications than is the Billroth I because it bypasses the duodenum and upper jejunum (the site of calcium absorption). Procedures that destroy the pylorus can result in rapid gastric emptying, which may contribute to the development of metabolic bone disease. Rapid gastric emptying not only reduces absorption time but also, when fats are malabsorbed, can lead to formation of insoluble calcium soaps.[27] Fat malabsorption can also lead to vitamin D malabsorption, which leads to impaired metabolism of calcium and phosphorus.

INTESTINAL SURGERY

Surgical resections of the small and large intestine are usually well tolerated. If excessive amounts of bowel are removed, nutritional consequences can arise depending on the location resected (see Table 22-3). If more than 50% of the small intestine is removed, short bowel syndrome may occur. This syndrome is characterized by severe diarrhea or steatorrhea, malabsorption, and malnutrition. Often the patient may require long-term parenteral nutrition to maintain his or her nutritional status and fluid and electrolyte balance (see Chapter 17).

PANCREATICODUODENECTOMY (WHIPPLE PROCEDURE)

In cases of ampullary, duodenal, and pancreatic malignancies, a pancreaticoduodenectomy may be performed. This procedure, one of the most difficult and technically demanding in GI surgery, involves resecting the distal stomach, the distal common duct, the pancreatic head, and the duodenum. Three anastomoses—pancreaticojejunostomy, choledochojejunostomy, and gastrojejunostomy (Billroth II)—must be performed. In the past few years a pyloric sparing Whipple procedure has become more prominent, resulting in a Billroth I anastomosis. This procedure carries fewer postoperative nutrition concerns than the other, which results in a Billroth II anastomosis (Figure 22-4).

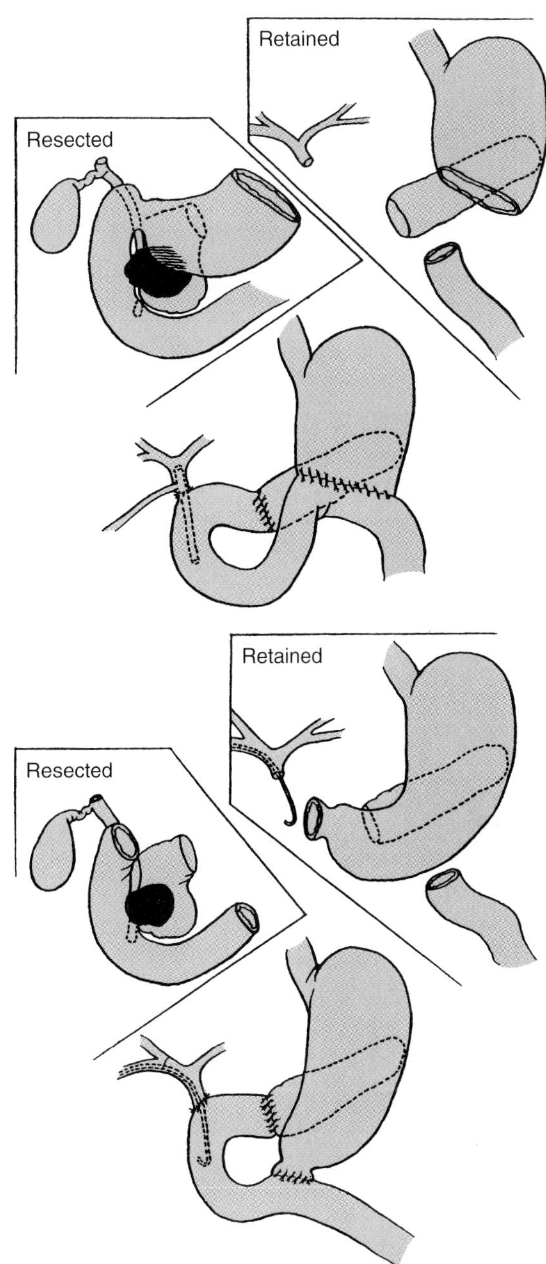

FIGURE 22-4 Whipple procedure. (*From Hardy JD, ed:* Hardy's textbook of surgery, *ed 2, Philadelphia, 1988, JB Lippincott.*)

ILEOSTOMY AND COLOSTOMY

In cases of intestinal lesions, obstruction, or inflammatory bowel disease of the entire colon or when diversion of fecal matter is required, an ileostomy or a colostomy may be the treatment of choice. These procedures involve the creation of an artificial anus on the abdominal wall by incision into the colon or ileum and bringing it out to the surface, forming a stoma (Figure 22-5). A pouch is placed externally over the stoma to collect the fecal matter. In general patients with ostomies should eat regular diets. Foods that are gas forming or difficult to digest may be avoided to reduce undesired side effects. In the case of high-output ostomies (>800 ml/day), patients may need to avoid hypertonic, simple sugar–containing liquids and foods, fatty foods, and foods with a high amount of insoluble fiber to reduce outputs.

BARIATRIC SURGERY

In the past several years, surgery for the treatment of obesity has become more prevalent. Probably the most common procedure for weight loss in the world is the vertical banded gastroplasty (VBG), or gastric stapling (Figure 22-6, *A*). This technique is performed under general anesthesia and requires about 4 to 5 days in the hospital postoperatively. The VBG procedure limits food intake by creating a small pouch (½ oz) in the upper stomach with a narrow outlet (½ inch) reinforced by a mesh band to prevent stretching. The pouch fills quickly and empties slowly with solid food, producing a feeling of fullness. Overeating results in pain or vomiting, thus restricting food intake. This procedure is preferred for those people who engage in "bulk" or "binge" eating. The disadvantage of this procedure is that weight loss is not as great as that with other procedures. It does not restrict the intake of high-caloric liquids, and the pouch can stretch with overeating. As a result, 20% of people do not lose weight, and only half of people lose at least 50% of their excess weight with a VBG.

The Roux-en-Y gastric bypass (Figure 22-6, *B*) is a combination of gastric stapling and intestinal bypass. It promotes weight loss by (1) restricting the amount of food a person can ingest by reducing the holding capacity of the stomach and (2) interfering with the complete absorption of nutrients by shortening the length of small intestine through which the food travels. Unlike the VBG, this procedure discourages the intake of high-calorie sweets by producing nausea, diarrhea, and other unpleasant symptoms. With this procedure a small gastric pouch (15 ml) is made near where the stomach and esophagus

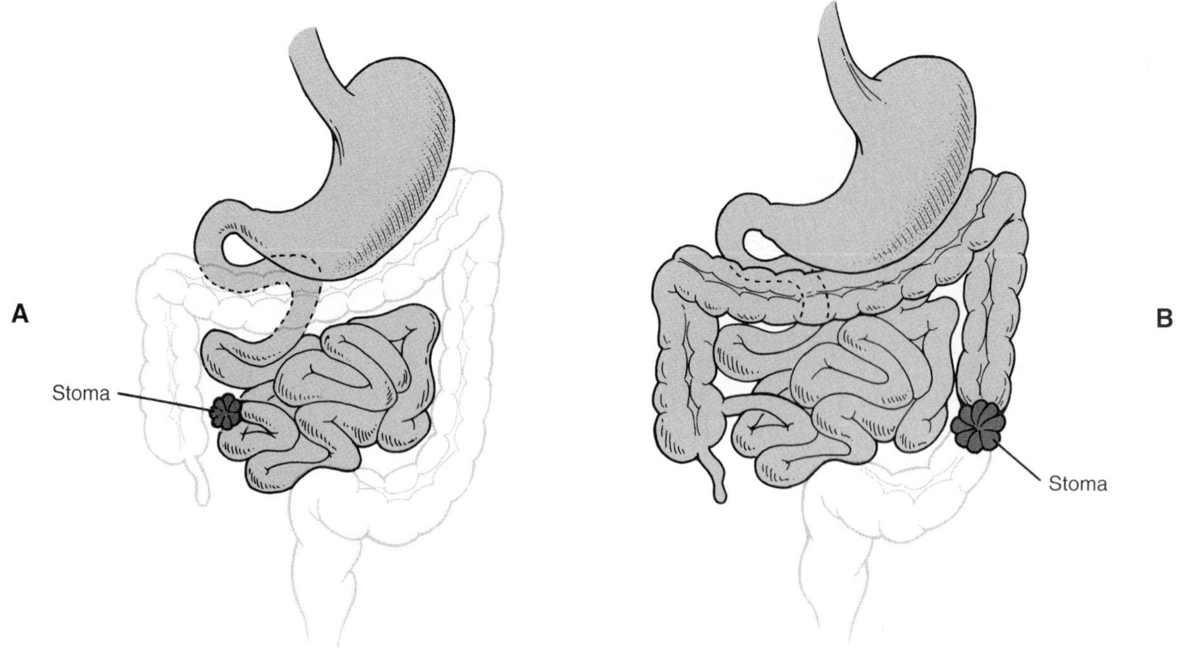

FIGURE 22-5 A, Ileostomy. B, Colostomy.

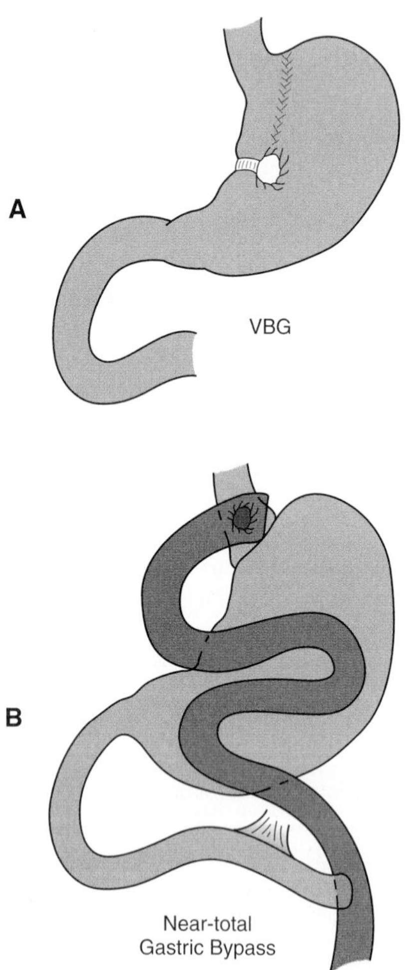

FIGURE 22-6 A, Vertical banded gastroplasty (VBG). B, Roux-en-Y gastric bypass.

meet. The small pouch and the remainder of the stomach are divided from each other with staples. An opening is made in the pouch where a portion of the small intestine is connected. This new connection between the pouch and the small intestine is called a Roux-en-Y limb. Food then travels down the esophagus and bypasses nearly all of the stomach and the first 2 ft of the small intestine. The gallbladder is removed to prevent complications related to gallstones, which tend to form during rapid weight loss. This procedure is intended for people who "graze" during the day on high-calorie and sugar-containing foods as well as eating large amounts. See Box 22-6 for a sample meal plan after gastric bypass surgery.

Like any major abdominal operation, these bariatric surgical procedures carry risks such as bleeding, infection, bowel blockage due to scar tissue formation, hernia through the incision, and anesthesia risks. The most serious risk is leakage of fluid from the stomach or intestines resulting in abdominal infection and reoperation. There are additional risks directly related to being obese; these include blood clots in the legs or lungs, pneumonia, and cardiac complications. Less-immediate risks are ulcers in the stomach or intestine, dumping syndrome, bezoar formation, obstruction of stoma, and malnutrition from too rapid weight loss and loss of vitamins and minerals. From 10 to 15 per 100 people experience some complications from the gastric bypass; death may occur from complications in 1 or 2 per 100 patients. Because this procedure is not risk free, strict criteria for eligibility should be made. Generally those who have at least 100 lb excess body weight (or a body mass index of $\geq$40 kg/m^2) and have significant obesity-related medical problems and for whom all other serious attempts

BOX 22-6 Postoperative Diet for Gastric Bypass Procedure for Morbid Obesity

Stage I: Clear liquids	Begin once liquids allowed; continue for 2-3 meals
Stage II: Gastric bypass liquids	Begin after clear liquids tolerated; continue for 3-4 weeks
Stage III: Pureed	Begin after postoperative week 4; continue for 1-2 weeks
Stage IV: Soft, solids	Begin after postoperative week 6; continue indefinitely

Gastric Bypass Liquids

Nonfat milk
Blenderized soups
100% Fruit juice (diluted ½ water, ½ juice)
Vegetable juice (e.g., V8, tomato)
Sugar-Free Carnation Instant Breakfast powder mixed with nonfat milk
Grits, oatmeal, cream of wheat, mashed potatoes (thinned down enough that it could go through a straw)
Nonfat, sugar-free milkshakes
Thinned baby food
Sugar-free drinks (e.g., sodas, tea)

Eating Guidelines

Small meals: each "feeding" should be ≤4 oz total (½ cup)
6-8 "feedings" per day to consume adequate nutrients
60 minutes between meals and drinking fluids
Eat slowly and chew food well; each "feeding" should last at least 30 minutes
Avoid sugars (sucrose, honey, corn syrup, fructose) and sugar-containing beverages and foods/candy
Low-fat foods only (avoid fried foods, gravies, excessive margarine, butter, high-fat meats, and breads)
Eat high-protein foods (milk, yogurt, soft meats, eggs)
Avoid soft, calorie-dense foods (e.g., ice cream, chocolate, cheese, cookies)
Avoid obstructive foods (e.g., tough, fibrous red meat, bread made from refined flour, celery, popcorn, nuts, seeds, membranes of citrus fruits)
Take a daily complete multivitamin (liquid or chewable)
Calcium supplements (1500 mg/day)

Sample Menu (after 8 weeks)

Breakfast	Lunch	Dinner
Banana, ¼ medium	Broiled chicken breast, 2 oz	Baked or broiled fish , 2 oz
Scrambled egg, 1 egg	Carrots, boiled, ¼ cup	Green beans, ¼ cup
Toast, white, ½ slice	Margarine, 1 tsp	Potato, baked, ½ small
Margarine, ½ tsp	Pasta salad, ¼ cup	Margarine, ½ tsp
Morning Snack	**Afternoon Snack**	**Evening Snack**
Graham crackers, 2	Canned fruit, water packed, ½ cup	Cheese, American, 1 oz
Pudding, sugar-free made with nonfat milk, ½ cup		Saltine crackers, 2 squares

*Consume nonfat milk or yogurt between meals, throughout the day. Drink/eat no more than 2-3 oz at a time for a daily total of 2 cups.

at weight reduction have failed may be candidates. A thorough medical and nutritional/behavioral evaluation is necessary to determine eligibility.

OTHER RELATED DISEASES

Enteric Fistulas

Enteric fistulas are abnormal communications between a portion of the intestinal tract and another organ (internal) or between the intestinal tract and the surface of the body (external or enterocutaneous).[27] The most common sites of origin are the pancreas and the large and small intestines. The majority of enteric fistulas result from surgical wound dehiscence or necrosis from bowel ischemia. Inflammatory bowel disease, cancer, trauma, and radiation to the abdomen can also lead to fistula development.

Several metabolic complications can arise as a result of an enteric fistula, including fluid and electrolyte losses, malnutrition, and sepsis. The route of nutritional intervention depends on the location of the fistula. Proximal fistulas may require a patient to be placed on parenteral nutrition if enteral access distal to the fistula cannot be

bariatrics The field of medicine that focuses on the treatment and the control of obesity and diseases associated with obesity.

bezoar A hard ball of hair or vegetable fiber that may develop within the stomach and intestines; can cause an obstruction, requiring removal. Formed because of reduced gastric motility, decreased gastric mixing and churning, and reduced gastric secretions.

TO PROBE FURTHER
Metabolic Response to Injury

Stressed patients undergo several metabolic phases as a series of "ebb and flow" states reflecting a patient's response to the severity of the stress. The initial ebb phase occurs immediately after the injury and is associated with shock. If the injured patient survives, the ebb phase evolves into the flow phase. Listed below are the hormonal, metabolic, and clinical outcome comparisons between the two phases.

Ebb Phase	Flow Phase
Hormonal	**Hormonal and Nonhormonal**
↑ Glucagon	↑ Counterregulatory hormones (epinephrine, norepinephrine, glucagon, cortisol)
↑ Adrenocorticotropic hormone (ACTH)	↑ Insulin
	↑ Catecholamines
	↑ Cytokines (tumor necrosis factor-alpha, interleukins-1, -2, and -6)
Metabolic	**Metabolic**
Circulatory insufficiency ↑ heart rate (vascular constriction)	Hyperglycemia
↓ Digestive enzyme production	↓ Protein synthesis/↑ amino acid efflux
↓ Urine production	↑ Gluconeogenesis
	↑ Glycogenolysis
	↑↑ Urea nitrogen excretion/net (−) nitrogen balance
Clinical Outcomes	**Clinical Outcomes**
Hemodynamic instability	Fluid and electrolyte imbalances
	Mild metabolic acidosis
	↑ Resting energy expenditure

Clinical efforts in the ebb phase are focused on maintaining heart action and blood circulation. The flow state is a hyperdynamic phase in which substrates are mobilized for energy production while increased cellular activity and hormonal stimulation are noted.

There is an energy expenditure distinction for each phase, making the goals of nutrition therapy variable depending on the stage in question. During the ebb phase there is a decrease in metabolic needs. Typically due to hemodynamic instability and need for resuscitation, nutrition intervention is not pursued during this phase. The flow phase brings hypermetabolism, yielding increased proteolysis and nitrogen loss, accelerated gluconeogenesis, hyperglycemia and increased glucose utilization, and retention of salt and water. The mobilization of protein, fat, and glycogen is believed to be mediated through the release of cytokines such as tumor necrosis factor-alpha, interleukins-1, -2, and -6, and the counterregulatory hormones such as epinephrine, norepinephrine, glucagon, and cortisol. Circulating levels of insulin are also elevated in most metabolically stressed patients, but the responsiveness of tissues to insulin, especially skeletal muscle, is severely blunted. This relative insulin resistance is believed to be due to the effects of the counterregulatory hormones. The hormonal milieu normalizes only after the injury or metabolic stress has resolved. As long as the patient is in a hyperdynamic catabolic state, optimal nutrition support is needed, but can only at best approach zero nitrogen balance in attempts to minimize further protein wasting.

References

Cresci G, Martindale R: Nutrition in critical illness. In Berdanier C et al, eds: *Handbook of nutrition and food,* Boca Raton, FL, 2002, CRC Press.

Cresci G: Metabolic stress. In Matarese L, Gottschlich M, eds: *Contemporary nutrition support practice,* ed 2, Philadelphia, 2003, WB Saunders.

achieved. This is because eating, and thus nutrients in the proximal bowel, stimulates GI secretions, thereby complicating fistula management and the likelihood of spontaneous fistula closure. Fistulas located in the distal bowel, particularly the colon, may have low output (<500 ml/day) and thus allow for oral intake of low residue or even elemental feedings. High-output fistulas (>500 ml/day) most likely will not close spontaneously and require surgical correction.

Chylous Ascites and Chylothorax

Chylous leaks into the peritoneal and thoracic cavities can follow surgical injury or trauma to the lymphatic ducts and obstruction due to cancer or congenital anomalies.

Leakage of chyle into the abdominal or thoracic cavity can cause ascites, pleural effusions, abdominal pain, anorexia, hypoalbuminemia, hyponatremia, hypocalcemia, hypocholesterolemia, and elevated alkaline phosphatase.[27] Chylous leaks may resolve with conservative management alone, although surgical repair can be required to ligate the duct. Conservative management involves reducing the chyle flow, which is normally 1500 to 5500 ml/day. Dietary intake (fat and fluid), blood pressure, and portal blood flow contribute to the production of chyle. Dietary manipulation is the main means of reducing chyle flow. Because dietary long-chain triglycerides (LCTs) are incorporated into chylomicrons, restriction of these fats in the diet is imperative. Depending on the severity of the chyle leak and the patient's response, the patient may be allowed oral dietary intake with no LCT, enteral feeding with no LCT, or parenteral nutrition. Medium-chain triglycerides (MCTs) are allowed enterally because these are absorbed directly via the portal vein, not the lymphatic system. A diet without or limited to less than 4% of calories as LCTs is not advised for more than 10 to 14 days because it lacks essential fatty acids (linoleic and linolenic acid) and the patient can develop a deficiency. Resolution of lymphatic leaks conservatively can take up to 6 weeks; therefore adequate nutrition during this period is important to maintain nutrition status.

Nutritional Needs During Metabolic Stress

Trauma and burn patients exhibit similar metabolic alterations as previously described (see *To Probe Further* box), except that the metabolic alterations often occur to a much greater extent. Few traumatic injuries result in a hypermetabolic state comparable to that of a major burn. An understanding of the etiology of the metabolic response and the implications on nutritional requirements is necessary with traumatic and burn injuries for a nutrition care plan to be designed to minimize the effects of hypermetabolism and hypercatabolism and for support immunocompetence to be developed.

BURN WOUNDS

The size and depth of the burn wound affect its healing process and overall prognosis (Figure 22-7). Burns are usually classified by degree using the "rule of nines."

1. *First-degree burns:* erythema involving cell necrosis above the basal layer of the epidermis
2. *Second-degree burns:* erythema and blistering, and necrosis within the dermis
3. *Third-degree burns:* full-thickness skin loss, including fat layer
4. *Fourth-degree burns:* exposed bone and tendon

Burns of first- and second-degree depths generally reepithelialize without surgical intervention. Third-degree burns will not heal independent of excision and grafting. Fourth-degree burns typically involve the use of muscle flaps because skin grafting onto bone is not a viable therapy option.

The extent of the burn directly affects fluid resuscitation, surgical needs, immunocompetence, metabolic sequelae, and nutrition intervention. Second- and third-degree burns covering 15% to 20% or more of the total body surface area (TBSA), or 10% in children and elderly persons, usually cause extensive fluid loss and require intravenous fluid and electrolyte replacement therapy. Burns of severe depth covering more than 50% of the TBSA are often fatal, especially in infants and the elderly. Thermal injury permits the loss of heat, water, nitrogen, whole proteins, and micronutrients through the open wound. The loss of the protective skin barrier allows microorganisms to access subcutaneous tissue and potentiates systemic infectious processes, which contribute to the postburn hypermetabolic state. Loss of plasma volume and electrolytes through the open wound predispose the burned patient to acid-base imbalance and cardiovascular, pulmonary, and renal instability. Adequate fluid and electrolyte resuscitation during the first 24 to 48 hours of postburn hypovolemia is essential for hemodynamic stability. Extensive fluid shifts, unique to burn injury, drive the characteristic edema process of resuscitation by increasing intracellular and interstitial fluid volumes. Fluids given during the resuscitative period should be titrated in accordance with urine output to prevent both overresuscitation and underresuscitation. The replacement of extracellular sodium chloride, most commonly in the form of lactated Ringer's solution, is obligatory for successful resuscitation.[28]

Nutrition Therapy After Burn Injury

Thermal injury induces hypermetabolism of varying intensity and duration depending on the extent and depth of the body surface affected, the presence of infection, and the efficacy of early treatment. Energy requirements peak at approximately postburn day 12 and typically slowly normalize as the percentage of open wound decreases with reepithelialization or skin grafting.

Energy. Burn patients require individualized nutrition plans to provide optimal energy and protein to accelerate

chyle The fat-containing, creamy white fluid that is formed in the lacteals of the intestine during digestion, transported through the lymphatics, and enters the venous circulation via the thoracic duct.

erythema Redness of the skin produced by coagulation of the capillaries.

lactated Ringer's solution Sterile solution of calcium chloride, potassium chloride, sodium chloride, and sodium lactate in water administered to replenish fluid and electrolytes.

rule of nines Describes the percentage of the body surface represented by various anatomic areas. For example: each upper limb, 9%; each lower limb, 18%; anterior and posterior trunk, each 18%; head and neck, 9%; and perineum and genitalia, 1%.

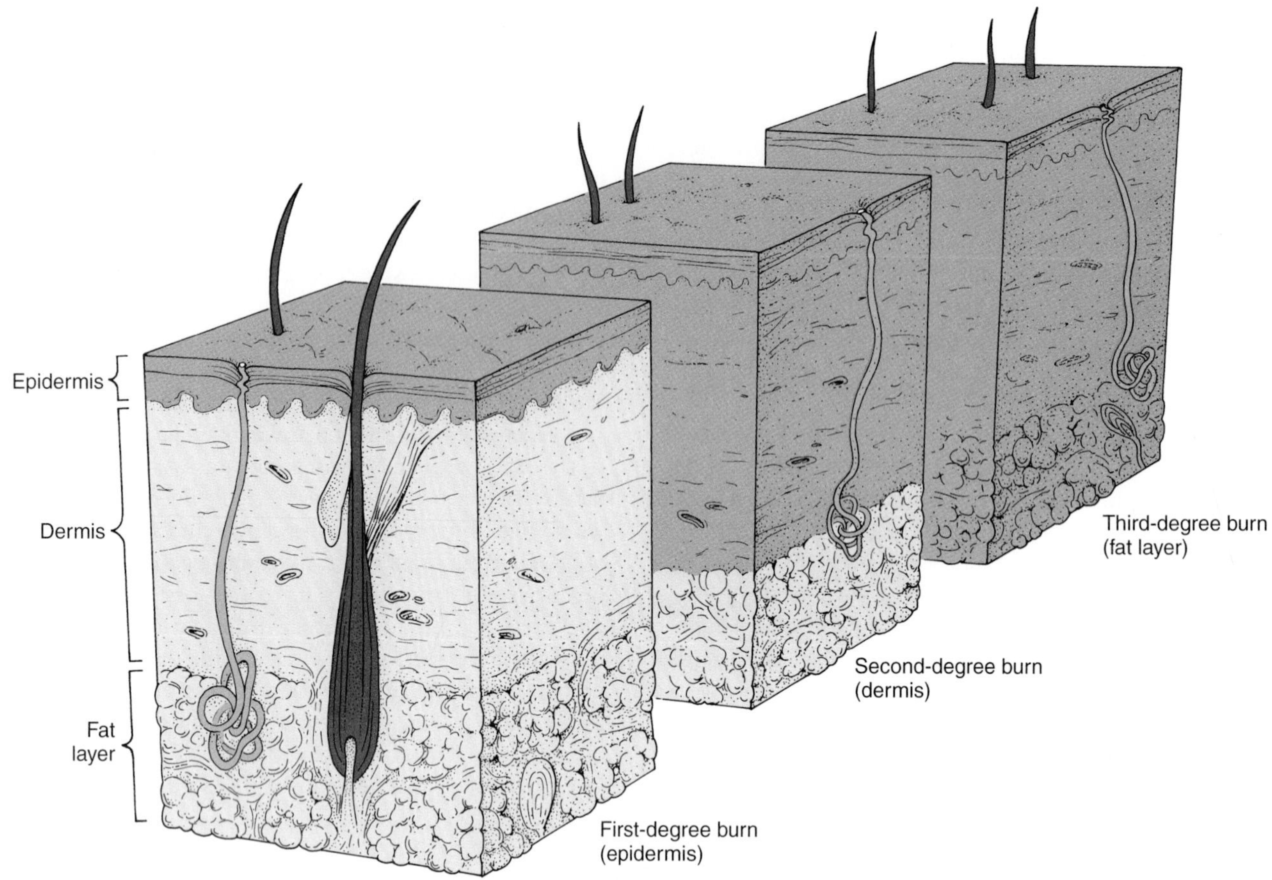

FIGURE 22-7 Depth of skin area involved in burns.

muscle and protein synthesis and minimize proteolysis. There are numerous predictive equations to estimate energy needs. Several studies have reviewed the accuracy of predictive equations in determining energy requirements in burn patients. The consensus appears that predictive equations tend to overestimate energy expenditure, and the preferred method of determining energy requirements is by using indirect calorimetry. If indirect calorimetry is not available in the clinical situation, it is suggested that resting energy expenditure can be estimated as 50% to 60% above the Harris-Benedict equation for burns of more than 20% of TBSA.[29]

Carbohydrate. During the flow phase of metabolic stress, hyperglycemia is present due to the increased glucagon-to-insulin ratio that activates gluconeogenesis. Tissue insulin resistance further exacerbates glucose intolerance. Despite these metabolic aberrations, carbohydrate should be the primary energy source provided for the burned patient. For burns exceeding 25% TBSA, carbohydrate should compose 60% to 65% of the calories.[28] Patients should be monitored closely for hyperglycemia and glucosuria with exogenous insulin provided to maintain blood glucose levels at less than 180 mg/dl.[6] Complications of hyperglycemia include osmotic diuresis with resulting dehydration and hypovolemia, lipogenesis, fatty liver, and carbon dioxide retention inhibiting ventilatory weaning.

Protein. Trauma, burns, and sepsis initiate a cascade of events that leads to accelerated protein degradation, decreased rates of synthesis of selected proteins, and increased amino acid catabolism and nitrogen loss. Clinical consequences of these metabolic alterations may increase morbidity and mortality rates of patients, causing serious organ dysfunction and impaired host defenses. Therefore trauma and burn patients require increased amounts of protein in attempts to minimize endogenous proteolysis as well as to support the large losses from wound exudate. Providing 20% to 25% of calories as protein to those with burns of greater than 25% TBSA promotes improved nutrition laboratory values, immunity, nitrogen balance, and survival.[30] Overall recommendations are to provide 1.5 to 2.0, rarely up to 3.0, g protein/kg body weight/day in attempts to minimize protein losses. Providing these higher levels of protein requires continuous monitoring of fluid status, blood urea nitrogen, and serum creatinine because of the high renal solute load. In addition to the quantity of protein provided, the protein quality is also significant. The use of high-biologic protein, such as whey or casein rather than soy, is preferred for burn patients. Whey protein has been further endorsed over casein due to its beneficial effects on burned children, improvement in tube feeding tolerance, enhanced solubility at low gastric pH, greater digestibility, and improved nitrogen retention. Pharmacologic doses of the single amino acids arginine and glutamine have also been explored as to their benefit in critical illness and burns.

Fat. Lipid is an important component of a trauma or burn patient's diet for many reasons, one being an iso-osmotic concentrated energy source at 9 calories/g. Dietary lipid is also a carrier for fat-soluble vitamins as well as a provider of the essential fatty acids linoleic and linolenic acid. Even though lipids are required in critical illness, excess lipid can be detrimental. Excessive lipid administration has been associated with hyperlipidemia, fatty liver immune suppression, and impaired clotting ability. For burn and multiple trauma patients, the recommended amount of total fat delivery is 12% to 15% of total calories. A minimum of 4% of calories in the diet should consist of essential fatty acids to prevent deficiencies, which often equates to about 10% of total calories as fat because most sources do not solely contain essential fatty acid. Formulations supplemented with fish oil, a rich source of n-3 fatty acids (eicosapentaenoic acid [EPA] and docosahexaenoic acid [DHA]) and canola oil (α-linolenic acid) are of particular interest for their potential antiinflammatory and immune enhancing benefits.[29]

Vitamins and minerals. Micronutrients function as coenzymes and cofactors in metabolic pathways at the cellular level. With the increased energy and protein demands associated with traumatic and burn injury, one would expect there to also be increased need for vitamins and minerals. In addition, increased nutrient losses from open wounds and altered metabolism, absorption, and excretion would also be suspect for requirements beyond that of the Recommended Dietary Allowances. Various vitamins and minerals have also been found to aid with wound healing, immune function, and other biologic functions. Unfortunately, little concrete data are available to support exact requirements during these hypermetabolic states. However, in addition to a daily multivitamin burn patients may benefit from additional vitamin A (5000 IU/1000 calories of enteral nutrition), vitamin C (500 mg twice daily), and zinc (45 mg elemental zinc/day).

Nutrient Delivery

Oral intake is generally adequate in children and adults with burns of less than 25% TBSA and in young children and infants with less than 15% TBSA. Adequate oral intake can be achieved by providing patient food preferences, high-calorie, high-protein supplements, and modular calorie and protein enhancement of foods.[28] However, patients with burns of greater than 25% TBSA often require enteral tube feeding. Gastric feedings are frequently interrupted in burn patients for multiple reasons such as the presence of gastric ileus, dressing changes, physical therapy, prone positioning, respiratory treatments, and surgery. Enteral feeding is well tolerated in burn patients when delivered in the small intestine because the small bowel maintains its absorptive capacity. Therefore a nasoenteric feeding tube is preferred. Small bowel feeding may also reduce the incidence of aspiration. Enteral nutrient delivery as soon as postinjury allows during the resuscitative period should be initiated. Early enteral feedings, within the first 6 hours after the burn, have been shown to decrease the level of catabolic hormones, improve nitrogen balance, maintain gut mucosal integrity, lower the incidence of diarrhea, and decrease hospital stay.[31] A full-strength, intact protein formula at low rate (20 to 30 ml/hr) advanced by 5 to 20 ml/hr to the desired volume is typically tolerated.[28] Parenteral nutrition is indicated only if enteral nutrition is not tolerated or grossly inadequate because it has been associated with metabolic and immunologic complications.[31] Whenever possible, low rate enteral feedings should accompany parenteral nutrition to prevent villous atrophy.

TO SUM UP

The nutritional status of the patient should be addressed before the patient is even considered for surgery. If the patient has any nutrient deficiencies, these should be corrected before surgery, if time allows. Postoperatively, the patient should be provided with nutrition as soon as feasible to improve surgical outcomes.

Postoperative nutrition may be provided in a number of ways. The oral route is preferred; however, often it is not feasible or adequate to support metabolic needs. Enteral or parenteral nutrition may be provided for those unable to achieve adequate nutrient intake and absorption orally. Enteral feeding is preferred over parenteral. Because alimentary tract surgery often alters the flow of nutrients resulting in several potential metabolic and nutrition complications, postoperative diets are described to help minimize these effects.

■ Questions for Review

1. Discuss the requirements for energy, protein, vitamins, and minerals and means of providing them during the various stages of surgery (preoperative, immediately preoperative, postoperative).
2. Describe the potential nutrition consequences that may result after surgery of the head and neck, esophagus, stomach, and intestine.
3. Develop a menu plan for a patient undergoing gastric bypass surgery for morbid obesity; include all phases of the diet progression.

4. Describe the metabolic alterations that occur during metabolic stress.
5. Develop a nutrition care plan for a patient sustaining third-degree burns covering 40% TBSA.

■ References

1. Klein S et al: Nutrition support in clinical practice: review of published data and recommendations for future research directions, *J Parenter Enteral Nutr* 21:133, 1997.
2. Vitello J: Prevalence of malnutrition in hospitalized patients remains high, *J Am Coll Nutr* 12:589, 1993.
3. Naber T et al: Prevalence of malnutrition in nonsurgical hospitalized patients and its association with disease complication, *Am J Clin Nutr* 66:1232, 1997.
4. Coats K et al: Hospital-associated malnutrition: a reevaluation 12 years later, *J Am Diet Assoc* 93:27, 1993.
5. Kelly I et al: Still hungry in hospital: identifying malnutrition in acute hospital admissions, *Q J Med* 93:93, 2000.
6. A.S.P.E.N. Board of Directors. Guidelines for the use of parenteral and enteral nutrition in adult and pediatric patients, *J Parenter Enteral Nutr* 26, 2002.
7. VA TPN Cooperative Study: Perioperative total parenteral nutrition in surgical patients, *N Engl J Med* 325:525, 1991.
8. Cerra B et al: Applied nutrition in ICU patients: a consensus statement of the American College of Chest Physicians, *Chest* 111:769, 1997.
9. Klein C, Stanek G, Willes C: Overfeeding macronutrients to critically ill adults: metabolic complications, *J Am Diet Assoc* 98:795, 1998.
10. Pomposelli JJ et al: Early postoperative glucose control predicts nosocomial infection rate in diabetic patients, *J Parenter Enteral Nutr* 22:77, 1998.
11. Pomposelli JJ, Bistrian BR: Is total parenteral nutrition immunosuppressive? *New Horiz* 2:224, 1994.
12. Flancbaum L et al: Comparison of indirect calorimetry, the Fick method, and prediction equations in estimating the energy requirements of critically ill patients, *Am J Clin Nutr* 69:461, 1999.
13. Chiolero R, Revelly JP, Tappy L: Energy metabolism in sepsis and injury, *Nutrition* 13(suppl):45S, 1997.
14. Barton RG: Nutrition support in critical illness, *Nutr Clin Pract* 10:129, 1994.
15. Cutts M et al: Predicting energy needs in ventilator-dependent critically ill patients: effect of adjusting weight for edema or adiposity, *Am J Clin Nutr* 66:1250, 1997.
16. Marik P, Varon J: The obese patient in the ICU, *Chest* 113:492, 1998.
17. Ireton-Jones CS et al: Equations for estimation of energy expenditures in patients with burns with special reference to ventilatory status, *J Burn Care Rehab* 13:330, 1992.
18. Patino J et al: Hypocaloric support in the critically ill, *World J Surg* 23:553, 1999.
19. Cresci GA, Martindale RG: Nutrition support in trauma. In *The science and practice of nutrition support,* ed 3, Dubuque, Iowa, 2001, Kendall/Hunt.
20. Campbell W et al: Increased protein requirements in elderly people: new data and retrospective reassessments, *Am J Clin Nutr* 60:501, 1994.
21. Dabrowski G, Rombeau J: Practical nutritional management in the trauma intensive care unit, *Surg Clin North Am* 80:92, 2000.
22. Whitmire S: Fluid and electrolytes. In *The science and practice of nutrition support,* ed 3, Dubuque, Iowa, 2001, Kendall/Hunt.
23. Kiele AM et al: Two phase randomized controlled clinical trial of prospective oral dietary supplements in surgical patients, *Gut* 40:343, 1997.
24. Jeffery KM et al: The clear liquid diet is no longer a necessity in the routine postoperative management of surgical patients, *Am Surg* 62:167, 1996.
25. Lipman T: Grains or veins: is enteral nutrition really better than parenteral nutrition? A look at the evidence, *J Parenter Enteral Nutr* 22:167, 1998.
26. Heyland DK et al: Should immunonutrition become routine in critically ill patients? A systematic review of the evidence, *JAMA* 286:944, 2001.
27. Sullivan M, Alonso E: Gastrointestinal and pancreatic disease. In Matarese L, Gottschlich M, eds: *Contemporary nutrition support practice,* Philadelphia, 1998, WB Saunders.
28. Mayes T, Gottschlich M: Burns and wound healing. In *The science and practice of nutrition support,* ed 3, Dubuque, Iowa, 2001, Kendall/Hunt.
29. Khorram-Sefat R et al: Long-term measurements of energy expenditure in severe burn injury, *West J Surg* 23:115, 1999.
30. Alexander JW et al: Beneficial effects of aggressive protein feeding in severely burned children, *Ann Surg* 192:505, 1980.
31. Rose J et al: Advances in burn care. In Cameron J et al, eds: *Advances in surgery, vol 30,* Chicago, 1996, Mosby–Year Book.

■ Further Reading

Cerra FB: How nutrition intervention changes what getting sick means, *J Parenter Enteral Nutr* 14(suppl 5):164, 1990.

This article provides a good review of three basic factors that influence what is observed at an ill patient's bedside when considering the effects of nutrition intervention: (1) the disease process inherent in the metabolic response to injury, (2) the presence of starvation, and (3) the presence of the nutritional intervention.

Hustler DA: Nutritional monitoring of a pediatric burn patient, *Nutr Clin Pract* 6:11, 1991.

This experienced dietitian-specialist on a burn-center team provides a case report of a young boy who sustained mostly full-thickness burns over 56% of his total body surface area. She describes in detail the challenge of initial evaluation and therapy, constant close monitoring, and appropriate responses to changing needs.

Tynes JJ et al: Diet tolerance and stool frequency in patients with ileoanal reservoirs, *J Am Diet Assoc* 92(7):861, 1992.

This brief report of a survey of patients with ileoanal reservoirs provides much helpful background information about this recently developed alternative surgical procedure to the ileostomy, with practical guidance for nutritional management and patient counseling.

CASE STUDY The patient with esophageal cancer

Mr. Smith is a 54-year-old accountant who was seen by his family physician for pain with swallowing and difficulty swallowing solid foods for the past 6 weeks. This has resulted in continued weight loss and fatigue. Mr. Smith was referred to the gastrointestinal medicine service for further evaluation. After a series of tests that included endoscopy and biopsy, Mr. Smith was found to have esophageal cancer with the tumor lying in the mid-esophagus. He was then referred to the gastrointestinal surgery service for surgical evaluation.

A medical history revealed Mr. Smith to smoke 2 packs of cigarettes per day, to drink 3 martinis per day, and to be cachectic. A referral was sent to the dietitian for nutrition evaluation and recommendations for optimizing his nutritional status for surgery. A nutrition history revealed that during the past 6 weeks, his diet had progressively decreased in consistency to where he could tolerate only liquids and some soft solid foods such as mashed potatoes, oatmeal, and applesauce. At a height of 178 cm, Mr. Smith's weight had dropped from 80 to 63 kg, leaving him at 79% of his usual body weight. His blood work revealed a serum albumin level of 3.0 g/dl and prealbumin of 13.2 mg/dl. He no longer could stand long enough to make himself a meal and had to take a bath rather than shower because he became too tired. He was not currently taking any medications because he could not swallow them. His current diet order was a full liquid diet.

Assessment of calorie and protein requirements estimated that Mr. Smith required approximately 1800 kcalories (basal energy expenditure + 25%) and 75 to 95 g of protein (1.2 to 1.5 g/kg) daily. Because he could eat some solid foods, the dietitian changed him to a soft diet. She modified his diet so that it contained soft, high protein–containing solids and liquids that he stated he could eat and ordered a 48-hour calorie count. A liquid multivitamin was also provided. Mr. Smith was now able to eat enough calories and protein for 14 days preoperatively that he gained 3 kg; his albumin increased to 3.1 g/dl and prealbumin increased to 17 mg/dl.

He underwent an esophagectomy with a gastric pull-up. A feeding jejunostomy tube was placed intraoperatively. He was started on low-rate enteral feedings on postoperative day 2, which were gradually advanced to his goal requirements over the next 2 days. He was not allowed to eat until postoperative day 7 after a swallowing study for anastomotic evaluation. Once his diet was initiated and tolerated, his tube feedings were provided nocturnally because he was not able to consume 100% of his nutrition needs orally. He was discharged home with an oral postgastrectomy diet and nocturnal tube feedings to provide about 50% of his nutrition needs for 10 days, at which time his nutrition would be reevaluated.

QUESTIONS FOR ANALYSIS

1. Evaluate the preoperative nutrition assessment data. Why were the particular energy and protein assessment factors chosen?
2. What dietary modifications accompany a postgastrectomy diet?
3. Why was Mr. Smith placed on a postgastrectomy diet when his stomach was not resected?
4. At what point should his enteral tube feedings be discontinued?

Issues & ANSWERS

Immunonutrition

It is known that malnutrition leads to suppressed immune responses. Providing nutrition support using standard enteral formulations has shown improvements in various clinical indices of nutritional status when adequate calories and protein are given; however, there is a lack of demonstrated effect on morbidity and mortality. During the past two decades the field of immunology has exploded and expanded into nearly every area of medicine, including nutrition. Certain dietary components have been classified as "immune-enhancing nutrients." Compared with standard nutrients, an immune-enhancing nutrient is a substance that provides positive effects on the immune system when provided in certain quantities. Of the many immune-enhancing nutrients identified in human clinical trials, the ones that appear to be most beneficial are L-arginine, L-glutamine, nucleotides, omega-3 fatty acids (EPA and DHA), and various vitamins and minerals (zinc and vitamins A, E, and C). Several special enteral nutrient formulations have been categorized as immune-enhancing formulations (IEFs). Each of these formulas contains various combinations and/or levels of these immune-enhancing nutrients.

Glutamine

Glutamine is known to be a major fuel source for rapidly dividing cells such as enterocytes, reticulocytes, and lymphocytes. In normal metabolic states, glutamine is a nonessential amino acid. However, during times of metabolic stress, glutamine is implicated as being conditionally essential because it is needed for maintenance of gut metabolism, structure, and function. Despite the accelerated skeletal muscle release of amino acids, blood glutamine levels are not increased after burns. In fact, decreased plasma glutamine levels have been reported after severe burn, multiple trauma, or multiple organ failure.

A number of studies have shown beneficial effects with supplemental glutamine, its precursors (ornithine α-ketoglutarate and α-ketoglutarate), or glutamine dipeptides (alanine-glutamine, glycine-glutamine). These studies deliver glutamine in pharmacologic doses of 25% to 35% of the dietary protein. Supplemental glutamine has been shown to have multiple benefits to include increased nitrogen retention and muscle mass, maintenance of the GI mucosa, and its permeability, preserved immune function and reduced infections, and preserved organ glutathione levels. These protective effects of glutamine supplementation could have significant effects on morbidity and mortality rates in trauma and burn patients. Safety and cost-effectiveness of glutamine supplementation in trauma and burns continue to be researched.

Arginine

Arginine, like glutamine, is considered a conditionally essential amino acid. Arginine is the specific precursor for nitric oxide production as well as a potent secretagogue for anabolic hormones such as insulin, prolactin, and growth hormone. Under normal circumstances, arginine is considered a nonessential amino acid because it is adequately synthesized endogenously via the urea cycle. However, research suggests that during times of metabolic stress, optimal amounts of arginine are not synthesized to promote tissue regeneration or positive nitrogen balance.

Studies in animal and humans have investigated the effects of supplemental arginine in various injury models. Positive outcomes from supplementation include improved nitrogen balance, wound healing, and immune function and increased anabolic hormones, insulin and growth hormone. The outcomes are of special interest in the posttrauma and postburn patient during the flow phase when enhancement of these processes would yield the greatest advantage. However, despite these positive effects, caution with excessive arginine supplementation is warranted in burn patients because of its potential adverse effects on nitric oxide production.

Lipid

Even though lipids are required, excess lipid can be detrimental. Excessive lipid administration has been associated with hyperlipidemia, fatty liver immunosuppression, and impaired clotting ability. All of the long-chain fatty acids share the same enzyme systems because they are elongated and desaturated with each pathway competitive in nature based on substrate availability. Dietary fatty acids modulate the phospholipid cell membrane composition and the type and quantities of eicosanoids produced. Prostaglandins of the 3 series (PGE_3) and series 5 leukotrienes have proved to be anti-inflammatory and immune-enhancing agents. Also, PGE_3 is a potent vasodilator. These concepts have received considerable attention for the potential of n-3 fatty acids to enhance immune function and reduce acute and chronic inflammation.

In most standard enteral formulations, the fat source is predominantly n-6 fatty acids with a portion coming from MCTs. Formulations supplemented with fish oil, a rich source of n-3 fatty acids (EPA and DHA) and canola oil (α-linolenic acid), are available. Clinical trials utilizing these formulations have shown positive benefits in patients with psoriasis, rheumatoid arthritis, burns, sepsis, and trauma. These benefits are thought to be due to alterations in eicosanoid and leukotriene production, with decreased arachidonic acid metabolites (e.g., PGE_2), as well as increased production of the less biologically active trienoic prostaglandins and pentaenoic leukotrienes.

Clinical outcomes with immune-enhancing formulas

Trauma outcomes. IEFs have been used in trauma patients and are associated with decreased incidence of intraabdominal abscess, multiple organ failure, infections, and systemic inflammatory response syndrome (SIRS), as well as decreased hospital length of stay and days of therapeutic antibiotic use.

Intensive care unit/sepsis outcomes. This study population involves a very heterogeneous group, making data interpretation difficult. This population involves differing severity and pathology of various disease states. Studies conducted with this population have differences in study design and methods of reporting data, adding to the complexity of comparing results between investigations. A few studies have been conducted with various diagnoses, such as cardiac failure, pulmonary failure, transplantation, trauma, and GI surgery. Positive outcomes in the form of decreased incidence of infections, requirement for mechanical ventilation, incidence of bacteremia, and length of stay were reported when using IEFs.

Surgery outcomes. Research in surgical populations using IEFs has been performed with preoperative, postoperative, or combined nutritional therapies. The majority of the procedures performed in these studies involved upper GI cancer or head and neck cancer surgery. Significantly improved outcomes in the IEF groups include fewer infections and wound complications, decreased severity of complications, and shorter postoperative and hospital length of stay.

Other populations (burns, head injury, HIV/AIDS). Study of the use of IEFs in these patient populations is limited. Currently only two studies investigating the effect of IEFs on immune function and nutritional status of AIDS patients have been published. Improved weight gain was found in one of the studies when IEF was provided but not in the other study. Burn patients appear to benefit when provided with IEFs, exhibiting decreased infections and length of hospital stay. Head injury patients theoretically should benefit from IEFs because of severe hypermetabolism and the likelihood of infectious complications. However, there are no clinical data available to support this theory. More research using IEFs in these populations is needed.

REFERENCES

Hillhouse J: Immune-enhancing enteral formulas: effect on patient outcome, *Support Line* 23:16, 2001.

Martindale R, Cresci G: The use of immune enhancing diets in burns, *J Parenter Enteral Nutr* 25(suppl):S24, 2001.

Sax H: Effect of immune enhancing formulas in general surgery patients, *J Parenter Enteral Nutr* 25(suppl):S19, 2001.

Schloerb P: Immune-enhancing diets: products, components, and their rationales, *J Parenter Enteral Nutr* 25(suppl):S3, 2001.

Chapter

23

Nutrition and Acquired Immunodeficiency Syndrome (AIDS)

Deborah A. Cohen

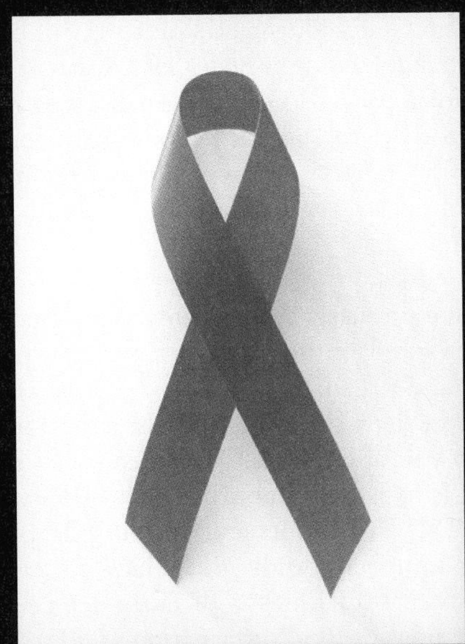

Chapter Outline

In this chapter of our clinical series we focus on acquired immunodeficiency syndrome (AIDS). This modern-day plague has eluded medical science's search for a cure and left countless numbers of infected and dying young adults and children in its wake.

Here we examine the background of the AIDS epidemic and the nature of the human immunodeficiency virus-1 (HIV-1). We review the current state of medical management and its relation to nutritional status in the course of the disease. As knowledge of the disease process has grown during the past two decades, it has become increasingly evident that nutritional support plays a vital role in the care of HIV-infected and AIDS patients.

Evolution of HIV and the AIDS Epidemic

In the late 1970s, physicians on the east and west coasts of the United States, centered in New York City and San Francisco, became puzzled about an uncommon medical problem appearing among their patients.[1] No known cause of immune suppression could be found. Nonetheless they were suffering and dying from complications of common infections, largely pneumonia, ordinarily handled easily by the human immune system and the usual antibiotics or other antibacterial drugs. Its virus source and pandemic effects were soon to become alarmingly evident worldwide.

EVOLUTION OF HIV

Social Change

Where did this new deadly virus come from, and how did it gain such strength? Apparently, HIV represents not a new virus but an old one that in recent years has grown deadly in humans as it gained strength during the social upheavals of the 1960s and 1970s. The uprooting effect of this rapid social change and urbanization allowed the virus to spread rapidly through world populations and to reproduce aggressively in its human host.

Parasite Nature of Virus

No virus can have a life of its own; by their structure and nature, all viruses are parasites. They are mere shreds of genetic material, a small packet of genetic information encased in a protein coat. They contain only a small chromosome of nucleic acids (RNA or DNA), usually with fewer than five genes (see Chapter 24). They can live only through a host, whom they invade and infect. There they hijack the host's cell machinery to run off a multitude of copies of themselves. Their purpose is to make as many self-copies as they can. Today's viruses are those that succeeded in that task over time and are, like all plants and animals, simply descendants of earlier forms. Scientists agree that the human immunodeficiency viruses HIV-1 and HIV-2 are genetically similar to viruses found in African primates such as monkeys and apes (SIV [simian immunodeficiency virus]) and were probably transmitted to humans in an earlier age.

The earliest known case of AIDS was recently identified in an African blood sample collected in 1959 from a Bantu man who lived in the Democratic Republic of Congo, an area from which the current epidemic is believed to have spread.[2] This sample is the oldest HIV infection discovered so far, indicating that it predates the time at which the virus divided into several of the current varieties that now infect different parts of the world. Over the years HIV has mutated into many different subtypes. Africa is home to 70% of the adults and 80% of the children living with HIV infection in the world.[3] Although the course of the present worldwide epidemic is difficult to predict, there is a growing sense of guarded optimism among the leading scientists based on the current research agenda, especially among the increasing number of young, newly trained scientists with new ideas and a changing U.S. culture of AIDS research that embraces more cooperative team attitudes.[4-7]

DISEASE PROGRESSION

The individual clinical course of HIV infection varies substantially. Four distinct stages mark the progression of the disease and are usually referred to as (1) asymptomatic stage, (2) early symptomatic stage, (3) late symptomatic stage, and (4) advanced HIV disease stage.

Primary HIV Infection

HIV infects cells that express the $CD4^+$ receptor on their surface, including T-helper cells, monocytes, macrophages, and dendritic cells. After initial attachment to the $CD4^+$ molecule, HIV fuses with and then enters the cell's cytoplasm, sheds its envelope coat, and releases its contents. Reverse transcription takes place creating viral DNA, which is integrated into the host DNA.[8] The virus may then remain dormant or become activated, at which time new virions are reassembled and shed from the cell into the circulation to infect another host cell. Lymphoid tissue (lymph nodes, adenoids, tonsil, spleen) contain the highest concentration of HIV-infected cells during the latent period, which can last up to 10 years before clinical manifestation of the disease occurs.

About 5 to 30 days (median, 14 days) after initial exposure and infection, a mild flu-like syndrome (fever, adenopathy, sore throat, rash, myalgia, arthralgia, diarrhea, nausea, and vomiting) may occur, lasting about 1 week. Antibody tests for HIV do not usually test positive at this time. This brief response corresponds to the process of *seroconversion,* the development of antibodies to the viral infection. Subsequent HIV testing will be positive. Signs of enlarged lymph nodes, or persistent generalized lymphadenopathy (PGL), persist in about 30% of cases. An extended asymptomatic period usually continues for the next 10 to 12 years. However, this seemingly inactive period of relative wellness can be deceiving.

Asymptomatic Stage

During the asymptomatic stage of infection, viral replication continues and cellular destruction takes place in many tissues and organs of the body.[8] There also is a steady decline in the $CD4^+$ T-cell levels, a drop of 40 to 80/μl for every year of infection. With the use of viral load measurement, it has been established that HIV load correlates with $CD4^+$ cell counts and with disease progression. Healthy, uninfected individuals have a $CD4^+$ cell count of 500 to 1500/μl of blood. Early detection and treatment may prevent local propagation of HIV.

Early Symptomatic Stage

After the extended asymptomatic HIV-positive stage, which may last as long as 12 years, a period of associated infectious illnesses begins. This stage develops when $CD4^+$ cell counts drop to about 500/μl and HIV viral loads increases to greater than 10,000/ml.[9] At this point, even the most common infections, known as *opportunistic infections,* have an open opportunity to take affect, spread, and cause systemic disease. Common symptoms observed during this pre-AIDS period include candidiasis, herpes zoster, cervical dysplasia, pelvic inflammatory disease, listeriosis, and peripheral neuropathy.

Late Symptomatic Stage

The late symptomatic stage begins when the $CD4^+$ T-cell count in blood falls to less than 200/μl and viral load counts increase to greater than 100,000/ml.[10] Diseases such as tuberculosis or Kaposi's sarcoma (the most common AIDS-associated malignancy) occur; at counts below $200/mm^3$, *Pneumocystis carinii* pneumonia and *Toxoplasma gondii* (protozoan parasites able to infect a number of body organs) appear; and at counts under $50/mm^3$, cytomegalovirus (CMV) or lymphoma can flourish.[11] When the virus finally destroys sufficient white cells and the $CD4^+$ count decreases to less than 50/μl, the immune system is severely impaired, resulting in multiple opportunistic infections and malignancies. Death usually occurs in less than 1 year.

U.S. PUBLIC HEALTH SERVICE RESPONSIBILITIES

In any major epidemic, the U.S. Public Health Service and its related agencies have the major task of monitoring and stopping the spread of a disease. Thus they carry responsibilities in two major areas: (1) surveillance, including testing and counseling; and (2) community education and prevention through interrupting its spread, vaccine research, and treatment.

Surveillance

Throughout the AIDS epidemic, as knowledge of this new disease and its nature has grown, the U.S. Centers for Disease Control and Prevention (CDC) in Atlanta has worked with state and territorial health departments and has been involved in constant worldwide knowledge exchange, to conduct accurate and comprehensive AIDS surveillance in the United States.[11] Since the mid-1980s, such seroprevalence studies have provided a massive amount of information about HIV spread in various population groups and have helped CDC develop early classification guidelines for medical teams caring for HIV-infected patients. The periodic CDC revisions of surveillance criteria reflect advances in the care and understanding of disease caused by HIV infection. In accord with current knowledge and the evolution of the HIV epidemic among demographic groups, the CDC has expanded the AIDS surveillance definition to include any HIV-seropositive person with a $CD4^+$ (specific T-lymphocyte subset analysis) cell count of less than 200 cells/μl of blood.[11]

Because of the tremendous life-changing import of a positive HIV-1 test result to the individual and his or her family and loved ones, public health testing programs have developed a coordinated pretest and posttest counseling component, especially in clinics serving high-risk areas.[12] First, a brief pretest interview assesses personal knowledge of HIV infection, provides risk-reduction education, and offers the HIV test. Then those who accept the HIV testing are given a 2-week return appointment for a longer follow-up review of test results and counseling concerning healthcare and personal needs.

Education and Prevention

The U.S. Department of Health and Human Services (DHHS), through its Public Health Service and Food and Drug Administration (FDA) divisions, has provided national health promotion and disease prevention objectives for the year 2010 that call for the expansion of HIV education and prevention efforts.[13] Wide community involvement in the community-based process of developing any health promotion or disease prevention program is essential for its successful outcome. This need has been shown, for example, in the mobilizing of community leadership and resources to plan and implement interventions in other health problems such as heart disease or changing lifestyle habits (e.g., smoking) that contribute to lung disease.

The community-support need is particularly true with HIV infection. Despite its burdening social stigma, it is reaching into all communities in some form, cutting short the lives of children, adolescents, and young adults in ever-increasing numbers. Such a deadly pandemic warrants mobilization and coordination of the most realistic and effective preventive strategies possible for all ethnic and socioeconomic community groups

lymphoma General term applied to any neoplastic disorder (cancer) of the lymphoid tissue.

pandemic A widespread epidemic, distributed through a region, a continent, or the world.

parasite An organism that lives on or in an organism of another species, known as the host, from whom all life cycle nourishment is obtained.

virus Minute infectious agent, characterized by lack of independent metabolism and by the ability to reproduce with genetic continuity only with living host cells. They range in decreasing size from about 200 nanometers (nm) down to only 15 nm. (A nanometer is a linear measure equal to one billionth of a meter; it is also called a millimicron.) Each particle (virion) consists basically of nucleic acids (genetic material) and a protein shell, which protects and contains the genetic material and any enzymes present.

to change sexual risk-taking behavior at all levels—local, national, and international.[14] New drugs are continually being developed, but prevention of the spread of the disease is key.[14]

Nature of the Disease Process

ACTION OF HIV ON THE IMMUNE SYSTEM

HIV-1 and HIV-2 are members of a class of viruses called **retrovirus** because their unique life cycle involves a reverse transcription of RNA into DNA in the cell nucleus, which is then integrated into the host cell DNA.[2] The virus consists of an outer envelope with attached surface proteins covering the outer protective shell and an inner shell that contains the small strands of RNA genetic material and enzymes, including the reverse transcriptase. Of the virus's nine genes, four apparently less essential ones are poorly understood. After entering the body, the virus attaches to host cells, mostly the actively replicating T-helper ($CD4^+$) white blood cells, major lymphocytes of the body's immune system. There it integrates itself into the host cell's DNA copying system, infecting and eventually killing the host cell. Rapidly increasing masses of virus particles erupt from the dying cells in small buds to immediately infect new cells.

METHODS OF TRANSMISSION AND GROUPS AT RISK

Throughout the world, sexual behavior is central to the epidemic spread of HIV infection and AIDS. An estimated 71% of HIV infections worldwide are a result of heterosexual behavior and 15% are a result of homosexual behavior; only a relatively small proportion of cases are a result of intravenous drug use with contaminated needles.[2] In 1997, it was estimated that there were between 650,000 and 900,000 cases of AIDS in the United States. Approximately 40,000 individuals are infected and die of the disease yearly. The CDC of the Public Health Service indicated that AIDS cases by type of transmission reported in 1999 were as follows.[15]

- 46% Male homosexual/bisexual behavior
- 30% Heterosexuals
- 18% Injecting drug users
- 1% Perinatal transmission
- <1% Blood transfusions
- <1% Hemophiliacs

The remaining cases were listed as "no risk reported." Women and young people, particularly nonwhites, are increasingly at risk. Persons in the South and Northeast accounted for higher percentages of reported cases than the previous year.[14]

Mother-to-child HIV transmission has been drastically reduced in the United States in recent years—from a high of 2500 in 1992 to fewer than 400 perinatal HIV infections annually. HIV can be transmitted through breast milk, and therefore HIV-infected women are advised to avoid breastfeeding their infants.[14]

Groups at Risk

Persons at greatest risk of HIV infection are those who, if sexually active, are not consistently practicing responsible and safer sexual behavior, which consists of (1) consistent and correct condom use for protection (the regular Latex male sheath, the female polyurethane condom, or a cervical cap approved for use by the FDA), and (2) reduction in high-risk sexual practices such as avoidance of sex with multiple partners and persons at risk for HIV.[14] Others at risk are injection drug users who share needles. Because the public-donated blood supply for transfusions has been thoroughly cleared of HIV infection through a rigorous double-testing program, this route of infection risk by blood units for medical purposes has virtually been eliminated.

DIAGNOSIS OF HIV INFECTION

Testing Procedures

HIV infection is diagnosed by detection of the virus or serologic response to the virus. HIV infection can be identified by the detection of specific antibodies, as is done in the routine screening of blood and blood products for transfusion and in most epidemiologic studies. The recommended procedure for virus detection is a two-step process. The first step is enzyme-linked immunosorbent assay (ELISA) screening. Second, suspected positive samples from the ELISA screening are followed with Western blot testing for confirmation. Both of these tests are highly sensitive and specific, and both are used to confirm the results before informing the individual. Because a positive test is such a personal and life-changing event, most experienced physicians caring for HIV-infected patients repeat all positive tests again, even when they have been confirmed by Western blotting, before informing the individual. Requirements for the testing procedure include pretest and posttest counseling to cover such issues as the following.

- Medical significance of the test, whether positive or negative
- Limitations of the test
- Information about HIV-1 and AIDS, how they are spread, and how to prevent their spread
- Medical, nutritional, and psychosocial care availability
- Confidentiality concept involved with documentation in the medical record; possible social and legal results of testing, personal needs and support system

Viral load assays are used to assess prognosis, determine the need for antiretroviral therapy and type of antiretroviral therapy to use, and monitor the progression of the disease. Viral load is inversely correlated with the $CD4^+$ cell count.

Clinical Symptoms and Illnesses

The early clinical symptoms that may follow initial exposure to the virus add further confirmation to the HIV-seropositive testing procedures. These initial symptoms, as well as possible associated illnesses and diseases that characterize the later HIV stages, have been generally described earlier in discussion of the basic disease progression. Some examples of these common opportunistic infections that manifest depending on $CD4^+$ cell count range are listed in Table 23-1.

TABLE 23-1 Common Infectious Complications of AIDS

Microorganism	Nutritional Implications
Parasites	
Pneumocystis carinii	Dyspnea, fever, weight loss
Toxoplasma gondii	Fever
Cryptosporidium	Malabsorption, diarrhea
Isospora belli	Diarrhea
Microspora	Malabsorption, diarrhea
Entamoeba histolytica	Diarrhea
Giardia lamblia	Diarrhea
Acanthamoeba	Meningoencephalitis
Bacteria	
Campylobacter	Abdominal pain, cramping, bloody diarrhea, fever
Legionella	Fever
Listeria monocytogenes	Fever
Mycobacterium avium-intracellulare	Fever, weight loss, diarrhea, malabsorption
Salmonella	Diarrhea, bacteremia
Shigella	Abdominal pain, bloody diarrhea, fever
Fungi	
Aspergillus	Fungemia, fevers, weight loss
Candida albicans	Thrush, stomatitis, esophagitis, nausea
Cryptococcus neoformans	Fever, nausea, vomiting
Histoplasma capsulatum	Fever, weight loss, dysphagia
Viruses	
Cytomegalovirus	Esophagitis, colitis, diarrhea
Herpes simplex virus	Ulcerative mucocutaneous lesions, stomatitis, esophagitis, pneumonia
Epstein-Barr virus	Oral hairy leukoplakia
Hepatitis B	Nausea, vomiting, fever
Herpes zoster	Mucocutaneous lesions

Modified from *Manual of clinical dietetics*, ed 6, Chicago, 2000, American Dietetic Association; Gold JWM: HIV-1 infection: diagnosis and management, *Med Clin North Am* 76(1):1, 1992; Bernard EM et al: Pneumocystosis, *Med Clin North Am* 76(1):107, 1992; and Ralten DJ: Nutrition and HIV infection: a review and evaluation of the extent of knowledge of the relationship between nutrition and HIV infection, *Nutr Clin Prac* 6(3):1S, 1991.

BASIC ROLE OF NUTRITION IN HIV DISEASE PROCESS

Nutrition support plays a vital role throughout the HIV disease process in three basic areas. First, it is a vital component of care for the involuntary weight loss and body tissue wasting caused by the disease effects on metabolism, reflected in the severe state of protein-energy malnutrition. Second, and fundamental in all conditions associated with the body's basic immune system (see extended discussion in Chapter 24), nutrition is an intimate and integral component of care through the specific roles of key nutrients in maintaining the body's immunocompetence. Furthermore, for many of the associated diseases, individual nutritional status influences the impact of morbidity and mortality regardless of the disease process. Third, many of the new drug therapies, especially the protease inhibitors, cause lipodystrophy, reduced levels of high-density lipoprotein cholesterol, hypertriglyceridemia, hyperglycemia, and insulin resistance. Long-term consequences include an elevated risk of cardiovascular disease in this population.

Medical Management

BASIC CURRENT GOALS

The medical management of HIV-1 infection in all of its stages is constantly evolving as medical research seeks to eliminate, or at least suppress, the virus. Intensive current research is aimed at preventing the progressive immunodeficiency, stopping HIV-1 transmission to uninfected persons, and restoring depressed immune function to normal to prevent AIDS-associated complications. Thus the present basic medical management objectives are to (1) delay progression of the infection and improve the patient's immune system, (2) prevent opportunistic illnesses, and (3) recognize the infection early and provide rapid treatment for any complications of immune deficiency, including infections and cancers.

INITIAL EVALUATION: AIDS TEAM

The initial medical evaluation of a newly diagnosed HIV-infected patient is critical. It requires ongoing comprehensive care by the AIDS team of professional medical, nutritional, nursing, and psychosocial healthcare specialists.

retrovirus Any of a family of single-strand RNA viruses having an envelope and containing a reverse coding enzyme that allows for a reversal of genetic transcription from RNA to DNA rather than the usual DNA to RNA, the newly transcribed viral DNA then being incorporated into the host cell's DNA strand for the production of new RNA retroviruses.

BOX 23-1 Initial Evaluation of Newly Diagnosed HIV-Infected Patients

Routine history and physical examination include
- History of exposure to infectious complications of AIDS
- Assessment of baseline mental status
- Baseline laboratory studies
    - CBC, differential, platelets
    - Biochemistry screening profile
    - Urinalysis
    - Chest radiographic examination
    - Tuberculin test with anergy panel
    - Serologic test for syphilis
    - Toxoplasma serology
    - T-lymphocyte subsets
    - Hepatitis B serology (optional)
- Nutritional assessment, counseling, support, and follow-up
- Psychosocial and financial status assessment

Referral to and involvement in psychosocial support include
- Social worker, nurse, psychologist or psychiatrist, patient support group, community support group, and agencies
- Rehabilitation program for substance abusers
- Planning for family members and children, including issues of testing and providing for their care

Modified from Gold JWM: HIV-1 infection: diagnosis and management, *Med Clin North Am* 76(1):1, 1992.

Box 23-1 outlines an initial evaluation guide for beginning the care of a person with newly identified HIV-1 infection. These guidelines emphasize the special coordinated care by all members of the AIDS team and the importance of personal nutritional and psychosocial support.

ANTIRETROVIRAL DRUG THERAPY

As of the end of 2000, there were 15 FDA-approved antiretroviral drugs available in the United States. Antiretroviral therapy consists of three classifications of agents: (1) nucleoside reverse transcriptase inhibitors (NRTIs) such as zidovudine (AZT) and didanosine (ddI), (2) nonnucleoside reverse transcriptase inhibitors (NNRTIs) such as nevirapine (NVP), and (3) protease inhibitors (PIs) such as saquinavir, indinavir, and ritonavir. Antiretroviral agents are commonly given as part of a two- or three-drug regimen, or "cocktail," known as highly active antiretroviral therapy, or HAART. Guidelines set by the International AIDS Society-USA (IAS-USA) recommend treatment of patients with viral loads greater than 30,000 copies/ml regardless of $CD4^+$ cell count, of patients with viral loads between 5000 and 30,000 copies/ml who have $CD4^+$ cell counts below 500/μl, and of patients with $CD4^+$ cell counts below 350 cells/μl regardless of viral load.[16]

Nucleoside Reverse Transcriptase Inhibitors

These agents are nucleoside analogs that become phosphorylated by the host enzymes, after which they are incorporated into the newly formed DNA. Transcription ceases, thus halting replication of the virus before incorporating into the host genome.[17] The following is a list of the currently available NRTIs.

Generic Name	Trade Name
1. Zidovudine (AZT, ZDV)	Retrovir
2. Didanosine (ddI)	Videx
3. Zalcitabine (ddC)	HIVID
4. Lamivudine (3TC)	Epivir
5. Stavudine (d4T)	Zerit
6. Abacavir (ABC)	Ziagen

Nonnucleoside Reverse Transcriptase Inhibitors

These agents work by binding directly to the reverse transcriptase, which causes a confirmational change in the enzyme, rendering it nonfunctional.[18]

Generic Name	Trade Name
1. Nevirapine (NVP)	Viramune
2. Delaviridine (DLV)	Rescriptor
3. Efavirenz (EFV)	Sustiva

Protease Inhibitors

These antiretrovirals work by preventing cleavage of the protein precursors by inhibiting the protease enzyme. The resultant proteins that are formed cannot be packaged into mature virus and therefore are not virulent.[19] Studies have shown that PIs can reduce the amount of virus in the blood. The following is a list of the currently available PIs.

Generic Name	Trade Name
1. Saquinavir	Invirase, Fortovase
2. Indinavir	Crixivan
3. Ritonavir	Norvir
4. Nelfinavir	Viracept
5. Amprenavir	Agenerase
6. Lopinavir/ritonavir (LPV/RTV)	Kaletra

Rigid adherence to the drug regimens is crucial to the therapeutic efficacy of the drugs. Noncompliance, because of either the side effects, which can be severe, or the round-the-clock administration that is required, increases the risk of drug resistance. There are many side effects from these drugs, which may contribute to noncompliance with the drug regimens as listed in Table 23-2. Side effects such as nausea and diarrhea may require diet modifications (see Chapter 24). The efficacy of NNRTIs and NRTIs has been found to diminish over time because the

TABLE 23-2 Protease Inhibitor Drug-Nutrient Side Effects and Interactions

Protease Inhibitor Drugs	Drug Side Effects	Comments
Saquinavir (Invirase)	Diarrhea, nausea, abdominal cramps	Take after a high-kcalorie, high-fat meal for best absorption; grapefruit juice decreases absorption
Indinavir (Crixivan)	Taste changes, nausea, vomiting, diarrhea, elevated blood cholesterol, hypertriglyceridemia, and hyperglycemia	Best absorbed on an empty stomach or a nonfat light snack Increase fluids to about 24 oz/day (consider weight and age) High-calorie diet
Ritonavir (Norvir)	Diarrhea, nausea, vomiting; elevated liver function tests, anorexia, abnormal feelings in mouth (burning, prickling); hypercholesterolemia, hypertriglyceridemia	Take with high-kcalorie, high-fat foods
Nelfinavir (Viracept)	Nausea, diarrhea, loose stools	Take with food
Amprenavir (Agenerase)	Nausea, vomiting, diarrhea, flatulence	Do not take with a high-fat meal
Nevirapine* (Viramune)	Skin rash, mouth sores, general fatigue; elevated liver function tests	May take with food or an empty stomach

NOTE: All protease inhibitors have the potential for causing hypercholesterolemia, hypertriglyceridemia, and hyperglycemia, along with body composition changes (lipodystrophy).

NOTE: A high-fat/high-calorie meal is defined as 1006 kcalories, 48 g protein, 57 g fat, 60 g carbohydrate (the nutritional breakdown for this meal for the best absorption rates).

Adapted from Heller LS, Shattuck L: Nutrition support with children with HIV/AIDS, *J Am Diet Assoc* 97(5):473, 1997. Some data from *http://www.apla.org/apla/nutrition/factsheets/indexp.html.* Nutritional considerations for protease inhibitors.

*Nevirapine is in the drug category of nonnucleoside reverse transcriptase inhibitors.

virus has the ability to mutate and thus becomes resistant to the drugs currently available. The use of combination therapy, or "cocktails," with two or three of the drugs that have complementary actions, achieves more effective results over longer periods of time, especially in reducing reservoirs of infection hidden in lymph tissues.[20,21] To keep HIV levels as low as possible, it is recommended that PIs be taken with at least two other anti-HIV drugs, the combination known as HAART. However, this multidrug therapy, requiring dozens of pills daily along with a long list of sometimes unbearable side effects, and their often complicated medication-meal schedules, is very expensive, often costing upward of $15,000 per year.[22]

Self-Testing Monitoring Kits

The growing AIDS-related market has led to the development of self-testing kits used by patients and their physicians to help make treatment decisions. Most of these monitors measure levels of white blood cells with a $CD4^+$ receptor, the receiving point used by surface protein of the HIV to infect cells. These measures indicate how much damage has been done to the immune system.

CONTINUING VACCINE AND RESEARCH AND DEVELOPMENTS

A safe and effective vaccine against HIV is essential for the global control of the AIDS pandemic. Vaccine development is an extremely lengthy and costly process. There are many political and social hurdles and obstacles that must be overcome, including the question as to who will pay for such an enormous venture. In addition, a vaccine must be safe, effective, stable at a wide range of temperatures, and effective against more than one strain of HIV/AIDS. Although funding for HIV vaccine research has increased more than 100% from fiscal year 1997 to fiscal year 2000, an effective vaccine has yet to be developed.[23]

Global Perspective

Worldwide, more than 50 million people have been infected with HIV/AIDS and 16 million have died, surpassing tuberculosis and malaria as the leading infectious cause of death worldwide, according to data released by the Joint United Nations Programme on HIV/AIDS (UNAIDS) and the World Heath Organization (WHO).[24] In 1999, a record 2.8 million people died—more than any prior year—and an estimated 5.4 million people contracted HIV. Of people living with HIV infection, 95% live in developing countries, with more than two thirds of the total living in sub-Saharan Africa. Four of five HIV-positive women and 87% of HIV-positive children in the world live in Africa.[24] HIV is spreading rapidly in South Africa, Zimbabwe, Botswana, and India. China, Cambodia, Myanmar, Thailand, Vietnam, and Latin America are showing increasing levels of HIV infection.[24] The social ramifications are significant; millions of children are becoming orphans each year.

Undoubtedly the epidemiology and treatment of HIV-1 infection will change rapidly over the next few years. Patients will live longer and have improved quality of life. Nonetheless, with longer life and treatment for known complications, new complications will probably appear, such as uncommon infections, neurologic disease, or wasting syndromes. The medical management of AIDS will continue to require highly involved healthcare professionals and patients, as well as community support.

BASIC APPROACH: INDIVIDUAL STATUS AND NEEDS

Although answers will eventually come to many of our puzzling questions, HIV infection is still an elusive, epidemic, terminal disease, and its treatment varies according to individual status and needs—medical, nutritional, and psychosocial. Research breakthroughs will help light the course, but in every case, healthcare professionals and patients must remain highly involved, seeking the best possible individual care each step of the way.

There are many causes of malnutrition in HIV infection. Thus at any point, nutritional recommendations and support must be individualized and integrated with other therapies. Nutritional care plans must provide a comprehensive view of the disease process through each stage, specific drug use, and the patient's wishes. All patients diagnosed as HIV infected should be considered to be at nutritional risk. Although the patient may be in an earlier, asymptomatic period, the disease process, its complications, or treatments will eventually take their toll on the person's nutritional status. The nutritional status of any HIV-infected person may be compromised in numerous ways. At all times, each patient must be viewed within the context of his or her own disease and individual lifestyle.

HIV WASTING

Severe Malnutrition and Weight Loss

Before the development of antiretroviral agents, weight loss and cachexia were a predominant and eventual outcome of HIV disease. Multiple pathologic processes contribute to the weight loss commonly seen in patients with AIDS, including the drug regimens, malignancies, fevers, enteropathy, opportunistic infections (OIs), increased resting energy metabolism, lack of finances for food, and depression. Weight loss tends to be episodic; acute episodes of weight loss was found to be associated with acute OIs, whereas chronic weight loss was found to be associated with gastrointestinal disease and malabsorption.[25] Malnutrition itself suppresses cellular immune function. So striking is this chronic, relentless body wasting of AIDS that early in the AIDS epidemic outbreak in Uganda, Africa, it was given the name "slim disease."[26] Body wasting in AIDS is characterized by loss of body cell mass, primarily muscle protein. Death occurs when body weight reaches two thirds of normal weight and body cell mass reaches half of normal values. This designation implies that death may be more often a result of malnutrition, specifically negative nitrogen balance, than the direct effects of infection or malignancy.[27] Also, the attendant diseases of the wasting process play a major role in the decreased quality of life, debilitating weakness, and fatigue seen in patients with AIDS.

Factors Contributing to Wasting

The wasting seen in persons with HIV infection or AIDS may be a result of any of the following processes, alone or in any combination.

1. *Inadequate food intake.* Both clinicians and persons with HIV infection and AIDS indicate, from their combined clinical observations and personal experience, that an important factor in the profound weight loss is severe anorexia. This state is probably related to both the patient's personal life-changing situation and the body's physiologic changes from the disease. Anorexia and its resulting decreased food intake, insufficient to meet body needs, clearly contribute to the body wasting.[28]
2. *Anorexia:* Pharmacologic appetite stimulants, such as megestrol acetate (Megace) and dronabinol, have shown promising results. Megestrol acetate is a derivative of progesterone that was found to increase appetite in women who were given the medication as an adjunct to their oncologic therapy for breast cancer. Studies have shown megestrol acetate to enhance appetite, improve weight gain, and enhance sense of well-being in both cancer and HIV/AIDS patients.[29] An increase in fat mass rather than lean body mass may occur because megestrol acetate lowers the level of serum testosterone in patients with AIDS,[30] an effect that is not reversed by testosterone supplementation. Overall, megestrol acetate is generally well tolerated, especially in the liquid form; however, its costs can be prohibitive. Megestrol acetate may cause an exacerbation of hyperglycemia, and therefore should not be prescribed to diabetics or those experiencing hyperglycemia secondary to medications. Dronabinol (Marinol) is another pharmacologic agent useful for anorexia as well as helpful in treating nausea and vom-

iting. Side effects include altered mental status, anxiety, confusion, emotional lability, and hallucinations, which may be undesirable in older patients and patients whose job requires mental acuity. Dronabinol has not been shown to be more effective than megestrol acetate in the treatment of anorexia.

3. *Malabsorption of nutrients.* From early reports, as well as continuing clinical experience, diarrhea and malabsorption have been common in persons with HIV infection and AIDS. Diarrhea and malabsorption have been related to food (especially lactose) intolerances, antiretroviral therapy, other medications used to treat OIs, villous atrophy resulting from malnutrition or repeated bowel infections, low serum albumin levels, zinc deficiency or excess, and inadequate or absent digestive enzymes or bile salts.[31]
4. *Altered metabolism.* Many persons with HIV infection and AIDS have a tendency to have an increased resting energy metabolism and become hypermetabolic, especially during an acute infectious episode. Other metabolic abnormalities include the depletion of body cell mass, depletion of total body nitrogen, and body composition changes that occur with HAART.

TREATMENT OF HIV WASTING

Nutrition Assessment

The initial nutrition assessment must be comprehensive to provide the baseline information necessary for beginning and continuing nutritional care, including nutritional supplementation, early in the course of the disease.[32,33] Table 23-3 provides guidelines the team clinical dietitian uses to calculate daily calorie and protein needs, assess weight changes, and evaluate biochemical data. The calculations and evaluations are required especially for selected patients—children and adults—on special nutritional support therapies, either enteral or parenteral.[34]

A nutrition assessment should be conducted for all patients at all stages of HIV-related diseases to monitor status routinely and identify potential problems early.

Initially, nutrition assessment and intervention will help in devising practical medication-meal schedules, provide medical nutrition therapy to preserve lean body mass and prevent weight loss, identify potential symptoms that may interfere with adequate food intake, and monitor anthropometric and biochemical indices as indicated in Table 23-4.

Further, person-centered nutritional care required for all HIV-infected patients is evident in ongoing nutrition assessment (see *Practical Application* box). Special attention is given to any taste and smell losses, which reduce appetite and food intake. These losses in appetite may be aided by increased flavor enhancement in food preparation.[35] This type of detailed initial nutrition interview includes investigation of the patient's medical history, physical and anthropometric data, biochemical indices, full medication review, living situation, dietary intake, general socioeconomic status, and assistance needs. All patients, at first contact with a health professional, should be referred to the HIV/AIDS team clinical dietitian for screening to evaluate the degree of any nutrition problems.[36] Thus together with the patient, a plan for personal ongoing nutritional care and support can be initiated.

TABLE 23-3 Estimated Energy and Protein Requirements

Adults: minimum 35-40 kcalories/kg and 1-2 g protein/kg

Children: Recommended Dietary Allowances

Age	Energy (kcalorie/kg)	Protein (g/kg)
0-6 mo	108	2.2
6-12 mo	98	1.6
1-3 yr	102	1.2
4-6 yr	90	1.1
7-10 yr	70	1.0

Formula for catch-up growth:

$$\text{Kcalorie/kg and protein g/kg} = \frac{\text{RDA for weight/age} \times \text{median weight/height}}{\text{actual weight}}$$

Modified from Henderson R: Nutrition support of persons living with human immunodeficiency virus infection. In Matarese LE, Gottschlich MM, eds: *Contemporary nutrition support practice: a clinical guide,* Philadelphia, 1998, WB Saunders.

Micronutrients and Antioxidant Therapy

The role of micronutrients, that is, vitamins and minerals, in therapeutic amounts as part of the treatment of AIDS is the focus of much current research. Ongoing studies have focused on the antioxidant capacities of six basic micronutrients—vitamins A, C, and E and beta carotene and the trace minerals iron and zinc[37] (Table 23-5). Studies have shown an increase in oxidative stress resulting from metabolic overproduction of reactive oxygen intermediates, and a weakened antioxidant defense system in HIV-positive individuals.[38] Supplementation with megadoses of vitamins and minerals is increasingly common, and although persons with HIV/AIDS do have increased needs, a megadose of certain micronutrients (selenium, zinc) may be detrimental to the immune system. More research is needed in this area to obtain a more accurate assessment of the need for vitamins, minerals, and antioxidants.

Alternative Therapies

Persons with HIV infection and AIDS are particularly vulnerable to alternative therapies and supplements. In

TABLE 23-4 Nutritional Assessment Parameters

	Extent of Malnutrition (Adults)		
	Mild	Moderate*	Severe*
Albumin (g/dl)	3.0-3.5	2.4-2.9	<2.4
Transferrin (mg/dl)	150-200	100-150	<100
Thyroxine binding prealbumin (g/L)	1.0-1.5	0.5-1.0	<0.5
Ideal body weight (%)	80-90	70-79	<69
Usual body weight (%)	85-95	75-84	<74
Weight loss/unit time	<5%/mo <7.5%/3 mo <10%/6 mo	<2%/wk >5%/mo >7.5%/3 mo >10%/6 mo	>2%/wk

Anthropometry	Normal Male	Normal Female
Triceps skinfold (mm)	12.5	16.5
Mid-arm circumference (cm)	29.3	28.5

Adapted from: © 2000, American Dietetic Association. "*Manual of Clinical Dietetics,* 6e." Used with permission; and Hickey MS: Nutritional support of patients with AIDS, *Surg Clin North Am* 71(3):645, 1991.
*Nutritional therapy indicated.

PRACTICAL APPLICATION
The ABCDs of Nutrition Assessment in AIDS

The initial nutrition assessment visit with an HIV-infected patient is an important beginning point for the continuing nutritional care that is to follow. This encounter serves both informational and relational functions. It provides the necessary baseline information for planning practical individual nutrition support. More important, it establishes the essential provider-patient relationship, the human context within which this continuing nutritional care and support will be provided as needed. The basic ABCDs of nutrition assessment will provide a practical guide with special assessment (the letters "E" and "F") added for HIV-infected patients.

ANTHROPOMETRY
- Age, sex, height
- Weight: current, usual, percent of usual, ideal, percent of ideal, weight loss over defined time period
- Mid-upper-arm measures: circumference, triceps skinfold thickness; calculated mid-arm muscle circumference

BIOCHEMICAL INDICES
- Serum proteins: albumin, prealbumin, transferrin
- Liver function tests (evaluate liver function)
- Blood urea nitrogen, serum electrolytes (evaluate renal function)
- Urinary urea nitrogen excretion over 24 hours (nitrogen balance)
- Creatinine height index
- Complete blood cell count (evaluate for anemia)
- Fasting glucose (evaluate for hyperglycemia or hypoglycemia)

CLINICAL OBSERVATIONS
- General signs of nutritional status
- Drug effects

DIET EVALUATION
- Usual intake, current intake, restrictions, modifications (use both 24-hour recall and food diaries)
- Nutrition supplements, vitamin-mineral supplements
- Food allergies, intolerances
- Activity level (general kcalories expended per day)
- Support system (caregivers to help with nutrition care plan)

ENVIRONMENTAL, BEHAVIORAL, AND PSYCHOLOGIC ASSESSMENT
- Living situation, personal support
- Food environment, types of meals, eating assistance needed

FINANCIAL ASSESSMENT
- Medical insurance
- Income, financial support through caregivers
- Current medical and other expenses
- Ability to afford food, enteral supplements, added vitamins-minerals

References
Fields-Gardner C: Position of the American Dietetic Association and the Canadian Dietetic Association: Nutrition intervention in the care of persons with human immunodeficiency virus infection, *J Am Diet Assoc* 94(9):1042, 1994.

Trujillo EB et al: Assessment of nutritional status, nutrient intake, and nutrition support in AIDS patients, *J Am Diet Assoc* 92(4):477, 1992.

TABLE 23-5 Micronutrients Immune Response Deficiency and Supplement Effects

Micronutrient	Immune Response Deficiency	Supplement Effects
Vitamins		
Vitamin A	Impaired response; increased infections and subsequent mortality	Improves immunity; excess is toxic
Beta carotene	Impaired immunity, increased cancer risk	Enhances response, CD41T-cells
B vitamins	Reduced lymphoid tissue	Vitamin B_{12} enhances skin test, mitogen response; vitamin B_6 does not enhance above reactions
Vitamin C	Impaired phagocytosis	May enhance immune function
Vitamin E	T-, B-cell dysfunction	Enhances immunity, skin test response, and function
Minerals		
Copper	Impaired function of macrophages	Good repletion, but excess can be toxic
Iron	Reduced immune response	Excess can harm
Selenium	Low intake, cancer risk	Repletion contributes to survival; excess can impair immunity
Zinc	Loss of T-cell immunity	Improves with moderate supplementation; excess can harm

Modified from Cunningham-Rundles S et al: Micronutrient and cytokine interaction in congenital pediatric HIV infection, *J Nutr* 126(10S):2674S, 1996.

1990, it was estimated that in the United States approximately 425 million visits were made to alternative practitioners, representing $13.7 billion in expenditures, including $10.3 billion in out-of-pocket expenses.[39] Alternative treatments used by persons with HIV infection and AIDS include, but are not limited to, Ayurvedic medicine, homeopathic medicine, traditional Chinese medicine, acupuncture, chiropractic, massage therapy, reflexology, therapeutic touch, and Qi gong. A full description of these therapies is beyond the scope of this chapter; however, it may be found in other resources. Herbal therapies are also commonly used among this population. Hundreds, and maybe thousands, of herbal preparations are consumed by millions of people in the United States. Herbals targeted toward persons with HIV/AIDS include bitter melon, compound Q, curcumin, astragalus, echinacea, milk thistle, Siberian ginseng, SPV-30, aloe vera, alpha lipoic acid, Iscador, NAC (*N*-acetylcysteine), and shark cartilage. A significant interaction has been described between the herbal therapy St. John's Wort *(Hypericum perforatum)*, which is commonly taken for depression, and the PI indinavir (Crixivan). St John's Wort decreases blood levels of indinavir by 49% to 99%.[40] The FDA warns that St John's Wort may also significantly reduce blood concentrations of all HIV PIs and possibly other drugs, including those antiretrovirals in the NNRTI class. A description of these and other commonly used herbals, along with their mechanisms of actions and side effects, can be found in a variety of pharmacology and pharmaceutical textbooks, Office of Dietary Supplements within the National Institutes of Health, and the FDA publications.

Nutrition Intervention

The major goals of medical nutrition therapy during HIV infection, as recommended by the HIV/AIDS Practice Group of the American Dietetic Association,[41] are as follows.

1. To optimize nutrition status, immunity, and overall well-being
2. To prevent the development of specific nutrient deficiencies
3. To prevent loss of weight and lean body mass
4. To maximize the effectiveness of medical and pharmacologic treatments
5. To minimize healthcare costs

It is the position of the American Dietetic Association and the Canadian Dietetic Association that nutrition intervention, medical nutrition therapy, and education should be components of the total healthcare provided to persons infected with HIV.[41] Suggested guidelines for developing such patient-centered care plans are outlined in Box 23-2. For those persons receiving nutrition support in special enteral or parenteral forms, the dietitian should work with the HIV/AIDS team physician, and other members of the nutrition support team, to develop an appropriate feeding mode, using enteral means or parenteral feeding via peripheral or central veins (see Chapter 17).

Treatment of HIV-Associated Wasting

For some patients, control of viral load with antiretroviral agents is accompanied by weight gain. However, weight gain may be accompanied by adipose tissue gain, versus lean body mass. The primary goal should be repletion of lean body cell mass. The first step is to improve

BOX 23-2 Guidelines for Developing Patient-Centered Care Plans

Symptom Management

Loss of Appetite

- Eat a snack of small meal every 2-3 hours because large portions may fill you up too much
- Eat more food in the morning when your appetite is best
- Eat favorite foods whenever you feel like it
- Eat foods that contain a lot of protein and calories (peanut butter and jelly sandwiches, milkshakes, pizza)
- Avoid low-calorie foods or low-fat/fat-free foods
- Take medicines with juice, chocolate milk, or an instant breakfast drink instead of water, unless your physician or nurse tells you not to
- Try 10-15 minutes of mild exercise before eating to stimulate your appetite
- If fatigue is a problem, keep easy to prepare foods on hand, such as frozen meals, canned soups, and eggs; have family members or friends prepare foods or arrange for home delivery of foods

Nausea and Vomiting

- Avoid fried, greasy, spicy, and very sweet foods
- Eat bland, well-cooked, easy-to-digest foods such as rice, noodles, potatoes, chicken, turkey, custard, yogurt, and oatmeal
- Try eating dry, salty foods such as crackers and toast first thing in the morning and sipping on flat sodas and weak ginger or mint tea throughout the day to calm your stomach
- If food odors are a problem, eat cold or lukewarm food and stay out of the kitchen while foods are being cooked

Nausea and Vomiting—cont'd

- Avoid eating your favorite foods while nauseated
- Do not lie down for 2 hours after eating meals

Sore Mouth or Throat

- Eat foods that are soft and smooth in texture such as mashed potatoes, yogurt, pudding, custards, oatmeal, and scrambled eggs
- Avoid spicy acidic, hard and hot foods—they can irritate your mouth
- Cold foods such as ice cream and Popsicles can be soothing to your mouth
- Add gravies or cream sauces to meats and vegetables before eating to make them easier to swallow
- Soak dry foods such as bread and cookies in milk or other beverage before eating
- Use a straw to drink beverages and soup to help ease discomfort

Diarrhea

- Avoid foods that may make diarrhea worse such as milk and milk products, greasy and fatty foods, high fiber foods and foods that cause gas, and carbonated, caffeinated and alcoholic beverages
- Eat foods that may help control diarrhea such as bananas, applesauce, rice and gummy bears
- Eat well-cooked, easy-to digest foods like canned peaches, cooked carrots, baked chicken and fish, potatoes, and noodles
- Drink 8 or more glasses of fluids such as sports drinks, apple juice, and broth each day
- Eat foods that are high in minerals such as potatoes, bananas, fish and meat
- Try a BRAT diet—bananas, rice, applesauce, and toast—for a couple of days

Adapted from ***MEDSURG Nursing,*** 1998, Volume 7, Number 5, pg. 261. Reprinted with permission from the publisher, Janetti Publications, Inc., East Holly Avenue, Box 56, Pitman, NJ 08071-0056. Phone (856) 256-2300; Fax (856) 589-7463. (For a sample issue of the journal, contact the publisher.)

nutritional intake—adequate calories and protein, vitamins and minerals, and medical nutritional supplements as necessary.

HAART-associated metabolic and body composition changes. Although HAART has revolutionized the medical treatment of HIV and AIDS and reduced the incidence of malnutrition and infections, the adverse effects of HAART continue to be a major obstacle to patient compliance and a limiting factor that drives the cost-benefit ratio for pharmacologic therapy. Lipodystrophy and its related fat distribution complications have become the major nutrition issues in patients being treated with PIs. *Lipodystrophy syndrome* consists of changes in body shape that are caused by abnormal redistribution of fat. Fat accumulates in the abdominal area (truncal and visceral obesity), in the axillary pads, and in the dorsocervical pads ("buffalo hump") but decreases in the legs, arms, and nasolabial and cheek pads.[42] Lipodystrophy, although not life threatening, can cause varying degrees of depression, anxiety, social withdrawal, and low self-esteem, which can ultimately lead to poor medication compliance. Many patients discontinue therapy, risking the progression of HIV infection. HAART can also cause hyperlipidemia (especially hypertriglyceridemia and hypercholesterolemia) and insulin resistance, which can significantly increase the risk of developing cardiovascular disease. This is a major concern and potentially a major deterrent to early or continuous therapy. Overall, the risk of myocardial infarction in HIV-infected patients taking PIs appears to be 2- to 3-fold higher than in the general population.[43] Persons on HAART are also at increased risk of developing diabetes, hypertension, and osteoporosis.

Obtaining baseline anthropometrics (waist-hip ratio, bioelectric impedance analysis, skinfold measurements) and serial measurements (i.e., at each clinic visit) is important for monitoring changes in body composition. Baseline measurements of triglycerides, total cholesterol and lipoproteins (HDL, LDL, VLDL), blood glucose, and blood pressure should be obtained. They should also be obtained at each clinic visit to monitor for changes. Diet, exercise, and pharmacologic agents are useful in the treatment of lipodystrophy syndrome. Patients with abnormal LDL, HDL, and total cholesterol levels may benefit from following the American Heart Association's Step I or Step II diet (see Chapter 19 for details), which emphasize grains, cereals, legumes, fruits, vegetables, lean meats, poultry, fish, and low-fat dairy products. Diet-resistant hyperlipidemia may need to be controlled with lipid-lowering agents. Currently, researchers are trying to determine which drugs can be used safely and effectively in persons on anti-HIV drugs. Individuals with insulin resistance and hyperglycemia will need counseling for carbohydrate counting (see Chapter 20). An individual with hypertriglyceridemia will need to limit intake of simple carbohydrates and alcohol. Exercise, especially weight training, may help prevent muscle wasting in the arms, legs, and buttocks, whereas aerobic exercise may help control abdominal visceral fat accumulation. Clinical trials are ongoing to determine actual benefits.

Use of anabolic agents in HIV and AIDS. The use of anabolic agents has been recommended as an effective way of improving gains in lean body mass. Anabolic agents such as oxandrolone and nandrolone decanoate are known to promote protein anabolism and are generally safe when taken as prescribed.[44] Recombinant human growth hormone (rhGH), whose trade name is Serostim, is the most extensively studied anabolic agent; it has also been shown to significantly improve lean body mass and nitrogen balance in the treatment of HIV/AIDS wasting.[45] Human growth hormone therapy may help control some of the body composition changes seen in some individuals with lipodystrophy. There are many potential side effects of anabolic agents, including gynecomastia, testicular atrophy and decreased fertility, salt retention, lipid and carbohydrate abnormalities, and acne. In addition, anabolic agents are frequently very expensive (approximately $18,000 per year); however, Medicaid has approved reimbursement for this treatment.[46] Resistance or weight training is strongly recommended as a safe and effective method for maintaining and improving lean body mass in all individuals who are physically able to exercise.

NUTRITION COUNSELING, EDUCATION, AND SUPPORTIVE STRATEGIES

Counseling Principles

An adolescent client once aptly defined a counselor as "someone to talk to while I make up my mind." Client-centered counseling in the care of persons with HIV infection and AIDS must be just that. Professionals and patients must remain involved throughout the progressive course of the disease because the patient's wishes and needs are ultimately paramount in various treatments and decisions about care. The basic goal of nutrition counseling is to make the fewest possible changes in the person's lifestyle and food patterns necessary to promote optimal nutritional status while providing maximum comfort and quality of life. In this person-centered care process, several counseling principles are particularly pertinent.

1. *Motivation.* Changed behavior in any area requires the motivation, desire, and ability to achieve one's goals. Until the patient perceives food patterns and behaviors as appropriate goals, it is best to wait for a better time and begin with establishing a general supportive climate in which to continue working together. Any specific obstacle raised by the patient, such as time, physical limitations, money, or increased anxiety, can be met with related suggestions to think about. Priorities among needs should be recognized in the care plan, and items should be introduced according to order of importance and immediacy of the patient's nutritional problems.
2. *Rationale.* Any diet or food behavior change, with possible benefits and risks, must be clearly explained to the patient. The question "Why?" is always important to everybody.
3. *Provider-patient agreement.* In the best interests of all concerned, the patient and healthcare provider must agree to the change. Any change should be structured around daily routines and include any caregivers as needed. The nutrition counselor should provide any needed information and encouragement throughout the process.
4. *Manageable steps.* All information given and actions agreed on should proceed in manageable steps, as small as necessary, in order of complexity and difficulty. Information overload can discourage anyone. But here the particular stress load at any point can be intolerable for the patient. At such points of stress, patients are also more vulnerable to the lure of unproved HIV/AIDS therapies (see *To Probe Further* box).

TO PROBE FURTHER
Are Persons With HIV/AIDS Vulnerable to Nutritional Quackery?

People with chronic diseases, such as AIDS, that lack curative therapy and have poor prognoses are susceptible to claims of unproved therapies and nutrition quackery. Some of the nutritional quackery that is being touted as treatments for HIV infection includes the following questionable practices.

MEGADOSES OF NUTRIENTS

Large doses of vitamins A and C, selenium, and zinc have been recommended to restore cell-mediated immunity by increasing T-cell number and activity. The value of such large doses has not been established in controlled clinical studies. In fact, the opposite is true; megadoses of these nutrients can be dangerous. Chronic intakes of vitamin A in excess of 25,000 IU/day can be toxic, especially to the liver. Doses of vitamin C above 2000 mg can cause diarrhea, nausea, and gastrointestinal upset; increase the risk of kidney stones; and cause a urine test to test falsely positive for diabetes. Chronic intakes of excess zinc, as little as 25 mg/day, can cause gastrointestinal distress, nausea, and impaired immune function. Selenium is also toxic in high chronic doses. It is recommended for persons with HIV/AIDS to take two multivitamin/mineral supplements per day to ensure intake of 200% of the RDA for vitamins and minerals.

DR. BERGER'S IMMUNE POWER DIET

In his book, Berger (1985) states that poor health is caused by "immune hypersensitivity" to many foods such as milk, wheat, corn, yeast, soy, sugar, and eggs. He suggests a 21-day elimination diet for foods believed to cause allergies, followed by a reintroduction phase and then a maintenance diet, to prevent food sensitivities and "revitalize" the immune system. The usefulness of this diet has not been tested or proved by scientific studies. The diet promoted in Berger's book (high in fruits and vegetables and low in fat and calcium) may cause malnutrition, and the suggestion that moldy food be consumed to test for allergy to molds is dangerous to persons who are immunocompromised. His claims are unsubstantiated.

ANTIVIRAL AL 721

This compound, developed in Israel and approved by the FDA for clinical trials, is composed of "active lipids" (AL) mixed in a ratio of 70% neutral lipid, 20% lecithin, and 10% phosphatidylethanolamine—hence the 721 designation. It has been hypothesized that 721 can reduce or inhibit HIV infection. Clinical trials found little toxicity but no consistent trends in T-cell quantification or HIV cultures. AL 721 made at home from soy or egg yolk lecithin or obtained already mixed may be impure and can spoil easily if stored improperly.

YEAST-FREE DIET (ANTICANDIDIASIS DIET)

Candida infection, which causes oral and esophageal thrush, is common in individuals who are immunocompromised. The authors of this diet suggest that certain persons have "candidiasis hypersensitivity" and that by following the diet (restricted in carbohydrates, yeast, sugar, processed foods, fruits [initially], and milk), this disorder can be successfully treated. The American Academy of Allergy, Asthma, and Immunology has been strongly critical of these concepts. Because the diet is limited in carbohydrates, an individual may develop ketosis, which can cause nausea and headache. This diet may also be too low in calories for individuals with HIV infection/AIDS.

COLONIC THERAPY

Colonic irrigation is touted to detoxify the large intestine to reduce the body of poisons and wastes. Not only is the procedure expensive, but it is not FDA approved for "cleansing" the body of wastes. Colon cleansing is only approved and medically indicated before a colonoscopy/sigmoidoscopy. There is also great potential for harm because colonic irrigation can cause severe cramps, pain, perforation of the large intestine resulting in serious infection, and electrolyte losses, especially potassium. There is no medically substantiated reason for a person with HIV infection/AIDS (or anyone, for that matter) to have a colonic irrigation.

MACROBIOTIC DIET

A macrobiotic diet is based on an Oriental philosophy that it will restore balance and harmony between Yin and Yang forces and thereby improve health. However, it is very low in fat and high in fiber: 50% (by volume) whole-grain cereals, 20% to 30% vegetables, 10% to 15% cooked beans or seaweed; and 5% miso (fermented soy paste) or tamari broth soup. This regimen can produce protein-calorie malnutrition and provides inadequate intake of riboflavin, niacin, and calcium in adults, as well as pyridoxine and vitamins B_{12} and D in children (in addition to those nutrients mentioned for adults).

These diets and other alternative therapies require further study in controlled clinical trials.

References

Anderson JA: Position statement on candidiasis hypersensitivity, *J Allerg Immunol* 78:271, 1986.

Jarvis WT: *Colonic irrigation,* Peabody, Mass, 1995, National Council Against Health Fraud, 1995.

Raiten DJ: Nutrition and HIV infection: a review and evaluation of the extant knowledge of the relationship between nutrition and HIV infection, *Nutr Clin Pract* 6(3):S1, 1991.

Personal Food Management Skills

The patient's living situation and general practical skills in planning, purchasing, and preparing food must be considered. Any need for information and guidance in developing skills in any aspect of procuring food, or in sources of needed help, should be provided.

Community Programs

Information may be needed about any available community food programs, such as Meals-on-Wheels, for delivery of prepared meals at times when the patient is too ill to get out for food. A number of these programs in various hard-hit inner cities on the east and west coasts of the United States, for example, as well as in central cities, have developed to meet these needs, and in some cases they also provide home health and nutritional care services.[47-50] Also, information may need to be provided about food assistance programs such as Food Stamps or Food Commodities (see Chapter 10), for which the lower-income person may qualify.

Psychosocial Support

Every aspect of care provided should be given within a form and context that also provides genuine psychosocial support. All healthcare providers working with HIV-infected patients must be particularly sensitive to the special psychologic and social issues that confront persons with AIDS. Major stress areas may include issues relating to autonomy and dependency, a sense of uncertainty and fear of the unknown, grief, change and loss, fear of symptoms, fears of abandonment, and spiritual questions that arise when someone confronts a life-threatening illness. Common emotions are hostility, denial, withdrawal, depression, anxiety, guilt, and confusion. All of these at one time or another may significantly influence treatment. Healthcare providers must always be aware and assess how the patient and caregivers are relating to the disease, using assistance of social workers, clinical psychologists, or psychiatrists as needed.[51,52] Stress reduction groups, including exercise training, are helpful, as they have proved to be in other life-threatening situations such as patients with cancer or coronary heart disease.[53]

Most important, however, healthcare workers must examine their own values and fears regarding sexual orientation, sexual behavior, intravenous drug use, and fears of AIDS transmission. Preconceived judgments are easily picked up by patients and threaten the provider-patient relationship. Before they can be effective with patients, all healthcare workers must first confront their own fears and prejudices and learn to let go of such judgmental behavior.

TO SUM UP

The viral evolution and current worldwide spread of HIV infection have reached epidemic proportions and are still growing. The disease progression follows three distinct stages: HIV infection, AIDS-related complex (ARC) with associated opportunistic illnesses, and full-blown AIDS with complicating diseases leading to death. This overall disease progression from initial infection to death lasts about 10 to 12 years. The Public Health Service and the CDC of the U.S. Department of Health and Human Services (DHHS) have responsibilities for monitoring the disease and providing leadership in research and treatment development, based on collaborative information exchange with scientists worldwide.

During the initial decade of the epidemic in the 1980s, scientists learned the nature and life cycle of the new mutation of HIV and its transmission modes and population groups at risk. Development of diagnostic testing procedures has enabled population surveillance and individual detection of disease and personal care to proceed. A fundamental role of nutrition support in this personal care of HIV-infected individuals has become evident.

Medical management of HIV infection, which is without a vaccine or cure, involves supportive treatment of associated illnesses and complicating diseases. In the terminal HIV stage, the virus eventually gains sufficient strength to destroy the white blood cells of the host's immune system, and death follows. New drugs to slow the disease progression are under development.

Current ongoing research involves study of the role of micronutrients in oxidation processes in the cell. Nutritional management focuses on providing personal individual nutrition support to counteract the severe body wasting and malnutrition characteristic of the disease. The process of nutritional care involves comprehensive nutrition assessment and evaluation of personal needs, planning care with each patient and caregivers, and meeting practical food needs. Throughout the care process, nutrition counseling, education, and strategic services also help provide psychosocial support to each patient.

■ Questions for Review

1. Describe the evolutionary history of HIV-1 and its current worldwide epidemic spread. How is it transmitted, and why do you think it has spread so rapidly? Identify major population groups at risk.
2. Describe the nature of the AIDS virus and its action in the human body. What is a retrovirus?
3. Describe the progression of HIV infection in terms of its stages of development from initial infection to death.
4. Identify the drugs currently used in the medical management of HIV/AIDS, and describe any associated actions, side effects, or toxicities that may relate to dietary management.
5. Discuss the etiologies of HIV wasting and its medical and nutritional therapies.
6. Outline the basic parts of a comprehensive initial nutrition assessment of a patient with HIV infection/AIDS.

7. Describe the general process of planning nutritional care on the basis of the patient assessment information and the main types of nutrition problems in HIV infection/AIDS. Devise a related plan of action for each type of problem. Can you give an example of how you might follow up to see what worked or did not work and make adjustments accordingly?

■ References

1. Piot P: AIDS: a global response (editorial), *Science* 272 (5270):1855, 1996.
2. Tuofu Z et al: An African HIV-1 sequence from 1959 and implications for the origin of the epidemic, *Nature* 391 (6667):594, 1998.
3. AIDS Epidemic Update, Joint United Nations Programme of HIV/AIDS (UNAIDS) Dec 2000.
4. Cohen J: The changing of the guard, *Science* 272(5270): 1876, 1996.
5. Holmberg SD: The estimated prevalence and incidence of HIV in 96 large US metropolitan areas, *Am J Public Health* 86(5):642, 1996.
6. Stein Z, Susser M: AIDS—an update on global dynamics (editorial), *Am J Public Health* 97(6):901, 1997.
7. Cohen J: AIDS therapy: failure isn't what it used to be . . . but neither is success, *Science* 279(5354):1133, 1998.
8. Flaskerud JH, Ungvarski PJ: Overview and update of HIV disease. In Ungvarski PJ, Flaskerud JH, eds: *HIV/AIDS: a guide to primary care management,* ed 4, Philadelphia, 1999, WB Saunders.
9. Sax P: Viral load testing, *AIDS Clin Care* 8(4):31-32, 1996.
10. Ryan F: *Virus X: tracking the new killer plaques,* Boston, 1997, Little, Brown.
11. Gold JWM: HIV-1 infection, *Med Clin North Am* 76(1):1992.
12. Otten MW et al: Changes in sexually transmitted disease rates after HIV testing and posttest counseling, Miami, 1988 to 1989, *Am J Public Health* 83(4):529-533, 1993.
13. U.S Department of Health and Human Services: *Healthy people 2010,* ed 2, 2 vols, Washington, DC, 2000, U.S. Government Printing Office, available at *http://www.health.gov/healthypeople.*
14. Centers for Disease Control and Prevention, Public Health Service: *HIV prevention strategic plan through 2005,* Atlanta, 2001, Centers for Disease Control and Prevention.
15. Centers for Disease Control and Prevention, Public Health Service: Guidelines for national human immunodeficiency virus case surveillance, including monitoring for immunodeficiency virus infection and acquired immunodeficiency syndrome, *MMWR* 48(RR13):1, 1999.
16. Carpenter CCJ: Antiretroviral therapy in adults: updated recommendations of the International AIDS Society-USA Panel, *JAMA* 283(3):381, 2000.
17. Samuel R, Suh B: Antiretroviral therapy 2000, *Arch Pharmacol Res* 23(5):425, 2000.
18. Miller V et al: Clinical experience with non-nucleoside reverse transcriptase inhibitors, *AIDS* 11(suppl A):S157, 1997.
19. Flexner C: HIV-protease inhibitors, *N Engl J Med* 338(18): 1281, 1998.
20. Cohen J: Stubborn HIV reservoirs vulnerable to new treatments, *Science* 276(5314):898, 1997.
21. Cavert W et al: Kinetics of response in lymphoid tissues to antiretroviral therapy of HIV-1 infection, *Science* 276(5314): 960, 1997.
22. Office of AIDS Research, NIH: *Research overview, 2000,* Bethesda, Md, 2000, National Institutes of Health.
23. HIV/AIDS: Confronting the Global Pandemic—Canada's Contribution, Toronto, June 1-2, 2000 (conference).
24. Temesgen Z: Overview of HIV infection, *Ann Allergy Asthma Immunol* 83:1, 1999.
25. Macallan DC: Wasting in HIV infection and AIDS, *J Nutr* 129(1):S238, 1999.
26. Serwadda D et al: Slim disease: a new disease in Uganda and its association with HTLV-III infection, *Lancet* 2:849, 1985.
27. Macallan DC et al: Energy expenditure and wasting in human immunodeficiency virus infection, *N Engl J Med* 333(2):83, 1995.
28. American Gastroenterological Association Medical Position Statement: Guidelines for the management of malnutrition and cachexia, chronic diarrhea, and hepatobiliary disease in patients with HIV infection, *Gastroenterology* 111:1722, 1996.
29. Oster MH et al: Megestrol acetate in patients with AIDS and cachexia, *Ann Intern Med* 121(6):400, 1994.
30. Engelson ES et al: Effects of megestrol acetate therapy upon body composition and serum testosterone in patients with AIDS (abstract), *Clin Res* 42:281A, 1994.
31. Adinolfi AJ: Symptom management in HIV/AIDS. In Durham JD, Lashley FR, eds: *The person with HIV/AIDS: a nursing perspective,* ed 3, New York, 2000, Springer.
32. Stack JA et al: High-energy, high-protein, oral, liquid, nutrition supplementation in patients with HIV infection: effect on weight status in relation to incidence of secondary infection, *J Am Diet Assoc* 96(4):337, 1996.
33. Chlebowski RT et al: Dietary intake and counseling, weight maintenance, and the course of HIV infection, *J Am Diet Assoc* 95(4):428, 1995.
34. Heller LS, Shattuck D: Nutrition support for children with HIV/AIDS, *J Am Diet Assoc* 97(5):473, 1997.
35. Graham CS et al: Taste and smell losses in HIV infected patients, *Physiol Behav* 58(2):287, 1995.
36. Fields-Gardner C et al: *A clinician's guide to nutrition and HIV and AIDS,* Chicago, 1997, The American Dietetic Association.
37. Kotler DP: Antioxidant therapy and HIV infection: 1998, *Am J Clin Nutr* 67:7, 1998.
38. Los Angeles County Commission on HIV Health Services: *Guidelines for implementing HIV/AIDS medical nutrition therapy protocols,* Los Angeles, Oct 1997, The Commission.
39. Anastasi JK: Alternative and complementary therapies. In Flaskerud JH, Ungvarski PJ, eds: *HIV/AIDS: a guide to primary care management,* ed 4, Philadelphia, 1999, WB Saunders.
40. Piscitelli SC et al: Indinavir concentrations and St. John's Wort, *Lancet* 355(9203):547, 2000.
41. Young JS: HIV and medical nutrition therapy, *J Am Diet Assoc* 97(10):S161, 1997.

42. Kotler DP: *Lipodystrophy—it just gets more complicated,* 8th Annual Conference on Retroviruses and Opportunistic Infections, Chicago, Feb 6, 2001.
43. Scerola D et al: Reversal of cachexia in patient treated with potent antiviral therapy, *AIDS Read* 10(6):365, 2000.
44. Loss JC: The use of anabolic agents in HIV disease, *Support Line* 21(3):23, June 1999.
45. Schambelan M, Mulligan K, Grunfeld C: Recombinant growth hormone in patients with HIV-associated wasting: a randomized, placebo-controlled trial, *Ann Intern Med* 125: 873, 1996.
46. FDC Reports: *Serono serostim required on state Medicaid formularies, HCFA says,* vol 66, Chevy Chase, Md, 1999, FDC Reports.
47. Luder E et al: Assessment of nutritional, clinical, and immunologic status of HIV-infected, inner-city patients with multiple risk factors, *J Am Diet Assoc* 95(6):655, 1995.
48. Topping CM et al: A community-based, interagency approach by dietitians to provide meals, medical nutrition therapy, and education to clients with HIV/AIDS, *J Am Diet Assoc* 95(6):683, 1995.
49. Kraak VI: Home-delivered meal programs for homebound people with HIV/AIDS, *J Am Diet Assoc* 95(4):476, 1995.
50. Udine LM, Rorthkopf MM: Utilization of home health care services in HIV infection: a pilot study in Ohio, *J Am Diet Assoc* 94(1):83, 1994.
51. Antoni MH et al: Cognitive-behavior stress management intervention buffers distress responses and immunologic change following notification of HIV-1 seropositivity, *J Consult Clin Psychol* 59(6):906, 1991.
52. Jacobsberg LB, Perry S: Psychiatric disturbances, *Med Clin North Am* 76(1):99, 1992.
53. LaPerriere A et al: Aerobic exercise training in an AIDS risk group, *Int J Sports Med* 12(suppl 1):S53, 1991.

■ Further Reading

Nowak MA, McMichael AJ: How HIV defeats the immune system, *Sci Am* 273(2):58, 1995.

This article provides interesting background in a case study, and its accompanying editorial, of perinatal transmission of AIDS at birth with apparent clearance afterward, in a boy now 5 years old and in kindergarten, and a discussion of the controversial question of breast-feeding by HIV-positive mothers.

■ Websites of Interest

http://www.napwa.org National Association of People with AIDS

http://www.amfar.org American Foundation for AIDS Research (AmFAR)

http://hiv.medscape.com/Home/Topics/AIDS/directories/dir-AIDS.ConfSummaries.htm Medscape

http://www.cdc.gov/hiv/dhap.htm Centers for Disease Control and Prevention, Division of HIV/AIDS Prevention (DHAP)

http://www.niaid.nih.gov/daids/default.htm National Institute of Allergy and Infectious Diseases (NIAID), Division of Acquired Immunodeficiency Syndrome (DAIDS)

http://www.nih.gov/od/oar National Institutes of Health Office of AIDS Research

http://www.aidsnutrition.org AIDS Nutrition Services Alliance (ANSA)

http://www.daair.org Direct AIDS Alternative Information Resources (DAAIR)

http://www.aids.org/immune/atn.nsf/homepage AIDS Treatment News-Online

http://www.natap.org National AIDS Treatment Advocacy Project

http://www.eatright.org American Dietetic Association

CASE STUDY AIDS in a young man

David is a 32-year-old man who was recently admitted to the hospital with a history of weight loss, painful difficulty swallowing, and watery diarrhea. He has been in a long-term, monogamous relationship with his partner for 6 years. David works as an accountant at a large firm. Six months ago, David started to notice he was losing weight involuntarily and he began having large-volume, loose stools. He developed thrush in his mouth about 3 months before admission, which caused the odynophagia. About 1 week before admission, a high temperature developed in David that did not respond to analgesics. He also complained of shortness of breath, chest tightness, and a dry cough. Physical examination revealed a weight loss of 25 pounds and oral candidiasis; the chest radiographic examination was positive for *Pneumocystis carinii* pneumonia (PCP). David was admitted to receive intravenous antibiotics (trimethoprim-sulfamethoxazole [TMP-SMX]) and intravenous fluconazole, an antifungal. A stool culture revealed cytomegalovirus (CMV), and therefore intravenous ganciclovir, an antiviral agent, was initiated. David's oral intake was noted to be extremely poor; he also developed severe nausea and vomiting as a result of the medications and the infectious processes. His average daily volume of diarrhea also increased to 1800 ml/day. Results of the nutritional assessment were as follows.

Height (cm)	177.8 cm
Weight (kg)	61.4
Usual weight (kg)	72.7
Percent weight loss	15.5
Body weight (percent of usual)	84
Triceps skinfold:	25th percentile
Midarm muscle circumference:	25th percentile
$CD4^+$	118
Serum potassium (mEq/dl)	3.1
Blood glucose (mg/dl)	70
Blood urea nitrogen (mg/dl)	32
Creatinine (mg/dl)	0.4
Serum albumin (mg/dl)	2.8
Serum osmolality	325
Calculated BEE	2450 calories/day

QUESTIONS FOR ANALYSIS

1. Name and describe the nutritional complications of oral candidiasis, gastrointestinal CMV infection, and PCP. How does the treatment affect nutritional status?
2. Based on the laboratory and anthropometric data, does David appear to be malnourished? What is your specific, objective evidence? What type of malnutrition does he exhibit?
3. Assess David's hydration status. What data could help you determine this?
4. What are the acute or immediate nutritional goals? What about long-term goals?
5. What type of nutritional support (enteral or parenteral) would you administer to David to prevent further nutritional depletion?

Issues & ANSWERS

Special Considerations for Children With AIDS

Malnutrition, particularly inadequate calories and protein, and dehydration are serious issues in children with AIDS. In adults, the disease affects nutrition status. In children, not only is nutritional status affected, but also growth and development can be significantly impaired resulting in growth failure. There is a strong relationship between early nutritional status—poor growth, cachexia, poor oral intake, decreased absorption of nutrients and increased energy expenditure—and mortality risk.

Nutritional assessments should be performed routinely in all children with AIDS so that any problems can be identified and treated as they occur and nutritional deficits can be minimized. Assessments should include evaluation of anthropometrics, visceral protein stores, red blood cell indices and electrolytes. Appetite, intake and feeding ability should also be assessed. Developmental delays can also increase the risk for developing failure to thrive.

Providing adequate calories to maintain linear growth and support weight gain can be difficult as a result of chronic infections, fever, and medications. In 1994 the CDC revised the criteria for wasting in HIV-infected children under 13 years of age and they are as follows.

1. Persistent weight loss of more than 10% of baseline
2. Decrease of at least 2 percentiles on the weight-for-age chart in children younger than 1 year of age *or*
3. Two consecutive measurements more than 30 days apart of less than the fifth percentile on the weight-for-height chart and chronic diarrhea (>2 loose stools daily for >30 days) or documented or constant fever for more than 30 days.

Diarrhea and malabsorption can result in dehydration, which can be very serious in infants and young children and the onset may occur suddenly. To prevent dehydration, offer Popsicles, Jell-O, juices and other beverages often. Oral rehydration fluids, such as Pedialyte, will also help to replace electrolytes lost with acute or chronic diarrhea.

Suggestions for provide supplemental calories and nutrient intake are as follows.

- Use a calorie-dense formula (24 to 27 kilocalories [kcalories]/oz) for infants. Add glucose polymers or medium-chain triglycerides to formulas or reduce the amount of water added to powdered formulas to boost calories.
- Try liquid medical nutritional supplements, such as Pediasure, to provide supplemental calories.
- Add fats such as butter, margarine, or mayonnaise to foods to boost calories.
- Encourage nutrient-dense snacks such as raisins and peanuts or peanut butter.
- For the older, lactose-tolerant child, add skim milk powder to whole milk to boost calories and proteins.
- Make adjustments in diet consistency and temperatures to overcome eating difficulties associated with disease complications and any other eating problems.
- For lactose-intolerant children with AIDS, use soy-based infant formulas instead of milk.
- Add Lactaid (the enzyme lactase) to milk for better tolerance and digestion.
- Use low-lactose dairy foods such as yogurt and mild cheddar cheese, if tolerated.

Vitamin and mineral supplements in amounts 1 or 2 times the Recommended Dietary Allowance (RDA) may ensure adequate intake of these nutrients and contribute to meet the increased requirements which occur during hypermetabolic states. Attention should also be given to drug-nutrient interactions and other effects of these drugs have on nutritional status.

Caregivers need to be particularly careful about food safety and sanitation. Safe food preparation is as important for children as it is for adults with HIV/AIDS and the same food safety guidelines also apply.

Proper procedures and sanitary formula preparation must be followed for infants being bottle-fed. Infants should not be put to bed with a bottle of milk or juice, as they are easily contaminated. Unpasteurized milk and milk products should never be given, as they may be a source of Salmonella and other microorganisms that can cause intestinal infections.

Children should never be fed any food directly from a jar to avoid possible bacterial contamination of the remaining food from the child's mouth. Fruits and vegetables should be peeled or cooked, and meat, chicken and fish should be well cooked. All utensils and dishes should be washed in a dishwasher or in hot sudsy water.

REFERENCES

Ball CS: Global issues in pediatric nutrition AIDS, *Nutrition* 14(10): 767-770, 1998.

Beisel WR: Nutrition in pediatric HIV infection, *J Nutr* 126(10 suppl):2611S-2615S, 1996.

Fields-Gardner C: Nutrition in pediatric HIV disease, *BETA* vol 37, 1998.

Grossman M: Special problems in the child with AIDS. In Sande MA, Volberding PA, eds: *The medical management of AIDS*, ed 2, Philadelphia, 1990, WB Saunders.

Nutrition Intervention in the Care of Persons with HIV-Position of the American Dietetic Association and Dietitians of Canada, *J Am Diet Assoc* 100:708-717, 2000.

Raiten DJ: Nutrition and HIV infection: a review and evaluation of the extant knowledge of the relationship between nutrition and HIV infection, *Nutr Clin Pract* 6(3):S1, 1991.

Chapter

24

Nutrition and Cancer

Susan Emery

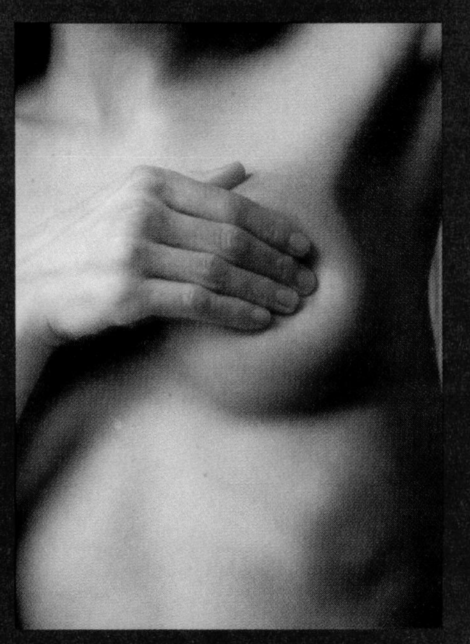

Chapter Outline

This chapter focuses on cancer, one of the major diseases in the Western world. We examine the nature of the cancer process and its treatments and seek to relate these processes to the nutritional factors involved.

Here we look at nutrition and cancer in two basic areas: its role in cancer development and prevention and its role in cancer therapy and rehabilitation. Cancer development and its prevention are discussed in relation to the interplay of environment, the body's defense system, and the nutritional factors that govern each. During medical therapy for the disease process, nutrition support plays a large role in the effectiveness of therapy and quality of life. To understand these nutritional relationships we must understand the nature of cancer as a growth process, the physiologic basis of cancer and the structure and function of cells, and the body's defense systems in immunity and in the healing process.

The Process of Cancer Development

MULTIPLE FORMS OF CANCER

The health toll of cancer continues to extract its price in human disease and death, despite ongoing efforts by the scientific and healthcare communities. In 1971, the United States first initiated a nationwide moratorium to fight the disease with the National Cancer Act. In 1995, the Assistant Secretary for Health and the Surgeon General chaired an initiative called Healthy People 2000. This program, co-coordinated by the U.S. Department of Health and Human Services and the National Cancer Institute of the National Institutes of Health (NIH), began a national initiative on health goals and objectives. It sought to focus the attacks on cancer into several priority areas. Building on these initiatives, *Healthy People 2010* was launched in 1999. It is a set of health objectives for the nation to achieve during the first decade of the new century.[1]

In its latest report the NIH statistical cancer review program Surveillance, Epidemiology, and End Results (SEER) has indicated an overall decline in the incidence of cancer by 0.8% per year between 1990 and 1997.[2] However, when reported in aggregate, due in large part to an older and expanding population, the incidence expressed in numbers of cases of overall cancer deaths continues to increase.[3] The World Health Organization estimates that 35% of human cancers in the Western world are diet related.[4]

The American Cancer Society estimates that in 2001, approximately 553,400 Americans will die from cancer. In its multiple forms cancer has become one of our major health problems, second only to heart disease, and accounts for about 23% of the total deaths in the United States each year.[3]

Breast cancer is the most common form of cancer among women in the United States. The incidence of breast cancer has continued to rise for the past two decades.[5] Prostate cancer is the leading cancer diagnosed among men in the United States.[5] Cancer of the lung is the second most common cancer and the leading cause of cancer death among both men and women.[5]

Difficulties in the study of cancer have arisen from its varying nature and multiple forms. The word cancer is a general term used to designate any one of many malignant tumors, or neoplasms (new growths), forming in various body tissue sites. There are many different forms of cancer, varying world wide and changing with population migrations. There are multiple causes and often conflicting research results because of the large number of variables involved. We would be more correct, then, to use the plural term *cancers* in discussing this great variety of neoplasms.

To better understand cancer development we should view it as a growth process that has its physiologic basis in the structure and function of cells. Because nutrition is fundamental to all tissue growth, we need to look briefly at the cancer cell to understand the relationship of nutritional factors to cancer. This "misguided cell" and its tumor tissue represent normal cell growth that has gone wild.

THE CANCER CELL

The molecular mechanisms that influence the conversion of a normal cell into a cancerous cell have been extensively studied and continually evolve on the basis of new scientific theories. It was originally thought that the scientific basis of all cancers was a single metabolic disturbance in cell replication caused by some sort of mutation. However, in the latter half of the twentieth century, it was determined that because the normal cell cycle of division and replication is governed by multiple signals, the loss of the controlled state as it occurs during neoplastic development must proceed through multiple steps.[6] In fact, it is now generally understood that cancer develops through a series of four distinct steps: initiation, promotion, development and progression.[7]

In adult humans about 3 to 4 million cells complete the normal life-sustaining process of cell division every second, in large part without mistake, guided by a genetic code unique to each living being. How are the process and rate of cell reproduction maintained so precisely in normal cells? And, more important, why is this normal, precise regulation of cell reproduction and function lost in cancer cells, and why do cancer cells then remain mutant and malformed, functionally imperfect, incapable of normal cell life?

The first part of the answer lies in the nature of the cell's genetic material and its regulating components. The specific genetic material in the cell's nucleus is arranged as chromosomes, containing deoxyribonucleic acid (DNA). Specific sites along the chromosome threads are called *genes*. Each gene carries specific information that controls synthesis of specific proteins and transmits genetic heritage. A single chromosome thread is made up of hundreds of genes arranged end to end, and each gene of DNA is made up of about 600 to several thousand smaller subunits called *nucleotides*. The nucleic acids, DNA and its companion ribonucleic acid (RNA), compose the controlling system by which both the cell and thus the organism sustain life. The structure of DNA is that of a very large polynucleotide made up of many individual mononucleotides, each one of which has three parts: (1) a sugar (deoxyribose), (2) a phosphate, and (3) a specific nitrogenous base—adenine, cytosine, guanine, or thymine. It is the ladderlike pairing of these nitrogenous bases, as shown in Figure 24-1,

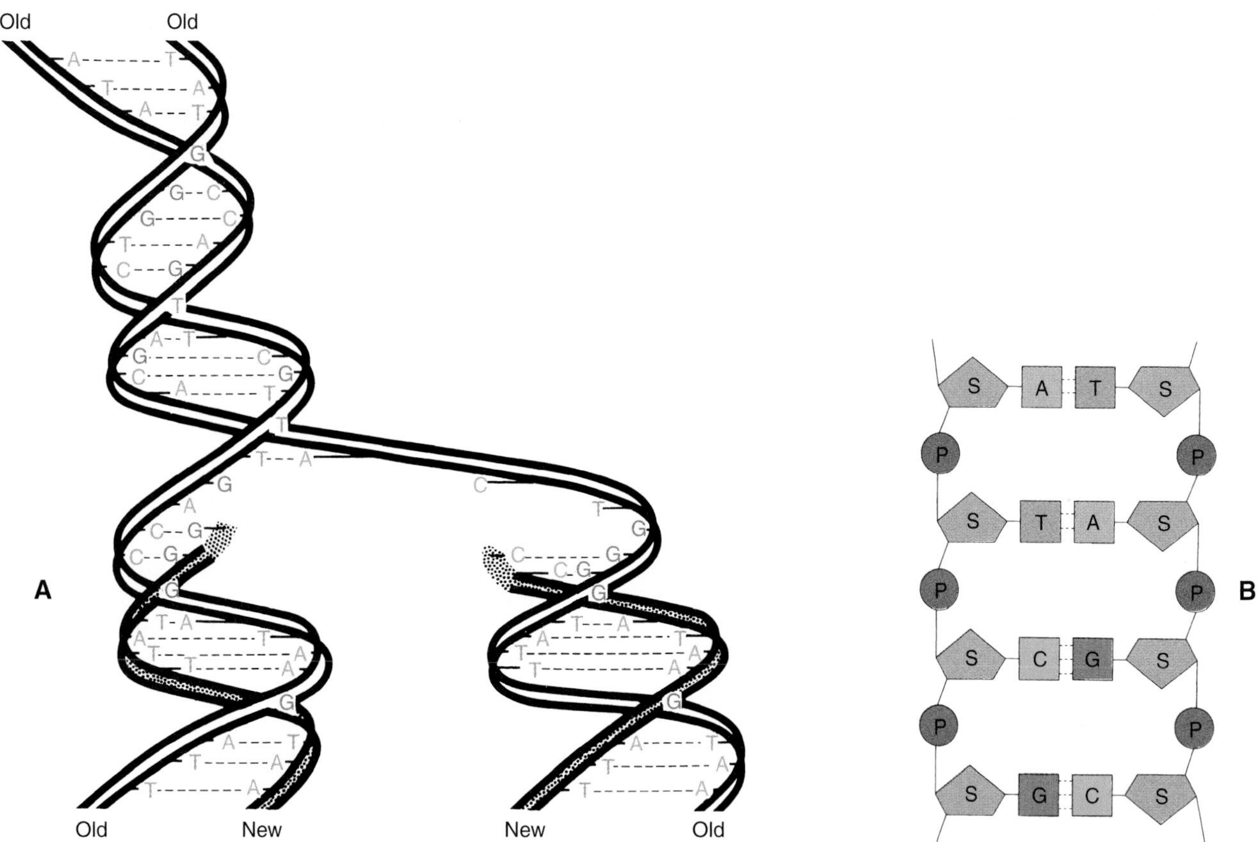

FIGURE 24-1 DNA structure. A, The "unzipping" of DNA to form new RNA strands. Note the cross-links connecting the strands: *A,* adenine; *T,* thymine; *C,* cytosine; *G,* guanine. B, Diagram of a portion of DNA structure. An enlargement of a four-bar twist of the DNA molecule.

that incorporates the "genetic code" and enables the DNA to transmit messages to guide protein structure. The DNA appears as a twisted ladder or spiral staircase in structure and thus is called a *helix,* the Greek word that means "coil."

GENE CONTROL OF CELL REPRODUCTION AND FUNCTION

The Normal Cell

New cells are created by the division of preexisting cells; a process in which the preexisting cell's genetic pattern is exactly replicated in the new cell. Normally each particular cell's structure and function operate in an orderly manner under gene control, directing the cell's specific processes of protein synthesis. Gene action, however, may be switched on and off, depending on the position of a cell in the body, the stage of body development, and the external environment. Specific regulator genes control such function by producing a repressor substance as needed to regulate operator genes and structural genes. This orderly regulation of induction and repression in cell activity, however, may be lost with mutation of these regulatory genes. Control is also lost when a specific gene for some reason moves from its position to another location on the chromosome. There are four types of such mutated genes presently thought to contribute to tumor development: oncogenes, tumor suppressor genes, DNA repair genes, and genes that influence programmed cell death.[6]

---

cancer A malignant cellular tumor with properties of tissue invasion and spreading to other parts of the body.

malignant melanoma A tumor tending to become progressively worse, composed of melanin (the dark pigment of the skin and other body tissues), usually arising from the skin and aggravated by excessive sun exposure.

neoplasm Any new tissue growth that is abnormal, uncontrolled, and progressive.

oncogene Any of various genes that, when activated as by radiation or a virus, may cause a normal cell to become cancerous; viral genetic material carrying the potential of cancer and passed from parent to offspring.

The Cancer Cell

A cell may become malignant when one of these potentially cancer-causing genes is translocated and reinserted into a highly active part of the DNA. This has been shown to occur, for example, in patients with Burkitt's lymphoma and the blood cancer acute nonlymphocytic leukemia (i.e., the cancer cell appears to be derived from a normal cell that has mutated and lost control over cell reproduction).

Cancer Tumor Types

On this basis of cell nature and differentiation, it is possible to classify cancer tumor types according to the type of originating tissue; for example, those arising from connective tissues are called sarcomas and those arising from epithelial tissues are called carcinomas. We can also classify tumor types by the extent or degree of cell tissue change. Tumor stages are defined in relation to rate of growth, degree of autonomy, and invasiveness.

Relation to the Aging Process

Because the incidence of cancer increases with age, a relationship exists between cancer development and the aging process in cells, tissues, and organ systems.

CAUSES OF CANCER CELL DEVELOPMENT

It is thus evident that the basic cause of cancers is a mutation of the genes that govern normal cell reproduction.

Chemical and Environmental Carcinogens

One of the first indications that chemical carcinogens exist in the environment came from a British investigator, Percival Pott, when he discovered that chimney sweeps had an increased incidence of scrotal cancer; it was determined that the common denominator among the cancer victims were exposure to soot.[8] Chemical carcinogens interfere with the structure or function of regulatory genes by binding to DNA bases, in such a way that the likelihood that it will undergo a mutation during DNA repair or replication is increased. This mutation can thus lead to neoplastic transformation.[8] Exposure to such agents may be by individual choice, as in cigarette smoking, which accounts for nearly 90% of all lung cancers,[5] making tobacco smoke the single most lethal carcinogen in the United States. Smoking also causes cancer in other primary sites such as the larynx, oral cavity, and oropharynx. Smoking contributes to cancer of the upper respiratory tract, esophagus, bladder, and pancreas, with the degree of malignancy depending on the frequency of smoking and duration of the habit, especially when started at a young age. Although the prevalence of cigarette smoking among people 18 years of age and over has decreased since 1987, the prevalence of smoking among the vulnerable age group of children and teenagers continues to rise with inevitable long-term mortality risks.

Other exposure comes via general environmental substances, such as pesticide residues, water and air pollutants, food additives and contaminants, and occupational hazards. However, many of our natural environmental agents can carry more hazard potential, depending on the dose. The principle that "the dose makes the poison" applies to all substances, including carcinogens, natural or synthetic. These potentially carcinogenic substances may cause cancer by either mutation, altering the regulation of gene function, or by activating a dormant virus.

Radiation

Radiation that is sufficient to damage DNA causes breakage and incorrect rejoining of chromosomes. Such radiation damage may be ionizing, such as from x-rays, radioactive materials, and atomic exhausts or wastes, or it may be nonionizing, such as from sunlight. Ultraviolet radiation in sunlight is one of the most prominent sources of environmental carcinogens. It is highly genotoxic but does not penetrate the skin.. Our longtime pursuit of the bronzed-god look has taken a large toll: sun-related skin cancer rates has risen rapidly in the United States and Europe, afflicting younger and younger persons. The common forms on the head and neck—basal cell carcinoma and squamous cell carcinoma—are easily cured by surgical removal. However, a far more lethal form, malignant melanoma, occurs in the skin cells that produce the pigment melanin and will account for approximately 7800 deaths in 2001 alone.[3] In the United States the incidence varies with latitude, with the greater number occurring in the southern states. It is thought that exposure to high levels of sunlight in childhood is a strong determinant of risk for the development of melanoma; however, sun exposure in adulthood also plays a role.[9] The rising incidence probably results from increased recreational exposure to sunlight as well as the potential "greenhouse effect" of decreased protective ozone layers.[10]

Oncogenic Viruses

Although oncogenes were first found in viruses, their evolutionary history indicates that they are also present and functioning in normal vertebrate cells in the form of proto-oncogenes. It is their abnormal expression, or activation by mutation, that can lead to cancerous growth. Viruses may be thought of as a major risk factor for cancer development, exceeded only by tobacco use.

A virus is little more than a packet of genetic information encased in a protein coat (see Chapter 23). It contains a small chromosome, DNA or RNA, with a relatively small number of genes, usually fewer than five and never more than several hundred. In contrast, cells of complex organisms have tens of thousands of genes. Generally, when viruses produce disease, they act as parasites, taking over the cell machinery to replicate themselves. Numerous oncogenic, or tumor-producing, viruses have been identified. A tumor virus is a type of transforming virus that is capable of producing tumors only in hosts in which the virus can replicate. They transform cells by integrating a DNA copy of the virus (termed a *provirus*) into the host cell genome. If a proto-oncogene is contained in the region, the provirus integration then alters the structure or function of the proto-oncogene and thereby promotes tumor development.[8] Human papilloma virus (HPV) is now recognized as the main cause of cervical cancer.[11] Retroviruses are implicated in a number of mammary tumors and skin cancer.[12] Other viruses implicated in the causes of cancer include the Epstein-Barr virus (lymphomas), hepatitis B and C (hepatocellular carcinoma), and human immunodeficiency virus (Kaposi's sarcoma).

Epidemiologic Factors

Studies of cancer distribution and occurrence in relation to such factors as race, diet, region, sex, age, heredity, and occupation show variable and conflicting results. It is becoming increasingly clear, for example, that racial differences in cancer incidence between blacks and whites in the United States are great, with more cancer cases among blacks than among whites. However, it is also clear that these differences have nothing to do with race but have much to do with poverty, which has implications for nutritional status, healthcare, education, and resources. The world incidence of cancer does vary a great deal from country to country, and that of specific cancer types varies from 6- to 300-fold, with incidence rates in the United States being appreciably greater than those in many other countries.

Also, racial incidence of cancer seems to change as population groups migrate and acquire the different cancer characteristics of the new population. Although specific dietary factors have been hard to pinpoint in the cause of cancer, worldwide epidemiologic studies show significant correlation of death from breast cancer, for example, with the consumption of fat in the diet; and of liver cancer with the consumption of alcohol.

STRESS FACTORS

The idea that emotions may play a part in malignancy is not new. Galen, a second-century Greek physician, wrote of such relationships, as have many different kinds of "healers" since that time. However, these relationships are difficult to measure. Even with great technologic and scientific advances, Western medicine holds fast to its basic tenet that a thing must be measurable under controlled conditions to be said to exist.

Nonetheless, increasing observations are being made of relationships between cancer and less-measurable factors of stress. Clinicians and researchers have reported that psychic trauma, especially the loss of a central relationship, seems to carry with it a strong cancer correlation. The cause of a possible relationship between such trauma and cancer may lie in two physiologic areas: (1) damage to the thymus gland and the immune system and (2) neuroendocrine effects mediated through the hypothalamus, pituitary, and adrenal cortex. This automatic "cascade of physiologic events" triggered by stress may well provide the neurologic currency that converts anxiety to malignancy. Such a stressful state may also make a person more vulnerable to other factors that are present, influencing the integrity of the immune system, food behaviors, and the nutritional status. Once cancer occurs, however, patients with cancer have many options for easing their distress and improving the quality of their lives through supportive relations and current positive medical approaches to pain management.[13,14]

The Body's Defense System

COMPONENTS OF THE IMMUNE SYSTEM

The human body's defense system is remarkably efficient and complex. Several components of special type cells protect not only against external invaders such as bacteria and viruses but also against internal "aliens" such as malignant tumor cells. These malignant cells from developing tumors in the body can spread invading cells into other body tissues and form secondary tumors, or metastases, that become life threatening.

Two major populations of cells provide the immune system's primary line of defense for detecting and destroying malignant cells that arise daily in the body. These cells mediate specific cellular immunity and humoral immunity, as well as providing supportive backup biologic systems. These two populations of lymphoid cells, or lymphocytes, a type of white blood cell, develop early in life from a common stem cell in fetal liver and bone marrow (Figure 24-2). They then differentiate and populate the peripheral lymphoid organs during the latter stages of gestation. One type is called T cells, traced from the thymus-derived cells. The other type, B cells, is preprocessed by the liver and bone marrow.

T Cells

After precursor cells migrate to the thymus, the T-cell population is differentiated in this small gland, which lies posterior to the sternum and anterior to the great vessels

carcinoma A malignant new growth made up of epithelial cells, infiltrating the surrounding tissue and spreading to other parts of the body.
radiation A highly controlled treatment for cancer, using radioactive substances in limited, controlled exposure to kill cancerous cells.
sarcoma A tumor, usually malignant, arising from connective tissue.

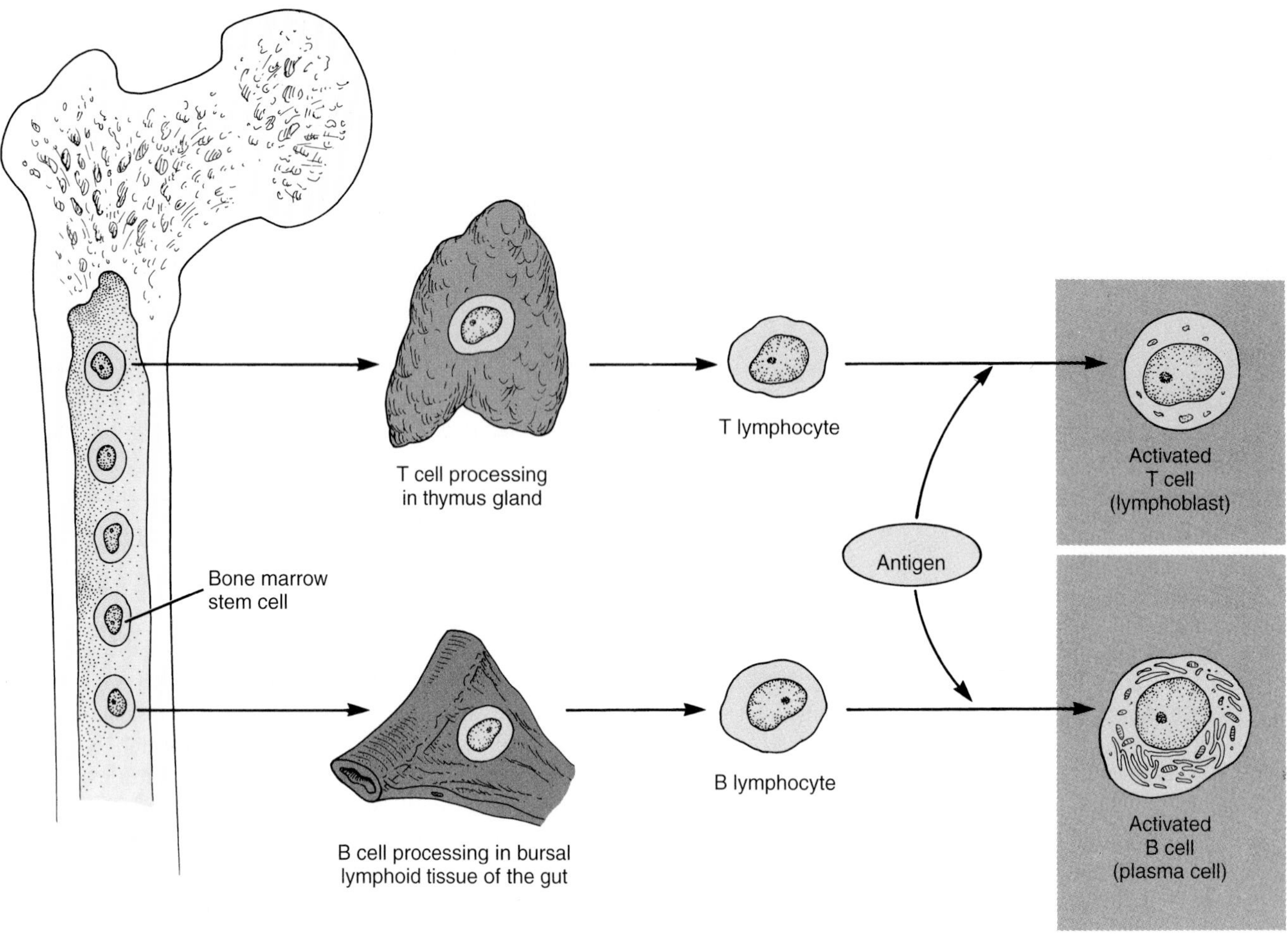

FIGURE 24-2 Development of the T and B cells, lymphocyte components of the body's immune system.

partially covering the trachea. The majority of the circulating small lymphocytes in blood, lymph, and certain areas of the lymph nodes and spleen are T cells. These cells recognize invading antigens by means of specific specialized receptors on their surfaces. When T cells meet an antigen—a foreign intruder, a "non-self," or an alien substance such as abnormal cancer cells—they proliferate and initiate specific cellular immune responses: (1) they activate the phagocytes, special cells that have intracellular killing and degrading mechanisms for destroying invaders; and (2) they cause an inflammatory response through chemical mediators released by the antigen-stimulated T cells. In the early 1970s, Burnet[15] proposed the theory of immune surveillance of cancer wherein most cancer tumors are rejected by the immune system and the occasional failure to do so leads to cancer development. It was subsequently discovered that most tumors express tumor antigens that can then be targets for rejection responses. Furthermore, T cells recognize these antigens in a different way than antibodies recognize them.[16] Harnessing this ability in the patient with cancer, scientists developed gene therapy, which has been used to create these cytotoxic T-lymphocytes specific for specific tumor types. Many strategies are being developed to deploy this immune-mediated destruction of tumors. For example, bone marrow transplantation has developed to infuse T cells from healthy donors against well-defined tumor antigens into the blood of patients with cancer with that specific tumor type.

B Cells

The B-cell population matures first in the bone marrow and then, after migration, in the solid peripheral lymphoid tissues of the body—the lymph nodes, spleen, and gut. These cells are responsible for synthesis and secretion of specialized protein known as antibodies. When the B cells contact an antigen, they increase and initiate specific humoral immune responses: (1) they produce specific antibodies or immunoglobulins in the blood and (2) they produce a particular antibody secretion, immunoglobulin A, in the bowel and upper respiratory mucosa. This combination of antigen and antibody then activates the complement system, which attracts phagocytes and initiates the inflammatory response for healing.

RELATION TO NUTRITION

Immune System

The integrity of the body's immune system components requires nutritional support. Acute starvation causes thymic atrophy and has immunosuppressive effects.[17,18] Severely malnourished persons show changes in the structure and function of the immune system with atrophy of the liver, bowel wall, bone marrow, spleen, lymphoid tissue, and diaphragm muscles.[19] Sound nutrition can help to maintain normal immunity and combats sustained attacks in malignancy The early use of vigorous nutrition support for patients with cancer may help to provide recovery of normal nutritional status, including immunocompetence, thereby improving their response to therapy and prognosis.[20]

The Healing Process

Tissue integrity, essential for the healing process, is maintained through protein synthesis. Such strength of tissue is a front line of the body's defense system. This process of healing requires optimal nutritional intake to support (1) cell function and structure of all its parts involving DNA, RNA, amino acids, and proteins and (2) the integrity of all of the immune system components.

Impact of Cancer Therapy on Nutrition

Current cancer therapy takes four major forms: surgery, radiation, chemotherapy, and bone marrow transplantation. Medical treatments for cancer entail physiologic stress. These results include toxic tissue effects, often with damage to cell DNA structure and changes in normal body function. Thus the benefit achieved is not without attendant problems. Nutritional support seeks to alleviate these problems and to enhance the potential success for cancer therapy.

SURGERY

Operable Tumors

The early diagnosis of operable tumors has led to successful surgical treatment of a large number of patients with cancer. The success of any surgery depends in large measure on the sound nutritional status of the patient (see Chapter 22); this is especially true of patients with cancer because their general condition may be weakened. The prevention of problems through early detection and surgical treatment has significantly increased cancer cure rates. Surgical treatment may also be used with other forms of therapy for removal of single metastases or for prevention and alleviation of symptoms. Optimal nutritional status preoperatively and maximal nutritional support postoperatively are fundamental to the healing process.

Medical Nutrition Therapy of the Oncology Surgery Patient

Nutritional therapy of the patient with cancer undergoing surgery takes on two goals: (1) to support the general healing process and overall body metabolism and (2) to modify the diet or feeding regimen in appropriate ways to compensate for the surgical site involved. Beyond the regular nutritional needs surrounding any surgical procedure and its healing process, gastrointestinal surgery poses special problems for normal eating and digesting and absorbing of food nutrients (Table 24-1).

Clinical Examples include esophageal and stomach resections.

1. *Head and neck surgery,* or resections in the oropharyngeal area, is sometimes necessitated by the presence of cancer. In such cases food intake is greatly affected. A creative variety of food forms and semiliquid textures as well as modes of feeding must be devised. Often the mechanical problems of food ingestion make long-term tube feeding necessary (see Chapter 17).
2. *Gastrectomy* may cause numerous postgastrectomy "dumping" problems requiring frequent, small, low-carbohydrate feedings (see Chapter 22). Vagotomy contributes to gastric stasis. Various intestinal resections or tumor excisions may cause steatorrhea because of general malabsorption, fistulas, or stenosis.
3. *Pancreatectomy* causes the loss of digestive enzymes with ensuing malabsorption and weight loss; it also induces insulin-dependent diabetes mellitus.

RADIATION

After the discovery of radiation in the 19th century, scientists soon found that it could damage body tissue. Continued study of its use and control revealed that normal tissue could largely withstand an amount of radiation that would damage and destroy cancer tissue. The subsequent role of radiation in cancer treatment has developed around the controlled use with two types of tumors: (1) those responsive to radiation therapy, or radiotherapy, within a dose level tolerable to health of normal tissue and (2) those that can be targeted without damage to overlying vital organ tissue.

Forms of Radiation Therapy

Radiation therapy damages the DNA of cells; therefore the cells cannot continue to divide and grow. Radiation used in cancer therapy is produced from three main sources. (1) In external beam irradiation (or x-ray), radiation is directed at the patient externally from a linear

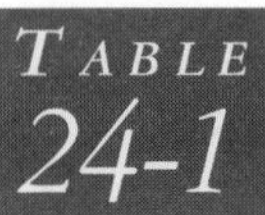

Nutrition-Related Side Effects of Cancer Treatment

Treatment Modality	Nutrition-Related Side Effects
Surgery	
Radical resection of oropharyngeal area	Chewing and swallowing difficulties
Esophagectomy	Gastric stasis, hypochlorhydria, steatorrhea, and diarrhea secondary to vagotomy, early satiety, regurgitation
Gastrectomy	Dumping syndrome, malabsorption, achlorhydria, lack of intrinsic factor and R protein, hypoglycemia, and early satiety
Intestinal Resection	
Jejunum	Decreased efficiency of absorption and many nutrients
Ileum	Vitamin B_{12} deficiency, bile salt losses with diarrhea or steatorrhea, hyperoxaluria and renal stones, calcium and magnesium depletion, and fat-soluble vitamin deficiencies
Massive bowel resection	Life-threatening malabsorption, malnutrition, metabolic acidosis, and dehydration
Ileostomy and colostomy	Complication of salt and water balance
Blind-loop syndrome	Vitamin B_{12} malabsorption
Pancreatectomy	Malabsorption and diabetes mellitus
Radiation Therapy	
Oropharyngeal area	Destruction of sense of taste and smell, xerostomia and odynophagia, oral mucositis and ulceration, loss of teeth, and osteonecrosis
Thorax and mediastinum	Esophagitis with dysphagia; fibrosis with esophageal stricture
Abdomen and pelvis	Bowel damage, acute and chronic, with diarrhea, malabsorption, stenosis and obstruction, ulceration and fistula formation
Chemotherapy	Nausea and vomiting (cisplatin, cyclophosphamide, carmustine, mitomycin), anorexia (carmustine, cyclophosphamide, doxorubicin, 5-fluorouracil), diarrhea (methotrexate, 5-fluorouracil, L-asparaginase, doxorubicin), oral ulceration (methotrexate, bleomycin, doxorubicin, dactinomycin), constipation (vincristine), gastrointestinal ulceration (methotrexate, ara-C, procarbazine hydrochloride), abdominal or epigastric pain (methotrexate, cyclophosphamide, dactinomycin), and monoamine oxidase inhibition (procarbazine hydrochloride)

Adapted from Shils ME: Nutrition and diet in cancer. In Shils ME, Young VR, eds: *Modern nutrition in health and disease,* Philadelphia, 1988, Lea & Febiger.

accelerator. This type of radiation frequently causes nutrition-related side effects. (2) In brachytherapy, highly radioactive isotopes, such as cobalt 60, are placed directly into or next to the tumor to deliver a highly localized dose. Nutritional side effects do not generally occur from this type of radiotherapy. (3) In stereotaxis, radiation is delivered in a narrow beam to difficult-to-reach places such as brain tumors.

Medical Nutrition Therapy of the Radiation Oncology Patient

Radiotherapy may be used alone or in conjunction with other therapies both for curative and palliative care for approximately 50% of all patients with cancer at some time during the course of their disease. Radiation enteritis will influence nutritional status and therapy a great deal, depending on the site and intensity of treatment.

Clinical examples include irradiation to the head, neck, and abdominal cavity.

1. *Head and neck* irradiation will affect the oral mucosa and salivary secretions, as well as the esophagus, influencing taste sensations and sensitivity to food temperature and texture. Common side effects include mucositis, xerostomia, loss of taste, and alteration in or loss of smell. Other means of tempting appetite through food appearance and aroma, as well as texture, must be developed. Nutritional management may be further compounded by the curtailment of food intake caused by anorexia and nausea. The esophagitis from head and neck radiation may be so severe as to cause esophageal fibrosis or stricture. In this scenario, dilatation of the esophagus is sometimes attempted, to create a passageway large enough to swallow a bolus of food; but if unsuccessful, a feeding tube often becomes necessary for nutritional support.
2. *Abdomen* irradiation may produce denuded bowel mucosa, loss of villi, and absorbing surface area with tissue edema and congestion; vascular changes occur as a result of intimal thickening, thrombosis, ulcer formation, or inflammation. In the intestinal wall there may be fibrosis, stenosis, necrosis, or ulceration. General malabsorption or fistulas may develop, as well as hemorrhage, obstruction, and diarrhea, all contributing to nutritional problems.

CHEMOTHERAPY

Drug Development

Chemotherapy refers to the use of chemical agents to treat cancer in a systemic manner; these agents are delivered intravenously and therefore elicit their effects throughout the body. Many of the most effective chemotherapy agents currently in use have been developed only within the past few years. The therapeutic use of a chemotherapy agent is based on two general principles related to rate and mode of action.

Rate of Action

The so-called cell or log (logarithm)-kill hypothesis of the action of chemotherapeutic agents on tumors indicates that a single dose can be only as much as 99.9% effective in killing the tumor cells. Thus if as large a tumor as is compatible with life can be treated with a drug tolerable at a toxicity level that is 99.9% effective, the tumor is gradually reduced with successive doses that cause "fractional killing" with each dose. This process finally brings the tumor within the capability of the body's own immune system to take over and make the final kill and cure. The smaller the tumor, either because of early detection or initial treatment by surgery or radiation, the greater is the possible effectiveness of the chemotherapeutic agents. Also, two other principles of dosage rate for greater effectiveness are important: (1) aggressive use of maximal tolerable dosages in repeated series and (2) use of several drugs combined for a synergistic effect. Many malignancies such as leukemias, lymphomas, and testicular cancer are now successfully treated by such combination therapy.[21] However, most common cancers, such as breast, lung, colorectal, and prostate, require an overall program that involves surgery and radiation for a maximal cure rate.

Mode of Action

Chemotherapeutic agents are effective because they disrupt the normal processes in the cell responsible for cell growth and reproduction. Some agents interfere with DNA synthesis. Others disrupt DNA structure and RNA replication. Others prevent cell division through mitosis, cause hormonal imbalances, or make unavailable the specific amino acids necessary for protein synthesis. It is this diversity in mode of action that provides a basis for grouping drugs into certain classes of chemotherapeutic agents: (1) alkaloids, (2) alkylating agents, (3) antibiotics, (4) antimetabolites, (5) enzymes, and (6) hormones. They are usually used in combined therapy or as adjuvant therapy in conjunction with surgery or radiation.

Toxic Effects

Chemotherapeutic agents have the same effects on rapidly reproducing normal cells as they do on the rapidly reproducing cancer cells. Interference with normal function is most apparent in normal cells of the bone marrow, the gastrointestinal tract, and the hair follicles, accounting for a number of the toxic side effects and problems in nutritional management.

1. *Bone marrow effects* include interference with the production of red blood cells (anemia), white blood cells (infections), and platelets (bleeding). Many healthcare practitioners ascribe to the use of a neutropenic diet during these instances, in which potentially microbial contaminated food ingredients, such as raw, unwashed vegetables and other foods are eliminated.
2. *Gastrointestinal effects* include nausea and vomiting, stomatitis, anorexia, ulcers, and diarrhea.
3. *Hair follicle effects* include alopecia (baldness) and general hair loss.

Modes of Drug Use

Chemotherapy may be used alone or in conjunction with other treatments such as surgery or radiotherapy to increase the cure rate.

Chemotherapy Research

Researchers are working to find substances, in either food or drugs, that can prevent or halt cancer development. Their goal is to develop drugs or modify foods as a preventive strategy for people at high risk for cancer.[22] There is considerable evidence to suggest that many plant-derived extracts contain compounds that can inhibit the process of carcinogenesis effectively.[23] These chemical compounds produced by plants or in persons eating the plants are now termed phytochemicals (see discussion in Chapter 7). For example, members of this group of compounds include alpha- and beta-carotene found in carrots; beta-cryptoxanthin found in oranges, peaches, and tangerines; and lutein found in vegetables such as tomatoes, green beans, spinach, and other green vegetables. There are many of these phytochemicals, found in a wide variety of vegetables and fruits, that provide specific health benefits. Another group, called disease-preventive agents, is being studied. This group—the dithiolthiones found in cruciferous vegetables such as broccoli, cauliflower, and cabbage—are potential preventive agents.[23] Phytochemicals can inhibit carcinogenesis by inhibiting phase I and II enzymes, scavenging DNA reactive agents, suppressing the abnormal proliferation of preneoplastic lesions, and inhibiting certain properties of the cancer cell.[24,25] Moreover, the ingestion of specific beneficial bacteria, known as probiotics, may have anticarcinogenic effects in colon cancer.[26]

The major nutritional concerns during chemotherapy relate to (1) the gastrointestinal symptoms caused by the

---

palliative Care affording relief but not cure; useful for comfort when cure is still unknown or obscure.

stomatitis Inflammation of the oral mucosa, especially the buccal tissue lining the inside of the cheeks, but it also may involve the tongue, palate, floor of mouth, and the gums.

effect of the toxic drugs on the rapidly developing mucosal cells, (2) the anemia associated with bone marrow effects, and (3) the general systemic toxicity effect on appetite. Stomatitis, nausea, diarrhea, and malabsorption contribute to many food intolerances. Antiemetic drugs such as prochlorperazine (Compazine) may be used (Table 24-2); such drugs act on the vomiting center in the brain to prevent the nausea response. Prolonged vomiting seriously affects fluid and electrolyte balance, especially in elderly patients, and needs to be controlled. In patients with breast cancer, relief from nausea has been achieved with use of the antiemetic drug megestrol acetate (Megace), a synthetic female sex hormone similar to the natural hormone progesterone. However, results have shown that although megestrol acetate can increase appetite and weight gain in patients with cancer, it has no effect on lean body mass; rather weight gain appears to be related solely to increases in fat mass.[27,28] Two drugs that act as serotonin blockers, granisetron hydrochloride (Kytril) and ondansetron hydrochloride (Zofran), administered in combination therapy with dexamethasone, an adrenal cortical steroid, have been shown to control episodic nausea and vomiting.[29]

In some cases of chronic long-term drug therapy, special nutritional management restricting conditioned, or learned, food aversions to odors and colors has been effective. For example, patients receiving periodic treatments of the drug cisplatin (Platinol), who had a special diet of three meals a day of plain colorless, odorless foods, including items such as cottage cheese, applesauce, vanilla ice cream, and other predetermined foods, experienced little nausea and increased food intake.[30] The potential for the development of conditioned food aversions while on long-term chemotherapy is diminished by the use of food having little or no odor or color because the drug-related dysgeusis (perverted sense of taste) and dysosmia (impaired sense of smell) are correlated with visual olfactory stimulation factors.[30,31]

Certain chemotherapeutic drugs also have special effects. For example, monoamine oxidase (MAO) inhibitors may be used for the pretreatment relief of mental and emotional depression or for palliative therapy. These antidepressant drugs cause well-known pressor effects when used with tyramine-rich foods (Table 24-3). Thus these foods should be avoided when using such drugs.

Nutritional Therapy

THERAPEUTIC GOALS

In general, nutritional therapy deals with two types of cancer-related issues: (1) those alterations in nutritional status related to the disease process itself and (2) those related to medical treatment of the disease. The basic objectives of nutritional therapy in cancer are to (1) meet the increased metabolic demands of the disease and prevent catabolism as much as possible and (2) alleviate symptoms resulting from the disease and its treatment through adaptations of food and the feeding process.

ALTERATIONS IN NUTRITIONAL STATUS RELATED TO THE DISEASE PROCESS

The basic feeding challenges governing nutritional therapy are caused by general systemic effects of the neoplastic disease process and by specific responses related to the type of cancer.

General Systemic Effects of the Neoplastic Disease Process Affecting Nutritional Therapy

Malnutrition is the most common secondary diagnosis in patients with cancer and is a prognostic indicator for poor response to cancer therapy and shortened survival time.[32] The disease process causes three basic systemic effects: (1) anorexia, (2) altered metabolic state, and (3) negative nitrogen balance, which are often accompanied by a continuing weight loss. These effects may vary widely with individual patients, according to type and stage of the disease, from mild, scarcely discernible responses to the extreme forms of debilitating cachexia seen in advanced disease, and they are estimated to cause more than 50% of the cancer deaths.[33,34] Cachexia is not a local effect but rather arises from distant metabolic effects (i.e., it is a type of paraneoplastic syndrome). Although some have suggested that the tumor and host complete for nutrients, this is unlikely, given that some patients with cancer with very large tumors show no signs of cachexia.[34] This extreme weight loss and weakness are caused by abnormalities in fat, muscle, and glucose metabolism, mediated in part by natural body defense substances such as tumor necrosis factor and cytokines. First, there is evidence that the cancer's catabolic effects may be the result of an increase in fat breakdown, brought about by tumor necrosis factor.[34] Second, a reduced rate of somatic protein synthesis and an increased rate of protein degradation have been noted, also brought about by tumor necrosis factor. Third, there is evidence that the wasting in patients with cancer is caused in part by abnormalities in the metabolism of glucose.[34] The drug hydrazine sulfate seems to correct this metabolic error, allowing patients to conserve more energy and show modest improvements in survival, but no remissions have been documented.[35]

Anorexia is frequently accompanied by depression or discomfort during normal eating. This contributes further to a limited nutrient intake at the very time the disease process causes an increased metabolic rate and nutrient demand. Often this imbalance of decreased intake and increased demand creates a negative nitrogen balance, an indication of body-tissue wasting. Sometimes a true tissue loss of protein is masked by outward nitrogen equilibrium as the growing tumor retains nitrogen at the expense of the host, further compounding the problem.

TABLE 24-2 Medications Used to Control Nausea and Vomiting in Patients Receiving Chemotherapy

Antiemetics								
		Route						
Class	Drug	Oral	Rectal	Injectable	Mechanism of Action	Site of Action	Side Effects	Comments
Phenothiazines	Perphenazine (Trilafon)	×		×	DA	CTZ	EPS, sedation, hypotension	Prochlorperazine is the most effective agent in this class; perphenazine may be effective with high IV doses; prochlorperazine is available in sustained released capsule which should not be crushed
	Prochlorperazine (Compazine)	×	×	×				
	Promethazine (Phenergan)	×	×	×				
	Thiethylperazine (Torecan)	×	×	×				
Butyrophenones	Droperidol (Inapsine)	×		×	DA	CTZ	EPS, sedation	
	Haloperidol (Haldol)	×	×	×				
Substituted benzamide	Metoclopramide (Reglan)	×	×	×	DA or 5-HT_3 in high doses	CTZ	EPS, sedation, fatigue, diarrhea, nausea	Also used in early satiety and anorexia
Serotonin antagonists	Dolasetron (Anzemet)	×		×	5-HT_3	CTZ, PGSEC	Headache, diarrhea, constipation, ECG changes, somnolence	Increased effect with corticosteroids
	Granisetron (Kytril)	×		×			Headache, diarrhea, constipation, somnolence	
	Ondansetron (Zofran)	×		×				
Benzodiazepines	Lorazepam (Ativan)	×		×	BDZ	Unknown	Sedation, confusion, amnesia, slurred speech	Effective for anticipatory nausea/anxiety; lorazepam may be placed under the tongue
	Diazepam (Valium)	×		×				
Corticosteroids	Dexamethasone (Decadron)	×		×	Unknown	Unknown	Increased appetite, mood change, anxiety, euphoria, headache, metallic taste, hyperglycemia	Most effective when used with 5-HT_3
Anticholinergics	Scopolamine (TransDerm)		Patch		ACH	Emetic center	Urinary retention, dry eyes, constipation	Effective for nausea related to motion
Cannabinoids	Dronabinol (Marinol)	×			Unknown	CNS	Mood changes, increased appetite, hypotension, tachycardia	Well tolerated in younger patients; may crush

From Kennedy LD: Common supportive drug therapies used with oncology patients. In MacCallum PD, Polisena CG, eds: *The clinical guide to oncology nutrition,* Chicago, Ill: American Dietetic Association, 2000:168-181.

DA, Dopamine antagonist; *CTZ,* chemoreceptor trigger zone; *EPS,* extrapyramidal side effects; *5-HT_3*, serotonin$_3$ (5-hydroxytryptamine$_3$) antagonist; *PGSEC,* peripheral gastrointestinal stimulation to emetic center; *ECG,* electrocardiographic; *BDZ,* benzodiazepine; *ACH,* anticholinergic; *CNS,* central nervous system.

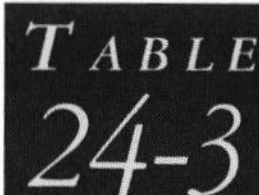

Tyramine-Restricted Diet

General Directions

- Designed for patients on monoamine oxidase inhibitors, drugs that have been reported to cause hypertensive crises when used with tyramine-rich foods. These include foods in which aging, protein breakdown, and putrefaction are used to increase flavor. Studies indicate that as little as 5 to 6 mg of tyramine may produce a response, and 25 mg is a dangerous dose.
- Food sources of other pressor amines such as histamine, dihydroxyphenylalanine, and hydroxytyramine are also avoided.
- Avoid all foods listed. Limited amounts of foods with a lower amount of tyramine, such as yeast bread, may be included in a specific diet.
- Avoid over-the-counter drugs such as decongestants, cold remedies, and antihistamines.

Foods to Avoid	Representative Tyramine Values (μg/g or ml)	Additional Foods to Avoid
Cheeses		Other aged cheeses
New York State cheddar	1416	Blue
Gruyère	516	Boursalt
Stilton	466	Brick
Emmentaler	225	Cheddars (other)
Brie	180	Gouda
Camembert	86	Mozzarella
Processed American	50	Parmesan
Wines		Provolone
Chianti	25.4	Romano
Sherry	3.6	Roquefort
Riesling	0.6	Yeast and products made with yeast
Sauternes	0.4	Homemade bread
Beer, ale (varies with brand)		Yeast extracts such as soup cubes, canned meats, and marmite
Highest	4.4	Italian broad beans with pod (fava beans)
Average	2.3	Meat
Least	1.8	Aged game
		Liver
		Canned meats with yeast extracts
		Fish (salted dried)
		Herring, cod, capelin
		Pickled herring
		Other
		Chocolate
		Cream (especially sour cream)
		Salad dressings
		Soy sauce
		Vanilla
		Yogurt

NUTRITIONAL EFFECTS RELATED TO THE TYPE OF CANCER

In addition to the generalized wasting syndrome known as cachexia discussed here, specific nutritional problems individually present themselves depending on the site or organ involved. Of foremost significance are tumors that cause obstruction or lesions in the gastrointestinal tract or adjacent tissue. In fact the cancer may reduce intake or absorption of nutrients via (1) altered oral intake, (2) malabsorption of nutrients and subsequent diarrhea, (3) functional and motility problems arising from surgical procedures or tumor growth, (4) fluid-and electrolyte imbalances, (5) hormonal imbalances (e.g., diabetes that has been caused by pancreatectomy for pancreatic cancer), and (6) anemia.

Abdominal radiation may cause intestinal damage, with tissue edema and congestion, decreased peristalsis, or endarteritis in small blood vessels.[36] The liver is somewhat more resistant to damage from radiation in adults, but children are more vulnerable than adults.

INDIVIDUALIZING NUTRITIONAL THERAPY FOR CANCER

Two important principles of nutritional therapy, vital in any sound nutrition practice but especially essential in care of patients with cancer, provide the basis for planning the nutritional care of each patient: (1) personal nutritional assessment and (2) vigorous nutrition therapy to maintain good nutritional status and support medical treatment.

Nutrition Screening and Assessment

It is far more difficult to replenish a nutritionally depleted patient than to maintain a good nutritional status from the outset of the disease process. Therefore a primary goal in nutritional therapy is to prevent a depleted state. Initial assessment for baseline data and regular monitoring thereafter during treatment are necessary. A detailed personal history is essential to determine individual needs, desires, and tolerances. To be valid, the interview should be conducted as a conversation, using verbal and nonverbal probes and pauses rather than a cross-fire of separate questions and answers (see Chapter 15).

Nutritional Therapy and Plan of Care

Based on careful individual nutritional assessment, the team clinical dietitian prepares a plan for optimal nutritional therapy to meet needs. This nutritional therapy outline is then incorporated into the nursing care plan as the clinical dietitian works with the nursing staff to carry it out. Primary care provided by the dietitian and the nurse on a regular basis is a necessary part of the oncology team practice. This early, vigorous care often makes the difference in the success rate of medical therapy. Thus working closely with the oncology nurse and physician, the clinical dietitian assesses personal needs, determines nutritional requirements, plans and manages nutritional care, monitors progress and responses to therapy, and makes adjustments in care according to status and tolerances.

Determining Nutritional Needs

Each of the nutrient factors related to tissue protein synthesis and energy metabolism requires careful attention. The increased needs for energy, protein, vitamins and minerals, and fluid are based on demands made by the disease and its treatment. Individual needs and food tolerances vary, but general guidelines are the same.

Energy. Great energy demands may be placed on the patient with cancer. These demands result from a hypermetabolic state that exists in some patients with cancer and from the tissue-healing requirements. Of this total dietary calorie value, sufficient carbohydrate (at least 45% to 50% of total calories) to spare protein for vital tissue synthesis is essential. For the adult patient with good nutritional status, approximately 25 to 30 kcalories/kg body weight/day will provide for maintenance needs. A more malnourished patient may require more calories, depending on the degree of malnutrition and body trauma. Carbohydrate should supply the majority of the energy intake, with fat making up about 30% of the total calories.

Providing a malnourished patient with cancer with nutritional support must be done with caution. Overfeeding must be avoided to minimize the risk of "refeeding syndrome," in which severe intracellular electrolyte and fluid shifts may occur.

Dietary fat. Some studies have related excessive dietary fat to cancer metastasis and effectiveness of cancer therapy.[37,38] However, in deciding whether to alter the components of the diet of the patient with cancer, it is important to note the patient's usual intake and recent intake and the relative efficacy of this diet change at the particular stage of disease of the patient. Certainly in early stages of cancer, a reduction in fat may be beneficial; however, in later states of disease, a primary goal of therapy is to increase the caloric density of the diet, and limiting fat will be counterproductive to that end!

Protein. Tissue protein synthesis, a necessary component of healing and rehabilitation, requires essential amino acids and nitrogen. Efficient protein use, which depends on an optimum protein/calorie ratio, promotes tissue building, prevents tissue wastage (catabolism), and helps make up tissue deficits. An adult patient with good nutritional status will need about 0.8 to 1.25 g of protein/kg body weight/day of protein to meet maintenance needs and ensure anabolism. A malnourished patient may need 2 to 3 times more protein to replenish tissue and restore positive nitrogen balance.

Vitamins and minerals. Adequate intakes of vitamins and trace elements are important for normal tissue function and healing and for maintenance of immune function. However, care must be given to avoiding megavitamin and trace mineral alternative therapy in cancer treatment. Excessive dosages for vitamins can have deleterious health effects, may interfere with immune function, and may accelerate the rate of growth of some cancers.[39] Key vitamins and minerals control protein and energy metabolism through their roles in cell enzyme systems. They also play a necessary part in structural development and tissue integrity. The B-complex vitamins in general serve as necessary coenzyme agents in energy and protein metabolism. Vitamins A and C are necessary for the development and integrity of body tissues. Vitamin A also has a significant role in protective immunity and cell differentiation; vitamin C has significant antioxidant, enzymatic, and immune biologic functions related to cancer.[40,41] Increased dietary consumption of vegetables and fruits is the best way to obtain these vitamins. Vitamins A, E, and D may alter the expression of certain oncogenes.[42] Vitamin D hormone ensures proper calcium and phosphorus metabolism in bone and blood serum. Vitamin E protects the integrity of cell wall materials and hence tissue integrity. Many minerals function in structural and enzymatic roles in vital metabolic and tissue-building processes. Thus an optimal intake of vitamins and minerals, at least to the Recommended Dietary Allowance (RDA) levels but frequently augmented with

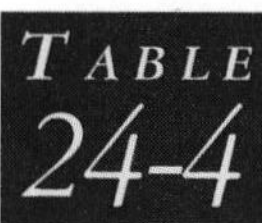

Alternative Therapy: Commonly Recommended Herbal Products

Herb	Claim	Efficacy	Safety	Current Recommendations
Chaparral	Analgesic Expectorant Diuretic Emetic Antiinflammatory	Studies have shown no anticancer effect.	Long-term use in rats led to lesions in mesentery, lymph nodes, and kidneys. One documented case of liver disease in humans. Removed from the Generally Recommended as Safe (GRAS) list.	Not recommended.
Echinacea	Immune stimulant Wound healer	Widely used in Germany to treat the common cold and respiratory and urinary tract infections. Needs more research.	Significant side effects have not been observed. Allergies are always possible.	May be used with caution. Not recommended for longer than 8 consecutive weeks. Not recommended during pregnancy or lactation.
Essiac	Developed by Canadian nurse Rene Cassie to treat cancer.	No anticancer effects.	Not safe for consumption and is illegal to distribute in the United States.	Not recommended.
Ginger	Digestive aid Stimulant Diuretic Antiemetic	Found to be useful in treating motion sickness. Antiemetic properties are due to the local action on the stomach, not on the central nervous system.	No toxicities have been reported. Very large overdoses may cause central nervous system depression and cardiac arrhythmias. Thrombocytopenia has been reported in people taking large doses.	May be used for temporary relief of nausea.
Hoxey herbs	Anticancer agent	No benefit has ever been documented. Note that the originator Harry Hoxey died of prostate cancer while treating himself with his formula.	Not recommended.	Not recommended.
Kombucha tea (Manchurian tea or Korgasok tea)	Immune system stimulator	Unsubstantiated claims of antitumor activity.	Home-brewed "mushroom" usually passed to friends and family members. Susceptible to microbial contamination. Acidosis, aspergillosis, nausea, vomiting, and jaundice have been reported.	Not recommended.
Milk thistle	Liver protector (active ingredient is silymarin)	Appears to protect undamaged liver cells from toxins. May be helpful in cirrhosis and hepatitis.	No adverse effects have been noted.	Safe for use. May have beneficial effects.

From Molseed L: Alternative therapies in oncology. In MacCallum PD, Polisena CG, eds: *The clinical guide to oncology nutrition,* Chicago, Ill: American Dietetic Association, 2000:150-159.

TABLE 24-4 Alternative Therapy: Commonly Recommended Herbal Products—cont'd

Herb	Claim	Efficacy	Safety	Current Recommendations
Mistletoe (American and European)	American—stimulates smooth muscle, increases blood pressure, increases uterine and intestinal contractions European—decreases blood pressure, antispasmodic, calmative agent	Extracts of the European form have been used as a palliative cancer treatment. There is little evidence supporting effectiveness.	Berries are poisonous, and some evidence suggests that the leaves may also be poisonous.	Not recommended.
Pau D'arco	Powerful tonic Blood builder Anticancer agent Also used to treat diabetes, rheumatism, and ulcers	Has been shown to have activity against cancer in animals but causes severe side effects in humans.	Toxic—induces nausea, vomiting, anemia, and bleeding in humans.	Not recommended.
Peppermint	Digestive aid Antispasmodic	Stimulates bile flow Stimulates tonus of the lower esophageal sphincter Appetite stimulant	Safe for adults. Not recommended for children due to increased choking reflex with menthol.	Safe for adults. Not recommended for children.
Pokeroot	Cathartic Emetic Narcotic Anticancer Dyspepsia Glandular swelling	No efficacy has been demonstrated for any claim except that it is a strong emetic and cathartic.	Extremely toxic. Causes gastroenteritis, hypotension, and hyporespiration. Fatal in children.	Not recommended.

From Molseed L: Alternative therapies in oncology. In MacCallum PD, Polisena CG, eds: *The clinical guide to oncology nutrition,* Chicago, Ill: American Dietetic Association, 2000:150-159.

supplements according to individual patient nutritional status, is indicated.

Fluids. Most adults require approximately 35 ml of water/kg/day, or between 1500 and 2000 ml/day. Adequate fluid intake is important for two reasons: (1) to replace gastrointestinal losses or losses caused by infection and fever and (2) to help the kidneys dispose of the metabolic breakdown products from the destroyed cancer cells as well as from the toxic drugs used in treatment. For example, some toxic drugs such as cyclophosphamide (Cytoxan) require as much as 2 to 3 L of forced fluids daily to prevent hemorrhagic cystitis.

Alternative therapy with herbal products. In recent years many cancer patients have turned toward herbal therapy as an alternative to chemotherapy, radiation, or surgery. Many herbal therapies have not been adequately tested and have been found to have toxic effects (Table 24-4).

The healthcare practitioner must have some basic understanding of the therapeutic claims and dangers of some of these herbal products. While many cancer patients should not have all hopes for a cure dashed, it behooves the healthcare team to caution their use of these products and point out those products that are unproven and could be unsafe.

Nutritional Management of Selected Cancer-Related Symptoms

The specific feeding method used depends on the individual patient's condition. However, the classic dictum of nutritional management should prevail: "If the gut works, use it." Details of available enteral and parenteral modes

PRACTICAL APPLICATION
Promoting Oral Intake in Patients With Cancer

Encouraging and maintaining adequate oral intake for patients with cancer represent one of the most difficult aspects of cancer treatment. It is time consuming and often frustrating but may be one of the most rewarding experiences in patient care. By identifying feeding problems, initiating appropriate interventions, and providing individual education, adequate oral nutrition is promoted. The dietitian is the key figure for coordinating the nutritional program, but its success requires the full support and cooperation of the entire healthcare team, especially the nurse.

The patient interview is one of the most important parts of the nutritional assessment. Information that helps identify adequacy of current nutritional intake and potential nutritional problems is obtained during the interview. The following list of questions may assist in gathering accurate information about the patient's ability to obtain oral nutrition:

- How would you describe your appetite?
- Has it changed recently?
- Are you eating differently than you have most of your life?
- Do you usually eat three meals each day? Has this changed recently?
- Are you nauseated or experiencing vomiting? Is this food or medication related? How long have you been experiencing this? How often do you vomit or feel nauseated?
- Do you have a bowel movement every day? Has this changed?
- Do you have diarrhea? If so, do you think this may be food related?
- Do food smells or cooking odors bother you?
- Do you have difficulty chewing?
- Do your dentures (if any) fit? Do you wear them?
- Do you have difficulty swallowing?
- Is your mouth dry? Does your saliva seem to be different? Is it thicker or decreased in amounts?
- Do you find it easier to drink liquids than to eat solid foods?
- What were you able to eat yesterday? (Obtain a brief 24-hour dietary recall.)
- Are you unable to eat certain foods right now?
- Do some foods taste different to you? Can you give an example?
- Have you ever taken any high-kcalorie, high-protein supplements? When? What kind? How often? Were you able to tolerate them?
- Do you take a multivitamin supplement?
- Do you have any food allergies or intolerances? Are these new, or have you always experienced these intolerances?
- Do you prepare your own meals? If so, do you ever feel too tired to prepare something to eat?

The success of the interview depends on the dietitian's professional competence, interviewing skills, and bedside manner. If the dietitian establishes a feeling of comfort and trust with the patient, the opportunity to accomplish successful dietary interventions is great.

References

Bloch AS: Nutrition and cancer: the paradox, *Diet Curr* 23(2):1996.

Marian M: Cancer cachexia: prevalence, mechanisms, and interventions, *Support Line* 20(2):3, 1998.

Nahikian-Nelms ML: Encouraging oral intake. In Bloch AS, ed: *Nutrition management of the cancer patient,* Rockville, Md, 1990, Aspen.

of nutritional support are provided in Chapter 17. If at all possible, an oral diet with supplementation is the most desired form of feeding, of course. A carefully designed personal plan of care based on nutrition assessment data and including adjustments in texture, temperature, food choices, and tolerances, as well as family food patterns, can often meet needs (see *Practical Application* box). Often the hospitalized patient's diet can be supplemented with familiar foods from home as the clinical nutritionist plans with the family. Personal food tolerances will vary according to the current treatment and nature of the disease. A number of adjustments in food texture, temperature, amount, timing, taste, appearance, and form can be made to help alleviate symptoms stemming from common problems in successive parts of the gastrointestinal tract.

Difficulties in eating may be caused by loss of appetite, problems in the mouth, or swallowing problems.

LOSS OF APPETITE

Anorexia is a major problem and curtails food intake when it is needed most. It is a general systemic effect of the cancer disease process itself, often further induced by the cancer treatment and progressively enhanced by personal anxiety, depression, and stress of the illness. Such a vicious cycle, if not countered by much effort, can lead to more malnutrition and the well-recognized starvation "cancer cachexia," a syndrome of emaciation, debilitation, and malnutrition (Table 24-5).[34]

A vigorous program of eating, not dependent on appetite for stimulus, must be planned and maintained with the patient and family. It is helpful sometimes to develop protein and caloric goals, discussing the role of nutrients and key foods in combating the disease and providing support for therapy. With such support both patient and family are better able to build a positive mental attitude

TABLE 24-5 Dietary Modifications for Nutrition-Related Side Effects of Cancer

Side Effect	Suggested Dietary Modifications
Anorexia	Provide small, frequent meals Offer high calorie, high protein, nutrient-dense foods Encourage consumption of the highest calorie, highest protein foods first at meals Suggest commercially available nutritional supplements, as tolerated Avoid foods with offensive odors Encourage favorite foods
Altered perception of taste and odor	Maximize use of herbs and seasonings to enhance flavor of foods If the flavor and aroma of red meats are offensive, avoid these foods and encourage intake of alternative protein-rich foods such as chicken, fish, cheese, eggs, and milk Serve cold foods and beverages more often than hot foods and beverages Vary appearance (i.e., color and texture) of foods Prepare and serve food in glass or porcelain rather than metal pans or dishes
Stomatitis and mucositis	Provide foods in liquid, semisolid, or pureed form Avoid tart, citric, or acidic foods and beverages Avoid extremes in temperature Avoid excessively seasoned and spicy foods Avoid dry, coarse foods; serve foods with sauces or gravies Encourage foods that melt or are liquid or soft textured at room temperature Avoid carbonated beverages
Xerostomia	Moisten foods with sauces, gravies, liquid, melted butter, mayonnaise, or yogurt Encourage naturally soft, most foods Encourage sipping of liquids throughout the day Avoid alcohol
Dysphagia	Provide foods in liquid, semisolid, or pureed form Maximize calorie and protein density of food as possible Use commercially available liquid nutritional supplements
Nausea and vomiting	Give small, frequent meals Give dry foods without added fats or sauces, such as dry toast Give liquids only between meals Avoid greasy, fried, high fat foods Avoid foods with strong odors
Diarrhea	Provide small, frequent meals Encourage plenty of liquids to prevent dehydration Avoid greasy, fried, high fat foods Consider limiting dietary lactose if these foods exacerbate symptoms Avoid high fiber foods Avoid gassy, cruciferous vegetables, such as broccoli and cauliflower Avoid caffeine

Adapted with permission from Dobbin M, Harmuller VW: Suggested management of nutrition-related symptoms. In MacCallum PD, Polisena CG, eds: *The clinical guide to oncology nutrition,* Chicago, Ill: American Dietetic Association, 2000:164-167.

toward the diet as an integral part of the treatment and are thus more able to accept responsibility for this aspect of therapy. Often this positive attitude of the vital role patients play in their own treatment is a means of gaining some sense of control of their own lives, a sense frequently lost in the bewildering world of cancer and its therapy.

The overall goal is to provide food with as much nutrient density as possible so that every bite will count. If appetite is better in the morning, a good breakfast should be emphasized. Food texture may be varied as tolerated, with appeal to sensory perceptions of color, aroma, and taste. A series of small meals with a wide variety of foods is better tolerated than regular larger meals. Getting some exercise before meals and maintaining surroundings that reduce stress may also help in the eating process.

MOUTH PROBLEMS

Eating difficulties may stem from sore mouth, stomatitis, or taste changes. Sore mouth often results from chemotherapy or from radiation to the head and neck area. It is increased by any state of malnutrition or from

TO PROBE FURTHER
When Does Feeding Become an Ethical Issue?

Plato believed that the moral person and the physician both should abide by the Hippocratic principle of medicine: "Above all, do no harm." In recent times others have returned to Plato's use of this medical model of ethics. Current writers assert that an ethic of care rests on the "premise of nonviolence—that no one should be hurt."

Technology such as enteral and parenteral nutrition may sometimes support a caring intent and compassionate spirit, whereas at other times such modern technology becomes a value in and of itself with its own standard of efficiency. Enteral and parenteral feeding techniques may be used to maintain indefinitely patients who are unable to take food orally.

Concerned ethical thinkers use the following moral principles for decisions in regard to life-sustaining treatment that encompasses enteral or parenteral nutrition: benefit to patient, respect for patient autonomy or self-determination, maintenance of moral integrity of health professionals, and justice in distributing scarce medical resources among eligible patients. They offer helpful views to guide clinicians in coming to a reasoned and defensible resolution of moral conflict.

ALTERNATIVES TO ARTIFICIAL NUTRITION

All options of nutritional support should be explored, not simply the consideration of "Give food or fluids" versus "Do not give food or fluids." Dietitians are particularly useful in identifying alternative feeding strategies. The full range of therapeutic options should be carefully explored instead of assuming that the choices are "Let the patient die" or "Keep the patient alive."

PATIENT PROGNOSIS FOR RECOVERY OF FUNCTIONS

A widely held ethically defensible view is that aggressive means of life prolongation becomes less morally desirable in proportion to the inability of the patient to regain what he or she considers to be useful function. The persistent vegetative state and permanent loss of consciousness are examples of extreme cases where recovery of function is not possible. Accurately determining the prognosis for recovery is essential.

TOTAL MANAGEMENT PLANS AND GOALS OF THERAPY

The patient's prognosis and nature of the illness might determine whether the goal of medical care is to attempt cure, to manage a chronic illness that cannot be cured so as to maintain maximal patient function, or to allow a terminally ill patient to die with maximal comfort and symptom control. Nutritional treatment may make sense within one plan of care but no sense at all in another.

WISHES OF THE PATIENT OR PATIENT SURROGATE

It is legally and ethically acceptable that in almost all cases the voluntary choice of an informed patient should override all other concerns. When the patient cannot choose, a surrogate or other substitute decision maker who is familiar with the patient's values and wishes may be consulted.

ABILITY OF THE PATIENT TO CHOOSE

It is important to assess the patient's ability to make the particular medical care choice that is relevant to the matter at hand. In some circumstances, expert psychiatric or psychologic evaluation is needed to determine this.

BENEFITS AND BURDENS OF ARTIFICIAL TREATMENT

The medical team often tends to overestimate the benefits and underestimate the burdens of the treatments they use routinely. When the means of administering nutrition become invasive and painful, then the burdens may become substantial. Restraining the patient or repeated blood draws to monitor the effects of total parenteral nutrition may be deemed burdens unacceptable to the patient. Patients may feel that being kept alive by artificial means is an indignity itself and that life is no longer useful or meaningful to them. Spiritual and emotional burdens should be assessed equally with physical burdens in making accurate assessments of the moral obligations to patients.

Modern medical technology has produced circumstances that caregivers and patients alike have never faced before. Decisions regarding nutrition and hydration in terminally ill patients are becoming more frequent. Ethical and moral questions do not always have black or white solutions; there are gray areas to consider. The ethical task for dietitians may be to achieve balance between what works and who cares.

References

Brody H, Noel MB: Dietitians' role in decisions to withhold nutrition and hydration, *J Am Diet Assoc* 91(5):580, 1991.

Dalton S: What are the sources and standards of ethical judgment in dietetics? *J Am Diet Assoc* 91(5):545, 1991.

Edelstein S, Anderson S: Bioethics and dietetics: education and attitudes, *J Am Diet Assoc* 91(5):546, 1991.

Wall MG et al: Feeding the terminally ill: dietitians attitudes and beliefs, *J Am Diet Assoc* 91(5):549, 1991.

infections such as candidiasis (thrush), with numerous ulcerations of the oral and throat mucosa. Frequent small meals and snacks—soft in texture, bland in nature, and cool or cold in temperature—are often better tolerated. There may also be alterations in the tongue's taste buds, causing taste distortion ("taste blindness") and inability to distinguish the basic tastes of salt, sweet, sour, or bitter, with consequent food aversions. Because the aversion is often toward basic protein foods, a high-protein, high-energy liquid drink supplement may be needed. Dental problems may also contribute to mouth difficulties and should be corrected. Salivary secretions are also affected by cancer treatment; therefore foods with a high liquid content should be used. Solid foods may be swallowed more easily with the use of sauces, gravies, broth, yogurt, or salad dressings. A food processor or blender can render foods in semisolid or liquid forms and make them easier to swallow. If the swallowing problem is especially severe because of tumor growth or therapy, guides for a special swallowing training program, including progressive food textures, exercises, and positions, can be followed.

GASTROINTESTINAL PROBLEMS

Eating difficulties may include nausea and vomiting, general indigestion, bloating, or specific surgery responses such as the postgastrectomy "dumping" syndrome (see Chapter 22). Nausea is often enhanced by foods that are hot, sweet, fatty, or spicy; these can be avoided according to individual tolerance. Other lower gastrointestinal problems may include general diarrhea, constipation, flatulence, or specific lactose intolerance or surgery responses, such as occur with intestinal resections and various ostomies. Helpful guidance for patients with colostomies, ileostomies, or ileoanal reservoirs is necessary (see Chapter 22). The effect of chemotherapy or radiation treatment on the mucosal cells secreting lactase contributes to lactose intolerance. In such cases a nutrient supplement formula that is lactose free or a soymilk formula should be used.

A number of commercial nutrient supplement products are available. A comparative review of these products will provide the basis for developing a formulary in the hospital setting for a limited number of such products (see Chapter 17). A food processor or blender can be used at home to produce creative solid and liquid food combinations from regular foods for interval liquid supplementation.

Patients with cancer need plenty of encouragement and a feeling of autonomy or personal control for the optimal success of a dietary plan. Sometimes it becomes necessary to make small attainable goals of specific foods and amounts to be consumed. If the patient can be made to view food as important as medication in their daily routine, better success will be likely.

FEEDING IN TERMINAL ILLNESS

Although many advances have been made in the detection and treatment of cancer, mortality rates for some cancers have not declined and have actually increased for some cancers.[3] In working with patients with cancer, one can automatically see that the progressive weight loss and malnutrition that occur, caused by the primary tumor and its spread, and lead to profound nutritional depletion cause a great deal of personal turmoil, increased morbidity, and overall reduced quality of life. For some patients a time comes when the spread of the disease overcomes the body's capacity to combat it. When the patient is no longer able to eat, enteral tube-feeding or parenteral feeding may be considered. Ultimately, however, ethical questions about continued feeding efforts are faced in many cases (see *To Probe Further* box). Answers lie with the patient, as long as possible, and with the family. But sensitive and supportive counseling is needed from the cancer team members, especially the clinical dietitian and the nurse responsible for administering the continued feeding and for personal care.

Nutrition and Cancer: The Final Analysis

What, then, are our overall final conclusions? As Bloch, an experienced oncology nutrition specialist, has well reminded us, we see that nutrition has a dual role in relation to cancer—both prevention and therapy.[29]

PREVENTIVE ROLE

Nutrition and health professionals have a major wellness role in maintaining health and preventing illness, especially in relation to cancer. This role is embodied in the American Cancer Society's new dietary guidelines.[43]

1. Choose most of the foods you eat from plant sources.
   - Eat five or more servings of fruits and vegetables each day.
   - Eat other foods from plant sources, such as breads, cereals, grain products, rice, pasta, or beans, several times each day.
2. Limit your intake of high-fat foods, particularly from animal sources. Choose foods low in fat. Limit consumption of meats, especially high-fat meats.

---

candidiasis Infection with the fungus of the genus *Candida,* generally caused by *C. albicans,* so named for the whitish appearance of its small lesions; usually a superficial infection in moist areas of the skin or inner mucous membranes.

3. Be physically active; achieve and maintain a healthy weight. Be at least moderately active for 30 minutes or more on most days of the week. Stay within your healthy weight range.
4. Limit consumption of alcoholic beverages, if you drink at all.

These guidelines are similar to the overall *Dietary Guidelines for Americans 2000* (see Chapter 1). They are displayed in the *Food Guide Pyramid* and emphasized in national and state health initiatives, including encouraging Americans to eat more servings of fruits and vegetables every day.[44] This emphasis stems from certain compounds found in plants, thus called phytochemicals ("plant chemicals"), which ongoing research indicates have promising effects in the chemoprevention of cancer.[23] As indicated, these compounds include food nutrients—vitamins A (and its analogues), C, and E—as well as nonnutritive substances such as indoles, isothiocyanates, dithiolthiones, and organosulfur.[24,25]

THERAPEUTIC ROLE

For the patient with cancer, the clinical dietitian must shift into a therapeutic role, in which the patient is central in diet planning during disease stages and therapy effects. Nutrition therapy must now focus constantly on proactive assessment with early and continuing preventive measures to intervene wisely before malnutrition occurs. For example, anticipate possible gastrointestinal needs or psychosocial situations that relate to appetite, eating various foods, or drug effects. Provide information concerning mouth care, symptoms experienced, or drug actions and effects. The cancer diagnosis need not be a ticket to starvation. With appropriate pain control and treatment for chemotherapy and radiation-induced side effects, patients with cancer can continue to eat well through the latter stages of their disease. The clinical dietitian and healthcare team should work closely together with the patient to plan meals and snacks based on food preferences and dislikes, subjective intolerance of certain foods, and difficulties in chewing and swallowing.

TO SUM UP

Cancer is a term applied to abnormal, malignant growths in various body tissue sites. The cancerous cell is derived from a normal cell that loses control over cell reproduction. Cancer cell development occurs via mutation, carcinogens, radiation, and oncogenic viruses. It is also influenced by many epidemiologic factors such as diet, alcohol, and smoking, as well as physical and psychologic stress factors. Cell development is mediated by the body's immune system, primarily its T cells, a type of white blood cell found in blood, lymph, and certain parts of the lymph nodes and spleen, and B cells, which manufacture and secrete antibodies.

Cancer therapy consists primarily of surgery, radiation, and chemotherapy. Supportive nutritional therapy for the patient with cancer should be highly individualized and depends on the response of each body system to the disease and to the treatment itself. It is based on a thorough nutritional assessment and provided by a number of routes—oral, tube feeding, peripheral vein, and total parenteral nutrition. The oral route is preferred if at all possible. Nutrient requirements and feeding mode must be designed for the specific physical and psychologic needs of individual patients.

■ Questions for Review

1. What is cancer? Identify and describe several major causes of cancer cell formation.
2. How does your body attempt to defend itself against cancer? What nutritional factors may diminish this ability?
3. List and describe the rationale and mode of action of the types of therapies used to treat cancer.
4. Differentiate those factors challenging cancer recovery that are associated with the disease versus the type of therapy used.
5. Outline the general procedure for the nutritional management of a patient with cancer.

■ References

1. U.S. Department of Health and Human Services: *Healthy people 2010,* ed 2, *With understanding and improving health and objectives for improving health,* 2 vols, Washington, DC, November 2000, U.S. Government Printing Office.
2. Ries LAG et al: The annual report to the nation on the status of cancer, with a special section on colorectal cancer, 1970-1997, *Cancer* 88:2398, 2000.
3. Greenlee RT et al: Cancer statistics 2001, *CA Cancer J Clin* 51:15, 2001.
4. Miller AB: *Diet in cancer prevention,* Online WHO Database, 2001, World Health Organization, accessible at *http://www.who.int/library/database/index.en.shtml.*
5. Miller et al: *Racial/ethnic patterns of cancer in the United States, 1988-1992,* Bethesda, Md, 1996, National Cancer Institute, Publication No. 956-4104.
6. Klein G: Fould's dangerous ideas revisited: the multistep development of tumors 40 years later, *Adv Cancer Res* 72:1, 1998.
7. Reif AE, Hearen T: Consensus on synergism between cigarette smoke and other environmental carcinogens in the causation of lung cancer, *Adv Cancer Res* 76:161, 1999.
8. Ross J: Structure and function of the gene. In Abeloff MD et al, eds: *Clinical oncology,* ed 2, New York, 2000, Churchill Livingstone.
9. Whiteman DC, Whiteman CA, Green AC: Childhood sun exposure as a risk factor for melanoma: a systematic review of epidemiologic studies, *Cancer Causes Control* 12:69, 2001.

10. deGruijl FR: Skin cancer and solar UV radiation, *Eur J Cancer* 35:2003, 1999.
11. Franco EL, Duarte-Franco E, Ferenczy A: Cervical cancer: epidemiology, prevention and the role of human papillomavirus infection, *CMAJ* 164:1017, 2001.
12. Sourvinos G, Tsatsanis C, Spandidos DA: Mechanisms of retrovirus-induced oncogenesis, *Folia Biol (Praha)* 46:226, 2000.
13. Holland JC: Cancer's psychological challenges, *Sci Am* 275 (3):158, 1996.
14. Foley KM: Controlling the pain of cancer, *Sci Am* 275(3): 164, 1996.
15. Burnet FM: Immunologic surveillance in neoplasia, *Transplant Rev* 7:3, 1971.
16. Boon T et al: T-lymphocyte response. In Abeloff MD et al, eds: *Clinical oncology,* ed 2, New York, 2000, Churchill Livingstone.
17. Matarese G: Leptin and the immune system: how nutritional status influences immune response, *Eur Cytokine Netw* 11:7, 2000.
18. Carlson GL: The influence of nutrition and sepsis upon wound healing, *J Wound Care* 8(9):471, 1999.
19. Dureil B, Matuszczak Y: Alteration in nutritional status and diaphragm muscle function, *Reprod Nutr Dev* 38:175, 1998.
20. Bozzetti F et al: Perioperative total parenteral nutrition in malnourished gastrointestinal cancer patients: a randomized clinical trial, *J Am Soc Parenter Enteral Nutr* 24:7, 2000.
21. Hellman S, Vokes EE: Advancing current treatments for cancer, *Sci Am* 275(3):118, 1996.
22. Watzl B, Watson RR: Role of alcohol abuse in nutrition immunosuppression, *J Nutr* 122:733, 1992.
23. Greenwald P: Chemoprevention of cancer, *Sci Am* 275(3): 96, 1996.
24. Kelloff GJ et al: Progress in cancer chemoprevention: development of diet-derived chemopreventive agents, *J Nutr* 130: 467S-471S, 2000.
25. Walaadkhan AR, Clemens MR: Effect of dietary phytochemicals on cancer development, *Int J Mol Med* 1(4):742-753, 1998.
26. Vanderhoof JA: Probiotics: future directions, *Amer J Clin Nutr* 73(suppl):1152S-1155S, 2001.
27. Aulas JJ: Alternative cancer treatments, *Sci Amer* 275(3): 162, 1996.
28. Loprinzi CL et al: Body composition changes in patients who gain weight while receiving megestrol acetate, *J Clin Oncol* 11:152, 1993.
29. Bloch AS: Nutrition and cancer: the paradox, *Diet Curr* 23(2):1, 1996.
30. Menashiam L et al: Improved food intake and reduced nausea and vomiting in patients given a restricted diet while receiving cisplatin chemotherapy, *J Am Diet Assoc* 92(2): 58-61, 1992.
31. Darbinian J, Coulston A: Impact of chemotherapy on the nutritional status of the cancer patient. In Bloch AS, ed: *Nutrition management of the cancer patient,* Rockville, Md, 1990, Aspen.
32. Wilson RL: Optimizing nutrition for patients with cancer, *Clin J Oncol Nurs* 4(1):23-28, 2000.
33. Tayek JA, Chlebowski RT: Metabolic response to chemotherapy in colon cancer patients, *J Parenter Enter Nutr* 16(suppl 6):65, 1992.
34. Shaw JHF et al: Leukine kinetics in patients with benign disease, non-weight losing cancer and cancer cachexia: studies at the whole body level and the response to nutritional support, *Surgery* 109:37, 1991.
35. Tisdale MJ: Wasting in cancer, *J Nutri* 129(1):243S, 1999.
36. Polisena GG: Nutrition concerns in the radiation therapy patient. In McCallum PD, Polisena CG, eds: *The clinical guide to oncology,* Chicago, 2000, American Dietetic Association.
37. Djuric Z et al: Effects of a low-fat diet on levels of oxidative damage to DNA in human peripheral nucleated blood cells, *J Natl Cancer Inst* 83(11):766, 1991.
38. Burns CP, Spector AA: Effects of lipids on cancer therapy, *Nutr Rev* 48(6):233, 1990.
39. Molseed L: Alternative therapies in oncology. In McCallum PD, Polisena CG, eds. *The clinical guide to oncology nutrition,* Chicago, 2000, American Dietetic Association.
40. Ross C: Vitamin A and protective immunity, *Nutr Today* 27(4):18, 1992.
41. Henson DE et al: Ascorbic acid: biologic functions and relation to cancer, *J Natl Cancer Inst* 83(8):547, 1991.
42. Prasad KN, Edwards-Prasad J: Expressions of some molecular cancer risk factors and their modification by vitamins, *J Am Coll Nutr* 9(1):28, 1990.
43. American Cancer Society: *Guidelines for nutrition in cancer prevention,* Atlanta, 1999, American Cancer Society.
44. Foerster SB et al: California's "5-a-Day—For Better Health" campaign: an innovative population-based effort to effect large-scale dietary change, *Am J Prev Med* 11:124, 1995.

■ Further Reading

Bloch AS, ed: *Nutrition management of the cancer patient,* Rockville, Md, 1990, Aspen.

This helpful reference by an experienced oncology dietitian and her contributors provides a comprehensive background for a better understanding of the complexities of caring for cancer patients.

Bloch AS, Thomson CA: Position of the American Dietetic Association: phytochemicals and functional foods, *J Am Diet Association* 95(4):493, 1995.

Steinmetz KA, Potter JD: Vegetables, fruit, and cancer prevention: a review, *J Am Diet Assoc* 96(10):1027, 1996.

These two statements, one an American Dietetic Association position paper and the other a review of the role of certain foods in cancer prevention, provide important information for counseling.

Kalman D, Villani LJ: Nutritional aspects of cancer-related fatigue, *J Am Diet Assoc* 97(6):650, 1997.

This article describes the fatigue associated with cancer and its treatment and ways in which all cancer team members may contribute to using nutrition management to minimize these side effects and broaden the patient's nutritional limits and food choices.

CASE STUDY Patient with cancer

Catherine is a 35-year-old mother of three young children. She was admitted to the hospital 3 weeks ago with multiple enterocutaneous fistulas. She weighed 52 kg (116 lb) on admission and is 165 cm (5 ft 6 in) tall. Catherine had undergone a hysterectomy 4 months before admission, after a recurrence of cervical cancer. During the chemotherapy that followed for 7 months, she had regular bouts with nausea and anorexia. Surgery was performed again. Her fistulas continued to drain for 2 weeks postoperatively, during which she tolerated clear liquids only. An intravenous drip of 10% glucose and 45% normal saline was ordered to supplement fluids and kcalories. This week she developed peritonitis and has had a fever with a temperature of 39° C (102° F) for the past 24 hours. Her weight has dropped to 41 kg (90 lb); drainage from the fistulas has become odorous. The patient was placed in isolation today and was advised by her physician that he intended to start her on TPN and conduct some more tests to determine her progress.

QUESTIONS FOR ANALYSIS

1. What types of nutritional assessment procedures would be used by the TPN team for planning Catherine's nutritional therapy? Explain the purpose of each.
2. Calculate Catherine's energy and protein needs, and account for increased needs.
3. Why did Catherine develop nausea and anorexia during chemotherapy? What are the implications of this for recovery? Outline a plan for evaluating and controlling nausea and vomiting in patients undergoing chemotherapy.
4. What personal concerns would you expect Catherine to have? What resources would you use to help her obtain the personal and physical support she probably needs?

Issues & ANSWERS

Toward the Prevention of Cancer

Studies of geographic, socioeconomic, chronologic, and immigration patterns of cancer distribution indicate that the vast majority of cases of cancer are primarily caused by environmental factors. The logical conclusion is that reduction of these causative factors may reduce or eliminate most forms of cancer.

The American Cancer Society suggests that two thirds of all cases of cancer in the United States are caused by only two factors: inhaled smoke and ingested food.

Tobacco, alone or in combination with alcohol, remains the most important cause of cancer, accounting for about one of every three cancer deaths in the United States. Cigarettes are the most important cause of tobacco-related cancer, but other forms of tobacco (chewing tobacco and snuff) are also established carcinogens. The cancer risk of ex-smokers remains elevated with lifetime nonsmokers. However, quitting smoking, even late in life after heavy long-term abuse, greatly reduces cancer risk when compared with the risk of continued smoking. Despite the rhetoric of tobacco companies, even regular smokers of low-tar cigarettes still have a much higher cancer risk than nonsmokers.

Alcohol, in addition to its synergistic effects with tobacco, increases risk of cancers of the oral cavity, pharynx, liver, and esophagus. Alcohol use has also been consistently linked to colorectal cancer and female breast cancer. Liquor, wine, and beer seem to be equal in effect on cancer risk.

Major incriminating dietary factors that appear now to be carcinogenic are the food changes that contrast current Western diets with those of our Paleolithic hunter-gatherer ancestors. We have reduced the amount of energy we obtain from starchy foods by one half to two thirds. We have decreased our intake of dietary fiber by 75%. We have more than doubled the proportion of energy we derive from fat and changed from mostly unsaturated fats to saturated fats. We have increased our salt intake fivefold. And sugar now accounts for one fifth of our total energy intake. The diet of our ancestors was energy dilute, whereas our modern diet is energy dense.

Many studies link what we eat and do not eat to the development of cancer. Direct relationships between preserved or salty foods and nasopharynx and stomach cancer have been consistently observed in case-control and correlational studies. The generous ingestion of fresh fruits and vegetables has consistently been found to decrease the risk of stomach cancer. Epidemiologic studies suggest a relation between high–animal fat, low-fiber intakes and colorectal cancer. The basis for this relationship lies in the decreased transit time through the colon associated with high-fiber diets and the increased water content in the intestinal lumen that dilutes other nutrients such as animal fat.

Considerable, although not yet conclusive, evidence exists that ascorbic acid has a protective effect against cancer of the esophagus, larynx, and oral cavity. Nutrients such as vitamin A, beta-carotene, vitamin E, and ascorbic acid are thought to lower cancer risk in patients with elevated risk for cancers of the lung, esophagus, colon, and skin. Clinical and laboratory studies support findings that adequate intakes of vitamin D and calcium are associated with reduced incidence of colorectal cancer. These studies did not necessarily use supplemental amounts of these nutrients in addition to the RDAs but were based more on low levels of intake of these nutrients, which would parallel the low levels of fresh fruit and vegetable intakes that are prevalent in our society.

The majority of the causes of cancer—such as tobacco, alcohol, animal fat, obesity, and ultraviolet light—are associated with lifestyle, that is, personal choices and not environmental causes. This fact reinforces the basic truth that the best cure is prevention. Lifestyle changes, including regular exercise, are the best prevention.

REFERENCES

Garland CF et al: Can colon cancer incidence and death rates be reduced with calcium and vitamin D? *Am J Clin Nutr* 54:193S, 1991.

Henderson BE et al: Toward the primary prevention of cancer, *Science* 254:1131, 1991.

Kalman DS, Villani LJ: Exercise and the cancer patient, *On-Line* 6(1):1, American Dietetic Association.

Leffell DJ, Brash DE: Sunlight and skin cancer, *Sci Am* 275(1):52, 1996.

Trichopoulos D et al: What causes cancer? *Sci Am* 275(3):80, 1996.

Willett WC et al: Strategies for minimizing cancer risk, *Sci Am* 275(3):88, 1996.

Wynder EL: Primary prevention of cancer: planning and policy considerations, *J Natl Cancer Inst* 83(7):475, 1991.

Chapter

25

Nutrition Therapy in Chronic Disabling Conditions and Rehabilitation

Marcia Silkroski

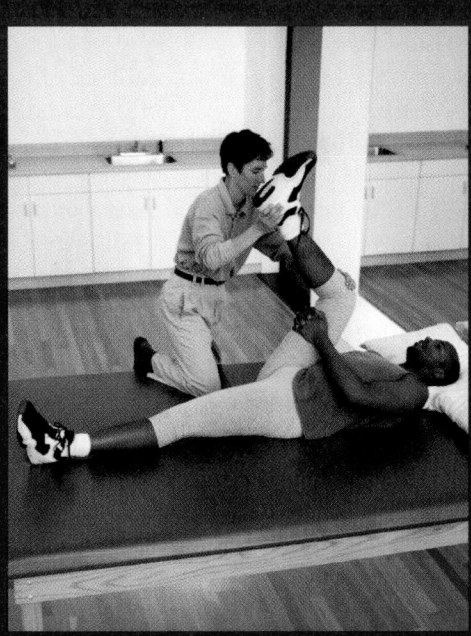

Chapter Outline

This chapter completes our clinical nutrition series. In addition to the primary care clinical problems we reviewed in the preceding chapters of this section, we conclude with a focus on chronic disabling diseases that require rehabilitative care.

Persons who have sustained severe injury or illness often require extended specialized care. These long-term needs result from the stress of disabling injury or illness, which carries added physical, mental, and social burdens. Such situations often involve profound trauma and devastating effects that call for tremendous coping resources.

In this final chapter, we examine the supportive role of nutrition therapy in the rehabilitative process. We look at musculoskeletal disease, neuromuscular disease, and progressive neurologic disorders. In each case we see that personalized nutrition care plays a vital role in the healing and restoring process. Such care demands special knowledge and skills and much personal strength.

Nutrition Therapy and Rehabilitation

GOALS OF SUPPORTIVE CARE

Positive goals guide care for those with chronic disabling disease or injury. Successful support is rooted in a positive philosophy based on the optimal potential of each person affected. This approach requires a specialized team working with the patient and family to meet individualized needs. It is built on clearly defined preventive and restorative personal care objectives. To the greatest degree possible within each situation, two goals are fundamental in planning care: (1) the prevention of further disability and (2) the restoration of potential function. Healthcare workers and their clients have developed many creative techniques of care to meet these twin goals. Both of these key principles involve nutrition therapy. Together with the other specialized therapists on the rehabilitation team, the registered dietitian functions as the nutrition specialist and carries numerous responsibilities.

1. *Nutrition assessment:* initial comprehensive evaluation
2. *Nutrition follow-up:* continuing reassessment at appropriate intervals
3. *Nutrition plan:* to meet fundamental nutrient and energy requirements, as well as any specialized requirements
4. *Coordination of community services:* referrals and communication to meet individual needs, home healthcare, rehabilitation, public health, vocational agencies, financial assistance, or other services
5. *Nutrition education and counseling:* work with the individual client, the family, and other caregivers to best understand and achieve the nutrition goals

TEAM APPROACH METHOD

In some devastating cases, obstacles may seem almost insurmountable. Chronic disease where there is no cure or a poor prognosis can be overwhelming to patients and their caregivers. Often the patient's initial reaction is one of defeat and resignation or withdrawal. The healthcare team can draw on its tremendous resources to meet the various needs of patients. Rehabilitation team specialists include the physician (physiatrist), clinical nutritionist, nurse, occupational therapist, physical therapist, psychologist, speech pathologist, and social worker. These sensitive and skilled specialists lend their particular expertise, bringing their unique training, insights, and resources to identify specific personal needs.

At all times, however, these healthcare specialists remember that the most important member of the team is the patient. They always work with, not for, the patient and family to help develop solutions. Goal setting is always personal. These three partners—the professional specialists, the client, and the family—form a greater healthcare team. It is always a shared, supportive undertaking, whatever the individual limitations or outcome. (See *To Probe Further* box for more ethical concerns.)

SOCIOECONOMIC AND PSYCHOLOGIC FACTORS

Social Attitudes

The general attitudes of society toward disabled persons vary between extremes of overprotection and avoidance. These social attitudes result mainly from years of negative conditioning and are not easily changed. Deformities or severe illness may make some people uncomfortable, perhaps because they sense their own vulnerability and mortality. Others may be unsure how to work with these individuals or choose to completely ignore them. Neither extreme is helpful, but at the same time, overprotection robs persons of their selfhood and smothers the will to fight against surrounding odds and develop self-acceptance. However, disabled persons do have varying special needs, and social avoidance of these needs creates additional problems in everyday living. There are doorways not made for wheelchairs, unmanageable stairs and curbing, lack of access to public transportation, and many more daily barriers.

Economic Problems

Care for a person with a disabling injury or severe illness can be a long and costly process. A major area of exploration for the healthcare team is one of financial resources. A skilled financial expert can work with insurance companies and the patient's personal finances to get the best care with the least possible monetary burden. Continuing long-term economic problems may revolve around employment capabilities or earning capacities, or the means for providing care.

Living Situation

Disabled persons face many practical problems of everyday living. Whether a person needs long-term hospital care or can maintain independent living, perhaps with an attendant, depends on a number of physical and situational factors. If the person can maintain a home, then the necessary special equipment for maximal self-care enables the person to do more things for themselves and helps preserve his or her sense of self-worth.[1] Depending on the disability, manipulating utensils, chewing, and swallowing may be problems. These issues often result in problems maintaining food quality, keeping desirable food temperatures, adequacy of intake, and ultimately malnutrition.

Psychologic Barriers

The positive resolution of many practical and emotional problems requires tremendous psychologic adjustment. Each person struggles with self-image and physical body

TO PROBE FURTHER
What Are the Ethical Concerns?

As with all areas of medicine, there is considerable debate over the ethical considerations of disability and rehabilitation. Issues such as life-sustaining treatment, withholding nutrition and hydration, and assisted death all fall under the main heading of quality of life. Since the time of Hippocrates, there have been many controversial definitions in the evolution of clinical ethics; however, it mainly means to search for the good and right option when one faces a choice about a potential action. Religious, cultural, and legal factors may all play a part in ethics, but do not singly affect the outcome.

The 1976 New Jersey Supreme Court decision that recognized the right of Karen Ann Quinlan's family to withdraw medical treatment that they believed she would not have wanted was a landmark in the advent of modern clinical ethics. One of the recommendations handed down by the justice system relating to this case, was that alternative means of resolving ethical dilemmas be developed by healthcare institutions, specifically mentioning an *ethics committee.* Also developed at this point was the *Quinlan formula* that aided professionals in resolving dilemmas of this nature.

Rehabilitation for catastrophic illness or injury is complex and labor intensive. It requires interaction between patient, caregivers, and staff to achieve the best possible outcome. Strong emotions and psychologic barriers are inevitable at the onset of hospitalization as well as throughout rehabilitation, often shaping the course of treatment. At the crux of ethical decision making is compassion for the individual, caring, and other humanistic qualities to create a healing environment.

Certainly it is helpful to have advance directives in place for each patient upon admission so that these decisions are clear, but this is not always the case. Other useful tools are clinical pathways that act as a roadmap, indicating which way to proceed based on a particular clinical situation. The ultimate goal is to care for a patient "holistically," considering all aspects and caring for him or her as an individual with decision-making capabilities either now or at a previous point in life.

References

In re Quinlan, 355 A.2d 647 (NJ 1976); *cert. denied,* 429 US, 1992.

Sakakihara Y: Ethical attitudes of Japanese physicians regarding life-sustaining treatment for children with severe neurological disabilities, *Brain Dev* 22(2):113, 2000.

Shevell M: Ethical issues in neurodevelopmental disabilities, *Curr Opin Pediatr* 11(6):508, 1999.

Stanley AL: Withholding artificially provided nutrition and hydration from disabled children: assessing their quality of life, *Clin Pediatr* 39(10):575, 2000.

trauma. It is no wonder that they often withdraw in defeat and exhaustion. Personality changes occur during rehabilitation processes that test both inner strength and physical stamina. Depending on personal resources and strengths, the person may or may not be able to function. Much of the healthcare team's keen insight and concern are directed toward supporting each person's efforts to meet individual needs. That many disabled persons do reach self-care goals in some measure is evident in the remarkable achievements some of them attain, despite or perhaps because of their difficulties.

SPECIAL NEEDS OF OLDER DISABLED PERSONS

America is aging. By 2050, the U.S. Census Bureau estimates that there will be more than 80 million people 65 years old or older living in the United States. During the next decade the most rapid population increase will be among those older than 85 years. With older age comes an increased number of disabled elderly persons. The U.S. Rehabilitation Services Administration, using a baseline of 1 disabled American in 10 Americans, estimates that the odds of being disabled increases to 1 in 3 after the age of 65 years. Increased services, including rehabilitation services, are needed, but rehabilitation needs of older persons differ from those of younger people. According to the National Institute on Aging (NIA), about 79% of people aged 70 years or older have at least one of seven potentially disabling conditions (arthritis, hypertension, heart disease, diabetes, respiratory diseases, stroke, and cancer).[2,3]

National Long-Term Care Survey Results

The good news is that during the past decade, there has been a sharp decline in the observed rate of disability for people 65 years old or older. In a landmark study,

advance directives Instructions for medical treatment given by a patient while he or she has decisional capacity to do so.

clinical pathways Clear standards or protocols for patient care that are designed to promote cost efficiency, better outcomes, and faster recovery.

disability A mental or physical impairment that prevents an individual from performing one or more gainful activities; not synonymous with handicap, which implies serious disadvantage.

researchers used the 1982 disability rates from the National Long-Term Care Survey (NLTCS) for people 65 years old or older to estimate the numbers of disabled persons in each future year using data from the Census Bureau projections. They then used subsequent waves of the NLTCS to determine the actual numbers of disabled persons and compared that with their estimates. Using this method, they observed 1.6 million fewer disabled older people in the United States in 1998 than there would have if the disability rate had not changed since 1982. These decreases in disability have been confirmed using multiple databases and have been shown to benefit both men and women and both minority and nonminority populations. The latest preliminary findings from the 1999 NLTCS suggest that the rate of decline in chronic disability is continuing and may be accelerating in a downward trend.[4] (See *Practical Application* box for more outcomes measurement data.)

Three life-changing events of aging determine needs: retirement, chronic illnesses, and general physical decline.

Vocational Rehabilitation

Without adequate planning, many older persons experience stressful disorientation with retirement. They have had a lifetime occupation of active involvement in a familiar working environment and now a sense of stability and identity is lacking. Supportive activities focus on vocational planning and the effective use of leisure time. At this point, many persons have not been accustomed to viewing leisure activities in a positive manner and need help in making this adjustment. In addition, vocational programs can help persons find gainful employment after they retire from work. They can also help retired healthy Americans find ways of contributing their wisdom and skills to others now working in the same field. In turn,

PRACTICAL APPLICATION
Outcomes Measurement

In the United States, the number of persons reporting disabling conditions between 1994 to 1995 was 54 million (*MMWR,* 2001). During 1996, direct medical costs for persons with disability were $260 billion. Rising healthcare costs are just one of the reasons behind developing outcome standards. A second rationale for developing outcome standards is for the practitioner to have a reliable tool to compare factual data to make an accurate assessment of a patient. Practically every specialty has a set of standards. In disability and rehabilitation, a commonly reported standard is the Functional Independence Measure (FIM). The FIM is an objective method of obtaining functional performance information from a patient. From this seven-point test, the observer can make a determination as far as the patient's length of stay or discharge plan. This information is essential in this age of cost containment. A traditional method of objective reporting is the activities of daily living (ADLs). ADLs include mobility around the home, getting to and from the toilet, transfer from chair, transfer from bed, feeding, dressing, and bathing. With either of these methods, a point system is used to determine a specific outcome, leaving less room for subjective interpretations that would otherwise be obtained strictly from an interview process with patient and caregivers. That is not to presume that subjective assessment does not have a place in patient care, but rather to point out the importance of objective methods in making logical conclusions about patient outcomes.

Other assessment methods that have been developed and are routinely used throughout hospitals and rehabilitation settings are the Glasgow Coma Scale score, the Revised Trauma Score, the Fugl-Meyer Assessment (FMA) and the Neurobehavioural Cognitive Status Examination (NCSE) for motor and cognitive abilities, Spinal Pain Independence Measure (SPIM) for patients with chronic low back pain disability; the Spinal Cord Independence Measure (SCIM) recently revised by Catz-Itzkovich, to more sensitively measure the functional performance of patient's with spinal cord lesions; the Office of Population Censuses and Surveys Scale (OPCS) and the Amputee Activity Score (AAS) to measure specifically the function for an amputee; and the Test of Playfulness (ToP) used primarily with children with disabilities, to measure interactions between the child and his or her environment and activity.

As with any assessment tool, reliability and validity between users is of primary significance. By choosing a method described above, the observer can easily assess a patient's disability and make a logical determination based on factual data.

References

Cameron D et al: The clinical utility of the test of playfulness, *Can J Occup Ther* 68(2):104, 2001.

Fong KN, Chan CC, Au DK: Relationship of motor and cognitive abilities to functional performance in stroke rehabilitation, *Brain Inj* 15(5):443-453, 2001.

Itzkovich M et al: Spinal Pain Independence Measure: a new scale for assessment of primary ADL dysfunction related to LBP, *Disabil Rehabil* 23(5):186, 2001.

Jagger C et al: Patterns of onset of disability in activities of daily living with age, *J Am Geriatr Soc* 49(4):404, 2001.

Panesar BS, Morrison P, Hunter J: A comparison of three measure of progress in early lower limb amputee rehabilitation, *Clin Rehabil* 15(2):157, 2001.

Prevalence of disabilities and associated health conditions among adults—United States, 1999, *MMWR Morb Mortal Wkly Rep* 50(7):120, 2001.

such activity can enhance the health and social assets of the older person.

Residual Disabilities From Illnesses

In the age period of 60 to 75 years (the young-old), rehabilitation is focused on problems of chronic diseases of aging—heart disease, hypertension, stroke, and cancer. Chronic illnesses may also be related to damaging health behaviors such as alcoholism, smoking, excessive calorie intake from foods high in fat and salt, and a sedentary lifestyle. Cardiovascular disease is the leading cause of disability in the United States today.[5] Survival after a heart attack or stroke occurs more often with modern medical care. Early efforts at rehabilitation help prevent disability, avoid complications, and restore reasonable function.

Physical Decline in Aging

In persons between 75 to 85 years of age and older (the old-old), disability increases sharply. Much of this increase comes from falls and resulting fractures, chronic brain failure, disorders in locomotion, impaired senses of perception, and increased problems with drug reactions and interactions. Older persons may have several different diseases and take a number of different drugs or receive a variety of medical treatments. In this age group, minor disabilities often result in major handicaps. Mental and physical dependency may require supportive care in the home or long-term care facility. Common health problems in both the young-old and old-old groups involve nutritional care as well. These problems include arthritis, cardiorespiratory and cardiovascular insufficiency, depression, sensory deprivation, infections, skin and foot disorders, and nutritional deficiencies from poor dentition and fad diets.

Disease and disability do not affect only the elderly. Many disabled groups include young people, and many older adults continue to be fit and healthy. However, the increasing age of the general population inevitably brings with it an increasing number of older adults with chronic disease and various disabilities of aging. Even minor disabilities may cause major handicaps in everyday living, and minor injuries may bring major debilitating results. In any case, the twin goals of rehabilitation care continue to be prevention of further disability and restoration of the maximal function available.

Principles of Nutrition Therapy

PREVENTION OF MALNUTRITION

Calories

The rehabilitative process of physical therapy involves hard work. The patient tires easily, and energy intake must be sufficient to meet the energy output demands. Excess calories must be avoided to prevent obesity, but sufficient energy for physical activity and tissue metabolism is essential.

Protein

General protein needs are based on maintaining strength of tissue structure and function. Tissue and organ integrity protects against catabolism, infections, negative nitrogen balance, and pressure sores. Dietary protein in optimal quantity (15% to 20%) and quality ensures the necessary supply of all essential amino acids required for tissue synthesis. In addition to these general needs, severe trauma such as that involved in spinal cord injury brings special needs to meet the catabolic response.

Carbohydrate

General energy needs are great. They are met by optimal dietary carbohydrate as the body's major fuel source (approximately 50% to 60% of calories). Severe trauma requires maximal carbohydrate, especially in the early stages after injury. Protein and fat help to provide needed energy but are primarily used for tissue rebuilding and integrity. Thus sufficient carbohydrate foods are important to provide the needed energy as well as to prevent protein catabolism and negative nitrogen balance.

Fat

Fat is a calorically dense form of energy that supplies essential fatty acids and adds palatability to the diet. The general dietary recommendation that fat supply about 25% to 30% of the total calories is sufficient.

Vitamins and Minerals

Optimal intake of vitamins and minerals is needed for metabolic activity and maintenance of tissue reserves. The normal Recommended Dietary Allowance (RDA) standards for age and sex are adequate in most cases. However, a deficiency state such as anemia indicates need for supplementation. In some rehabilitation centers, multivitamin preparations are given routinely to ensure adequate amounts.

RESTORATION OF EATING ABILITY

Normal Development of the Eating Process

In the normal growth and development of a child, the feeding and eating process develops through an overlapping and interdependent series of physical and psychologic stages. The usual activities of eating—swallowing, chewing, hand and utensil use—gradually develop with motor ability. The learning comes with much practice and

---

handicap A mental or physical defect that may or may not be congenital, which prevents the individual from participating in normal life activities; implies disadvantage.

pressure sores Long-term bed-bound or immobile patients risk the development of pressure sores at points of bony protuberances, where prolonged pressure of body weight in one position cuts off adequate blood circulation to that area, causing tissue death and ulceration.

---

patience. In a sense, the injured person must "start over" and relearn these basic skills.

Thus with an understanding of these normal patterns, the disabled person works with the professional team of occupational and physical therapists, nutritionists, and nurses to find adaptive procedures to restore basic eating ability. For each client, four aspects of the eating process will require individual attention: (1) the nature and degree of motor control, (2) eating position, (3) use of adaptive utensils, and (4) support of individual needs. For example, blind persons will need a description of the food served, its placement on the plate (named usually in a clockwise direction), and a follow-up training course in preparing food with a number of assistive tools and techniques.

NUTRITION BASE

The personal food plan must fulfill basic nutritional needs, in increased amounts to meet additional metabolic demands. In addition, appetite and motivation must be supported to accomplish the task. Sensory stimuli such as variety in food texture, temperature, color, and flavor can enhance appetite and help motivate the learning of new adapted modes of eating. Also, "comfort foods" or familiar ethnic dishes and well-liked foods can encourage the client with the sometimes frustrating and difficult process of relearning how to eat.

Independence in Daily Living

With each disabled person the goal is to achieve as much independence in daily living as possible. Maximal use is made of individual neuromotor resources and emotional reserves. Self-help devices are used as needed to aid these personal resources. A large number of creative devices are available.

A number of chronic conditions can illustrate various areas of need for nutrition therapy. Briefly reviewed here are examples of such conditions in three types of problems: (1) musculoskeletal disease, (2) neuromuscular injury and disease, and (3) progressive neurologic disorders.

Musculoskeletal Disease

RHEUMATOID ARTHRITIS

Clinical Characteristics

The general term *arthritis* comes from the Greek word *arthron,* meaning "joint." Its underlying chronic, systemic, inflammatory disease process usually occurs in the young adult years. The peak age for onset of disease is between 25 and 55. Women are affected 2.5 times more often than are men, and approximately 1% to 2% of the total population is affected.[6]

The cause of rheumatoid arthritis (RA) is unknown. There are infectious, genetic, and hormonal factors that may play a role. It is a severe type of autoimmune disorder in which the body's immune system acts against its own tissue. It mainly attacks the joints of the hands, arms, and feet, causing them to become extremely painful, stiff, and deformed. Severe disease is associated with larger joints such as the hips, and a life-threatening joint complication can occur when the cervical spine is affected. The precise triggering antigen is still unknown.

Joint damage occurs due to tissue change in the synosheaths. The synovium becomes inflamed and secrete more fluid, leaving the joint swollen and fatigued. Later the cartilage becomes rough and pitted, eventually affecting the underlying bone. Progressive joint deformity usually progresses rapidly, with joint destruction taking place 1 to 2 years after appearance of the disease.

This disability dramatically affects activities of daily living, especially the fundamental necessity of obtaining and eating food. There is hand and wrist involvement, including destruction of wrist ligaments and tendons, with weakened finger and handgrip strength, and limited finger movement (Figure 25-1). All of these changes limit the ability to self-feed, shop for, or prepare food. Also, elbow and shoulder involvement hinders bringing food to the mouth. Tissue damage at the temporomandibular joint (TMJ) of the jaw limits normal opening and closing of the mouth and may alter chewing ability. Other nonjoint problems—anemia of chronic disease, decrease in salivary secretions, dysphagia, and bone disease—further complicate nutrition problems, leading to overall malnutrition. In its juvenile form in children and adolescents, this resulting malnutrition can cause serious growth retardation.

Medical Management

Medical treatment may involve a number of drugs for control of the inflammatory process. Since the updated American College of Rheumatology (ACR) recommendations for the medical management of patients with lower limb osteoarthritis (OA), additional recommendations, newer epidemiologic studies, systematic reviews, and clinical trials have been published. Aspirin and other nonsteroidal anti-inflammatory drugs (NSAIDs) remain mainstays of medical therapy, with the use of enteric-coated preparations to avoid gastric irritation. Cyclooxygenase (COX)-2 inhibitors are now readily available as well. They are favorable because the risk of gastrointestinal bleeding with long-term use is significantly reduced. Currently there are two available COX-2 inhibitors on the market: rofecoxib (Vioxx) and celecoxib (Celebrex). Neutraceuticals such as glucosamine sulfate, for pain relief and function improvement, has been found to be effective first-line treatment for patients with mild to moderate pain due to OA. Glucosamine, although documented as slow to take effect, also does not contribute to the risk of gastrointestinal bleeding.[7-9]

If rest, exercise, and the use of NSAIDs are ineffective after several months, aggressive therapy with disease-

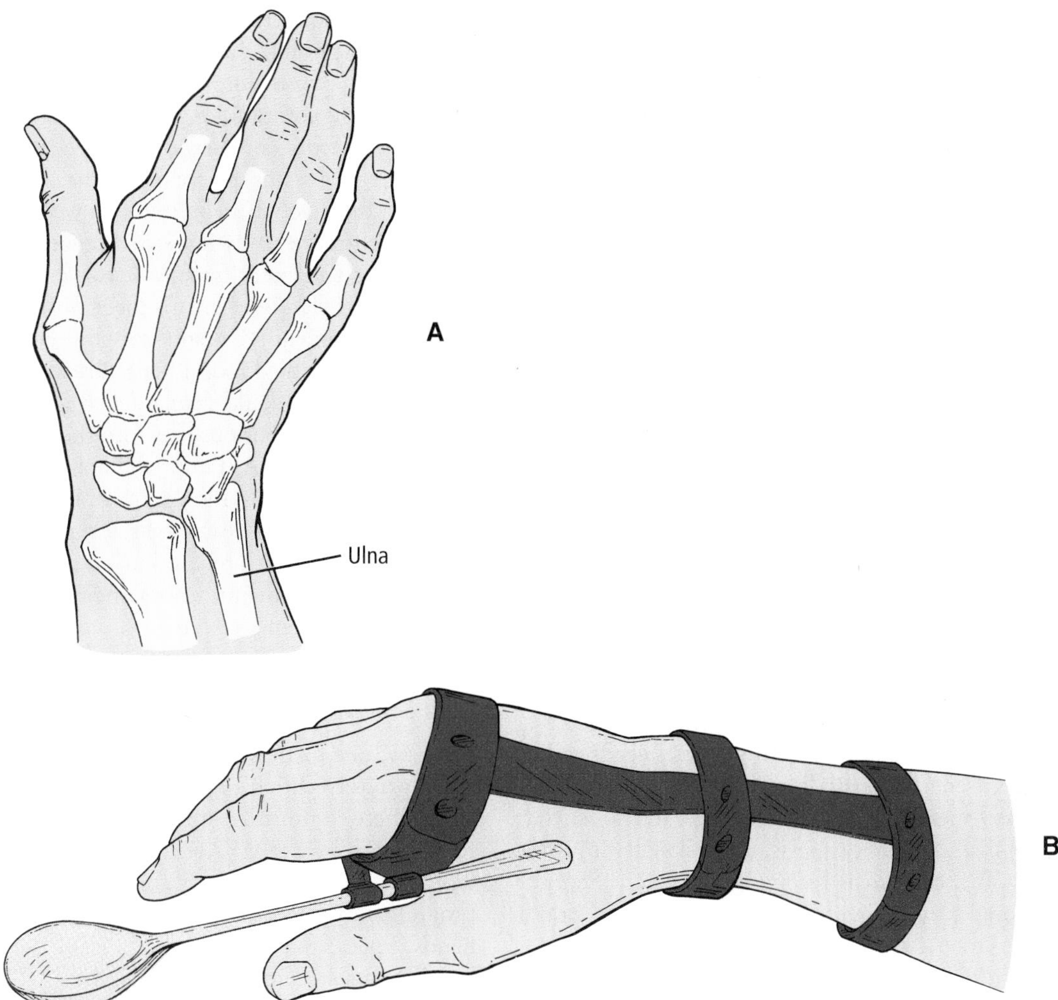

FIGURE 25-1 A, Arthritic hand showing ulnar drift. B, Self-help device for stirring food during preparation and for eating assistance.

modifying antirheumatic drugs (DMARDs) may be in order. Included in this group are gold compounds—injectable varieties like Myochrysine (gold sodium thiomalate) and Solganal (aurothioglucose), or oral medications such as Ridaura (auranofin)—D-penicillamine, antimalarial medications such as Plaquenil (hydroxychloroquine sulfate), and antineoplastic/anticancer drugs such as methotrexate. Weekly low-dose therapy with methotrexate, which acts as an antimetabolite to folic acid in DNA synthesis, is sometimes used but may cause the complicating viral condition herpes zoster.[10] Sometimes combination drug therapy is used as with cyclosporin and methotrexate.[11] Other options include steroid and immunosuppressive agents. When irreversible destruction of cartilage occurs in advanced stages of the disease, reconstructive joint surgery along with physical therapy and occupational therapy gives the best results.[12]

In the past few years, a promising medication called Enbrel (etanercept) has become a first-line agent for the treatment of RA. Etanercept acts by inhibiting the inflammatory protein called tumor necrosis factor (TNF). Other new medications include Remicade (infliximab) which also blocks TNF, and Arava (leflunomide), which works to block growth of new cells. Remicade is available as an intravenous injection on a regular basis, whereas Arava is taken as a daily oral medication.

herpes zoster An acute self-limiting viral inflammatory disease of posterior nerve roots causing skin eruptions in a lateral pattern across the back of the torso served by these nerves, accompanied by neuralgic pain; caused by the virus of chickenpox and commonly called *shingles*.

synosheath Protective pliable connective tissue surrounding the bony collagen mesh and fluid that come together in the synovial area between major bone heads in joints, which allows normal padded and lubricated joint movement and motion.

Nutritional Management

In all settings, the planning of nutrition therapy must begin with early assessment of individual patient status and needs, especially to detect any degree of malnutrition.[13] Initial history must then assess potential drug-nutrient food interactions. The history should include any "nonconventional" treatments for RA as well, such as dietary supplements and practices that may not be scientifically proved.[13] In addition, attention may be given to dietary modifications under study that have shown therapeutic promise. Results indicate that supplementation with the omega-3 fatty acids suppresses synthesis of cytokines with potent inflammatory activities.[14] However, the amount needed to produce this effect is far more than people can normally tolerate.

Special functional assessment of eating ability is needed. Classic guidelines for this assessment and training have been provided.[15] Such guidelines should include any swallowing problem from lack of salivary secretions and dysphagia. Standard nutrition assessment is essential. On the basis of these data, nutrition needs can be determined and monitored.

1. *Energy.* Energy needs vary widely and must be determined on an individual basis. In general, needs will involve basal energy expenditure plus added calories for increased metabolic activity factors (MAFs), such as stress of disease activity, sepsis, fever, skeletal injury, or surgery. If the client is receiving physical therapy, an additional physical activity factor is used. Total calories are increased as needed to achieve desirable weight gain during growth, or decreased if indicated for obese adults. Follow-up monitoring determines any needed adjustments in energy estimates.
2. *Protein.* Protein needs vary with protein status, surgical therapy, proteinuria, and nitrogen balance. A well-nourished adult patient needs about 0.5 to 1 g of protein/kg/day during quiet disease periods. An increase to 1.5 to 2 g/kg/day is needed during active inflammatory disease periods. The RDA standards for age and sex can guide protein needs for children to meet basic growth needs. States of malnutrition will require more.
3. *Vitamins and minerals.* Standard recommendations for vitamins and minerals are used. Specific supplementation may be used if needed, such as supplying calcium and vitamin D if bone disease is involved, or if the patient is undergoing steroid therapy.
4. *Special enteral and parenteral feeding.* Tube feeding may be used either to supplement oral intake or to supply total nutrition support. Parenteral nutrition support is reserved for preoperative and postoperative needs or when bowel rest is indicated.

Some researchers have investigated the potential for a vegetarian diet—more specifically a vegan diet—using uncooked foods to relieve the symptoms of RA. This is often referred to as the "living foods" diet. It consists of uncooked berries, fruits, vegetables, roots, nuts, germinated seeds, and sprouts, that is, rich sources of antioxidants, carotenoids, vitamins C and E, and flavonoids, and polyphenolic compounds such as quercetin, myricetin, and kaempherol. The diet is also high in fiber.[16]

Some reports have concluded that a large number of people subjectively benefited from a vegan diet.[17-19] However, much more study is needed regarding this mode of therapeutic treatment for RA. It is extremely difficult for young healthy individuals to meet protein and vital nutrient requirements (B_{12} and iron) following a vegan diet. Elderly and disabled individuals, already managing an array of obstacles, would face an even greater challenge to incorporate this laborious diet into their therapeutic plan.

The course of RA is unpredictable. The disease is usually progressive and some degree of permanent disability usually results. After years of disease, many persons are capable of self-care with rehabilitation training and are fully employable.[20] Continuing optimal nutrition therapy is important maintenance care.

OSTEOARTHRITIS

This milder form of arthritis in older adults is more appropriately called *degenerative joint disease (DJD)* because there is minimal inflammation involved. DJD affects approximately 44% of persons over the age of 40 years in the United States. It is chronic and may progress, limiting movement of affected joints, mainly the hands, knees, and hips. Marked disability is uncommon, but OA may become a chronic disabling disease in the elderly. There is no cure for the disease process, which ultimately destroys cartilage between the rubbing heads of bones in involved joints. However, damaged joints can be replaced by arthroplasty, surgical removal of the degenerated joint, and replacement of a joint made with metal or plastic components. Hip replacements have been performed since the early 1960s, and the technique is now being refined and applied to other joints. In general, appropriate pain-controlling medication and therapeutic nutrition for general health promotion help relieve symptoms. Glucosamine sulfate, a relatively new nutraceutical, is now being used to treat the pain associated with OA. It is gaining recognition and favor in the medical field because it is relatively inexpensive and has little to no side effects, yet it is able to stimulate proteoglycan synthesis by chondrocytes and has mild anti-inflammatory properties more effective than those of placebo in controlling symptoms.[9] Depending on the degree of hand joint involvement, self-feeding devices may assist eating.

OSTEOPOROSIS

The metabolic bone disorder osteoporosis is the most common skeletal disorder in the United States. According to the National Osteoporosis Foundation (NOF), 10 million

TABLE 25-1 Medications Used to Manage Osteoporosis

Medication	Comments
Estrogen replacement therapy (ERT)/hormone replacement therapy (HRT)	Available as pill, skin patch; low dose; increased risk of uterine cancer when taken alone—recommended to be taken with the hormone progestin for women who have an intact uterus to prevent cancer, although the issue of a relationship between breast cancer and estrogen is still to be determined
Alendronate sodium (Fosamax)	Classified as a bisphosphonate; best if taken on an empty stomach with a full glass of water; normally prescribed to be taken once a week
Risedronate (Actonel)	Classified as a bisphosphonate; taken daily on an empty stomach with a large glass of water
Raloxifene (Evista)	Classified as a selective estrogen receptor modulator (SERM); taken daily in pill form with or without meals; unlike estrogens, SERMs do not appear to stimulate uterine or breast tissue, thereby minimizing the risk for these types of cancer
Calcitonin (Miacalcin)	Naturally occurring hormone involved in calcium regulation and bone metabolism; protein available as injection or nasal spray
Parathyroid hormone (PTH)	Stimulates bone formation unlike the other anti-resorptive drugs mentioned above; treatment with PTH is still experimental; most effective when given 1-2 yr and followed by antiresorptive medications to maintain the benefits

Americans have osteoporosis and an additional 18 million have low bone mass, putting them at a high risk for developing osteoporosis. Osteoporosis is referred to as the "silent disease" because bone loss occurs without symptoms. The first sign of problem might not be until a person experiences a fracture. At this point, the disease is in the advanced stages and the damage can be profound.[21,22]

Osteoporosis is the result of the body not forming sufficient new bone or of the body reabsorbing too much bone, or both. The latter is typically a situation that occurs in old age. Calcium and phosphate are the two minerals responsible for normal bone formation. If calcium intake is not sufficient throughout the early years in life or if the body does not absorb sufficient calcium from the diet, bone tissue may suffer. Other causes of osteoporosis include hyperparathyroidism, hyperthyroidism, Cushing's syndrome, immobilization, bone malignancies, certain genetic disorders, and excessive corticosteroid use.

Approximately 80% of postmenopausal women of the United States have osteoporosis. Overall, one in two women and one in eight men over 50 will experience osteoporosis-related fractures. This is primarily because of the decline in estrogen production in women and androgen production in men. After age 70, osteoporosis affects men and women equally after a slow, steady rate of bone loss, and increasing fracture potential develops over many decades. These fractures in the elderly are a major cause of disabling illness and death. Bones of the vertebrae and the hip are most vulnerable, but hip fractures are more serious. In 1995, direct medical expenditures relating to osteoporotic fractures totaled $13.8 billion.[23]

The best line of defense against osteoporosis is prevention. Much of the research today is in the development of medications for prevention. Medical treatment of postmenopausal osteoporosis in women is most effectively managed with estrogen replacement therapy (ERT).[24]

Medical Management

A number of new medications for the prevention and treatment of osteoporosis are currently available and approved by the Food and Drug Administration (FDA). These include a variety of estrogens and hormone replacement therapies, alendronate, risedronate, and raloxifene. Calcitonin is approved for treatment of osteoporosis only. These are all classified as antiresorptive medications. They affect the bone remodeling cycle by slowing or stopping the bone resorption or breakdown. As a result, new formation continues at a greater rate than bone resorption, and bone density may increase. See Table 25-1 for a summary of medications currently in use for osteoporosis prevention and treatment.

Nutrition Management

The slow, steadily developing form of osteoporosis in men and women responds very readily to nutrition therapy. It includes a well-balanced diet with a calcium intake of at least 1000 mg/day (100% Daily Reference Value [DRV]), 400 IU of vitamin D (100% DRV), and regular physical

arthroplasty Plastic surgery of nonfunctioning body joints to form movable joints with replacement metal or plastic materials.

cytokines Substances, produced in tissues, that can cause inflammatory changes in tissue cells (e.g., tumor necrosis factor and interleukin-1).

TABLE 25-2 Recommended Daily Calcium and Vitamin D Intakes

Age	Calcium	Vitamin D
Birth-6 mo	210 mg (21% DV)	200 IU (50% DV)
6 mo-1 yr	270 mg (27% DV)	200 IU (50% DV)
1-3 yr	500 mg (50% DV)	200 IU (50% DV)
4-8 yr	800 mg (80% DV)	200 IU (50% DV)
9-18 yr	1300 mg (130% DV)	200 IU (50% DV)
19-50 yr	1000 mg (100% DV)	200 IU (50% DV)
51-70 yr	1200 mg (120% DV)	400 IU (100% DV)
71 and older	1200 mg (120% DV)	600 IU (150% DV)
Pregnant/lactating		
14-18 yr	1300 mg (130% DV)	200 IU (50% DV)
19-50 yr	1000 mg (100% DV)	200 IU (50% DV)

activity. Peak bone mass occurs around age 30, stimulated by physical activity. Bone mass then needs to be sustained through a healthy diet and physical activity.[25,26]

Percent DRV varies according to age, sex, and circumstances such as pregnancy and lactation; see Table 25-2 for the daily values of calcium. These amounts are based on the 1997 recommendations of the National Academy of Sciences (NAS). It is also important to note that the NAS suggests a tolerable upper intake level (UL) for calcium of 2500 mg/day and for vitamin D of no greater than 50 μg (2000 IU) daily for anyone over the age of 1. Appropriate ULs for those under age 1 have not been established yet. These ULs include the use of supplements as well as food for obtaining calcium and vitamin D. The body can properly handle about 500 mg of calcium at one time, whether from food or supplements.

Neuromuscular Injury and Disease

GROWING PROBLEM OF NEUROLOGIC INJURIES

According to the American Heart Association, traumatic injury is the leading cause of death in the first four decades of life. It is also the third leading cause of death for all ages.[27] In 1 year, automobile and industrial accidents, gunshot wounds, homicides, and sports injuries kill about 150,000 persons. There are an estimated 50 million Americans affected by diseases or disorders of the spinal cord and brain.[28] The lengthy list of disorders includes spinal cord injury, memory loss, addiction, schizophrenia, learning disability, depression, violence, stroke, brain injury, dementia, and suicide.

With current advances in emergency medicine, the number of persons surviving traumatic brain and spinal cord injury has increased dramatically. Proper nutrition therapy after these injuries in the acute care and rehabilitative setting is essential.

TRAUMATIC OR ACQUIRED BRAIN INJURY

An estimated 5.3 million Americans, a little more than 2% of the population, now live with disabilities resulting from a brain injury. Each year, 80,000 Americans experience the onset of long-term disability after a traumatic brain injury.[29] Vehicular crashes are the leading cause of brain injury (50%), followed by violence, mostly with firearms, and falls in the elderly. The cost of brain injury in the United States is estimated to be $48.3 billion annually. Hospitalization accounts for $31.7 billion, and fatal brain injuries cost the nation $16.6 billion each year.[30]

It is important to note two distinct types of brain injury.

1. *Traumatic brain injury (TBI).* This injury is an insult to the brain, not of a degenerative or congenital nature, caused by an external physical force that may produce a diminished or altered state of consciousness, which results in an impairment of cognitive abilities or physical functioning. It can also result in the disturbance of behavioral or emotional functioning.
2. *Acquired brain injury (ABI).* This is an injury to the brain that is not hereditary, congenital, or degenerative.

Postinjury Metabolic Alterations

The brain is the control center of body functions and activities. Thus brain injury brings an immediate cascade of systemic metabolic and protective responses that affect the entire body and its resources. The systemic inflammatory response is activated, and a sustained state of hypermetabolism develops. Ultimately, if the process continues unchecked, a sequence of organ failure follows. Any complication prolongs the hypermetabolic phase, and the increasing protein catabolism causes depletion of lean body mass.[31] Increased energy expenditure and urinary nitrogen excretion mark this increased metabolic demand in response to trauma.

Initial Nutrition Management

The immediate goals of the care team are control of the injury, maintenance of oxygen transport, and metabolic support. Nutrition support as soon as possible is vital to meet the hypermetabolic drain on the body tissue resources for increased energy, protein, and fluid demands. Regular monitoring of energy needs is essential, often more than once a day. Most trauma centers now use indirect calorimetry at the bedside with a mobile calorimeter unit.

Early nutrition support may be delivered via the enteral or parenteral route. Delayed gastric emptying after TBI has led some to advocate early percutaneous endoscopic gastrostomy or jejunal (PEG/PEJ) feeding.[32,33] Success has been reported using enteral feedings as early as 2 to 3 days after injury, primarily to keep bowel function intact.[34] Total parenteral nutrition (TPN) is a practical option because it can be started within the first 24 hours after injury and may be immediately adjusted to the nutrition requirements of each patient according to daily metabolic profile and urinary nitrogen analysis.[34-36] Providing TPN and enteral nutrition in combination therapy is commonly used in this population to preserve gut integrity while achieving nutrient requirements. TPN is gradually tapered when the enteral formula is well tolerated and considered adequate.[37]

Rehabilitative Nutrition

Nutritional rehabilitation for the person with TBI or ABI presents a complex of individual problems that require skilled and sensitive nutrition management. Individualized care plans are designed to focus on the immediate and long-range plans for the patient. To develop individual nutrition care plans, the rehabilitation dietitian works closely with other team members, such as the nurse, occupational therapist, speech pathologist, cognitive rehabilitation therapist, and physical therapist.[38] Together they assess the degree of dysphagia, difficulty with chewing and swallowing, level of language deficit and communication, and ability to perform basic activities of daily living skills, including food preparation and eating. Short- and long-range goals, as well as strategies to reach these goals, are developed along with many practical suggestions for adapting food forms and textures to meet eating problems.

SPINAL CORD INJURY

Postinjury Management

The cervical region of the spine at the neck is the most mobile portion and hence the most vulnerable site for spinal cord injuries.[39] Spinal cord damage disrupts the nerve transmission of impulses from the brain to peripheral nerves and muscles so that muscle function below the level of injury is lost—paralysis. The resultant immobilization leads to complicated illnesses. According to the Christopher Reeve Paralysis Foundation, there are an estimated 250,000 to 400,000 spinal cord–injured individuals living in the United States. Each year catastrophic spinal cord injury (SCI) in the United States affects some 11,000 new survivors. Because of advanced medical care, the number of survivors, and consequent costs, is increasing each year.

Most of these SCIs are a result of automobile accidents (44%); other factors include physical assaults (26%), falls (22%), and sports injuries (7%). Quadriplegia (loss of movement and sensation in both the arms and legs) and paraplegia (loss of movement and sensation in the lower body) affect 47% of the SCI population. SCIs cost the nation at least $9.7 billion per year for medical care, equipment, and disability support. Initial hospitalization (average 15 days acute care and then 44 days in rehabilitation), adaptive equipment, and home modification costs after injury average $140,000 per patient. Trauma and rehabilitation costs alone are almost $250,000 for each SCI individual.[40,41]

Nutrition Management

Protein-energy malnutrition is common in individuals with SCI. About half of the hospitalized patients and two thirds of the patients admitted to a rehabilitation unit exhibit clinical signs of malnutrition.[42-45] Malnutrition increases the risk for development of pressure sores, and fat mass excess due to immobility increases the cardiovascular and respiratory risks of these patients. They are predisposed for the development of diabetes mellitus and bony fractures as well.[46]

SCI patients are usually well nourished at the time of the sudden injury. Thus the goal of starting the feeding process as early as possible is to counteract the initial acute phase of spinal shock and to prevent the onset of a nutritional decline and secondary illness. Enteral feeding tubes placed beyond the pylorus usually make it possible to start nutrition support within 3 to 5 days. There is a wide variation in metabolic rate and energy needs, but they tend to be lower than those of other trauma patients as a result of decreased metabolic activity of denervated muscle.[44,45] The higher the injury to the spinal column, the greater is the denervated muscle mass and the lower is the measure of energy expenditure. Daily guidelines for energy needs are approximately 23 kilocalories (kcalories)/kg for quadriplegics and 28 kcalories/kg for paraplegics.[44]

Rehabilitation Nutrition

When the acute phase passes and the patient is stabilized, usually 2 to 3 months after injury, the extended rehabilitation training phase begins. This complex process is designed to restore the client to the best functional capacity possible to promote independent living.[47] The goal is to prevent and treat any complications associated with SCI. Combined therapies are used from the team of rehabilitation specialists: physiatrist, registered dietitian, registered nurse, physical therapist, occupational therapist, speech therapist, psychologist, social worker, and vocational counselor. Nutrition management involves individual assessment and care of (1) basic energy-nutrient needs and feeding capacities and (2) complications associated with the SCI.

Basic Nutrition Needs

Energy needs are based on sufficient calories to maintain an ideal body weight somewhat below that for a comparative person given in standard weight-height tables for healthy populations. For example, general weight goals for paraplegics have been recommended at 10 to 15 pounds below standard body weight, and for quadriplegics, 15 to 20 pounds below standard weight.[44,45] Excess weight gain is common in clients with SCI as a result of the decreased metabolic rate that persists from the preceding acute postinjury phase and the continued relative immobilization.[38] Obesity contributes to medical problems, as well as adding physical problems in the frequent turning necessary in bed to prevent bedsores and the transfers between bed to wheelchair. Adequate protein intake is essential for maintaining muscle mass and tissue integrity to prevent negative nitrogen balance, ulcer formation, or infection. Palatable high-protein supplements between meals may be needed to maintain an adequate intake. The client may be at risk for vitamin or mineral deficiencies if appetite and food intake are poor as a result of depression or fatigue. A standard multiple vitamin-mineral preparation is often recommended to ensure nutritional adequacy.

Associated Complications

Several nutrition-related complications in rehabilitation for patients with SCI require special attention:

1. *Pressure sores.* Pressure sores are caused by immobilization, loss of pressure sensation around bony prominences, decreased blood circulation, skin breakdown, and ulcer formation that is open to infection and difficult to heal. They occur in 60% of quadriplegic patients and 52% of paraplegics. Nutritional factors involved include anemia, which reduces oxygen supply to tissues; excessive weight loss, which reduces padding of bony prominences; and low levels of plasma proteins such as albumin, which lead to edema and loss of skin elasticity. The protein deficiency requires an increased protein intake. More severe ulcers require more intense nutrition intervention, with protein needs of 1.5 to 2 g/kg. Although not a panacea, vitamin C and zinc supplementation can aid in the healing process when combined with proper diet.[43,48]
2. *Hypercalciuria.* Immobility leads to an imbalance in calcium metabolism with a loss of bone calcium and its increased excretion in the urine. Over the long term this loss of bone calcium leads to osteoporosis, which has been found to be present and progressive in 88% of the patients with SCI, affecting the denervated musculoskeletal tissue below the level of injury.[49] A balance of calcium–vitamin D therapy, and a prudent control of excessive protein and sodium intakes, which cause increased calcium withdrawal, is indicated. Bone fractures result in about 7% of these patients.
3. *Kidney stones.* Hypercalciuria also contributes to formation of kidney stones. The neurogenic effects after SCI cause loss of normal bladder control, resulting in problems of urinary reflux, retention, incontinence, infection, and stone formation.[49] Regular catheterization is necessary to prevent accumulation of bacteria and solutes such as calcium and other particles that can easily form stones. A high fluid intake of 2 to 3 L/day must be a part of the overall nutrition care plan to dilute the urine and reduce the solute concentration.
4. *Neurogenic bowel.* Gastrointestinal complications from loss of normal neuromuscular controls include decreased peristalsis and loss of bowel control. A regularly scheduled program for emptying the bowel is necessary. Remedies vary but could include prune juice with lemon, glycerin suppositories, a high-fiber diet with ample fluid to prevent fecal impaction, and regular toileting. A daily schedule and accurate recording of results are recommended to promote regularity and limit the need for enemas or manual evacuation of stool.
5. *Depression.* During the initial days of shock and survival, the full impact of the disability is not comprehended. When transfer to the rehabilitation unit occurs and the full extent of the disability is realized, a period of depression, even anger, is a normal part of the personal grieving and healing process. Its severity and duration depend in large measure on the patient's personal strengths and resources, but it also requires the sensitive yet realistic support of family and the rehabilitation team for the serious and demanding work of rehabilitation to be successful. The nutritionist must help ensure that adequate energy, protein, and fluid intake is maintained. Optimum nutrition status is achieved with appetizing foods, especially when the patient's human spirit is low. Even subtle improvements in muscle mass and function from nutrition therapy can be a source of strength to mind and body.

CEREBROVASCULAR ACCIDENT—STROKE

Brain injury resulting from a stroke causes varying degrees of nerve damage and body paralysis. According to the American Heart Association, cerebrovascular disease from underlying atherosclerosis ranks third as a cause of death and second as a cause of disability in the United States. In recent years the incidence of strokes has declined, largely as a result of the improvement in control of hypertension and increased public education concerning hypertension. The length of time to recover from a stroke depends on its severity. From 50% to 70% of survivors regain functional independence, but 15% to 30% are permanently disabled. Institutional care is required by 20% at 3 months after onset. In 1997, $3.8 billion ($5955 per patient discharge) was paid to Medicare beneficiaries discharged from short-stay hospitals for stroke.[50] Dysphagia occurs in up to half of patients after a stroke; in most, it is transient with only about 1 in 10 patients having any swallowing problems at 6 months. Persistent dysphagia may be due to lack of bilateral cerebral hemisphere representation of the oral and pharyngeal musculature involved in swallowing.[51] Further rehabilitative care follows the same general goals and methods discussed in this chapter.

DEVELOPMENTAL DISABILITIES

During the developmental period of childhood, neuromuscular conditions such as cerebral palsy (CP), epilepsy, spina bifida, and Down syndrome cause eating problems that can contribute to poor growth and delayed development.

Cerebral Palsy

CP is a general term for nonprogressive disorders of muscle control of movements and posture. CP affects some 500,000 children and adults in the United States. Approximately 5000 infants are diagnosed with the condition each year. It is not a disease and it has no "cure" per se, although training and therapy can help to improve function. CP has many causes and usually results from brain damage that occurs during fetal development or shortly after birth, probably as a result of *hypoxia,* poor oxygen supply to the brain.[52,53] Other causes are premature birth, low birth weight, Rh or A-B-O blood type incompatibility between mother and infant, infection of the mother with German measles or other viral diseases in early pregnancy, and bacteria that directly or indirectly attack the infant's central nervous system.

Most affected children fall into three principal types: (1) spastic—muscles of one or more limbs permanently contracted, making normal movements very difficult or impossible; (2) athetoid—involuntary writhing movements; and (3) ataxic—disturbed sense of balance and depth perception. An individual may possess more than one type. These continuous involuntary movements increase energy needs, with research reports indicating increased resting metabolic rates that are approximately 15% higher than those of control subjects.[53-57] Because the immune system is often compromised in persons with developmental disabilities, they are at high risk for problems related to food safety. Thus all caregivers involved should have food safety training.[54,55]

Mental retardation, with an IQ below 70, occurs in about 75% of persons with CP, mostly in the spastic group. Important exceptions occur, mostly among those with the athetoid type. Some of these individuals are highly intelligent. Some features of the condition during childhood change, as the child grows older, often for the better with patience and skillful treatment.

Early nutrition therapy focuses mainly on feeding problems. When the infant or young child cannot obtain sufficient nourishment as a result of oral motor dysfunction, or when satisfactory oral feeding is interrupted for a prolonged period because of illness or surgery, enteral nutrition support via nasoenteric or gastrostomy tube feeding may be necessary. For patients with severe CP, tube feeding improves the quality of life for both the child and the family despite minor complications.[58,59]

TABLE 25-3 Equations for Estimating Stature From Knee Height*

Age/Sex Group	Equation
White Males	
6-18 yr	Stature = (knee height × 2.22) + 40.54
19-59 yr	Stature = (knee height × 1.88) + 71.85
White Females	
6-18 yr	Stature = (knee height × 2.15) + 43.21
19-59 yr	Stature = (knee height × 1.86) − (age × 0.05) + 70.25

Used with permission of Ross Products Division, Abbott Laboratories, Inc., Columbus, OH 43212. Modified from Estimating stature from knee height. In *Direction for the Ross Knee Height Caliper,* 1990, Ross Products Division, Abbott Laboratories, Inc.

*Equations are based on normal, healthy individuals. Stature and knee height are measured in centimeters.

Oral feeding can pose numerous problems, both functional and behavioral. Feeding problems of oral motor dysfunction (e.g., difficulties in sucking, swallowing, or chewing), gross motor/self-feeding impairment, lack of appetite, and food aversions can significantly reduce energy and nutrient intake, as can prolonged assisted feeding and use of pureed foods. In persons with severe physical and developmental difficulties, malnutrition and growth failure are common.[60]

Early and ongoing nutrition assessment, intervention, and counseling are essential components of rehabilitation team care. In cases where accurate height measures to assess growth are difficult because of joint contractures, spasticity, or inability to stand, reasonably accurate stature can be calculated from knee height measures, using the standard equations given in Table 25-3.[61,62] Growth retardation seen in children persists with age. Studies have shown that at age 2 years they are 2% shorter than their peers, and at 8 years of age they are more than 10% shorter.[61,62] As adults, persons with spastic CP need about 500 extra kcalories/day to cover the added energy need for *athetosis,* the continuous involuntary writhing motions of the disease.[57] Many still have feeding problems, but exercise helps promote better nutrition.[63] Other nutrition concerns are food intolerance, food allergies, drug-nutrient interactions, constipation, and reflux.[64]

Epilepsy

Epilepsy, literally "seizures," is a neuromuscular disorder in which abnormal electrical activity in the brain causes recurring transient seizures. Normally, the brain regulates

---

spina bifida A congenital defect in the fetal closing of the neural tube to form a portion of the lower spine, leaving the spine unclosed and the spinal cord open in various degrees of exposure and damage.

all human activities, thoughts, perceptions, and emotions through the regular orderly electrical excitation of its nerve cells, but in an epileptic state during a seizure, an unregulated, chaotic electrical discharge occurs. Seizures often appear spontaneously, or in some cases they may be set off by some stimulus such as a flashing light. This brain dysfunction may develop for no obvious reason, or there may be an inherited predisposition. In other cases, it may result from a wide variety of diseases or injuries such as birth trauma, a metabolic imbalance in the body, head injury, brain infection (meningitis, encephalitis), stroke, brain tumor, drug intoxication, or alcohol or drug withdrawal states.

According to the American Epilepsy Society, epilepsy and seizures affect about 2.3 million Americans and result in an estimated $12.5 billion in medical costs and lost or reduced earnings and production. Approximately 10% of all Americans will experience a seizure and 3% will have or will have had a diagnosis of epilepsy by age 80.

Usually the disorder starts in childhood or adolescence. It plateaus from ages 15 to 65 years and then rises again among the elderly.[65] About a third of these persons will outgrow the condition and do not need medication. Another third find their seizures well controlled by drug treatment and require less medication over time. The remaining third find that their condition remains the same or becomes more resistant to drug therapy.

Anticonvulsant drugs like valproic acid are the first line of treatment for epilepsy and in most cases do lessen seizure frequency. In cases of Lennox-Gastaut syndrome, a severe form of epilepsy that usually begins in early childhood and is difficult to treat, newer antiepileptic drugs such as lamotrigine (Lamictal) and topiramate have proved to be effective and well-tolerated treatments for associated seizures.[66,67] When medications fail to control seizure activity, other treatments are available such as vagal nerve stimulation (VNS) and the ketogenic diet.

VNS is currently approved for use in adults and children over the age of 12. A flat, round battery about the size of a silver dollar is surgically implanted in the chest wall. The therapy works by sending small regular pulses of electrical energy to the brain via the vagus nerve. Electrodes are threaded under the skin and wound around the vagus nerve in the neck. The healthcare team initially programs electrical impulses, and the patient has the option to activate the impulses if he or she feels a seizure about to occur. Although seizures are rarely eliminated completely, the majority of people who undergo VNS implantation experience fewer seizures and have a better sense of control. It still may be necessary to continue with antiepileptic medication.

Nutrition management of epilepsy functions in several areas of care. First, it helps to ensure an appropriate diet for normal growth during childhood and adolescence and for health maintenance in adulthood. Second, it seeks to ameliorate side effects of the anticonvulsant drugs used. Some of those most commonly used and their relation to food and nutrients are shown in Table 25-4.

TABLE 25-4 Anticonvulsant Drugs Used to Control Basic Types of Epilepsy and Their Nutrition-Related Side Effects

Most Commonly Used Drug	Drug Trade Name	Nutrition-Based Side Effects
Grand Mal (Tonic/Clonic) Seizures		
Phenytoin (adults)	Dilantin	Nausea, vomiting, and constipation; reduced taste sensation; vitamins D and K catabolism; reduced serum calcium, vitamins B_6 and B_{12}, folate, and serum magnesium levels; overgrowth of gums
Phenobarbital	Luminal	Increased appetite or anorexia, nausea, vomiting, vitamins D and K catabolism, reduced bone density
Primidone	Mysoline	Gastrointestinal upset, weight loss
Carbamazepine	Tegretol	Nausea, vomiting, diarrhea, abdominal pain, xerostomia (dry mouth), glossitis (sore tongue), stomatitis (sore mouth), increased blood urea nitrogen
Petit Mal (Absence of Seizures)		
Ethosuximide	Zarontin	Gastrointestinal upset, nausea, vomiting, anorexia, weight loss
Valproic acid	Depakene, Depakote	Nausea, vomiting, indigestion, diarrhea, abdominal pain, constipation, anorexia and weight loss, or increased appetite and weight gain
Clonazepam	Klonopin	Hyperactivity, short attention span, impulsive behavior, weight gain
Partial Seizures		
Phenytoin (adults)	Dilantin	Nausea, vomiting, and constipation; reduced taste sensation; vitamins D and K catabolism; reduced levels of serum calcium, vitamins B_6 and B_{12}, folate, and serum magnesium; overgrowth of gums
Phenobarbital	Luminal	Increased appetite or anorexia, nausea, vomiting, vitamins D and K catabolism, reduced bone density
Carbamazepine	Tegretol	Nausea, vomiting, diarrhea, abdominal pain, xerostomia (dry mouth), glossitis (sore tongue), stomatitis (sore mouth), increased blood urea nitrogen

Third, if a ketogenic diet is used, the clinical nutritionist is responsible for its calculations and education of staff, patient, and family in its use. This special high-fat, low-carbohydrate diet was developed to control epilepsy before current anticonvulsant drugs became widely available in the 1940s. It is still successfully used with some children possessing intractable myoclonic epilepsy that resists drug therapy.[68,69]

Details of the strict calculations required to achieve the necessary ratio of high fat to low carbohydrate ratios are outlined in The American Dietetic Association's *Manual of Clinical Dietetics.*[70]

Spina Bifida

Spina bifida is the most commonly occurring type of neural tube defect (NTD), a congenital malformation of the spine that contributes to serious developmental disabilities in the United States.[71] It develops during early embryonic life when the neural tube, which forms the spinal cord, does not close completely, leaving part of one or more vertebrae of the spinal cord exposed at birth. The vertebral canal usually closes within 4 weeks of conception. Thus this congenital defect can often be diagnosed early in the pregnancy by ultrasound scanning or by high levels of alpha-fetoprotein in the amniotic fluid or maternal blood; therefore appropriate genetic counseling can be provided for the parents. Recent discovery of the cell enzyme error involved indicates that folic acid (folate) and vitamin B_{12} supplementation at the time of conception through the first few months of pregnancy reduces a woman's risk that the baby will develop this devastating neural tube defect.[72,73] Many grains and cereals are now fortified with folate to prevent this condition.

The defect can occur anywhere along the spine but is more common in the lower back. One group study of children with myelomeningocele indicates that the neurologic damage that occurs depends on the severity and level of the lesion on the spine.[74] The incidence is about 1 per 1000 babies born, but it increases with either very young or old maternal age. A mother who has had one affected child is 10 times more likely to have another affected child.

There are three main forms of spina bifida.

1. *Spina bifida occulta.* This is the least serious and most common form. The name indicates an "unseen cleft in the spine." It often goes unnoticed in otherwise healthy children except for a small dimple over the area of the underlying abnormality.
2. *Myelomeningocele.* Also known as myelocele, this is the most severe form, and the child is usually severely disabled. Here the spinal cord *(myelo)* and its enveloping membranes *(meninges)* protrude from the spine in a sac *(cele).*
3. *Meningocele.* This form is less severe because the nerve tissue of the spinal cord is usually intact. Outer skin covers the bulging sac, and therefore there usually are no functional problems. Ideally, necessary surgical repairs are performed in the first few days of life.

Nutrition management of children with spina bifida focuses on growth pattern and individual degree of problems of growth retardation and short stature, low muscle mass and weakness, deformities or paralysis of lower extremities, and reduced ability to control bladder and bowels. Normal growth charts have been revised for use with nutrition assessment of these children.[75] Nutrition care plans give attention to the main problems of short stature and poor growth, increased weight, and constipation. Obesity is a particular problem because of several factors: (1) low basal metabolic rate related to lowered amount of lean body mass, (2) little physical activity related to the disabled condition and dependency on a wheelchair, and (3) use of food and overfeeding by parents or other caregivers to reward or show love or to counteract what is seen as frailty or weakness caused by the disability. All of these factors become part of ongoing nutrition counseling. Most children born with spina bifida live well into adulthood as a result of caring professionals and sophisticated medical techniques available today.

A growing concern is the development of a latex allergy, which is a common secondary condition associated with spina bifida. A latex allergy produces symptoms of watery eyes, wheezing, hives, rash, swelling, and, in severe cases, anaphylaxis. Research has shown that people with spina bifida are more susceptible because they are exposed to latex products early in life and repeatedly due to medical procedures. Some common products that contain latex are catheters, elastic bandages, baby bottle nipples, pacifiers, medical gloves, and balloons.

Down Syndrome

A chromosomal abnormality accounts for the mental retardation and characteristic appearance of children with Down syndrome, a condition first described in the previous century by the English physician John L.H. Down (1828-1896). Its cause remained a mystery until 1959, when modern researchers discovered that persons with Down syndrome had one too many chromosomes in each of their cells: 47 instead of the normal 46. Then because the extra chromosome is usually number 21, they gave it the alternate name of trisomy 21. The two parent chromosomes numbered 21 fail to separate into daughter cells during the first stage of sperm or egg cell formation, and some eggs or sperm are thus formed with an extra number 21 chromosome. If one of these takes part in fertilization, the resulting baby will have the extra chromosome and Down syndrome. This event is more likely if the mother is over 35 years of age, indicating that defective egg formation, rather than sperm formation, is usually the cause.

Down syndrome occurs in about 1 in 650 infants born. The rate rises steeply with increased maternal age

alpha-fetoprotein A fetal antigen in amniotic fluid that provides an early pregnancy test for fetal malformations such as neural tube defect.

to about 1 in 40 among mothers over 40 years. Currently there are more than 350,000 people living in the United States with this syndrome. The degree of mental retardation varies, with an IQ anywhere between 30 to 80, but all are capable of limited learning. Up to 50% of these individuals have congenital heart defects, which can be surgically corrected. More than 25% develop Alzheimer's disease after the age of 35, and 15% to 20% have a greater chance of developing a curable form of leukemia as a newborn and up to age 3.[76] Despite the complications associated with Down's syndrome, these children are usually affectionate, cheerful, and friendly and get along well with family and friends. They thrive to their full potential in a loving family.

Nutrition therapy focuses on delayed feeding skills; inappropriate, excessive, or inadequate intakes of food energy and nutrients; and poor eating habits. Diets need to be individualized because these children tend to gain excess weight if they are given the intakes recommended for most children.[76] Plans for increasing physical activity are important.

Progressive Neurologic Disorders

Progressive neurologic disorders, especially through the middle and older years of adulthood, have disabling effects on the personal lives of many individuals. Examples reviewed here illustrate some of these effects and nutrition approaches to providing support.

PARKINSON'S DISEASE

Parkinson's disease is a long-known neurologic disease, first described by the English physician James Parkinson (1755-1824) nearly two centuries ago, when in 1817 he described its characteristic symptoms in "An Essay on the Shaking Palsy."[77] According to the World Parkinson's Disease Association, more than 4 million people worldwide have Parkinson's disease. It is a common disorder reported in every race, region of the world, and age group, although the average age of onset is 55 years. Ten percent of cases affect those under age 40. The onset of motor symptoms usually occurs after the age of 40 years, rising in incidence with advancing age. Its underlying origin remains unknown, but some researchers speculate that the trigger may be related to some environmental factor such as a toxin.[78,79] Genetic factors are not the cause, but in some families genetic factors may predispose persons to the disease.

Another theory is iron status. Iron deficiency in early stages of life, despite correction with iron supplementation, may play a role in neurologic degeneration, although it is not possible to ascertain this information until an autopsy is performed. Iron deficiency in children has long been associated with retardation in growth and cognitive development. The effects of cognition are irreversible, even with treatment.[80] Iron is known to accumulate at sites of brain pathology of patients with Parkinson's disease; this is one theory behind the neurologic damage. Postmortem examination cannot distinguish whether iron accumulation caused the damage or resulted from damage.[81] A delicate balance of iron throughout life and how it affects the brain may be an area of research in the years to come.

Parkinson's disease affects the basal ganglia of the brain, a cluster of nerve cells at the central base of the brain. Signals from the brain's motor cortex pass, via the brainstem reticular formation and the spinal cord, to the muscles, which contract. Other signals pass through the basal ganglia, which provides a damping effect to help smooth and control the signal flow to reticular formation and the spinal cord, thus preventing uncoordinated muscle contraction responses. This damping effect is produced by the balancing action of two neurotransmitters: (1) dopamine, which is made in the basal ganglia and is necessary for the damping effect, stimulates the signal flow, and (2) acetylcholine, a widespread neurotransmitter in the body, inhibits it. In Parkinson's disease, degeneration of key parts of the basal ganglia causes a lack of dopamine within this part of the brain, thus preventing the basal ganglia from modifying nerve pathways that control muscle function.[82] The muscles become overly tense, causing joint rigidity and a general body stiffness, a fine constant tremor even at rest, and slow movements.

Medical Management

Although there is no cure for Parkinson's disease, drug management has helped to minimize the symptoms for many patients. A dramatic change in treatment came in the 1960s with the advent of the drug levodopa, which the body can transform into the needed dopamine. Dopamine itself cannot be used, because it does not cross the blood-brain barrier, as does levadopa.[83] The latest breakthrough in medications is entacapone (Comtan). This new class of Parkinson's medication is called a COMT (catechol-*O*-methyltransferase) inhibitor. COMT inhibitors are taken with levodopa. They prolong the duration of symptom relief by blocking the action of the enzyme, which breaks down levodopa before it reaches the brain. COMT inhibitors are usually started when a patient begins to experience a natural "wearing off" of the levodopa as the disease progresses. A more consistent exposure of levodopa to the brain aids in more independent function on the part of the patient. It improves the patient's ability to perform activities of daily living. See Box 25-1 for a list of medications commonly prescribed.

Current surgical research is investigating transplants of dopamine-secreting adrenal medulla tissue and the brain grafting of fetal dopamine neurons.[84,85] The new dis-

BOX 25-1 Medications to Treat Parkinson's Disease

- Levodopa
- Sinemet (levodopa/carbidopa)
- Symmetrel (amantadine hydrochloride)
- Anticholinergics (trihexyphenidyl, benztropine mesylate, procyclidine)
- Eldepryl (selegiline or deprenyl)
- Dopamine agonists: Parlodel (bromocriptine), Permax (pergolide), Mirapex (pramipexole), Requip (ropinirole)
- COMT inhibitors: Tasmar (tolcapone), Comtan (entacapone)

covery of a mutant form of the Parkinson's disease gene in several generations of a large Italian family with Greek origins has provided scientists with a major clue to the disease origins in the much larger number of patients with nonhereditary Parkinson's.[86,87]

Pallidotomy is a surgical procedure that fell out of favor with the development of levodopa; however, it has gained new popularity. Using magnetic resonance imaging (MRI), a surgeon is able to target the source of damaged cell tissue located in the globus pallidus and uses an electrode to destroy them. The risks include stroke, partial loss of vision, speech and swallowing difficulties, and confusion. Weight gain is a concern after pallidotomy.[88] Another option is deep brain stimulation. Like pallidotomy, this technique seeks to stop uncontrollable movements. Electrodes are implanted in the thalamus or globus pallidus and connected to a pacemaker-like device, which the patient can control.

Nutrition Management

The focus of nutrition therapy is on nutrition-related drug effects, eating problems, and malnutrition. Common side effects of levodopa include severe nausea that affects food intake. When the patient also takes anticholinergics, dryness of secretions is a major problem. Excessive intake of vitamin B_6 should be avoided because it interacts with levodopa and reduces the beneficial effect of the drug. Hand tremors make obtaining and preparing food, as well as eating movements of carrying food from the bowl or plate to the mouth, difficult. Thus, for example, soups should be avoided and more textured foods used. As the disease progresses, there may be problems with chewing, swallowing, or aspiration of small food items such as peas or nuts, as well as discomfort from constipation, flatulence, or delayed gastric emptying. Small frequent meals of increased carbohydrate and decreased fat, chewing thoroughly and eating slowly with special utensils as needed, with appropriate energy intake to maintain optimal weight and adequate fiber and fluid to prevent constipation, will be helpful.

As mentioned, levodopa should be taken on an empty stomach, because levodopa and protein use the same uptake in metabolism. Protein typically wins the competition; therefore levodopa is less affective. If nausea is severe, patients may possibly take a piece of bread or some crackers with the medication.

A very small percentage of patients are so extremely sensitive to the proteins in foods that they must undertake a protein-redistribution diet. This involves a special diet of daytime protein restriction to about 10 g.[89] The remaining protein foods such as meat and dairy products, to a day's total RDA intake (0.8 g/kg/day), are reserved for use in the evening meal and later snack. These beneficial effects of steady symptom control appear to result from a decrease during the day in the plasma concentration of dietary protein–derived large neutral amino acids that compete with levodopa for transport into the brain. Many of these patients report sleep disturbances with protein distribution and it is rarely recommended professionally.

Unintentional weight loss and body composition changes are common in Parkinson's disease patients. They are at greater nutritional risk than a matched population and should have continuing nutritional assessment and guidance to prevent this complication.[90]

HUNTINGTON'S CHOREA

First described in a landmark 1872 paper by American physician George Huntington (1850-1916), Huntington's chorea is an uncommon genetic disease in which degeneration of the basal ganglia of the brain results in chorea—rapid, jerky, involuntary movements, and dementia—progressive mental impairment. In 1993, a large group of scientists from six institutions discovered the defective gene that causes the disease, opening the way to future therapeutic interventions and possibly a cure.[91,92] Cases of symptomatic effects beginning in childhood are rare. This genetic disease is inherited in an autosomal dominant pattern with each child having a 50% chance of developing the condition. The highest concentration of persons world wide with Huntington's chorea in one family has been found and its gene linkage studied by Wexler's group in the little town of San Luis on the shores of Lake Maracaibo high in the Andes mountains of Venezuela.[92] In the United States, the disease develops in about 5 of 100,000 persons. Generally, the symptoms do not appear until middle adulthood (ages 35 to 50), so affected persons may have children before knowing that they have the disease. Continuing study has identified gene

chorea A wide variety of ceaseless involuntary movements that are rapid, complex, and jerky, yet appear to be well coordinated; characteristic movements of Huntington's disease.

mutation that causes an abnormal protein product the scientists have called *huntingtin*.[93]

Medical Management

As a result of recent advances in genetics, a test is now available for young adults whose parents have Huntington's chorea to learn, with 95% accuracy, if they carry the gene and thus have the disorder. This test can then help them decide whether to have children themselves. There is no known cure; therefore medical management helps to lessen the characteristic chorea, which affects face, arms, and trunk with random grimaces, twitches, and general clumsiness. The drug chlorpromazine (Thorazine), the most widely used antipsychotic drug for its tranquilizing effect (it suppresses brain centers that control abnormal emotions and behaviors), has been found to be useful. The mental impairment causes behavior changes, difficulty making decisions, apathy, irritability, and memory loss.

Nutrition Management

The excessive muscular activity requires adequate energy and nutrient intake to prevent malnutrition and excess weight loss. As the disease progresses, patients become cachectic and, despite adequate food intake, demonstrate a progressive catabolic state. Nutrition counseling involves planning energy-nutrient dense diets to combat malnutrition, usually 1.2 to 1.5 g of protein/kg of body weight.[94] Also helpful is assistance with dysphagia or feeding problems and the provision of adequate fiber to combat the drug side effect of constipation. Persons with advanced disease accompanied by dysphagia, marasmus, and depression may best be supported with an enteral formula. Bolus feedings via a PEG tube or other long-term enteral method is recommended due to the constant movement and risk of displacing the tube.

GUILLAIN-BARRÉ SYNDROME

Two twentieth-century French neurologists, Georges Guillain (1876-1961) and Jean Alexander Barré (1880-1965), first described this acute postinfectious polyneuritis. It is less commonly referred to as Landry's ascending paralysis. It is a rare form of damage to the peripheral nerves in which the myelin sheaths covering nerve axons, and sometimes the axons themselves, deteriorate, causing loss of nerve conduction and partial or complete paralysis. Nerve inflammation occurs particularly where their roots leave the spine, impairing both movement and sensation. Muscular weakness in the legs, often accompanied by numbness and tingling, progresses upward to trunk and arms, as well as face and head. A low-grade fever persists, and there may be urinary tract infection, respiratory failure requiring a ventilator, and personality changes. This acute syndrome is an autoimmune reaction, often following a viral infection or sometimes an immunization, such as the swine flu vaccine given readily in 1976. Recent study has indicated that infection with *Campylobacter jejuni* often precedes the Guillain-Barré syndrome and is associated with axonal degeneration, slow recovery, and, sometimes, severe residual disability.[95] This has been shown in approximately 1 to 2 cases per 2000 of *C. jejuni* infection. In general, the U.S. incidence is about 15 cases per 1 million per year.

Medical Management

Hospitalization for close monitoring of acute condition is essential, especially if a breathing difficulty occurs. In severe cases, plasmapheresis, in which blood plasma is withdrawn from the patient, treated to remove antibodies, and replaced, may be done. Most people recover completely without specific treatment other than general supportive care, but some are left with permanent weakness in affected areas. Disabilities in ambulation due to leg weakness and possibly feeding disabilities due to arm and trunk damage may need attention from professional staff.

Nutrition Management

During early acute phases, enteral or parenteral nutrition support may be necessary, with attention to increased energy and protein needs in the formula solutions. Respiratory distress requiring ventilator assistance can be problematic. In this case, it is crucial not to overfeed the patient. Popular high-fat formulations that claim to decrease CO_2 production can cause delayed gastric emptying and further gastrointestinal complications and therefore should be avoided.[96] Food consistency and texture may need to be adjusted in early oral feedings to accommodate any chewing and swallowing problems from weak facial and throat muscles. Continuing attention to energy and nutrient needs during convalescence is required to restore lost body weight and muscle mass.

AMYOTROPHIC LATERAL SCLEROSIS

Medical Management

Amyotrophic lateral sclerosis (ALS), named Lou Gehrig disease for the famous U.S. baseball player who developed ALS at the height of his successful Major League career, is the most common of the motor neuron diseases, affecting approximately 1 person in 10,000.[97] In these rare neuron disorders, nerves that control muscular activity degenerate within the brain and spinal cord. Researchers report the discovery of the gene causing a hereditary form of the disease.[98,99] The gene, superoxide dismutase-1 *(SOD1)*, controls the synthesis of an enzyme that helps cells get rid of highly toxic and destructive superoxide free radicals, which are produced by a variety of oxidative cell reactions.[100,101] If the enzyme was abnormal because of the defective ALS gene, free cell radicals might build up, causing the death of the motor neurons affected in ALS. As it is now, the relentless nerve degeneration of ALS progresses to involve the muscles of respiration and swallowing, usually killing its victims in about 3 years.[99-101] Identifying the responsible defective gene has led to more knowledge of how the progressive destructive course of ALS may be slowed, controlled, or prevented. Riluzole remains the only drug to slow disease progression, although interventions such as noninvasive ventilation and gastrostomy also extend survival.[102] The latest research on ALS detects a virus in the spinal cord. This is not new information by any stretch, but past reports of a virus being responsible for ALS were criticized for poor laboratory handling or technical errors.[103] Scientists are optimistic about the theory of a virus, because any virus has the potential for a vaccine (as with polio) or treatment with antiretroviral medications (as with HIV).

Nutrition Management

Nutrition therapy and counseling focus on increased energy intake and adjusting nutrient needs as the disease progresses. Weakness of hands and arms, as well as problems with chewing, swallowing, delayed or absent response of gag reflex, and risk of aspiration, will require eating assistance and modification of food textures. Frequent small meals are better tolerated. In advanced stages, enteral and parenteral nutrition support can supply needed energy and nutrients in a variety of individualized formulas.[104,105]

MULTIPLE SCLEROSIS

Multiple sclerosis (MS) is a progressive disease of the central nervous system in which scattered patches of insulating myelin, the fatty covering of nerve fibers in the brain and spinal cord that protects the neurons and facilitates the passage of neuromuscular impulses, are destroyed. In these denuded patches, nonfunctional plaques of scar tissue replace the myelin whereby nerve fiber can no longer conduct normal electrical impulses. The severity of the condition varies markedly among the person it affects. The precise cause of MS is unknown, but it is an autoimmune disease in which the body's defense system begins to treat the myelin tissue in the central nervous system as a foreign substance and gradually sets out to destroy it, with subsequent scarring left in its wake.

An as-yet-unknown genetic factor is probably involved because relatives of affected persons are 8 times more likely than others to develop the disease. Environment seems to play a role. MS is 5 times more common in temperate zones, such as the United States and Europe, than in the tropics. Perhaps it is induced by a virus picked up in the first 15 years of life in these temperate climates. Approximately two thirds of the persons affected experience the beginning symptoms between ages 20 to 40 years, more women than men are affected at a 2:1 ratio, and it is most commonly found in white populations. In the relatively high-risk temperate areas the incidence of MS is about 1 of every 1000 people.[106] Depending on how extensive the tissue involvement and which parts of the brain and spinal cord are affected, the effects of MS vary widely from mild periodic feelings of tingling, numbness, constriction, or stiffness in any part of the body to more severe disabling disease.

Medical Management

Physicians have lacked specific means of treatment while the search for a cure continues. Corticosteroid drugs have been used traditionally to alleviate symptoms of an acute attack. Currently, however, more specifically effective drugs are being used. The first one to be approved by the FDA was beta-interferon (Betaseron), followed by Avonex. Next came glatiramer acetate (Copaxone), developed in Israel and approved by the FDA for use in the United States.[107] These drugs reduce the frequency and severity of attacks. The latest drug to be approved is mitoxantrone (Novantrone). It is an injectable concentrate belonging to a group of medicines called antineoplastics. Before its approval for MS, it was used to treat certain cancers by suppressing the activity of B cells, T cells, and macrophages that are thought to lead to the attack of the myelin sheath. It is administered via intravenous infusion once every 3 months. It is important to note that this medication is currently approved only for secondary progressive forms or relapsing types of MS. Individuals with a primary progressive type of MS are not eligible to undergo treatment with this drug. Adjunct physical therapy helps maintain muscle strength and the ability to stay mobile and independent and remains a vital part of rehabilitation.

Nutrition Management

Individuals with MS respond to basic nutrition therapy that supplies adequate energy and nutrients to achieve optimal nutrition status. As discussed with other neuromuscular diseases, assistance with symptomatic gastrointestinal problems, elimination, and dysphagia is instituted as needed.[108] If steroid therapy is initiated, dietary sodium is reduced. Nasoenteric or gastrostomy tube feeding may be needed in advanced disease to provide enteral nutrition support and is generally well tolerated.[109]

There are no well-supported data that diet has a profound effect on treatment of MS; however, a low-fat, low-calorie, low–saturated fat diet may help to manage some symptoms associated with the disease.[110] Prevention of MS has been the debate for many years. Often the "diets" touted to prevent MS are confused by the general public as treatment regimens. For example, it has been suggested that high consumption of animal fat and low intake of fish

---

amyotrophic lateral sclerosis (ALS) A progressive neuromuscular disease characterized by the degeneration of the neurons of the spinal cord and the motor cells of the brainstem, causing a deficit of upper and lower motor neurons; death usually occurs in 2 to 3 years.

products and plant components may play a role in the "etiology" of MS,[111] but there is no evidence that eating high amounts of plant foods and fish products has any great affect on the prevention, prognosis, or progression of the disease.

MYASTHENIA GRAVIS

The neuromuscular disease myasthenia gravis (MG) occurs in about 14 of every 100,000 persons, eventually causing the affected person to become paralyzed as a result of the inability of the neuromuscular junctions to transmit nerve fiber signals to the voluntary muscles.[112] The most common form of MG is a chronic autoimmune disorder, in which the body's immune system attacks and gradually destroys the receptors in voluntary muscles that are responsible for picking up nerve impulses. As a result, the affected muscles respond only weakly or not at all to nerve impulses.

According to the Myasthenia Gravis Foundation of America, only about 2 to 5 new cases of this rare disease per 100,000 people are diagnosed annually. It affects more women than men in a ratio of 3:2. Although it can occur at any age, it usually occurs between ages 20 to 30 years in women and 50 to 70 years in men. Facial muscles are usually involved first, causing drooped eyelids, double vision, and sometimes a lack of facial animation with an absent stare appearance. Weak muscles of the face, throat, larynx, and neck cause difficulties in speaking and eating. As muscles in the arms and legs become involved, problems with other daily living activities such as food procurement and preparation, as well as dressing, combing the hair, and climbing stairs, also develop. In severe cases, respiratory muscles in the chest weaken and cause breathing difficulty.

Medical Management

Treatment may involve a thymectomy, that is, removal of the thymus gland, a small gland in the upper chest thought to be partly responsible for the abnormal antibody activity, especially if a small tumor is found there. Temporary relief may be obtained by regular plasmapheresis, exchanges of the patient's antibody-containing blood for antibody-free blood. These antibodies produced by the disease attack the receptors on the muscle cells that bind the acetylcholine neurotransmitter necessary for muscle contraction, thus effectively reducing stimulation of muscle cells and weakening muscle action. Anticholinesterase agents used to treat MG, such as neostigmine (Prostigmin) or pyridostigmine (Mestinon), increase the amount of the neurotransmitter acetylcholine at the nerve ending by blocking the action of the enzyme that normally breaks it down.[112,113] The blocking action of these drugs increases levels of the acetylcholine transmitter by allowing more of it to accumulate in the synaptic cleft between nerve and muscle fiber endings, thus permitting the remaining receptors to function more efficiently. Corticosteroids (prednisone) and immunosuppressants like azathioprine (Imuran) may be used to suppress the abnormal action of the immune system that occurs in MG. Intravenous immunoglobulins (IVIg) are sometimes used to affect the function or production of the abnormal antibodies as well.

Nutrition Management

Nutrition therapy has three main goals: (1) maintain optimal energy-nutrient intake for muscle strength and good nutritional status, (2) solve any associated eating problems, and (3) help counteract drug side effects of nausea and vomiting. The drugs described should be taken with liquid or food to lessen stomach irritation. Other suggestions are to adjust meal patterns to accommodate the individual. Provide the largest meal at breakfast, when the patient is more rested, and then frequent small meals throughout the day; take medications 1 hour before eating when strength is best; modify food texture to decrease excessive chewing; and supplement with enteral feedings as needed.

ALZHEIMER'S DISEASE

Alzheimer's disease was named for the German neurologist Alois Alzheimer (1864-1915), who in 1907 first described the characteristic neurofibrillary tangles found in the postmortem brain of a 51-year-old demented woman named Auguste who died in 1906.[114-117] Also referred to as senile dementia Alzheimer's type (SDAT), the disease is a form of progressive dementia in which nerve cells degenerate in the brain and the brain substance shrinks. The hallmark of the disease is the development of abnormal intracellular filaments in tangles of neurofibrils and extracellular deposits of amyloid-forming protein in senile plaques (amyloid plaques) and cerebral blood vessels, as first reported by Alzheimer. The density of these plaques has become the basis for the postmortem diagnosis of Alzheimer's disease; there is no absolute diagnostic test for the disease during life. Alzheimer's disease accounts for 60% to 80% of dementia cases over the age of 65 years. It afflicts 1 in 10 people over the age of 65 years and about half of the population over the age of 85 years.[117]

In addition to its human cost to patient and family, Alzheimer's disease levies a tremendous social and financial burden. Currently, more than 4 million Americans have been diagnosed. The Alzheimer's Association estimates that there may be 14 million cases in the United States by the year 2050 and 22 million cases worldwide. With the rapidly increasing elderly population of persons over 85 years, the healthcare problem of Alzheimer's disease is assuming enormous proportions.

Research into causes and treatment has greatly expanded in recent years. Current reports describe the dis-

TABLE 25-5 Alternative Treatments for Alzheimer's Disease

Product	Description
Vitamin E	Vitamin E is a lipid-soluble vitamin obtained naturally from foods or supplemented. Because of its antioxidative effect, it may aid in the breakdown of free radicals that may be the cause of damage to brain cells. There is no clear evidence that vitamin E can treat Alzheimer's disease; however, it is not thought to be harmful taken in moderation. The U.S. RDA for vitamin E is 30 IU/day.[126,127]
Ginkgo biloba	Ginkgo biloba is plant extract that has both antioxidant and anti-inflammatory properties to protect cell membranes and to regulate neurotransmitter function. Researchers have linked ginkgo biloba with possible improvement in cognition, activities of daily living, and social behavior, although further study is needed to fully understand its potential therapeutic value. One known risk associated with gingko is hemorrhaging if taken with other anticoagulants, because it is known to reduce the ability of the blood to clot.[128]
Huperzine A	Huperzine A is a moss extract traditionally used in Chinese medicine for centuries. It acts as an acetylcholinesterase inhibitor. It has been shown to be just as effective as the leading FDA-approved medications, but it is unregulated and manufactured under no uniform standards. Therefore it is not recommended and is considered dangerous.
Coenzyme Q10	Also known as ubiquinone, coenzyme Q10 is an antioxidant that occurs naturally in the body and is necessary for normal cell reactions. Little is known about coenzyme Q10 and its consideration to treat Alzheimer's disease.

covery of genes for early-onset familial Alzheimer's disease and the more common late-onset form.[118,119] One theory behind the development of SDAT is oxidative stress. Many researchers have investigated this area reviewing flavonoids, antioxidants, and dietary restriction as methods to both prevent the onset of Alzheimer's as well as treat it.[120-122] However, the direct cause remains unknown, and there is still no means of stopping the progressive years of mental and personal decline until death.

This declining progression of Alzheimer's disease has been divided into three broad stages: (1) stage 1, the early period of increasing forgetfulness and anxious depression; (2) stage 2, a middle period of severe memory loss for recent events, disorientation, and personality changes; and (3) stage 3, the final period of severe confusion, psychosis, memory loss, personal neglect, bed-bound, feeding problems, full-time nursing care, and finally death from an infection such as pneumonia.[123]

Medical Management

There is no treatment for the disease itself, except for suitable day-to-day nursing and social care for both the patient and the family. Keeping the patient well nourished, occupied, and physically active helps to lessen anxiety and personal distress, especially in the early stages when the person is sufficiently aware of his or her condition.[124] Some use of antianxiety medication often helps improve difficult behavior and enables the patient to sleep more restfully. Research into drug therapy continues. Family counseling and respite care are essential.

Several medications have met approval of the FDA to manage the symptoms of Alzheimer's disease.[125] These are donepezil (Aricept), rivastigmine (Exelon), tacrine (Cognex), and finally galantamine hydrobromide (Reminyl). A host of alternative treatments for Alzheimer's is also emerging with the millennial trend moving toward "natural medicine." In most cases, there is insufficient scientific evidence backing the majority of products available on the market. The latest news available on some of the more popular products is presented in Table 25-5.

Nutrition Management

Nutrition therapy in each stage of Alzheimer's disease becomes increasingly difficult and challenging. Adequate nutrition throughout the course of the disease is essential to improve physical well-being, help maximize the patient's functioning, and improve the quality of life. Nutrition-related changes occur at each progressive stage of the illness, as shown in Table 25-6, and illustrate the major goals of maintaining adequate nutrition and preventing malnutrition, and devising practical ways of dealing with feeding problems.[129] Because these patients tend to have lower body weight, they require higher energy intakes than normal elderly persons. They often require

amyloid A glycoprotein substance having a relation to starchlike structure but more a protein compound; an abnormal complex material forming characteristic brain deposits of fibrillary tangles always found in postmortem examinations of patients with Alzheimer's disease, the only means of definitive diagnosis; found in various body tissues that, when advanced, form lesions that destroy functional cells and injure the organ.

myasthenia gravis (MG) A progressive neuromuscular disease caused by faulty nerve conduction resulting from the presence of antibodies to acetylcholine receptors at the neuromuscular junction.

TABLE 25-6 Progression of Alzheimer's Disease

Stage	General Symptoms	Nutrition-Related Effects
1 (Early)	Loss of memory Decrease in social and vocational skills Careless work, housekeeping, finances Easily lost Personality changes Recognition of faces Well-oriented to time	Difficulty in shopping, cooking Forgetting to eat Changes in taste and smell Unusual food choices Degeneration of appetite regulation
2 (Middle)	Inability to recall names Disorientation to time Delusions Depression Agitation Language problems	Increased energy requirement from agitation Holding food in mouth Forgetting to swallow Losing ability to use utensils Use spoon only Eating with hands
3 (Final)	Complete disorientation Forgetting own name Not recognizing family Loss of verbal skills Loss of basic self-care skills Urinary and fecal incontinence Bed-bound	No recognition of food Refusal to eat or open mouth for feeding Need for nasogastric feeding

Data from Gray GE: Nutrition and dementia. Copyright by the American Dietetic Association. Reprinted with permission from the *Journal of the American Dietetic Association,* Vol 89(12):1795, 1989.

high-caloric supplements to help supply added nourishment. In general, they have more risk factors and major indicators of poor nutrition status than the overall elderly population.[130] Four major factors help promote optimal intake in long-term care.

1. Using skillful individual feeding techniques
2. Selecting appropriate food consistency
3. Providing adequate time in which to feed
4. Focusing on the midday meal when peak cognitive abilities occur

TO SUM UP

Individuals facing chronic disabling illness and injury confront a myriad of complex challenges, including social, financial, physical, and psychologic barriers. The team approach, involving family and friends in addition to health professionals, becomes an essential basis of care.

The basic principles of nutrition care involve the prevention of malnutrition and restoration of eating ability. The role of the nutritionist is to assess individual nutrition requirements to meet basal energy expenditure (BEE) needs, adjust for metabolic activity factors (MAFs) resulting from any underlying disease process, and consider the requirements to meet physical therapy and other activities. There must be sufficient intake to meet energy and macronutrient requirements. Vitamin and mineral supplements may be needed to guard against deficiencies.

To restore eating ability, the occupational therapist and nurse play significant roles in promoting adequate swallowing, chewing, and hand and utensil use skills. To meet individual nutrient needs, the nutritionist must assess eating skills, estimate eating desire (sensory stimuli, "comfort foods"), and help the client develop new ways of eating with various self-help devices.

Chronic disabling conditions that require special nutrition attention and modification to treat underlying disease effects include (1) musculoskeletal disease, such as various forms of arthritis; (2) neuromuscular injury and disease, caused by a sudden brain or spinal cord injury or a stroke, or by developmental disabilities resulting from cerebral palsy, epilepsy, or spina bifida; and (3) progressive neurologic disorders, such as Parkinson's and Huntington's diseases, ALS, multiple sclerosis, or dementia as seen in Alzheimer's disease.

■ Questions for Review

1. What are the two major goals of rehabilitative therapy for chronic disabling conditions? How do the basic principles of nutrition therapy help meet these goals?
2. Describe the functions of major nutrients in preventing or retarding the catabolic process that often occurs in long-term disabling illness or injury.
3. Select six of the different disease processes or injuries discussed that result in eating disabilities. Describe the

nature of the disease or injury and relate it to disability involved. Outline the medical and nutrition therapy used in each case, giving the rationale for the nutrition management.

References

1. Verbrugge LM et al: The great efficacy of personal and equipment assistance in reducing disability, *Am J Public Health* 87(3):384, 1997.
2. National Center for Health Statistics: *National vital statistics report, United States life tables, 1998,* The Center, February 2001, Washington, DC.
3. Federal Interagency Forum on Aging-Related Statistics: *Older Americans 2000: key indicators of well-being,* 2000, accessible at *http://www.nia.nih.gov/research/extramural/behavior/ifars.htm.*
4. Manton KG, Stallard E, Corder LS: The dynamics of dimensions of age-related disability 1982 to 1994 in the U.S. elderly population, *J Gerontol A Biol Sci Med Sci* 53(1):B59-70, 1998.
5. Doyle R: Stroke mortality in men ages 35 to 74, *Sci Am* 274(3):26, 1996.
6. Hootman J, Helmick C, Schappert S: Characteristics of chronic arthritis and other rheumatic condition-related ambulatory care visits, United States, 1997, *Ann Epidemiol* 10(7):454, 2000.
7. Hochberg MC: What a difference a year makes: reflections on the ACR recommendations for the medical management of osteoarthritis, *Curr Rheumatol Rep* 3:473, 2001.
8. Hochberg MC: Pharmacological therapy of osteoarthritis, *Best Pract Res Clin Rheumatol* 15:583, 2001.
9. Muller-Fassbender H et al: Glucosamine sulfate compared with ibuprofen in osteoarthritis of the knee, *Osteoarthritis Cartilage* 2:61, 1994.
10. Antonelli MAS et al: Herpes zoster in patients with rheumatoid arthritis treated with weekly, low-dose methotrexate, *Am J Med* 90:295, 1991.
11. Tugwell P et al: Combination therapy with cyclosporine and methotrexate in severe rheumatoid arthritis, *N Engl J Med* 333(3):137, 1995.
12. Harris ED: Rheumatoid arthritis: pathophysiology and implications for therapy, *N Engl J Med* 322(18):1277, 1990.
13. Wolman PG: Arthritis. In Gines DJ, ed: *Nutrition management in rehabilitation,* Rockville, Md, 1990, Aspen Publishers.
14. Kremer JM et al: Dietary fish oil and olive oil supplementation in patients with rheumatoid arthritis: clinical and immunologic effects, *Arthritis Rheum* 33(6):810, 1990.
15. Price ME, Dilorio C: Swallowing: a practice guide, *Am J Nurs* 90(7):42, 1990.
16. Agren JJ et al: Divergent changes in serum sterols during a strict uncooked vegan diet in patients with rheumatoid arthritis, *Br J Nutr* 85(2):137, 2001.
17. Muller H, de Toledo FW, Resch KL: Fasting followed by vegetarian diet in patients with rheumatoid arthritis: a systematic review, *Scand J Rheumatol* 30(1):1, 2001.
18. Hanninen O et al: Antioxidants in vegan diet and rheumatic disorders, *Toxicology* 155(1-3):45, 2000.
19. Hannimen O et al: Vegan diet in physiological health promotion, *Acta Physiol Hung* 86(3-4):171, 1999.
20. Westhoff G, Listing J, Zink A: Loss of physical independence in rheumatoid arthritis: interview data from a representative sample of patients in rheumatologic care, *Arthritis Care Res* 13(1):11, 2000.
21. Kanis JA et al: Risk of hip fracture according to the World Health Organization criteria for osteopenia and osteoporosis, *Bone* 27(5):585, 2000.
22. Turner LW, Faile PA, Tomlinson R: Osteoporosis diagnosis and fracture, *Orthop Nurs* 18(5):21, 1999.
23. Wolf RL et al: Update on the epidemiology of osteoporosis, *Curr Rheumatol Rep* 2(1):74, 2000.
24. Snelling AM et al: Modifiable and nonmodifiable factors associated with osteoporosis in postmenopausal women: results from the Third National Health and Nutrition Examination Survey, 1988-1994, *J Womens Health Gend Based Med* 10(1):57, 2001.
25. Prince RL, Kerr DA: What strategies can women use to optimise bone health at this stage of life? *Med J Aust* 173(suppl):S106, 2000.
26. Marchigiano G: Calcium intake in midlife women: one step in preventing osteoporosis, *Orthop Nurse* 18(5):11, 1999.
27. American Heart Association: *Leading causes of death: 1998, biostatistical fact sheet,* Dallas, 2001, The Association.
28. The Dana Alliance for Brain Initiatives, Christopher Reeve Paralysis Foundation: *The facts about spinal cord injury and central nervous system disorders,* 1999, accessible at *http://www.apacure.org.* Statistics published by the University of Alabama National Spinal Cord Injury Statistical Center.
29. TBI state demonstration grants, *J Head Trauma Rehabil* 15(1):750-760, 2000.
30. Lewin ICF: *The cost of disorders of the brain,* Washington, DC, 1992, The National Foundation for the Brain.
31. Pepe JL, Barba CA: The metabolic response to acute traumatic brain injury and implications for nutritional support, *J Head Trauma Rehabil* 14(5):462, 1999.
32. Klodell CT et al: Routine intragastric feeding following traumatic brain injury is safe and well tolerated, *Am J Surg* 179(3):168, 2000.
33. Yanagawa T et al: Nutritional support for head injured patients, *Cochrane Database Syst Rev* (2):CDC001530, 2000.
34. Kirby DF et al: Early enteral nutrition after brain injury by percutaneous endoscopic gastrojejunostomy, *J Parenter Enteral Nutr* 15(3):298, 1991.
35. Weakes E, Elia M: Observations on the patterns of 24-hour energy expenditure change in body composition and gastric emptying in head-injuries patients receiving nasogastric tube feeding, *J Parenter Enteral Nutr* 20(1):31, 1996.
36. Annis K et al: Nutritional support of the severe head-injured patient, *Nutr Clin Pract* 6(6):245, 1991.
37. Silkroski M: Transitional feeding. In *Tube feeding: practical guidelines and nursing protocols,* Gaithersburg, Md, 2001, Aspen Publishers.
38. Yankelson S: Traumatic brain injury. In Gines DJ, ed: *Nutrition management in rehabilitation,* Gaithersburg, Md, 1990, Aspen Publishers.
39. Chiles BW, Cooper PR: Acute spinal injury, *N Engl J Med* 334(8):514, 1996.

40. Rice DR, Max W: Annotation: The high cost of injuries in the United States, *Am J Public Health* 86(1):14, 1996.
41. Berkowitz et al: *Spinal cord injury: an analysis of medical and social costs.* The University of Alabama at Birmingham National Spinal Cord Injury Statistical Center; The National Spinal Cord Injury Association, New York, 1998, Demos Medical Publishing.
42. Cruse JM et al: Review of immune function, healing of pressure ulcers, and nutritional status in patients with spinal cord injury, *J Spinal Cord Med* 23(2):129, 2000.
43. Cruse JM et al: Facilitation of immune function, healing of pressure ulcers, and nutritional status in spinal cord injury patients, *Exp Mol Pathol* 68(1):384, 2000.
44. Monroe MB et al: Lower daily energy expenditure as measured by a respiratory chamber in subjects with spinal cord injury compared with control subjects, *Am J Clin Nutr* 68(6):1223, 1998.
45. Rodriguez DJ, Benzel EC, Clevenger FW: The metabolic response to spinal cord injury, *Spinal Cord* 35(9):599, 1997.
46. Desport JC et al: Total body water and percentage fat mass measurements using bioelectrical impedance analysis and anthropometry in spinal cord-injured patients, *Clin Nutr* 19(3):185, 2000.
47. Rouch W: Are pushy axons a key to spinal cord repair? *Science* 276(5321):1917, 1997.
48. Ruan CM et al: Magnetic resonance imaging of nonhealing pressure ulcers and myocutaneous flaps, *Arch Phys Med Rehabil* 79(9):1080, 1998.
49. Audran M, Legrand E: Hypercalciuria, *Joint Bone Spine* 67(6):509, 2000.
50. HCFA: *Health care financing review: statistical supplement,* Washington, DC, 1999, HCFA.
51. O'Neill PA: Swallowing and prevention of complications, *Br Med Bull* 56(2):457, 2000.
52. Johnson RK et al: Athetosis increases resting metabolic rate in adults with cerebral palsy, *J Am Diet Assoc* 96(2):145, 1996.
53. Johnson RK et al: Total energy expenditure in adults with cerebral palsy as assessed by doubly labeled water, *J Am Diet Assoc* 97(9):966, 1997.
54. Walter A et al: Food safety training needs exist for staff and consumers in a variety of community-based homes for people with developmental disabilities, *J Am Diet Assoc* 97(6):611, 1997.
55. Hogan SE, Evers SE: A multinational rehabilitation program for persons with severe physical and developmental disabilities, *J Am Diet Assoc* 97(2):162, 1997.
56. Lucas BL, Blyler E: Position of the American Dietetic Association: Nutrition in comprehensive program planning for persons with developmental disabilities, *J Am Diet Assoc* 97(2):189, 1997.
57. Stallings VA et al: Body composition in children with spastic quadriplegic cerebral palsy, *J Pediatr* 126:1883, 1995.
58. Smith SW, Camfield C, Camfield P: Living with cerebral palsy and tube feeding: a population-based follow up study, *J Pediatr* 135(3):307, 2000.
59. Harrington M, Lyman B: Special considerations for the pediatric patient. In Silkroski M, Guenter P, ed: *Tube feeding: practical guidelines and nursing protocols,* Gaithersburg, Md, 2001, Aspen Publishers.
60. Krick J et al: Pattern of growth in children with cerebral palsy, *J Am Diet Assoc* 96(7):680, 1996.
61. Ross Laboratories: Estimating stature from the knee height. In Ross Laboratories: *Directions for the Ross knee height caliper,* Columbus, Ohio, 1992, Ross.
62. Johnson RK, Ferrara MS: Estimating stature from knee height for persons with cerebral palsy: an evaluation of estimating equations, *J Am Diet Assoc* 91(10):1283, 1991.
63. Ferrang TM et al: Dietary and anthropomorphic assessment of adults with cerebral palsy, *J Am Diet Assoc* 92(9):1083, 1992.
64. Gonzalez L, Nazario CM, Gonzalez MJ: Nutrition related problems of pediatric patients with neuromuscular disorders, *P R Health Sci J* 19(1):35, 2000.
65. Brodie MJ, Dichter MA: Antiepileptic drugs, *N Engl J Med* 334(2):168, 1996.
66. Motte J et al: Lamotrigine for generalized seizures associated with the Lennox-Gastaut syndrome, *N Engl J Med* 337(25):1807, 1997.
67. Schmidt D, Bourgeois B: A risk-benefit assessment of therapies for Lennox-Gastaut syndrome, *Drug Saf* 22(6):467, 2000.
68. Gasch AT: Use of the traditional ketogenic diet for treatment of intractable epilepsy, *J Am Diet Assoc* 90(10):1433, 1990.
69. Edelstein SF, Chisholm M: Management of intractable childhood seizures using the non-MCT oil ketogenic diet in 20 patients, *J Am Diet Assoc* 96(11):1181, 1996.
70. Sutton M et al: Pediatric diets. In Chicago Dietetic Association and the South Suburban Dietetic Association: *Manual of clinical dietetics,* ed 4, Chicago, 1992, American Dietetic Association.
71. Lary JM, Edmonds LD: Prevalence of spina bifida at birth—United States, 1983-1990: a comparison of two surveillance systems, *MMWR* 45(SS-2):15, 1996.
72. Gross SM et al: Inadequate folic acid intakes are prevalent among young women with neural tube defects, *J Am Diet Assoc* 101(3):342, 2001.
73. Lucock M: Folic acid: nutritional biochemistry, molecular biology, and role in disease processes, *Mol Genet Metab* 71(1-2):121, 2000.
74. Atencio PL et al: Effect of level of lesion and quality of ambulation on growth chart measurements in children with myelomeningocele, *J Am Diet Assoc* 92(7):858, 1992.
75. Dustrude A, Prince A: Provision of optimal nutrition care in myelomeningocele, *Top Clin Nutr* 5(2):34, 1990.
76. Luke A et al: Nutrient intake and obesity in prepubescent children with Down syndrome, *J Am Diet Assoc* 96(12):1262, 1996.
77. Youdim MBH, Riederer P: Understanding Parkinson's disease, *Sci Am* 276(1):52, 1997.
78. Rajput AH: Frequency and cause of Parkinson's disease, *Can J Neurol Sci* 19:103, 1992.
79. Branddmann O et al: Association of the slow acetylator genotype for N-acetyltransferase 2, *Lancet* 350(Oct 18):1136, 1997.
80. Pinero D, Jones B, Beard J: Variations in dietary iron alter behavior in developing rats, *J Nutr* 131(2):311, 2001.
81. Shoham S, Youdim MB: Iron involvement in neural damage and microgliosis in models of neurodegenerative diseases, *Cell Mol Biol* 46(4):743, 2000.

82. Guyton AC: *Textbook of medical physiology,* ed 9, Philadelphia, 1996, WB Saunders.
83. Tsui JKC: Future treatment of Parkinson's disease, *Can J Neurol Sci* 19:160, 1992.
84. Lindvall O et al: Grafts of fetal dopamine neurons survive and improve motor function in Parkinson's disease, *Science* 247:574, 1990.
85. Fackelmann K: Fetal cells thrive in a Parkinsonian brain, *Sci News* 147(17):262, 1995.
86. Vogel G: Gene discovery offers tentative clues to Parkinson's, *Science* 276(5321):1973, 1997.
87. Polymeropoulos MH et al: Mutation in the α-synuclein gene identified in families with Parkinson's disease, *Science* 276(5321):2045, 1997.
88. Ondo WG et al: Weight gain following unilateral pallidotomy in Parkinson's disease, *Acta Neurol Scand* 101(2): 79, 2000.
89. Paré S et al: Effect of daytime protein restriction on nutrient intakes of free-living Parkinson's disease patients, *Am J Clin Nutr* 55:701, 1992.
90. Beyer PI et al: Weight change and body composition in patients with Parkinson's disease, *JAMA* 95(9):979, 1995.
91. Revkin A: Hunting down Huntington's, Discover 14(12): 98, 1993.
92. Wexler NS et al: Huntington's disease in Venezuela and gene kinkage, *Cytogenet Cell Genet* 37:605, 1984.
93. Barinaga M: An intriguing new lead on Huntington's disease, *Science* 271(5253):1233, 1996.
94. Huntington's disease. In Escott-Stump S, ed: *Nutrition and diagnosis-related care,* ed 4, Philadelphia, 1997, Lippincott Williams & Wilkins.
95. Rees JH et al: *Campylobacter jejuni* infection and Guillain-Barré syndrome, *N Engl J Med* 333(21):1374, 1995.
96. A.S.P.E.N. Board of Directors: Guidelines for the use of parenteral and enteral nutrition in adult and pediatric patients, *J Parenter Enteral Nutr* 17(4 suppl):1SA, 1993.
97. McNamara JO, Fridovich I: Did radicals strike Lou Gehrig? *Nature* 362(6415):20, 1993.
98. Rosen DR et al : Mutations in Cu/Zn superoxide dismutase gene are associated with familial amyotrophic lateral sclerosis, *Nature* 362(6415):59, 1993.
99. Marx J: Gene linked to Lou Gehrig's disease, *Science* 259(5100):1393, 1993.
100. Pennisi E: Free-radical scavenger gene tied to ALS, *Sci News* 143(10):148, 1993.
101. Wiedau-Pazas M et al: Altered reactivity of superoxide dismutase in familial amyotrophic lateral sclerosis, *Science* 271(5247):515, 1996.
102. Al-Chalabi A, Leigh PN: Recent advances in amyotrophic lateral sclerosis, *Curr Opin Neurol* 13(4):397, 2000.
103. Berger MM et al: Detection and cellular localization of enterovirus RNA sequences in spinal cord of patients with ALS, *Neurology* 54(1):20, 2000.
104. Hardiman O: Symptomatic treatment of respiratory and nutritional failure in amyotrophic lateral sclerosis, *J Neurol* 247(4):245, 2000.
105. Strong MJ, Rowe A, Rankin RN: Percutaneous gastrojejunostomy in amyotrophic lateral sclerosis, *J Neurol Sci* 169(1-2):128, 1999.
106. Johnson S: The possible role of gradual accumulation of copper, cadmium, lead and iron and gradual depletion of zinc, magnesium, selenium, vitamins B_2, B_6, D, and E and essential fatty acids in multiple sclerosis, *Med Hypotheses* 55(3):239, 2000.
107. Staff: New multiple sclerosis drug clears hurdle, *Sci News* 150(13):199, 1996.
108. Thomas FJ, Wiles CM: Dysphagia and nutritional status in multiple sclerosis, *J Neurol* 246(8):677, 1999.
109. Annoni JM et al: Percutaneous endoscopic gastrostomy in neurological rehabilitation: a report of six cases, *Disabil Rehabil* 20(8):308, 1998.
110. Timmerman GM, Stuifbergin AK: Eating patterns of women with multiple sclerosis, *J Neurosci Nurs* 31(3):152, 1999.
111. Ghadirian P et al: Nutritional factors in the aetiology of multiple sclerosis: a case-control study in Montreal, Canada, *Int J Epidemiol* 27(5):845, 1998.
112. Guyton AC, Hall JE: *Textbook of medical physiology,* ed 9, Philadelphia, 1996, WB Saunders.
113. Dobkin BH: Vital signs—standing tall, *Discover* 15(9):58, 1994.
114. Alzheimer A: Uber eine eigenartige Erkrankung der Hirnrinde, *Allgemeine Zeitschrift fur Psychiatrie* 64:146, 1907. (English translation, *Arch Neurol* 21:109, 1969.)
115. Campion EW: When a mind dies (editorial), *N Engl J Med* 334(12):791, 1996.
116. O'Brien C: Auguste D. and Alzheimer's disease, *Science* 273(5271):28, 1996.
117. Yankner BA, Mesulam M: *m*-Amyloid and the pathogenesis of Alzheimer's disease, *N Engl J Med* 325(26):1849, 1991.
118. Barinaga M: New Alzheimer's gene found, *Science* 2685 (219):1845, 1996.
119. Reiman EM et al: Preclinical evidence of Alzheimer's disease in persons homozygous for the e4 allele for apolipoprotein E, *N Engl J Med* 334(12):752, 1996.
120. Mattson MP: Existing data suggest that Alzheimer's disease is preventable, *Ann N Y Acad Sci* 924:153, 2000.
121. Commenges D et al: Intake of flavonoids and risk of dementia, *Eur J Epidemiol* 16(4):357, 2000.
122. Mattson MP: Emerging neuroprotective strategies for Alzheimer's disease: dietary restriction, telomerase activation, and stem cell therapy, *Exp Gerontol* 35(4):489, 2000.
123. Gray GE: Nutrition and dementia, *J Am Diet Assoc* 89(12):1795, 1989.
124. Rolland Y et al: Feasibility of regular physical exercise for patients with moderate to severe Alzheimer's disease, *J Nutr Health Aging* 4(2):109, 2000.
125. Marx J: Searching for drugs that combat Alzheimer's, *Science* 273(5271):29, 1996.
126. National Institutes of Medicine Update, *N Engl J Med* April 24, 1997.
127. Miller JW: Vitamin E and memory: is it vascular protection? *Nutr Rev* 58(4):109, 2000.
128. LeBars PL et al: A placebo-controlled, double-blind, randomized trial of an extract of Ginkgo biloba for dementia: North American EGb study group, *JAMA* 278(16):1327-1332, 1997.
129. Poehlman ET, Dvorak RV: Energy expenditure in Alzheimer's disease, *J Nutr Health Aging* 2(2):155, 1998.

130. Renvall NJ et al: Nutritional care of ambulatory residents in special care units for Alzheimer's patients, *J Nutr Elderly* 12(4):5, 1993.

Further Reading

In addition to the web listings and the references mentioned at the end of the text, the following is a summary of some additional resources that may prove helpful.

Thornton H, Jackson D, Turner-Stokes L: Accuracy of prediction of walking for young stroke patients by use of the FIM, *Physiother Res Int* 6(1):14, 2001.

This article scientifically evaluates the commonly used FIM, or Functional Independence Measure, for its precision and identifies factors influencing accuracy.

Halstead LS: The John Stanley Coulter lecture: the power of compassion and caring in rehabilitation healing, *Arch Phys Med Rehabil* 82(2):149, 2001.

This article is an excellent and timely review of the complementary and alternative side of medicine as it relates to rehabilitation. The authors review seven articles from the literature and provide examples of research-based interventions with potential for enhancing outcomes in traditional rehabilitation populations.

Ahronheim JC, Moreno JD, Zuckerman C: *Ethics in clinical practice,* ed 2, Gaithersburg, Md, 2000, Aspen Publishers.

This text is a must-have for any practicing clinician interested in the ethical questions facing our society today. It covers an array of topics and contains 31 case studies with detailed question and answer format following each case.

Shoham S, Youdim MB: Iron involvement in neural damage and microgliosis in models of neurodegenertive diseases, *Cell Mol Biol* 46(4):743, 2000.

This is an excellent article that explains the study of iron accumulation at sites of the brain. Among the diseases mentioned are Parkinson's disease, Huntington's chorea, and multiple sclerosis.

Yanagawa T et al: Nutritional support for head-injured patients (Cochrane Review). In: The Cochrane Library, 2, 2001, Oxford, Update Software.

This review from Japan suggests that early enteral feeding may be associated with better outcomes in terms of survival and disability. Because enteral nutrition support is commonly required for patients sustaining injury or with chronic illness, it is crucial that the caregiver have some understanding of its relevance.

Websites of Interest

http://www.alz.org Alzheimer's Association
http://www.aesnet.org American Epilepsy Society
http://www.americanheart.org American Heart Association and Stroke 2000 Statistical Update
http://www.biausa.org The Brain Injury Association
http://www.apacure.org Christopher Reeve Paralysis Foundation
http://www.efa.org Epilepsy Foundation of America
http://www.hdsa.org Huntington's Disease Society of America
http://www.myasthenia.org Myasthenia Gravis Foundation of America
http://www.nichcy.org National Information Center for Children and Youth with Disabilities (NICHCY)
http://www.nih.gov/nia National Institutes of Health, National Institute on Aging
http://www.nationalmssociety.org National Multiple Sclerosis Society
http://www.nof.org National Osteoporosis Foundation
http://www.spinalcord.org National Spinal Cord Injury Association
http://www.ed.gov/offices/OSERS/IDEA/index.html Office of Special Education Programs (OSEP) at the United States Department of Education
http://www.pdf.ofg Parkinson's Disease Foundation, Inc.
http://www.sbaa.org Spina Bifida Association of America
http://www.ucp.org United Cerebral Palsy
http://www.wfnals.org World Federation of Neurology
http://www.wpda.org World Parkinson's Disease Association

CASE STUDY

Managing nutritional status with homemade tube feeding formula

Charles, a 30-year-old white man with Baltic myoclonic epilepsy for 15 years, was ordered by the home care agency to have a nutrition consultation. He was unable to communicate and had a PEG tube for feeding and 24-hour nursing care at home. Charles had a stage III pressure ulcer and was on a therapeutic bed at a 45-degree angle. He was repositioned every 2 hours to aid in wound healing/prevent further decline. His medical history was significant for hemolytic anemia due to antiseizure medications, fevers, and electrolyte imbalances from fluid overload.

Charles was well supported by family and healthcare professionals. His family heritage was Italian, and his mother loved to cook and nurture her son. Therefore she prepared his tube feeding from scratch every few days. It consisted of a hearty soup that was pureed and put through a mesh strainer and was well tolerated by the patient.

Tube Feeding Formula

Water	Dry skim milk powder
Olive oil	Meatloaf mix
Garlic ground turkey/chicken	Yellow squash
Beans	Aloe vera
Tempeh	Tomato
Sweet potato	Apple
Zucchini	Eggplant
Tofu	Wheat germ
Flax seed	Rice
Soy protein	Liquid skim milk

He received approximately 2 quarts of feeding/day, which was estimated to provide 2300 calories and 75 g of protein.

He also received approximately 200 ml of water every 4 hours and the tube was flushed with 50 ml of water after all food and medications were administered. His fluid was restricted to no greater than 3000 ml/day, and the nurses indicated that it was sometimes difficult to achieve less than this amount due to his number of medications. Nursing provided range of motion exercises daily, but he received no other physical rehabilitative therapy.

His medications included phenobarbital q8h, 60 mg QD and 90 mg BID; valproic acid 120 mg q6h; Pepcid 20 mg BID; Klonopin 4 mg TID; Dilantin 100 mg q8h; Colace 15 ml QD; Proventil inhaler via trach q8h; folic acid 2 mg; KCl 30 mEq; Ferrum phosphate QD; and a bowel regimen with milk of magnesia and Dulcolax as needed.

His laboratory study results at the initial assessment included Ca 8.1 mg/dl ↓, Phos 2.8 mg/dl, Alb 2.7 g/dl ↓, H/H 10.5 g/dl ↓/30.2% ↓, Chol 115 mg/dl ↓, Na 128 mEq/l ↓, K 4.2 mEq/l, Gluc 59 mg/dl ↓, Dilantin 6.7 μg/ml ↓, Zn 22 μg/dl ↓, Fe 48 μg/dl.

Charles was 6 ft 0 in tall and weighed approximately 155 lb. It was suspected that he had lost weight in the last year, but the amount was unknown because he had no bed scale. His ideal weight was 172 lb. Estimated requirements for anabolism were 3017 calories, 126 g of protein, and approximately 3000 ml of fluid per day. In light of his pressure ulcer, moderately depleted visceral protein stores (partly dilutional), low cholesterol, and recent weight loss, the following was suggested to the family.

1. Use whole milk and additional oil instead of water when preparing food to increase calories.
2. If whole milk and additional oil are tolerated yet there is no weight change, increase to heavy cream to provide more calories but not additional volume from free water to prevent hyponatremia and fluid overload.
3. Add an MVI without Fe to ensure adequate nutrient intake.
4. Change the FePhos to $FeSO_4$.
5. Add 220 mg $ZnSO_4$ BID and an additional 500 mg vitamin C to facilitate wound healing.
6. Increase Dilantin: be sure to give it 1 hour after and 2 hours before feeding.
7. Keep accurate I/O reports.

Family and agency were instructed to call the registered dietitian with questions or concerns.

At a 6-month follow up, the dietitian found that all of the recommendations were instituted as suggested. Laboratory study results were as follows: Alb 3.0 g/dl ↓, Na 139 mEq/l, K 4.9 mEq/l, Cl 100 mEq/l, CO_2 31 mEq/l, BUN 12 mg/dl, Cr 0.3 mg/dl ↓, Glu 96 mg/dl, Chol 130 mg/dl ↓, H/H 11.6 g/dl ↓/33.0% ↓, Dilantin 11.5 μg/ml.

At this stage, Charles had a debridement of his stage III pressure ulcer and was granulating tissue well. He appeared to be gaining weight according to a subjective nursing assessment. His estimated weight at this juncture was 180 lb, and the nurses reported difficulty in turning him due to the weight gain. The tube feeding was unchanged except for the addition of heavy cream in place of milk. There was an increase in constipation and a recent urinary tract infection reported. He appeared nonedematous and comfortable. His abdomen was soft, but the family was complaining that he looked "pudgy." His estimated needs decreased to approximately 2300 calories and 95 g of protein per day with the 25-lb weight gain.

Lactulose was added to his bowel regimen as an as-needed medication; however, nurses reported using it almost daily because the other medications were not treating his high impactions. There was also a question of consistent care in turning him and giving bowel medications as prescribed. He continued to tolerate his homemade tube feeding without other apparent problems.

The dietitian recommended the following.

1. Continue medications and supplements as ordered.
2. Give 120 ml of warm prune juice via G-tube and flush with 50 ml of water.
3. Warm tube feeding rather than administering cold from refrigerator to aid in bowel stimulation.
4. Change to low-fat (2%) milk for preparing tube feeding.
5. Maintain adequate flushing to prevent dehydration and constipation, but keep careful I/O reports to prevent edema.
6. Ensure that all staff maintain a consistent turning schedule and range of motion activities.

QUESTIONS FOR ANALYSIS

1. What can the registered dietitian do if a question of inconsistent care becomes an issue in the home? With whom should she speak first?
2. What is the best way to calculate a homemade tube feeding formula? Did the homemade formula meet his needs and provide adequate nutrients? Was it necessary for the mother to prepare a tube feeding formula for her son?
3. How accurate are the estimated requirements if height and weight cannot be adequately obtained? Are there other methods the registered dietitian could have used to track his progress?
4. What other ways could the constipation have been managed? What do you feel was the greatest cause of the constipation?
5. Why did his serum albumin level remain low given the amount of protein he received from his tube feeding? Should the registered dietitian have ordered other laboratory studies to assess protein status?

Issues & ANSWERS

Special Education for Special Kids

Advances in technology, science, and medicine have made it possible for more children with disabilities to function in the public education system. More children are able to complete an education than ever before. By law, all eligible school-aged children and youth with disabilities are entitled to receive a free appropriate public education (FAPE). The federal law that supports special education and related service programming for children and youth with disabilities is called the Individuals with Disabilities Education Act (IDEA). IDEA was formerly known as EHA or Education for the Handicapped Act, which was enacted in 1975. EHA has a long history of amendments to improve the services that it covers, including special funding incentives for states to make FAPE available for all school-aged children with disabilities ages 3 through 5. Provisions were also included to help states develop early intervention programs for infants and toddlers with disabilities.

In 1990, among the amendments to the EHA was a name change to the IDEA. One primary purpose of the IDEA is to ensure that all children with disabilities have available to them a "free appropriate public education" that emphasizes special education and related services designed to meet their unique needs and prepare them for employment and independent living. This means that services are provided at public expense, under public supervision and direction, and without charge. Disabilities include mental retardation, hearing impairment or deafness, speech or language impairment, visual impairment or blindness, serious emotional disturbance, orthopedic impairment, autism, traumatic brain injury, or specific learning disability.

Special education is defined as instruction that is specially designed, at no cost to caregivers, to meet a child's unique needs. Specially designed means adapting the content, methodology, or delivery of instruction making it possible for the child to meet certain standards of education that apply to all children within the jurisdiction of the public agency. Special education can be conducted in the classroom, the home, hospital, institutions, and other settings. Special education must be provided to students in what is known as the least restrictive environment. Some related services also covered under this law include speech-language pathology and audiology; psychologic, physical and occupational therapy; therapeutic recreation; early identification and assessment of childhood disabilities, counseling services for students as well as parents or caregivers; orientation and mobility services; and social work in schools.

Final regulations currently guiding the school systems in how they design and implement their special education and related services were published in the 1997 IDEA Amendments document located in the Federal Register. Because state policies can vary widely, caregivers are encouraged to obtain a copy of their state's policy either through the school district or the state director of special education. The National Information Center for Children and Youth with Disabilities (NICHCY), located in Washington, DC, is another resource for caregivers and students. The IDEA, its amendments, and regulations, can be obtained by contacting The Office of Special Education Programs (OSEP) at the United States Department of Education.

REFERENCES

Assistance to states for the education of children with disabilities and the early intervention program for infants and toddlers with disabilities; Final regulations. United States Department of Education, *Federal Register* 64(48):12406-12671, March 12, 1999.

Family Educational Rights and Privacy Act (P.L. 93-380), *Code of Federal Regulations*, Title 34, Part 99, 1988.

Flippo KF, Inge KJ, Barcus JM: *Assistive technology: a resource for school, work, and community*, Baltimore, Md, 1995, Paul H. Brookes.

Individuals with Disabilities Education Act Amendments of 1997 (P.L. 105-17), 20 U.S.C. Chapter 33, Sections 1400-1485, 1997.

Report to accompany S. 717. Committee on Labor and Human Resources. Washington, DC, 1997, GPO.

APPENDIXES

Appendix

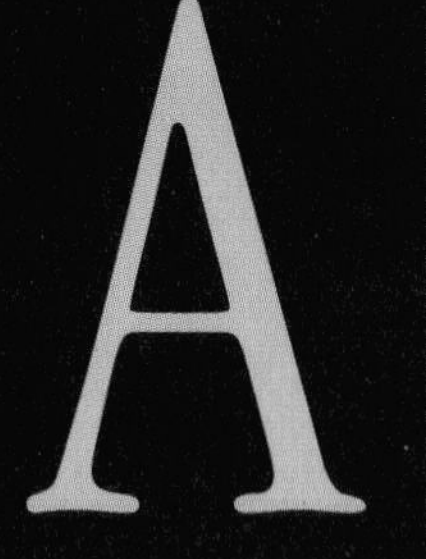

Food Composition Table

The following Food Composition Table was developed by SureQuest Systems, Inc., and includes all of the foods listed in *Mosby's NutriTrac Nutrition Analysis CD-ROM, Version III,* which accompanies every copy of this text. Please note, however, that you will be able to find some nutrient information in *Mosby's NutriTrac Nutrition Analysis CD-ROM* that is not listed here in the Food Composition Table.

USDA ID Code	Food Name	Weight in Grams*	Quantity of Units	Unit of Measure	Protein (gm)	Fat (gm)	Carbohydrate (gm)	Kcalories	Caffeine (gm)	Fiber (gm)	Cholesterol (mg)	Saturated Fat (gm)
	Babyfood, Applesauce	170.0000	3.000	Ounce	0.00	0.00	17.51	62.90	0.00	2.89	0.00	0.00
	Babyfood, Bananas w/ Tapioca	170.0000	3.000	Ounce	0.68	0.34	30.26	113.90	0.00	2.72	0.00	0.14
	Babyfood, Barley, Ppd w/ Whole Milk	28.3500	3.000	Ounce	1.30	0.94	4.62	31.47	0.00	0.00	0.00	0.00
	Babyfood, Beef	71.0000	3.000	Ounce	10.30	3.48	0.00	75.26	0.00	0.00	19.53	1.84
	Babyfood, Beef and Rice	170.0000	3.000	Ounce	8.50	4.93	14.96	139.40	0.00	0.00	0.00	0.00
	Babyfood, Beef Lasagna	170.0000	3.000	Ounce	7.14	3.57	17.00	130.90	0.00	0.00	0.00	0.00
	Babyfood, Beef Noodle	170.0000	3.000	Ounce	4.25	3.23	12.58	96.90	0.00	1.87	13.60	1.31
	Babyfood, Beef Stew	170.0000	3.000	Ounce	8.67	2.04	9.35	86.70	0.00	1.87	21.30	0.99
	Babyfood, Beets	224.0000	1.000	Cup	2.91	0.22	17.25	76.16	0.00	4.26	0.00	0.04
	Babyfood, Carrots	224.0000	1.000	Cup	1.79	0.45	16.13	71.68	0.00	3.81	0.00	0.09
	Babyfood, Chicken	71.0000	3.000	Ounce	10.44	6.82	0.00	105.79	0.00	0.00	41.68	1.75
	Babyfood, Chicken Noodle	170.0000	3.000	Ounce	4.03	2.01	14.94	93.50	0.00	1.53	15.30	0.58
	Babyfood, Chicken Soup	229.0000	1.000	Cup	3.66	3.89	16.49	114.50	0.00	2.52	9.16	0.64
	Babyfood, Chicken Sticks	71.0000	3.000	Ounce	10.37	10.22	0.99	133.48	0.00	0.14	55.38	2.90
	Babyfood, Cookies, Arrowroot	28.3500	1.000	Ounce	2.15	4.05	20.19	125.31	0.00	0.06	0.30	0.94
	Babyfood, Corn, Creamed	240.0000	1.000	Cup	3.36	0.96	39.12	156.00	0.00	5.04	2.40	0.17
	Babyfood, Cottage Cheese w/ Fruit	28.3500	3.000	Ounce	0.85	0.20	4.51	22.11	0.00	0.00	0.00	0.00
	Babyfood, Egg Yolks	28.3500	3.000	Ounce	2.84	4.90	0.28	57.55	0.00	0.00	208.37	1.47
	Babyfood, Egg Yolks and Bacon	170.0000	3.000	Ounce	4.25	8.50	10.54	134.30	0.00	1.53	159.80	2.79
	Babyfood, Fruit Dessert	170.0000	3.000	Ounce	0.51	0.00	29.24	107.10	0.00	1.02	0.00	0.00
	Babyfood, Green Beans	240.0000	1.000	Cup	2.88	0.24	13.68	60.00	0.00	4.56	0.00	0.05
	Babyfood, Ham	71.0000	3.000	Ounce	10.72	4.76	0.00	88.75	0.00	0.00	20.66	1.59
	Babyfood, Juice, Apple	131.0000	4.200	Fl Oz	0.00	0.13	15.33	61.57	0.00	0.13	0.00	0.03
	Babyfood, Juice, Mixed Fruit	127.0000	3.000	Ounce	0.13	0.13	14.73	59.69	0.00	0.13	0.00	0.03
	Babyfood, Juice, Orange	127.0000	3.000	Ounce	0.76	0.38	12.95	55.88	0.00	0.13	0.00	0.05
	Babyfood, Macaroni and Cheese	170.0000	3.000	Ounce	4.42	3.40	13.94	103.70	0.00	0.51	10.20	2.01
	Babyfood, Macaroni and Tomato and Beef	170.0000	3.000	Ounce	4.25	1.87	15.98	100.30	0.00	1.87	6.80	0.70
	Babyfood, Meat Sticks	71.0000	3.000	Ounce	9.51	10.37	0.78	130.64	0.00	0.14	49.70	4.13
	Babyfood, Mixed Vegetable	170.0000	3.000	Ounce	1.70	0.00	13.43	56.10	0.00	0.00	0.00	0.00
	Babyfood, Noodles and Chicken	170.0000	3.000	Ounce	2.89	3.74	15.47	108.80	0.00	1.87	0.00	0.00
	Babyfood, Peach Cobbler	220.0000	3.000	Ounce	0.66	0.00	40.26	147.40	0.00	1.54	0.00	0.00
	Babyfood, Peach Melba	28.3500	3.000	Ounce	0.09	0.00	4.65	17.01	0.00	0.00	0.00	0.00
	Babyfood, Peaches w/ Sugar	170.0000	3.000	Ounce	0.85	0.34	32.13	120.70	0.00	2.55	0.00	0.03
	Babyfood, Pears	170.0000	3.000	Ounce	0.51	0.17	19.72	73.10	0.00	6.12	0.00	0.02
	Babyfood, Peas, Buttered	28.3500	3.000	Ounce	0.99	0.37	3.20	17.01	0.00	0.00	0.00	0.00

The easiest way to look for a food is to use the "Search For" feature in *Mosby's NutriTrac Nutrition Analysis CD-ROM.* However, if you do not have access to a computer or your computer time is limited, you can easily look for a food using this Food Composition Table. The foods in the table are arranged alphabetically within groups.

The code number before each food listing corresponds to the food data bank in *Mosby's NutriTrac Nutrition Analysis CD-ROM.* When you input your dietary intake into the CD-ROM program, you may choose to use these code numbers. Alternatively, you may choose to enter your dietary intake into *Mosby's NutriTrac Nutrition Analysis CD-ROM* by typing the name or partial name of a food and using the "Search For" option.

Column heading key: *gm* = grams; *mg* = milligrams; *mcg* = micrograms; *re* = retinol equivalent.
*Please note that the "Weight in Grams" column provides the weight in grams of the serving or of one unit of measure. (For example, if a serving is 3 ounces, the "Weight in Grams" column may indicate the weight of 1 ounce.)

Monounsaturated Fat (gm)	Polyunsaturated Fat (gm)	Vitamin D (mg)	Vitamin K (mg)	Vitamin E (mg)	Vitamin A (re)	Vitamin C (mg)	Thiamin (mg)	Riboflavin (mg)	Niacin (mg)	Vitamin B_6 (mg)	Folate (mg)	Vitamin B_{12} (mcg)	Calcium (mg)	Iron (mg)	Magnesium (mg)	Phosphorus (mg)	Potassium (mg)	Sodium (mg)	Zinc (mg)
0.00	0.00	0.00	0.00	1.02	1.70	64.26	0.02	0.05	0.10	0.05	2.89	0.00	8.50	0.37	5.10	10.20	130.90	3.40	0.07
0.03	0.07	0.00	0.00	1.02	6.80	43.69	0.03	0.03	0.37	0.24	10.88	0.00	13.60	0.51	20.40	15.30	183.60	15.30	0.12
0.00	0.00	0.00	0.00	0.00	0.00	0.00	0.14	0.16	1.70	0.03	2.52	0.09	65.21	3.50	8.51	42.53	54.43	13.89	0.24
1.31	0.11	0.00	0.00	0.28	22.01	1.35	0.01	0.11	2.33	0.09	4.05	1.04	5.68	1.17	6.39	51.12	134.90	46.86	1.42
0.00	0.00	0.00	0.00	0.00	134.30	6.63	0.03	0.12	2.28	0.24	10.20	0.87	18.70	1.17	13.60	59.50	204.00	606.90	1.56
0.00	0.00	0.00	0.00	0.00	265.20	3.23	0.12	0.15	2.30	0.12	10.20	0.87	30.60	1.48	18.70	68.00	207.40	771.80	1.19
1.43	0.15	0.00	0.00	0.68	149.60	2.38	0.05	0.07	0.99	0.05	20.40	0.17	13.60	0.73	11.90	51.00	78.20	28.90	0.68
0.75	0.17	0.00	0.00	0.41	425.00	5.10	0.02	0.12	2.23	0.12	10.20	0.87	15.30	1.22	18.70	74.80	241.40	586.50	1.48
0.04	0.09	0.00	0.00	1.16	6.72	5.38	0.02	0.09	0.29	0.04	68.99	0.00	31.36	0.72	31.36	31.36	407.68	185.92	0.27
0.02	0.20	0.00	0.00	1.16	2645.44	12.32	0.04	0.09	1.12	0.18	38.75	0.00	51.52	0.87	24.64	44.80	452.48	109.76	0.40
3.07	1.65	0.00	0.00	0.28	8.52	1.07	0.01	0.11	2.43	0.13	7.88	0.28	39.05	0.70	7.81	63.90	86.62	36.21	0.72
0.80	0.46	0.00	0.00	0.31	294.10	0.17	0.05	0.07	1.19	0.09	11.90	0.02	35.70	0.65	11.90	134.30	66.30	132.60	0.68
0.98	2.06	0.00	0.00	0.55	393.88	2.29	0.05	0.07	0.66	0.09	11.91	0.27	84.73	0.62	11.45	54.96	151.14	36.64	0.50
4.45	2.12	0.00	0.00	0.28	2.13	1.21	0.01	0.14	1.43	0.07	7.88	0.28	51.83	1.11	9.94	85.91	75.26	340.09	0.72
2.55	0.24	0.00	0.00	0.00	0.00	1.56	0.14	0.12	1.63	0.01	9.92	0.02	9.07	0.85	6.24	32.89	44.23	104.90	0.15
0.29	0.43	0.00	0.00	1.25	19.20	5.28	0.02	0.12	1.20	0.10	30.48	0.05	43.20	0.65	19.20	79.20	194.40	124.80	0.55
0.00	0.00	0.00	0.00	0.17	0.57	6.75	0.00	0.01	0.01	0.00	1.45	0.02	8.79	0.04	1.13	11.06	11.91	14.46	0.05
1.96	0.64	0.00	0.00	0.22	106.60	0.40	0.02	0.08	0.01	0.05	26.11	0.44	21.55	0.78	1.98	81.36	21.83	11.06	0.54
3.76	1.09	0.00	0.00	0.46	47.60	1.53	0.09	0.14	0.46	0.05	6.97	0.15	47.60	0.80	8.50	85.00	59.50	81.60	0.46
0.00	0.00	0.00	0.00	0.39	40.80	5.10	0.03	0.02	0.24	0.05	5.95	0.00	15.30	0.36	8.50	13.60	161.50	22.10	0.09
0.00	0.12	0.00	0.00	1.25	103.20	20.16	0.05	0.24	0.77	0.10	78.48	0.00	156.00	2.59	52.80	45.60	307.20	4.80	0.46
2.26	0.65	0.00	0.00	0.28	7.10	1.49	0.10	0.13	2.02	0.14	1.49	0.07	3.55	0.72	7.81	63.19	149.10	47.57	1.21
0.00	0.04	0.00	0.00	0.79	2.62	75.85	0.01	0.03	0.10	0.04	0.13	0.00	5.24	0.75	3.93	6.55	119.21	3.93	0.04
0.01	0.05	0.00	0.00	0.25	5.08	80.77	0.03	0.01	0.15	0.05	8.51	0.00	10.16	0.43	6.35	6.35	128.27	5.08	0.04
0.06	0.08	0.00	0.00	0.76	7.62	79.38	0.06	0.04	0.30	0.06	33.53	0.00	15.24	0.22	11.43	13.97	233.68	1.27	0.08
0.90	0.22	0.00	0.00	0.41	5.10	2.21	0.10	0.10	0.94	0.03	18.70	0.05	86.70	0.51	11.90	100.30	74.80	129.20	0.54
0.77	0.14	0.00	0.00	0.41	185.30	2.55	0.09	0.10	1.28	0.09	15.30	0.41	23.80	0.61	11.90	74.80	122.40	28.90	0.61
4.60	1.13	0.00	0.00	0.28	14.91	1.70	0.04	0.12	1.05	0.06	6.32	0.21	24.14	0.98	7.81	73.13	80.94	388.37	1.35
0.00	0.00	0.00	0.00	0.00	414.80	5.61	0.02	0.03	0.70	0.14	11.39	0.00	28.90	0.53	17.00	37.40	190.40	15.30	0.41
0.00	0.00	0.00	0.00	0.00	221.00	1.36	0.07	0.07	1.16	0.03	5.78	0.15	44.20	0.83	18.70	56.10	100.30	44.20	0.54
0.00	0.00	0.00	0.00	0.51	30.80	45.10	0.02	0.04	0.57	0.02	2.42	0.00	8.80	0.22	4.40	13.20	123.20	19.80	0.07
0.00	0.00	0.00	0.00	0.00	5.67	7.37	0.00	0.01	0.08	0.00	0.54	0.00	3.12	0.09	0.57	1.42	26.37	2.55	0.08
0.12	0.15	0.00	0.00	1.02	30.60	32.13	0.02	0.05	1.11	0.03	6.63	0.00	8.50	0.46	8.50	18.70	263.50	8.50	0.10
0.03	0.03	0.00	0.00	1.02	5.10	37.40	0.02	0.05	0.32	0.02	6.46	0.00	13.60	0.43	15.30	20.40	195.50	3.40	0.14
0.00	0.00	0.00	0.00	0.00	11.62	3.60	0.02	0.02	0.39	0.00	10.26	0.00	12.76	0.29	0.00	0.00	33.17	1.42	0.00

USDA ID Code	Food Name	Weight in Grams*	Quantity of Units	Unit of Measure	Protein (gm)	Fat (gm)	Carbohydrate (gm)	Kcalories	Caffeine (gm)	Fiber (gm)	Cholesterol (mg)	Saturated Fat (gm)
	Babyfood, Plums w/ Tapioca	170.0000	3.000	Ounce	0.17	0.00	34.68	125.80	0.00	2.04	0.00	0.00
	Babyfood, Rice, Ppd w/ Whole Mil	28.3500	1.000	Ounce	1.11	1.02	4.73	32.60	0.00	0.02	3.21	0.66
	Babyfood, Rice, w/ Mixed Fruit	170.0000	3.000	Ounce	1.53	0.34	31.11	134.30	0.00	1.02	0.00	0.10
	Babyfood, Spaghetti and Tomato a	170.0000	3.000	Ounce	4.37	2.33	19.41	115.60	0.00	1.87	8.50	0.92
	Babyfood, Spinach, Creamed	28.3500	3.000	Ounce	0.85	0.40	1.81	11.91	0.00	0.51	0.00	0.00
	Babyfood, Split Pea and Ham	28.3500	3.000	Ounce	0.94	0.37	3.20	20.13	0.00	0.31	0.00	0.00
	Babyfood, Squash	224.0000	1.000	Cup	1.79	0.45	12.54	53.76	0.00	4.70	0.00	0.09
	Babyfood, Sweet potatoes	224.0000	1.000	Cup	2.46	0.22	31.14	134.40	0.00	3.36	0.00	0.04
	Babyfood, Teething Biscuits	28.3500	1.000	Ounce	3.03	1.19	21.66	111.13	0.00	0.40	0.00	0.43
	Babyfood, Tropical Fruit	113.0000	3.000	Ounce	0.23	0.00	18.53	67.80	0.00	0.00	0.00	0.00
	Babyfood, Turkey	71.0000	3.000	Ounce	10.93	5.04	0.00	91.59	0.00	0.00	37.70	1.64
	Babyfood, Turkey and Rice	170.0000	3.000	Ounce	4.03	1.56	16.27	95.20	0.00	1.70	6.80	0.41
	Babyfood, Turkey Sticks	71.0000	3.000	Ounce	9.73	10.08	0.99	129.22	0.00	0.36	46.15	2.94
	Bagels, Blueberry	56.7000	1.000	Each	5.96	0.90	30.28	155.92	0.00	1.30	0.00	0.12
	Bagels, Cinnamon-raisin	56.7000	1.000	Each	5.56	0.96	31.30	155.36	0.00	1.30	0.00	0.16
	Bagels, Cinnamon-raisin, Toasted	56.7000	1.000	Each	6.02	1.02	33.62	166.70	0.00	1.42	0.00	0.18
	Bagels, Egg	56.7000	1.000	Each	6.02	1.20	30.06	157.62	0.00	1.30	13.60	0.24
	Bagels, Egg, Toasted	66.0000	1.000	Each	7.52	1.45	37.62	197.34	0.00	0.00	17.16	0.30
	Bagels, Oat Bran	56.7000	1.000	Each	6.06	0.68	30.22	144.58	0.00	2.04	0.00	0.10
	Bagels, Oat Bran, Toasted	66.0000	1.000	Each	7.59	0.86	37.82	180.84	0.00	0.00	0.00	0.14
	Bagels, Plain	56.7000	1.000	Each	5.96	0.90	30.28	155.92	0.00	1.30	0.00	0.12
	Bagels, Plain, Toasted	66.0000	1.000	Each	7.46	1.12	37.95	194.70	0.00	0.00	0.00	0.16
	Biscuits, Plain or Buttermilk	56.7000	1.000	Each	7.04	9.36	27.50	206.38	0.00	0.74	0.56	1.42
	Cake, Angelfood	28.3500	1.000	Slice	1.67	0.23	16.39	73.14	0.00	0.43	0.00	0.03
	Cake, Boston Cream Pie	28.3500	1.000	Slice	0.68	2.41	12.16	71.44	0.00	0.40	10.49	0.69
	Cake, Carrot, w/ Cream Cheese Frosting	111.0000	1.000	Slice	5.11	29.30	52.39	483.96	0.00	0.00	59.94	5.43
	Cake, Chocolate w/ Chocolate Fro	28.3500	1.000	Slice	1.16	4.65	15.48	104.04	0.00	0.79	11.91	1.35
124	Cake, Chocolate, Double, Layer-S	79.0000	1.000	Piece	3.00	13.00	33.00	260.00	0.00	2.00	25.00	11.00
125	Cake, Chocolate, German, Layer-S	83.0000	1.000	Piece	4.00	15.00	34.00	280.00	0.00	2.00	30.00	11.00
126	Cake, Coconut Layer -Sara Lee	81.0000	1.000	Piece	3.00	14.00	34.00	280.00	0.00	2.00	30.00	12.00
	Cake, Fruitcake	28.3500	1.000	Slice	0.82	2.58	17.46	91.85	0.00	1.05	1.42	0.30
127	Cake, Fudge Golden Layer-Sara Le	80.0000	1.000	Piece	3.00	13.00	34.00	270.00	0.00	1.00	25.00	11.00
	Cake, German Chocolate, w/ Frost	111.0000	1.000	Slice	3.89	20.65	55.17	404.04	0.00	0.00	53.28	5.26
	Cake, Gingerbread	67.0000	1.000	Slice	2.68	6.83	33.97	207.03	0.00	2.14	23.45	1.74
	Cake, Pineapple Upside-down	28.3500	1.000	Slice	0.99	3.43	14.32	90.44	0.00	0.23	6.24	0.83
	Cake, Pound	30.0000	1.000	Slice	1.65	5.97	14.64	116.40	0.00	0.15	66.30	3.47
128	Cake, Pound, All Butter, Family	76.0000	1.000	Piece	4.00	17.00	36.00	310.00	0.00	0.50	75.00	9.00
129	Cake, Pound, All Butter-Sara Lee	76.0000	1.000	Piece	4.00	16.00	38.00	320.00	0.00	0.50	85.00	9.00
130	Cake, Pound, Chocolate Swirl-Sar	83.0000	1.000	Piece	5.00	16.00	42.00	330.00	0.00	0.50	75.00	8.00
131	Cake, Pound, Reduced, Fat-Sara L	76.0000	1.000	Piece	4.00	11.00	42.00	280.00	0.00	1.00	65.00	3.00
132	Cake, Pound, Strawberry Swirl-Sa	83.0000	1.000	Piece	4.00	11.00	44.00	290.00	0.00	0.50	60.00	3.00
	Cake, Sponge	28.3500	1.000	Slice	1.53	0.77	17.32	81.93	0.00	0.16	28.92	0.23
133	Cake, Vanilla Layer-Sara Lee	80.0000	1.000	Piece	2.00	13.00	31.00	250.00	0.00	0.00	35.00	10.00
	Cake, White, w/ Coconut Frosting	28.3500	1.000	Slice	1.25	2.92	17.92	100.93	0.00	0.28	0.28	1.11
134	Cake, White, w/o Frosting	74.0000	1.000	Slice	4.00	9.18	42.33	264.18	0.00	0.00	1.48	2.42
	Cake, Yellow, w/ Chocolate Frost	28.3500	1.000	Slice	1.08	4.93	15.71	107.45	0.00	0.51	15.59	1.32
	Cake, Yellow, w/ Vanilla Frostin	28.3500	1.000	Slice	0.99	4.11	16.67	105.75	0.00	0.09	15.59	0.67
169	Cheesecake, 25% Reduced Fat, Crm	120.0000	1.000	Piece	9.00	13.00	40.00	310.00	0.00	2.00	70.00	8.00
170	Cheesecake, Cherry Cream-Sara Le	135.0000	1.000	Piece	6.00	12.00	55.00	350.00	0.00	2.00	35.00	5.00
171	Cheesecake, Chocolate Chip-Sara	120.0000	1.000	Piece	8.00	21.00	47.00	410.00	0.00	2.00	65.00	14.00
	Cheesecake, Commercially Prepare	28.3500	1.000	Slice	1.56	6.38	7.23	91.00	0.00	0.12	15.59	2.81
172	Cheesecake, French-Sara Lee	111.0000	1.000	Piece	5.00	21.00	24.00	350.00	0.00	1.00	20.00	13.00
	Cheesecake, Homemade	85.0000	1.000	Slice	0.50	22.10	21.42	303.45	0.00	0.00	102.85	12.21
	Cheesecake, No-bake Type	28.3500	1.000	Slice	1.56	3.60	10.06	77.68	0.00	0.54	8.22	1.90
173	Cheesecake, Original Cream-Sara	121.0000	1.000	Piece	7.00	18.00	39.00	350.00	0.00	1.00	50.00	9.00

Monounsaturated Fat (gm)	Polyunsaturated Fat (gm)	Vitamin D (mg)	Vitamin K (mg)	Vitamin E (mg)	Vitamin A (re)	Vitamin C (mg)	Thiamin (mg)	Riboflavin (mg)	Niacin (mg)	Vitamin B_6 (mg)	Folate (mg)	Vitamin B_{12} (mcg)	Calcium (mg)	Iron (mg)	Magnesium (mg)	Phosphorus (mg)	Potassium (mg)	Sodium (mg)	Zinc (mg)
0.00	0.00	0.00	0.00	1.02	15.30	1.36	0.02	0.05	0.36	0.05	1.53	0.00	10.20	0.37	6.80	10.20	141.10	13.60	0.14
0.00	0.00	0.00	0.00	0.00	7.35	0.34	0.13	0.14	1.48	0.03	2.32	0.09	67.76	3.46	12.76	49.61	53.87	13.04	0.18
0.07	0.09	0.00	0.00	0.12	3.40	15.81	0.22	0.27	3.60	0.19	1.70	0.03	27.20	4.42	8.50	35.70	85.00	17.00	0.24
0.85	0.32	0.00	0.00	0.12	214.20	0.34	0.09	0.12	1.65	0.10	45.90	0.05	25.50	0.90	18.70	59.50	207.40	127.50	0.90
0.00	0.00	0.00	0.00	0.15	104.33	1.02	0.01	0.02	0.07	0.02	19.50	0.02	32.04	0.40	17.86	13.89	62.65	15.59	0.10
0.00	0.00	0.00	0.00	0.07	22.68	0.54	0.01	0.01	0.14	0.01	3.69	0.01	6.52	0.14	0.00	13.89	38.56	3.97	0.18
0.04	0.18	0.00	0.00	1.16	450.24	17.47	0.02	0.16	0.85	0.16	34.50	0.00	53.76	0.78	26.88	35.84	414.40	2.24	0.18
0.00	0.09	0.00	0.00	1.16	1487.36	21.50	0.07	0.07	0.85	0.25	23.07	0.00	35.84	0.87	26.88	53.76	544.32	49.28	0.25
0.41	0.24	0.00	0.00	0.12	3.40	2.58	0.07	0.15	1.23	0.03	13.89	0.02	74.56	1.01	9.92	46.49	91.57	102.63	0.26
0.00	0.00	0.00	0.00	0.00	2.26	21.24	0.01	0.03	0.09	0.03	3.73	0.00	11.30	0.29	5.65	9.04	65.54	7.91	0.06
1.87	1.25	0.00	0.00	0.28	7.10	1.70	0.01	0.18	2.47	0.12	8.59	0.76	19.88	0.96	8.52	67.45	127.80	51.12	1.28
0.51	0.39	0.00	0.00	0.27	319.60	0.51	0.05	0.07	1.17	0.09	13.60	0.03	40.80	0.70	15.30	62.90	146.20	136.00	0.80
3.32	2.57	0.00	0.00	0.28	4.26	1.07	0.01	0.11	1.24	0.06	8.02	0.71	51.12	0.88	11.36	73.13	64.61	342.93	1.30
0.08	0.40	0.00	0.00	0.02	0.00	0.00	0.30	0.18	2.58	0.02	49.90	0.00	41.96	2.02	16.44	54.44	57.26	302.78	0.50
0.10	0.38	0.00	0.00	0.08	0.00	0.40	0.22	0.16	1.74	0.04	51.04	0.00	10.78	2.16	15.88	56.70	83.92	182.58	0.64
0.10	0.40	0.00	0.00	0.10	3.96	0.34	0.18	0.16	1.68	0.04	43.66	0.00	11.34	2.32	13.04	47.06	92.42	196.18	0.46
0.24	0.36	0.00	0.00	0.00	18.72	0.34	0.30	0.14	1.96	0.06	49.90	0.10	7.38	2.26	14.18	47.62	38.56	286.34	0.44
0.30	0.46	0.00	0.00	0.00	21.12	0.33	0.30	0.15	2.20	0.06	11.22	0.11	9.24	2.82	17.82	59.40	48.18	358.38	0.55
0.14	0.28	0.00	0.00	0.08	0.00	0.12	0.18	0.20	1.68	0.02	45.92	0.00	6.80	1.74	17.58	62.38	65.20	287.46	0.52
0.18	0.35	0.00	0.00	0.00	0.00	0.07	0.19	0.22	1.89	0.13	23.10	0.00	8.58	2.18	40.92	116.82	144.54	359.70	1.48
0.08	0.40	0.00	0.00	0.02	0.00	0.00	0.30	0.18	2.58	0.02	49.90	0.00	41.96	2.02	16.44	54.44	57.26	302.78	0.50
0.09	0.49	0.00	0.00	0.00	0.00	0.00	0.31	0.20	2.91	0.03	11.22	0.00	12.54	2.52	20.46	67.98	71.94	378.84	0.62
3.92	3.52	0.00	0.00	1.66	0.56	0.00	0.24	0.16	1.90	0.02	33.46	0.08	27.78	1.88	9.64	243.82	127.00	596.48	0.28
0.02	0.10	0.00	0.00	0.00	0.00	0.00	0.03	0.14	0.25	0.01	9.92	0.02	39.69	0.15	3.40	9.07	26.37	212.34	0.02
1.29	0.29	0.00	0.00	0.30	6.52	0.06	0.12	0.08	0.05	0.01	4.25	0.05	6.52	0.11	1.70	13.89	11.06	40.82	0.05
7.24	15.10	0.00	0.00	0.00	426.24	1.22	0.15	0.17	1.13	0.08	13.32	0.11	27.75	1.39	19.98	78.81	124.32	273.06	0.54
2.48	0.52	0.00	0.00	0.00	7.09	0.03	0.01	0.04	0.16	0.01	4.82	0.04	12.19	0.62	9.64	34.59	56.70	94.69	0.20
0.00	0.00	0.00	0.00	0.00	20.00	0.00	0.00	0.00	0.00	0.00	0.00	0.00	40.00	1.00	0.00	0.00	0.00	180.00	0.00
0.00	0.00	0.00	0.00	0.00	20.00	0.00	0.00	0.00	0.00	0.00	0.00	0.00	40.00	0.70	0.00	0.00	0.00	160.00	0.00
0.00	0.00	0.00	0.00	0.00	0.00	0.00	0.00	0.00	0.00	0.00	0.00	0.00	40.00	1.00	0.00	0.00	0.00	170.00	0.00
1.19	0.94	0.00	0.00	0.47	1.13	0.14	0.01	0.03	0.22	0.01	5.39	0.00	9.36	0.59	4.54	14.74	43.38	76.55	0.08
0.00	0.00	0.00	0.00	0.00	20.00	0.00	0.00	0.00	0.00	0.00	0.00	0.00	40.00	0.50	0.00	0.00	0.00	130.00	0.00
8.71	5.46	0.00	0.00	0.00	23.31	0.00	0.11	0.14	1.10	0.02	4.44	0.10	53.28	1.22	18.87	173.16	150.96	368.52	0.49
3.75	0.90	0.00	0.00	0.00	10.72	0.07	0.13	0.12	1.05	0.03	6.70	0.05	46.23	2.22	10.72	112.56	161.47	306.86	0.27
1.47	0.93	0.00	0.00	0.38	18.43	0.34	0.04	0.05	0.34	0.01	7.37	0.02	34.02	0.42	3.69	23.25	31.75	90.44	0.09
1.77	0.32	0.00	0.00	0.00	46.80	0.00	0.04	0.07	0.39	0.01	12.30	0.08	10.50	0.41	3.30	41.10	35.70	119.40	0.14
0.00	0.00	0.00	0.00	0.00	80.00	0.00	0.00	0.00	0.00	0.00	0.00	0.00	20.00	1.20	0.00	0.00	0.00	310.00	0.00
0.00	0.00	0.00	0.00	0.00	80.00	0.00	0.00	0.00	0.00	0.00	0.00	0.00	20.00	0.70	0.00	0.00	0.00	280.00	0.00
0.00	0.00	0.00	0.00	0.00	40.00	0.00	0.00	0.00	0.00	0.00	0.00	0.00	60.00	1.20	0.00	0.00	0.00	350.00	0.00
0.00	0.00	0.00	0.00	0.00	60.00	0.00	0.00	0.00	0.00	0.00	0.00	0.00	20.00	1.00	0.00	0.00	0.00	350.00	0.00
0.00	0.00	0.00	0.00	0.00	20.00	0.00	0.00	0.00	0.00	0.00	0.00	0.00	40.00	0.70	0.00	0.00	0.00	140.00	0.00
0.27	0.13	0.00	0.00	0.08	13.04	0.00	0.07	0.08	0.55	0.01	11.06	0.07	19.85	0.77	3.12	38.84	28.07	69.17	0.14
0.00	0.00	0.00	0.00	0.00	0.00	0.00	0.00	0.00	0.00	0.00	0.00	0.00	20.00	0.50	0.00	0.00	0.00	140.00	0.00
1.05	0.61	0.00	0.00	0.20	3.12	0.03	0.04	0.05	0.30	0.01	6.24	0.02	25.52	0.33	3.40	19.85	28.07	80.51	0.09
3.93	2.33	0.00	0.00	0.00	11.84	0.15	0.14	0.18	1.13	0.02	5.18	0.06	96.20	1.12	8.88	68.82	70.30	241.98	0.24
2.72	0.60	0.00	0.00	0.64	9.36	0.00	0.03	0.05	0.35	0.01	6.24	0.05	10.49	0.59	8.51	45.64	50.46	95.54	0.18
1.73	1.46	0.00	0.00	0.00	5.39	0.00	0.03	0.02	0.14	0.01	7.65	0.04	17.58	0.30	1.70	40.54	15.03	97.52	0.07
0.00	0.00	0.00	0.00	0.00	60.00	0.00	0.00	0.00	0.00	0.00	0.00	0.00	100.00	1.00	0.00	0.00	0.00	310.00	0.00
0.00	0.00	0.00	0.00	0.00	20.00	15.00	0.00	0.00	0.00	0.00	0.00	0.00	40.00	0.70	0.00	0.00	0.00	320.00	0.00
0.00	0.00	0.00	0.00	0.00	60.00	1.20	0.00	0.00	0.00	0.00	0.00	0.00	60.00	1.20	0.00	0.00	0.00	300.00	0.00
2.45	0.45	0.00	0.00	0.45	41.39	0.11	0.01	0.05	0.06	0.01	5.10	0.05	14.46	0.18	3.12	26.37	25.52	58.68	0.14
0.00	0.00	0.00	0.00	0.00	20.00	1.20	0.00	0.00	0.00	0.00	0.00	0.00	40.00	0.50	0.00	0.00	0.00	280.00	0.00
6.87	1.75	0.00	0.00	0.00	272.85	0.34	0.03	0.18	0.34	0.04	10.20	0.21	49.30	1.06	6.80	81.60	86.70	240.55	0.47
1.28	0.23	0.00	0.00	0.00	28.07	0.14	0.03	0.07	0.14	0.01	8.51	0.09	48.76	0.13	5.39	66.34	59.82	107.73	0.13
0.00	0.00	0.00	0.00	0.00	20.00	0.00	0.00	0.00	0.00	0.00	0.00	0.00	80.00	0.50	0.00	0.00	0.00	320.00	0.00

USDA ID Code	Food Name	Weight in Grams*	Quantity of Units	Unit of Measure	Protein (gm)	Fat (gm)	Carbohydrate (gm)	Kcalories	Caffeine (gm)	Fiber (gm)	Cholesterol (mg)	Saturated Fat (gm)
	Cheesecake, Plain, w/ Cherry Top	90.0000	1.000	Slice	4.50	16.65	23.85	258.30	0.00	0.00	76.50	9.11
174	Cheesecake, Strawberry Cream-Sar	135.0000	1.000	Piece	6.00	12.00	49.00	330.00	0.00	2.00	40.00	5.00
175	Cheesecake, Strawberry French-Sa	123.0000	1.000	Piece	4.00	14.00	43.00	320.00	0.00	1.00	20.00	9.00
	Coffeecake	28.3500	1.000	Slice	1.93	6.61	13.24	118.50	0.00	0.57	9.07	1.64
198	Coffeecake, Butter Streusel-Sara	54.0000	1.000	Piece	4.00	12.00	25.00	220.00	0.00	0.50	35.00	6.00
	Coffeecake, Cheese	28.3500	1.000	Slice	1.98	4.31	12.56	96.11	0.00	0.28	24.10	1.53
199	Coffeecake, Cheese, Reduced Fat,	54.0000	1.000	Piece	3.00	6.00	28.00	180.00	0.00	0.00	20.00	1.50
200	Coffeecake, Crumb-Sara Lee	57.0000	1.000	Piece	3.00	9.00	32.00	220.00	0.00	0.50	15.00	1.50
	Coffeecake, Fruit	28.3500	1.000	Slice	1.47	2.89	14.60	88.17	0.00	0.71	1.98	0.71
201	Coffeecake, Pecan-Sara Lee	54.0000	1.000	Piece	4.00	12.00	24.00	230.00	0.00	0.50	25.00	4.50
202	Coffeecake, Raspberry-Sara Lee	54.0000	1.000	Piece	3.00	8.00	27.00	220.00	0.00	0.50	15.00	2.50
	Cream Puffs, Shell, w/ Custard F	28.3500	1.000	Each	1.90	4.39	6.49	73.14	0.00	0.11	37.99	1.04
	Crisp, Apple	282.0000	1.000	Cup	5.08	10.15	91.09	459.66	0.00	0.00	0.00	2.03
	Croissant, Apple	28.3500	1.000	Ounce	2.10	2.47	10.52	72.01	0.00	0.71	8.79	1.41
	Croissant, Butter	28.3500	1.000	Ounce	2.32	5.95	12.98	115.10	0.00	0.74	18.99	3.31
	Croissant, Cheese	28.3500	1.000	Ounce	2.61	5.93	13.32	117.37	0.00	0.74	16.16	3.01
	Croissant, Chocolate	56.0000	1.000	Medium	5.21	14.07	25.15	234.61	0.00	2.20	38.00	8.07
218	Croissants, Petite-Sara Lee	57.0000	2.000	Each	6.00	11.00	26.00	230.00	0.00	1.00	3.00	4.00
219	Croissants, Sara Lee	43.0000	1.000	Each	4.00	8.00	20.00	170.00	0.00	1.00	4.00	3.00
	Danish Pastry, Cheese	28.3500	1.000	Small	2.27	6.21	10.55	106.03	0.00	0.27	4.54	1.92
	Danish Pastry, Cinnamon	28.3500	1.000	Small	1.98	6.35	12.64	114.25	0.00	0.37	5.95	1.61
	Danish Pastry, Fruit	28.3500	1.000	Small	1.53	5.24	13.55	105.18	0.00	0.54	32.32	1.38
	Danish Pastry, Lemon	28.3500	1.000	Small	1.53	5.24	13.55	105.18	0.00	0.54	11.34	0.80
	Danish Pastry, Nut	28.3500	1.000	Small	2.01	7.14	12.96	121.91	0.00	0.57	13.04	1.65
	Danish Pastry, Raspberry	28.3500	1.000	Small	1.53	5.24	13.55	105.18	0.00	0.54	11.34	0.80
	Doughnuts, Chocolate, Sugared or	28.3500	1.000	Each	1.28	5.64	16.27	118.22	0.28	0.62	16.16	1.45
	Doughnuts, French Crullers, Glaz	28.3500	1.000	Each	0.88	5.19	16.87	116.80	0.00	0.34	3.12	1.32
	Doughnuts, Glazed	28.3500	1.000	Each	1.81	6.46	12.56	114.25	0.00	0.34	1.70	1.65
	Doughnuts, Plain	28.3500	1.000	Each	1.42	6.49	14.09	119.35	0.00	0.43	10.49	1.03
	Doughnuts, Plain, Chocolate-coat	28.3500	1.000	Each	1.42	8.79	13.61	134.38	0.57	0.57	17.29	2.30
	Doughnuts, Plain, Sugared or Gla	28.3500	1.000	Each	1.47	6.49	14.40	120.77	0.00	0.43	9.07	1.68
	Doughnuts, w/ Creme Filling	28.3500	1.000	Each	1.81	6.95	8.51	102.34	0.00	0.22	6.80	1.54
	Doughnuts, w/ Jelly Filling	28.3500	1.000	Each	1.67	5.30	11.06	96.39	0.00	0.24	7.37	1.37
	Doughnuts, Whole Wheat, Sugared	28.3500	1.000	Each	1.79	5.47	12.08	102.06	0.00	0.63	5.67	0.86
	Eclairs, Custard-filled w/ Choco	28.3500	1.000	Small	1.81	4.45	6.86	74.28	0.57	0.17	36.00	1.17
612	Mousse, Chocolate-Sara Lee	122.0000	1.000	Piece	5.00	25.00	37.00	400.00	0.00	2.00	30.00	20.00
	Muffins, Banana Nut	95.0000	1.000	Each	6.00	12.00	53.00	340.00	0.00	2.00	35.00	0.90
	Muffins, Blueberry	28.3500	1.000	Small	1.56	1.84	13.61	78.53	0.00	0.74	8.51	0.40
	Muffins, Corn	28.3500	1.000	Small	1.67	2.38	14.43	86.47	0.00	0.96	7.37	0.38
	Muffins, Oat Bran	28.3500	1.000	Small	1.98	2.10	13.69	76.55	0.00	1.30	0.00	0.31
	Muffins, Plain	28.3500	1.000	Small	1.96	3.23	11.74	83.92	0.00	0.77	11.06	0.61
	Muffins, Wheat Bran	65.0000	1.000	Large	4.62	7.93	27.24	183.95	0.00	0.00	21.45	1.47
	Pie, Apple	28.3500	1.000	Small Sl	0.68	3.54	10.52	75.13	0.00	0.00	0.00	0.86
641	Pie, Apple, 45% Reduced Fat-Sara	128.0000	1.000	Slice	4.00	8.00	51.00	290.00	0.00	2.00	4.00	1.50
642	Pie, Apple, Dutch, Homestyle-Sar	131.0000	1.000	Slice	3.00	15.00	53.00	350.00	0.00	2.00	0.00	3.00
643	Pie, Apple, Homestyle-Sara Lee	131.0000	1.000	Slice	3.00	16.00	46.00	340.00	0.00	1.00	0.00	3.50
	Pie, Banana Cream	28.3500	1.000	Small Sl	1.25	3.86	9.33	76.26	0.00	0.20	14.46	1.07
	Pie, Blueberry	28.3500	1.000	Small Sl	0.51	2.84	9.89	65.77	0.00	0.29	0.00	0.48
644	Pie, Blueberry, Homestyle-Sara L	131.0000	1.000	Slice	3.50	15.00	54.00	360.00	0.00	2.00	0.00	3.50
	Pie, Butterscotch Pudding	127.0000	1.000	Slice	5.97	18.16	42.29	354.33	0.00	0.00	77.47	5.09
	Pie, Cherry	28.3500	1.000	Small Sl	0.57	3.12	11.28	73.71	0.00	0.23	0.00	0.73
	Pie, Cherry, Fast Food	28.3500	1.000	Small	0.85	4.56	12.08	89.59	0.00	0.74	0.00	0.70
645	Pie, Cherry, Homestyle-Sara Lee	131.0000	1.000	Slice	3.00	16.00	42.00	320.00	0.00	2.00	0.00	3.50
	Pie, Chocolate Creme	28.3500	1.000	Small Sl	0.74	5.50	9.53	86.18	0.00	0.57	1.42	1.41
	Pie, Chocolate Mousse	28.3500	1.000	Small Sl	0.99	4.37	8.39	73.71	0.28	0.00	9.92	2.32

Monounsaturated Fat (gm)	Polyunsaturated Fat (gm)	Vitamin D (mg)	Vitamin K (mg)	Vitamin E (mg)	Vitamin A (re)	Vitamin C (mg)	Thiamin (mg)	Riboflavin (mg)	Niacin (mg)	Vitamin B_6 (mg)	Folate (mg)	Vitamin B_{12} (mcg)	Calcium (mg)	Iron (mg)	Magnesium (mg)	Phosphorus (mg)	Potassium (mg)	Sodium (mg)	Zinc (mg)
5.21	1.38	0.00	0.00	0.00	216.90	0.63	0.03	0.14	0.32	0.04	9.00	0.15	38.70	1.11	6.30	63.90	83.70	182.70	0.36
0.00	0.00	0.00	0.00	0.00	0.00	18.00	0.00	0.00	0.00	0.00	0.00	0.00	40.00	0.70	0.00	0.00	0.00	320.00	0.00
0.00	0.00	0.00	0.00	0.00	0.00	12.00	0.00	0.00	0.00	0.00	0.00	0.00	40.00	0.50	0.00	0.00	0.00	230.00	0.00
3.68	0.88	0.00	0.00	0.97	9.36	0.09	0.06	0.07	0.48	0.01	17.29	0.05	15.31	0.54	6.24	30.62	34.87	99.51	0.23
0.00	0.00	0.00	0.00	0.00	60.00	0.00	0.00	0.00	0.00	0.00	0.00	0.00	20.00	0.50	0.00	0.00	0.00	240.00	0.00
2.02	0.47	0.00	0.00	0.44	24.66	0.03	0.03	0.04	0.19	0.02	11.06	0.10	16.73	0.18	4.25	28.63	81.93	96.11	0.17
0.00	0.00	0.00	0.00	0.00	0.00	0.00	0.00	0.00	0.00	0.00	0.00	0.00	40.00	0.50	0.00	0.00	0.00	230.00	0.00
0.00	0.00	0.00	0.00	0.00	0.00	0.00	0.00	0.00	0.00	0.00	0.00	0.00	20.00	0.50	0.00	0.00	0.00	210.00	0.00
1.58	0.42	0.00	0.00	0.24	5.67	0.23	0.01	0.05	0.73	0.01	13.32	0.01	12.76	0.69	4.82	33.45	25.52	109.15	0.18
0.00	0.00	0.00	0.00	0.00	20.00	0.00	0.00	0.00	0.00	0.00	0.00	0.00	20.00	0.70	0.00	0.00	0.00	170.00	0.00
0.00	0.00	0.00	0.00	0.00	0.00	0.00	0.00	0.00	0.00	0.00	0.00	0.00	0.00	0.50	0.00	0.00	0.00	220.00	0.00
1.85	1.18	0.00	0.00	0.63	56.42	0.09	0.03	0.08	0.24	0.02	7.94	0.10	18.71	0.33	3.40	30.90	32.60	96.67	0.17
4.31	2.99	0.00	0.00	0.00	87.42	6.49	0.24	0.20	2.19	0.12	14.10	0.00	78.96	2.12	19.74	70.50	273.54	513.24	0.45
0.68	0.18	0.00	0.00	0.00	27.78	0.14	0.07	0.05	0.45	0.01	16.16	0.06	8.51	0.31	3.69	16.44	25.52	77.68	0.29
1.57	0.31	0.00	0.00	0.12	52.73	0.06	0.11	0.07	0.62	0.02	17.58	0.05	10.49	0.58	4.54	29.77	33.45	210.92	0.21
1.85	0.67	0.00	0.00	0.29	55.85	0.06	0.15	0.09	0.61	0.02	20.98	0.09	15.03	0.61	6.80	36.86	37.42	157.34	0.27
3.31	0.89	0.00	0.00	0.00	76.41	0.11	0.22	0.15	1.22	0.02	16.11	0.16	23.89	1.18	10.89	63.20	69.69	376.34	0.43
0.00	0.00	0.00	0.00	0.00	40.00	0.00	0.00	0.00	0.00	0.00	0.00	0.00	40.00	1.00	0.00	0.00	0.00	200.00	0.00
0.00	0.00	0.00	0.00	0.00	40.00	0.00	0.00	0.00	0.00	0.00	0.00	0.00	20.00	0.70	0.00	0.00	0.00	200.00	0.00
3.21	0.73	0.00	0.00	0.72	12.76	0.03	0.05	0.07	0.57	0.01	17.01	0.05	9.92	0.45	4.25	30.62	27.78	127.58	0.20
3.55	0.83	0.00	0.00	0.84	0.85	0.03	0.09	0.07	0.81	0.01	17.58	0.03	20.13	0.56	5.39	30.33	35.44	105.18	0.20
2.84	0.67	0.00	0.00	0.70	6.24	1.11	0.07	0.06	0.56	0.01	9.36	0.03	13.04	0.50	4.25	25.23	23.53	100.36	0.15
1.68	0.43	0.00	0.00	0.42	15.03	1.11	0.02	0.03	0.22	0.01	4.54	0.03	13.04	0.21	4.25	25.23	23.53	100.36	0.15
3.88	1.21	0.00	0.00	1.03	3.97	0.48	0.06	0.07	0.65	0.03	23.53	0.06	26.65	0.51	9.07	31.19	26.93	102.91	0.25
1.68	0.43	0.00	0.00	0.42	17.01	1.11	0.02	0.03	0.22	0.01	4.54	0.03	13.04	0.21	4.25	25.23	23.53	100.36	0.15
3.20	0.70	0.00	0.00	0.76	3.12	0.03	0.01	0.02	0.13	0.01	10.77	0.03	60.39	0.64	9.64	45.93	30.05	96.39	0.16
2.96	0.65	0.00	0.00	0.70	0.85	0.00	0.05	0.07	0.60	0.01	9.92	0.01	7.37	0.69	3.40	34.87	22.11	97.81	0.07
3.65	0.82	0.00	0.00	0.87	1.13	0.03	0.10	0.06	0.81	0.02	12.19	0.03	12.19	0.58	6.24	26.37	30.62	96.96	0.22
2.64	2.23	0.00	0.00	1.09	4.82	0.06	0.06	0.07	0.52	0.02	13.32	0.08	12.47	0.55	5.67	76.26	36.00	154.79	0.16
4.96	1.07	0.00	0.00	1.18	3.12	0.06	0.04	0.03	0.37	0.01	8.22	0.07	9.92	0.70	11.34	57.27	55.57	121.62	0.17
3.60	0.82	0.00	0.00	0.00	0.85	0.03	0.07	0.06	0.43	0.01	13.04	0.07	17.01	0.30	4.82	33.17	28.92	113.97	0.12
3.42	0.87	0.00	0.00	0.78	5.39	0.00	0.10	0.04	0.64	0.02	18.14	0.04	7.09	0.52	5.67	21.55	22.68	87.60	0.23
2.90	0.67	0.00	0.00	0.70	4.54	0.00	0.09	0.04	0.61	0.03	17.58	0.06	7.09	0.50	5.67	24.10	22.40	83.07	0.21
2.30	2.01	0.00	0.00	1.02	4.25	0.06	0.06	0.07	0.52	0.03	5.67	0.05	13.89	0.31	6.24	29.48	41.96	100.64	0.19
1.84	1.12	0.00	0.00	0.60	54.15	0.09	0.03	0.08	0.23	0.02	7.94	0.10	17.86	0.33	4.25	30.33	33.17	95.54	0.17
0.00	0.00	0.00	0.00	0.00	40.00	0.00	0.00	0.00	0.00	0.00	0.00	0.00	60.00	1.20	0.00	0.00	0.00	190.00	0.00
1.50	2.40	0.00	0.00	0.00	21.00	0.03	0.18	0.12	0.04	0.01	13.20	0.00	44.00	1.01	16.10	108.20	371.00	210.00	0.20
0.56	0.71	0.00	0.00	0.30	2.55	0.31	0.04	0.03	0.31	0.01	12.76	0.16	16.16	0.46	4.54	55.85	34.87	126.72	0.14
0.60	0.91	0.00	0.00	0.52	10.21	0.00	0.08	0.09	0.58	0.02	17.58	0.03	20.98	0.80	9.07	80.51	19.56	147.70	0.15
0.48	1.17	0.00	0.00	0.37	0.00	0.00	0.07	0.03	0.12	0.05	14.74	0.00	17.86	1.19	44.51	106.60	143.73	111.42	0.52
0.78	1.62	0.00	0.00	0.00	11.34	0.09	0.08	0.09	0.65	0.01	14.46	0.04	56.70	0.68	4.82	43.38	34.30	132.39	0.16
1.91	4.09	0.00	0.00	0.00	162.50	5.07	0.22	0.29	2.62	0.21	33.80	0.09	121.55	2.72	50.70	185.25	206.70	382.20	1.79
1.53	0.95	0.00	0.00	0.00	3.40	0.48	0.04	0.03	0.35	0.01	6.80	0.00	1.98	0.32	1.98	7.94	22.40	59.82	0.05
0.00	0.00	0.00	0.00	0.00	0.00	0.00	0.00	0.00	0.00	0.00	0.00	0.00	20.00	1.20	0.00	0.00	0.00	400.00	0.00
0.00	0.00	0.00	0.00	0.00	0.00	1.20	0.00	0.00	0.00	0.00	0.00	0.00	0.00	1.00	0.00	0.00	0.00	350.00	0.00
0.00	0.00	0.00	0.00	0.00	0.00	1.20	0.00	0.00	0.00	0.00	0.00	0.00	0.00	0.70	0.00	0.00	0.00	310.00	0.00
1.62	0.93	0.00	0.00	0.42	19.85	0.45	0.04	0.06	0.30	0.04	7.65	0.07	21.26	0.29	4.54	26.08	46.78	68.04	0.14
1.20	1.00	0.00	0.00	0.57	9.64	0.77	0.00	0.01	0.09	0.01	6.24	0.00	2.27	0.09	1.42	6.52	14.18	92.14	0.05
0.00	0.00	0.00	0.00	0.00	0.00	2.40	0.00	0.00	0.00	0.00	0.00	0.00	0.00	0.70	0.00	0.00	0.00	340.00	0.00
7.64	4.35	0.00	0.00	0.00	106.68	0.64	0.18	0.27	1.26	0.07	13.97	0.38	128.27	1.64	21.59	134.62	220.98	335.28	0.69
1.66	0.58	0.00	0.00	0.43	15.31	0.26	0.01	0.01	0.06	0.01	6.24	0.00	3.40	0.14	2.27	8.22	22.96	69.74	0.05
2.11	1.53	0.00	0.00	0.00	4.82	0.37	0.04	0.03	0.41	0.01	5.10	0.02	6.24	0.35	2.84	12.19	18.43	106.03	0.07
0.00	0.00	0.00	0.00	0.00	80.00	0.00	0.00	0.00	0.00	0.00	0.00	0.00	0.00	0.70	0.00	0.00	0.00	290.00	0.00
3.15	0.68	0.00	0.00	0.77	0.00	0.00	0.01	0.03	0.19	0.01	3.69	0.00	10.21	0.30	5.95	19.28	36.00	38.56	0.07
1.44	0.23	0.00	0.00	0.00	28.63	0.14	0.01	0.04	0.17	0.01	7.37	0.06	21.83	0.31	9.07	65.49	80.80	130.41	0.17

USDA ID Code	Food Name	Weight in Grams*	Quantity of Units	Unit of Measure	Protein (gm)	Fat (gm)	Carbohydrate (gm)	Kcalories	Caffeine (gm)	Fiber (gm)	Cholesterol (mg)	Saturated Fat (gm)
646	Pie, Chocolate Silk Supreme-Sara	136.0000	1.000	Slice	4.00	32.00	49.00	500.00	0.00	2.00	4.00	16.00
647	Pie, Coconut Cream -Sara Lee	136.0000	1.000	Slice	4.00	31.00	47.00	480.00	0.00	2.00	0.00	14.00
	Pie, Coconut Creme	28.3500	1.000	Small Sl	0.60	4.71	10.55	84.48	0.00	0.37	0.00	1.98
	Pie, Coconut Custard	28.3500	1.000	Small Sl	1.67	3.74	8.56	73.71	0.00	0.51	9.92	1.66
	Pie, Egg Custard	28.3500	1.000	Small Sl	1.56	3.29	5.90	59.54	0.00	0.45	9.36	0.67
	Pie, Fruit, Fried	28.3500	1.000	Small Sl	0.85	4.56	12.08	89.59	0.00	0.74	0.00	0.70
	Pie, Lemon Meringue	28.3500	1.000	Small Sl	0.43	2.47	13.38	75.98	0.00	0.34	12.76	0.50
648	Pie, Lemon Meringue-Sara Lee	142.0000	1.000	Slice	2.00	11.00	59.00	350.00	0.00	5.00	0.00	2.50
	Pie, Lemon, Fried	28.3500	1.000	Small	0.85	4.56	12.08	89.59	0.00	0.74	0.00	0.70
	Pie, Mince Meat	28.3500	1.000	Small Sl	0.74	3.06	13.61	81.93	0.00	0.74	0.00	0.76
649	Pie, Mince, Homestyle-Sara Lee	131.0000	1.000	Slice	3.00	17.00	56.00	390.00	0.00	3.00	0.00	4.00
650	Pie, Peach, Homestyle-Sara Lee	131.0000	1.000	Slice	3.00	14.00	46.00	320.00	0.00	2.00	0.00	3.00
	Pie, Pecan	28.3500	1.000	Small Sl	1.13	5.24	16.22	113.40	0.00	0.99	9.07	1.01
651	Pie, Pecan, Homestyle-Sara Lee	121.0000	1.000	Slice	5.00	24.00	70.00	520.00	0.00	3.00	45.00	4.50
	Pie, Pumpkin	28.3500	1.000	Small Sl	1.11	2.69	7.74	59.54	0.00	0.77	5.67	0.51
652	Pie, Pumpkin, Homestyle-Sara Lee	131.0000	1.000	Slice	4.00	11.00	37.00	260.00	0.00	2.00	30.00	2.50
653	Pie, Raspberry, Homestyle-Sara L	131.0000	1.000	Slice	3.00	19.00	48.00	380.00	0.00	2.00	4.00	4.50
	Pie, Vanilla Creme	28.3500	1.000	Small Sl	1.36	4.08	9.24	78.81	0.00	0.17	17.58	1.14
696	Shortcake, Strawberry-Sara Lee	71.0000	1.000	Piece	2.00	7.00	27.00	180.00	0.00	0.50	15.00	5.00
	Strudel, Apple	28.3500	1.000	Small	0.94	3.18	11.65	77.68	0.00	0.62	1.70	0.58
	Sweet Rolls w/ Raisins and Nuts	57.0000	1.000	Each	3.76	7.30	29.58	196.08	0.00	0.00	13.11	1.35
	Sweet Rolls, Cheese	28.3500	1.000	Small	2.01	5.19	12.39	102.06	0.00	0.34	21.55	1.72
	Sweet Rolls, Cinnamon w/ Raisins	28.3500	1.000	Small	1.76	4.65	14.43	105.46	0.00	0.68	18.71	0.87
729	Sweet Rolls, Cinnamon, Deluxe-Sa	76.0000	1.000	Roll	5.00	15.00	41.00	370.00	0.00	1.00	40.00	9.00
	Beef Broth and Tomato Juice, Cnd	168.0000	5.500	Fl Oz	1.01	0.17	14.28	62.16	0.00	0.17	0.00	0.05
	Beer, Dark	29.5000	12.000	Fl Oz	0.09	0.00	1.10	12.18	0.00	0.06	0.00	0.00
	Beer, Killians	29.5000	12.000	Fl Oz	0.09	0.00	1.10	12.18	0.00	0.06	0.00	0.00
	Beer, Light	354.0000	12.000	Fl Oz	0.71	0.00	4.60	99.12	0.00	0.00	0.00	0.00
	Beer, Regular	356.0000	12.000	Fl Oz	1.07	0.00	13.17	145.96	0.00	0.71	0.00	0.00
	Beverage, Strawberry Flavor	266.0000	1.000	Cup	7.98	8.25	32.72	234.08	0.00	0.00	31.92	5.08
	Bloody Mary	29.7000	1.000	Fl Oz	0.15	0.03	0.98	23.17	0.00	0.00	0.00	0.00
	Choc Mix, Hot, No Sugar-Swiss M	20.0000	1.000	Packet	3.00	1.50	13.00	70.00	4.00	0.00	0.00	0.00
	Choc Mix, Hot, No Sugar, Fat Fre	15.0000	1.000	Packet	4.00	0.00	9.00	50.00	4.00	0.00	0.00	0.00
	Coffee, Brewed	237.0000	1.000	Cup	0.24	0.00	0.95	4.74	137.46	0.00	0.00	0.00
	Coffee, Brewed, Decaf.	29.6000	6.000	Fl Oz	0.03	0.00	0.12	0.59	0.18	0.00	0.00	0.00
	Coffee, Instant, Cappuccino Flav	29.3000	6.000	Fl Oz	0.06	0.32	1.64	9.38	12.16	0.00	0.00	0.28
	Coffee, Instant, Decaffeinated	179.0000	6.000	Fl Oz	0.18	0.00	0.72	3.58	1.79	0.00	0.00	0.00
	Coffee, Instant, Mocha Flavor	29.3000	6.000	Fl Oz	0.09	0.29	1.32	7.91	6.83	0.00	0.00	0.25
	Coffee, Instant, Regular	179.0000	6.000	Fl Oz	0.18	0.00	0.72	3.58	57.28	0.00	0.00	0.00
203	Cola	369.0000	12.000	Fl Oz	0.10	0.10	38.50	151.00	7.60	0.00	0.00	0.00
	Cola, Diet	369.0000	12.000	Fl Oz	0.20	0.00	0.30	2.00	7.60	0.00	0.00	0.00
	Crystal Lite	29.5750	8.000	Fl Oz	0.00	0.00	0.00	0.63	0.00	0.00	0.00	0.00
	Gatorade Thirst Quencher	244.0000	8.000	Fl Oz	0.00	0.00	14.00	50.00	0.00	0.00	0.00	0.00
	Gatorlode High Carb, Loading Rec	354.0000	11.600	Fl Oz	0.00	0.00	71.00	280.00	0.00	0.00	0.00	0.00
	Gatorpro Sports Nutrition Sup.	336.0000	11.000	Fl Oz	17.00	6.00	59.00	360.00	0.00	0.00	0.00	0.50
	Juice Drink, Cranberry-apple, Bo	245.0000	1.000	Cup	0.25	0.00	41.90	164.15	0.00	0.25	0.00	0.00
	Juice Drink, Cranberry-apricot,	245.0000	1.000	Cup	0.49	0.00	39.69	156.80	0.00	0.25	0.00	0.00
	Juice Drink, Cranberry-grape, Bo	245.0000	1.000	Cup	0.49	0.25	34.30	137.20	0.00	0.25	0.00	0.07
	Juice Drink, Grape, Cnd	250.0000	1.000	Cup	0.25	0.00	32.25	125.00	0.00	0.25	0.00	0.00
	Juice Drink, Orange and Apricot,	250.0000	1.000	Cup	0.75	0.25	31.75	127.50	0.00	0.25	0.00	0.03
	Juice Drink, Pineapple and Grape	250.0000	1.000	Cup	0.50	0.25	29.00	117.50	0.00	0.25	0.00	0.03
	Juice Drink, Pineapple and Orang	250.0000	1.000	Cup	3.25	0.00	29.50	125.00	0.00	0.25	0.00	0.00
	Juice, Apple, Unsweetened	248.0000	1.000	Cup	0.15	0.27	28.97	116.56	0.00	0.25	0.00	0.05
	Juice, Carrot, Cnd	236.0000	1.000	Cup	2.24	0.35	21.92	94.40	0.00	1.89	0.00	0.07
	Juice, Clam and Tomato, Cnd	166.0000	5.500	Fl Oz	1.00	0.33	18.18	79.68	0.00	0.33	0.00	0.08

Monounsaturated Fat (gm)	Polyunsaturated Fat (gm)	Vitamin D (mg)	Vitamin K (mg)	Vitamin E (mg)	Vitamin A (re)	Vitamin C (mg)	Thiamin (mg)	Riboflavin (mg)	Niacin (mg)	Vitamin B_6 (mg)	Folate (mg)	Vitamin B_{12} (mcg)	Calcium (mg)	Iron (mg)	Magnesium (mg)	Phosphorus (mg)	Potassium (mg)	Sodium (mg)	Zinc (mg)
0.00	0.00	0.00	0.00	0.00	0.00	0.00	0.00	0.00	0.00	0.00	0.00	0.00	40.00	1.20	0.00	0.00	0.00	440.00	0.00
0.00	0.00	0.00	0.00	0.00	0.00	0.00	0.00	0.00	0.00	0.00	0.00	0.00	40.00	0.70	0.00	0.00	0.00	430.00	0.00
2.06	0.44	0.00	0.00	0.53	0.00	0.00	0.01	0.02	0.06	0.02	1.98	0.03	8.22	0.23	5.67	24.10	18.43	72.29	0.13
1.56	0.33	0.00	0.00	0.00	7.65	0.17	0.03	0.04	0.11	0.00	3.69	0.03	22.96	0.23	5.10	34.59	49.61	94.97	0.19
1.36	1.05	0.00	0.00	0.53	18.99	0.17	0.01	0.06	0.08	0.01	5.67	0.12	22.68	0.16	3.12	31.75	30.05	68.04	0.15
2.11	1.53	0.00	0.00	0.84	0.85	0.37	0.04	0.03	0.41	0.01	5.10	0.02	6.24	0.35	2.84	12.19	18.43	106.03	0.07
0.76	1.03	0.00	0.00	0.62	14.74	0.91	0.02	0.06	0.18	0.01	3.69	0.05	15.88	0.17	4.25	29.77	25.23	41.39	0.14
0.00	0.00	0.00	0.00	0.00	0.00	0.00	0.00	0.00	0.00	0.00	0.00	0.00	0.00	1.00	0.00	0.00	0.00	460.00	0.00
2.11	1.53	0.00	0.00	0.00	0.85	0.00	0.04	0.03	0.41	0.01	5.10	0.02	6.24	0.35	2.84	12.19	18.43	106.03	0.07
1.32	0.81	0.00	0.00	0.53	0.57	1.67	0.04	0.03	0.34	0.02	6.52	0.00	6.24	0.42	3.97	11.91	57.55	72.01	0.06
0.00	0.00	0.00	0.00	0.00	0.00	2.40	0.00	0.00	0.00	0.00	0.00	0.00	20.00	1.00	0.00	0.00	0.00	450.00	0.00
0.00	0.00	0.00	0.00	0.00	40.00	21.00	0.00	0.00	0.00	0.00	0.00	0.00	0.00	1.00	0.00	0.00	0.00	250.00	0.00
3.04	0.90	0.00	0.00	0.52	13.32	0.31	0.03	0.03	0.07	0.01	7.65	0.03	4.82	0.29	5.10	21.83	20.98	120.20	0.16
0.00	0.00	0.00	0.00	0.00	0.00	0.00	0.00	0.00	0.00	0.00	0.00	0.00	20.00	0.70	0.00	0.00	0.00	480.00	0.00
1.14	0.89	0.00	0.00	0.48	105.46	0.28	0.02	0.04	0.05	0.02	5.67	0.07	17.01	0.22	4.25	20.13	43.66	79.95	0.13
0.00	0.00	0.00	0.00	0.00	150.00	0.00	0.00	0.00	0.00	0.00	0.00	0.00	60.00	1.00	0.00	0.00	0.00	460.00	0.00
0.00	0.00	0.00	0.00	0.00	0.00	4.80	0.00	0.00	0.00	0.00	0.00	0.00	0.00	1.00	0.00	0.00	0.00	330.00	0.00
1.71	0.98	0.00	0.00	0.38	24.10	0.14	0.04	0.06	0.28	0.01	7.37	0.09	25.52	0.29	3.69	29.48	35.72	73.71	0.15
0.00	0.00	0.00	0.00	0.00	0.00	9.00	0.00	0.00	0.00	0.00	0.00	0.00	20.00	0.20	0.00	0.00	0.00	140.00	0.00
0.93	1.51	0.00	0.00	0.87	2.55	0.48	0.01	0.01	0.09	0.01	3.97	0.06	4.25	0.12	2.55	9.36	42.24	76.26	0.05
2.66	2.85	0.00	0.00	0.00	60.42	0.34	0.16	0.16	1.33	0.05	17.67	0.06	36.48	1.46	15.96	62.70	123.12	185.25	0.38
2.57	0.58	0.00	0.00	0.00	21.83	0.06	0.04	0.04	0.24	0.02	12.19	0.09	33.45	0.22	5.39	27.78	38.84	101.21	0.18
1.36	2.12	0.00	0.00	1.22	18.14	0.57	0.09	0.08	0.67	0.03	14.74	0.04	20.41	0.45	4.82	21.55	31.47	108.58	0.17
0.00	0.00	0.00	0.00	0.00	60.00	0.00	0.00	0.00	0.00	0.00	0.00	0.00	20.00	0.70	0.00	0.00	0.00	300.00	0.00
0.05	0.03	0.00	0.00	0.00	21.84	1.51	0.00	0.05	0.27	0.03	7.22	0.08	18.48	0.97	5.04	21.84	161.28	220.08	0.03
0.00	0.00	0.00	0.00	0.00	0.00	0.00	0.00	0.01	0.14	0.02	1.78	0.01	1.49	0.01	1.78	3.56	7.43	1.49	0.01
0.00	0.00	0.00	0.00	0.00	0.00	0.00	0.00	0.01	0.14	0.02	1.78	0.01	1.49	0.01	1.78	3.56	7.43	1.49	0.01
0.00	0.00	0.00	0.00	0.00	0.00	0.00	0.04	0.11	1.38	0.11	14.51	0.04	17.70	0.14	17.70	42.48	63.72	10.62	0.11
0.00	0.00	0.00	0.00	0.00	0.00	0.00	0.04	0.11	1.60	0.18	21.36	0.07	17.80	0.11	21.36	42.72	89.00	17.80	0.07
2.37	0.29	0.00	0.00	0.00	74.48	2.39	0.11	0.43	0.21	0.11	12.24	0.88	292.60	0.21	31.92	228.76	369.74	127.68	0.93
0.00	0.01	0.00	0.00	0.00	10.10	4.10	0.01	0.01	0.13	0.02	3.95	0.00	2.08	0.11	2.38	4.16	43.36	66.53	0.03
0.00	0.00	0.00	0.00	0.00	0.00	0.00	0.00	0.00	0.00	0.00	0.00	0.00	80.00	0.40	0.00	0.00	0.00	220.00	0.00
0.00	0.00	0.00	0.00	0.00	0.00	0.00	0.00	0.00	0.00	0.00	0.00	0.00	80.00	0.20	0.00	0.00	0.00	180.00	0.00
0.00	0.00	0.00	0.00	0.00	0.00	0.00	0.00	0.00	0.52	0.00	0.24	0.00	4.74	0.12	11.85	2.37	127.98	4.74	0.05
0.00	0.00	0.00	0.00	0.00	0.00	0.00	0.00	0.00	0.07	0.00	0.03	0.00	0.59	0.01	1.48	0.30	15.98	0.59	0.01
0.02	0.01	0.00	0.00	0.00	0.00	0.00	0.00	0.00	0.05	0.00	0.00	0.00	1.17	0.02	1.47	4.10	18.17	15.82	0.01
0.00	0.00	0.00	0.00	0.00	0.00	0.00	0.00	0.02	0.50	0.00	0.00	0.00	5.37	0.07	7.16	5.37	62.65	5.37	0.05
0.02	0.01	0.00	0.00	0.00	0.00	0.00	0.00	0.00	0.04	0.00	0.00	0.00	1.17	0.04	1.47	4.40	18.46	5.57	0.02
0.00	0.00	0.00	0.00	0.00	0.00	0.00	0.00	0.00	0.50	0.00	0.00	0.00	5.37	0.09	7.16	5.37	64.44	5.37	0.05
0.00	0.00	0.00	0.00	0.00	0.00	0.00	0.00	0.00	0.00	0.00	0.00	0.00	0.00	0.13	3.00	46.00	4.00	14.00	0.05
0.00	0.00	0.00	0.00	0.00	0.00	0.00	0.00	0.00	0.00	0.00	0.00	0.00	0.00	0.11	4.00	30.00	0.00	21.00	0.28
0.00	0.00	0.00	0.00	0.00	0.00	0.75	0.00	0.00	0.00	0.00	0.00	0.00	0.00	0.00	0.00	0.00	0.00	0.00	0.00
0.00	0.00	0.00	0.00	0.00	0.00	0.00	0.00	0.00	0.00	0.00	0.00	0.00	0.00	0.00	0.00	0.00	30.00	110.00	0.00
0.00	0.00	0.00	0.00	0.00	0.00	18.00	0.11	0.39	4.50	0.45	0.00	0.00	0.00	0.00	0.00	0.00	0.00	0.00	0.00
0.00	0.00	0.05	0.00	3.50	160.00	50.00	1.10	0.50	6.00	0.64	63.00	0.80	280.00	3.00	70.00	400.00	1310.00	300.00	3.60
0.00	0.00	0.00	0.00	0.00	0.00	78.40	0.02	0.05	0.15	0.05	0.49	0.00	17.15	0.15	4.90	7.35	66.15	4.90	0.10
0.00	0.00	0.00	0.00	0.00	112.70	0.00	0.02	0.02	0.29	0.05	1.47	0.00	22.05	0.37	7.35	12.25	149.45	4.90	0.10
0.00	0.05	0.00	0.00	0.00	0.00	78.40	0.02	0.05	0.29	0.07	1.72	0.00	19.60	0.02	7.35	9.80	58.80	7.35	0.10
0.00	0.00	0.00	0.00	0.00	0.00	40.00	0.03	0.03	0.25	0.05	2.00	0.00	7.50	0.25	10.00	10.00	87.50	2.50	0.08
0.08	0.05	0.00	0.00	0.00	145.00	50.00	0.05	0.03	0.50	0.08	14.50	0.00	12.50	0.25	10.00	20.00	200.00	5.00	0.13
0.03	0.08	0.00	0.00	0.00	10.00	115.00	0.08	0.05	0.68	0.10	26.25	0.00	17.50	0.78	15.00	15.00	152.50	35.00	0.15
0.00	0.00	0.00	0.00	0.00	132.50	56.25	0.08	0.05	0.53	0.13	27.25	0.00	12.50	0.68	15.00	10.00	115.00	7.50	0.15
0.02	0.07	0.00	0.00	0.02	0.00	103.17	0.05	0.05	0.00	0.07	0.25	0.00	17.36	0.92	7.44	17.36	295.12	7.44	0.07
0.02	0.17	0.00	0.00	0.02	2584.20	20.06	0.21	0.14	0.92	0.52	8.97	0.00	56.64	1.09	33.04	99.12	689.12	68.44	0.42
0.02	0.03	0.00	0.00	0.00	36.52	6.81	0.07	0.05	0.32	0.13	26.39	50.80	19.92	1.00	36.52	129.48	149.40	600.92	1.79

USDA ID Code	Food Name	Weight in Grams*	Quantity of Units	Unit of Measure	Protein (gm)	Fat (gm)	Carbohydrate (gm)	Kcalories	Caffeine (gm)	Fiber (gm)	Cholesterol (mg)	Saturated Fat (gm)
	Juice, Cranberry, Bottled	252.5860	0.750	Cup	0.00	0.25	36.37	143.97	0.00	0.00	0.00	0.00
	Juice, Grape, Cnd Or Bottle, Uns	253.0000	1.000	Cup	1.42	0.20	37.85	154.33	0.00	0.25	0.00	0.08
	Juice, Grapefruit, Cnd. Sweetene	250.0000	1.000	Cup	1.45	0.23	27.83	115.00	0.00	0.25	0.00	0.03
	Juice, Grapefruit, Cnd. Unsweete	247.0000	1.000	Cup	1.28	0.25	22.13	93.86	0.00	0.25	0.00	0.02
	Juice, Grapefruit, Pink, Fresh	247.0000	1.000	Cup	1.24	0.25	22.72	96.33	0.00	0.00	0.00	0.02
	Juice, Grapefruit, White, Fresh	247.0000	1.000	Cup	1.24	0.25	22.72	96.33	0.00	0.25	0.00	0.02
	Juice, Guava	239.9120	0.750	Cup	0.00	0.00	21.63	87.86	0.00	0.00	0.00	0.00
	Juice, Mango	239.9120	0.750	Cup	0.00	0.00	21.63	87.86	0.00	0.00	0.00	0.00
	Juice, Orange, Fresh	248.0000	1.000	Cup	1.74	0.50	25.79	111.60	0.00	0.50	0.00	0.05
	Juice, Orange, From Concentrate	249.0000	1.000	Cup	1.69	0.15	26.84	112.05	0.00	0.50	0.00	0.02
	Juice, Orange, w/ Added Calcium	248.5900	0.750	Cup	1.69	0.15	26.80	111.87	0.00	0.50	0.00	0.02
	Juice, Passion-fruit, Purple, Fr	247.0000	1.000	Cup	0.96	0.12	33.59	125.97	0.00	0.49	0.00	0.00
	Juice, Passion-fruit, Yellow, Fr	247.0000	1.000	Cup	1.65	0.44	35.69	148.20	0.00	0.49	0.00	0.05
	Juice, Pineapple, Cnd	250.0000	1.000	Cup	0.80	0.20	34.45	140.00	0.00	0.50	0.00	0.03
	Juice, Prune, Cnd	256.0000	1.000	Cup	1.56	0.08	44.67	181.76	0.00	2.56	0.00	0.00
	Juice, Tangerine, Cnd Sweetened	249.0000	1.000	Cup	1.25	0.50	29.88	124.50	0.00	0.50	0.00	0.02
	Juice, Tangerine, Fresh	247.0000	1.000	Cup	1.24	0.49	24.95	106.21	0.00	0.49	0.00	0.05
	Juice, Tomato, Cnd w/ Added Salt	243.0000	1.000	Cup	1.85	0.15	10.28	41.31	0.00	0.97	0.00	0.02
	Juice, Tomato, Cnd w/o Salt	243.0000	1.000	Cup	1.85	0.15	10.28	41.31	0.00	1.94	0.00	0.02
	Juice, Tropical Fruit, Blend	247.0000	1.000	Cup	0.00	0.00	28.90	113.62	0.00	0.25	0.00	0.00
558	Juice, V-8 Splash, Berry Blend	240.0000	8.000	Fl Oz	0.00	0.00	28.00	110.00	0.00	0.00	0.00	0.00
559	Juice, V-8 Splash, Strawberry Ki	240.0000	8.000	Fl Oz	0.00	0.00	28.00	110.00	0.00	0.00	0.00	0.00
560	Juice, V-8 Splash, Tropical Blen	240.0000	8.000	Fl Oz	0.00	0.00	30.00	120.00	0.00	0.00	0.00	0.00
	Juice, V-8, Low Salt	243.0000	8.000	Fl Oz	1.60	0.00	8.20	40.00	0.00	0.25	0.00	0.00
	Juice, Vegetable, Cnd.	242.0000	1.000	Cup	1.52	0.22	11.01	45.98	0.00	1.94	0.00	0.02
	Kool-Aid	236.0000	8.000	Fl Oz	0.00	0.00	25.10	98.00	0.00	0.00	0.00	0.00
	Lemonade Flavor Drink	266.0000	1.000	Cup	0.00	0.00	28.73	111.72	0.00	0.00	0.00	0.05
	Lemonade, Low Calorie	237.0000	1.000	Cup	0.00	0.00	1.19	4.74	0.00	0.00	0.00	0.00
	Lemonade, Pink	247.0000	1.000	Cup	0.25	0.00	25.94	98.80	0.00	0.00	0.00	0.02
	Lemonade, White	248.0000	1.000	Cup	0.25	0.00	26.04	99.20	0.00	0.25	0.00	0.02
	Liqueur, Coffee w/ Cream, 34 Pro	47.0000	1.500	Fl Oz	1.32	7.38	9.82	153.69	7.05	0.00	7.05	4.54
	Liqueur, Coffee, 53 Proof	52.0000	1.500	Fl Oz	0.05	0.16	24.34	174.72	13.52	0.00	0.00	0.06
	Liqueur, Coffee, 63 Proof	52.0000	1.500	Fl Oz	0.05	0.16	16.74	160.16	13.52	0.00	0.00	0.06
	Liqueur, Creme De Menthe, 72 Pro	50.0000	1.500	Fl Oz	0.00	0.15	20.80	185.50	0.00	0.00	0.00	0.01
	Liquor Drink, Bourbon and Soda	29.0000	1.000	Fl Oz	0.00	0.00	0.00	26.10	0.00	0.00	0.00	0.00
	Liquor Drink, Daiquiri	60.0000	2.000	Fl Oz	0.06	0.06	4.08	111.60	0.00	0.00	0.00	0.01
	Liquor Drink, Daiquiri, Bottled	207.0000	6.800	Fl Oz	0.00	0.00	32.50	258.75	0.00	0.00	0.00	0.00
	Liquor Drink, Gin and Tonic	30.0000	1.000	Fl Oz	0.00	0.00	2.10	22.80	0.00	0.00	0.00	0.00
	Liquor Drink, Manhattan	28.5000	6.000	Fl Oz	0.03	0.00	0.91	63.84	0.00	0.00	0.00	0.00
	Liquor Drink, Margarita	29.5750	6.000	Fl Oz	0.00	0.00	4.50	28.75	0.00	0.00	0.00	0.00
	Liquor Drink, Martini	28.2000	6.000	Fl Oz	0.00	0.00	0.08	62.89	0.00	0.00	0.00	0.00
	Liquor Drink, Pina Colada	141.0000	4.500	Fl Oz	0.56	2.68	39.90	262.26	0.00	0.85	0.00	1.23
	Liquor Drink, Screwdriver	30.4000	6.000	Fl Oz	0.15	0.00	2.61	24.93	0.00	0.00	0.00	0.00
	Liquor Drink, Tom Collins	29.6000	1.000	Fl Oz	0.00	0.00	0.38	16.28	0.00	0.00	0.00	0.00
	Liquor Drink, Whiskey Sour	29.9000	1.000	Fl Oz	0.06	0.03	1.67	40.66	0.00	0.00	0.00	0.01
	Liquor, Distilled, All 100 Proof	42.0000	1.500	Fl Oz	0.00	0.00	0.00	123.90	0.00	0.00	0.00	0.00
	Liquor, Distilled, All 80 Proof	42.0000	1.500	Fl Oz	0.00	0.00	0.00	97.02	0.00	0.00	0.00	0.00
	Liquor, Distilled, All 86 Proof	42.0000	1.500	Fl Oz	0.00	0.00	0.04	105.00	0.00	0.00	0.00	0.00
	Liquor, Distilled, All 90 Proof	42.0000	1.000	Jigger	0.00	0.00	0.00	110.46	0.00	0.00	0.00	0.00
	Liquor, Distilled, All 94 Proof	42.0000	1.500	Fl Oz	0.00	0.00	0.00	115.50	0.00	0.00	0.00	0.00
	Liquor, Vodka, 80 Proof	42.0000	1.500	Fl Oz	0.00	0.00	0.00	97.02	0.00	0.00	0.00	0.00
	Punch Drink, Fruit, Cnd	248.0000	1.000	Cup	0.00	0.00	29.51	116.56	0.00	0.25	0.00	0.00
	Shake, Chocolate	458.0000	22.000	Fl Oz	15.57	16.95	93.89	581.66	13.74	3.66	59.54	10.58
	Shake, Chocolate, Thick	300.0000	1.330	Cup	9.15	8.10	63.45	355.83	6.00	0.90	31.50	5.04
	Shake, Strawberry	283.0000	10.000	Fl Oz	9.62	7.92	53.49	319.79	0.00	1.13	31.13	4.90

Monounsaturated Fat (gm)	Polyunsaturated Fat (gm)	Vitamin D (mg)	Vitamin K (mg)	Vitamin E (mg)	Vitamin A (re)	Vitamin C (mg)	Thiamin (mg)	Riboflavin (mg)	Niacin (mg)	Vitamin B_6 (mg)	Folate (mg)	Vitamin B_{12} (mcg)	Calcium (mg)	Iron (mg)	Magnesium (mg)	Phosphorus (mg)	Potassium (mg)	Sodium (mg)	Zinc (mg)
0.00	0.00	0.00	0.00	0.00	0.00	89.42	0.02	0.02	0.09	0.05	0.51	0.00	7.58	0.38	5.05	5.05	45.47	5.05	0.18
0.00	0.05	0.00	0.00	0.00	2.53	0.25	0.08	0.10	0.66	0.18	6.58	0.00	22.77	0.61	25.30	27.83	333.96	7.59	0.13
0.03	0.05	0.00	0.00	0.13	0.00	67.25	0.10	0.05	0.80	0.05	26.00	0.00	20.00	0.90	25.00	27.50	405.00	5.00	0.15
0.02	0.05	0.00	0.00	0.12	2.47	72.12	0.10	0.05	0.57	0.05	25.69	0.00	17.29	0.49	24.70	27.17	377.91	2.47	0.22
0.02	0.05	0.00	0.00	0.00	108.68	93.86	0.10	0.05	0.49	0.10	25.19	0.00	22.23	0.49	29.64	37.05	400.14	2.47	0.12
0.02	0.05	0.00	0.05	0.12	2.47	93.86	0.10	0.05	0.49	0.10	25.19	0.00	22.23	0.49	29.64	37.05	400.14	2.47	0.12
0.00	0.00	0.00	0.00	0.00	0.00	40.55	0.00	0.00	0.00	0.00	0.00	0.00	0.00	0.00	0.00	0.00	0.00	23.65	0.00
0.00	0.00	0.00	0.00	0.00	0.00	40.55	0.00	0.00	0.00	0.00	0.00	0.00	0.00	0.00	0.00	0.00	0.00	23.65	0.00
0.10	0.10	0.00	0.10	0.22	49.60	124.00	0.22	0.07	0.99	0.10	75.14	0.00	27.28	0.50	27.28	42.16	496.00	2.48	0.12
0.02	0.02	0.00	0.00	0.47	19.92	96.86	0.20	0.05	0.50	0.10	109.06	0.00	22.41	0.25	24.90	39.84	473.10	2.49	0.12
0.02	0.03	0.00	0.00	0.00	19.89	96.70	0.20	0.04	0.50	0.11	108.88	0.00	298.31	0.25	24.86	39.77	472.32	2.49	0.12
0.02	0.07	0.00	0.00	0.12	177.84	73.61	0.00	0.32	3.61	0.12	17.29	0.00	9.88	0.59	41.99	32.11	686.66	14.82	0.12
0.05	0.27	0.00	0.00	0.12	595.27	44.95	0.00	0.25	5.53	0.15	19.76	0.00	9.88	0.89	41.99	61.75	686.66	14.82	0.15
0.03	0.08	0.00	0.00	0.05	0.00	26.75	0.15	0.05	0.65	0.25	57.75	0.00	42.50	0.65	32.50	20.00	335.00	2.50	0.28
0.05	0.03	0.00	0.00	0.03	0.00	10.50	0.05	0.18	2.02	0.56	1.02	0.00	30.72	3.02	35.84	64.00	706.56	10.24	0.54
0.05	0.07	0.00	0.00	0.22	104.58	54.78	0.15	0.05	0.25	0.07	11.45	0.00	44.82	0.50	19.92	34.86	443.22	2.49	0.07
0.10	0.10	0.00	0.00	0.22	103.74	76.57	0.15	0.05	0.25	0.10	11.36	0.00	44.46	0.49	19.76	34.58	439.66	2.47	0.07
0.02	0.05	0.00	0.00	2.21	136.08	44.47	0.12	0.07	1.63	0.27	48.36	0.00	21.87	1.41	26.73	46.17	534.60	877.23	0.34
0.02	0.05	0.00	0.00	2.21	136.08	44.47	0.12	0.07	1.63	0.27	48.36	0.00	21.87	1.41	26.73	46.17	534.60	24.30	0.34
0.00	0.00	0.00	0.00	0.00	2.47	108.43	0.02	0.02	0.05	0.02	2.22	0.00	9.88	0.22	4.94	2.47	32.11	9.88	0.10
0.00	0.00	0.00	0.00	0.00	0.00	0.00	0.00	0.00	0.00	0.00	0.00	0.00	0.00	0.00	0.00	0.00	0.00	25.00	0.00
0.00	0.00	0.00	0.00	0.00	0.00	0.00	0.00	0.00	0.00	0.00	0.00	0.00	0.00	0.00	0.00	0.00	0.00	10.00	0.00
0.00	0.00	0.00	0.00	0.00	0.00	0.00	0.00	0.00	0.00	0.00	0.00	0.00	0.00	0.00	0.00	0.00	0.00	20.00	0.00
0.00	0.00	0.00	0.00	0.00	62.50	39.00	0.04	0.05	0.00	0.00	0.00	0.00	31.00	1.20	0.00	0.00	439.00	41.00	0.00
0.02	0.10	0.00	0.00	0.77	283.14	67.03	0.10	0.07	1.77	0.34	51.06	0.00	26.62	1.02	26.62	41.14	467.06	653.40	0.48
0.00	0.00	0.00	0.00	0.00	0.00	6.00	0.00	0.00	0.00	0.00	0.00	0.00	15.00	0.00	0.00	8.00	1.00	8.00	0.00
0.00	0.00	0.00	0.00	0.00	0.00	34.05	0.00	0.00	0.00	0.00	0.00	0.00	29.26	0.05	2.66	2.66	2.66	18.62	0.08
0.00	0.00	0.00	0.00	0.00	0.00	5.93	0.00	0.00	0.00	0.00	0.24	0.00	49.77	0.09	2.37	23.70	0.00	7.11	0.07
0.00	0.02	0.00	0.07	0.00	0.00	9.63	0.02	0.05	0.05	0.02	5.43	0.00	7.41	0.40	4.94	4.94	37.05	7.41	0.10
0.00	0.02	0.00	0.00	0.00	4.96	9.67	0.02	0.05	0.05	0.02	5.46	0.00	7.44	0.40	4.96	4.96	37.20	7.44	0.10
2.10	0.31	0.00	0.00	0.12	20.21	0.00	0.00	0.03	0.04	0.01	0.00	0.06	7.52	0.06	0.94	23.50	15.04	43.24	0.08
0.01	0.06	0.00	0.00	0.00	0.00	0.00	0.00	0.01	0.07	0.00	0.00	0.00	0.52	0.03	1.56	3.12	15.60	4.16	0.02
0.01	0.06	0.00	0.00	0.00	0.00	0.00	0.00	0.01	0.07	0.00	0.00	0.00	0.52	0.03	1.56	3.12	15.60	4.16	0.02
0.01	0.09	0.00	0.00	0.00	0.00	0.00	0.00	0.00	0.00	0.00	0.00	0.00	0.00	0.04	0.00	0.00	0.00	2.50	0.02
0.00	0.00	0.00	0.00	0.00	0.00	0.00	0.00	0.00	0.01	0.00	0.00	0.00	0.87	0.01	0.29	0.58	0.58	4.06	0.02
0.01	0.01	0.00	0.00	0.00	0.00	0.96	0.01	0.00	0.02	0.01	1.20	0.00	1.80	0.09	1.20	3.60	12.60	3.00	0.04
0.00	0.00	0.00	0.00	0.00	0.00	2.69	0.00	0.00	0.02	0.00	1.66	0.00	0.00	0.02	2.07	4.14	22.77	82.80	0.06
0.00	0.00	0.00	0.00	0.00	0.00	0.12	0.00	0.00	0.00	0.00	0.15	0.00	0.60	0.01	0.30	0.30	1.50	1.20	0.02
0.00	0.00	0.00	0.00	0.00	0.00	0.00	0.00	0.00	0.03	0.00	0.03	0.00	0.57	0.03	0.57	2.00	7.41	0.86	0.01
0.00	0.00	0.00	0.00	0.00	0.00	0.00	0.00	0.00	0.00	0.00	0.00	0.00	0.00	0.00	0.00	0.00	0.00	11.88	0.00
0.00	0.00	0.00	0.00	0.00	0.00	0.00	0.00	0.00	0.00	0.00	0.06	0.00	0.56	0.03	0.56	0.85	5.08	0.85	0.01
0.23	0.49	0.00	0.00	0.00	0.00	6.63	0.04	0.01	0.17	0.07	14.38	0.00	11.28	0.31	11.28	9.87	100.11	8.46	0.18
0.00	0.00	0.00	0.00	0.00	1.82	9.48	0.02	0.00	0.05	0.01	10.67	0.00	2.13	0.02	2.43	4.26	46.51	0.30	0.01
0.00	0.00	0.00	0.00	0.00	0.00	0.50	0.00	0.00	0.00	0.00	0.21	0.00	1.18	0.00	0.30	0.30	2.37	5.03	0.02
0.00	0.01	0.00	0.00	0.00	0.30	3.77	0.06	0.00	0.04	0.01	1.55	0.00	1.79	0.02	1.20	2.09	15.85	3.29	0.01
0.00	0.00	0.00	0.00	0.00	0.00	0.00	0.00	0.00	0.00	0.00	0.00	0.00	0.00	0.02	0.00	1.68	0.84	0.42	0.02
0.00	0.00	0.00	0.00	0.00	0.00	0.00	0.00	0.00	0.00	0.00	0.00	0.00	0.00	0.02	0.00	1.68	0.84	0.42	0.02
0.00	0.00	0.00	0.00	0.00	0.00	0.00	0.00	0.00	0.00	0.00	0.00	0.00	0.00	0.02	0.00	1.68	0.84	0.42	0.02
0.00	0.00	0.00	0.00	0.00	0.00	0.00	0.00	0.00	0.00	0.00	0.00	0.00	0.00	0.02	0.00	1.68	0.84	0.42	0.02
0.00	0.00	0.00	0.00	0.00	0.00	0.00	0.00	0.00	0.00	0.00	0.00	0.00	0.00	0.02	0.00	1.68	0.84	0.42	0.02
0.00	0.00	0.00	0.00	0.00	0.00	0.00	0.00	0.00	0.00	0.00	0.00	0.00	0.00	0.00	0.00	2.10	0.42	0.42	0.00
0.00	0.00	0.00	0.00	0.00	2.48	73.41	0.05	0.05	0.05	0.00	3.22	0.00	19.84	0.52	4.96	2.48	62.00	54.56	0.30
4.95	0.64	1.83	0.00	0.32	105.34	1.83	0.27	1.15	0.73	0.23	16.03	1.56	517.54	1.42	77.86	467.16	916.00	444.26	1.88
2.34	0.30	0.00	0.00	0.30	63.00	0.00	0.15	0.66	0.36	0.09	14.70	0.96	396.00	0.93	48.00	378.00	672.00	333.00	1.44
0.00	0.00	0.57	0.00	0.00	82.07	2.26	0.14	0.57	0.51	0.11	8.49	0.88	319.79	0.31	36.79	283.00	515.06	234.89	1.02

USDA ID Code	Food Name	Weight in Grams*	Quantity of Units	Unit of Measure	Protein (gm)	Fat (gm)	Carbohydrate (gm)	Kcalories	Caffeine (gm)	Fiber (gm)	Cholesterol (mg)	Saturated Fat (gm)
	Shake, Vanilla	458.0000	22.000	Fl Oz	16.03	13.74	81.98	508.38	0.00	1.83	50.38	8.52
	Shakes, Vanilla, Thick	313.0000	1.330	Cup	12.08	9.48	55.56	349.97	0.00	0.00	36.93	5.92
709	Snapple, cranberry raspberry	240.0000	8.000	Fl Oz	0.00	0.00	29.00	120.00	0.00	0.00	0.00	0.00
710	Snapple, cranberry raspberry, Di	30.0000	8.000	Fl Oz	0.00	0.00	2.00	10.00	0.00	0.00	0.00	0.00
711	Snapple, grape, white, Diet	30.0000	8.000	Fl Oz	0.00	0.00	2.00	10.00	0.00	0.00	0.00	0.00
712	Snapple, grapeade	240.0000	8.000	Fl Oz	0.00	0.00	29.00	120.00	0.00	0.00	0.00	0.00
713	Snapple, kiwi strawberry	240.0000	8.000	Fl Oz	0.00	0.00	26.00	100.00	0.00	0.00	0.00	0.00
714	Snapple, mango madness	240.0000	8.000	Fl Oz	0.00	0.00	29.00	120.00	0.00	0.00	0.00	0.00
715	Snapple, pink lemonade	240.0000	8.000	Fl Oz	0.00	0.00	29.00	120.00	0.00	0.00	0.00	0.00
704	Snapple, Tea, Iced, lemon	240.0000	8.000	Fl Oz	0.00	0.00	25.00	100.00	0.00	0.00	0.00	0.00
705	Snapple, Tea, Iced, peach	240.0000	8.000	Fl Oz	0.00	0.00	26.00	100.00	0.00	0.00	0.00	0.00
706	Snapple, Tea, Iced, peach, Diet	30.0000	8.000	Fl Oz	0.00	0.00	1.00	0.00	0.00	0.00	0.00	0.00
707	Snapple, Tea, Iced, raspberry	240.0000	8.000	Fl Oz	0.00	0.00	26.00	100.00	0.00	0.00	0.00	0.00
708	Snapple, Tea, Iced, raspberry, D	30.0000	8.000	Fl Oz	0.00	0.00	1.00	0.00	0.00	0.00	0.00	0.00
	Soda, Club	474.0000	16.000	Fl Oz	0.00	0.00	0.00	0.00	0.00	0.00	0.00	0.00
	Soda, Cream	494.0000	16.000	Fl Oz	0.00	0.00	65.70	251.94	0.00	0.00	0.00	0.00
	Soda, Dr. Pepper	491.0000	16.000	Fl Oz	0.00	0.49	51.06	201.31	49.10	0.00	0.00	0.34
	Soda, Ginger Ale	488.0000	16.000	Fl Oz	0.00	0.00	42.46	165.92	0.00	0.00	0.00	0.00
	Soda, Ginger Ale, Diet	366.0000	12.000	Fl Oz	0.00	0.00	0.00	0.00	0.00	0.00	0.00	0.00
	Soda, Grape	372.0000	12.000	Fl Oz	0.00	0.00	41.66	159.96	0.00	0.00	0.00	0.00
	Soda, Grape Drink, Cnd	250.0000	1.000	Cup	0.00	0.00	28.75	112.50	0.00	0.00	0.00	0.00
716	Soda, Lemon-lime	355.0000	12.000	Fl Oz	0.00	0.00	38.40	149.00	0.00	0.00	0.00	0.00
	Soda, Lemon-lime, Diet	355.0000	12.000	Fl Oz	0.00	0.00	0.00	0.00	0.00	0.00	0.00	0.00
	Soda, Mountain Dew	360.0000	12.000	Fl Oz	0.00	0.00	44.40	179.00	54.00	0.00	0.00	0.00
	Soda, Orange Drink, Cnd	248.0000	1.000	Cup	0.00	0.00	31.99	126.48	0.00	0.25	0.00	0.00
	Soda, Root Beer	493.0000	16.000	Fl Oz	0.00	0.00	52.26	202.13	0.00	0.00	0.00	0.00
	Soda, Root Beer, Diet	355.0000	12.000	Fl Oz	0.00	0.00	0.36	0.00	0.00	0.00	0.00	0.00
719	Starbucks-Caffe Americano	340.8000	12.000	Fl Oz	0.00	0.00	2.00	10.00	0.00	0.00	0.00	0.00
720	Starbucks-Caffe Latte w/nonfat m	340.8000	12.000	Fl Oz	12.00	0.50	17.00	120.00	0.00	0.00	0.00	0.00
721	Starbucks-Caffe Latte w/whole mi	340.8000	12.000	Fl Oz	11.00	11.00	17.00	210.00	0.00	0.00	0.00	0.00
722	Starbucks-Caffe Mocha w/nonfat mi	340.8000	12.000	Fl Oz	12.00	12.00	32.00	260.00	0.00	0.00	0.00	0.00
723	Starbucks-Caffe Mocha w/whole mil	340.8000	12.000	Fl Oz	12.00	21.00	31.00	340.00	0.00	0.00	0.00	0.00
724	Starbucks-Cappuccino w/nonfat mi	340.8000	12.000	Fl Oz	7.00	0.00	11.00	80.00	0.00	0.00	0.00	0.00
725	Starbucks-Cappuccino w/whole mil	340.8000	12.000	Fl Oz	7.00	7.00	11.00	140.00	0.00	0.00	0.00	0.00
726	Starbucks-Coffee Frappuccino	340.8000	12.000	Fl Oz	6.00	3.00	39.00	200.00	0.00	0.00	0.00	0.00
727	Starbucks-Coffee, Drip	340.8000	12.000	Fl Oz	1.00	0.00	1.00	10.00	0.00	0.00	0.00	0.00
	Tea, Brewed	237.0000	1.000	Cup	0.00	0.00	0.71	2.37	47.40	0.00	0.00	0.00
	Tea, Herb, Brewed	237.0000	1.000	Cup	0.00	0.00	0.47	2.37	0.00	0.00	0.00	0.00
	Tea, Iced, Bottled, All Flavors	236.6000	1.000	Cup	0.00	0.00	28.59	118.30	44.00	0.00	0.00	0.00
	Tea, Iced, Bottled, All Flavors,	236.6000	1.000	Cup	0.00	0.00	0.99	0.00	54.00	0.00	0.00	0.00
	Tea, Instant, Sweetened	259.0000	1.000	Cup	0.26	0.00	22.02	88.06	28.49	0.00	0.00	0.00
	Tea, Instant, Unsweetened	237.0000	1.000	Cup	0.00	0.00	0.47	2.37	30.81	0.00	0.00	0.00
	Tequila Sunrise	31.2000	6.000	Fl Oz	0.09	0.03	2.68	34.32	0.00	0.00	0.00	0.00
	Thirst Quencher Drink, Bottled	241.0000	1.000	Cup	0.00	0.00	15.18	60.25	0.00	0.00	0.00	0.00
	Water, Bottled, Perrier	192.0000	6.500	Fl Oz	0.00	0.00	0.00	0.00	0.00	0.00	0.00	0.00
	Water, Municipal	240.0000	8.000	Fl Oz	0.00	0.00	0.00	0.00	0.00	0.00	0.00	0.00
785	Water, Spring-Aquafina	240.0000	8.000	Fl Oz	0.00	0.00	0.00	0.00	0.00	0.00	0.00	0.00
786	Water, Spring-Avalon	240.0000	8.000	Fl Oz	0.00	0.00	0.00	0.00	0.00	0.00	0.00	0.00
787	Water, Spring-Dannon	240.0000	8.000	Fl Oz	0.00	0.00	0.00	0.00	0.00	0.00	0.00	0.00
788	Water, Spring-Deer Park	240.0000	8.000	Fl Oz	0.00	0.00	0.00	0.00	0.00	0.00	0.00	0.00
789	Water, Spring-Evian	240.0000	8.000	Fl Oz	0.00	0.00	0.00	0.00	0.00	0.00	0.00	0.00
790	Water, Spring-Naya	240.0000	8.000	Fl Oz	0.00	0.00	0.00	0.00	0.00	0.00	0.00	0.00
	Water, Tonic	488.0000	16.000	Fl Oz	0.00	0.00	42.94	165.92	0.00	0.00	0.00	0.00
	Wine, Dessert, Dry, 3.5 Oz Glass	103.0000	1.000	Glass	0.21	0.00	4.22	129.78	0.00	0.00	0.00	0.00
	Wine, Dessert, Sweet, 3.5 Oz Gla	103.0000	1.000	Glass	0.21	0.00	12.15	157.59	0.00	0.00	0.00	0.00

Monounsaturated Fat (gm)	Polyunsaturated Fat (gm)	Vitamin D (mg)	Vitamin K (mg)	Vitamin E (mg)	Vitamin A (re)	Vitamin C (mg)	Thiamin (mg)	Riboflavin (mg)	Niacin (mg)	Vitamin B_6 (mg)	Folate (mg)	Vitamin B_{12} (mcg)	Calcium (mg)	Iron (mg)	Magnesium (mg)	Phosphorus (mg)	Potassium (mg)	Sodium (mg)	Zinc (mg)
3.94	0.50	0.92	0.00	0.27	146.56	3.66	0.23	0.82	0.87	0.23	15.11	1.65	558.76	0.41	54.96	467.16	796.92	375.56	1.65
2.75	0.34	0.00	0.00	0.31	87.64	0.00	0.09	0.63	0.47	0.13	20.66	1.63	457.29	0.31	36.81	360.58	571.85	298.60	1.22
0.00	0.00	0.00	0.00	0.00	0.00	0.00	0.00	0.00	0.00	0.00	0.00	0.00	0.00	0.00	0.00	0.00	0.00	10.00	0.00
0.00	0.00	0.00	0.00	0.00	0.00	0.00	0.00	0.00	0.00	0.00	0.00	0.00	0.00	0.00	0.00	0.00	0.00	10.00	0.00
0.00	0.00	0.00	0.00	0.00	0.00	0.00	0.00	0.00	0.00	0.00	0.00	0.00	0.00	0.00	0.00	0.00	0.00	10.00	0.00
0.00	0.00	0.00	0.00	0.00	0.00	0.00	0.00	0.00	0.00	0.00	0.00	0.00	0.00	0.00	0.00	0.00	0.00	10.00	0.00
0.00	0.00	0.00	0.00	0.00	0.00	0.00	0.00	0.00	0.00	0.00	0.00	0.00	0.00	0.00	0.00	0.00	0.00	10.00	0.00
0.00	0.00	0.00	0.00	0.00	0.00	0.00	0.00	0.00	0.00	0.00	0.00	0.00	0.00	0.00	0.00	0.00	0.00	10.00	0.00
0.00	0.00	0.00	0.00	0.00	0.00	0.00	0.00	0.00	0.00	0.00	0.00	0.00	0.00	0.00	0.00	0.00	0.00	10.00	0.00
0.00	0.00	0.00	0.00	0.00	0.00	0.00	0.00	0.00	0.00	0.00	0.00	0.00	0.00	0.00	0.00	0.00	0.00	0.00	0.00
0.00	0.00	0.00	0.00	0.00	0.00	0.00	0.00	0.00	0.00	0.00	0.00	0.00	0.00	0.00	0.00	0.00	0.00	0.00	0.00
0.00	0.00	0.00	0.00	0.00	0.00	0.00	0.00	0.00	0.00	0.00	0.00	0.00	0.00	0.00	0.00	0.00	0.00	10.00	0.00
0.00	0.00	0.00	0.00	0.00	0.00	0.00	0.00	0.00	0.00	0.00	0.00	0.00	0.00	0.00	0.00	0.00	0.00	0.00	0.00
0.00	0.00	0.00	0.00	0.00	0.00	0.00	0.00	0.00	0.00	0.00	0.00	0.00	0.00	0.00	0.00	0.00	0.00	10.00	0.00
0.00	0.00	0.00	0.00	0.00	0.00	0.00	0.00	0.00	0.00	0.00	0.00	0.00	23.70	0.05	4.74	0.00	9.48	99.54	0.47
0.00	0.00	0.00	0.00	0.00	0.00	0.00	0.00	0.00	0.00	0.00	0.00	0.00	24.70	0.25	4.94	0.00	4.94	59.28	0.35
0.00	0.00	0.00	0.00	0.00	0.00	0.00	0.00	0.00	0.00	0.00	0.00	0.00	14.73	0.20	0.00	54.01	4.91	49.10	0.20
0.00	0.00	0.00	0.05	0.00	0.00	0.00	0.00	0.00	0.00	0.00	0.00	0.00	14.64	0.88	4.88	0.00	4.88	34.16	0.24
0.00	0.00	0.00	0.00	0.00	0.00	0.00	0.00	0.00	0.00	0.00	0.00	0.00	0.00	0.00	0.00	0.00	0.00	2.50	0.00
0.00	0.00	0.00	0.00	0.00	0.00	0.00	0.00	0.00	0.00	0.00	0.00	0.00	11.16	0.30	3.72	0.00	3.72	55.80	0.26
0.00	0.00	0.00	0.00	0.00	0.00	85.25	0.00	0.00	0.08	0.03	0.75	0.00	7.50	0.43	5.00	2.50	12.50	15.00	0.28
0.00	0.00	0.00	0.00	0.00	0.00	0.00	0.00	0.00	0.10	0.00	0.00	0.00	9.00	0.25	2.00	1.00	4.00	41.00	0.18
0.00	0.00	0.00	0.00	0.00	0.00	0.00	0.00	0.00	0.00	0.00	0.00	0.00	0.00	0.00	0.00	0.00	0.00	2.50	0.00
0.00	0.00	0.00	0.00	0.00	0.00	0.00	0.00	0.00	0.00	0.00	0.00	0.00	0.00	0.00	0.00	0.00	10.00	31.00	0.00
0.00	0.00	0.00	0.00	0.00	4.96	84.57	0.02	0.00	0.07	0.02	5.46	0.00	14.88	0.69	4.96	2.48	44.64	39.68	0.22
0.00	0.00	0.00	0.00	0.00	0.00	0.00	0.00	0.00	0.00	0.00	0.00	0.00	24.65	0.25	4.93	0.00	4.93	64.09	0.35
0.00	0.00	0.00	0.00	0.00	0.00	0.00	0.00	0.00	0.00	0.00	0.00	0.00	0.00	0.00	0.00	0.00	0.00	2.50	0.00
0.00	0.00	0.00	0.00	0.00	0.00	0.00	0.00	0.00	0.00	0.00	0.00	0.00	0.00	0.00	0.00	0.00	0.00	105.00	0.00
0.00	0.00	0.00	0.00	0.00	0.00	0.00	0.00	0.00	0.00	0.00	0.00	0.00	0.00	0.00	0.00	0.00	0.00	170.00	0.00
0.00	0.00	0.00	0.00	0.00	0.00	0.00	0.00	0.00	0.00	0.00	0.00	0.00	0.00	0.00	0.00	0.00	0.00	160.00	0.00
0.00	0.00	0.00	0.00	0.00	0.00	0.00	0.00	0.00	0.00	0.00	0.00	0.00	0.00	0.00	0.00	0.00	0.00	170.00	0.00
0.00	0.00	0.00	0.00	0.00	0.00	0.00	0.00	0.00	0.00	0.00	0.00	0.00	0.00	0.00	0.00	0.00	0.00	160.00	0.00
0.00	0.00	0.00	0.00	0.00	0.00	0.00	0.00	0.00	0.00	0.00	0.00	0.00	0.00	0.00	0.00	0.00	0.00	110.00	0.00
0.00	0.00	0.00	0.00	0.00	0.00	0.00	0.00	0.00	0.00	0.00	0.00	0.00	0.00	0.00	0.00	0.00	0.00	105.00	0.00
0.00	0.00	0.00	0.00	0.00	0.00	0.00	0.00	0.00	0.00	0.00	0.00	0.00	0.00	0.00	0.00	0.00	0.00	170.00	0.00
0.00	0.00	0.00	0.00	0.00	0.00	0.00	0.00	0.00	0.00	0.00	0.00	0.00	0.00	0.00	0.00	0.00	0.00	10.00	0.00
0.00	0.00	0.00	0.12	0.00	0.00	0.00	0.00	0.02	0.00	0.00	12.32	0.00	0.00	0.05	7.11	2.37	87.69	7.11	0.05
0.00	0.02	0.00	0.00	0.00	0.00	0.00	0.02	0.00	0.00	0.00	1.42	0.00	4.74	0.19	2.37	0.00	21.33	2.37	0.09
0.00	0.00	0.00	0.00	0.00	0.00	0.00	0.00	0.00	0.00	0.00	0.00	0.00	0.00	0.00	0.00	0.00	0.00	9.86	0.00
0.00	0.00	0.00	0.00	0.00	0.00	0.00	0.00	0.00	0.00	0.00	0.00	0.00	0.00	0.00	0.00	0.00	0.00	0.00	0.00
0.00	0.03	0.00	0.00	0.00	0.00	0.00	0.00	0.05	0.10	0.00	9.58	0.00	5.18	0.05	5.18	2.59	49.21	7.77	0.08
0.00	0.00	0.00	0.00	0.00	0.00	0.00	0.00	0.00	0.09	0.00	0.71	0.00	4.74	0.05	4.74	2.37	47.40	7.11	0.07
0.01	0.01	0.00	0.00	0.00	3.12	6.02	0.01	0.00	0.06	0.02	3.31	0.00	1.87	0.09	2.18	3.12	32.45	1.25	0.02
0.00	0.00	0.00	0.00	0.00	0.00	0.00	0.02	0.00	0.00	0.00	0.00	0.00	0.00	0.12	2.41	21.69	26.51	96.40	0.05
0.00	0.00	0.00	0.00	0.00	0.00	0.00	0.00	0.00	0.00	0.00	0.00	0.00	26.88	0.00	0.00	0.00	0.00	1.92	0.00
0.00	0.00	0.00	0.00	0.00	0.00	0.00	0.00	0.00	0.00	0.00	0.00	0.00	0.00	0.00	0.00	0.00	0.00	0.00	0.00
0.00	0.00	0.00	0.00	0.00	0.00	0.00	0.00	0.00	0.00	0.00	0.00	0.00	0.00	0.00	0.00	0.00	0.00	0.00	0.00
0.00	0.00	0.00	0.00	0.00	0.00	0.00	0.00	0.00	0.00	0.00	0.00	0.00	0.00	0.00	0.00	0.00	0.00	0.00	0.00
0.00	0.00	0.00	0.00	0.00	0.00	0.00	0.00	0.00	0.00	0.00	0.00	0.00	0.00	0.00	0.00	0.00	0.00	0.00	0.00
0.00	0.00	0.00	0.00	0.00	0.00	0.00	0.00	0.00	0.00	0.00	0.00	0.00	0.00	0.00	0.00	0.00	0.00	0.00	0.00
0.00	0.00	0.00	0.00	0.00	0.00	0.00	0.00	0.00	0.00	0.00	0.00	0.00	0.00	0.00	0.00	0.00	0.00	0.00	0.00
0.00	0.00	0.00	0.00	0.00	0.00	0.00	0.00	0.00	0.00	0.00	0.00	0.00	0.00	0.00	0.00	0.00	0.00	0.00	0.00
0.00	0.00	0.00	0.00	0.00	0.00	0.00	0.00	0.00	0.00	0.00	0.00	0.00	4.88	0.05	0.00	0.00	0.00	19.52	0.49
0.00	0.00	0.00	0.00	0.00	0.00	0.00	0.02	0.02	0.22	0.00	0.41	0.00	8.24	0.25	9.27	9.27	94.76	9.27	0.07
0.00	0.00	0.00	0.00	0.00	0.00	0.00	0.02	0.02	0.22	0.00	0.41	0.00	8.24	0.25	9.27	9.27	94.76	9.27	0.07

USDA ID Code	Food Name	Weight in Grams*	Quantity of Units	Unit of Measure	Protein (gm)	Fat (gm)	Carbohydrate (gm)	Kcalories	Caffeine (gm)	Fiber (gm)	Cholesterol (mg)	Saturated Fat (gm)
	Wine, Table, All, 3.5 Oz Glass	103.0000	1.000	Glass	0.21	0.00	1.44	72.10	0.00	0.00	0.00	0.00
	Wine, Table, Red, 3.5 Oz Glass	103.0000	1.000	Glass	0.21	0.00	1.75	74.16	0.00	0.00	0.00	0.00
	Wine, Table, Rose, 3.5 Oz Glass	103.0000	1.000	Glass	0.21	0.00	1.44	73.13	0.00	0.00	0.00	0.00
	Wine, Table, White, 3.5 Oz Glass	103.0000	1.000	Glass	0.10	0.00	0.82	70.04	0.00	0.00	0.00	0.00
	Barley, Cooked	184.0000	1.000	Cup	22.96	4.23	135.20	651.36	0.00	31.83	0.00	0.88
61	Bread Sticks, Plain	10.0000	1.000	Stick	1.20	0.95	6.84	41.20	0.00	0.00	0.00	0.14
	Bread Stuffing, Plain	232.0000	1.000	Cup	8.82	16.70	51.50	389.76	0.00	0.00	0.00	3.39
	Bread, Banana	60.0000	1.000	Slice	2.58	7.08	33.06	202.80	0.00	0.00	25.80	1.83
	Bread, Cornbread	28.3500	1.000	Slice	1.90	2.01	12.33	75.41	0.00	0.00	11.34	0.44
	Bread, Cracked-wheat	28.3500	1.000	Slice	2.47	1.11	14.03	73.71	0.00	1.56	0.00	0.26
	Bread, Cracked-wheat, Toasted	23.0000	1.000	Slice	2.19	0.97	12.37	65.09	0.00	0.00	0.00	0.23
	Bread, Dinner Roll, Egg	28.3500	1.000	Each	2.69	1.81	14.74	87.03	0.00	1.05	14.18	0.45
	Bread, Dinner Roll, French	28.3500	1.000	Each	2.44	1.22	14.23	78.53	0.00	0.91	0.00	0.27
	Bread, Dinner Roll, Oat Bran	28.3500	1.000	Each	2.69	1.30	11.40	66.91	0.00	1.16	0.00	0.18
	Bread, Dinner Roll, Plain	86.0000	1.000	Each	7.22	6.28	43.34	258.00	0.00	2.58	0.86	1.51
	Bread, Dinner Roll, Rye	43.0000	1.000	Large	4.43	1.46	22.83	122.98	0.00	2.09	0.00	0.26
	Bread, Dinner Roll, Wheat	28.3500	1.000	Each	2.44	1.79	13.04	77.40	0.00	1.07	0.00	0.43
	Bread, Dinner Roll, Whole-wheat	43.0000	1.000	Each	3.74	2.02	21.97	114.38	0.00	3.24	0.00	0.36
	Bread, Egg	28.3500	1.000	Slice	2.69	1.70	13.55	81.36	0.00	0.65	14.46	0.45
	Bread, Egg, Toasted	28.3500	1.000	Slice	2.98	1.87	14.91	89.30	0.00	0.71	15.88	0.46
	Bread, French or Vienna	28.3500	1.000	Slice	2.49	0.85	14.71	77.68	0.00	0.85	0.00	0.18
	Bread, French or Vienna, Toasted	28.3500	1.000	Slice	2.72	0.94	15.99	84.48	0.00	0.94	0.00	0.20
	Bread, Italian	28.3500	1.000	Slice	2.49	0.99	14.18	76.83	0.00	0.77	0.00	0.24
	Bread, Italian, Toasted	27.0000	1.000	Slice	2.62	1.05	14.85	80.46	0.00	0.00	0.00	0.25
	Bread, Lo Cal, Oat Bran	28.3500	1.000	Slice	2.27	0.91	11.71	56.98	0.00	3.40	0.00	0.13
	Bread, Lo Cal, Oat Bran, Toasted	28.3500	1.000	Slice	2.69	1.08	13.95	67.76	0.00	4.05	0.00	0.15
	Bread, Lo Cal, Oatmeal	28.3500	1.000	Slice	2.15	0.99	12.28	59.54	0.00	0.00	0.00	0.17
	Bread, Lo Cal, Oatmeal, Toasted	19.0000	1.000	Slice	1.71	0.80	9.79	47.69	0.00	0.00	0.00	0.14
	Bread, Lo Cal, Rye	28.3500	1.000	Slice	2.58	0.82	11.48	57.55	0.00	3.40	0.00	0.10
	Bread, Lo Cal, Rye, Toasted	19.0000	1.000	Slice	2.05	0.65	9.16	45.79	0.00	0.00	0.19	0.08
	Bread, Lo Cal, Wheat	28.3500	1.000	Slice	2.58	0.65	12.36	56.13	0.00	3.40	0.00	0.10
	Bread, Lo Cal, Wheat, Toasted	19.0000	1.000	Slice	2.05	0.51	9.86	44.84	0.00	0.00	0.00	0.08
	Bread, Lo Cal, White	28.3500	1.000	Slice	2.47	0.71	12.56	58.68	0.00	2.75	0.00	0.16
	Bread, Lo Cal, White, Toasted	19.0000	1.000	Slice	1.96	0.57	10.01	46.93	0.00	0.00	0.00	0.12
	Bread, Mixed-grain	28.3500	1.000	Slice	2.84	1.08	13.15	70.88	0.00	1.81	0.00	0.23
	Bread, Mixed-grain, Toasted	28.3500	1.000	Slice	3.09	1.16	14.29	77.11	0.00	1.87	0.00	0.25
	Bread, Oat Bran	28.3500	1.000	Slice	2.95	1.25	11.28	66.91	0.00	1.28	0.00	0.20
	Bread, Oat Bran, Toasted	28.3500	1.000	Slice	3.23	1.36	12.39	73.43	0.00	1.39	0.00	0.22
	Bread, Oatmeal	28.3500	1.000	Slice	2.38	1.25	13.75	76.26	0.00	1.13	0.00	0.20
	Bread, Oatmeal, Toasted	28.3500	1.000	Slice	2.61	1.36	14.94	82.78	0.00	1.22	0.00	0.22
	Bread, Pita, White, Enriched	60.0000	1.000	Pita	5.46	0.72	33.42	165.00	0.00	1.32	0.00	0.10
	Bread, Pita, Whole-wheat	64.0000	1.000	Pita	6.27	1.66	35.20	170.24	0.00	4.74	0.00	0.26
	Bread, Pumpernickel	28.3500	1.000	Slice	2.47	0.88	13.47	70.88	0.00	1.84	0.00	0.12
	Bread, Pumpernickel, Toasted	28.3500	1.000	Slice	2.69	0.96	14.80	77.96	0.00	2.01	0.00	0.14
	Bread, Pumpkin	60.0000	1.000	Slice	2.40	7.68	30.72	198.60	0.00	0.00	26.40	1.23
	Bread, Raisin	28.3500	1.000	Slice	2.24	1.25	14.83	77.68	0.00	1.22	0.00	0.31
	Bread, Raisin, Toasted	28.3500	1.000	Slice	2.44	1.36	16.13	84.20	0.00	1.33	0.00	0.33
	Bread, Rice Bran	28.3500	1.000	Slice	2.52	1.30	12.33	68.89	0.00	1.39	0.00	0.20
	Bread, Rice Bran, Toasted	28.3500	1.000	Slice	2.75	1.42	13.41	74.84	0.00	1.50	0.00	0.22
	Bread, Rolls, Hard (includes Kai	28.3500	1.000	Each	2.81	1.22	14.94	83.07	0.00	0.65	0.00	0.17
	Bread, Rye	28.3500	1.000	Slice	2.41	0.94	13.69	73.43	0.00	1.64	0.00	0.18
	Bread, Rye, Toasted	28.3500	1.000	Slice	2.66	1.02	15.05	80.51	0.00	1.81	0.00	0.20
	Bread, Wheat (includes Wheat Ber	28.3500	1.000	Slice	2.58	1.16	13.38	73.71	0.00	1.22	0.00	0.25
	Bread, Wheat Bran	28.3500	1.000	Slice	9 2.49	0.96	13.55	70.31	0.00	1.13	0.00	0.22
	Bread, Wheat Bran, Toasted	33.0000	1.000	Slice	3.20	1.22	17.33	90.09	0.00	0.00	0.00	0.28

Monounsaturated Fat (gm)	Polyunsaturated Fat (gm)	Vitamin D (mg)	Vitamin K (mg)	Vitamin E (mg)	Vitamin A (re)	Vitamin C (mg)	Thiamin (mg)	Riboflavin (mg)	Niacin (mg)	Vitamin B_6 (mg)	Folate (mg)	Vitamin B_{12} (mcg)	Calcium (mg)	Iron (mg)	Magnesium (mg)	Phosphorus (mg)	Potassium (mg)	Sodium (mg)	Zinc (mg)
0.00	0.00	0.00	0.00	0.00	0.00	0.00	0.00	0.02	0.07	0.02	1.13	0.01	8.24	0.42	10.30	14.42	91.67	8.24	0.07
0.00	0.00	0.00	0.00	0.00	0.00	0.00	0.01	0.03	0.08	0.03	2.06	0.01	8.24	0.44	13.39	14.42	115.36	5.15	0.09
0.00	0.00	0.00	0.00	0.00	0.00	0.00	0.00	0.02	0.07	0.02	1.13	0.01	8.24	0.39	10.30	15.45	101.97	5.15	0.06
0.00	0.00	0.00	0.00	0.00	0.00	0.00	0.00	0.01	0.07	0.01	0.21	0.00	9.27	0.33	10.30	14.42	82.40	5.15	0.07
0.55	2.04	0.00	0.00	1.10	3.68	0.00	1.20	0.53	8.46	0.59	34.96	0.00	60.72	6.62	244.72	485.76	831.68	22.08	5.10
0.37	0.36	0.00	0.00	0.00	0.00	0.00	0.06	0.06	0.53	0.01	3.00	0.00	2.20	0.43	3.20	12.10	12.40	65.70	0.09
7.40	4.89	0.00	0.00	0.00	160.08	3.94	0.39	0.33	3.69	0.12	39.44	0.00	148.48	3.80	34.80	113.68	303.92	1069.52	0.74
3.02	1.77	0.00	0.00	0.00	14.40	1.02	0.10	0.12	0.87	0.09	6.60	0.05	10.80	0.84	8.40	33.60	78.60	118.80	0.22
0.52	0.91	0.00	0.00	0.00	15.31	0.09	0.08	0.08	0.64	0.03	18.14	0.04	70.59	0.71	7.09	47.91	41.67	186.54	0.17
0.54	0.19	0.00	0.00	0.17	0.00	0.00	0.10	0.07	1.04	0.09	17.29	0.01	12.19	0.80	14.74	43.38	50.18	152.52	0.35
0.48	0.17	0.00	0.00	0.00	0.00	0.00	0.07	0.05	0.83	0.07	6.90	0.01	10.81	0.70	13.11	38.18	44.16	134.55	0.31
0.83	0.32	0.00	0.00	0.20	2.27	0.00	0.15	0.15	0.93	0.01	29.77	0.07	16.73	1.00	7.09	28.63	29.48	154.51	0.32
0.56	0.24	0.00	0.00	0.13	0.00	0.00	0.15	0.09	1.23	0.01	26.93	0.00	25.80	0.77	5.67	23.81	32.32	172.65	0.26
0.42	0.45	0.00	0.00	0.20	0.00	0.00	0.13	0.08	1.40	0.01	26.93	0.00	24.10	1.17	9.36	32.60	34.30	117.09	0.29
3.18	1.04	0.00	0.00	0.76	0.00	0.09	0.42	0.28	3.47	0.04	81.70	0.05	102.34	2.69	19.78	99.76	114.38	448.06	0.66
0.53	0.31	0.00	0.00	0.15	0.43	0.00	0.16	0.12	1.68	0.03	36.98	0.00	12.90	1.16	23.22	68.37	77.40	383.56	0.42
0.88	0.31	0.00	0.00	0.27	0.00	0.00	0.12	0.08	1.15	0.02	14.46	0.00	49.90	1.01	10.21	29.48	32.60	96.39	0.26
0.52	0.93	0.00	0.00	0.58	0.00	0.00	0.11	0.06	1.58	0.09	12.90	0.00	45.58	1.04	36.55	96.32	116.96	205.54	0.86
0.65	0.31	0.00	0.00	0.17	6.52	0.00	0.12	0.12	1.37	0.02	29.77	0.03	26.37	0.86	5.39	30.05	32.60	139.48	0.22
0.85	0.33	0.00	0.00	0.24	6.52	0.00	0.11	0.12	1.36	0.02	25.23	0.03	28.92	0.95	5.95	33.17	35.72	153.09	0.24
0.35	0.20	0.00	0.00	0.08	0.00	0.00	0.15	0.09	1.35	0.01	26.93	0.00	21.26	0.72	7.65	29.77	32.04	172.65	0.25
0.37	0.21	0.00	0.00	0.07	0.00	0.00	0.13	0.09	1.32	0.01	22.96	0.00	22.96	0.78	8.51	32.32	34.59	187.39	0.27
0.23	0.39	0.00	0.00	0.10	0.00	0.00	0.13	0.08	1.24	0.01	26.93	0.00	22.11	0.83	7.65	29.20	31.19	165.56	0.24
0.24	0.41	0.00	0.00	0.00	0.00	0.00	0.11	0.08	1.17	0.01	6.21	0.00	22.95	0.87	8.10	30.78	32.67	173.34	0.26
0.19	0.47	0.00	0.00	0.13	0.00	0.00	0.10	0.06	1.07	0.03	18.71	0.00	16.16	0.89	15.59	39.41	28.92	99.51	0.30
0.23	0.56	0.00	0.00	0.15	0.00	0.00	0.10	0.06	1.14	0.03	15.88	0.00	19.28	1.06	15.59	40.82	34.59	118.50	0.34
0.23	0.38	0.00	0.00	0.00	0.28	0.06	0.10	0.08	0.86	0.01	15.59	0.03	32.60	0.65	6.80	28.35	35.15	110.00	0.24
0.19	0.31	0.00	0.00	0.00	0.19	0.04	0.06	0.06	0.62	0.01	5.32	0.03	26.03	0.52	6.46	26.98	34.58	87.78	0.21
0.19	0.21	0.00	0.00	0.07	0.00	0.11	0.10	0.07	0.72	0.02	13.61	0.01	21.55	0.88	6.24	22.11	27.78	114.82	0.19
0.15	0.17	0.00	0.00	0.00	0.00	0.02	0.07	0.05	0.51	0.01	3.61	0.02	17.29	0.70	3.99	18.81	22.23	91.77	0.17
0.07	0.27	0.00	0.00	0.03	0.00	0.03	0.12	0.09	1.10	0.04	20.13	0.00	22.68	0.84	11.06	28.92	34.59	144.87	0.32
0.06	0.22	0.00	0.00	0.00	0.00	0.02	0.08	0.06	0.79	0.03	4.37	0.01	18.24	0.67	6.46	20.71	27.93	115.52	0.19
0.31	0.16	0.00	0.00	0.04	0.28	0.14	0.12	0.08	1.03	0.01	26.93	0.08	26.65	0.90	6.52	34.30	21.55	128.43	0.38
0.24	0.13	0.00	0.00	0.00	0.19	0.08	0.07	0.06	0.74	0.01	5.51	0.06	21.28	0.72	5.89	30.21	17.29	102.41	0.30
0.43	0.26	0.00	0.00	0.19	0.00	0.09	0.12	0.10	1.24	0.09	22.68	0.02	25.80	0.98	15.03	49.90	57.83	138.06	0.36
0.47	0.28	0.00	0.00	0.19	0.00	0.09	0.10	0.09	1.21	0.09	19.28	0.02	28.07	1.07	16.44	54.15	62.94	150.26	0.39
0.45	0.48	0.00	0.00	0.18	0.00	0.00	0.14	0.10	1.37	0.02	22.96	0.00	18.43	0.88	9.92	39.97	41.67	115.38	0.25
0.50	0.53	0.00	0.00	0.12	0.00	0.00	0.12	0.10	1.36	0.01	19.56	0.00	20.13	0.97	9.64	32.89	34.87	127.01	0.30
0.45	0.48	0.00	0.00	0.17	0.57	0.00	0.11	0.07	0.89	0.02	17.58	0.01	18.71	0.77	10.49	35.72	40.26	169.82	0.29
0.49	0.52	0.00	0.00	0.10	0.57	0.09	0.10	0.07	0.87	0.02	15.03	0.01	20.41	0.83	11.62	38.84	43.66	184.56	0.31
0.07	0.32	0.00	0.00	0.02	0.00	0.00	0.36	0.20	2.78	0.02	57.00	0.00	51.60	1.57	15.60	58.20	72.00	321.60	0.50
0.22	0.68	0.00	0.00	0.58	0.00	0.00	0.22	0.05	1.82	0.17	22.40	0.00	9.60	1.96	44.16	115.20	108.80	340.48	0.97
0.26	0.35	0.00	0.00	0.12	0.00	0.00	0.09	0.09	0.88	0.04	22.68	0.00	19.28	0.81	15.31	50.46	58.97	190.23	0.42
0.29	0.39	0.00	0.00	0.17	0.00	0.00	0.08	0.09	0.87	0.03	19.28	0.00	20.98	0.89	17.01	55.28	64.64	209.22	0.46
1.85	4.11	0.00	0.00	0.00	334.20	0.60	0.09	0.10	0.79	0.02	6.60	0.05	10.80	0.99	7.80	31.80	55.20	187.80	0.20
0.65	0.19	0.00	0.00	0.14	0.00	0.03	0.10	0.11	0.98	0.02	24.66	0.00	18.71	0.82	7.37	30.90	64.35	110.57	0.20
0.71	0.21	0.00	0.00	0.23	0.00	0.11	0.08	0.11	0.96	0.02	20.98	0.00	20.41	0.89	7.94	33.45	69.74	120.20	0.22
0.47	0.50	0.00	0.00	0.24	0.00	0.00	0.18	0.09	1.93	0.08	18.43	0.00	19.56	1.02	22.68	50.46	60.95	124.74	0.37
0.51	0.54	0.00	0.00	0.22	0.00	0.00	0.16	0.08	1.89	0.06	15.59	0.00	21.26	1.11	21.55	49.33	60.10	135.51	0.39
0.32	0.49	0.00	0.00	0.09	0.00	0.00	0.14	0.10	1.20	0.01	26.93	0.00	26.93	0.93	7.65	28.35	30.62	154.22	0.27
0.37	0.23	0.00	0.00	0.10	0.28	0.11	0.12	0.10	1.08	0.02	24.38	0.00	20.70	0.80	11.34	35.44	47.06	187.11	0.32
0.41	0.25	0.00	0.00	0.17	0.00	0.06	0.11	0.09	1.07	0.02	20.70	0.00	22.68	0.88	12.19	39.12	51.88	205.54	0.35
0.49	0.26	0.00	0.00	0.15	0.00	0.00	0.12	0.08	1.17	0.03	21.83	0.00	29.77	0.94	13.04	42.53	56.98	150.26	0.29
0.46	0.18	0.00	0.00	0.13	0.00	0.00	0.11	0.08	1.25	0.05	19.56	0.00	20.98	0.87	22.96	52.45	64.35	137.78	0.38
0.59	0.24	0.00	0.00	0.00	0.00	0.00	0.12	0.09	1.44	0.06	6.60	0.00	26.73	1.11	29.37	67.32	82.17	176.22	0.49

USDA ID Code	Food Name	Weight in Grams*	Quantity of Units	Unit of Measure	Protein (gm)	Fat (gm)	Carbohydrate (gm)	Kcalories	Caffeine (gm)	Fiber (gm)	Cholesterol (mg)	Saturated Fat (gm)
	Bread, Wheat, Toasted	28.3500	1.000	Slice	2.81	1.25	14.54	79.95	0.00	1.50	0.00	0.27
62	Bread, White	25.0000	1.000	Slice	2.05	0.90	12.38	66.75	0.00	0.58	0.25	0.20
63	Bread, White, Toasted	23.0000	1.000	Slice	2.07	0.92	12.51	67.39	0.00	0.00	0.23	0.21
	Bread, Whole Wheat	28.3500	1.000	Slice	2.75	1.19	13.07	69.74	0.00	1.96	0.00	0.26
	Bread, Whole Wheat, Toasted	28.3500	1.000	Slice	2.61	1.67	15.99	86.47	0.00	1.90	0.00	0.25
	Breadsticks, Sesame Sticks, Whea	28.3500	1.000	Ounce	3.09	10.40	13.18	153.37	0.00	0.79	0.00	1.84
	Buns, Hamburger or Hot Dog, Mixe	28.3500	1.000	Each	5.44	3.40	25.25	149.12	0.00	2.16	0.00	0.78
	Buns, Hamburger or Hot Dog, Plai	28.3500	1.000	Each	4.82	2.90	28.52	162.16	0.00	1.54	0.00	0.68
	Cornstarch	128.0000	1.000	Cup	0.33	0.06	116.83	487.68	0.00	1.15	0.00	0.01
	Couscous, Cooked	157.0000	1.000	Cup	5.95	0.25	36.46	175.84	0.00	2.20	0.00	0.05
	Crackers, Cheese, Regular	62.0000	1.000	Cup	6.26	15.69	36.08	311.86	0.00	1.49	8.06	5.81
206	Crackers, Cheese, w/Peanut Butte	7.0000	1.000	Each	0.88	1.62	3.99	33.74	0.00	0.08	0.35	0.36
	Crackers, Crack Pepper, Fat Free	2.1400	7.000	Each	0.29	0.00	1.85	8.56	0.00	0.07	0.00	0.00
207	Crackers, Crispbread, Rye	10.0000	1.000	Each	0.79	0.13	8.22	36.60	0.00	1.62	0.00	0.01
	Crackers, Graham Snacks, Cinn.,	0.6700	20.000	Each	0.04	0.00	0.58	2.46	0.00	0.02	0.00	0.00
208	Crackers, Graham, Plain or Honey	7.0000	1.000	Each	0.48	0.71	5.38	29.61	0.00	0.19	0.00	0.18
	Crackers, Matzo, Egg	28.3500	1.000	Each	3.49	0.60	22.28	110.85	0.00	0.79	23.53	0.16
	Crackers, Matzo, Egg and Onion	28.3500	1.000	Each	2.84	1.11	21.86	110.85	0.00	1.42	12.76	0.27
	Crackers, Matzo, Plain	28.3500	1.000	Each	2.84	0.40	23.73	111.98	0.00	0.85	0.00	0.07
	Crackers, Matzo, Whole-wheat	28.3500	1.000	Each	3.71	0.43	22.37	99.51	0.00	3.35	0.00	0.07
	Crackers, Melba Toast, Plain	30.0000	1.000	Cup	3.63	0.96	22.98	117.00	0.00	1.89	0.00	0.14
209	Crackers, Melba Toast, Plain, w/	5.0000	1.000	Each	0.61	0.16	3.83	19.50	0.00	0.00	0.00	0.02
	Crackers, Melba Toast, Rye	14.1750	1.000	Each	1.64	0.48	10.96	55.14	0.00	1.13	0.00	0.06
	Crackers, Melba Toast, Wheat	14.1750	1.000	Each	1.83	0.33	10.83	53.01	0.00	1.05	0.00	0.05
	Crackers, Ritz	62.0000	1.000	Cup	4.59	15.69	37.82	311.24	0.00	0.99	0.00	2.34
	Crackers, Ritz, Low Sodium	62.0000	1.000	Cup	4.59	15.69	37.82	311.24	0.00	0.99	0.00	2.34
	Crackers, Rye, w/ Cheese Filling	14.1750	1.000	Each	1.30	3.16	8.62	68.18	0.00	0.51	1.28	0.85
210	Crackers, Rye, Wafers, Plain	25.0000	1.000	Each	2.40	0.23	20.10	83.50	0.00	0.00	0.00	0.03
	Crackers, Rye, Wafers, Seasoned	14.1750	1.000	Each	1.28	1.30	10.46	54.01	0.00	2.96	0.00	0.18
211	Crackers, Saltines	3.0000	1.000	Each	0.28	0.35	2.15	13.02	0.00	0.08	0.00	0.06
	Crackers, Saltines, Fat Free	3.0000	1.000	Each	0.40	0.00	2.40	12.00	0.00	0.00	0.00	0.00
212	Crackers, Saltines, Low Salt	3.0000	1.000	Each	0.28	0.35	2.15	13.02	0.00	0.00	0.00	0.06
	Crackers, w/ Cheese Filling, Sna	14.1750	1.000	Each	1.32	2.99	8.75	67.61	0.00	0.26	0.28	0.87
	Crackers, w/Peanut Butter Fillin	14.1750	1.000	Each	1.57	3.39	8.32	69.17	0.00	0.39	0.00	0.79
	Crackers, Wheat, Fat Free - Snac	3.0000	5.000	Each	0.40	0.00	2.40	12.00	0.00	0.20	0.00	0.00
213	Crackers, Wheat, Low Salt	2.0000	1.000	Each	0.17	0.41	1.30	9.46	0.00	0.00	0.00	0.07
214	Crackers, Wheat, Regular	2.0000	1.000	Each	0.17	0.41	1.30	9.46	0.00	0.11	0.00	0.07
	Crackers, Wheat, w/ Cheese Filli	14.1750	1.000	Each	1.39	3.54	8.25	70.45	0.00	0.44	0.99	0.59
	Crackers, Wheat, w/Peanut Butter	14.1750	1.000	Each	1.91	3.78	7.63	70.17	0.00	0.62	0.00	0.65
215	Crackers, Whole-wheat	4.0000	1.000	Each	0.35	0.69	2.74	17.72	0.00	0.42	0.00	0.12
216	Crackers, Whole-wheat, Low Salt	4.0000	1.000	Each	0.35	0.69	2.74	17.72	0.00	0.00	0.00	0.12
	Croutons, Plain	30.0000	1.000	Cup	3.57	1.98	22.05	122.10	0.00	1.53	0.00	0.45
	Croutons, Seasoned	40.0000	1.000	Cup	4.32	7.32	25.40	186.00	0.00	2.00	2.80	2.10
	English Muffins, Mixed-grain	56.7000	1.000	Each	5.16	1.02	26.26	133.24	0.00	1.58	0.00	0.14
	English Muffins, Mixed-grain, To	56.7000	1.000	Each	5.62	1.08	28.52	144.58	0.00	1.72	0.00	0.14
	English Muffins, Plain	56.7000	1.000	Each	4.36	1.02	26.08	133.24	0.00	1.54	0.00	0.14
	English Muffins, Plain, Toasted	56.7000	1.000	Each	4.76	1.14	28.36	144.58	0.00	1.64	0.00	0.16
	English Muffins, Raisin-cinnamon	56.7000	1.000	Each	4.26	1.44	27.62	137.78	0.00	1.64	0.00	0.22
	English Muffins, Raisin-cinnamon	56.7000	1.000	Each	4.62	1.64	30.06	149.68	0.00	1.76	0.00	0.24
	English Muffins, Wheat	56.7000	1.000	Each	4.94	1.14	25.40	126.44	0.00	2.62	0.00	0.16
	English Muffins, Wheat, Toasted	56.7000	1.000	Each	5.32	1.20	27.62	137.78	0.00	2.86	0.00	0.18
	English Muffins, Whole-wheat	56.7000	1.000	Each	4.98	1.20	22.90	115.10	0.00	3.80	0.00	0.18
	English Muffins, Whole-wheat, To	56.7000	1.000	Each	5.44	1.30	25.00	125.30	0.00	4.14	0.00	0.20
	Flour, White	125.0000	1.000	Cup	12.91	1.23	95.39	455.00	0.00	3.38	0.00	0.20
	Flour, Whole Grain	120.0000	1.000	Cup	16.44	2.24	87.08	406.80	0.00	14.64	0.00	0.38

Monounsaturated Fat (gm)	Polyunsaturated Fat (gm)	Vitamin D (mg)	Vitamin K (mg)	Vitamin E (mg)	Vitamin A (re)	Vitamin C (mg)	Thiamin (mg)	Riboflavin (mg)	Niacin (mg)	Vitamin B_6 (mg)	Folate (mg)	Vitamin B_{12} (mcg)	Calcium (mg)	Iron (mg)	Magnesium (mg)	Phosphorus (mg)	Potassium (mg)	Sodium (mg)	Zinc (mg)
0.53	0.28	0.00	0.00	0.17	0.00	0.00	0.10	0.08	1.14	0.03	18.43	0.00	32.32	1.02	14.18	46.21	61.80	163.30	0.32
0.40	0.19	0.00	0.00	0.00	0.00	0.00	0.12	0.09	0.99	0.02	8.50	0.00	27.00	0.76	6.00	23.50	29.75	134.50	0.16
0.41	0.19	0.00	0.00	0.00	0.00	0.00	0.10	0.08	0.90	0.01	5.98	0.00	27.37	0.77	5.98	23.69	30.13	136.16	0.16
0.48	0.28	0.00	0.00	0.24	0.00	0.00	0.10	0.06	1.09	0.05	14.18	0.00	20.41	0.94	24.38	64.92	71.44	149.40	0.55
0.36	0.92	0.00	0.00	0.45	0.00	0.00	0.08	0.07	1.12	0.06	16.16	0.00	10.21	0.96	25.23	58.12	97.81	108.01	0.47
3.09	4.94	0.00	0.00	1.11	2.55	0.00	0.03	0.02	0.44	0.03	6.24	0.00	48.20	0.21	12.76	39.12	50.18	421.85	0.33
1.62	0.66	0.00	0.00	0.32	0.00	0.00	0.26	0.18	2.54	0.06	53.86	0.00	53.86	2.24	24.94	69.18	90.72	259.68	0.60
0.48	1.42	0.00	0.00	0.88	0.00	0.06	0.28	0.18	2.22	0.02	53.86	0.04	78.82	1.80	11.34	49.84	79.94	317.52	0.36
0.02	0.03	0.00	0.00	0.00	0.00	0.00	0.00	0.00	0.00	0.00	0.00	0.00	2.56	0.60	3.84	16.64	3.84	11.52	0.08
0.04	0.10	0.00	0.00	0.02	0.00	0.00	0.10	0.04	1.54	0.08	23.55	0.00	12.56	0.60	12.56	34.54	91.06	7.85	0.41
7.51	1.53	0.00	0.00	1.64	18.60	0.00	0.35	0.27	2.90	0.34	49.60	0.29	93.62	2.96	22.32	135.16	89.90	616.90	0.70
0.85	0.31	0.00	0.00	0.00	0.00	0.00	0.03	0.02	0.46	0.10	1.75	0.00	5.53	0.20	4.06	22.68	17.15	69.44	0.08
0.00	0.00	0.00	0.00	0.00	0.00	0.00	0.00	0.00	0.00	0.00	0.00	0.00	3.42	0.06	0.00	0.00	0.00	21.40	0.00
0.02	0.06	0.00	0.00	0.00	0.00	0.00	0.02	0.01	0.10	0.02	2.20	0.00	3.10	0.24	7.80	26.90	31.90	26.40	0.24
0.00	0.00	0.00	0.00	0.00	0.00	0.00	0.00	0.00	0.00	0.00	0.00	0.00	0.00	0.01	0.00	0.00	0.00	2.01	0.00
0.35	0.11	0.00	0.00	0.00	0.00	0.00	0.02	0.02	0.29	0.00	1.19	0.00	1.68	0.26	2.10	7.28	9.45	42.35	0.06
0.17	0.13	0.00	0.00	0.00	3.69	0.03	0.22	0.18	1.44	0.01	33.17	0.05	11.34	0.77	6.80	41.96	42.53	5.95	0.21
0.28	0.28	0.00	0.00	0.00	1.98	0.06	0.16	0.12	1.39	0.03	44.79	0.06	10.21	1.24	8.51	25.23	23.53	80.80	0.21
0.04	0.17	0.00	0.00	0.02	0.00	0.00	0.11	0.08	1.10	0.03	33.17	0.00	3.69	0.90	7.09	25.23	31.75	0.57	0.19
0.05	0.18	0.00	0.00	0.38	0.00	0.00	0.10	0.08	1.53	0.05	9.92	0.00	6.52	1.32	37.99	86.47	89.59	0.57	0.74
0.23	0.38	0.00	0.00	0.02	0.00	0.00	0.12	0.08	1.23	0.03	37.20	0.00	27.90	1.11	17.70	58.80	60.60	248.70	0.60
0.04	0.06	0.00	0.00	0.00	0.00	0.00	0.02	0.01	0.21	0.00	1.30	0.00	4.65	0.19	2.95	9.80	10.10	0.95	0.10
0.13	0.19	0.00	0.00	0.09	0.00	0.00	0.07	0.04	0.67	0.01	12.05	0.00	11.06	0.52	5.53	25.94	27.36	127.43	0.19
0.08	0.13	0.00	0.00	0.00	0.00	0.00	0.06	0.04	0.72	0.01	18.71	0.00	6.10	0.64	7.94	23.39	20.98	118.64	0.21
6.60	5.92	0.00	0.00	2.80	0.00	0.00	0.25	0.21	2.51	0.03	47.74	0.00	74.40	2.23	16.74	141.36	82.46	525.14	0.42
6.60	5.92	0.00	0.00	2.80	0.00	0.00	0.25	0.21	2.51	0.03	47.74	0.00	74.40	2.23	16.74	141.36	220.10	231.26	0.42
1.74	0.41	0.00	0.00	0.00	5.53	0.06	0.09	0.07	0.51	0.01	11.48	0.02	31.47	0.35	5.24	48.05	48.48	147.99	0.10
0.04	0.10	0.00	0.00	0.00	0.50	0.03	0.11	0.07	0.40	0.07	11.25	0.00	10.00	1.49	30.25	83.50	123.75	198.50	0.70
0.46	0.51	0.00	0.00	0.00	0.14	0.01	0.05	0.03	0.35	0.03	7.37	0.00	6.24	0.43	15.03	43.52	64.35	125.73	0.36
0.19	0.06	0.00	0.00	0.00	0.00	0.00	0.02	0.01	0.16	0.00	0.93	0.00	3.57	0.16	0.81	3.15	3.84	39.06	0.02
0.00	0.00	0.00	0.00	0.00	0.00	0.00	0.00	0.00	0.00	0.00	0.00	0.00	0.00	0.12	0.00	0.00	25.60	36.00	0.00
0.19	0.06	0.00	0.00	0.00	0.00	0.00	0.02	0.01	0.16	0.00	0.93	0.00	3.57	0.16	0.81	3.15	21.72	19.08	0.02
1.59	0.36	0.00	0.00	0.37	2.69	0.01	0.06	0.10	0.53	0.01	11.91	0.01	36.43	0.34	5.10	57.55	60.81	198.59	0.09
1.79	0.62	0.00	0.00	0.53	0.00	0.00	0.06	0.05	0.83	0.02	11.91	0.00	13.75	0.43	7.51	34.16	31.61	133.53	0.15
0.00	0.00	0.00	0.00	0.00	0.00	0.00	0.00	0.00	0.00	0.00	0.00	0.00	4.80	0.08	0.00	0.00	9.00	34.00	0.00
0.23	0.06	0.00	0.00	0.00	0.00	0.00	0.01	0.01	0.10	0.00	0.36	0.00	0.98	0.09	1.24	4.40	4.06	5.66	0.03
0.23	0.06	0.00	0.00	0.00	0.00	0.00	0.01	0.01	0.10	0.00	0.36	0.00	0.98	0.09	1.24	4.40	3.66	15.90	0.03
1.47	1.30	0.00	0.00	0.00	1.28	0.21	0.05	0.06	0.45	0.04	9.07	0.02	28.92	0.37	7.65	54.15	43.38	129.42	0.12
1.67	1.26	0.00	0.00	0.00	0.00	0.00	0.06	0.04	0.83	0.02	9.92	0.00	24.10	0.38	5.39	49.19	42.10	114.39	0.12
0.38	0.11	0.00	0.00	0.00	0.00	0.00	0.01	0.00	0.18	0.01	1.12	0.00	2.00	0.12	3.96	11.80	11.88	26.36	0.09
0.38	0.11	0.00	0.00	0.00	0.00	0.00	0.01	0.00	0.18	0.01	1.12	0.00	2.00	0.12	3.96	11.80	11.88	9.88	0.09
0.92	0.38	0.00	0.00	0.00	0.00	0.00	0.19	0.08	1.63	0.01	39.60	0.00	22.80	1.22	9.30	34.50	37.20	209.40	0.27
3.80	0.95	0.00	0.00	0.87	4.00	0.00	0.20	0.17	1.86	0.03	35.20	0.06	38.40	1.13	16.80	56.00	72.40	495.20	0.38
0.48	0.32	0.00	0.00	0.16	0.00	0.00	0.24	0.18	2.02	0.02	45.36	0.00	111.14	1.72	23.24	45.92	88.46	235.88	0.78
0.52	0.54	0.00	0.00	0.70	0.56	0.00	0.20	0.18	2.00	0.06	37.98	0.00	120.78	1.86	27.22	91.86	95.82	256.86	0.60
0.18	0.50	0.00	0.00	0.10	0.00	0.00	0.24	0.16	2.20	0.02	45.92	0.02	98.66	1.42	11.90	75.42	74.28	263.08	0.40
0.18	0.54	0.00	0.00	0.10	0.00	0.06	0.22	0.16	2.16	0.02	41.96	0.02	107.16	1.54	12.48	82.22	81.08	285.76	0.44
0.28	0.78	0.00	0.00	0.24	0.00	0.18	0.22	0.16	2.02	0.04	45.92	0.00	83.34	1.38	8.50	39.12	117.94	253.44	0.56
0.32	0.82	0.00	0.00	0.10	0.00	0.18	0.18	0.16	3.96	0.04	39.12	0.00	90.16	1.50	9.64	47.62	128.14	275.56	0.62
0.16	0.48	0.00	0.00	0.28	0.00	0.00	0.24	0.16	1.90	0.06	31.18	0.00	100.92	1.62	20.98	60.66	105.46	216.60	0.60
0.18	0.52	0.00	0.00	0.20	0.00	0.00	0.22	0.16	1.86	0.06	26.04	0.00	109.44	1.76	23.82	70.88	114.54	235.30	0.70
0.28	0.48	0.00	0.00	0.40	0.00	0.00	0.18	0.08	1.94	0.10	27.78	0.00	150.26	1.38	40.26	159.90	119.08	361.18	0.90
0.32	0.52	0.00	0.00	0.44	0.00	0.00	0.14	0.08	1.90	0.10	20.98	0.00	163.12	1.50	43.66	174.06	129.28	392.36	0.98
0.11	0.51	0.00	0.63	0.08	0.00	0.00	0.99	0.61	7.38	0.05	192.50	0.00	18.75	5.80	27.50	135.00	133.75	2.50	0.88
0.28	0.94	0.00	1.32	1.48	0.00	0.00	0.54	0.26	7.64	0.41	52.80	0.00	40.80	4.66	165.60	415.20	486.00	6.00	3.52

USDA ID Code	Food Name	Weight in Grams*	Quantity of Units	Unit of Measure	Protein (gm)	Fat (gm)	Carbohydrate (gm)	Kcalories	Caffeine (gm)	Fiber (gm)	Cholesterol (mg)	Saturated Fat (gm)
	Grits	165.0000	1.000	Cup	2.44	1.45	23.53	118.80	0.00	4.13	0.00	0.20
	Hominy, Cnd, Yellow	160.0000	1.000	Cup	2.37	1.41	22.82	115.20	0.00	4.00	0.00	0.19
	Hush Puppies	152.0000	1.000	Cup	11.70	20.52	69.92	512.24	0.00	4.26	68.40	3.21
	Macaroni, Ckd, Enriched	140.0000	1.000	Cup	6.68	0.94	39.68	197.40	0.00	1.82	0.00	0.14
	Macaroni, Ckd, Unenriched	140.0000	1.000	Cup	6.68	0.94	39.68	197.40	0.00	1.82	0.00	0.14
	Macaroni, Vegetable, Ckd, Enrich	134.0000	1.000	Cup	6.07	0.15	35.66	171.52	0.00	5.76	0.00	0.03
	Macaroni, Whole-wheat, Ckd	140.0000	1.000	Cup	7.46	0.76	37.16	173.60	0.00	3.92	0.00	0.14
	Noodles, Chinese, Chow Mein	45.0000	1.000	Cup	3.77	13.84	25.89	237.15	0.00	1.76	0.00	1.97
	Noodles, Egg, Ckd, Enriched	160.0000	1.000	Cup	7.60	2.35	39.74	212.80	0.00	1.76	52.80	0.50
	Noodles, Egg, Ckd, Unenriched	160.0000	1.000	Cup	7.60	2.35	39.74	212.80	0.00	0.00	52.80	0.50
	Noodles, Egg, Spinach, Ckd, Enri	160.0000	1.000	Cup	8.06	2.51	38.80	211.20	0.00	3.68	52.80	0.58
	Noodles, Japanese, Soba, Ckd	114.0000	1.000	Cup	5.77	0.11	24.44	112.86	0.00	0.00	0.00	0.02
	Noodles, Ramen	86.0000	1.000	Each	10.00	16.00	52.00	380.00	0.00	2.00	0.00	8.00
615	Noodles, Rice Stick	56.0000	2.000	Ounce	0.00	0.00	48.00	193.00	0.00	0.00	0.00	0.00
616	Noodles, Rice, dry	28.0000	0.500	Cup	2.30	3.00	21.40	121.00	0.00	0.40	0.00	0.60
	Pasta, Ckd, Enriched, w/ Added S	140.0000	1.000	Cup	6.68	0.94	39.68	197.40	0.00	2.38	0.00	0.14
	Pasta, Ckd, Enriched, w/o Added	140.0000	1.000	Cup	6.68	0.94	39.68	197.40	0.00	2.38	0.00	0.14
	Pasta, Fresh-refrigerated, Plain	57.0000	2.000	Ounce	2.94	0.60	14.21	74.67	0.00	0.00	18.81	0.09
	Pasta, Fresh-refrigerated, Spina	57.0000	2.000	Ounce	2.88	0.54	14.27	74.10	0.00	0.00	18.81	0.13
	Pasta, Homemade, Made w/ Egg, Ck	57.0000	2.000	Ounce	3.01	0.99	13.42	74.10	0.00	0.00	23.37	0.23
	Pasta, Homemade, Made w/o Egg, C	57.0000	2.000	Ounce	2.49	0.56	14.32	70.68	0.00	0.00	0.00	0.08
	Pasta, Spinach, Ckd	140.0000	1.000	Cup	6.41	0.88	36.61	182.00	0.00	0.00	0.00	0.13
	Pasta, Whole-wheat, Ckd	140.0000	1.000	Cup	7.46	0.76	37.16	173.60	0.00	6.30	0.00	0.14
690	Rice, Basmati	45.0000	0.250	Cup	3.00	0.00	34.00	150.00	0.00	0.00	0.00	0.00
	Rice, Brown, Long-grain, Ckd	195.0000	1.000	Cup	5.03	1.76	44.77	216.45	0.00	3.51	0.00	0.35
	Rice, Brown, Medium-grain, Ckd	195.0000	1.000	Cup	4.52	1.62	45.84	218.40	0.00	3.51	0.00	0.33
691	Rice, Dirty Rice, mix	38.0000	3.000	Tbsp	3.00	0.00	29.00	130.00	0.00	0.00	0.00	0.00
693	Rice, Jasmine	45.0000	0.250	Cup	3.00	0.00	34.00	150.00	0.00	0.00	0.00	0.00
	Rice, w/ Red Beans	28.3500	2.000	Ounce	3.98	0.50	19.89	94.50	0.00	3.48	0.00	0.00
	Rice, White, Long-grain, Ckd	158.0000	1.000	Cup	4.25	0.44	44.51	205.40	0.00	0.63	0.00	0.13
	Rice, White, Long-grain, Instant	165.0000	1.000	Cup	3.40	0.26	35.10	161.70	0.00	0.99	0.00	0.07
	Rice, White, Medium-grain, Ckd	186.0000	1.000	Cup	4.43	0.39	53.18	241.80	0.00	0.56	0.00	0.11
	Rice, White, Short-grain, Ckd	186.0000	1.000	Cup	4.39	0.35	53.44	241.80	0.00	0.00	0.00	0.09
	Rice, White, w/ Pasta, Ckd	202.0000	1.000	Cup	5.13	5.70	43.29	246.44	0.00	5.05	2.02	1.09
	Rice, Wild, Ckd	164.0000	1.000	Cup	6.54	0.56	35.00	165.64	0.00	2.95	0.00	0.08
	Rice, Wild, Uncle Ben's	56.0000	1.000	Cup	6.00	0.50	41.00	190.00	0.00	1.00	0.00	0.00
	Sesame Breadsticks, Wheat-based,	28.3500	1.000	Ounce	3.09	10.40	13.18	153.37	0.00	0.00	0.00	1.84
	Tabouli	28.3500	1.000	Ounce	1.00	2.00	2.00	30.00	0.00	1.00	0.00	0.00
	Taco Shells, Baked	28.3500	1.000	Ounce	2.04	6.41	17.69	132.68	0.00	2.13	0.00	0.92
	Taco Shells, Baked, w/o Added Sa	28.3500	1.000	Ounce	2.04	6.41	17.69	132.68	0.00	2.13	0.00	0.92
739	Tempeh	166.0000	1.000	Cup	31.46	12.75	28.27	330.34	0.00	0.00	0.00	1.84
	Tortillas, Corn	28.3500	1.000	Each	1.62	0.71	13.21	62.94	0.00	1.47	0.00	0.09
	Tortillas, Corn, w/o Added Salt	28.3500	1.000	Each	1.62	0.71	13.21	62.94	0.00	1.47	0.00	0.09
	Tortillas, Flour	28.3500	1.000	Each	2.47	2.01	15.76	92.14	0.00	0.94	0.00	0.50
	Tortillas, Flour, w/o Added Salt	28.3500	1.000	Each	2.47	2.01	15.76	92.14	0.00	0.94	0.00	0.50
	biscuit	28.3500	1.000	Each	1.73	2.61	8.22	62.94	0.00	0.00	15.88	0.56
	Cereal, Bran 100%	66.0000	1.000	Cup	8.25	3.30	48.11	177.54	0.00	19.54	0.00	0.59
	Cereal, 100% Natural Cereal, Pla	48.0000	0.500	Cup	5.05	7.90	32.95	213.12	0.00	3.60	0.48	3.47
	Cereal, 100% Natural Cereal, w/	110.0000	1.000	Cup	11.22	20.35	72.38	496.10	0.00	7.26	0.00	13.68
	Cereal, 100% Natural Cereal, w/a	104.0000	1.000	Cup	10.71	19.55	69.78	477.36	0.00	6.86	0.00	15.46
	Cereal, 100% Natural Cereal, w/o	48.0000	0.500	Cup	5.05	7.90	32.95	213.12	0.00	3.60	0.48	3.47
136	Cereal, 100% Natural Crl, w/oats	51.0000	0.500	Cup	4.84	7.28	35.83	218.28	0.00	3.67	0.51	3.19
	Cereal, All-bran	30.0000	0.500	Cup	3.66	0.93	22.77	79.20	0.00	9.69	0.00	0.21
137	Cereal, All-Bran with Extra Fibe	30.0000	0.500	Cup	3.69	0.93	22.68	52.80	0.00	15.33	0.00	0.17
	Cereal, Almond Crunch	55.0000	1.000	Cup	4.35	0.83	46.92	198.00	0.00	4.62	0.00	0.17

Monounsaturated Fat (gm)	Polyunsaturated Fat (gm)	Vitamin D (mg)	Vitamin K (mg)	Vitamin E (mg)	Vitamin A (re)	Vitamin C (mg)	Thiamin (mg)	Riboflavin (mg)	Niacin (mg)	Vitamin B_6 (mg)	Folate (mg)	Vitamin B_{12} (mcg)	Calcium (mg)	Iron (mg)	Magnesium (mg)	Phosphorus (mg)	Potassium (mg)	Sodium (mg)	Zinc (mg)
0.38	0.66	0.00	0.00	0.08	0.00	0.00	0.00	0.02	0.05	0.02	1.65	0.00	16.50	1.02	26.40	57.75	14.85	346.50	1.73
0.37	0.64	0.00	0.00	0.00	17.60	0.00	0.00	0.02	0.05	0.02	1.60	0.00	16.00	0.99	25.60	56.00	14.40	336.00	1.68
4.96	10.97	0.00	0.00	3.62	65.36	0.30	0.53	0.50	4.23	0.15	112.48	0.29	422.56	4.62	36.48	287.28	218.88	1015.36	1.00
0.11	0.38	0.00	0.00	0.04	0.00	0.00	0.28	0.14	2.34	0.06	98.00	0.00	9.80	1.96	25.20	75.60	43.40	1.40	0.74
0.11	0.38	0.00	0.00	0.04	0.00	0.00	0.03	0.03	0.56	0.06	9.80	0.00	9.80	0.70	25.20	75.60	43.40	1.40	0.74
0.01	0.05	0.00	0.00	0.05	6.70	0.00	0.15	0.08	1.43	0.03	87.10	0.00	14.74	0.66	25.46	67.00	41.54	8.04	0.59
0.11	0.29	0.00	0.00	0.14	0.00	0.00	0.15	0.07	0.99	0.11	7.00	0.00	21.00	1.48	42.00	124.60	61.60	4.20	1.13
3.46	7.80	0.00	0.00	0.07	4.05	0.00	0.26	0.19	2.68	0.05	40.50	0.00	9.00	2.13	23.40	72.45	54.00	197.55	0.63
0.69	0.66	0.00	0.00	0.00	9.60	0.00	0.30	0.13	2.38	0.06	102.40	0.14	19.20	2.54	30.40	110.40	44.80	264.00	0.99
0.69	0.66	0.00	0.00	0.00	9.60	0.00	0.05	0.03	0.64	0.06	11.20	0.14	19.20	0.96	30.40	110.40	44.80	264.00	0.99
0.78	0.56	0.00	0.00	0.08	22.40	0.00	0.40	0.19	2.35	0.18	102.40	0.22	30.40	1.74	38.40	91.20	59.20	19.20	1.01
0.03	0.03	0.00	0.00	0.00	0.00	0.00	0.10	0.03	0.58	0.05	7.98	0.00	4.56	0.55	10.26	28.50	39.90	68.40	0.14
0.00	0.00	0.00	0.00	0.00	0.00	0.00	0.00	0.00	0.00	0.00	0.00	0.00	0.00	1.60	0.00	0.00	0.00	1560.00	0.00
0.00	0.00	0.00	0.00	0.00	0.00	0.00	0.00	0.00	0.00	0.00	0.00	0.00	0.00	0.00	0.00	0.00	0.00	100.00	0.00
0.00	0.00	0.00	0.00	0.00	0.00	0.00	0.00	0.00	0.00	0.00	0.00	0.00	17.00	0.83	0.00	0.00	0.00	378.00	0.00
0.11	0.38	0.00	0.00	0.00	0.00	0.00	0.28	0.14	2.34	0.06	98.00	0.00	9.80	1.96	25.20	75.60	43.40	140.00	0.74
0.11	0.38	0.00	0.00	0.08	0.00	0.00	0.28	0.14	2.34	0.06	98.00	0.00	9.80	1.96	25.20	75.60	43.40	1.40	0.74
0.07	0.25	0.00	0.00	0.00	3.42	0.00	0.12	0.09	0.56	0.02	36.48	0.08	3.42	0.65	10.26	35.91	13.68	3.42	0.32
0.17	0.12	0.00	0.00	0.00	7.98	0.00	0.10	0.07	0.58	0.06	36.48	0.08	10.26	0.63	13.68	32.49	21.09	3.42	0.36
0.29	0.30	0.00	0.00	0.00	9.69	0.00	0.10	0.10	0.72	0.02	24.51	0.06	5.70	0.66	7.98	29.64	11.97	47.31	0.25
0.11	0.29	0.00	0.00	0.00	0.00	0.00	0.10	0.09	0.76	0.02	24.51	0.00	3.42	0.64	7.98	22.80	10.83	42.18	0.21
0.10	0.36	0.00	0.00	0.00	21.00	0.00	0.14	0.14	2.14	0.14	16.80	0.00	42.00	1.46	86.80	151.20	81.20	19.60	1.51
0.11	0.29	0.00	0.00	0.07	0.00	0.00	0.15	0.07	0.99	0.11	7.00	0.00	21.00	1.48	42.00	124.60	61.60	4.20	1.13
0.00	0.00	0.00	0.00	0.00	0.00	0.00	0.00	0.00	0.00	0.00	0.00	0.00	0.00	0.00	0.00	0.00	0.00	0.00	0.00
0.64	0.62	0.00	0.00	1.40	0.00	0.00	0.20	0.06	2.98	0.29	7.80	0.00	19.50	0.82	83.85	161.85	83.85	9.75	1.23
0.59	0.59	0.00	0.00	0.00	0.00	0.00	0.20	0.02	2.59	0.29	7.80	0.00	19.50	1.03	85.80	150.15	154.05	1.95	1.21
0.00	0.00	0.00	0.00	0.00	0.00	0.00	0.00	0.00	0.00	0.00	0.00	0.00	0.00	0.00	0.00	0.00	0.00	680.00	0.00
0.00	0.00	0.00	0.00	0.00	0.00	0.00	0.00	0.00	0.00	0.00	0.00	0.00	0.00	0.00	0.00	0.00	0.00	0.00	0.00
0.00	0.00	0.00	0.00	0.00	49.74	2.98	0.11	0.00	1.42	0.00	0.00	0.00	23.87	0.75	0.00	0.00	0.00	392.92	0.00
0.14	0.13	0.00	0.00	0.08	0.00	0.00	0.25	0.02	2.34	0.14	91.64	0.00	15.80	1.90	18.96	67.94	55.30	1.58	0.77
0.08	0.07	0.00	0.00	0.08	0.00	0.00	0.13	0.08	1.45	0.02	67.65	0.00	13.20	1.04	8.25	23.10	6.60	4.95	0.40
0.13	0.11	0.00	0.00	0.00	0.00	0.00	0.32	0.04	3.42	0.09	107.88	0.00	5.58	2.77	24.18	68.82	53.94	0.00	0.78
0.11	0.09	0.00	0.00	0.00	0.00	0.00	0.30	0.04	2.77	0.11	109.74	0.00	1.86	2.72	14.88	61.38	48.36	0.00	0.74
2.26	1.92	0.00	0.00	0.00	0.00	0.40	0.24	0.16	3.60	0.20	88.88	0.12	16.16	1.90	24.24	74.74	84.84	1147.36	0.57
0.08	0.34	0.00	0.00	0.38	0.00	0.00	0.08	0.15	2.12	0.23	42.64	0.00	4.92	0.98	52.48	134.48	165.64	4.92	2.20
0.00	0.00	0.00	0.00	0.00	0.00	2.40	0.00	0.00	0.00	0.00	0.00	0.00	24.00	1.00	0.00	0.00	0.00	620.00	0.00
3.09	4.94	0.00	0.00	0.00	2.55	0.00	0.03	0.02	0.44	0.03	6.24	0.00	48.20	0.21	12.76	39.12	50.18	8.22	0.33
0.00	0.00	0.00	0.00	0.00	100.00	12.00	0.00	0.00	0.00	0.00	0.00	0.00	0.00	0.40	0.00	0.00	0.00	75.00	0.00
2.53	2.41	0.00	0.00	1.03	0.00	0.00	0.07	0.01	0.38	0.09	29.77	0.00	45.36	0.71	29.77	70.31	50.75	104.04	0.40
2.53	2.41	0.00	0.00	1.03	0.00	0.00	0.07	0.01	0.38	0.09	29.77	0.00	45.36	0.71	29.77	70.31	50.75	4.25	0.40
2.81	7.19	0.00	0.00	0.00	114.54	0.00	0.22	0.18	7.69	0.50	86.32	1.66	154.38	3.75	116.20	341.96	609.22	9.96	3.01
0.18	0.32	0.00	0.00	0.04	0.00	0.00	0.03	0.02	0.43	0.06	32.32	0.00	49.61	0.40	18.43	89.02	43.66	45.64	0.27
0.18	0.32	0.00	0.00	0.04	0.00	0.00	0.03	0.02	0.43	0.06	32.32	0.00	49.61	0.40	18.43	89.02	43.66	3.12	0.27
1.07	0.30	0.00	0.00	0.26	0.00	0.00	0.15	0.08	1.01	0.01	34.87	0.00	35.44	0.94	7.37	35.15	37.14	135.51	0.20
1.07	0.30	0.00	0.00	0.26	0.00	0.00	0.15	0.08	1.01	0.01	34.87	0.00	11.06	0.94	7.37	35.15	37.14	135.51	0.20
0.66	1.18	0.00	0.00	0.00	14.46	0.62	0.06	0.08	0.43	0.01	10.21	0.06	58.40	0.49	4.54	42.81	39.12	116.80	0.15
0.57	1.87	0.00	0.00	1.53	0.00	62.70	1.58	1.78	20.92	2.11	46.86	6.27	46.20	8.12	312.18	801.24	652.08	457.38	5.74
3.48	1.04	0.00	0.00	0.55	0.48	0.14	0.17	0.08	0.85	0.09	12.00	0.05	46.08	1.44	50.40	148.80	210.72	12.96	1.15
3.72	1.71	0.00	0.00	0.77	6.60	0.00	0.31	0.65	2.09	0.17	45.10	0.15	159.50	3.12	124.30	347.60	537.90	47.30	2.11
1.83	1.33	0.00	0.00	0.73	6.24	1.04	0.33	0.57	1.87	0.11	16.64	0.30	157.04	2.89	71.76	350.48	513.76	52.00	2.00
3.48	1.04	0.00	0.00	0.55	0.48	0.14	0.17	0.08	0.85	0.09	12.00	0.05	46.08	1.44	50.40	148.80	210.72	12.96	1.15
3.17	0.82	0.00	0.00	0.51	0.51	0.31	0.14	0.09	0.77	0.08	11.73	0.05	38.76	1.67	47.94	149.94	213.69	11.22	1.08
0.18	0.54	0.03	0.00	0.55	225.30	15.00	0.39	0.42	5.01	0.51	90.00	1.50	105.90	4.50	128.70	294.00	341.70	60.90	3.75
0.18	0.58	0.00	0.00	0.64	259.80	17.31	0.42	0.48	5.76	0.57	120.00	1.74	115.50	5.19	119.70	287.40	300.00	126.90	4.32
0.22	0.44	0.00	0.00	3.00	47.30	0.00	0.52	0.59	7.00	0.69	99.00	2.10	26.40	5.99	48.95	129.80	170.50	284.35	1.43

USDA ID Code	Food Name	Weight in Grams*	Quantity of Units	Unit of Measure	Protein (gm)	Fat (gm)	Carbohydrate (gm)	Kcalories	Caffeine (gm)	Fiber (gm)	Cholesterol (mg)	Saturated Fat (gm)
138	Cereal, Almond Crunch w/Raisins	58.0000	1.000	Cup	5.00	2.50	46.00	210.00	0.00	5.00	0.00	0.00
	Cereal, Alpha-Bits	34.0000	1.000	Cup	2.58	0.78	29.44	133.28	0.00	1.46	0.00	0.13
139	Cereal, Apple Cinnamon Squares	55.0000	0.750	Cup	3.96	0.99	44.06	182.05	0.00	4.73	0.00	0.22
	Cereal, Apple Jacks	30.0000	1.000	Cup	1.44	0.39	26.84	115.50	0.00	0.57	0.00	0.09
	Cereal, Apple Raisin Crisp	55.0000	1.000	Cup	3.47	0.50	46.70	184.80	0.00	4.40	0.00	0.11
	Cereal, Basic 4	55.0000	1.000	Cup	4.18	2.84	41.97	200.75	0.00	3.36	0.00	0.42
	Cereal, Berry Berry-Kix	30.0000	0.750	Cup	1.31	1.16	26.13	120.00	0.00	0.18	0.00	0.20
	Cereal, Blueberry Squares	55.0000	0.750	Cup	4.18	0.99	43.78	181.50	0.00	4.84	0.00	0.22
140	Cereal, Boo Berry	30.0000	1.000	Cup	1.00	0.50	27.00	120.00	0.00	0.00	0.00	0.00
141	Cereal, Bran Buds	30.0000	0.330	Cup	2.82	0.72	23.97	82.80	0.00	11.97	0.00	0.12
	Cereal, Bran Flakes, 40%, Kello	29.0000	0.750	Cup	3.02	0.64	23.16	94.83	0.00	4.61	0.00	0.12
	Cereal, Bran Flakes, 40%, Post	47.0000	1.000	Cup	5.31	0.75	37.27	152.28	0.00	9.17	0.00	0.00
	Cereal, Bran Flakes, 40%, Ralsto	49.0000	1.000	Cup	5.64	0.69	39.10	158.76	0.00	6.91	0.00	0.00
	Cereal, Bran Flakes, Kellogg's	29.0000	0.750	Cup	3.02	0.64	23.16	94.83	0.00	4.61	0.00	0.12
	Cereal, Bran Flakes, Post	47.0000	1.000	Cup	5.31	0.75	37.27	152.28	0.00	9.17	0.00	0.12
142	Cereal, Bran, Frosted	30.0000	0.750	Cup	2.37	0.33	25.41	101.40	0.00	3.36	0.00	0.03
	Cereal, Brown Sugar Squares, Toa	55.0000	1.250	Cup	5.23	1.05	44.99	189.20	0.00	5.12	0.00	0.18
	Cereal, C.W. Post, Plain	97.0000	1.000	Cup	7.95	12.80	72.65	420.98	0.00	7.18	0.18	1.67
	Cereal, C.W. Post, w/ Raisins	103.0000	1.000	Cup	8.86	14.73	73.95	445.99	0.00	13.60	0.20	10.97
	Cereal, Cap'n Crunch	27.0000	0.750	Cup	1.35	1.37	23.04	107.19	0.00	0.86	0.00	0.37
	Cereal, Cap'n Crunch's Crunchber	26.0000	0.750	Cup	1.26	1.28	22.26	103.74	0.00	0.57	0.00	0.35
	Cereal, Cap'n Crunch's Peanut Bu	27.0000	0.750	Cup	1.95	2.32	21.51	112.32	0.00	0.78	0.00	0.52
	Cereal, Cheerios	30.0000	1.000	Cup	3.14	1.77	22.86	109.50	0.00	2.64	0.00	0.35
	Cereal, Cheerios, Apple Cinnamon	30.0000	0.750	Cup	1.86	1.63	25.05	117.90	0.00	1.59	0.00	0.30
143	Cereal, Cheerios, Frosted	30.0000	1.000	Cup	2.00	1.00	25.00	120.00	0.00	1.00	0.00	0.00
	Cereal, Cheerios, Honey Nut	30.0000	1.000	Cup	2.78	1.24	24.26	114.90	0.00	1.56	0.00	0.23
	Cereal, Cheerios, Multigrain	30.0000	1.000	Cup	2.56	1.09	24.45	111.90	0.00	1.92	0.00	0.25
	Cereal, Chex, Bran	49.0000	1.000	Cup	5.05	1.37	39.05	156.31	0.00	7.94	0.00	0.20
	Cereal, Chex, Corn	30.0000	1.000	Cup	2.18	0.37	25.61	112.80	0.00	0.54	0.00	0.07
	Cereal, Chex, Rice	31.0000	1.250	Cup	1.92	0.16	27.18	117.18	0.00	0.28	0.00	0.04
	Cereal, Chex, Wheat	30.0000	1.000	Cup	3.16	0.68	24.21	103.80	0.00	3.30	0.00	0.12
	Cereal, Cinnamon Mini Buns	30.0000	0.750	Cup	1.47	0.63	26.61	115.20	0.00	0.66	0.00	0.15
	Cereal, Cinnamon Oatmeal Squares	60.0000	1.000	Cup	7.57	2.57	47.15	231.60	0.00	4.56	0.00	0.50
	Cereal, Cinnamon Toast Crunch	30.0000	0.750	Cup	1.68	3.04	23.84	124.20	0.00	1.50	0.00	0.50
	Cereal, Cocoa Krispies	31.0000	0.750	Cup	1.55	0.81	27.25	120.28	1.24	0.40	0.00	0.59
	Cereal, Cocoa Puffs	30.0000	1.000	Cup	1.14	0.90	26.72	118.80	0.00	0.18	0.00	0.20
	Cereal, Cookie-crisp, Choc Chip	30.0000	1.000	Cup	1.53	1.08	26.25	120.00	0.60	0.42	0.00	0.60
	Cereal, Corn Bran	27.0000	0.750	Cup	1.86	0.89	22.73	89.91	0.00	4.81	0.00	0.21
144	Cereal, Corn Flakes, Country	30.0000	1.000	Cup	1.83	0.50	25.96	114.00	0.00	0.45	0.00	0.15
	Cereal, Corn Flakes, Honey and N	55.0000	1.250	Cup	4.02	2.48	45.98	222.75	0.00	0.88	0.00	0.50
145	Cereal, Corn Flakes, Honey Crunc	30.0000	0.750	Cup	5.00	1.00	44.00	190.00	0.00	5.00	0.00	0.00
	Cereal, Corn Flakes, Kellogg's	28.0000	1.000	Cup	1.84	0.20	24.22	102.20	0.00	0.78	0.00	0.06
	Cereal, Corn Flakes, Low Sodium	25.0000	1.000	Cup	1.93	0.08	22.20	99.75	0.00	0.28	0.00	0.01
	Cereal, Corn Flakes, Ralston Pur	25.0000	1.000	Cup	1.95	0.10	21.65	97.50	0.00	0.48	0.00	0.00
	Cereal, Corn Pops	31.0000	1.000	Cup	1.15	0.18	28.43	118.11	0.00	0.43	0.00	0.06
146	Cereal, Count Chocula	30.0000	1.000	Cup	1.00	1.00	26.00	120.00	0.00	0.00	0.00	0.00
	Cereal, Cracklin' Oat Bran	55.0000	0.750	Cup	4.61	6.97	40.10	224.95	0.00	6.55	0.00	2.92
	Cereal, Cream Of Rice, Ckd	244.0000	1.000	Cup	2.20	0.24	28.06	126.88	0.00	0.24	0.00	0.05
	Cereal, Cream Of Wheat, Instant	241.0000	1.000	Cup	4.34	0.48	31.57	154.24	0.00	2.89	0.00	0.07
	Cereal, Cream Of Wheat, Quick	239.0000	1.000	Cup	3.59	0.48	26.77	129.06	0.00	1.20	0.00	0.07
	Cereal, Cream Of Wheat, Regular	251.0000	1.000	Cup	3.77	0.50	27.61	133.03	0.00	1.76	0.00	0.08
	Cereal, Crisp Rice, Low Sodium	26.0000	1.000	Cup	1.43	0.08	23.66	104.52	0.00	0.36	0.00	0.02
	Cereal, Crispex	29.0000	1.000	Cup	2.15	0.29	25.00	108.46	0.00	0.64	0.00	0.09
	Cereal, Crispy Rice	28.0000	1.000	Cup	1.79	0.11	24.81	110.88	0.00	0.34	0.00	0.03
	Cereal, Crispy Wheats 'n Raisins	55.0000	1.000	Cup	4.47	0.76	44.33	191.40	0.00	3.41	0.00	0.15

Monounsaturated Fat (gm)	Polyunsaturated Fat (gm)	Vitamin D (mg)	Vitamin K (mg)	Vitamin E (mg)	Vitamin A (re)	Vitamin C (mg)	Thiamin (mg)	Riboflavin (mg)	Niacin (mg)	Vitamin B_6 (mg)	Folate (mg)	Vitamin B_{12} (mcg)	Calcium (mg)	Iron (mg)	Magnesium (mg)	Phosphorus (mg)	Potassium (mg)	Sodium (mg)	Zinc (mg)
1.50	1.00	0.05	0.00	3.00	500.00	0.00	0.53	0.60	7.00	0.70	0.10	2.10	20.00	6.30	60.00	150.00	200.00	230.00	1.50
0.26	0.29	0.00	0.00	0.02	450.16	0.00	0.44	0.51	5.98	0.61	120.02	1.80	9.86	3.23	20.06	61.54	65.96	215.90	1.80
0.28	0.50	0.00	0.00	0.59	0.00	0.00	0.39	0.44	5.00	0.50	110.00	1.49	20.90	16.23	48.40	154.00	166.00	19.80	1.49
0.12	0.18	0.00	0.00	0.05	225.30	15.00	0.39	0.42	5.01	0.51	105.90	0.00	3.30	4.50	8.70	30.00	31.80	134.40	3.75
0.17	0.22	0.00	0.00	0.46	233.75	0.00	0.39	0.44	5.17	0.50	110.00	1.54	14.85	1.87	9.90	85.80	85.25	373.45	1.54
0.99	1.10	0.00	0.00	0.68	375.10	14.96	0.37	0.42	5.00	0.50	99.55	0.00	309.65	4.50	40.15	231.55	161.70	322.85	3.75
0.46	0.06	0.00	0.00	0.17	225.30	15.00	0.38	0.43	5.00	0.50	99.90	0.00	66.00	4.50	5.70	37.20	23.70	184.50	3.75
0.22	0.55	0.00	0.00	0.85	0.00	0.00	0.39	0.44	5.12	0.50	110.00	1.54	19.25	16.50	51.15	161.70	183.15	20.35	1.54
0.00	0.00	0.00	0.00	0.00	0.00	15.00	0.38	0.43	5.00	0.50	100.00	0.00	20.00	4.50	0.00	20.00	15.00	210.00	3.75
0.15	0.45	0.00	0.00	0.48	225.30	15.00	0.39	0.42	5.01	0.51	90.00	0.00	20.10	4.50	83.40	166.20	269.70	199.80	6.45
0.12	0.41	0.03	0.00	5.37	362.79	14.99	0.38	0.44	5.00	0.49	102.37	1.45	13.92	8.12	60.03	149.93	175.16	226.20	3.75
0.00	0.00	0.00	0.00	0.54	622.28	0.00	0.61	0.70	8.27	0.85	165.91	2.49	20.68	7.47	101.52	296.10	250.51	430.99	2.49
0.00	0.00	0.00	0.00	0.00	648.76	25.97	0.64	0.74	8.62	0.88	172.97	2.60	22.54	7.79	117.60	272.93	286.16	456.19	2.04
0.12	0.41	0.00	0.00	5.37	362.79	14.99	0.38	0.44	5.00	0.49	102.37	1.45	13.92	8.12	60.03	149.93	175.16	226.20	3.75
0.11	0.37	0.00	0.00	0.54	622.28	0.00	0.61	0.71	8.27	0.85	165.91	2.49	20.68	13.44	101.52	296.10	250.51	430.99	2.49
0.09	0.21	0.00	0.00	0.23	217.80	14.52	0.36	0.42	4.83	0.48	90.00	1.44	9.30	4.35	37.80	92.40	122.10	206.40	3.63
0.15	0.43	0.00	0.00	3.00	51.15	0.00	0.55	0.61	7.15	0.72	110.00	2.15	18.70	6.44	59.40	194.15	213.95	1.65	1.54
6.00	4.66	0.00	0.00	0.68	1284.28	0.00	1.26	1.46	17.07	1.75	342.41	5.14	46.56	15.42	66.93	224.07	197.88	166.84	1.64
1.67	1.38	0.00	0.00	0.72	1363.72	0.00	1.34	1.55	18.13	1.85	363.59	5.46	50.47	16.38	74.16	231.75	260.59	160.68	1.64
0.27	0.19	0.00	0.00	0.14	3.51	0.00	0.38	0.42	5.00	0.50	100.17	0.00	5.40	4.50	9.45	28.62	34.56	208.44	3.75
0.26	0.20	0.00	0.00	0.18	4.68	0.03	0.37	0.42	5.00	0.50	100.10	0.01	6.50	4.50	9.88	29.64	36.66	190.32	4.01
0.82	0.53	0.00	0.00	0.15	3.78	0.00	0.38	0.42	5.00	0.50	100.17	0.00	2.70	4.50	18.63	51.84	62.10	203.85	3.75
0.64	0.22	0.03	0.00	0.21	375.30	15.00	0.38	0.43	5.00	0.50	99.90	0.00	55.20	8.10	32.70	114.00	88.50	284.10	3.75
0.64	0.21	0.00	0.00	0.30	225.30	15.00	0.38	0.43	5.00	0.50	99.90	0.00	35.40	4.50	20.10	65.10	60.00	150.30	3.75
0.00	0.00	0.00	0.00	0.00	750.00	15.00	0.38	0.43	5.00	0.50	100.00	0.00	20.00	4.50	16.00	60.00	60.00	210.00	3.75
0.48	0.19	0.03	0.00	0.31	225.30	15.00	0.38	0.43	5.00	0.50	99.90	0.00	20.40	4.50	29.40	102.90	85.20	258.90	3.75
0.30	0.15	0.00	0.00	0.19	225.30	15.00	0.38	0.43	5.00	0.50	99.90	0.00	57.00	8.10	29.70	114.30	97.20	254.10	3.75
0.25	0.67	0.00	0.00	0.56	10.78	25.97	0.64	0.26	8.62	0.88	172.97	2.60	29.40	13.99	69.09	172.97	216.09	345.45	6.48
0.09	0.20	0.00	0.00	0.10	0.00	6.00	0.38	0.00	5.00	0.50	99.90	1.50	100.20	9.00	8.40	21.60	32.40	288.90	0.37
0.05	0.05	0.00	0.00	0.00	0.00	6.01	0.38	0.02	5.00	0.50	99.82	1.50	103.54	9.00	9.30	35.34	35.96	291.40	0.00
0.11	0.28	0.00	0.00	0.44	0.00	3.60	0.23	0.04	3.00	0.30	60.00	0.90	60.00	9.00	33.60	109.50	116.10	268.50	0.74
0.18	0.30	0.00	0.00	0.05	225.30	15.00	0.39	0.42	5.01	0.51	90.00	0.00	3.90	4.50	11.10	24.00	36.60	207.60	3.75
0.86	1.07	0.00	0.00	2.22	165.00	6.60	0.41	0.46	5.48	0.55	109.80	0.00	41.40	14.55	70.20	181.80	250.20	266.40	4.11
0.93	0.53	0.00	0.00	0.28	225.30	15.00	0.38	0.43	5.00	0.50	99.90	0.00	42.30	4.50	13.50	74.40	44.10	210.30	3.75
0.09	0.12	0.00	0.00	0.14	225.06	15.00	0.37	0.43	4.99	0.50	93.00	0.00	4.03	1.80	11.47	29.45	60.14	210.18	1.49
0.35	0.05	0.00	0.00	0.14	0.00	15.00	0.38	0.43	5.00	0.50	99.90	0.00	33.00	4.50	6.60	42.60	52.20	180.60	3.75
0.22	0.16	0.00	0.00	0.08	0.00	0.00	0.39	0.27	5.28	0.54	105.90	1.59	5.70	4.77	8.40	24.00	29.40	206.70	3.17
0.23	0.27	0.00	0.00	0.14	3.78	0.00	0.08	0.42	5.00	0.50	100.17	0.00	20.52	7.56	14.31	35.64	56.16	253.26	3.75
0.09	0.03	0.00	0.00	0.08	225.30	15.00	0.38	0.43	5.00	0.50	99.90	0.00	53.40	8.10	7.20	39.30	40.50	283.80	3.75
1.16	0.83	1.25	0.00	0.14	225.50	15.02	0.39	0.44	5.01	0.50	110.00	0.00	5.50	4.51	4.95	36.30	59.95	370.15	0.39
0.50	0.00	0.05	0.00	3.00	500.00	0.00	0.53	0.60	7.00	0.70	0.10	2.10	0.00	6.30	60.00	200.00	210.00	5.00	1.50
0.03	0.11	0.02	0.00	0.04	210.28	14.00	0.36	0.39	4.68	0.48	98.84	0.00	1.12	8.68	3.36	10.92	25.48	297.92	0.17
0.02	0.03	0.00	0.00	0.03	9.50	0.00	0.00	0.05	0.11	0.02	1.75	0.00	10.75	0.56	3.25	12.25	18.25	2.50	0.07
0.00	0.00	0.00	0.00	0.00	9.50	0.00	0.13	0.03	1.05	0.02	1.75	0.00	1.75	0.63	2.75	9.75	22.00	239.00	0.06
0.06	0.03	0.00	0.00	0.03	232.81	15.50	0.40	0.43	5.18	0.53	109.43	0.00	2.48	1.86	2.48	6.51	22.63	123.07	1.55
0.00	0.00	0.00	0.00	0.00	0.00	15.00	0.38	0.43	5.00	0.50	100.00	1.50	20.00	4.50	0.00	20.00	65.00	190.00	3.75
3.25	0.75	0.05	0.00	0.36	253.00	16.83	0.42	0.48	5.61	0.56	152.90	0.00	24.75	2.04	76.45	186.45	254.65	195.25	1.65
0.00	0.00	0.00	0.00	0.00	0.00	0.00	0.00	0.00	0.98	0.07	7.32	0.00	7.32	0.49	7.32	41.48	48.80	422.12	0.39
0.00	0.00	0.00	0.00	0.00	0.00	0.00	0.24	0.00	1.69	0.02	149.42	0.00	60.25	12.05	14.46	43.38	48.20	363.91	0.41
0.00	0.00	0.00	0.00	0.00	0.00	0.00	0.24	0.00	1.43	0.02	107.55	0.00	50.19	10.28	11.95	100.38	45.41	463.66	0.33
0.00	0.00	0.00	0.00	0.00	0.00	0.00	0.25	0.00	1.51	0.03	45.18	0.00	50.20	10.29	10.04	42.67	42.67	336.34	0.33
0.02	0.03	0.00	0.00	0.03	0.00	0.00	0.00	0.05	0.36	0.04	2.86	0.00	17.42	0.80	10.14	27.04	20.28	2.60	0.39
0.06	0.12	0.02	0.00	0.12	225.33	14.99	0.38	0.44	4.99	0.49	87.00	0.00	3.48	1.80	6.96	26.68	35.09	240.12	1.51
0.04	0.03	0.00	0.00	0.03	371.00	14.81	0.52	0.59	6.92	0.69	138.32	0.08	5.04	0.70	11.76	30.52	26.60	205.52	0.46
0.12	0.17	0.00	0.00	0.57	375.10	0.00	0.37	0.42	5.00	0.50	99.55	0.00	69.30	4.50	42.35	140.25	229.90	284.90	1.08

USDA ID Code	Food Name	Weight in Grams*	Quantity of Units	Unit of Measure	Protein (gm)	Fat (gm)	Carbohydrate (gm)	Kcalories	Caffeine (gm)	Fiber (gm)	Cholesterol (mg)	Saturated Fat (gm)
147	Cereal, Crunchy Pecan-Great Grai	53.0000	0.660	Cup	5.00	6.00	38.00	220.00	0.00	4.00	0.00	1.00
	Cereal, Fiber One	30.0000	0.500	Cup	2.78	0.84	24.01	61.50	0.00	14.25	0.00	0.13
	Cereal, Fortified Oat Flakes	48.0000	1.000	Cup	8.98	0.72	34.75	177.12	0.00	1.44	0.00	0.00
148	Cereal, Frankenberry	30.0000	1.000	Cup	1.00	1.00	27.00	120.00	0.00	0.00	0.00	0.00
149	Cereal, French Toast Crunch	30.0000	0.750	Cup	1.00	1.50	26.00	120.00	0.00	0.00	0.00	0.00
	Cereal, Frosted Flakes	31.0000	0.750	Cup	1.21	0.16	28.27	119.35	0.00	0.62	0.00	0.06
150	Cereal, Frosted Flakes, Cocoa-Ke	31.0000	0.750	Cup	1.00	0.00	28.00	120.00	0.00	0.00	0.00	0.00
	Cereal, Frosted Mini-Wheats	55.0000	1.000	Cup	5.17	0.88	45.38	186.45	0.00	5.89	0.00	0.17
	Cereal, Fruit Loops	30.0000	1.000	Cup	1.47	0.87	26.46	117.30	0.00	0.57	0.00	0.39
	Cereal, Fruity Pebbles	32.0000	1.000	Cup	1.28	1.66	27.55	129.60	0.00	0.42	0.00	1.37
	Cereal, Golden Grahams	30.0000	0.750	Cup	1.60	1.08	25.69	115.50	0.00	0.93	0.00	0.18
	Cereal, Graham Crackos	30.0000	1.000	Cup	2.25	0.18	25.92	108.30	0.00	1.83	0.00	0.00
151	Cereal, Granola Low Fat w/Raisin	60.0000	0.500	Cup	5.00	3.00	47.00	220.00	0.00	3.00	0.00	1.00
152	Cereal, Granola Low Fat-Kellogg'	50.0000	0.500	Cup	4.00	3.00	39.00	190.00	0.00	3.00	0.00	0.50
	Cereal, Granola w/ Almonds-Sun C	57.0000	0.500	Cup	6.71	10.27	38.30	266.19	0.00	2.96	0.00	1.27
	Cereal, Granola, Low Fat-Kellog	82.4590	1.000	Cup	7.50	4.50	64.47	314.84	0.00	4.50	0.00	1.50
	Cereal, Granola, Homemade	122.0000	1.000	Cup	17.93	30.01	64.66	569.74	0.00	12.81	0.00	5.80
	Cereal, Granola, w/ raisins, Low	55.0000	0.670	Cup	4.51	2.75	43.67	201.85	0.00	3.30	0.00	0.94
	Cereal, Granola, w/o raisins, L	55.0000	0.500	Cup	4.62	3.25	44.17	213.40	0.00	3.25	0.00	0.50
	Cereal, Granola, w/raisins&dates	31.0000	0.500	Cup	3.02	4.23	22.38	135.16	0.00	1.86	0.00	0.64
	Cereal, Granola-Nature Valley	55.0000	0.750	Cup	5.80	9.69	36.23	248.05	0.00	3.52	0.00	1.27
	Cereal, Grape-nuts	109.0000	1.000	Cup	12.75	0.44	89.38	389.13	0.00	10.90	0.00	0.06
	Cereal, Grape-nuts Flakes	39.0000	1.000	Cup	3.94	0.36	26.55	116.20	0.00	3.21	0.00	0.00
	Cereal, Great Grains	79.4600	1.000	Cup	1.13	9.00	56.97	329.84	0.00	6.00	0.00	1.50
	Cereal, Heartland Natural Cereal	115.0000	1.000	Cup	11.62	17.71	78.55	499.10	0.00	7.02	0.00	4.52
	Cereal, Heartland Natural Cereal	110.0000	1.000	Cup	10.67	15.62	75.90	467.50	0.00	6.05	0.00	3.98
	Cereal, Heartland Natural Cereal	105.0000	1.000	Cup	10.92	17.12	71.30	463.05	0.00	7.46	0.00	6.23
153	Cereal, Honey Bunches of Oats	30.0000	0.750	Cup	2.00	1.50	25.00	120.00	0.00	1.00	0.00	0.50
154	Cereal, Honey Bunches of Oats w/	31.0000	0.750	Cup	3.00	3.00	24.00	130.00	0.00	1.00	0.00	0.50
	Cereal, Honey Graham Oh!	27.0000	0.750	Cup	1.35	1.91	22.75	111.78	0.00	0.70	0.00	0.55
155	Cereal, Honey Nut Clusters	55.0000	1.000	Cup	4.00	2.50	46.00	210.00	0.00	3.00	0.00	0.00
	Cereal, Honeybran	35.0000	1.000	Cup	3.08	0.74	28.63	119.35	0.00	3.89	0.00	0.26
	Cereal, Honeycomb	22.0000	1.000	Cup	1.28	0.40	19.60	86.02	0.00	0.62	0.00	0.00
	Cereal, Just Right	55.0000	1.000	Cup	4.24	1.49	46.04	204.05	0.00	2.81	0.00	0.11
	Cereal, Just Right, Fruit & Nut	55.0000	1.000	Cup	4.13	1.60	44.28	192.50	0.00	2.75	0.00	0.28
156	Cereal, King Vitamin	31.0000	1.500	Cup	2.30	1.10	26.10	120.00	0.00	1.20	0.00	0.30
	Cereal, Kix	30.0000	1.330	Cup	1.96	0.62	25.91	114.30	0.00	0.81	0.00	0.17
	Cereal, Life	32.0000	0.750	Cup	3.15	1.28	25.18	121.28	0.00	2.05	0.00	0.24
	Cereal, Life, Cinnamon	50.0000	1.000	Cup	4.36	1.74	40.40	189.50	0.00	2.95	0.00	0.33
	Cereal, Lucky Charms	30.0000	1.000	Cup	2.15	1.08	25.17	116.10	0.00	1.20	0.00	0.22
	Cereal, Malt-o-meal, Plain and C	240.0000	1.000	Cup	3.60	0.24	25.92	122.40	2.40	0.96	0.00	0.05
	Cereal, Maypo, Ckd w/ water, w/	240.0000	1.000	Cup	5.76	2.40	31.92	170.40	0.00	5.76	0.00	0.46
	Cereal, Maypo, Ckd w/ water, w/o	240.0000	1.000	Cup	5.76	2.40	31.92	170.40	0.00	5.76	0.00	0.43
157	Cereal, Mueslix Raisin&Almond Cr	55.0000	0.660	Cup	5.00	3.00	41.00	200.00	0.00	4.00	0.00	0.00
	Cereal, Mueslix, Apple & Almond	55.0000	0.750	Cup	5.39	4.95	40.87	210.65	0.00	4.68	0.00	1.05
	Cereal, Nut & Honey Crunch	55.0000	1.250	Cup	4.02	2.48	45.98	222.75	0.00	0.88	0.00	0.50
158	Cereal, Nutri-Grain Almond Raisi	49.0000	1.250	Cup	4.00	2.50	38.00	180.00	0.00	4.00	0.00	0.00
	Cereal, Nutri-grain, Barley	41.0000	1.000	Cup	4.47	0.33	33.95	152.52	0.00	2.38	0.00	0.00
	Cereal, Nutri-grain, Corn	42.0000	1.000	Cup	3.36	0.97	35.45	160.02	0.00	2.60	0.00	0.00
	Cereal, Nutri-grain, Rye	40.0000	1.000	Cup	3.48	0.28	33.88	143.60	0.00	2.56	0.00	0.00
	Cereal, Nutri-grain, Wheat	30.0000	0.750	Cup	3.03	0.99	24.00	100.50	0.00	3.78	0.00	0.06
	Cereal, Oat Bran Cereal	57.0000	1.250	Cup	8.54	2.95	41.39	212.61	0.00	5.99	0.00	0.54
	Cereal, Oat Flakes	48.0000	1.000	Cup	7.87	0.96	36.10	180.48	0.00	1.44	0.00	0.16
	Cereal, Oatmeal Cereal, Honey Nu	49.0000	1.000	Cup	4.89	2.71	38.96	190.61	0.00	3.33	0.49	0.52
	Cereal, Oatmeal Raisin Crisp	55.0000	1.000	Cup	4.35	2.45	43.70	204.05	0.00	3.52	0.00	0.39

Monounsaturated Fat (gm)	Polyunsaturated Fat (gm)	Vitamin D (mg)	Vitamin K (mg)	Vitamin E (mg)	Vitamin A (re)	Vitamin C (mg)	Thiamin (mg)	Riboflavin (mg)	Niacin (mg)	Vitamin B_6 (mg)	Folate (mg)	Vitamin B_{12} (mcg)	Calcium (mg)	Iron (mg)	Magnesium (mg)	Phosphorus (mg)	Potassium (mg)	Sodium (mg)	Zinc (mg)
0.00	0.00	0.00	0.00	0.00	1250.00	0.00	0.38	0.43	5.00	0.50	100.00	1.50	20.00	2.70	40.00	150.00	120.00	150.00	1.20
0.14	0.06	0.00	0.00	0.33	0.00	9.00	0.38	0.43	5.00	0.50	99.90	0.00	58.50	4.50	68.10	168.30	216.90	142.50	1.24
0.00	0.00	0.00	0.00	0.34	635.52	0.00	0.62	0.72	8.45	0.86	169.44	2.54	68.16	13.73	57.60	176.16	343.20	429.12	1.50
0.50	0.00	0.00	0.00	0.00	0.00	15.00	0.38	0.43	5.00	0.50	100.00	1.50	20.00	4.50	0.00	20.00	15.00	210.00	3.75
0.00	0.00	0.00	0.00	0.00	750.00	15.00	0.38	0.43	5.00	0.50	100.00	0.00	60.00	4.50	0.00	40.00	20.00	170.00	3.75
0.03	0.09	0.03	0.00	0.04	225.06	15.00	0.37	0.43	4.99	0.50	93.00	0.00	0.62	4.50	2.79	8.06	20.46	199.95	0.16
0.00	0.00	0.03	0.00	0.00	750.00	15.00	0.38	0.43	5.00	0.50	0.10	1.50	0.00	4.50	0.00	0.00	20.00	210.00	0.00
0.11	0.61	0.00	0.00	0.50	0.00	0.00	0.39	0.44	5.01	0.50	102.30	1.49	19.80	61.23	55.55	159.50	183.15	1.65	1.49
0.21	0.27	0.03	0.00	0.11	211.20	14.07	0.39	0.42	5.01	0.51	90.00	0.00	3.30	4.23	8.70	20.70	31.50	140.70	3.75
0.10	0.08	0.00	0.00	0.03	423.68	0.00	0.42	0.48	5.63	0.58	112.96	1.70	3.84	2.02	9.28	18.88	24.32	177.60	1.70
0.28	0.16	0.03	0.00	0.23	225.30	15.00	0.38	0.43	5.00	0.50	99.90	0.00	14.40	4.50	9.30	36.00	52.80	274.50	3.75
0.00	0.00	0.00	0.00	0.02	397.20	15.90	0.39	0.45	5.28	0.54	105.90	0.00	13.80	1.89	24.90	65.70	108.30	195.90	1.59
0.50	1.50	0.03	0.00	8.00	750.00	3.60	0.38	0.43	5.00	0.50	0.10	1.50	20.00	1.80	40.00	150.00	170.00	150.00	3.75
0.50	2.00	0.03	0.00	0.00	750.00	2.40	0.38	0.43	5.00	0.50	0.10	1.50	20.00	1.80	40.00	100.00	120.00	120.00	3.75
3.33	1.81	0.00	0.00	1.19	0.00	0.06	0.18	0.10	0.54	0.07	19.38	0.04	49.02	2.48	51.87	167.58	221.16	18.81	1.14
0.00	0.00	0.02	0.00	0.00	224.89	0.00	0.56	0.64	7.12	0.75	74.96	0.75	35.98	1.50	52.47	179.91	254.87	202.40	5.62
9.60	12.90	0.00	0.00	15.71	4.88	1.71	0.90	0.34	2.50	0.39	104.92	0.00	98.82	5.12	217.16	563.64	656.36	29.28	4.95
0.66	1.16	0.00	0.00	5.53	206.25	0.00	0.33	0.39	4.57	0.44	110.00	1.38	24.20	1.93	45.65	127.05	155.65	123.75	3.47
0.66	2.09	0.00	0.00	5.53	253.00	0.00	0.44	0.50	5.61	0.55	110.00	1.71	22.55	2.04	46.75	134.75	137.50	134.75	4.24
1.42	0.80	0.00	0.00	0.48	0.00	0.12	0.09	0.07	0.26	0.04	9.61	0.06	23.87	1.29	26.04	91.76	132.68	7.75	0.50
6.49	1.87	0.00	0.00	3.88	0.00	0.00	0.17	0.06	0.61	0.08	8.25	0.00	41.25	1.72	52.25	160.05	182.60	89.10	1.11
0.06	0.19	1.00	0.00	0.27	1443.16	0.00	1.42	1.64	19.18	1.96	384.77	5.78	10.36	31.17	73.03	273.59	364.06	757.55	2.40
0.00	0.00	0.00	0.00	0.08	429.73	0.00	0.42	0.49	5.71	0.58	114.57	1.72	12.98	9.28	35.70	96.72	112.95	183.06	0.65
0.00	0.00	0.02	0.00	0.00	374.81	0.00	0.56	0.64	7.12	0.75	74.96	0.75	35.98	2.25	52.47	179.91	179.91	224.89	1.80
4.80	7.08	0.00	0.00	0.81	6.90	1.15	0.36	0.16	1.61	0.20	64.40	0.00	74.75	4.34	147.20	416.30	385.25	293.25	3.04
4.22	6.24	0.00	0.00	0.77	6.60	1.10	0.32	0.14	1.54	0.20	44.00	0.00	66.00	4.02	140.80	376.20	414.70	225.50	2.83
3.97	5.68	0.00	0.00	0.74	6.30	1.05	0.35	0.15	1.79	0.17	56.70	0.00	66.15	5.39	137.55	380.10	384.30	213.15	2.74
0.00	0.00	0.00	0.00	0.00	1250.00	0.00	0.38	0.43	5.00	0.50	100.00	1.50	0.00	2.70	16.00	40.00	50.00	190.00	0.30
0.00	0.00	0.00	0.00	0.00	1250.00	0.00	0.38	0.43	5.00	0.50	100.00	1.50	0.00	2.70	24.00	60.00	65.00	180.00	0.30
1.06	0.28	0.00	0.00	0.11	301.32	12.04	0.38	0.47	5.02	0.50	100.44	0.00	12.42	4.51	12.69	41.85	45.09	0.00	3.76
0.00	0.00	0.00	0.00	0.00	0.00	9.00	0.38	0.43	5.00	0.50	100.00	0.00	40.00	4.50	32.00	100.00	130.00	270.00	0.60
0.08	0.26	0.00	0.00	0.81	463.40	18.55	0.46	0.53	6.16	0.63	23.45	1.86	16.10	5.57	45.85	131.95	150.50	202.30	0.90
0.00	0.00	0.02	0.00	0.09	291.28	0.00	0.29	0.33	3.87	0.40	77.66	1.17	3.74	2.09	7.48	21.78	70.40	123.86	1.17
0.28	1.05	0.00	0.00	2.24	375.65	0.00	0.39	0.44	5.01	0.50	102.30	1.49	14.30	16.23	34.10	106.15	121.00	337.70	0.88
0.77	0.55	0.00	0.00	3.00	344.30	0.00	0.33	0.39	4.57	0.44	110.00	1.38	0.00	14.85	33.00	108.90	155.65	265.65	1.05
0.40	0.30	0.00	0.00	0.00	1044.00	13.00	0.39	0.44	5.20	0.52	104.00	1.57	4.00	8.74	26.00	79.00	86.00	260.00	3.91
0.15	0.04	0.03	0.00	0.08	375.30	15.00	0.38	0.43	5.00	0.50	99.90	0.00	43.50	8.10	9.30	42.00	41.10	263.10	3.75
0.41	0.56	0.00	0.00	0.16	1.28	0.00	0.40	0.45	5.33	0.53	106.88	0.00	97.60	8.96	31.04	135.68	79.04	174.40	4.00
0.57	0.77	0.00	0.00	0.23	1.50	0.10	0.63	0.71	8.38	0.84	167.50	0.00	134.50	74.54	41.50	181.00	113.00	220.00	6.29
0.39	0.15	0.03	0.00	0.13	225.30	15.00	0.38	0.43	5.00	0.50	99.90	0.00	32.40	4.50	19.50	75.60	54.00	203.10	3.75
0.00	0.00	0.00	0.00	0.00	0.00	0.00	0.48	0.24	5.76	0.02	4.80	0.00	4.80	9.60	4.80	24.00	31.20	324.00	0.17
0.00	0.00	0.00	0.00	0.00	703.20	28.80	0.72	0.72	9.36	0.96	9.60	2.88	124.80	8.40	50.40	247.20	211.20	259.20	1.49
0.74	0.89	0.00	0.00	1.68	703.20	28.80	0.72	0.72	9.36	0.96	9.60	2.88	124.80	8.40	50.40	247.20	211.20	9.60	1.49
2.00	1.00	0.20	0.00	8.00	200.00	20.00	0.38	0.43	5.00	0.50	0.10	1.50	20.00	4.50	40.00	150.00	240.00	160.00	3.75
2.59	1.05	0.00	0.00	5.78	233.75	0.00	0.39	0.44	5.17	0.50	110.00	1.27	33.55	4.68	62.70	175.45	209.00	270.05	3.14
1.16	0.83	0.00	0.00	0.14	225.50	15.02	0.39	0.44	5.01	0.50	110.00	0.00	5.50	4.51	4.95	36.30	59.95	370.15	0.39
1.00	1.50	0.00	0.00	8.00	0.00	0.00	0.38	0.43	5.00	0.50	0.10	1.50	150.00	1.40	16.00	200.00	190.00	170.00	3.75
0.00	0.00	0.00	0.00	10.82	542.84	21.73	0.53	0.62	7.22	0.74	144.73	2.17	11.07	1.45	32.39	126.28	107.83	277.16	5.41
0.00	0.00	0.00	0.00	11.09	556.08	22.26	0.55	0.63	7.39	0.76	148.26	2.23	1.26	0.89	26.88	120.54	97.86	276.36	5.54
0.00	0.00	0.00	0.00	10.56	529.60	21.20	0.52	0.60	7.04	0.72	141.20	2.12	8.40	1.13	30.40	104.00	71.60	272.00	5.28
0.24	0.69	0.00	0.00	5.40	0.00	15.00	0.39	0.42	5.01	0.51	90.00	1.50	9.60	0.99	24.30	108.30	109.50	220.80	3.75
0.96	1.21	0.00	0.00	2.10	155.61	6.21	0.39	0.44	5.19	0.52	103.74	0.00	30.21	15.96	99.18	306.09	257.07	205.20	3.89
0.28	0.36	0.00	0.00	0.34	635.52	0.00	0.62	0.72	8.45	0.86	169.44	2.54	68.16	13.73	57.60	176.16	228.00	220.32	2.54
1.15	0.75	0.00	0.00	2.01	150.43	5.98	0.37	0.42	5.00	0.50	99.96	0.02	26.95	4.50	53.41	166.11	184.73	165.62	3.92
1.16	0.36	0.00	0.00	1.36	225.50	0.00	0.37	0.42	5.01	0.50	100.10	0.00	37.95	4.50	44.55	117.15	211.75	223.85	3.75

USDA ID Code	Food Name	Weight in Grams*	Quantity of Units	Unit of Measure	Protein (gm)	Fat (gm)	Carbohydrate (gm)	Kcalories	Caffeine (gm)	Fiber (gm)	Cholesterol (mg)	Saturated Fat (gm)
	Cereal, Oatmeal Squares	56.0000	1.000	Cup	7.27	2.59	43.32	216.16	0.00	4.26	0.00	0.48
	Cereal, Oatmeal, Dry	2.5000	1.000	Tbsp	0.34	0.20	1.73	9.95	0.00	0.17	0.00	0.03
	Cereal, Oatmeal, Prepared	28.3500	1.000	Ounce	1.42	1.16	4.34	32.89	0.00	0.31	3.21	0.64
	Cereal, Oats Granola, Toasted	55.0000	0.750	Cup	5.80	9.69	36.23	238.05	0.00	3.52	0.00	1.27
	Cereal, Oats, Instant, Plain	234.0000	1.000	Cup	5.85	2.34	23.87	138.06	0.00	3.98	0.00	0.42
	Cereal, Oats, Instant, w/ apples	149.0000	1.000	Pkt.	3.19	1.42	26.15	125.16	0.00	2.53	0.00	0.30
	Cereal, Oats, Instant, w/ bran &	195.0000	1.000	Pkt.	4.88	1.95	30.42	157.95	0.00	5.46	0.00	0.35
	Cereal, Oats, Instant, w/ cinn a	240.0000	1.000	Cup	7.20	2.88	52.32	264.00	0.00	3.84	0.00	0.53
	Cereal, Oats, Instant, w/ maple	155.0000	1.000	Pkt.	4.17	1.78	31.40	153.45	0.00	2.64	0.00	0.36
	Cereal, Oats, Instant, w/ raisin	240.0000	1.000	Cup	6.48	2.64	48.48	244.80	0.00	3.36	0.00	0.50
	Cereal, Oats, Reg and Quick and	234.0000	1.000	Cup	6.08	2.34	25.27	145.08	0.00	3.98	0.00	0.42
159	Cereal, Organic Frst Ultra Mini	55.0000	0.750	Cup	4.00	1.00	46.00	190.00	0.00	7.00	0.00	0.00
160	Cereal, Organic Mini Cr Wheat-Ba	55.0000	0.750	Cup	5.00	1.00	45.00	190.00	0.00	8.00	0.00	0.00
	Cereal, Peanut Butter Puffs-Rees	30.0000	0.750	Cup	2.57	3.20	22.98	129.30	0.00	0.39	0.00	0.64
	Cereal, Product 19	30.0000	1.000	Cup	2.67	0.39	24.96	109.80	0.00	0.99	0.00	0.03
	Cereal, Puffed Rice	14.0000	1.000	Cup	0.98	0.13	12.29	53.62	0.00	0.20	0.00	0.05
	Cereal, Puffed Wheat	15.0000	1.250	Cup	2.44	0.32	11.46	54.90	0.00	1.14	0.00	0.02
161	Cereal, Puffins-Barbara	27.0000	0.750	Cup	2.00	1.00	23.00	90.00	0.00	5.00	0.00	0.00
	Cereal, Quisp	27.0000	1.000	Cup	1.35	1.49	22.97	108.81	0.00	0.68	0.00	0.41
	Cereal, Raisin Bran, Total-Gener	55.0000	1.000	Cup	4.00	1.01	42.75	178.20	0.00	5.01	0.00	0.23
	Cereal, Raisin Bran-Kellogg's	61.0000	1.000	Cup	5.61	1.46	47.09	186.05	0.00	8.17	0.00	0.00
	Cereal, Raisin Bran-Post	56.0000	1.000	Cup	5.21	1.06	42.34	171.92	0.00	7.90	0.00	0.18
	Cereal, Raisin Bran-Ralston Puri	56.0000	1.000	Cup	4.37	0.28	46.48	178.08	0.00	7.50	0.00	0.04
	Cereal, Raisin Nut Bran	55.0000	1.000	Cup	5.16	4.40	41.45	209.00	0.00	5.06	0.00	0.72
	Cereal, Raisin Squares	55.0000	0.750	Cup	4.40	1.54	42.90	187.00	0.00	5.17	0.00	0.17
162	Cereal, Raisins, Dates & Pecans-	54.0000	0.660	Cup	4.00	5.00	39.00	210.00	0.00	4.00	0.00	0.50
	Cereal, Raisins, Rice and Rye	46.0000	1.000	Cup	2.62	0.14	39.28	154.56	0.00	2.62	0.00	0.00
	Cereal, Rice Krispies	33.0000	1.250	Cup	2.08	0.36	28.55	124.41	0.00	0.36	0.00	0.13
163	Cereal, Rice Krispies, Apple-Cin	30.0000	0.750	Cup	1.53	0.51	26.70	111.90	0.00	0.45	0.00	0.00
	Cereal, Rice, Puffed	14.0000	1.000	Cup	0.88	0.07	12.57	56.28	0.00	0.24	0.00	0.02
	Cereal, Shredded Wheat, Large	23.6000	1.000	Biscuit	2.57	0.39	19.19	84.96	0.00	2.31	0.00	0.07
	Cereal, Shredded Wheat, Small	30.0000	1.000	Cup	3.30	0.50	24.12	107.10	0.00	2.94	0.00	0.08
164	Cereal, Smacks Kellogg's	27.0000	0.750	Cup	2.00	0.50	24.00	100.00	0.00	1.00	0.00	0.00
	Cereal, S'mores Grahams	30.0000	0.750	Cup	1.68	1.20	25.59	117.00	0.00	0.84	0.00	0.18
	Cereal, Special K	31.0000	1.000	Cup	6.36	0.28	22.44	114.70	0.00	0.96	0.00	0.00
	Cereal, Super Sugar Crisp	33.0000	1.000	Cup	2.15	0.30	29.77	123.42	0.00	0.50	0.00	0.05
	Cereal, Tasteeos	24.0000	1.000	Cup	3.07	0.67	18.98	94.32	0.00	2.54	0.00	0.23
	Cereal, Team	42.0000	1.000	Cup	2.69	0.76	36.04	164.22	0.00	0.55	0.00	0.00
165	Cereal, Temptations, Fr. Vanilla	30.0000	0.750	Cup	2.13	1.65	24.72	119.40	0.00	0.78	0.00	1.05
166	Cereal, Temptations, Honey Roast	30.0000	1.000	Cup	1.80	2.25	24.42	122.40	0.00	0.69	0.00	0.51
	Cereal, Toasties	23.0000	1.000	Cup	1.84	0.05	19.73	89.01	0.00	0.78	0.00	0.01
168	Cereal, Total	30.0000	0.750	Cup	2.99	0.70	23.88	105.30	0.00	2.64	0.00	0.18
	Cereal, Triples	30.0000	1.000	Cup	2.38	1.01	24.98	116.10	0.00	0.84	0.00	0.29
	Cereal, Trix	30.0000	1.000	Cup	0.95	1.71	26.04	122.40	0.00	0.72	0.00	0.41
	Cereal, Waffelos	30.0000	1.000	Cup	1.68	1.26	25.89	121.50	0.00	0.00	0.00	0.00
167	Cereal, Weetabix	35.0000	2.000	Biscuits	4.00	1.00	28.00	120.00	0.00	4.00	0.00	0.00
	Cereal, Wheat Germ, Toasted	28.3500	1.000	Oz.	8.25	3.03	14.06	108.30	0.00	3.66	0.00	0.52
	Cereal, Wheat 'n Raisin Chex	54.0000	1.000	Cup	5.08	0.43	42.98	185.22	0.00	3.56	0.00	0.00
	Cereal, Wheatena, Ckd w/ water	243.0000	1.000	Cup	4.86	1.22	28.67	136.08	0.00	6.56	0.00	0.19
	Cereal, Wheatena, Ckd w/ water,	243.0000	1.000	Cup	4.86	1.22	28.67	136.08	0.00	6.56	0.00	0.22
	Cereal, Wheaties	30.0000	1.000	Cup	3.24	0.93	23.79	110.10	0.00	2.10	0.00	0.20
	Cereal, Whole Wheat Hot Natural	242.0000	1.000	Cup	4.84	0.97	33.15	150.04	0.00	3.87	0.00	0.15
	French Toast, Frozen, Ready-to-h	28.3500	1.000	Slice	2.10	1.73	9.10	60.39	0.00	0.31	23.25	0.43
	French Toast, Made w/ Lowfat (2%	28.3500	1.000	Slice	2.18	3.06	7.09	64.92	0.00	0.00	32.89	0.77
	French Toast, Made w/ Whole Milk	65.0000	1.000	Slice	5.01	7.35	16.19	150.80	0.00	0.00	76.05	1.95

Monounsaturated Fat (gm)	Polyunsaturated Fat (gm)	Vitamin D (mg)	Vitamin K (mg)	Vitamin E (mg)	Vitamin A (re)	Vitamin C (mg)	Thiamin (mg)	Riboflavin (mg)	Niacin (mg)	Vitamin B_6 (mg)	Folate (mg)	Vitamin B_{12} (mcg)	Calcium (mg)	Iron (mg)	Magnesium (mg)	Phosphorus (mg)	Potassium (mg)	Sodium (mg)	Zinc (mg)
0.81	1.05	0.00	0.00	2.28	169.12	6.78	0.42	0.48	5.63	0.56	112.56	0.00	35.84	15.68	70.00	185.92	227.92	263.20	4.22
0.06	0.07	0.00	0.00	0.01	0.05	0.08	0.07	0.07	0.90	0.00	0.88	0.00	18.33	1.19	3.63	12.48	11.75	0.83	0.09
0.00	0.00	0.00	0.00	0.00	7.40	0.37	0.14	0.16	1.70	0.02	2.84	0.09	62.37	3.44	9.92	45.36	57.83	13.04	0.26
6.49	1.87	0.00	0.00	3.88	0.00	0.00	0.17	0.06	0.61	0.08	8.25	0.00	41.25	1.72	52.25	160.05	182.60	189.10	1.11
0.75	0.87	0.00	0.00	0.28	599.04	0.00	0.70	0.37	7.23	0.98	128.70	0.00	215.28	8.33	56.16	175.50	131.04	376.74	1.15
0.51	0.58	0.00	0.00	0.12	305.45	0.30	0.30	0.34	4.08	0.40	93.87	0.00	104.30	3.89	29.80	113.24	105.79	120.69	0.70
0.00	0.00	0.00	0.00	0.00	479.70	0.00	0.57	0.64	8.13	0.76	156.00	0.00	173.55	7.62	56.55	206.70	235.95	247.65	1.35
0.96	1.01	0.00	0.00	0.53	705.60	0.00	0.84	0.50	8.42	1.15	228.00	0.00	256.80	9.89	76.80	216.00	156.00	417.60	1.44
0.62	0.74	0.00	0.00	0.17	302.25	0.00	0.29	0.34	4.03	0.40	80.60	0.00	105.40	3.86	38.75	131.75	111.60	234.05	0.90
0.84	0.94	0.00	0.00	0.24	669.60	0.00	0.77	0.55	8.33	1.13	228.00	0.00	252.00	10.01	55.20	201.60	228.00	343.20	1.08
0.75	0.87	0.00	0.00	0.00	4.68	0.00	0.26	0.05	0.30	0.05	9.36	0.00	18.72	1.59	56.16	177.84	131.04	374.40	1.15
0.00	0.00	0.00	0.00	0.00	0.00	0.00	0.00	0.00	0.00	0.00	0.00	0.00	0.00	0.00	0.00	0.00	0.00	200.00	0.00
0.00	0.00	0.00	0.00	0.00	0.00	0.00	0.00	0.00	0.00	0.00	0.00	0.00	0.00	0.00	0.00	0.00	0.00	240.00	0.00
1.43	0.60	0.00	0.00	0.57	225.30	15.00	0.38	0.43	5.00	0.50	99.90	0.00	21.00	4.50	15.90	43.20	61.50	177.30	3.75
0.15	0.21	0.03	0.00	22.20	225.30	60.00	1.50	1.71	20.01	2.01	390.00	6.00	2.70	18.00	12.30	33.00	40.50	216.00	15.00
0.03	0.05	0.00	0.00	0.01	0.00	0.00	0.06	0.01	0.88	0.00	1.40	0.00	1.26	0.41	4.20	16.52	16.24	0.70	0.15
0.05	0.16	0.00	0.00	0.10	0.15	0.00	0.06	0.04	1.79	0.02	5.10	0.06	3.60	0.70	19.95	49.65	54.60	0.75	0.46
0.00	0.00	0.00	0.00	0.00	0.00	0.00	0.00	0.00	0.00	0.00	0.00	0.00	0.00	0.00	0.00	0.00	0.00	190.00	0.00
0.33	0.21	0.00	0.00	0.14	3.24	0.00	0.38	0.43	5.09	0.51	101.79	0.00	5.13	4.58	13.77	42.39	36.18	194.40	3.82
0.17	0.17	0.00	0.00	29.98	375.10	0.00	1.50	1.70	20.02	2.00	399.85	6.35	238.15	18.00	44.55	258.50	287.10	239.80	15.00
0.24	0.79	0.04	0.00	0.56	250.10	0.00	0.43	0.49	5.55	0.55	122.00	1.65	35.38	5.00	89.06	214.11	436.76	353.80	4.15
0.15	0.50	0.05	0.00	1.30	741.44	0.00	0.73	0.84	9.86	1.01	197.68	2.97	26.32	8.90	95.20	234.64	344.96	365.12	2.97
0.04	0.13	0.00	0.00	1.30	556.08	1.68	0.56	0.62	7.39	0.73	148.40	2.24	26.88	27.33	84.56	247.52	287.28	486.08	1.67
1.93	0.46	0.00	0.00	2.03	0.00	0.00	0.37	0.42	5.00	0.50	99.55	0.00	73.70	4.50	53.90	162.80	218.35	245.85	1.11
0.11	0.50	0.00	0.00	0.29	0.00	0.00	0.39	0.44	5.17	0.50	110.00	1.54	18.70	16.83	47.85	159.50	259.60	3.30	1.54
0.00	0.00	0.00	0.00	0.00	1500.00	0.00	0.45	0.51	6.00	0.60	120.00	1.80	20.00	3.60	40.00	150.00	150.00	150.00	1.20
0.00	0.00	0.00	0.00	0.25	467.82	0.46	0.46	0.55	6.26	0.64	124.66	1.89	10.12	5.61	19.78	49.68	143.52	349.60	4.69
0.10	0.17	0.03	0.00	0.04	247.83	16.50	0.43	0.46	5.51	0.56	116.49	0.00	3.30	1.98	15.84	43.56	42.24	353.76	0.60
0.00	0.51	0.00	0.00	0.13	233.10	15.51	0.39	0.45	5.16	0.51	90.00	0.00	2.10	1.86	7.80	24.90	30.90	222.90	0.33
0.00	0.00	0.00	0.00	0.00	0.00	0.00	0.36	0.25	4.94	0.01	2.66	0.00	0.84	4.44	3.50	13.72	15.82	0.42	0.14
0.06	0.21	0.00	0.00	0.13	0.00	0.00	0.07	0.07	1.08	0.06	11.80	0.00	9.68	0.74	40.12	85.67	77.17	0.47	0.59
0.08	0.26	0.00	0.00	0.16	0.00	0.00	0.08	0.08	1.58	0.08	15.00	0.00	11.40	1.27	39.60	105.90	108.30	3.00	0.99
0.00	0.00	0.03	0.00	0.00	750.00	15.00	0.38	0.43	5.00	0.50	0.10	1.50	0.00	1.80	8.00	40.00	40.00	50.00	0.30
0.39	0.15	0.00	0.00	0.22	225.30	15.00	0.38	0.43	5.00	0.50	99.90	0.00	14.40	4.50	10.80	40.50	48.00	212.40	3.75
0.00	0.22	1.25	0.00	0.08	225.06	15.00	0.53	0.59	7.01	0.71	93.00	0.00	4.65	8.71	17.67	50.84	54.56	249.86	3.75
0.06	0.12	0.00	0.00	0.12	436.92	0.00	0.43	0.50	5.81	0.59	116.49	1.75	6.93	2.08	19.80	43.89	47.85	50.82	1.75
0.17	0.18	0.00	0.00	0.17	317.76	12.72	0.31	0.36	4.22	0.43	84.72	1.27	11.04	6.86	26.16	95.76	71.04	182.88	0.69
0.00	0.00	0.00	0.00	0.10	556.08	22.26	0.55	0.63	7.39	0.76	6.72	2.23	6.30	2.57	18.48	65.10	70.98	259.56	0.58
0.36	0.24	0.00	0.00	0.83	259.80	17.31	0.42	0.48	5.76	0.57	120.00	0.00	10.80	5.19	6.90	20.40	40.80	207.00	0.21
1.17	0.57	0.00	0.00	0.14	232.80	15.51	0.39	0.45	5.16	0.51	90.00	0.00	0.60	4.65	2.70	7.50	28.80	248.40	0.12
0.01	0.02	0.00	0.00	0.06	304.52	0.00	0.30	0.35	4.05	0.41	81.91	1.22	0.92	0.61	3.45	10.12	26.68	241.04	0.07
0.14	0.08	0.03	0.00	23.49	375.30	60.00	1.50	1.70	20.10	2.00	399.90	7.67	258.30	18.00	32.10	210.90	96.90	198.60	15.00
0.27	0.03	0.00	0.00	0.14	375.30	15.00	0.38	0.43	5.00	0.50	99.90	0.00	41.10	8.10	6.90	35.40	30.60	191.40	3.75
0.90	0.29	0.03	0.00	0.60	225.30	15.00	0.38	0.43	5.00	0.50	99.90	0.00	32.10	4.50	3.60	26.10	17.70	196.80	3.75
0.00	0.00	0.00	0.00	0.00	397.20	15.90	0.39	0.45	5.28	0.54	3.30	1.59	8.40	4.77	6.30	244.50	26.40	124.80	0.24
0.00	0.00	0.00	0.00	0.00	0.00	0.00	0.00	0.00	0.00	0.00	0.00	0.00	0.00	0.00	0.00	0.00	120.00	130.00	0.00
0.43	1.88	0.00	0.00	5.14	0.00	1.70	0.47	0.23	1.59	0.28	99.79	0.00	12.76	2.58	90.72	324.89	268.48	1.13	4.73
0.00	0.00	0.00	0.00	0.31	0.00	1.62	0.54	0.59	7.13	0.70	143.10	2.16	24.30	7.72	52.92	163.08	226.80	305.64	1.19
0.17	0.61	0.00	0.00	0.90	0.00	0.00	0.02	0.05	1.34	0.05	17.01	0.00	9.72	1.36	48.60	145.80	187.11	4.86	1.68
0.00	0.00	0.00	0.00	0.00	0.00	0.00	0.02	0.05	1.34	0.05	17.01	0.00	9.72	1.36	48.60	145.80	187.11	578.34	1.68
0.22	0.15	0.03	0.00	0.37	225.30	15.00	0.38	0.43	5.00	0.50	99.90	0.00	54.60	8.10	31.80	95.40	104.10	222.30	0.71
0.00	0.00	0.00	0.00	0.00	0.00	0.00	0.17	0.12	2.15	0.17	26.62	0.00	16.94	1.50	53.24	166.98	171.82	563.86	1.16
0.58	0.35	0.00	0.00	0.19	15.31	0.09	0.08	0.11	0.77	0.14	14.74	0.48	30.33	0.63	4.82	39.41	37.99	140.33	0.22
1.28	0.73	0.00	0.00	0.00	37.42	0.09	0.06	0.09	0.46	0.02	12.19	0.09	28.35	0.47	4.82	33.17	37.99	135.80	0.19
3.03	1.70	0.00	0.00	0.00	80.60	0.20	0.13	0.21	1.06	0.05	14.95	0.20	64.35	1.09	11.05	76.05	86.45	310.70	0.44

USDA ID Code	Food Name	Weight in Grams*	Quantity of Units	Unit of Measure	Protein (gm)	Fat (gm)	Carbohydrate (gm)	Kcalories	Caffeine (gm)	Fiber (gm)	Cholesterol (mg)	Saturated Fat (gm)
546	Instant Breakfast, Caffe Mocha-Ca	37.0000	1.300	Ounce	4.50	0.50	28.00	130.00	0.00	0.40	3.00	0.00
547	Instant Breakfast, Choc Malt, No	20.0000	0.700	Ounce	4.50	1.50	11.00	70.00	0.00	1.00	3.00	1.00
548	Instant Breakfast, Choc, Creamy	37.0000	1.300	Ounce	4.50	1.00	28.00	130.00	0.00	1.00	2.00	0.00
549	Instant Breakfast, Choc, No Suga	21.0000	0.720	Ounce	4.50	1.00	12.00	70.00	0.00	1.00	3.00	0.50
550	Instant Breakfast, Chocolate Mal	36.0000	1.250	Ounce	4.50	1.50	26.00	130.00	0.00	1.00	3.00	0.50
551	Instant Breakfast, Chocolate Mal	35.0000	1.200	Ounce	5.70	0.50	25.10	126.00	0.00	0.00	0.00	0.00
552	Instant Breakfast, Chocolate-Pil	35.0000	1.200	Ounce	5.70	0.50	25.70	130.00	0.00	0.00	0.00	0.00
553	Instant Breakfast, Strawberry, N	20.0000	0.700	Ounce	4.50	0.00	12.00	70.00	0.00	0.00	3.00	0.00
554	Instant Breakfast, Strawberry-Ca	36.0000	1.260	Ounce	4.50	0.00	28.00	130.00	0.00	0.00	0.00	0.00
555	Instant Breakfast, Strawberry-Pi	35.0000	1.200	Ounce	5.40	0.20	26.00	130.00	0.00	0.00	0.00	0.00
556	Instant Breakfast, Vanilla, Fren	36.0000	1.260	Ounce	4.50	0.00	27.00	130.00	0.00	0.00	3.00	0.00
557	Instant Breakfast, Vanilla-Pills	35.0000	1.200	Ounce	5.40	0.20	27.30	133.00	0.00	0.00	0.00	0.00
	Pancakes, Buttermilk	28.3500	1.000	Each	1.93	2.64	8.14	64.35	0.00	0.00	16.44	0.52
	Pancakes, Dietary	22.0000	1.000	3 In.	1.12	0.18	9.28	43.78	0.00	0.00	0.00	0.03
	Pancakes, Plain	28.3500	1.000	Each	1.81	2.75	8.02	64.35	0.00	0.00	16.73	0.60
	Pancakes, Plain, Frozen	28.3500	1.000	Each	1.47	0.94	12.36	64.92	0.00	0.51	2.55	0.22
	Pancakes, Whole-wheat	28.3500	1.000	Each	2.41	1.84	8.33	58.97	0.00	0.80	17.29	0.50
	Waffles, Buttermilk	75.0000	1.000	Each	6.23	10.20	24.75	216.75	0.00	0.00	50.25	1.88
	Waffles, Plain, Frozen, Toasted	28.3500	1.000	Each	1.76	2.32	11.54	74.84	0.00	0.65	6.80	0.41
	Waffles, Plain, Homemade	28.3500	1.000	Each	2.24	4.00	9.33	82.50	0.00	0.00	19.56	0.81
	Cheese Spread, American, Past.	28.3500	1.000	Ounce	4.65	6.02	2.47	82.35	0.00	0.00	15.65	3.78
	Cheese, American, Pasteurized Pr	28.3500	1.000	Ounce	6.28	8.86	0.45	106.44	0.00	0.00	26.76	5.58
	Cheese, Blue	28.3500	1.500	Ounce	6.07	8.15	0.66	100.09	0.00	0.00	21.32	5.29
	Cheese, Brick	132.0000	1.000	Cup	30.68	39.18	3.68	489.61	0.00	0.00	124.61	24.76
	Cheese, Brie	240.0000	1.500	Cup	49.80	66.43	1.08	800.76	0.00	0.00	240.00	41.78
	Cheese, Caraway	28.3500	1.500	Ounce	7.14	8.28	0.87	106.60	0.00	0.00	26.37	5.27
	Cheese, Cheddar	132.0000	1.000	Cup	32.87	43.74	1.69	531.41	0.00	0.00	138.47	27.84
	Cheese, Cheddar, Non-Fat	28.3500	1.500	Ounce	8.10	0.00	2.03	45.56	0.00	0.00	4.05	0.00
	Cheese, Cheddar, Reduced Fat	28.3500	1.500	Ounce	8.00	5.00	1.00	80.00	0.00	0.00	15.00	3.00
	Cheese, Colby	132.0000	1.000	Cup	31.36	42.39	3.39	519.62	0.00	0.00	125.27	26.69
	Cheese, Cottage, Creamed	113.0000	4.000	Ounce	14.11	5.10	3.03	116.79	0.00	0.00	16.84	3.22
	Cheese, Cottage, Creamed, w/ Fru	226.0000	1.000	Cup	22.37	7.68	30.06	279.40	0.00	0.00	25.31	4.86
	Cheese, Cottage, Fat Free	226.0000	0.500	Cup	26.00	0.00	0.00	140.00	0.00	0.00	20.00	0.00
	Cheese, Cottage, Lowfat, 1% Fat	226.0000	1.000	Cup	28.00	2.31	6.15	163.62	0.00	0.00	9.94	1.47
	Cheese, Cottage, Lowfat, 2% Fat	226.0000	1.000	Cup	31.05	4.36	8.20	202.68	0.00	0.00	18.98	2.76
	Cheese, Cottage, Uncreamed, Dry	145.0000	1.000	Cup	25.04	0.61	2.68	122.66	0.00	0.00	9.72	0.39
	Cheese, Cream	232.0000	1.000	Cup	17.52	80.90	6.17	809.77	0.00	0.00	254.50	50.97
	Cheese, Cream, Fat Free	17.5080	2.000	Tbsp	2.50	0.00	1.00	17.51	0.00	0.00	2.50	0.00
	Cheese, Cream, Light	16.0140	2.000	Tbsp	1.50	2.50	1.00	35.03	0.00	0.00	7.51	1.75
	Cheese, Cream, w/ Strawberry	30.0000	1.000	Ounce	4.00	0.00	2.00	35.00	0.00	0.00	3.00	0.00
	Cheese, Edam	28.3500	1.000	Ounce	7.08	7.88	0.41	101.10	0.00	0.00	25.29	4.98
	Cheese, Fat Free Slices, White	21.2630	1.000	Slice	5.00	0.00	2.00	30.00	0.00	0.00	0.00	0.00
	Cheese, Fat Free Slices, Yellow	21.2630	1.000	Slice	5.00	0.00	2.00	30.00	0.00	0.00	0.00	0.00
	Cheese, Feta	150.0000	1.000	Cup	21.32	31.92	6.14	395.34	0.00	0.00	133.50	22.43
	Cheese, Fontina	132.0000	1.000	Cup	33.79	41.10	2.05	513.52	0.00	0.00	153.12	25.34
	Cheese, Goat, Hard Type	28.3500	1.000	Ounce	8.65	10.09	0.62	128.14	0.00	0.00	29.77	6.98
	Cheese, Goat, Semisoft Type	28.3500	1.000	Ounce	6.12	8.46	0.72	103.19	0.00	0.00	22.40	5.85
	Cheese, Goat, Soft Type	28.3500	1.000	Ounce	5.25	5.98	0.25	75.98	0.00	0.00	13.04	4.13
	Cheese, Gouda	28.3500	1.500	Ounce	7.07	7.78	0.63	101.01	0.00	0.00	32.32	4.99
	Cheese, Gruyere	132.0000	1.000	Cup	39.35	42.69	0.48	545.09	0.00	0.00	145.20	24.96
	Cheese, Limburger	134.0000	1.000	Cup	26.87	36.52	0.66	438.23	0.00	0.00	120.60	22.45
	Cheese, Monterey	132.0000	1.000	Cup	32.31	39.97	0.90	492.78	0.00	0.00	117.48	25.17
	Cheese, Monterey, Reduced Fat	28.3500	1.500	Ounce	8.00	5.00	1.00	80.00	0.00	0.00	15.00	3.00
	Cheese, Mozzarella, Part Skim Mi	28.3500	1.500	Ounce	6.88	4.51	0.79	72.08	0.00	0.00	16.39	2.87
	Cheese, Mozzarella, Part Skim Mi	132.0000	1.000	Cup	36.26	22.60	4.14	369.51	0.00	0.00	71.28	14.36

Monounsaturated Fat (gm)	Polyunsaturated Fat (gm)	Vitamin D (mg)	Vitamin K (mg)	Vitamin E (mg)	Vitamin A (re)	Vitamin C (mg)	Thiamin (mg)	Riboflavin (mg)	Niacin (mg)	Vitamin B_6 (mg)	Folate (mg)	Vitamin B_{12} (mcg)	Calcium (mg)	Iron (mg)	Magnesium (mg)	Phosphorus (mg)	Potassium (mg)	Sodium (mg)	Zinc (mg)
0.00	0.00	0.00	0.00	0.00	1750.00	27.00	0.30	0.14	5.00	0.40	100.00	0.60	350.00	4.50	80.00	250.00	340.00	100.00	3.00
0.00	0.00	0.00	0.00	0.00	1750.00	27.00	0.30	0.10	5.00	0.40	100.00	0.60	250.00	4.50	80.00	250.00	290.00	115.00	3.00
0.00	0.00	0.00	0.00	0.00	1750.00	27.00	0.30	0.14	5.00	0.40	100.00	0.60	300.00	4.50	80.00	250.00	350.00	100.00	3.00
0.00	0.00	0.00	0.00	0.00	1750.00	27.00	0.30	0.10	5.00	0.40	100.00	0.60	300.00	4.50	80.00	250.00	350.00	95.00	3.00
0.00	0.00	0.00	0.00	0.00	1750.00	27.00	0.30	0.07	5.00	0.40	100.00	0.60	250.00	4.50	80.00	250.00	250.00	130.00	3.00
0.00	0.00	0.00	0.00	0.00	1684.00	23.00	0.47	0.41	5.80	0.00	0.00	0.00	335.00	5.60	0.00	125.00	263.00	119.00	0.00
0.00	0.00	0.00	0.00	0.00	1681.00	23.00	0.46	0.35	5.80	0.00	0.00	0.00	91.00	5.64	0.00	89.00	256.00	141.00	0.00
0.00	0.00	0.00	0.00	0.00	1750.00	27.00	0.30	0.14	5.00	0.40	100.00	0.60	350.00	4.50	80.00	250.00	250.00	95.00	3.00
0.00	0.00	0.00	0.00	0.00	1750.00	27.00	0.30	0.14	5.00	0.40	100.00	0.60	350.00	4.50	80.00	250.00	250.00	160.00	3.00
0.00	0.00	0.00	0.00	0.00	1681.00	23.00	0.44	0.32	5.80	0.00	0.00	0.00	91.00	5.40	0.00	70.00	250.00	130.00	0.00
0.00	0.00	0.00	0.00	0.00	1750.00	27.00	0.30	0.14	5.00	0.40	100.00	0.60	300.00	4.50	80.00	250.00	350.00	100.00	3.00
0.00	0.00	0.00	0.00	0.00	1686.00	23.00	0.33	0.23	4.70	0.00	0.00	0.00	79.00	5.10	0.00	111.00	229.00	198.00	0.00
0.67	1.27	0.00	0.00	0.00	8.51	0.11	0.06	0.08	0.45	0.01	10.77	0.05	44.51	0.48	4.25	39.41	41.11	147.99	0.18
0.03	0.08	0.00	0.00	0.00	2.20	0.00	0.04	0.02	0.37	0.00	1.10	0.00	12.76	0.39	5.94	74.80	84.92	57.64	0.15
0.70	1.26	0.00	0.00	0.00	15.31	0.09	0.06	0.08	0.45	0.01	10.77	0.06	62.09	0.51	4.54	45.08	37.42	124.46	0.16
0.34	0.27	0.00	0.00	0.11	8.22	0.09	0.11	0.13	1.14	0.02	14.18	0.05	17.58	0.99	3.97	105.46	20.70	144.30	0.19
0.49	0.68	0.00	0.00	0.00	18.14	0.14	0.06	0.15	0.65	0.03	8.22	0.08	70.88	0.88	13.04	105.75	79.10	162.16	0.29
2.52	5.09	0.00	0.00	0.00	26.25	0.38	0.20	0.27	1.55	0.04	11.25	0.16	136.50	1.63	13.50	123.75	128.25	450.75	0.56
0.91	0.79	0.00	0.00	0.24	103.19	0.00	0.11	0.14	1.26	0.26	12.76	0.71	65.77	1.27	6.24	119.07	36.29	223.11	0.16
1.00	1.92	0.00	0.00	0.00	18.43	0.11	0.07	0.10	0.59	0.02	13.04	0.07	72.29	0.65	5.39	53.87	45.08	144.87	0.19
1.76	0.18	0.00	0.00	0.00	53.58	0.00	0.01	0.12	0.04	0.03	1.98	0.11	159.30	0.09	8.09	248.06	68.58	460.69	0.73
2.54	0.28	0.00	0.00	0.00	82.22	0.00	0.01	0.10	0.02	0.02	2.21	0.20	174.49	0.11	6.31	125.87	45.93	184.28	0.85
2.21	0.23	0.00	0.00	0.18	64.64	0.00	0.01	0.11	0.29	0.05	10.32	0.35	149.57	0.09	6.50	109.83	72.66	395.57	0.75
11.35	1.03	0.00	0.00	0.66	398.64	0.00	0.01	0.46	0.16	0.09	26.80	1.66	889.28	0.57	32.10	595.32	179.26	738.67	3.43
19.22	1.99	0.00	0.00	1.58	436.80	0.00	0.17	1.25	0.91	0.58	156.00	3.96	441.60	1.20	48.00	451.20	364.80	1510.56	5.71
2.35	0.24	0.00	0.00	0.00	81.93	0.00	0.01	0.13	0.05	0.02	5.16	0.08	190.88	0.18	6.27	138.92	26.37	195.62	0.83
12.39	1.24	0.40	0.00	0.48	366.96	0.00	0.04	0.50	0.11	0.09	24.02	1.10	952.12	0.90	36.67	675.97	129.89	819.06	4.11
0.00	0.00	0.00	0.00	0.00	60.75	0.00	0.00	0.00	0.00	0.00	0.00	0.00	243.00	0.00	0.00	0.00	0.00	283.50	0.00
0.00	0.00	0.00	0.00	0.00	60.00	0.00	0.00	0.00	0.00	0.00	0.00	0.00	240.00	0.00	0.00	0.00	23.00	180.00	0.00
12.25	1.25	0.00	0.00	0.46	363.00	0.00	0.03	0.50	0.12	0.11	24.02	1.10	903.67	1.00	34.08	602.58	166.98	797.54	4.05
1.46	0.16	0.00	0.00	0.14	54.24	0.00	0.02	0.18	0.15	0.08	13.79	0.70	67.80	0.16	5.94	148.93	95.26	457.42	0.42
2.19	0.25	0.00	0.00	0.20	81.36	0.00	0.05	0.29	0.23	0.11	21.92	1.11	107.58	0.25	9.42	236.17	151.19	914.85	0.66
0.00	0.00	0.00	0.00	0.00	0.00	0.00	0.00	0.00	0.00	0.00	0.00	0.00	240.00	0.00	0.00	0.00	0.00	840.00	0.00
0.66	0.07	0.00	0.00	0.25	24.86	0.00	0.05	0.38	0.29	0.16	28.02	1.42	137.63	0.32	12.07	302.39	193.23	917.56	0.86
1.24	0.14	0.00	0.00	0.14	45.20	0.00	0.05	0.43	0.32	0.18	29.61	1.60	154.81	0.36	13.56	340.13	217.41	917.56	0.95
0.16	0.03	0.00	0.00	0.16	11.60	0.00	0.04	0.20	0.23	0.12	21.46	1.20	45.97	0.33	5.71	150.80	46.98	18.56	0.68
22.83	2.95	0.00	0.00	2.18	886.24	0.00	0.05	0.46	0.23	0.12	30.62	0.97	185.37	2.78	14.94	242.21	277.01	685.56	1.25
0.00	0.00	0.00	0.00	0.00	50.02	0.00	0.00	0.00	0.00	0.00	0.00	0.00	60.03	0.00	0.00	0.00	0.00	90.04	0.00
0.00	0.00	0.00	0.00	0.00	40.03	0.00	0.00	0.00	0.00	0.00	0.00	0.00	24.02	0.00	0.00	0.00	0.00	75.06	0.00
0.00	0.00	0.00	0.00	0.00	10.00	0.00	0.00	0.00	0.00	0.00	0.00	0.00	24.00	0.00	0.00	0.00	0.00	200.00	0.00
2.30	0.19	0.26	0.00	0.21	71.73	0.00	0.01	0.11	0.02	0.02	4.59	0.44	207.24	0.12	8.44	151.84	53.21	273.58	1.06
0.00	0.00	0.00	0.00	0.00	40.00	0.00	0.00	0.00	0.00	0.00	0.00	0.00	120.00	0.00	0.00	0.00	18.00	310.00	0.00
0.00	0.00	0.00	0.00	0.00	40.00	0.00	0.00	0.00	0.00	0.00	0.00	0.00	120.00	0.00	0.00	0.00	18.00	310.00	0.00
6.93	0.89	0.00	0.00	0.05	192.00	0.00	0.23	1.26	1.49	0.63	48.00	2.54	738.75	0.98	28.82	505.80	92.70	1674.15	4.32
11.47	2.18	0.00	0.00	0.46	382.80	0.00	0.03	0.26	0.20	0.11	7.92	2.22	726.00	0.30	18.48	457.12	83.82	1056.00	4.62
2.30	0.24	0.00	0.00	0.22	135.23	0.00	0.04	0.34	0.68	0.02	1.13	0.03	253.73	0.53	15.31	206.67	13.61	98.09	0.45
1.93	0.20	0.00	0.00	0.18	113.40	0.00	0.02	0.19	0.33	0.02	0.57	0.06	84.48	0.46	8.22	106.31	44.79	146.00	0.19
1.36	0.14	0.00	0.00	0.13	80.23	0.00	0.02	0.11	0.12	0.07	3.40	0.05	39.69	0.54	4.54	72.58	7.37	104.33	0.26
2.20	0.19	0.00	0.00	0.10	49.33	0.00	0.01	0.09	0.02	0.02	5.93	0.44	198.39	0.07	8.22	154.88	34.16	232.27	1.11
13.25	2.28	0.00	0.00	0.46	397.32	0.00	0.08	0.37	0.15	0.11	13.73	2.11	1334.52	0.22	47.40	799.00	106.92	443.52	5.15
11.54	0.67	0.00	0.00	0.86	423.44	0.00	0.11	0.67	0.21	0.12	77.05	1.39	665.58	0.17	28.14	526.62	171.52	1072.00	2.81
11.55	1.19	0.00	0.00	0.45	333.96	0.00	0.03	0.51	0.12	0.11	24.02	1.10	985.25	0.95	35.65	586.08	106.52	707.92	3.96
0.00	0.00	0.00	0.00	0.00	60.00	0.00	0.00	0.00	0.00	0.00	0.00	0.00	240.00	0.00	0.00	0.00	18.00	180.00	0.00
1.28	0.13	0.00	0.00	0.12	50.18	0.00	0.01	0.09	0.03	0.02	2.49	0.23	183.06	0.06	6.58	131.26	23.73	132.11	0.78
6.40	0.67	0.00	0.00	0.61	252.12	0.00	0.03	0.45	0.16	0.11	13.07	1.23	965.32	0.33	34.68	691.81	125.19	696.56	4.13

USDA ID Code	Food Name	Weight in Grams*	Quantity of Units	Unit of Measure	Protein (gm)	Fat (gm)	Carbohydrate (gm)	Kcalories	Caffeine (gm)	Fiber (gm)	Cholesterol (mg)	Saturated Fat (gm)
	Cheese, Mozzarella, Stick	28.0000	1.000	Each	8.00	5.00	0.00	80.00	0.00	0.00	15.00	3.00
	Cheese, Mozzarella, Substitute	113.0000	1.000	Cup	12.96	13.81	26.75	280.24	0.00	0.00	0.00	4.19
	Cheese, Mozzarella, Whole Milk	112.0000	1.000	Cup	21.75	24.19	2.49	315.15	0.00	0.00	87.81	14.73
	Cheese, Mozzarella, Whole Milk,	28.3500	1.000	Ounce	6.12	6.99	0.70	90.26	0.00	0.00	25.34	4.41
	Cheese, Muenster	132.0000	1.000	Cup	30.90	39.65	1.48	486.22	0.00	0.00	126.19	25.23
	Cheese, Parmesan, Grated	100.0000	1.000	Cup	41.56	30.02	3.74	455.81	0.00	0.00	78.70	19.07
	Cheese, Parmesan, Grated, Fat Fr	5.0020	1.000	Tbsp	0.67	0.00	0.67	5.00	0.00	0.00	1.67	0.00
	Cheese, Parmesan, Piece	28.3500	1.000	Ounce	10.14	7.32	0.91	111.18	0.00	0.00	19.19	4.65
	Cheese, Parmesan, Shredded	5.0000	1.000	Tbsp	1.89	1.37	0.17	20.75	0.00	0.00	3.60	0.87
	Cheese, Pepper	132.0000	1.000	Cup	32.31	39.97	0.90	492.78	0.00	0.00	117.48	25.17
	Cheese, Provolone	132.0000	1.000	Cup	33.77	35.14	2.82	463.98	0.00	0.00	90.95	22.55
	Cheese, Ricotta, Part Skim Milk	246.0000	1.000	Cup	28.02	19.46	12.64	339.63	0.00	0.00	75.77	12.13
	Cheese, Ricotta, Whole Milk	246.0000	1.000	Cup	27.70	31.93	7.48	427.89	0.00	0.00	124.48	20.42
	Cheese, Romano	28.3500	1.000	Ounce	9.02	7.64	1.03	109.61	0.00	0.00	29.48	4.85
	Cheese, Roquefort	28.3500	1.000	Ounce	6.11	8.69	0.57	104.62	0.00	0.00	25.52	5.46
	Cheese, Swiss, Domestic	132.0000	1.000	Cup	37.53	36.23	4.46	496.00	0.00	0.00	121.04	23.47
	Cheese, Swiss, Pasteurized Proce	140.0000	1.000	Cup	34.62	35.01	2.94	466.98	0.00	0.00	118.72	22.47
	Cream Substitute, Non-dairy, Liq	240.0000	1.000	Cup	2.40	23.93	27.31	325.56	0.00	0.00	0.00	4.66
	Cream Substitute, Non-dairy, Pow	94.0000	1.000	Cup	4.50	33.35	51.59	513.69	0.00	0.00	0.00	30.58
	Cream, Half and Half, Cream and	242.0000	1.000	Cup	7.16	27.83	10.41	315.50	0.00	0.00	89.30	17.33
	Cream, Light, Coffee or Table	240.0000	1.000	Cup	6.48	46.34	8.78	469.03	0.00	0.00	158.64	28.85
	Cream, Medium, 25% Fat	15.0000	1.000	Tbsp	0.37	3.75	0.52	36.56	0.00	0.00	13.12	2.33
	Cream, Whipped, Pressurized	60.0000	1.000	Cup	1.92	13.33	7.49	154.39	0.00	0.00	45.60	8.30
	Cream, Whipping, Heavy	119.5000	1.000	Cup	2.45	44.22	3.33	412.01	0.00	0.00	163.83	27.52
	Cream, Whipping, Light	120.0000	1.000	Cup	2.60	37.09	3.55	350.90	0.00	0.00	133.20	23.21
	Dessert Topping, Non-dairy	75.0000	1.000	Cup	0.94	18.98	17.29	238.71	0.00	0.00	0.00	16.34
	Egg Substitute, Frozen	240.0000	1.000	Cup	27.10	26.66	7.68	383.57	0.00	0.00	4.80	4.63
	Egg Substitute, Liquid	251.0000	1.000	Cup	30.12	8.31	1.61	210.99	0.00	0.00	2.51	1.66
	Egg White Only, w/o Yolk	243.0000	1.000	Cup	25.56	0.00	2.50	121.50	0.00	0.00	0.00	0.00
	Eggnog	254.0000	1.000	Cup	9.68	19.00	34.39	341.91	0.00	0.00	149.10	11.28
	Eggnog, Reduced Fat	246.0000	1.000	Cup	12.00	8.00	48.00	320.00	0.00	0.00	90.00	5.00
	Eggs, Chicken, Whole, Ckd, Fried	46.0000	1.000	Large	6.23	6.90	0.63	91.54	0.00	0.00	211.14	1.92
	Eggs, Chicken, Whole, Ckd, Hard-	136.0000	1.000	Cup	17.11	14.43	1.52	210.80	0.00	0.00	576.64	4.45
	Eggs, Chicken, Whole, Ckd, Omele	15.2000	1.000	Tbsp	1.57	1.74	0.16	23.10	0.00	0.00	53.20	0.48
	Eggs, Chicken, Whole, Ckd, Poach	50.0000	1.000	Large	6.22	4.99	0.61	74.50	0.00	0.00	211.50	1.55
	Eggs, Chicken, Whole, Ckd, Scram	220.0000	1.000	Cup	24.40	26.86	4.84	365.20	0.00	0.00	774.40	8.10
264	Eggs, Chicken, Whole, Fresh, and	50.0000	1.000	Large	6.25	5.01	0.61	74.50	0.00	0.00	212.50	1.55
	Frozen Yogurt	148.0000	0.500	Cup	6.00	12.00	48.00	320.00	0.00	0.00	20.00	4.00
444	Frozen Yogurt Bar, Banana/Straw-	71.0000	1.000	Each	2.00	0.00	20.00	90.00	0.00	0.00	0.00	0.00
445	Frozen Yogurt Bar, Rasp/Vanilla-	71.0000	1.000	Each	2.00	0.00	20.00	90.00	0.00	0.00	0.00	0.00
446	Frozen Yogurt Bar, Straw Daiquir	70.0000	1.000	Each	2.00	1.00	18.00	90.00	0.00	0.00	15.00	0.50
447	Frozen Yogurt Bar, Toc/Cherry-Ha	71.0000	1.000	Each	3.00	0.00	21.00	100.00	0.00	0.00	0.00	0.00
448	Frozen Yogurt Bar, Toc/Vanilla-H	71.0000	1.000	Each	3.00	0.00	20.00	90.00	0.00	0.00	0.00	0.00
449	Frozen Yogurt, Capp., No Fat-Ben	95.0000	0.500	Cup	4.00	0.00	26.00	120.00	0.00	0.00	0.00	0.00
450	Frozen Yogurt, Cherry Garcia-Ben	95.0000	0.500	Cup	4.00	2.50	27.00	140.00	0.00	0.00	5.00	2.00
451	Frozen Yogurt, Cherry Vanilla-Ha	93.0000	0.500	Cup	6.00	0.00	30.00	140.00	0.00	0.00	0.00	0.00
452	Frozen Yogurt, Choc Chip Cookie	95.0000	0.500	Cup	4.00	3.00	34.00	180.00	0.00	0.00	10.00	2.00
453	Frozen Yogurt, Choc Fudge Browni	95.0000	0.500	Cup	4.00	1.00	32.00	150.00	0.00	0.00	0.00	0.00
454	Frozen Yogurt, Chocolate, No Fat	95.0000	0.500	Cup	4.00	0.00	25.00	120.00	0.00	0.00	0.00	0.00
	Frozen Yogurt, Chocolate, Soft-s	72.0000	0.500	Cup	2.88	4.32	17.93	115.20	2.16	1.58	3.60	2.61
455	Frozen Yogurt, Chocolate-Haagen-	93.0000	0.500	Cup	6.00	0.00	28.00	140.00	0.00	0.00	0.00	0.00
456	Frozen Yogurt, Coffee Fudge, No	95.0000	0.500	Cup	4.00	0.00	25.00	120.00	0.00	0.00	0.00	0.00
457	Frozen Yogurt, Coffee-Haagen-Daz	93.0000	0.500	Cup	6.00	0.00	29.00	140.00	0.00	0.00	0.00	0.00
	Frozen Yogurt, Fat Free	133.9160	0.500	Cup	7.99	0.00	43.97	199.87	0.00	0.00	0.00	0.00
	Frozen Yogurt, Low Fat	148.0000	0.500	Cup	6.00	6.00	48.00	280.00	0.00	0.00	20.00	4.00

Monounsaturated Fat (gm)	Polyunsaturated Fat (gm)	Vitamin D (mg)	Vitamin K (mg)	Vitamin E (mg)	Vitamin A (re)	Vitamin C (mg)	Thiamin (mg)	Riboflavin (mg)	Niacin (mg)	Vitamin B_6 (mg)	Folate (mg)	Vitamin B_{12} (mcg)	Calcium (mg)	Iron (mg)	Magnesium (mg)	Phosphorus (mg)	Potassium (mg)	Sodium (mg)	Zinc (mg)
0.00	0.00	0.00	0.00	0.00	40.00	0.00	0.00	0.00	0.00	0.00	0.00	0.00	240.00	0.00	0.00	0.00	0.00	170.00	0.00
7.05	1.97	0.00	0.00	2.24	493.81	0.11	0.03	0.50	0.36	0.06	12.43	0.92	689.30	0.45	46.33	658.79	514.15	774.05	2.17
7.36	0.86	0.00	0.00	0.39	269.92	0.00	0.02	0.27	0.09	0.07	7.84	0.73	579.04	0.20	20.81	415.18	75.15	417.87	2.48
1.99	0.22	0.00	0.00	0.19	77.68	0.00	0.01	0.08	0.03	0.02	2.21	0.21	162.98	0.06	5.86	116.89	21.15	117.65	0.70
11.50	0.87	0.00	0.00	0.62	417.12	0.00	0.01	0.42	0.13	0.08	15.97	1.94	946.84	0.54	36.10	617.36	177.41	828.56	3.71
8.73	0.66	0.00	0.00	0.80	173.00	0.00	0.05	0.39	0.32	0.11	8.00	1.40	1375.70	0.95	50.80	807.10	107.10	1861.50	3.19
0.00	0.00	0.00	0.00	0.00	0.00	0.00	0.00	0.00	0.00	0.00	0.00	0.00	16.01	0.00	0.00	0.00	10.00	15.01	0.00
2.13	0.16	0.20	0.00	0.23	42.24	0.00	0.01	0.09	0.08	0.03	1.96	0.34	335.52	0.23	12.39	196.86	26.14	454.03	0.78
0.44	0.03	0.00	0.00	0.00	8.65	0.00	0.00	0.02	0.01	0.01	0.40	0.07	62.65	0.04	2.54	36.75	4.85	84.80	0.16
11.55	1.19	0.00	0.00	0.45	333.96	0.00	0.03	0.51	0.12	0.11	24.02	1.10	985.25	0.95	35.65	586.08	106.52	707.92	3.96
9.75	1.02	0.00	0.00	0.46	348.48	0.00	0.03	0.42	0.21	0.09	13.73	1.93	997.79	0.69	36.41	654.85	182.56	1155.66	4.26
5.68	0.64	0.00	0.00	0.52	277.98	0.00	0.05	0.47	0.20	0.05	32.23	0.71	669.12	1.08	36.33	449.20	307.50	306.76	3.30
8.93	0.96	0.00	0.00	0.86	329.64	0.00	0.02	0.49	0.25	0.10	30.01	0.84	509.22	0.93	27.80	388.93	257.32	206.89	2.85
2.22	0.17	0.00	0.00	0.21	39.97	0.00	0.01	0.10	0.02	0.03	1.93	0.32	301.59	0.22	11.60	215.46	24.47	340.20	0.73
2.40	0.37	0.00	0.00	0.00	84.77	0.00	0.01	0.17	0.21	0.03	13.89	0.18	187.62	0.16	8.37	111.16	25.71	512.85	0.59
9.60	1.28	1.45	0.00	0.66	333.96	0.00	0.03	0.49	0.12	0.11	8.45	2.22	1268.39	0.22	47.40	798.07	146.12	343.20	5.15
9.87	0.87	0.00	0.00	0.95	320.60	0.00	0.01	0.39	0.06	0.06	8.26	1.72	1080.66	0.85	40.77	1066.10	301.70	1918.42	5.05
18.12	0.07	0.00	0.00	3.89	21.60	0.00	0.00	0.00	0.00	0.00	0.00	0.00	22.32	0.07	0.79	154.08	457.20	190.08	0.05
0.91	0.01	0.00	0.00	0.25	18.80	0.00	0.00	0.16	0.00	0.00	0.00	0.00	20.96	1.08	3.82	396.68	763.09	170.23	0.48
8.03	1.04	0.00	0.00	0.27	258.94	2.08	0.10	0.36	0.19	0.10	6.05	0.80	253.86	0.17	24.61	230.38	313.63	98.49	1.23
13.39	1.73	0.00	0.00	0.36	436.80	1.82	0.07	0.36	0.14	0.07	5.52	0.53	230.88	0.10	20.76	191.76	292.08	95.04	0.65
1.08	0.14	0.00	0.00	0.09	34.80	0.11	0.00	0.02	0.01	0.00	0.34	0.03	13.53	0.01	1.26	10.59	17.17	5.55	0.04
3.85	0.50	0.00	0.00	0.36	124.20	0.00	0.02	0.04	0.04	0.02	1.56	0.17	60.60	0.03	6.47	53.58	88.38	78.00	0.22
12.77	1.64	0.35	0.00	0.75	503.10	0.69	0.02	0.13	0.05	0.04	4.42	0.22	77.20	0.04	8.40	74.57	90.10	44.93	0.27
10.91	1.06	0.00	0.00	0.72	354.00	0.73	0.02	0.16	0.05	0.04	4.44	0.24	83.28	0.04	8.68	73.32	116.16	41.16	0.30
1.22	0.39	0.00	0.00	0.14	64.50	0.00	0.00	0.00	0.00	0.00	0.00	0.00	4.73	0.09	1.34	5.78	13.65	18.98	0.02
5.86	14.98	0.00	0.00	5.06	324.00	1.13	0.29	0.94	0.34	0.31	39.36	0.82	174.72	4.75	35.90	172.08	511.92	478.56	2.35
2.26	4.02	0.00	0.00	1.23	542.16	0.00	0.28	0.75	0.28	0.00	37.40	0.75	133.03	5.27	21.89	303.71	828.30	444.27	3.26
0.00	0.00	0.00	0.05	0.00	0.00	0.00	0.02	1.09	0.22	0.00	7.29	0.49	14.58	0.07	26.73	31.59	347.49	398.52	0.02
5.66	0.86	0.00	0.00	0.58	203.20	3.81	0.08	0.48	0.28	0.13	2.29	1.14	330.20	0.51	46.99	277.88	419.61	138.18	1.17
0.00	0.00	0.00	0.00	0.00	160.00	2.40	0.00	0.00	0.00	0.00	0.00	0.00	480.00	0.40	0.00	0.00	0.00	280.00	0.00
2.75	1.28	0.00	0.00	0.75	114.08	0.00	0.03	0.24	0.04	0.06	17.48	0.42	25.30	0.72	5.06	89.24	60.72	162.38	0.55
5.55	1.92	0.00	0.00	1.43	228.48	0.00	0.10	0.69	0.08	0.16	59.84	1.51	68.00	1.62	13.60	233.92	171.36	168.64	1.43
0.69	0.32	0.00	0.00	0.20	28.42	0.00	0.01	0.06	0.01	0.02	4.41	0.11	6.38	0.18	1.37	22.50	15.35	41.04	0.14
1.90	0.68	0.00	0.00	0.53	95.00	0.00	0.03	0.22	0.03	0.06	17.50	0.40	24.50	0.72	5.00	88.50	60.00	140.00	0.55
10.49	4.73	0.00	0.00	2.88	429.00	0.44	0.11	0.97	0.18	0.26	66.00	1.69	156.20	2.64	26.40	374.00	303.60	616.00	2.20
1.90	0.68	0.02	25.00	1.03	95.50	0.00	0.03	0.25	0.04	0.07	23.50	0.50	24.50	0.72	5.00	89.00	60.50	63.00	0.55
0.00	0.00	0.00	0.00	0.00	40.00	0.00	0.00	0.00	0.00	0.00	0.00	0.00	192.00	0.00	0.00	0.00	0.00	100.00	0.00
0.00	0.00	0.00	0.00	0.00	0.00	0.00	0.00	0.00	0.00	0.00	0.00	0.00	0.00	0.00	0.00	0.00	0.00	15.00	0.00
0.00	0.00	0.00	0.00	0.00	0.00	0.00	0.00	0.00	0.00	0.00	0.00	0.00	0.00	0.00	0.00	0.00	0.00	15.00	0.00
0.00	0.00	0.00	0.00	0.00	0.00	0.00	0.00	0.00	0.00	0.00	0.00	0.00	0.00	0.00	0.00	0.00	0.00	20.00	0.00
0.00	0.00	0.00	0.00	0.00	0.00	0.00	0.00	0.00	0.00	0.00	0.00	0.00	0.00	0.00	0.00	0.00	0.00	40.00	0.00
0.00	0.00	0.00	0.00	0.00	0.00	0.00	0.00	0.00	0.00	0.00	0.00	0.00	0.00	0.00	0.00	0.00	0.00	45.00	0.00
0.00	0.00	0.00	0.00	0.00	0.00	0.00	0.00	0.00	0.00	0.00	0.00	0.00	0.00	0.00	0.00	0.00	0.00	65.00	0.00
0.00	0.00	0.00	0.00	0.00	0.00	0.00	0.00	0.00	0.00	0.00	0.00	0.00	0.00	0.00	0.00	0.00	0.00	65.00	0.00
0.00	0.00	0.00	0.00	0.00	0.00	0.00	0.00	0.00	0.00	0.00	0.00	0.00	0.00	0.00	0.00	0.00	0.00	40.00	0.00
0.00	0.00	0.00	0.00	0.00	0.00	0.00	0.00	0.00	0.00	0.00	0.00	0.00	0.00	0.00	0.00	0.00	0.00	110.00	0.00
0.00	0.00	0.00	0.00	0.00	0.00	0.00	0.00	0.00	0.00	0.00	0.00	0.00	0.00	0.00	0.00	0.00	0.00	80.00	0.00
0.00	0.00	0.00	0.00	0.00	0.00	0.00	0.00	0.00	0.00	0.00	0.00	0.00	0.00	0.00	0.00	0.00	0.00	65.00	0.00
1.26	0.16	0.00	0.00	0.10	30.96	0.22	0.03	0.15	0.22	0.05	7.92	0.21	105.84	0.90	19.44	100.08	187.92	70.56	0.35
0.00	0.00	0.00	0.00	0.00	0.00	0.00	0.00	0.00	0.00	0.00	0.00	0.00	0.00	0.00	0.00	0.00	0.00	45.00	0.00
0.00	0.00	0.00	0.00	0.00	0.00	0.00	0.00	0.00	0.00	0.00	0.00	0.00	0.00	0.00	0.00	0.00	0.00	65.00	0.00
0.00	0.00	0.00	0.00	0.00	0.00	0.00	0.00	0.00	0.00	0.00	0.00	0.00	0.00	0.00	0.00	0.00	0.00	45.00	0.00
0.00	0.00	0.00	0.00	0.00	39.97	0.00	0.00	0.00	0.00	0.00	0.00	0.00	191.88	0.00	0.00	0.00	0.00	139.91	0.00
0.00	0.00	0.00	0.00	0.00	40.00	0.00	0.00	0.00	0.00	0.00	0.00	0.00	192.00	0.00	0.00	0.00	0.00	100.00	0.00

USDA ID Code	Food Name	Weight in Grams*	Quantity of Units	Unit of Measure	Protein (gm)	Fat (gm)	Carbohydrate (gm)	Kcalories	Caffeine (gm)	Fiber (gm)	Cholesterol (mg)	Saturated Fat (gm)
458	Frozen Yogurt, Low Fat-Ben & Jer	106.0000	0.500	Cup	4.00	3.00	31.00	170.00	0.00	0.00	10.00	2.00
459	Frozen Yogurt, Peach Melba, Tang	95.0000	0.500	Cup	3.00	0.00	29.00	130.00	0.00	0.00	0.00	0.00
460	Frozen Yogurt, Raspberry, Black,	95.0000	0.500	Cup	3.00	0.00	27.00	120.00	0.00	1.00	0.00	0.00
461	Frozen Yogurt, Vanilla Fudge, No	95.0000	0.500	Cup	4.00	0.00	31.00	140.00	0.00	1.00	0.00	0.00
462	Frozen Yogurt, Vanilla Fudge-Haa	93.0000	0.500	Cup	6.00	0.00	34.00	160.00	0.00	0.00	0.00	0.00
463	Frozen Yogurt, Vanilla Rasp Swir	96.0000	0.500	Cup	4.00	0.00	28.00	130.00	0.00	0.00	0.00	0.00
464	Frozen Yogurt, Vanilla w/ Heath	95.0000	0.500	Cup	4.00	5.00	29.00	180.00	0.00	0.00	10.00	2.50
465	Frozen Yogurt, Vanilla, No Fat-B	95.0000	0.500	Cup	4.00	0.00	26.00	120.00	0.00	0.00	0.00	0.00
	Frozen Yogurt, Vanilla, Soft-ser	72.0000	0.500	Cup	2.88	4.03	17.42	114.48	0.00	0.00	1.44	2.46
466	Frozen Yogurt, Vanilla-Haagen-Da	93.0000	0.500	Cup	6.00	0.00	29.00	140.00	0.00	0.00	0.00	0.00
	Ice Cream - fat free	72.0000	0.500	Cup	4.00	0.00	23.00	100.00	0.00	0.00	0.00	0.00
469	Ice Cream Bar, Choc/Dark Choc-Ha	102.0000	1.000	Each	5.00	24.00	28.00	350.00	0.00	2.00	85.00	15.00
470	Ice Cream Bar, Coffee/Almond Cru	106.0000	1.000	Each	5.00	26.00	27.00	360.00	0.00	1.00	100.00	15.00
471	Ice Cream Bar, Straw/White Choc-	97.0000	1.000	Each	4.00	23.00	24.00	320.00	0.00	0.00	70.00	14.00
472	Ice Cream Bar, Vanilla & Almonds	106.0000	1.000	Each	6.00	27.00	26.00	370.00	0.00	1.00	90.00	14.00
473	Ice Cream Bar, Vanilla/Dark Choc	102.0000	1.000	Each	5.00	24.00	27.00	350.00	0.00	1.00	85.00	15.00
474	Ice Cream Bar, Vanilla/Milk Choc	100.0000	1.000	Each	5.00	24.00	24.00	330.00	0.00	0.00	90.00	14.00
	Ice Cream Cones, Cake or Wafer-t	28.3500	1.000	Ounce	2.30	1.96	22.40	118.22	0.00	0.85	0.00	0.35
	Ice Cream Cones, Sugar, Rolled-t	28.3500	1.000	Ounce	2.24	1.08	23.84	113.97	0.00	0.47	0.00	0.16
	Ice Cream Sandwich	63.0000	1.000	Each	3.00	6.00	27.00	170.00	0.00	1.00	10.00	3.00
476	Ice Cream Sandwich, Vanilla/Choc	80.0000	1.000	Each	4.00	13.00	31.00	260.00	0.00	1.00	65.00	8.00
477	Ice Cream Sandwich, Vanilla/Dark	83.0000	1.000	Each	4.00	20.00	23.00	290.00	0.00	2.00	70.00	12.00
475	Ice Cream Sandwich, Vanilla-Haag	80.0000	1.000	Each	4.00	13.00	32.00	260.00	0.00	0.00	65.00	8.00
478	Ice Cream, Bailey's Irish Cream-	102.0000	0.500	Cup	5.00	17.00	23.00	270.00	0.00	0.00	115.00	10.00
479	Ice Cream, Brownies a la Mode-Ha	99.0000	0.500	Cup	4.00	18.00	26.00	280.00	0.00	0.00	100.00	11.00
480	Ice Cream, Butter Pecan-Ben & Je	106.0000	0.500	Cup	4.00	21.00	15.00	250.00	0.00	1.00	80.00	9.00
481	Ice Cream, Butter Pecan-Haagen-D	106.0000	0.500	Cup	5.00	23.00	20.00	310.00	0.00	0.00	110.00	11.00
482	Ice Cream, Cappuccino Choc Chunk	106.0000	0.500	Cup	3.00	15.00	22.00	220.00	0.00	1.00	65.00	10.00
483	Ice Cream, Cappuccino Commotion-	103.0000	0.500	Cup	5.00	21.00	25.00	310.00	0.00	1.00	100.00	12.00
484	Ice Cream, Caramel Cone Explosio	103.0000	0.500	Cup	5.00	20.00	27.00	310.00	0.00	0.00	95.00	12.00
485	Ice Cream, Cherry Garcia-Ben & J	106.0000	0.500	Cup	3.00	13.00	21.00	200.00	0.00	0.00	65.00	8.00
486	Ice Cream, Cherry Vanilla-Haagen	101.0000	0.500	Cup	4.00	15.00	23.00	240.00	0.00	0.00	100.00	9.00
487	Ice Cream, Choc Chip Cookie Doug	106.0000	0.500	Cup	4.00	14.00	27.00	230.00	0.00	0.00	65.00	8.00
488	Ice Cream, Choc Choc Chip-Haagen	106.0000	0.500	Cup	5.00	20.00	26.00	300.00	0.00	2.00	100.00	12.00
489	Ice Cream, Choc Choc, Belgian-Ha	102.0000	0.500	Cup	5.00	21.00	29.00	330.00	0.00	3.00	85.00	12.00
490	Ice Cream, Choc Fudge Brownie, L	92.0000	0.500	Cup	7.00	2.50	34.00	190.00	0.00	1.00	8.00	1.50
491	Ice Cream, Choc Fudge Brownie-Be	106.0000	0.500	Cup	4.00	11.00	27.00	220.00	0.00	2.00	40.00	7.00
492	Ice Cream, Choc Mint Chip-Haagen	106.0000	0.500	Cup	5.00	20.00	25.00	300.00	0.00	4.00	95.00	11.00
493	Ice Cream, Choc PB, Deep-Haagen-	102.0000	0.500	Cup	8.00	24.00	26.00	350.00	0.00	4.00	80.00	11.00
494	Ice Cream, Choc Peanut Butter Do	106.0000	0.500	Cup	4.00	16.00	23.00	240.00	0.00	1.00	50.00	6.00
495	Ice Cream, Choc Raspberry Swirl-	106.0000	0.500	Cup	3.00	11.00	28.00	220.00	0.00	2.00	35.00	7.00
496	Ice Cream, Choc, Deep Dark, Egg	106.0000	0.500	Cup	3.00	12.00	24.00	200.00	0.00	2.00	45.00	7.00
	Ice Cream, Chocolate	58.0000	3.500	Fl Oz	2.20	6.38	16.36	125.28	1.74	0.70	19.72	3.94
497	Ice Cream, Chocolate, Low Fat-Ha	92.0000	0.500	Cup	7.00	2.50	29.00	170.00	0.00	0.00	8.00	4.00
498	Ice Cream, Chocolate-Haagen-Daz	106.0000	0.500	Cup	5.00	18.00	22.00	270.00	0.00	1.00	115.00	11.00
499	Ice Cream, Chubby Hubby-Ben & Je	106.0000	0.500	Cup	6.00	17.00	24.00	260.00	0.00	2.00	50.00	8.00
500	Ice Cream, Chunky Monkey-Ben & J	106.0000	0.500	Cup	3.00	16.00	24.00	240.00	0.00	1.00	55.00	8.00
501	Ice Cream, Coconut Almond Fudge	106.0000	0.500	Cup	5.00	20.00	19.00	260.00	0.00	2.00	60.00	11.00
502	Ice Cream, Coffee Fudge, Low Fat	92.0000	0.500	Cup	5.00	2.50	32.00	170.00	0.00	0.00	25.00	1.50
503	Ice Cream, Coffee Mocha Chip-Haa	106.0000	0.500	Cup	4.00	19.00	25.00	290.00	0.00	0.00	110.00	12.00
504	Ice Cream, Coffee Ole-Ben & Jerr	106.0000	0.500	Cup	3.00	13.00	18.00	180.00	0.00	0.00	70.00	8.00
505	Ice Cream, Coffee w/ Heath Crunc	106.0000	0.500	Cup	3.00	16.00	24.00	240.00	0.00	0.00	60.00	9.00
506	Ice Cream, Coffee-Haagen-Daz	106.0000	0.500	Cup	5.00	18.00	21.00	270.00	0.00	0.00	120.00	11.00
507	Ice Cream, Cookie Dough Dynamo-H	103.0000	0.500	Cup	4.00	19.00	29.00	300.00	0.00	0.00	95.00	12.00
508	Ice Cream, Cookie, Sweet Cream-B	106.0000	0.500	Cup	3.00	14.00	22.00	220.00	0.00	1.00	65.00	8.00

Monounsaturated Fat (gm)	Polyunsaturated Fat (gm)	Vitamin D (mg)	Vitamin K (mg)	Vitamin E (mg)	Vitamin A (re)	Vitamin C (mg)	Thiamin (mg)	Riboflavin (mg)	Niacin (mg)	Vitamin B_6 (mg)	Folate (mg)	Vitamin B_{12} (mcg)	Calcium (mg)	Iron (mg)	Magnesium (mg)	Phosphorus (mg)	Potassium (mg)	Sodium (mg)	Zinc (mg)
0.00	0.00	0.00	0.00	0.00	0.00	1.20	0.00	0.00	0.00	0.00	0.00	0.00	120.00	0.20	0.00	0.00	0.00	70.00	0.00
0.00	0.00	0.00	0.00	0.00	0.00	0.00	0.00	0.00	0.00	0.00	0.00	0.00	0.00	0.00	0.00	0.00	0.00	55.00	0.00
0.00	0.00	0.00	0.00	0.00	0.00	0.00	0.00	0.00	0.00	0.00	0.00	0.00	0.00	0.00	0.00	0.00	0.00	50.00	0.00
0.00	0.00	0.00	0.00	0.00	0.00	0.00	0.00	0.00	0.00	0.00	0.00	0.00	0.00	0.00	0.00	0.00	0.00	75.00	0.00
0.00	0.00	0.00	0.00	0.00	0.00	0.00	0.00	0.00	0.00	0.00	0.00	0.00	0.00	0.00	0.00	0.00	0.00	100.00	0.00
0.00	0.00	0.00	0.00	0.00	0.00	0.00	0.00	0.00	0.00	0.00	0.00	0.00	0.00	0.00	0.00	0.00	0.00	30.00	0.00
0.00	0.00	0.00	0.00	0.00	0.00	0.00	0.00	0.00	0.00	0.00	0.00	0.00	0.00	0.00	0.00	0.00	0.00	100.00	0.00
0.00	0.00	0.00	0.00	0.00	0.00	0.00	0.00	0.00	0.00	0.00	0.00	0.00	0.00	0.00	0.00	0.00	0.00	65.00	0.00
1.14	0.15	0.00	0.00	0.04	41.04	0.58	0.03	0.16	0.21	0.06	4.32	0.21	102.96	0.22	10.08	92.88	151.92	62.64	0.30
0.00	0.00	0.00	0.00	0.00	0.00	0.00	0.00	0.00	0.00	0.00	0.00	0.00	0.00	0.00	0.00	0.00	0.00	45.00	0.00
0.00	0.00	0.00	0.00	0.00	0.00	0.00	0.00	0.00	0.00	0.00	0.00	0.00	120.00	0.00	0.00	0.00	0.00	65.00	0.00
0.00	0.00	0.00	0.00	0.00	0.00	0.00	0.00	0.00	0.00	0.00	0.00	0.00	0.00	0.00	0.00	0.00	0.00	60.00	0.00
0.00	0.00	0.00	0.00	0.00	0.00	0.00	0.00	0.00	0.00	0.00	0.00	0.00	0.00	0.00	0.00	0.00	0.00	85.00	0.00
0.00	0.00	0.00	0.00	0.00	0.00	0.00	0.00	0.00	0.00	0.00	0.00	0.00	0.00	0.00	0.00	0.00	0.00	75.00	0.00
0.00	0.00	0.00	0.00	0.00	0.00	0.00	0.00	0.00	0.00	0.00	0.00	0.00	0.00	0.00	0.00	0.00	0.00	80.00	0.00
0.00	0.00	0.00	0.00	0.00	0.00	0.00	0.00	0.00	0.00	0.00	0.00	0.00	0.00	0.00	0.00	0.00	0.00	65.00	0.00
0.00	0.00	0.00	0.00	0.00	0.00	0.00	0.00	0.00	0.00	0.00	0.00	0.00	0.00	0.00	0.00	0.00	0.00	75.00	0.00
0.52	0.92	0.00	0.00	0.49	0.00	0.00	0.07	0.10	1.26	0.01	28.92	0.00	7.09	1.02	7.37	27.50	31.75	40.54	0.19
0.42	0.41	0.00	0.00	0.13	0.00	0.00	0.14	0.12	1.44	0.01	23.53	0.00	12.47	1.26	8.79	29.20	41.11	90.72	0.21
0.00	0.00	0.00	0.00	0.00	20.00	0.00	0.00	0.00	0.00	0.00	0.00	0.00	48.00	0.40	0.00	0.00	0.00	140.00	0.00
0.00	0.00	0.00	0.00	0.00	0.00	0.00	0.00	0.00	0.00	0.00	0.00	0.00	0.00	0.00	0.00	0.00	0.00	120.00	0.00
0.00	0.00	0.00	0.00	0.00	0.00	0.00	0.00	0.00	0.00	0.00	0.00	0.00	0.00	0.00	0.00	0.00	0.00	45.00	0.00
0.00	0.00	0.00	0.00	0.00	0.00	0.00	0.00	0.00	0.00	0.00	0.00	0.00	0.00	0.00	0.00	0.00	0.00	125.00	0.00
0.00	0.00	0.00	0.00	0.00	0.00	0.00	0.00	0.00	0.00	0.00	0.00	0.00	0.00	0.00	0.00	0.00	0.00	85.00	0.00
0.00	0.00	0.00	0.00	0.00	0.00	0.00	0.00	0.00	0.00	0.00	0.00	0.00	0.00	0.00	0.00	0.00	0.00	115.00	0.00
0.00	0.00	0.00	0.00	0.00	0.00	0.00	0.00	0.00	0.00	0.00	0.00	0.00	0.00	0.00	0.00	0.00	0.00	135.00	0.00
0.00	0.00	0.00	0.00	0.00	0.00	0.00	0.00	0.00	0.00	0.00	0.00	0.00	0.00	0.00	0.00	0.00	0.00	160.00	0.00
0.00	0.00	0.00	0.00	0.00	0.00	0.00	0.00	0.00	0.00	0.00	0.00	0.00	0.00	0.00	0.00	0.00	0.00	50.00	0.00
0.00	0.00	0.00	0.00	0.00	0.00	0.00	0.00	0.00	0.00	0.00	0.00	0.00	0.00	0.00	0.00	0.00	0.00	105.00	0.00
0.00	0.00	0.00	0.00	0.00	0.00	0.00	0.00	0.00	0.00	0.00	0.00	0.00	0.00	0.00	0.00	0.00	0.00	130.00	0.00
0.00	0.00	0.00	0.00	0.00	0.00	0.00	0.00	0.00	0.00	0.00	0.00	0.00	0.00	0.00	0.00	0.00	0.00	50.00	0.00
0.00	0.00	0.00	0.00	0.00	0.00	0.00	0.00	0.00	0.00	0.00	0.00	0.00	0.00	0.00	0.00	0.00	0.00	75.00	0.00
0.00	0.00	0.00	0.00	0.00	0.00	0.00	0.00	0.00	0.00	0.00	0.00	0.00	0.00	0.00	0.00	0.00	0.00	85.00	0.00
0.00	0.00	0.00	0.00	0.00	0.00	0.00	0.00	0.00	0.00	0.00	0.00	0.00	0.00	0.00	0.00	0.00	0.00	70.00	0.00
0.00	0.00	0.00	0.00	0.00	0.00	0.00	0.00	0.00	0.00	0.00	0.00	0.00	0.00	0.00	0.00	0.00	0.00	60.00	0.00
0.00	0.00	0.00	0.00	0.00	0.00	0.00	0.00	0.00	0.00	0.00	0.00	0.00	0.00	0.00	0.00	0.00	0.00	110.00	0.00
0.00	0.00	0.00	0.00	0.00	0.00	0.00	0.00	0.00	0.00	0.00	0.00	0.00	0.00	0.00	0.00	0.00	0.00	75.00	0.00
0.00	0.00	0.00	0.00	0.00	0.00	0.00	0.00	0.00	0.00	0.00	0.00	0.00	0.00	0.00	0.00	0.00	0.00	65.00	0.00
0.00	0.00	0.00	0.00	0.00	0.00	0.00	0.00	0.00	0.00	0.00	0.00	0.00	0.00	0.00	0.00	0.00	0.00	100.00	0.00
0.00	0.00	0.00	0.00	0.00	0.00	0.00	0.00	0.00	0.00	0.00	0.00	0.00	0.00	0.00	0.00	0.00	0.00	65.00	0.00
0.00	0.00	0.00	0.00	0.00	0.00	0.00	0.00	0.00	0.00	0.00	0.00	0.00	0.00	0.00	0.00	0.00	0.00	35.00	0.00
0.00	0.00	0.00	0.00	0.00	0.00	0.00	0.00	0.00	0.00	0.00	0.00	0.00	0.00	0.00	0.00	0.00	0.00	35.00	0.00
1.86	0.24	0.00	0.00	0.19	69.02	0.41	0.02	0.11	0.13	0.03	9.28	0.17	63.22	0.54	16.82	62.06	144.42	44.08	0.34
0.00	0.00	0.00	0.00	0.00	0.00	0.00	0.00	0.00	0.00	0.00	0.00	0.00	0.00	0.00	0.00	0.00	0.00	50.00	0.00
0.00	0.00	0.00	0.00	0.00	0.00	0.00	0.00	0.00	0.00	0.00	0.00	0.00	0.00	0.00	0.00	0.00	0.00	75.00	0.00
0.00	0.00	0.00	0.00	0.00	0.00	0.00	0.00	0.00	0.00	0.00	0.00	0.00	0.00	0.00	0.00	0.00	0.00	140.00	0.00
0.00	0.00	0.00	0.00	0.00	0.00	0.00	0.00	0.00	0.00	0.00	0.00	0.00	0.00	0.00	0.00	0.00	0.00	40.00	0.00
0.00	0.00	0.00	0.00	0.00	0.00	0.00	0.00	0.00	0.00	0.00	0.00	0.00	0.00	0.00	0.00	0.00	0.00	70.00	0.00
0.00	0.00	0.00	0.00	0.00	0.00	0.00	0.00	0.00	0.00	0.00	0.00	0.00	0.00	0.00	0.00	0.00	0.00	95.00	0.00
0.00	0.00	0.00	0.00	0.00	0.00	0.00	0.00	0.00	0.00	0.00	0.00	0.00	0.00	0.00	0.00	0.00	0.00	90.00	0.00
0.00	0.00	0.00	0.00	0.00	0.00	0.00	0.00	0.00	0.00	0.00	0.00	0.00	0.00	0.00	0.00	0.00	0.00	45.00	0.00
0.00	0.00	0.00	0.00	0.00	0.00	0.00	0.00	0.00	0.00	0.00	0.00	0.00	0.00	0.00	0.00	0.00	0.00	110.00	0.00
0.00	0.00	0.00	0.00	0.00	0.00	0.00	0.00	0.00	0.00	0.00	0.00	0.00	0.00	0.00	0.00	0.00	0.00	85.00	0.00
0.00	0.00	0.00	0.00	0.00	0.00	0.00	0.00	0.00	0.00	0.00	0.00	0.00	0.00	0.00	0.00	0.00	0.00	140.00	0.00
0.00	0.00	0.00	0.00	0.00	0.00	0.00	0.00	0.00	0.00	0.00	0.00	0.00	0.00	0.00	0.00	0.00	0.00	110.00	0.00

USDA ID Code	Food Name	Weight in Grams*	Quantity of Units	Unit of Measure	Protein (gm)	Fat (gm)	Carbohydrate (gm)	Kcalories	Caffeine (gm)	Fiber (gm)	Cholesterol (mg)	Saturated Fat (gm)
509	Ice Cream, Cookies & Cream, Midn	102.0000	0.500	Cup	5.00	18.00	29.00	300.00	0.00	1.00	90.00	11.00
510	Ice Cream, Cookies & Cream-Haage	102.0000	0.500	Cup	5.00	17.00	23.00	270.00	0.00	0.00	110.00	11.00
511	Ice Cream, Cool Britannia-Ben &	106.0000	0.500	Cup	3.00	12.00	23.00	200.00	0.00	0.00	55.00	8.00
512	Ice Cream, De Leche Caramel-Haag	106.0000	0.500	Cup	5.00	17.00	28.00	290.00	0.00	0.00	100.00	10.00
513	Ice Cream, DiSaronno Amaretto-Ha	103.0000	0.500	Cup	4.00	15.00	26.00	260.00	0.00	0.00	95.00	9.00
514	Ice Cream, Fudge Chunk, NY Super	106.0000	0.500	Cup	4.00	17.00	23.00	240.00	0.00	2.00	40.00	9.00
	Ice Cream, Light	67.0000	0.500	Cup	3.00	4.50	18.00	130.00	0.00	0.00	35.00	2.50
	Ice Cream, Low Fat-Haagen Daz	92.0000	0.500	Cup	7.00	2.50	29.00	170.00	0.00	0.00	0.00	0.00
	Ice Cream, Low Fat-Starbucks	99.0000	0.500	Cup	5.00	3.00	31.00	170.00	0.00	0.00	10.00	1.50
515	Ice Cream, Macadamia Nut Brittle	106.0000	0.500	Cup	4.00	20.00	25.00	300.00	0.00	0.00	110.00	11.00
516	Ice Cream, Malted Milk Ball-Ben	106.0000	0.500	Cup	3.00	14.00	22.00	220.00	0.00	0.00	65.00	9.00
517	Ice Cream, Maple Walnut-Ben & Je	106.0000	0.500	Cup	4.00	18.00	18.00	240.00	0.00	1.00	60.00	8.00
518	Ice Cream, Mint Chip-Haagen-Daz	106.0000	0.500	Cup	4.00	19.00	26.00	290.00	0.00	0.00	105.00	12.00
519	Ice Cream, Mint Choc Chunk-Ben &	106.0000	0.500	Cup	3.00	15.00	22.00	220.00	0.00	1.00	65.00	10.00
520	Ice Cream, Mint Choc Cookie-Ben	106.0000	0.500	Cup	3.00	14.00	23.00	220.00	0.00	1.00	65.00	8.00
521	Ice Cream, Mocha Fudge-Ben & Jer	106.0000	0.500	Cup	3.00	13.00	22.00	200.00	0.00	0.00	60.00	7.00
522	Ice Cream, Peanut Butter Cup-Ben	106.0000	0.500	Cup	5.00	18.00	21.00	260.00	0.00	1.00	60.00	9.00
523	Ice Cream, Pistachio Pistachio-B	106.0000	0.500	Cup	4.00	17.00	16.00	220.00	0.00	1.00	70.00	8.00
524	Ice Cream, Praline Pecan-Ben & J	106.0000	0.500	Cup	3.00	17.00	26.00	250.00	0.00	0.00	70.00	8.00
525	Ice Cream, Pralines & Cream-Haag	102.0000	0.500	Cup	4.00	18.00	27.00	290.00	0.00	0.00	95.00	9.00
526	Ice Cream, Rainforest Crunch-Ben	106.0000	0.500	Cup	4.00	18.00	19.00	240.00	0.00	0.00	70.00	9.00
527	Ice Cream, Rum Raisin-Haagen-Daz	106.0000	0.500	Cup	4.00	17.00	22.00	270.00	0.00	0.00	110.00	10.00
	Ice Cream, Strawberry	58.0000	3.500	Fl Oz	1.86	4.87	16.01	111.36	0.00	0.17	16.82	3.01
528	Ice Cream, Strawberry Cheesecake	103.0000	0.500	Cup	4.00	16.00	27.00	270.00	0.00	0.00	100.00	10.00
529	Ice Cream, Strawberry, Low Fat-H	92.0000	0.500	Cup	5.00	2.00	28.00	150.00	0.00	0.00	15.00	1.00
530	Ice Cream, Strawberry-Ben & Jerr	106.0000	0.500	Cup	2.00	10.00	19.00	170.00	0.00	1.00	55.00	6.00
531	Ice Cream, Strawberry-Haagen-Daz	106.0000	0.500	Cup	4.00	16.00	23.00	250.00	0.00	0.00	95.00	10.00
	Ice Cream, Vanilla	58.0000	3.500	Fl Oz	2.03	6.38	13.69	116.58	0.00	0.00	25.52	3.94
532	Ice Cream, Vanilla Bean-Ben & J	106.0000	0.500	Cup	3.00	13.00	18.00	190.00	0.00	0.00	75.00	8.00
533	Ice Cream, Vanilla Caramel Fudge	106.0000	0.500	Cup	2.00	12.00	24.00	180.00	0.00	0.00	70.00	7.00
534	Ice Cream, Vanilla Caramel, Low	92.0000	0.500	Cup	6.00	2.50	32.00	180.00	0.00	0.00	20.00	1.50
535	Ice Cream, Vanilla Choc Chip-Haa	106.0000	0.500	Cup	5.00	20.00	26.00	310.00	0.00	0.00	105.00	12.00
536	Ice Cream, Vanilla Choc Chunk-Be	106.0000	0.500	Cup	3.00	15.00	22.00	220.00	0.00	1.00	65.00	10.00
537	Ice Cream, Vanilla Fudge Brownie	106.0000	0.500	Cup	4.00	12.00	23.00	210.00	0.00	0.00	60.00	7.00
538	Ice Cream, Vanilla Fudge-Haagen-	106.0000	0.500	Cup	5.00	18.00	26.00	290.00	0.00	0.00	100.00	12.00
539	Ice Cream, Vanilla Swiss Almond-	106.0000	0.500	Cup	6.00	21.00	23.00	310.00	0.00	1.00	105.00	11.00
540	Ice Cream, Vanilla w/ Heath Crun	106.0000	0.500	Cup	3.00	17.00	24.00	240.00	0.00	0.00	65.00	9.00
541	Ice Cream, Vanilla, French, Coff	106.0000	0.500	Cup	5.00	18.00	21.00	270.00	0.00	0.00	120.00	11.00
	Ice Cream, Vanilla, French, Soft	86.0000	0.500	Cup	3.53	11.18	19.09	184.90	0.00	0.00	78.26	6.43
543	Ice Cream, Vanilla, Low Fat-Haag	92.0000	0.500	Cup	7.00	2.50	29.00	170.00	0.00	0.00	20.00	1.50
	Ice Cream, Vanilla, Rich	74.0000	0.500	Cup	2.59	11.99	16.58	178.34	0.00	0.00	45.14	7.38
542	Ice Cream, Vanilla-Haagen-Daz	106.0000	0.500	Cup	5.00	18.00	21.00	270.00	0.00	0.00	120.00	11.00
544	Ice Cream, Wavy Gravy-Ben & Jerr	106.0000	0.500	Cup	5.00	19.00	22.00	260.00	0.00	2.00	55.00	7.00
545	Ice Cream, White Russian-Ben & J	106.0000	0.500	Cup	3.00	13.00	18.00	190.00	0.00	0.00	70.00	8.00
	Ice Cream-Starbucks	99.0000	0.500	Cup	4.00	13.00	30.00	250.00	0.00	0.00	60.00	8.00
	Milk Substitutes, Fluid w/ hydr	244.0000	1.000	Cup	4.27	8.32	15.03	149.96	0.00	0.00	0.49	1.88
	Milk Substitutes, Fluid, w/ laur	244.0000	1.000	Cup	4.27	8.32	15.03	149.96	0.00	0.00	0.49	7.42
	Milk, Buttermilk	245.0000	1.000	Cup	8.11	2.16	11.74	99.00	0.00	0.00	8.57	1.35
	Milk, Chocolate Drink, Lowfat, 1	250.0000	1.000	Cup	8.10	2.50	26.10	157.58	5.00	1.25	7.25	1.55
	Milk, Chocolate Drink, Lowfat, 2	250.0000	1.000	Cup	8.03	5.00	26.00	178.85	5.00	1.25	17.00	3.10
	Milk, Chocolate Drink, Whole	250.0000	1.000	Cup	7.93	8.48	25.85	208.38	5.00	2.00	30.50	5.25
	Milk, Chocolate Homemade Hot Coc	250.0000	1.000	Cup	9.78	5.83	29.48	192.50	5.00	2.00	20.00	3.60
	Milk, Condensed, Sweetened, Cnd	306.0000	1.000	Cup	24.20	26.62	166.46	981.59	0.00	0.00	103.73	16.80
	Milk, Evaporated, Cnd	31.5000	1.000	Fl Oz	2.15	2.38	3.16	42.33	0.00	0.00	9.26	1.45
	Milk, Evaporated, Skim, Cnd	256.0000	1.000	Cup	19.33	0.51	29.06	199.48	0.00	0.00	9.22	0.31

Monounsaturated Fat (gm)	Polyunsaturated Fat (gm)	Vitamin D (mg)	Vitamin K (mg)	Vitamin E (mg)	Vitamin A (re)	Vitamin C (mg)	Thiamin (mg)	Riboflavin (mg)	Niacin (mg)	Vitamin B_6 (mg)	Folate (mg)	Vitamin B_{12} (mcg)	Calcium (mg)	Iron (mg)	Magnesium (mg)	Phosphorus (mg)	Potassium (mg)	Sodium (mg)	Zinc (mg)
0.00	0.00	0.00	0.00	0.00	0.00	0.00	0.00	0.00	0.00	0.00	0.00	0.00	0.00	0.00	0.00	0.00	0.00	140.00	0.00
0.00	0.00	0.00	0.00	0.00	0.00	0.00	0.00	0.00	0.00	0.00	0.00	0.00	0.00	0.00	0.00	0.00	0.00	115.00	0.00
0.00	0.00	0.00	0.00	0.00	0.00	0.00	0.00	0.00	0.00	0.00	0.00	0.00	0.00	0.00	0.00	0.00	0.00	55.00	0.00
0.00	0.00	0.00	0.00	0.00	0.00	0.00	0.00	0.00	0.00	0.00	0.00	0.00	0.00	0.00	0.00	0.00	0.00	110.00	0.00
0.00	0.00	0.00	0.00	0.00	0.00	0.00	0.00	0.00	0.00	0.00	0.00	0.00	0.00	0.00	0.00	0.00	0.00	80.00	0.00
0.00	0.00	0.00	0.00	0.00	0.00	0.00	0.00	0.00	0.00	0.00	0.00	0.00	0.00	0.00	0.00	0.00	0.00	50.00	0.00
0.00	0.00	0.00	0.00	0.00	0.00	0.00	0.00	0.00	0.00	0.00	0.00	0.00	80.00	0.00	0.00	0.00	0.00	50.00	0.00
0.00	0.00	0.00	0.00	0.00	0.00	0.00	0.00	0.00	0.00	0.00	0.00	0.00	160.00	0.00	0.00	0.00	0.00	50.00	0.00
0.00	0.00	0.00	0.00	0.00	0.00	0.00	0.00	0.00	0.00	0.00	0.00	0.00	80.00	0.00	0.00	0.00	0.00	65.00	0.00
0.00	0.00	0.00	0.00	0.00	0.00	0.00	0.00	0.00	0.00	0.00	0.00	0.00	0.00	0.00	0.00	0.00	0.00	120.00	0.00
0.00	0.00	0.00	0.00	0.00	0.00	0.00	0.00	0.00	0.00	0.00	0.00	0.00	0.00	0.00	0.00	0.00	0.00	60.00	0.00
0.00	0.00	0.00	0.00	0.00	0.00	0.00	0.00	0.00	0.00	0.00	0.00	0.00	0.00	0.00	0.00	0.00	0.00	40.00	0.00
0.00	0.00	0.00	0.00	0.00	0.00	0.00	0.00	0.00	0.00	0.00	0.00	0.00	0.00	0.00	0.00	0.00	0.00	105.00	0.00
0.00	0.00	0.00	0.00	0.00	0.00	0.00	0.00	0.00	0.00	0.00	0.00	0.00	0.00	0.00	0.00	0.00	0.00	50.00	0.00
0.00	0.00	0.00	0.00	0.00	0.00	0.00	0.00	0.00	0.00	0.00	0.00	0.00	0.00	0.00	0.00	0.00	0.00	110.00	0.00
0.00	0.00	0.00	0.00	0.00	0.00	0.00	0.00	0.00	0.00	0.00	0.00	0.00	0.00	0.00	0.00	0.00	0.00	45.00	0.00
0.00	0.00	0.00	0.00	0.00	0.00	0.00	0.00	0.00	0.00	0.00	0.00	0.00	0.00	0.00	0.00	0.00	0.00	95.00	0.00
0.00	0.00	0.00	0.00	0.00	0.00	0.00	0.00	0.00	0.00	0.00	0.00	0.00	0.00	0.00	0.00	0.00	0.00	70.00	0.00
0.00	0.00	0.00	0.00	0.00	0.00	0.00	0.00	0.00	0.00	0.00	0.00	0.00	0.00	0.00	0.00	0.00	0.00	90.00	0.00
0.00	0.00	0.00	0.00	0.00	0.00	0.00	0.00	0.00	0.00	0.00	0.00	0.00	0.00	0.00	0.00	0.00	0.00	180.00	0.00
0.00	0.00	0.00	0.00	0.00	0.00	0.00	0.00	0.00	0.00	0.00	0.00	0.00	0.00	0.00	0.00	0.00	0.00	105.00	0.00
0.00	0.00	0.00	0.00	0.00	0.00	0.00	0.00	0.00	0.00	0.00	0.00	0.00	0.00	0.00	0.00	0.00	0.00	75.00	0.00
0.00	0.00	0.00	0.00	0.00	45.24	4.47	0.03	0.15	0.10	0.03	6.96	0.17	69.60	0.12	8.12	58.00	109.04	34.80	0.20
0.00	0.00	0.00	0.00	0.00	0.00	0.00	0.00	0.00	0.00	0.00	0.00	0.00	0.00	0.00	0.00	0.00	0.00	150.00	0.00
0.00	0.00	0.00	0.00	0.00	0.00	0.00	0.00	0.00	0.00	0.00	0.00	0.00	0.00	0.00	0.00	0.00	0.00	40.00	0.00
0.00	0.00	0.00	0.00	0.00	0.00	0.00	0.00	0.00	0.00	0.00	0.00	0.00	0.00	0.00	0.00	0.00	0.00	35.00	0.00
0.00	0.00	0.00	0.00	0.00	0.00	0.00	0.00	0.00	0.00	0.00	0.00	0.00	0.00	0.00	0.00	0.00	0.00	80.00	0.00
1.84	0.24	0.00	0.00	0.00	67.86	0.35	0.02	0.14	0.07	0.03	2.90	0.23	74.24	0.05	8.12	60.90	115.42	46.40	0.40
0.00	0.00	0.00	0.00	0.00	0.00	0.00	0.00	0.00	0.00	0.00	0.00	0.00	0.00	0.00	0.00	0.00	0.00	45.00	0.00
0.00	0.00	0.00	0.00	0.00	0.00	0.00	0.00	0.00	0.00	0.00	0.00	0.00	0.00	0.00	0.00	0.00	0.00	50.00	0.00
0.00	0.00	0.00	0.00	0.00	0.00	0.00	0.00	0.00	0.00	0.00	0.00	0.00	0.00	0.00	0.00	0.00	0.00	120.00	0.00
0.00	0.00	0.00	0.00	0.00	0.00	0.00	0.00	0.00	0.00	0.00	0.00	0.00	0.00	0.00	0.00	0.00	0.00	90.00	0.00
0.00	0.00	0.00	0.00	0.00	0.00	0.00	0.00	0.00	0.00	0.00	0.00	0.00	0.00	0.00	0.00	0.00	0.00	50.00	0.00
0.00	0.00	0.00	0.00	0.00	0.00	0.00	0.00	0.00	0.00	0.00	0.00	0.00	0.00	0.00	0.00	0.00	0.00	80.00	0.00
0.00	0.00	0.00	0.00	0.00	0.00	0.00	0.00	0.00	0.00	0.00	0.00	0.00	0.00	0.00	0.00	0.00	0.00	110.00	0.00
0.00	0.00	0.00	0.00	0.00	0.00	0.00	0.00	0.00	0.00	0.00	0.00	0.00	0.00	0.00	0.00	0.00	0.00	90.00	0.00
0.00	0.00	0.00	0.00	0.00	0.00	0.00	0.00	0.00	0.00	0.00	0.00	0.00	0.00	0.00	0.00	0.00	0.00	110.00	0.00
0.00	0.00	0.00	0.00	0.00	0.00	0.00	0.00	0.00	0.00	0.00	0.00	0.00	0.00	0.00	0.00	0.00	0.00	85.00	0.00
3.00	0.39	0.00	0.00	0.32	132.44	0.69	0.04	0.15	0.09	0.04	7.74	0.43	112.66	0.18	10.32	99.76	152.22	52.46	0.45
0.00	0.00	0.00	0.00	0.00	0.00	0.00	0.00	0.00	0.00	0.00	0.00	0.00	0.00	0.00	0.00	0.00	0.00	50.00	0.00
3.45	0.44	0.00	0.00	0.00	136.16	0.52	0.03	0.12	0.06	0.03	3.70	0.27	86.58	0.04	8.14	70.30	117.66	41.44	0.30
0.00	0.00	0.00	0.00	0.00	0.00	0.00	0.00	0.00	0.00	0.00	0.00	0.00	0.00	0.00	0.00	0.00	0.00	85.00	0.00
0.00	0.00	0.00	0.00	0.00	0.00	0.00	0.00	0.00	0.00	0.00	0.00	0.00	0.00	0.00	0.00	0.00	0.00	90.00	0.00
0.00	0.00	0.00	0.00	0.00	0.00	0.00	0.00	0.00	0.00	0.00	0.00	0.00	0.00	0.00	0.00	0.00	0.00	45.00	0.00
0.00	0.00	0.00	0.00	0.00	0.00	0.00	0.00	0.00	0.00	0.00	0.00	0.00	120.00	0.00	0.00	0.00	0.00	15.00	0.00
4.88	1.20	0.00	0.00	2.56	0.00	0.00	0.02	0.22	0.00	0.00	0.00	0.00	79.30	0.95	15.57	181.05	278.89	191.05	2.88
0.44	0.02	0.00	0.00	0.00	0.00	0.00	0.02	0.22	0.00	0.00	0.00	0.00	79.30	0.95	15.57	181.05	278.89	191.05	2.88
0.61	0.07	0.00	0.00	0.15	19.60	2.40	0.07	0.37	0.15	0.07	12.25	0.54	285.18	0.12	26.83	218.54	370.69	257.01	1.03
0.75	0.10	2.50	0.00	0.08	147.50	2.33	0.10	0.43	0.33	0.10	12.00	0.85	286.75	0.60	33.33	256.50	425.50	151.75	1.03
1.48	0.18	2.50	0.00	0.13	142.50	2.30	0.10	0.40	0.33	0.10	12.00	0.85	284.00	0.60	33.00	254.25	422.00	150.50	1.03
2.48	0.30	2.50	0.00	0.23	72.50	2.28	0.10	0.40	0.33	0.10	11.75	0.83	280.25	0.60	32.58	251.25	417.25	149.00	1.03
1.70	0.23	0.00	0.00	0.25	137.50	2.50	0.10	0.43	0.38	0.13	15.00	0.93	315.00	1.15	70.00	292.50	500.00	127.50	1.48
7.44	1.04	0.00	0.00	0.64	247.86	7.96	0.28	1.29	0.64	0.15	34.27	1.35	867.51	0.58	78.49	775.10	1136.48	388.62	2.88
0.74	0.08	0.00	0.00	0.00	17.01	0.59	0.02	0.10	0.06	0.02	2.49	0.05	82.15	0.06	7.62	63.79	95.48	33.33	0.24
0.15	0.03	5.12	0.00	0.03	299.52	3.17	0.13	0.79	0.44	0.15	22.02	0.61	741.12	0.74	69.12	498.94	848.64	294.40	2.30

USDA ID Code	Food Name	Weight in Grams*	Quantity of Units	Unit of Measure	Protein (gm)	Fat (gm)	Carbohydrate (gm)	Kcalories	Caffeine (gm)	Fiber (gm)	Cholesterol (mg)	Saturated Fat (gm)
	Milk, Light, 1% Fat	244.0000	1.000	Cup	8.03	2.59	11.66	102.14	0.00	0.00	9.76	1.61
	Milk, Malted, Beverage	265.0000	1.000	Cup	10.34	9.81	27.30	235.85	0.00	0.00	37.10	5.95
	Milk, Malted, Chocolate Flavor,	265.0000	1.000	Cup	9.01	9.01	29.95	227.90	7.95	0.00	34.45	5.53
	Milk, Non-Fat, Skim	245.0000	1.000	Cup	8.35	0.44	11.88	85.53	0.00	0.00	4.41	0.29
	Milk, Reduced, 2% Fat	244.0000	1.000	Cup	8.13	4.68	11.71	121.19	0.00	0.00	18.30	2.93
583	Milk, Rice, Enriched Brown-Rice	240.0000	8.000	Fl Oz	1.00	2.00	25.00	120.00	0.00	0.00	0.00	0.00
584	Milk, Soy	240.0000	1.000	Cup	6.60	4.58	4.34	79.00	0.00	3.12	0.00	0.51
	Milk, Whole, 3.3% Fat	244.0000	1.000	Cup	8.03	8.15	11.37	149.91	0.00	0.00	33.18	5.08
	Milk, Whole, 3.7% Fat	244.0000	1.000	Cup	8.00	8.93	11.35	156.57	0.00	0.00	34.89	5.56
	Sour Cream	230.0000	1.000	Cup	7.27	48.21	9.82	492.80	0.00	0.00	102.12	30.02
	Sour Cream, Fat Free	16.0140	1.000	Tbsp	0.50	0.00	2.50	12.51	0.00	0.00	2.50	0.00
	Sour Cream, Imitation, Non-dairy	230.0000	1.000	Cup	5.52	44.90	15.25	479.46	0.00	0.00	0.00	40.92
	Sour Cream, Light	16.0140	1.000	Tbsp	0.92	1.14	0.92	16.01	0.00	0.00	4.58	0.69
	Sour Cream, Non-Fat	16.0000	2.000	Tbsp	0.50	0.00	2.50	12.50	0.00	0.00	2.50	0.00
	Yogurt, 99% Fat Free-Dannon	227.0000	8.000	Ounce	9.00	3.00	45.00	240.00	0.00	0.00	15.00	1.50
834	Yogurt, Apl Cin., Non Fat, Chunk	170.0000	6.000	Ounce	7.00	0.00	33.00	160.00	0.00	0.00	5.00	0.00
835	Yogurt, Apple Cin, Fruit on Bott	227.0000	8.000	Ounce	9.00	3.00	46.00	240.00	0.00	1.00	15.00	1.50
836	Yogurt, Apple Cobbler, Smooth &	227.0000	8.000	Ounce	8.00	2.00	46.00	230.00	0.00	0.00	20.00	1.00
837	Yogurt, Apple Pie a la Mode, Non	227.0000	8.000	Ounce	7.00	0.00	22.00	120.00	0.00	0.00	10.00	0.00
838	Yogurt, Ban Crm/Straw, Double De	170.0000	6.000	Ounce	7.00	1.00	32.00	160.00	0.00	0.00	10.00	0.50
839	Yogurt, Banana Cream Pie, Light-	227.0000	8.000	Ounce	8.00	0.00	16.00	100.00	0.00	0.00	5.00	0.00
840	Yogurt, Bav Crm/Rasp, Double Del	170.0000	6.000	Ounce	7.00	1.00	34.00	170.00	0.00	0.00	10.00	0.50
841	Yogurt, Bavarian & Peach, Light	170.0000	6.000	Ounce	5.00	0.00	18.00	90.00	0.00	0.00	0.00	0.00
842	Yogurt, Berries, Mixed, Fruit on	227.0000	8.000	Ounce	9.00	3.00	45.00	240.00	0.00	1.00	15.00	1.50
843	Yogurt, Berry Banana Split, Non	227.0000	8.000	Ounce	8.00	0.00	21.00	120.00	0.00	0.00	10.00	0.00
844	Yogurt, Berry, Mixed, Fruit on B	125.0000	4.400	Ounce	5.00	1.50	25.00	130.00	0.00	0.00	10.00	1.00
845	Yogurt, Berry, Mixed, Lowfat-Bre	227.0000	8.000	Ounce	9.00	2.50	43.00	230.00	0.00	0.00	15.00	1.50
846	Yogurt, Berry, Tropical, Non Fat	170.0000	6.000	Ounce	7.00	0.00	32.00	160.00	0.00	0.00	5.00	0.00
847	Yogurt, Blackberry Pie, Light-Da	227.0000	8.000	Ounce	8.00	0.00	16.00	100.00	0.00	0.00	5.00	0.00
848	Yogurt, Blueberries N' Cream, No	227.0000	8.000	Ounce	8.00	0.00	23.00	120.00	0.00	0.00	10.00	0.00
849	Yogurt, Blueberries/Crm, Smooth	227.0000	8.000	Ounce	9.00	2.00	46.00	240.00	0.00	0.00	20.00	1.00
850	Yogurt, Blueberry, Blended-Breye	125.0000	4.400	Ounce	4.00	1.00	25.00	130.00	0.00	0.00	10.00	0.50
851	Yogurt, Blueberry, Danimals-Dann	125.0000	4.400	Ounce	6.00	1.00	24.00	130.00	0.00	0.00	5.00	0.50
852	Yogurt, Blueberry, Fruit on Bott	227.0000	8.000	Ounce	9.00	3.00	46.00	240.00	0.00	1.00	15.00	1.50
853	Yogurt, Blueberry, Light-Dannon	227.0000	8.000	Ounce	8.00	0.00	18.00	100.00	0.00	0.00	5.00	0.00
854	Yogurt, Blueberry, Lowfat -Breye	227.0000	8.000	Ounce	9.00	2.50	43.00	230.00	0.00	0.00	15.00	1.50
855	Yogurt, Blueberry, Non Fat, Blen	125.0000	4.400	Ounce	5.00	0.00	25.00	120.00	0.00	0.00	5.00	0.00
856	Yogurt, Blueberry, Non Fat, Chun	170.0000	6.000	Ounce	7.00	0.00	32.00	160.00	0.00	0.00	5.00	0.00
857	Yogurt, Boysenberry, Fruit on B	227.0000	8.000	Ounce	9.00	3.00	45.00	240.00	0.00	1.00	15.00	1.50
858	Yogurt, Cappuccino, Light-Dannon	227.0000	8.000	Ounce	8.00	0.00	16.00	100.00	0.00	0.00	5.00	0.00
859	Yogurt, Car Apl Cinn, Double Del	170.0000	6.000	Ounce	7.00	1.00	47.00	220.00	0.00	0.00	10.00	0.50
860	Yogurt, Car Praline, Double Deli	170.0000	6.000	Ounce	7.00	1.00	47.00	200.00	0.00	0.00	10.00	0.50
861	Yogurt, Caramel Apple Crunch, Li	227.0000	8.000	Ounce	8.00	0.00	25.00	140.00	0.00	0.00	5.00	0.00
862	Yogurt, Cheesck/Straw, Double De	170.0000	6.000	Ounce	7.00	1.00	33.00	170.00	0.00	0.00	10.00	0.50
863	Yogurt, Cheescke/Cher, Double De	170.0000	6.000	Ounce	7.00	1.00	34.00	170.00	0.00	0.00	10.00	0.50
864	Yogurt, Cheeseck & Cherry, Light	170.0000	6.000	Ounce	5.00	0.00	18.00	90.00	0.00	0.00	0.00	0.00
865	Yogurt, Cheeseck & Straw, Light	170.0000	6.000	Ounce	5.00	0.00	17.00	90.00	0.00	0.00	0.00	0.00
866	Yogurt, Cherr Van, Sprinklin' Ra	116.0000	4.000	Ounce	5.00	1.50	24.00	130.00	0.00	0.00	5.00	0.50
867	Yogurt, Cherry Bon-Bon, Non Fat-	227.0000	8.000	Ounce	8.00	0.00	22.00	120.00	0.00	0.00	10.00	0.00
868	Yogurt, Cherry Van, Non Fat, Chu	170.0000	6.000	Ounce	7.00	0.00	31.00	160.00	0.00	0.00	5.00	0.00
869	Yogurt, Cherry Vanilla Crm, Non	227.0000	8.000	Ounce	8.00	0.00	22.00	120.00	0.00	0.00	10.00	0.00
870	Yogurt, Cherry Vanilla, Light-Da	227.0000	8.000	Ounce	8.00	0.00	18.00	100.00	0.00	0.00	5.00	0.00
871	Yogurt, Cherry, Black Jubilee, N	227.0000	8.000	Ounce	8.00	0.00	23.00	120.00	0.00	0.00	10.00	0.00
872	Yogurt, Cherry, Black, Lowfat-Br	227.0000	8.000	Ounce	9.00	2.50	44.00	240.00	0.00	0.00	15.00	1.50
873	Yogurt, Cherry, Danimals-Dannon	125.0000	4.400	Ounce	6.00	1.00	23.00	120.00	0.00	0.00	5.00	0.50

Monounsaturated Fat (gm)	Polyunsaturated Fat (gm)	Vitamin D (mg)	Vitamin K (mg)	Vitamin E (mg)	Vitamin A (re)	Vitamin C (mg)	Thiamin (mg)	Riboflavin (mg)	Niacin (mg)	Vitamin B_6 (mg)	Folate (mg)	Vitamin B_{12} (mcg)	Calcium (mg)	Iron (mg)	Magnesium (mg)	Phosphorus (mg)	Potassium (mg)	Sodium (mg)	Zinc (mg)
0.76	0.10	2.44	0.00	0.10	143.96	2.37	0.10	0.41	0.22	0.10	12.44	0.90	300.12	0.12	33.72	234.73	380.88	123.22	0.95
2.78	0.56	0.00	0.00	0.00	95.40	2.92	0.20	0.59	1.31	0.19	21.73	1.03	355.10	0.27	53.00	302.10	530.00	222.60	1.14
2.57	0.38	0.00	0.00	0.00	79.50	2.65	0.13	0.44	0.63	0.14	16.43	0.93	304.75	0.61	47.70	265.00	498.20	172.25	1.09
0.12	0.02	2.45	9.80	0.10	149.45	2.40	0.10	0.34	0.22	0.10	12.74	0.93	302.33	0.10	27.83	247.21	405.72	126.18	0.98
1.37	0.17	2.44	0.00	0.17	139.08	2.32	0.10	0.41	0.22	0.10	12.44	0.88	296.70	0.12	33.35	232.04	376.74	121.76	0.95
0.00	0.00	0.00	0.00	0.00	0.00	0.00	0.00	0.00	0.00	0.00	0.00	0.00	0.00	0.00	0.00	0.00	0.00	90.00	0.00
0.78	1.90	0.00	0.00	0.00	23.06	0.00	0.38	0.16	0.35	0.09	3.60	0.00	9.60	1.39	45.60	117.60	338.40	28.80	0.55
2.37	0.29	2.44	9.76	0.24	75.64	2.29	0.10	0.39	0.20	0.10	12.20	0.88	291.34	0.12	32.79	227.90	369.66	119.56	0.93
2.59	0.34	0.00	0.00	0.24	82.96	3.59	0.10	0.39	0.20	0.10	12.20	0.88	290.36	0.12	32.70	227.16	368.44	119.07	0.93
13.92	1.79	0.00	0.00	1.31	448.50	1.98	0.09	0.35	0.16	0.05	24.84	0.69	267.72	0.14	25.83	195.27	331.20	122.59	0.62
0.00	0.00	0.00	0.00	0.00	30.03	0.00	0.00	0.00	0.00	0.00	0.00	0.00	36.03	0.00	0.00	0.00	0.00	17.51	0.00
1.36	0.14	0.00	0.00	0.35	0.00	0.00	0.00	0.00	0.00	0.00	0.00	0.00	5.75	0.90	14.67	102.35	369.15	234.60	2.71
0.00	0.00	0.00	0.00	0.00	18.30	0.00	0.00	0.00	0.00	0.00	0.00	0.00	21.96	0.00	0.00	0.00	27.45	9.15	0.00
0.00	0.00	0.00	0.00	0.00	30.00	0.00	0.00	0.00	0.00	0.00	0.00	0.00	36.00	0.00	0.00	0.00	0.00	17.50	0.00
0.00	0.00	0.00	0.00	0.00	0.00	12.00	0.00	0.00	0.00	0.00	0.00	0.00	280.00	0.00	0.00	0.00	0.00	140.00	0.00
0.00	0.00	0.00	0.00	0.00	0.00	0.00	0.00	0.00	0.00	0.00	0.00	0.00	0.00	0.00	0.00	0.00	320.00	100.00	0.00
0.00	0.00	0.00	0.00	0.00	0.00	0.00	0.00	0.00	0.00	0.00	0.00	0.00	0.00	0.00	0.00	0.00	460.00	140.00	0.00
0.00	0.00	0.00	0.00	0.00	0.00	0.00	0.00	0.00	0.00	0.00	0.00	0.00	0.00	0.00	0.00	0.00	390.00	140.00	0.00
0.00	0.00	0.00	0.00	0.00	0.00	0.00	0.00	0.00	0.00	0.00	0.00	0.00	0.00	0.00	0.00	0.00	300.00	105.00	0.00
0.00	0.00	0.00	0.00	0.00	0.00	0.00	0.00	0.00	0.00	0.00	0.00	0.00	0.00	0.00	0.00	0.00	330.00	100.00	0.00
0.00	0.00	0.00	0.00	0.00	0.00	0.00	0.00	0.00	0.00	0.00	0.00	0.00	0.00	0.00	0.00	0.00	360.00	130.00	0.00
0.00	0.00	0.00	0.00	0.00	0.00	0.00	0.00	0.00	0.00	0.00	0.00	0.00	0.00	0.00	0.00	0.00	330.00	125.00	0.00
0.00	0.00	0.00	0.00	0.00	0.00	0.00	0.00	0.00	0.00	0.00	0.00	0.00	0.00	0.00	0.00	0.00	240.00	75.00	0.00
0.00	0.00	0.00	0.00	0.00	0.00	0.00	0.00	0.00	0.00	0.00	0.00	0.00	0.00	0.00	0.00	0.00	450.00	150.00	0.00
0.00	0.00	0.00	0.00	0.00	0.00	0.00	0.00	0.00	0.00	0.00	0.00	0.00	0.00	0.00	0.00	0.00	320.00	105.00	0.00
0.00	0.00	0.00	0.00	0.00	0.00	0.00	0.00	0.00	0.00	0.00	0.00	0.00	0.00	0.00	0.00	0.00	250.00	80.00	0.00
0.00	0.00	0.00	0.00	0.00	0.00	0.00	0.00	0.00	0.00	0.00	0.00	0.00	0.00	0.00	0.00	0.00	440.00	125.00	0.00
0.00	0.00	0.00	0.00	0.00	0.00	0.00	0.00	0.00	0.00	0.00	0.00	0.00	0.00	0.00	0.00	0.00	340.00	110.00	0.00
0.00	0.00	0.00	0.00	0.00	0.00	0.00	0.00	0.00	0.00	0.00	0.00	0.00	0.00	0.00	0.00	0.00	360.00	135.00	0.00
0.00	0.00	0.00	0.00	0.00	0.00	0.00	0.00	0.00	0.00	0.00	0.00	0.00	0.00	0.00	0.00	0.00	310.00	100.00	0.00
0.00	0.00	0.00	0.00	0.00	0.00	0.00	0.00	0.00	0.00	0.00	0.00	0.00	0.00	0.00	0.00	0.00	380.00	125.00	0.00
0.00	0.00	0.00	0.00	0.00	0.00	0.00	0.00	0.00	0.00	0.00	0.00	0.00	0.00	0.00	0.00	0.00	180.00	60.00	0.00
0.00	0.00	0.00	0.00	0.00	0.00	0.00	0.00	0.00	0.00	0.00	0.00	0.00	0.00	0.00	0.00	0.00	270.00	100.00	0.00
0.00	0.00	0.00	0.00	0.00	0.00	0.00	0.00	0.00	0.00	0.00	0.00	0.00	0.00	0.00	0.00	0.00	460.00	140.00	0.00
0.00	0.00	0.00	0.00	0.00	0.00	0.00	0.00	0.00	0.00	0.00	0.00	0.00	0.00	0.00	0.00	0.00	370.00	130.00	0.00
0.00	0.00	0.00	0.00	0.00	0.00	0.00	0.00	0.00	0.00	0.00	0.00	0.00	0.00	0.00	0.00	0.00	430.00	125.00	0.00
0.00	0.00	0.00	0.00	0.00	0.00	0.00	0.00	0.00	0.00	0.00	0.00	0.00	0.00	0.00	0.00	0.00	260.00	105.00	0.00
0.00	0.00	0.00	0.00	0.00	0.00	0.00	0.00	0.00	0.00	0.00	0.00	0.00	0.00	0.00	0.00	0.00	310.00	110.00	0.00
0.00	0.00	0.00	0.00	0.00	0.00	0.00	0.00	0.00	0.00	0.00	0.00	0.00	0.00	0.00	0.00	0.00	450.00	150.00	0.00
0.00	0.00	0.00	0.00	0.00	0.00	0.00	0.00	0.00	0.00	0.00	0.00	0.00	0.00	0.00	0.00	0.00	350.00	135.00	0.00
0.00	0.00	0.00	0.00	0.00	0.00	0.00	0.00	0.00	0.00	0.00	0.00	0.00	0.00	0.00	0.00	0.00	330.00	200.00	0.00
0.00	0.00	0.00	0.00	0.00	0.00	0.00	0.00	0.00	0.00	0.00	0.00	0.00	0.00	0.00	0.00	0.00	330.00	200.00	0.00
0.00	0.00	0.00	0.00	0.00	0.00	0.00	0.00	0.00	0.00	0.00	0.00	0.00	0.00	0.00	0.00	0.00	350.00	170.00	0.00
0.00	0.00	0.00	0.00	0.00	0.00	0.00	0.00	0.00	0.00	0.00	0.00	0.00	0.00	0.00	0.00	0.00	340.00	100.00	0.00
0.00	0.00	0.00	0.00	0.00	0.00	0.00	0.00	0.00	0.00	0.00	0.00	0.00	0.00	0.00	0.00	0.00	340.00	100.00	0.00
0.00	0.00	0.00	0.00	0.00	0.00	0.00	0.00	0.00	0.00	0.00	0.00	0.00	0.00	0.00	0.00	0.00	250.00	75.00	0.00
0.00	0.00	0.00	0.00	0.00	0.00	0.00	0.00	0.00	0.00	0.00	0.00	0.00	0.00	0.00	0.00	0.00	250.00	75.00	0.00
0.00	0.00	0.00	0.00	0.00	0.00	0.00	0.00	0.00	0.00	0.00	0.00	0.00	0.00	0.00	0.00	0.00	250.00	85.00	0.00
0.00	0.00	0.00	0.00	0.00	0.00	0.00	0.00	0.00	0.00	0.00	0.00	0.00	0.00	0.00	0.00	0.00	300.00	105.00	0.00
0.00	0.00	0.00	0.00	0.00	0.00	0.00	0.00	0.00	0.00	0.00	0.00	0.00	0.00	0.00	0.00	0.00	360.00	100.00	0.00
0.00	0.00	0.00	0.00	0.00	0.00	0.00	0.00	0.00	0.00	0.00	0.00	0.00	0.00	0.00	0.00	0.00	320.00	105.00	0.00
0.00	0.00	0.00	0.00	0.00	0.00	0.00	0.00	0.00	0.00	0.00	0.00	0.00	0.00	0.00	0.00	0.00	380.00	130.00	0.00
0.00	0.00	0.00	0.00	0.00	0.00	0.00	0.00	0.00	0.00	0.00	0.00	0.00	0.00	0.00	0.00	0.00	330.00	100.00	0.00
0.00	0.00	0.00	0.00	0.00	0.00	0.00	0.00	0.00	0.00	0.00	0.00	0.00	0.00	0.00	0.00	0.00	450.00	125.00	0.00
0.00	0.00	0.00	0.00	0.00	0.00	0.00	0.00	0.00	0.00	0.00	0.00	0.00	0.00	0.00	0.00	0.00	270.00	95.00	0.00

USDA ID Code	Food Name	Weight in Grams*	Quantity of Units	Unit of Measure	Protein (gm)	Fat (gm)	Carbohydrate (gm)	Kcalories	Caffeine (gm)	Fiber (gm)	Cholesterol (mg)	Saturated Fat (gm)
874	Yogurt, Cherry, Fruit on Bottom-	227.0000	8.000	Ounce	9.00	3.00	45.00	240.00	0.00	0.00	15.00	1.50
875	Yogurt, Cherry, Non Fat, Blended	125.0000	4.400	Ounce	5.00	0.00	23.00	110.00	0.00	0.00	5.00	0.00
877	Yogurt, Choc _clair, Double Deli	170.0000	6.000	Ounce	8.00	1.00	45.00	220.00	0.00	0.00	10.00	0.50
876	Yogurt, Choc Chscake, Double Del	170.0000	6.000	Ounce	8.00	1.00	45.00	220.00	0.00	0.00	10.00	0.50
878	Yogurt, Choc, White & Rasp, Ligh	170.0000	6.000	Ounce	5.00	0.00	17.00	90.00	0.00	0.00	0.00	0.00
879	Yogurt, Choc, White, Rasp, Light	227.0000	8.000	Ounce	8.00	0.00	16.00	100.00	0.00	0.00	5.00	0.00
880	Yogurt, Choc/Straw, Double Delig	170.0000	6.000	Ounce	8.00	1.00	45.00	210.00	0.00	0.00	10.00	0.50
881	Yogurt, Coconut Crm Pie, Light-D	227.0000	8.000	Ounce	8.00	0.00	16.00	100.00	0.00	0.00	5.00	0.00
882	Yogurt, Coffee, Lowfat-Dannon	227.0000	8.000	Ounce	10.00	3.00	36.00	210.00	0.00	0.00	15.00	2.00
883	Yogurt, Cookies 'N Cream, Light-	227.0000	8.000	Ounce	8.00	0.00	24.00	130.00	0.00	0.00	5.00	0.00
884	Yogurt, Cranberry Raspberry, Low	227.0000	8.000	Ounce	10.00	3.00	36.00	210.00	0.00	0.00	15.00	2.00
885	Yogurt, Creme Caramel, Light-Dan	227.0000	8.000	Ounce	8.00	0.00	16.00	100.00	0.00	0.00	5.00	0.00
	Yogurt, Fruit, Fat Free	247.9570	1.000	Cup	10.21	0.00	48.13	233.37	0.00	0.00	7.29	0.00
	Yogurt, Fruit, Fat Free, Light	247.9570	1.000	Cup	10.00	0.00	19.00	109.98	0.00	0.00	5.00	0.00
	Yogurt, Fruit, Lowfat, 10 Gm Pro	245.0000	1.000	Cup	10.71	2.65	46.67	249.61	0.00	0.00	10.29	1.72
	Yogurt, Fruit, Lowfat, 11 Gm Pro	227.0000	1.000	Cup	11.03	3.20	42.22	238.65	0.00	0.00	12.49	2.07
	Yogurt, Fruit, Lowfat, 9 Gm Prot	245.0000	1.000	Cup	9.75	2.82	45.67	243.14	0.00	0.00	11.03	1.81
886	Yogurt, Key Lime Pie, Non Fat-Br	227.0000	8.000	Ounce	8.00	0.00	22.00	120.00	0.00	0.00	10.00	0.00
887	Yogurt, Lem Mer Pie, Double Deli	170.0000	6.000	Ounce	6.00	1.00	37.00	180.00	0.00	0.00	10.00	0.50
888	Yogurt, Lemon Blueberry Cobbler,	227.0000	8.000	Ounce	8.00	0.00	24.00	140.00	0.00	0.00	5.00	0.00
889	Yogurt, Lemon Chiffon, Light Non	227.0000	8.000	Ounce	7.00	0.00	22.00	120.00	0.00	0.00	10.00	0.00
890	Yogurt, Lemon Chiffon, Light-Dan	227.0000	8.000	Ounce	8.00	0.00	16.00	100.00	0.00	0.00	5.00	0.00
891	Yogurt, Lemon Ice, Danimals-Dann	125.0000	4.400	Ounce	6.00	1.00	22.00	120.00	0.00	0.00	5.00	0.50
892	Yogurt, Lemon, Lowfat-Dannon	227.0000	8.000	Ounce	10.00	3.00	36.00	210.00	0.00	0.00	15.00	2.00
893	Yogurt, Light, Strawberry Kiwi-D	227.0000	8.000	Ounce	8.00	0.00	17.00	100.00	0.00	0.00	5.00	0.00
	Yogurt, Light-Dannon	227.0000	8.000	Ounce	9.00	0.00	45.00	240.00	0.00	0.00	15.00	1.50
	Yogurt, No Sugar w/ Granola, Non	227.0000	8.000	Ounce	9.00	0.00	26.00	140.00	0.00	0.00	5.00	0.00
894	Yogurt, Orange Van, Smooth & Crm	227.0000	8.000	Ounce	9.00	2.00	45.00	230.00	0.00	0.00	20.00	1.00
895	Yogurt, Orange, Fruit on Bottom-	227.0000	8.000	Ounce	9.00	3.00	45.00	240.00	0.00	0.00	15.00	1.50
896	Yogurt, Peach, Blended-Breyer's	125.0000	4.400	Ounce	4.00	1.00	26.00	130.00	0.00	0.00	10.00	0.50
897	Yogurt, Peach, Fruit on Bottom-D	227.0000	8.000	Ounce	9.00	3.00	45.00	240.00	0.00	0.00	15.00	1.50
898	Yogurt, Peach, Light-Dannon	227.0000	8.000	Ounce	8.00	0.00	18.00	100.00	0.00	0.00	5.00	0.00
901	Yogurt, Peach, Lowfat-Breyer's	227.0000	8.000	Ounce	9.00	2.50	43.00	240.00	0.00	0.00	15.00	1.50
899	Yogurt, Peach, Non Fat, Blended-	125.0000	4.400	Ounce	5.00	0.00	23.00	110.00	0.00	0.00	5.00	0.00
900	Yogurt, Peach, Non Fat, Chunky F	170.0000	6.000	Ounce	7.00	0.00	33.00	160.00	0.00	0.00	5.00	0.00
902	Yogurt, Peaches N' Crm, Light No	227.0000	8.000	Ounce	8.00	0.00	22.00	120.00	0.00	0.00	10.00	0.00
903	Yogurt, Peaches/Crm, Smooth & Cr	227.0000	8.000	Ounce	9.00	2.00	45.00	230.00	0.00	0.00	20.00	1.00
904	Yogurt, Pina Co, Non Fat, Chunky	170.0000	6.000	Ounce	7.00	0.00	32.00	160.00	0.00	0.00	5.00	0.00
905	Yogurt, Pineapple, Lowfat-Breyer	227.0000	8.000	Ounce	9.00	2.50	45.00	240.00	0.00	0.00	15.00	1.50
906	Yogurt, Plain Lowfat-Dannon	227.0000	8.000	Ounce	12.00	4.00	16.00	140.00	0.00	0.00	20.00	2.50
907	Yogurt, Plain Non Fat-Dannon	227.0000	8.000	Ounce	12.00	0.00	16.00	110.00	0.00	0.00	5.00	0.00
	Yogurt, Plain, Fat Free	247.9570	1.000	Cup	13.00	0.00	17.00	119.98	0.00	0.00	5.00	0.00
	Yogurt, Plain, Lowfat, 12 Gm Pro	245.0000	1.000	Cup	12.86	3.80	17.25	155.06	0.00	0.00	14.95	2.45
	Yogurt, Plain, Skim Milk, 13 Gm	245.0000	1.000	Cup	14.04	0.44	18.82	136.64	0.00	0.00	4.41	0.29
	Yogurt, Plain, Whole Milk, 8 Gm	245.0000	1.000	Cup	8.50	7.96	11.42	150.48	0.00	0.00	31.12	5.15
908	Yogurt, Rasp N' Cream, Light Non	227.0000	8.000	Ounce	8.00	0.00	22.00	120.00	0.00	0.00	10.00	0.00
909	Yogurt, Rasp/Cream, Smooth & Crm	227.0000	8.000	Ounce	9.00	2.00	45.00	230.00	0.00	0.00	20.00	1.00
910	Yogurt, Raspberry w/Granola, Lig	227.0000	8.000	Ounce	8.00	0.00	25.00	140.00	0.00	0.00	5.00	0.00
911	Yogurt, Raspberry, Fruit on Bott	227.0000	8.000	Ounce	9.00	3.00	45.00	240.00	0.00	1.00	15.00	1.50
912	Yogurt, Raspberry, Light-Dannon	227.0000	8.000	Ounce	8.00	0.00	17.00	100.00	0.00	0.00	5.00	0.00
913	Yogurt, Raspberry, Non Fat, Blen	125.0000	4.400	Ounce	5.00	0.00	24.00	110.00	0.00	0.00	5.00	0.00
914	Yogurt, Raspberry, Red, Lowfat-B	227.0000	8.000	Ounce	9.00	2.50	43.00	230.00	0.00	0.00	15.00	1.50
915	Yogurt, Raspberry, Wild, Danimal	125.0000	4.400	Ounce	6.00	1.00	22.00	120.00	0.00	0.00	5.00	0.50
916	Yogurt, Smooth & Crmy, Black Che	227.0000	8.000	Ounce	9.00	2.00	46.00	240.00	0.00	0.00	20.00	1.00
917	Yogurt, Straw Ban Spl, Smooth &	227.0000	8.000	Ounce	8.00	2.00	48.00	240.00	0.00	0.00	20.00	1.00

Monounsaturated Fat (gm)	Polyunsaturated Fat (gm)	Vitamin D (mg)	Vitamin K (mg)	Vitamin E (mg)	Vitamin A (re)	Vitamin C (mg)	Thiamin (mg)	Riboflavin (mg)	Niacin (mg)	Vitamin B_6 (mg)	Folate (mg)	Vitamin B_{12} (mcg)	Calcium (mg)	Iron (mg)	Magnesium (mg)	Phosphorus (mg)	Potassium (mg)	Sodium (mg)	Zinc (mg)
0.00	0.00	0.00	0.00	0.00	0.00	0.00	0.00	0.00	0.00	0.00	0.00	0.00	0.00	0.00	0.00	0.00	480.00	140.00	0.00
0.00	0.00	0.00	0.00	0.00	0.00	0.00	0.00	0.00	0.00	0.00	0.00	0.00	0.00	0.00	0.00	0.00	250.00	75.00	0.00
0.00	0.00	0.00	0.00	0.00	0.00	0.00	0.00	0.00	0.00	0.00	0.00	0.00	0.00	0.00	0.00	0.00	350.00	150.00	0.00
0.00	0.00	0.00	0.00	0.00	0.00	0.00	0.00	0.00	0.00	0.00	0.00	0.00	0.00	0.00	0.00	0.00	350.00	150.00	0.00
0.00	0.00	0.00	0.00	0.00	0.00	0.00	0.00	0.00	0.00	0.00	0.00	0.00	0.00	0.00	0.00	0.00	230.00	80.00	0.00
0.00	0.00	0.00	0.00	0.00	0.00	0.00	0.00	0.00	0.00	0.00	0.00	0.00	0.00	0.00	0.00	0.00	360.00	135.00	0.00
0.00	0.00	0.00	0.00	0.00	0.00	0.00	0.00	0.00	0.00	0.00	0.00	0.00	0.00	0.00	0.00	0.00	350.00	150.00	0.00
0.00	0.00	0.00	0.00	0.00	0.00	0.00	0.00	0.00	0.00	0.00	0.00	0.00	0.00	0.00	0.00	0.00	350.00	130.00	0.00
0.00	0.00	0.00	0.00	0.00	0.00	0.00	0.00	0.00	0.00	0.00	0.00	0.00	0.00	0.00	0.00	0.00	510.00	160.00	0.00
0.00	0.00	0.00	0.00	0.00	0.00	0.00	0.00	0.00	0.00	0.00	0.00	0.00	0.00	0.00	0.00	0.00	350.00	150.00	0.00
0.00	0.00	0.00	0.00	0.00	0.00	0.00	0.00	0.00	0.00	0.00	0.00	0.00	0.00	0.00	0.00	0.00	510.00	160.00	0.00
0.00	0.00	0.00	0.00	0.00	0.00	0.00	0.00	0.00	0.00	0.00	0.00	0.00	0.00	0.00	0.00	0.00	370.00	135.00	0.00
0.00	0.00	0.00	0.00	0.00	0.00	0.00	0.00	0.00	0.00	0.00	0.00	0.00	437.57	0.00	0.00	0.00	422.99	153.15	0.00
0.00	0.00	0.00	0.00	0.00	0.00	15.00	0.00	0.00	0.00	0.00	0.00	0.00	419.93	0.20	0.00	0.00	509.91	159.97	0.00
0.74	0.07	0.00	0.00	0.07	26.95	1.62	0.10	0.44	0.25	0.10	22.79	1.15	372.16	0.17	35.70	292.53	476.53	143.08	1.81
0.89	0.09	0.00	0.00	0.00	34.05	1.68	0.09	0.45	0.25	0.11	23.61	1.18	383.40	0.16	36.77	301.23	491.00	147.32	1.86
0.78	0.07	0.00	0.00	0.07	29.40	1.47	0.07	0.39	0.22	0.10	20.83	1.05	338.84	0.15	32.51	266.32	433.90	130.34	1.64
0.00	0.00	0.00	0.00	0.00	0.00	0.00	0.00	0.00	0.00	0.00	0.00	0.00	0.00	0.00	0.00	0.00	300.00	100.00	0.00
0.00	0.00	0.00	0.00	0.00	0.00	0.00	0.00	0.00	0.00	0.00	0.00	0.00	0.00	0.00	0.00	0.00	300.00	170.00	0.00
0.00	0.00	0.00	0.00	0.00	0.00	0.00	0.00	0.00	0.00	0.00	0.00	0.00	0.00	0.00	0.00	0.00	360.00	140.00	0.00
0.00	0.00	0.00	0.00	0.00	0.00	0.00	0.00	0.00	0.00	0.00	0.00	0.00	0.00	0.00	0.00	0.00	310.00	100.00	0.00
0.00	0.00	0.00	0.00	0.00	0.00	0.00	0.00	0.00	0.00	0.00	0.00	0.00	0.00	0.00	0.00	0.00	360.00	130.00	0.00
0.00	0.00	0.00	0.00	0.00	0.00	0.00	0.00	0.00	0.00	0.00	0.00	0.00	0.00	0.00	0.00	0.00	270.00	100.00	0.00
0.00	0.00	0.00	0.00	0.00	0.00	0.00	0.00	0.00	0.00	0.00	0.00	0.00	0.00	0.00	0.00	0.00	510.00	160.00	0.00
0.00	0.00	0.00	0.00	0.00	0.00	0.00	0.00	0.00	0.00	0.00	0.00	0.00	0.00	0.00	0.00	0.00	380.00	140.00	0.00
0.00	0.00	0.00	0.00	0.00	0.00	12.00	0.00	0.00	0.00	0.00	0.00	0.00	280.00	0.00	0.00	0.00	0.00	130.00	0.00
0.00	0.00	0.00	0.00	0.00	0.00	2.40	0.00	0.00	0.00	0.00	0.00	0.00	280.00	0.40	0.00	0.00	0.00	125.00	0.00
0.00	0.00	0.00	0.00	0.00	0.00	0.00	0.00	0.00	0.00	0.00	0.00	0.00	0.00	0.00	0.00	0.00	380.00	125.00	0.00
0.00	0.00	0.00	0.00	0.00	0.00	0.00	0.00	0.00	0.00	0.00	0.00	0.00	0.00	0.00	0.00	0.00	470.00	135.00	0.00
0.00	0.00	0.00	0.00	0.00	0.00	0.00	0.00	0.00	0.00	0.00	0.00	0.00	0.00	0.00	0.00	0.00	180.00	65.00	0.00
0.00	0.00	0.00	0.00	0.00	0.00	0.00	0.00	0.00	0.00	0.00	0.00	0.00	0.00	0.00	0.00	0.00	450.00	140.00	0.00
0.00	0.00	0.00	0.00	0.00	0.00	0.00	0.00	0.00	0.00	0.00	0.00	0.00	0.00	0.00	0.00	0.00	370.00	130.00	0.00
0.00	0.00	0.00	0.00	0.00	0.00	0.00	0.00	0.00	0.00	0.00	0.00	0.00	0.00	0.00	0.00	0.00	440.00	125.00	0.00
0.00	0.00	0.00	0.00	0.00	0.00	0.00	0.00	0.00	0.00	0.00	0.00	0.00	0.00	0.00	0.00	0.00	240.00	75.00	0.00
0.00	0.00	0.00	0.00	0.00	0.00	0.00	0.00	0.00	0.00	0.00	0.00	0.00	0.00	0.00	0.00	0.00	330.00	100.00	0.00
0.00	0.00	0.00	0.00	0.00	0.00	0.00	0.00	0.00	0.00	0.00	0.00	0.00	0.00	0.00	0.00	0.00	340.00	115.00	0.00
0.00	0.00	0.00	0.00	0.00	0.00	0.00	0.00	0.00	0.00	0.00	0.00	0.00	0.00	0.00	0.00	0.00	390.00	125.00	0.00
0.00	0.00	0.00	0.00	0.00	0.00	0.00	0.00	0.00	0.00	0.00	0.00	0.00	0.00	0.00	0.00	0.00	330.00	110.00	0.00
0.00	0.00	0.00	0.00	0.00	0.00	0.00	0.00	0.00	0.00	0.00	0.00	0.00	0.00	0.00	0.00	0.00	430.00	125.00	0.00
0.00	0.00	0.00	0.00	0.00	0.00	0.00	0.00	0.00	0.00	0.00	0.00	0.00	0.00	0.00	0.00	0.00	590.00	170.00	0.00
0.00	0.00	0.00	0.00	0.00	0.00	0.00	0.00	0.00	0.00	0.00	0.00	0.00	0.00	0.00	0.00	0.00	550.00	150.00	0.00
0.00	0.00	0.00	0.00	0.00	0.00	3.60	0.00	0.25	0.00	0.00	0.00	0.00	479.92	0.00	0.00	0.21	599.90	169.97	0.00
1.05	0.10	0.00	0.00	0.10	39.20	1.96	0.10	0.51	0.27	0.12	27.44	1.37	447.37	0.20	42.75	351.58	572.81	171.99	2.18
0.12	0.02	0.00	0.00	0.02	4.90	2.13	0.12	0.56	0.29	0.12	29.89	1.49	487.80	0.22	46.80	383.43	624.51	187.43	2.38
2.18	0.22	0.00	0.00	0.22	73.50	1.30	0.07	0.34	0.20	0.07	18.13	0.91	295.72	0.12	28.37	232.51	378.77	113.68	1.45
0.00	0.00	0.00	0.00	0.00	0.00	0.00	0.00	0.00	0.00	0.00	0.00	0.00	0.00	0.00	0.00	0.00	330.00	105.00	0.00
0.00	0.00	0.00	0.00	0.00	0.00	0.00	0.00	0.00	0.00	0.00	0.00	0.00	0.00	0.00	0.00	0.00	400.00	135.00	0.00
0.00	0.00	0.00	0.00	0.00	0.00	0.00	0.00	0.00	0.00	0.00	0.00	0.00	0.00	0.00	0.00	0.00	380.00	150.00	0.00
0.00	0.00	0.00	0.00	0.00	0.00	0.00	0.00	0.00	0.00	0.00	0.00	0.00	0.00	0.00	0.00	0.00	460.00	150.00	0.00
0.00	0.00	0.00	0.00	0.00	0.00	0.00	0.00	0.00	0.00	0.00	0.00	0.00	0.00	0.00	0.00	0.00	370.00	150.00	0.00
0.00	0.00	0.00	0.00	0.00	0.00	0.00	0.00	0.00	0.00	0.00	0.00	0.00	0.00	0.00	0.00	0.00	250.00	75.00	0.00
0.00	0.00	0.00	0.00	0.00	0.00	0.00	0.00	0.00	0.00	0.00	0.00	0.00	0.00	0.00	0.00	0.00	450.00	125.00	0.00
0.00	0.00	0.00	0.00	0.00	0.00	0.00	0.00	0.00	0.00	0.00	0.00	0.00	0.00	0.00	0.00	0.00	270.00	90.00	0.00
0.00	0.00	0.00	0.00	0.00	0.00	0.00	0.00	0.00	0.00	0.00	0.00	0.00	0.00	0.00	0.00	0.00	390.00	130.00	0.00
0.00	0.00	0.00	0.00	0.00	0.00	0.00	0.00	0.00	0.00	0.00	0.00	0.00	0.00	0.00	0.00	0.00	390.00	125.00	0.00

USDA ID Code	Food Name	Weight in Grams*	Quantity of Units	Unit of Measure	Protein (gm)	Fat (gm)	Carbohydrate (gm)	Kcalories	Caffeine (gm)	Fiber (gm)	Cholesterol (mg)	Saturated Fat (gm)
918	Yogurt, Straw Cheesck, Light Non	227.0000	8.000	Ounce	8.00	0.00	22.00	120.00	0.00	0.00	10.00	0.00
919	Yogurt, Straw Chscke, Smooth & C	227.0000	8.000	Ounce	9.00	2.00	46.00	240.00	0.00	0.00	20.00	1.00
920	Yogurt, Straw Sundae, Light Duet	170.0000	6.000	Ounce	5.00	0.00	17.00	90.00	0.00	0.00	0.00	0.00
924	Yogurt, Straw/Ban, Sprinklin' Ra	116.0000	4.000	Ounce	5.00	1.50	24.00	130.00	0.00	0.00	5.00	0.50
921	Yogurt, Straw-Ban, Fruit on Bot	227.0000	8.000	Ounce	9.00	3.00	43.00	240.00	0.00	1.00	15.00	1.50
922	Yogurt, Straw-Ban, Non Fat, Blen	125.0000	4.400	Ounce	5.00	0.00	23.00	110.00	0.00	0.00	5.00	0.00
923	Yogurt, Straw-Ban, Non Fat, Chun	170.0000	6.000	Ounce	7.00	0.00	32.00	160.00	0.00	0.00	5.00	0.00
925	Yogurt, Strawberry Banana, Light	227.0000	8.000	Ounce	8.00	0.00	17.00	100.00	0.00	0.00	5.00	0.00
926	Yogurt, Strawberry Banana, Lowfa	227.0000	8.000	Ounce	9.00	2.50	44.00	240.00	0.00	0.00	15.00	1.50
927	Yogurt, Strawberry, Blended-Brey	125.0000	4.400	Ounce	4.00	1.00	26.00	130.00	0.00	0.00	10.00	0.50
928	Yogurt, Strawberry, Danimals-Dan	125.0000	4.400	Ounce	6.00	1.00	24.00	130.00	0.00	0.00	5.00	0.50
929	Yogurt, Strawberry, Fruit on Bot	227.0000	8.000	Ounce	9.00	3.00	45.00	240.00	0.00	1.00	15.00	1.50
931	Yogurt, Strawberry, Light-Dannon	227.0000	8.000	Ounce	8.00	0.00	17.00	100.00	0.00	0.00	5.00	0.00
932	Yogurt, Strawberry, Lowfat-Breye	227.0000	8.000	Ounce	9.00	2.50	43.00	230.00	0.00	0.00	15.00	1.50
933	Yogurt, Strawberry, Non Fat, Ble	125.0000	4.400	Ounce	5.00	0.00	23.00	110.00	0.00	0.00	5.00	0.00
934	Yogurt, Strawberry, Non Fat, Chu	170.0000	6.000	Ounce	7.00	0.00	32.00	160.00	0.00	0.00	5.00	0.00
937	Yogurt, Strawberry, Non Fat-Brey	227.0000	8.000	Ounce	8.00	0.00	22.00	120.00	0.00	0.00	10.00	0.00
935	Yogurt, Strawberry, Smooth & Crm	227.0000	8.000	Ounce	9.00	2.00	45.00	230.00	0.00	0.00	20.00	1.00
936	Yogurt, Strawberry, Sprinklin' R	116.0000	4.000	Ounce	5.00	1.50	24.00	130.00	0.00	0.00	5.00	0.50
938	Yogurt, Tangerine Chiffon, Light	227.0000	8.000	Ounce	8.00	0.00	16.00	100.00	0.00	0.00	5.00	0.00
939	Yogurt, Tropical Punch, Danimals	125.0000	4.400	Ounce	6.00	1.00	25.00	130.00	0.00	0.00	5.00	0.50
940	Yogurt, Van/Cherry, Magic Crysta	116.0000	4.000	Ounce	5.00	1.00	21.00	110.00	0.00	0.00	5.00	0.50
941	Yogurt, Van/Orange, Magic Crysta	116.0000	4.000	Ounce	5.00	1.00	21.00	110.00	0.00	0.00	5.00	0.50
942	Yogurt, Van/Peach/Apr, Double De	170.0000	6.000	Ounce	7.00	1.00	33.00	170.00	0.00	0.00	10.00	0.50
943	Yogurt, Vanilla, Danimals-Dannon	125.0000	4.000	Ounce	6.00	1.00	23.00	120.00	0.00	0.00	5.00	0.50
944	Yogurt, Vanilla, Light-Dannon	227.0000	8.000	Ounce	8.00	0.00	16.00	100.00	0.00	0.00	5.00	0.00
	Yogurt, Vanilla, Lowfat, 11 Gm P	245.0000	1.000	Cup	12.08	3.06	33.81	209.33	0.00	0.00	12.01	1.98
945	Yogurt, Vanilla, Lowfat-Breyer's	227.0000	8.000	Ounce	10.00	3.00	38.00	220.00	0.00	0.00	20.00	2.00
946	Yogurt, Vanilla, Lowfat-Dannon	227.0000	8.000	Ounce	10.00	3.00	36.00	210.00	0.00	0.00	15.00	2.00
947	Yogurt, Vanilla/Straw, Double De	170.0000	6.000	Ounce	7.00	1.00	33.00	170.00	0.00	0.00	10.00	0.50
	Butter, w/ Salt	5.0000	1.000	Pat	0.05	4.06	0.01	35.85	0.00	0.00	10.95	2.53
	Butter, w/o Salt	5.0000	1.000	Pat	0.04	4.06	0.00	35.85	0.00	0.00	10.95	2.52
	Butter, Whipped	3.8000	1.000	Pat	0.03	3.08	0.00	27.24	0.00	0.00	8.32	1.92
	Lard	12.8000	1.000	Tbsp	0.00	12.80	0.00	115.46	0.00	0.00	12.16	5.02
	Margarine, Hard, Corn & soybn	4.7000	1.000	Tbsp	0.04	3.78	0.04	33.78	0.00	0.00	0.00	0.71
	Margarine, Hard, Corn (hydr)	4.7000	1.000	Tbsp	0.04	3.78	0.04	33.78	0.00	0.00	0.00	0.62
	Margarine, Imitation (appx 40% F	4.8000	1.000	Tbsp	0.02	1.86	0.02	16.57	0.00	0.00	0.00	0.37
	Margarine, Regular, w/ Salt Adde	4.7000	1.000	Tbsp	0.04	3.78	0.04	33.78	0.00	0.00	0.00	0.74
	Margarine, Regular, w/o Added Sa	4.7000	1.000	Tbsp	0.02	3.77	0.02	33.56	0.00	0.00	0.00	0.71
	Margarine, Soft, w/ Salt Added	227.0000	1.000	Cup	1.82	182.51	1.14	1626.23	0.00	0.00	0.00	31.33
	Margarine, Soft, w/o Added Salt	4.7000	1.000	Tbsp	0.04	3.77	0.04	33.67	0.00	0.00	0.00	0.65
	Mayonnaise	14.7000	1.000	Tbsp	0.13	4.91	3.51	57.29	0.00	0.00	3.82	0.72
	Mayonnaise, Fat Free	15.0070	1.000	Tbsp	0.00	0.00	3.00	10.00	0.00	0.00	0.00	0.00
	Mayonnaise, Light	15.0070	1.000	Tbsp	0.00	2.00	1.00	25.01	0.00	0.00	5.00	0.00
	Oil, Olive	13.5000	1.000	Tbsp	0.00	13.50	0.00	119.34	0.00	0.00	0.00	1.82
	Oil, Peanut	13.5000	1.000	Tbsp	0.00	13.50	0.00	119.34	0.00	0.00	0.00	2.28
	Oil, Sesame	13.6000	1.000	Tbsp	0.00	13.60	0.00	120.22	0.00	0.00	0.00	1.93
	Oil, Soybean	13.6000	1.000	Tbsp	0.00	13.60	0.00	120.22	0.00	0.00	0.00	1.96
	Oil, Soybean, (hydr)	13.6000	1.000	Tbsp	0.00	13.60	0.00	120.22	0.00	0.00	0.00	2.03
	Oil, Soybean, (hydr) & cottonsee	13.6000	1.000	Tbsp	0.00	13.60	0.00	120.22	0.00	0.00	0.00	2.45
	Oil, Vegetable Corn	13.6000	1.000	Tbsp	0.00	13.60	0.00	120.22	0.00	0.00	0.00	1.73
	Oil, Vegetable, Canola	14.0000	1.000	Tbsp	0.00	14.00	0.00	123.76	0.00	0.00	0.00	0.99
	Oil, Vegetable, Cocoa Butter	13.6000	1.000	Tbsp	0.00	13.60	0.00	120.22	0.00	0.00	0.00	8.12
	Oil, Vegetable, Cottonseed	13.6000	1.000	Tbsp	0.00	13.60	0.00	120.22	0.00	0.00	0.00	3.52
	Oil, Vegetable, Palm	13.6000	1.000	Tbsp	0.00	13.60	0.00	120.22	0.00	0.00	0.00	6.70

Monounsaturated Fat (gm)	Polyunsaturated Fat (gm)	Vitamin D (mg)	Vitamin K (mg)	Vitamin E (mg)	Vitamin A (re)	Vitamin C (mg)	Thiamin (mg)	Riboflavin (mg)	Niacin (mg)	Vitamin B_6 (mg)	Folate (mg)	Vitamin B_{12} (mcg)	Calcium (mg)	Iron (mg)	Magnesium (mg)	Phosphorus (mg)	Potassium (mg)	Sodium (mg)	Zinc (mg)
0.00	0.00	0.00	0.00	0.00	0.00	0.00	0.00	0.00	0.00	0.00	0.00	0.00	0.00	0.00	0.00	0.00	320.00	100.00	0.00
0.00	0.00	0.00	0.00	0.00	0.00	0.00	0.00	0.00	0.00	0.00	0.00	0.00	0.00	0.00	0.00	0.00	400.00	125.00	0.00
0.00	0.00	0.00	0.00	0.00	0.00	0.00	0.00	0.00	0.00	0.00	0.00	0.00	0.00	0.00	0.00	0.00	250.00	75.00	0.00
0.00	0.00	0.00	0.00	0.00	0.00	0.00	0.00	0.00	0.00	0.00	0.00	0.00	0.00	0.00	0.00	0.00	250.00	80.00	0.00
0.00	0.00	0.00	0.00	0.00	0.00	0.00	0.00	0.00	0.00	0.00	0.00	0.00	0.00	0.00	0.00	0.00	480.00	140.00	0.00
0.00	0.00	0.00	0.00	0.00	0.00	0.00	0.00	0.00	0.00	0.00	0.00	0.00	0.00	0.00	0.00	0.00	240.00	75.00	0.00
0.00	0.00	0.00	0.00	0.00	0.00	0.00	0.00	0.00	0.00	0.00	0.00	0.00	0.00	0.00	0.00	0.00	350.00	105.00	0.00
0.00	0.00	0.00	0.00	0.00	0.00	0.00	0.00	0.00	0.00	0.00	0.00	0.00	0.00	0.00	0.00	0.00	380.00	140.00	0.00
0.00	0.00	0.00	0.00	0.00	0.00	0.00	0.00	0.00	0.00	0.00	0.00	0.00	0.00	0.00	0.00	0.00	470.00	125.00	0.00
0.00	0.00	0.00	0.00	0.00	0.00	0.00	0.00	0.00	0.00	0.00	0.00	0.00	0.00	0.00	0.00	0.00	180.00	60.00	0.00
0.00	0.00	0.00	0.00	0.00	0.00	0.00	0.00	0.00	0.00	0.00	0.00	0.00	0.00	0.00	0.00	0.00	270.00	90.00	0.00
0.00	0.00	0.00	0.00	0.00	0.00	0.00	0.00	0.00	0.00	0.00	0.00	0.00	0.00	0.00	0.00	0.00	460.00	140.00	0.00
0.00	0.00	0.00	0.00	0.00	0.00	0.00	0.00	0.00	0.00	0.00	0.00	0.00	0.00	0.00	0.00	0.00	380.00	140.00	0.00
0.00	0.00	0.00	0.00	0.00	0.00	0.00	0.00	0.00	0.00	0.00	0.00	0.00	0.00	0.00	0.00	0.00	440.00	125.00	0.00
0.00	0.00	0.00	0.00	0.00	0.00	0.00	0.00	0.00	0.00	0.00	0.00	0.00	0.00	0.00	0.00	0.00	230.00	80.00	0.00
0.00	0.00	0.00	0.00	0.00	0.00	0.00	0.00	0.00	0.00	0.00	0.00	0.00	0.00	0.00	0.00	0.00	360.00	115.00	0.00
0.00	0.00	0.00	0.00	0.00	0.00	0.00	0.00	0.00	0.00	0.00	0.00	0.00	0.00	0.00	0.00	0.00	320.00	100.00	0.00
0.00	0.00	0.00	0.00	0.00	0.00	0.00	0.00	0.00	0.00	0.00	0.00	0.00	0.00	0.00	0.00	0.00	400.00	125.00	0.00
0.00	0.00	0.00	0.00	0.00	0.00	0.00	0.00	0.00	0.00	0.00	0.00	0.00	0.00	0.00	0.00	0.00	250.00	85.00	0.00
0.00	0.00	0.00	0.00	0.00	0.00	0.00	0.00	0.00	0.00	0.00	0.00	0.00	0.00	0.00	0.00	0.00	360.00	130.00	0.00
0.00	0.00	0.00	0.00	0.00	0.00	0.00	0.00	0.00	0.00	0.00	0.00	0.00	0.00	0.00	0.00	0.00	270.00	95.00	0.00
0.00	0.00	0.00	0.00	0.00	0.00	0.00	0.00	0.00	0.00	0.00	0.00	0.00	0.00	0.00	0.00	0.00	240.00	85.00	0.00
0.00	0.00	0.00	0.00	0.00	0.00	0.00	0.00	0.00	0.00	0.00	0.00	0.00	0.00	0.00	0.00	0.00	240.00	85.00	0.00
0.00	0.00	0.00	0.00	0.00	0.00	0.00	0.00	0.00	0.00	0.00	0.00	0.00	0.00	0.00	0.00	0.00	330.00	100.00	0.00
0.00	0.00	0.00	0.00	0.00	0.00	0.00	0.00	0.00	0.00	0.00	0.00	0.00	0.00	0.00	0.00	0.00	270.00	90.00	0.00
0.00	0.00	0.00	0.00	0.00	0.00	0.00	0.00	0.00	0.00	0.00	0.00	0.00	0.00	0.00	0.00	0.00	350.00	130.00	0.00
0.83	0.10	0.00	0.00	0.07	31.85	1.84	0.10	0.49	0.27	0.12	25.73	1.30	419.69	0.17	40.25	329.77	537.29	161.21	2.03
0.00	0.00	0.00	0.00	0.00	0.00	0.00	0.00	0.00	0.00	0.00	0.00	0.00	0.00	0.00	0.00	0.00	480.00	135.00	0.00
0.00	0.00	0.00	0.00	0.00	0.00	0.00	0.00	0.00	0.00	0.00	0.00	0.00	0.00	0.00	0.00	0.00	510.00	160.00	0.00
0.00	0.00	0.00	0.00	0.00	0.00	0.00	0.00	0.00	0.00	0.00	0.00	0.00	0.00	0.00	0.00	0.00	340.00	100.00	0.00
1.17	0.15	0.00	0.00	0.08	37.70	0.00	0.00	0.00	0.00	0.00	0.15	0.01	1.20	0.01	0.10	1.15	1.30	41.30	0.00
1.17	0.15	0.00	0.00	0.08	37.70	0.00	0.00	0.00	0.00	0.00	0.14	0.01	1.18	0.01	0.10	1.14	1.30	0.55	0.00
0.89	0.11	0.00	0.00	0.06	28.65	0.00	0.00	0.00	0.00	0.00	0.11	0.00	0.89	0.01	0.08	0.87	0.99	31.41	0.00
5.77	1.43	0.00	0.00	0.15	0.00	0.00	0.00	0.00	0.00	0.00	0.00	0.00	0.01	0.00	0.00	0.00	0.00	0.00	0.01
1.73	1.18	0.00	0.00	0.52	37.55	0.01	0.00	0.00	0.00	0.00	0.06	0.00	1.41	0.00	0.12	1.08	1.99	44.34	0.00
2.15	0.85	0.00	0.00	0.55	37.55	0.01	0.00	0.00	0.00	0.00	0.06	0.00	1.41	0.00	0.12	1.08	1.99	44.34	0.00
0.75	0.66	0.00	0.00	0.11	38.35	0.00	0.00	0.00	0.00	0.00	0.03	0.00	0.85	0.00	0.07	0.66	1.21	46.06	0.00
1.68	1.19	0.00	0.00	0.60	37.55	0.01	0.00	0.00	0.00	0.00	0.06	0.00	1.41	0.00	0.12	1.08	1.99	44.34	0.00
1.72	1.18	0.00	0.00	0.60	37.55	0.00	0.00	0.00	0.00	0.00	0.03	0.00	0.82	0.00	0.07	0.63	1.16	0.10	0.00
64.69	78.54	0.00	0.00	27.24	1813.73	0.32	0.02	0.07	0.05	0.02	2.38	0.18	60.16	0.00	5.24	46.08	85.58	2448.54	0.00
1.75	1.21	0.00	0.00	0.41	37.55	0.01	0.00	0.00	0.00	0.00	0.05	0.00	1.25	0.00	0.11	0.95	1.77	1.29	0.00
1.32	2.65	0.00	0.00	0.59	12.35	0.00	0.00	0.00	0.00	0.00	0.92	0.03	2.06	0.03	0.29	3.82	1.32	104.48	0.03
0.00	0.00	0.00	0.00	0.00	0.00	0.00	0.00	0.00	0.00	0.00	0.00	0.00	0.00	0.00	0.00	0.00	10.00	105.05	0.00
0.00	0.00	0.00	0.00	0.00	0.00	0.00	0.00	0.00	0.00	0.00	0.00	0.00	0.00	0.00	0.00	0.00	5.00	130.06	0.00
9.95	1.13	0.00	7.83	1.67	0.00	0.00	0.00	0.00	0.00	0.00	0.00	0.00	0.02	0.05	0.00	0.16	0.00	0.01	0.01
6.24	4.32	0.00	0.27	1.74	0.00	0.00	0.00	0.00	0.00	0.00	0.00	0.00	0.01	0.00	0.01	0.00	0.00	0.01	0.00
5.40	5.67	0.00	1.63	0.56	0.00	0.00	0.00	0.00	0.00	0.00	0.00	0.00	0.00	0.00	0.00	0.00	0.00	0.00	0.00
3.17	7.87	0.00	0.00	2.47	0.00	0.00	0.00	0.00	0.00	0.00	0.00	0.00	0.01	0.00	0.00	0.03	0.00	0.00	0.00
5.85	5.11	0.00	0.00	2.47	0.00	0.00	0.00	0.00	0.00	0.00	0.00	0.00	0.00	0.00	0.00	0.00	0.00	0.00	0.00
4.01	6.54	0.00	0.00	3.84	0.00	0.00	0.00	0.00	0.00	0.00	0.00	0.00	0.00	0.00	0.00	0.00	0.00	0.00	0.00
3.29	7.98	0.00	0.68	2.87	0.00	0.00	0.00	0.00	0.00	0.00	0.00	0.00	0.00	0.00	0.00	0.00	0.00	0.00	0.00
8.25	4.14	0.00	116.20	2.93	0.00	0.00	0.00	0.00	0.00	0.00	0.00	0.00	0.00	0.00	0.00	0.00	0.00	0.00	0.00
4.47	0.41	0.00	0.00	0.24	0.00	0.00	0.00	0.00	0.00	0.00	0.00	0.00	0.00	0.00	0.00	0.00	0.00	0.00	0.00
2.42	7.06	0.00	0.00	5.20	0.00	0.00	0.00	0.00	0.00	0.00	0.00	0.00	0.00	0.00	0.00	0.00	0.00	0.00	0.00
5.03	1.26	0.00	1.09	2.96	0.00	0.00	0.00	0.00	0.00	0.00	0.00	0.00	0.00	0.00	0.00	0.02	0.00	0.00	0.00

USDA ID Code	Food Name	Weight in Grams*	Quantity of Units	Unit of Measure	Protein (gm)	Fat (gm)	Carbohydrate (gm)	Kcalories	Caffeine (gm)	Fiber (gm)	Cholesterol (mg)	Saturated Fat (gm)
	Oil, Vegetable, Palm Kernel	13.6000	1.000	Tbsp	0.00	13.60	0.00	117.23	0.00	0.00	0.00	11.08
	Oil, Vegetable, Safflower, Linol	13.6000	1.000	Tbsp	0.00	13.60	0.00	120.22	0.00	0.00	0.00	0.84
	Oil, Vegetable, Safflower, Oleic	13.6000	1.000	Tbsp	0.00	13.60	0.00	120.22	0.00	0.00	0.00	0.84
	Oil, Vegetable, Sunflower	14.0000	1.000	Tbsp	0.00	14.00	0.00	123.76	0.00	0.00	0.00	1.37
	Salad Dressing, Blue Cheese	16.0140	2.000	Tbsp	0.50	3.50	2.50	45.04	0.00	0.00	5.00	2.00
	Salad Dressing, Blue Cheese, Fat	17.5080	2.000	Tbsp	0.25	0.00	6.00	25.01	0.00	0.00	0.00	0.00
	Salad Dressing, Ceasar	17.1200	2.000	Tbsp	0.17	17.12	1.31	155.00	0.00	0.00	1.11	3.22
	Salad Dressing, French	12.3000	1.000	Pkt	0.07	5.04	2.15	52.85	0.00	0.00	0.00	1.17
	Salad Dressing, French, Fat Free	17.5080	2.000	Tbsp	0.00	0.00	6.00	25.01	0.00	0.00	0.00	0.00
	Salad Dressing, French, Low Fat	16.3000	1.000	Tbsp	0.03	0.95	3.54	21.87	0.00	0.00	0.00	0.13
	Salad Dressing, Honey Mustard	31.2000	2.000	Tbsp	0.05	6.33	14.22	102.11	0.00	0.23	0.00	1.33
	Salad Dressing, Italian	14.7000	1.000	Tbsp	0.10	7.10	1.50	68.69	0.00	0.00	0.00	1.03
	Salad Dressing, Italian, Creamy	29.4000	2.000	Tbsp	0.03	16.12	2.33	147.43	0.00	0.00	1.22	2.43
	Salad Dressing, Italian, Fat Fre	15.5100	2.000	Tbsp	0.00	0.00	1.00	5.00	0.00	0.00	0.00	0.00
	Salad Dressing, Italian, Low Cal	15.0000	1.000	Tbsp	0.02	1.47	0.74	15.81	0.00	0.02	0.90	0.20
	Salad Dressing, Peppercorn	26.8000	2.000	Tbsp	0.02	16.22	1.10	151.22	0.00	0.00	13.11	3.11
	Salad Dressing, Poppy Seed	29.4000	2.000	Tbsp	0.02	12.31	6.41	130.44	0.00	0.00	0.00	2.33
	Salad Dressing, Ranch	14.5190	2.000	Tbsp	0.00	9.01	1.00	85.11	0.00	0.00	2.50	1.50
	Salad Dressing, Ranch, Fat Free	17.5080	2.000	Tbsp	0.00	0.00	5.50	25.01	0.00	0.00	0.00	0.00
	Salad Dressing, Raspberry Vinegr	14.7000	2.000	Tbsp	0.10	7.10	1.50	68.69	0.00	0.00	0.00	1.03
	Salad Dressing, Russian	15.3000	1.000	Tbsp	0.24	7.77	1.59	75.58	0.00	0.00	2.75	1.12
	Salad Dressing, Russian, Low Cal	16.3000	1.000	Tbsp	0.08	0.65	4.50	23.05	0.00	0.05	0.98	0.10
	Salad Dressing, Sesame Seed	15.3000	1.000	Tbsp	0.47	6.92	1.32	67.79	0.00	0.15	0.00	0.95
	Salad Dressing, Thousand Island	15.6000	1.000	Tbsp	0.14	5.57	2.37	58.86	0.00	0.00	4.06	0.94
	Salad Dressing, Thousand Island,	17.5080	2.000	Tbsp	0.00	0.00	5.50	22.51	0.00	0.00	0.00	0.00
	Salad Dressing, Thousand Island,	15.3000	1.000	Tbsp	0.12	1.64	2.48	24.27	0.00	0.18	2.30	0.24
	Salad Dressing, Vinegar and Oil	15.6000	1.000	Tbsp	0.00	7.82	0.39	70.01	0.00	0.00	0.00	1.42
	Apples, Cnd, Sweetened	204.0000	1.000	Cup	0.37	1.00	34.07	136.68	0.00	3.47	0.00	0.16
	Apples, Dehydrated, Sulfured	60.0000	0.250	Cup	0.79	0.35	56.12	207.60	0.00	7.44	0.00	0.06
	Apples, Fresh, w/ Skin	125.0000	1.000	Cup	0.24	0.45	19.06	73.75	0.00	3.38	0.00	0.08
	Apples, Fresh, w/o Skin	110.0000	1.000	Cup	0.17	0.34	16.32	62.70	0.00	2.09	0.00	0.06
	Applesauce, Sweetened	255.0000	1.000	Cup	0.46	0.46	50.77	193.80	0.00	3.06	0.00	0.08
	Applesauce, Unsweetened	244.0000	1.000	Cup	0.41	0.12	27.55	104.92	0.00	2.93	0.00	0.02
	Apricots, Cnd, Heavy Syrup Pack	258.0000	1.000	Cup	1.32	0.23	55.34	214.14	0.00	4.13	0.00	0.03
	Apricots, Cnd, Juice Pack	244.0000	1.000	Cup	1.54	0.10	30.11	117.12	0.00	3.90	0.00	0.00
	Apricots, Cnd, Light Syrup Pack	253.0000	1.000	Cup	1.34	0.13	41.72	159.39	0.00	4.05	0.00	0.00
	Apricots, Cnd, Water Pack	243.0000	1.000	Cup	1.73	0.39	15.53	65.61	0.00	3.89	0.00	0.02
	Apricots, Dehydrated, Sulfured	119.0000	0.500	Cup	5.83	0.74	98.64	380.80	0.00	0.00	0.00	0.05
	Apricots, Dried, Sulfured	130.0000	1.000	Cup	4.75	0.60	80.28	309.40	0.00	11.70	0.00	0.04
	Apricots, Fresh	155.0000	1.000	Cup	2.17	0.60	17.24	74.40	0.00	3.72	0.00	0.05
	Apricots, Frozen, Sweetened	242.0000	1.000	Cup	1.69	0.24	60.74	237.16	0.00	5.32	0.00	0.02
	Artichoke, Boiled, Hearts w/ Sal	84.0000	0.500	Cup	2.92	0.13	9.39	42.00	0.00	4.54	0.00	0.03
	Artichoke, Boiled, Hearts w/o Sa	84.0000	0.500	Cup	2.92	0.13	9.39	42.00	0.00	4.54	0.00	0.03
	Asparagus, Ckd	90.0000	0.500	Cup	2.33	0.28	3.81	21.60	0.00	1.89	0.00	0.06
	Asparagus, Cnd	242.0000	1.000	Cup	5.18	1.57	6.00	45.98	0.00	3.87	0.00	0.36
	Asparagus, Fresh	134.0000	1.000	Cup	3.06	0.27	6.08	30.82	0.00	2.81	0.00	0.07
	Asparagus, Frz, Ckd	180.0000	1.000	Cup	5.31	0.76	8.77	50.40	0.00	2.88	0.00	0.18
	Avocados, Fresh	150.0000	1.000	Cup	2.97	22.98	11.09	241.50	0.00	7.50	0.00	3.66
	Bamboo Shoots, Cnd	131.0000	1.000	Cup	2.25	0.52	4.22	24.89	0.00	1.83	0.00	0.12
	Bamboo Shoots, Fresh	151.0000	1.000	Cup	3.93	0.45	7.85	40.77	0.00	3.32	0.00	0.11
	Banana, Dehydrated, Chips	100.0000	1.000	Cup	3.89	1.81	88.28	346.00	0.00	7.50	0.00	0.70
	Bananas, Fresh	225.0000	1.000	Cup	2.32	1.08	52.72	207.00	0.00	5.40	0.00	0.43
	Bean Sprouts	133.3330	0.500	Cup	17.47	9.47	12.53	166.67	0.00	0.00	0.00	0.00
	Beans, Green, Cnd	135.0000	1.000	Cup	1.55	0.14	6.08	27.00	0.00	2.57	0.00	0.03
	Beans, Green, Fresh	110.0000	1.000	Cup	2.00	0.13	7.85	34.10	0.00	3.74	0.00	0.03

Monounsaturated Fat (gm)	Polyunsaturated Fat (gm)	Vitamin D (mg)	Vitamin K (mg)	Vitamin E (mg)	Vitamin A (re)	Vitamin C (mg)	Thiamin (mg)	Riboflavin (mg)	Niacin (mg)	Vitamin B_6 (mg)	Folate (mg)	Vitamin B_{12} (mcg)	Calcium (mg)	Iron (mg)	Magnesium (mg)	Phosphorus (mg)	Potassium (mg)	Sodium (mg)	Zinc (mg)
1.55	0.22	0.00	0.00	0.52	0.00	0.00	0.00	0.00	0.00	0.00	0.00	0.00	0.00	0.00	0.00	0.00	0.00	0.00	0.00
1.95	10.15	0.00	0.95	5.86	0.00	0.00	0.00	0.00	0.00	0.00	0.00	0.00	0.00	0.00	0.00	0.00	0.00	0.00	0.00
10.15	1.95	0.00	0.00	4.68	0.00	0.00	0.00	0.00	0.00	0.00	0.00	0.00	0.00	0.00	0.00	0.00	0.00	0.00	0.00
11.70	0.53	0.00	0.00	0.00	0.00	0.00	0.00	0.00	0.00	0.00	0.00	0.00	0.00	0.00	0.00	0.00	0.00	0.00	0.00
0.00	0.00	0.00	0.00	0.00	0.00	0.00	0.00	0.00	0.00	0.00	0.00	0.00	12.01	0.00	0.00	0.00	0.00	235.20	0.00
0.00	0.00	0.00	0.00	0.20	0.00	0.00	0.00	0.00	0.00	0.00	0.00	0.00	0.00	0.00	0.00	0.00	0.00	170.08	0.00
2.22	5.89	0.00	0.00	0.77	0.44	0.00	0.00	0.00	0.00	0.00	0.00	0.00	12.01	0.00	0.00	0.00	0.00	317.33	0.00
0.98	2.67	0.00	0.00	1.04	15.99	0.00	0.00	0.00	0.00	0.00	0.52	0.02	1.35	0.05	0.00	1.72	9.72	168.51	0.01
0.00	0.00	0.00	0.00	0.00	50.02	0.00	0.00	0.00	0.00	0.00	0.00	0.00	0.00	0.00	0.00	0.00	0.00	150.07	0.00
0.23	0.55	0.00	0.00	0.19	21.19	0.00	0.00	0.00	0.00	0.00	0.00	0.00	1.79	0.07	0.00	2.28	12.88	128.28	0.03
1.64	3.22	0.00	0.00	0.98	0.00	0.30	0.00	0.00	0.00	0.00	0.00	0.00	10.11	0.11	0.00	0.00	0.00	74.33	0.00
1.65	4.12	0.00	0.00	1.52	3.53	0.00	0.00	0.00	0.00	0.00	0.72	0.02	1.47	0.03	0.09	0.74	2.21	115.69	0.02
1.77	4.13	0.00	0.00	0.43	9.77	0.00	0.00	0.00	0.00	0.00	0.00	0.00	0.74	0.05	0.00	0.00	0.00	2.33	0.00
0.00	0.00	0.00	0.00	0.00	0.00	0.00	0.00	0.00	0.00	0.00	0.00	0.00	0.00	0.00	0.00	0.00	0.00	145.10	0.00
0.30	0.90	0.00	0.00	0.23	0.00	0.00	0.00	0.00	0.00	0.00	0.00	0.00	0.30	0.03	0.00	0.75	2.25	118.05	0.02
1.77	4.11	0.00	0.00	0.00	0.00	0.30	0.00	0.00	0.00	0.00	0.00	0.00	0.22	0.02	0.00	0.00	0.00	285.32	0.00
1.33	2.88	0.00	0.00	0.00	0.00	0.30	0.00	0.00	0.00	0.00	0.00	0.00	0.22	0.02	0.00	0.00	0.00	127.11	0.00
0.00	0.00	0.00	0.00	0.00	0.00	0.00	0.00	0.00	0.00	0.00	0.00	0.00	0.00	0.00	0.00	0.00	0.00	135.18	0.00
0.00	0.00	0.00	0.00	0.30	0.00	0.00	0.00	0.00	0.00	0.00	0.00	0.00	0.00	0.00	0.00	0.00	0.00	155.07	0.00
1.65	4.12	0.00	0.00	1.52	3.53	0.00	0.00	0.00	0.00	0.00	0.72	0.02	1.47	0.03	0.09	0.73	2.20	115.69	0.02
1.81	4.50	0.00	0.00	1.56	31.67	0.92	0.01	0.01	0.09	0.00	1.59	0.05	2.91	0.09	0.23	5.66	24.02	132.80	0.07
0.15	0.37	0.00	0.00	0.12	2.61	0.98	0.00	0.00	0.00	0.00	0.57	0.02	3.10	0.10	0.07	6.03	25.59	141.48	0.02
1.82	3.84	0.00	0.00	0.77	31.67	0.00	0.00	0.00	0.00	0.00	0.00	0.00	2.91	0.09	0.00	5.66	24.02	153.00	0.02
1.29	3.09	0.00	0.00	0.18	14.98	0.00	0.00	0.00	0.00	0.00	0.98	0.03	1.72	0.09	0.31	2.65	17.63	109.20	0.02
0.00	0.00	0.00	0.00	0.00	0.00	0.00	0.00	0.00	0.00	0.00	0.00	0.00	0.00	0.00	0.00	0.00	0.00	150.07	0.00
0.37	0.95	0.00	0.00	0.18	14.69	0.00	0.00	0.00	0.00	0.00	0.85	0.03	1.68	0.09	0.11	2.60	17.29	153.00	0.02
2.31	3.76	0.00	0.00	1.37	0.00	0.00	0.00	0.00	0.00	0.00	0.00	0.00	0.00	0.00	0.00	0.00	1.17	0.08	0.00
0.04	0.29	0.00	0.00	0.02	10.20	0.82	0.02	0.02	0.14	0.08	0.61	0.00	8.16	0.47	4.08	10.20	138.72	6.12	0.06
0.01	0.10	0.00	0.00	2.15	4.80	1.32	0.03	0.08	0.41	0.17	0.60	0.00	11.40	1.20	13.20	33.00	384.00	74.40	0.17
0.03	0.14	0.00	5.00	0.40	6.25	7.13	0.03	0.01	0.10	0.06	3.50	0.00	8.75	0.23	6.25	8.75	143.75	0.00	0.05
0.01	0.10	0.00	0.51	0.09	4.40	4.40	0.02	0.01	0.10	0.06	0.44	0.00	4.40	0.08	3.30	7.70	124.30	0.00	0.04
0.03	0.13	0.00	0.00	0.03	2.55	4.34	0.03	0.08	0.48	0.08	1.53	0.00	10.20	0.89	7.65	17.85	155.55	7.65	0.10
0.00	0.02	0.00	0.00	0.02	7.32	2.93	0.02	0.07	0.46	0.07	1.46	0.00	7.32	0.29	7.32	17.08	183.00	4.88	0.07
0.10	0.05	0.00	0.00	0.00	319.92	7.22	0.05	0.05	1.08	0.13	4.39	0.00	23.22	1.11	20.64	33.54	345.72	28.38	0.26
0.05	0.02	0.00	0.00	2.17	412.36	11.96	0.05	0.05	0.83	0.12	4.15	0.00	29.28	0.73	24.40	48.80	402.60	9.76	0.27
0.05	0.03	0.00	0.00	2.25	333.96	6.83	0.05	0.05	0.76	0.13	4.30	0.00	27.83	0.99	20.24	32.89	349.14	10.12	0.28
0.17	0.07	0.00	0.00	2.16	313.47	8.26	0.05	0.05	0.97	0.12	4.13	0.00	19.44	0.78	17.01	31.59	466.56	7.29	0.27
0.32	0.14	0.00	0.00	0.00	1507.73	11.31	0.05	0.18	4.26	0.62	5.24	0.00	72.59	7.51	74.97	186.83	2201.50	15.47	1.19
0.26	0.12	0.00	0.00	1.95	941.20	3.12	0.01	0.20	3.90	0.21	13.39	0.00	58.50	6.11	61.10	152.10	1791.40	13.00	0.96
0.26	0.12	0.00	0.00	1.38	404.55	15.50	0.05	0.06	0.93	0.08	13.33	0.00	21.70	0.84	12.40	29.45	458.80	1.55	0.40
0.10	0.05	0.00	0.00	2.15	406.56	21.78	0.05	0.10	1.94	0.15	4.11	0.00	24.20	2.18	21.78	45.98	554.18	9.68	0.24
0.00	0.06	0.00	0.00	0.16	15.12	8.40	0.06	0.06	0.84	0.09	42.84	0.00	37.80	1.08	50.40	72.24	297.36	278.04	0.41
0.00	0.06	0.00	0.00	0.16	15.12	8.40	0.06	0.06	0.84	0.09	42.84	0.00	37.80	1.08	50.40	72.24	297.36	79.80	0.41
0.01	0.13	0.00	0.00	0.00	48.60	9.72	0.11	0.12	0.97	0.11	131.40	0.00	18.00	0.66	9.00	48.60	144.00	216.00	0.38
0.05	0.68	0.00	0.00	1.04	128.26	44.53	0.15	0.24	2.30	0.27	231.35	0.00	38.72	4.43	24.20	104.06	416.24	694.54	0.97
0.01	0.12	0.00	52.26	2.68	77.72	17.69	0.19	0.17	1.57	0.17	171.52	0.00	28.14	1.17	24.12	75.04	365.82	2.68	0.62
0.02	0.32	0.00	0.00	2.25	147.60	43.92	0.13	0.18	1.87	0.04	242.46	0.00	41.40	1.15	23.40	99.00	392.40	7.20	1.01
14.42	2.94	0.00	0.00	2.01	91.50	11.85	0.17	0.18	2.88	0.42	92.85	0.00	16.50	1.53	58.50	61.50	898.50	15.00	0.63
0.01	0.24	0.00	0.00	0.50	1.31	1.44	0.04	0.04	0.18	0.18	4.19	0.00	10.48	0.42	5.24	32.75	104.80	9.17	0.85
0.02	0.20	0.00	0.00	1.51	3.02	6.04	0.23	0.11	0.91	0.36	10.72	0.00	19.63	0.76	4.53	89.09	804.83	6.04	1.66
0.15	0.34	0.00	0.00	0.00	31.00	7.00	0.18	0.24	2.80	0.44	14.00	0.00	22.00	1.15	108.00	74.00	1491.00	3.00	0.61
0.09	0.20	0.00	1.13	0.61	18.00	20.48	0.11	0.23	1.22	1.31	42.98	0.00	13.50	0.70	65.25	45.00	891.00	2.25	0.36
0.00	0.00	0.00	0.00	0.00	2.67	16.00	0.56	0.25	1.47	0.22	169.87	0.00	109.33	0.53	128.00	288.00	756.00	333.33	2.80
0.00	0.07	0.00	0.00	0.19	47.25	6.48	0.03	0.08	0.27	0.05	42.93	0.00	35.10	1.22	17.55	25.65	147.15	353.70	0.39
0.01	0.07	0.00	30.80	0.45	73.70	17.93	0.09	0.12	0.83	0.08	40.15	0.00	40.70	1.14	27.50	41.80	229.90	6.60	0.26

USDA ID Code	Food Name	Weight in Grams*	Quantity of Units	Unit of Measure	Protein (gm)	Fat (gm)	Carbohydrate (gm)	Kcalories	Caffeine (gm)	Fiber (gm)	Cholesterol (mg)	Saturated Fat (gm)
	Beans, Green, Fzn	135.0000	1.000	Cup	2.01	0.23	8.71	37.80	0.00	4.05	0.00	0.05
	Beans, Lima, Fzn	311.0000	1.250	Cup	20.68	0.93	60.49	326.55	0.00	18.66	0.00	0.22
	Beans, Yellow, Cnd	135.0000	1.000	Cup	1.55	0.14	6.08	27.00	0.00	1.76	0.00	0.03
	Beans, Yellow, Fresh	110.0000	1.000	Cup	2.00	0.13	7.85	34.10	0.00	3.74	0.00	0.03
	Beets, Ckd	85.0000	0.500	Cup	1.43	0.15	8.47	37.40	0.00	1.70	0.00	0.03
	Blueberries, Cnd, Heavy Syrup	256.0000	1.000	Cup	1.66	0.84	56.47	225.28	0.00	3.84	0.00	0.08
	Blueberries, Fresh	145.0000	1.000	Cup	0.97	0.55	20.49	81.20	0.00	3.92	0.00	0.04
	Blueberries, Frozen, Sweetened	230.0000	1.000	Cup	0.92	0.30	50.49	186.30	0.00	4.83	0.00	0.02
	Blueberries, Frozen, Unsweetened	155.0000	1.000	Cup	0.65	0.99	18.86	79.05	0.00	4.19	0.00	0.08
	Broccoli, Ckd	280.0000	1.000	Cup	8.34	0.98	14.17	78.40	0.00	8.12	0.00	0.14
	Broccoli, Flower Clusters, Fresh	71.0000	1.000	Cup	2.12	0.25	3.72	19.88	0.00	0.00	0.00	0.04
	Broccoli, Frz, Chopped, Ckd	184.0000	1.000	Cup	5.70	0.22	9.84	51.52	0.00	5.52	0.00	0.04
	Brussels Sprouts, Ckd	21.0000	1.000	Each	0.54	0.11	1.82	8.19	0.00	0.55	0.00	0.02
	Cabbage, Chinese (pak-choi)	70.0000	1.000	Cup	1.05	0.14	1.56	9.10	0.00	0.70	0.00	0.02
	Cabbage, Ckd		1.000	Head	12.87	5.43	56.29	277.64	0.00	29.03	0.00	0.63
	Cabbage, Fresh	908.0000	1.000	Head	10.99	1.63	48.76	217.92	0.00	20.88	0.00	0.18
	Carrots, Baby, Fresh	15.0000	1.000	Large	0.13	0.08	1.22	5.70	0.00	0.27	0.00	0.01
135	Carrots, Ckd	156.0000	1.000	Cup	1.70	0.28	16.35	70.20	0.00	5.15	0.00	0.05
	Carrots, Cnd, Reg Pk	228.0000	1.000	Cup	1.46	0.43	12.63	57.00	0.00	3.42	0.00	0.09
	Carrots, Fresh	128.0000	1.000	Cup	1.32	0.24	12.98	55.04	0.00	3.84	0.00	0.04
	Carrots, Frz, Ckd	146.0000	0.500	Cup	1.74	0.16	12.05	52.56	0.00	5.11	0.00	0.03
	Cauliflower, Ckd, Boiled	62.0000	0.500	Cup	1.14	0.28	2.55	14.26	0.00	1.67	0.00	0.04
	Cauliflower, Fresh	100.0000	0.500	Cup	1.98	0.21	5.20	25.00	0.00	2.50	0.00	0.03
	Cauliflower, Frz, Ckd	180.0000	1.000	Cup	2.90	0.40	6.75	34.20	0.00	4.86	0.00	0.05
	Celery, Ckd	150.0000	1.000	Cup	1.25	0.24	6.02	27.00	0.00	2.40	0.00	0.06
	Celery, Fresh	120.0000	1.000	Cup	0.90	0.17	4.38	19.20	0.00	2.04	0.00	0.05
	Cherries, Sour, Red, Cnd, Heavy	256.0000	1.000	Cup	1.87	0.26	59.57	232.96	0.00	2.82	0.00	0.05
	Cherries, Sour, Red, Cnd, Light	252.0000	1.000	Cup	1.86	0.25	48.64	189.00	0.00	2.02	0.00	0.05
	Cherries, Sour, Red, Cnd, Water	244.0000	1.000	Cup	1.88	0.24	21.81	87.84	0.00	2.68	0.00	0.05
	Cherries, Sour, Red, Cnd, X-heav	261.0000	1.000	Cup	1.85	0.23	76.29	297.54	0.00	2.09	0.00	0.05
	Cherries, Sour, Red, Fresh	155.0000	1.000	Cup	1.55	0.47	18.88	77.50	0.00	2.48	0.00	0.11
	Cherries, Sweet, Cnd, Heavy Syru	253.0000	1.000	Cup	1.52	0.38	53.81	209.99	0.00	3.80	0.00	0.08
	Cherries, Sweet, Cnd, Juice Pack	250.0000	1.000	Cup	2.28	0.05	34.53	135.00	0.00	3.75	0.00	0.00
	Cherries, Sweet, Cnd, Light Syru	252.0000	1.000	Cup	1.54	0.38	43.57	168.84	0.00	3.78	0.00	0.08
	Cherries, Sweet, Cnd, Water Pack	248.0000	1.000	Cup	1.91	0.32	29.16	114.08	0.00	3.72	0.00	0.07
	Cherries, Sweet, Cnd, X-heavy Sy	261.0000	1.000	Cup	1.54	0.39	68.46	266.22	0.00	3.92	0.00	0.08
	Cherries, Sweet, Fresh	117.0000	1.000	Cup	1.40	1.12	19.36	84.24	0.00	2.69	0.00	0.26
	Cherries, Sweet, Frozen, Sweeten	259.0000	1.000	Cup	2.98	0.34	57.91	230.51	0.00	5.44	0.00	0.08
	Chives, Raw	1.0000	1.000	Tsp	0.03	0.01	0.04	0.30	0.00	0.03	0.00	0.00
	Coleslaw	8.0000	1.000	Tbsp	0.10	0.21	0.99	5.52	0.00	0.12	0.64	0.03
	Collards, Ckd	190.0000	1.000	Cup	4.01	0.68	9.31	49.40	0.00	5.32	0.00	0.10
	Collards, Fresh	36.0000	1.000	Cup	0.88	0.15	2.05	10.80	0.00	1.30	0.00	0.02
	Collards, Frz, Chopped, Ckd	170.0000	1.000	Cup	5.05	0.70	12.09	61.20	0.00	4.76	0.00	0.10
	Corn, Ckd	140.0000	1.000	Cup	3.68	1.02	39.07	176.40	0.00	6.72	0.00	0.14
	Corn, Sweet, White, Ckd	77.0000	1.000	Cup	2.56	0.99	19.33	83.16	0.00	2.08	0.00	0.15
	Corn, Sweet, White, Cnd	164.0000	1.000	Cup	4.30	1.64	30.49	132.84	0.00	3.28	0.00	0.25
	Corn, Sweet, White, Cnd, Cream S	256.0000	1.000	Cup	4.45	1.08	46.41	184.32	0.00	3.07	0.00	0.18
	Corn, Sweet, White, Fresh	154.0000	1.000	Cup	4.96	1.82	29.29	132.44	0.00	4.16	0.00	0.28
	Corn, Sweet, Yellow, Ckd	164.0000	1.000	Cup	5.44	2.10	41.18	177.12	0.00	4.59	0.00	0.33
	Corn, Sweet, Yellow, Cnd, Brine	164.0000	1.000	Cup	4.30	1.64	30.49	132.84	0.00	3.28	0.00	0.25
	Corn, Sweet, Yellow, Cnd, Cream	256.0000	1.000	Cup	4.45	1.08	46.41	184.32	0.00	3.07	0.00	0.18
	Corn, Sweet, Yellow, Fresh	154.0000	1.000	Cup	4.96	1.82	29.29	132.44	0.00	4.16	0.00	0.28
	Crabapples, Fresh	110.0000	1.000	Cup	0.44	0.33	21.95	83.60	0.00	0.00	0.00	0.06
	Cranberries, Fresh	110.0000	1.000	Cup	0.43	0.22	13.95	53.90	0.00	4.62	0.00	0.02
	Cranberry Sauce, Cnd, Sweetened	277.0000	1.000	Cup	0.55	0.42	107.75	418.27	0.00	2.77	0.00	0.03

Monounsaturated Fat (gm)	Polyunsaturated Fat (gm)	Vitamin D (mg)	Vitamin K (mg)	Vitamin E (mg)	Vitamin A (re)	Vitamin C (mg)	Thiamin (mg)	Riboflavin (mg)	Niacin (mg)	Vitamin B_6 (mg)	Folate (mg)	Vitamin B_{12} (mcg)	Calcium (mg)	Iron (mg)	Magnesium (mg)	Phosphorus (mg)	Potassium (mg)	Sodium (mg)	Zinc (mg)
0.01	0.11	0.00	0.00	0.19	54.00	5.54	0.05	0.12	0.51	0.08	31.05	0.00	66.15	1.19	32.40	41.85	170.10	12.15	0.65
0.06	0.47	0.00	0.00	1.99	52.87	18.04	0.22	0.19	2.39	0.37	48.21	0.00	87.08	6.10	174.16	348.32	1278.21	90.19	1.71
0.00	0.07	0.00	0.00	0.39	14.85	6.48	0.03	0.08	0.27	0.05	42.93	0.00	35.10	1.22	17.55	25.65	147.15	338.85	0.39
0.01	0.07	0.00	0.00	0.00	12.10	17.93	0.09	0.12	0.83	0.08	40.15	0.00	40.70	1.14	27.50	41.80	229.90	6.60	0.26
0.03	0.05	0.00	0.00	0.26	3.40	3.06	0.03	0.03	0.28	0.06	68.00	0.00	13.60	0.67	19.55	32.30	259.25	65.45	0.30
0.13	0.36	0.00	1.28	2.56	15.36	2.82	0.08	0.13	0.28	0.10	4.10	0.00	12.80	0.84	10.24	25.60	102.40	7.68	0.18
0.07	0.25	0.00	0.00	1.45	14.50	18.85	0.07	0.07	0.52	0.06	9.28	0.00	8.70	0.25	7.25	14.50	129.05	8.70	0.16
0.05	0.14	0.00	0.00	1.63	9.20	2.30	0.05	0.12	0.58	0.14	15.41	0.00	13.80	0.90	4.60	16.10	138.00	2.30	0.14
0.14	0.43	0.00	0.00	1.55	12.40	3.88	0.05	0.06	0.81	0.09	10.39	0.00	12.40	0.28	7.75	17.05	83.70	1.55	0.11
0.06	0.48	0.00	0.00	4.73	389.20	208.88	0.17	0.31	1.60	0.39	140.00	0.00	128.80	2.35	67.20	165.20	817.60	72.80	1.06
0.01	0.12	0.00	0.00	1.18	213.00	66.17	0.05	0.09	0.45	0.11	50.41	0.00	34.08	0.62	17.75	46.86	230.75	19.17	0.28
0.02	0.11	0.00	0.00	3.04	347.76	73.78	0.11	0.15	0.85	0.24	103.78	0.00	93.84	1.12	36.80	101.20	331.20	44.16	0.55
0.01	0.05	0.00	0.00	0.18	15.12	13.02	0.02	0.02	0.13	0.04	12.60	0.00	7.56	0.25	4.20	11.76	66.57	4.41	0.07
0.01	0.07	0.00	0.00	0.08	210.00	31.50	0.03	0.05	0.35	0.14	45.99	0.00	73.50	0.56	13.30	25.90	176.40	45.50	0.13
0.38	2.52	0.00	0.00	1.39	164.06	253.66	0.76	0.76	3.53	1.39	252.40	0.00	391.22	2.15	100.96	189.30	1224.14	100.96	1.14
0.09	0.82	0.00	0.00	0.00	118.04	463.08	0.45	0.27	2.72	0.91	514.84	0.00	426.76	5.08	136.20	208.84	2233.68	163.44	1.63
0.00	0.04	0.00	0.00	0.00	225.15	1.26	0.00	0.01	0.13	0.01	4.95	0.00	3.45	0.12	1.80	5.70	41.85	5.25	0.02
0.01	0.14	0.00	0.00	0.66	3829.80	3.59	0.05	0.09	0.79	0.38	21.68	0.00	48.36	0.97	20.28	46.80	354.12	102.96	0.47
0.02	0.21	0.00	0.00	0.96	3139.56	6.16	0.05	0.07	1.25	0.25	20.98	0.00	57.00	1.46	18.24	54.72	408.12	551.76	0.59
0.01	0.10	0.00	16.64	0.59	3600.64	11.90	0.13	0.08	1.19	0.19	17.92	0.00	34.56	0.64	19.20	56.32	413.44	44.80	0.26
0.01	0.07	0.00	0.00	0.61	2584.20	4.09	0.04	0.06	0.64	0.19	15.77	0.00	40.88	0.69	14.60	37.96	230.68	86.14	0.35
0.02	0.14	0.00	0.00	0.02	1.24	27.47	0.02	0.03	0.25	0.11	27.28	0.00	9.92	0.20	5.58	19.84	88.04	9.30	0.11
0.01	0.10	0.00	191.00	0.04	2.00	46.40	0.06	0.06	0.53	0.22	57.00	0.00	22.00	0.44	15.00	44.00	303.00	30.00	0.28
0.04	0.18	0.00	0.00	0.07	3.60	56.34	0.07	0.09	0.56	0.16	73.80	0.00	30.60	0.74	16.20	43.20	250.20	32.40	0.23
0.05	0.12	0.00	0.00	0.54	19.50	9.15	0.06	0.08	0.48	0.14	33.00	0.00	63.00	0.63	18.00	37.50	426.00	136.50	0.21
0.04	0.08	0.00	0.00	0.43	15.60	8.40	0.06	0.06	0.38	0.11	33.60	0.00	48.00	0.48	13.20	30.00	344.40	104.40	0.16
0.08	0.08	0.00	0.00	0.33	181.76	5.12	0.05	0.10	0.44	0.10	19.46	0.00	25.60	3.33	15.36	25.60	238.08	17.92	0.15
0.08	0.08	0.00	0.00	0.00	183.96	5.04	0.05	0.10	0.43	0.10	19.40	0.00	25.20	3.33	15.12	25.20	239.40	17.64	0.18
0.07	0.07	0.00	0.00	0.32	183.00	5.12	0.05	0.10	0.44	0.10	19.52	0.00	26.84	3.34	14.64	24.40	239.12	17.08	0.17
0.08	0.08	0.00	0.00	0.00	182.70	4.96	0.05	0.10	0.42	0.10	19.31	0.00	26.10	3.29	13.05	23.49	237.51	18.27	0.16
0.12	0.14	0.00	0.00	0.20	198.40	15.50	0.05	0.06	0.62	0.06	11.63	0.00	24.80	0.50	13.95	23.25	268.15	4.65	0.16
0.10	0.13	0.00	0.00	0.15	37.95	9.11	0.05	0.10	1.01	0.08	10.63	0.00	22.77	0.89	22.77	45.54	366.85	7.59	0.25
0.03	0.03	0.00	0.00	0.25	32.50	6.25	0.05	0.05	1.03	0.08	10.50	0.00	35.00	1.45	30.00	55.00	327.50	7.50	0.25
0.10	0.13	0.00	0.00	0.33	40.32	9.32	0.05	0.10	1.01	0.08	10.58	0.00	22.68	0.91	22.68	45.36	372.96	7.56	0.25
0.07	0.10	0.00	0.00	0.32	39.68	5.46	0.05	0.10	1.02	0.07	10.42	0.00	27.28	0.89	22.32	37.20	324.88	2.48	0.20
0.10	0.13	0.00	0.00	0.00	39.15	9.40	0.05	0.10	1.02	0.08	10.96	0.00	23.49	0.91	20.88	44.37	370.62	7.83	0.26
0.30	0.34	0.00	0.00	0.15	24.57	8.19	0.06	0.07	0.47	0.05	4.91	0.00	17.55	0.46	12.87	22.23	262.08	0.00	0.07
0.10	0.10	0.00	0.00	0.34	49.21	2.59	0.08	0.13	0.47	0.10	10.88	0.00	31.08	0.91	25.90	41.44	515.41	2.59	0.10
0.00	0.00	0.00	0.00	0.00	4.35	0.58	0.00	0.00	0.01	0.00	1.05	0.00	0.92	0.02	0.42	0.58	2.96	0.03	0.01
0.06	0.11	0.00	0.00	0.00	6.56	2.62	0.01	0.00	0.02	0.01	2.12	0.00	3.60	0.05	0.80	2.56	14.48	1.84	0.02
0.06	0.32	0.00	0.00	1.67	594.70	34.58	0.08	0.21	1.10	0.25	176.70	0.00	226.10	0.87	32.30	49.40	494.00	17.10	0.80
0.01	0.07	0.00	0.00	0.81	137.52	12.71	0.02	0.05	0.27	0.06	59.76	0.00	52.20	0.07	3.24	3.60	60.84	7.20	0.05
0.03	0.36	0.00	0.00	0.85	1016.60	44.88	0.09	0.20	1.09	0.19	129.37	0.00	357.00	1.90	51.00	45.90	426.70	85.00	0.46
0.27	0.46	0.00	0.00	0.46	8.40	0.00	0.07	0.03	0.78	0.08	8.40	0.00	1.40	0.35	50.40	106.40	43.40	0.00	0.88
0.28	0.46	0.00	0.00	0.07	0.00	4.77	0.17	0.05	1.24	0.05	35.73	0.00	1.54	0.47	24.64	79.31	191.73	13.09	0.37
0.48	0.77	0.00	0.00	0.15	0.00	13.94	0.05	0.13	1.97	0.08	79.70	0.00	8.20	1.41	32.80	106.60	319.80	529.72	0.64
0.31	0.51	0.00	0.00	0.23	0.00	11.78	0.08	0.13	2.46	0.15	114.69	0.00	7.68	0.97	43.52	130.56	343.04	729.60	1.36
0.54	0.86	0.00	0.00	0.14	0.00	10.47	0.31	0.09	2.62	0.09	70.53	0.00	3.08	0.80	56.98	137.06	415.80	23.10	0.69
0.61	0.98	0.00	0.00	0.15	36.08	10.17	0.36	0.11	2.64	0.10	76.10	0.00	3.28	1.00	52.48	168.92	408.36	27.88	0.79
0.48	0.77	0.00	0.00	0.25	26.24	13.94	0.05	0.13	1.97	0.08	79.70	0.00	8.20	1.41	32.80	106.60	319.80	350.96	0.64
0.31	0.51	0.00	0.00	0.23	25.60	11.78	0.08	0.13	2.46	0.15	114.69	0.00	7.68	0.97	43.52	130.56	343.04	729.60	1.36
0.54	0.86	0.00	10.78	0.14	43.12	10.47	0.31	0.09	2.62	0.09	70.53	0.00	3.08	0.80	56.98	137.06	415.80	23.10	0.69
0.01	0.10	0.00	0.00	0.00	4.40	8.80	0.03	0.02	0.11	0.00	0.00	0.00	19.80	0.40	7.70	16.50	213.40	1.10	0.00
0.03	0.10	0.00	0.00	0.11	5.50	14.85	0.03	0.02	0.11	0.08	1.87	0.00	7.70	0.22	5.50	9.90	78.10	1.10	0.14
0.06	0.19	0.00	3.88	0.28	5.54	5.54	0.06	0.06	0.28	0.03	2.77	0.00	11.08	0.61	8.31	16.62	72.02	80.33	0.14

USDA ID Code	Food Name	Weight in Grams*	Quantity of Units	Unit of Measure	Protein (gm)	Fat (gm)	Carbohydrate (gm)	Kcalories	Caffeine (gm)	Fiber (gm)	Cholesterol (mg)	Saturated Fat (gm)
	Cranberry-orange Relish, Cnd	275.0000	1.000	Cup	0.83	0.28	127.05	489.50	0.00	0.00	0.00	0.03
	Cucumber, Fresh	52.0000	0.500	Cup	0.36	0.07	1.44	6.76	0.00	0.42	0.00	0.02
	Dates, Domestic, Natural and Dry	178.0000	1.000	Cup	3.51	0.80	130.85	489.50	0.00	13.35	0.00	0.34
	Eggplant, Ckd	99.0000	1.000	Cup	0.82	0.23	6.57	27.72	0.00	2.48	0.00	0.04
	Eggplant, Fresh	82.0000	1.000	Cup	0.84	0.15	4.98	21.32	0.00	2.05	0.00	0.02
	Endive, Raw	25.0000	0.500	Cup	0.31	0.05	0.84	4.25	0.00	0.78	0.00	0.01
	Fruit Salad, Heavy Syrup	255.0000	1.000	Cup	0.87	0.18	48.73	186.15	0.00	2.55	0.00	0.03
	Fruit Salad, Juice Pack	249.0000	1.000	Cup	1.27	0.07	32.49	124.50	0.00	2.49	0.00	0.00
	Fruit Salad, Light Syrup	252.0000	1.000	Cup	0.86	0.18	38.15	146.16	0.00	2.52	0.00	0.03
	Fruit Salad, Water Pack	245.0000	1.000	Cup	0.86	0.17	19.28	73.50	0.00	2.45	0.00	0.02
	Fruit, Heavy Syrup	248.0000	1.000	Cup	0.97	0.17	46.90	181.04	0.00	2.48	0.00	0.02
	Fruit, Juice Pack	237.0000	1.000	Cup	1.09	0.02	28.11	109.02	0.00	2.37	0.00	0.00
	Fruit, Light Syrup	242.0000	1.000	Cup	0.97	0.17	36.13	137.94	0.00	2.42	0.00	0.02
	Fruit, Mixed, Dried	293.0000	1.250	Cup	7.21	1.44	187.70	711.99	0.00	22.85	0.00	0.12
	Fruit, Mixed, Frzn, Swtnd, Thawd	250.0000	1.000	Cup	3.55	0.45	60.58	245.00	0.00	4.75	0.00	0.08
	Fruit, Mixed, Hvy Syrup	255.0000	1.000	Cup	0.94	0.26	47.84	183.60	0.00	2.55	0.00	0.03
	Fruit, Water Pack	237.0000	1.000	Cup	1.00	0.12	20.17	75.84	0.00	2.37	0.00	0.02
	Garlic, Raw	3.0000	1.000	Clove	0.19	0.02	0.99	4.47	0.00	0.06	0.00	0.00
	Grapefruit, Fresh, Pink & Red	230.0000	1.000	Cup	1.27	0.23	17.66	69.00	0.00	0.00	0.00	0.02
	Grapefruit, Fresh, White	230.0000	1.000	Cup	1.59	0.23	19.34	75.90	0.00	2.53	0.00	0.02
	Grapefruit, Sections, Cnd, Juice	249.0000	1.000	Cup	1.74	0.22	22.93	92.13	0.00	1.00	0.00	0.02
	Grapefruit, Sections, Cnd, Light	254.0000	1.000	Cup	1.42	0.25	39.22	152.40	0.00	1.02	0.00	0.03
	Grapefruit, Sections, Cnd, Water	244.0000	1.000	Cup	1.42	0.24	22.33	87.84	0.00	0.98	0.00	0.02
	Grapes, Fresh	92.0000	1.000	Cup	0.58	0.32	15.78	61.64	0.00	0.92	0.00	0.10
	Kiwifruit, Fresh	177.0000	1.000	Cup	1.75	0.78	26.34	107.97	0.00	6.02	0.00	0.05
	Leeks, Ckd	124.0000	1.000	Leek	1.00	0.25	9.45	38.44	0.00	1.24	0.00	0.04
	Leeks, Fresh	89.0000	1.000	Cup	1.34	0.27	12.59	54.29	0.00	1.60	0.00	0.04
	Lemons, Fresh, w/o Peel	212.0000	1.000	Cup	2.33	0.64	19.76	61.48	0.00	5.94	0.00	0.08
	Lettuce, Butterhead, Fresh	55.0000	1.000	Cup	0.71	0.12	1.28	7.15	0.00	0.55	0.00	0.02
	Lettuce, Iceberg, Fresh	55.0000	1.000	Cup	0.56	0.10	1.15	6.60	0.00	0.77	0.00	0.02
	Lettuce, Looseleaf, Fresh	10.0000	1.000	Leaf	0.13	0.03	0.35	1.80	0.00	0.19	0.00	0.00
	Lettuce, Romaine, Fresh	10.0000	1.000	Leaf	0.16	0.02	0.24	1.40	0.00	0.17	0.00	0.00
	Lime, Raw	67.0000	1.000	Medium	0.47	0.13	7.06	20.10	0.00	1.88	0.00	0.02
	Mangos, Fresh	165.0000	0.500	Cup	0.84	0.45	28.05	107.25	0.00	2.97	0.00	0.12
	Melon Balls, Frozen, Unthawed	173.0000	1.000	Cup	1.45	0.43	13.74	57.09	0.00	1.21	0.00	0.10
	Melons, Cantaloupe, Fresh	177.0000	1.000	Cup	1.56	0.50	14.80	61.95	0.00	1.42	0.00	0.12
	Melons, Casaba, Fresh	170.0000	1.000	Cup	1.53	0.17	10.54	44.20	0.00	1.36	0.00	0.05
	Melons, Honeydew, Fresh	177.0000	1.000	Cup	0.81	0.18	16.25	61.95	0.00	1.06	0.00	0.05
	Mushrooms, Ckd	156.0000	1.000	Cup	3.39	0.73	8.02	42.12	0.00	3.43	0.00	0.09
	Mushrooms, Cnd, Drained Solids	156.0000	1.000	Cup	2.92	0.45	7.74	37.44	0.00	3.74	0.00	0.06
	Mushrooms, Enoki, Fresh	5.0000	1.000	Large	0.12	0.02	0.35	1.70	0.00	0.13	0.00	0.00
	Mushrooms, Fresh	70.0000	1.000	Cup	2.03	0.23	2.86	17.50	0.00	0.84	0.00	0.04
	Mushrooms, Shiitake, Ckd	145.0000	1.000	Cup	2.26	0.32	20.71	79.75	0.00	3.05	0.00	0.09
	Mushrooms, Shiitake, Dried	3.6000	1.000	Medium	0.34	0.04	2.71	10.66	0.00	0.41	0.00	0.01
	Nectar, Apricot, Cnd, w/ Added V	251.0000	1.000	Cup	0.93	0.23	36.12	140.56	0.00	1.51	0.00	0.03
	Nectar, Apricot, Cnd, w/o Vit C	251.0000	1.000	Cup	0.93	0.23	36.12	140.56	0.00	1.51	0.00	0.03
	Nectar, Papaya, Cnd.	250.0000	1.000	Cup	0.43	0.38	36.28	142.50	0.00	1.50	0.00	0.13
	Nectar, Peach, Cnd, wo/ Added Vi	249.0000	1.000	Cup	0.67	0.05	34.66	134.46	0.00	1.49	0.00	0.00
	Nectarine, Raw	136.0000	1.000	Medium	1.28	0.63	16.02	66.64	0.00	2.18	0.00	0.07
	Okra, Ckd	80.0000	0.500	Cup	1.50	0.14	5.77	25.60	0.00	2.00	0.00	0.04
	Okra, Fresh	100.0000	1.000	Cup	2.00	0.10	7.63	33.00	0.00	3.20	0.00	0.03
	Okra, Frz, Ckd	255.0000	1.250	Cup	5.30	0.77	14.66	71.40	0.00	7.14	0.00	0.20
	Okra, Frz, Unprepared	284.0000	1.250	Cup	4.80	0.71	18.86	85.20	0.00	6.25	0.00	0.20
	Olives, Green	3.0000	5.000	Each	0.00	0.50	0.00	5.00	0.00	0.00	0.00	0.00
	Olives, Ripe, Canned (jumbo-supe	8.3000	1.000	Jumbo	0.08	0.57	0.47	6.72	0.00	0.21	0.00	0.08

Monounsaturated Fat (gm)	Polyunsaturated Fat (gm)	Vitamin D (mg)	Vitamin K (mg)	Vitamin E (mg)	Vitamin A (re)	Vitamin C (mg)	Thiamin (mg)	Riboflavin (mg)	Niacin (mg)	Vitamin B_6 (mg)	Folate (mg)	Vitamin B_{12} (mcg)	Calcium (mg)	Iron (mg)	Magnesium (mg)	Phosphorus (mg)	Potassium (mg)	Sodium (mg)	Zinc (mg)
0.00	0.00	0.00	0.00	0.00	19.25	49.50	0.08	0.06	0.28	0.00	0.00	0.00	30.25	0.55	11.00	22.00	104.50	88.00	0.00
0.00	0.03	0.00	2.60	0.04	10.92	2.76	0.01	0.01	0.11	0.02	6.76	0.00	7.28	0.14	5.72	10.40	74.88	1.04	0.10
0.27	0.05	0.00	0.00	0.18	8.90	0.00	0.16	0.18	3.92	0.34	22.43	0.00	56.96	2.05	62.30	71.20	1160.56	5.34	0.52
0.02	0.09	0.00	0.00	0.03	5.94	1.29	0.08	0.02	0.59	0.09	14.26	0.00	5.94	0.35	12.87	21.78	245.52	2.97	0.15
0.02	0.07	0.00	0.00	0.02	6.56	1.39	0.04	0.02	0.49	0.07	15.58	0.00	5.74	0.22	11.48	18.04	177.94	2.46	0.11
0.00	0.02	0.00	0.00	0.11	51.25	1.63	0.02	0.02	0.10	0.01	35.50	0.00	13.00	0.21	3.75	7.00	78.50	5.50	0.20
0.03	0.08	0.00	0.00	1.17	127.50	6.12	0.05	0.05	0.89	0.08	6.38	0.00	15.30	0.71	12.75	22.95	204.00	15.30	0.18
0.02	0.02	0.00	0.00	0.00	149.40	8.22	0.02	0.02	0.90	0.07	6.47	0.00	27.39	0.62	19.92	34.86	288.84	12.45	0.35
0.03	0.08	0.00	0.00	0.00	108.36	6.30	0.03	0.05	0.93	0.08	6.55	0.00	17.64	0.73	12.60	22.68	206.64	15.12	0.18
0.02	0.07	0.00	0.00	0.00	107.80	4.66	0.05	0.05	0.91	0.07	6.37	0.00	17.15	0.74	12.25	22.05	191.10	7.35	0.20
0.02	0.07	0.00	0.00	0.72	49.60	4.71	0.05	0.05	0.92	0.12	6.45	0.00	14.88	0.72	12.40	27.28	218.24	14.88	0.20
0.00	0.00	0.00	0.00	0.47	73.47	6.40	0.02	0.05	0.95	0.12	5.93	0.00	18.96	0.50	16.59	33.18	225.15	9.48	0.21
0.02	0.07	0.00	0.00	0.70	50.82	4.60	0.05	0.05	0.92	0.12	6.53	0.00	14.52	0.70	12.10	26.62	215.38	14.52	0.22
0.67	0.32	0.00	0.00	0.00	714.92	11.13	0.12	0.47	5.65	0.47	11.43	0.00	111.34	7.94	114.27	225.61	2332.28	52.74	1.47
0.08	0.20	0.00	0.00	0.00	80.00	187.50	0.05	0.10	1.00	0.08	19.00	0.00	17.50	0.70	15.00	30.00	327.50	7.50	0.13
0.05	0.10	0.00	0.00	0.00	48.45	175.95	0.05	0.10	1.53	0.10	7.65	0.00	2.55	0.92	12.75	25.50	214.20	10.20	0.18
0.02	0.05	0.00	0.00	0.69	59.25	4.98	0.05	0.02	0.85	0.12	6.40	0.00	11.85	0.59	16.59	26.07	222.78	9.48	0.21
0.00	0.01	0.00	0.00	0.00	0.00	0.94	0.01	0.00	0.02	0.04	0.09	0.00	5.43	0.05	0.75	4.59	12.03	0.51	0.04
0.02	0.05	0.00	0.00	0.00	59.80	87.63	0.07	0.05	0.44	0.09	28.06	0.00	25.30	0.28	18.40	20.70	296.70	0.00	0.16
0.02	0.05	0.00	0.00	0.58	2.30	76.59	0.09	0.05	0.62	0.09	23.00	0.00	27.60	0.14	20.70	18.40	340.40	0.00	0.16
0.02	0.05	0.00	0.00	0.62	0.00	84.41	0.07	0.05	0.62	0.05	21.91	0.00	37.35	0.52	27.39	29.88	420.81	17.43	0.20
0.03	0.05	0.00	0.00	0.64	0.00	54.10	0.10	0.05	0.61	0.05	21.59	0.00	35.56	1.02	25.40	25.40	327.66	5.08	0.20
0.02	0.05	0.00	0.00	0.61	0.00	53.19	0.10	0.05	0.61	0.05	21.47	0.00	36.60	1.00	24.40	24.40	322.08	4.88	0.22
0.01	0.09	0.00	0.00	0.31	9.20	3.68	0.08	0.06	0.28	0.10	3.59	0.00	12.88	0.27	4.60	9.20	175.72	1.84	0.04
0.07	0.42	0.00	0.00	1.98	31.86	173.46	0.04	0.09	0.89	0.16	67.26	0.00	46.02	0.73	53.10	70.80	587.64	8.85	0.30
0.00	0.14	0.00	0.00	0.00	6.20	5.21	0.04	0.02	0.25	0.14	30.13	0.00	37.20	1.36	17.36	21.08	107.88	12.40	0.07
0.00	0.15	0.00	0.00	0.82	8.90	10.68	0.05	0.03	0.36	0.20	57.05	0.00	52.51	1.87	24.92	31.15	160.20	17.80	0.11
0.02	0.19	0.00	0.00	0.51	6.36	112.36	0.08	0.04	0.21	0.17	22.47	0.00	55.12	1.27	16.96	33.92	292.56	4.24	0.13
0.01	0.07	0.00	0.00	0.24	53.35	4.40	0.03	0.03	0.17	0.03	40.32	0.00	17.60	0.17	7.15	12.65	141.35	2.75	0.09
0.01	0.06	0.00	62.15	0.15	18.15	2.15	0.03	0.02	0.10	0.02	30.80	0.00	10.45	0.28	4.95	11.00	86.90	4.95	0.12
0.00	0.02	0.00	0.00	0.04	19.00	1.80	0.01	0.01	0.04	0.01	4.98	0.00	6.80	0.14	1.10	2.50	26.40	0.90	0.03
0.00	0.01	0.00	0.00	0.04	26.00	2.40	0.01	0.01	0.05	0.01	13.57	0.00	3.60	0.11	0.60	4.50	29.00	0.80	0.03
0.01	0.04	0.00	0.00	0.16	0.67	19.49	0.02	0.01	0.13	0.03	5.49	0.00	22.11	0.40	4.02	12.06	68.34	1.34	0.07
0.17	0.08	0.00	0.00	1.85	641.85	45.71	0.10	0.10	0.96	0.21	23.10	0.00	16.50	0.21	14.85	18.15	257.40	3.30	0.07
0.02	0.17	0.00	0.00	0.26	306.21	10.73	0.29	0.03	1.11	0.19	44.46	0.00	17.30	0.50	24.22	20.76	484.40	53.63	0.29
0.02	0.19	0.00	0.00	0.27	569.94	74.69	0.07	0.04	1.01	0.21	30.09	0.00	19.47	0.37	19.47	30.09	546.93	15.93	0.28
0.00	0.07	0.00	0.00	0.26	5.10	27.20	0.10	0.03	0.68	0.20	28.90	0.00	8.50	0.68	13.60	11.90	357.00	20.40	0.27
0.00	0.07	0.00	0.00	0.27	7.08	43.90	0.14	0.04	1.06	0.11	10.62	0.00	10.62	0.12	12.39	17.70	479.67	17.70	0.12
0.02	0.28	0.00	0.00	0.19	0.00	6.24	0.11	0.47	6.96	0.16	28.39	0.00	9.36	2.71	18.72	135.72	555.36	3.12	1.36
0.02	0.17	0.00	0.00	0.19	0.00	0.00	0.14	0.03	2.48	0.09	19.19	0.00	17.16	1.23	23.40	102.96	201.24	663.00	1.12
0.00	0.01	0.00	0.00	0.00	0.05	0.60	0.00	0.01	0.18	0.00	1.50	0.00	0.05	0.04	0.80	5.65	19.05	0.15	0.03
0.01	0.10	1.33	5.60	0.08	0.00	1.61	0.06	0.29	2.83	0.07	8.40	0.03	3.50	0.73	7.00	72.80	259.00	2.80	0.51
0.10	0.04	0.00	0.00	0.17	0.00	0.44	0.06	0.25	2.18	0.23	30.31	0.00	4.35	0.64	20.30	42.05	169.65	5.80	1.93
0.01	0.01	1.49	0.00	0.00	0.00	0.13	0.01	0.05	0.51	0.03	5.88	0.00	0.40	0.06	4.75	10.58	55.22	0.47	0.28
0.10	0.05	0.00	0.00	0.00	331.32	136.54	0.03	0.03	0.65	0.05	3.26	0.00	17.57	0.95	12.55	22.59	286.14	7.53	0.23
0.10	0.05	0.00	0.00	0.20	331.32	1.51	0.03	0.03	0.65	0.05	3.26	0.00	17.57	0.95	12.55	22.59	286.14	7.53	0.23
0.10	0.10	0.00	0.00	0.05	27.50	7.50	0.03	0.00	0.38	0.03	5.25	0.00	25.00	0.85	7.50	0.00	77.50	12.50	0.38
0.02	0.02	0.00	0.00	0.02	64.74	13.20	0.00	0.02	0.72	0.02	3.49	0.00	12.45	0.47	9.96	14.94	99.60	17.43	0.20
0.24	0.31	0.00	0.00	1.21	100.64	7.34	0.02	0.06	1.35	0.03	5.03	0.00	6.80	0.10	10.88	21.76	288.32	0.00	0.12
0.02	0.04	0.00	0.00	0.55	46.40	13.04	0.10	0.05	0.70	0.15	36.56	0.00	50.40	0.36	45.60	44.80	257.60	4.00	0.44
0.02	0.03	0.00	0.00	0.69	66.00	21.10	0.20	0.06	1.00	0.22	87.80	0.00	81.00	0.80	57.00	63.00	303.00	8.00	0.60
0.13	0.20	0.00	0.00	1.76	130.05	31.11	0.26	0.31	2.01	0.13	371.28	0.00	244.80	1.71	130.05	117.30	596.70	7.65	1.58
0.11	0.20	0.00	0.00	1.96	130.64	35.22	0.26	0.31	2.02	0.11	419.18	0.00	230.04	1.62	122.12	119.28	599.24	8.52	1.51
0.00	0.00	0.00	0.00	0.00	0.00	0.00	0.00	0.00	0.00	0.00	0.00	0.00	0.00	0.00	0.00	0.00	0.00	13.00	0.00
0.42	0.05	0.00	0.00	0.25	2.91	0.12	0.00	0.00	0.00	0.00	0.00	0.00	7.80	0.28	0.33	0.25	0.75	74.53	0.02

USDA ID Code	Food Name	Weight in Grams*	Quantity of Units	Unit of Measure	Protein (gm)	Fat (gm)	Carbohydrate (gm)	Kcalories	Caffeine (gm)	Fiber (gm)	Cholesterol (mg)	Saturated Fat (gm)
	Olives, Ripe, Canned (small-extr	8.4000	1.000	Tbsp	0.07	0.90	0.53	9.66	0.00	0.27	0.00	0.12
	Onions, Ckd	210.0000	1.000	Cup	2.86	0.40	21.32	92.40	0.00	2.94	0.00	0.06
	Onions, Cnd, Solid & Liquid	63.0000	1.000	Onion	0.54	0.06	2.53	11.97	0.00	0.76	0.00	0.01
	Onions, Fresh	160.0000	1.000	Cup	1.86	0.26	13.81	60.80	0.00	2.88	0.00	0.05
	Oranges, Fresh	180.0000	1.000	Cup	1.69	0.22	21.15	84.60	0.00	4.32	0.00	0.04
	Papayas, Fresh	140.0000	1.000	Cup	0.85	0.20	13.73	54.60	0.00	2.52	0.00	0.06
	Parsnips, Ckd, w/ Salt	78.0000	0.500	Cup	1.03	0.23	15.23	63.18	0.00	3.12	0.00	0.04
	Parsnips, Ckd, w/o Salt	78.0000	0.500	Cup	1.03	0.23	15.23	63.18	0.00	3.12	0.00	0.04
	Parsnips, Fresh	133.0000	1.000	Cup	1.60	0.40	23.93	99.75	0.00	6.52	0.00	0.07
	Peaches, Cnd, Heavy Syrup Pack	262.0000	1.000	Cup	1.18	0.26	52.24	193.88	0.00	3.41	0.00	0.03
	Peaches, Cnd, Juice Pack	250.0000	1.000	Cup	1.58	0.08	28.93	110.00	0.00	3.25	0.00	0.00
	Peaches, Cnd, Light Syrup Pack	251.0000	1.000	Cup	1.13	0.08	36.52	135.54	0.00	3.26	0.00	0.00
	Peaches, Cnd, Water Pack	244.0000	1.000	Cup	1.07	0.15	14.91	58.56	0.00	3.17	0.00	0.02
	Peaches, Cnd, X-heavy Syrup Pack	262.0000	1.000	Cup	1.23	0.08	68.28	251.52	0.00	2.62	0.00	0.00
	Peaches, Cnd, X-light Syrup	247.0000	1.000	Cup	0.99	0.25	27.42	103.74	0.00	2.47	0.00	0.02
	Peaches, Dehydrated, Sulfured	116.0000	1.000	Cup	5.67	1.19	96.49	377.00	0.00	0.00	0.00	0.13
	Peaches, Dried, Sulfured	160.0000	1.000	Cup	5.78	1.22	98.13	382.40	0.00	13.12	0.00	0.13
	Peaches, Fresh	170.0000	1.000	Cup	1.19	0.15	18.87	73.10	0.00	3.40	0.00	0.02
	Peaches, Frozen, Sliced, Sweeten	250.0000	1.000	Cup	1.58	0.33	59.95	235.00	0.00	4.50	0.00	0.03
	Pears, Asian, Fresh	122.0000	1.000	Medium	0.61	0.28	12.99	51.24	0.00	4.39	0.00	0.01
	Pears, Cnd, Heavy Syrup Pack	266.0000	1.000	Cup	0.53	0.35	50.99	196.84	0.00	4.26	0.00	0.03
	Pears, Cnd, Juice Pack	248.0000	1.000	Cup	0.84	0.17	32.09	124.00	0.00	3.97	0.00	0.00
	Pears, Cnd, Light Syrup Pack	251.0000	1.000	Cup	0.48	0.08	38.08	143.07	0.00	4.02	0.00	0.00
	Pears, Cnd, Water Pack	244.0000	1.000	Cup	0.46	0.07	19.06	70.76	0.00	3.90	0.00	0.00
	Pears, Cnd, X-heavy Syrup Pack	266.0000	1.000	Cup	0.51	0.35	67.17	258.02	0.00	4.26	0.00	0.03
	Pears, Cnd, X-light Syrup Pack	247.0000	1.000	Cup	0.74	0.25	30.13	116.09	0.00	3.95	0.00	0.02
	Pears, Fresh	165.0000	1.000	Cup	0.64	0.66	24.93	97.35	0.00	3.96	0.00	0.03
	Peas and Carrots, Cnd	255.0000	1.000	Cup	5.53	0.69	21.62	96.90	0.00	5.10	0.00	0.13
	Peas and Carrots, Frz, Ckd	278.0000	1.250	Cup	8.59	1.17	28.13	133.44	0.00	8.62	0.00	0.22
	Peas and Onions, Cnd	120.0000	1.000	Cup	3.94	0.46	10.28	61.20	0.00	2.76	0.00	0.08
	Peas and Onions, Frz, Ckd	180.0000	1.000	Cup	4.57	0.36	15.53	81.00	0.00	3.96	0.00	0.07
	Peas, Edible-podded, Fresh	98.0000	1.000	Cup	2.74	0.20	7.41	41.16	0.00	2.55	0.00	0.04
	Peas, Green, Ckd	160.0000	1.000	Cup	8.58	0.35	25.02	134.40	0.00	8.80	0.00	0.06
	Peas, Green, Cnd	170.0000	1.000	Cup	7.51	0.60	21.39	117.30	0.00	6.97	0.00	0.10
	Peas, Green, Cnd, Seasoned	227.0000	1.000	Cup	7.01	0.61	21.00	113.50	0.00	4.54	0.00	0.11
	Peas, Green, Fresh	145.0000	1.000	Cup	7.86	0.58	20.97	117.45	0.00	7.40	0.00	0.10
	Peas, Green, Frz, Ckd	253.0000	1.250	Cup	13.03	0.68	36.08	197.34	0.00	13.92	0.00	0.13
	Peppers, Hot Chili, Green, Cnd	73.0000	1.000	Each	0.66	0.07	3.72	15.33	0.00	0.95	0.00	0.01
	Peppers, Hot Chili, Green, Fresh	45.0000	1.000	Each	0.90	0.09	4.26	18.00	0.00	0.68	0.00	0.01
	Peppers, Hot Chili, Red, Cnd	73.0000	1.000	Each	0.66	0.07	3.72	15.33	0.00	0.95	0.00	0.01
	Peppers, Hot Chili, Red, Fresh	45.0000	1.000	Each	0.90	0.09	4.26	18.00	0.00	0.68	0.00	0.01
	Peppers, Jalapeno, Cnd	136.0000	1.000	Cup	1.25	1.28	6.42	36.72	0.00	3.54	0.00	0.14
	Peppers, Sweet, Green, Fresh	149.0000	1.000	Cup	1.33	0.28	9.58	40.23	0.00	2.68	0.00	0.04
	Peppers, Sweet, Red, Fresh	149.0000	1.000	Cup	1.33	0.28	9.58	40.23	0.00	2.98	0.00	0.04
	Peppers, Sweet, Yellow, Fresh	186.0000	1.000	Large	1.86	0.39	11.76	50.22	0.00	1.67	0.00	0.06
	Persimmon, Japanese, Raw	168.0000	1.000	Medium	0.97	0.32	31.23	117.60	0.00	6.05	0.00	0.03
	Pickle, Cucumber ,Sour	155.0000	1.000	Cup	0.51	0.31	3.49	17.05	0.00	1.86	0.00	0.08
	Pickle, Cucumber, Dill	143.0000	1.000	Cup	0.89	0.27	5.91	25.74	0.00	1.72	0.00	0.07
	Pickle, Cucumber, Dill, Low Sodi	65.0000	1.000	Slice	0.40	0.12	2.68	11.70	0.00	0.78	0.00	0.03
	Pickle, Cucumber, Sour, Low Sodi	143.0000	1.000	Cup	0.47	0.29	3.22	15.73	0.00	1.72	0.00	0.07
	Pickle, Cucumber, Sweet	160.0000	1.000	Cup	0.59	0.42	50.90	187.20	0.00	1.76	0.00	0.11
	Pickle, Cucumber, Sweet, Low Sod	160.0000	1.000	Cup	0.59	0.42	50.90	187.20	0.00	1.76	0.00	0.11
	Pineapple, Cnd, Heavy Syrup Pack	254.0000	1.000	Cup	0.89	0.28	51.31	198.12	0.00	2.03	0.00	0.03
	Pineapple, Cnd, Juice Pack	249.0000	1.000	Cup	1.05	0.20	39.09	149.40	0.00	1.99	0.00	0.02
	Pineapple, Cnd, Light Syrup Pack	252.0000	1.000	Cup	0.91	0.30	33.89	131.04	0.00	2.02	0.00	0.03

Monounsaturated Fat (gm)	Polyunsaturated Fat (gm)	Vitamin D (mg)	Vitamin K (mg)	Vitamin E (mg)	Vitamin A (re)	Vitamin C (mg)	Thiamin (mg)	Riboflavin (mg)	Niacin (mg)	Vitamin B_6 (mg)	Folate (mg)	Vitamin B_{12} (mcg)	Calcium (mg)	Iron (mg)	Magnesium (mg)	Phosphorus (mg)	Potassium (mg)	Sodium (mg)	Zinc (mg)
0.66	0.08	0.00	0.00	0.25	3.36	0.08	0.00	0.00	0.00	0.00	0.00	0.00	7.39	0.28	0.34	0.25	0.67	73.25	0.02
0.06	0.15	0.00	0.00	0.27	0.00	10.92	0.08	0.04	0.36	0.27	31.50	0.00	46.20	0.50	23.10	73.50	348.60	6.30	0.44
0.01	0.03	0.00	0.00	0.04	0.00	2.71	0.02	0.01	0.04	0.09	6.11	0.00	28.35	0.08	3.78	17.64	69.93	233.73	0.18
0.03	0.10	0.00	0.83	0.21	0.00	10.24	0.06	0.03	0.24	0.19	30.40	0.00	32.00	0.35	16.00	52.80	251.20	4.80	0.30
0.04	0.05	0.00	2.43	0.43	37.80	95.76	0.16	0.07	0.50	0.11	54.54	0.00	72.00	0.18	18.00	25.20	325.80	0.00	0.13
0.06	0.04	0.00	0.00	1.57	39.20	86.52	0.04	0.04	0.48	0.03	53.20	0.00	33.60	0.14	14.00	7.00	359.80	4.20	0.10
0.09	0.04	0.00	0.00	0.00	0.00	10.14	0.06	0.04	0.56	0.07	45.40	0.00	28.86	0.45	22.62	53.82	286.26	191.88	0.20
0.09	0.04	0.00	0.00	0.78	0.00	10.14	0.06	0.04	0.56	0.07	45.40	0.00	28.86	0.45	22.62	53.82	286.26	7.80	0.20
0.15	0.07	0.00	0.00	0.00	0.00	22.61	0.12	0.07	0.93	0.12	88.84	0.00	47.88	0.78	38.57	94.43	498.75	13.30	0.78
0.10	0.13	0.00	0.00	2.33	86.46	7.34	0.03	0.05	1.60	0.05	8.38	0.00	7.86	0.71	13.10	28.82	241.04	15.72	0.24
0.03	0.05	0.00	7.50	3.75	95.00	9.00	0.03	0.05	1.45	0.05	8.50	0.00	15.00	0.68	17.50	42.50	320.00	10.00	0.28
0.03	0.05	0.00	0.00	2.23	87.85	6.02	0.03	0.08	1.48	0.05	8.28	0.00	7.53	0.90	12.55	27.61	243.47	12.55	0.23
0.05	0.07	0.00	0.00	2.17	129.32	7.08	0.02	0.05	1.27	0.05	8.30	0.00	4.88	0.78	12.20	24.40	241.56	7.32	0.22
0.03	0.03	0.00	0.00	0.00	34.06	3.14	0.03	0.05	1.36	0.05	8.12	0.00	7.86	0.76	13.10	28.82	217.46	20.96	0.24
0.10	0.12	0.00	0.00	0.00	66.69	7.41	0.05	0.05	1.98	0.05	8.15	0.00	12.35	0.74	12.35	27.17	182.78	12.35	0.22
0.44	0.58	0.00	0.00	0.00	164.72	12.30	0.05	0.13	5.60	0.19	7.66	0.00	44.08	6.39	66.12	187.92	1567.16	11.60	0.90
0.45	0.59	0.00	0.00	0.00	345.60	7.68	0.00	0.34	7.01	0.11	0.48	0.00	44.80	6.50	67.20	190.40	1593.60	11.20	0.91
0.05	0.09	0.00	0.00	1.19	91.80	11.22	0.03	0.07	1.68	0.03	5.78	0.00	8.50	0.19	11.90	20.40	334.90	0.00	0.24
0.13	0.15	0.00	0.00	2.23	70.00	235.50	0.03	0.10	1.63	0.05	8.00	0.00	7.50	0.93	12.50	27.50	325.00	15.00	0.13
0.06	0.07	0.00	0.00	0.61	0.00	4.64	0.01	0.01	0.27	0.02	9.76	0.00	4.88	0.00	9.76	13.42	147.62	0.00	0.02
0.08	0.08	0.00	0.00	1.33	0.00	2.93	0.03	0.05	0.64	0.03	3.19	0.00	13.30	0.59	10.64	18.62	172.90	13.30	0.21
0.02	0.05	0.00	1.14	1.24	2.48	3.97	0.02	0.02	0.50	0.02	2.98	0.00	22.32	0.72	17.36	29.76	238.08	9.92	0.22
0.03	0.03	0.00	0.00	1.26	0.00	1.76	0.03	0.05	0.38	0.03	3.01	0.00	12.55	0.70	10.04	17.57	165.66	12.55	0.20
0.02	0.02	0.00	0.00	1.22	0.00	2.44	0.02	0.02	0.12	0.02	2.93	0.00	9.76	0.51	9.76	17.08	129.32	4.88	0.22
0.08	0.08	0.00	0.00	0.00	0.00	2.93	0.03	0.05	0.64	0.03	3.19	0.00	13.30	0.59	10.64	18.62	170.24	13.30	0.21
0.05	0.05	0.00	0.00	0.00	0.00	4.94	0.02	0.05	0.99	0.02	2.96	0.00	17.29	0.49	12.35	17.29	111.15	4.94	0.17
0.13	0.15	0.00	0.00	0.83	3.30	6.60	0.03	0.07	0.17	0.03	12.05	0.00	18.15	0.41	9.90	18.15	206.25	0.00	0.20
0.05	0.33	0.00	0.00	0.00	1471.35	16.83	0.18	0.13	1.48	0.23	46.67	0.00	58.65	1.91	35.70	117.30	255.00	663.00	1.48
0.11	0.56	0.00	0.00	0.89	2157.28	22.52	0.64	0.17	3.20	0.25	72.28	0.00	63.94	2.61	44.48	136.22	439.24	189.04	1.25
0.05	0.22	0.00	0.00	0.00	19.20	3.60	0.12	0.08	1.54	0.23	31.92	0.00	20.40	1.04	19.20	61.20	115.20	530.40	0.70
0.04	0.16	0.00	0.00	0.27	63.00	12.42	0.27	0.13	1.87	0.16	35.82	0.00	25.20	1.69	23.40	61.20	210.60	66.60	0.52
0.02	0.09	0.00	0.00	0.38	13.72	58.80	0.15	0.08	0.59	0.16	40.87	0.00	42.14	2.04	23.52	51.94	196.00	3.92	0.26
0.03	0.16	0.00	0.00	0.62	96.00	22.72	0.42	0.24	3.23	0.35	101.28	0.00	43.20	2.46	62.40	187.20	433.60	4.80	1.90
0.05	0.27	0.00	0.00	0.65	130.90	16.32	0.20	0.14	1.24	0.10	75.31	0.00	34.00	1.62	28.90	113.90	294.10	428.40	1.21
0.05	0.30	0.00	0.00	0.00	97.61	26.11	0.23	0.16	1.57	0.23	64.92	0.00	34.05	2.72	34.05	122.58	276.94	576.58	1.48
0.06	0.28	0.00	0.00	0.57	92.80	58.00	0.39	0.19	3.03	0.25	94.25	0.00	36.25	2.13	47.85	156.60	353.80	7.25	1.80
0.05	0.33	0.00	0.00	0.43	169.51	25.05	0.71	0.25	3.74	0.28	148.26	0.00	60.72	3.97	73.37	227.70	425.04	220.11	2.38
0.01	0.04	0.00	0.00	0.50	44.53	49.64	0.01	0.04	0.58	0.11	7.30	0.00	5.11	0.37	10.22	12.41	136.51	856.29	0.12
0.00	0.05	0.00	0.00	0.31	34.65	109.13	0.04	0.04	0.43	0.13	10.53	0.00	8.10	0.54	11.25	20.70	153.00	3.15	0.14
0.01	0.04	0.00	0.00	0.50	867.97	49.64	0.01	0.04	0.58	0.11	7.30	0.00	5.11	0.37	10.22	12.41	136.51	856.29	0.12
0.00	0.05	0.00	0.00	0.31	483.75	109.13	0.04	0.04	0.43	0.13	10.53	0.00	8.10	0.54	11.25	20.70	153.00	3.15	0.14
0.07	0.69	0.00	0.00	0.94	231.20	13.60	0.05	0.05	0.54	0.26	19.04	0.00	31.28	2.56	20.40	24.48	262.48	2272.56	0.46
0.01	0.15	0.00	0.00	1.03	93.87	133.06	0.10	0.04	0.76	0.37	32.78	0.00	13.41	0.69	14.90	28.31	263.73	2.98	0.18
0.01	0.15	0.00	0.00	1.03	849.30	283.10	0.10	0.04	0.76	0.37	32.78	0.00	13.41	0.69	14.90	28.31	263.73	2.98	0.18
0.00	0.00	0.00	0.00	0.00	44.64	341.31	0.06	0.06	1.66	0.32	48.36	0.00	20.46	0.86	22.32	44.64	394.32	3.72	0.32
0.06	0.07	0.00	0.00	0.99	364.56	12.60	0.05	0.03	0.17	0.17	12.60	0.00	13.44	0.25	15.12	28.56	270.48	1.68	0.19
0.00	0.12	0.00	0.00	0.25	23.25	1.55	0.00	0.02	0.00	0.02	1.10	0.00	0.00	0.62	6.20	21.70	35.65	1872.40	0.03
0.00	0.11	0.00	0.00	0.23	47.19	2.72	0.01	0.04	0.09	0.01	1.43	0.00	12.87	0.76	15.73	30.03	165.88	1833.26	0.20
0.00	0.05	0.00	0.00	0.00	21.45	1.24	0.01	0.02	0.04	0.01	0.65	0.00	5.85	0.34	7.15	13.65	75.40	11.70	0.09
0.00	0.11	0.00	0.00	0.07	21.45	1.43	0.00	0.01	0.00	0.01	1.02	0.00	0.00	0.57	5.72	20.02	32.89	25.74	0.03
0.00	0.18	0.00	0.00	0.26	20.80	1.92	0.02	0.05	0.27	0.03	1.60	0.00	6.40	0.94	6.40	19.20	51.20	1502.40	0.13
0.00	0.18	0.00	0.00	0.26	20.80	1.92	0.02	0.05	0.27	0.03	1.60	0.00	6.40	0.94	6.40	19.20	51.20	28.80	0.13
0.03	0.10	0.00	0.00	0.25	2.54	18.80	0.23	0.08	0.74	0.18	11.68	0.00	35.56	0.97	40.64	17.78	264.16	2.54	0.30
0.02	0.07	0.00	0.00	0.25	9.96	23.66	0.25	0.05	0.70	0.17	11.95	0.00	34.86	0.70	34.86	14.94	303.78	2.49	0.25
0.03	0.10	0.00	0.00	0.25	2.52	18.90	0.23	0.08	0.73	0.18	11.84	0.00	35.28	0.98	40.32	17.64	264.60	2.52	0.30

USDA ID Code	Food Name	Weight in Grams*	Quantity of Units	Unit of Measure	Protein (gm)	Fat (gm)	Carbohydrate (gm)	Kcalories	Caffeine (gm)	Fiber (gm)	Cholesterol (mg)	Saturated Fat (gm)
	Pineapple, Cnd, Water Pack	246.0000	1.000	Cup	1.06	0.22	20.42	78.72	0.00	1.97	0.00	0.02
	Pineapple, Cnd, X-heavy Syrup Pa	260.0000	1.000	Cup	0.88	0.29	55.90	215.80	0.00	2.08	0.00	0.03
	Pineapple, Fresh	155.0000	1.000	Cup	0.60	0.67	19.20	75.95	0.00	1.86	0.00	0.05
	Plantain, Raw	179.0000	1.000	Medium	2.33	0.66	57.08	218.38	0.00	4.12	0.00	0.26
	Plums, Cnd, Purple, Heavy Syrup	258.0000	1.000	Cup	0.93	0.26	59.96	229.62	0.00	2.58	0.00	0.03
	Plums, Cnd, Purple, Juice Pack	252.0000	1.000	Cup	1.29	0.05	38.18	146.16	0.00	2.52	0.00	0.00
	Plums, Cnd, Purple, Light Syrup	252.0000	1.000	Cup	0.93	0.25	41.03	158.76	0.00	2.52	0.00	0.03
	Plums, Cnd, Purple, Water Pack	249.0000	1.000	Cup	0.97	0.02	27.46	102.09	0.00	2.49	0.00	0.00
	Plums, Cnd, Purple, X-heavy Syru	261.0000	1.000	Cup	0.94	0.26	68.67	263.61	0.00	2.61	0.00	0.03
	Plums, Fresh	165.0000	0.500	Cup	1.30	1.02	21.47	90.75	0.00	2.48	0.00	0.08
	Potato Pancakes, Home-prepared	76.0000	1.000	Each	4.68	11.58	21.77	206.72	0.00	1.52	72.96	2.31
	Potato Puffs, Frz, Prepared	128.0000	1.000	Cup	4.29	13.73	39.01	284.16	0.00	4.10	0.00	6.53
	Potato Salad	250.0000	1.000	Cup	6.70	20.50	27.93	357.50	0.00	3.25	170.00	3.58
	Potatoes, Au Gratin, Home-prepar	245.0000	1.000	Cup	12.40	18.60	27.61	323.40	0.00	4.41	36.75	8.65
	Potatoes, Baked w/o Skin	61.0000	0.500	Cup	1.20	0.06	13.15	56.73	0.00	0.92	0.00	0.02
	Potatoes, Baked, Skin only	58.0000	1.000	Each	2.49	0.06	26.72	114.84	0.00	4.58	0.00	0.02
	Potatoes, Baked, w/ Skin	202.0000	1.000	Medium	4.65	0.20	50.96	220.18	0.00	4.85	0.00	0.06
	Potatoes, Boiled, Ckd In Skin w/	78.0000	0.500	Cup	1.46	0.08	15.70	67.86	0.00	1.40	0.00	0.02
	Potatoes, Boiled, Ckd w/o Skin	78.0000	0.500	Cup	1.33	0.08	15.61	67.08	0.00	1.40	0.00	0.02
	Potatoes, Boiled, Skin only	34.0000	1.000	Each	0.97	0.03	5.85	26.52	0.00	1.12	0.00	0.01
	Potatoes, Cnd, Drained Solids	180.0000	1.000	Cup	2.54	0.38	24.50	108.00	0.00	4.14	0.00	0.09
	Potatoes, Cnd, Solids and Liquid	300.0000	1.000	Cup	3.60	0.33	29.67	132.00	0.00	4.20	0.00	0.09
	Potatoes, Hashed Brown	156.0000	1.000	Cup	3.78	21.70	33.26	326.04	0.00	3.12	0.00	8.47
	Potatoes, Mashed, Home-prepared	210.0000	1.000	Cup	4.07	1.24	36.86	161.70	0.00	4.20	4.20	0.69
	Potatoes, Mashed, Prepared From	210.0000	1.000	Cup	3.99	11.76	31.54	237.30	0.00	4.83	8.40	3.07
	Potatoes, Microwaved w/o Skin	78.0000	0.500	Cup	1.64	0.08	18.16	78.00	0.00	1.25	0.00	0.02
	Potatoes, Microwaved, Skin only	58.0000	1.000	Each	2.55	0.06	17.19	76.56	0.00	3.19	0.00	0.02
	Potatoes, Microwaved, w/ Skin	202.0000	1.000	Medium	4.93	0.20	48.74	212.10	0.00	4.65	0.00	0.06
	Potatoes, O'brien, Home-prepared	194.0000	1.000	Cup	4.56	2.48	30.01	157.14	0.00	0.00	7.76	1.55
	Potatoes, Scalloped	245.0000	1.000	Cup	7.03	9.02	26.41	210.70	0.00	4.66	14.70	3.38
	Prunes, Dehydrated	132.0000	1.000	Cup	4.88	0.96	117.57	447.48	0.00	0.00	0.00	0.08
	Prunes, Dried, Stewed, w/ Added	248.0000	1.000	Cup	2.70	0.55	81.54	307.52	0.00	9.42	0.00	0.05
	Prunes, Dried, Stewed, w/o Added	248.0000	1.000	Cup	2.90	0.57	69.64	265.36	0.00	16.37	0.00	0.05
	Prunes, Dried, Uncooked	170.0000	1.000	Cup	4.44	0.88	106.64	406.30	0.00	12.07	0.00	0.07
	Pumpkin, Ckd	245.0000	1.000	Cup	1.76	0.17	11.98	49.00	0.00	2.70	0.00	0.10
	Pumpkin, Cnd, w/o Salt	245.0000	1.000	Cup	2.70	0.69	19.80	83.30	0.00	7.11	0.00	0.37
	Radishes, Fresh	116.0000	1.000	Cup	0.70	0.63	4.16	23.20	0.00	1.86	0.00	0.03
	Radishes, Oriental, Ckd	147.0000	0.500	Cup	0.98	0.35	5.04	24.99	0.00	2.35	0.00	0.10
	Radishes, Oriental, Dried	116.0000	1.000	Cup	9.16	0.84	73.51	314.36	0.00	0.00	0.00	0.26
	Radishes, Oriental, Fresh	338.0000	1.000	Each	2.03	0.34	13.89	60.84	0.00	5.41	0.00	0.10
	Radishes, White Icicle, Fresh	50.0000	0.500	Cup	0.55	0.05	1.32	7.00	0.00	0.70	0.00	0.02
	Raisins, Golden Seedless	165.0000	1.000	Cup	5.59	0.76	131.21	498.30	0.00	6.60	0.00	0.25
	Raisins, Seeded	165.0000	1.000	Cup	4.16	0.89	129.48	488.40	0.00	11.22	0.00	0.30
	Raisins, Seedless	165.0000	1.000	Cup	5.31	0.76	130.56	495.00	0.00	6.60	0.00	0.25
	Raspberries, Cnd, Red, Heavy Syr	256.0000	1.000	Cup	2.12	0.31	59.80	232.96	0.00	8.45	0.00	0.03
	Raspberries, Fresh	123.0000	1.000	Cup	1.12	0.68	14.23	60.27	0.00	8.36	0.00	0.02
	Raspberries, Frozen, Red, Sweete	250.0000	1.000	Cup	1.75	0.40	65.40	257.50	0.00	11.00	0.00	0.03
	Sauerkraut, Cnd, Solid & Liquid	142.0000	1.000	Cup	1.29	0.20	6.08	26.98	0.00	3.55	0.00	0.06
	Shallots, Freeze-dried	0.9000	1.000	Tbsp	0.11	0.00	0.73	3.13	0.00	0.00	0.00	0.00
	Shallots, Fresh	10.0000	1.000	Tbsp	0.25	0.01	1.68	7.20	0.00	0.00	0.00	0.00
	Spinach, Ckd	180.0000	1.000	Cup	5.35	0.47	6.75	41.40	0.00	4.32	0.00	0.07
	Spinach, Cnd, Drained Solids	214.0000	1.000	Cup	6.01	1.07	7.28	49.22	0.00	5.14	0.00	0.17
	Spinach, Cnd, Reg Pk, Solid & Li	234.0000	1.000	Cup	4.94	0.87	6.83	44.46	0.00	3.74	0.00	0.14
	Spinach, Fresh	30.0000	1.000	Cup	0.86	0.11	1.05	6.60	0.00	0.81	0.00	0.02
	Spinach, Frz, Ckd	220.0000	1.250	Cup	6.91	0.46	11.75	61.60	0.00	6.60	0.00	0.07

Monounsaturated Fat (gm)	Polyunsaturated Fat (gm)	Vitamin D (mg)	Vitamin K (mg)	Vitamin E (mg)	Vitamin A (re)	Vitamin C (mg)	Thiamin (mg)	Riboflavin (mg)	Niacin (mg)	Vitamin B_6 (mg)	Folate (mg)	Vitamin B_{12} (mcg)	Calcium (mg)	Iron (mg)	Magnesium (mg)	Phosphorus (mg)	Potassium (mg)	Sodium (mg)	Zinc (mg)
0.02	0.07	0.00	0.00	0.25	4.92	18.94	0.22	0.07	0.74	0.17	11.81	0.00	36.90	0.98	44.28	9.84	312.42	2.46	0.30
0.03	0.10	0.00	0.00	0.00	2.60	18.98	0.23	0.08	0.73	0.18	11.96	0.00	36.40	0.99	39.00	18.20	265.20	2.60	0.29
0.08	0.23	0.00	0.00	0.16	3.10	23.87	0.14	0.06	0.65	0.14	16.43	0.00	10.85	0.57	21.70	10.85	175.15	1.55	0.12
0.06	0.12	0.00	0.00	0.48	202.27	32.94	0.09	0.10	1.23	0.54	39.38	0.00	5.37	1.07	66.23	60.86	893.21	7.16	0.25
0.18	0.05	0.00	0.00	1.81	67.08	1.03	0.05	0.10	0.75	0.08	6.45	0.00	23.22	2.17	12.90	33.54	234.78	49.02	0.18
0.03	0.03	0.00	0.00	1.76	254.52	7.06	0.05	0.15	1.18	0.08	6.55	0.00	25.20	0.86	20.16	37.80	388.08	2.52	0.28
0.18	0.05	0.00	0.00	1.76	65.52	1.01	0.05	0.10	0.76	0.08	6.55	0.00	22.68	2.17	12.60	32.76	234.36	50.40	0.20
0.02	0.00	0.00	0.00	1.74	226.59	6.72	0.05	0.10	0.92	0.07	6.47	0.00	17.43	0.40	12.45	32.37	313.74	2.49	0.20
0.18	0.05	0.00	0.00	0.00	65.25	1.04	0.05	0.10	0.76	0.08	6.53	0.00	23.49	2.14	13.05	31.32	232.29	49.59	0.18
0.68	0.21	0.00	0.00	0.99	52.80	15.68	0.07	0.17	0.83	0.13	3.63	0.00	6.60	0.17	11.55	16.50	283.80	0.00	0.17
3.53	4.97	0.00	0.00	0.00	10.64	16.72	0.11	0.13	1.63	0.29	17.48	0.14	18.24	1.19	25.08	84.36	597.36	386.08	0.63
5.58	1.02	0.00	0.00	0.06	2.56	8.83	0.26	0.09	2.76	0.29	21.12	0.00	38.40	2.00	24.32	61.44	486.40	954.88	0.38
6.20	9.35	0.00	0.00	0.00	82.50	25.00	0.20	0.15	2.23	0.35	16.75	0.00	47.50	1.63	37.50	130.00	635.00	1322.50	0.78
6.35	2.65	0.00	0.00	0.00	93.10	24.26	0.15	0.29	2.43	0.42	26.95	0.00	291.55	1.57	49.00	276.85	970.20	1060.85	1.69
0.00	0.02	0.00	0.13	0.02	0.00	7.81	0.07	0.01	0.85	0.18	5.55	0.00	3.05	0.21	15.25	30.50	238.51	3.05	0.18
0.00	0.02	0.00	0.00	0.02	0.00	7.83	0.07	0.06	1.78	0.35	12.53	0.00	19.72	4.08	24.94	58.58	332.34	12.18	0.28
0.00	0.08	0.00	1.07	0.10	0.00	26.06	0.22	0.06	3.33	0.71	22.22	0.00	20.20	2.75	54.54	115.14	844.36	16.16	0.65
0.00	0.03	0.00	0.00	0.04	0.00	10.14	0.09	0.02	1.12	0.23	7.80	0.00	3.90	0.24	17.16	34.32	295.62	3.12	0.23
0.00	0.03	0.00	0.00	0.04	0.00	5.77	0.08	0.02	1.02	0.21	6.94	0.00	6.24	0.24	15.60	31.20	255.84	3.90	0.21
0.00	0.01	0.00	0.00	0.00	0.00	1.77	0.01	0.01	0.41	0.08	3.30	0.00	15.30	2.06	10.20	18.36	138.38	4.76	0.15
0.02	0.16	0.00	0.00	0.09	0.00	9.18	0.13	0.02	1.66	0.34	11.16	0.00	9.00	2.27	25.20	50.40	412.20	394.20	0.50
0.00	0.15	0.00	0.00	0.12	0.00	22.80	0.09	0.06	2.67	0.42	13.50	0.00	117.00	2.16	42.00	66.00	615.00	651.00	1.17
9.69	2.50	0.00	0.00	0.30	0.00	8.89	0.11	0.03	3.12	0.44	12.01	0.00	12.48	1.26	31.20	65.52	500.76	37.44	0.47
0.32	0.13	0.00	0.00	0.11	12.60	14.07	0.19	0.08	2.35	0.48	17.22	0.00	54.60	0.57	37.80	100.80	627.90	636.30	0.61
4.85	3.26	0.00	0.00	0.00	44.10	20.37	0.23	0.11	1.41	0.02	15.54	0.00	102.90	0.46	37.80	117.60	489.30	697.20	0.38
0.00	0.03	0.00	0.00	0.00	0.00	11.78	0.10	0.02	1.27	0.25	9.67	0.00	3.90	0.32	19.50	85.02	320.58	5.46	0.26
0.00	0.02	0.00	0.00	0.00	0.00	8.87	0.04	0.05	1.29	0.28	9.63	0.00	26.68	3.45	21.46	47.56	377.00	9.28	0.30
0.00	0.08	0.00	0.00	0.00	0.00	30.50	0.24	0.06	3.45	0.69	24.24	0.00	22.22	2.50	54.54	212.10	902.94	16.16	0.73
0.68	0.12	0.00	0.00	0.00	110.58	32.40	0.16	0.12	1.96	0.41	16.10	0.00	69.84	0.91	34.92	97.00	516.04	420.98	0.58
3.31	1.84	0.00	0.00	0.00	46.55	25.97	0.17	0.22	2.57	0.44	26.95	0.00	139.65	1.40	46.55	154.35	926.10	820.75	0.98
0.63	0.21	0.00	0.00	0.00	232.32	0.00	0.16	0.22	3.96	0.99	2.51	0.00	95.04	4.65	84.48	147.84	1396.56	6.60	0.99
0.35	0.12	0.00	0.00	0.00	71.92	6.70	0.05	0.22	1.69	0.50	0.25	0.00	52.08	2.58	47.12	81.84	773.76	4.96	0.55
0.37	0.12	0.00	0.00	0.00	76.88	7.19	0.05	0.25	1.79	0.55	0.25	0.00	57.04	2.75	49.60	86.80	828.32	4.96	0.60
0.58	0.19	0.00	0.00	2.47	338.30	5.61	0.14	0.27	3.33	0.44	6.29	0.00	86.70	4.22	76.50	134.30	1266.50	6.80	0.90
0.02	0.00	0.00	0.00	2.60	264.60	11.52	0.07	0.20	1.00	0.10	20.83	0.00	36.75	1.40	22.05	73.50	563.50	2.45	0.56
0.10	0.05	0.00	36.75	2.60	5404.70	10.29	0.05	0.12	0.91	0.15	30.14	0.00	63.70	3.41	56.35	85.75	504.70	12.25	0.42
0.02	0.06	0.00	0.00	0.00	1.16	26.45	0.01	0.06	0.35	0.08	31.32	0.00	24.36	0.34	10.44	20.88	269.12	27.84	0.35
0.06	0.16	0.00	0.00	0.00	0.00	22.20	0.00	0.03	0.22	0.06	25.58	0.00	24.99	0.22	13.23	35.28	418.95	19.11	0.19
0.14	0.38	0.00	0.00	0.00	0.00	0.00	0.31	0.79	3.94	0.72	341.85	0.00	729.64	7.81	197.20	236.64	4053.04	322.48	2.47
0.07	0.17	0.00	0.00	0.00	0.00	74.36	0.07	0.07	0.68	0.17	95.32	0.00	91.26	1.35	54.08	77.74	767.26	70.98	0.51
0.01	0.03	0.00	0.00	0.00	0.00	14.50	0.02	0.01	0.15	0.04	7.00	0.00	13.50	0.40	4.50	14.00	140.00	8.00	0.07
0.03	0.23	0.00	0.00	1.16	6.60	5.28	0.02	0.31	1.88	0.53	5.45	0.00	87.45	2.95	57.75	189.75	1230.90	19.80	0.53
0.03	0.26	0.00	0.00	1.16	0.00	8.91	0.18	0.30	1.83	0.31	5.45	0.00	46.20	4.27	49.50	123.75	1361.25	46.20	0.30
0.03	0.23	0.00	0.00	1.16	1.65	5.45	0.26	0.15	1.35	0.41	5.45	0.00	80.85	3.43	54.45	160.05	1239.15	19.80	0.45
0.03	0.18	0.00	0.00	1.15	7.68	22.27	0.05	0.08	1.13	0.10	26.88	0.00	28.16	1.08	30.72	23.04	240.64	7.68	0.41
0.06	0.38	0.00	0.00	0.55	15.99	30.75	0.04	0.11	1.11	0.07	31.98	0.00	27.06	0.70	22.14	14.76	186.96	0.00	0.57
0.05	0.23	0.00	0.00	1.13	15.00	41.25	0.05	0.13	0.58	0.08	65.00	0.00	37.50	1.63	32.50	42.50	285.00	2.50	0.45
0.01	0.09	0.00	0.00	0.14	2.84	20.87	0.03	0.03	0.20	0.18	33.65	0.00	42.60	2.09	18.46	28.40	241.40	938.62	0.27
0.00	0.00	0.00	0.00	0.00	50.49	0.35	0.00	0.00	0.01	0.02	1.05	0.00	1.65	0.05	0.94	2.66	14.85	0.53	0.02
0.00	0.00	0.00	0.00	0.00	11.90	0.80	0.01	0.00	0.02	0.04	3.42	0.00	3.70	0.12	2.10	6.00	33.40	1.20	0.04
0.02	0.20	0.00	0.00	1.73	1474.20	17.64	0.18	0.43	0.88	0.43	262.44	0.00	244.80	6.43	156.60	100.80	838.80	126.00	1.37
0.02	0.45	0.00	0.00	2.78	1878.92	30.60	0.04	0.30	0.83	0.21	209.29	0.00	271.78	4.92	162.64	94.16	740.44	57.78	0.98
0.02	0.37	0.00	0.00	2.50	1504.62	31.59	0.05	0.26	0.63	0.19	135.72	0.00	194.22	3.70	131.04	74.88	538.20	746.46	0.98
0.00	0.05	0.00	79.80	0.57	201.60	8.43	0.02	0.06	0.22	0.06	58.32	0.00	29.70	0.81	23.70	14.70	167.40	23.70	0.16
0.02	0.20	0.00	0.00	2.11	1711.60	27.06	0.13	0.37	0.92	0.33	236.50	0.00	321.20	3.34	151.80	105.60	655.60	189.20	1.54

USDA ID Code	Food Name	Weight in Grams*	Quantity of Units	Unit of Measure	Protein (gm)	Fat (gm)	Carbohydrate (gm)	Kcalories	Caffeine (gm)	Fiber (gm)	Cholesterol (mg)	Saturated Fat (gm)
	Spinach, Frz, Unprepared	156.0000	1.000	Cup	4.56	0.48	6.24	37.44	0.00	4.68	0.00	0.08
	Squash, Acorn, Ckd, w/o Salt	205.0000	1.000	Cup	2.30	0.29	29.89	114.80	0.00	9.02	0.00	0.06
	Squash, Butternut, Ckd, w/o Salt	205.0000	1.000	Cup	1.85	0.18	21.50	82.00	0.00	0.00	0.00	0.04
	Squash, Spaghetti, Ckd. w/o Salt	155.0000	1.000	Cup	1.02	0.40	10.01	41.85	0.00	2.17	0.00	0.09
	Squash, Summer, Ckd	180.0000	0.500	Cup	1.64	0.56	7.76	36.00	0.00	2.52	0.00	0.11
	Squash, Summer, Fresh	113.0000	0.500	Cup	1.33	0.24	4.92	22.60	0.00	2.15	0.00	0.05
	Squash, Winter, Baked	205.0000	1.000	Cup	1.82	1.29	17.94	79.95	0.00	5.74	0.00	0.27
	Squash, Winter, Fresh	116.0000	1.000	Cup	1.68	0.27	10.21	42.92	0.00	1.74	0.00	0.06
	Squash, Zucchini, Baby, Fresh	16.0000	1.000	Large	0.43	0.06	0.50	3.36	0.00	0.18	0.00	0.01
	Strawberries, Fresh	152.0000	1.000	Cup	0.93	0.56	10.67	45.60	0.00	3.50	0.00	0.03
	Strawberries, Frozen, Sweetened	255.0000	1.000	Cup	1.35	0.33	66.10	244.80	0.00	4.85	0.00	0.03
	Strawberries, Frozen, Unsweetene	221.0000	1.000	Cup	0.95	0.24	20.18	77.35	0.00	4.64	0.00	0.02
	Sweet Potatoes, Baked In Skin	200.0000	1.000	Cup	3.44	0.22	48.54	206.00	0.00	6.00	0.00	0.04
	Sweet Potatoes, Boiled, w/o Skin	328.0000	1.000	Cup	5.41	0.98	79.64	344.40	0.00	5.90	0.00	0.20
	Sweet Potatoes, Candied	105.0000	1.000	Piece	0.91	3.41	29.25	143.85	0.00	2.52	8.40	1.42
	Sweet Potatoes, Mashed	255.0000	1.000	Cup	5.05	0.51	59.16	257.55	0.00	4.34	0.00	0.10
	Sweet Potatoes, Syrup Pack, Drai	196.0000	1.000	Cup	2.51	0.63	49.71	211.68	0.00	5.88	0.00	0.14
	Tangerines, Cnd, Juice Pack	249.0000	1.000	Cup	1.54	0.07	23.83	92.13	0.00	1.74	0.00	0.00
	Tangerines, Cnd, Light Syrup Pac	252.0000	1.000	Cup	1.13	0.25	40.80	153.72	0.00	1.76	0.00	0.03
	Tangerines, Fresh	195.0000	1.000	Cup	1.23	0.37	21.82	85.80	0.00	4.48	0.00	0.04
	Tator Tots	2.8350	10.000	Each	0.30	0.50	2.00	14.00	0.00	0.30	0.00	0.10
	Tomatillos, Fresh	34.0000	1.000	Slice	0.33	0.35	1.98	10.88	0.00	0.65	0.00	0.05
	Tomatoes, Cherry	149.0000	1.000	Cup	1.27	0.49	6.91	31.29	0.00	1.64	0.00	0.07
	Tomatoes, Ckd, Boiled	240.0000	1.000	Cup	2.57	0.98	13.99	64.80	0.00	2.40	0.00	0.14
	Tomatoes, Ckd, Stewed	101.0000	1.000	Cup	1.98	2.71	13.18	79.79	0.00	1.72	0.00	0.53
	Tomatoes, Cnd, Stewed	255.0000	1.000	Cup	2.42	0.33	17.29	71.40	0.00	2.55	0.00	0.05
	Tomatoes, Cnd, w/ Green Chilies	241.0000	1.000	Cup	1.66	0.19	8.72	36.15	0.00	0.00	0.00	0.02
	Tomatoes, Cnd, Wedges In Tomato	261.0000	1.000	Cup	2.06	0.42	16.47	67.86	0.00	0.00	0.00	0.05
	Tomatoes, Cnd, Whole, Reg Pk	240.0000	1.000	Cup	2.21	0.31	10.49	45.60	0.00	2.40	0.00	0.05
	Tomatoes, Fresh	149.0000	1.000	Cup	1.27	0.49	6.91	31.29	0.00	1.64	0.00	0.07
	Tomatoes, Green, Fresh	180.0000	1.000	Cup	2.16	0.36	9.18	43.20	0.00	1.98	0.00	0.05
	Tomatoes, Sun-dried	54.0000	0.250	Cup	7.62	1.60	30.11	139.32	0.00	6.64	0.00	0.23
	Tomatoes, Sun-dried, Packed In O	110.0000	1.000	Cup	5.57	15.49	25.66	234.30	0.00	6.38	0.00	2.08
	Turnips, Ckd	156.0000	1.000	Cup	1.11	0.12	7.64	32.76	0.00	3.12	0.00	0.02
	Turnips, Fresh	130.0000	1.000	Cup	1.17	0.13	8.10	35.10	0.00	2.34	0.00	0.01
	Vegetables, Mixed, Cnd	163.0000	1.000	Cup	4.22	0.41	15.09	76.61	0.00	4.89	0.00	0.08
	Vegetables, Mixed, Frz	275.0000	1.250	Cup	7.87	0.41	36.00	162.25	0.00	12.10	0.00	0.08
	Veggie Burger	90.0000	1.000	Each	18.00	4.00	8.00	140.00	0.00	5.00	0.00	1.50
	Watercress, Raw	2.5000	1.000	Sprig	0.06	0.00	0.03	0.28	0.00	0.04	0.00	0.00
	Watermelon	154.0000	1.000	Cup	0.95	0.66	11.06	49.28	0.00	0.77	0.00	0.08
	Yam, Baked	136.0000	1.000	Cup	2.03	0.19	37.54	157.76	0.00	5.30	0.00	0.04
	Bacon	19.0000	3.000	Slice	5.79	9.36	0.11	109.44	0.00	0.00	16.15	3.31
	Bacon, Canadian-style Bacon, Gri	46.5000	2.000	Slice	11.27	3.92	0.63	86.03	0.00	0.00	26.97	1.32
	Bacon, Turkey	14.0000	1.000	Slice	3.00	2.00	0.00	25.00	0.00	0.00	10.00	0.50
	Barbecue Loaf, Lunch Meat	23.0000	1.000	Slice	3.64	2.05	1.47	39.79	0.00	0.00	8.51	0.73
	Beans, Baked, Cnd, Vegetarian	254.0000	1.000	Cup	12.17	1.14	52.10	236.22	0.00	12.70	0.00	0.30
	Beans, Baked, Cnd, w/ Beef	266.0000	1.000	Cup	16.97	9.18	44.98	321.86	0.00	0.00	58.52	4.47
	Beans, Baked, Cnd, w/ Franks	259.0000	1.000	Cup	17.48	17.02	39.86	367.78	0.00	17.87	15.54	6.09
	Beans, Baked, Cnd, w/ Pork	253.0000	1.000	Cup	13.13	3.92	50.55	268.18	0.00	13.92	17.71	1.52
	Beans, Baked, Home Prepared	253.0000	1.000	Cup	14.02	13.03	54.12	382.03	0.00	13.92	12.65	4.93
	Beans, Black, Ckd	172.0000	1.000	Cup	15.24	0.93	40.78	227.04	0.00	14.96	0.00	0.24
	Beans, Garbanzo, Cnd	240.0000	1.000	Cup	11.88	2.74	54.29	285.60	0.00	10.56	0.00	0.29
	Beans, Kidney, Cnd	256.0000	1.000	Cup	13.31	0.79	38.09	207.36	0.00	8.96	0.00	0.13
1	Beans, Lentils	198.0000	1.000	Cup	17.87	0.74	39.87	231.00	0.00	5.46	0.00	0.11
	Beans, Lima, Cnd	241.0000	1.000	Cup	11.88	0.41	35.93	190.39	0.00	11.57	0.00	0.10

Monounsaturated Fat (gm)	Polyunsaturated Fat (gm)	Vitamin D (mg)	Vitamin K (mg)	Vitamin E (mg)	Vitamin A (re)	Vitamin C (mg)	Thiamin (mg)	Riboflavin (mg)	Niacin (mg)	Vitamin B_6 (mg)	Folate (mg)	Vitamin B_{12} (mcg)	Calcium (mg)	Iron (mg)	Magnesium (mg)	Phosphorus (mg)	Potassium (mg)	Sodium (mg)	Zinc (mg)
0.02	0.20	0.00	215.28	1.50	1210.56	37.91	0.12	0.23	0.69	0.22	186.58	0.00	173.16	3.20	90.48	63.96	503.88	115.44	0.69
0.02	0.12	0.00	0.00	0.00	88.15	22.14	0.35	0.02	1.80	0.39	38.34	0.00	90.20	1.91	88.15	92.25	895.85	8.20	0.35
0.02	0.08	0.00	0.00	0.00	1435.00	30.96	0.14	0.04	1.99	0.25	39.36	0.00	84.05	1.23	59.45	55.35	582.20	8.20	0.27
0.03	0.20	0.00	0.00	0.19	17.05	5.43	0.06	0.03	1.26	0.16	12.40	0.00	32.55	0.53	17.05	21.70	181.35	27.90	0.31
0.04	0.23	0.00	0.00	0.22	52.20	9.90	0.07	0.07	0.92	0.13	36.18	0.00	48.60	0.65	43.20	70.20	345.60	1.80	0.70
0.02	0.10	0.00	0.00	0.14	22.60	16.72	0.07	0.05	0.62	0.12	28.93	0.00	22.60	0.52	25.99	39.55	220.35	2.26	0.29
0.10	0.55	0.00	0.00	0.25	729.80	19.68	0.18	0.04	1.44	0.14	57.40	0.00	28.70	0.68	16.40	41.00	895.85	2.05	0.53
0.02	0.10	0.00	0.00	0.14	470.96	14.27	0.12	0.03	0.93	0.09	25.17	0.00	35.96	0.67	24.36	37.12	406.00	4.64	0.15
0.00	0.03	0.00	0.00	0.00	7.84	5.46	0.01	0.01	0.11	0.02	3.20	0.00	3.36	0.13	5.28	14.88	73.44	0.48	0.13
0.08	0.29	0.00	21.28	0.21	4.56	86.18	0.03	0.11	0.35	0.09	26.90	0.00	21.28	0.58	15.20	28.88	252.32	1.52	0.20
0.05	0.15	0.00	0.00	0.36	5.10	105.57	0.05	0.13	1.02	0.08	38.00	0.00	28.05	1.50	17.85	33.15	249.90	7.65	0.15
0.04	0.11	0.00	0.00	0.60	8.84	91.05	0.04	0.09	1.02	0.07	37.13	0.00	35.36	1.66	24.31	28.73	327.08	4.42	0.29
0.00	0.10	0.00	0.00	0.56	4364.00	49.20	0.14	0.26	1.20	0.48	45.20	0.00	56.00	0.90	40.00	110.00	696.00	20.00	0.58
0.03	0.43	0.00	0.00	0.92	5592.40	56.09	0.16	0.46	2.10	0.79	36.41	0.00	68.88	1.84	32.80	88.56	603.52	42.64	0.89
0.66	0.16	0.00	0.00	0.00	439.95	7.04	0.02	0.04	0.41	0.04	11.97	0.00	27.30	1.19	11.55	27.30	198.45	73.50	0.16
0.03	0.23	0.00	0.00	0.69	3858.15	13.26	0.08	0.23	2.45	0.61	27.29	0.00	76.50	3.39	61.20	132.60	535.50	191.25	0.54
0.02	0.27	0.00	0.00	0.55	1403.36	21.17	0.06	0.08	0.67	0.12	15.48	0.00	33.32	1.86	23.52	49.00	378.28	76.44	0.31
0.02	0.02	0.00	0.00	1.25	211.65	85.16	0.20	0.07	1.12	0.10	11.45	0.00	27.39	0.67	27.39	24.90	331.17	12.45	1.27
0.05	0.05	0.00	0.00	0.86	211.68	49.90	0.13	0.10	1.13	0.10	11.59	0.00	17.64	0.93	20.16	25.20	196.56	15.12	0.60
0.06	0.08	0.00	0.00	0.47	179.40	60.06	0.21	0.04	0.31	0.14	39.78	0.00	27.30	0.20	23.40	19.50	306.15	1.95	0.47
0.00	0.00	0.00	0.00	0.00	0.00	0.00	0.00	0.00	0.00	0.00	0.00	0.00	0.00	0.00	0.00	0.00	24.00	24.00	0.00
0.05	0.14	0.00	0.00	0.13	3.74	3.98	0.01	0.01	0.63	0.02	2.38	0.00	2.38	0.21	6.80	13.26	91.12	0.34	0.07
0.07	0.21	0.00	0.00	0.57	92.38	38.74	0.09	0.07	0.94	0.12	22.35	0.00	7.45	0.67	16.39	35.76	330.78	13.41	0.13
0.14	0.41	0.00	0.00	0.91	177.60	54.72	0.17	0.14	1.80	0.24	31.20	0.00	14.40	1.34	33.60	74.40	669.60	26.40	0.26
1.06	0.89	0.00	0.00	1.28	67.67	18.38	0.11	0.08	1.12	0.09	11.11	0.00	26.26	1.07	15.15	38.38	249.47	459.55	0.18
0.05	0.13	0.00	0.00	0.97	137.70	29.07	0.13	0.10	1.81	0.05	13.77	0.00	84.15	1.86	30.60	51.00	606.90	563.55	0.43
0.02	0.07	0.00	0.00	0.00	93.99	14.94	0.07	0.05	1.54	0.24	21.93	0.00	48.20	0.63	26.51	33.74	257.87	966.41	0.31
0.05	0.18	0.00	0.00	0.00	151.38	38.63	0.16	0.08	1.77	0.31	26.36	0.00	67.86	1.20	28.71	60.03	655.11	566.37	0.42
0.05	0.12	0.00	0.00	0.77	144.00	34.08	0.12	0.07	1.78	0.22	18.72	0.00	72.00	1.32	28.80	45.60	530.40	355.20	0.38
0.07	0.21	0.00	34.27	0.57	92.38	28.46	0.09	0.07	0.94	0.12	22.35	0.00	7.45	0.67	16.39	35.76	330.78	13.41	0.13
0.05	0.14	0.00	84.60	0.68	115.20	42.12	0.11	0.07	0.90	0.14	15.84	0.00	23.40	0.92	18.00	50.40	367.20	23.40	0.13
0.26	0.60	0.00	0.00	0.01	46.98	21.17	0.29	0.26	4.89	0.18	36.72	0.00	59.40	4.91	104.76	192.24	1850.58	1131.30	1.07
9.53	2.27	0.00	0.00	0.00	141.90	111.98	0.21	0.42	3.99	0.35	25.30	0.00	51.70	2.95	89.10	152.90	1721.50	292.60	0.86
0.02	0.06	0.00	0.00	0.05	0.00	18.10	0.05	0.03	0.47	0.11	14.35	0.00	34.32	0.34	12.48	29.64	210.60	78.00	0.31
0.01	0.07	0.00	0.00	0.04	0.00	27.30	0.05	0.04	0.52	0.12	18.85	0.00	39.00	0.39	14.30	35.10	248.30	87.10	0.35
0.03	0.20	0.00	0.00	0.98	1898.95	8.15	0.08	0.08	0.95	0.13	38.47	0.00	44.01	1.71	26.08	68.46	474.33	242.87	0.67
0.03	0.19	0.00	0.00	0.99	1177.00	8.80	0.19	0.33	2.34	0.19	52.25	0.00	68.75	2.26	60.50	140.25	464.75	96.25	1.35
0.00	0.50	0.00	0.00	0.00	0.00	0.00	0.25	0.00	4.00	0.00	0.00	0.00	96.00	1.50	0.00	0.00	0.00	380.00	7.50
0.00	0.00	0.00	0.00	0.03	11.75	1.08	0.00	0.00	0.01	0.00	0.23	0.00	3.00	0.01	0.53	1.50	8.25	1.03	0.00
0.17	0.23	0.00	0.00	0.23	56.98	14.78	0.12	0.03	0.31	0.22	3.39	0.00	12.32	0.26	16.94	13.86	178.64	3.08	0.11
0.01	0.08	0.00	0.00	0.22	0.00	16.46	0.14	0.04	0.75	0.31	21.76	0.00	19.04	0.71	24.48	66.64	911.20	10.88	0.27
4.50	1.10	0.00	0.00	0.10	0.00	0.00	0.13	0.06	1.39	0.05	0.95	0.33	2.28	0.31	4.56	63.84	92.34	303.24	0.62
1.88	0.38	0.00	0.00	0.12	0.00	0.00	0.38	0.09	3.22	0.21	1.86	0.36	4.65	0.38	9.77	137.64	181.35	718.89	0.79
0.00	0.00	0.00	0.00	0.00	0.00	0.00	0.00	0.00	0.00	0.00	0.00	0.00	0.00	0.00	0.00	0.00	0.00	170.00	0.00
0.95	0.19	0.21	0.00	0.00	1.61	0.00	0.08	0.06	0.52	0.06	2.07	0.39	12.65	0.27	3.91	30.36	75.67	306.82	0.57
0.10	0.48	0.00	0.00	1.35	43.18	7.87	0.38	0.15	1.09	0.33	60.71	0.00	127.00	0.74	81.28	264.16	751.84	1008.38	3.56
3.70	0.56	0.00	0.00	0.00	55.86	4.79	0.13	0.13	2.50	0.24	115.44	0.00	119.70	4.26	66.50	215.46	851.20	1263.50	3.19
7.33	2.18	0.00	0.00	1.22	38.85	5.96	0.16	0.16	2.33	0.13	77.70	0.00	124.32	4.48	72.52	269.36	608.65	1113.70	4.84
1.70	0.51	0.00	0.00	0.00	45.54	5.06	0.13	0.10	1.14	0.15	91.84	0.00	134.09	4.30	86.02	273.24	781.77	1047.42	3.69
5.39	1.87	0.00	0.00	0.00	0.00	2.78	0.35	0.13	1.04	0.23	122.45	0.00	154.33	5.03	108.79	275.77	905.74	1067.66	1.85
0.09	0.40	0.00	0.00	0.00	1.72	0.00	0.41	0.10	0.88	0.12	255.94	0.00	46.44	3.61	120.40	240.80	610.60	407.64	1.93
0.62	1.22	0.00	0.00	0.00	4.80	9.12	0.07	0.07	0.34	1.13	160.32	0.00	76.80	3.24	69.60	216.00	412.80	717.60	2.54
0.05	0.44	0.00	0.00	0.00	0.00	3.07	0.28	0.18	1.28	0.18	125.95	0.00	69.12	3.15	79.36	268.80	657.92	888.32	1.41
0.13	0.35	0.00	0.00	0.00	2.00	2.90	0.34	0.15	2.10	0.35	357.90	0.00	37.00	6.59	71.00	356.00	731.00	4.00	2.50
0.05	0.17	0.00	0.00	0.00	0.00	0.00	0.14	0.07	0.63	0.22	121.46	0.00	50.61	4.36	93.99	178.34	530.20	809.76	1.57

USDA ID Code	Food Name	Weight in Grams*	Quantity of Units	Unit of Measure	Protein (gm)	Fat (gm)	Carbohydrate (gm)	Kcalories	Caffeine (gm)	Fiber (gm)	Cholesterol (mg)	Saturated Fat (gm)
	Beans, Navy, Cnd	262.0000	1.000	Cup	19.73	1.13	53.58	296.06	0.00	13.36	0.00	0.29
	Beans, Pinto, Cnd	240.0000	1.000	Cup	11.66	1.94	36.60	206.40	0.00	11.04	0.00	0.41
	Beans, Refried, Cnd	15.8000	1.000	Tbsp	0.87	0.20	2.45	14.85	0.00	0.84	1.26	0.07
	Beans, Refried, Lowfat, Cnd	268.0000	0.500	Cup	16.00	0.00	42.00	240.00	0.00	14.00	0.00	0.00
2	Beans, Refried, No Fat	128.0000	0.500	Cup	7.30	0.50	19.50	92.00	0.00	6.20	0.00	0.00
	Beef, Corned, Brisket, Ckd	85.0000	3.000	Ounce	15.44	16.13	0.40	213.35	0.00	0.00	83.30	5.39
	Beef, Corned, Loaf, Jellied	28.3500	1.000	Slice	6.49	1.73	0.00	43.38	0.00	0.00	13.32	0.74
	Beef, Cured, Lunch Meat, Jellied	28.3500	1.000	Slice	5.39	0.94	0.00	31.47	0.00	0.00	9.64	0.40
	Beef, Cured, Smoked, Chopped Bee	28.3500	1.000	Slice	5.72	1.25	0.53	37.71	0.00	0.00	13.04	0.51
	Beef, Cured, Thin-sliced	21.0000	5.000	Slice	5.90	0.81	1.20	37.17	0.00	0.00	8.61	0.35
	Beef, Filet, Tnderloin, Broiled	85.0000	3.000	Ounce	23.55	9.75	0.00	188.70	0.00	0.00	70.55	3.68
	Beef, Ground, Extra Lean, Broile	85.0000	3.000	Ounce	21.59	13.88	0.00	217.60	0.00	0.00	71.40	5.46
	Beef, Ground, Extra Lean, Pan-fr	85.0000	3.000	Ounce	21.22	13.96	0.00	216.75	0.00	0.00	68.85	5.48
	Beef, Ground, Lean, Broiled	85.0000	3.000	Ounce	21.01	15.69	0.00	231.20	0.00	0.00	73.95	6.16
	Beef, Ground, Lean, Pan-fried	85.0000	3.000	Ounce	20.60	16.20	0.00	233.75	0.00	0.00	71.40	6.37
	Beef, Ground, Regular, Broiled	85.0000	3.000	Ounce	20.46	17.59	0.00	245.65	0.00	0.00	76.50	6.91
	Beef, Ground, Regular, Pan-fried	85.0000	3.000	Ounce	20.33	19.18	0.00	260.10	0.00	0.00	75.65	7.53
	Beef, Liver, Ckd, Braised	85.0000	3.000	Ounce	20.72	4.16	2.90	136.85	0.00	0.00	330.65	1.62
	Beef, Liver, Ckd, Pan-fried	85.0000	3.000	Ounce	22.71	6.80	6.67	184.45	0.00	0.00	409.70	2.27
	Beef, Loaved, Lunch Meat	28.3500	1.000	Slice	4.08	7.43	0.82	87.32	0.00	0.00	18.14	3.17
	Beef, Steaks and Roasts, Ckd, 1/	28.3500	3.000	Ounce	7.07	7.62	0.00	98.94	0.00	0.00	25.80	3.15
	Beef, Steaks and Roasts, Ckd, Fa	85.0000	3.000	Ounce	23.23	14.76	0.00	232.05	0.00	0.00	73.95	5.82
	Beef, Steaks and Roasts, Ckd., 1	85.0000	3.000	Ounce	22.05	18.31	0.00	259.25	0.00	0.00	74.80	7.26
	Beef, Thin Sliced	21.0000	5.000	Slice	5.90	0.81	1.20	37.17	0.00	0.00	8.61	0.35
	Bologna, Beef, Lunch Meat	23.0000	1.000	Slice	2.81	6.56	0.18	71.76	0.00	0.00	13.34	2.78
	Bologna, Lunch Meat	23.0000	1.000	Slice	3.52	4.57	0.17	56.81	0.00	0.00	13.57	1.58
	Bologna, Turkey	21.0000	1.000	Slice	2.88	3.19	0.20	41.79	0.00	0.00	20.79	1.06
	Buffalo (Chicken) Wings	22.7500	4.000	Each	4.50	3.00	0.50	47.50	0.00	0.00	25.00	0.75
	Chicken Roll, Light Meat	28.3500	3.000	Ounce	5.54	2.09	0.69	45.08	0.00	0.00	14.18	0.57
	Chicken Salad Sandwich Spread	28.3500	3.000	Ounce	3.30	3.83	2.10	56.70	0.00	0.00	8.51	0.98
	Chicken Spread, Cnd	28.3500	3.000	Ounce	4.37	3.32	1.53	54.43	0.00	0.00	14.74	0.96
	Chicken, Back, Meat & Skin, Ckd,	72.0000	3.000	Ounce	15.82	15.78	7.38	238.32	0.00	0.00	63.36	4.20
	Chicken, Back, Meat & Skin, Ckd,	44.0000	3.000	Ounce	12.23	9.13	2.86	145.64	0.00	0.00	39.16	2.47
	Chicken, Back, Meat & Skin, Ckd,	32.0000	3.000	Ounce	8.30	6.71	0.00	96.00	0.00	0.00	28.16	1.86
	Chicken, Back, Meat & Skin, Ckd,	36.0000	3.000	Ounce	7.98	6.53	0.00	92.88	0.00	0.00	28.08	1.81
	Chicken, Back, Meat Only, Ckd, F	35.0000	3.000	Ounce	10.50	5.36	1.99	100.80	0.00	0.00	32.55	1.44
	Chicken, Back, Meat Only, Ckd, R	24.0000	3.000	Ounce	6.77	3.16	0.00	57.36	0.00	0.00	21.60	0.86
	Chicken, Back, Meat Only, Ckd, S	26.0000	3.000	Ounce	6.58	2.91	0.00	54.34	0.00	0.00	22.10	0.79
	Chicken, Breast, Meat & Skin, Ck	84.0000	3.000	Ounce	20.87	11.09	7.55	218.40	0.00	0.25	71.40	2.96
	Chicken, Breast, Meat & Skin, Ck	59.0000	3.000	Ounce	18.79	5.23	0.97	130.98	0.00	0.06	52.51	1.45
	Chicken, Breast, Meat & Skin, Ck	58.0000	3.000	Ounce	17.28	4.51	0.00	114.26	0.00	0.00	48.72	1.27
	Chicken, Breast, Meat & Skin, Ck	66.0000	3.000	Ounce	18.08	4.90	0.00	121.44	0.00	0.00	49.50	1.37
	Chicken, Breast, Meat Only, Ckd,	52.0000	3.000	Ounce	17.39	2.45	0.27	97.24	0.00	0.00	47.32	0.67
	Chicken, Breast, Meat Only, Ckd,	52.0000	3.000	Ounce	16.13	1.86	0.00	85.80	0.00	0.00	44.20	0.53
	Chicken, Breast, Meat Only, Ckd,	57.0000	3.000	Ounce	16.52	1.73	0.00	86.07	0.00	0.00	43.89	0.48
	Chicken, Cnd	142.0000	5.000	Fl Oz	30.91	11.29	0.00	234.30	0.00	0.00	88.04	3.12
	Chicken, Dark Meat, Meat & Skin,	167.0000	3.000	Ounce	36.49	31.13	15.66	497.66	0.00	0.00	148.63	8.27
	Chicken, Dark Meat, Meat & Skin,	110.0000	3.000	Ounce	29.94	18.60	4.49	313.50	0.00	0.00	101.20	5.04
	Chicken, Dark Meat, Meat & Skin,	101.0000	3.000	Ounce	26.23	15.94	0.00	255.53	0.00	0.00	91.91	4.41
	Chicken, Dark Meat, Meat & Skin,	110.0000	3.000	Ounce	25.85	16.13	0.00	256.30	0.00	0.00	90.20	4.47
	Chicken, Dark Meat, Meat Only, C	91.0000	3.000	Ounce	26.38	10.57	2.36	217.49	0.00	0.00	87.36	2.84
	Chicken, Dark Meat, Meat Only, C	81.0000	3.000	Ounce	22.17	7.88	0.00	166.05	0.00	0.00	75.33	2.15
	Chicken, Dark Meat, Meat Only, C	86.0000	3.000	Ounce	22.33	7.72	0.00	165.12	0.00	0.00	75.68	2.11
	Chicken, Drumstick, Meat & Skin,	43.0000	3.000	Ounce	9.44	6.77	3.56	115.24	0.00	0.13	36.98	1.78
	Chicken, Drumstick, Meat & Skin,	29.0000	3.000	Ounce	7.82	3.98	0.47	71.05	0.00	0.03	26.10	1.06

Monounsaturated Fat (gm)	Polyunsaturated Fat (gm)	Vitamin D (mg)	Vitamin K (mg)	Vitamin E (mg)	Vitamin A (re)	Vitamin C (mg)	Thiamin (mg)	Riboflavin (mg)	Niacin (mg)	Vitamin B_6 (mg)	Folate (mg)	Vitamin B_{12} (mcg)	Calcium (mg)	Iron (mg)	Magnesium (mg)	Phosphorus (mg)	Potassium (mg)	Sodium (mg)	Zinc (mg)
0.10	0.50	0.00	0.00	1.00	0.00	1.83	0.37	0.16	1.28	0.26	163.23	0.00	123.14	4.85	123.14	351.08	754.56	1173.76	2.02
0.38	0.70	0.00	0.00	2.26	4.80	2.16	0.24	0.14	0.70	0.17	144.48	0.00	103.20	3.50	64.80	220.80	583.20	705.60	1.66
0.09	0.02	0.00	0.00	0.00	0.00	0.95	0.00	0.00	0.05	0.02	1.74	0.00	5.53	0.26	5.21	13.59	42.19	47.24	0.18
0.00	0.00	0.00	0.00	0.00	0.00	0.00	0.00	0.00	0.00	0.00	0.00	0.00	0.00	2.00	0.00	0.00	0.00	960.00	0.00
0.00	0.00	0.00	0.00	0.00	0.00	0.00	0.00	0.00	0.00	0.00	0.00	0.00	43.00	1.92	0.00	0.00	0.00	480.00	0.00
7.84	0.57	0.00	0.00	0.14	0.00	0.00	0.03	0.14	2.58	0.20	5.10	1.39	6.80	1.58	10.20	106.25	123.25	963.90	3.89
0.76	0.09	0.00	0.00	0.05	0.00	0.00	0.00	0.03	0.50	0.03	2.27	0.36	3.12	0.58	3.12	20.70	28.63	270.18	1.16
0.41	0.05	0.00	0.00	0.00	0.00	0.00	0.04	0.08	1.37	0.07	1.98	1.46	2.84	0.98	5.10	39.41	113.97	374.79	1.01
0.52	0.07	0.00	0.00	0.00	0.00	0.00	0.02	0.05	1.30	0.10	2.27	0.49	2.27	0.81	5.95	51.31	106.88	356.64	1.11
0.35	0.04	0.00	0.00	0.03	0.00	0.00	0.02	0.04	1.11	0.07	2.31	0.54	2.31	0.57	3.99	35.28	90.09	302.19	0.84
3.81	0.44	0.00	0.00	0.00	0.00	0.00	0.09	0.26	2.90	0.25	7.65	2.30	5.95	3.13	22.95	203.15	332.35	51.85	4.07
6.08	0.52	0.00	0.00	0.15	0.00	0.00	0.05	0.23	4.22	0.23	7.65	1.84	5.95	2.00	17.85	136.85	266.05	59.50	4.63
6.11	0.52	0.00	0.00	0.15	0.00	0.00	0.05	0.22	4.00	0.23	7.65	1.70	5.95	2.01	17.85	136.00	265.20	59.50	4.61
6.87	0.59	0.00	0.00	0.17	0.00	0.00	0.04	0.18	4.39	0.22	7.65	2.00	9.35	1.79	17.85	134.30	255.85	65.45	4.56
7.09	0.60	0.00	0.00	0.17	0.00	0.00	0.04	0.19	4.07	0.24	7.65	1.93	8.50	1.85	17.00	135.15	254.15	65.45	4.42
7.70	0.65	0.00	0.00	0.20	0.00	0.00	0.03	0.16	4.90	0.23	7.65	2.49	9.35	2.07	17.00	144.50	248.20	70.55	4.40
8.40	0.71	0.00	0.00	0.20	0.00	0.00	0.03	0.17	4.96	0.20	7.65	2.30	9.35	2.08	17.00	145.35	255.00	71.40	4.31
0.55	0.91	0.00	0.00	0.00	9011.70	19.55	0.17	3.48	9.11	0.77	184.45	60.35	5.95	5.75	17.00	343.40	199.75	59.50	5.16
1.38	1.45	0.00	0.00	0.54	9119.65	19.55	0.18	3.52	12.27	1.22	187.00	95.03	9.35	5.34	19.55	391.85	309.40	90.10	4.63
3.47	0.25	0.00	0.00	0.06	0.00	0.00	0.03	0.06	1.04	0.05	1.42	1.10	3.12	0.66	3.97	33.74	58.97	376.77	0.72
3.41	0.29	0.00	0.00	0.00	0.00	0.00	0.02	0.06	0.98	0.09	1.98	0.68	2.84	0.74	5.95	54.72	81.36	16.73	1.56
6.30	0.54	0.00	0.00	0.15	0.00	0.00	0.07	0.19	3.13	0.28	5.95	2.13	7.65	2.32	19.55	179.35	274.55	52.70	5.15
7.84	0.66	0.00	0.00	0.17	0.00	0.00	0.07	0.18	3.09	0.28	5.95	2.07	8.50	2.23	18.70	172.55	266.05	52.70	4.97
0.35	0.04	0.00	0.00	0.04	0.00	0.00	0.02	0.04	1.11	0.07	2.31	0.54	2.31	0.57	3.99	35.28	90.09	302.19	0.84
3.17	0.25	0.16	0.00	0.04	0.00	0.00	0.01	0.03	0.55	0.03	1.15	0.33	2.76	0.38	2.76	20.24	36.11	225.63	0.50
2.25	0.49	0.00	0.00	0.06	0.00	8.12	0.12	0.04	0.90	0.06	1.15	0.21	2.53	0.18	3.22	31.97	64.63	272.32	0.47
1.01	0.90	0.00	0.00	0.00	0.00	0.00	0.01	0.03	0.74	0.05	1.47	0.06	17.64	0.32	2.94	27.51	41.79	184.38	0.37
0.00	0.00	0.00	0.00	0.00	15.00	0.30	0.00	0.00	0.00	0.00	0.00	0.00	6.00	0.10	0.00	0.00	0.00	225.00	0.00
0.84	0.45	0.00	0.00	0.08	6.80	0.00	0.02	0.04	1.50	0.06	0.57	0.04	12.19	0.27	5.39	44.51	64.64	165.56	0.20
0.92	1.76	0.00	0.00	0.00	11.91	0.34	0.01	0.02	0.47	0.03	1.42	0.11	2.84	0.17	2.84	9.36	51.88	106.88	0.29
1.38	0.71	0.00	0.00	0.00	7.09	0.00	0.00	0.03	0.78	0.04	0.85	0.04	35.44	0.66	3.40	25.23	30.05	109.43	0.33
6.42	3.74	0.00	0.00	0.00	25.92	0.00	0.09	0.15	4.20	0.17	14.40	0.19	18.72	1.07	13.68	98.64	129.60	228.24	1.41
3.60	2.12	0.00	0.00	0.00	16.28	0.00	0.05	0.11	3.21	0.13	6.60	0.12	10.56	0.71	10.12	73.04	99.44	39.60	1.09
2.65	1.48	0.00	0.00	0.09	31.68	0.00	0.02	0.06	2.15	0.09	1.92	0.09	6.72	0.45	6.40	49.28	67.20	27.84	0.72
2.57	1.44	0.00	0.00	0.10	31.68	0.00	0.01	0.05	1.56	0.05	1.80	0.06	6.48	0.44	5.76	43.20	52.20	23.04	0.69
2.01	1.27	0.00	0.00	0.00	10.15	0.00	0.04	0.09	2.69	0.12	3.15	0.11	9.10	0.58	8.75	61.60	87.85	34.65	0.98
1.16	0.73	0.00	0.00	0.06	6.72	0.00	0.02	0.05	1.70	0.08	1.68	0.07	5.76	0.33	5.28	39.60	56.88	23.04	0.64
1.05	0.68	0.00	0.00	0.07	7.02	0.00	0.01	0.04	1.19	0.05	1.82	0.05	5.46	0.33	4.42	33.80	41.08	17.42	0.62
4.59	2.59	0.00	0.00	0.89	16.80	0.00	0.10	0.13	8.84	0.36	12.60	0.25	16.80	1.05	20.16	155.40	168.84	231.00	0.80
2.07	1.16	0.00	0.00	0.00	8.85	0.00	0.05	0.08	8.11	0.34	3.54	0.20	9.44	0.70	17.70	137.47	152.81	44.84	0.65
1.76	0.96	0.00	0.00	0.16	15.66	0.00	0.04	0.07	7.37	0.32	2.32	0.19	8.12	0.62	15.66	124.12	142.10	41.18	0.59
1.91	1.04	0.00	0.00	0.18	15.84	0.00	0.03	0.08	5.15	0.19	1.98	0.14	8.58	0.61	14.52	102.96	117.48	40.92	0.64
0.89	0.56	0.00	0.00	0.22	3.64	0.00	0.04	0.07	7.69	0.33	2.08	0.19	8.32	0.59	16.12	127.92	143.52	41.08	0.56
0.64	0.40	0.00	0.00	0.14	3.12	0.00	0.04	0.06	7.13	0.31	2.08	0.18	7.80	0.54	15.08	118.56	133.12	38.48	0.52
0.59	0.38	0.00	0.00	0.15	3.42	0.00	0.02	0.07	4.83	0.19	1.71	0.13	7.41	0.50	13.68	94.05	106.59	35.91	0.55
4.47	2.49	0.00	0.00	0.30	48.28	2.84	0.03	0.18	8.99	0.50	5.68	0.41	19.88	2.24	17.04	157.62	195.96	714.26	2.00
12.66	7.40	0.00	0.00	0.00	51.77	0.00	0.20	0.37	9.37	0.42	30.06	0.45	35.07	2.40	33.40	242.15	308.95	492.65	3.47
7.33	4.30	0.00	0.00	0.00	34.10	0.00	0.11	0.26	7.52	0.35	12.10	0.33	18.70	1.65	26.40	193.60	253.00	97.90	2.86
6.25	3.52	0.00	0.00	0.00	58.58	0.00	0.07	0.21	6.42	0.31	7.07	0.29	15.15	1.37	22.22	169.68	222.20	87.87	2.51
6.33	3.56	0.00	0.00	0.00	59.40	0.00	0.06	0.20	4.96	0.19	6.60	0.22	15.40	1.44	19.80	146.30	182.60	77.00	2.49
3.93	2.52	0.00	0.00	0.00	21.84	0.00	0.08	0.23	6.43	0.34	8.19	0.30	16.38	1.36	22.75	170.17	230.23	88.27	2.65
2.88	1.83	0.00	0.00	0.22	17.82	0.00	0.06	0.19	5.31	0.29	6.48	0.26	12.15	1.08	18.63	144.99	194.40	75.33	2.27
2.80	1.80	0.00	0.00	0.23	18.06	0.00	0.05	0.17	4.08	0.18	6.02	0.19	12.04	1.17	17.20	122.98	155.66	63.64	2.29
2.76	1.63	0.00	0.00	0.00	11.18	0.00	0.05	0.09	2.19	0.12	7.74	0.12	7.31	0.58	8.60	63.21	79.98	115.67	1.00
1.57	0.94	0.00	0.00	0.00	7.25	0.00	0.02	0.07	1.75	0.10	2.90	0.09	3.48	0.39	6.67	51.04	66.41	25.81	0.84

USDA ID Code	Food Name	Weight in Grams*	Quantity of Units	Unit of Measure	Protein (gm)	Fat (gm)	Carbohydrate (gm)	Kcalories	Caffeine (gm)	Fiber (gm)	Cholesterol (mg)	Saturated Fat (gm)
	Chicken, Drumstick, Meat & Skin,	31.0000	3.000	Ounce	8.38	3.46	0.00	66.96	0.00	0.00	28.21	0.95
	Chicken, Drumstick, Meat & Skin,	34.0000	3.000	Ounce	8.61	3.62	0.00	69.36	0.00	0.00	28.22	0.99
	Chicken, Drumstick, Meat Only, C	25.0000	3.000	Ounce	7.16	2.02	0.00	48.75	0.00	0.00	23.50	0.53
	Chicken, Drumstick, Meat Only, C	26.0000	3.000	Ounce	7.36	1.47	0.00	44.72	0.00	0.00	24.18	0.38
	Chicken, Drumstick, Meat Only, C	28.0000	3.000	Ounce	7.70	1.60	0.00	47.32	0.00	0.00	24.64	0.42
	Chicken, Giblets, Ckd, Fried	13.0000	3.000	Ounce	4.23	1.75	0.57	36.01	0.00	0.00	57.98	0.49
	Chicken, Giblets, Ckd, Simmered	14.0000	3.000	Ounce	3.62	0.67	0.13	21.98	0.00	0.00	55.02	0.21
	Chicken, Heart, Ckd, Simmered	1.0000	3.000	Ounce	0.26	0.08	0.00	1.85	0.00	0.00	2.42	0.02
	Chicken, Leg, Meat & Skin, Ckd,	95.0000	3.000	Ounce	20.68	15.36	8.28	259.35	0.00	0.29	85.50	4.07
	Chicken, Leg, Meat & Skin, Ckd,	67.0000	3.000	Ounce	17.98	9.67	1.68	170.18	0.00	0.07	62.98	2.61
	Chicken, Leg, Meat & Skin, Ckd,	69.0000	3.000	Ounce	17.91	9.29	0.00	160.08	0.00	0.00	63.48	2.57
	Chicken, Leg, Meat & Skin, Ckd,	75.0000	3.000	Ounce	18.13	9.69	0.00	165.00	0.00	0.00	63.00	2.68
	Chicken, Leg, Meat Only, Ckd, Fr	56.0000	3.000	Ounce	15.89	5.22	0.36	116.48	0.00	0.00	55.44	1.39
	Chicken, Leg, Meat Only, Ckd, Ro	57.0000	3.000	Ounce	15.41	4.81	0.00	108.87	0.00	0.00	53.58	1.31
	Chicken, Leg, Meat Only, Ckd, St	60.0000	3.000	Ounce	15.76	4.84	0.00	111.00	0.00	0.00	53.40	1.32
	Chicken, Liver, Ckd, Simmered	6.0000	3.000	Ounce	1.46	0.33	0.05	9.42	0.00	0.00	37.86	0.11
	Chicken, Meat Only, Ckd, Fried	140.0000	1.000	Cup	42.80	12.77	2.37	306.60	0.00	0.14	131.60	3.44
	Chicken, Meat Only, Roasted	8.7000	1.000	Tbsp	2.52	0.64	0.00	16.53	0.00	0.00	7.74	0.18
	Chicken, Meat Only, Stewed	8.7000	1.000	Tbsp	2.37	0.58	0.00	15.40	0.00	0.00	7.22	0.16
	Chicken, Thigh, Meat & Skin, Ckd	52.0000	3.000	Ounce	11.24	8.60	4.72	144.04	0.00	0.16	48.36	2.29
	Chicken, Thigh, Meat & Skin, Ckd	38.0000	3.000	Ounce	10.17	5.69	1.21	99.56	0.00	0.04	36.86	1.55
	Chicken, Thigh, Meat & Skin, Ckd	37.0000	3.000	Ounce	9.27	5.73	0.00	91.39	0.00	0.00	34.41	1.60
	Chicken, Thigh, Meat & Skin, Ckd	41.0000	3.000	Ounce	9.54	6.04	0.00	95.12	0.00	0.00	34.44	1.69
	Chicken, Thigh, Meat Only, Ckd,	31.0000	3.000	Ounce	8.74	3.19	0.37	67.58	0.00	0.00	31.62	0.86
	Chicken, Thigh, Meat Only, Ckd,	31.0000	3.000	Ounce	8.04	3.37	0.00	64.79	0.00	0.00	29.45	0.94
	Chicken, Thigh, Meat Only, Ckd,	33.0000	3.000	Ounce	8.25	3.23	0.00	64.35	0.00	0.00	29.70	0.89
	Chicken, Wing, Meat & Skin, Ckd,	29.0000	3.000	Ounce	5.76	6.32	3.17	93.96	0.00	0.09	22.91	1.69
	Chicken, Wing, Meat & Skin, Ckd,	19.0000	3.000	Ounce	4.96	4.21	0.45	60.99	0.00	0.02	15.39	1.15
	Chicken, Wing, Meat & Skin, Ckd,	21.0000	3.000	Ounce	5.64	4.09	0.00	60.90	0.00	0.00	17.64	1.14
	Chicken, Wing, Meat & Skin, Ckd,	24.0000	3.000	Ounce	5.47	4.04	0.00	59.76	0.00	0.00	16.80	1.13
	Chicken, Wing, Meat Only, Ckd, F	12.0000	3.000	Ounce	3.62	1.10	0.00	25.32	0.00	0.00	10.08	0.30
	Chicken, Wing, Meat Only, Ckd, R	13.0000	3.000	Ounce	3.96	1.06	0.00	26.39	0.00	0.00	11.05	0.29
	Chicken, Wing, Meat Only, Ckd, S	14.0000	3.000	Ounce	3.81	1.01	0.00	25.34	0.00	0.00	10.36	0.28
189	Chili w/ Beans, Cnd	255.0000	0.500	Cup	14.56	14.00	30.37	285.60	0.00	11.22	43.35	6.00
	Cornish Game Hen	110.0000	0.500	Bird	25.63	4.26	0.00	147.40	0.00	0.00	116.60	1.09
	Duck, Domesticated, Meat & Skin,	140.0000	1.000	Cup	26.59	39.69	0.00	471.80	0.00	0.00	117.60	13.54
	Duck, Domesticated, Meat Only, R	100.0000	3.000	Ounce	23.48	11.20	0.00	201.00	0.00	0.00	89.00	4.17
	Gardenburger	90.0000	1.000	Each	18.00	4.00	8.00	140.00	0.00	5.00	0.00	2.00
	Ham and Cheese Loaf(or Roll), Lu	28.3500	1.000	Slice	4.71	5.73	0.41	73.43	0.00	0.00	16.16	2.13
	Ham and Cheese Spread, Lunch Mea	15.0000	1.000	Tbsp	2.43	2.78	0.34	36.75	0.00	0.00	9.15	1.29
	Ham Salad Spread	15.0000	1.000	Tbsp	1.30	2.33	1.60	32.40	0.00	0.00	5.55	0.76
	Ham, Approx 11% Fat, Sliced	28.3500	1.000	Slice	4.98	3.00	0.88	51.60	0.00	0.00	16.16	0.96
	Ham, Chopped, Not Cnd	21.0000	1.000	Slice	3.60	3.62	0.00	48.09	0.00	0.00	10.71	1.20
	Ham, Chopped, Spiced, Cnd	21.0000	1.000	Slice	3.37	3.95	0.06	50.19	0.00	0.00	10.29	1.32
	Ham, Extra Lean, Appx 5% Fat	28.3500	1.000	Slice	5.49	1.41	0.27	37.14	0.00	0.00	13.32	0.46
	Ham, Minced	21.0000	1.000	Slice	3.42	4.34	0.39	55.23	0.00	0.00	14.70	1.51
	Hamburger Patty, Meatless	90.0000	1.000	Each	18.00	4.00	8.00	140.00	0.00	5.00	0.00	1.50
	Hot Dog, Beef	45.0000	1.000	Each	5.40	12.83	0.81	141.75	0.00	0.00	27.45	5.42
	Hot Dog, Chicken	28.3500	1.000	Ounce	3.67	5.52	1.92	72.86	0.00	0.00	28.63	1.57
	Hot Dog, Fat Free	50.0000	1.000	Each	7.00	0.00	2.00	40.00	0.00	0.00	15.00	0.00
	Hot Dog, Turkey	28.3500	1.000	Ounce	4.05	5.02	0.42	64.07	0.00	0.00	30.33	1.67
	Hummus, Fresh	15.0000	1.000	Tbsp	0.74	1.27	3.03	25.65	0.00	0.77	0.00	0.19
	Lamb, Ground, Ckd, Broiled	85.0000	3.000	Ounce	21.04	16.70	0.00	240.55	0.00	0.00	82.45	6.90
	Lamb, Leg, Shank, Meat and Fat,	85.0000	3.000	Ounce	22.45	10.58	0.00	191.25	0.00	0.00	76.50	4.33
	Lamb, Leg, Shank, Meat Only, Ckd	85.0000	3.000	Ounce	23.94	5.67	0.00	153.00	0.00	0.00	73.95	2.02

Monounsaturated Fat (gm)	Polyunsaturated Fat (gm)	Vitamin D (mg)	Vitamin K (mg)	Vitamin E (mg)	Vitamin A (re)	Vitamin C (mg)	Thiamin (mg)	Riboflavin (mg)	Niacin (mg)	Vitamin B_6 (mg)	Folate (mg)	Vitamin B_{12} (mcg)	Calcium (mg)	Iron (mg)	Magnesium (mg)	Phosphorus (mg)	Potassium (mg)	Sodium (mg)	Zinc (mg)
1.32	0.78	0.00	0.00	0.08	9.30	0.00	0.02	0.07	1.86	0.11	2.48	0.10	3.72	0.41	7.13	54.25	70.99	27.90	0.89
1.38	0.81	0.00	0.00	0.09	9.18	0.00	0.02	0.06	1.43	0.06	2.38	0.07	3.74	0.45	6.80	47.94	62.56	25.84	0.90
0.74	0.49	0.00	0.00	0.12	4.50	0.00	0.02	0.06	1.54	0.10	2.25	0.09	3.00	0.33	6.00	46.50	62.25	24.00	0.81
0.49	0.36	0.00	0.00	0.07	4.68	0.00	0.02	0.06	1.58	0.10	2.34	0.09	3.12	0.34	6.24	47.84	63.96	24.70	0.83
0.54	0.38	0.00	0.00	0.08	4.76	0.00	0.01	0.06	1.20	0.06	2.24	0.07	3.08	0.38	5.88	42.00	55.72	22.40	0.85
0.57	0.44	0.00	0.00	0.00	465.27	1.13	0.01	0.20	1.43	0.08	49.27	1.73	2.34	1.34	3.25	37.18	42.90	14.69	0.82
0.17	0.15	0.00	0.00	0.18	312.06	1.12	0.01	0.13	0.57	0.05	52.64	1.42	1.68	0.90	2.80	32.06	22.12	8.12	0.64
0.02	0.02	0.00	0.00	0.00	0.09	0.02	0.00	0.01	0.03	0.00	0.80	0.07	0.19	0.09	0.20	1.99	1.32	0.48	0.07
6.25	3.66	0.00	0.00	0.00	25.65	0.00	0.11	0.21	5.16	0.26	17.10	0.27	17.10	1.33	19.00	144.40	179.55	265.05	2.06
3.81	2.23	0.00	0.00	0.00	18.76	0.00	0.06	0.16	4.39	0.23	7.37	0.21	8.71	0.96	16.08	121.94	156.11	58.96	1.80
3.62	2.07	0.00	0.00	0.19	26.91	0.00	0.05	0.14	4.28	0.23	4.83	0.21	8.28	0.92	15.87	120.06	155.25	60.03	1.79
3.78	2.15	0.00	0.00	0.20	27.00	0.00	0.04	0.14	3.44	0.14	4.50	0.15	8.25	1.01	15.00	104.25	132.00	54.75	1.82
1.92	1.24	0.00	0.00	0.00	11.20	0.00	0.04	0.14	3.75	0.22	5.04	0.19	7.28	0.78	14.00	108.08	142.24	53.76	1.67
1.74	1.12	0.00	0.00	0.15	10.83	0.00	0.05	0.13	3.60	0.21	4.56	0.18	6.84	0.75	13.68	104.31	137.94	51.87	1.63
1.76	1.13	0.00	0.00	0.16	10.80	0.00	0.04	0.13	2.88	0.13	4.80	0.14	6.60	0.84	12.60	89.40	114.00	46.80	1.67
0.08	0.05	0.00	0.00	0.09	294.78	0.95	0.01	0.11	0.27	0.03	46.20	1.16	0.84	0.51	1.26	18.72	8.40	3.06	0.26
4.69	3.01	0.00	0.00	0.64	25.20	0.00	0.13	0.28	13.52	0.67	9.80	0.48	23.80	1.89	37.80	287.00	359.80	127.40	3.14
0.23	0.15	0.00	0.00	0.02	1.39	0.00	0.01	0.02	0.80	0.04	0.52	0.03	1.31	0.11	2.18	16.97	21.14	7.48	0.18
0.21	0.13	0.00	0.00	0.02	1.31	0.00	0.00	0.01	0.53	0.02	0.52	0.02	1.22	0.10	1.83	13.05	15.66	6.09	0.17
3.48	2.03	0.00	0.00	0.00	15.08	0.00	0.06	0.12	2.97	0.14	9.88	0.15	9.36	0.75	10.92	80.60	99.84	149.76	1.06
2.23	1.30	0.00	0.00	0.00	11.02	0.00	0.03	0.09	2.64	0.13	4.56	0.11	5.32	0.57	9.50	71.06	90.06	33.44	0.96
2.28	1.27	0.00	0.00	0.10	17.76	0.00	0.03	0.08	2.36	0.11	2.59	0.11	4.44	0.50	8.14	64.38	82.14	31.08	0.87
2.39	1.33	0.00	0.00	0.11	18.04	0.00	0.02	0.08	2.00	0.07	2.46	0.08	4.51	0.56	7.79	56.99	69.70	29.11	0.92
1.18	0.75	0.00	0.00	0.00	6.51	0.00	0.03	0.08	2.21	0.12	2.79	0.10	4.03	0.45	8.06	61.69	80.29	29.45	0.86
1.29	0.77	0.00	0.00	0.08	6.20	0.00	0.02	0.07	2.02	0.11	2.48	0.10	3.72	0.41	7.44	56.73	73.78	27.28	0.80
1.22	0.74	0.00	0.00	0.09	6.27	0.00	0.02	0.07	1.72	0.07	2.31	0.07	3.63	0.47	6.93	49.17	60.39	24.75	0.85
2.60	1.47	0.00	0.00	0.00	9.86	0.00	0.03	0.04	1.53	0.09	5.22	0.07	5.80	0.37	4.64	35.09	40.02	92.80	0.40
1.69	0.94	0.00	0.00	0.00	7.22	0.00	0.01	0.03	1.27	0.08	1.14	0.05	2.85	0.24	3.61	28.50	33.63	14.63	0.33
1.60	0.87	0.00	0.00	0.06	9.87	0.00	0.01	0.03	1.40	0.09	0.63	0.06	3.15	0.27	3.99	31.71	38.64	17.22	0.38
1.58	0.86	0.00	0.00	0.06	9.60	0.00	0.01	0.02	1.11	0.05	0.72	0.04	2.88	0.27	3.84	29.04	33.36	16.08	0.39
0.37	0.25	0.00	0.00	0.00	2.16	0.00	0.01	0.02	0.87	0.07	0.48	0.04	1.80	0.14	2.52	19.68	24.96	10.92	0.25
0.34	0.23	0.00	0.00	0.04	2.34	0.00	0.01	0.02	0.95	0.08	0.52	0.04	2.08	0.15	2.73	21.58	27.30	11.96	0.28
0.32	0.22	0.00	0.00	0.04	2.24	0.00	0.01	0.02	0.73	0.04	0.42	0.03	1.82	0.16	2.52	18.76	21.42	10.22	0.28
5.95	0.92	0.00	0.00	1.87	86.70	4.34	0.12	0.27	0.91	0.34	57.89	0.00	119.85	8.75	114.75	392.70	930.75	1331.10	5.10
1.36	1.03	0.00	0.00	0.29	22.00	0.66	0.08	0.25	6.90	0.39	2.20	0.33	14.30	0.85	20.90	163.90	275.00	69.30	1.68
18.06	5.11	0.00	0.00	0.98	88.20	0.00	0.24	0.38	6.76	0.25	8.40	0.42	15.40	3.78	22.40	218.40	285.60	82.60	2.60
3.70	1.43	0.00	0.00	0.70	23.00	0.00	0.26	0.47	5.10	0.25	10.00	0.40	12.00	2.70	20.00	203.00	252.00	65.00	2.60
0.00	1.00	0.00	0.00	0.00	0.00	0.00	0.00	0.00	4.00	0.00	0.00	0.00	96.00	2.00	0.00	0.00	0.00	380.00	8.00
2.63	0.62	0.31	0.00	0.08	6.52	0.00	0.17	0.05	0.98	0.07	0.85	0.23	16.44	0.26	4.54	71.73	83.35	380.74	0.57
1.06	0.21	0.00	0.00	0.00	13.65	0.00	0.05	0.03	0.32	0.02	0.45	0.11	32.55	0.11	2.70	74.25	24.30	179.55	0.34
1.08	0.41	0.00	0.00	0.26	0.00	0.00	0.07	0.02	0.32	0.02	0.15	0.11	1.20	0.09	1.50	18.00	22.50	136.80	0.17
1.40	0.34	0.00	0.00	0.08	0.00	0.00	0.24	0.07	1.49	0.10	0.85	0.24	1.98	0.28	5.39	70.02	94.12	373.37	0.61
1.72	0.44	0.00	0.00	0.00	0.00	0.00	0.13	0.04	0.81	0.07	0.21	0.19	1.47	0.17	3.36	32.55	66.99	287.91	0.41
1.93	0.43	0.00	0.00	0.05	0.00	0.42	0.11	0.04	0.67	0.07	0.21	0.15	1.47	0.20	2.73	29.19	59.64	286.65	0.38
0.67	0.14	0.00	0.00	0.08	0.00	0.00	0.26	0.06	1.37	0.13	1.13	0.21	1.98	0.22	4.82	61.80	99.22	405.12	0.55
2.01	0.52	0.00	0.00	0.00	0.00	0.00	0.15	0.04	0.87	0.05	0.21	0.20	2.10	0.17	3.36	32.97	65.31	261.45	0.40
0.00	0.50	0.00	0.00	0.00	0.00	0.00	0.25	0.00	4.00	0.00	0.00	0.00	96.00	1.50	0.00	0.00	0.00	380.00	7.50
6.13	0.62	0.41	0.00	0.09	0.00	0.00	0.02	0.05	1.09	0.05	1.80	0.69	9.00	0.64	1.35	39.15	74.70	461.70	0.98
2.40	1.15	0.00	0.00	0.06	10.77	0.00	0.02	0.03	0.88	0.09	1.13	0.07	26.93	0.57	2.84	30.33	23.81	388.40	0.29
0.00	0.00	0.00	0.00	0.00	0.00	0.00	0.00	0.00	0.00	0.00	0.00	0.00	0.00	0.20	0.00	0.00	0.00	460.00	0.00
1.58	1.42	0.00	0.00	0.18	0.00	0.00	0.01	0.05	1.17	0.07	2.27	0.08	30.05	0.52	3.97	37.99	50.75	404.27	0.88
0.53	0.48	0.00	0.00	0.15	0.30	1.19	0.01	0.01	0.06	0.06	8.91	0.00	7.50	0.24	4.35	16.80	26.10	36.60	0.17
7.07	1.19	0.00	0.00	0.21	0.00	0.00	0.09	0.21	5.70	0.12	16.15	2.22	18.70	1.52	20.40	170.85	288.15	68.85	3.97
4.50	0.75	0.00	0.00	0.14	0.00	0.00	0.09	0.23	5.57	0.14	18.70	2.27	8.50	1.68	21.25	168.30	277.10	55.25	3.96
2.48	0.37	0.00	0.00	0.15	0.00	0.00	0.09	0.24	5.43	0.14	20.40	2.30	6.80	1.75	22.10	176.80	290.70	56.10	4.27

USDA ID Code	Food Name	Weight in Grams*	Quantity of Units	Unit of Measure	Protein (gm)	Fat (gm)	Carbohydrate (gm)	Kcalories	Caffeine (gm)	Fiber (gm)	Cholesterol (mg)	Saturated Fat (gm)
	Lamb, Leg, Sirloin, Meat and Fat	85.0000	3.000	Ounce	20.94	17.57	0.00	248.20	0.00	0.00	82.45	7.43
	Lamb, Leg, Sirloin, Meat Only, C	85.0000	3.000	Ounce	24.10	7.79	0.00	173.40	0.00	0.00	78.20	2.79
	Lamb, Leg, Whole, Meat and Fat,	85.0000	3.000	Ounce	21.72	14.01	0.00	219.30	0.00	0.00	79.05	5.86
	Lamb, Leg, Whole, Meat Only, Ckd	85.0000	3.000	Ounce	24.06	6.58	0.00	162.35	0.00	0.00	75.65	2.35
	Lamb, Loin, Meat and Fat, Ckd, B	64.0000	3.000	Ounce	16.11	14.77	0.00	202.24	0.00	0.00	64.00	6.29
	Lamb, Loin, Meat and Fat, Ckd, R	85.0000	3.000	Ounce	19.17	20.05	0.00	262.65	0.00	0.00	80.75	8.70
	Lamb, Loin, Meat Only, Ckd, Broi	46.0000	3.000	Ounce	13.80	4.48	0.00	99.36	0.00	0.00	43.70	1.60
	Lamb, Loin, Meat Only, Ckd, Roas	85.0000	3.000	Ounce	22.60	8.30	0.00	171.70	0.00	0.00	73.95	3.16
	Lamb, Meat and Fat, Ckd	85.0000	3.000	Ounce	20.84	17.80	0.00	249.90	0.00	0.00	82.45	7.51
	Lamb, Meat Only, Ckd	85.0000	3.000	Ounce	23.99	8.09	0.00	175.10	0.00	0.00	78.20	2.89
	Lamb, Rib, Meat and Fat, Ckd, Br	85.0000	3.000	Ounce	18.81	25.15	0.00	306.85	0.00	0.00	84.15	10.80
	Lamb, Rib, Meat and Fat, Ckd, Ro	85.0000	3.000	Ounce	17.95	25.35	0.00	305.15	0.00	0.00	82.45	10.85
	Lamb, Rib, Meat Only, Ckd, Broil	85.0000	3.000	Ounce	23.58	11.01	0.00	199.75	0.00	0.00	77.35	3.95
	Lamb, Rib, Meat Only, Ckd, Roast	85.0000	3.000	Ounce	22.24	11.31	0.00	197.20	0.00	0.00	74.80	4.05
	Lunch Meat, Dutch Brand Loaf	28.3500	1.000	Slice	3.80	5.05	1.58	68.04	0.00	0.00	13.32	1.80
	Lunch Meat, Honey Loaf	28.3500	1.000	Slice	4.47	1.27	1.51	36.29	0.00	0.00	9.64	0.41
	Lunch Meat, Olive Loaf	28.3500	1.000	Slice	3.36	4.68	2.60	66.62	0.00	0.00	10.77	1.66
	Lunch Meat, Olive Loaf, Pork	28.3500	1.000	Slice	3.35	4.68	2.61	66.62	0.00	0.00	10.77	1.66
	Lunch Meat, Pickle and Pimento L	28.3500	1.000	Slice	3.26	5.98	1.67	74.28	0.00	0.00	10.49	2.23
	Lunch Meat, Pickle and Pimiento	28.3500	1.000	Slice	3.26	5.98	1.67	74.28	0.00	0.00	10.49	2.22
	Lunch Meat, Picnic Loaf	28.3500	1.000	Slice	4.23	4.72	1.35	65.77	0.00	0.00	10.77	1.72
	Pastrami, Beef, Cured	28.3500	1.000	Slice	4.89	8.27	0.86	98.94	0.00	0.00	26.37	2.95
	Pastrami, Turkey	28.3500	1.000	Slice	5.21	1.76	0.47	39.97	0.00	0.00	15.31	0.51
	Pork, Backribs	85.0000	3.000	Ounce	20.62	25.14	0.00	314.50	0.00	0.00	100.30	9.34
	Pork, Braunschweiger	28.3500	3.000	Ounce	3.83	9.10	0.89	101.78	0.00	0.00	44.23	3.09
	Pork, Cnd, Lunch Meat	21.0000	1.000	Slice	2.63	6.36	0.44	70.14	0.00	0.00	13.02	2.27
	Pork, Ground, Ckd	85.0000	3.000	Ounce	21.84	17.65	0.00	252.45	0.00	0.00	79.90	6.56
	Pork, Ham and Cheese Loaf or Rol	28.3500	3.000	Ounce	4.71	5.73	0.41	73.43	0.00	0.00	16.16	2.13
	Pork, Ham Patties, Grilled	59.5000	3.000	Ounce	7.91	18.36	1.01	203.49	0.00	0.00	42.84	6.60
	Pork, Ham Salad Spread	28.3500	3.000	Ounce	2.46	4.40	3.02	61.24	0.00	0.00	10.49	1.43
	Pork, Ham, Chopped, Cnd	28.3500	3.000	Ounce	4.55	5.34	0.08	67.76	0.00	0.00	13.89	1.78
	Pork, Ham, Cnd, Extra Lean (appx	85.0000	3.000	Ounce	17.99	4.15	0.44	115.60	0.00	0.00	25.50	1.36
	Pork, Ham, Cnd, Extra Lean and R	85.0000	3.000	Ounce	17.80	7.17	0.42	141.95	0.00	0.00	34.85	2.39
	Pork, Ham, Cnd, Extra Lean and R	28.3500	1.000	Ounce	5.09	2.11	0.00	40.82	0.00	0.00	10.77	0.69
	Pork, Ham, Cnd, Regular (approx	85.0000	3.000	Ounce	17.45	12.92	0.36	192.10	0.00	0.00	52.70	4.28
	Pork, Ham, Extra Lean (5% Fat),	85.0000	3.000	Ounce	17.79	4.70	1.28	123.25	0.00	0.00	45.05	1.54
	Pork, Ham, Extra Lean (5% Fat),	28.3500	3.000	Ounce	5.49	1.41	0.27	37.14	0.00	0.00	13.32	0.46
	Pork, Ham, Extra Lean and Reg, R	85.0000	3.000	Ounce	18.67	6.51	0.43	140.25	0.00	0.00	48.45	2.22
	Pork, Ham, Extra Lean and Reg, U	28.3500	1.000	Slice	5.18	2.38	0.65	45.93	0.00	0.00	15.03	0.77
	Pork, Ham, Meat and Fat, Roasted	85.0000	3.000	Ounce	18.33	14.25	0.00	206.55	0.00	0.00	52.70	5.08
	Pork, Ham, Meat Only, Roasted	85.0000	3.000	Ounce	21.29	4.68	0.00	133.45	0.00	0.00	46.75	1.56
	Pork, Ham, Regular (11% Fat), Ro	85.0000	3.000	Ounce	19.23	7.67	0.00	151.30	0.00	0.00	50.15	2.65
	Pork, Ham, Regular (11% Fat), Un	28.3500	3.000	Ounce	4.98	3.00	0.88	51.60	0.00	0.00	16.16	0.96
	Pork, Spareribs, Meat and Fat, C	85.0000	3.000	Ounce	24.70	25.76	0.00	337.45	0.00	0.00	102.85	9.45
	Pork, Tenderloin, Meat and Fat,	76.0000	3.000	Ounce	22.69	6.16	0.00	152.76	0.00	0.00	71.44	2.23
	Pork, Tenderloin, Meat Only, Ckd	73.0000	3.000	Ounce	22.21	4.62	0.00	136.51	0.00	0.00	68.62	1.64
	Salami, Turkey	28.3500	1.000	Slice	4.64	3.91	0.16	55.57	0.00	0.00	23.25	1.14
	Sausage, Beerwurst, Pork	6.0000	1.000	Slice	0.85	1.13	0.12	14.28	0.00	0.00	3.54	0.38
	Sausage, Bockwurst	28.3500	1.000	Ounce	3.78	7.82	0.14	87.03	0.00	0.00	16.73	2.87
	Sausage, Bratwurst	28.3500	1.000	Ounce	3.99	7.33	0.59	85.33	0.00	0.00	17.01	2.64
	Sausage, Italian, Ckd	67.0000	1.000	Link	13.42	17.22	1.01	216.41	0.00	0.00	52.26	6.08
	Sausage, Kielbasa, Kolbassy	26.0000	1.000	Slice	3.45	7.06	0.56	80.60	0.00	0.00	17.42	2.58
	Sausage, Knockwurst	28.3500	1.000	Ounce	3.37	7.87	0.50	87.32	0.00	0.00	16.44	2.89
	Sausage, Link, Pork and Beef	16.0000	1.000	Small	2.14	4.85	0.23	53.76	0.00	0.00	11.36	1.70
	Sausage, Pepperoni	5.5000	1.000	Slice	1.15	2.42	0.16	27.34	0.00	0.00	4.35	0.89

Monounsaturated Fat (gm)	Polyunsaturated Fat (gm)	Vitamin D (mg)	Vitamin K (mg)	Vitamin E (mg)	Vitamin A (re)	Vitamin C (mg)	Thiamin (mg)	Riboflavin (mg)	Niacin (mg)	Vitamin B_6 (mg)	Folate (mg)	Vitamin B_{12} (mcg)	Calcium (mg)	Iron (mg)	Magnesium (mg)	Phosphorus (mg)	Potassium (mg)	Sodium (mg)	Zinc (mg)
7.40	1.27	0.00	0.00	0.11	0.00	0.00	0.09	0.24	5.63	0.12	14.45	2.15	9.35	1.70	18.70	155.55	255.85	57.80	3.51
3.42	0.51	0.00	0.00	0.14	0.00	0.00	0.10	0.26	5.33	0.14	17.85	2.19	6.80	1.87	21.25	172.55	283.05	60.35	4.12
5.92	1.00	0.00	0.00	0.13	0.00	0.00	0.09	0.23	5.60	0.13	17.00	2.20	9.35	1.68	20.40	162.35	266.05	56.10	3.74
2.88	0.43	0.00	0.00	0.15	0.00	0.00	0.09	0.25	5.39	0.14	19.55	2.24	6.80	1.80	22.10	175.10	287.30	57.80	4.20
6.21	1.08	0.00	0.00	0.08	0.00	0.00	0.06	0.16	4.54	0.08	11.52	1.58	12.80	1.16	15.36	125.44	209.28	49.28	2.23
8.23	1.59	0.00	0.00	0.09	0.00	0.00	0.09	0.20	6.04	0.09	16.15	1.88	15.30	1.80	19.55	153.00	209.10	54.40	2.90
1.96	0.29	0.00	0.00	0.07	0.00	0.00	0.05	0.13	3.15	0.07	11.04	1.16	8.74	0.92	12.88	103.96	172.96	38.64	1.90
3.36	0.73	0.00	0.00	0.14	0.00	0.00	0.09	0.23	5.81	0.14	21.25	1.84	14.45	2.07	22.95	175.10	226.95	56.10	3.45
7.50	1.28	0.00	0.00	0.12	0.00	0.00	0.09	0.21	5.66	0.11	15.30	2.17	14.45	1.60	19.55	159.80	263.50	61.20	3.79
3.54	0.53	0.00	0.00	0.16	0.00	0.00	0.09	0.24	5.37	0.14	19.55	2.22	12.75	1.74	22.10	178.50	292.40	64.60	4.48
10.30	2.01	0.00	0.00	0.10	0.00	0.00	0.08	0.19	5.95	0.09	11.90	2.16	16.15	1.60	19.55	151.30	229.50	64.60	3.40
10.64	1.84	0.00	0.00	0.09	0.00	0.00	0.08	0.18	5.74	0.09	12.75	1.90	18.70	1.36	17.00	141.10	230.35	62.05	2.97
4.43	1.00	0.00	0.00	0.15	0.00	0.00	0.09	0.21	5.57	0.13	17.85	2.24	13.60	1.88	24.65	181.05	266.05	72.25	4.48
4.96	0.74	0.00	0.00	0.13	0.00	0.00	0.08	0.20	5.24	0.13	18.70	1.84	17.85	1.50	19.55	165.75	267.75	68.85	3.80
2.36	0.54	0.28	0.00	0.06	0.00	0.00	0.09	0.08	0.68	0.07	0.57	0.37	23.81	0.35	5.95	45.93	106.60	354.38	0.49
0.57	0.13	0.26	0.00	0.06	0.00	0.00	0.14	0.07	0.89	0.09	2.27	0.31	4.82	0.38	4.82	40.54	97.24	374.22	0.69
2.23	0.55	0.00	0.00	0.00	5.67	2.49	0.08	0.07	0.52	0.07	0.57	0.36	30.90	0.15	5.39	36.00	84.20	420.71	0.39
2.23	0.55	0.31	0.00	0.07	5.67	0.00	0.09	0.07	0.52	0.07	0.57	0.36	30.90	0.15	5.39	36.00	84.20	420.71	0.39
2.72	0.73	0.00	0.00	0.00	1.98	3.83	0.08	0.07	0.58	0.05	1.42	0.33	26.93	0.29	5.10	39.69	96.39	393.78	0.40
2.72	0.73	0.31	0.00	0.07	1.98	0.00	0.08	0.07	0.58	0.05	1.42	0.33	26.93	0.29	5.10	39.69	96.39	393.78	0.40
2.18	0.54	0.34	0.00	0.00	0.00	0.00	0.10	0.07	0.65	0.09	0.57	0.43	13.32	0.29	4.25	35.44	75.69	329.99	0.62
4.10	0.28	0.00	0.00	0.07	0.00	0.00	0.03	0.05	1.44	0.05	1.98	0.50	2.55	0.54	5.10	42.53	64.64	347.85	1.21
0.58	0.45	0.00	0.00	0.06	0.00	0.00	0.02	0.07	1.00	0.08	1.42	0.07	2.55	0.47	3.97	56.70	73.71	296.26	0.61
11.44	1.97	0.00	0.00	0.00	2.55	0.26	0.37	0.17	3.02	0.26	2.55	0.54	38.25	1.17	17.85	165.75	267.75	85.85	2.86
4.23	1.06	0.00	0.00	0.00	1196.37	2.72	0.07	0.43	2.37	0.09	12.47	5.70	2.55	2.65	3.12	47.63	56.42	324.04	0.80
3.00	0.75	0.00	0.00	0.05	0.00	0.21	0.08	0.04	0.66	0.04	1.26	0.19	1.26	0.15	2.10	17.22	45.15	270.69	0.31
7.86	1.59	0.00	0.00	0.22	1.70	0.60	0.60	0.19	3.58	0.33	5.10	0.46	18.70	1.10	20.40	192.10	307.70	62.05	2.73
2.63	0.62	0.00	0.00	0.00	6.52	7.12	0.17	0.05	0.98	0.07	0.85	0.23	16.44	0.26	4.54	71.73	83.35	380.74	0.57
8.73	1.98	0.00	0.00	0.15	0.00	0.00	0.21	0.11	1.93	0.10	1.79	0.42	5.36	0.96	5.95	60.10	145.18	632.49	1.13
2.04	0.77	0.00	0.00	0.00	0.00	1.70	0.12	0.03	0.59	0.04	0.28	0.22	2.27	0.17	2.84	34.02	42.53	258.55	0.31
2.60	0.58	0.00	0.00	0.00	0.00	0.51	0.15	0.05	0.91	0.09	0.28	0.20	1.98	0.27	3.69	39.41	80.51	386.98	0.52
2.12	0.37	0.00	0.00	0.22	0.00	0.00	0.88	0.21	4.16	0.38	4.25	0.60	5.10	0.78	17.85	177.65	295.80	964.75	1.90
3.45	0.77	0.00	0.00	0.22	0.00	0.00	0.82	0.21	4.28	0.34	4.25	0.71	5.95	0.91	17.00	187.85	298.35	907.80	1.97
1.01	0.22	0.00	0.00	0.07	0.00	0.00	0.25	0.07	1.30	0.13	1.70	0.23	1.70	0.26	4.54	58.68	94.69	361.75	0.52
6.01	1.51	0.00	0.00	0.00	0.00	11.90	0.70	0.22	4.51	0.26	4.25	0.90	6.80	1.16	14.45	206.55	303.45	799.85	2.13
2.23	0.46	0.00	0.00	0.22	0.00	0.00	0.64	0.17	3.42	0.34	2.55	0.55	6.80	1.26	11.90	166.60	243.95	1022.55	2.45
0.67	0.14	0.00	0.00	0.07	0.00	7.46	0.26	0.06	1.37	0.13	1.13	0.21	1.98	0.22	4.82	61.80	99.23	405.12	0.55
3.18	0.91	0.00	0.00	0.22	0.00	0.00	0.63	0.24	4.52	0.30	2.55	0.58	6.80	1.19	16.15	210.80	307.70	1177.25	2.24
1.12	0.26	0.00	0.00	0.07	0.00	0.00	0.25	0.07	1.44	0.11	0.85	0.23	1.98	0.26	5.10	66.91	84.20	362.31	0.58
6.70	1.54	0.00	0.00	0.22	0.00	0.00	0.51	0.19	3.79	0.32	2.55	0.54	5.95	0.74	16.15	181.90	243.10	1008.95	1.97
2.15	0.54	0.00	0.00	0.22	0.00	0.00	0.58	0.21	4.27	0.40	3.40	0.60	5.95	0.80	18.70	192.95	268.60	1127.95	2.18
3.77	1.20	0.00	0.00	0.22	0.00	0.00	0.62	0.28	5.23	0.26	2.55	0.60	6.80	1.14	18.70	238.85	347.65	1275.00	2.10
1.40	0.34	0.00	0.00	0.07	0.00	7.85	0.24	0.07	1.49	0.10	0.85	0.24	1.98	0.28	5.39	70.02	94.12	373.37	0.61
11.46	2.32	0.00	0.00	0.22	2.55	0.00	0.35	0.32	4.66	0.30	3.40	0.92	39.95	1.57	20.40	221.85	272.00	79.05	3.91
2.54	0.56	0.00	0.00	0.00	1.52	0.76	0.74	0.29	3.84	0.40	4.56	0.74	3.80	1.06	26.60	220.40	337.44	48.64	2.20
1.88	0.41	0.00	0.00	0.00	1.46	0.73	0.72	0.28	3.75	0.39	4.38	0.73	3.65	1.04	26.28	215.35	329.23	47.45	2.15
1.29	1.00	0.00	0.00	0.00	0.00	0.00	0.02	0.05	1.00	0.07	1.13	0.06	5.67	0.46	4.25	30.05	69.17	284.63	0.51
0.54	0.14	0.05	0.00	0.00	0.00	0.00	0.03	0.01	0.20	0.02	0.18	0.05	0.48	0.05	0.78	6.18	15.18	74.40	0.10
3.69	0.84	0.00	0.00	0.04	1.70	0.00	0.12	0.05	1.17	0.07	1.70	0.23	4.54	0.18	5.10	41.39	76.55	313.27	0.44
3.46	0.78	0.31	0.00	0.07	0.00	0.28	0.14	0.05	0.91	0.06	0.57	0.27	12.47	0.37	4.25	42.24	60.10	157.91	0.65
8.01	2.20	0.00	0.00	0.17	0.00	1.34	0.42	0.15	2.79	0.22	3.35	0.87	16.08	1.01	12.06	113.90	203.68	617.74	1.60
3.36	0.80	0.00	0.00	0.06	0.00	0.00	0.06	0.05	0.75	0.05	1.30	0.42	11.44	0.38	4.16	38.48	70.46	279.76	0.53
3.63	0.83	0.00	0.00	0.16	0.00	0.00	0.10	0.04	0.77	0.05	0.57	0.33	3.12	0.26	3.12	27.78	56.42	286.34	0.47
2.27	0.52	0.20	0.00	0.04	0.00	0.00	0.04	0.03	0.52	0.03	0.32	0.24	1.60	0.23	1.92	17.12	30.24	151.20	0.34
1.16	0.24	0.00	0.00	0.01	0.00	0.00	0.02	0.01	0.27	0.01	0.22	0.14	0.55	0.08	0.88	6.55	19.09	112.20	0.14

USDA ID Code	Food Name	Weight in Grams*	Quantity of Units	Unit of Measure	Protein (gm)	Fat (gm)	Carbohydrate (gm)	Kcalories	Caffeine (gm)	Fiber (gm)	Cholesterol (mg)	Saturated Fat (gm)
	Sausage, Polish-style	28.3500	1.000	Ounce	4.00	8.14	0.46	92.42	0.00	0.00	19.85	2.93
	Sausage, Pork, Links or Bulk, Ck	13.0000	1.000	Link	2.55	4.05	0.13	47.97	0.00	0.00	10.79	1.41
	Sausage, Pork, Smoked Link, Gril	28.3500	3.000	Ounce	6.29	9.00	0.60	110.28	0.00	0.00	19.28	3.21
	Sausage, Salami, Beef and Pork,	10.0000	1.000	Slice	2.29	3.44	0.26	41.80	0.00	0.00	7.90	1.22
	Sausage, Salami, Beef, Ckd	23.0000	1.000	Slice	3.46	4.76	0.65	60.26	0.00	0.00	14.95	2.07
	Sausage, Smoked Link, Pork	16.0000	1.000	Small	3.55	5.07	0.34	62.24	0.00	0.00	10.88	1.81
	Sausage, Smoked, Beef, Cured,	28.3500	1.000	Ounce	4.00	7.63	0.69	88.45	0.00	0.00	18.99	3.24
	Sausage, Turkey	28.3500	3.000	Ounce	4.00	2.50	1.50	45.00	0.00	0.00	15.00	1.25
743	Tofu Pups-Light Life	42.0000	1.000	Each	8.00	2.50	2.00	60.00	0.00	0.00	0.00	1.00
744	Tofu Rella, Garlic Herb	28.0000	1.000	Ounce	6.00	5.00	3.00	80.00	0.00	0.00	0.00	1.00
745	Tofu Rella, Monterey Style	28.0000	1.000	Ounce	6.00	5.00	3.00	80.00	0.00	0.00	0.00	1.00
746	Tofu Wieners-Yves	38.0000	1.000	Each	9.00	0.50	2.00	45.00	0.00	0.00	0.00	0.00
	Turkey Breast Meat	21.0000	1.000	Slice	4.73	0.33	0.00	23.10	0.00	0.00	8.61	0.10
	Turkey Burger, Breaded, Battered	28.0000	3.000	Ounce	3.92	5.04	4.40	79.24	0.00	0.14	17.36	1.31
749	Turkey Burger, Grilled	82.0000	3.000	Ounce	22.44	10.78	0.00	192.70	0.00	0.00	83.64	2.78
	Turkey Lunch Meat	28.3500	1.000	Slice	5.37	1.44	0.10	36.29	0.00	0.00	15.88	0.48
	Turkey Roast, Roasted	135.0000	1.000	Cup	28.78	7.80	4.14	209.25	0.00	0.00	71.55	2.57
	Turkey Roll, Light and Dark Meat	28.3500	3.000	Ounce	5.14	1.98	0.60	42.24	0.00	0.00	15.59	0.58
	Turkey Roll, Light Meat	28.3500	3.000	Ounce	5.30	2.05	0.15	41.67	0.00	0.00	12.19	0.57
	Turkey Sticks, Breaded, Battered	64.0000	2.250	Ounce	9.09	10.82	10.88	178.56	0.00	0.00	40.96	2.80
	Turkey Thigh, Prebasted, Meat &	314.0000	3.000	Ounce	59.03	26.82	0.00	492.98	0.00	0.00	194.68	8.32
	Turkey, Back, Meat & Skin, Ckd,	34.0000	3.000	Ounce	9.04	4.89	0.00	82.62	0.00	0.00	30.94	1.42
	Turkey, Breast, Meat & Skin, Ckd	112.0000	3.000	Ounce	32.16	8.30	0.00	211.68	0.00	0.00	82.88	2.35
	Turkey, Ckd, Roasted, Meat & Ski	260.0000	3.000	Ounce	72.75	24.57	0.18	533.00	0.00	0.00	247.00	7.20
	Turkey, Dark Meat, Ckd, Roasted	91.0000	3.000	Ounce	26.00	6.57	0.00	170.17	0.00	0.00	77.35	2.20
	Turkey, Dark Meat, Meat & Skin,	104.0000	3.000	Ounce	28.59	12.00	0.00	229.84	0.00	0.00	92.56	3.63
	Turkey, Giblets, Ckd, Simmered,	10.0000	3.000	Ounce	2.66	0.51	0.21	16.70	0.00	0.00	41.80	0.15
	Turkey, Ground, Ckd	82.0000	3.000	Ounce	22.44	10.78	0.00	192.70	0.00	0.00	83.64	2.78
	Turkey, Leg, Meat & Skin, Ckd, R	71.0000	3.000	Ounce	19.79	6.97	0.00	147.68	0.00	0.00	60.35	2.17
	Turkey, Light Meat, Ckd, Roasted	117.0000	3.000	Ounce	34.98	3.77	0.00	183.69	0.00	0.00	80.73	1.21
	Turkey, Light Meat, Meat & Skin,	136.0000	3.000	Ounce	38.86	11.33	0.00	267.92	0.00	0.00	103.36	3.18
	Turkey, Meat & Skin, Ckd, Roaste	140.0000	1.000	Cup	39.34	13.62	0.00	291.20	0.00	0.00	114.80	3.98
	Turkey, Meat Only, Ckd, Roasted	140.0000	1.000	Cup	41.05	6.96	0.00	238.00	0.00	0.00	106.40	2.30
	Turkey, Thin Sliced	28.3500	3.000	Ounce	6.38	0.45	0.00	31.19	0.00	0.00	11.62	0.14
	Turkey, Wing, Meat & Skin, Ckd,	24.0000	3.000	Ounce	6.57	2.98	0.00	54.96	0.00	0.00	19.44	0.81
	Veal, Meat and Fat, Ckd	85.0000	3.000	Ounce	25.59	9.68	0.00	196.35	0.00	0.00	96.90	3.64
	Veal, Meat Only, Ckd	85.0000	3.000	Ounce	27.12	5.59	0.00	166.60	0.00	0.00	100.30	1.56
	Venison, Ckd, Roasted	85.0000	3.000	Ounce	25.68	2.71	0.00	134.30	0.00	0.00	95.20	1.06
	Alfalfa Seeds, Sprouted, Fresh	3.0000	1.000	Tbsp	0.12	0.02	0.11	0.87	0.00	0.08	0.00	0.00
	Almond Butter, w/ salt	16.0000	1.000	Tbsp	2.43	9.46	3.40	101.28	0.00	0.59	0.00	0.90
	Almond Butter, w/o salt	16.0000	1.000	Tbsp	2.43	9.46	3.40	101.28	0.00	0.59	0.00	0.90
	Almonds, Toasted, Unblanched	141.9600	0.500	Cup	28.93	72.07	32.52	836.14	0.00	15.90	0.00	6.83
	Brazil Nuts, Dried, Unblanched	28.3500	1.000	Ounce	4.07	18.77	3.63	185.98	0.00	1.53	0.00	4.58
	Cashews, Dry Roasted	28.3500	1.000	Ounce	4.34	13.14	9.27	162.73	0.00	0.85	0.00	2.60
	Cashews, Oil Roasted	28.3500	1.000	Ounce	4.58	13.67	8.09	163.30	0.00	1.08	0.00	2.70
467	Hazelnuts, Dry Roasted	28.0000	1.000	Ounce	2.80	18.80	5.10	188.00	0.00	2.00	0.00	1.40
468	Hazelnuts, Oil Roasted	28.0000	1.000	Ounce	4.00	18.00	5.40	187.00	0.00	1.80	0.00	1.30
	Macadamias, Dried	28.3500	1.000	Ounce	2.24	21.48	3.92	203.55	0.00	2.44	0.00	3.42
	Macadamias, Oil Roasted	112.0000	0.500	Cup	9.60	83.60	15.60	769.00	0.00	10.40	0.00	13.60
	Peanut Butter, Chunk Style, w/ S	32.0000	2.000	Tbsp	7.70	15.98	6.91	188.48	0.00	2.11	0.00	3.07
	Peanut Butter, Chunk Style, w/o	32.0000	2.000	Tbsp	7.70	15.98	6.91	188.48	0.00	2.11	0.00	3.07
	Peanut Butter, Reduced Fat, Crea	18.0000	2.000	Tbsp	4.00	6.00	7.50	95.00	0.00	1.00	0.00	1.25
638	Peanut Butter, Reduced Fat, Crun	18.0000	2.000	Tbsp	4.00	6.00	7.50	95.00	0.00	1.00	0.00	1.25
	Peanut Butter, Smooth Style, w/	32.0000	2.000	Tbsp	8.07	16.33	6.17	189.76	0.00	1.89	0.00	3.31
	Peanut Butter, Smooth Style, w/o	32.0000	2.000	Tbsp	8.07	16.33	6.17	189.76	0.00	1.89	0.00	3.31

Monounsaturated Fat (gm)	Polyunsaturated Fat (gm)	Vitamin D (mg)	Vitamin K (mg)	Vitamin E (mg)	Vitamin A (re)	Vitamin C (mg)	Thiamin (mg)	Riboflavin (mg)	Niacin (mg)	Vitamin B_6 (mg)	Folate (mg)	Vitamin B_{12} (mcg)	Calcium (mg)	Iron (mg)	Magnesium (mg)	Phosphorus (mg)	Potassium (mg)	Sodium (mg)	Zinc (mg)
3.83	0.87	0.00	0.00	0.00	0.00	0.28	0.14	0.04	0.98	0.05	0.57	0.28	3.40	0.41	3.97	38.56	67.19	248.35	0.55
1.81	0.50	0.00	0.00	0.02	0.00	0.26	0.10	0.03	0.59	0.04	0.26	0.22	4.16	0.16	2.21	23.92	46.93	168.22	0.33
4.15	1.07	0.00	0.00	0.09	0.00	0.51	0.20	0.07	1.28	0.10	1.42	0.46	8.51	0.33	5.39	45.93	95.26	425.25	0.80
1.71	0.32	0.00	0.00	0.03	0.00	0.00	0.06	0.03	0.49	0.05	0.20	0.19	0.80	0.15	1.70	14.20	37.80	186.00	0.32
2.17	0.24	0.28	0.00	0.04	0.00	0.00	0.02	0.04	0.75	0.04	0.46	0.70	2.07	0.50	3.22	25.99	51.52	270.48	0.50
2.34	0.60	0.00	0.00	0.04	0.00	0.32	0.11	0.04	0.72	0.06	0.80	0.26	4.80	0.19	3.04	25.92	53.76	240.00	0.45
3.68	0.30	0.00	0.00	0.00	0.00	0.00	0.01	0.04	0.90	0.03	1.13	0.53	1.98	0.50	3.69	29.77	49.90	320.64	0.79
0.00	0.00	0.00	0.00	0.00	10.00	6.00	0.00	0.00	0.00	0.00	0.00	0.00	12.00	1.75	0.00	0.00	0.00	300.00	0.00
0.00	0.00	0.00	0.00	0.00	0.00	0.00	0.00	0.00	0.00	0.00	0.00	0.00	0.00	0.00	0.00	0.00	0.00	140.00	0.00
0.00	0.00	0.00	0.00	0.00	0.00	0.00	0.00	0.00	0.00	0.00	0.00	0.00	0.00	0.00	0.00	0.00	0.00	280.00	0.00
0.00	0.00	0.00	0.00	0.00	0.00	0.00	0.00	0.00	0.00	0.00	0.00	0.00	0.00	0.00	0.00	0.00	0.00	280.00	0.00
0.00	0.00	0.00	0.00	0.00	0.00	0.00	0.00	0.00	0.00	0.00	0.00	0.00	0.00	0.00	0.00	0.00	0.00	240.00	0.00
0.09	0.06	0.00	0.00	0.02	0.00	0.00	0.01	0.02	1.75	0.08	0.84	0.42	1.47	0.08	4.20	48.09	58.38	300.51	0.24
2.09	1.32	0.00	0.00	0.67	3.08	0.00	0.03	0.05	0.64	0.06	7.84	0.06	3.92	0.62	4.20	75.60	77.00	224.00	0.40
4.01	2.65	0.00	0.00	0.28	0.00	0.00	0.04	0.14	3.95	0.32	5.74	0.27	20.50	1.58	19.68	160.72	221.40	87.74	2.35
0.33	0.43	0.00	0.00	0.18	0.00	0.00	0.01	0.07	1.00	0.07	1.70	0.07	2.84	0.78	4.54	54.15	92.14	282.37	0.83
1.62	2.24	0.00	0.00	0.51	0.00	0.00	0.07	0.22	8.46	0.36	6.75	2.05	6.75	2.20	29.70	329.40	402.30	918.00	3.43
0.65	0.50	0.00	0.00	0.10	0.00	0.00	0.03	0.08	1.36	0.08	1.42	0.07	9.07	0.38	5.10	47.63	76.55	166.13	0.57
0.71	0.49	0.00	0.00	0.00	0.00	0.00	0.03	0.06	1.98	0.09	1.13	0.07	11.34	0.36	4.54	51.88	71.16	138.63	0.44
4.43	2.81	0.00	0.00	0.00	7.68	0.00	0.06	0.12	1.34	0.13	18.56	0.15	8.96	1.41	9.60	149.76	166.40	536.32	0.93
7.94	7.38	0.00	0.00	0.00	0.00	0.00	0.25	0.82	7.57	0.72	18.84	0.75	25.12	4.74	53.38	536.94	756.74	1372.18	12.94
1.70	1.26	0.00	0.00	0.20	0.00	0.00	0.02	0.07	1.17	0.10	2.72	0.12	11.22	0.74	7.48	64.26	88.40	24.82	1.33
2.74	2.02	0.00	0.00	0.00	0.00	0.00	0.07	0.15	7.13	0.54	6.72	0.40	23.52	1.57	30.24	235.20	322.56	70.56	2.27
7.93	6.29	0.00	0.00	0.00	176.80	0.26	0.16	0.55	12.84	1.04	52.00	3.33	67.60	5.23	62.40	520.00	707.20	174.20	8.19
1.49	1.97	0.00	0.00	0.58	0.00	0.00	0.05	0.23	3.32	0.33	8.19	0.34	29.12	2.12	21.84	185.64	263.90	71.89	4.06
3.80	3.21	0.00	0.00	0.63	0.00	0.00	0.06	0.25	3.67	0.33	9.36	0.37	34.32	2.36	23.92	203.84	284.96	79.04	4.33
0.12	0.12	0.00	0.00	0.15	179.50	0.17	0.01	0.09	0.45	0.03	34.50	2.40	1.30	0.67	1.70	20.40	20.00	5.90	0.37
4.01	2.65	0.00	0.00	0.28	0.00	0.00	0.04	0.14	3.95	0.32	5.74	0.27	20.50	1.58	19.68	160.72	221.40	87.74	2.35
2.04	1.93	0.00	0.00	0.44	0.00	0.00	0.04	0.17	2.53	0.23	6.39	0.26	22.72	1.63	16.33	141.29	198.80	54.67	3.03
0.66	1.01	0.00	0.00	0.11	0.00	0.00	0.07	0.15	8.00	0.63	7.02	0.43	22.23	1.58	32.76	256.23	356.85	74.88	2.39
3.86	2.73	0.00	0.00	0.18	0.00	0.00	0.08	0.18	8.55	0.64	8.16	0.48	28.56	1.92	35.36	282.88	387.60	85.68	2.77
4.47	3.47	0.00	0.00	0.48	0.00	0.00	0.08	0.25	7.13	0.57	9.80	0.49	36.40	2.51	35.00	284.20	392.00	95.20	4.14
1.44	2.00	0.00	0.00	0.46	0.00	0.00	0.08	0.25	7.62	0.64	9.80	0.52	35.00	2.49	36.40	298.20	417.20	98.00	4.34
0.13	0.08	0.00	0.00	0.03	0.00	0.00	0.01	0.03	2.36	0.10	1.13	0.57	1.98	0.11	5.67	64.92	78.81	405.69	0.32
1.12	0.71	0.00	0.00	0.04	0.00	0.00	0.01	0.03	1.38	0.10	1.44	0.08	5.76	0.35	6.00	47.28	63.84	14.64	0.50
3.74	0.68	0.00	0.00	0.34	0.00	0.00	0.05	0.27	6.77	0.26	12.75	1.33	18.70	0.98	22.10	203.15	276.25	73.95	4.05
2.00	0.50	0.00	0.00	0.36	0.00	0.00	0.05	0.29	7.16	0.28	13.60	1.40	20.40	0.99	23.80	212.50	287.30	75.65	4.33
0.75	0.53	0.00	0.00	0.00	0.00	0.00	0.15	0.51	5.70	0.00	0.00	0.00	5.95	3.80	20.40	192.10	284.75	45.90	2.34
0.00	0.01	0.00	0.00	0.00	0.48	0.25	0.00	0.00	0.01	0.00	1.08	0.00	0.96	0.03	0.81	2.10	2.37	0.18	0.03
6.14	1.98	0.00	0.00	3.24	0.00	0.11	0.02	0.10	0.46	0.01	10.43	0.00	43.20	0.59	48.48	83.68	121.28	72.00	0.49
6.14	1.98	0.00	0.00	3.25	0.00	0.11	0.02	0.10	0.46	0.01	10.43	0.00	43.20	0.59	48.48	83.68	121.28	1.76	0.49
46.80	15.12	0.00	0.00	22.71	0.00	0.99	0.19	0.85	4.02	0.11	91.00	0.00	401.75	6.98	432.98	780.78	1097.35	15.62	6.98
6.53	6.84	0.00	0.00	2.15	0.00	0.20	0.28	0.03	0.46	0.07	1.13	0.00	49.90	0.96	63.79	170.10	170.10	0.57	1.30
7.75	2.22	0.00	0.00	0.16	0.00	0.00	0.06	0.06	0.40	0.07	19.62	0.00	12.76	1.70	73.71	138.92	160.18	181.44	1.59
8.06	2.31	0.00	0.00	0.44	0.00	0.00	0.12	0.05	0.51	0.07	19.19	0.00	11.62	1.16	72.29	120.77	150.26	177.47	1.35
14.70	1.80	0.00	0.00	0.00	20.00	0.00	0.06	0.06	0.80	0.18	21.00	0.00	55.00	0.96	84.00	92.00	131.00	1.00	0.71
14.10	1.70	0.00	0.00	0.00	20.00	0.00	0.06	0.06	0.80	0.18	21.00	0.00	56.00	0.97	84.00	92.00	132.00	1.00	0.71
16.69	0.43	0.00	0.00	0.15	0.00	0.34	0.34	0.05	0.70	0.08	3.12	0.00	24.10	1.05	36.86	53.30	104.33	1.42	0.37
66.00	1.77	0.00	0.00	0.55	0.00	0.00	0.40	0.15	2.71	0.27	16.00	0.00	80.00	2.41	156.78	156.00	440.86	8.00	1.47
7.54	4.53	0.00	0.00	0.00	0.00	0.00	0.04	0.04	4.38	0.14	29.44	0.00	13.12	0.61	50.88	101.44	239.04	155.52	0.89
7.54	4.53	0.00	0.00	3.20	0.00	0.00	0.04	0.04	4.38	0.14	29.44	0.00	13.12	0.61	50.88	101.44	239.04	5.44	0.89
0.00	0.00	0.00	0.00	0.00	0.00	0.00	0.00	0.00	2.38	0.06	6.00	0.00	0.00	0.20	26.25	0.00	360.50	125.00	0.45
0.00	0.00	0.00	0.00	0.00	0.00	0.00	0.00	0.00	2.38	0.06	6.00	0.00	0.00	0.20	26.25	0.00	360.50	110.00	0.45
7.77	4.41	0.00	0.04	3.20	0.00	0.00	0.03	0.04	4.29	0.14	23.68	0.00	12.16	0.59	50.88	118.08	214.08	149.44	0.93
7.77	4.41	0.00	0.00	3.20	0.00	0.00	0.03	0.04	4.29	0.14	23.68	0.00	12.16	0.59	50.88	118.08	214.08	5.44	0.93

USDA ID Code	Food Name	Weight in Grams*	Quantity of Units	Unit of Measure	Protein (gm)	Fat (gm)	Carbohydrate (gm)	Kcalories	Caffeine (gm)	Fiber (gm)	Cholesterol (mg)	Saturated Fat (gm)
	Peanut Kernels, Oil Roasted	112.0000	0.500	Cup	37.94	70.99	27.26	836.64	0.00	12.67	0.00	9.85
	Peanuts, All Types, Ckd, Boiled,	28.0000	33.000	Each	3.78	6.16	5.95	89.04	0.00	2.46	0.00	0.86
	Peanuts, All Types, Dry-roasted,	1.0000	1.000	Each	0.24	0.50	0.22	5.85	0.00	0.08	0.00	0.07
	Peanuts, All Types, Dry-roasted,	1.0000	1.000	Each	0.24	0.50	0.22	5.85	0.00	0.08	0.00	0.07
	Peanuts, All Types, Fresh	28.3500	1.000	Ounce	7.31	13.96	4.58	160.74	0.00	2.41	0.00	1.94
	Peanuts, All Types, Oil-roasted,	0.9000	1.000	Each	0.24	0.44	0.17	5.23	0.00	0.08	0.00	0.06
	Peanuts, All Types, Oil-roasted,	28.0000	32.000	Each	7.38	13.80	5.30	162.68	0.00	1.93	0.00	1.92
	Peanuts, Dry Roasted	28.3500	1.000	Ounce	4.90	14.59	7.19	168.40	0.00	2.55	0.00	1.96
	Peanuts, Oil Roasted	28.3500	1.000	Ounce	4.40	15.92	6.31	174.35	0.00	1.56	0.00	2.58
	Peanuts, Spanish, Fresh	28.3500	1.000	Ounce	7.41	14.06	4.48	161.60	0.00	2.69	0.00	2.17
	Peanuts, Spanish, Oil-roasted, w	28.3500	1.000	Ounce	7.94	13.90	4.95	164.15	0.00	2.52	0.00	2.14
	Peanuts, Spanish, Oil-roasted, w	28.3500	1.000	Ounce	7.94	13.90	4.95	164.15	0.00	2.52	0.00	2.14
	Peanuts, Valencia, Fresh	28.3500	1.000	Ounce	7.11	13.49	5.93	161.60	0.00	2.47	0.00	2.08
	Peanuts, Valencia, Oil-roasted,	28.3500	1.000	Ounce	7.67	14.53	4.62	166.98	0.00	2.52	0.00	2.24
	Peanuts, Valencia, Oil-roasted,	28.3500	1.000	Ounce	7.67	14.53	4.62	166.98	0.00	2.52	0.00	2.24
	Peanuts, Virginia, Fresh	28.3500	1.000	Ounce	7.14	13.82	4.69	159.61	0.00	2.41	0.00	1.80
	Peanuts, Virginia, Oil-roasted,	28.3500	1.000	Ounce	7.33	13.78	5.63	163.86	0.00	2.52	0.00	1.80
	Peanuts, Virginia, Oil-roasted,	28.3500	1.000	Ounce	7.33	13.78	5.63	163.86	0.00	2.52	0.00	1.80
	Pecans, Dried	28.3500	1.000	Ounce	2.60	20.40	3.93	195.90	0.00	2.72	0.00	1.75
	Pine Nuts	1.8000	10.000	Each	0.43	0.91	0.26	10.19	0.00	0.08	0.00	0.14
	Pistachios, Dried	18.0000	30.000	Each	3.69	7.77	5.25	99.18	0.00	1.80	0.00	0.95
	Pistachios, Dry Roasted	28.3500	1.000	Ounce	6.02	12.96	7.69	160.74	0.00	2.92	0.00	1.57
	Sausage, Meatless	25.0000	1.000	Link	4.63	4.54	2.46	64.00	0.00	0.70	0.00	0.73
	Seeds, Sesame, Toasted, w/o salt	28.3500	1.000	Ounce	4.81	13.61	7.38	160.75	0.00	4.79	0.00	1.91
	Seeds, Sesame, Toasted, w/salt	28.3500	1.000	Ounce	4.81	13.61	7.38	160.75	0.00	4.79	0.00	1.91
	Seeds, Sunflower, Dried	46.0000	1.000	Cup	10.48	22.80	8.63	262.20	0.00	4.83	0.00	2.39
	Seeds, Sunflower, Dry Roasted, w	28.3500	1.000	Ounce	5.48	14.12	6.82	165.00	0.00	2.55	0.00	1.48
	Seeds, Sunflower, Dry Roasted, w	28.3500	1.000	Ounce	5.48	14.12	6.82	165.00	0.00	3.15	0.00	1.48
	Seeds, Sunflower, Oil Roasted, w	28.3500	1.000	Ounce	6.06	16.29	4.18	174.35	0.00	1.93	0.00	1.71
	Seeds, Sunflower, Oil Roasted, w	28.3500	1.000	Ounce	6.06	16.29	4.18	174.35	0.00	1.93	0.00	1.71
	Seeds, Sunflower, Toasted, w/ Sa	28.3500	1.000	Ounce	4.88	16.10	5.84	175.49	0.00	3.26	0.00	1.69
	Seeds, Sunflower, Toasted, w/o S	28.3500	1.000	Ounce	4.88	16.10	5.84	175.49	0.00	3.26	0.00	1.69
	Sesame Butter, Tahini, Toasted	15.0000	1.000	Tbsp	2.55	8.06	3.18	89.25	0.00	1.40	0.00	1.13
	Soybeans, Boiled	10.7000	1.000	Tbsp	1.78	0.96	1.06	18.51	0.00	0.64	0.00	0.14
	Soybeans, Dry Roasted	172.0000	1.000	Cup	68.08	37.19	56.28	774.00	0.00	13.93	0.00	5.38
	Tofu, Fresh, Firm	81.0000	1.000	Ounce	6.51	3.61	2.41	62.37	0.00	0.32	0.00	0.53
	Tofu, Fresh, Regular	17.6000	1.000	Ounce	1.15	0.65	0.32	10.74	0.00	0.04	0.00	0.09
	Tofu, Fried	13.0000	1.000	Piece	2.23	2.62	1.37	35.23	0.00	0.51	0.00	0.38
	Tofu, Fried, Prepared w/ Calcium	13.0000	1.000	Piece	2.23	2.62	1.37	35.23	0.00	0.51	0.00	0.38
	Tofu, Okara	122.0000	1.000	Cup	3.93	2.11	15.30	93.94	0.00	0.00	0.00	0.23
	Tofu, Salted and Fermented (fuyu	11.0000	1.000	Block	0.90	0.88	0.57	12.76	0.00	0.00	0.00	0.13
	Walnuts, Black, Dried	7.8000	1.000	Tbsp	1.90	4.41	0.94	47.35	0.00	0.39	0.00	0.28
	Walnuts, English, Dried	28.0000	0.500	Cup	4.26	18.26	3.84	183.12	0.00	1.88	0.00	1.72
	Apples, Escalloped-Stouffer's	170.0960	1.000	Each	0.00	4.00	41.00	200.00	0.00	0.00	0.00	0.00
	Bean, Green, Mushroom Casserole-	134.6590	1.000	Each	5.00	10.00	13.00	160.00	0.00	0.00	0.00	0.00
	Beef Ribs w/Barbecue Sauce, Bone	311.8430	1.000	Each	28.00	6.00	40.00	330.00	0.00	0.00	70.00	2.00
	Beef Roast, Tender, Top Shelf-Ho	283.4930	1.000	Each	28.00	6.00	19.00	240.00	0.00	0.00	60.00	2.00
	Beef Sirloin Tips w/ Mushroom Gr	269.3190	1.000	Each	22.00	5.00	43.00	310.00	0.00	0.00	35.00	2.00
	Beef Sirloin Tips-Healthy Choice	318.9300	1.000	Each	22.00	7.00	29.00	270.00	0.00	0.00	65.00	3.00
	Beef Stew, Micro Cup-Hormel	212.6200	1.000	Each	13.00	15.00	11.00	230.00	0.00	0.00	45.00	5.00
	Beef Stroganoff w/ Parsley Noodl	276.4060	1.000	Each	24.00	20.00	28.00	390.00	0.00	0.00	0.00	0.00
	Beef, Chipped, Creamed-Stouffer'	28.3500	1.000	Ounce	2.10	3.30	1.60	45.00	0.00	0.00	13.00	0.00
	Beef, Oriental, w/ Veg., Lean Cu	244.5130	1.000	Each	20.00	9.00	31.00	290.00	0.00	0.00	40.00	2.00
	Beef, Pot Roast, Yankee-Healthy	311.8430	1.000	Each	19.00	4.00	36.00	260.00	0.00	0.00	55.00	2.00
	Beef, Sirloin, w/ Barbecue Sauce	311.8430	1.000	Each	17.00	4.00	44.00	280.00	0.00	0.00	25.00	2.00

Monounsaturated Fat (gm)	Polyunsaturated Fat (gm)	Vitamin D (mg)	Vitamin K (mg)	Vitamin E (mg)	Vitamin A (re)	Vitamin C (mg)	Thiamin (mg)	Riboflavin (mg)	Niacin (mg)	Vitamin B_6 (mg)	Folate (mg)	Vitamin B_{12} (mcg)	Calcium (mg)	Iron (mg)	Magnesium (mg)	Phosphorus (mg)	Potassium (mg)	Sodium (mg)	Zinc (mg)
35.23	22.44	0.00	0.00	10.67	0.00	0.00	0.36	0.16	20.56	0.37	181.01	0.00	126.72	2.64	266.40	744.48	982.08	623.52	9.55
3.06	1.95	0.00	0.00	0.89	0.00	0.00	0.07	0.02	1.47	0.04	20.89	0.00	15.40	0.28	28.56	55.44	50.40	210.28	0.51
0.25	0.16	0.00	0.00	0.07	0.00	0.00	0.00	0.00	0.14	0.00	1.45	0.00	0.54	0.02	1.76	3.58	6.58	8.13	0.03
0.25	0.16	0.00	0.00	0.08	0.00	0.00	0.00	0.00	0.14	0.00	1.45	0.00	0.54	0.02	1.76	3.58	6.58	0.06	0.03
6.93	4.41	0.00	0.00	2.59	0.00	0.00	0.18	0.04	3.42	0.10	67.98	0.00	26.08	1.30	47.63	106.60	199.87	5.10	0.93
0.22	0.14	0.00	0.00	0.07	0.00	0.00	0.00	0.00	0.13	0.00	1.13	0.00	0.79	0.02	1.67	4.65	6.14	3.90	0.06
6.85	4.36	0.00	0.00	2.07	0.00	0.00	0.07	0.03	4.00	0.07	35.20	0.00	24.64	0.51	51.80	144.76	190.96	1.68	1.86
8.90	3.05	0.00	0.00	1.70	0.28	0.11	0.06	0.06	1.33	0.09	14.29	0.00	19.85	1.05	63.79	123.32	169.25	189.66	1.08
9.40	3.25	0.00	0.00	1.70	0.57	0.14	0.14	0.14	0.56	0.05	15.99	0.00	30.05	0.73	71.16	127.29	154.22	198.45	1.32
6.33	4.88	0.00	0.00	0.00	0.00	0.00	0.19	0.04	4.52	0.10	68.04	0.00	30.05	1.11	53.30	110.00	210.92	6.24	0.60
6.26	4.82	0.00	0.00	0.00	0.00	0.00	0.09	0.03	4.23	0.07	35.69	0.00	28.35	0.65	47.63	109.71	220.00	122.76	0.57
6.26	4.82	0.00	0.00	0.00	0.00	0.00	0.09	0.03	4.23	0.07	35.69	0.00	28.35	0.65	47.63	109.71	220.00	1.70	0.57
6.07	4.68	0.00	0.00	0.00	0.00	0.00	0.18	0.09	3.65	0.10	69.60	0.00	17.58	0.59	52.16	95.26	94.12	0.28	0.95
6.54	5.04	0.00	0.00	0.00	0.00	0.00	0.03	0.04	4.07	0.07	35.58	0.00	15.31	0.47	45.36	90.44	173.50	218.86	0.87
6.54	5.04	0.00	0.00	0.00	0.00	0.00	0.03	0.04	4.07	0.07	35.58	0.00	15.31	0.47	45.36	90.44	173.50	1.70	0.87
7.17	4.17	0.00	0.00	0.00	0.00	0.00	0.18	0.04	3.51	0.10	67.67	0.00	25.23	0.72	48.48	107.73	195.62	2.84	1.26
7.15	4.16	0.00	0.00	0.00	0.00	0.00	0.08	0.03	4.17	0.07	35.55	0.00	24.38	0.47	53.30	143.45	184.84	122.76	1.88
7.15	4.16	0.00	0.00	0.00	0.00	0.00	0.08	0.03	4.17	0.07	35.55	0.00	24.38	0.47	53.30	143.45	184.84	1.70	1.88
11.56	6.12	0.00	0.00	1.04	2.27	0.31	0.19	0.04	0.33	0.06	6.24	0.00	19.85	0.72	34.30	78.53	116.24	0.00	1.28
0.34	0.38	0.00	0.00	0.06	0.05	0.03	0.01	0.00	0.06	0.00	1.03	0.00	0.47	0.17	4.19	9.14	10.78	0.07	0.08
4.08	2.35	0.00	0.00	0.83	9.90	0.90	0.16	0.03	0.23	0.31	9.18	0.00	19.26	0.77	21.78	88.20	175.86	0.18	0.40
6.83	3.92	0.00	0.00	1.21	15.03	0.65	0.24	0.05	0.41	0.48	14.18	0.00	30.62	1.19	34.02	137.50	292.86	120.77	0.65
1.13	2.32	0.00	0.00	0.53	16.00	0.00	0.59	0.10	2.80	0.21	6.50	0.00	15.75	0.93	9.00	56.25	57.75	222.00	0.37
5.14	5.97	0.00	0.00	0.64	1.99	0.00	0.34	0.13	1.54	0.04	27.16	0.00	37.14	2.21	98.09	219.43	115.10	11.06	2.90
5.14	5.97	0.00	0.00	0.64	1.99	0.00	0.34	0.13	1.54	0.04	27.16	0.00	37.14	2.21	98.09	219.43	115.10	166.70	2.90
4.35	15.06	0.00	0.00	23.12	2.30	0.64	1.05	0.12	2.07	0.35	104.60	0.00	53.36	3.11	162.84	324.30	316.94	1.38	2.33
2.70	9.32	0.00	0.00	14.25	0.00	0.40	0.03	0.07	2.00	0.23	67.30	0.00	19.85	1.08	36.57	327.44	240.98	221.13	1.50
2.70	9.32	0.00	0.00	14.25	0.00	0.40	0.03	0.07	2.00	0.23	67.30	0.00	19.85	1.08	36.57	327.44	240.98	0.85	1.50
3.11	10.76	0.00	0.00	11.34	1.42	0.40	0.09	0.08	1.17	0.22	66.34	0.00	15.88	1.90	36.00	322.91	136.93	170.95	1.48
3.11	10.76	0.00	0.00	14.25	1.42	0.40	0.09	0.08	1.17	0.22	66.34	0.00	15.88	1.90	36.00	322.91	136.93	0.85	1.48
3.07	10.63	0.00	0.00	0.00	0.00	0.40	0.09	0.08	1.19	0.23	67.42	0.00	16.16	1.93	36.57	328.29	139.20	173.79	1.50
3.07	10.63	0.00	0.00	0.00	0.00	0.40	0.09	0.08	1.19	0.23	67.42	0.00	16.16	1.93	36.57	328.29	139.20	0.85	1.50
3.05	3.54	0.00	0.00	0.34	1.05	0.00	0.18	0.07	0.82	0.02	14.66	0.00	63.90	1.34	14.25	109.80	62.10	17.25	0.69
0.21	0.54	0.00	0.00	0.21	0.11	0.18	0.02	0.03	0.04	0.02	5.76	0.00	10.91	0.55	9.20	26.22	55.11	0.11	0.12
8.22	21.00	0.00	0.00	0.00	3.44	7.91	0.74	1.31	1.82	0.40	351.91	0.00	240.80	6.79	392.16	1116.28	2346.08	3.44	8.20
0.80	2.04	0.00	0.00	0.00	0.81	0.16	0.07	0.08	0.01	0.05	26.73	0.00	131.22	1.17	37.26	119.07	142.56	6.48	0.82
0.14	0.37	0.00	0.00	0.00	0.18	0.04	0.01	0.01	0.10	0.01	7.74	0.00	19.54	0.20	4.75	16.19	21.12	1.41	0.11
0.58	1.48	0.00	0.00	0.00	0.00	0.00	0.02	0.01	0.01	0.01	3.48	0.00	48.36	0.63	7.80	37.31	18.98	2.08	0.26
0.58	1.48	0.00	0.00	0.00	0.00	0.00	0.02	0.01	0.01	0.01	3.48	0.00	124.93	0.63	12.35	37.31	18.98	2.08	0.26
0.37	0.93	0.00	0.00	0.00	0.00	0.00	0.02	0.02	0.12	0.15	32.21	0.00	97.60	1.59	31.72	73.20	259.86	10.98	0.68
0.19	0.50	0.00	0.00	0.00	1.87	0.02	0.02	0.01	0.04	0.01	3.20	0.00	5.06	0.22	5.72	8.03	8.25	316.03	0.17
0.99	2.92	0.00	0.00	0.20	2.34	0.25	0.02	0.01	0.05	0.04	5.11	0.00	4.52	0.24	15.76	36.19	40.87	0.08	0.27
2.50	13.21	0.00	0.00	0.82	1.12	0.36	0.10	0.04	0.53	0.15	27.44	0.00	29.12	0.81	44.24	96.88	123.48	0.56	0.87
0.00	0.00	0.00	0.00	0.00	0.00	30.00	0.03	0.00	0.00	0.00	0.00	0.00	0.00	0.00	0.00	0.00	90.00	15.00	0.00
0.00	0.00	0.00	0.00	0.00	40.00	2.40	0.06	0.17	0.38	0.00	0.00	0.00	64.00	0.20	0.00	0.00	200.00	550.00	0.00
0.00	2.00	0.00	0.00	0.00	60.00	4.80	0.23	0.26	2.85	0.00	0.00	0.00	48.00	1.00	0.00	220.00	670.00	530.00	0.00
2.00	1.00	0.00	0.00	0.00	400.00	2.40	0.75	0.43	5.70	0.00	0.00	0.00	16.00	1.50	42.00	0.00	933.00	880.00	4.50
0.00	0.00	0.00	0.00	0.00	60.00	2.40	0.00	0.03	0.38	0.00	0.00	0.00	0.00	0.20	0.00	0.00	80.00	500.00	0.00
0.00	2.00	0.00	0.00	0.00	700.00	42.00	0.15	0.17	2.85	0.00	0.00	0.00	16.00	1.00	0.00	190.00	520.00	360.00	0.00
4.00	0.00	0.00	0.00	0.28	320.00	2.40	0.05	0.10	2.28	0.00	0.00	0.00	16.00	0.90	21.00	0.00	487.00	1140.00	2.40
0.00	0.00	0.00	0.00	0.00	40.00	1.20	0.12	0.34	2.85	0.00	0.00	0.00	48.00	1.50	0.00	0.00	300.00	1090.00	0.00
0.00	0.00	0.00	0.00	0.00	0.00	0.00	0.00	0.00	0.21	0.00	0.00	0.00	184.00	0.02	0.00	0.00	57.00	176.00	0.00
0.00	0.00	0.00	0.00	0.00	150.00	1.20	0.09	0.17	2.85	0.00	0.00	0.00	16.00	1.00	0.00	0.00	400.00	590.00	0.00
0.00	0.00	0.00	0.00	0.00	100.00	9.00	0.15	0.17	1.52	0.00	0.00	0.00	32.00	1.00	0.00	150.00	350.00	400.00	0.00
0.00	1.00	0.00	0.00	0.00	0.00	0.00	0.00	0.00	0.00	0.00	0.00	0.00	0.00	0.00	0.00	190.00	630.00	240.00	0.00

USDA ID Code	Food Name	Weight in Grams*	Quantity of Units	Unit of Measure	Protein (gm)	Fat (gm)	Carbohydrate (gm)	Kcalories	Caffeine (gm)	Fiber (gm)	Cholesterol (mg)	Saturated Fat (gm)
	Burritos, Beef and Bean (medium)	148.8340	1.000	Each	12.00	7.00	42.00	270.00	0.00	0.00	15.00	3.00
	Burritos, Beef and Bean (mild)-H	148.8340	1.000	Each	11.00	5.00	45.00	250.00	0.00	0.00	10.00	1.00
	Burritos,Chicken Con Queso (mil	148.8340	1.000	Each	15.00	8.00	40.00	280.00	0.00	0.00	20.00	2.00
	Cabbage, Stuffed, no Sauce-Stouf	28.3500	1.000	Ounce	2.00	2.10	3.10	39.00	0.00	0.00	5.00	0.00
	Cabbage, Stuffed, w/ Meat, Lean	269.3190	1.000	Each	13.00	6.00	26.00	210.00	0.00	0.00	30.00	2.00
	Cabbage, Stuffed-Stouffer's	28.3500	1.000	Ounce	1.40	1.40	2.70	29.00	0.00	0.00	4.00	0.00
	Cacciatore, Chicken, Lean Cuisin	308.2990	1.000	Each	22.00	7.00	31.00	280.00	0.00	0.00	45.00	2.00
	Cacciatore, Chicken, Top Shelf-H	283.4930	1.000	Each	21.00	3.00	25.00	210.00	0.00	0.00	50.00	0.00
	Cannelloni, Beef, w/ Sauce, Lean	272.8620	1.000	Each	14.00	3.00	28.00	200.00	0.00	0.00	25.00	1.00
	Cannelloni, Cheese, Lean Cuisine	258.6880	1.000	Each	23.00	8.00	27.00	270.00	0.00	0.00	25.00	4.00
	Chicken a la King w/ Rice-Stouff	269.3190	1.000	Each	18.00	5.00	38.00	270.00	0.00	0.00	0.00	0.00
	Chicken a la King, Top Shelf-Hor	5283.4930	1.000	Each	18.00	10.00	49.00	360.00	0.00	0.00	37.00	4.00
	Chicken a la King-Swanson	250.0000	1.000	Each	16.80	20.16	15.12	319.15	0.00	0.00	0.00	0.00
	Chicken a la Orange, Lean Cuisin	226.7950	1.000	Each	27.00	4.00	33.00	280.00	0.00	0.00	55.00	1.00
	Chicken a la Orange-Healthy Choi	255.1440	1.000	Each	20.00	2.00	36.00	240.00	0.00	0.00	45.00	2.00
	Chicken and Dumplings-Stouffer's	220.0000	1.000	Each	14.74	16.30	24.06	302.65	0.00	0.00	69.84	0.00
	Chicken and Dumplings-Swanson	200.0000	1.000	Each	10.35	10.35	17.87	206.94	0.00	0.00	0.00	0.00
	Chicken and Pasta Divan-Healthy	340.1920	1.000	Each	25.00	4.00	41.00	300.00	0.00	0.00	50.00	2.00
	Chicken and Veg. Oriental-Stouff	220.0000	1.000	Each	11.64	9.31	13.97	186.25	0.00	0.00	31.04	0.00
	Chicken and Veg. w/ Vermicelli,	333.1050	1.000	Each	18.00	5.00	30.00	240.00	0.00	0.00	30.00	1.00
	Chicken and Vegetables-Healthy C	326.0170	1.000	Each	20.00	1.00	31.00	210.00	0.00	0.00	35.00	0.00
	Chicken Classica-Stouffer's	28.3500	1.000	Ounce	1.80	0.70	2.30	22.00	0.00	0.00	5.00	0.00
	Chicken Dijon-Healthy Choice	311.8430	1.000	Each	21.00	3.00	40.00	250.00	0.00	0.00	40.00	1.00
	Chicken Divan-Stouffer's	226.7950	1.000	Each	24.00	10.00	11.00	220.00	0.00	0.00	0.00	0.00
	Chicken in BBQ Sauce, Lean Cuisi	248.0570	1.000	Each	20.00	6.00	32.00	260.00	0.00	0.00	50.00	1.00
	Chicken Italiano, Lean Cuisine-S	255.1440	1.000	Each	22.00	6.00	33.00	270.00	0.00	0.00	40.00	1.00
	Chicken Italienne-Stouffer's	28.3500	1.000	Ounce	2.20	0.90	1.20	22.00	0.00	0.00	7.00	0.00
	Chicken Oriental, Lean Cuisine-S	255.1440	1.000	Each	22.00	7.00	31.00	280.00	0.00	0.00	35.00	2.00
	Chicken Oriental-Healthy Choice	318.9300	1.000	Each	19.00	1.00	32.00	200.00	0.00	0.00	35.00	0.00
	Chicken Parmigiana-Healthy Choic	326.0170	1.000	Each	22.00	4.00	45.00	280.00	0.00	0.00	45.00	2.00
186	Chicken Piccata, Lemon Herb-Smar	238.0000	8.500	Ounce	11.00	2.00	34.00	200.00	0.00	3.00	25.00	0.50
	Chicken Stir Fry w/ Broccoli-Hea	340.1920	1.000	Each	21.00	6.00	35.00	280.00	0.00	0.00	55.00	3.00
	Chicken Tenderloins, Lean Cuisin	269.3190	1.000	Each	29.00	5.00	19.00	240.00	0.00	0.00	60.00	2.00
	Chicken w/ Barbecue Sauce-Health	361.4540	1.000	Each	24.00	6.00	65.00	410.00	0.00	0.00	55.00	2.00
	Chicken w/ Spanish Rice, Breast	283.4930	1.000	Each	27.00	15.00	38.00	400.00	0.00	0.00	75.00	7.00
	Chicken, Breast, Glazed, Top She	283.4930	1.000	Each	19.00	2.00	19.00	170.00	0.00	0.00	35.00	1.00
	Chicken, Creamed-Stouffer's	28.3500	1.000	Ounce	2.80	3.50	1.20	48.00	0.00	0.00	14.00	0.00
	Chicken, Escalloped, and Noodles	283.4930	1.000	Each	21.00	24.00	30.00	420.00	0.00	0.00	0.00	0.00
	Chicken, Fiesta -Weight Watchers	240.9750	1.000	Each	12.00	2.00	38.00	220.00	0.00	5.00	25.00	0.50
	Chicken, Glazed, w/ Veg. Lean Cu	240.9690	1.000	Each	21.00	7.00	24.00	250.00	0.00	0.00	50.00	2.00
	Chicken, Glazed-Healthy Choice	240.9690	1.000	Each	21.00	3.00	27.00	220.00	0.00	0.00	45.00	1.00
	Chicken, Glazed-Stouffer's	28.3500	1.000	Ounce	2.90	1.10	1.00	26.00	0.00	0.00	9.00	0.00
	Chicken, Herb Roasted -Healthy C	347.2790	1.000	Each	22.00	5.00	50.00	300.00	0.00	0.00	40.00	2.00
	Chicken, Honey Mustard, Lean Cui	212.6200	1.000	Each	18.00	4.00	30.00	230.00	0.00	0.00	40.00	1.00
	Chicken, Honey Mustard-Healthy C	269.3190	1.000	Each	26.00	4.00	41.00	310.00	0.00	0.00	45.00	1.00
187	Chicken, Honey Mustard-Smart One	238.0000	8.500	Ounce	11.00	2.00	37.00	200.00	0.00	3.00	30.00	0.50
	Chicken, Mandarin-Healthy Choice	311.8430	1.000	Each	23.00	2.00	39.00	260.00	0.00	0.00	50.00	0.00
	Chicken, Mexicali-Stouffer's	28.3500	1.000	Ounce	1.40	0.80	1.80	20.00	0.00	0.00	5.00	0.00
	Chicken, Oriental, w/ Spicy Pean	269.3190	1.000	Each	33.00	5.00	40.00	340.00	0.00	0.00	45.00	1.00
	Chicken, Oven Baked, Lean Cuisin	226.7950	1.000	Each	17.00	5.00	21.00	200.00	0.00	0.00	35.00	2.00
	Chicken, Salsa -Healthy Choice	318.9300	1.000	Each	20.00	2.00	36.00	240.00	0.00	0.00	50.00	1.00
	Chicken, Southwestern Style-Heal	354.3670	1.000	Each	25.00	5.00	51.00	340.00	0.00	0.00	60.00	2.00
	Chicken, Sweet and Sour-Healthy	326.0170	1.000	Each	20.00	2.00	52.00	280.00	0.00	0.00	35.00	0.00
188	Chicken, Szechwan Veg, Spicy & H	252.0000	9.000	Ounce	11.00	2.00	39.00	220.00	0.00	3.00	10.00	0.50
	Chicken, Teriyaki-Healthy Choice	347.2790	1.000	Each	24.00	4.00	39.00	290.00	0.00	0.00	55.00	1.00

Monounsaturated Fat (gm)	Polyunsaturated Fat (gm)	Vitamin D (mg)	Vitamin K (mg)	Vitamin E (mg)	Vitamin A (re)	Vitamin C (mg)	Thiamin (mg)	Riboflavin (mg)	Niacin (mg)	Vitamin B_6 (mg)	Folate (mg)	Vitamin B_{12} (mcg)	Calcium (mg)	Iron (mg)	Magnesium (mg)	Phosphorus (mg)	Potassium (mg)	Sodium (mg)	Zinc (mg)
0.00	3.00	0.00	0.00	0.00	20.00	3.60	0.38	0.17	1.90	0.00	0.00	0.00	48.00	1.50	0.00	180.00	270.00	520.00	0.00
0.00	2.00	0.00	0.00	0.00	20.00	1.20	0.38	0.17	2.85	0.00	0.00	0.00	32.00	2.00	0.00	130.00	330.00	450.00	0.00
0.00	3.00	0.00	0.00	0.00	20.00	6.00	0.45	0.34	2.85	0.00	0.00	0.00	80.00	1.50	0.00	170.00	260.00	500.00	0.00
0.00	0.00	0.00	0.00	0.00	0.00	0.60	0.00	0.00	0.08	0.00	0.00	0.00	72.00	0.04	0.00	0.00	48.00	150.00	0.00
0.00	1.00	0.00	0.00	0.00	80.00	6.00	0.12	0.17	3.80	0.00	0.00	0.00	64.00	1.50	0.00	0.00	600.00	560.00	0.00
0.00	0.00	0.00	0.00	0.00	0.00	3.00	0.00	0.00	0.06	0.00	0.00	0.00	48.00	0.02	0.00	0.00	51.00	145.00	0.00
0.00	1.00	0.00	0.00	0.00	100.00	9.00	0.23	0.17	5.70	0.00	0.00	0.00	32.00	0.80	0.00	0.00	560.00	570.00	0.00
0.00	0.00	0.00	0.00	0.46	100.00	2.40	0.15	0.26	6.65	0.00	0.00	0.00	80.00	1.00	0.00	0.00	0.00	810.00	0.00
0.00	0.00	0.00	0.00	0.00	350.00	6.00	0.12	0.17	2.85	0.00	0.00	0.00	120.00	1.50	0.00	0.00	800.00	490.00	0.00
0.00	0.00	0.00	0.00	0.00	60.00	21.00	0.12	0.26	1.52	0.00	0.00	0.00	240.00	0.40	0.00	0.00	400.00	590.00	0.00
0.00	0.00	0.00	0.00	0.00	20.00	1.20	0.09	0.17	2.85	0.00	0.00	0.00	160.00	0.80	0.00	32.00	260.00	800.00	0.00
4.00	2.00	0.00	0.00	0.17	250.00	1.20	0.12	0.17	8.55	0.00	0.00	0.00	48.00	0.20	28.00	0.00	476.00	890.00	1.20
0.00	0.00	0.00	0.00	0.00	0.00	0.00	0.05	0.23	3.19	0.00	0.00	0.00	53.75	0.34	0.00	0.00	0.00	1159.01	0.00
0.00	0.00	0.00	0.00	0.00	80.00	12.00	0.23	0.17	9.50	0.00	0.00	0.00	32.00	0.40	0.00	0.00	490.00	290.00	0.00
0.00	0.00	0.00	0.00	0.00	150.00	27.00	0.15	0.10	5.70	0.00	0.00	0.00	16.00	0.80	0.00	230.00	430.00	220.00	0.00
0.00	0.00	0.00	0.00	0.00	0.00	0.00	0.00	0.01	0.44	0.00	0.00	0.00	1.06	0.16	0.00	0.00	248.33	659.63	0.00
0.00	0.00	0.00	0.00	0.00	75.25	0.00	0.03	0.10	1.79	0.00	0.00	0.00	15.05	0.38	0.00	0.00	0.00	921.83	0.00
0.00	1.00	0.00	0.00	0.00	800.00	72.00	0.38	0.26	4.75	0.00	0.00	0.00	120.00	1.00	0.00	270.00	500.00	520.00	0.00
0.00	0.00	0.00	0.00	0.00	0.00	4.66	0.00	0.00	0.59	0.00	0.00	0.00	372.49	0.08	0.00	0.00	349.21	1078.68	0.00
0.00	1.00	0.00	0.00	0.00	150.00	6.00	0.30	0.26	5.70	0.00	0.00	0.00	64.00	1.00	0.00	0.00	500.00	500.00	0.00
0.00	0.00	0.00	0.00	0.00	150.00	9.00	0.30	0.17	3.80	0.00	0.00	0.00	32.00	1.50	0.00	190.00	390.00	490.00	0.00
0.00	0.00	0.00	0.00	0.00	0.00	1.20	0.00	0.00	0.10	0.00	0.00	0.00	112.00	0.01	0.00	0.00	50.00	83.00	0.00
0.00	0.00	0.00	0.00	0.00	100.00	9.00	0.23	0.14	9.50	0.00	0.00	0.00	16.00	1.00	0.00	300.00	350.00	470.00	0.00
0.00	0.00	0.00	0.00	0.00	60.00	3.60	0.45	0.17	3.80	0.00	0.00	0.00	200.00	2.00	0.00	32.00	490.00	610.00	0.00
0.00	2.00	0.00	0.00	0.00	250.00	18.00	0.15	0.17	5.70	0.00	0.00	0.00	48.00	0.80	0.00	0.00	650.00	500.00	0.00
0.00	2.00	0.00	0.00	0.00	100.00	24.00	0.30	0.26	5.70	0.00	0.00	0.00	80.00	0.80	0.00	0.00	600.00	590.00	0.00
0.00	0.00	0.00	0.00	0.00	0.00	1.20	0.00	0.00	0.10	0.00	0.00	0.00	48.00	0.01	0.00	0.00	57.00	128.00	0.00
0.00	2.00	0.00	0.00	0.00	40.00	6.00	0.23	0.17	6.65	0.00	0.00	0.00	32.00	1.00	0.00	0.00	470.00	480.00	0.00
0.00	0.00	0.00	0.00	0.00	250.00	36.00	0.15	0.14	7.60	0.00	0.00	0.00	32.00	0.80	0.00	200.00	400.00	440.00	0.00
0.00	0.00	0.00	0.00	0.00	900.00	12.00	0.15	0.17	9.50	0.00	0.00	0.00	80.00	1.00	0.00	260.00	500.00	370.00	0.00
0.00	0.00	0.00	0.00	0.00	0.00	0.00	0.00	0.00	0.00	0.00	0.00	0.00	0.00	0.00	0.00	0.00	0.00	460.00	0.00
0.00	0.00	0.00	0.00	0.00	20.00	0.00	0.23	0.34	2.85	0.00	0.00	0.00	48.00	1.50	0.00	260.00	630.00	500.00	0.00
0.00	1.00	0.00	0.00	0.00	200.00	4.80	0.23	0.34	7.60	0.00	0.00	0.00	120.00	0.40	0.00	0.00	750.00	490.00	0.00
0.00	2.00	0.00	0.00	0.00	100.00	12.00	0.12	0.14	8.55	0.00	0.00	0.00	48.00	1.50	0.00	250.00	670.00	550.00	0.00
4.00	3.00	0.00	0.00	0.07	100.00	3.60	0.09	0.26	7.60	0.00	0.00	0.00	80.00	0.40	35.00	0.00	584.00	810.00	1.65
1.00	1.00	0.00	0.00	0.76	400.00	3.60	0.06	0.17	7.60	0.00	0.00	0.00	32.00	0.40	35.00	0.00	804.00	780.00	1.05
0.00	0.00	0.00	0.00	0.00	0.00	0.00	0.00	0.00	0.10	0.00	0.00	0.00	352.00	0.01	0.00	0.00	37.00	119.00	0.00
0.00	0.00	0.00	0.00	0.00	20.00	0.00	0.15	0.34	3.80	0.00	0.00	0.00	80.00	0.80	0.00	0.00	300.00	840.00	0.00
0.00	0.00	0.00	0.00	0.00	450.00	42.00	0.00	0.00	0.00	0.00	0.00	0.00	72.00	1.50	0.00	0.00	490.00	480.00	0.00
0.00	4.00	0.00	0.00	0.00	20.00	3.60	0.15	0.17	7.60	0.00	0.00	0.00	16.00	0.20	0.00	0.00	580.00	590.00	0.00
0.00	1.00	0.00	0.00	0.00	0.00	1.20	0.15	0.14	6.65	0.00	0.00	0.00	0.00	0.60	0.00	240.00	370.00	510.00	0.00
0.00	0.00	0.00	0.00	0.00	0.00	0.00	0.00	0.00	0.23	0.00	0.00	0.00	24.00	0.01	0.00	0.00	45.00	105.00	0.00
0.00	1.00	0.00	0.00	0.00	250.00	24.00	0.15	0.14	7.60	0.00	0.00	0.00	32.00	0.80	0.00	280.00	370.00	560.00	0.00
0.00	1.00	0.00	0.00	0.00	200.00	2.40	0.15	0.17	3.80	0.00	0.00	0.00	16.00	0.40	0.00	0.00	340.00	540.00	0.00
0.00	0.00	0.00	0.00	0.00	100.00	3.60	0.15	0.03	1.52	0.00	0.00	0.00	16.00	0.80	0.00	0.00	110.00	520.00	0.00
0.00	0.00	0.00	0.00	0.00	0.00	0.00	0.00	0.00	0.00	0.00	0.00	0.00	0.00	0.00	0.00	0.00	0.00	370.00	0.00
0.00	0.00	0.00	0.00	0.00	250.00	9.00	0.15	0.17	4.75	0.00	0.00	0.00	16.00	1.00	0.00	200.00	400.00	400.00	0.00
0.00	0.00	0.00	0.00	0.00	0.00	4.20	0.00	0.00	0.11	0.00	0.00	0.00	88.00	0.02	0.00	0.00	68.00	48.00	0.00
0.00	1.00	0.00	0.00	0.00	0.00	2.40	0.00	0.00	0.38	0.00	0.00	0.00	0.00	0.20	0.00	0.00	50.00	470.00	0.00
0.00	0.00	0.00	0.00	0.00	350.00	6.00	0.15	0.17	7.60	0.00	0.00	0.00	16.00	0.80	0.00	0.00	550.00	480.00	0.00
0.00	0.00	0.00	0.00	0.00	200.00	66.00	0.23	0.17	3.80	0.00	0.00	0.00	64.00	0.60	0.00	200.00	540.00	450.00	0.00
0.00	2.00	0.00	0.00	0.00	0.00	0.00	0.00	0.00	0.00	0.00	0.00	0.00	0.00	0.00	0.00	260.00	560.00	550.00	0.00
0.00	0.00	0.00	0.00	0.00	250.00	30.00	0.15	0.17	8.55	0.00	0.00	0.00	32.00	1.00	0.00	220.00	480.00	320.00	0.00
0.00	0.00	0.00	0.00	0.00	0.00	0.00	0.00	0.00	0.00	0.00	0.00	0.00	0.00	0.00	0.00	0.00	0.00	730.00	0.00
0.00	2.00	0.00	0.00	0.00	20.00	6.00	0.09	0.10	7.60	0.00	0.00	0.00	32.00	0.80	0.00	250.00	520.00	560.00	0.00

USDA ID Code	Food Name	Weight in Grams*	Quantity of Units	Unit of Measure	Protein (gm)	Fat (gm)	Carbohydrate (gm)	Kcalories	Caffeine (gm)	Fiber (gm)	Cholesterol (mg)	Saturated Fat (gm)
	Chili Beef Soup-Healthy Choice	212.6200	1.000	Each	11.00	1.00	22.00	150.00	0.00	0.00	15.00	0.00
	Chili Con Carne w/ Beans-Stouffe	248.0570	1.000	Each	20.00	10.00	28.00	280.00	0.00	0.00	0.00	0.00
	Chili Mac, Micro Cup-Hormel	212.6200	1.000	Each	10.00	9.00	18.00	192.00	0.00	0.00	22.00	4.00
	Chili no Beans, Micro Cup-Hormel	209.0760	1.000	Each	18.00	17.00	15.00	290.00	0.00	0.00	60.00	8.00
	Chili w/ Beans Soup-Stouffer's	283.9200	1.000	Cup	14.02	9.01	25.04	240.36	0.00	0.00	30.04	0.00
	Chili w/ Beans, Chunky -Hormel	253.1620	1.000	Cup	17.86	16.67	29.77	345.30	0.00	0.00	59.53	0.00
	Chili w/ Beans, Micro Cup-Hormel	209.0760	1.000	Each	15.00	11.00	23.00	250.00	0.00	0.00	49.00	4.00
	Chili w/ Beans-Hormel	253.1620	1.000	Cup	17.86	17.86	32.15	357.20	0.00	0.00	65.49	5.95
	Chili w/o Beans-Hormel	253.1620	1.000	Cup	19.05	32.15	16.67	428.64	0.00	0.00	71.44	13.10
	Chili, Fat Free	240.0000	0.500	Cup	14.00	0.00	30.00	160.00	0.00	14.00	0.00	0.00
	Chili, Hot, no Beans-Hormel	212.6200	1.000	Each	16.00	27.00	14.00	360.00	0.00	0.00	60.00	11.00
	Chili, Hot, w/ Beans, Micro Cup-	209.0760	1.000	Each	15.00	11.00	24.00	250.00	0.00	0.00	49.00	4.00
	Chili, Hot, w/ Beans-Hormel	212.6200	1.000	Each	15.00	15.00	27.00	300.00	0.00	0.00	55.00	5.00
	Chili, Three Bean-Stouffer's	283.9200	1.000	Cup	10.02	5.01	32.05	210.32	0.00	0.00	20.03	0.00
	Chow Mein w/ Rice, Chicken, Lean	255.1440	1.000	Each	14.00	5.00	34.00	240.00	0.00	0.00	30.00	1.00
	Chow Mein w/ Rice, Chicken-Stouf	304.7550	1.000	Each	13.00	5.00	39.00	250.00	0.00	0.00	0.00	0.00
	Chow Mein, Beef	247.0000	1.000	Cup	10.00	1.50	15.00	110.00	0.00	4.00	10.00	1.00
	Chow Mein, Chicken -Weight Watch	255.1500	1.000	Each	12.00	2.00	34.00	200.00	0.00	3.00	25.00	0.50
	Chow Mein, Chicken-Healthy Choic	240.9690	1.000	Each	18.00	3.00	31.00	220.00	0.00	0.00	45.00	1.00
190	Chow Mein, Chicken-Smart Ones	252.0000	9.000	Ounce	12.00	2.00	34.00	200.00	0.00	3.00	25.00	0.50
	Chow Mein, Vegetable-Stouffer's	28.3500	1.000	Ounce	0.30	0.70	1.60	14.00	0.00	0.00	0.00	0.00
	Corn Pudding-Stouffer's	28.3500	1.000	Ounce	1.20	1.70	4.50	38.00	0.00	0.00	15.00	0.00
	Corn Souffle-Stouffer's	170.0960	1.000	Each	7.00	11.00	27.00	240.00	0.00	0.00	0.00	0.00
	Corned Beef Hash-Hormel	253.1620	1.000	Cup	26.79	26.79	17.86	419.71	0.00	0.00	80.37	8.93
	Egg Roll	85.0000	1.000	Each	7.00	5.00	21.00	160.00	0.00	2.00	10.00	1.00
	Enchiladas, Beef and Bean, Lean	262.2310	1.000	Each	15.00	6.00	32.00	240.00	0.00	0.00	45.00	3.00
	Enchiladas, Beef -Healthy Choice	379.1720	1.000	Each	15.00	5.00	66.00	370.00	0.00	0.00	30.00	2.00
	Enchiladas, Cheese-Stouffer's	276.4060	1.000	Each	23.00	29.00	33.00	490.00	0.00	0.00	0.00	0.00
	Enchiladas, Chicken Suiza-Weight	255.1500	1.000	Each	15.00	8.00	28.00	250.00	0.00	4.00	25.00	3.00
	Enchiladas, Chicken, Lean Cuisin	279.9500	1.000	Each	17.00	9.00	34.00	290.00	0.00	0.00	55.00	3.00
	Enchiladas, Chicken, Nacho Grand	255.1500	1.000	Each	15.00	8.00	42.00	290.00	0.00	4.00	20.00	2.50
	Enchiladas, Chicken-Healthy Choi	269.3190	1.000	Each	14.00	9.00	44.00	310.00	0.00	0.00	35.00	3.00
	Enchiladas, Chicken-Stouffer's	283.4930	1.000	Each	21.00	31.00	31.00	490.00	0.00	0.00	0.00	0.00
	Fajitas, Chicken-Healthy Choice	198.4450	1.000	Each	17.00	3.00	25.00	200.00	0.00	0.00	35.00	1.00
442	Fettuccini Alfredo w/Broccoli-Sm	238.0000	8.500	Ounce	10.00	6.00	34.00	230.00	0.00	3.00	20.00	3.00
443	Fettuccini, Chicken-Smart Ones	280.0000	10.000	Ounce	19.00	7.00	39.00	290.00	0.00	4.00	50.00	2.00
	Fettucini Alfredo with Broccoli-	240.9750	1.000	Each	15.00	6.00	24.00	220.00	0.00	6.00	15.00	2.50
	Fettucini Alfredo, Lean Cuisine-	255.1440	1.000	Each	14.00	7.00	41.00	280.00	0.00	0.00	15.00	3.00
	Fettucini Alfredo-Stouffer's	141.7460	1.000	Each	8.00	14.00	22.00	245.00	0.00	0.00	0.00	0.00
	Fettucini Primavera, Lean Cuisin	283.4930	1.000	Each	14.00	8.00	32.00	260.00	0.00	0.00	45.00	3.00
	Fettucini Sauce (Alfredo Style)-	283.9200	1.000	Cup	14.02	67.10	11.02	701.05	0.00	0.00	180.27	0.00
	Fettucini w/ Turkey and Vegetabl	354.3670	1.000	Each	29.00	6.00	45.00	350.00	0.00	0.00	60.00	3.00
	Fettucini, Chicken -Weight Watch	233.8900	1.000	Each	22.00	9.00	25.00	280.00	0.00	2.00	40.00	3.00
	Fettucini, Chicken, Lean Cuisine	255.1440	1.000	Each	23.00	6.00	33.00	280.00	0.00	0.00	35.00	3.00
	Fettucini, Chicken-Healthy Choic	240.9690	1.000	Each	19.00	7.00	39.00	240.00	0.00	0.00	45.00	2.00
	Fish Divan, Filet of, Lean Cuisi	294.1240	1.000	Each	27.00	5.00	13.00	210.00	0.00	0.00	65.00	2.00
	Fish Florentine, Filet of, Lean	272.8620	1.000	Each	26.00	7.00	13.00	220.00	0.00	0.00	65.00	3.00
	Fish, Breaded-Healthy Choice	9.7450	1.000	Stick	1.00	0.50	1.75	15.00	0.00	0.00	2.50	0.00
	Fish, Lemon Pepper -Healthy Choi	304.7550	1.000	Each	13.00	5.00	52.00	300.00	0.00	0.00	40.00	1.00
	Ham and Asparagus Bake-Stouffer'	269.3190	1.000	Each	18.00	35.00	32.00	520.00	0.00	0.00	0.00	0.00
	Hamburger Helper, Beef Noodle	220.0000	1.000	Cup	4.00	10.50	23.00	260.00	0.00	1.00	5.00	4.00
	Hamburger Helper, Cheesy Italian	220.0000	1.000	Cup	5.00	21.00	30.00	330.00	0.00	1.00	5.00	2.00
	Hamburger Helper, Chili Mac	220.0000	1.000	Cup	3.00	16.00	30.00	290.00	0.00	1.00	4.00	4.00
	Heartland Medley-Stouffer's	28.3500	1.000	Ounce	1.40	0.40	1.80	17.00	0.00	0.00	3.00	0.00
580	Lasagna Florentine-Smart Ones	280.0000	10.000	Ounce	10.00	2.00	34.00	200.00	0.00	5.00	10.00	0.00

Monounsaturated Fat (gm)	Polyunsaturated Fat (gm)	Vitamin D (mg)	Vitamin K (mg)	Vitamin E (mg)	Vitamin A (re)	Vitamin C (mg)	Thiamin (mg)	Riboflavin (mg)	Niacin (mg)	Vitamin B_6 (mg)	Folate (mg)	Vitamin B_{12} (mcg)	Calcium (mg)	Iron (mg)	Magnesium (mg)	Phosphorus (mg)	Potassium (mg)	Sodium (mg)	Zinc (mg)
0.00	0.00	0.00	0.00	0.00	20.00	6.00	0.09	0.03	0.38	0.00	0.00	0.00	16.00	0.60	0.00	0.00	290.00	560.00	0.00
0.00	0.00	0.00	0.00	0.00	200.00	15.00	0.15	0.26	2.85	0.00	0.00	0.00	64.00	2.00	0.00	0.00	700.00	910.00	0.00
4.00	0.00	0.00	0.00	0.17	210.00	0.00	0.08	0.17	2.09	0.00	0.00	0.00	0.00	1.50	35.00	0.00	443.00	977.00	2.10
8.00	1.00	0.00	0.00	0.01	400.00	0.00	0.08	0.24	2.47	0.00	0.00	0.00	48.00	1.60	35.00	0.00	507.00	830.00	3.90
0.00	0.00	0.00	0.00	0.00	0.00	0.00	0.00	0.00	0.57	0.00	0.00	0.00	0.00	0.30	0.00	0.00	711.07	991.49	0.00
0.00	0.00	0.00	0.00	0.00	0.00	0.00	0.00	0.00	0.00	0.00	0.00	0.00	0.00	0.00	0.00	0.00	0.00	928.73	0.00
4.00	0.00	0.00	0.00	18.90	190.00	0.00	0.14	0.15	1.71	0.00	0.00	0.00	48.00	1.90	45.50	0.00	677.00	977.00	2.70
7.14	1.19	0.00	0.00	0.01	250.04	0.00	0.11	0.20	2.04	0.00	0.00	0.00	57.15	1.91	58.34	0.00	913.25	1226.40	2.50
15.48	1.19	0.00	0.00	0.60	785.85	0.00	0.11	0.26	2.94	0.00	0.00	0.00	47.63	1.67	41.67	0.00	591.77	1023.98	3.21
0.00	0.00	0.00	0.00	0.00	2000.00	24.00	0.00	0.00	0.00	0.00	0.00	0.00	48.00	2.00	0.00	0.00	0.00	320.00	0.00
13.00	1.00	0.00	0.00	10.56	330.00	0.00	0.05	0.22	2.47	0.00	0.00	0.00	40.00	1.40	35.00	0.00	497.00	860.00	2.70
4.00	0.00	0.00	0.00	1.95	190.00	0.00	0.14	0.15	1.71	0.00	0.00	0.00	48.00	1.90	45.50	0.00	677.00	977.00	2.70
6.00	1.00	0.00	0.00	0.00	210.00	0.00	0.09	0.17	1.71	0.00	0.00	0.00	48.00	1.80	49.00	0.00	777.00	1030.00	2.25
0.00	0.00	0.00	0.00	0.00	0.00	6.01	0.00	0.01	0.57	0.00	0.00	0.00	1.20	0.40	0.00	0.00	891.34	861.29	0.00
0.00	1.00	0.00	0.00	0.00	60.00	6.00	0.15	0.17	4.75	0.00	0.00	0.00	32.00	0.60	0.00	0.00	350.00	530.00	0.00
0.00	0.00	0.00	0.00	0.00	80.00	12.00	0.03	0.17	1.90	0.00	0.00	0.00	16.00	0.40	0.00	0.00	340.00	720.00	0.00
0.00	0.00	0.00	0.00	0.00	40.00	12.00	0.00	0.00	0.00	0.00	0.00	0.00	24.00	0.40	0.00	0.00	0.00	760.00	0.00
0.00	0.00	0.00	0.00	0.00	300.00	36.00	0.00	0.00	0.00	0.00	0.00	0.00	48.00	0.40	0.00	0.00	360.00	570.00	0.00
0.00	1.00	0.00	0.00	0.00	80.00	3.60	0.15	0.14	3.80	0.00	0.00	0.00	16.00	0.80	0.00	290.00	290.00	440.00	0.00
0.00	0.00	0.00	0.00	0.00	0.00	0.00	0.00	0.00	0.00	0.00	0.00	0.00	0.00	0.00	0.00	0.00	0.00	570.00	0.00
0.00	0.00	0.00	0.00	0.00	0.00	0.60	0.00	0.00	0.02	0.00	0.00	0.00	24.00	0.01	0.00	0.00	26.00	156.00	0.00
0.00	0.00	0.00	0.00	0.00	0.00	0.60	0.00	0.00	0.06	0.00	0.00	0.00	88.00	0.02	0.00	0.00	51.00	125.00	0.00
0.00	0.00	0.00	0.00	0.00	60.00	0.00	0.15	0.26	1.14	0.00	0.00	0.00	48.00	0.40	0.00	0.00	200.00	760.00	0.00
17.86	0.00	0.00	0.00	0.43	0.00	0.00	0.00	0.15	3.39	0.00	0.00	0.00	71.44	1.79	31.26	0.00	625.11	991.24	4.02
0.00	0.00	0.00	0.00	0.00	100.00	1.20	0.00	0.00	0.00	0.00	0.00	0.00	24.00	0.20	0.00	0.00	0.00	350.00	0.00
0.00	1.00	0.00	0.00	0.00	80.00	6.00	0.23	0.26	1.90	0.00	0.00	0.00	80.00	1.00	0.00	0.00	470.00	480.00	0.00
0.00	2.00	0.00	0.00	0.00	250.00	24.00	0.30	0.26	1.90	0.00	0.00	0.00	120.00	1.00	0.00	260.00	600.00	450.00	0.00
0.00	0.00	0.00	0.00	0.00	150.00	6.00	0.09	0.34	1.52	0.00	0.00	0.00	480.00	0.80	0.00	0.00	400.00	550.00	0.00
0.00	0.00	0.00	0.00	0.00	40.00	1.20	0.00	0.00	0.00	0.00	0.00	0.00	360.00	0.80	0.00	0.00	470.00	570.00	0.00
0.00	2.00	0.00	0.00	0.00	250.00	6.00	0.23	0.34	2.85	0.00	0.00	0.00	120.00	1.50	0.00	0.00	450.00	500.00	0.00
0.00	0.00	0.00	0.00	0.00	300.00	12.00	0.00	0.00	0.00	0.00	0.00	0.00	360.00	0.60	0.00	0.00	600.00	560.00	0.00
0.00	1.00	0.00	0.00	0.00	80.00	21.00	0.15	0.17	4.75	0.00	0.00	0.00	80.00	0.80	0.00	160.00	380.00	480.00	0.00
0.00	0.00	0.00	0.00	0.00	60.00	2.40	0.09	0.34	2.85	0.00	0.00	0.00	240.00	0.60	0.00	0.00	420.00	860.00	0.00
0.00	1.00	0.00	0.00	0.00	150.00	9.00	0.23	0.17	3.80	0.00	0.00	0.00	64.00	1.50	0.00	210.00	360.00	310.00	0.00
0.00	0.00	0.00	0.00	0.00	0.00	0.00	0.00	0.00	0.00	0.00	0.00	0.00	0.00	0.00	0.00	0.00	0.00	450.00	0.00
0.00	0.00	0.00	0.00	0.00	0.00	0.00	0.00	0.00	0.00	0.00	0.00	0.00	0.00	0.00	0.00	0.00	0.00	590.00	0.00
0.00	0.00	0.00	0.00	0.00	60.00	1.20	0.00	0.00	0.00	0.00	0.00	0.00	300.00	1.50	0.00	0.00	510.00	540.00	0.00
0.00	0.00	0.00	0.00	0.00	0.00	0.00	0.30	0.43	1.52	0.00	0.00	0.00	200.00	0.80	0.00	0.00	270.00	570.00	0.00
0.00	0.00	0.00	0.00	0.00	0.00	0.00	0.15	0.26	0.95	0.00	0.00	0.00	120.00	0.40	0.00	0.00	100.00	400.00	0.00
0.00	0.00	0.00	0.00	0.00	400.00	18.00	0.30	0.43	1.52	0.00	0.00	0.00	240.00	0.80	0.00	0.00	400.00	510.00	0.00
0.00	0.00	0.00	0.00	0.00	0.00	0.00	0.00	0.01	0.00	0.00	0.00	0.00	2.72	0.00	0.00	0.00	340.51	1812.72	0.00
0.00	2.00	0.00	0.00	0.00	150.00	0.00	0.45	0.51	3.80	0.00	0.00	0.00	120.00	1.50	0.00	310.00	450.00	480.00	0.00
0.00	0.00	0.00	0.00	0.00	40.00	0.00	0.00	0.00	0.00	0.00	0.00	0.00	240.00	1.00	0.00	0.00	730.00	590.00	0.00
0.00	0.00	0.00	0.00	0.00	0.00	0.00	0.30	0.43	5.70	0.00	0.00	0.00	120.00	0.80	0.00	0.00	420.00	500.00	0.00
0.00	2.00	0.00	0.00	0.00	0.00	0.00	0.23	0.17	2.85	0.00	0.00	0.00	64.00	1.00	0.00	210.00	190.00	370.00	0.00
0.00	1.00	0.00	0.00	0.00	20.00	27.00	0.15	0.34	1.90	0.00	0.00	0.00	120.00	0.40	0.00	0.00	800.00	490.00	0.00
0.00	2.00	0.00	0.00	0.00	500.00	1.20	0.15	0.34	1.90	0.00	0.00	0.00	120.00	0.40	0.00	0.00	780.00	590.00	0.00
0.00	0.13	0.00	0.00	0.00	0.00	0.00	0.01	0.02	0.10	0.00	0.00	0.00	0.00	0.10	0.00	0.00	20.00	31.25	0.00
0.00	2.00	0.00	0.00	0.00	80.00	48.00	0.23	0.14	1.14	0.00	0.00	0.00	32.00	0.60	0.00	180.00	410.00	370.00	0.00
0.00	0.00	0.00	0.00	0.00	60.00	36.00	0.53	0.51	2.85	0.00	0.00	0.00	160.00	0.80	0.00	0.00	360.00	1100.00	0.00
0.00	0.00	0.00	0.00	0.00	60.00	0.00	0.23	0.17	3.80	0.00	0.00	0.00	24.00	1.00	0.00	0.00	240.00	900.00	0.00
0.00	0.00	0.00	0.00	0.00	60.00	0.00	0.30	0.34	3.80	0.00	0.00	0.00	120.00	1.50	0.00	0.00	400.00	900.00	0.00
0.00	0.00	0.00	0.00	0.00	200.00	0.00	0.30	0.26	4.75	0.00	0.00	0.00	24.00	1.50	0.00	0.00	0.00	900.00	0.00
0.00	0.00	0.00	0.00	0.00	0.00	0.60	0.00	0.00	0.06	0.00	0.00	0.00	40.00	0.02	0.00	0.00	60.00	85.00	0.00
0.00	0.00	0.00	0.00	0.00	0.00	0.00	0.00	0.00	0.00	0.00	0.00	0.00	0.00	0.00	0.00	0.00	0.00	590.00	0.00

USDA ID Code	Food Name	Weight in Grams*	Quantity of Units	Unit of Measure	Protein (gm)	Fat (gm)	Carbohydrate (gm)	Kcalories	Caffeine (gm)	Fiber (gm)	Cholesterol (mg)	Saturated Fat (gm)
	Lasagna Florentine-Weight Watche	283.5000	1.000	Each	13.00	2.00	37.00	210.00	0.00	5.00	10.00	0.50
	Lasagna w/ Meat Sauce, Lean Cuis	290.5810	1.000	Each	20.00	6.00	36.00	280.00	0.00	0.00	25.00	3.00
	Lasagna w/ Meat Sauce-Healthy Ch	283.4930	1.000	Each	18.00	5.00	37.00	260.00	0.00	0.00	20.00	2.00
581	Lasagna w/ Meat Sauce-Smart Ones	252.0000	9.000	Ounce	13.00	2.00	43.00	240.00	0.00	4.00	10.00	0.50
	Lasagna w/ Meat Sauce-Weight Wat	290.5900	1.000	Each	24.00	7.00	34.00	290.00	0.00	7.00	15.00	2.50
	Lasagna, Cheese, Italian -Weight	311.8500	1.000	Each	29.00	8.00	28.00	300.00	0.00	7.00	25.00	3.00
	Lasagna, Italian, Top Shelf-Horm	283.4930	1.000	Each	23.00	16.00	30.00	350.00	0.00	0.00	60.00	8.00
	Lasagna, Micro Cup-Hormel	212.6200	1.000	Each	8.00	13.00	25.00	250.00	0.00	0.00	23.00	6.00
	Lasagna, Vegetable-Stouffer's	274.0420	1.000	Each	23.00	20.00	33.00	400.00	0.00	0.00	0.00	0.00
	Lasagna, Zucchini, Lean Cuisine-	311.8430	1.000	Each	17.00	6.00	34.00	260.00	0.00	0.00	20.00	2.00
	Lasagna, Zucchini-Healthy Choice	326.0170	1.000	Each	14.00	3.00	41.00	250.00	0.00	0.00	15.00	2.00
	Lasagna-Stouffer's	283.4930	1.000	Each	18.00	12.00	40.00	340.00	0.00	0.00	0.00	0.00
	Linguini w/ Clam Sauce, Lean Cui	272.8620	1.000	Each	17.00	8.00	36.00	280.00	0.00	0.00	30.00	2.00
	Macaroni and Beef in Sauce, Lean	283.4930	1.000	Each	14.00	6.00	35.00	250.00	0.00	0.00	25.00	1.00
	Macaroni and Beef w/ Tomatoes-St	326.0170	1.000	Each	21.00	12.00	38.00	340.00	0.00	0.00	0.00	0.00
	Macaroni and Beef-Healthy Choice	240.9690	1.000	Each	12.00	3.00	32.00	200.00	0.00	0.00	15.00	1.00
	Macaroni and Cheese	111.9120	1.000	Cup	1.00	12.99	43.97	359.72	0.00	15.99	39.97	7.99
	Macaroni and Cheese, Deluxe Ligh	90.0000	1.000	Serving	14.00	4.50	48.00	290.00	0.00	0.00	15.00	2.50
	Macaroni and Cheese, Kraft	70.0000	1.000	Serving	12.00	18.50	50.00	420.00	0.00	0.00	15.00	5.00
	Macaroni and Cheese, Lean Cuisin	255.1440	1.000	Each	15.00	9.00	37.00	290.00	0.00	0.00	30.00	4.00
	Macaroni and Cheese, Micro Cup-H	212.6200	1.000	Each	12.00	11.00	28.00	260.00	0.00	0.00	45.00	6.00
	Macaroni and Cheese, Nacho-Healt	255.1440	1.000	Each	13.00	5.00	44.00	280.00	0.00	0.00	20.00	3.00
	Macaroni and Cheese-Healthy Choi	255.1440	1.000	Each	12.00	6.00	45.00	280.00	0.00	0.00	20.00	3.00
	Macaroni and Cheese-Stouffer's	170.0960	1.000	Each	11.00	13.00	23.00	250.00	0.00	0.00	0.00	0.00
	Macaroni and Cheese-Weight Watch	255.1500	1.000	Each	11.00	7.00	49.00	300.00	0.00	7.00	20.00	2.00
	Manicotti, Cheese-Healthy Choice	262.2310	1.000	Each	15.00	3.00	34.00	220.00	0.00	0.00	30.00	2.00
	Manicotti, Cheese-Stouffer's	28.3500	1.000	Ounce	1.60	1.30	2.60	29.00	0.00	0.00	4.00	0.00
	Meatballs, Swedish, w/ Pasta, Le	258.6880	1.000	Each	23.00	8.00	31.00	290.00	0.00	0.00	55.00	3.00
	Meatballs, Swedish, w/ Pasta-Sto	262.2310	1.000	Each	24.00	21.00	32.00	420.00	0.00	0.00	0.00	0.00
582	Meatballs, Swedish-Smart Ones	252.0000	9.000	Ounce	19.00	10.00	33.00	300.00	0.00	2.00	50.00	4.00
	Meatloaf w/ Mac. and Cheese, Lea	265.7750	1.000	Each	26.00	8.00	26.00	280.00	0.00	0.00	55.00	3.00
	Meatloaf-Healthy Choice	340.1920	1.000	Each	17.00	8.00	48.00	340.00	0.00	0.00	40.00	3.00
	Meatloaf-Stouffer's	28.3500	1.000	Ounce	4.40	3.40	2.10	57.00	0.00	0.00	15.00	0.00
585	Morningstar Farms- Buffalo Wings	85.0000	5.000	Each	13.00	9.00	16.00	200.00	0.00	3.00	0.00	1.50
586	Morningstar Farms- Burger, Bean,	78.0000	1.000	Each	11.00	1.00	16.00	110.00	0.00	5.00	0.00	0.00
587	Morningstar Farms- Burger, Veggi	67.0000	1.000	Each	14.00	8.00	40.00	120.00	0.00	2.00	0.00	3.50
588	Morningstar Farms- Burger/Cheese	128.0000	1.000	Each	14.00	8.00	40.00	290.00	0.00	2.00	0.00	3.50
589	Morningstar Farms- Burgers, Bett	78.0000	1.000	Each	13.00	0.00	8.00	80.00	0.00	3.00	0.00	0.00
590	Morningstar Farms- Chik Nuggets	86.0000	4.000	Each	13.00	4.00	17.00	160.00	0.00	5.00	0.00	0.50
591	Morningstar Farms- Chik Patties	71.0000	1.000	Each	9.00	6.00	15.00	150.00	0.00	2.00	0.00	1.00
592	Morningstar Farms- Corn Dogs, Me	71.0000	1.000	Each	7.00	4.00	22.00	150.00	0.00	3.00	0.00	0.50
593	Morningstar Farms- Corn Dogs, Mi	71.0000	1.000	Each	11.00	4.50	21.00	150.00	0.00	1.00	0.00	0.50
594	Morningstar Farms- Crumbles, Bur	55.0000	0.660	Cup	10.00	2.50	4.00	80.00	0.00	2.00	0.00	0.00
595	Morningstar Farms- Crumbles, Sau	55.0000	0.660	Cup	11.00	3.00	5.00	90.00	0.00	2.00	0.00	0.00
596	Morningstar Farms- Eggs, Better'	57.0000	0.250	Cup	5.00	0.00	0.00	20.00	0.00	0.00	0.00	0.00
597	Morningstar Farms- Garden Grille	71.0000	1.000	Each	6.00	2.50	18.00	120.00	0.00	4.00	0.00	1.00
598	Morningstar Farms- Grillers	64.0000	1.000	Each	15.00	6.00	5.00	140.00	0.00	2.00	0.00	1.00
599	Morningstar Farms- Ham/Cheese Sd	128.0000	1.000	Each	15.00	7.00	25.00	300.00	0.00	1.00	0.00	2.50
600	Morningstar Farms- Harvest Burge	90.0000	1.000	Each	17.00	4.50	8.00	140.00	0.00	5.00	0.00	1.50
601	Morningstar Farms- Harvest Burge	90.0000	1.000	Each	18.00	4.00	8.00	140.00	0.00	5.00	0.00	1.50
602	Morningstar Farms- Harvest Burge	90.0000	1.000	Each	16.00	4.00	9.00	140.00	0.00	5.00	0.00	1.50
603	Morningstar Farms- Links, Breakf	45.0000	2.000	Each	8.00	2.00	2.00	60.00	0.00	2.00	0.00	0.50
604	Morningstar Farms- Meatless, Gro	55.0000	0.500	Cup	10.00	0.00	4.00	60.00	0.00	2.00	0.00	0.00
605	Morningstar Farms- Patties, Brea	38.0000	1.000	Each	10.00	0.00	3.00	38.00	0.00	2.00	0.00	0.50
606	Morningstar Farms- Patties, Gard	67.0000	1.000	Each	10.00	2.50	9.00	100.00	0.00	4.00	0.00	0.50

Monounsaturated Fat (gm)	Polyunsaturated Fat (gm)	Vitamin D (mg)	Vitamin K (mg)	Vitamin E (mg)	Vitamin A (re)	Vitamin C (mg)	Thiamin (mg)	Riboflavin (mg)	Niacin (mg)	Vitamin B_6 (mg)	Folate (mg)	Vitamin B_{12} (mcg)	Calcium (mg)	Iron (mg)	Magnesium (mg)	Phosphorus (mg)	Potassium (mg)	Sodium (mg)	Zinc (mg)
0.00	0.00	0.00	0.00	0.00	300.00	15.00	0.00	0.00	0.00	0.00	0.00	0.00	300.00	1.50	0.00	0.00	440.00	420.00	0.00
0.00	0.00	0.00	0.00	0.00	100.00	6.00	0.15	0.26	2.85	0.00	0.00	0.00	120.00	1.00	0.00	0.00	700.00	560.00	0.00
0.00	1.00	0.00	0.00	0.00	150.00	2.40	0.30	0.26	1.90	0.00	0.00	0.00	80.00	1.50	0.00	210.00	500.00	420.00	0.00
0.00	0.00	0.00	0.00	0.00	0.00	0.00	0.00	0.00	0.00	0.00	0.00	0.00	0.00	0.00	0.00	0.00	0.00	520.00	0.00
0.00	0.00	0.00	0.00	0.00	250.00	12.00	0.00	0.00	0.00	0.00	0.00	0.00	480.00	1.50	0.00	0.00	720.00	580.00	0.00
0.00	0.00	0.00	0.00	0.00	350.00	15.00	0.00	0.00	0.00	0.00	0.00	0.00	780.00	1.50	0.00	0.00	720.00	560.00	0.00
5.00	1.00	0.00	0.00	0.70	100.00	2.40	0.30	0.51	3.80	0.00	0.00	0.00	240.00	1.50	49.00	0.00	728.00	840.00	3.15
4.00	2.00	0.00	0.00	0.00	100.00	1.80	0.12	0.20	1.90	0.00	0.00	0.00	40.00	0.80	24.50	0.00	331.00	949.00	1.05
0.00	0.00	0.00	0.00	0.00	250.00	0.00	0.12	0.43	0.76	0.00	0.00	0.00	160.00	0.60	0.00	0.00	350.00	760.00	0.00
0.00	0.00	0.00	0.00	0.00	150.00	6.00	0.15	0.26	1.90	0.00	0.00	0.00	200.00	0.80	0.00	0.00	650.00	520.00	0.00
0.00	0.00	0.00	0.00	0.00	350.00	6.00	0.38	0.26	1.90	0.00	0.00	0.00	200.00	1.50	0.00	250.00	830.00	400.00	0.00
0.00	0.00	0.00	0.00	0.00	150.00	6.00	0.15	0.34	6.65	0.00	0.00	0.00	200.00	1.00	0.00	0.00	570.00	840.00	0.00
0.00	2.00	0.00	0.00	0.00	0.00	0.00	0.30	0.17	1.90	0.00	0.00	0.00	32.00	1.50	0.00	0.00	90.00	560.00	0.00
0.00	1.00	0.00	0.00	0.00	100.00	3.60	0.15	0.17	2.85	0.00	0.00	0.00	48.00	1.50	0.00	0.00	450.00	540.00	0.00
0.00	0.00	0.00	0.00	0.00	60.00	6.00	0.06	0.10	1.90	0.00	0.00	0.00	32.00	0.80	0.00	0.00	300.00	1440.00	0.00
0.00	0.00	0.00	0.00	0.00	200.00	15.00	0.30	0.26	0.00	0.00	0.00	0.00	32.00	1.00	0.00	0.00	530.00	420.00	0.00
0.00	0.00	0.00	0.00	0.00	99.92	0.00	0.00	0.00	0.00	0.00	0.00	0.00	239.81	1.50	0.00	0.00	0.00	1029.19	0.00
0.00	0.00	0.00	0.00	0.00	0.00	0.00	0.00	0.00	0.00	0.00	0.00	0.00	160.00	1.50	0.00	0.00	0.00	810.00	0.00
0.00	0.00	0.00	0.00	0.00	0.00	0.00	0.00	0.00	0.00	0.00	0.00	0.00	120.00	1.50	0.00	0.00	0.00	760.00	0.00
0.00	0.00	0.00	0.00	0.00	0.00	0.00	0.30	0.43	1.52	0.00	0.00	0.00	200.00	0.80	0.00	0.00	160.00	550.00	0.00
3.00	1.00	0.00	0.00	0.00	80.00	6.00	0.09	0.26	1.14	0.00	0.00	0.00	80.00	0.60	24.50	0.00	209.00	650.00	1.05
0.00	0.00	0.00	0.00	0.00	0.00	0.00	0.60	0.51	0.00	0.00	0.00	0.00	160.00	0.80	0.00	0.00	420.00	560.00	0.00
0.00	1.00	0.00	0.00	0.00	0.00	0.00	0.30	0.26	1.14	0.00	0.00	0.00	120.00	1.00	0.00	230.00	220.00	520.00	0.00
0.00	0.00	0.00	0.00	0.00	20.00	0.00	0.15	0.26	0.38	0.00	0.00	0.00	160.00	0.40	0.00	0.00	140.00	640.00	0.00
0.00	0.00	0.00	0.00	0.00	100.00	0.00	0.00	0.00	0.00	0.00	0.00	0.00	300.00	1.00	0.00	0.00	410.00	570.00	0.00
0.00	0.00	0.00	0.00	0.00	250.00	6.00	0.30	0.26	1.90	0.00	0.00	0.00	120.00	1.50	0.00	210.00	590.00	310.00	0.00
0.00	0.00	0.00	0.00	0.00	0.00	2.40	0.00	0.00	0.04	0.00	0.00	0.00	296.01	0.02	0.00	0.00	45.00	108.00	0.00
0.00	1.00	0.00	0.00	0.00	20.00	0.00	0.23	0.34	3.80	0.00	0.00	0.00	48.00	1.50	0.00	0.00	450.00	550.00	0.00
0.00	0.00	0.00	0.00	0.00	20.00	1.20	0.15	0.26	2.85	0.00	0.00	0.00	48.00	1.50	0.00	0.00	350.00	740.00	0.00
0.00	0.00	0.00	0.00	0.00	0.00	0.00	0.00	0.00	0.00	0.00	0.00	0.00	0.00	0.00	0.00	0.00	0.00	510.00	0.00
0.00	1.00	0.00	0.00	0.00	60.00	9.00	0.23	0.43	3.80	0.00	0.00	0.00	120.00	2.00	0.00	0.00	550.00	540.00	0.00
0.00	1.00	0.00	0.00	0.00	0.00	0.00	0.00	0.00	0.00	0.00	0.00	0.00	0.00	0.00	0.00	240.00	690.00	560.00	0.00
0.00	0.00	0.00	0.00	0.00	0.00	0.00	0.00	0.00	0.13	0.00	0.00	0.00	48.00	0.06	0.00	0.00	4.40	193.00	0.00
2.50	5.00	0.00	0.00	0.00	0.00	0.00	1.05	0.17	3.00	0.20	0.00	1.20	40.00	2.70	0.00	0.00	390.00	730.00	0.00
0.00	0.00	0.00	0.00	0.00	0.00	0.00	0.00	0.00	0.00	0.00	0.00	0.00	40.00	1.80	0.00	0.00	350.00	470.00	0.00
3.00	1.50	0.00	0.00	0.00	0.00	0.00	0.00	0.00	0.00	0.00	0.00	0.00	100.00	1.08	0.00	0.00	130.00	400.00	0.00
3.00	1.50	0.00	0.00	0.00	0.00	0.00	0.00	0.00	0.00	0.00	0.00	0.00	60.00	1.08	0.00	0.00	130.00	400.00	0.00
0.00	0.00	0.00	0.00	0.00	0.00	0.00	0.00	0.00	0.00	0.00	0.00	0.00	20.00	1.80	0.00	0.00	390.00	360.00	0.00
1.00	2.50	0.00	0.00	0.00	0.00	0.00	0.90	0.17	2.00	0.20	0.00	1.50	20.00	1.80	0.00	0.00	330.00	670.00	0.00
1.50	3.50	0.00	0.00	0.00	0.00	0.00	0.60	0.10	0.40	0.16	0.00	0.90	0.00	0.72	0.00	0.00	150.00	570.00	0.00
1.00	2.50	0.00	0.00	0.00	0.00	0.00	0.00	0.00	0.00	0.00	0.00	0.00	0.00	1.08	0.00	0.00	60.00	500.00	0.00
2.50	1.50	0.00	0.00	0.00	0.00	0.00	0.00	0.00	0.00	0.00	0.00	0.00	0.00	1.08	0.00	0.00	90.00	580.00	0.00
0.50	2.00	0.00	0.00	0.00	0.00	0.00	0.30	0.10	4.00	0.30	0.00	1.80	20.00	1.80	0.00	0.00	120.00	210.00	0.00
0.50	2.00	0.00	0.00	0.00	0.00	0.00	1.80	0.17	4.00	0.40	0.00	1.80	20.00	1.80	0.00	0.00	80.00	370.00	0.00
0.00	0.00	0.60	0.00	1.20	225.00	0.00	0.03	0.34	0.00	0.08	0.02	0.60	20.00	0.72	0.00	0.00	75.00	90.00	0.60
1.00	0.50	0.00	0.00	0.00	0.00	0.00	0.00	0.00	0.00	0.00	0.00	0.00	60.00	1.80	0.00	0.00	130.00	280.00	0.00
2.00	3.00	0.00	0.00	0.00	0.00	0.00	1.80	0.17	2.00	0.40	0.00	2.70	40.00	1.08	0.00	0.00	130.00	260.00	0.00
3.00	1.50	0.00	0.00	0.00	0.00	0.00	0.00	0.00	0.00	0.00	0.00	0.00	60.00	1.08	0.00	0.00	100.00	520.00	0.00
0.50	0.50	0.00	0.00	0.00	0.00	0.00	0.30	0.14	4.00	0.30	0.00	1.50	80.00	2.70	0.00	0.00	440.00	370.00	6.75
0.00	0.50	0.00	0.00	0.00	0.00	0.00	0.30	0.14	4.00	0.30	0.00	1.50	80.00	2.70	0.00	0.00	430.00	370.00	7.50
0.00	0.50	0.00	0.00	0.00	0.00	0.00	0.30	0.14	4.00	0.30	0.00	1.20	80.00	2.70	0.00	0.00	450.00	370.00	6.75
0.50	1.00	0.00	0.00	0.00	0.00	0.00	1.80	0.14	2.00	0.30	0.00	3.60	0.00	1.44	0.00	0.00	60.00	340.00	0.00
0.00	0.00	0.00	0.00	0.00	0.00	0.00	0.45	0.14	3.00	0.30	0.00	1.80	20.00	1.80	0.00	0.00	100.00	260.00	0.00
0.50	2.00	0.00	0.00	0.00	0.00	0.00	1.80	0.10	2.00	0.20	0.00	1.50	0.00	1.80	0.00	0.00	110.00	270.00	0.00
0.50	1.50	0.00	0.00	0.00	60.04	0.00	0.00	0.00	0.00	0.00	0.00	0.00	40.00	0.72	0.00	0.00	180.00	350.00	0.00

USDA ID Code	Food Name	Weight in Grams*	Quantity of Units	Unit of Measure	Protein (gm)	Fat (gm)	Carbohydrate (gm)	Kcalories	Caffeine (gm)	Fiber (gm)	Cholesterol (mg)	Saturated Fat (gm)
607	Morningstar Farms- Pizza, Pepper	128.0000	1.000	Each	12.00	7.00	42.00	280.00	0.00	5.00	0.00	3.00
608	Morningstar Farms- Quarter Prime	96.0000	1.000	Each	24.00	2.00	6.00	140.00	0.00	3.00	0.00	0.00
609	Morningstar Farms- Scramblers	57.0000	0.250	Cup	6.00	0.00	2.00	35.00	0.00	0.00	0.00	0.00
610	Morningstar Farms- Strips, Break	16.0000	2.000	Each	2.00	4.50	2.00	60.00	0.00	1.00	0.00	0.50
611	Morningstar Farms- Veggie Dog	57.0000	1.000	Each	11.00	0.50	6.00	57.00	0.00	1.00	0.00	0.00
	Muffin, Banana Nut -Healthy Choi	70.8730	1.000	Each	3.00	6.00	32.00	180.00	0.00	0.00	0.00	0.00
	Muffin,English, Sandwich-Healthy	120.4840	1.000	Each	16.00	3.00	30.00	200.00	0.00	0.00	20.00	1.00
	Noodles and Chicken, Micro Cup-H	212.6200	1.000	Each	7.00	7.00	19.00	174.00	0.00	0.00	29.00	2.00
	Noodles Romanoff-Stouffer's	283.9200	1.000	Cup	17.03	25.04	36.05	440.66	0.00	0.00	40.06	0.00
614	Noodles, Kung Pao & Veg-Smart On	280.0000	10.000	Ounce	8.00	10.00	35.00	260.00	0.00	5.00	5.00	1.50
	Omelet, Turkey Sausage, on Engli	134.6590	1.000	Each	16.00	4.00	30.00	210.00	0.00	0.00	20.00	2.00
	Omelet, Western Style, on Englis	134.6590	1.000	Each	16.00	3.00	29.00	200.00	0.00	0.00	15.00	2.00
624	Pasta Accents, White Cheddar Sce	181.0000	1.750	Cup	9.00	9.00	37.00	270.00	0.00	3.00	10.00	2.50
625	Pasta Accents-Alfredo	160.0000	2.000	Cup	9.00	8.00	25.00	210.00	0.00	4.00	5.00	2.50
626	Pasta Accents-Crmy Cheddar	190.0000	2.330	Cup	9.00	8.00	36.00	250.00	0.00	5.00	15.00	3.00
627	Pasta Accents-Florentine	206.0000	2.000	Cup	13.00	9.00	44.00	310.00	0.00	5.00	20.00	3.00
628	Pasta Accents-Garden Herb	195.0000	2.000	Cup	9.00	7.00	32.00	230.00	0.00	7.00	15.00	4.00
629	Pasta Accents-Garlic Seasoning	188.0000	2.000	Cup	7.00	10.00	36.00	260.00	0.00	3.00	15.00	5.00
630	Pasta Accents-Lasagna Style	188.0000	2.000	Cup	9.00	10.00	33.00	260.00	0.00	4.00	10.00	3.00
631	Pasta Accents-Oriental Style	201.0000	2.500	Cup	8.00	10.00	35.00	260.00	0.00	4.00	20.00	4.00
632	Pasta Accents-Primavera	200.0000	2.250	Cup	12.00	9.00	39.00	290.00	0.00	4.00	5.00	2.50
	Pasta Accents-Primavera	175.0000	1.000	Serving	9.00	10.00	27.00	230.00	0.00	0.00	0.00	0.00
633	Pasta and Spinach Romano-Smart O	291.0000	10.400	Ounce	11.00	8.00	32.00	240.00	0.00	4.00	5.00	3.50
	Pasta Florentine-Stouffer's	283.9200	0.500	Cup	16.02	21.03	32.05	380.57	0.00	0.00	50.07	0.00
	Pasta Italiano, Vegetable-Health	283.4930	1.000	Each	7.00	1.00	46.00	220.00	0.00	0.00	0.00	0.00
	Pasta Italiano-Healthy Choice	340.1920	1.000	Each	16.00	5.00	59.00	350.00	0.00	0.00	30.00	2.00
	Pasta Roma-Stouffer's	283.9200	0.500	Cup	16.02	7.01	31.05	260.39	0.00	0.00	30.04	0.00
	Pasta Shells w/ Tomato Sauce-Hea	340.1920	1.000	Each	24.00	3.00	53.00	330.00	0.00	0.00	35.00	2.00
	Pasta Shells, Cheese w/ Sauce-St	262.2310	1.000	Each	17.00	13.00	28.00	300.00	0.00	0.00	0.00	0.00
	Pasta w/ Chicken, Cacciatore-Hea	354.3670	1.000	Each	26.00	3.00	47.00	310.00	0.00	0.00	35.00	0.00
	Pasta w/ Chicken, Teriyaki-Healt	357.9100	1.000	Each	24.00	3.00	58.00	350.00	0.00	0.00	45.00	1.00
634	Pasta w/ Tomato Basil Sauce-Smar	268.8000	9.600	Ounce	12.00	9.00	33.00	260.00	0.00	5.00	10.00	3.50
	Pasta, Angel Hair, Lean Cuisine-	283.4930	1.000	Each	10.00	5.00	38.00	240.00	0.00	0.00	10.00	1.00
635	Pasta, Bowtie & Mushroom Marsala	270.0000	9.650	Ounce	13.00	9.00	36.00	280.00	0.00	5.00	10.00	3.50
636	Pasta, Crmy Rigatoni w/ Brocc &	252.0000	9.000	Ounce	14.00	2.00	40.00	230.00	0.00	4.00	20.00	0.50
637	Pasta, Penne w/ Sun-dried Tomato	280.0000	10.000	Ounce	12.00	9.00	41.00	290.00	0.00	4.00	15.00	3.00
639	Penne Pollo-Smart Ones	280.0000	10.000	Ounce	22.00	5.00	40.00	290.00	0.00	3.00	35.00	2.00
640	Penne, Spicy, & Ricotta-Smart On	285.6000	10.200	Ounce	12.00	6.00	45.00	280.00	0.00	5.00	5.00	2.00
	Pepper, Stuffed, Single Serving-	283.4930	1.000	Each	10.00	8.00	28.00	220.00	0.00	0.00	0.00	0.00
	Peppers, Stuffed Green-Stouffer'	219.7070	1.000	Each	9.00	8.00	22.00	200.00	0.00	0.00	0.00	0.00
654	Pizza Combo, Deluxe-Smart Ones	184.0000	6.570	Ounce	23.00	11.00	47.00	380.00	0.00	6.00	40.00	3.50
	Pizza, Cheese, 4 - DiGiorno	139.0000	1.000	Slice	16.00	11.00	39.00	320.00	0.00	3.11	25.10	6.10
	Pizza, Cheese, Microwave for One	104.0000	1.000	Each	10.00	11.00	25.00	240.00	0.00	1.00	15.00	3.50
	Pizza, Cheese, Party - Totino's	277.0000	1.000	Slice	15.00	5.00	33.00	320.00	0.00	2.00	20.00	5.00
	Pizza, French Bread, Cheese-Heal	159.4650	1.000	Each	19.00	4.00	46.00	290.00	0.00	0.00	15.00	2.00
	Pizza, French Bread, Cheese-Stou	145.2900	1.000	Each	16.00	14.00	40.00	350.00	0.00	0.00	0.00	0.00
	Pizza, French Bread, Deluxe-Heal	180.7270	1.000	Each	23.00	7.00	41.00	330.00	0.00	0.00	35.00	3.00
	Pizza, French Bread, Deluxe-Stou	173.6390	1.000	Each	21.00	19.00	40.00	420.00	0.00	0.00	0.00	0.00
	Pizza, French Bread, Double Chee	166.5520	1.000	Each	22.00	18.00	43.00	420.00	0.00	0.00	0.00	0.00
	Pizza, French Bread, Hamburger-S	173.6390	1.000	Each	23.00	18.00	39.00	410.00	0.00	0.00	0.00	0.00
	Pizza, French Bread, Pepperoni-H	170.0960	1.000	Each	20.00	7.00	38.00	310.00	0.00	0.00	30.00	3.00
	Pizza, French Bread, Pepperoni-S	159.4650	1.000	Each	19.00	19.00	39.00	400.00	0.00	0.00	0.00	0.00
	Pizza, French Bread, Sausage-Sto	170.0960	1.000	Each	20.00	21.00	40.00	430.00	0.00	0.00	0.00	0.00
	Pizza, French Bread, Vegetable D	180.7270	1.000	Each	18.00	20.00	41.00	420.00	0.00	0.00	0.00	0.00
	Pizza, Meat, 3 - DiGiorno	154.0000	1.000	Slice	19.00	16.00	40.00	380.00	0.00	3.11	40.00	8.00

Monounsaturated Fat (gm)	Polyunsaturated Fat (gm)	Vitamin D (mg)	Vitamin K (mg)	Vitamin E (mg)	Vitamin A (re)	Vitamin C (mg)	Thiamin (mg)	Riboflavin (mg)	Niacin (mg)	Vitamin B_6 (mg)	Folate (mg)	Vitamin B_{12} (mcg)	Calcium (mg)	Iron (mg)	Magnesium (mg)	Phosphorus (mg)	Potassium (mg)	Sodium (mg)	Zinc (mg)
2.50	1.50	0.00	0.00	0.00	0.00	0.00	0.00	0.00	0.00	0.00	0.00	0.00	40.00	1.80	0.00	0.00	180.00	420.00	0.00
1.00	1.00	0.00	0.00	0.00	0.00	9.00	0.75	0.34	2.00	0.50	0.00	5.40	60.00	2.70	0.00	0.00	210.00	370.00	0.00
0.00	0.00	0.40	0.00	0.00	225.00	0.00	0.30	0.34	0.00	0.12	0.00	1.80	20.00	1.08	0.00	0.00	60.00	95.00	0.60
1.00	3.00	0.00	0.00	0.00	0.00	0.00	0.75	0.03	0.04	0.08	0.00	0.24	0.00	0.36	0.00	0.00	15.00	220.00	0.00
0.00	0.00	0.00	0.00	0.00	0.00	0.00	0.00	0.00	0.00	0.00	0.00	0.00	0.00	0.72	0.00	0.00	60.00	580.00	0.00
0.00	3.00	0.00	0.00	0.00	0.00	0.00	0.15	0.14	0.76	0.00	0.00	0.00	80.00	1.00	0.00	160.00	250.00	80.00	0.00
0.00	1.00	0.00	0.00	0.00	60.00	3.60	0.45	0.43	2.85	0.00	0.00	0.00	120.00	2.00	0.00	220.00	200.00	510.00	0.00
3.00	2.00	0.00	0.00	0.00	270.00	8.40	0.08	0.12	1.71	0.00	0.00	0.00	32.00	0.70	21.00	0.00	254.00	1009.00	0.75
0.00	0.00	0.00	0.00	0.00	0.00	0.00	0.00	0.01	0.19	0.00	0.00	0.00	1.60	0.20	0.00	0.00	260.39	1992.99	0.00
0.00	0.00	0.00	0.00	0.00	0.00	0.00	0.00	0.00	0.00	0.00	0.00	0.00	0.00	0.00	0.00	0.00	0.00	690.00	0.00
0.00	1.00	0.00	0.00	0.00	60.00	0.00	0.38	0.51	2.85	0.00	0.00	0.00	160.00	2.00	0.00	250.00	590.00	470.00	0.00
0.00	0.00	0.00	0.00	0.00	100.00	3.60	0.45	0.51	1.90	0.00	0.00	0.00	160.00	2.00	0.00	240.00	220.00	480.00	0.00
0.00	0.00	0.00	0.00	0.00	0.00	0.00	0.00	0.00	0.00	0.00	0.00	0.00	0.00	0.00	0.00	0.00	0.00	750.00	0.00
0.00	0.00	0.00	0.00	0.00	0.00	0.00	0.00	0.00	0.00	0.00	0.00	0.00	0.00	0.00	0.00	0.00	0.00	480.00	0.00
0.00	0.00	0.00	0.00	0.00	0.00	0.00	0.00	0.00	0.00	0.00	0.00	0.00	0.00	0.00	0.00	0.00	0.00	700.00	0.00
0.00	0.00	0.00	0.00	0.00	0.00	0.00	0.00	0.00	0.00	0.00	0.00	0.00	0.00	0.00	0.00	0.00	0.00	910.00	0.00
0.00	0.00	0.00	0.00	0.00	0.00	0.00	0.00	0.00	0.00	0.00	0.00	0.00	0.00	0.00	0.00	0.00	0.00	750.00	0.00
0.00	0.00	0.00	0.00	0.00	0.00	0.00	0.00	0.00	0.00	0.00	0.00	0.00	0.00	0.00	0.00	0.00	0.00	640.00	0.00
0.00	0.00	0.00	0.00	0.00	0.00	0.00	0.00	0.00	0.00	0.00	0.00	0.00	0.00	0.00	0.00	0.00	0.00	540.00	0.00
0.00	0.00	0.00	0.00	0.00	0.00	0.00	0.00	0.00	0.00	0.00	0.00	0.00	0.00	0.00	0.00	0.00	0.00	580.00	0.00
0.00	0.00	0.00	0.00	0.00	0.00	0.00	0.00	0.00	0.00	0.00	0.00	0.00	0.00	0.00	0.00	0.00	0.00	530.00	0.00
0.00	0.00	0.00	0.00	0.00	0.00	20.00	0.00	0.00	0.00	0.00	0.00	0.00	160.00	1.20	0.00	0.00	0.00	450.00	0.00
0.00	0.00	0.00	0.00	0.00	0.00	0.00	0.00	0.00	0.00	0.00	0.00	0.00	0.00	0.00	0.00	0.00	0.00	510.00	0.00
0.00	0.00	0.00	0.00	0.00	0.00	0.54	0.00	0.01	0.19	0.00	0.00	0.00	3.45	0.10	0.00	0.00	400.60	891.34	0.00
0.00	0.00	0.00	0.00	0.00	250.00	0.00	0.45	0.26	1.52	0.00	0.00	0.00	32.00	2.50	0.00	0.00	380.00	330.00	0.00
0.00	3.00	0.00	0.00	0.00	60.00	0.00	0.53	0.51	2.85	0.00	0.00	0.00	48.00	2.00	0.00	180.00	540.00	530.00	0.00
0.00	0.00	0.00	0.00	0.00	0.00	6.01	0.11	0.01	0.95	0.00	0.00	0.00	1.04	0.30	0.00	0.00	600.90	781.17	0.00
0.00	0.00	0.00	0.00	0.00	100.00	21.00	0.53	0.43	2.85	0.00	0.00	0.00	320.00	1.50	0.00	240.00	640.00	470.00	0.00
0.00	0.00	0.00	0.00	0.00	150.00	9.00	0.12	0.26	1.90	0.00	0.00	0.00	280.00	1.00	0.00	0.00	480.00	820.00	0.00
0.00	1.00	0.00	0.00	0.00	100.00	6.00	0.45	0.43	6.65	0.00	0.00	0.00	32.00	1.50	0.00	250.00	660.00	430.00	0.00
0.00	2.00	0.00	0.00	0.00	100.00	6.00	0.30	0.34	3.80	0.00	0.00	0.00	48.00	1.50	0.00	200.00	390.00	370.00	0.00
0.00	0.00	0.00	0.00	0.00	0.00	0.00	0.00	0.00	0.00	0.00	0.00	0.00	0.00	0.00	0.00	0.00	0.00	360.00	0.00
0.00	1.00	0.00	0.00	0.00	250.00	6.00	0.30	0.34	2.85	0.00	0.00	0.00	80.00	1.50	0.00	0.00	500.00	410.00	0.00
0.00	0.00	0.00	0.00	0.00	0.00	0.00	0.00	0.00	0.00	0.00	0.00	0.00	0.00	0.00	0.00	0.00	0.00	560.00	0.00
0.00	0.00	0.00	0.00	0.00	0.00	0.00	0.00	0.00	0.00	0.00	0.00	0.00	0.00	0.00	0.00	0.00	0.00	670.00	0.00
0.00	0.00	0.00	0.00	0.00	0.00	0.00	0.00	0.00	0.00	0.00	0.00	0.00	0.00	0.00	0.00	0.00	0.00	560.00	0.00
0.00	0.00	0.00	0.00	0.00	0.00	0.00	0.00	0.00	0.00	0.00	0.00	0.00	0.00	0.00	0.00	0.00	0.00	620.00	0.00
0.00	0.00	0.00	0.00	0.00	0.00	0.00	0.00	0.00	0.00	0.00	0.00	0.00	0.00	0.00	0.00	0.00	0.00	370.00	0.00
0.00	0.00	0.00	0.00	0.00	20.00	6.00	0.23	0.17	2.85	0.00	0.00	0.00	32.00	1.00	0.00	0.00	400.00	1010.00	0.00
0.00	0.00	0.00	0.00	0.00	60.00	6.00	0.12	0.14	2.85	0.00	0.00	0.00	32.00	0.80	0.00	0.00	380.00	650.00	0.00
0.00	0.00	0.00	0.00	0.00	0.00	0.00	0.00	0.00	0.00	0.00	0.00	0.00	0.00	0.00	0.00	0.00	0.00	550.00	0.00
0.00	1.00	0.00	0.00	0.00	138.30	0.00	0.50	0.30	3.00	0.00	0.00	0.00	350.00	0.90	0.00	200.00	330.00	870.00	0.00
0.00	1.00	0.00	0.00	0.00	0.00	0.00	0.00	0.00	0.00	0.00	0.00	0.00	220.00	1.50	0.00	180.00	290.00	530.00	0.00
0.00	1.00	0.00	0.00	0.00	0.00	0.00	0.00	0.00	0.00	0.00	0.00	0.00	300.00	1.50	0.00	200.00	330.00	630.00	0.00
0.00	1.00	0.00	0.00	0.00	20.00	0.00	0.45	0.26	2.85	0.00	0.00	0.00	240.00	2.00	0.00	240.00	310.00	390.00	0.00
0.00	0.00	0.00	0.00	0.00	60.00	3.60	0.45	0.34	2.85	0.00	0.00	0.00	200.00	1.50	0.00	0.00	300.00	630.00	0.00
0.00	1.00	0.00	0.00	0.00	80.00	0.00	0.45	0.34	3.80	0.00	0.00	0.00	200.00	2.50	0.00	280.00	350.00	500.00	0.00
0.00	0.00	0.00	0.00	0.00	100.00	6.00	0.45	0.43	3.80	0.00	0.00	0.00	160.00	1.50	0.00	0.00	350.00	950.00	0.00
0.00	0.00	0.00	0.00	0.00	40.00	6.00	0.45	0.51	3.80	0.00	0.00	0.00	360.00	1.50	0.00	0.00	320.00	850.00	0.00
0.00	0.00	0.00	0.00	0.00	60.00	6.00	0.38	0.34	3.80	0.00	0.00	0.00	160.00	1.50	0.00	0.00	340.00	650.00	0.00
0.00	1.00	0.00	0.00	0.00	150.00	0.00	0.53	0.34	3.80	0.00	0.00	0.00	160.00	2.50	0.00	240.00	350.00	470.00	0.00
0.00	0.00	0.00	0.00	0.00	100.00	6.00	0.53	0.43	3.80	0.00	0.00	0.00	160.00	1.50	0.00	0.00	300.00	880.00	0.00
0.00	0.00	0.00	0.00	0.00	80.00	6.00	0.60	0.43	3.80	0.00	0.00	0.00	160.00	1.50	0.00	0.00	340.00	840.00	0.00
0.00	0.00	0.00	0.00	0.00	250.00	3.60	0.45	0.43	3.80	0.00	0.00	0.00	280.00	1.50	0.00	0.00	230.00	830.00	0.00
0.00	1.00	0.00	0.00	0.00	138.30	0.00	0.50	0.30	3.00	0.00	0.00	0.00	330.00	1.00	0.00	200.00	330.00	1100.00	0.00

USDA ID Code	Food Name	Weight in Grams*	Quantity of Units	Unit of Measure	Protein (gm)	Fat (gm)	Carbohydrate (gm)	Kcalories	Caffeine (gm)	Fiber (gm)	Cholesterol (mg)	Saturated Fat (gm)
	Pizza, Pepperoni	154.0000	1.000	Slice	19.00	24.00	40.00	450.00	0.00	2.00	35.00	9.00
	Pizza, Pepperoni -Weight Watcher	157.6260	1.000	Each	23.00	12.00	46.00	390.00	0.00	4.00	45.00	4.00
	Pizza, Pepperoni, Microwave for	104.0000	1.000	Each	10.00	16.00	25.00	280.00	0.00	1.00	15.00	3.50
	Pizza, Pepperoni, Party - Totino	289.0000	1.000	Slice	14.00	21.00	33.00	380.00	0.00	2.00	20.00	5.00
	Pizza, Sausage & Pepperoni - Tom	132.0000	1.000	Slice	19.00	19.00	25.00	340.00	0.00	2.00	45.00	9.00
	Pizza, Sausage & Pepperoni, Supr	122.0000	1.000	Slice	13.00	20.00	28.00	340.00	0.00	2.00	25.00	7.00
	Pizza, Special Deluxe - Red Baro	129.0000	1.000	Slice	13.00	18.00	32.00	340.00	0.00	2.00	25.00	7.00
	Pizza, Supreme, Party - Totino's	309.0000	1.000	Slice	15.00	20.00	34.00	380.00	0.00	2.00	20.00	4.50
	Pizzas, French Bread, Bacon, Can	163.0080	1.000	Each	18.00	15.00	40.00	370.00	0.00	0.00	0.00	0.00
	Pot Pie, Beef -Swanson	198.4450	1.000	Pie	12.00	19.00	36.00	370.00	0.00	0.00	0.00	0.00
	Pot Pie, Beef-Stouffer's	283.4930	1.000	Each	18.00	27.00	37.00	460.00	0.00	0.00	0.00	0.00
	Pot Pie, Chicken -Swanson	198.4450	1.000	Each	11.00	22.00	35.00	380.00	0.00	0.00	0.00	0.00
	Pot Pie, Chicken-Stouffer's	283.4930	1.000	Each	16.00	27.00	32.00	440.00	0.00	0.00	0.00	0.00
	Pot Pie, Macaroni and Cheese -Sw	198.4450	1.000	Each	7.00	8.00	24.00	200.00	0.00	0.00	0.00	0.00
	Pot Pie, Turkey -Swanson	198.0000	1.000	Each	5.54	10.58	18.14	191.49	0.00	0.00	0.00	0.00
	Pot Pie, Turkey-Stouffer's	283.4930	1.000	Each	16.00	24.00	33.00	410.00	0.00	0.00	0.00	0.00
	Potato Casserole, Garden-Healthy	262.2310	1.000	Each	12.00	4.00	23.00	180.00	0.00	0.00	20.00	2.00
	Potato, Baked, Broccoli and Chee	283.5000	1.000	Each	12.00	7.00	34.00	230.00	0.00	6.00	10.00	2.00
	Potato, Baked, w/ Sour Cream, Le	294.1240	1.000	Each	9.00	5.00	38.00	230.00	0.00	0.00	15.00	2.00
672	Potato, Bkd, Broccoli & Chse -Sm	280.0000	10.000	Ounce	12.00	7.00	35.00	250.00	0.00	6.00	15.00	2.00
	Potatoes Au Gratin-Stouffer's	163.0080	1.000	Each	5.00	9.00	17.00	170.00	0.00	0.00	0.00	0.00
	Potatoes, Scalloped, and Ham, Mi	212.6200	1.000	Each	8.00	16.00	21.00	260.00	0.00	0.00	33.00	6.00
	Potatoes, Scalloped-Stouffer's	163.0080	1.000	Each	4.00	6.00	16.00	130.00	0.00	0.00	0.00	0.00
	Primavera, Chicken-Stouffer's	28.3500	1.000	Ounce	1.60	0.60	1.20	17.00	0.00	0.00	5.00	0.00
689	Ravioli Florentine-Smart Ones	238.0000	8.500	Ounce	9.00	2.00	43.00	220.00	0.00	4.00	5.00	0.50
	Ravioli, Baked Cheese, Lean Cuis	240.9690	1.000	Each	13.00	8.00	30.00	240.00	0.00	0.00	55.00	3.00
	Ravioli, Baked Cheese-Healthy Ch	255.1440	1.000	Each	14.00	2.00	44.00	250.00	0.00	0.00	20.00	1.00
	Ravioli, Beef	243.9350	1.000	Cup	9.00	5.00	35.99	229.94	0.00	4.00	19.99	2.50
	Ravioli, Beef, Micro Cup-Hormel	212.6200	1.000	Each	9.00	11.00	34.00	270.00	0.00	0.00	20.00	4.00
	Ravioli, Cheese	243.9350	1.000	Cup	9.00	3.00	37.99	219.94	0.00	4.00	15.00	1.50
	Ravioli, Cheese-Stouffer's	28.3500	1.000	Ounce	2.80	1.90	6.40	54.00	0.00	0.00	14.00	0.00
	Rice, Confetti-Stouffer's	28.3500	1.000	Ounce	0.50	0.30	4.80	24.00	0.00	0.00	1.00	0.00
692	Rice, Hunan & Vegetables-Smart O	289.5000	10.340	Ounce	7.00	7.00	39.00	250.00	0.00	8.00	5.00	2.00
694	Rice, Sante Fe and Beans-Smart O	280.0000	10.000	Ounce	12.00	9.00	41.00	290.00	0.00	10.00	5.00	4.00
	Rice, Wild - Rice-a-Roni	56.0000	1.000	Cup	5.00	1.00	43.00	240.00	0.00	1.00	0.00	0.00
	Rigatoni Bake, Lean Cuisine-Stou	276.4060	1.000	Each	18.00	8.00	27.00	250.00	0.00	0.00	25.00	3.00
	Rigatoni in Meat Sauce-Healthy C	269.3190	1.000	Each	16.00	6.00	34.00	260.00	0.00	0.00	30.00	2.00
	Rigatoni w/ Meat Sauce-Stouffer'	283.9200	0.500	Cup	16.02	11.02	31.05	290.44	0.00	0.00	30.04	0.00
695	Risotto w/Cheese & Mushrooms-Sma	280.0000	10.000	Ounce	11.00	8.00	44.00	290.00	0.00	4.00	20.00	4.00
	Sauce, Cheddar Cheese-Stouffer's	283.9200	1.000	Cup	26.04	60.09	22.03	731.10	0.00	0.00	130.20	0.00
	Sauce, Marinara-Stouffer's	283.9200	1.000	Cup	3.00	11.02	18.03	180.27	0.00	0.00	0.00	0.00
	Sauce, Newburg, Supreme-Stouffer	283.9200	1.000	Cup	7.01	41.06	20.03	480.72	0.00	0.00	120.18	0.00
	Sauce, Pesto-Stouffer's	283.9200	0.250	Cup	35.05	61.09	21.03	771.16	0.00	0.00	70.11	0.00
	Sauce, Veloute, Supreme-Stouffer	307.5800	1.000	Cup	8.68	49.91	20.61	564.18	0.00	0.00	97.65	0.00
	Shells, Cheese Stuffed-Stouffer'	28.3500	1.000	Ounce	1.50	0.90	3.40	28.00	0.00	0.00	3.00	0.00
	Shrimp Marinara-Healthy Choice	297.6680	1.000	Each	10.00	1.00	51.00	260.00	0.00	0.00	60.00	0.00
697	Shrimp Marinara-Smart Ones	252.0000	9.000	Ounce	9.00	2.00	35.00	190.00	0.00	4.00	40.00	0.50
	Shrimp Marinara-Weight Watchers	255.1500	1.000	Each	9.00	2.00	35.00	190.00	0.00	4.00	40.00	0.50
717	Spaghetti Marinara-Smart Ones	252.0000	9.000	Ounce	9.00	7.00	46.00	280.00	0.00	5.00	5.00	1.50
	Spaghetti w/ Meat Sauce, Lean Cu	326.0170	1.000	Each	15.00	6.00	45.00	290.00	0.00	0.00	20.00	2.00
	Spaghetti w/ Meat Sauce, Top She	283.4930	1.000	Each	14.00	6.00	37.00	260.00	0.00	0.00	20.00	2.00
	Spaghetti w/ Meat Sauce-Healthy	283.4930	1.000	Each	14.00	6.00	42.00	280.00	0.00	0.00	20.00	2.00
718	Spaghetti w/ Meat Sauce-Smart On	280.0000	10.000	Ounce	17.00	6.00	41.00	290.00	0.00	4.00	15.00	2.00
	Spaghetti w/ Meat Sauce-Stouffer	364.9980	1.000	Each	16.00	12.00	38.00	320.00	0.00	0.00	0.00	0.00
	Spaghetti w/ Meatballs, Micro Cu	212.6200	1.000	Each	10.00	7.00	27.00	210.00	0.00	0.00	20.00	3.00

Monounsaturated Fat (gm)	Polyunsaturated Fat (gm)	Vitamin D (mg)	Vitamin K (mg)	Vitamin E (mg)	Vitamin A (re)	Vitamin C (mg)	Thiamin (mg)	Riboflavin (mg)	Niacin (mg)	Vitamin B_6 (mg)	Folate (mg)	Vitamin B_{12} (mcg)	Calcium (mg)	Iron (mg)	Magnesium (mg)	Phosphorus (mg)	Potassium (mg)	Sodium (mg)	Zinc (mg)
0.00	1.00	0.00	0.00	0.00	90.00	0.00	0.00	0.00	0.00	0.00	0.00	0.00	330.00	1.90	0.00	200.00	330.00	920.00	0.00
0.00	0.00	0.00	0.00	0.00	80.00	4.80	0.00	0.00	0.00	0.00	0.00	0.00	540.00	1.00	0.00	0.00	320.00	650.00	0.00
0.00	1.00	0.00	0.00	0.00	0.00	0.00	0.00	0.00	0.00	0.00	0.00	0.00	200.00	1.50	0.00	180.00	290.00	710.00	0.00
0.00	1.00	0.00	0.00	0.00	0.00	0.00	0.00	0.00	0.00	0.00	0.00	0.00	280.00	1.50	0.00	200.00	330.00	920.00	0.00
0.00	1.00	0.00	0.00	0.00	150.00	1.20	0.00	0.00	0.00	0.00	0.00	0.00	350.00	0.90	0.00	200.00	330.00	820.00	0.00
0.00	1.00	0.00	0.00	0.00	40.00	2.40	0.00	0.00	0.00	0.00	0.00	0.00	200.00	1.50	0.00	200.00	330.00	610.00	0.00
0.00	1.00	0.00	0.00	0.00	78.00	0.00	0.00	0.00	0.00	0.00	0.00	0.00	220.00	2.70	0.00	200.00	330.00	690.00	0.00
0.00	1.00	0.00	0.00	0.00	0.00	0.00	0.00	0.00	0.00	0.00	0.00	0.00	280.00	1.50	0.00	200.00	330.00	890.00	0.00
0.00	0.00	0.00	0.00	0.00	80.00	6.00	0.60	0.43	3.80	0.00	0.00	0.00	160.00	1.00	0.00	0.00	300.00	1070.00	0.00
0.00	0.00	0.00	0.00	0.00	250.00	0.00	0.23	0.17	2.85	0.00	0.00	0.00	16.00	1.50	0.00	0.00	0.00	730.00	0.00
0.00	0.00	0.00	0.00	0.00	700.00	2.40	0.30	0.43	3.80	0.00	0.00	0.00	32.00	1.50	0.00	0.00	300.00	1130.00	0.00
0.00	0.00	0.00	0.00	0.00	400.00	0.00	0.23	0.17	2.85	0.00	0.00	0.00	16.00	1.00	0.00	0.00	0.00	760.00	0.00
0.00	0.00	0.00	0.00	0.00	500.00	1.20	0.30	0.43	4.75	0.00	0.00	0.00	80.00	1.00	0.00	0.00	320.00	750.00	0.00
0.00	0.00	0.00	0.00	0.00	80.00	0.00	0.09	0.17	0.76	0.00	0.00	0.00	120.00	0.60	0.00	0.00	0.00	740.00	0.00
0.00	0.00	0.00	0.00	0.00	176.37	0.00	0.11	0.09	1.44	0.00	0.00	0.00	8.06	0.50	0.00	0.00	0.00	362.82	0.00
0.00	0.00	0.00	0.00	0.00	250.00	0.00	0.30	0.43	3.80	0.00	0.00	0.00	80.00	1.00	0.00	0.00	290.00	750.00	0.00
0.00	0.00	0.00	0.00	0.00	0.00	0.00	0.00	0.00	0.00	0.00	0.00	0.00	0.00	0.00	0.00	0.00	600.00	360.00	0.00
0.00	0.00	0.00	0.00	0.00	200.00	9.00	0.00	0.00	0.00	0.00	0.00	0.00	300.00	0.80	0.00	0.00	830.00	510.00	0.00
0.00	0.00	0.00	0.00	0.00	350.00	30.00	0.23	0.26	1.14	0.00	0.00	0.00	160.00	0.60	0.00	0.00	900.00	570.00	0.00
0.00	0.00	0.00	0.00	0.00	0.00	0.00	0.00	0.00	0.00	0.00	0.00	0.00	0.00	0.00	0.00	0.00	0.00	590.00	0.00
0.00	0.00	0.00	0.00	0.00	20.00	3.60	0.00	0.10	0.76	0.00	0.00	0.00	48.00	0.80	0.00	0.00	260.00	670.00	0.00
8.00	2.00	0.00	0.00	0.39	0.00	11.40	0.09	0.10	2.09	0.00	0.00	0.00	32.00	0.40	21.00	0.00	425.00	768.00	0.90
0.00	0.00	0.00	0.00	0.00	0.00	2.40	0.03	0.14	0.76	0.00	0.00	0.00	80.00	0.20	0.00	0.00	375.00	610.00	0.00
0.00	0.00	0.00	0.00	0.00	0.00	1.20	0.00	0.00	0.06	0.00	0.00	0.00	48.00	0.01	0.00	0.00	40.00	119.00	0.00
0.00	0.00	0.00	0.00	0.00	0.00	0.00	0.00	0.00	0.00	0.00	0.00	0.00	0.00	0.00	0.00	0.00	0.00	490.00	0.00
0.00	0.00	0.00	0.00	0.00	60.00	36.00	0.06	0.26	1.14	0.00	0.00	0.00	160.00	0.80	0.00	0.00	380.00	590.00	0.00
0.00	0.00	0.00	0.00	0.00	500.00	4.80	0.30	0.26	1.90	0.00	0.00	0.00	200.00	1.50	0.00	240.00	590.00	420.00	0.00
0.00	0.00	0.00	0.00	0.00	149.96	2.40	0.00	0.00	0.00	0.00	0.00	0.00	0.00	1.50	0.00	0.00	0.00	1149.69	0.00
5.00	1.00	0.00	0.00	0.50	100.00	11.40	0.15	0.27	2.47	0.00	0.00	0.00	48.00	0.90	28.00	0.00	359.00	920.00	1.05
0.00	0.00	0.00	0.00	0.00	59.98	1.20	0.00	0.00	0.00	0.00	0.00	0.00	23.99	1.50	0.00	0.00	0.00	1279.66	0.00
0.00	0.00	0.00	0.00	0.00	0.00	0.00	0.00	0.00	0.02	0.00	0.00	0.00	336.01	0.01	0.00	0.00	16.00	52.00	0.00
0.00	0.00	0.00	0.00	0.00	0.00	0.00	0.00	0.00	0.04	0.00	0.00	0.00	24.00	0.00	0.00	0.00	14.00	136.00	0.00
0.00	0.00	0.00	0.00	0.00	0.00	0.00	0.00	0.00	0.00	0.00	0.00	0.00	0.00	0.00	0.00	0.00	0.00	630.00	0.00
0.00	0.00	0.00	0.00	0.00	0.00	0.00	0.00	0.00	0.00	0.00	0.00	0.00	0.00	0.00	0.00	0.00	0.00	670.00	0.00
0.00	0.00	0.00	0.00	0.00	80.00	6.00	0.15	0.10	1.52	0.00	0.00	0.00	48.00	0.80	0.00	0.00	0.00	1110.00	0.00
0.00	1.00	0.00	0.00	0.00	200.00	6.00	0.23	0.34	3.80	0.00	0.00	0.00	160.00	1.50	0.00	0.00	620.00	430.00	0.00
0.00	0.00	0.00	0.00	0.00	200.00	2.40	0.30	0.26	2.85	0.00	0.00	0.00	120.00	1.50	0.00	200.00	700.00	540.00	0.00
0.00	0.00	0.00	0.00	0.00	0.00	48.07	0.00	0.01	0.76	0.00	0.00	0.00	2.08	0.30	0.00	0.00	620.93	851.28	0.00
0.00	0.00	0.00	0.00	0.00	0.00	0.00	0.00	0.00	0.00	0.00	0.00	0.00	0.00	0.00	0.00	0.00	0.00	540.00	0.00
0.00	0.00	0.00	0.00	0.00	0.00	0.00	0.00	0.01	0.00	0.00	0.00	0.00	6.33	0.10	0.00	0.00	340.51	1392.09	0.00
0.00	0.00	0.00	0.00	0.00	0.00	66.10	0.00	0.00	0.38	0.00	0.00	0.00	0.00	0.20	0.00	0.00	681.02	1221.83	0.00
0.00	0.00	0.00	0.00	0.00	0.00	0.00	0.00	0.01	0.00	0.00	0.00	0.00	1.84	0.00	0.00	0.00	370.56	1051.58	0.00
0.00	0.00	0.00	0.00	0.00	0.00	12.02	0.00	0.02	0.38	0.00	0.00	0.00	5.69	0.30	0.00	0.00	620.93	1362.04	0.00
0.00	0.00	0.00	0.00	0.00	0.00	0.00	0.00	0.01	0.00	0.00	0.00	0.00	2.26	0.00	0.00	0.00	368.89	1410.45	0.00
0.00	0.00	0.00	0.00	0.00	0.00	0.60	0.00	0.00	0.06	0.00	0.00	0.00	248.01	0.02	0.00	0.00	53.00	59.00	0.00
0.00	0.00	0.00	0.00	0.00	100.00	114.00	0.23	0.14	1.14	0.00	0.00	0.00	48.00	1.50	0.00	130.00	390.00	320.00	0.00
0.00	0.00	0.00	0.00	0.00	0.00	0.00	0.00	0.00	0.00	0.00	0.00	0.00	0.00	0.00	0.00	0.00	0.00	470.00	0.00
0.00	0.00	0.00	0.00	0.00	150.00	6.00	0.00	0.00	0.00	0.00	0.00	0.00	120.00	1.00	0.00	0.00	440.00	400.00	0.00
0.00	0.00	0.00	0.00	0.00	0.00	0.00	0.00	0.00	0.00	0.00	0.00	0.00	0.00	0.00	0.00	0.00	0.00	690.00	0.00
0.00	2.00	0.00	0.00	0.00	100.00	6.00	0.30	0.34	3.80	0.00	0.00	0.00	48.00	2.00	0.00	0.00	500.00	500.00	0.00
2.00	1.00	0.00	0.00	0.11	100.00	2.40	0.23	0.26	3.80	0.00	0.00	0.00	48.00	1.50	45.50	0.00	879.00	980.00	2.40
0.00	2.00	0.00	0.00	0.00	250.00	4.80	0.38	0.26	1.90	0.00	0.00	0.00	48.00	2.00	0.00	160.00	540.00	480.00	0.00
0.00	0.00	0.00	0.00	0.00	0.00	0.00	0.00	0.00	0.00	0.00	0.00	0.00	0.00	0.00	0.00	0.00	0.00	560.00	0.00
0.00	12.00	0.00	0.00	0.00	150.00	6.00	0.15	0.17	3.80	0.00	0.00	0.00	80.00	1.50	0.00	0.00	800.00	560.00	0.00
3.00	1.00	0.00	0.00	0.00	140.00	3.60	0.12	0.26	2.28	0.00	0.00	0.00	32.00	1.10	24.50	0.00	341.00	930.00	1.05

USDA ID Code	Food Name	Weight in Grams*	Quantity of Units	Unit of Measure	Protein (gm)	Fat (gm)	Carbohydrate (gm)	Kcalories	Caffeine (gm)	Fiber (gm)	Cholesterol (mg)	Saturated Fat (gm)
	Spaghetti w/ Meatballs-Stouffer'	276.4060	1.000	Each	14.00	9.00	37.00	290.00	0.00	0.00	0.00	0.00
	Spinach Souffle-Stouffer's	170.0960	1.000	Each	9.00	15.00	11.00	220.00	0.00	0.00	0.00	0.00
	Spinach, Creamed-Stouffer's	127.5720	1.000	Each	4.00	16.00	8.00	190.00	0.00	0.00	0.00	0.00
	Steak, Green Pepper, w/ Rice-Sto	297.6680	1.000	Each	20.00	10.00	35.00	310.00	0.00	0.00	0.00	0.00
	Steak, Green Pepper-Stouffer's	28.3500	1.000	Ounce	2.60	1.40	1.30	28.00	0.00	0.00	7.00	0.00
728	Steak, Pepper-Smart Ones	280.0000	10.000	Ounce	18.00	4.50	33.00	240.00	0.00	4.00	35.00	1.50
	Steak, Salisbury, Grilled -Weigh	240.9750	1.000	Each	19.00	9.00	24.00	250.00	0.00	4.00	30.00	3.00
	Steak, Salisbury, Top Shelf-Horm	283.4930	1.000	Each	25.00	15.00	22.00	320.00	0.00	0.00	70.00	7.00
	Steak, Salisbury, w/ Mushroom Gr	311.8430	1.000	Each	21.00	6.00	35.00	280.00	0.00	0.00	55.00	3.00
	Stew, Beef, Dinty Moore -Hormel	253.1620	1.000	Cup	12.28	14.51	17.86	245.58	0.00	0.00	33.49	6.70
	Stew, Chicken, Dinty Moore -Horm	253.1620	1.000	Cup	13.10	21.43	17.86	309.58	0.00	0.00	95.25	4.76
	Stew, Meatball, Dinty Moore -Hor	253.1620	1.000	Cup	12.28	17.86	15.63	267.90	0.00	0.00	33.49	7.81
	Stew, Vegetable, Dinty Moore -Ho	253.1620	1.000	Cup	5.58	6.70	22.33	173.02	0.00	0.00	15.63	2.23
	Stuff'n, Old-Fashion-Stouffer's	283.9200	0.500	Cup	11.02	37.06	61.09	620.93	0.00	0.00	10.02	0.00
	Sweet Potatoes, Whipped-Stouffer	283.9200	0.500	Cup	3.00	18.03	60.09	410.61	0.00	0.00	60.09	0.00
	Taco Shells, Chi-Chi's-Hormel	20.0000	1.000	Each	1.41	4.94	11.99	98.77	0.00	0.00	0.00	0.00
	Tetrazzini, Turkey-Healthy Choic	357.9100	1.000	Each	23.00	6.00	49.00	340.00	0.00	0.00	40.00	3.00
	Tetrazzini, Turkey-Stouffer's	283.4930	1.000	Each	22.00	23.00	26.00	400.00	0.00	0.00	0.00	0.00
	Tortellini w/ Egg Pasta, Cheese-	145.2900	1.000	Each	11.29	8.47	22.22	211.64	0.00	0.00	63.49	0.00
	Tortellini w/ Egg Pasta, Chicken	28.3500	1.000	Ounce	3.10	1.50	6.20	51.00	0.00	0.00	20.00	0.00
	Tortellini w/ Spinach Pasta, Che	28.3500	1.000	Ounce	3.00	2.40	5.70	56.00	0.00	0.00	19.00	0.00
	Tortellini, Beef	257.8940	1.000	Cup	5.00	1.00	45.98	229.91	0.00	9.00	14.99	0.00
	Tortellini, Cheese in Alfredo Sa	251.6000	1.000	Each	26.00	37.00	35.00	580.00	0.00	0.00	0.00	0.00
	Tortellini, Cheese w/ Tomato Sau	262.2310	1.000	Each	18.00	15.00	39.00	360.00	0.00	0.00	0.00	0.00
747	Tuna Noodle Casserole-Smart Ones	266.0000	9.500	Ounce	13.00	7.00	39.00	270.00	0.00	4.00	40.00	3.50
	Tuna Noodle Casserole-Stouffer's	283.4930	1.000	Each	17.00	15.00	33.00	280.00	0.00	0.00	0.00	0.00
	Turkey and Gravy-Stouffer's	255.0000	1.000	Each	11.99	2.47	2.12	77.60	0.00	0.00	23.28	0.00
	Turkey Breast, Sliced, w/ Gravy	283.4930	1.000	Each	27.00	4.00	30.00	270.00	0.00	0.00	50.00	2.00
	Turkey Breast, Sliced, w/ Gravy-	340.1920	1.000	Each	19.00	3.00	46.00	290.00	0.00	0.00	20.00	1.00
748	Turkey Breast, Stuffed-Smart One	280.0000	10.000	Ounce	13.00	7.00	37.00	260.00	0.00	5.00	20.00	2.00
	Turkey Dijon, Lean Cuisine-Stouf	269.3190	1.000	Each	20.00	6.00	20.00	210.00	0.00	0.00	45.00	2.00
	Turkey Dijonnaise-Stouffer's	260.0000	1.000	Each	8.47	5.29	7.05	112.88	0.00	0.00	28.22	0.00
	Turkey Medallions, Roast -Weight	240.9750	1.000	Each	10.00	2.00	34.00	190.00	0.00	4.00	20.00	0.50
750	Turkey Medallions, Rst, /Mush-Sm	238.0000	8.500	Ounce	10.00	2.00	32.00	190.00	0.00	2.00	20.00	0.50
	Turkey, Breast of -Healthy Choic	297.6680	1.000	Each	21.00	5.00	39.00	290.00	0.00	0.00	45.00	2.00
	Turkey, Homestyle w/ Vegetables-	269.3190	1.000	Each	26.00	2.00	34.00	260.00	0.00	0.00	30.00	0.00
	Turkey, Roasted, and Mushrooms i	240.9690	1.000	Each	18.00	3.00	26.00	200.00	0.00	0.00	40.00	1.00
	Turkey, Sliced, w/ Dressing, Lea	223.2510	1.000	Each	16.00	5.00	23.00	200.00	0.00	0.00	25.00	1.00
	Vegetables, Italian Style-Stouff	28.3500	1.000	Ounce	0.30	0.30	1.60	10.00	0.00	0.00	0.00	0.00
	Welsh Rarebit-Stouffer's	141.7460	1.000	Each	13.00	20.00	9.00	270.00	0.00	0.00	0.00	0.00
791	Worthington- Beef, Smoked, Meatl	57.0000	6.000	Slices	11.00	6.00	6.00	120.00	0.00	3.00	0.00	1.00
792	Worthington- Bolono	57.0000	3.000	Slices	10.00	3.50	2.00	80.00	0.00	2.00	0.00	1.00
793	Worthington- Burger, Vegetarian	55.0000	0.250	Cup	9.00	2.00	2.00	60.00	0.00	1.00	0.00	0.00
795	Worthington- Chicken Roll, Meatl	55.0000	1.000	Slice	9.00	4.50	1.00	80.00	0.00	1.00	0.00	1.00
796	Worthington- Chicken Slices, Mea	57.0000	2.000	Slices	9.00	4.50	1.00	80.00	0.00	1.00	0.00	1.00
797	Worthington- Chicken, Diced, Mea	55.0000	0.250	Cup	10.00	0.00	2.00	50.00	0.00	1.00	0.00	0.00
794	Worthington- Chic-Ketts	55.0000	2.000	Slices	13.00	7.00	2.00	120.00	0.00	2.00	0.00	1.00
798	Worthington- Chik Patties, Crisp	71.0000	1.000	Each	8.00	6.00	15.00	150.00	0.00	2.00	0.00	1.00
799	Worthington- Chik Stiks	47.0000	1.000	Each	9.00	7.00	3.00	110.00	0.00	2.00	0.00	1.00
800	Worthington- Chik, Diced	55.0000	0.250	Cup	7.00	0.00	1.00	40.00	0.00	1.00	0.00	0.00
801	Worthington- Chik, Sliced	90.0000	3.000	Slices	14.00	0.50	2.00	70.00	0.00	2.00	0.00	0.00
802	Worthington- Chili	230.0000	1.000	Cup	19.00	15.00	21.00	290.00	0.00	9.00	0.00	2.50
803	Worthington- Chili, Low Fat	230.0000	1.000	Cup	18.00	1.00	21.00	170.00	0.00	11.00	0.00	0.00
804	Worthington- Choplets	92.0000	2.000	Slices	17.00	1.50	3.00	90.00	0.00	2.00	0.00	1.00
805	Worthington- Choplets, Multigrai	92.0000	2.000	Slices	15.00	2.00	5.00	100.00	0.00	4.00	0.00	0.50

Monounsaturated Fat (gm)	Polyunsaturated Fat (gm)	Vitamin D (mg)	Vitamin K (mg)	Vitamin E (mg)	Vitamin A (re)	Vitamin C (mg)	Thiamin (mg)	Riboflavin (mg)	Niacin (mg)	Vitamin B_6 (mg)	Folate (mg)	Vitamin B_{12} (mcg)	Calcium (mg)	Iron (mg)	Magnesium (mg)	Phosphorus (mg)	Potassium (mg)	Sodium (mg)	Zinc (mg)
0.00	0.00	0.00	0.00	0.00	100.00	6.00	0.30	0.26	3.80	0.00	0.00	0.00	64.00	1.50	0.00	0.00	550.00	790.00	0.00
0.00	0.00	0.00	0.00	0.00	200.00	6.00	0.12	0.34	0.38	0.00	0.00	0.00	120.00	0.40	0.00	0.00	345.00	820.00	0.00
0.00	0.00	0.00	0.00	0.00	400.00	6.00	0.03	0.17	0.00	0.00	0.00	0.00	80.00	0.40	0.00	0.00	400.00	400.00	0.00
0.00	0.00	0.00	0.00	0.00	40.00	6.00	0.15	0.17	3.80	0.00	0.00	0.00	16.00	1.00	0.00	0.00	410.00	700.00	0.00
0.00	0.00	0.00	0.00	0.00	0.00	3.60	0.00	0.00	0.10	0.00	0.00	0.00	48.00	0.02	0.00	0.00	51.00	164.00	0.00
0.00	0.00	0.00	0.00	0.00	0.00	0.00	0.00	0.00	0.00	0.00	0.00	0.00	0.00	0.00	0.00	0.00	0.00	690.00	0.00
0.00	0.00	0.00	0.00	0.00	60.00	0.00	0.00	0.00	0.00	0.00	0.00	0.00	120.00	1.50	0.00	0.00	450.00	590.00	0.00
8.00	1.00	0.00	0.00	0.03	0.00	3.60	0.03	0.26	4.75	0.00	0.00	0.00	16.00	1.50	35.00	0.00	801.00	910.00	5.70
0.00	0.00	0.00	0.00	0.00	0.00	0.00	0.00	0.00	0.00	0.00	0.00	0.00	0.00	0.00	0.00	260.00	630.00	500.00	0.00
5.58	1.12	0.00	0.00	0.00	814.87	2.68	0.03	0.13	2.55	0.00	0.00	0.00	26.79	1.00	23.44	0.00	588.27	971.15	2.85
7.14	8.33	0.00	0.00	0.00	476.27	2.14	0.05	0.28	3.62	0.00	0.00	0.00	38.10	0.71	25.00	0.00	609.63	1012.08	1.25
7.81	1.12	0.00	0.00	2.59	279.06	1.34	0.07	0.15	3.18	0.00	0.00	0.00	26.79	1.23	27.35	0.00	586.04	1093.93	2.68
1.12	2.23	0.00	0.00	0.60	714.41	2.01	0.08	0.09	1.70	0.00	0.00	0.00	35.72	0.67	31.26	0.00	509.01	948.82	0.84
0.00	0.00	0.00	0.00	0.00	0.00	0.84	0.01	0.01	0.74	0.00	0.00	0.00	0.00	0.33	0.00	0.00	200.30	1121.68	0.00
0.00	0.00	0.00	0.00	0.00	0.00	0.00	0.00	0.00	0.19	0.00	0.00	0.00	0.00	0.10	0.00	0.00	400.60	1111.67	0.00
0.00	0.00	0.00	0.00	0.09	0.00	0.00	0.06	0.07	0.54	0.00	0.00	0.00	0.00	0.14	0.00	0.00	0.00	3.53	0.00
0.00	2.00	0.00	0.00	0.00	0.00	72.00	0.23	0.34	3.80	0.00	0.00	0.00	80.00	1.00	0.00	250.00	510.00	490.00	0.00
0.00	0.00	0.00	0.00	0.00	20.00	0.00	0.15	0.43	2.85	0.00	0.00	0.00	80.00	0.80	0.00	0.00	300.00	960.00	0.00
0.00	0.00	0.00	0.00	0.00	0.00	0.00	0.00	0.00	0.20	0.00	0.00	0.00	1.52	0.07	0.00	0.00	70.55	271.61	0.00
0.00	0.00	0.00	0.00	0.00	0.00	0.00	0.00	0.00	0.13	0.00	0.00	0.00	72.00	0.03	0.00	0.00	31.00	57.00	0.00
0.00	0.00	0.00	0.00	0.00	0.00	0.00	0.00	0.00	0.06	0.00	0.00	0.00	0.00	0.02	0.00	0.00	26.00	79.00	0.00
0.00	0.00	0.00	0.00	0.00	149.94	3.60	0.00	0.00	0.00	0.00	0.00	0.00	95.96	1.50	0.00	0.00	0.00	769.68	0.00
0.00	0.00	0.00	0.00	0.00	40.00	3.60	0.30	0.51	1.90	0.00	0.00	0.00	320.00	0.80	0.00	0.00	270.00	830.00	0.00
0.00	0.00	0.00	0.00	0.00	150.00	6.00	0.23	0.34	1.90	0.00	0.00	0.00	240.00	1.00	0.00	0.00	420.00	720.00	0.00
0.00	0.00	0.00	0.00	0.00	0.00	0.00	0.00	0.00	0.00	0.00	0.00	0.00	0.00	0.00	0.00	0.00	0.00	670.00	0.00
0.00	0.00	0.00	0.00	0.00	20.00	0.00	0.15	0.34	3.80	0.00	0.00	0.00	120.00	0.60	0.00	0.00	380.00	1090.00	0.00
0.00	0.00	0.00	0.00	0.00	0.00	0.42	0.00	0.00	0.87	0.00	0.00	0.00	84.66	0.03	0.00	0.00	405.65	296.30	0.00
0.00	1.00	0.00	0.00	0.00	150.00	0.00	0.30	0.34	7.60	0.00	0.00	0.00	48.00	1.00	0.00	310.00	590.00	530.00	0.00
0.00	1.00	0.00	0.00	0.00	150.00	27.00	0.15	0.10	1.52	0.00	0.00	0.00	16.00	0.60	0.00	0.00	360.00	520.00	0.00
0.00	0.00	0.00	0.00	0.00	0.00	0.00	0.00	0.00	0.00	0.00	0.00	0.00	0.00	0.00	0.00	0.00	0.00	680.00	0.00
0.00	0.00	0.00	0.00	0.00	400.00	2.40	0.23	0.34	4.75	0.00	0.00	0.00	120.00	0.40	0.00	0.00	640.00	590.00	0.00
0.00	0.00	0.00	0.00	0.00	0.00	0.63	0.00	0.00	0.27	0.00	0.00	0.00	0.00	0.07	0.00	0.00	176.37	356.27	0.00
0.00	0.00	0.00	0.00	0.00	100.00	4.80	0.00	0.00	0.00	0.00	0.00	0.00	24.00	1.00	0.00	0.00	220.00	530.00	0.00
0.00	0.00	0.00	0.00	0.00	0.00	0.00	0.00	0.00	0.00	0.00	0.00	0.00	0.00	0.00	0.00	0.00	0.00	530.00	0.00
0.00	0.00	0.00	0.00	0.00	40.00	48.00	0.45	0.26	5.70	0.00	0.00	0.00	32.00	1.00	0.00	270.00	540.00	420.00	0.00
0.00	0.00	0.00	0.00	0.00	100.00	4.80	0.03	0.07	0.00	0.00	0.00	0.00	32.00	0.00	0.00	0.00	100.00	550.00	0.00
0.00	1.00	0.00	0.00	0.00	200.00	0.00	0.12	0.14	2.85	0.00	0.00	0.00	16.00	0.80	0.00	150.00	260.00	380.00	0.00
0.00	2.00	0.00	0.00	0.00	500.00	6.00	0.23	0.26	4.75	0.00	0.00	0.00	32.00	0.80	0.00	0.00	400.00	590.00	0.00
0.00	0.00	0.00	0.00	0.00	0.00	1.80	0.00	0.00	0.02	0.00	0.00	0.00	72.00	0.01	0.00	0.00	62.00	147.00	0.00
0.00	0.00	0.00	0.00	0.00	40.00	0.00	0.03	0.34	0.00	0.00	0.00	0.00	280.00	0.20	0.00	0.00	140.00	460.00	0.00
2.50	2.50	0.00	0.00	0.00	0.00	0.00	1.80	0.14	3.00	0.30	0.00	1.80	0.00	1.08	0.00	0.00	150.00	730.00	0.00
1.00	1.50	0.00	0.00	0.00	0.00	0.00	0.60	0.14	0.40	0.40	0.00	0.90	40.00	1.80	0.00	0.00	120.00	720.00	0.00
0.50	1.00	0.00	0.00	0.00	0.00	0.00	0.12	0.07	1.60	0.20	0.00	1.20	0.00	1.80	0.00	0.00	25.00	270.00	0.00
1.00	2.50	0.00	0.00	0.00	0.00	0.00	0.30	0.14	1.20	2.00	0.00	0.90	0.00	1.80	0.00	0.00	270.00	360.00	0.00
1.00	2.50	0.00	0.00	0.00	0.00	0.00	0.30	0.14	1.20	0.20	0.00	0.90	0.00	1.80	0.00	0.00	280.00	370.00	0.00
0.00	0.00	0.00	0.00	0.00	0.00	0.00	0.15	0.14	2.00	0.20	0.00	0.90	0.00	1.44	0.00	0.00	200.00	400.00	0.00
1.50	4.00	0.00	0.00	0.00	0.00	0.00	0.43	0.14	0.80	0.12	0.00	1.20	0.00	1.80	0.00	0.00	30.00	390.00	0.00
1.50	3.50	0.00	0.00	0.00	0.00	0.00	1.20	0.10	0.40	0.20	0.00	0.60	0.00	0.72	0.00	0.00	200.00	600.00	0.00
2.50	3.50	0.00	0.00	0.00	0.00	0.00	0.30	0.03	2.00	0.30	0.00	2.10	0.00	0.72	0.00	0.00	60.00	360.00	0.00
0.00	0.00	0.00	0.00	0.00	0.00	0.00	0.06	0.10	4.00	0.08	0.00	0.24	0.00	1.08	0.00	0.00	100.00	270.00	0.00
0.00	0.00	0.00	0.00	0.00	0.00	0.00	0.12	0.26	7.00	0.12	0.00	0.48	20.00	1.80	0.00	0.00	170.00	430.00	0.00
3.50	9.00	0.00	0.00	0.00	0.00	0.00	0.06	0.07	2.00	0.70	0.00	1.50	40.00	3.60	0.00	0.00	420.00	1130.00	0.00
0.00	0.00	0.00	0.00	0.00	150.00	0.00	0.00	0.00	0.00	0.00	0.00	0.00	40.00	1.80	0.00	0.00	480.00	870.00	0.00
0.00	0.00	0.00	0.00	0.00	0.00	0.00	0.00	0.00	0.00	0.00	0.00	0.00	0.00	0.36	0.00	0.00	40.00	500.00	0.00
0.50	1.00	0.00	0.00	0.00	0.00	0.00	0.00	0.00	0.00	0.00	0.00	0.00	0.00	0.72	0.00	0.00	30.00	390.00	0.00

USDA ID Code	Food Name	Weight in Grams*	Quantity of Units	Unit of Measure	Protein (gm)	Fat (gm)	Carbohydrate (gm)	Kcalories	Caffeine (gm)	Fiber (gm)	Cholesterol (mg)	Saturated Fat (gm)
806	Worthington- Corned Beef, Meatle	57.0000	4.000	Slices	10.00	9.00	5.00	140.00	0.00	2.00	0.00	1.00
807	Worthington- Croquettes, Golden	85.0000	4.000	Each	14.00	10.00	14.00	210.00	0.00	3.00	0.00	1.50
808	Worthington- Fillets	85.0000	2.000	Each	16.00	10.00	8.00	180.00	0.00	4.00	0.00	2.00
809	Worthington- FriChik	90.0000	2.000	Each	10.00	8.00	1.00	120.00	0.00	1.00	0.00	1.00
810	Worthington- FriChik, Low Fat	85.0000	2.000	Each	10.00	3.00	2.00	80.00	0.00	1.00	0.00	0.00
811	Worthington- FriPats	64.0000	1.000	Each	14.00	6.00	4.00	130.00	0.00	3.00	0.00	1.00
812	Worthington- Leanies	40.0000	1.000	Each	7.00	7.00	2.00	100.00	0.00	1.00	0.00	1.00
813	Worthington- Links, Super	48.0000	1.000	Each	7.00	8.00	2.00	110.00	0.00	1.00	0.00	1.00
814	Worthington- Links, Veja	31.0000	1.000	Each	5.00	3.00	1.00	50.00	0.00	0.00	0.00	0.50
815	Worthington- Numete	55.0000	1.000	Slice	6.00	10.00	5.00	130.00	0.00	3.00	0.00	2.50
816	Worthington- Prosage Links	45.0000	2.000	Each	8.00	2.50	2.00	60.00	0.00	2.00	0.00	0.50
817	Worthington- Prosage Patties	38.0000	1.000	Each	9.00	3.00	3.00	80.00	0.00	2.00	0.00	0.50
818	Worthington- Prosage Roll, Froze	55.0000	1.000	Slice	10.00	10.00	2.00	140.00	0.00	2.00	0.00	2.00
819	Worthington- Protose	55.0000	1.000	Slice	13.00	7.00	5.00	130.00	0.00	3.00	0.00	1.00
820	Worthington- Roast, Dinner	85.0000	1.000	Slice	12.00	12.00	5.00	180.00	0.00	3.00	0.00	1.50
821	Worthington- Salami, Meatless	57.0000	3.000	Slices	12.00	8.00	2.00	130.00	0.00	2.00	0.00	1.00
822	Worthington- Saucettes	38.0000	1.000	Each	6.00	6.00	1.00	90.00	0.00	1.00	0.00	1.00
823	Worthington- Skallops, Vegetable	85.0000	0.500	Cup	15.00	1.50	3.00	90.00	0.00	3.00	0.00	0.50
824	Worthington- Slices, Savory	84.0000	3.000	Slices	10.00	9.00	6.00	150.00	0.00	3.00	0.00	3.50
825	Worthington- Stakelets	71.0000	1.000	Each	12.00	8.00	6.00	140.00	0.00	2.00	0.00	1.00
826	Worthington- Stakes, Prime	92.0000	1.000	Each	10.00	7.00	4.00	120.00	0.00	4.00	0.00	1.00
827	Worthington- Steaks, Vegetable	72.0000	2.000	Slices	15.00	1.50	3.00	80.00	0.00	3.00	0.00	0.50
828	Worthington- Stew, Country	240.0000	1.000	Cup	13.00	9.00	20.00	210.00	0.00	5.00	0.00	1.00
829	Worthington- Stripples	16.0000	2.000	Each	2.00	4.50	2.00	60.00	0.00	1.00	0.00	0.50
830	Worthington- Tuno	55.0000	0.500	Cup	6.00	6.00	2.00	80.00	0.00	1.00	0.00	1.00
831	Worthington- Turkee Slices	94.0000	3.000	Slices	13.00	12.00	3.00	170.00	0.00	2.00	0.00	1.50
832	Worthington- Turkey, Smoked, Mea	57.0000	3.000	Slices	10.00	0.00	3.00	140.00	0.00	2.00	0.00	2.00
833	Worthington- Wham	45.0000	2.000	Slices	7.00	5.00	1.00	80.00	0.00	0.00	0.00	1.00
948	Ziti Mozzarella-Smart Ones	252.0000	9.000	Ounce	11.00	6.00	45.00	280.00	0.00	4.00	5.00	1.50
	Arby's-Beef, Roast, Regular	155.9210	1.000	Each	24.68	15.70	38.14	388.12	0.00	1.12	58.33	4.04
	Arby's-Beef, Roast, Super	240.9690	1.000	Each	25.74	22.66	51.49	515.92	0.00	1.65	41.19	8.75
	Arby's-Beef'N Cheddar Sandwich	194.0000	1.000	Each	35.27	19.84	29.76	443.11	0.00	1.21	84.88	9.92
	Arby's-Chicken BBQ, Grilled	201.0000	1.000	Each	23.00	13.00	47.00	388.00	0.00	2.00	43.00	3.00
	Arby's-Chicken Breast Fillet San	204.0000	1.000	Each	25.50	27.72	53.22	546.59	0.00	1.77	100.89	5.65
	Arby's-Chicken Cordon Bleu	240.0000	1.000	Each	38.00	33.00	46.00	623.00	0.00	5.00	77.00	5.65
	Arby's-Chicken Fingers	102.0000	1.000	Each	16.00	16.00	20.00	290.00	0.00	0.50	32.00	2.00
	Arby's-Chicken, Grilled, Delux	230.0000	1.000	Each	23.00	20.00	47.00	430.00	0.00	3.00	61.00	4.00
	Arby's-Chicken, Roast, Delux	195.0000	1.000	Each	20.00	6.00	33.00	276.00	0.00	4.00	33.00	2.00
	Arby's-Chowder, Clam, Boston	226.7950	1.000	Each	10.00	11.00	18.00	207.00	0.00	1.40	28.00	4.00
	Arby's-Fish Fillet Sandwich	221.0000	1.000	Each	23.00	27.00	50.00	526.00	0.00	0.00	43.80	7.00
	Arby's-French Fries	70.8730	1.000	Order	2.10	13.20	29.80	246.00	0.00	0.00	0.00	3.00
	Arby's-French Fries, Curly	99.2230	1.000	Order	4.20	17.70	43.20	337.00	0.00	0.00	0.00	7.40
	Arby's-Ham'N Cheese Sandwich	170.0960	1.000	Each	24.47	18.64	38.45	411.26	0.00	1.17	67.57	7.46
	Arby's-Soup, Broccoli, Cream Of	226.7950	1.000	Each	9.00	8.00	19.00	180.00	0.00	1.80	3.00	5.00
	Arby's-Soup, Cheese, Wisconsin	226.7950	1.000	Each	9.00	19.00	19.00	287.00	0.00	1.80	31.00	8.00
	Arby's-Turkey Sub	277.0000	1.000	Each	32.86	28.17	53.99	598.60	0.00	0.00	82.16	6.22
10	Boston Market-Apples, Cinnamon,	181.0000	0.750	Cup	0.00	4.50	56.00	250.00	0.00	3.00	0.00	0.00
11	Boston Market-Beans, BBQ Baked	201.0000	0.750	Cup	11.00	9.00	53.00	330.00	0.00	9.00	10.00	0.00
12	Boston Market-Brownie	95.0000	1.000	Each	6.00	27.00	47.00	450.00	0.00	3.00	80.00	0.00
13	Boston Market-Caesar, no dressin	225.0000	8.000	Ounce	19.00	13.00	14.00	240.00	0.00	4.00	25.00	0.00
14	Boston Market-Chicken Salad Sand	327.0000	1.000	Each	38.00	33.00	63.00	680.00	0.00	5.00	145.00	0.00
15	Boston Market-Chicken Salad, Chu	158.0000	0.750	Cup	27.00	30.00	3.00	390.00	0.00	1.00	145.00	0.00
16	Boston Market-Chicken Sandwich w	352.0000	1.000	Each	46.00	32.00	71.00	760.00	0.00	12.00	160.00	0.00
17	Boston Market-Chicken Sandwich,	281.0000	1.000	Each	39.00	3.50	61.00	430.00	0.00	11.00	95.00	0.00
18	Boston Market-Chicken, Dark Meat	125.0000	1.000	Each	31.00	22.00	2.00	330.00	0.00	1.00	180.00	0.00

Monounsaturated Fat (gm)	Polyunsaturated Fat (gm)	Vitamin D (mg)	Vitamin K (mg)	Vitamin E (mg)	Vitamin A (re)	Vitamin C (mg)	Thiamin (mg)	Riboflavin (mg)	Niacin (mg)	Vitamin B_6 (mg)	Folate (mg)	Vitamin B_{12} (mcg)	Calcium (mg)	Iron (mg)	Magnesium (mg)	Phosphorus (mg)	Potassium (mg)	Sodium (mg)	Zinc (mg)
2.00	6.00	0.00	0.00	0.00	0.00	0.00	1.80	0.07	1.20	0.30	0.00	1.80	0.00	1.08	0.00	0.00	60.00	520.00	0.00
2.50	6.00	0.00	0.00	0.00	0.00	0.00	0.45	0.07	2.00	0.30	0.00	2.70	40.00	1.44	0.00	0.00	190.00	600.00	0.00
3.50	4.50	0.00	0.00	0.00	0.00	0.00	0.68	0.14	0.80	0.40	0.00	2.70	0.00	1.80	0.00	0.00	130.00	750.00	0.00
2.00	5.00	0.00	0.00	0.00	0.00	0.00	0.09	0.14	0.80	0.16	0.00	2.40	0.00	1.08	0.00	0.00	150.00	430.00	0.00
1.00	2.00	0.00	0.00	0.00	0.00	0.00	0.09	0.14	0.80	0.16	0.00	2.40	0.00	1.08	0.00	0.00	150.00	430.00	0.00
1.50	3.50	0.00	0.00	0.00	0.00	0.00	1.80	0.17	3.00	0.60	0.00	1.20	60.00	1.08	0.00	0.00	125.00	320.00	0.00
1.50	4.50	0.00	0.00	0.00	0.00	0.00	0.23	0.14	0.80	0.20	0.00	0.90	20.00	0.72	0.00	0.00	40.00	430.00	0.00
2.00	4.50	0.00	0.00	0.00	0.00	0.00	0.09	0.10	0.80	0.12	0.00	1.20	0.00	0.00	0.00	0.00	30.00	350.00	0.00
1.50	1.00	0.00	0.00	0.00	0.00	0.00	0.12	0.10	1.60	0.16	0.00	0.48	0.00	0.72	0.00	0.00	20.00	190.00	0.00
4.50	2.50	0.00	0.00	0.00	0.00	0.00	0.09	0.07	0.40	0.20	0.00	0.60	0.00	1.08	0.00	0.00	160.00	270.00	0.00
0.50	1.50	0.00	0.00	0.00	0.00	0.00	1.80	0.14	2.00	0.30	0.00	3.60	0.00	1.44	0.00	0.00	60.00	340.00	0.00
0.50	2.00	0.00	0.00	0.00	0.00	0.00	0.45	0.10	0.40	0.30	0.00	1.50	0.00	1.08	0.00	0.00	100.00	300.00	0.00
3.50	4.50	0.00	0.00	0.00	0.00	0.00	1.05	0.17	1.60	0.20	0.00	0.90	0.00	1.80	0.00	0.00	80.00	390.00	0.00
3.00	2.50	0.00	0.00	0.00	0.00	0.00	0.15	0.14	1.20	0.20	0.00	1.20	0.00	1.80	0.00	0.00	50.00	280.00	0.00
5.00	5.00	0.00	0.00	0.00	0.00	0.00	1.80	0.23	6.00	0.60	0.00	1.50	40.00	0.36	0.00	0.00	55.00	580.00	0.00
1.00	6.00	0.00	0.00	0.00	0.00	0.00	0.75	0.14	1.20	0.20	0.00	0.60	20.00	1.44	0.00	0.00	95.00	930.00	0.00
1.50	3.50	0.00	0.00	0.00	0.00	0.00	0.60	0.07	4.00	0.12	0.00	0.36	0.00	1.08	0.00	0.00	25.00	200.00	0.00
0.50	0.00	0.00	0.00	0.00	0.00	0.00	0.00	0.00	0.00	0.00	0.00	0.00	0.00	0.72	0.00	0.00	10.00	410.00	0.00
4.00	1.50	0.00	0.00	0.00	0.00	0.00	0.23	0.17	1.60	0.30	0.00	1.50	0.00	1.44	0.00	0.00	40.00	540.00	0.00
5.00	2.00	0.00	0.00	0.00	0.00	0.00	1.50	0.14	3.00	0.30	0.00	1.50	40.00	1.08	0.00	0.00	95.00	480.00	0.00
1.50	4.00	0.00	0.00	0.00	0.00	0.00	0.12	0.14	2.00	0.40	0.00	0.90	0.00	0.36	0.00	0.00	80.00	440.00	0.00
0.00	0.00	0.00	0.00	0.00	0.00	0.00	0.53	0.10	4.00	0.20	0.00	3.00	0.00	3.60	0.00	0.00	20.00	300.00	0.00
2.00	5.00	0.00	0.00	0.00	675.45	0.00	1.80	0.23	4.00	0.90	0.00	3.60	60.00	5.40	0.00	0.00	270.00	830.00	0.00
1.00	2.50	0.00	0.00	0.00	0.00	0.00	0.75	0.03	0.40	0.08	0.00	0.24	0.00	0.36	0.00	0.00	15.00	220.00	0.00
1.50	3.00	0.00	0.00	0.00	0.00	0.00	0.15	0.03	1.20	0.30	0.00	2.10	20.00	1.08	0.00	0.00	35.00	290.00	0.00
2.50	8.00	0.00	0.00	0.00	0.00	0.00	1.80	0.14	1.20	0.20	0.00	1.50	0.00	1.44	0.00	0.00	45.00	580.00	0.00
3.50	4.00	0.00	0.00	0.00	0.00	0.00	1.80	0.17	2.00	0.30	0.00	2.10	0.00	1.80	0.00	0.00	70.00	620.00	0.00
1.00	3.00	0.00	0.00	0.00	0.00	0.00	1.80	0.14	1.60	0.20	0.00	1.20	0.00	1.08	0.00	0.00	90.00	430.00	0.00
0.00	0.00	0.00	0.00	0.00	0.00	0.00	0.00	0.00	0.00	0.00	0.00	0.00	0.00	0.00	0.00	0.00	0.00	430.00	0.00
7.63	1.91	0.00	0.00	0.22	70.67	2.24	0.43	0.35	6.62	0.30	44.87	1.37	60.57	4.71	34.77	268.09	354.47	888.41	3.81
8.44	5.56	0.00	0.00	0.41	0.00	0.00	0.65	0.62	9.68	0.49	42.22	4.42	118.42	6.59	59.73	413.97	517.98	821.77	11.02
4.08	3.86	0.00	0.00	0.44	63.93	1.32	0.42	0.51	6.50	0.37	45.19	2.26	201.72	5.62	44.09	442.01	380.28	1801.11	5.95
2.00	1.00	0.00	0.00	0.00	16.63	0.00	0.50	0.43	16.41	0.72	35.48	0.38	123.07	3.88	51.00	321.52	365.87	1002.00	1.88
10.64	11.42	0.00	0.00	2.88	16.63	0.00	0.50	0.43	16.41	0.72	35.48	0.38	123.07	3.88	51.00	321.52	365.87	1129.76	1.88
10.64	11.42	0.00	0.00	2.88	16.63	0.00	0.50	0.43	16.41	0.72	35.48	0.38	123.07	3.88	51.00	321.52	365.87	1594.00	1.88
4.00	4.10	0.00	0.00	1.40	2.60	0.00	0.00	0.00	0.00	0.09	17.00	0.19	92.00	1.90	22.00	140.00	190.00	677.00	0.30
2.00	1.00	0.00	0.00	0.00	16.63	0.00	0.50	0.43	16.41	0.72	35.48	0.38	123.07	3.88	51.00	321.52	365.87	848.00	1.88
2.00	1.00	0.00	0.00	0.00	16.63	0.00	0.50	0.43	16.41	0.72	35.48	0.38	123.07	3.88	51.00	321.52	365.87	777.00	1.88
5.00	2.00	0.00	0.00	0.10	100.00	4.00	0.06	0.22	0.90	0.12	9.00	9.38	170.00	1.40	20.00	143.00	319.00	1157.00	0.70
9.20	10.60	0.00	0.00	0.00	0.00	1.20	0.35	0.31	5.32	0.00	0.00	0.00	72.00	2.10	0.00	0.00	450.00	872.00	0.00
5.50	4.70	0.00	0.00	0.00	0.00	3.60	0.06	0.00	1.90	0.00	0.00	0.00	0.00	0.60	0.00	0.00	240.00	114.00	0.00
7.60	1.50	0.00	0.00	0.00	0.00	0.00	0.06	0.07	1.90	0.00	0.00	0.00	16.00	0.80	0.00	0.00	724.00	167.00	0.00
7.81	1.63	0.00	0.00	1.28	111.84	3.50	0.36	0.57	3.15	0.23	82.72	0.63	151.46	3.84	18.64	177.09	337.86	899.41	1.63
2.00	1.00	0.00	0.00	1.40	50.00	9.00	0.11	0.42	0.80	0.18	46.00	0.59	237.00	0.80	55.00	193.00	455.00	1113.00	0.70
8.00	3.00	0.00	0.00	0.40	90.00	2.00	0.03	0.24	0.70	0.05	7.00	0.00	252.00	1.30	7.00	241.00	441.00	1129.00	1.10
7.04	8.22	0.00	0.00	0.00	0.00	0.00	0.53	0.40	9.39	0.00	0.00	0.00	93.90	3.17	0.00	0.00	0.00	1431.95	0.00
0.00	0.00	0.00	0.00	0.00	0.00	0.00	0.00	0.00	0.00	0.00	0.00	0.00	0.00	0.00	0.00	0.00	0.00	45.00	0.00
0.00	0.00	0.00	0.00	0.00	0.00	0.00	0.00	0.00	0.00	0.00	0.00	0.00	0.00	0.00	0.00	0.00	0.00	630.00	0.00
0.00	0.00	0.00	0.00	0.00	0.00	0.00	0.00	0.00	0.00	0.00	0.00	0.00	0.00	0.00	0.00	0.00	0.00	190.00	0.00
0.00	0.00	0.00	0.00	0.00	0.00	0.00	0.00	0.00	0.00	0.00	0.00	0.00	0.00	0.00	0.00	0.00	0.00	780.00	0.00
0.00	0.00	0.00	0.00	0.00	0.00	0.00	0.00	0.00	0.00	0.00	0.00	0.00	0.00	0.00	0.00	0.00	0.00	1350.00	0.00
0.00	0.00	0.00	0.00	0.00	0.00	0.00	0.00	0.00	0.00	0.00	0.00	0.00	0.00	0.00	0.00	0.00	0.00	790.00	0.00
0.00	0.00	0.00	0.00	0.00	0.00	0.00	0.00	0.00	0.00	0.00	0.00	0.00	0.00	0.00	0.00	0.00	0.00	1810.00	0.00
0.00	0.00	0.00	0.00	0.00	0.00	0.00	0.00	0.00	0.00	0.00	0.00	0.00	0.00	0.00	0.00	0.00	0.00	860.00	0.00
0.00	0.00	0.00	0.00	0.00	0.00	0.00	0.00	0.00	0.00	0.00	0.00	0.00	0.00	0.00	0.00	0.00	0.00	460.00	0.00

USDA ID Code	Food Name	Weight in Grams*	Quantity of Units	Unit of Measure	Protein (gm)	Fat (gm)	Carbohydrate (gm)	Kcalories	Caffeine (gm)	Fiber (gm)	Cholesterol (mg)	Saturated Fat (gm)
19	Boston Market-Chicken, Dark Meat	95.0000	1.000	Each	28.00	10.00	1.00	210.00	0.00	1.00	150.00	0.00
22	Boston Market-Chicken, w/ skin,	227.0000	1.000	Each	74.00	37.00	2.00	630.00	0.00	2.00	370.00	0.00
20	Boston Market-Chicken, White Mea	140.0000	1.000	Each	31.00	3.50	0.00	160.00	0.00	0.00	95.00	0.00
21	Boston Market-Chicken, White Mea	152.0000	1.000	Each	43.00	17.00	2.00	330.00	0.00	1.00	175.00	0.00
23	Boston Market-Coleslaw	184.0000	0.750	Cup	2.00	16.00	32.00	280.00	0.00	3.00	25.00	0.00
24	Boston Market-Cookie, Chocolate	79.0000	1.000	Each	4.00	17.00	48.00	340.00	0.00	1.00	25.00	0.00
25	Boston Market-Cookie, Oatmeal Ra	79.0000	1.000	Each	4.00	13.00	48.00	320.00	0.00	1.00	25.00	0.00
26	Boston Market-Corn Bread	68.0000	1.000	Each	3.00	6.00	33.00	200.00	0.00	1.00	25.00	0.00
27	Boston Market-Corn, Buttered	146.0000	0.750	Cup	6.00	4.00	39.00	190.00	0.00	4.00	0.00	0.00
28	Boston Market-Cranberry Relish	225.0000	0.750	Cup	2.00	5.00	84.00	370.00	0.00	5.00	0.00	0.00
29	Boston Market-Fruit Salad	156.0000	0.750	Cup	1.00	0.50	17.00	70.00	0.00	2.00	0.00	0.00
30	Boston Market-Gravy, Chicken	28.0000	1.000	Ounce	0.00	1.00	2.00	15.00	0.00	0.00	0.00	0.00
31	Boston Market-Ham Sandwich w/ Ch	337.0000	1.000	Each	38.00	35.00	71.00	760.00	0.00	5.00	100.00	0.00
32	Boston Market-Ham Sandwich, plai	266.0000	1.000	Each	25.00	9.00	66.00	450.00	0.00	4.00	45.00	0.00
33	Boston Market-Ham, Hearth Honey	142.0000	5.000	Ounce	25.00	9.00	9.00	210.00	0.00	0.00	75.00	0.00
34	Boston Market-Ham/Turkey Club w/	379.0000	1.000	Each	47.00	43.00	79.00	890.00	0.00	4.00	150.00	0.00
35	Boston Market-Ham/Turkey Club, p	266.0000	1.000	Each	29.00	6.00	64.00	430.00	0.00	4.00	55.00	0.00
36	Boston Market-Macaroni & Cheese	192.0000	0.750	Cup	12.00	10.00	36.00	280.00	0.00	1.00	20.00	0.00
37	Boston Market-Meatloaf Sandwich	383.0000	1.000	Each	46.00	33.00	95.00	860.00	0.00	6.00	165.00	0.00
38	Boston Market-Meatloaf w/ Brown	198.0000	7.000	Ounce	30.00	22.00	19.00	390.00	0.00	1.00	120.00	0.00
39	Boston Market-Meatloaf, plain	351.0000	1.000	Each	40.00	21.00	86.00	690.00	0.00	6.00	120.00	0.00
40	Boston Market-Meatloaf/Chunky To	227.0000	8.000	Ounce	30.00	18.00	22.00	370.00	0.00	5.00	120.00	0.00
41	Boston Market-Pot Pie, Chicken,	425.0000	1.000	Each	34.00	34.00	78.00	750.00	0.00	6.00	115.00	0.00
42	Boston Market-Potatoes, Mashed	161.0000	0.660	Cup	3.00	8.00	25.00	180.00	0.00	4.00	25.00	0.00
43	Boston Market-Potatoes, Mashed &	189.0000	0.750	Cup	3.00	9.00	27.00	200.00	0.00	4.00	25.00	0.00
44	Boston Market-Potatoes, New	131.0000	0.750	Cup	3.00	3.00	25.00	140.00	0.00	2.00	0.00	0.00
45	Boston Market-Rice Pilaf	145.0000	0.660	Cup	5.00	5.00	32.00	180.00	0.00	2.00	0.00	0.00
46	Boston Market-Salad, Caesar, Chi	369.0000	13.000	Ounce	45.00	47.00	16.00	670.00	0.00	3.00	120.00	0.00
47	Boston Market-Salad, Caesar, Ent	283.0000	10.000	Ounce	20.00	43.00	16.00	520.00	0.00	3.00	40.00	0.00
48	Boston Market-Salad, Caesar, Sid	113.0000	4.000	Ounce	8.00	17.00	6.00	210.00	0.00	1.00	20.00	0.00
49	Boston Market-Salad, Pasta, Med.	156.0000	0.750	Cup	4.00	10.00	16.00	170.00	0.00	2.00	10.00	0.00
50	Boston Market-Salad, Tortellini	156.0000	0.750	Cup	14.00	24.00	29.00	380.00	0.00	2.00	90.00	0.00
51	Boston Market-Soup, Chicken	257.0000	1.000	Cup	9.00	3.00	4.00	80.00	0.00	2.00	25.00	0.00
52	Boston Market-Soup, Chicken Tort	238.0000	1.000	Cup	10.00	11.00	19.00	220.00	0.00	2.00	35.00	0.00
53	Boston Market-Spinach, Creamed	181.0000	0.750	Cup	10.00	24.00	13.00	300.00	0.00	2.00	75.00	0.00
54	Boston Market-Squash, Butternut	193.0000	0.750	Cup	2.00	6.00	25.00	160.00	0.00	3.00	15.00	0.00
55	Boston Market-Stuffing	174.0000	0.750	Cup	6.00	12.00	44.00	310.00	0.00	3.00	0.00	0.00
56	Boston Market-Turkey Breast, Rot	142.0000	5.000	Ounce	36.00	1.00	1.00	170.00	0.00	0.00	100.00	0.00
57	Boston Market-Turkey Sandwich w/	337.0000	1.000	Each	45.00	28.00	68.00	710.00	0.00	4.00	110.00	0.00
58	Boston Market-Turkey Sandwich, p	266.0000	1.000	Each	32.00	3.50	61.00	400.00	0.00	4.00	60.00	0.00
59	Boston Market-Vegetables, Steame	105.0000	0.660	Cup	2.00	0.50	7.00	35.00	0.00	3.00	0.00	0.00
60	Boston Market-Zucchini Marinara	146.0000	0.750	Cup	2.00	4.00	10.00	80.00	0.00	2.00	0.00	0.00
	Burger King-Biscuit With Bacon,	171.0000	1.000	Each	19.00	31.00	39.00	280.00	0.00	1.00	225.00	10.00
	Burger King-Biscuit with Sausage	151.0000	1.000	Each	16.00	40.00	41.00	360.00	0.00	1.00	45.00	13.00
	Burger King-Cheeseburger	138.0000	1.000	Each	23.00	16.00	28.00	380.00	0.00	1.00	65.00	9.00
	Burger King-Cheeseburger, Bacon	218.0000	1.000	Each	44.00	39.00	28.00	640.00	0.00	1.00	145.00	18.00
	Burger King-Cheeseburger, Double	210.0000	1.000	Each	41.00	36.00	28.00	600.00	0.00	1.00	135.00	17.00
	Burger King-Chicken Salad, Broil	302.0000	1.000	Each	21.00	10.00	7.00	90.00	0.00	3.00	60.00	4.00
	Burger King-Chicken Sandwich	229.0000	1.000	Each	26.00	43.00	54.00	710.00	0.00	2.00	60.00	9.00
	Burger King-Chicken Sandwich- BK	248.0000	1.000	Each	30.00	29.00	41.00	550.00	0.00	2.00	80.00	6.00
	Burger King-Chicken Tenders - 8	117.0000	1.000	Each	21.00	17.00	19.00	310.00	0.00	3.00	50.00	4.00
	Burger King-Coca Cola Classic -	360.0000	1.000	Each	0.00	0.00	70.00	280.00	3.08	0.00	0.00	0.00
	Burger King-Coke, Diet - medium	360.0000	1.000	Each	0.00	0.00	0.00	1.00	3.08	0.00	0.00	0.00
	Burger King-Croissan'Wich, w/ sa	176.0000	1.000	Each	22.00	46.00	25.00	600.00	0.00	1.00	260.00	16.00
	Burger King-Dressing, French	30.0000	1.000	Each	0.00	10.00	11.00	140.00	0.00	0.00	0.00	2.00

Monounsaturated Fat (gm)	Polyunsaturated Fat (gm)	Vitamin D (mg)	Vitamin K (mg)	Vitamin E (mg)	Vitamin A (re)	Vitamin C (mg)	Thiamin (mg)	Riboflavin (mg)	Niacin (mg)	Vitamin B_6 (mg)	Folate (mg)	Vitamin B_{12} (mcg)	Calcium (mg)	Iron (mg)	Magnesium (mg)	Phosphorus (mg)	Potassium (mg)	Sodium (mg)	Zinc (mg)
0.00	0.00	0.00	0.00	0.00	0.00	0.00	0.00	0.00	0.00	0.00	0.00	0.00	0.00	0.00	0.00	0.00	0.00	320.00	0.00
0.00	0.00	0.00	0.00	0.00	0.00	0.00	0.00	0.00	0.00	0.00	0.00	0.00	0.00	0.00	0.00	0.00	0.00	960.00	0.00
0.00	0.00	0.00	0.00	0.00	0.00	0.00	0.00	0.00	0.00	0.00	0.00	0.00	0.00	0.00	0.00	0.00	0.00	350.00	0.00
0.00	0.00	0.00	0.00	0.00	0.00	0.00	0.00	0.00	0.00	0.00	0.00	0.00	0.00	0.00	0.00	0.00	0.00	530.00	0.00
0.00	0.00	0.00	0.00	0.00	0.00	0.00	0.00	0.00	0.00	0.00	0.00	0.00	0.00	0.00	0.00	0.00	0.00	520.00	0.00
0.00	0.00	0.00	0.00	0.00	0.00	0.00	0.00	0.00	0.00	0.00	0.00	0.00	0.00	0.00	0.00	0.00	0.00	240.00	0.00
0.00	0.00	0.00	0.00	0.00	0.00	0.00	0.00	0.00	0.00	0.00	0.00	0.00	0.00	0.00	0.00	0.00	0.00	260.00	0.00
0.00	0.00	0.00	0.00	0.00	0.00	0.00	0.00	0.00	0.00	0.00	0.00	0.00	0.00	0.00	0.00	0.00	0.00	390.00	0.00
0.00	0.00	0.00	0.00	0.00	0.00	0.00	0.00	0.00	0.00	0.00	0.00	0.00	0.00	0.00	0.00	0.00	0.00	130.00	0.00
0.00	0.00	0.00	0.00	0.00	0.00	0.00	0.00	0.00	0.00	0.00	0.00	0.00	0.00	0.00	0.00	0.00	0.00	5.00	0.00
0.00	0.00	0.00	0.00	0.00	0.00	0.00	0.00	0.00	0.00	0.00	0.00	0.00	0.00	0.00	0.00	0.00	0.00	10.00	0.00
0.00	0.00	0.00	0.00	0.00	0.00	0.00	0.00	0.00	0.00	0.00	0.00	0.00	0.00	0.00	0.00	0.00	0.00	170.00	0.00
0.00	0.00	0.00	0.00	0.00	0.00	0.00	0.00	0.00	0.00	0.00	0.00	0.00	0.00	0.00	0.00	0.00	0.00	1880.00	0.00
0.00	0.00	0.00	0.00	0.00	0.00	0.00	0.00	0.00	0.00	0.00	0.00	0.00	0.00	0.00	0.00	0.00	0.00	1600.00	0.00
0.00	0.00	0.00	0.00	0.00	0.00	0.00	0.00	0.00	0.00	0.00	0.00	0.00	0.00	0.00	0.00	0.00	0.00	1490.00	0.00
0.00	0.00	0.00	0.00	0.00	0.00	0.00	0.00	0.00	0.00	0.00	0.00	0.00	0.00	0.00	0.00	0.00	0.00	2310.00	0.00
0.00	0.00	0.00	0.00	0.00	0.00	0.00	0.00	0.00	0.00	0.00	0.00	0.00	0.00	0.00	0.00	0.00	0.00	1330.00	0.00
0.00	0.00	0.00	0.00	0.00	0.00	0.00	0.00	0.00	0.00	0.00	0.00	0.00	0.00	0.00	0.00	0.00	0.00	760.00	0.00
0.00	0.00	0.00	0.00	0.00	0.00	0.00	0.00	0.00	0.00	0.00	0.00	0.00	0.00	0.00	0.00	0.00	0.00	2270.00	0.00
0.00	0.00	0.00	0.00	0.00	0.00	0.00	0.00	0.00	0.00	0.00	0.00	0.00	0.00	0.00	0.00	0.00	0.00	1040.00	0.00
0.00	0.00	0.00	0.00	0.00	0.00	0.00	0.00	0.00	0.00	0.00	0.00	0.00	0.00	0.00	0.00	0.00	0.00	1610.00	0.00
0.00	0.00	0.00	0.00	0.00	0.00	0.00	0.00	0.00	0.00	0.00	0.00	0.00	0.00	0.00	0.00	0.00	0.00	1170.00	0.00
0.00	0.00	0.00	0.00	0.00	0.00	0.00	0.00	0.00	0.00	0.00	0.00	0.00	0.00	0.00	0.00	0.00	0.00	2380.00	0.00
0.00	0.00	0.00	0.00	0.00	0.00	0.00	0.00	0.00	0.00	0.00	0.00	0.00	0.00	0.00	0.00	0.00	0.00	390.00	0.00
0.00	0.00	0.00	0.00	0.00	0.00	0.00	0.00	0.00	0.00	0.00	0.00	0.00	0.00	0.00	0.00	0.00	0.00	560.00	0.00
0.00	0.00	0.00	0.00	0.00	0.00	0.00	0.00	0.00	0.00	0.00	0.00	0.00	0.00	0.00	0.00	0.00	0.00	100.00	0.00
0.00	0.00	0.00	0.00	0.00	0.00	0.00	0.00	0.00	0.00	0.00	0.00	0.00	0.00	0.00	0.00	0.00	0.00	600.00	0.00
0.00	0.00	0.00	0.00	0.00	0.00	0.00	0.00	0.00	0.00	0.00	0.00	0.00	0.00	0.00	0.00	0.00	0.00	1860.00	0.00
0.00	0.00	0.00	0.00	0.00	0.00	0.00	0.00	0.00	0.00	0.00	0.00	0.00	0.00	0.00	0.00	0.00	0.00	1420.00	0.00
0.00	0.00	0.00	0.00	0.00	0.00	0.00	0.00	0.00	0.00	0.00	0.00	0.00	0.00	0.00	0.00	0.00	0.00	560.00	0.00
0.00	0.00	0.00	0.00	0.00	0.00	0.00	0.00	0.00	0.00	0.00	0.00	0.00	0.00	0.00	0.00	0.00	0.00	490.00	0.00
0.00	0.00	0.00	0.00	0.00	0.00	0.00	0.00	0.00	0.00	0.00	0.00	0.00	0.00	0.00	0.00	0.00	0.00	530.00	0.00
0.00	0.00	0.00	0.00	0.00	0.00	0.00	0.00	0.00	0.00	0.00	0.00	0.00	0.00	0.00	0.00	0.00	0.00	470.00	0.00
0.00	0.00	0.00	0.00	0.00	0.00	0.00	0.00	0.00	0.00	0.00	0.00	0.00	0.00	0.00	0.00	0.00	0.00	1410.00	0.00
0.00	0.00	0.00	0.00	0.00	0.00	0.00	0.00	0.00	0.00	0.00	0.00	0.00	0.00	0.00	0.00	0.00	0.00	790.00	0.00
0.00	0.00	0.00	0.00	0.00	0.00	0.00	0.00	0.00	0.00	0.00	0.00	0.00	0.00	0.00	0.00	0.00	0.00	580.00	0.00
0.00	0.00	0.00	0.00	0.00	0.00	0.00	0.00	0.00	0.00	0.00	0.00	0.00	0.00	0.00	0.00	0.00	0.00	1140.00	0.00
0.00	0.00	0.00	0.00	0.00	0.00	0.00	0.00	0.00	0.00	0.00	0.00	0.00	0.00	0.00	0.00	0.00	0.00	850.00	0.00
0.00	0.00	0.00	0.00	0.00	0.00	0.00	0.00	0.00	0.00	0.00	0.00	0.00	0.00	0.00	0.00	0.00	0.00	1390.00	0.00
0.00	0.00	0.00	0.00	0.00	0.00	0.00	0.00	0.00	0.00	0.00	0.00	0.00	0.00	0.00	0.00	0.00	0.00	1070.00	0.00
0.00	0.00	0.00	0.00	0.00	0.00	0.00	0.00	0.00	0.00	0.00	0.00	0.00	0.00	0.00	0.00	0.00	0.00	35.00	0.00
0.00	0.00	0.00	0.00	0.00	0.00	0.00	0.00	0.00	0.00	0.00	0.00	0.00	0.00	0.00	0.00	0.00	0.00	470.00	0.00
0.00	0.00	0.00	0.00	0.00	0.00	0.00	0.00	0.00	0.00	0.00	0.00	0.00	0.00	0.00	0.00	0.00	0.00	1530.00	0.00
0.00	0.00	0.00	0.00	0.00	0.00	0.00	0.00	0.00	0.00	0.00	0.00	0.00	0.00	0.00	0.00	0.00	0.00	1390.00	0.00
0.00	0.00	0.00	0.00	0.00	0.00	0.00	0.00	0.00	0.00	0.00	0.00	0.00	0.00	0.00	0.00	0.00	0.00	770.00	0.00
14.50	6.22	0.00	0.00	1.55	73.54	8.29	0.31	0.40	8.39	0.38	32.11	3.36	161.59	4.14	39.36	386.37	479.59	1240.00	6.63
12.24	2.23	0.00	0.00	2.00	111.25	6.68	0.24	0.34	5.45	0.27	34.49	2.01	210.27	3.34	34.49	339.33	382.72	1060.00	4.45
0.00	0.00	0.00	0.00	0.00	0.00	0.00	0.00	0.00	0.00	0.00	0.00	0.00	0.00	0.00	0.00	0.00	0.00	110.00	0.00
0.00	0.00	0.00	0.00	0.00	0.00	0.00	0.00	0.00	0.00	0.00	0.00	0.00	0.00	0.00	0.00	0.00	0.00	1400.00	0.00
0.00	0.00	0.00	0.00	0.00	0.00	0.00	0.00	0.00	0.00	0.00	0.00	0.00	0.00	0.00	0.00	0.00	0.00	4803.00	0.00
0.00	0.00	0.00	0.00	0.00	0.00	0.00	0.00	0.00	0.00	0.00	0.00	0.00	0.00	0.00	0.00	0.00	0.00	710.00	0.00
0.00	0.00	0.00	0.00	0.00	0.00	0.00	0.00	0.00	0.00	0.00	0.00	0.00	0.00	0.00	0.00	0.00	0.00	0.00	0.00
0.00	0.00	0.00	0.00	0.00	0.00	0.00	0.00	0.00	0.00	0.00	0.00	0.00	0.00	0.00	0.00	0.00	0.00	0.00	0.00
0.00	0.00	0.00	0.00	0.00	0.00	0.00	0.00	0.00	0.00	0.00	0.00	0.00	0.00	0.00	0.00	0.00	0.00	1140.00	0.00
0.00	0.00	0.00	0.00	0.00	0.00	0.00	0.00	0.00	0.00	0.00	0.00	0.00	0.00	0.00	0.00	0.00	0.00	190.00	0.00

USDA ID Code	Food Name	Weight in Grams*	Quantity of Units	Unit of Measure	Protein (gm)	Fat (gm)	Carbohydrate (gm)	Kcalories	Caffeine (gm)	Fiber (gm)	Cholesterol (mg)	Saturated Fat (gm)
	Burger King-Dressing, Italian, R	30.0000	1.000	Each	0.00	0.50	3.00	15.00	0.00	0.00	0.00	0.00
	Burger King-Dressing, Ranch	30.0000	1.000	Each	0.00	19.00	2.00	180.00	0.00	0.00	10.00	4.00
	Burger King-Dressing, Thousand I	30.0000	1.000	Each	0.00	12.00	7.00	140.00	0.00	0.00	15.00	3.00
	Burger King-Fish Sandwich, BK Bi	255.0000	1.000	Each	26.00	41.00	56.00	700.00	0.00	3.00	90.00	6.00
	Burger King-French Fries, Coated	102.0000	1.000	Each	3.00	17.00	43.00	340.00	0.00	3.00	0.00	5.00
	Burger King-French Fries, Medium	116.0000	1.000	Each	5.00	20.00	43.00	180.00	0.00	3.00	0.00	5.00
	Burger King-French Toast Sticks	141.0000	1.000	Each	4.00	27.00	60.00	500.00	0.00	1.00	0.00	27.00
	Burger King-Hamburger	126.0000	1.000	Each	20.00	15.00	28.00	330.00	0.00	1.00	55.00	6.00
	Burger King-Hash Browns	71.0000	1.000	Each	2.00	12.00	25.00	110.00	0.00	2.00	0.00	3.00
	Burger King-Jam, Grape	12.0000	1.000	Each	0.00	0.00	8.00	30.00	0.00	0.00	0.00	0.00
	Burger King-Jam, Strawberry	12.0000	1.000	Each	0.00	0.00	8.00	30.00	0.00	0.00	0.00	0.00
	Burger King-Ketchup	14.0000	1.000	Each	0.00	0.00	4.00	15.00	0.00	0.00	0.00	0.00
	Burger King-Onion Rings	124.0000	1.000	Each	4.00	14.00	41.00	310.00	0.00	6.00	0.00	2.00
	Burger King-Pie, Apple, Dutch	113.0000	1.000	Each	3.00	15.00	39.00	300.00	0.00	2.00	0.00	3.00
	Burger King-Salad w/ 1000 Island	176.0000	1.000	Each	2.00	12.00	9.00	145.00	0.00	0.00	17.00	0.00
	Burger King-Salad w/ Bleu Cheese	176.0000	1.000	Each	3.00	16.00	7.00	184.00	0.00	0.00	22.00	0.00
	Burger King-Salad w/ Dressing, H	176.0000	1.000	Each	3.00	13.00	8.00	159.00	0.00	0.00	11.00	0.00
	Burger King-Salad w/ French	176.0000	1.000	Each	2.00	11.00	13.00	152.00	0.00	0.00	0.00	0.00
	Burger King-Salad w/ Italian, Go	176.0000	1.000	Each	2.00	14.00	7.00	162.00	0.00	0.00	0.00	0.00
	Burger King-Salad w/ Italian, Re	176.0000	1.000	Each	2.00	1.00	7.00	42.00	0.00	0.00	0.00	0.00
	Burger King-Salad, Garden	255.0000	1.000	Each	6.00	5.00	8.00	100.00	0.00	4.00	15.00	3.00
	Burger King-Salad, Side	133.0000	1.000	Each	3.00	3.00	4.00	60.00	0.00	2.00	5.00	2.00
	Burger King-Sauce, Dipping, Barb	28.0000	1.000	Each	0.00	0.00	9.00	35.00	0.00	0.00	0.00	0.00
	Burger King-Sauce, Dipping, Hone	28.0000	1.000	Each	0.00	0.00	21.00	80.00	0.00	0.00	0.00	0.00
	Burger King-Sauce, Dipping, Swee	28.0000	1.000	Each	0.00	0.00	11.00	45.00	0.00	0.00	0.00	0.00
	Burger King-Shake, Chocolate, Me	397.0000	1.000	Each	12.00	10.00	75.00	440.00	0.00	4.00	30.00	6.00
	Burger King-Shake, Vanilla, Medi	397.0000	1.000	Each	13.00	9.00	73.00	430.00	0.00	2.00	30.00	5.00
	Burger King-Whopper	270.0000	1.000	Each	27.00	39.00	45.00	640.00	0.00	3.00	90.00	11.00
	Burger King-Whopper Jr.	164.0000	1.000	Each	21.00	24.00	29.00	420.00	0.00	2.00	60.00	8.00
	Burger King-Whopper Jr. w/ chees	177.0000	1.000	Each	23.00	28.00	29.00	460.00	0.00	2.00	75.00	10.00
	Burger King-Whopper w/ Cheese, D	375.0000	1.000	Each	52.00	63.00	46.00	960.00	0.00	3.00	195.00	24.00
	Burger King-Whopper, Double	351.0000	1.000	Each	33.00	46.00	46.00	730.00	0.00	3.00	115.00	16.00
177	Chick-fil-A-Chicken Club, Chargr	232.0000	1.000	Each	33.00	12.00	38.00	390.00	0.00	2.00	70.00	5.00
178	Chick-fil-A-Chicken Salad Sandwi	167.0000	1.000	Each	25.00	5.00	42.00	320.00	0.00	1.00	10.00	2.00
179	Chick-fil-A-Chicken Sandwich	167.0000	1.000	Each	24.00	9.00	27.00	290.00	0.00	1.00	50.00	0.00
180	Chick-fil-A-Chicken, Chargrilled	150.0000	1.000	Each	27.00	3.00	36.00	280.00	0.00	1.00	40.00	1.00
176	Chick-fil-A-Chick-n-Strips	119.0000	4.000	Each	29.00	8.00	10.00	230.00	0.00	1.00	20.00	2.00
181	Chick-fil-A-Nuggets	110.0000	8.000	Each	28.00	14.00	12.00	290.00	0.00	0.00	60.00	3.00
182	Chick-fil-A-Salad, Ceasar, Chick	241.0000	1.000	Serving	33.00	10.00	5.00	240.00	0.00	2.00	90.00	7.00
184	Chick-fil-A-Salad, Garden w/ Chi	289.0000	1.000	Serving	30.00	8.00	7.00	200.00	0.00	3.00	80.00	3.00
183	Chick-fil-A-Salad, Garden w/ Chi	334.0000	1.000	Serving	32.00	17.00	21.00	370.00	0.00	4.00	113.00	6.00
185	Chick-fil-A-Soup, Chicken Breast	215.0000	1.000	Serving	16.00	1.00	10.00	110.00	0.00	1.00	45.00	0.00
	Fast Food-Beef, Roast Sandwich w	176.0000	1.000	Each	32.23	18.00	45.37	473.44	0.00	0.00	77.44	9.03
	Fast Food-Beef, Roast Sandwich,	139.0000	1.000	Each	21.50	13.76	33.44	346.11	0.00	0.00	51.43	3.60
	Fast Food-Biscuit w/ Egg	136.0000	1.000	Each	11.12	20.20	24.17	315.52	0.00	0.00	232.56	6.17
	Fast Food-Biscuit w/ Egg and Bac	150.0000	1.000	Each	17.00	31.10	28.59	457.50	0.00	0.75	352.50	7.95
	Fast Food-Biscuit w/ Egg and Ham	192.0000	1.000	Each	20.43	27.03	30.32	441.60	0.00	0.77	299.52	5.91
	Fast Food-Biscuit w/ Egg and Sau	180.0000	1.000	Each	19.15	38.70	41.15	581.40	0.00	0.90	302.40	14.98
	Fast Food-Biscuit w/ Egg, Cheese	144.0000	1.000	Each	16.26	31.39	33.42	476.64	0.00	0.00	260.64	11.40
	Fast Food-Biscuit w/ Ham	113.0000	1.000	Each	13.39	18.42	43.79	386.46	0.00	0.79	24.86	11.41
	Fast Food-Biscuit w/ Sausage	124.0000	1.000	Each	12.11	31.78	40.04	484.84	0.00	1.36	34.72	14.22
	Fast Food-Biscuit w/ Steak	141.0000	1.000	Each	13.10	25.99	44.39	455.43	0.00	0.00	25.38	6.94
	Fast Food-Biscuit, Plain	74.0000	1.000	Each	4.31	13.35	34.43	276.02	0.00	0.00	5.18	8.74
	Fast Food-Brownie	60.0000	1.000	Each	2.74	10.10	38.97	243.00	1.20	0.00	9.60	3.13
	Fast Food-Burrito w/ Beans	217.0000	2.000	Each	14.06	13.50	71.44	447.02	0.00	0.00	4.34	6.88

Monounsaturated Fat (gm)	Polyunsaturated Fat (gm)	Vitamin D (mg)	Vitamin K (mg)	Vitamin E (mg)	Vitamin A (re)	Vitamin C (mg)	Thiamin (mg)	Riboflavin (mg)	Niacin (mg)	Vitamin B_6 (mg)	Folate (mg)	Vitamin B_{12} (mcg)	Calcium (mg)	Iron (mg)	Magnesium (mg)	Phosphorus (mg)	Potassium (mg)	Sodium (mg)	Zinc (mg)
0.00	0.00	0.00	0.00	0.00	0.00	0.00	0.00	0.00	0.00	0.00	0.00	0.00	0.00	0.00	0.00	0.00	0.00	50.00	0.00
0.00	0.00	0.00	0.00	0.00	0.00	0.00	0.00	0.00	0.00	0.00	0.00	0.00	0.00	0.00	0.00	0.00	0.00	170.00	0.00
0.00	0.00	0.00	0.00	0.00	0.00	0.00	0.00	0.00	0.00	0.00	0.00	0.00	0.00	0.00	0.00	0.00	0.00	190.00	0.00
0.00	0.00	0.00	0.00	0.00	0.00	0.00	0.00	0.00	0.00	0.00	0.00	0.00	0.00	0.00	0.00	0.00	0.00	980.00	0.00
0.00	0.00	0.00	0.00	0.00	0.00	0.00	0.00	0.00	0.00	0.00	0.00	0.00	0.00	0.00	0.00	0.00	0.00	680.00	0.00
0.00	0.00	0.00	0.00	0.00	0.00	0.00	0.00	0.00	0.00	0.00	0.00	0.00	0.00	0.00	0.00	0.00	0.00	240.00	0.00
0.00	0.00	0.00	0.00	0.00	0.00	0.00	0.00	0.00	0.00	0.00	0.00	0.00	0.00	0.00	0.00	0.00	0.00	490.00	0.00
0.00	0.00	0.00	0.00	0.00	0.00	0.00	0.00	0.00	0.00	0.00	0.00	0.00	0.00	0.00	0.00	0.00	0.00	530.00	0.00
0.00	0.00	0.00	0.00	0.00	0.00	0.00	0.00	0.00	0.00	0.00	0.00	0.00	0.00	0.00	0.00	0.00	0.00	320.00	0.00
0.00	0.00	0.00	0.00	0.00	0.00	0.00	0.00	0.00	0.00	0.00	0.00	0.00	0.00	0.00	0.00	0.00	0.00	0.00	0.00
0.00	0.00	0.00	0.00	0.00	0.00	0.00	0.00	0.00	0.00	0.00	0.00	0.00	0.00	0.00	0.00	0.00	0.00	5.00	0.00
0.00	0.00	0.00	0.00	0.00	0.00	0.00	0.00	0.00	0.00	0.00	0.00	0.00	0.00	0.00	0.00	0.00	0.00	180.00	0.00
0.00	0.00	0.00	0.00	0.00	0.00	0.00	0.00	0.00	0.00	0.00	0.00	0.00	0.00	0.00	0.00	0.00	0.00	810.00	0.00
0.00	0.00	0.00	0.00	0.00	0.00	0.00	0.00	0.00	0.00	0.00	0.00	0.00	0.00	0.00	0.00	0.00	0.00	230.00	0.00
0.00	0.00	0.00	0.00	0.00	0.00	25.80	0.00	0.00	0.19	0.00	0.00	0.00	336.00	0.14	98.00	528.00	405.00	251.00	0.08
0.00	0.00	0.00	0.00	0.00	0.00	25.20	0.00	0.00	0.19	0.00	0.00	0.00	528.00	0.13	101.50	664.00	382.00	333.00	0.09
0.00	0.00	0.00	0.00	0.00	0.00	25.20	0.00	0.00	0.19	0.00	0.00	0.00	352.00	0.13	94.50	592.00	402.00	293.00	0.08
0.00	0.00	0.00	0.00	0.00	0.00	25.80	0.00	0.00	0.19	0.00	0.00	0.00	320.00	0.14	98.00	480.00	410.00	330.00	0.07
0.00	0.00	0.00	0.00	0.00	0.00	5.20	0.00	0.00	0.19	0.00	0.00	0.00	320.00	0.13	98.00	480.00	389.00	292.00	0.06
0.00	0.00	0.00	0.00	0.00	0.00	25.20	0.00	0.00	0.19	0.00	0.00	0.00	320.00	0.14	105.00	472.00	390.00	430.00	0.06
0.00	0.00	0.00	0.00	0.00	0.00	0.00	0.00	0.00	0.00	0.00	0.00	0.00	0.00	0.00	0.00	0.00	0.00	115.00	0.00
0.00	0.00	0.00	0.00	0.00	0.00	0.00	0.00	0.00	0.00	0.00	0.00	0.00	0.00	0.00	0.00	0.00	0.00	55.00	0.00
0.00	0.00	0.00	0.00	0.00	0.00	0.00	0.00	0.00	0.00	0.00	0.00	0.00	0.00	0.00	0.00	0.00	0.00	400.00	0.00
0.00	0.00	0.00	0.00	0.00	0.00	0.00	0.00	0.00	0.00	0.00	0.00	0.00	0.00	0.00	0.00	0.00	0.00	20.00	0.00
0.00	0.00	0.00	0.00	0.00	0.00	0.00	0.00	0.00	0.00	0.00	0.00	0.00	0.00	0.00	0.00	0.00	0.00	50.00	0.00
0.00	0.00	0.00	0.00	0.00	0.00	0.00	0.00	0.00	0.00	0.00	0.00	0.00	0.00	0.00	0.00	0.00	0.00	330.00	0.00
0.00	0.00	0.00	0.00	0.00	0.00	0.00	0.00	0.00	0.00	0.00	0.00	0.00	0.00	0.00	0.00	0.00	0.00	330.00	0.00
14.99	2.39	0.00	0.00	4.24	208.55	14.12	0.02	0.03	5.65	0.34	33.67	3.05	112.96	6.52	54.31	338.89	564.81	870.00	5.76
0.00	0.00	0.00	0.00	0.00	0.00	0.00	0.00	0.00	0.00	0.00	0.00	0.00	0.00	0.00	0.00	0.00	0.00	530.00	0.00
0.00	0.00	0.00	0.00	0.00	0.00	0.00	0.00	0.00	0.00	0.00	0.00	0.00	0.00	0.00	0.00	0.00	0.00	770.00	0.00
0.00	0.00	0.00	0.00	0.00	0.00	0.00	0.00	0.00	0.00	0.00	0.00	0.00	0.00	0.00	0.00	0.00	0.00	1420.00	0.00
0.00	0.00	0.00	0.00	0.00	0.00	0.00	0.00	0.00	0.00	0.00	0.00	0.00	0.00	0.00	0.00	0.00	0.00	1350.00	0.00
0.00	0.00	0.00	0.00	0.00	0.00	0.00	0.00	0.00	0.00	0.00	0.00	0.00	0.00	0.00	0.00	0.00	0.00	980.00	0.00
0.00	0.00	0.00	0.00	0.00	0.00	0.00	0.00	0.00	0.00	0.00	0.00	0.00	0.00	0.00	0.00	0.00	0.00	810.00	0.00
0.00	0.00	0.00	0.00	0.00	0.00	0.00	0.00	0.00	0.00	0.00	0.00	0.00	0.00	0.00	0.00	0.00	0.00	870.00	0.00
0.00	0.00	0.00	0.00	0.00	0.00	0.00	0.00	0.00	0.00	0.00	0.00	0.00	0.00	0.00	0.00	0.00	0.00	640.00	0.00
0.00	0.00	0.00	0.00	0.00	0.00	0.00	0.00	0.00	0.00	0.00	0.00	0.00	0.00	0.00	0.00	0.00	0.00	810.00	0.00
0.00	0.00	0.00	0.00	0.00	0.00	0.00	0.00	0.00	0.00	0.00	0.00	0.00	0.00	0.00	0.00	0.00	0.00	770.00	0.00
0.00	0.00	0.00	0.00	0.00	700.00	6.00	0.00	0.00	0.00	0.00	0.00	0.00	350.00	2.70	0.00	0.00	0.00	990.00	0.00
0.00	0.00	0.00	0.00	0.00	1100.00	18.00	0.00	0.00	0.00	0.00	0.00	0.00	170.00	0.90	0.00	0.00	0.00	790.00	0.00
0.00	0.00	0.00	0.00	0.00	1200.00	15.00	0.00	0.00	0.00	0.00	0.00	0.00	170.00	0.72	0.00	0.00	0.00	725.00	0.00
0.00	0.00	0.00	0.00	0.00	0.00	0.00	0.00	0.00	0.00	0.00	0.00	0.00	0.00	0.00	0.00	0.00	0.00	760.00	0.00
3.66	3.50	0.00	0.00	0.00	45.76	0.00	0.39	0.46	5.90	0.33	63.36	2.06	183.04	5.05	40.48	401.28	344.96	1633.28	5.37
6.81	1.71	0.00	0.00	0.00	20.85	2.09	0.38	0.31	5.87	0.26	56.99	1.22	54.21	4.23	30.58	239.08	315.53	792.30	3.39
8.19	4.22	0.00	0.00	0.00	178.16	0.00	0.34	0.34	0.71	0.08	61.20	0.75	153.68	3.13	20.40	184.96	160.48	654.16	1.10
13.44	7.47	0.00	0.00	2.12	52.50	2.70	0.14	0.23	2.40	0.14	60.00	1.04	189.00	3.74	24.00	238.50	250.50	999.00	1.64
10.96	7.70	0.00	0.00	2.21	240.00	0.00	0.67	0.60	2.00	0.27	65.28	1.19	220.80	4.55	30.72	316.80	318.72	1382.40	2.23
16.40	4.45	0.00	0.00	2.77	163.80	0.00	0.50	0.45	3.60	0.20	64.80	1.37	154.80	3.96	25.20	489.60	320.40	1141.20	2.16
14.23	3.50	0.00	0.00	0.00	165.60	1.58	0.30	0.43	2.30	0.10	53.28	1.05	164.16	2.55	20.16	459.36	230.40	1260.00	1.54
4.84	1.04	0.00	0.00	2.24	33.90	0.11	0.51	0.32	3.48	0.14	38.42	0.03	160.46	2.72	22.60	553.70	196.62	1432.84	1.65
12.82	3.03	0.00	0.00	3.08	13.64	0.12	0.40	0.29	3.27	0.11	45.88	0.51	127.72	2.58	19.84	446.40	198.40	1071.36	1.55
11.08	6.42	0.00	0.00	0.00	15.51	0.14	0.35	0.39	4.16	0.16	63.45	0.94	115.62	4.30	26.79	204.45	234.06	795.24	2.66
3.41	0.52	0.00	0.00	0.00	24.42	0.00	0.27	0.18	1.62	0.03	5.92	0.10	89.54	1.63	8.88	260.48	86.58	583.86	0.29
3.83	2.64	0.00	0.00	0.00	2.40	3.18	0.07	0.13	0.58	0.02	17.40	0.16	25.20	1.29	16.20	87.60	83.40	153.00	0.55
4.73	1.19	0.00	0.00	0.00	32.55	1.95	0.63	0.61	4.06	0.30	86.80	1.09	112.84	4.51	86.80	97.65	653.17	985.18	1.52

USDA ID Code	Food Name	Weight in Grams*	Quantity of Units	Unit of Measure	Protein (gm)	Fat (gm)	Carbohydrate (gm)	Kcalories	Caffeine (gm)	Fiber (gm)	Cholesterol (mg)	Saturated Fat (gm)
	Fast Food-Burrito w/ Beans and C	186.0000	2.000	Each	15.07	11.70	54.96	377.58	0.00	0.00	27.90	6.84
	Fast Food-Burrito w/ Beans and C	204.0000	2.000	Each	16.38	14.67	58.08	412.08	0.00	0.00	32.64	7.61
	Fast Food-Burrito w/ Beans and M	231.0000	2.000	Each	22.48	17.81	66.02	508.20	0.00	0.00	48.51	8.32
	Fast Food-Burrito w/ Beans, Chee	336.0000	2.000	Each	33.30	22.98	85.18	661.92	0.00	0.00	157.92	11.19
	Fast Food-Burrito w/ Beans, Chee	203.0000	2.000	Each	14.58	13.30	39.69	330.89	0.00	0.00	123.83	7.15
	Fast Food-Burrito w/ Beef	220.0000	2.000	Each	26.60	20.81	58.52	523.60	0.00	0.00	63.80	10.45
	Fast Food-Burrito w/ Beef and Ch	201.0000	2.000	Each	21.51	16.54	49.45	426.12	0.00	0.00	54.27	8.00
	Fast Food-Burrito w/ Beef, Chees	304.0000	2.000	Each	40.92	24.78	63.72	632.32	0.00	0.00	170.24	10.40
	Fast Food-Burrito w/ Fruit (Appl	74.0000	1.000	Each	2.50	9.52	34.98	230.88	0.00	0.00	3.70	4.57
	Fast Food-Cheeseburger, Large, D	258.0000	1.000	Each	37.98	43.65	39.65	704.34	0.00	0.00	141.90	17.67
	Fast Food-Cheeseburger, Large, S	185.0000	1.000	Each	30.14	32.99	47.42	608.65	0.00	0.00	96.20	14.84
	Fast Food-Cheeseburger, Large, S	195.0000	1.000	Each	32.00	36.76	37.13	608.40	0.00	0.00	111.15	16.24
	Fast Food-Cheeseburger, Large, S	219.0000	1.000	Each	28.19	32.94	38.39	562.83	0.00	0.00	87.60	15.05
	Fast Food-Cheeseburger, Regular,	228.0000	1.000	Each	29.73	35.27	53.12	649.80	0.00	0.00	93.48	12.77
	Fast Food-Cheeseburger, Regular,	102.0000	1.000	Each	14.77	15.15	31.75	319.26	0.00	0.00	49.98	6.47
	Fast Food-Cheeseburger, Regular,	154.0000	1.000	Each	17.83	19.79	28.14	358.82	0.00	0.00	52.36	9.19
	Fast Food-Cheeseburger, Triple P	304.0000	1.000	Each	56.06	50.95	26.69	796.48	0.00	0.00	161.12	21.71
	Fast Food-Chicken Fillet Sandwic	228.0000	1.000	Each	29.41	38.76	41.59	631.56	0.00	0.00	77.52	12.45
	Fast Food-Chicken Fillet Sandwic	182.0000	1.000	Each	24.12	29.45	38.69	515.06	0.00	0.00	60.06	8.54
	Fast Food-Chicken Nuggets, Plain	17.7000	1.000	Piece	3.01	3.44	2.55	53.28	0.00	0.00	10.27	0.78
	Fast Food-Chicken Nuggets, w/ Ba	130.0000	6.000	Each	17.15	17.97	25.03	330.20	0.00	0.00	61.10	5.58
	Fast Food-Chicken Nuggets, w/ Ho	115.0000	6.000	Each	16.77	17.54	26.88	328.90	0.00	0.00	60.95	5.50
	Fast Food-Chicken Nuggets, w/ Mu	130.0000	6.000	Each	17.42	18.94	20.85	322.40	0.00	0.00	61.10	5.72
	Fast Food-Chicken Nuggets, w/ Sw	130.0000	6.000	Each	16.95	17.95	28.95	345.80	0.00	0.00	61.10	5.51
	Fast Food-Chili Con Carne	253.0000	1.000	Cup	24.62	8.27	21.94	255.53	0.00	0.00	134.09	3.44
	Fast Food-Chimichanga, w/ Beef	174.0000	1.000	Each	19.61	19.68	42.80	424.56	0.00	0.00	8.70	8.51
	Fast Food-Chimichanga, w/ Beef a	183.0000	1.000	Each	20.06	23.44	39.33	442.86	0.00	0.00	51.24	11.18
	Fast Food-Clams, Breaded and Fri	115.0000	0.750	Cup	12.82	26.40	38.81	450.80	0.00	0.00	87.40	6.60
	Fast Food-Cookies, Chocolate Chi	55.0000	1.000	Box	2.89	12.14	36.22	232.65	6.05	0.00	11.55	5.34
	Fast Food-Corn On The Cob w/ But	146.0000	1.000	Each	4.47	3.43	31.94	154.76	0.00	0.00	5.84	1.65
	Fast Food-Crab, Soft-shell, Frie	125.0000	1.000	Each	10.99	17.86	31.20	333.75	0.00	0.00	45.00	4.40
	Fast Food-Croissant w/Egg and Ch	127.0000	1.000	Each	12.79	24.70	24.31	368.30	0.00	0.00	215.90	14.07
	Fast Food-Croissant w/Egg, Chees	160.0000	1.000	Each	20.30	38.16	24.72	523.20	0.00	0.00	216.00	18.22
	Fast Food-Croissant w/Egg, Chees	129.0000	1.000	Each	16.23	28.35	23.65	412.80	0.00	0.00	215.43	15.43
	Fast Food-Croissant w/Egg, Chees	152.0000	1.000	Each	18.92	33.58	24.20	474.24	0.00	0.00	212.80	17.48
	Fast Food-Danish Pastry, Cheese	91.0000	1.000	Each	5.83	24.62	28.69	353.08	0.00	0.00	20.02	5.12
	Fast Food-Danish Pastry, Cinnamo	88.0000	1.000	Each	4.80	16.72	46.85	349.36	0.00	0.00	27.28	3.48
	Fast Food-Danish Pastry, Fruit	94.0000	1.000	Each	4.76	15.93	45.06	334.64	0.00	0.00	18.80	3.32
	Fast Food-Egg and Cheese Sandwic	146.0000	1.000	Each	15.61	19.42	25.93	340.18	0.00	0.00	290.54	6.63
	Fast Food-Egg, Scrambled	94.0000	2.000	Eggs	13.01	15.21	1.96	199.28	0.00	0.00	400.44	5.78
	Fast Food-Enchilada w/ Cheese	163.0000	1.000	Each	9.63	18.84	28.54	319.48	0.00	0.00	44.01	10.60
	Fast Food-Enchilada w/ Cheese an	192.0000	1.000	Each	11.92	17.64	30.47	322.56	0.00	0.00	40.32	9.04
	Fast Food-Enchirito w/ Cheese, B	193.0000	1.000	Each	17.89	16.08	33.79	343.54	0.00	0.00	50.18	7.95
	Fast Food-Fish Fillet, Battered	91.0000	1.000	Each	13.34	11.18	15.44	211.12	0.00	0.46	30.94	2.57
	Fast Food-Fish Sandwich w/ Tarta	158.0000	1.000	Each	16.94	22.77	41.02	431.34	0.00	0.00	55.30	5.23
	Fast Food-Fish Sandwich w/ Tarta	183.0000	1.000	Each	20.61	28.60	47.63	523.38	0.00	0.00	67.71	8.14
	Fast Food-French Toast w/ Butter	135.0000	2.000	Slice	10.34	18.77	36.05	356.40	0.00	0.00	116.10	7.75
	Fast Food-Frijoles w/ Cheese	167.0000	1.000	Cup	11.37	7.78	28.71	225.45	0.00	0.00	36.74	4.07
	Fast Food-Ham and Cheese Sandwic	146.0000	1.000	Each	20.69	15.48	33.35	351.86	0.00	0.00	58.40	6.44
	Fast Food-Ham, Egg, and Cheese S	143.0000	1.000	Each	19.25	16.30	30.95	347.49	0.00	0.00	245.96	7.41
	Fast Food-Hamburger, Double Patt	226.0000	1.000	Each	34.28	26.56	40.27	540.14	0.00	0.00	122.04	10.51
	Fast Food-Hamburger, Double Patt	215.0000	1.000	Each	31.82	32.47	38.74	576.20	0.00	0.00	103.20	12.00
	Fast Food-Hamburger, Double Patt	176.0000	1.000	Each	29.92	27.90	42.93	543.84	0.00	0.00	98.56	10.38
	Fast Food-Hamburger, Large, Sing	218.0000	1.000	Each	25.83	27.36	40.00	512.30	0.00	0.00	87.20	10.42
	Fast Food-Hamburger, Single Patt	106.0000	1.000	Each	12.32	9.77	34.25	272.42	0.00	2.33	29.68	3.56

Monounsaturated Fat (gm)	Polyunsaturated Fat (gm)	Vitamin D (mg)	Vitamin K (mg)	Vitamin E (mg)	Vitamin A (re)	Vitamin C (mg)	Thiamin (mg)	Riboflavin (mg)	Niacin (mg)	Vitamin B_6 (mg)	Folate (mg)	Vitamin B_{12} (mcg)	Calcium (mg)	Iron (mg)	Magnesium (mg)	Phosphorus (mg)	Potassium (mg)	Sodium (mg)	Zinc (mg)
2.49	1.79	0.00	0.00	0.00	238.08	1.67	0.22	0.71	3.57	0.24	74.40	0.89	213.90	2.27	79.98	180.42	496.62	1166.22	1.64
5.37	0.96	0.00	0.00	0.00	20.40	1.22	0.45	0.71	4.39	0.29	95.88	1.16	99.96	4.55	71.40	114.24	579.36	1044.48	3.41
7.02	1.22	0.00	0.00	0.00	64.68	1.85	0.53	0.83	5.41	0.37	115.50	1.73	106.26	4.90	83.16	140.91	656.04	1335.18	3.83
8.47	1.28	0.00	0.00	0.00	383.04	6.72	0.54	1.21	7.69	0.40	164.64	1.98	288.96	7.69	97.44	285.60	809.76	2059.68	6.08
4.47	1.02	0.00	0.00	0.00	150.22	5.08	0.30	0.71	3.86	0.22	75.11	1.10	129.92	3.74	50.75	140.07	410.06	990.64	2.35
7.41	0.86	0.00	0.00	0.00	28.60	1.10	0.24	0.92	6.45	0.31	129.80	1.96	83.60	6.09	81.40	173.80	739.20	1491.60	4.73
6.07	0.98	0.00	0.00	0.00	46.23	1.61	0.40	0.80	5.09	0.30	96.48	1.29	86.43	4.44	60.30	140.70	498.48	1115.55	4.32
9.94	2.22	0.00	0.00	0.00	112.48	3.65	0.61	1.25	8.33	0.36	139.84	2.07	221.92	7.81	69.92	316.16	665.76	2091.52	7.90
3.42	1.06	0.00	0.00	0.00	37.00	0.74	0.17	0.18	1.86	0.07	24.42	0.51	15.54	1.07	7.40	14.80	104.34	211.64	0.40
17.36	4.70	0.00	0.00	0.00	54.18	1.03	0.36	0.49	7.25	0.41	74.82	3.41	239.94	5.91	51.60	394.74	595.98	1148.10	6.68
12.75	2.44	0.56	0.00	0.00	148.00	0.00	0.48	0.57	11.17	0.28	74.00	2.53	90.65	5.46	38.85	421.80	643.80	1589.15	5.55
14.49	2.71	0.00	0.00	0.00	79.95	2.15	0.31	0.41	6.63	0.31	85.80	2.34	161.85	4.74	44.85	399.75	331.50	1043.25	6.83
12.61	2.04	0.00	0.00	1.18	129.21	7.88	0.39	0.46	7.38	0.28	81.03	2.56	205.86	4.66	43.80	310.98	444.57	1108.14	4.60
12.63	6.36	0.00	0.00	1.98	84.36	2.74	0.57	0.43	8.34	0.27	91.20	2.07	168.72	4.72	36.48	348.84	389.88	921.12	4.13
5.77	1.54	0.31	0.00	0.00	36.72	0.00	0.40	0.40	3.70	0.09	54.06	0.97	140.76	2.44	21.42	195.84	164.22	499.80	2.37
7.16	1.48	0.00	0.00	0.00	70.84	2.31	0.32	0.23	6.38	0.15	64.68	1.23	181.72	2.65	26.18	215.60	229.46	976.36	2.62
21.52	3.16	0.00	0.00	0.00	85.12	2.74	0.61	0.64	11.46	0.61	69.92	5.90	282.72	8.30	60.80	541.12	820.80	1212.96	10.88
13.66	9.94	0.00	0.00	0.00	127.68	2.96	0.41	0.46	9.07	0.41	109.44	0.46	257.64	3.63	43.32	405.84	332.88	1238.04	2.90
10.41	8.39	0.00	0.00	0.00	30.94	8.92	0.33	0.24	6.81	0.20	100.10	0.38	60.06	4.68	34.58	232.96	353.08	957.32	1.87
1.75	0.77	0.00	0.00	0.23	0.00	0.00	0.02	0.03	1.25	0.05	5.13	0.05	2.30	0.16	4.07	48.32	50.98	85.67	0.17
8.76	2.39	0.00	0.00	0.00	46.80	0.78	0.10	0.16	7.02	0.34	29.90	0.30	20.80	1.46	24.70	214.50	318.50	829.40	1.12
8.61	2.22	0.00	0.00	0.00	29.90	0.46	0.09	0.15	6.81	0.31	29.90	0.30	17.25	1.32	19.55	202.40	255.30	537.05	1.08
9.04	2.91	0.00	0.00	0.00	32.50	0.39	0.12	0.16	6.94	0.31	29.90	0.31	24.70	1.48	26.00	218.40	279.50	790.40	1.14
8.65	2.24	0.00	0.00	0.00	72.80	0.78	0.10	0.20	6.86	0.33	29.90	0.36	20.80	1.48	23.40	210.60	276.90	677.30	1.09
3.42	0.53	0.00	0.00	0.00	166.98	1.52	0.13	1.14	2.48	0.33	45.54	1.14	68.31	5.19	45.54	197.34	690.69	1006.94	3.57
8.07	1.13	0.00	0.00	0.00	15.66	4.70	0.49	0.64	5.78	0.28	83.52	1.51	62.64	4.54	62.64	123.54	586.38	910.02	4.96
9.44	0.73	0.00	0.00	0.00	126.27	2.75	0.38	0.86	4.67	0.22	91.50	1.30	237.90	3.84	60.39	186.66	203.13	957.09	3.37
11.44	6.77	0.00	0.00	0.00	36.80	0.00	0.21	0.26	2.86	0.03	42.55	1.10	20.70	3.05	31.05	238.05	265.65	833.75	1.63
5.05	1.03	0.00	0.00	0.37	14.85	0.55	0.09	0.19	1.39	0.03	33.00	0.10	19.80	1.47	16.50	52.25	81.95	188.10	0.34
1.01	0.61	0.00	0.00	0.00	96.36	6.86	0.25	0.10	2.18	0.32	43.80	0.00	4.38	0.88	40.88	108.04	359.16	29.20	0.91
7.69	4.88	0.00	0.00	0.00	3.75	0.75	0.10	0.08	1.75	0.15	20.00	4.48	55.00	1.81	25.00	131.25	162.50	1117.50	1.06
7.54	1.37	0.00	0.00	0.00	255.27	0.13	0.19	0.38	1.51	0.10	46.99	0.77	243.84	2.20	21.59	347.98	173.99	551.18	1.75
14.26	3.01	0.00	0.00	0.00	108.80	0.16	0.99	0.32	4.00	0.11	43.20	0.90	144.00	3.04	24.00	289.60	283.20	1115.20	2.14
9.17	1.75	0.00	0.00	0.00	119.97	2.19	0.35	0.34	2.19	0.12	45.15	0.86	150.93	2.19	23.22	276.06	201.24	888.81	1.90
11.40	2.36	0.00	0.00	0.00	117.04	11.40	0.52	0.30	3.19	0.23	45.60	1.00	144.40	2.13	25.84	335.92	272.08	1080.72	2.17
15.60	2.42	0.00	0.00	0.00	42.77	2.64	0.26	0.21	2.55	0.05	54.60	0.23	70.07	1.85	15.47	80.08	116.48	319.41	0.63
10.60	1.65	0.00	0.00	0.00	5.28	2.55	0.26	0.19	2.20	0.05	54.56	0.22	36.96	1.80	14.08	73.92	95.92	326.48	0.48
10.10	1.57	0.00	0.00	0.00	24.44	1.60	0.29	0.21	1.80	0.06	31.02	0.24	21.62	1.40	14.10	68.62	109.98	332.76	0.48
8.26	2.58	0.00	0.00	0.00	181.04	1.46	0.26	0.57	2.07	0.13	97.82	1.14	224.84	2.98	21.90	302.22	188.34	804.46	1.65
5.54	1.85	1.60	0.00	1.58	251.92	3.10	0.08	0.49	0.20	0.18	52.64	0.95	53.58	2.43	13.16	227.48	138.18	210.56	1.56
6.31	0.81	0.00	0.00	0.00	185.82	0.98	0.08	0.42	1.91	0.39	65.20	0.75	324.37	1.32	50.53	133.66	239.61	784.03	2.51
6.14	1.38	0.00	0.00	0.00	142.08	1.34	0.10	0.40	2.52	0.27	67.20	1.02	228.48	3.07	82.56	167.04	574.08	1319.04	2.69
6.52	0.33	0.00	0.00	0.00	133.17	4.63	0.17	0.69	2.99	0.21	59.83	1.62	218.09	2.39	71.41	223.88	559.70	1250.64	2.76
2.35	5.71	0.00	0.00	0.00	10.92	0.00	0.10	0.10	1.91	0.09	15.47	1.01	16.38	1.92	21.84	155.61	291.20	484.12	0.40
7.69	8.25	0.00	0.00	0.87	30.02	2.84	0.33	0.22	3.40	0.11	85.32	1.07	83.74	2.61	33.18	211.72	339.70	614.62	1.00
8.91	9.42	0.92	0.00	1.83	96.99	2.75	0.46	0.42	4.23	0.11	91.50	1.08	184.83	3.50	36.60	311.10	353.19	938.79	1.17
7.07	2.44	0.00	0.00	0.00	145.80	0.14	0.58	0.50	3.92	0.05	72.90	0.36	72.90	1.89	16.20	145.80	176.85	513.00	0.59
2.62	0.70	0.00	0.00	0.00	70.14	1.50	0.13	0.33	1.49	0.20	111.89	0.68	188.71	2.24	85.17	175.35	604.54	881.76	1.74
6.75	1.37	0.00	0.00	0.29	75.92	2.77	0.31	0.48	2.69	0.20	75.92	0.54	129.94	3.24	16.06	151.84	290.54	770.88	1.37
5.75	1.69	0.00	0.00	0.59	148.72	2.72	0.43	0.56	4.20	0.16	75.79	1.23	211.64	3.10	25.74	346.06	210.21	1005.29	1.99
10.33	2.80	0.00	0.00	0.00	11.30	1.13	0.36	0.38	7.57	0.54	76.84	4.07	101.70	5.85	49.72	314.14	569.52	791.00	5.67
14.13	2.77	0.00	0.00	0.00	4.30	1.08	0.34	0.41	6.73	0.37	83.85	3.33	92.45	5.55	45.15	283.80	526.75	741.75	5.81
12.11	2.34	0.70	0.00	1.32	0.00	0.00	0.33	0.37	8.25	0.32	77.44	2.92	86.24	4.56	36.96	234.08	362.56	554.40	5.72
11.42	2.20	0.00	0.00	0.00	32.70	2.62	0.41	0.37	7.28	0.33	82.84	2.38	95.92	4.93	43.60	233.26	479.60	824.04	4.88
3.40	1.01	0.00	0.00	0.01	9.54	2.23	0.29	0.23	3.91	0.12	51.94	1.09	126.14	2.71	23.32	114.48	251.22	534.24	2.25

USDA ID Code	Food Name	Weight in Grams*	Quantity of Units	Unit of Measure	Protein (gm)	Fat (gm)	Carbohydrate (gm)	Kcalories	Caffeine (gm)	Fiber (gm)	Cholesterol (mg)	Saturated Fat (gm)
	Fast Food-Hamburger, Single Patt	90.0000	1.000	Each	12.32	11.82	30.51	274.50	0.00	0.00	35.10	4.14
	Fast Food-Hamburger, Triple Patt	259.0000	1.000	Each	49.99	41.47	28.59	691.53	0.00	0.00	142.45	15.93
	Fast Food-Hot Dog w/ Chili	114.0000	1.000	Each	13.51	13.44	31.29	296.40	0.00	0.00	51.30	4.86
	Fast Food-Hot Dog w/ Corn Flour	175.0000	1.000	Each	16.80	18.90	55.79	460.25	0.00	0.00	78.75	5.16
	Fast Food-Hot Dog, Plain	98.0000	1.000	Each	10.39	14.54	18.03	242.06	0.00	0.00	44.10	5.11
	Fast Food-Ice Milk, Vanilla, Sof	103.0000	1.000	Each	3.89	6.12	24.11	163.77	0.00	0.10	27.81	3.53
	Fast Food-Muffin, English w/ But	63.0000	1.000	Each	4.87	5.76	30.36	189.00	0.00	0.00	12.60	2.43
	Fast Food-Muffin, English w/ Che	115.0000	1.000	Each	15.34	24.27	29.16	393.30	0.00	1.50	58.65	9.86
	Fast Food-Muffin, English w/ Egg	137.0000	1.000	Each	16.69	12.59	26.74	289.07	0.00	1.51	234.27	4.67
	Fast Food-Muffin, English w/ Egg	165.0000	1.000	Each	21.66	30.86	30.97	486.75	0.00	0.00	273.90	12.42
	Fast Food-Nachos w/ Cheese	113.0000	7.000	Each	9.10	18.95	36.33	345.78	0.00	0.00	18.08	7.79
	Fast Food-Nachos w/ Cheese and J	204.0000	7.000	Each	16.81	34.15	60.08	607.92	0.00	0.00	83.64	14.01
	Fast Food-Nachos w/ Cheese, Bean	255.0000	7.000	Each	19.79	30.70	55.82	568.65	0.00	0.00	20.40	12.50
	Fast Food-Nachos w/ Cinnamon and	109.0000	7.000	Each	7.19	35.98	63.39	591.87	0.00	0.00	39.24	18.21
	Fast Food-Onion Rings, Breaded a	83.0000	1.000	Order	3.70	15.51	31.32	275.56	0.00	0.00	14.11	6.96
	Fast Food-Oysters, Battered or B	139.0000	6.000	Each	12.54	17.93	39.88	368.35	0.00	0.00	108.42	4.57
	Fast Food-Pancakes w/ Butter and	232.0000	2.000	Each	8.26	13.99	90.90	519.68	0.00	0.00	58.00	5.85
	Fast Food-Pie, Fried, Fruit (App	85.0000	1.000	Each	2.41	14.37	33.05	266.05	0.00	0.00	12.75	6.51
	Fast Food-Pizza w/ Cheese	63.0000	1.000	Slice	7.68	3.21	20.50	140.49	0.00	0.00	9.45	1.54
	Fast Food-Pizza w/ Cheese, Sausa	79.0000	1.000	Slice	13.01	5.36	21.29	184.07	0.00	0.00	20.54	1.53
	Fast Food-Pizza w/ Pepperoni	71.0000	1.000	Slice	10.12	6.96	19.87	181.05	0.00	0.00	14.20	2.24
	Fast Food-Potato, Baked w/ Chees	296.0000	1.000	Piece	14.62	28.74	46.50	473.60	0.00	0.00	17.76	10.57
	Fast Food-Potato, Baked w/ Chees	299.0000	1.000	Piece	18.42	25.89	44.43	451.49	0.00	0.00	29.90	10.14
	Fast Food-Potato, Baked w/ Chees	339.0000	1.000	Piece	13.66	21.42	46.58	403.41	0.00	0.00	20.34	8.51
	Fast Food-Potato, Baked w/ Chees	395.0000	1.000	Piece	23.23	21.84	55.85	481.90	0.00	0.00	31.60	13.04
	Fast Food-Potato, Baked w/ Sour	302.0000	1.000	Piece	6.67	22.32	50.01	392.60	0.00	0.00	24.16	10.03
	Fast Food-Potato, French Fried I	115.0000	1.000	Large	4.59	18.50	44.36	358.80	0.00	0.00	20.70	8.52
	Fast Food-Potato, French Fried I	115.0000	1.000	Large	4.59	18.50	44.36	357.65	0.00	0.00	16.10	7.63
	Fast Food-Potato, French Fried I	85.0000	1.000	Small	3.66	15.67	33.84	290.70	0.00	2.98	0.00	3.27
	Fast Food-Potato, Mashed	80.0000	0.330	Cup	1.85	0.97	12.90	66.40	0.00	0.00	1.60	0.38
	Fast Food-Potatoes, Hashed Brown	72.0000	0.500	Cup	1.94	9.22	16.15	151.20	0.00	0.00	9.36	4.33
	Fast Food-Salad, w/o Dressing	104.0000	0.750	Cup	1.30	0.07	3.35	16.64	0.00	0.00	0.00	0.01
	Fast Food-Salad, w/o Dressing, w	217.0000	1.500	Cup	8.77	5.79	4.75	101.99	0.00	0.00	97.65	2.97
	Fast Food-Salad, w/o Dressing, w	218.0000	1.500	Cup	17.44	2.18	3.73	104.64	0.00	0.00	71.94	0.59
	Fast Food-Salad, w/o Dressing, w	417.0000	1.500	Cup	16.43	20.85	31.98	379.47	0.00	0.00	50.04	2.59
	Fast Food-Salad, w/o Dressing, w	236.0000	1.500	Cup	14.51	2.48	6.61	106.20	0.00	0.00	179.36	0.66
	Fast Food-Scallops, Breaded and	144.0000	6.000	Each	15.75	19.40	38.49	385.92	0.00	0.00	108.00	4.88
	Fast Food-Shrimp, Breaded and Fr	164.0000	7.000	Each	18.88	24.90	40.00	454.28	0.00	0.00	200.08	5.38
	Fast Food-Steak Sandwich	204.0000	1.000	Each	30.33	14.08	51.96	459.00	0.00	0.00	73.44	3.81
	Fast Food-Submarine Sandwich w/	228.0000	1.000	Each	21.84	18.63	51.05	456.00	0.00	0.00	36.48	6.82
	Fast Food-Submarine Sandwich w/	216.0000	1.000	Each	28.64	12.96	44.30	410.40	0.00	0.00	73.44	7.08
	Fast Food-Submarine Sandwich w/	256.0000	1.000	Each	29.70	27.98	55.37	583.68	0.00	0.00	48.64	5.32
	Fast Food-Sundae, Caramel	155.0000	1.000	Each	7.30	9.27	49.31	303.80	0.00	0.00	24.80	4.51
	Fast Food-Sundae, Hot Fudge	158.0000	1.000	Each	5.64	8.63	47.67	284.40	1.58	0.00	20.54	5.02
	Fast Food-Sundae, Strawberry	153.0000	1.000	Each	6.26	7.85	44.65	267.75	0.00	0.00	21.42	3.73
	Fast Food-Taco	171.0000	1.000	Small	20.66	20.55	26.73	369.36	0.00	0.00	56.43	11.37
	Fast Food-Taco Salad	198.0000	1.500	Cup	13.23	14.77	23.58	279.18	0.00	0.00	43.56	6.83
	Fast Food-Taco Salad w/ Chili Co	261.0000	1.500	Cup	17.41	13.13	26.57	289.71	0.00	0.00	5.22	6.00
	Fast Food-Tostada w/ Guacamole	261.0000	2.000	Each	12.48	23.26	32.02	360.18	0.00	0.00	39.15	9.87
	Fast Food-Tostada, w/ Beans and	144.0000	1.000	Piece	9.60	9.86	26.52	223.20	0.00	0.00	30.24	5.37
	Fast Food-Tostada, w/ Beans, Bee	225.0000	1.000	Piece	16.09	16.94	29.66	333.00	0.00	0.00	74.25	11.48
	Fast Food-Tostada, w/ Beef and C	163.0000	1.000	Piece	18.99	16.35	22.77	314.59	0.00	0.00	40.75	10.40
	Hardee's-Beef, Roast, Big	163.0080	1.000	Each	21.90	13.38	38.93	364.94	0.00	1.09	54.74	6.08
	Hardee's-Beef, Roast, Sandwich	141.7460	1.000	Each	18.65	11.19	38.54	323.28	0.00	0.99	43.52	4.97
	Hardee's-Big Cheese	141.7500	1.000	Each	30.00	30.00	28.00	495.00	0.00	0.00	0.00	0.00

Monounsaturated Fat (gm)	Polyunsaturated Fat (gm)	Vitamin D (mg)	Vitamin K (mg)	Vitamin E (mg)	Vitamin A (re)	Vitamin C (mg)	Thiamin (mg)	Riboflavin (mg)	Niacin (mg)	Vitamin B_6 (mg)	Folate (mg)	Vitamin B_{12} (mcg)	Calcium (mg)	Iron (mg)	Magnesium (mg)	Phosphorus (mg)	Potassium (mg)	Sodium (mg)	Zinc (mg)
5.45	0.92	0.27	0.00	0.50	0.00	0.00	0.33	0.27	3.72	0.06	53.10	0.89	63.00	2.40	18.90	102.60	144.90	387.00	2.00
18.23	2.75	0.00	0.00	0.00	15.54	1.30	0.31	0.54	10.96	0.62	75.11	4.92	64.75	8.31	54.39	393.68	784.77	712.25	10.75
6.60	1.19	0.00	0.00	0.00	5.70	2.74	0.22	0.40	3.74	0.05	72.96	0.30	19.38	3.28	10.26	191.52	166.44	479.94	0.78
9.12	3.50	0.00	0.00	0.00	36.75	0.00	0.28	0.70	4.17	0.09	103.25	0.44	101.50	6.18	17.50	166.25	262.50	973.00	1.31
6.85	1.71	0.00	0.00	0.00	0.00	0.10	0.24	0.27	3.65	0.05	48.02	0.51	23.52	2.31	12.74	97.02	143.08	670.32	1.98
1.81	0.36	0.21	0.00	0.38	51.50	1.13	0.05	0.26	0.31	0.06	12.36	0.21	153.47	0.15	15.45	139.05	168.92	91.67	0.57
1.53	1.35	0.00	0.00	0.13	33.39	0.76	0.25	0.32	2.61	0.04	56.70	0.02	102.69	1.59	13.23	85.05	69.30	386.19	0.42
10.09	2.69	0.00	0.00	0.49	86.25	1.27	0.70	0.25	4.14	0.15	66.70	0.68	167.90	2.25	24.15	186.30	215.05	1036.15	1.68
4.67	1.56	1.10	0.00	0.85	156.18	1.78	0.49	0.45	3.33	0.15	43.84	0.67	150.70	2.44	23.29	269.89	198.65	728.84	1.56
12.75	3.32	0.00	0.00	0.00	171.60	1.49	0.84	0.50	4.46	0.20	54.45	1.37	196.35	3.47	29.70	287.10	293.70	1135.20	2.36
7.99	2.24	0.00	0.00	0.00	91.53	1.24	0.19	0.37	1.54	0.20	10.17	0.82	272.33	1.28	55.37	275.72	171.76	815.86	1.79
14.40	4.02	0.00	0.00	0.00	471.24	1.02	0.12	0.49	2.84	0.37	18.36	1.02	620.16	2.45	108.12	393.72	293.76	1736.04	2.90
10.99	5.69	0.00	0.00	0.00	469.20	4.85	0.23	0.69	3.34	0.41	38.25	1.02	385.05	2.78	96.90	387.60	451.35	1800.30	3.65
11.84	4.13	0.00	0.00	0.00	10.90	7.96	0.19	0.45	3.92	0.17	7.63	1.72	85.02	2.89	19.62	32.70	78.48	439.27	0.59
6.65	0.66	0.00	0.00	0.33	0.83	0.58	0.08	0.10	0.92	0.06	54.78	0.12	73.04	0.85	15.77	86.32	129.48	429.94	0.35
6.92	4.64	0.00	0.00	0.00	108.42	4.17	0.31	0.35	4.42	0.03	30.58	1.01	27.80	4.46	23.63	195.99	182.09	676.93	15.64
5.27	1.95	0.00	0.00	1.39	69.60	3.48	0.39	0.56	3.39	0.12	51.04	0.23	127.60	2.62	48.72	475.60	250.56	1104.32	1.02
5.83	1.16	0.00	0.00	0.37	33.15	1.11	0.10	0.08	0.98	0.03	4.25	0.08	12.75	0.88	7.65	37.40	51.00	324.70	0.17
0.99	0.49	0.00	0.00	0.00	73.71	1.26	0.18	0.16	2.48	0.04	34.65	0.33	116.55	0.58	15.75	112.77	109.62	335.79	0.81
2.54	0.92	0.00	0.00	0.00	101.12	1.58	0.21	0.17	1.96	0.09	32.39	0.36	101.12	1.53	18.17	131.14	178.54	382.36	1.11
3.14	1.16	0.00	0.00	0.00	54.67	1.63	0.13	0.23	3.05	0.06	36.92	0.18	64.61	0.94	8.52	75.26	152.65	266.96	0.52
10.72	6.04	0.00	0.00	0.00	227.92	26.05	0.24	0.21	3.34	0.71	26.64	0.18	310.80	3.02	65.12	319.68	1166.24	381.84	1.89
9.72	4.75	0.00	0.00	0.00	173.42	28.70	0.27	0.24	3.98	0.75	29.90	0.33	307.97	3.14	68.77	346.84	1178.06	971.75	2.15
7.70	4.17	0.00	0.00	0.00	277.98	48.48	0.27	0.27	3.59	0.78	61.02	0.34	335.61	3.32	77.97	345.78	1440.75	484.77	2.03
6.83	0.91	0.00	0.00	0.00	173.80	31.60	0.28	0.36	4.19	0.95	47.40	0.24	410.80	6.12	110.60	497.70	1572.10	699.15	3.79
7.88	3.32	0.00	0.00	0.00	277.84	33.82	0.27	0.18	3.71	0.79	33.22	0.21	105.70	3.11	69.46	184.22	1383.16	181.20	0.91
8.03	0.93	0.00	0.00	0.02	3.45	6.10	0.16	0.05	2.60	0.30	37.95	0.14	18.40	1.55	37.95	152.95	818.80	187.45	0.60
8.23	1.99	0.00	0.00	0.00	3.45	6.10	0.16	0.05	2.60	0.30	37.95	0.14	18.40	1.55	37.95	152.95	818.80	187.45	0.60
9.05	2.66	0.00	0.00	1.04	0.00	9.86	0.07	0.03	2.42	0.31	32.30	0.00	11.90	0.66	33.15	109.65	585.65	168.30	0.40
0.28	0.23	0.00	0.00	0.00	8.00	0.32	0.07	0.04	0.96	0.18	6.40	0.04	16.80	0.38	14.40	44.00	235.20	181.60	0.26
3.86	0.47	0.00	0.00	0.12	2.88	5.47	0.08	0.01	1.07	0.17	7.92	0.01	7.20	0.48	15.84	69.12	267.12	290.16	0.22
0.00	0.03	0.00	0.00	0.00	118.56	24.13	0.03	0.05	0.57	0.08	38.48	0.00	13.52	0.66	11.44	40.56	178.88	27.04	0.22
1.76	0.48	0.00	0.00	0.00	115.01	9.77	0.09	0.17	0.98	0.11	84.63	0.30	99.82	0.67	23.87	132.37	371.07	119.35	1.00
0.68	0.57	0.00	0.00	0.00	95.92	17.44	0.11	0.13	5.89	0.44	67.58	0.20	37.06	1.09	32.70	170.04	446.90	209.28	0.89
4.84	9.09	0.00	0.00	0.00	638.01	38.36	0.29	0.21	3.54	0.33	187.65	1.71	70.89	3.17	50.04	204.33	600.48	1572.09	1.67
0.83	0.50	0.00	0.00	0.00	77.88	9.20	0.12	0.17	1.16	0.14	87.32	3.78	59.00	0.90	37.76	160.48	403.56	488.52	1.27
12.56	0.60	0.00	0.00	0.00	41.76	0.00	0.20	0.85	0.00	0.07	53.28	0.43	18.72	2.04	31.68	292.32	293.76	918.72	1.08
17.38	0.64	0.00	0.00	0.00	36.08	0.00	0.21	0.90	0.00	0.07	36.08	0.15	83.64	2.95	39.36	344.40	183.68	1446.48	1.21
5.34	3.35	0.00	0.00	0.00	44.88	5.51	0.41	0.37	7.30	0.37	89.76	1.57	91.80	5.16	48.96	297.84	524.28	797.64	4.53
8.23	2.28	0.00	0.00	0.00	79.80	12.31	1.00	0.80	5.49	0.14	86.64	1.09	189.24	2.51	68.40	287.28	394.44	1650.72	2.58
1.84	2.61	0.00	0.00	0.00	49.68	5.62	0.41	0.41	5.96	0.32	71.28	1.81	41.04	2.81	66.96	192.24	330.48	844.56	4.38
13.41	7.30	0.00	0.00	0.00	40.96	3.58	0.46	0.33	11.34	0.23	102.40	1.61	74.24	2.64	79.36	220.16	335.36	1292.80	1.87
3.04	1.01	0.31	0.00	0.90	68.20	3.41	0.06	0.29	0.95	0.05	12.40	0.60	189.10	0.22	27.90	217.00	317.75	195.30	0.82
2.34	0.81	0.47	0.00	0.66	56.88	2.37	0.06	0.30	1.07	0.13	9.48	0.65	206.98	0.58	33.18	227.52	395.00	181.70	0.95
2.66	1.03	0.46	0.00	0.78	58.14	1.99	0.06	0.28	0.90	0.08	18.36	0.64	160.65	0.32	24.48	154.53	270.81	91.80	0.66
6.58	0.96	0.00	0.00	0.00	147.06	2.22	0.15	0.44	3.21	0.24	68.40	1.04	220.59	2.41	70.11	203.49	473.67	801.99	3.93
5.17	1.74	0.00	0.00	0.00	77.22	3.56	0.10	0.36	2.46	0.22	83.16	0.63	192.06	2.28	51.48	142.56	415.80	762.30	2.69
4.54	1.54	0.00	0.00	0.00	214.02	3.39	0.16	0.50	2.53	0.52	91.35	0.73	245.34	2.66	52.20	153.99	391.50	884.79	3.29
8.48	3.05	0.00	0.00	0.00	216.63	3.65	0.13	0.57	1.98	0.26	114.84	0.99	422.82	1.62	73.08	232.29	649.89	798.66	4.07
3.05	0.75	0.00	0.00	0.00	84.96	1.30	0.10	0.33	1.32	0.16	43.20	0.69	210.24	1.89	59.04	116.64	403.20	542.88	1.90
3.51	0.61	0.00	0.00	0.00	173.25	4.05	0.09	0.50	2.86	0.25	85.50	1.13	189.00	2.45	67.50	173.25	490.50	870.75	3.17
3.34	0.98	0.00	0.00	0.00	96.17	2.61	0.10	0.55	3.15	0.23	74.98	1.17	216.79	2.87	63.57	179.30	572.13	896.50	3.68
6.08	2.43	0.00	0.00	0.24	0.00	0.00	0.36	0.41	6.57	0.34	29.20	2.98	80.29	4.50	40.14	279.79	389.27	1070.50	7.42
4.97	2.49	0.00	0.00	0.25	0.00	0.00	0.32	0.36	5.72	0.30	24.87	2.60	69.63	3.85	34.81	243.70	323.28	907.67	6.47
0.00	0.00	0.00	0.00	0.00	0.00	0.00	0.00	0.00	0.00	0.00	0.00	0.00	0.00	0.00	0.00	0.00	0.00	1251.00	0.00

USDA ID Code	Food Name	Weight in Grams*	Quantity of Units	Unit of Measure	Protein (gm)	Fat (gm)	Carbohydrate (gm)	Kcalories	Caffeine (gm)	Fiber (gm)	Cholesterol (mg)	Saturated Fat (gm)
	Hardee's-Big Deluxe	248.1000	1.000	Each	31.00	41.00	46.00	675.00	0.00	0.00	0.00	0.00
	Hardee's-Big Twin	141.7460	1.000	Each	18.84	20.48	27.86	368.70	0.00	1.39	45.06	9.01
	Hardee's-Biscuit	77.9610	1.000	Each	5.00	13.00	35.00	275.00	0.00	0.00	0.00	0.00
	Hardee's-Cheeseburger	100.6310	1.000	Each	17.00	17.00	29.00	335.00	0.00	0.00	0.00	0.00
	Hardee's-Chicken Fillet	191.3580	1.000	Each	27.00	26.00	42.00	510.00	0.00	0.00	0.00	0.00
	Hardee's-Fish Sandwich, Big	191.3580	1.000	Each	20.00	26.00	49.00	514.00	0.00	0.00	0.00	0.00
	Hardee's-Ham & Cheese, Hot	141.7460	1.000	Each	23.00	15.00	37.00	376.00	0.00	0.00	0.00	0.00
	Hardee's-Hamburger	100.0630	1.000	Each	17.00	13.00	29.00	305.00	0.00	0.00	0.00	0.00
	Hardee's-Hot Dog	50.0000	1.000	Each	11.00	22.00	26.00	346.00	0.00	0.00	0.00	0.00
	Jack In The Box-Breakfast Jack	126.0000	1.000	Each	18.74	13.54	29.16	313.44	0.00	0.00	189.52	5.31
	Jack In The Box-Cheeseburger, Ba	242.0000	1.000	Each	35.00	45.00	41.00	705.00	0.00	0.00	113.00	14.90
	Jack In The Box-Cheesecake	99.0000	1.000	Each	8.00	18.00	29.00	309.00	0.00	0.00	63.00	9.40
	Jack In The Box-French Fries, Re	109.0000	1.000	Order	4.00	17.00	45.00	351.00	0.00	0.00	0.00	4.00
	Jack In The Box-French Fries, Sm	68.0000	1.000	Order	3.00	11.00	28.00	219.00	0.00	0.00	0.00	2.50
	Jack In The Box-Jumbo Jack	222.0000	1.000	Each	25.27	26.17	40.61	497.24	0.00	0.00	72.20	10.29
	Jack In The Box-Jumbo Jack w/ Ch	242.0000	1.000	Each	28.47	31.14	40.04	558.74	0.00	0.00	97.87	13.35
	K.F.C.-Breast, Center, Original	103.0000	1.000	Each	25.18	15.26	9.16	260.93	0.00	0.08	86.98	3.81
	K.F.C.-Chicken Sandwich, Colonel	166.0000	1.000	Each	20.80	27.00	39.00	482.00	0.00	1.40	47.00	6.00
	K.F.C.-Drumstick, Original Recip	57.0000	1.000	Each	11.57	11.57	4.96	168.52	0.00	0.00	58.65	2.48
	K.F.C.-French Fries	77.0000	1.000	Order	3.20	12.00	31.00	244.00	0.00	0.00	2.00	3.00
	K.F.C.-Potatoes, Mashed, and Gra	98.0000	1.000	Each	2.40	2.00	12.00	71.00	0.00	0.00	0.00	1.00
	K.F.C.-Thigh, Original Recipe	95.0000	1.000	Each	15.97	23.95	11.18	324.12	0.00	0.08	102.98	6.39
	K.F.C.-Wing, Original Recipe	53.0000	1.000	Each	11.80	11.00	5.00	172.00	0.00	0.00	59.00	3.00
	McDonald's-Arch Deluxe	239.0000	1.000	Each	28.00	31.00	39.00	550.00	0.00	4.00	90.00	11.00
	McDonald's-Arch Deluxe w/Bacon	247.0000	1.000	Each	32.00	34.00	39.00	590.00	0.00	4.00	100.00	12.00
	McDonald's-Big Mac	215.0000	1.000	Each	25.00	32.00	43.00	560.00	0.00	0.00	103.00	10.10
	McDonald's-Biscuit w/ Spread	75.0000	1.000	Each	5.00	13.00	32.00	260.00	0.00	1.00	1.00	3.00
	McDonald's-Biscuit, Bacon, Egg a	153.0000	1.000	Each	18.00	28.00	36.00	470.00	0.00	1.00	235.00	8.04
	McDonald's-Biscuit, Sausage	118.0000	1.000	Each	11.00	31.00	35.00	470.00	0.00	0.00	44.00	8.00
	McDonald's-Biscuit, Sausage w/ E	175.0000	1.000	Each	19.00	28.00	27.00	440.00	0.00	0.00	260.00	10.00
	McDonald's-Burrito, Breakfast	117.0000	1.000	Each	13.00	19.00	23.00	320.00	0.00	1.00	195.00	7.00
	McDonald's-Cheeseburger	116.0000	1.000	Each	15.00	13.00	35.00	320.00	0.00	0.00	50.00	5.00
	McDonald's-Chicken McNuggets	18.5000	1.000	Each	3.33	2.50	2.83	45.00	0.00	0.00	9.17	0.58
	McDonald's-Chicken Sld, Grilled,	257.0000	1.000	Each	21.00	1.50	7.00	120.00	0.00	0.00	45.00	0.00
	McDonald's-Chicken, Crispy, Delu	223.0000	1.000	Each	26.00	25.00	43.00	0.00	0.00	3.00	55.00	4.00
	McDonald's-Chicken, Grilled, Del	223.0000	1.000	Each	27.00	20.00	38.00	300.00	0.00	3.00	50.00	1.00
	McDonald's-Cookies, McDonaldland	56.6990	1.000	Each	3.00	5.00	32.00	180.00	0.00	0.00	0.00	1.00
	McDonald's-Danish, Apple	105.0000	1.000	Each	5.00	16.00	51.00	360.00	0.00	1.60	25.00	4.00
	McDonald's-Danish, Cheese, Iced	110.0000	1.000	Each	7.00	22.00	47.00	410.00	0.00	0.00	47.00	6.00
	McDonald's-Eggs, Scrambled	100.0000	1.000	Each	12.00	10.00	1.00	140.00	0.00	0.00	425.00	3.00
	McDonald's-Fish Filet Deluxe	141.0000	1.000	Each	27.00	28.00	54.00	560.00	0.00	1.09	49.65	5.16
	McDonald's-French Fries, Large	122.0000	1.000	Order	6.00	22.00	57.00	450.00	0.00	0.00	0.00	5.00
	McDonald's-French Fries, Small	68.0000	1.000	Order	3.00	12.00	26.00	220.00	0.00	0.00	0.00	2.50
	McDonald's-French Fries, Super S	176.0000	1.000	Each	8.00	26.00	68.00	540.00	0.00	6.00	0.00	4.50
	McDonald's-Hamburger	102.0000	1.000	Each	13.00	9.00	34.00	260.00	0.00	0.00	30.00	3.50
	McDonald's-Hotcakes w/ Margarine	174.0000	1.000	Each	13.00	19.00	100.00	570.00	0.00	0.00	15.00	3.00
	McDonald's-Ice Crm Cone, Vanilla	90.0000	1.000	Each	4.00	4.50	23.00	150.00	0.00	0.00	20.00	3.00
	McDonald's-McMuffin, Egg	135.0000	1.000	Each	17.61	10.76	27.39	283.70	0.00	1.37	221.09	3.72
	McDonald's-McMuffin, Sausage	135.0000	1.000	Each	15.00	20.00	27.00	345.00	0.00	0.00	57.00	7.00
	McDonald's-McMuffin, Sausage w/	159.0000	1.000	Each	21.00	25.00	27.00	430.00	0.00	0.00	270.00	8.00
	McDonald's-Muffin, Apple Bran, L	114.0000	1.000	Each	6.00	3.00	61.00	300.00	0.00	3.00	0.00	0.50
	McDonald's-Muffin, English w/ Sp	58.0000	1.000	Each	5.00	4.00	26.00	170.00	0.00	1.60	9.00	2.40
	McDonald's-Potatoes, Hash Brown	53.0000	1.000	Each	1.00	7.00	15.00	130.00	0.00	0.00	0.00	1.00
	McDonald's-Quarter Pounder	166.0000	1.000	Each	23.00	21.00	37.00	420.00	0.00	0.00	85.00	8.00
	McDonald's-Quarter Pounder w/ Ch	200.0000	1.000	Each	28.00	30.00	38.00	530.00	0.00	2.00	95.00	13.00

Monounsaturated Fat (gm)	Polyunsaturated Fat (gm)	Vitamin D (mg)	Vitamin K (mg)	Vitamin E (mg)	Vitamin A (re)	Vitamin C (mg)	Thiamin (mg)	Riboflavin (mg)	Niacin (mg)	Vitamin B_6 (mg)	Folate (mg)	Vitamin B_{12} (mcg)	Calcium (mg)	Iron (mg)	Magnesium (mg)	Phosphorus (mg)	Potassium (mg)	Sodium (mg)	Zinc (mg)
0.00	0.00	0.00	0.00	0.00	0.00	0.00	0.00	0.00	0.00	0.00	0.00	0.00	0.00	0.00	0.00	0.00	0.00	1063.00	0.00
7.37	4.10	0.00	0.00	0.74	13.93	2.46	0.23	0.25	5.49	0.22	27.86	1.86	65.55	3.28	28.68	161.41	229.42	475.22	3.77
0.00	0.00	0.00	0.00	0.00	0.00	0.00	0.00	0.00	0.00	0.00	0.00	0.00	0.00	0.00	0.00	0.00	0.00	650.00	0.00
0.00	0.00	0.00	0.00	0.00	0.00	2.00	0.51	0.32	5.50	0.00	0.00	0.00	0.00	0.00	0.00	0.00	0.00	789.00	0.00
0.00	0.00	0.00	0.00	0.00	0.00	0.00	0.00	0.00	0.00	0.00	0.00	0.00	0.00	0.00	0.00	0.00	0.00	360.00	0.00
0.00	0.00	0.00	0.00	0.00	0.00	0.00	0.00	0.00	0.00	0.00	0.00	0.00	0.00	0.00	0.00	0.00	0.00	314.00	0.00
0.00	0.00	0.00	0.00	0.00	0.00	0.00	0.00	0.00	0.00	0.00	0.00	0.00	0.00	0.00	0.00	0.00	0.00	1067.00	0.00
0.00	0.00	0.00	0.00	0.00	0.00	2.00	0.55	0.58	6.40	0.00	0.00	0.00	0.00	0.00	0.00	0.00	0.00	682.00	0.00
0.00	0.00	0.00	0.00	0.00	0.00	0.00	0.00	0.00	0.00	0.00	0.00	0.00	0.00	0.00	0.00	0.00	0.00	744.00	0.00
5.21	2.60	0.00	0.00	0.14	138.50	3.12	0.43	0.49	5.31	0.15	0.00	1.15	184.31	2.60	24.99	322.81	197.85	1079.85	1.87
15.70	8.70	0.00	0.00	0.60	70.00	7.80	0.24	0.48	8.36	0.00	0.00	0.00	200.00	2.80	0.00	0.00	0.00	1240.00	0.00
7.40	1.60	0.00	0.00	0.32	0.00	0.00	0.05	0.24	1.90	0.00	0.00	0.00	88.00	0.30	0.00	0.00	0.00	208.00	0.00
7.00	0.00	0.00	0.00	5.31	0.00	25.80	0.18	0.03	3.61	0.00	0.00	0.00	0.00	0.70	0.00	0.00	0.00	194.00	0.00
7.00	0.00	0.00	0.00	10.36	0.00	16.20	0.11	0.00	2.28	0.00	0.00	0.00	0.00	0.40	0.00	0.00	0.00	121.00	0.00
11.37	2.17	0.00	0.00	0.18	66.78	3.61	0.42	0.31	10.47	0.27	0.00	2.42	120.93	4.06	39.71	235.54	444.00	1023.37	3.79
11.21	1.78	0.00	0.00	0.21	195.74	4.45	0.46	0.34	10.05	0.28	0.00	2.71	242.89	4.09	43.60	365.67	443.96	1482.25	4.27
3.59	1.53	0.00	0.00	0.46	15.26	0.00	0.08	0.13	14.04	0.59	3.81	0.35	16.02	1.22	30.52	238.04	264.75	602.74	1.14
3.90	9.00	0.00	0.00	2.30	14.00	0.00	0.39	0.27	10.64	0.59	29.00	0.31	100.00	3.10	41.00	261.00	297.00	1060.00	1.50
3.06	1.65	0.00	0.00	0.41	14.04	0.00	0.05	0.13	3.39	0.20	4.96	0.18	6.61	0.74	13.22	99.13	129.70	267.65	1.65
7.00	1.00	0.00	0.00	0.00	0.00	15.60	0.15	0.05	1.90	0.00	0.00	0.00	0.00	0.30	0.00	0.00	0.00	139.00	0.00
0.00	0.00	0.00	0.00	0.00	0.00	0.00	0.00	0.03	1.14	0.00	0.00	0.00	16.00	0.20	0.00	0.00	0.00	339.00	0.00
5.59	3.19	0.00	0.00	0.48	27.94	0.00	0.09	0.23	6.55	0.32	7.98	0.29	12.77	1.44	23.15	176.43	223.53	549.24	2.39
6.00	2.00	0.00	0.00	0.00	0.00	0.00	0.03	0.07	2.85	0.00	0.00	0.00	24.00	0.30	0.00	0.00	0.00	383.00	0.00
0.00	0.00	0.00	0.00	0.00	10.00	0.00	0.00	0.00	0.00	0.00	0.00	0.00	6.00	25.00	0.00	0.00	0.00	1010.00	0.00
0.00	0.00	0.00	0.00	0.00	10.00	0.00	0.00	0.00	0.00	0.00	0.00	0.00	6.00	6.00	0.00	0.00	0.00	1150.00	0.00
20.10	1.50	0.00	0.00	0.00	106.00	2.00	0.48	0.41	6.80	0.27	21.00	1.80	256.00	4.00	38.00	314.00	237.00	950.00	4.70
9.00	1.00	0.00	0.00	1.80	0.00	0.00	0.23	0.10	1.52	0.03	6.00	0.10	75.00	1.30	14.00	168.00	100.00	730.00	0.70
15.79	1.96	0.00	0.00	1.47	156.92	0.00	0.35	0.32	2.45	0.17	17.65	0.58	181.44	2.55	30.40	442.33	232.44	1250.00	1.67
17.00	3.00	0.00	0.00	0.00	0.00	0.00	0.45	0.17	3.80	0.00	0.00	0.00	64.00	1.00	0.00	0.00	0.00	1080.00	0.00
20.00	3.00	0.00	0.00	0.00	60.00	0.00	0.45	0.34	3.80	0.00	0.00	0.00	80.00	2.00	0.00	0.00	0.00	1210.00	0.00
0.00	0.00	0.00	0.00	0.00	10.00	15.00	0.00	0.00	0.00	0.00	0.00	0.00	8.00	10.00	0.00	0.00	0.00	600.00	0.00
7.70	1.00	0.00	0.00	0.50	118.00	2.00	0.29	0.21	3.90	0.12	18.00	0.94	199.00	2.30	21.00	177.00	223.00	750.00	2.10
1.67	0.25	0.00	0.00	0.00	0.00	0.00	0.02	0.02	1.27	0.00	0.00	0.00	0.00	0.10	0.00	0.00	0.00	96.67	0.00
0.00	0.00	0.00	0.00	0.00	120.00	40.00	0.00	0.00	0.00	0.00	0.00	0.00	4.00	8.00	0.00	0.00	0.00	240.00	0.00
0.00	0.00	0.00	0.00	0.00	6.00	8.00	0.00	0.00	0.00	0.00	0.00	0.00	6.00	15.00	0.00	0.00	0.00	1060.00	0.00
0.00	0.00	0.00	0.00	0.00	6.00	8.00	0.00	0.00	0.00	0.00	0.00	0.00	6.00	15.00	0.00	0.00	0.00	930.00	0.00
7.00	1.00	0.00	0.00	0.00	0.00	0.00	0.23	0.17	1.90	0.00	0.00	0.00	0.00	1.00	0.00	0.00	0.00	190.00	0.00
11.00	2.00	0.00	0.00	3.80	35.00	15.00	0.30	0.17	2.20	0.03	3.00	0.00	14.00	1.40	8.00	31.00	69.00	290.00	0.20
13.00	2.00	0.00	0.00	0.00	40.00	0.00	0.30	0.26	1.90	0.00	0.00	0.00	32.00	0.80	0.00	0.00	0.00	420.00	0.00
5.00	2.00	0.00	0.00	0.00	100.00	0.00	0.06	0.26	0.00	0.00	0.00	0.00	48.00	1.00	0.00	0.00	0.00	290.00	0.00
10.13	10.72	0.00	0.00	0.00	43.69	0.00	0.30	0.14	2.68	0.10	19.86	0.81	163.84	1.79	26.81	227.39	148.94	1060.00	0.89
15.00	2.00	0.00	0.00	0.00	0.00	15.00	0.23	0.00	2.85	0.00	0.00	0.00	0.00	0.60	0.00	0.00	0.00	290.00	0.00
8.00	1.00	0.00	0.00	0.00	0.00	9.00	0.15	0.00	1.90	0.00	0.00	0.00	0.00	0.20	0.00	0.00	0.00	110.00	0.00
0.00	0.00	0.00	0.00	0.00	0.00	0.00	0.00	0.00	0.00	0.00	0.00	0.00	35.00	8.00	0.00	0.00	0.00	350.00	0.00
5.00	1.00	0.00	0.00	0.00	40.00	4.00	0.30	0.17	3.80	0.00	0.00	0.00	15.00	1.50	0.00	0.00	0.00	580.00	0.00
5.00	5.00	0.00	0.00	0.00	40.00	0.00	0.30	0.34	2.85	0.00	0.00	0.00	80.00	1.00	0.00	0.00	0.00	750.00	0.00
0.00	0.00	0.00	0.00	0.00	6.00	2.00	0.00	0.00	0.00	0.00	0.00	0.00	10.00	2.00	0.00	0.00	0.00	75.00	0.00
5.97	1.27	0.00	0.00	1.76	146.74	0.98	0.46	0.32	3.62	0.16	43.04	0.78	250.43	2.74	32.28	312.07	208.37	723.91	1.76
11.00	2.00	0.00	0.00	0.00	40.00	0.00	0.53	0.26	4.75	0.00	0.00	0.00	160.00	1.50	0.00	0.00	0.00	770.00	0.00
14.00	3.00	0.00	0.00	0.00	100.00	0.00	0.53	0.43	4.75	0.00	0.00	0.00	200.00	2.00	0.00	0.00	0.00	920.00	0.00
0.00	0.00	0.00	0.00	0.00	0.00	0.00	0.00	0.00	0.00	0.00	0.00	0.00	10.00	8.00	0.00	0.00	0.00	380.00	0.00
2.00	1.00	0.00	0.00	0.10	37.00	0.00	0.33	0.14	2.50	0.10	51.00	0.00	151.00	1.60	12.00	60.00	74.00	285.00	0.40
4.00	2.00	0.00	0.00	0.00	0.00	1.20	0.06	0.00	0.76	0.00	0.00	0.00	0.00	0.00	0.00	0.00	0.00	330.00	0.00
11.00	1.00	0.00	0.00	0.00	40.00	3.60	0.38	0.26	6.65	0.00	0.00	0.00	120.00	2.00	0.00	0.00	0.00	645.00	0.00
0.00	0.00	0.00	0.00	0.00	10.00	4.00	0.00	0.00	0.00	0.00	0.00	0.00	15.00	25.00	0.00	0.00	0.00	1290.00	0.00

USDA ID Code	Food Name	Weight in Grams*	Quantity of Units	Unit of Measure	Protein (gm)	Fat (gm)	Carbohydrate (gm)	Kcalories	Caffeine (gm)	Fiber (gm)	Cholesterol (mg)	Saturated Fat (gm)
	McDonald's-Salad, Garden	189.0000	1.000	Each	4.00	2.00	6.00	50.00	0.00	0.00	65.00	0.60
	McDonald's-Shake, Chocolate Lowf	294.1240	1.000	Each	11.04	1.71	66.25	321.23	0.00	0.00	10.04	0.70
	McDonald's-Shake, Strawberry Low	294.1240	1.000	Each	11.00	9.00	60.00	360.00	0.00	0.00	10.00	0.60
	McDonald's-Shake, Vanilla Lowfat	294.1240	1.000	Each	11.00	9.00	60.00	360.00	0.00	0.00	10.00	0.60
	McDonald's-Sweet Roll, Cinnamon	95.0000	1.000	Each	7.00	20.00	47.00	400.00	0.00	2.00	75.00	5.00
	Subway-BLT- 6" white	191.0000	1.000	Each	14.00	10.00	38.00	311.00	0.00	3.00	16.00	3.00
	Subway-BMT- 6" Italian	213.0000	1.000	Each	44.00	55.00	83.00	982.00	0.00	5.00	133.00	20.00
	Subway-BMT- 6" Wheat	253.0000	1.000	Each	21.00	22.00	45.00	460.00	0.00	3.00	56.00	7.00
	Subway-BMT-Classic Italian - 6"	246.0000	1.000	Each	21.00	21.00	39.00	445.00	0.00	3.00	56.00	8.00
	Subway-Bologna - Deli Sandwich	171.0000	1.000	Each	10.00	12.00	38.00	292.00	0.00	2.00	20.00	4.00
	Subway-Chicken Breast, Roasted	246.0000	1.000	Each	26.00	6.00	41.00	332.00	0.00	3.00	48.00	1.00
	Subway-Chicken Taco Sub - 6" whi	286.0000	1.000	Each	24.00	16.00	43.00	421.00	0.00	3.00	52.00	5.00
	Subway-Club - 6" white	246.0000	1.000	Each	21.00	5.00	40.00	297.00	0.00	3.00	26.00	1.00
	Subway-Club Sandwich - 12" Itali	213.0000	1.000	Each	46.00	22.00	83.00	693.00	0.00	5.00	84.00	7.00
	Subway-Club Sandwich - 12" Wheat	220.0000	1.000	Each	47.00	23.00	89.00	722.00	0.00	6.00	84.00	7.00
	Subway-Cold Cut Combo - 12" Ital	184.0000	1.000	Each	46.00	40.00	83.00	853.00	0.00	5.00	166.00	12.00
	Subway-Cold Cut Combo - 12" Whea	184.0000	1.000	Each	48.00	41.00	88.00	853.00	0.00	6.00	166.00	12.00
	Subway-Cold Cut Trio - 6" white	246.0000	1.000	Each	19.00	13.00	39.00	362.00	0.00	3.00	64.00	4.00
	Subway-Ham - 6" white	232.0000	1.000	Each	18.00	5.00	39.00	287.00	0.00	3.00	28.00	1.00
	Subway-Ham - Deli Sandwich	171.0000	1.000	Each	11.00	4.00	37.00	234.00	0.00	2.00	14.00	1.00
	Subway-Ham and Cheese - 12" Ital	184.0000	1.000	Each	38.00	18.00	81.00	643.00	0.00	5.00	73.00	7.00
	Subway-Ham and Cheese Combo - 12	239.0000	1.000	Each	19.00	5.00	45.00	302.00	0.00	3.00	28.00	1.00
	Subway-Italian, Spicy - 12" Ital	213.0000	1.000	Each	42.00	63.00	83.00	1043.00	0.00	5.00	137.00	23.00
	Subway-Italian, Spicy - 6" white	232.0000	1.000	Each	20.00	24.00	38.00	467.00	0.00	3.00	57.00	9.00
	Subway-Meat Ball Sandwich - 12"	215.0000	1.000	Each	42.00	44.00	96.00	918.00	0.00	3.00	88.00	17.00
	Subway-Meat Ball Sandwich - 12"	224.0000	1.000	Each	44.00	45.00	101.00	947.00	0.00	0.00	88.00	17.00
	Subway-Meatballs - 6" white	260.0000	1.000	Each	18.00	16.00	44.00	404.00	0.00	3.00	33.00	6.00
	Subway-Melt - 6" white	251.0000	1.000	Each	22.00	12.00	40.00	366.00	0.00	3.00	42.00	5.00
	Subway-Pizza Sub - 6" white	250.0000	1.000	Each	19.00	22.00	41.00	448.00	0.00	3.00	50.00	9.00
	Subway-Roast Beef - 12" Italian	184.0000	1.000	Each	42.00	23.00	84.00	689.00	0.00	5.00	83.00	8.00
	Subway-Roast Beef - 12" Wheat	189.0000	1.000	Each	41.00	24.00	89.00	717.00	0.00	6.00	75.00	8.00
	Subway-Roast Beef - 6" white	232.0000	1.000	Each	19.00	5.00	39.00	288.00	0.00	3.00	20.00	1.00
	Subway-Roast Beef - Deli Sandwic	180.0000	1.000	Each	13.00	4.00	38.00	245.00	0.00	2.00	13.00	1.00
	Subway-Salad, Club	331.0000	1.000	Each	14.00	3.00	12.00	126.00	0.00	1.00	26.00	1.00
	Subway-Salad, Cold Cut Trio	330.0000	1.000	Each	13.00	11.00	11.00	191.00	0.00	1.00	64.00	3.00
	Subway-Salad, Roast Beef	316.0000	1.000	Each	12.00	3.00	11.00	117.00	0.00	1.00	20.00	1.00
	Subway-Salad, Seafood & Crab	331.0000	1.000	Each	13.00	17.00	10.00	244.00	0.00	2.00	34.00	3.00
	Subway-Salad, Turkey Breast	316.0000	1.000	Each	11.00	2.00	12.00	316.00	0.00	1.00	19.00	1.00
	Subway-Salad, Veggie Delite	260.0000	1.000	Each	2.00	1.00	10.00	51.00	0.00	1.00	0.00	0.00
	Subway-Seafood - 12" Italian	210.0000	1.000	Each	29.00	57.00	94.00	986.00	0.00	0.00	56.00	11.00
	Subway-Seafood - 12" Wheat	219.0000	1.000	Each	31.00	58.00	100.00	1015.00	0.00	2.50	56.00	11.00
	Subway-Seafood & Crab - 6" white	246.0000	1.000	Each	19.00	19.00	38.00	415.00	0.00	3.00	34.00	3.00
	Subway-Steak & Cheese - 6" white	257.0000	1.000	Each	29.00	10.00	41.00	383.00	0.00	3.00	70.00	6.00
	Subway-Steak and Cheese - 12" It	213.0000	1.000	Each	43.00	32.00	83.00	765.00	0.00	6.00	82.00	12.00
	Subway-Tuna - 6" white	246.0000	1.000	Each	18.00	32.00	38.00	527.00	0.00	3.00	36.00	5.00
	Subway-Tuna - Deli Sandwich, lit	178.0000	1.000	Each	11.00	9.00	38.00	279.00	0.00	2.00	16.00	2.00
	Subway-Turkey Breast - 12" Wheat	192.0000	1.000	Each	42.00	20.00	88.00	674.00	0.00	7.00	67.00	6.00
	Subway-Turkey Breast - 6" white	232.0000	1.000	Each	17.00	4.00	40.00	273.00	0.00	3.00	19.00	1.00
	Subway-Turkey Breast - Deli sand	180.0000	1.000	Each	12.00	4.00	38.00	235.00	0.00	2.00	12.00	1.00
	Subway-Turkey Breast & Ham - 6"	232.0000	1.000	Each	18.00	5.00	39.00	280.00	0.00	3.00	24.00	1.00
	Subway-Veggie Delight - 6" white	175.0000	1.000	Each	9.00	3.00	38.00	222.00	0.00	3.00	0.00	0.00
	Subway-Veggie Delite - 6" wheat	182.0000	1.000	Each	9.00	3.00	44.00	237.00	0.00	3.00	0.00	0.00
	Taco Bell-Burrito Supreme	198.0000	1.000	Each	20.00	22.00	55.00	440.00	0.00	3.00	33.00	8.00
	Taco Bell-Burrito Supreme, Light	248.0000	1.000	Each	20.00	8.00	50.00	350.00	0.00	0.00	25.00	0.00
	Taco Bell-Burrito, 7-Layer, Ligh	276.0000	1.000	Each	19.00	9.00	67.00	440.00	0.00	0.00	5.00	0.00

Monounsaturated Fat (gm)	Polyunsaturated Fat (gm)	Vitamin D (mg)	Vitamin K (mg)	Vitamin E (mg)	Vitamin A (re)	Vitamin C (mg)	Thiamin (mg)	Riboflavin (mg)	Niacin (mg)	Vitamin B_6 (mg)	Folate (mg)	Vitamin B_{12} (mcg)	Calcium (mg)	Iron (mg)	Magnesium (mg)	Phosphorus (mg)	Potassium (mg)	Sodium (mg)	Zinc (mg)
1.00	0.40	0.00	0.00	0.00	900.00	21.00	0.09	0.10	0.38	0.00	0.00	0.00	32.00	0.80	0.00	0.00	0.00	70.00	0.00
0.90	0.10	0.00	0.00	0.00	92.35	0.00	0.13	0.50	0.40	0.00	0.00	0.00	333.27	0.80	0.00	0.00	0.00	240.92	0.00
0.60	0.10	0.00	0.00	0.00	60.00	0.00	0.12	0.51	0.38	0.00	0.00	0.00	280.00	0.00	0.00	0.00	0.00	170.00	0.00
0.60	0.10	0.00	0.00	0.00	60.00	0.00	0.12	0.51	0.00	0.00	0.00	0.00	280.00	0.00	0.00	0.00	0.00	170.00	0.00
0.00	0.00	0.00	0.00	0.00	10.00	0.00	0.00	0.00	0.00	0.00	0.00	0.00	8.00	8.00	0.00	0.00	0.00	340.00	0.00
0.00	0.00	0.00	0.00	0.00	601.00	15.00	0.00	0.00	0.00	0.00	0.00	0.00	27.00	3.00	0.00	0.00	0.00	945.00	0.00
24.00	7.00	0.00	0.00	5.10	67.00	5.00	0.27	0.34	5.10	0.48	63.00	2.33	64.00	4.30	66.00	308.00	917.00	3139.00	6.10
25.00	7.00	0.00	0.00	0.00	753.00	15.00	0.00	0.00	0.00	0.00	0.00	0.00	44.00	4.00	0.00	0.00	1002.00	3199.00	0.00
0.00	0.00	0.00	0.00	0.00	753.00	15.00	0.00	0.00	0.00	0.00	0.00	0.00	44.00	4.00	0.00	0.00	0.00	1652.00	0.00
0.00	0.00	0.00	0.00	0.00	565.00	14.00	0.00	0.00	0.00	0.00	0.00	0.00	39.00	3.00	0.00	0.00	0.00	744.00	0.00
0.00	0.00	0.00	0.00	0.00	617.00	15.00	0.00	0.00	0.00	0.00	0.00	0.00	35.00	3.00	0.00	0.00	0.00	967.00	0.00
0.00	0.00	0.00	0.00	0.00	1044.00	18.00	0.00	0.00	0.00	0.00	0.00	0.00	118.00	4.00	0.00	0.00	0.00	1264.00	0.00
0.00	0.00	0.00	0.00	0.00	601.00	15.00	0.00	0.00	0.00	0.00	0.00	0.00	29.00	4.00	0.00	0.00	0.00	1341.00	0.00
8.00	4.00	0.00	0.00	1.30	74.00	20.00	0.48	0.33	12.50	0.58	47.00	0.95	58.00	3.10	66.00	384.00	971.00	2717.00	2.50
9.00	4.00	0.00	0.00	4.20	83.00	15.00	0.49	0.35	9.30	0.46	43.00	0.44	96.00	3.20	40.00	247.00	1055.00	2777.00	1.40
15.00	10.00	0.00	0.00	0.90	87.00	17.00	0.36	0.33	3.80	0.20	39.00	1.23	227.00	2.90	28.00	315.00	876.00	2218.00	2.70
15.00	10.00	0.00	0.00	0.90	90.00	18.00	0.37	0.35	3.90	0.21	41.00	1.28	235.00	3.00	29.00	327.00	1010.00	2278.00	2.80
0.00	0.00	0.00	0.00	0.00	649.00	16.00	0.00	0.00	0.00	0.00	0.00	0.00	49.00	4.00	0.00	0.00	0.00	1401.00	0.00
0.00	0.00	0.00	0.00	0.00	601.00	15.00	0.00	0.00	0.00	0.00	0.00	0.00	28.00	3.00	0.00	0.00	0.00	1308.00	0.00
0.00	0.00	0.00	0.00	0.00	565.00	14.00	0.00	0.00	0.00	0.00	0.00	0.00	24.00	3.00	0.00	0.00	0.00	773.00	0.00
8.00	4.00	0.00	0.00	3.80	174.00	17.00	0.53	0.39	3.60	0.34	45.00	0.76	304.00	2.20	50.00	527.00	834.00	1710.00	2.80
8.00	4.00	0.00	0.00	0.00	0.00	0.00	0.00	0.00	0.00	0.00	0.00	0.00	35.00	3.00	0.00	0.00	918.00	1319.00	0.00
28.00	7.00	0.00	0.00	0.00	0.00	0.00	0.00	0.00	0.00	0.00	0.00	0.00	0.00	0.00	0.00	0.00	880.00	2282.00	0.00
0.00	0.00	0.00	0.00	0.00	845.00	15.00	0.00	0.00	0.00	0.00	0.00	0.00	40.00	4.00	0.00	0.00	0.00	1592.00	0.00
17.00	4.00	0.00	0.00	1.00	72.00	19.00	0.33	0.39	9.40	0.40	35.00	3.21	78.00	5.00	47.00	263.00	1210.00	2022.00	6.20
18.00	4.00	0.00	0.00	0.00	0.00	0.00	0.00	0.00	0.00	0.00	0.00	0.00	0.00	0.00	0.00	0.00	1498.00	2082.00	0.00
0.00	0.00	0.00	0.00	0.00	712.00	16.00	0.00	0.00	0.00	0.00	0.00	0.00	32.00	4.00	0.00	0.00	0.00	1035.00	0.00
0.00	0.00	0.00	0.00	0.00	777.00	15.00	0.00	0.00	0.00	0.00	0.00	0.00	93.00	4.00	0.00	0.00	0.00	1735.00	0.00
0.00	0.00	0.00	0.00	0.00	1190.00	16.00	0.00	0.00	0.00	0.00	0.00	0.00	103.00	4.00	0.00	0.00	0.00	1609.00	0.00
9.00	4.00	0.00	0.00	4.40	58.00	5.00	0.23	0.29	4.40	0.42	54.00	2.01	55.00	3.70	57.00	266.00	910.00	2288.00	5.30
9.00	4.00	0.00	0.00	4.50	59.00	5.00	0.24	0.30	4.50	0.43	56.00	2.07	56.00	3.80	59.00	273.00	994.00	2348.00	5.40
0.00	0.00	0.00	0.00	0.00	601.00	15.00	0.00	0.00	0.00	0.00	0.00	0.00	25.00	4.00	0.00	0.00	0.00	928.00	0.00
0.00	0.00	0.00	0.00	0.00	565.00	14.00	0.00	0.00	0.00	0.00	0.00	0.00	23.00	3.00	0.00	0.00	0.00	638.00	0.00
0.00	0.00	0.00	0.00	0.00	1363.00	32.00	0.00	0.00	0.00	0.00	0.00	0.00	26.00	2.00	0.00	0.00	0.00	1067.00	0.00
0.00	0.00	0.00	0.00	0.00	1412.00	33.00	0.00	0.00	0.00	0.00	0.00	0.00	46.00	2.00	0.00	0.00	0.00	1127.00	0.00
0.00	0.00	0.00	0.00	0.00	1363.00	32.00	0.00	0.00	0.00	0.00	0.00	0.00	23.00	2.00	0.00	0.00	0.00	654.00	0.00
0.00	0.00	0.00	0.00	0.00	1366.00	32.00	0.00	0.00	0.00	0.00	0.00	0.00	25.00	2.00	0.00	0.00	0.00	575.00	0.00
0.00	0.00	0.00	0.00	0.00	1363.00	32.00	0.00	0.00	0.00	0.00	0.00	0.00	28.00	2.00	0.00	0.00	0.00	1117.00	0.00
0.00	0.00	0.00	0.00	0.00	1363.00	32.00	0.00	0.00	0.00	0.00	0.00	0.00	23.00	1.00	0.00	0.00	0.00	308.00	0.00
15.00	28.00	0.00	0.00	2.50	107.00	5.00	0.51	0.38	7.00	0.26	91.00	6.54	230.00	4.40	32.00	336.00	641.00	2027.00	5.30
16.00	28.00	0.00	0.00	0.00	0.00	0.00	0.00	0.00	0.00	0.00	0.00	0.00	0.00	0.00	0.00	0.00	557.00	1967.00	0.00
0.00	0.00	0.00	0.00	0.00	604.00	15.00	0.00	0.00	0.00	0.00	0.00	0.00	28.00	3.00	0.00	0.00	0.00	849.00	0.00
0.00	0.00	0.00	0.00	0.00	877.00	18.00	0.00	0.00	0.00	0.00	0.00	0.00	88.00	5.00	0.00	0.00	0.00	1106.00	0.00
12.00	4.00	0.00	0.00	0.80	119.00	6.00	0.33	0.46	5.10	0.38	36.00	2.54	231.00	4.20	43.00	456.00	909.00	1556.00	6.80
0.00	0.00	0.00	0.00	0.00	627.00	15.00	0.00	0.00	0.00	0.00	0.00	0.00	32.00	3.00	0.00	0.00	0.00	875.00	0.00
0.00	0.00	0.00	0.00	0.00	628.00	14.00	0.00	0.00	0.00	0.00	0.00	0.00	26.00	3.00	0.00	0.00	0.00	583.00	0.00
7.00	7.00	0.00	0.00	0.00	0.00	0.00	0.00	0.00	0.00	0.00	0.00	0.00	0.00	0.00	0.00	0.00	605.00	2520.00	0.00
0.00	0.00	0.00	0.00	0.00	601.00	15.00	0.00	0.00	0.00	0.00	0.00	0.00	30.00	4.00	0.00	0.00	0.00	1391.00	0.00
0.00	0.00	0.00	0.00	0.00	565.00	14.00	0.00	0.00	0.00	0.00	0.00	0.00	26.00	3.00	0.00	0.00	0.00	944.00	0.00
0.00	0.00	0.00	0.00	0.00	601.00	15.00	0.00	0.00	0.00	0.00	0.00	0.00	29.00	3.00	0.00	0.00	0.00	1350.00	0.00
0.00	0.00	0.00	0.00	0.00	601.00	15.00	0.00	0.00	0.00	0.00	0.00	0.00	25.00	0.00	0.00	0.00	0.00	3.00	0.00
0.00	0.00	0.00	0.00	0.00	601.00	15.00	0.00	0.00	0.00	0.00	0.00	0.00	32.00	3.00	0.00	0.00	0.00	593.00	0.00
0.00	2.00	0.00	0.00	0.00	0.00	26.00	0.40	2.10	3.60	0.00	0.00	0.00	190.00	4.00	0.00	0.00	501.00	1181.00	0.00
0.00	0.00	0.00	0.00	0.00	600.00	9.00	0.00	0.00	0.00	0.00	0.00	0.00	96.00	1.50	0.00	0.00	0.00	1160.00	0.00
0.00	0.00	0.00	0.00	0.00	350.00	4.80	0.00	0.00	0.00	0.00	0.00	0.00	300.00	2.50	0.00	0.00	0.00	1130.00	0.00

USDA ID Code	Food Name	Weight in Grams*	Quantity of Units	Unit of Measure	Protein (gm)	Fat (gm)	Carbohydrate (gm)	Kcalories	Caffeine (gm)	Fiber (gm)	Cholesterol (mg)	Saturated Fat (gm)
	Taco Bell-Burrito, Bean	206.0000	1.000	Each	15.00	14.00	63.00	387.00	0.00	3.00	9.00	4.00
	Taco Bell-Burrito, Bean, Light	198.0000	1.000	Each	14.00	6.00	55.00	330.00	0.00	0.00	5.00	0.00
	Taco Bell-Burrito, Beef	206.0000	1.000	Each	25.00	21.00	48.00	431.00	0.00	2.00	57.00	8.00
	Taco Bell-Burrito, Chicken, Ligh	170.0000	1.000	Each	12.00	6.00	45.00	290.00	0.00	0.00	30.00	0.00
	Taco Bell-Burrito, Chicken, Supr	248.0000	1.000	Each	18.00	10.00	62.00	410.00	0.00	0.00	65.00	0.00
730	Taco Bell-Cinnamon Twists	28.0000	1.000	Ounce	1.00	6.00	19.00	140.00	0.00	0.00	0.00	0.00
731	Taco Bell-Gordita, Beef, Supreme	154.0000	5.500	Ounce	14.00	13.00	31.00	300.00	0.00	3.00	35.00	6.00
732	Taco Bell-Gordita, Chicken, Gril	154.0000	5.500	Ounce	17.00	14.00	28.00	300.00	0.00	3.00	45.00	5.00
733	Taco Bell-Gordita, Steak, Grille	154.0000	5.500	Ounce	17.00	14.00	27.00	310.00	0.00	3.00	35.00	5.00
734	Taco Bell-MexiMelt, Beef, Big	133.0000	4.750	Ounce	16.00	15.00	23.00	290.00	0.00	4.00	45.00	7.00
	Taco Bell-Nachos	106.0000	1.000	Order	7.00	18.00	37.00	346.00	0.00	1.00	9.00	6.00
	Taco Bell-Nachos Bell Grande	287.0000	1.000	Order	22.00	35.00	61.00	649.00	0.00	4.00	36.00	12.00
735	Taco Bell-Nachos Supreme, Beef ,	98.0000	3.500	Ounce	14.00	24.00	45.00	220.00	0.00	9.00	30.00	8.00
	Taco Bell-Pintos 'N Cheese	128.0000	1.000	Each	9.00	9.00	19.00	190.00	0.00	2.00	16.00	4.00
	Taco Bell-Pizza, Mexican	223.0000	1.000	Each	21.00	37.00	40.00	575.00	0.00	3.00	52.00	11.00
	Taco Bell-Salad, Taco	575.0000	1.000	Each	34.00	61.00	55.00	905.00	0.00	4.00	80.00	19.00
	Taco Bell-Salad, Taco w/o Shell	520.0000	1.000	Each	28.00	31.00	22.00	484.00	0.00	3.00	80.00	14.00
	Taco Bell-Salad, Taco, Light	464.0000	1.000	Each	30.00	9.00	35.00	330.00	0.00	0.00	50.00	0.00
	Taco Bell-Salsa	10.0000	1.000	Each	1.00	0.00	4.00	18.00	0.00	0.40	0.00	0.00
	Taco Bell-Taco	78.0000	1.000	Each	10.00	11.00	11.00	183.00	0.00	1.00	32.00	5.00
736	Taco Bell-Taco, Double Decker	140.0000	5.000	Ounce	14.00	15.00	38.00	340.00	0.00	9.00	25.00	5.00
	Taco Bell-Taco, Light	78.0000	1.000	Each	11.00	5.00	11.00	140.00	0.00	1.00	20.00	4.00
	Taco Bell-Taco, Soft	92.0000	1.000	Each	12.00	12.00	18.00	225.00	0.00	2.00	32.00	5.00
	Taco Bell-Taco, Soft, Chicken, L	120.0000	1.000	Each	9.00	5.00	26.00	180.00	0.00	0.00	30.00	0.00
	Taco Bell-Taco, Soft, Light	99.0000	1.000	Each	13.00	5.00	19.00	180.00	0.00	2.00	25.00	4.00
737	Taco Bell-Taco, Soft, Steak, Gri	126.0000	4.500	Ounce	15.00	10.00	20.00	230.00	0.00	2.00	25.00	2.50
738	Taco Bell-Taco, Soft, Steak, Gri	161.0000	5.750	Ounce	16.00	14.00	24.00	290.00	0.00	3.00	35.00	5.00
	Taco Bell-Taco, Soft, Supreme, L	128.0000	1.000	Each	14.00	5.00	23.00	200.00	0.00	0.00	25.00	0.00
	Taco Bell-Taco, Supreme, Light	106.0000	1.000	Each	14.00	5.00	23.00	160.00	0.00	0.00	20.00	0.00
	Taco Bell-Tostada	156.0000	1.000	Each	9.00	11.00	27.00	243.00	0.00	2.00	16.00	4.00
	Wendy's-Cheesburger Deluxe, Jr.	180.0000	1.000	Each	18.00	17.00	36.00	360.00	0.00	3.00	50.00	6.00
	Wendy's-Cheesburger, Bacon, Jr.	166.0000	1.000	Each	20.00	19.00	34.00	380.00	0.00	2.00	60.00	7.00
	Wendy's-Cheesburger, Jr.	130.0000	1.000	Each	17.00	13.00	34.00	320.00	0.00	2.00	45.00	6.00
	Wendy's-Cheesburger, Kids' Meal	123.0000	1.000	Each	17.00	13.00	33.00	320.00	0.00	2.00	45.00	6.00
	Wendy's-Chicken Club Sandwich	216.0000	1.000	Each	31.00	20.00	44.00	470.00	0.00	2.00	70.00	4.00
	Wendy's-Chicken, Breaded, Sandwi	208.0000	1.000	Each	28.00	18.00	44.00	440.00	0.00	2.00	60.00	3.50
	Wendy's-Chicken, Grilled, Sandwi	189.0000	1.000	Each	27.00	8.00	35.00	310.00	0.00	2.00	65.00	1.50
	Wendy's-Chicken, Spicy, Sandwich	213.0000	1.000	Each	28.00	15.00	43.00	410.00	0.00	2.00	65.00	2.50
	Wendy's-Chili, Large	340.0000	1.000	Each	28.00	9.00	31.00	290.00	0.00	0.00	60.00	4.00
	Wendy's-Chili, Small	227.0000	1.000	Each	19.00	6.00	21.00	190.00	0.00	0.00	40.00	2.00
	Wendy's-French Fries, Biggie	170.0000	1.000	Order	7.00	23.00	61.00	450.00	0.00	0.00	0.00	5.00
	Wendy's-French Fries, Medium	136.0000	1.000	Order	5.00	17.00	50.00	360.00	0.00	0.00	0.00	4.00
	Wendy's-French Fries, Small	91.0000	1.000	Order	3.00	12.00	33.00	240.00	0.00	0.00	0.00	2.00
	Wendy's-Frosty Dairy Dessert, La	402.2200	1.000	Each	15.00	17.00	91.00	570.00	0.00	0.00	70.00	9.00
	Wendy's-Frosty Dairy Dessert, Me	321.7760	1.000	Each	12.00	13.00	76.00	460.00	0.00	0.00	55.00	7.00
	Wendy's-Frosty Dairy Dessert, Sm	241.3320	1.000	Each	9.00	10.00	57.00	340.00	0.00	0.00	40.00	5.00
	Wendy's-Hamburger, Bacon, Big Cl	285.0000	1.000	Each	34.00	30.00	46.00	580.00	0.00	3.00	100.00	12.00
	Wendy's-Hamburger, Big Classic	251.0000	1.000	Each	27.00	23.00	44.00	480.00	0.00	0.00	75.00	7.00
	Wendy's-Hamburger, Jr.	118.0000	1.000	Each	15.00	10.00	34.00	270.00	0.00	2.00	30.00	3.50
	Wendy's-Hamburger, Kids' Meal	111.0000	1.000	Each	15.00	10.00	33.00	270.00	0.00	2.00	30.00	3.50
	Wendy's-Hamburger, Single w/ eve	219.0000	1.000	Each	25.00	20.00	37.00	420.00	0.00	3.00	70.00	6.00
	Wendy's-Hamburger, Single, Plain	133.0000	1.000	Each	24.00	16.00	31.00	360.00	0.00	2.00	65.00	6.00
	Wendy's-Potato, Bkd w/ Bacon and	380.0000	1.000	Each	17.00	17.00	75.00	510.00	0.00	0.00	15.00	4.00
	Wendy's-Potato, Bkd w/ Broccoli	411.0000	1.000	Each	9.00	14.00	77.00	450.00	0.00	0.00	0.00	2.00
	Wendy's-Potato, Bkd w/ Cheese	383.0000	1.000	Each	14.00	24.00	74.00	550.00	0.00	0.00	30.00	8.00

Monounsaturated Fat (gm)	Polyunsaturated Fat (gm)	Vitamin D (mg)	Vitamin K (mg)	Vitamin E (mg)	Vitamin A (re)	Vitamin C (mg)	Thiamin (mg)	Riboflavin (mg)	Niacin (mg)	Vitamin B_6 (mg)	Folate (mg)	Vitamin B_{12} (mcg)	Calcium (mg)	Iron (mg)	Magnesium (mg)	Phosphorus (mg)	Potassium (mg)	Sodium (mg)	Zinc (mg)
0.00	2.00	0.00	0.00	0.00	0.00	53.00	0.40	2.00	2.80	0.00	0.00	0.00	190.00	4.00	0.00	0.00	495.00	1148.00	0.00
0.00	0.00	0.00	0.00	0.00	300.00	2.40	0.00	0.00	0.00	0.00	0.00	0.00	120.00	2.00	0.00	0.00	0.00	1340.00	0.00
0.00	2.00	0.00	0.00	0.00	0.00	2.00	0.40	0.30	3.20	0.00	0.00	0.00	150.00	3.00	0.00	0.00	380.00	1311.00	0.00
0.00	0.00	0.00	0.00	0.00	200.00	3.60	0.00	0.00	0.00	0.00	0.00	0.00	72.00	1.50	0.00	0.00	0.00	900.00	0.00
0.00	0.00	0.00	0.00	0.00	250.00	4.80	0.00	0.00	0.00	0.00	0.00	0.00	72.00	1.50	0.00	0.00	0.00	1190.00	0.00
0.00	0.00	0.00	0.00	0.00	0.00	0.00	0.00	0.00	0.00	0.00	0.00	0.00	0.00	0.00	0.00	0.00	0.00	190.00	0.00
0.00	0.00	0.00	0.00	0.00	0.00	0.00	0.00	0.00	0.00	0.00	0.00	0.00	0.00	0.00	0.00	0.00	0.00	390.00	0.00
0.00	0.00	0.00	0.00	0.00	0.00	0.00	0.00	0.00	0.00	0.00	0.00	0.00	0.00	0.00	0.00	0.00	0.00	540.00	0.00
0.00	0.00	0.00	0.00	0.00	0.00	0.00	0.00	0.00	0.00	0.00	0.00	0.00	0.00	0.00	0.00	0.00	0.00	550.00	0.00
0.00	0.00	0.00	0.00	0.00	0.00	0.00	0.00	0.00	0.00	0.00	0.00	0.00	0.00	0.00	0.00	0.00	0.00	850.00	0.00
0.00	2.00	0.00	0.00	0.00	0.00	2.00	0.00	0.20	0.60	0.00	0.00	0.00	191.00	1.00	0.00	0.00	159.00	399.00	0.00
0.00	3.00	0.00	0.00	0.00	0.00	58.00	0.10	0.30	2.20	0.00	0.00	0.00	297.00	3.00	0.00	0.00	674.00	997.00	0.00
0.00	0.00	0.00	0.00	0.00	0.00	0.00	0.00	0.00	0.00	0.00	0.00	0.00	0.00	0.00	0.00	0.00	0.00	810.00	0.00
0.00	1.00	0.00	0.00	0.00	0.00	52.00	0.10	0.20	0.40	0.00	0.00	0.00	156.00	1.00	0.00	0.00	384.00	642.00	0.00
0.00	10.00	0.00	0.00	0.00	0.00	31.00	0.30	0.30	3.00	0.00	0.00	0.00	257.00	4.00	0.00	0.00	408.00	1031.00	0.00
0.00	12.00	0.00	0.00	0.00	0.00	75.00	0.50	0.60	4.80	0.00	0.00	0.00	320.00	6.00	0.00	0.00	673.00	910.00	0.00
0.00	2.00	0.00	0.00	0.00	0.00	74.00	0.20	0.40	3.20	0.00	0.00	0.00	290.00	4.00	0.00	0.00	612.00	680.00	0.00
0.00	0.00	0.00	0.00	0.00	1200.00	27.00	0.00	0.00	0.00	0.00	0.00	0.00	120.00	1.50	0.00	0.00	0.00	1610.00	0.00
0.00	0.00	0.00	0.00	0.00	0.00	0.00	0.00	0.10	0.00	0.00	0.00	0.00	36.00	1.00	0.00	0.00	376.00	376.00	0.00
0.00	1.00	0.00	0.00	0.00	0.00	1.00	0.10	0.10	1.20	0.00	0.00	0.00	84.00	1.00	0.00	0.00	159.00	276.00	0.00
0.00	0.00	0.00	0.00	0.00	0.00	0.00	0.00	0.00	0.00	0.00	0.00	0.00	0.00	0.00	0.00	0.00	0.00	750.00	0.00
0.00	1.00	0.00	0.00	0.00	40.00	0.00	0.10	0.10	1.20	0.00	0.00	0.00	0.00	0.00	0.00	0.00	159.00	276.00	0.00
0.00	1.00	0.00	0.00	0.00	0.00	1.00	0.40	0.20	2.80	0.00	0.00	0.00	116.00	2.00	0.00	0.00	196.00	554.00	0.00
0.00	0.00	0.00	0.00	0.00	150.00	4.80	0.00	0.00	0.00	0.00	0.00	0.00	48.00	0.80	0.00	0.00	0.00	570.00	0.00
0.00	1.00	0.00	0.00	0.00	40.00	0.00	0.40	0.20	2.80	0.00	0.00	0.00	48.00	0.60	0.00	0.00	196.00	554.00	0.00
0.00	0.00	0.00	0.00	0.00	0.00	0.00	0.00	0.00	0.00	0.00	0.00	0.00	0.00	0.00	0.00	0.00	0.00	1020.00	0.00
0.00	0.00	0.00	0.00	0.00	0.00	0.00	0.00	0.00	0.00	0.00	0.00	0.00	0.00	0.00	0.00	0.00	0.00	1040.00	0.00
0.00	0.00	0.00	0.00	0.00	100.00	2.40	0.00	0.00	0.00	0.00	0.00	0.00	48.00	0.60	0.00	0.00	0.00	610.00	0.00
0.00	0.00	0.00	0.00	0.00	100.00	2.40	0.00	0.00	0.00	0.00	0.00	0.00	0.00	0.00	0.00	0.00	0.00	340.00	0.00
0.00	1.00	0.00	0.00	0.00	0.00	45.00	0.10	0.20	0.60	0.00	0.00	0.00	180.00	2.00	0.00	0.00	401.00	596.00	0.00
0.00	0.00	0.00	0.00	0.00	10.00	10.00	0.00	0.00	0.00	0.00	0.00	0.00	18.00	19.00	0.00	0.00	0.00	890.00	0.00
0.00	0.00	0.00	0.00	0.00	8.00	10.00	0.00	0.00	0.00	0.00	0.00	0.00	17.00	19.00	0.00	0.00	0.00	850.00	0.00
0.00	0.00	0.00	0.00	0.00	6.00	2.00	0.00	0.00	0.00	0.00	0.00	0.00	17.00	18.00	0.00	0.00	0.00	830.00	0.00
0.00	0.00	0.00	0.00	0.00	6.00	0.00	0.00	0.00	0.00	0.00	0.00	0.00	17.00	18.00	0.00	0.00	0.00	830.00	0.00
7.00	9.00	0.00	0.00	0.00	20.00	9.00	0.60	0.43	15.20	0.00	0.00	0.00	80.00	8.00	0.00	0.00	470.00	970.00	0.00
0.00	0.00	0.00	0.00	0.00	4.00	10.00	0.00	0.00	0.00	0.00	0.00	0.00	10.00	16.00	0.00	0.00	0.00	840.00	0.00
0.00	0.00	0.00	0.00	0.00	4.00	10.00	0.00	0.00	0.00	0.00	0.00	0.00	10.00	15.00	0.00	0.00	0.00	790.00	0.00
0.00	0.00	0.00	0.00	0.00	4.00	10.00	0.00	0.00	0.00	0.00	0.00	0.00	11.00	15.00	0.00	0.00	0.00	1280.00	0.00
2.00	1.00	0.00	0.00	0.00	150.00	12.00	0.15	0.17	2.85	0.00	0.00	0.00	80.00	4.50	0.00	0.00	660.00	1000.00	0.00
1.00	1.00	0.00	0.00	0.00	100.00	6.00	0.09	0.14	1.90	0.00	0.00	0.00	64.00	3.00	0.00	0.00	440.00	670.00	0.00
15.00	1.00	0.00	0.00	0.00	0.00	12.00	0.30	0.07	3.80	0.00	0.00	0.00	16.00	0.80	0.00	0.00	950.00	280.00	0.00
12.00	1.00	0.00	0.00	0.00	0.00	9.00	0.23	0.03	2.85	0.00	0.00	0.00	16.00	0.60	0.00	0.00	760.00	220.00	0.00
8.00	1.00	0.00	0.00	0.00	0.00	6.00	0.15	0.03	1.90	0.00	0.00	0.00	0.00	0.40	0.00	0.00	510.00	150.00	0.00
4.00	1.00	0.00	0.00	0.00	100.00	0.00	0.23	1.36	0.76	0.00	0.00	0.00	400.00	1.00	0.00	0.00	1040.00	330.00	0.00
3.00	1.00	0.00	0.00	0.00	100.00	0.00	0.15	1.02	0.76	0.00	0.00	0.00	320.00	0.80	0.00	0.00	830.00	260.00	0.00
3.00	0.00	0.00	0.00	0.00	80.00	0.00	0.12	0.77	0.38	0.00	0.00	0.00	240.00	0.60	0.00	0.00	630.00	200.00	0.00
0.00	0.00	0.00	0.00	0.00	15.00	25.00	0.00	0.00	0.00	0.00	0.00	0.00	25.00	30.00	0.00	0.00	0.00	1460.00	0.00
8.00	7.00	0.00	0.00	0.00	60.00	12.00	0.45	0.26	6.65	0.00	0.00	0.00	120.00	3.50	0.00	0.00	500.00	850.00	0.00
0.00	0.00	0.00	0.00	0.00	2.00	2.00	0.00	0.00	0.00	0.00	0.00	0.00	11.00	17.00	0.00	0.00	0.00	610.00	0.00
0.00	0.00	0.00	0.00	0.00	2.00	0.00	0.00	0.00	0.00	0.00	0.00	0.00	11.00	17.00	0.00	0.00	0.00	610.00	0.00
7.00	7.00	0.00	0.00	0.00	60.00	9.00	0.38	0.17	6.65	0.00	0.00	0.00	80.00	3.00	0.00	0.00	430.00	920.00	0.00
7.00	2.00	0.00	0.00	0.00	0.00	0.00	0.38	0.17	5.70	0.00	0.00	0.00	80.00	3.00	0.00	0.00	280.00	580.00	0.00
3.00	8.00	0.00	0.00	0.00	100.00	36.00	0.45	0.17	6.65	0.00	0.00	0.00	80.00	2.50	0.00	0.00	1370.00	1170.00	0.00
3.00	7.00	0.00	0.00	0.00	200.00	60.00	0.30	0.14	4.75	0.00	0.00	0.00	80.00	2.50	0.00	0.00	1310.00	450.00	0.00
6.00	7.00	0.00	0.00	0.00	150.00	36.00	0.30	0.17	3.80	0.00	0.00	0.00	240.00	2.00	0.00	0.00	1210.00	640.00	0.00

USDA ID Code	Food Name	Weight in Grams*	Quantity of Units	Unit of Measure	Protein (gm)	Fat (gm)	Carbohydrate (gm)	Kcalories	Caffeine (gm)	Fiber (gm)	Cholesterol (mg)	Saturated Fat (gm)
	White Castle-Cheeseburger Sandwi	64.8000	1.000	Each	7.80	11.20	15.53	199.58	0.00	2.70	0.00	0.00
	White Castle-Chicken Sandwich	63.7860	1.000	Each	7.99	7.45	20.49	185.75	0.00	1.73	0.00	0.00
	White Castle-Fish Sandwich, w/o	59.3330	1.000	Each	5.78	4.98	20.87	155.44	0.00	1.41	0.00	0.00
	White Castle-French Fries	96.8300	1.000	Order	2.49	14.70	37.73	301.14	0.00	4.64	0.00	0.00
	White Castle-Hamburger Sandwich	58.5000	1.000	Each	5.88	7.94	15.38	161.27	0.00	2.13	0.00	0.00
	White Castle-Onion Chips	92.1350	1.000	Each	3.72	16.55	38.83	328.66	0.00	3.52	0.00	0.00
	White Castle-Onion Rings	60.1700	1.000	Each	2.91	13.38	26.62	245.49	0.00	2.61	0.00	0.00
	White Castle-Sausage and Egg San	96.2500	1.000	Each	12.55	22.02	16.05	322.37	0.00	3.03	0.00	0.00
	White Castle-Sausage Sandwich	48.6670	1.000	Each	6.67	12.29	13.30	196.10	0.00	1.95	0.00	0.00
65	Bruegger's Bagels-Bagel, Blueber	101.0000	1.000	Each	10.00	2.00	60.00	300.00	0.00	2.00	0.00	0.00
66	Bruegger's Bagels-Bagel, Cinnamo	101.0000	1.000	Each	10.00	1.50	60.00	290.00	0.00	3.00	0.00	0.00
67	Bruegger's Bagels-Bagel, Egg	101.0000	1.000	Each	10.00	1.00	57.00	280.00	0.00	3.00	25.00	0.50
68	Bruegger's Bagels-Bagel, Everyth	104.0000	1.000	Each	11.00	2.00	58.00	290.00	0.00	2.00	0.00	0.00
69	Bruegger's Bagels-Bagel, Garlic	102.0000	1.000	Each	10.00	1.50	57.00	280.00	0.00	2.00	0.00	0.00
70	Bruegger's Bagels-Bagel, Honey G	103.0000	1.000	Each	11.00	2.50	58.00	300.00	0.00	3.00	0.00	0.50
71	Bruegger's Bagels-Bagel, Onion	102.0000	1.000	Each	10.00	1.50	57.00	280.00	0.00	2.00	0.00	0.00
72	Bruegger's Bagels-Bagel, Plain	101.0000	1.000	Each	10.00	1.50	56.00	280.00	0.00	2.00	0.00	0.00
73	Bruegger's Bagels-Bagel, Poppy S	102.0000	1.000	Each	11.00	1.50	57.00	280.00	0.00	2.00	0.00	0.00
74	Bruegger's Bagels-Bagel, Pumpern	101.0000	1.000	Each	11.00	1.50	56.00	280.00	0.00	4.00	0.00	0.00
75	Bruegger's Bagels-Bagel, Salt	102.0000	1.000	Each	10.00	1.50	55.00	270.00	0.00	2.00	0.00	0.00
76	Bruegger's Bagels-Bagel, Sesame	103.0000	1.000	Each	11.00	2.50	57.00	290.00	0.00	2.00	0.00	0.50
77	Bruegger's Bagels-Bagel, Sun-dri	101.0000	1.000	Each	10.00	1.50	56.00	280.00	0.00	3.00	0.00	0.00
64	Bruegger's Bagels-BLT Sandwich	187.0000	1.000	Each	18.00	18.00	61.00	480.00	0.00	3.00	35.00	7.00
78	Bruegger's Bagels-Brownie	0.0000	1.000	Each	3.00	16.00	27.00	250.00	0.00	1.00	60.00	7.00
79	Bruegger's Bagels-Bruegger Bar	94.0000	1.000	Each	5.00	36.00	39.00	490.00	0.00	2.00	5.00	11.00
80	Bruegger's Bagels-Brueggeroons	71.0000	1.000	Each	4.00	18.00	39.00	320.00	0.00	5.00	0.00	16.00
81	Bruegger's Bagels-Cheese, Veggie	244.0000	8.000	Ounce	5.10	13.00	16.00	200.00	0.00	3.20	15.00	4.50
82	Bruegger's Bagels-Chicken Fajita	250.0000	1.000	Each	28.00	10.00	66.00	460.00	0.00	3.00	80.00	4.50
83	Bruegger's Bagels-Chicken Salad,	116.0000	0.500	Cup	24.00	3.00	4.00	140.00	0.00	1.00	95.00	1.00
84	Bruegger's Bagels-Chicken, Aztec	241.0000	8.000	Ounce	8.00	3.50	14.00	120.00	0.00	2.00	15.00	0.50
85	Bruegger's Bagels-Chile Cilantro	246.0000	8.000	Ounce	8.00	7.00	28.00	200.00	0.00	7.00	0.00	1.00
86	Bruegger's Bagels-Chili, The Big	244.0000	8.000	Ounce	13.00	7.00	26.00	220.00	0.00	6.00	20.00	1.50
87	Bruegger's Bagels-Chowder, Bacon	241.0000	8.000	Ounce	4.00	9.00	25.00	190.00	0.00	1.00	10.00	2.50
88	Bruegger's Bagels-Chowder, Clam	241.0000	8.000	Ounce	8.00	7.00	18.00	170.00	0.00	1.00	10.00	2.00
89	Bruegger's Bagels-Cream Cheese,	27.0000	2.000	Tbsp	1.00	8.00	1.00	90.00	0.00	0.00	20.00	5.00
90	Bruegger's Bagels-Cream Cheese,	30.0000	2.000	Tbsp	2.00	10.00	1.00	100.00	0.00	0.00	30.00	6.00
91	Bruegger's Bagels-Cream Cheese,	26.0000	2.000	Tbsp	2.00	4.50	2.00	60.00	0.00	0.00	15.00	3.00
92	Bruegger's Bagels-Crm Chse, Chiv	26.0000	2.000	Tbsp	2.00	9.00	2.00	100.00	0.00	0.00	25.00	4.50
93	Bruegger's Bagels-Crm Chse, Cucu	28.0000	2.000	Tbsp	2.00	9.00	2.00	100.00	0.00	0.00	25.00	4.50
94	Bruegger's Bagels-Crm Chse, Gard	28.0000	2.000	Tbsp	1.00	8.00	1.00	80.00	0.00	0.00	25.00	5.00
95	Bruegger's Bagels-Crm Chse, Gard	27.0000	2.000	Tbsp	2.00	4.50	2.00	60.00	0.00	0.00	15.00	3.00
96	Bruegger's Bagels-Crm Chse, Herb	27.0000	2.000	Tbsp	2.00	4.50	3.00	60.00	0.00	0.00	15.00	3.00
97	Bruegger's Bagels-Crm Chse, Hone	27.0000	2.000	Tbsp	2.00	9.00	3.00	90.00	0.00	0.00	20.00	5.00
98	Bruegger's Bagels-Crm Chse, Jala	30.0000	2.000	Tbsp	1.00	8.00	1.00	80.00	0.00	0.00	20.00	5.00
99	Bruegger's Bagels-Crm Chse, Salm	29.0000	2.000	Tbsp	2.00	9.00	1.00	90.00	0.00	0.00	20.00	5.00
100	Bruegger's Bagels-Crm Chse, Stra	25.0000	2.000	Tbsp	2.00	4.50	5.00	70.00	0.00	0.00	15.00	3.00
101	Bruegger's Bagels-Crm Chse, Sun	27.0000	2.000	Tbsp	2.00	4.50	2.00	60.00	0.00	0.00	15.00	3.00
102	Bruegger's Bagels-Crm Chse, Wild	30.0000	2.000	Tbsp	1.00	8.00	3.00	90.00	0.00	0.00	20.00	5.00
103	Bruegger's Bagels-Cucumber Dill	236.0000	1.000	Each	18.00	15.00	62.00	450.00	0.00	4.00	40.00	8.00
104	Bruegger's Bagels-Garden Veggie,	227.0000	8.000	Ounce	2.00	1.50	11.00	60.00	0.00	2.00	0.00	0.00
105	Bruegger's Bagels-Gumbo, Cajun	241.0000	8.000	Ounce	3.00	4.50	17.00	120.00	0.00	2.00	0.00	1.00
106	Bruegger's Bagels-Hummus	71.0000	1.000	Scoop	5.00	9.00	13.00	150.00	0.00	4.00	0.00	1.50
107	Bruegger's Bagels-Javahhccino	280.0000	12.000	Fl Oz	9.00	3.00	35.00	210.00	0.00	0.00	10.00	3.00
108	Bruegger's Bagels-Kinnow Bruegge	227.0000	8.000	Fl Oz	1.00	0.00	35.00	140.00	0.00	0.00	0.00	0.00
109	Bruegger's Bagels-Leonardo da Ve	220.0000	1.000	Each	19.00	11.00	62.00	420.00	0.00	3.00	30.00	6.00

Monounsaturated Fat (gm)	Polyunsaturated Fat (gm)	Vitamin D (mg)	Vitamin K (mg)	Vitamin E (mg)	Vitamin A (re)	Vitamin C (mg)	Thiamin (mg)	Riboflavin (mg)	Niacin (mg)	Vitamin B_6 (mg)	Folate (mg)	Vitamin B_{12} (mcg)	Calcium (mg)	Iron (mg)	Magnesium (mg)	Phosphorus (mg)	Potassium (mg)	Sodium (mg)	Zinc (mg)
0.00	0.00	0.00	0.00	0.00	0.00	0.00	0.00	0.00	0.00	0.00	0.00	0.00	0.00	0.00	0.00	0.00	0.00	361.00	0.00
0.00	0.00	0.00	0.00	0.00	0.00	0.00	0.00	0.00	0.00	0.00	0.00	0.00	0.00	0.00	0.00	0.00	0.00	497.00	0.00
0.00	0.00	0.00	0.00	0.00	0.00	0.00	0.00	0.00	0.00	0.00	0.00	0.00	0.00	0.00	0.00	0.00	0.00	201.00	0.00
0.00	0.00	0.00	0.00	0.00	0.00	0.00	0.00	0.00	0.00	0.00	0.00	0.00	0.00	0.00	0.00	0.00	0.00	193.00	0.00
0.00	0.00	0.00	0.00	0.00	0.00	0.00	0.00	0.00	0.00	0.00	0.00	0.00	0.00	0.00	0.00	0.00	0.00	266.00	0.00
0.00	0.00	0.00	0.00	0.00	0.00	0.00	0.00	0.00	0.00	0.00	0.00	0.00	0.00	0.00	0.00	0.00	0.00	823.00	0.00
0.00	0.00	0.00	0.00	0.00	0.00	0.00	0.00	0.00	0.00	0.00	0.00	0.00	0.00	0.00	0.00	0.00	0.00	566.00	0.00
0.00	0.00	0.00	0.00	0.00	0.00	0.00	0.00	0.00	0.00	0.00	0.00	0.00	0.00	0.00	0.00	0.00	0.00	698.00	0.00
0.00	0.00	0.00	0.00	0.00	0.00	0.00	0.00	0.00	0.00	0.00	0.00	0.00	0.00	0.00	0.00	0.00	0.00	488.00	0.00
0.50	0.50	0.00	0.00	0.00	0.00	0.00	0.00	0.00	0.00	0.00	0.00	0.00	0.00	0.00	0.00	0.00	0.00	480.00	0.00
0.00	0.50	0.00	0.00	0.00	0.00	0.00	0.00	0.00	0.00	0.00	0.00	0.00	0.00	0.00	0.00	0.00	0.00	400.00	0.00
0.50	0.50	0.00	0.00	0.00	0.00	0.00	0.00	0.00	0.00	0.00	0.00	0.00	0.00	0.00	0.00	0.00	0.00	510.00	0.00
0.00	1.00	0.00	0.00	0.00	0.00	0.00	0.00	0.00	0.00	0.00	0.00	0.00	0.00	0.00	0.00	0.00	0.00	700.00	0.00
0.00	0.50	0.00	0.00	0.00	0.00	0.00	0.00	0.00	0.00	0.00	0.00	0.00	0.00	0.00	0.00	0.00	0.00	440.00	0.00
0.50	1.50	0.00	0.00	0.00	0.00	0.00	0.00	0.00	0.00	0.00	0.00	0.00	0.00	0.00	0.00	0.00	0.00	390.00	0.00
0.00	0.50	0.00	0.00	0.00	0.00	0.00	0.00	0.00	0.00	0.00	0.00	0.00	0.00	0.00	0.00	0.00	0.00	430.00	0.00
0.00	1.00	0.00	0.00	0.00	0.00	0.00	0.00	0.00	0.00	0.00	0.00	0.00	0.00	0.00	0.00	0.00	0.00	430.00	0.00
0.00	1.00	0.00	0.00	0.00	0.00	0.00	0.00	0.00	0.00	0.00	0.00	0.00	0.00	0.00	0.00	0.00	0.00	440.00	0.00
0.00	0.50	0.00	0.00	0.00	0.00	0.00	0.00	0.00	0.00	0.00	0.00	0.00	0.00	0.00	0.00	0.00	0.00	390.00	0.00
0.00	0.50	0.00	0.00	0.00	0.00	0.00	0.00	0.00	0.00	0.00	0.00	0.00	0.00	0.00	0.00	0.00	0.00	1670.00	0.00
1.00	1.00	0.00	0.00	0.00	0.00	0.00	0.00	0.00	0.00	0.00	0.00	0.00	0.00	0.00	0.00	0.00	0.00	440.00	0.00
0.00	1.00	0.00	0.00	0.00	0.00	0.00	0.00	0.00	0.00	0.00	0.00	0.00	0.00	0.00	0.00	0.00	0.00	490.00	0.00
0.00	0.00	0.00	0.00	0.00	0.00	0.00	0.00	0.00	0.00	0.00	0.00	0.00	0.00	0.00	0.00	0.00	0.00	820.00	0.00
0.00	0.00	0.00	0.00	0.00	0.00	0.00	0.00	0.00	0.00	0.00	0.00	0.00	0.00	0.00	0.00	0.00	0.00	95.00	0.00
0.00	0.00	0.00	0.00	0.00	0.00	0.00	0.00	0.00	0.00	0.00	0.00	0.00	0.00	0.00	0.00	0.00	0.00	440.00	0.00
0.00	0.00	0.00	0.00	0.00	0.00	0.00	0.00	0.00	0.00	0.00	0.00	0.00	0.00	0.00	0.00	0.00	0.00	140.00	0.00
0.00	0.00	0.00	0.00	0.00	0.00	0.00	0.00	0.00	0.00	0.00	0.00	0.00	0.00	0.00	0.00	0.00	0.00	1010.00	0.00
0.00	0.00	0.00	0.00	0.00	0.00	0.00	0.00	0.00	0.00	0.00	0.00	0.00	0.00	0.00	0.00	0.00	0.00	830.00	0.00
0.00	0.00	0.00	0.00	0.00	0.00	0.00	0.00	0.00	0.00	0.00	0.00	0.00	0.00	0.00	0.00	0.00	0.00	440.00	0.00
0.00	0.00	0.00	0.00	0.00	0.00	0.00	0.00	0.00	0.00	0.00	0.00	0.00	0.00	0.00	0.00	0.00	0.00	570.00	0.00
0.00	0.00	0.00	0.00	0.00	0.00	0.00	0.00	0.00	0.00	0.00	0.00	0.00	0.00	0.00	0.00	0.00	0.00	620.00	0.00
0.00	0.00	0.00	0.00	0.00	0.00	0.00	0.00	0.00	0.00	0.00	0.00	0.00	0.00	0.00	0.00	0.00	0.00	810.00	0.00
0.00	0.00	0.00	0.00	0.00	0.00	0.00	0.00	0.00	0.00	0.00	0.00	0.00	0.00	0.00	0.00	0.00	0.00	700.00	0.00
0.00	0.00	0.00	0.00	0.00	0.00	0.00	0.00	0.00	0.00	0.00	0.00	0.00	0.00	0.00	0.00	0.00	0.00	1230.00	0.00
0.00	0.00	0.00	0.00	0.00	0.00	0.00	0.00	0.00	0.00	0.00	0.00	0.00	0.00	0.00	0.00	0.00	0.00	110.00	0.00
0.00	0.00	0.00	0.00	0.00	0.00	0.00	0.00	0.00	0.00	0.00	0.00	0.00	0.00	0.00	0.00	0.00	0.00	120.00	0.00
0.00	0.00	0.00	0.00	0.00	0.00	0.00	0.00	0.00	0.00	0.00	0.00	0.00	0.00	0.00	0.00	0.00	0.00	130.00	0.00
0.00	0.00	0.00	0.00	0.00	0.00	0.00	0.00	0.00	0.00	0.00	0.00	0.00	0.00	0.00	0.00	0.00	0.00	85.00	0.00
0.00	0.00	0.00	0.00	0.00	0.00	0.00	0.00	0.00	0.00	0.00	0.00	0.00	0.00	0.00	0.00	0.00	0.00	85.00	0.00
0.00	0.00	0.00	0.00	0.00	0.00	0.00	0.00	0.00	0.00	0.00	0.00	0.00	0.00	0.00	0.00	0.00	0.00	120.00	0.00
0.00	0.00	0.00	0.00	0.00	0.00	0.00	0.00	0.00	0.00	0.00	0.00	0.00	0.00	0.00	0.00	0.00	0.00	160.00	0.00
0.00	0.00	0.00	0.00	0.00	0.00	0.00	0.00	0.00	0.00	0.00	0.00	0.00	0.00	0.00	0.00	0.00	0.00	150.00	0.00
0.00	0.00	0.00	0.00	0.00	0.00	0.00	0.00	0.00	0.00	0.00	0.00	0.00	0.00	0.00	0.00	0.00	0.00	90.00	0.00
0.00	0.00	0.00	0.00	0.00	0.00	0.00	0.00	0.00	0.00	0.00	0.00	0.00	0.00	0.00	0.00	0.00	0.00	100.00	0.00
0.00	0.00	0.00	0.00	0.00	0.00	0.00	0.00	0.00	0.00	0.00	0.00	0.00	0.00	0.00	0.00	0.00	0.00	120.00	0.00
0.00	0.00	0.00	0.00	0.00	0.00	0.00	0.00	0.00	0.00	0.00	0.00	0.00	0.00	0.00	0.00	0.00	0.00	60.00	0.00
0.00	0.00	0.00	0.00	0.00	0.00	0.00	0.00	0.00	0.00	0.00	0.00	0.00	0.00	0.00	0.00	0.00	0.00	160.00	0.00
0.00	0.00	0.00	0.00	0.00	0.00	0.00	0.00	0.00	0.00	0.00	0.00	0.00	0.00	0.00	0.00	0.00	0.00	100.00	0.00
0.00	0.00	0.00	0.00	0.00	0.00	0.00	0.00	0.00	0.00	0.00	0.00	0.00	0.00	0.00	0.00	0.00	0.00	630.00	0.00
0.00	0.00	0.00	0.00	0.00	0.00	0.00	0.00	0.00	0.00	0.00	0.00	0.00	0.00	0.00	0.00	0.00	0.00	690.00	0.00
0.00	0.00	0.00	0.00	0.00	0.00	0.00	0.00	0.00	0.00	0.00	0.00	0.00	0.00	0.00	0.00	0.00	0.00	930.00	0.00
0.00	0.00	0.00	0.00	0.00	0.00	0.00	0.00	0.00	0.00	0.00	0.00	0.00	0.00	0.00	0.00	0.00	0.00	140.00	0.00
0.00	0.00	0.00	0.00	0.00	0.00	0.00	0.00	0.00	0.00	0.00	0.00	0.00	0.00	0.00	0.00	0.00	0.00	150.00	0.00
0.00	0.00	0.00	0.00	0.00	0.00	0.00	0.00	0.00	0.00	0.00	0.00	0.00	0.00	0.00	0.00	0.00	0.00	0.00	0.00
0.00	0.00	0.00	0.00	0.00	0.00	0.00	0.00	0.00	0.00	0.00	0.00	0.00	0.00	0.00	0.00	0.00	0.00	690.00	0.00

USDA ID Code	Food Name	Weight in Grams*	Quantity of Units	Unit of Measure	Protein (gm)	Fat (gm)	Carbohydrate (gm)	Kcalories	Caffeine (gm)	Fiber (gm)	Cholesterol (mg)	Saturated Fat (gm)
110	Bruegger's Bagels-Mediterranean	231.0000	1.000	Each	20.00	24.00	74.00	610.00	0.00	8.00	30.00	11.00
111	Bruegger's Bagels-Olivia De Hami	239.0000	1.000	Each	29.00	17.00	62.00	520.00	0.00	3.00	75.00	8.00
112	Bruegger's Bagels-Soup, Chicken	241.0000	8.000	Ounce	10.00	3.50	25.00	170.00	0.00	1.00	40.00	1.00
113	Bruegger's Bagels-Soup, Garden S	247.0000	8.000	Ounce	4.00	6.00	19.00	150.00	0.00	3.00	10.00	3.00
114	Bruegger's Bagels-Soup, Marcello	241.0000	8.000	Ounce	4.00	1.00	18.00	90.00	0.00	2.00	0.00	0.00
115	Bruegger's Bagels-Soup, Turkey L	227.0000	8.000	Ounce	14.00	2.50	17.00	150.00	0.00	7.00	20.00	0.50
116	Bruegger's Bagels-Stew, Ratatoui	244.0000	8.000	Ounce	2.00	9.00	12.00	140.00	0.00	3.00	0.00	1.50
117	Bruegger's Bagels-Strawberry Bru	227.0000	8.000	Fl Oz	0.00	0.00	39.00	150.00	0.00	0.00	0.00	0.00
118	Bruegger's Bagels-Tuna Salad	116.0000	0.500	Cup	12.00	19.00	9.00	260.00	0.00	2.00	30.00	3.00
119	Bruegger's Bagels-Turkey Club Sa	258.0000	1.000	Each	27.00	31.00	58.00	620.00	0.00	3.00	55.00	5.00
120	Bruegger's Bagels-Turkey Orzo, T	241.0000	8.000	Ounce	8.00	3.00	13.00	110.00	0.00	1.00	15.00	0.50
121	Bruegger's Bagels-Turkey, Herby	235.0000	1.000	Each	30.00	13.00	67.00	510.00	0.00	3.00	45.00	5.00
122	Bruegger's Bagels-Turkey, Hot Sh	234.0000	1.000	Each	26.00	8.00	68.00	450.00	0.00	3.00	3.00	3.50
123	Bruegger's Bagels-Turkey, Santa	264.0000	1.000	Each	27.00	9.00	63.00	450.00	0.00	3.00	45.00	4.00
220	Denny's-All American Slam	368.5500	1.000	Serving	38.00	62.00	9.00	712.00	0.00	1.00	686.00	20.00
221	Denny's-Bacon, 4 Strips	28.3500	4.000	Each	12.00	18.00	1.00	162.00	0.00	0.00	36.00	5.00
222	Denny's-Bagel, Dry	85.0000	1.000	Each	9.00	1.00	46.00	235.00	0.00	0.00	0.00	0.00
223	Denny's-Big Texas Chicken Fajita	481.0000	1.000	Serving	49.00	70.00	25.00	1217.00	0.00	8.00	518.00	19.00
224	Denny's-Biscuit & Sausage Gravy	198.4500	1.000	Serving	8.00	21.00	45.00	398.00	0.00	0.00	12.00	6.00
225	Denny's-Biscuit, Buttered	85.0000	1.000	Each	5.00	11.00	39.00	272.00	0.00	0.00	0.00	4.00
226	Denny's-Buttermilk Hotcakes (3)	141.7500	3.000	Each	12.00	7.00	95.00	491.00	0.00	3.00	0.00	1.00
227	Denny's-Chicken Fried Steak & Eg	226.8000	1.000	Serving	22.00	36.00	9.00	430.00	0.00	4.00	440.00	12.00
228	Denny's-Chicken Fried Steak Skil	737.0000	1.000	Serving	60.00	104.00	119.00	1745.00	0.00	26.00	607.00	28.00
229	Denny's-Cinnamon Swirl French To	340.0000	1.000	Serving	23.00	49.00	124.00	1030.00	0.00	4.00	280.00	21.00
230	Denny's-Cinnamon Swirl Slam	368.5500	1.000	Serving	38.00	78.00	68.00	1105.00	0.00	2.00	635.00	26.00
231	Denny's-Country Fried Potatoes	170.0000	1.000	Serving	3.00	35.00	23.00	515.00	0.00	9.00	8.00	8.00
232	Denny's-Egg Beaters, Egg Substit	56.7000	1.000	Serving	5.00	5.00	1.00	71.00	0.00	0.00	1.00	1.00
233	Denny's-Eggs Benedict	425.2500	1.000	Serving	34.00	46.00	34.00	695.00	0.00	1.00	515.00	11.00
234	Denny's-English Muffin, Dry, 1mu	113.4000	1.000	Each	5.00	1.00	24.00	125.00	0.00	1.00	0.00	0.00
235	Denny's-Flour Tortillas and Sals	156.0000	1.000	Serving	6.00	8.00	50.50	281.00	0.00	4.00	0.00	1.50
236	Denny's-French Slam	397.0000	1.000	Serving	44.00	71.00	58.00	1029.00	0.00	2.00	777.00	20.00
237	Denny's-French Toast (2)	199.0000	2.000	Each	16.00	24.00	54.00	507.00	0.00	3.00	219.00	6.00
238	Denny's-Grand Slam Slugger	340.0000	1.000	Serving	32.00	46.00	58.00	789.00	0.00	2.00	487.00	14.00
239	Denny's-Grits	113.0000	0.500	Cup	2.00	0.00	18.00	80.00	0.00	0.00	0.00	0.00
241	Denny's-Ham, Grilled, sliced	85.0000	3.000	Ounce	15.00	3.00	2.00	94.00	0.00	0.00	23.00	1.00
240	Denny's-Ham'nCheddar Omelette	283.5000	1.000	Each	37.00	45.00	4.00	581.00	0.00	0.00	672.00	8.00
242	Denny's-Hashed Browns	113.4000	1.000	Serving	2.00	14.00	20.00	218.00	0.00	2.00	0.00	2.00
243	Denny's-Kelloggs Dry Cereal	28.3500	1.000	Serving	2.00	0.00	23.00	100.00	0.00	1.00	0.00	0.00
244	Denny's-Lumberjack Slam	538.6500	1.000	Serving	54.00	70.00	118.00	1259.00	0.00	5.00	481.00	18.00
245	Denny's-Meat Lover's Skillet	425.2500	1.000	Serving	41.00	93.00	24.00	1147.00	0.00	7.00	460.00	26.00
246	Denny's-Oatmeal N' Fixins	538.6500	1.000	Serving	13.00	6.00	95.00	460.00	0.00	7.00	11.00	3.00
247	Denny's-One Egg	56.7000	1.000	Each	6.00	10.00	0.50	120.00	0.00	0.00	210.00	3.00
248	Denny's-Original Grand Slam	283.5000	1.000	Serving	34.00	50.00	65.00	795.00	0.00	2.00	460.00	14.00
249	Denny's-Pork Chop & Eggs	354.3800	1.000	Serving	55.00	47.00	6.00	673.00	0.00	0.00	571.00	13.00
250	Denny's-Quaker Oatmeal	113.4000	0.500	Cup	5.00	2.00	18.00	100.00	0.00	3.00	0.00	0.00
251	Denny's-Sausage Gravy	113.4000	1.000	Serving	3.00	10.00	6.00	126.00	0.00	0.00	12.00	2.00
252	Denny's-Sausage, 4 Links	85.0000	4.000	Each	16.00	32.00	0.00	354.00	0.00	0.00	64.00	12.00
253	Denny's-Sirloin Steak & Eggs	255.0000	1.000	Serving	43.00	49.00	1.00	622.00	0.00	1.00	572.00	18.00
254	Denny's-T-bone Steak & Eggs	397.0000	1.000	Serving	73.00	77.00	1.00	991.00	0.00	1.00	657.00	31.00
255	Denny's-Toast, Dry, 1slice	28.3500	1.000	Slice	3.00	1.00	17.00	90.00	0.00	1.00	0.00	0.00
256	Denny's-Two Egg Breakfast	312.0000	1.000	Serving	31.00	67.00	24.00	825.00	0.00	2.00	538.00	17.00
257	Denny's-Ultimate Omelette	368.5500	1.000	Each	30.00	47.00	9.00	594.00	0.00	2.00	639.00	12.00
258	Denny's-Veggie-Cheese Omelette	340.0000	1.000	Each	26.00	39.00	9.00	480.00	0.00	2.00	644.00	13.00
	Dunkin' Donuts-Apple Filled w/ C	79.0000	1.000	Each	5.00	11.00	33.00	250.00	0.00	1.00	0.00	0.00
	Dunkin' Donuts-Bavarian Filled w	79.0000	1.000	Each	5.00	11.00	32.00	240.00	0.00	2.00	0.00	0.00

Monounsaturated Fat (gm)	Polyunsaturated Fat (gm)	Vitamin D (mg)	Vitamin K (mg)	Vitamin E (mg)	Vitamin A (re)	Vitamin C (mg)	Thiamin (mg)	Riboflavin (mg)	Niacin (mg)	Vitamin B_6 (mg)	Folate (mg)	Vitamin B_{12} (mcg)	Calcium (mg)	Iron (mg)	Magnesium (mg)	Phosphorus (mg)	Potassium (mg)	Sodium (mg)	Zinc (mg)
0.00	0.00	0.00	0.00	0.00	0.00	0.00	0.00	0.00	0.00	0.00	0.00	0.00	0.00	0.00	0.00	0.00	0.00	840.00	0.00
0.00	0.00	0.00	0.00	0.00	0.00	0.00	0.00	0.00	0.00	0.00	0.00	0.00	0.00	0.00	0.00	0.00	0.00	1500.00	0.00
0.00	0.00	0.00	0.00	0.00	0.00	0.00	0.00	0.00	0.00	0.00	0.00	0.00	0.00	0.00	0.00	0.00	0.00	1150.00	0.00
0.00	0.00	0.00	0.00	0.00	0.00	0.00	0.00	0.00	0.00	0.00	0.00	0.00	0.00	0.00	0.00	0.00	0.00	1050.00	0.00
0.00	0.00	0.00	0.00	0.00	0.00	0.00	0.00	0.00	0.00	0.00	0.00	0.00	0.00	0.00	0.00	0.00	0.00	890.00	0.00
0.00	0.00	0.00	0.00	0.00	0.00	0.00	0.00	0.00	0.00	0.00	0.00	0.00	0.00	0.00	0.00	0.00	0.00	820.00	0.00
0.00	0.00	0.00	0.00	0.00	0.00	0.00	0.00	0.00	0.00	0.00	0.00	0.00	0.00	0.00	0.00	0.00	0.00	1100.00	0.00
0.00	0.00	0.00	0.00	0.00	0.00	0.00	0.00	0.00	0.00	0.00	0.00	0.00	0.00	0.00	0.00	0.00	0.00	5.00	0.00
0.00	0.00	0.00	0.00	0.00	0.00	0.00	0.00	0.00	0.00	0.00	0.00	0.00	0.00	0.00	0.00	0.00	0.00	580.00	0.00
0.00	0.00	0.00	0.00	0.00	0.00	0.00	0.00	0.00	0.00	0.00	0.00	0.00	0.00	0.00	0.00	0.00	0.00	1420.00	0.00
0.00	0.00	0.00	0.00	0.00	0.00	0.00	0.00	0.00	0.00	0.00	0.00	0.00	0.00	0.00	0.00	0.00	0.00	940.00	0.00
0.00	0.00	0.00	0.00	0.00	0.00	0.00	0.00	0.00	0.00	0.00	0.00	0.00	0.00	0.00	0.00	0.00	0.00	1100.00	0.00
0.00	0.00	0.00	0.00	0.00	0.00	0.00	0.00	0.00	0.00	0.00	0.00	0.00	0.00	0.00	0.00	0.00	0.00	1090.00	0.00
0.00	0.00	0.00	0.00	0.00	0.00	0.00	0.00	0.00	0.00	0.00	0.00	0.00	0.00	0.00	0.00	0.00	0.00	1040.00	0.00
0.00	0.00	0.00	0.00	0.00	390.00	25.80	0.00	0.00	0.00	0.00	0.00	0.00	240.00	3.60	0.00	0.00	0.00	1281.00	0.00
0.00	0.00	0.00	0.00	0.00	0.00	6.00	0.00	0.00	0.00	0.00	0.00	0.00	0.00	0.36	0.00	0.00	0.00	640.00	0.00
0.00	0.00	0.00	0.00	0.00	0.00	0.00	0.00	0.00	0.00	0.00	0.00	0.00	0.00	14.94	0.00	0.00	0.00	495.00	0.00
0.00	0.00	0.00	0.00	0.00	530.00	28.20	0.00	0.00	0.00	0.00	0.00	0.00	220.00	3.06	0.00	0.00	0.00	1817.00	0.00
0.00	0.00	0.00	0.00	0.00	0.00	0.00	0.00	0.00	0.00	0.00	0.00	0.00	0.60	0.18	0.00	0.00	0.00	1267.00	0.00
0.00	0.00	0.00	0.00	0.00	0.00	0.00	0.00	0.00	0.00	0.00	0.00	0.00	0.00	0.00	0.00	0.00	0.00	790.00	0.00
0.00	0.00	0.00	0.00	0.00	0.00	0.00	0.00	0.00	0.00	0.00	0.00	0.00	150.00	1.80	0.00	0.00	0.00	0.00	0.00
0.00	0.00	0.00	0.00	0.00	220.00	0.00	0.00	0.00	0.00	0.00	0.00	0.00	550.00	0.54	0.00	0.00	0.00	861.00	0.00
0.00	0.00	0.00	0.00	0.00	140.00	36.00	0.00	0.00	0.00	0.00	0.00	0.00	130.00	8.10	0.00	0.00	0.00	6184.00	0.00
0.00	0.00	0.00	0.00	0.00	370.00	0.00	0.00	0.00	0.00	0.00	0.00	0.00	180.00	6.48	0.00	0.00	0.00	675.00	0.00
0.00	0.00	0.00	0.00	0.00	540.00	0.00	0.00	0.00	0.00	0.00	0.00	0.00	150.00	5.58	0.00	0.00	0.00	1374.00	0.00
0.00	0.00	0.00	0.00	0.00	0.00	0.00	0.00	0.00	0.00	0.00	0.00	0.00	60.00	1.08	0.00	0.00	0.00	805.00	0.00
0.00	0.00	0.00	0.00	0.00	370.00	0.00	0.00	0.00	0.00	0.00	0.00	0.00	20.00	1.08	0.00	0.00	0.00	138.00	0.00
0.00	0.00	0.00	0.00	0.00	530.00	0.00	0.00	0.00	0.00	0.00	0.00	0.00	190.00	3.96	0.00	0.00	0.00	1718.00	0.00
0.00	0.00	0.00	0.00	0.00	0.00	0.00	0.00	0.00	0.00	0.00	0.00	0.00	80.00	1.80	0.00	0.00	0.00	0.00	0.00
0.00	0.00	0.00	0.00	0.00	150.00	21.00	0.00	0.00	0.00	0.00	0.00	0.00	200.00	2.70	0.00	0.00	0.00	1031.00	0.00
0.00	0.00	0.00	0.00	0.00	530.00	0.00	0.00	0.00	0.00	0.00	0.00	0.00	120.00	5.58	0.00	0.00	0.00	1428.00	0.00
0.00	0.00	0.00	0.00	0.00	130.00	0.00	0.00	0.00	0.00	0.00	0.00	0.00	130.00	3.60	0.00	0.00	0.00	594.00	0.00
0.00	0.00	0.00	0.00	0.00	140.00	0.00	0.00	0.00	0.00	0.00	0.00	0.00	250.00	4.68	0.00	0.00	0.00	1438.00	0.00
0.00	0.00	0.00	0.00	0.00	0.00	0.00	0.00	0.00	0.00	0.00	0.00	0.00	0.00	0.72	0.00	0.00	0.00	520.00	0.00
0.00	0.00	0.00	0.00	0.00	0.00	0.00	0.00	0.00	0.00	0.00	0.00	0.00	0.00	0.72	0.00	0.00	0.00	761.00	0.00
0.00	0.00	0.00	0.00	0.00	390.00	0.00	0.00	0.00	0.00	0.00	0.00	0.00	380.00	2.88	0.00	0.00	0.00	1180.00	0.00
0.00	0.00	0.00	0.00	0.00	30.00	6.60	0.00	0.00	0.00	0.00	0.00	0.00	10.00	0.36	0.00	0.00	0.00	424.00	0.00
0.00	0.00	0.00	0.00	0.00	350.00	9.60	0.00	0.00	0.00	0.00	0.00	0.00	0.00	3.42	0.00	0.00	0.00	276.00	0.00
0.00	0.00	0.00	0.00	0.00	370.00	7.80	0.00	0.00	0.00	0.00	0.00	0.00	230.00	5.22	0.00	0.00	0.00	4028.00	0.00
0.00	0.00	0.00	0.00	0.00	470.00	4.20	0.00	0.00	0.00	0.00	0.00	0.00	220.00	3.42	0.00	0.00	0.00	2507.00	0.00
0.00	0.00	0.00	0.00	0.00	80.00	12.00	0.00	0.00	0.00	0.00	0.00	0.00	250.00	2.70	0.00	0.00	0.00	87.00	0.00
0.00	0.00	0.00	0.00	0.00	20.00	3.60	0.00	0.00	0.00	0.00	0.00	0.00	0.00	0.72	0.00	0.00	0.00	120.00	0.00
0.00	0.00	0.00	0.00	0.00	330.00	0.00	0.00	0.00	0.00	0.00	0.00	0.00	160.00	3.42	0.00	0.00	0.00	2237.00	0.00
0.00	0.00	0.00	0.00	0.00	150.00	0.00	0.00	0.00	0.00	0.00	0.00	0.00	50.00	3.06	0.00	0.00	0.00	1582.00	0.00
0.00	0.00	0.00	0.00	0.00	0.00	0.00	0.00	0.00	0.00	0.00	0.00	0.00	10.00	0.90	0.00	0.00	0.00	175.00	0.00
0.00	0.00	0.00	0.00	0.00	0.00	0.00	0.00	0.00	0.00	0.00	0.00	0.00	10.00	0.18	0.00	0.00	0.00	477.00	0.00
0.00	0.00	0.00	0.00	0.00	4.00	0.00	0.00	0.00	0.00	0.00	0.00	0.00	10.00	1.26	0.00	0.00	0.00	944.00	0.00
0.00	0.00	0.00	0.00	0.00	160.00	1.80	0.00	0.00	0.00	0.00	0.00	0.00	130.00	5.94	0.00	0.00	0.00	632.00	0.00
0.00	0.00	0.00	0.00	0.00	150.00	2.40	0.00	0.00	0.00	0.00	0.00	0.00	200.00	10.80	0.00	0.00	0.00	1003.00	0.00
0.00	0.00	0.00	0.00	0.00	0.00	0.00	0.00	0.00	0.00	0.00	0.00	0.00	30.00	0.72	0.00	0.00	0.00	166.00	0.00
0.00	0.00	0.00	0.00	0.00	170.00	7.80	0.00	0.00	0.00	0.00	0.00	0.00	80.00	3.24	0.00	0.00	0.00	1765.00	0.00
0.00	0.00	0.00	0.00	0.00	320.00	55.20	0.00	0.00	0.00	0.00	0.00	0.00	80.00	3.60	0.00	0.00	0.00	939.00	0.00
0.00	0.00	0.00	0.00	0.00	390.00	16.20	0.00	0.00	0.00	0.00	0.00	0.00	280.00	2.70	0.00	0.00	0.00	535.00	0.00
0.00	0.00	0.00	0.00	0.00	0.00	0.00	0.00	0.00	0.00	0.00	0.00	0.00	0.00	0.00	0.00	0.00	0.00	280.00	0.00
0.00	0.00	0.00	0.00	0.00	0.00	0.00	0.00	0.00	0.00	0.00	0.00	0.00	0.00	0.00	0.00	0.00	0.00	260.00	0.00

USDA ID Code	Food Name	Weight in Grams*	Quantity of Units	Unit of Measure	Protein (gm)	Fat (gm)	Carbohydrate (gm)	Kcalories	Caffeine (gm)	Fiber (gm)	Cholesterol (mg)	Saturated Fat (gm)
	Dunkin' Donuts-Blueberry Filled	67.0000	1.000	Each	4.00	8.00	29.00	210.00	0.00	2.00	0.00	0.00
	Dunkin' Donuts-Buttermilk Ring,	74.0000	1.000	Each	4.00	14.00	37.00	290.00	0.00	1.00	10.00	0.00
	Dunkin' Donuts-Cake Ring, Plain	62.0000	1.000	Each	4.00	17.00	25.00	270.00	0.00	1.00	0.00	0.00
	Dunkin' Donuts-Chocolate Rings,	71.0000	1.000	Each	3.50	21.00	34.00	324.00	0.00	1.90	0.00	0.00
	Dunkin' Donuts-Coffee Roll, Glaz	81.0000	1.000	Each	5.00	12.00	37.00	280.00	0.00	2.00	0.00	0.00
	Dunkin' Donuts-Cookie, Chocolate	43.0000	1.000	Each	3.00	10.00	25.00	200.00	0.00	1.00	30.00	0.00
	Dunkin' Donuts-Cookie, Chocolate	43.0000	1.000	Each	3.00	11.00	23.00	210.00	0.00	2.00	30.00	0.00
	Dunkin' Donuts-Cookie, Oatmeal P	46.0000	1.000	Each	3.00	9.00	28.00	200.00	0.00	1.00	25.00	0.00
	Dunkin' Donuts-Croissant, Almond	105.0000	1.000	Each	8.00	27.00	38.00	420.00	0.00	3.00	0.00	0.00
	Dunkin' Donuts-Croissant, Chocol	94.0000	1.000	Each	7.00	29.00	38.00	440.00	0.00	3.00	0.00	0.00
	Dunkin' Donuts-Croissant, Plain	72.0000	1.000	Each	7.00	19.00	27.00	310.00	0.00	2.00	0.00	0.00
	Dunkin' Donuts-Cruller, Glazed F	38.0000	1.000	Each	2.00	8.00	16.00	140.00	0.00	0.00	30.00	0.00
	Dunkin' Donuts-Filled, Jelly	67.0000	1.000	Each	4.00	9.00	31.00	220.00	0.00	1.00	0.00	0.00
	Dunkin' Donuts-Filled, Lemon	79.0000	1.000	Each	4.00	12.00	33.00	260.00	0.00	1.00	0.00	0.00
	Dunkin' Donuts-Muffin, Apple 'n	100.0000	1.000	Each	6.00	8.00	52.00	300.00	0.00	2.00	25.00	0.00
	Dunkin' Donuts-Muffin, Banana Nu	103.0000	1.000	Each	7.00	10.00	49.00	310.00	0.00	3.00	30.00	0.00
	Dunkin' Donuts-Muffin, Blueberry	101.0000	1.000	Each	6.00	8.00	46.00	280.00	0.00	2.00	30.00	0.00
	Dunkin' Donuts-Muffin, Bran w/ R	104.0000	1.000	Each	6.00	9.00	51.00	310.00	0.00	4.00	15.00	0.00
	Dunkin' Donuts-Muffin, Corn	96.0000	1.000	Each	7.00	12.00	51.00	340.00	0.00	1.00	40.00	0.00
	Dunkin' Donuts-Muffin, Cranberry	98.0000	1.000	Each	6.00	9.00	44.00	290.00	0.00	2.00	25.00	0.00
	Dunkin' Donuts-Muffin, Oat Bran	100.0000	1.000	Each	7.00	11.00	50.00	330.00	0.00	3.00	0.00	0.00
	Dunkin' Donuts-Yeast Ring, Choco	55.0000	1.000	Each	4.00	10.00	25.00	200.00	0.00	1.00	0.00	0.00
	Dunkin' Donuts-Yeast Ring, Glaze	55.0000	1.000	Each	4.00	9.00	26.00	200.00	0.00	1.00	0.00	0.00
265	Einstein Bros.-Almond Delight	360.0000	12.000	Fl Oz	8.00	4.50	29.00	190.00	0.00	0.00	20.00	3.00
266	Einstein Bros.-Almond Delight, I	480.0000	16.000	Fl Oz	7.00	4.00	28.00	180.00	0.00	0.00	15.00	2.50
267	Einstein Bros.-Almond Delight, N	360.0000	12.000	Fl Oz	8.00	0.00	29.00	150.00	0.00	0.00	5.00	0.00
268	Einstein Bros.-Americano	240.0000	8.000	Fl Oz	0.00	0.00	0.00	0.00	0.00	0.00	0.00	0.00
269	Einstein Bros.-Americano, Iced	360.0000	8.000	Fl Oz	0.00	0.00	0.00	0.00	0.00	0.00	0.00	0.00
270	Einstein Bros.-Bagel Chips, Blue	28.0000	1.000	Each	3.00	1.00	19.00	90.00	0.00	1.00	0.00	0.00
271	Einstein Bros.-Bagel Chips, Cinn	28.0000	1.000	Each	3.00	1.00	19.00	90.00	0.00	1.00	0.00	0.00
272	Einstein Bros.-Bagel Chips, Plai	28.0000	1.000	Each	3.00	0.00	18.00	90.00	0.00	1.00	0.00	0.00
273	Einstein Bros.-Bagel Chips, Sour	28.0000	1.000	Each	3.00	1.00	18.00	90.00	0.00	1.00	0.00	0.00
274	Einstein Bros.-Bagel Chips, Sun-	28.0000	1.000	Each	3.00	1.00	17.00	90.00	0.00	1.00	0.00	0.00
275	Einstein Bros.-Bagel Chips, Sunf	28.0000	1.000	Each	3.00	2.00	18.00	100.00	0.00	1.00	0.00	0.00
276	Einstein Bros.-Bagel, Blueberry,	113.0000	1.000	Each	11.00	1.00	77.00	350.00	0.00	3.00	0.00	0.00
277	Einstein Bros.-Bagel, Choc Chip	113.0000	1.000	Each	11.00	3.00	76.00	370.00	0.00	3.00	0.00	2.00
278	Einstein Bros.-Bagel, Cinnamon R	113.0000	1.000	Each	11.00	1.00	78.00	350.00	0.00	2.00	0.00	0.00
279	Einstein Bros.-Bagel, Cinnamon S	106.0000	1.000	Each	10.00	1.00	74.00	330.00	0.00	2.00	0.00	0.00
280	Einstein Bros.-Bagel, Cranberry	113.0000	1.000	Each	10.00	1.00	78.00	350.00	0.00	3.00	0.00	0.00
281	Einstein Bros.-Bagel, Egg	106.0000	1.000	Each	11.00	3.00	69.00	340.00	0.00	2.00	35.00	1.00
282	Einstein Bros.-Bagel, Everything	111.0000	1.000	Each	13.00	2.00	75.00	340.00	0.00	2.00	0.00	0.00
283	Einstein Bros.-Bagel, Garlic, Ch	119.0000	1.000	Each	13.00	3.00	79.00	380.00	0.00	4.00	0.00	1.00
284	Einstein Bros.-Bagel, Honey 8 Gr	106.0000	1.000	Each	11.00	1.00	69.00	320.00	0.00	4.00	0.00	0.00
285	Einstein Bros.-Bagel, Jalapeno	106.0000	1.000	Each	11.00	1.00	71.00	330.00	0.00	2.00	0.00	0.00
286	Einstein Bros.-Bagel, Nutty Bana	113.0000	1.000	Each	11.00	3.00	74.00	360.00	0.00	2.00	0.00	1.00
287	Einstein Bros.-Bagel, Onion, Chp	106.0000	1.000	Each	11.00	1.00	71.00	330.00	0.00	2.00	0.00	0.00
288	Einstein Bros.-Bagel, Plain	106.0000	1.000	Each	11.00	1.00	71.00	320.00	0.00	2.00	0.00	0.00
289	Einstein Bros.-Bagel, Poppy Dip'	111.0000	1.000	Each	12.00	2.00	74.00	350.00	0.00	2.00	0.00	0.00
290	Einstein Bros.-Bagel, Pumpernick	106.0000	1.000	Each	11.00	1.00	68.00	320.00	0.00	3.00	0.00	0.00
291	Einstein Bros.-Bagel, Rye, Marbl	113.0000	1.000	Each	11.00	2.00	73.00	340.00	0.00	3.00	0.00	0.00
292	Einstein Bros.-Bagel, Salt	111.0000	1.000	Each	11.00	1.00	73.00	330.00	0.00	2.00	0.00	0.00
293	Einstein Bros.-Bagel, Sesame Dip	117.0000	1.000	Each	11.00	5.00	75.00	380.00	0.00	3.00	0.00	1.00
294	Einstein Bros.-Bagel, Spinach He	106.0000	1.000	Each	11.00	1.00	68.00	310.00	0.00	3.00	0.00	0.00
295	Einstein Bros.-Bagel, Sun-dried	106.0000	1.000	Each	11.00	1.00	69.00	320.00	0.00	3.00	0.00	0.00
296	Einstein Bros.-Bagel, Sunflower	106.0000	1.000	Each	12.00	5.00	66.00	350.00	0.00	3.00	0.00	1.00

Monounsaturated Fat (gm)	Polyunsaturated Fat (gm)	Vitamin D (mg)	Vitamin K (mg)	Vitamin E (mg)	Vitamin A (re)	Vitamin C (mg)	Thiamin (mg)	Riboflavin (mg)	Niacin (mg)	Vitamin B_6 (mg)	Folate (mg)	Vitamin B_{12} (mcg)	Calcium (mg)	Iron (mg)	Magnesium (mg)	Phosphorus (mg)	Potassium (mg)	Sodium (mg)	Zinc (mg)
0.00	0.00	0.00	0.00	0.00	0.00	0.00	0.00	0.00	0.00	0.00	0.00	0.00	0.00	0.00	0.00	0.00	0.00	240.00	0.00
0.00	0.00	0.00	0.00	0.00	0.00	0.00	0.00	0.00	0.00	0.00	0.00	0.00	0.00	0.00	0.00	0.00	0.00	370.00	0.00
0.00	0.00	0.00	0.00	0.00	0.00	0.00	0.00	0.00	0.00	0.00	0.00	0.00	0.00	0.00	0.00	0.00	0.00	330.00	0.00
0.00	0.00	0.00	0.00	0.00	0.00	0.00	0.00	0.00	0.00	0.00	0.00	0.00	0.00	0.00	0.00	0.00	0.00	383.00	0.00
0.00	0.00	0.00	0.00	0.00	0.00	0.00	0.00	0.00	0.00	0.00	0.00	0.00	0.00	0.00	0.00	0.00	0.00	310.00	0.00
0.00	0.00	0.00	0.00	0.00	0.00	0.00	0.00	0.00	0.00	0.00	0.00	0.00	0.00	0.00	0.00	0.00	0.00	110.00	0.00
0.00	0.00	0.00	0.00	0.00	0.00	0.00	0.00	0.00	0.00	0.00	0.00	0.00	0.00	0.00	0.00	0.00	0.00	100.00	0.00
0.00	0.00	0.00	0.00	0.00	0.00	0.00	0.00	0.00	0.00	0.00	0.00	0.00	0.00	0.00	0.00	0.00	0.00	100.00	0.00
0.00	0.00	0.00	0.00	0.00	0.00	0.00	0.00	0.00	0.00	0.00	0.00	0.00	0.00	0.00	0.00	0.00	0.00	280.00	0.00
0.00	0.00	0.00	0.00	0.00	0.00	0.00	0.00	0.00	0.00	0.00	0.00	0.00	0.00	0.00	0.00	0.00	0.00	220.00	0.00
0.00	0.00	0.00	0.00	0.00	0.00	0.00	0.00	0.00	0.00	0.00	0.00	0.00	0.00	0.00	0.00	0.00	0.00	240.00	0.00
0.00	0.00	0.00	0.00	0.00	0.00	0.00	0.00	0.00	0.00	0.00	0.00	0.00	0.00	0.00	0.00	0.00	0.00	130.00	0.00
0.00	0.00	0.00	0.00	0.00	0.00	0.00	0.00	0.00	0.00	0.00	0.00	0.00	0.00	0.00	0.00	0.00	0.00	230.00	0.00
0.00	0.00	0.00	0.00	0.00	0.00	0.00	0.00	0.00	0.00	0.00	0.00	0.00	0.00	0.00	0.00	0.00	0.00	280.00	0.00
0.00	0.00	0.00	0.00	0.00	0.00	0.00	0.00	0.00	0.00	0.00	0.00	0.00	0.00	0.00	0.00	0.00	0.00	360.00	0.00
0.00	0.00	0.00	0.00	0.00	0.00	0.00	0.00	0.00	0.00	0.00	0.00	0.00	0.00	0.00	0.00	0.00	0.00	410.00	0.00
0.00	0.00	0.00	0.00	0.00	0.00	0.00	0.00	0.00	0.00	0.00	0.00	0.00	0.00	0.00	0.00	0.00	0.00	340.00	0.00
0.00	0.00	0.00	0.00	0.00	0.00	0.00	0.00	0.00	0.00	0.00	0.00	0.00	0.00	0.00	0.00	0.00	0.00	560.00	0.00
0.00	0.00	0.00	0.00	0.00	0.00	0.00	0.00	0.00	0.00	0.00	0.00	0.00	0.00	0.00	0.00	0.00	0.00	560.00	0.00
0.00	0.00	0.00	0.00	0.00	0.00	0.00	0.00	0.00	0.00	0.00	0.00	0.00	0.00	0.00	0.00	0.00	0.00	360.00	0.00
0.00	0.00	0.00	0.00	0.00	0.00	0.00	0.00	0.00	0.00	0.00	0.00	0.00	0.00	0.00	0.00	0.00	0.00	450.00	0.00
0.00	0.00	0.00	0.00	0.00	0.00	0.00	0.00	0.00	0.00	0.00	0.00	0.00	0.00	0.00	0.00	0.00	0.00	190.00	0.00
0.00	0.00	0.00	0.00	0.00	0.00	0.00	0.00	0.00	0.00	0.00	0.00	0.00	0.00	0.00	0.00	0.00	0.00	230.00	0.00
0.00	0.00	0.00	0.00	0.00	0.00	0.00	0.00	0.00	0.00	0.00	0.00	0.00	0.00	0.00	0.00	0.00	0.00	130.00	0.00
0.00	0.00	0.00	0.00	0.00	0.00	0.00	0.00	0.00	0.00	0.00	0.00	0.00	0.00	0.00	0.00	0.00	0.00	120.00	0.00
0.00	0.00	0.00	0.00	0.00	0.00	0.00	0.00	0.00	0.00	0.00	0.00	0.00	0.00	0.00	0.00	0.00	0.00	135.00	0.00
0.00	0.00	0.00	0.00	0.00	0.00	0.00	0.00	0.00	0.00	0.00	0.00	0.00	0.00	0.00	0.00	0.00	0.00	0.00	0.00
0.00	0.00	0.00	0.00	0.00	0.00	0.00	0.00	0.00	0.00	0.00	0.00	0.00	0.00	0.00	0.00	0.00	0.00	0.00	0.00
0.00	0.00	0.00	0.00	0.00	0.00	0.00	0.00	0.00	0.00	0.00	0.00	0.00	0.00	0.00	0.00	0.00	0.00	105.00	0.00
0.00	0.00	0.00	0.00	0.00	0.00	0.00	0.00	0.00	0.00	0.00	0.00	0.00	0.00	0.00	0.00	0.00	0.00	120.00	0.00
0.00	0.00	0.00	0.00	0.00	0.00	0.00	0.00	0.00	0.00	0.00	0.00	0.00	0.00	0.00	0.00	0.00	0.00	140.00	0.00
0.00	0.00	0.00	0.00	0.00	0.00	0.00	0.00	0.00	0.00	0.00	0.00	0.00	0.00	0.00	0.00	0.00	0.00	120.00	0.00
0.00	0.00	0.00	0.00	0.00	0.00	0.00	0.00	0.00	0.00	0.00	0.00	0.00	0.00	0.00	0.00	0.00	0.00	130.00	0.00
0.00	0.00	0.00	0.00	0.00	0.00	0.00	0.00	0.00	0.00	0.00	0.00	0.00	0.00	0.00	0.00	0.00	0.00	190.00	0.00
0.00	0.00	0.00	0.00	0.00	0.00	0.00	0.00	0.00	0.00	0.00	0.00	0.00	0.00	0.00	0.00	0.00	0.00	510.00	0.00
0.00	0.00	0.00	0.00	0.00	0.00	0.00	0.00	0.00	0.00	0.00	0.00	0.00	0.00	0.00	0.00	0.00	0.00	500.00	0.00
0.00	0.00	0.00	0.00	0.00	0.00	0.00	0.00	0.00	0.00	0.00	0.00	0.00	0.00	0.00	0.00	0.00	0.00	490.00	0.00
0.00	0.00	0.00	0.00	0.00	0.00	0.00	0.00	0.00	0.00	0.00	0.00	0.00	0.00	0.00	0.00	0.00	0.00	490.00	0.00
0.00	0.00	0.00	0.00	0.00	0.00	0.00	0.00	0.00	0.00	0.00	0.00	0.00	0.00	0.00	0.00	0.00	0.00	490.00	0.00
0.00	0.00	0.00	0.00	0.00	0.00	0.00	0.00	0.00	0.00	0.00	0.00	0.00	0.00	0.00	0.00	0.00	0.00	510.00	0.00
0.00	0.00	0.00	0.00	0.00	0.00	0.00	0.00	0.00	0.00	0.00	0.00	0.00	0.00	0.00	0.00	0.00	0.00	820.00	0.00
0.00	0.00	0.00	0.00	0.00	0.00	0.00	0.00	0.00	0.00	0.00	0.00	0.00	0.00	0.00	0.00	0.00	0.00	680.00	0.00
0.00	0.00	0.00	0.00	0.00	0.00	0.00	0.00	0.00	0.00	0.00	0.00	0.00	0.00	0.00	0.00	0.00	0.00	510.00	0.00
0.00	0.00	0.00	0.00	0.00	0.00	0.00	0.00	0.00	0.00	0.00	0.00	0.00	0.00	0.00	0.00	0.00	0.00	510.00	0.00
0.00	0.00	0.00	0.00	0.00	0.00	0.00	0.00	0.00	0.00	0.00	0.00	0.00	0.00	0.00	0.00	0.00	0.00	510.00	0.00
0.00	0.00	0.00	0.00	0.00	0.00	0.00	0.00	0.00	0.00	0.00	0.00	0.00	0.00	0.00	0.00	0.00	0.00	500.00	0.00
0.00	0.00	0.00	0.00	0.00	0.00	0.00	0.00	0.00	0.00	0.00	0.00	0.00	0.00	0.00	0.00	0.00	0.00	520.00	0.00
0.00	0.00	0.00	0.00	0.00	0.00	0.00	0.00	0.00	0.00	0.00	0.00	0.00	0.00	0.00	0.00	0.00	0.00	680.00	0.00
0.00	0.00	0.00	0.00	0.00	0.00	0.00	0.00	0.00	0.00	0.00	0.00	0.00	0.00	0.00	0.00	0.00	0.00	730.00	0.00
0.00	0.00	0.00	0.00	0.00	0.00	0.00	0.00	0.00	0.00	0.00	0.00	0.00	0.00	0.00	0.00	0.00	0.00	690.00	0.00
0.00	0.00	0.00	0.00	0.00	0.00	0.00	0.00	0.00	0.00	0.00	0.00	0.00	0.00	0.00	0.00	0.00	0.00	1790.00	0.00
0.00	0.00	0.00	0.00	0.00	0.00	0.00	0.00	0.00	0.00	0.00	0.00	0.00	0.00	0.00	0.00	0.00	0.00	680.00	0.00
0.00	0.00	0.00	0.00	0.00	0.00	0.00	0.00	0.00	0.00	0.00	0.00	0.00	0.00	0.00	0.00	0.00	0.00	520.00	0.00
0.00	0.00	0.00	0.00	0.00	0.00	0.00	0.00	0.00	0.00	0.00	0.00	0.00	0.00	0.00	0.00	0.00	0.00	520.00	0.00
0.00	0.00	0.00	0.00	0.00	0.00	0.00	0.00	0.00	0.00	0.00	0.00	0.00	0.00	0.00	0.00	0.00	0.00	710.00	0.00

USDA ID Code	Food Name	Weight in Grams*	Quantity of Units	Unit of Measure	Protein (gm)	Fat (gm)	Carbohydrate (gm)	Kcalories	Caffeine (gm)	Fiber (gm)	Cholesterol (mg)	Saturated Fat (gm)
297	Einstein Bros.-Bagel, Veggie Con	106.0000	1.000	Each	11.00	1.00	70.00	320.00	0.00	2.00	0.00	0.00
298	Einstein Bros.-Brownie, Choc Cho	79.5200	2.800	Ounce	3.00	15.00	51.00	346.00	0.00	2.00	18.00	4.00
299	Einstein Bros.-Caf_ Au Lait	360.0000	12.000	Fl Oz	6.00	3.50	9.00	100.00	0.00	0.00	15.00	2.00
300	Einstein Bros.-Caf_ Au Lait, Non	360.0000	12.000	Fl Oz	6.00	0.00	10.00	70.00	0.00	0.00	5.00	0.00
301	Einstein Bros.-Caf_ Latte, Iced	480.0000	16.000	Fl Oz	8.00	4.50	12.00	120.00	0.00	0.00	20.00	3.00
302	Einstein Bros.-Caf_ Latte, Non F	360.0000	12.000	Fl Oz	9.00	0.00	14.00	100.00	0.00	0.00	5.00	0.00
303	Einstein Bros.-Caf_ Latte, Reg	360.0000	12.000	Fl Oz	9.00	5.00	13.00	140.00	0.00	0.00	20.00	3.50
304	Einstein Bros.-Cappuccino	360.0000	12.000	Fl Oz	6.00	3.50	9.00	90.00	0.00	0.00	15.00	2.00
305	Einstein Bros.-Cappuccino, Non F	360.0000	12.000	Fl Oz	6.00	0.00	9.00	60.00	0.00	0.00	5.00	0.00
306	Einstein Bros.-Cheese Melt, Gril	213.0000	1.000	Each	25.00	12.00	74.00	500.00	0.00	3.00	35.00	7.00
307	Einstein Bros.-Chicken Salad, Re	113.6000	4.000	Ounce	16.00	7.00	4.00	150.00	0.00	0.00	45.00	1.50
308	Einstein Bros.-Chili, Turkey, Lo	198.8000	7.000	Ounce	6.00	2.50	9.00	80.00	0.00	3.00	20.00	0.00
309	Einstein Bros.-Chili, Vegetarian	198.8000	7.000	Ounce	3.00	2.00	23.00	120.00	0.00	4.00	0.00	0.00
310	Einstein Bros.-Chix Salad Bagel	324.0000	1.000	Each	28.00	9.00	79.00	510.00	0.00	4.00	45.00	2.00
311	Einstein Bros.-Choc, Hot, Lower	360.0000	12.000	Fl Oz	9.00	7.00	39.00	260.00	0.00	0.00	5.00	6.00
312	Einstein Bros.-Chocolate, Hot, R	360.0000	12.000	Fl Oz	9.00	11.00	39.00	290.00	0.00	0.00	20.00	8.00
313	Einstein Bros.-Chowder, Corn, Am	198.8000	7.000	Ounce	5.00	6.00	25.00	180.00	0.00	2.00	5.00	1.50
314	Einstein Bros.-Chowder, NE Clam	198.8000	7.000	Ounce	9.00	9.00	15.00	170.00	0.00	1.00	25.00	2.50
315	Einstein Bros.-Cinnamon Bun, Ice	142.0000	5.000	Ounce	11.00	16.00	89.00	545.00	0.00	3.00	20.00	5.00
316	Einstein Bros.-Coffee, Reg	360.0000	12.000	Fl Oz	0.00	0.00	0.00	0.00	0.00	0.00	0.00	0.00
317	Einstein Bros.-Coleslaw, Low Fat	113.6000	4.000	Ounce	2.00	3.50	13.00	90.00	0.00	2.00	5.00	0.50
318	Einstein Bros.-Coleslaw, Low Fat	113.6000	4.000	Ounce	1.00	3.50	13.00	90.00	0.00	2.00	5.00	0.50
319	Einstein Bros.-Cookie, Black & W	113.6000	4.000	Ounce	3.00	12.00	68.00	390.00	0.00	1.00	15.00	3.00
320	Einstein Bros.-Cookie, Chocolate	113.6000	4.000	Ounce	6.00	24.00	68.00	510.00	0.00	2.00	35.00	9.00
321	Einstein Bros.-Cookie, Oatmeal R	113.6000	4.000	Ounce	7.00	18.00	70.00	470.00	0.00	3.00	40.00	4.00
322	Einstein Bros.-Cookie, Peanut Bu	113.6000	4.000	Ounce	10.00	31.00	55.00	540.00	0.00	3.00	40.00	6.00
323	Einstein Bros.-Cookie, Sugar	113.6000	4.000	Ounce	6.00	28.00	28.00	530.00	0.00	1.00	45.00	7.00
324	Einstein Bros.-Cream Cheese, Ch	30.0000	2.000	Tbsp	2.00	9.00	2.00	100.00	0.00	0.00	30.00	6.00
325	Einstein Bros.-Cream Cheese, Pl	30.0000	2.000	Tbsp	2.00	5.00	2.00	60.00	0.00	0.00	15.00	3.00
326	Einstein Bros.-Cream Cheese, Cra	30.0000	2.000	Tbsp	2.00	8.00	5.00	100.00	0.00	0.00	25.00	6.00
327	Einstein Bros.-Cream Cheese, Gar	30.0000	2.000	Tbsp	2.00	9.00	2.00	100.00	0.00	0.00	30.00	6.00
328	Einstein Bros.-Cream Cheese, Jal	30.0000	2.000	Tbsp	2.00	8.00	2.00	90.00	0.00	0.00	25.00	6.00
329	Einstein Bros.-Cream Cheese, Map	30.0000	2.000	Tbsp	2.00	9.00	5.00	100.00	0.00	0.00	25.00	6.00
330	Einstein Bros.-Cream Cheese, Pla	30.0000	2.000	Tbsp	2.00	10.00	2.00	100.00	0.00	0.00	30.00	7.00
331	Einstein Bros.-Cream Cheese, Sal	30.0000	2.000	Tbsp	2.00	8.00	2.00	90.00	0.00	0.00	25.00	6.00
332	Einstein Bros.-Cream Cheese, Str	30.0000	2.000	Tbsp	2.00	8.00	5.00	100.00	0.00	0.00	25.00	6.00
333	Einstein Bros.-Cream Cheese, Sun	30.0000	2.000	Tbsp	2.00	9.00	2.00	100.00	0.00	0.00	30.00	6.00
334	Einstein Bros.-Cream Cheese, Veg	30.0000	2.000	Tbsp	2.00	5.00	2.00	60.00	0.00	0.00	16.00	4.00
335	Einstein Bros.-Cream Cheese, Wil	30.0000	2.000	Tbsp	2.00	5.00	6.00	70.00	0.00	0.00	15.00	4.00
336	Einstein Bros.-Cream Cheese-Hone	30.0000	2.000	Tbsp	2.00	9.00	5.00	100.00	0.00	0.00	25.00	6.00
337	Einstein Bros.-Egg, Scr, & Bacon	225.0000	1.000	Each	30.00	23.00	72.00	620.00	0.00	2.00	395.00	10.00
338	Einstein Bros.-Egg, Scr, & Ham B	248.0000	1.000	Each	34.00	18.00	74.00	590.00	0.00	2.00	405.00	8.00
339	Einstein Bros.-Egg, Scr, & Sausa	250.0000	1.000	Each	31.00	30.00	72.00	690.00	0.00	2.00	415.00	12.00
340	Einstein Bros.-Egg, Scr, & Turk	257.0000	1.000	Each	37.00	19.00	72.00	604.00	0.00	2.00	409.00	8.00
341	Einstein Bros.-Egg, Scr, Bagel S	212.0000	1.000	Each	27.00	16.00	72.00	540.00	0.00	2.00	385.00	7.00
342	Einstein Bros.-Espresso	45.0000	1.500	Fl Oz	0.00	0.00	0.00	1.00	0.00	0.00	0.00	0.00
343	Einstein Bros.-Fruit & Yogurt Cu	227.2000	8.000	Ounce	6.00	1.00	32.00	160.00	0.00	4.00	0.00	0.00
344	Einstein Bros.-Fruit Salad	227.2000	8.000	Ounce	1.00	0.50	25.00	110.00	0.00	2.00	0.00	0.00
345	Einstein Bros.-Fruit Salad, Ruby	113.6000	4.000	Ounce	0.00	0.00	23.00	90.00	0.00	1.00	0.00	0.00
346	Einstein Bros.-Fusilli w/ Olives	170.4000	6.000	Ounce	6.00	23.00	33.00	360.00	0.00	3.00	0.00	3.00
347	Einstein Bros.-Ham /Cheese Bagel	275.0000	1.000	Each	32.00	15.00	79.00	580.00	0.00	3.00	70.00	6.00
348	Einstein Bros.-Ham, Deli, Bagel	305.0000	1.000	Each	37.00	17.00	78.00	620.00	0.00	3.00	85.00	10.00
349	Einstein Bros.-Hummus	30.0000	2.000	Tbsp	2.00	3.50	6.00	60.00	0.00	1.00	0.00	0.50
350	Einstein Bros.-Hummus Bagel Sand	248.0000	1.000	Each	15.00	8.00	86.00	480.00	0.00	5.00	0.00	1.00
351	Einstein Bros.-Hummus, Carrot	57.0000	4.000	Tbsp	3.00	2.00	9.00	60.00	0.00	2.00	0.00	0.00

Monounsaturated Fat (gm)	Polyunsaturated Fat (gm)	Vitamin D (mg)	Vitamin K (mg)	Vitamin E (mg)	Vitamin A (re)	Vitamin C (mg)	Thiamin (mg)	Riboflavin (mg)	Niacin (mg)	Vitamin B_6 (mg)	Folate (mg)	Vitamin B_{12} (mcg)	Calcium (mg)	Iron (mg)	Magnesium (mg)	Phosphorus (mg)	Potassium (mg)	Sodium (mg)	Zinc (mg)
0.00	0.00	0.00	0.00	0.00	0.00	0.00	0.00	0.00	0.00	0.00	0.00	0.00	0.00	0.00	0.00	0.00	0.00	490.00	0.00
0.00	0.00	0.00	0.00	0.00	0.00	0.00	0.00	0.00	0.00	0.00	0.00	0.00	0.00	0.00	0.00	0.00	0.00	193.00	0.00
0.00	0.00	0.00	0.00	0.00	0.00	0.00	0.00	0.00	0.00	0.00	0.00	0.00	0.00	0.00	0.00	0.00	0.00	95.00	0.00
0.00	0.00	0.00	0.00	0.00	0.00	0.00	0.00	0.00	0.00	0.00	0.00	0.00	0.00	0.00	0.00	0.00	0.00	100.00	0.00
0.00	0.00	0.00	0.00	0.00	0.00	0.00	0.00	0.00	0.00	0.00	0.00	0.00	0.00	0.00	0.00	0.00	0.00	125.00	0.00
0.00	0.00	0.00	0.00	0.00	0.00	0.00	0.00	0.00	0.00	0.00	0.00	0.00	0.00	0.00	0.00	0.00	0.00	140.00	0.00
0.00	0.00	0.00	0.00	0.00	0.00	0.00	0.00	0.00	0.00	0.00	0.00	0.00	0.00	0.00	0.00	0.00	0.00	140.00	0.00
0.00	0.00	0.00	0.00	0.00	0.00	0.00	0.00	0.00	0.00	0.00	0.00	0.00	0.00	0.00	0.00	0.00	0.00	95.00	0.00
0.00	0.00	0.00	0.00	0.00	0.00	0.00	0.00	0.00	0.00	0.00	0.00	0.00	0.00	0.00	0.00	0.00	0.00	95.00	0.00
0.00	0.00	0.00	0.00	0.00	0.00	0.00	0.00	0.00	0.00	0.00	0.00	0.00	0.00	0.00	0.00	0.00	0.00	970.00	0.00
0.00	0.00	0.00	0.00	0.00	0.00	0.00	0.00	0.00	0.00	0.00	0.00	0.00	0.00	0.00	0.00	0.00	0.00	540.00	0.00
0.00	0.00	0.00	0.00	0.00	0.00	0.00	0.00	0.00	0.00	0.00	0.00	0.00	0.00	0.00	0.00	0.00	0.00	320.00	0.00
0.00	0.00	0.00	0.00	0.00	0.00	0.00	0.00	0.00	0.00	0.00	0.00	0.00	0.00	0.00	0.00	0.00	0.00	730.00	0.00
0.00	0.00	0.00	0.00	0.00	0.00	0.00	0.00	0.00	0.00	0.00	0.00	0.00	0.00	0.00	0.00	0.00	0.00	1060.00	0.00
0.00	0.00	0.00	0.00	0.00	0.00	0.00	0.00	0.00	0.00	0.00	0.00	0.00	0.00	0.00	0.00	0.00	0.00	160.00	0.00
0.00	0.00	0.00	0.00	0.00	0.00	0.00	0.00	0.00	0.00	0.00	0.00	0.00	0.00	0.00	0.00	0.00	0.00	160.00	0.00
0.00	0.00	0.00	0.00	0.00	0.00	0.00	0.00	0.00	0.00	0.00	0.00	0.00	0.00	0.00	0.00	0.00	0.00	670.00	0.00
0.00	0.00	0.00	0.00	0.00	0.00	0.00	0.00	0.00	0.00	0.00	0.00	0.00	0.00	0.00	0.00	0.00	0.00	820.00	0.00
0.00	0.00	0.00	0.00	0.00	0.00	0.00	0.00	0.00	0.00	0.00	0.00	0.00	0.00	0.00	0.00	0.00	0.00	656.00	0.00
0.00	0.00	0.00	0.00	0.00	0.00	0.00	0.00	0.00	0.00	0.00	0.00	0.00	0.00	0.00	0.00	0.00	0.00	0.00	0.00
0.00	0.00	0.00	0.00	0.00	0.00	0.00	0.00	0.00	0.00	0.00	0.00	0.00	0.00	0.00	0.00	0.00	0.00	300.00	0.00
0.00	0.00	0.00	0.00	0.00	0.00	0.00	0.00	0.00	0.00	0.00	0.00	0.00	0.00	0.00	0.00	0.00	0.00	300.00	0.00
0.00	0.00	0.00	0.00	0.00	0.00	0.00	0.00	0.00	0.00	0.00	0.00	0.00	0.00	0.00	0.00	0.00	0.00	260.00	0.00
0.00	0.00	0.00	0.00	0.00	0.00	0.00	0.00	0.00	0.00	0.00	0.00	0.00	0.00	0.00	0.00	0.00	0.00	390.00	0.00
0.00	0.00	0.00	0.00	0.00	0.00	0.00	0.00	0.00	0.00	0.00	0.00	0.00	0.00	0.00	0.00	0.00	0.00	360.00	0.00
0.00	0.00	0.00	0.00	0.00	0.00	0.00	0.00	0.00	0.00	0.00	0.00	0.00	0.00	0.00	0.00	0.00	0.00	620.00	0.00
0.00	0.00	0.00	0.00	0.00	0.00	0.00	0.00	0.00	0.00	0.00	0.00	0.00	0.00	0.00	0.00	0.00	0.00	420.00	0.00
0.00	0.00	0.00	0.00	0.00	0.00	0.00	0.00	0.00	0.00	0.00	0.00	0.00	0.00	0.00	0.00	0.00	0.00	130.00	0.00
0.00	0.00	0.00	0.00	0.00	0.00	0.00	0.00	0.00	0.00	0.00	0.00	0.00	0.00	0.00	0.00	0.00	0.00	110.00	0.00
0.00	0.00	0.00	0.00	0.00	0.00	0.00	0.00	0.00	0.00	0.00	0.00	0.00	0.00	0.00	0.00	0.00	0.00	80.00	0.00
0.00	0.00	0.00	0.00	0.00	0.00	0.00	0.00	0.00	0.00	0.00	0.00	0.00	0.00	0.00	0.00	0.00	0.00	135.00	0.00
0.00	0.00	0.00	0.00	0.00	0.00	0.00	0.00	0.00	0.00	0.00	0.00	0.00	0.00	0.00	0.00	0.00	0.00	140.00	0.00
0.00	0.00	0.00	0.00	0.00	0.00	0.00	0.00	0.00	0.00	0.00	0.00	0.00	0.00	0.00	0.00	0.00	0.00	80.00	0.00
0.00	0.00	0.00	0.00	0.00	0.00	0.00	0.00	0.00	0.00	0.00	0.00	0.00	0.00	0.00	0.00	0.00	0.00	100.00	0.00
0.00	0.00	0.00	0.00	0.00	0.00	0.00	0.00	0.00	0.00	0.00	0.00	0.00	0.00	0.00	0.00	0.00	0.00	210.00	0.00
0.00	0.00	0.00	0.00	0.00	0.00	0.00	0.00	0.00	0.00	0.00	0.00	0.00	0.00	0.00	0.00	0.00	0.00	80.00	0.00
0.00	0.00	0.00	0.00	0.00	0.00	0.00	0.00	0.00	0.00	0.00	0.00	0.00	0.00	0.00	0.00	0.00	0.00	100.00	0.00
0.00	0.00	0.00	0.00	0.00	0.00	0.00	0.00	0.00	0.00	0.00	0.00	0.00	0.00	0.00	0.00	0.00	0.00	150.00	0.00
0.00	0.00	0.00	0.00	0.00	0.00	0.00	0.00	0.00	0.00	0.00	0.00	0.00	0.00	0.00	0.00	0.00	0.00	90.00	0.00
0.00	0.00	0.00	0.00	0.00	0.00	0.00	0.00	0.00	0.00	0.00	0.00	0.00	0.00	0.00	0.00	0.00	0.00	80.00	0.00
0.00	0.00	0.00	0.00	0.00	0.00	0.00	0.00	0.00	0.00	0.00	0.00	0.00	0.00	0.00	0.00	0.00	0.00	950.00	0.00
0.00	0.00	0.00	0.00	0.00	0.00	0.00	0.00	0.00	0.00	0.00	0.00	0.00	0.00	0.00	0.00	0.00	0.00	1120.00	0.00
0.00	0.00	0.00	0.00	0.00	0.00	0.00	0.00	0.00	0.00	0.00	0.00	0.00	0.00	0.00	0.00	0.00	0.00	980.00	0.00
0.00	0.00	0.00	0.00	0.00	0.00	0.00	0.00	0.00	0.00	0.00	0.00	0.00	0.00	0.00	0.00	0.00	0.00	1070.00	0.00
0.00	0.00	0.00	0.00	0.00	0.00	0.00	0.00	0.00	0.00	0.00	0.00	0.00	0.00	0.00	0.00	0.00	0.00	750.00	0.00
0.00	0.00	0.00	0.00	0.00	0.00	0.00	0.00	0.00	0.00	0.00	0.00	0.00	0.00	0.00	0.00	0.00	0.00	0.00	0.00
0.00	0.00	0.00	0.00	0.00	0.00	0.00	0.00	0.00	0.00	0.00	0.00	0.00	0.00	0.00	0.00	0.00	0.00	95.00	0.00
0.00	0.00	0.00	0.00	0.00	0.00	0.00	0.00	0.00	0.00	0.00	0.00	0.00	0.00	0.00	0.00	0.00	0.00	10.00	0.00
0.00	0.00	0.00	0.00	0.00	0.00	0.00	0.00	0.00	0.00	0.00	0.00	0.00	0.00	0.00	0.00	0.00	0.00	20.00	0.00
0.00	0.00	0.00	0.00	0.00	0.00	0.00	0.00	0.00	0.00	0.00	0.00	0.00	0.00	0.00	0.00	0.00	0.00	290.00	0.00
0.00	0.00	0.00	0.00	0.00	0.00	0.00	0.00	0.00	0.00	0.00	0.00	0.00	0.00	0.00	0.00	0.00	0.00	1400.00	0.00
0.00	0.00	0.00	0.00	0.00	0.00	0.00	0.00	0.00	0.00	0.00	0.00	0.00	0.00	0.00	0.00	0.00	0.00	1690.00	0.00
0.00	0.00	0.00	0.00	0.00	0.00	0.00	0.00	0.00	0.00	0.00	0.00	0.00	0.00	0.00	0.00	0.00	0.00	65.00	0.00
0.00	0.00	0.00	0.00	0.00	0.00	0.00	0.00	0.00	0.00	0.00	0.00	0.00	0.00	0.00	0.00	0.00	0.00	640.00	0.00
0.00	0.00	0.00	0.00	0.00	0.00	0.00	0.00	0.00	0.00	0.00	0.00	0.00	0.00	0.00	0.00	0.00	0.00	260.00	0.00

USDA ID Code	Food Name	Weight in Grams*	Quantity of Units	Unit of Measure	Protein (gm)	Fat (gm)	Carbohydrate (gm)	Kcalories	Caffeine (gm)	Fiber (gm)	Cholesterol (mg)	Saturated Fat (gm)
352	Einstein Bros.-Hummus, Carrot, S	248.0000	1.000	Each	15.00	3.00	83.00	420.00	0.00	5.00	0.00	0.00
353	Einstein Bros.-Intellicino, Iced	480.0000	16.000	Fl Oz	6.00	7.00	13.00	140.00	0.00	0.00	15.00	4.00
354	Einstein Bros.-Intellicino, Low	360.0000	12.000	Fl Oz	7.00	3.50	15.00	120.00	0.00	0.00	5.00	2.50
355	Einstein Bros.-Intellicino, Reg	360.0000	12.000	Fl Oz	7.00	7.00	14.00	150.00	0.00	0.00	15.00	4.50
356	Einstein Bros.-Lox & Bagel	318.0000	1.000	Each	26.00	24.00	77.00	630.00	0.00	3.00	75.00	13.00
357	Einstein Bros.-Mocha, Iced	480.0000	16.000	Fl Oz	7.00	6.00	33.00	210.00	0.00	0.00	15.00	4.00
358	Einstein Bros.-Mocha, Low Fat, R	360.0000	12.000	Fl Oz	8.00	2.50	34.00	190.00	0.00	0.00	5.00	2.00
359	Einstein Bros.-Mocha, Reg	360.0000	12.000	Fl Oz	8.00	6.00	34.00	230.00	0.00	0.00	15.00	4.50
360	Einstein Bros.-Muffin, Apple Dat	56.8000	2.000	Ounce	3.00	2.00	35.00	160.00	0.00	2.00	0.00	0.00
361	Einstein Bros.-Muffin, Banana	56.8000	2.000	Ounce	3.00	12.00	25.00	220.00	0.00	0.00	40.00	2.00
362	Einstein Bros.-Muffin, Blueberry	56.8000	2.000	Ounce	3.00	10.00	25.00	200.00	0.00	0.00	40.00	2.00
363	Einstein Bros.-Muffin, Chocolate	56.8000	2.000	Ounce	3.00	13.00	28.00	240.00	0.00	0.00	40.00	3.00
364	Einstein Bros.-Muffin, Cran Oran	56.8000	2.000	Ounce	4.00	0.50	27.00	130.00	0.00	1.00	0.00	0.00
365	Einstein Bros.-Muffin, Lemon Pop	56.8000	2.000	Ounce	3.00	3.00	28.00	150.00	0.00	0.00	0.00	0.00
366	Einstein Bros.-Muffin, Wildberry	56.8000	2.000	Ounce	3.00	0.50	26.00	120.00	0.00	1.00	0.00	0.00
368	Einstein Bros.-Pastrami, Turkey,	305.0000	1.000	Each	37.00	16.00	78.00	600.00	0.00	3.00	85.00	9.00
369	Einstein Bros.-Pastrami, Turkey,	347.0000	1.000	Each	45.00	34.00	77.00	790.00	0.00	3.00	90.00	19.00
367	Einstein Bros.-PB&J Bagel Sandwi	172.0000	1.000	Each	18.00	17.00	99.00	595.00	0.00	4.00	0.00	2.00
370	Einstein Bros.-Peanut Butter, Cr	32.0000	2.000	Tbsp	7.00	16.00	8.00	190.00	0.00	2.00	0.00	2.00
371	Einstein Bros.-Pizza Melt, 3 Che	234.0000	1.000	Each	32.00	18.00	78.00	600.00	0.00	3.00	55.00	10.00
372	Einstein Bros.-Pizza Melt, Peppe	263.0000	1.000	Each	38.00	30.00	79.00	740.00	0.00	3.00	85.00	15.00
373	Einstein Bros.-Pizza Melt, Tomat	277.0000	1.000	Each	32.00	18.00	80.00	610.00	0.00	3.00	55.00	10.00
374	Einstein Bros.-Reuben Bagel Sand	319.0000	1.000	Each	42.00	33.00	82.00	790.00	0.00	5.00	100.00	12.00
375	Einstein Bros.-Salad, Caesar, Ch	269.8000	9.500	Ounce	26.00	37.00	11.00	480.00	0.00	2.00	75.00	8.00
376	Einstein Bros.-Salad, Caesar, La	198.8000	7.000	Ounce	9.00	35.00	10.00	390.00	0.00	2.00	25.00	7.00
377	Einstein Bros.-Salad, Caesar, Re	99.4000	3.500	Ounce	5.00	18.00	7.00	210.00	0.00	1.00	15.00	4.00
378	Einstein Bros.-Salad, Clairemont	113.6000	4.000	Ounce	1.00	4.00	9.00	70.00	0.00	2.00	0.00	0.00
379	Einstein Bros.-Salad, Pasta, Gre	255.6000	9.000	Ounce	12.00	30.00	35.00	270.00	0.00	3.00	45.00	9.00
380	Einstein Bros.-Salad, Pasta, Zit	113.6000	4.000	Ounce	4.00	11.00	20.00	200.00	0.00	2.00	0.00	2.00
381	Einstein Bros.-Salad, Potato & D	113.6000	4.000	Ounce	2.00	0.50	20.00	150.00	0.00	1.00	0.00	0.00
382	Einstein Bros.-Salad, Potato & M	113.6000	4.000	Ounce	2.00	2.50	19.00	110.00	0.00	2.00	0.00	0.00
383	Einstein Bros.-Salad, Potato, Id	113.6000	4.000	Ounce	2.00	7.00	19.00	150.00	0.00	1.00	5.00	1.50
384	Einstein Bros.-Salad, Potato, Ol	113.6000	4.000	Ounce	3.00	8.00	16.00	140.00	0.00	1.00	40.00	1.50
385	Einstein Bros.-Scone, Blueberry	99.4000	3.500	Ounce	8.00	8.50	49.00	295.00	0.00	1.50	20.00	4.50
386	Einstein Bros.-Scone, Cheddar Ch	99.4000	3.500	Ounce	8.00	15.00	37.00	310.00	0.00	2.00	35.00	8.00
387	Einstein Bros.-Scone, Cinnamon	99.4000	3.500	Ounce	8.00	11.00	50.00	325.00	0.00	1.50	20.00	5.50
388	Einstein Bros.-Soup, Bean, Black	198.8000	7.000	Ounce	3.00	1.00	11.00	70.00	0.00	2.00	0.00	0.00
389	Einstein Bros.-Soup, Bean, Monte	198.8000	7.000	Ounce	5.00	2.00	19.00	120.00	0.00	5.00	0.00	0.00
390	Einstein Bros.-Soup, Cheddar & B	198.8000	7.000	Ounce	5.00	10.00	14.00	170.00	0.00	1.00	15.00	3.00
391	Einstein Bros.-Soup, Chicken & R	198.8000	7.000	Ounce	7.00	10.00	15.00	180.00	0.00	0.00	15.00	2.50
392	Einstein Bros.-Soup, Chicken Noo	198.8000	7.000	Ounce	6.00	2.50	13.00	100.00	0.00	1.00	15.00	1.00
393	Einstein Bros.-Soup, Oriental Se	170.4000	6.000	Ounce	7.00	20.00	46.00	390.00	0.00	3.00	0.00	2.50
394	Einstein Bros.-Soup, Pasta Fagio	198.8000	7.000	Ounce	2.00	1.00	11.00	60.00	0.00	1.00	0.00	0.00
395	Einstein Bros.-Soup, Potato, Iri	198.8000	7.000	Ounce	5.00	8.00	19.00	170.00	0.00	1.00	5.00	2.50
396	Einstein Bros.-Soup, Tomato Flor	198.8000	7.000	Ounce	2.00	1.50	14.00	80.00	0.00	2.00	0.00	1.00
397	Einstein Bros.-Soup, Veg, Farmer	198.8000	7.000	Ounce	2.00	0.50	7.00	40.00	0.00	2.00	0.00	0.00
398	Einstein Bros.-Spread, Apricot	28.0000	2.000	Tbsp	0.00	0.00	19.00	75.00	0.00	0.00	0.00	0.00
399	Einstein Bros.-Spread, Butter	14.0000	1.000	Tbsp	0.00	11.00	0.00	100.00	0.00	0.00	30.00	8.00
400	Einstein Bros.-Spread, Butter/Ma	10.0000	1.000	Tbsp	0.00	7.00	0.00	60.00	0.00	0.00	0.00	1.50
401	Einstein Bros.-Spread, Grape Fru	28.0000	2.000	Tbsp	0.00	0.00	19.00	75.00	0.00	0.00	0.00	0.00
402	Einstein Bros.-Spread, Strawberr	28.0000	2.000	Tbsp	0.00	0.00	19.00	75.00	0.00	0.00	0.00	0.00
403	Einstein Bros.-Steamer, Non Fat,	360.0000	12.000	Fl Oz	9.00	0.00	29.00	160.00	0.00	0.00	5.00	0.00
404	Einstein Bros.-Steamer, Reg	360.0000	12.000	Fl Oz	6.00	5.00	30.00	200.00	0.00	0.00	20.00	3.50
405	Einstein Bros.-Syrup, Almond Fla	31.0000	2.000	Tbsp	0.00	0.00	18.00	80.00	0.00	0.00	0.00	0.00
406	Einstein Bros.-Syrup, Caramel Fl	31.0000	2.000	Tbsp	0.00	0.00	18.00	80.00	0.00	0.00	0.00	0.00

Monounsaturated Fat (gm)	Polyunsaturated Fat (gm)	Vitamin D (mg)	Vitamin K (mg)	Vitamin E (mg)	Vitamin A (re)	Vitamin C (mg)	Thiamin (mg)	Riboflavin (mg)	Niacin (mg)	Vitamin B_6 (mg)	Folate (mg)	Vitamin B_{12} (mcg)	Calcium (mg)	Iron (mg)	Magnesium (mg)	Phosphorus (mg)	Potassium (mg)	Sodium (mg)	Zinc (mg)
0.00	0.00	0.00	0.00	0.00	0.00	0.00	0.00	0.00	0.00	0.00	0.00	0.00	0.00	0.00	0.00	0.00	0.00	780.00	0.00
0.00	0.00	0.00	0.00	0.00	0.00	0.00	0.00	0.00	0.00	0.00	0.00	0.00	0.00	0.00	0.00	0.00	0.00	140.00	0.00
0.00	0.00	0.00	0.00	0.00	0.00	0.00	0.00	0.00	0.00	0.00	0.00	0.00	0.00	0.00	0.00	0.00	0.00	140.00	0.00
0.00	0.00	0.00	0.00	0.00	0.00	0.00	0.00	0.00	0.00	0.00	0.00	0.00	0.00	0.00	0.00	0.00	0.00	135.00	0.00
0.00	0.00	0.00	0.00	0.00	0.00	0.00	0.00	0.00	0.00	0.00	0.00	0.00	0.00	0.00	0.00	0.00	0.00	1240.00	0.00
0.00	0.00	0.00	0.00	0.00	0.00	0.00	0.00	0.00	0.00	0.00	0.00	0.00	0.00	0.00	0.00	0.00	0.00	120.00	0.00
0.00	0.00	0.00	0.00	0.00	0.00	0.00	0.00	0.00	0.00	0.00	0.00	0.00	0.00	0.00	0.00	0.00	0.00	130.00	0.00
0.00	0.00	0.00	0.00	0.00	0.00	0.00	0.00	0.00	0.00	0.00	0.00	0.00	0.00	0.00	0.00	0.00	0.00	135.00	0.00
0.00	0.00	0.00	0.00	0.00	0.00	0.00	0.00	0.00	0.00	0.00	0.00	0.00	0.00	0.00	0.00	0.00	0.00	210.00	0.00
0.00	0.00	0.00	0.00	0.00	0.00	0.00	0.00	0.00	0.00	0.00	0.00	0.00	0.00	0.00	0.00	0.00	0.00	170.00	0.00
0.00	0.00	0.00	0.00	0.00	0.00	0.00	0.00	0.00	0.00	0.00	0.00	0.00	0.00	0.00	0.00	0.00	0.00	180.00	0.00
0.00	0.00	0.00	0.00	0.00	0.00	0.00	0.00	0.00	0.00	0.00	0.00	0.00	0.00	0.00	0.00	0.00	0.00	180.00	0.00
0.00	0.00	0.00	0.00	0.00	0.00	0.00	0.00	0.00	0.00	0.00	0.00	0.00	0.00	0.00	0.00	0.00	0.00	260.00	0.00
0.00	0.00	0.00	0.00	0.00	0.00	0.00	0.00	0.00	0.00	0.00	0.00	0.00	0.00	0.00	0.00	0.00	0.00	220.00	0.00
0.00	0.00	0.00	0.00	0.00	0.00	0.00	0.00	0.00	0.00	0.00	0.00	0.00	0.00	0.00	0.00	0.00	0.00	260.00	0.00
0.00	0.00	0.00	0.00	0.00	0.00	0.00	0.00	0.00	0.00	0.00	0.00	0.00	0.00	0.00	0.00	0.00	0.00	1590.00	0.00
0.00	0.00	0.00	0.00	0.00	0.00	0.00	0.00	0.00	0.00	0.00	0.00	0.00	0.00	0.00	0.00	0.00	0.00	1780.00	0.00
0.00	0.00	0.00	0.00	0.00	0.00	0.00	0.00	0.00	0.00	0.00	0.00	0.00	0.00	0.00	0.00	0.00	0.00	663.00	0.00
0.00	0.00	0.00	0.00	0.00	0.00	0.00	0.00	0.00	0.00	0.00	0.00	0.00	0.00	0.00	0.00	0.00	0.00	140.00	0.00
0.00	0.00	0.00	0.00	0.00	0.00	0.00	0.00	0.00	0.00	0.00	0.00	0.00	0.00	0.00	0.00	0.00	0.00	1200.00	0.00
0.00	0.00	0.00	0.00	0.00	0.00	0.00	0.00	0.00	0.00	0.00	0.00	0.00	0.00	0.00	0.00	0.00	0.00	1780.00	0.00
0.00	0.00	0.00	0.00	0.00	0.00	0.00	0.00	0.00	0.00	0.00	0.00	0.00	0.00	0.00	0.00	0.00	0.00	1210.00	0.00
0.00	0.00	0.00	0.00	0.00	0.00	0.00	0.00	0.00	0.00	0.00	0.00	0.00	0.00	0.00	0.00	0.00	0.00	1920.00	0.00
0.00	0.00	0.00	0.00	0.00	0.00	0.00	0.00	0.00	0.00	0.00	0.00	0.00	0.00	0.00	0.00	0.00	0.00	1150.00	0.00
0.00	0.00	0.00	0.00	0.00	0.00	0.00	0.00	0.00	0.00	0.00	0.00	0.00	0.00	0.00	0.00	0.00	0.00	900.00	0.00
0.00	0.00	0.00	0.00	0.00	0.00	0.00	0.00	0.00	0.00	0.00	0.00	0.00	0.00	0.00	0.00	0.00	0.00	500.00	0.00
0.00	0.00	0.00	0.00	0.00	0.00	0.00	0.00	0.00	0.00	0.00	0.00	0.00	0.00	0.00	0.00	0.00	0.00	120.00	0.00
0.00	0.00	0.00	0.00	0.00	0.00	0.00	0.00	0.00	0.00	0.00	0.00	0.00	0.00	0.00	0.00	0.00	0.00	960.00	0.00
0.00	0.00	0.00	0.00	0.00	0.00	0.00	0.00	0.00	0.00	0.00	0.00	0.00	0.00	0.00	0.00	0.00	0.00	350.00	0.00
0.00	0.00	0.00	0.00	0.00	0.00	0.00	0.00	0.00	0.00	0.00	0.00	0.00	0.00	0.00	0.00	0.00	0.00	150.00	0.00
0.00	0.00	0.00	0.00	0.00	0.00	0.00	0.00	0.00	0.00	0.00	0.00	0.00	0.00	0.00	0.00	0.00	0.00	340.00	0.00
0.00	0.00	0.00	0.00	0.00	0.00	0.00	0.00	0.00	0.00	0.00	0.00	0.00	0.00	0.00	0.00	0.00	0.00	210.00	0.00
0.00	0.00	0.00	0.00	0.00	0.00	0.00	0.00	0.00	0.00	0.00	0.00	0.00	0.00	0.00	0.00	0.00	0.00	250.00	0.00
0.00	0.00	0.00	0.00	0.00	0.00	0.00	0.00	0.00	0.00	0.00	0.00	0.00	0.00	0.00	0.00	0.00	0.00	560.00	0.00
0.00	0.00	0.00	0.00	0.00	0.00	0.00	0.00	0.00	0.00	0.00	0.00	0.00	0.00	0.00	0.00	0.00	0.00	670.00	0.00
0.00	0.00	0.00	0.00	0.00	0.00	0.00	0.00	0.00	0.00	0.00	0.00	0.00	0.00	0.00	0.00	0.00	0.00	535.00	0.00
0.00	0.00	0.00	0.00	0.00	0.00	0.00	0.00	0.00	0.00	0.00	0.00	0.00	0.00	0.00	0.00	0.00	0.00	460.00	0.00
0.00	0.00	0.00	0.00	0.00	0.00	0.00	0.00	0.00	0.00	0.00	0.00	0.00	0.00	0.00	0.00	0.00	0.00	680.00	0.00
0.00	0.00	0.00	0.00	0.00	0.00	0.00	0.00	0.00	0.00	0.00	0.00	0.00	0.00	0.00	0.00	0.00	0.00	770.00	0.00
0.00	0.00	0.00	0.00	0.00	0.00	0.00	0.00	0.00	0.00	0.00	0.00	0.00	0.00	0.00	0.00	0.00	0.00	1070.00	0.00
0.00	0.00	0.00	0.00	0.00	0.00	0.00	0.00	0.00	0.00	0.00	0.00	0.00	0.00	0.00	0.00	0.00	0.00	910.00	0.00
0.00	0.00	0.00	0.00	0.00	0.00	0.00	0.00	0.00	0.00	0.00	0.00	0.00	0.00	0.00	0.00	0.00	0.00	320.00	0.00
0.00	0.00	0.00	0.00	0.00	0.00	0.00	0.00	0.00	0.00	0.00	0.00	0.00	0.00	0.00	0.00	0.00	0.00	450.00	0.00
0.00	0.00	0.00	0.00	0.00	0.00	0.00	0.00	0.00	0.00	0.00	0.00	0.00	0.00	0.00	0.00	0.00	0.00	650.00	0.00
0.00	0.00	0.00	0.00	0.00	0.00	0.00	0.00	0.00	0.00	0.00	0.00	0.00	0.00	0.00	0.00	0.00	0.00	870.00	0.00
0.00	0.00	0.00	0.00	0.00	0.00	0.00	0.00	0.00	0.00	0.00	0.00	0.00	0.00	0.00	0.00	0.00	0.00	390.00	0.00
0.00	0.00	0.00	0.00	0.00	0.00	0.00	0.00	0.00	0.00	0.00	0.00	0.00	0.00	0.00	0.00	0.00	0.00	8.00	0.00
0.00	0.00	0.00	0.00	0.00	0.00	0.00	0.00	0.00	0.00	0.00	0.00	0.00	0.00	0.00	0.00	0.00	0.00	100.00	0.00
0.00	0.00	0.00	0.00	0.00	0.00	0.00	0.00	0.00	0.00	0.00	0.00	0.00	0.00	0.00	0.00	0.00	0.00	75.00	0.00
0.00	0.00	0.00	0.00	0.00	0.00	0.00	0.00	0.00	0.00	0.00	0.00	0.00	0.00	0.00	0.00	0.00	0.00	3.00	0.00
0.00	0.00	0.00	0.00	0.00	0.00	0.00	0.00	0.00	0.00	0.00	0.00	0.00	0.00	0.00	0.00	0.00	0.00	17.00	0.00
0.00	0.00	0.00	0.00	0.00	0.00	0.00	0.00	0.00	0.00	0.00	0.00	0.00	0.00	0.00	0.00	0.00	0.00	140.00	0.00
0.00	0.00	0.00	0.00	0.00	0.00	0.00	0.00	0.00	0.00	0.00	0.00	0.00	0.00	0.00	0.00	0.00	0.00	150.00	0.00
0.00	0.00	0.00	0.00	0.00	0.00	0.00	0.00	0.00	0.00	0.00	0.00	0.00	0.00	0.00	0.00	0.00	0.00	10.00	0.00
0.00	0.00	0.00	0.00	0.00	0.00	0.00	0.00	0.00	0.00	0.00	0.00	0.00	0.00	0.00	0.00	0.00	0.00	10.00	0.00

USDA ID Code	Food Name	Weight in Grams*	Quantity of Units	Unit of Measure	Protein (gm)	Fat (gm)	Carbohydrate (gm)	Kcalories	Caffeine (gm)	Fiber (gm)	Cholesterol (mg)	Saturated Fat (gm)
407	Einstein Bros.-Syrup, Caramel Fl	31.0000	2.000	Tbsp	0.00	0.00	18.00	80.00	0.00	0.00	0.00	0.00
408	Einstein Bros.-Syrup, Caramel, S	31.0000	2.000	Tbsp	0.00	0.00	0.00	0.00	0.00	0.00	0.00	0.00
409	Einstein Bros.-Syrup, Choc-Hersh	31.0000	2.000	Tbsp	1.00	0.00	24.00	100.00	0.00	0.00	0.00	0.00
410	Einstein Bros.-Syrup, Raspberry	31.0000	2.000	Tbsp	0.00	0.00	18.00	80.00	0.00	0.00	0.00	0.00
411	Einstein Bros.-Syrup, Vanilla, S	31.0000	2.000	Tbsp	0.00	0.00	0.00	0.00	0.00	0.00	0.00	0.00
412	Einstein Bros.-Tabouli, Southwes	284.0000	10.000	Ounce	6.00	1.00	29.00	150.00	0.00	8.00	0.00	0.00
413	Einstein Bros.-Teas, Hot	360.0000	12.000	Fl Oz	0.00	0.00	0.00	1.00	0.00	0.00	0.00	0.00
428	Einstein Bros.-topping, Chocolat	2.5000	0.500	Tsp	0.00	0.00	2.00	10.00	0.00	0.00	0.00	0.00
429	Einstein Bros.-topping, Cinnamon	2.5000	0.500	Tsp	0.00	0.00	2.00	10.00	0.00	0.00	0.00	0.00
414	Einstein Bros.-Topping, Nutmeg	2.5000	0.500	Tsp	0.00	0.00	2.00	10.00	0.00	0.00	0.00	0.00
415	Einstein Bros.-Topping, On Top D	31.0000	2.000	Tbsp	0.00	1.50	2.00	20.00	0.00	0.00	0.00	1.00
416	Einstein Bros.-Topping, Vanilla	2.5000	0.500	Tsp	0.00	0.00	2.00	10.00	0.00	0.00	0.00	0.00
417	Einstein Bros.-Tuna Melt	375.0000	1.000	Each	52.00	36.00	78.00	840.00	0.00	3.00	120.00	19.00
418	Einstein Bros.-Tuna Salad	113.6000	4.000	Ounce	21.00	6.00	3.00	150.00	0.00	0.00	30.00	1.00
419	Einstein Bros.-Tuna Salad Bagel	324.0000	1.000	Each	31.00	8.00	78.00	510.00	0.00	4.00	30.00	1.50
420	Einstein Bros.-Turkey, Deli Smok	305.0000	1.000	Each	35.00	16.00	75.00	590.00	0.00	3.00	65.00	9.00
421	Einstein Bros.-Turkey, Smoked, B	275.0000	1.000	Each	30.00	14.00	75.00	550.00	0.00	3.00	45.00	6.00
422	Einstein Bros.-Turkey, Tasty, Ba	279.0000	1.000	Each	26.00	21.00	77.00	600.00	0.00	3.00	90.00	12.00
423	Einstein Bros.-Veg Out Bagel San	248.0000	1.000	Each	14.00	6.00	78.00	420.00	0.00	3.00	20.00	3.00
424	Einstein Bros.-Veggie Cup	170.4000	6.000	Ounce	1.00	20.00	11.00	230.00	0.00	3.00	5.00	3.00
425	Einstein Bros.-Whipped Cream, Li	31.0000	2.000	Tbsp	0.00	2.00	2.00	30.00	0.00	0.00	10.00	1.50
426	Einstein Bros.-Whitefish Bagel S	245.0000	1.000	Each	23.00	22.00	75.00	590.00	0.00	4.00	45.00	4.00
427	Einstein Bros.-Whitefish Salad	56.8000	2.000	Ounce	8.00	14.00	1.00	160.00	0.00	1.00	30.00	2.00
561	Krispy Kreme-Cinnamon Bun	61.0000	1.000	Each	5.00	11.00	26.00	220.00	0.00	4.00	0.00	3.00
562	Krispy Kreme-Cruller, Fudge Iced	48.0000	1.000	Each	2.00	14.00	26.00	240.00	0.00	0.00	0.00	4.00
563	Krispy Kreme-Cruller, Glazed	43.0000	1.000	Each	2.00	14.00	22.00	220.00	0.00	0.00	0.00	3.00
564	Krispy Kreme-Doughnut, Blueberry	59.0000	1.000	Each	4.00	9.00	26.00	200.00	0.00	2.00	0.00	3.00
565	Krispy Kreme-Doughnut, Cake, Blu	67.0000	1.000	Each	2.00	15.00	37.00	300.00	0.00	1.00	0.00	3.00
566	Krispy Kreme-Doughnut, Cake, Dev	54.0000	1.000	Each	2.00	13.00	29.00	240.00	0.00	3.00	0.00	3.00
567	Krispy Kreme-Doughnut, Cake, Fud	56.0000	1.000	Each	3.00	12.00	28.00	230.00	0.00	0.00	0.00	3.00
568	Krispy Kreme-Doughnut, Cake, Sug	52.0000	1.000	Each	3.00	11.00	26.00	220.00	0.00	0.00	0.00	3.00
569	Krispy Kreme-Doughnut, Cake, Tra	48.0000	1.000	Each	3.00	11.00	22.00	200.00	0.00	0.00	0.00	3.00
570	Krispy Kreme-Doughnut, Cinnamon	66.0000	1.000	Each	4.00	9.00	29.00	210.00	0.00	3.00	0.00	3.00
571	Krispy Kreme-Doughnut, Creme Fil	65.0000	1.000	Each	4.00	14.00	32.00	270.00	0.00	2.00	0.00	3.00
572	Krispy Kreme-Doughnut, Crm Fille	65.0000	1.000	Each	4.00	14.00	32.00	270.00	0.00	2.00	0.00	3.00
573	Krispy Kreme-Doughnut, Custard F	76.0000	1.000	Each	4.00	9.00	38.00	250.00	0.00	3.00	0.00	3.00
574	Krispy Kreme-Doughnut, Fdg Iced	54.0000	1.000	Each	3.00	10.00	31.00	220.00	0.00	0.00	0.00	2.50
575	Krispy Kreme-Doughnut, Fudge Ice	57.0000	1.000	Each	3.00	14.00	30.00	260.00	0.00	1.00	0.00	5.00
576	Krispy Kreme-Doughnut, Lemon Fil	64.0000	1.000	Each	4.00	10.00	28.00	210.00	0.00	0.00	0.00	3.00
577	Krispy Kreme-Doughnut, Maple Ice	51.0000	1.000	Each	3.00	9.00	28.00	200.00	0.00	2.00	0.00	2.50
578	Krispy Kreme-Doughnut, Raspberry	57.0000	1.000	Each	4.00	10.00	28.00	210.00	0.00	0.00	0.00	3.00
579	Krispy Kreme-Doughnut, Yeast, Gl	39.0000	1.000	Each	2.00	10.00	17.00	170.00	0.00	0.00	0.00	2.50
	Pizza Hut-Pizza, Cheese, Hand To	70.0000	1.000	Slice	17.00	10.00	27.50	259.00	0.00	0.00	27.50	6.80
	Pizza Hut-Pizza, Cheese, Pan	70.0000	1.000	Slice	15.00	9.00	28.50	246.00	0.00	0.00	17.00	4.50
	Pizza Hut-Pizza, Cheese, Thin'n	70.0000	1.000	Slice	14.00	8.50	18.50	199.00	0.00	0.00	16.50	5.20
	Pizza Hut-Pizza, Pepperoni, Hand	70.0000	1.000	Slice	14.00	11.50	25.00	250.00	0.00	0.00	25.00	6.45
	Pizza Hut-Pizza, Pepperoni, Pan	70.0000	1.000	Slice	14.50	11.00	31.00	270.00	0.00	0.00	21.00	4.50
	Pizza Hut-Pizza, Pepperoni, Pers	250.0000	1.000	Each	37.00	29.00	76.00	675.00	0.00	0.00	53.00	12.50
	Pizza Hut-Pizza, Pepperoni, Thin	70.0000	1.000	Slice	13.00	10.00	18.00	206.50	0.00	0.00	23.00	5.30
	Pizza Hut-Pizza, Super Sprm, Thi	70.0000	1.000	Slice	14.50	10.50	22.00	231.50	0.00	0.00	28.00	5.15
	Pizza Hut-Pizza, Super Supreme,	70.0000	1.000	Slice	16.50	12.50	27.00	278.00	0.00	0.00	27.00	6.50
	Pizza Hut-Pizza, Super Supreme,	70.0000	1.000	Slice	16.50	13.00	26.50	281.50	0.00	0.00	27.50	6.00
	Pizza Hut-Pizza, Supreme, Hand T	70.0000	1.000	Slice	16.00	13.00	25.00	270.00	0.00	0.00	27.50	6.10
	Pizza Hut-Pizza, Supreme, Pan	70.0000	1.000	Slice	16.00	15.00	26.50	294.50	0.00	0.00	24.00	7.00
	Pizza Hut-Pizza, Supreme, Person	250.0000	1.000	Each	33.00	28.00	76.00	647.00	0.00	0.00	49.00	11.20

Monounsaturated Fat (gm)	Polyunsaturated Fat (gm)	Vitamin D (mg)	Vitamin K (mg)	Vitamin E (mg)	Vitamin A (re)	Vitamin C (mg)	Thiamin (mg)	Riboflavin (mg)	Niacin (mg)	Vitamin B_6 (mg)	Folate (mg)	Vitamin B_{12} (mcg)	Calcium (mg)	Iron (mg)	Magnesium (mg)	Phosphorus (mg)	Potassium (mg)	Sodium (mg)	Zinc (mg)
0.00	0.00	0.00	0.00	0.00	0.00	0.00	0.00	0.00	0.00	0.00	0.00	0.00	0.00	0.00	0.00	0.00	0.00	10.00	0.00
0.00	0.00	0.00	0.00	0.00	0.00	0.00	0.00	0.00	0.00	0.00	0.00	0.00	0.00	0.00	0.00	0.00	0.00	20.00	0.00
0.00	0.00	0.00	0.00	0.00	0.00	0.00	0.00	0.00	0.00	0.00	0.00	0.00	0.00	0.00	0.00	0.00	0.00	25.00	0.00
0.00	0.00	0.00	0.00	0.00	0.00	0.00	0.00	0.00	0.00	0.00	0.00	0.00	0.00	0.00	0.00	0.00	0.00	10.00	0.00
0.00	0.00	0.00	0.00	0.00	0.00	0.00	0.00	0.00	0.00	0.00	0.00	0.00	0.00	0.00	0.00	0.00	0.00	20.00	0.00
0.00	0.00	0.00	0.00	0.00	0.00	0.00	0.00	0.00	0.00	0.00	0.00	0.00	0.00	0.00	0.00	0.00	0.00	690.00	0.00
0.00	0.00	0.00	0.00	0.00	0.00	0.00	0.00	0.00	0.00	0.00	0.00	0.00	0.00	0.00	0.00	0.00	0.00	0.00	0.00
0.00	0.00	0.00	0.00	0.00	0.00	0.00	0.00	0.00	0.00	0.00	0.00	0.00	0.00	0.00	0.00	0.00	0.00	0.00	0.00
0.00	0.00	0.00	0.00	0.00	0.00	0.00	0.00	0.00	0.00	0.00	0.00	0.00	0.00	0.00	0.00	0.00	0.00	0.00	0.00
0.00	0.00	0.00	0.00	0.00	0.00	0.00	0.00	0.00	0.00	0.00	0.00	0.00	0.00	0.00	0.00	0.00	0.00	10.00	0.00
0.00	0.00	0.00	0.00	0.00	0.00	0.00	0.00	0.00	0.00	0.00	0.00	0.00	0.00	0.00	0.00	0.00	0.00	5.00	0.00
0.00	0.00	0.00	0.00	0.00	0.00	0.00	0.00	0.00	0.00	0.00	0.00	0.00	0.00	0.00	0.00	0.00	0.00	0.00	0.00
0.00	0.00	0.00	0.00	0.00	0.00	0.00	0.00	0.00	0.00	0.00	0.00	0.00	0.00	0.00	0.00	0.00	0.00	1610.00	0.00
0.00	0.00	0.00	0.00	0.00	0.00	0.00	0.00	0.00	0.00	0.00	0.00	0.00	0.00	0.00	0.00	0.00	0.00	540.00	0.00
0.00	0.00	0.00	0.00	0.00	0.00	0.00	0.00	0.00	0.00	0.00	0.00	0.00	0.00	0.00	0.00	0.00	0.00	1080.00	0.00
0.00	0.00	0.00	0.00	0.00	0.00	0.00	0.00	0.00	0.00	0.00	0.00	0.00	0.00	0.00	0.00	0.00	0.00	1490.00	0.00
0.00	0.00	0.00	0.00	0.00	0.00	0.00	0.00	0.00	0.00	0.00	0.00	0.00	0.00	0.00	0.00	0.00	0.00	1310.00	0.00
0.00	0.00	0.00	0.00	0.00	0.00	0.00	0.00	0.00	0.00	0.00	0.00	0.00	0.00	0.00	0.00	0.00	0.00	1330.00	0.00
0.00	0.00	0.00	0.00	0.00	0.00	0.00	0.00	0.00	0.00	0.00	0.00	0.00	0.00	0.00	0.00	0.00	0.00	690.00	0.00
0.00	0.00	0.00	0.00	0.00	0.00	0.00	0.00	0.00	0.00	0.00	0.00	0.00	0.00	0.00	0.00	0.00	0.00	340.00	0.00
0.00	0.00	0.00	0.00	0.00	0.00	0.00	0.00	0.00	0.00	0.00	0.00	0.00	0.00	0.00	0.00	0.00	0.00	0.00	0.00
0.00	0.00	0.00	0.00	0.00	0.00	0.00	0.00	0.00	0.00	0.00	0.00	0.00	0.00	0.00	0.00	0.00	0.00	1140.00	0.00
0.00	0.00	0.00	0.00	0.00	0.00	0.00	0.00	0.00	0.00	0.00	0.00	0.00	0.00	0.00	0.00	0.00	0.00	410.00	0.00
0.00	0.00	0.00	0.00	0.00	0.00	0.00	0.00	0.00	0.00	0.00	0.00	0.00	0.00	0.00	0.00	0.00	0.00	160.00	0.00
0.00	0.00	0.00	0.00	0.00	0.00	0.00	0.00	0.00	0.00	0.00	0.00	0.00	0.00	0.00	0.00	0.00	0.00	160.00	0.00
0.00	0.00	0.00	0.00	0.00	0.00	0.00	0.00	0.00	0.00	0.00	0.00	0.00	0.00	0.00	0.00	0.00	0.00	150.00	0.00
0.00	0.00	0.00	0.00	0.00	0.00	0.00	0.00	0.00	0.00	0.00	0.00	0.00	0.00	0.00	0.00	0.00	0.00	160.00	0.00
0.00	0.00	0.00	0.00	0.00	0.00	0.00	0.00	0.00	0.00	0.00	0.00	0.00	0.00	0.00	0.00	0.00	0.00	300.00	0.00
0.00	0.00	0.00	0.00	0.00	0.00	0.00	0.00	0.00	0.00	0.00	0.00	0.00	0.00	0.00	0.00	0.00	0.00	180.00	0.00
0.00	0.00	0.00	0.00	0.00	0.00	0.00	0.00	0.00	0.00	0.00	0.00	0.00	0.00	0.00	0.00	0.00	0.00	280.00	0.00
0.00	0.00	0.00	0.00	0.00	0.00	0.00	0.00	0.00	0.00	0.00	0.00	0.00	0.00	0.00	0.00	0.00	0.00	250.00	0.00
0.00	0.00	0.00	0.00	0.00	0.00	0.00	0.00	0.00	0.00	0.00	0.00	0.00	0.00	0.00	0.00	0.00	0.00	280.00	0.00
0.00	0.00	0.00	0.00	0.00	0.00	0.00	0.00	0.00	0.00	0.00	0.00	0.00	0.00	0.00	0.00	0.00	0.00	150.00	0.00
0.00	0.00	0.00	0.00	0.00	0.00	0.00	0.00	0.00	0.00	0.00	0.00	0.00	0.00	0.00	0.00	0.00	0.00	150.00	0.00
0.00	0.00	0.00	0.00	0.00	0.00	0.00	0.00	0.00	0.00	0.00	0.00	0.00	0.00	0.00	0.00	0.00	0.00	150.00	0.00
0.00	0.00	0.00	0.00	0.00	0.00	0.00	0.00	0.00	0.00	0.00	0.00	0.00	0.00	0.00	0.00	0.00	0.00	150.00	0.00
0.00	0.00	0.00	0.00	0.00	0.00	0.00	0.00	0.00	0.00	0.00	0.00	0.00	0.00	0.00	0.00	0.00	0.00	95.00	0.00
0.00	0.00	0.00	0.00	0.00	0.00	0.00	0.00	0.00	0.00	0.00	0.00	0.00	0.00	0.00	0.00	0.00	0.00	105.00	0.00
0.00	0.00	0.00	0.00	0.00	0.00	0.00	0.00	0.00	0.00	0.00	0.00	0.00	0.00	0.00	0.00	0.00	0.00	150.00	0.00
0.00	0.00	0.00	0.00	0.00	0.00	0.00	0.00	0.00	0.00	0.00	0.00	0.00	0.00	0.00	0.00	0.00	0.00	100.00	0.00
0.00	0.00	0.00	0.00	0.00	0.00	0.00	0.00	0.00	0.00	0.00	0.00	0.00	0.00	0.00	0.00	0.00	0.00	160.00	0.00
0.00	0.00	0.00	0.00	0.00	0.00	0.00	0.00	0.00	0.00	0.00	0.00	0.00	0.00	0.00	0.00	0.00	0.00	95.00	0.00
3.20	0.00	0.00	0.00	0.00	50.00	4.80	0.24	0.25	2.57	0.00	0.00	0.30	300.00	1.50	31.50	220.00	198.00	638.00	2.33
4.50	0.00	0.00	0.00	0.00	45.00	3.60	0.28	0.30	2.47	0.00	0.00	0.30	252.00	1.50	26.25	188.00	160.00	470.00	2.03
3.30	0.00	0.00	0.00	0.00	35.00	2.40	0.20	0.20	2.28	0.00	0.00	0.25	264.00	0.90	21.00	188.00	130.50	433.50	1.80
5.05	0.00	0.00	0.00	0.00	50.00	3.60	0.27	0.26	2.66	0.00	0.00	0.33	176.00	1.40	26.25	156.00	207.50	633.50	1.88
6.50	0.00	0.00	0.00	0.00	50.00	4.20	0.32	0.25	2.57	0.00	0.00	0.30	208.00	1.75	24.50	176.00	202.50	563.50	2.10
16.50	0.00	0.00	0.00	0.00	120.00	10.20	0.56	0.66	7.79	0.00	0.00	0.44	584.00	3.20	52.50	360.00	408.00	1335.00	3.75
4.70	0.00	0.00	0.00	0.00	35.00	3.00	0.21	0.21	2.47	0.00	0.00	0.25	180.00	0.90	19.25	148.00	143.50	493.00	1.73
5.35	0.00	0.00	0.00	0.00	50.00	4.20	0.29	0.22	2.57	0.00	0.00	0.35	184.00	1.35	26.25	168.00	231.50	668.00	2.25
6.00	0.00	0.00	0.00	0.00	55.00	6.00	0.35	0.29	3.52	0.00	0.00	0.41	176.00	1.90	33.25	168.00	258.00	824.00	2.40
7.00	0.00	0.00	0.00	0.00	60.00	5.40	0.38	0.33	3.04	0.00	0.00	0.40	216.00	1.85	31.50	188.00	266.00	723.50	2.70
6.90	0.00	0.00	0.00	0.00	55.00	6.00	0.35	0.26	3.42	0.00	0.00	0.40	192.00	2.25	35.00	184.00	289.00	735.00	2.85
8.00	0.00	0.00	0.00	0.00	60.00	4.80	0.41	0.40	2.85	0.00	0.00	0.38	200.00	1.40	33.25	184.00	290.00	831.50	2.78
16.80	0.00	0.00	0.00	0.00	120.00	10.80	0.59	0.66	7.60	0.00	0.00	0.46	416.00	3.70	52.50	320.00	487.00	1313.00	3.75

USDA ID Code	Food Name	Weight in Grams*	Quantity of Units	Unit of Measure	Protein (gm)	Fat (gm)	Carbohydrate (gm)	Kcalories	Caffeine (gm)	Fiber (gm)	Cholesterol (mg)	Saturated Fat (gm)
	Pizza Hut-Pizza, Supreme, Thin'n	70.0000	1.000	Slice	14.00	11.00	20.50	229.50	0.00	0.00	21.00	5.50
	Red Lobster-Calamari, Brded and	141.7460	1.000	Each	13.00	21.00	30.00	360.00	0.00	0.00	140.00	5.60
	Red Lobster-Catfish, Lunch Porti	141.7460	1.000	Each	20.00	10.00	0.00	170.00	0.00	0.00	85.00	2.50
	Red Lobster-Chicken Breast, Skin	113.3970	1.000	Each	26.00	3.00	0.00	140.00	0.00	0.00	70.00	1.00
	Red Lobster-Cod, Atlantic, Lunch	141.7460	1.000	Each	23.00	1.00	0.00	100.00	0.00	0.00	70.00	0.30
	Red Lobster-Crab Legs, King, Lun	453.5900	1.000	Each	32.00	2.00	6.00	170.00	0.00	0.00	100.00	0.50
	Red Lobster-Crab Legs, Snow, Lun	453.5900	1.000	Each	33.00	2.00	1.00	150.00	0.00	0.00	130.00	0.60
	Red Lobster-Flounder, Lunch Port	141.7460	1.000	Each	21.00	1.00	1.00	100.00	0.00	0.00	70.00	0.30
	Red Lobster-Grouper, Lunch Porti	141.7460	1.000	Each	26.00	1.00	0.00	110.00	0.00	0.00	65.00	0.30
	Red Lobster-Haddock, Lunch Porti	141.7460	1.000	Each	24.00	1.00	2.00	110.00	0.00	0.00	85.00	0.30
	Red Lobster-Halibut, Lunch Porti	141.7460	1.000	Each	25.00	1.00	1.00	110.00	0.00	0.00	60.00	0.30
	Red Lobster-Hamburger, Lunch Por	151.1810	1.000	Each	37.00	28.00	0.00	410.00	0.00	0.00	130.00	11.00
	Red Lobster-Langostino, Lunch Po	141.7460	1.000	Each	26.00	1.00	2.00	120.00	0.00	0.00	210.00	0.20
	Red Lobster-Lobster, Live Maine	510.2880	1.000	Each	36.00	8.00	5.00	240.00	0.00	0.00	310.00	1.90
	Red Lobster-Lobster, Rock, Lunch	368.5410	1.000	Each	49.00	3.00	2.00	230.00	0.00	0.00	200.00	0.70
	Red Lobster-Mackerel, Lunch Port	141.7460	1.000	Each	20.00	12.00	1.00	190.00	0.00	0.00	100.00	3.60
	Red Lobster-Monkfish, Lunch Port	141.7460	1.000	Each	24.00	1.00	0.00	110.00	0.00	0.00	80.00	0.20
	Red Lobster-Perch, Atlantic Ocea	141.7460	1.000	Each	24.00	4.00	1.00	130.00	0.00	0.00	75.00	1.10
	Red Lobster-Pollock, Lunch Porti	141.7460	1.000	Each	28.00	1.00	1.00	120.00	0.00	0.00	90.00	0.30
	Red Lobster-Rockfish, Red, Lunch	141.7460	1.000	Each	21.00	1.00	0.00	90.00	0.00	0.00	85.00	0.30
	Red Lobster-Salmon, Norwegian, L	141.7460	1.000	Each	27.00	12.00	3.00	230.00	0.00	0.00	80.00	2.70
	Red Lobster-Salmon, Sockeye, Lun	141.7460	1.000	Each	28.00	4.00	3.00	160.00	0.00	0.00	50.00	1.10
	Red Lobster-Scallops, Deep Sea,	141.7460	1.000	Each	26.00	2.00	2.00	130.00	0.00	0.00	50.00	0.40
	Red Lobster-Shrimp, Lunch Portio	198.4450	1.000	Each	25.00	2.00	0.00	120.00	0.00	0.00	230.00	0.50
	Red Lobster-Snapper, Red, Lunch	141.7460	1.000	Each	25.00	1.00	0.00	110.00	0.00	0.00	70.00	0.40
	Red Lobster-Sole, Lemon, Lunch P	141.7460	1.000	Each	27.00	1.00	1.00	120.00	0.00	0.00	65.00	0.30
	Red Lobster-Steak, Strip, Lunch	255.1440	1.000	Each	47.00	40.00	0.00	560.00	0.00	0.00	150.00	17.00
	Red Lobster-Swordfish, Lunch Por	141.7460	1.000	Each	17.00	4.00	0.00	100.00	0.00	0.00	100.00	1.20
	Red Lobster-Trout, Rainbow, Lunc	141.7460	1.000	Each	23.00	9.00	0.00	170.00	0.00	0.00	90.00	2.50
	Red Lobster-Tuna, Yellow Fin, Lu	141.7460	1.000	Each	32.00	2.00	6.00	180.00	0.00	0.00	70.00	0.50
	Anchovy, European, Cnd In Oil	28.3500	3.000	Ounce	8.19	2.75	0.00	59.54	0.00	0.00	24.10	0.62
	Bass, Freshwater, Ckd, Dry Heat	62.0000	1.000	Each	14.99	2.93	0.00	90.52	0.00	0.00	53.94	0.62
	Bass, Striped, Ckd, Dry Heat	124.0000	1.000	Each	28.19	3.71	0.00	153.76	0.00	0.00	127.72	0.81
	Bluefish, Ckd, Dry Heat	117.0000	1.000	Each	30.06	6.36	0.00	186.03	0.00	0.00	88.92	1.37
	Catfish, Channel, Farmed, Ckd, D	143.0000	1.000	Each	26.77	11.47	0.00	217.36	0.00	0.00	91.52	2.56
	Catfish, Channel, Wild, Ckd, Dry	143.0000	1.000	Each	26.41	4.08	0.00	150.15	0.00	0.00	102.96	1.06
	Catfish, Fried	87.0000	1.000	Each	15.74	11.60	6.99	199.23	0.00	0.65	70.47	2.86
	Caviar, Black and Red, Granular	16.0000	1.000	Tbsp	3.94	2.86	0.64	40.32	0.00	0.00	94.08	0.65
	Clam, Ckd, Breaded and Fried	85.0000	3.000	Ounce	12.10	9.48	8.78	171.70	0.00	0.00	51.85	2.28
	Clam, Ckd, Moist Heat	85.0000	3.000	Ounce	21.72	1.66	4.36	125.80	0.00	0.00	56.95	0.16
	Clam, Cnd, Drained Solids	160.0000	1.000	Cup	40.88	3.12	8.21	236.80	0.00	0.00	107.20	0.30
	Cod, Atlantic, Ckd, Dry Heat	180.0000	1.000	Each	41.09	1.55	0.00	189.00	0.00	0.00	99.00	0.31
	Cod, Atlantic, Cnd	312.0000	1.000	Can	71.01	2.68	0.00	327.60	0.00	0.00	171.60	0.53
	Crab, Alaska King, Ckd, Moist He	134.0000	1.000	Leg	25.93	2.06	0.00	129.98	0.00	0.00	71.02	0.17
	Crab, Alaska King, Imitation	85.0000	3.000	Ounce	10.22	1.11	8.69	86.70	0.00	0.00	17.00	0.22
	Crab, Blue, Ckd, Moist Heat	118.0000	1.000	Cup	23.84	2.09	0.00	120.36	0.00	0.00	118.00	0.27
	Crab, Blue, Cnd	135.0000	1.000	Cup	27.70	1.66	0.00	133.65	0.00	0.00	120.15	0.34
	Crab, Blue, Crab Cakes	60.0000	1.000	Cake	12.13	4.51	0.29	93.00	0.00	0.00	90.00	0.89
	Crab, Dungeness, Ckd, Moist Heat	85.0000	3.000	Ounce	18.97	1.05	0.81	93.50	0.00	0.00	64.60	0.14
	Crab, Queen, Ckd, Moist Heat	85.0000	3.000	Ounce	20.16	1.28	0.00	97.75	0.00	0.00	60.35	0.15
217	Crawfish, Boiled	85.0000	3.000	oz	20.33	1.15	0.00	97.00	0.00	0.00	151.00	0.20
	Crayfish, Farmed, Ckd, Moist Hea	85.0000	3.000	Ounce	14.89	1.11	0.00	73.95	0.00	0.00	116.45	0.19
	Crayfish, Wild, Ckd, Moist Heat	85.0000	3.000	Ounce	14.25	1.02	0.00	69.70	0.00	0.00	113.05	0.15
	Fish Fillets and Sticks, Fried	57.0000	1.000	Piece	8.92	6.97	13.54	155.04	0.00	0.00	63.84	1.80
	Flounder, Ckd, Dry Heat	127.0000	1.000	Each	30.68	1.94	0.00	148.59	0.00	0.00	86.36	0.46

Monounsaturated Fat (gm)	Polyunsaturated Fat (gm)	Vitamin D (mg)	Vitamin K (mg)	Vitamin E (mg)	Vitamin A (re)	Vitamin C (mg)	Thiamin (mg)	Riboflavin (mg)	Niacin (mg)	Vitamin B_6 (mg)	Folate (mg)	Vitamin B_{12} (mcg)	Calcium (mg)	Iron (mg)	Magnesium (mg)	Phosphorus (mg)	Potassium (mg)	Sodium (mg)	Zinc (mg)
5.50	0.00	0.00	0.00	0.00	50.00	4.80	0.30	0.25	2.57	0.00	0.00	0.30	172.00	1.65	29.75	160.00	272.00	664.00	2.33
0.00	1.50	0.00	0.00	0.00	0.00	0.00	0.23	0.14	1.52	0.00	0.00	2.00	0.00	0.60	21.00	360.00	0.00	1150.00	0.90
0.00	1.90	0.00	0.00	0.00	0.00	0.00	0.30	0.14	1.90	0.00	0.00	0.04	0.00	0.00	21.00	160.00	0.00	50.00	0.30
0.00	1.00	0.00	0.00	0.00	0.00	0.00	0.06	0.10	11.40	0.00	0.00	0.08	0.00	0.40	21.00	160.00	0.00	60.00	0.90
0.00	0.60	0.00	0.00	0.00	0.00	0.00	0.03	0.07	0.76	0.00	0.00	0.60	0.00	0.00	28.00	200.00	0.00	200.00	0.30
0.00	1.60	0.00	0.00	0.00	0.00	0.00	0.09	0.17	1.90	0.00	0.00	1.60	48.00	0.00	70.00	320.00	0.00	900.00	6.00
0.00	1.80	0.00	0.00	0.00	0.00	0.00	0.03	0.10	1.90	0.00	0.00	1.60	80.00	0.20	70.00	200.00	0.00	1630.00	6.00
0.00	0.70	0.00	0.00	0.00	0.00	0.00	0.03	0.00	1.52	0.00	0.00	0.30	16.00	0.00	21.00	48.00	0.00	95.00	0.30
0.00	0.50	0.00	0.00	0.00	0.00	0.00	0.06	0.03	1.52	0.00	0.00	0.08	32.00	0.00	28.00	200.00	0.00	70.00	0.30
0.00	1.10	0.00	0.00	0.00	0.00	0.00	0.03	0.07	2.85	0.00	0.00	0.20	0.00	0.00	21.00	160.00	0.00	180.00	0.30
0.00	0.70	0.00	0.00	0.00	0.00	0.00	0.15	0.00	2.85	0.00	0.00	0.30	0.00	0.00	28.00	240.00	0.00	105.00	0.00
0.00	1.00	0.00	0.00	0.00	0.00	0.00	0.06	0.34	7.60	0.00	0.00	1.20	0.00	1.50	28.00	200.00	0.00	115.00	7.50
0.00	0.60	0.00	0.00	0.00	0.00	0.00	0.12	0.00	1.14	0.00	0.00	2.00	16.00	0.80	35.00	160.00	0.00	410.00	1.50
0.00	4.10	0.00	0.00	0.00	0.00	0.00	0.15	0.17	2.85	0.00	0.00	2.00	320.00	0.80	52.50	320.00	0.00	550.00	6.75
0.00	1.40	0.00	0.00	0.00	0.00	0.00	0.00	0.07	3.80	0.00	0.00	0.50	48.00	0.00	87.50	400.00	0.00	1090.00	6.00
0.00	5.40	0.00	0.00	0.00	0.00	0.00	0.15	0.43	5.70	0.00	0.00	0.80	16.00	0.80	21.00	200.00	0.00	250.00	1.20
0.00	0.70	0.00	0.00	0.00	40.00	0.00	0.06	0.14	0.76	0.00	0.00	0.20	0.00	1.00	14.00	64.00	0.00	95.00	0.30
0.00	1.20	0.00	0.00	0.00	0.00	0.00	0.06	0.10	1.52	0.00	0.00	0.30	0.00	0.00	21.00	160.00	0.00	190.00	0.30
0.00	1.00	0.00	0.00	0.00	0.00	0.00	0.06	0.17	0.38	0.00	0.00	1.00	0.00	0.00	28.00	160.00	0.00	90.00	0.30
0.00	0.50	0.00	0.00	0.00	0.00	0.00	0.09	0.10	0.76	0.00	0.00	0.60	0.00	0.00	21.00	120.00	0.00	95.00	0.30
0.00	4.60	0.00	0.00	0.00	0.00	0.00	0.23	0.07	6.65	0.00	0.00	0.20	16.00	0.00	35.00	240.00	0.00	60.00	0.30
0.00	1.80	0.00	0.00	0.00	0.00	0.00	0.38	0.14	7.60	0.00	0.00	2.00	0.00	0.00	35.00	280.00	0.00	60.00	0.30
0.00	1.50	0.00	0.00	0.00	0.00	0.00	0.00	0.10	1.90	0.00	0.00	0.40	0.00	0.00	52.50	240.00	0.00	260.00	1.50
0.00	1.10	0.00	0.00	0.00	0.00	0.00	0.00	0.03	1.90	0.00	0.00	0.50	32.00	0.00	35.00	120.00	0.00	110.00	1.50
0.00	0.60	0.00	0.00	0.00	0.00	0.00	0.06	0.03	4.75	0.00	0.00	0.30	0.00	0.00	21.00	120.00	0.00	140.00	0.30
0.00	0.40	0.00	0.00	0.00	0.00	0.00	0.06	0.10	0.38	0.00	0.00	0.40	0.00	0.00	21.00	64.00	0.00	90.00	0.30
0.00	2.00	0.00	0.00	0.00	0.00	0.00	0.15	0.34	7.60	0.00	0.00	1.20	0.00	2.00	35.00	280.00	0.00	115.00	9.00
0.00	1.00	0.00	0.00	0.00	20.00	0.00	0.06	0.07	3.80	0.00	0.00	0.30	0.00	0.00	28.00	80.00	0.00	140.00	0.60
0.00	4.00	0.00	0.00	0.00	0.00	0.00	0.12	0.17	2.85	0.00	0.00	1.00	80.00	0.00	21.00	200.00	0.00	90.00	0.90
0.00	1.60	0.00	0.00	0.00	0.00	0.00	0.06	0.03	13.30	0.00	0.00	1.60	0.00	0.60	35.00	240.00	0.00	70.00	0.30
1.07	0.73	0.00	0.00	1.42	5.95	0.00	0.02	0.10	5.64	0.06	3.54	0.25	65.77	1.31	19.56	71.44	154.22	1039.88	0.69
1.14	0.84	0.00	0.00	0.00	21.70	1.30	0.06	0.06	0.94	0.09	10.54	1.43	63.86	1.18	23.56	158.72	282.72	55.80	0.51
1.05	1.25	0.00	0.00	0.00	38.44	0.00	0.15	0.05	3.17	0.43	12.40	5.47	23.56	1.34	63.24	314.96	406.72	109.12	0.63
2.69	1.59	0.00	0.00	0.00	161.46	0.00	0.08	0.12	8.48	0.54	2.34	7.28	10.53	0.73	49.14	340.47	558.09	90.09	1.22
5.95	1.99	0.00	0.00	0.00	21.45	1.14	0.60	0.10	3.59	0.23	10.01	4.00	12.87	1.17	37.18	350.35	459.03	114.40	1.50
1.57	0.92	0.00	0.00	0.00	21.45	1.14	0.33	0.10	3.42	0.16	14.30	4.15	15.73	0.50	40.04	434.72	599.17	71.50	0.87
4.88	2.90	0.00	0.00	0.00	6.96	0.00	0.06	0.11	1.98	0.17	26.10	1.65	38.28	1.24	23.49	187.92	295.80	243.60	0.75
0.74	1.19	0.93	0.00	1.12	89.60	0.00	0.03	0.10	0.02	0.05	8.00	3.20	44.00	1.90	48.00	56.96	28.96	240.00	0.15
3.87	2.44	0.00	0.00	0.00	76.50	8.50	0.09	0.20	1.75	0.05	30.60	34.23	53.55	11.82	11.90	159.80	277.10	309.40	1.24
0.14	0.47	0.00	0.00	0.00	145.35	18.79	0.13	0.37	2.85	0.09	24.48	84.06	78.20	23.77	15.30	287.30	533.80	95.20	2.32
0.27	0.88	0.00	0.00	1.60	273.60	35.36	0.24	0.69	5.36	0.18	46.08	158.22	147.20	44.74	28.80	540.80	1004.80	179.20	4.37
0.22	0.52	0.00	0.00	0.54	25.20	1.80	0.16	0.14	4.52	0.50	14.58	1.89	25.20	0.88	75.60	248.40	439.20	140.40	1.04
0.37	0.90	6.55	0.00	0.62	43.68	3.12	0.28	0.25	7.83	0.87	25.27	3.28	65.52	1.53	127.92	811.20	1647.36	680.16	1.81
0.25	0.72	0.00	0.00	0.00	12.06	10.18	0.07	0.08	1.80	0.24	68.34	15.41	79.06	1.02	84.42	375.20	351.08	1436.48	10.21
0.17	0.57	0.00	0.00	0.09	17.00	0.00	0.03	0.03	0.15	0.03	1.36	1.36	11.05	0.33	36.55	239.70	76.50	714.85	0.28
0.33	0.80	0.00	0.00	1.18	2.36	3.89	0.12	0.06	3.89	0.21	59.94	8.61	122.72	1.07	38.94	243.08	382.32	329.22	4.98
0.30	0.59	0.00	0.00	1.35	2.70	3.65	0.11	0.11	1.85	0.20	57.38	0.62	136.35	1.13	52.65	351.00	504.90	449.55	5.43
1.69	1.36	0.00	0.00	0.00	48.60	1.68	0.05	0.05	1.74	0.10	31.80	3.56	63.00	0.65	19.80	127.80	194.40	198.00	2.45
0.18	0.35	0.00	0.00	0.00	26.35	3.06	0.05	0.17	3.08	0.14	35.70	8.82	50.15	0.37	49.30	148.75	346.80	321.30	4.65
0.28	0.46	0.00	0.00	0.00	44.20	6.12	0.09	0.20	2.46	0.14	35.70	8.82	28.05	2.45	53.55	108.80	170.00	587.35	3.05
0.32	0.28	0.00	0.00	0.00	0.00	2.80	0.00	0.07	2.49	0.00	0.00	2.94	26.00	2.67	27.00	280.00	298.00	58.00	1.42
0.21	0.35	0.00	0.00	0.00	12.75	0.43	0.04	0.07	1.42	0.11	9.35	2.64	43.35	0.94	28.05	204.85	202.30	82.45	1.26
0.20	0.31	0.00	0.00	1.28	12.75	0.77	0.04	0.08	1.94	0.07	37.40	1.83	51.00	0.71	28.05	229.50	251.60	79.90	1.50
2.89	1.81	0.00	0.00	0.78	17.67	0.00	0.07	0.10	1.21	0.03	10.37	1.03	11.40	0.42	14.25	103.17	148.77	331.74	0.38
0.30	0.83	0.00	0.00	2.40	13.97	0.00	0.10	0.14	2.77	0.30	11.68	3.19	22.86	0.43	73.66	367.03	436.88	133.35	0.80

USDA ID Code	Food Name	Weight in Grams*	Quantity of Units	Unit of Measure	Protein (gm)	Fat (gm)	Carbohydrate (gm)	Kcalories	Caffeine (gm)	Fiber (gm)	Cholesterol (mg)	Saturated Fat (gm)
	Grouper, Ckd, Dry Heat	202.0000	1.000	Each	50.18	2.63	0.00	238.36	0.00	0.00	94.94	0.61
	Haddock, Ckd, Dry Heat	150.0000	1.000	Each	36.36	1.40	0.00	168.00	0.00	0.00	111.00	0.26
	Haddock, Smoked	28.3500	1.000	Ounce	7.15	0.27	0.00	32.89	0.00	0.00	21.83	0.05
	Halibut, Ckd, Dry Heat	159.0000	3.000	Ounce	42.44	4.67	0.00	222.60	0.00	0.00	65.19	0.67
	Halibut, Greenland, Ckd, Dry Hea	159.0000	3.000	Ounce	29.29	28.21	0.00	380.01	0.00	0.00	93.81	4.93
	Herring, Ckd, Dry Heat	143.0000	1.000	Each	32.93	16.57	0.00	290.29	0.00	0.00	110.11	3.75
	Herring, Kippered	28.3500	1.000	Ounce	6.97	3.51	0.00	61.52	0.00	0.00	23.25	0.79
	Herring, Pacific, Ckd, Dry Heat	144.0000	1.000	Each	30.25	25.62	0.00	360.00	0.00	0.00	142.56	6.00
	Herring, Pickled	140.0000	1.000	Cup	19.87	25.20	13.50	366.80	0.00	0.00	18.20	3.33
	Lobster, Northern, Ckd, Moist He	145.0000	1.000	Cup	29.73	0.86	1.86	142.10	0.00	0.00	104.40	0.16
	Lobster, Spiny, Ckd, Moist Heat	163.0000	1.000	Lobster	43.05	3.16	5.09	233.09	0.00	0.00	146.70	0.49
	Mackerel, Ckd, Dry Heat	88.0000	1.000	Each	20.99	15.67	0.00	230.56	0.00	0.00	66.00	3.68
	Mullet, Striped, Ckd, Dry Heat	93.0000	1.000	Each	23.07	4.52	0.00	139.50	0.00	0.00	58.59	1.33
	Mussel, Blue, Ckd, Moist Heat	85.0000	3.000	Ounce	20.23	3.81	6.28	146.20	0.00	0.00	47.60	0.72
	Oyster, Eastern, Breaded and Fri	85.0000	3.000	Ounce	7.45	10.69	9.88	167.45	0.00	0.00	68.85	2.72
	Oyster, Eastern, Cnd	162.0000	1.000	Cup	11.44	4.00	6.33	111.78	0.00	0.00	89.10	1.02
	Oysters, Raw	85.0000	3.000	Ounce	4.44	1.32	4.70	50.15	0.00	0.00	21.25	0.37
	Perch, Atlantic, Ckd, Dry Heat	50.0000	1.000	Each	11.94	1.05	0.00	60.50	0.00	0.00	27.00	0.16
	Perch, Ckd, Dry Heat	46.0000	1.000	Each	11.44	0.54	0.00	53.82	0.00	0.00	52.90	0.11
	Pike, Northern, Ckd, Dry Heat	155.0000	3.000	Ounce	38.27	1.36	0.00	175.15	0.00	0.00	77.50	0.23
	Pike, Walleye, Ckd, Dry Heat	124.0000	1.000	Each	30.43	1.93	0.00	147.56	0.00	0.00	136.40	0.40
	Pollock, Atlantic, Ckd, Dry Heat	151.0000	3.000	Ounce	37.63	1.90	0.00	178.18	0.00	0.00	137.41	0.26
655	Pompano, Cooked	85.0000	3.000	Ounce	20.14	10.32	0.00	179.35	0.00	0.00	54.40	3.82
	Pompano, Florida, Ckd, Dry Heat	88.0000	1.000	Each	20.85	10.68	0.00	185.68	0.00	0.00	56.32	3.96
	Rockfish, Pacific, Ckd, Dry Heat	149.0000	1.000	Each	35.82	2.99	0.00	180.29	0.00	0.00	65.56	0.70
	Roughy, Orange, Ckd, Dry Heat	85.0000	3.000	Ounce	16.02	0.77	0.00	75.65	0.00	0.00	22.10	0.02
	Salmon, Atlantic, Wild, Ckd, Dry	154.0000	3.000	Ounce	39.18	12.52	0.00	280.28	0.00	0.00	109.34	1.94
	Salmon, Chinook, Ckd, Dry Heat	154.0000	3.000	Ounce	39.61	20.61	0.00	355.74	0.00	0.00	130.90	4.94
	Salmon, Chum, Ckd, Dry Heat	154.0000	3.000	Ounce	39.76	7.44	0.00	237.16	0.00	0.00	146.30	1.66
	Salmon, Cnd	369.0000	1.000	Can	75.53	26.97	0.00	564.57	0.00	0.00	162.36	6.05
	Salmon, Coho, Farmed, Ckd, Dry H	143.0000	1.000	Each	34.75	11.77	0.00	254.54	0.00	0.00	90.09	2.77
	Salmon, Coho, Wild, Ckd, Dry Hea	178.0000	3.000	Ounce	41.74	7.65	0.00	247.42	0.00	0.00	97.90	1.87
	Salmon, Coho, Wild, Ckd, Moist H	155.0000	3.000	Ounce	42.41	11.63	0.00	285.20	0.00	0.00	88.35	2.48
	Salmon, Pink, Ckd, Dry Heat	124.0000	3.000	Ounce	31.69	5.48	0.00	184.76	0.00	0.00	83.08	0.89
	Sardine, Atlantic, Cnd In Oil	149.0000	1.000	Cup	36.68	17.06	0.00	309.92	0.00	0.00	211.58	2.28
	Scallop, Breaded and Fried	31.0000	2.000	Large	5.60	3.39	3.14	66.65	0.00	0.00	18.91	0.83
	Scallop, Imitation	85.0000	3.000	Ounce	10.85	0.35	9.03	84.15	0.00	0.00	18.70	0.07
	Scallops, Sauteed	28.3500	3.000	Ounce	9.67	0.33	0.67	50.00	0.00	0.00	20.00	0.00
	Sea Bass, Ckd, Dry Heat	101.0000	1.000	Each	23.87	2.59	0.00	125.24	0.00	0.00	53.53	0.67
	Shark, Ckd, Batter-dipped and Fr	85.0000	3.000	Ounce	15.83	11.75	5.43	193.80	0.00	0.00	50.15	2.73
	Shrimp, Ckd, Breaded and Fried	85.0000	3.000	Ounce	18.18	10.44	9.75	205.70	0.00	0.32	150.45	1.78
	Shrimp, Ckd, Moist Heat	85.0000	3.000	Ounce	17.77	0.92	0.00	84.15	0.00	0.00	165.75	0.25
	Shrimp, Cnd	128.0000	1.000	Cup	29.54	2.51	1.32	153.60	0.00	0.00	221.44	0.47
	Shrimp, Fresh	6.0000	1.000	Slice	1.22	0.10	0.05	6.36	0.00	0.00	9.12	0.02
	Shrimp, Imitation	85.0000	3.000	Ounce	10.53	1.25	7.76	85.85	0.00	0.00	30.60	0.25
	Smelt, Rainbow, Ckd, Dry Heat	85.0000	3.000	Ounce	19.21	2.64	0.00	105.40	0.00	0.00	76.50	0.49
	Snapper, Ckd, Dry Heat	170.0000	1.000	Each	44.71	2.92	0.00	217.60	0.00	0.00	79.90	0.63
	Squid, Fried	85.0000	3.000	Ounce	15.25	6.36	6.62	148.75	0.00	0.00	221.00	1.60
	Sunfish, Ckd, Dry Heat	37.0000	1.000	Each	9.20	0.33	0.00	42.18	0.00	0.00	31.82	0.07
	Swordfish, Ckd, Dry Heat	106.0000	1.000	Piece	26.91	5.45	0.00	164.30	0.00	0.00	53.00	1.49
	Trout, Ckd, Dry Heat	62.0000	1.000	Each	16.51	5.25	0.00	117.80	0.00	0.00	45.88	0.91
	Trout, Rainbow, Farmed, Ckd, Dry	71.0000	1.000	Each	17.23	5.11	0.00	119.99	0.00	0.00	48.28	1.50
	Trout, Rainbow, Wild, Ckd, Dry H	143.0000	1.000	Each	32.78	8.32	0.00	214.50	0.00	0.00	98.67	2.32
	Tuna Salad	205.0000	1.000	Cup	32.88	18.98	19.29	383.35	0.00	0.00	26.65	3.16
	Tuna, Light Meat, Cnd In Oil	171.0000	1.000	Can	49.81	14.04	0.00	338.58	0.00	0.00	30.78	2.62

Monounsaturated Fat (gm)	Polyunsaturated Fat (gm)	Vitamin D (mg)	Vitamin K (mg)	Vitamin E (mg)	Vitamin A (re)	Vitamin C (mg)	Thiamin (mg)	Riboflavin (mg)	Niacin (mg)	Vitamin B_6 (mg)	Folate (mg)	Vitamin B_{12} (mcg)	Calcium (mg)	Iron (mg)	Magnesium (mg)	Phosphorus (mg)	Potassium (mg)	Sodium (mg)	Zinc (mg)
0.55	0.81	0.00	0.00	0.00	101.00	0.00	0.16	0.02	0.77	0.71	20.60	1.39	42.42	2.30	74.74	288.86	959.50	107.06	1.03
0.23	0.47	0.00	0.00	0.00	28.50	0.00	0.06	0.08	6.95	0.53	19.95	2.09	63.00	2.03	75.00	361.50	598.50	130.50	0.72
0.05	0.09	0.00	0.00	0.11	6.24	0.00	0.01	0.01	1.44	0.11	4.34	0.45	13.89	0.40	15.31	71.16	117.65	216.31	0.14
1.54	1.49	0.00	0.00	1.73	85.86	0.00	0.11	0.14	11.32	0.64	21.94	2.18	95.40	1.70	170.13	453.15	915.84	109.71	0.84
17.08	2.78	0.00	0.00	0.00	28.62	0.00	0.11	0.16	3.05	0.78	1.59	1.53	6.36	1.35	52.47	333.90	546.96	163.77	0.81
6.85	3.92	0.00	0.00	1.92	44.33	1.00	0.16	0.43	5.89	0.50	16.45	18.79	105.82	2.02	58.63	433.29	599.17	164.45	1.82
1.45	0.83	0.85	0.00	0.28	11.06	0.28	0.04	0.09	1.25	0.12	3.88	5.30	23.81	0.43	13.04	92.14	126.72	260.25	0.39
12.69	4.48	0.00	0.00	0.00	50.40	0.00	0.10	0.37	4.06	0.75	8.64	13.85	152.64	2.07	59.04	420.48	780.48	136.80	0.98
16.73	2.35	23.80	0.00	1.40	361.20	0.00	0.06	0.20	4.62	0.24	3.36	5.98	107.80	1.71	11.20	124.60	96.60	1218.00	0.74
0.23	0.13	0.00	0.00	1.45	37.70	0.00	0.01	0.10	1.55	0.12	16.10	4.51	88.45	0.57	50.75	268.25	510.40	551.00	4.23
0.57	1.24	0.00	0.00	0.00	9.78	3.42	0.02	0.10	7.99	0.28	1.63	6.59	102.69	2.30	83.13	373.27	339.04	370.01	11.85
6.17	3.78	0.00	0.00	0.00	47.52	0.35	0.14	0.36	6.03	0.40	1.32	16.72	13.20	1.38	85.36	244.64	352.88	73.04	0.83
1.28	0.86	0.00	0.00	0.00	39.06	1.12	0.09	0.09	5.86	0.46	9.11	0.23	28.83	1.31	30.69	226.92	425.94	66.03	0.82
0.86	1.03	0.00	0.00	0.00	77.35	11.56	0.26	0.36	2.55	0.09	64.26	20.40	28.05	5.71	31.45	242.25	227.80	313.65	2.27
4.00	2.81	0.00	0.00	0.00	76.50	3.23	0.13	0.17	1.40	0.05	26.35	13.29	52.70	5.91	49.30	135.15	207.40	354.45	74.06
0.41	1.20	0.00	0.00	1.38	145.80	8.10	0.24	0.28	2.01	0.16	14.42	30.99	72.90	10.85	87.48	225.18	370.98	181.44	47.34
0.13	0.50	0.00	0.00	0.00	6.80	4.00	0.09	0.06	1.08	0.05	15.30	13.77	37.40	4.91	28.05	79.05	105.40	151.30	32.23
0.40	0.28	0.00	0.00	0.00	7.00	0.40	0.07	0.07	1.22	0.14	5.20	0.58	68.50	0.59	19.50	138.50	175.00	48.00	0.31
0.09	0.22	0.00	0.00	0.00	4.60	0.78	0.04	0.06	0.87	0.06	2.67	1.01	46.92	0.53	17.48	118.22	158.24	36.34	0.66
0.31	0.40	0.00	0.00	0.00	37.20	5.89	0.11	0.12	4.34	0.22	26.82	3.57	113.15	1.10	62.00	437.10	513.05	75.95	1.33
0.47	0.71	0.00	0.00	0.00	29.76	0.00	0.38	0.25	3.47	0.17	21.08	2.86	174.84	2.07	47.12	333.56	618.76	80.60	0.98
0.21	0.94	0.00	0.00	0.00	18.12	0.00	0.08	0.35	6.01	0.50	4.53	5.56	116.27	0.89	129.86	427.33	688.56	166.10	0.91
2.82	1.24	0.00	0.00	0.00	0.00	0.00	0.58	0.13	3.23	0.20	14.71	1.02	36.55	0.57	26.35	289.85	540.60	64.60	0.59
2.92	1.28	0.00	0.00	0.00	31.68	0.00	0.60	0.13	3.34	0.20	15.22	1.06	37.84	0.59	27.28	300.08	559.68	66.88	0.61
0.67	0.88	0.00	0.00	1.86	98.34	0.00	0.06	0.12	5.84	0.40	15.50	1.79	17.88	0.79	50.66	339.72	774.80	114.73	0.79
0.53	0.02	0.00	0.00	0.00	20.40	0.00	0.10	0.15	3.10	0.30	6.80	1.96	32.30	0.20	32.30	217.60	327.25	68.85	0.82
4.16	5.02	0.00	0.00	0.00	20.02	0.00	0.43	0.75	15.52	1.45	44.66	4.70	23.10	1.59	56.98	394.24	967.12	86.24	1.26
8.84	4.10	0.00	0.00	0.00	229.46	6.31	0.06	0.23	15.48	0.71	53.90	4.42	43.12	1.40	187.88	571.34	777.70	92.40	0.86
3.05	1.77	0.00	0.00	0.00	52.36	0.00	0.14	0.34	13.14	0.71	7.70	5.33	21.56	1.09	43.12	559.02	847.00	98.56	0.92
11.66	6.97	0.00	0.00	5.90	195.57	0.00	0.07	0.70	20.22	1.11	36.16	1.11	881.91	3.91	107.01	1202.94	1391.13	1985.22	3.76
5.18	2.80	0.00	0.00	0.00	84.37	2.15	0.14	0.16	10.57	0.82	20.02	4.53	17.16	0.56	48.62	474.76	657.80	74.36	0.67
2.81	2.26	0.00	0.00	1.44	69.42	2.49	0.14	0.25	14.15	1.01	23.14	8.90	80.10	1.09	58.74	573.16	772.52	103.24	1.00
4.19	3.91	0.00	0.00	0.00	49.60	1.55	0.19	0.25	12.06	0.87	13.95	6.94	71.30	1.10	54.25	461.90	705.25	82.15	0.81
1.49	2.15	0.00	0.00	0.00	50.84	0.00	0.25	0.09	10.58	0.29	6.20	4.29	21.08	1.23	40.92	365.80	513.36	106.64	0.88
5.77	7.67	10.13	0.00	0.45	99.83	0.00	0.12	0.34	7.82	0.25	17.58	13.32	569.18	4.35	58.11	730.10	591.53	752.45	1.95
1.40	0.89	0.00	0.00	0.00	6.82	0.71	0.01	0.03	0.47	0.04	11.47	0.41	13.02	0.25	18.29	73.16	103.23	143.84	0.33
0.05	0.18	0.00	0.00	0.00	17.00	0.00	0.01	0.02	0.26	0.03	1.36	1.36	6.80	0.26	36.55	239.70	87.55	675.75	0.28
0.00	0.00	0.00	0.00	0.00	0.00	0.60	0.00	0.00	0.00	0.00	0.00	0.00	8.00	0.00	0.00	0.00	0.00	91.67	0.00
0.55	0.96	0.00	0.00	0.00	64.64	0.00	0.13	0.15	1.92	0.46	5.86	0.30	13.13	0.37	53.53	250.48	331.28	87.87	0.53
5.05	3.15	0.00	0.00	0.00	45.90	0.00	0.06	0.09	2.36	0.26	12.75	1.03	42.50	0.94	36.55	164.90	131.75	103.70	0.41
3.24	4.33	0.00	0.00	0.00	47.60	1.28	0.11	0.12	2.61	0.09	6.89	1.59	56.95	1.07	34.00	185.30	191.25	292.40	1.17
0.17	0.37	0.00	0.00	0.43	56.10	1.87	0.03	0.03	2.20	0.11	2.98	1.27	33.15	2.63	28.90	116.45	154.70	190.40	1.33
0.37	0.97	0.00	0.00	1.19	23.04	2.94	0.04	0.05	3.53	0.14	2.30	1.43	75.52	3.51	52.48	298.24	268.80	216.32	1.61
0.02	0.04	0.23	0.00	0.05	3.24	0.12	0.00	0.00	0.15	0.01	0.18	0.07	3.12	0.14	2.22	12.30	11.10	8.88	0.07
0.19	0.64	0.00	0.00	0.00	17.00	0.00	0.02	0.03	0.14	0.03	1.36	1.36	16.15	0.51	36.55	239.70	75.65	599.25	0.28
0.70	0.97	0.00	0.00	0.00	14.45	0.00	0.01	0.13	1.50	0.14	3.91	3.37	65.45	0.98	32.30	250.75	316.20	65.45	1.80
0.54	1.00	0.00	0.00	0.00	59.50	2.72	0.09	0.00	0.60	0.78	9.86	5.95	68.00	0.41	62.90	341.70	887.40	96.90	0.75
2.34	1.82	0.00	0.00	0.00	9.35	3.57	0.05	0.39	2.21	0.05	11.90	1.05	33.15	0.86	32.30	213.35	237.15	260.10	1.48
0.06	0.12	0.00	0.00	0.00	6.29	0.37	0.03	0.03	0.54	0.05	6.29	0.85	38.11	0.57	14.06	85.47	166.13	38.11	0.74
2.10	1.25	0.00	0.00	0.00	43.46	1.17	0.04	0.13	12.50	0.40	2.44	2.14	6.36	1.10	36.04	357.22	391.14	121.90	1.56
2.59	1.19	0.00	0.00	0.00	11.78	0.31	0.27	0.26	3.58	0.14	9.30	4.64	34.10	1.19	17.36	194.68	287.06	41.54	0.53
1.49	1.65	0.00	0.00	0.00	61.06	2.34	0.17	0.06	6.24	0.28	17.04	3.53	61.06	0.23	22.72	188.86	313.11	29.82	0.35
2.50	2.62	0.00	0.00	0.00	21.45	2.86	0.21	0.14	8.25	0.50	27.17	9.01	122.98	0.54	44.33	384.67	640.64	80.08	0.73
5.92	8.45	0.00	0.00	0.00	55.35	4.51	0.06	0.14	13.74	0.16	16.40	2.46	34.85	2.05	38.95	364.90	364.90	824.10	1.15
5.04	4.94	0.00	0.00	0.00	39.33	0.00	0.07	0.21	21.20	0.19	9.06	3.76	22.23	2.38	53.01	531.81	353.97	85.50	1.54

USDA ID Code	Food Name	Weight in Grams*	Quantity of Units	Unit of Measure	Protein (gm)	Fat (gm)	Carbohydrate (gm)	Kcalories	Caffeine (gm)	Fiber (gm)	Cholesterol (mg)	Saturated Fat (gm)
	Tuna, Light Meat, Cnd In Water	165.0000	1.000	Can	42.09	1.35	0.00	191.40	0.00	0.00	49.50	0.38
	Tuna, Light, Cnd In Water	154.0000	1.000	Cup	39.29	1.26	0.00	178.64	0.00	0.00	46.20	0.35
	Tuna, Skipjack, Ckd, Dry Heat	154.0000	3.000	Ounce	43.44	1.99	0.00	203.28	0.00	0.00	92.40	0.65
	Tuna, White Meat, Cnd In Oil	178.0000	1.000	Can	47.22	14.38	0.00	331.08	0.00	0.00	55.18	2.94
	Tuna, White Meat, Cnd In Water	172.0000	1.000	Can	40.63	5.11	0.00	220.16	0.00	0.00	72.24	1.36
	Tuna, Yellowfin, Ckd, Dry Heat	85.0000	3.000	Ounce	25.47	1.04	0.00	118.15	0.00	0.00	49.30	0.26
	Whitefish, Ckd, Dry Heat	154.0000	1.000	Each	37.68	11.57	0.00	264.88	0.00	0.00	118.58	1.79
	Whitefish, Smoked	136.0000	1.000	Cup	31.82	1.26	0.00	146.88	0.00	0.00	44.88	0.31
	Yellowtail, Ckd, Dry Heat	146.0000	3.000	Ounce	43.32	9.81	0.00	273.02	0.00	0.00	103.66	0.00
	Yellowtail, Fresh	187.0000	3.000	Ounce	43.27	9.80	0.00	273.02	0.00	0.00	102.85	2.39
	Brownies	28.3500	1.000	Ounce	1.36	4.62	18.12	114.82	0.57	0.60	4.82	1.20
	Candy Bar, Almond Joy	20.0000	1.000	Small Ba	0.84	5.36	11.66	93.40	0.00	0.96	0.80	3.46
	Candy Bar, Alpine White, w/ Almo	35.0000	1.000	Bar	3.50	12.92	17.64	197.40	0.00	1.89	4.20	6.67
	Candy Bar, Butterfinger Bar	174.0000	1.000	Cup	21.66	32.47	114.07	835.20	6.96	4.18	1.74	18.03
	Candy Bar, Chocolate Bar - Krack	41.0000	1.000	Each	2.71	11.77	25.26	217.71	7.38	0.90	7.79	7.42
	Candy Bar, Chocolate, Milk - Sym	42.0000	1.000	Each	3.02	13.78	24.33	232.26	0.00	0.80	9.24	0.00
	Candy Bar, Chocolate, Special Da	41.0000	1.000	Each	2.01	13.28	24.85	226.32	29.93	2.05	0.41	8.32
	Candy Bar, Chocolate-Mr. Goodbar	49.0000	1.000	Each	5.24	17.10	25.33	267.05	9.80	1.72	3.92	7.30
	Candy Bar, Chunky Bar	35.0000	1.000	Each	3.15	10.22	19.99	173.25	10.15	1.68	3.85	8.13
	Candy Bar, Fifth Avenue Bar	57.0000	1.000	Each	5.13	12.14	37.68	280.44	3.99	1.25	3.42	4.50
	Candy Bar, Milky Way	23.0000	1.000	Each	1.04	3.70	16.49	97.29	1.84	0.39	3.22	1.79
	Candy Bar, Mounds	53.0000	1.000	Each	2.01	13.30	31.22	252.81	9.01	3.13	1.06	10.76
	Candy Bar, Nestle Crunch	40.0000	1.000	Each	2.40	10.52	26.08	208.80	9.60	1.04	5.20	6.08
	Candy Bar, Peanut Bar	28.3500	1.000	Ounce	4.39	9.55	13.44	147.99	0.00	1.62	0.00	1.33
	Candy Bar, Peanut Butter Cups -	7.0000	1.000	Miniatur	0.72	2.19	3.82	37.87	0.70	0.22	0.35	0.78
	Candy Bar, Snickers	57.0000	1.000	Each	4.56	14.01	33.75	273.03	3.99	1.43	7.41	5.12
	Candy Bar, Three Musketeers	23.0000	1.000	Each	0.74	2.97	17.66	95.68	2.53	0.37	2.53	1.50
	Candy Bar, Twix	57.0000	1.000	Each	2.62	13.90	37.38	284.43	1.71	0.63	2.85	5.07
	Candy Bar, Wafer Bar - Kit Kat	42.0000	1.000	Each	2.98	10.71	26.88	215.88	5.04	0.80	2.52	6.85
	Candy, Butterscotch	28.3500	1.000	Ounce	0.03	0.99	27.02	111.98	0.00	0.00	2.55	0.31
	Candy, Caramels	71.0000	1.000	Package	3.27	5.75	54.67	271.22	0.00	0.85	4.97	4.67
	Candy, Goobers	39.0000	1.000	Package	5.34	13.07	18.99	200.07	8.58	2.38	3.51	4.76
	Candy, Gumdrops	182.0000	1.000	Cup	0.00	0.00	180.00	702.52	0.00	0.00	0.00	0.00
	Candy, Jellybeans	11.0000	10.000	Each	0.00	0.06	10.24	40.37	0.00	0.00	0.00	0.02
	Candy, Lollipop	28.3500	1.000	Ounce	0.00	0.06	27.78	111.70	0.00	0.00	0.00	0.00
	Candy, M&M's Almond	42.0000	1.000	Pkg	4.00	13.00	25.00	230.00	0.00	2.00	5.00	4.00
	Candy, M&M's Peanut	170.0000	1.000	Cup	16.10	44.61	102.78	877.20	18.70	5.78	15.30	17.56
	Candy, M&M's Plain	208.0000	1.000	Cup	9.01	43.95	148.12	1023.36	37.44	5.20	29.12	27.21
	Candy, Peanut Brittle	28.3500	1.000	Ounce	2.13	5.41	19.65	128.43	0.00	0.57	3.69	1.42
	Candy, Praline	39.0000	1.000	Piece	1.09	9.48	24.18	177.06	0.00	0.00	0.00	0.73
	Candy, Raisinets	45.0000	1.000	Package	2.12	7.16	32.04	185.40	11.25	2.30	1.80	3.30
	Candy, Reese's Pieces	47.0000	0.250	Cup	6.49	9.92	28.86	230.77	0.00	1.36	0.94	8.51
	Candy, Skittles Bite Size	205.0000	1.000	Cup	0.39	8.96	185.81	830.25	0.00	0.00	0.00	1.78
	Candy, Taffy	15.0000	1.000	Piece	0.02	0.50	13.71	56.40	0.00	0.00	1.35	0.31
	Candy, Toffee	12.0000	1.000	Piece	0.13	3.94	7.72	65.04	0.00	0.00	12.60	2.45
	Candy, Truffles	12.0000	1.000	Piece	0.68	4.12	5.40	58.56	0.00	0.00	6.24	2.58
	Candy, Twizzlers Strawberry	71.0000	1.000	Package	2.41	1.14	54.95	237.14	0.00	0.99	0.00	0.28
	Candy, York Peppermint Pattie (l	42.0000	1.000	Lg Patty	0.92	2.98	33.64	165.06	0.00	0.84	0.42	1.81
	Candy, York Peppermint Pattie (s	14.0000	1.000	Sm Patty	0.31	0.99	11.21	55.02	0.00	0.28	0.14	0.60
	Chips, Bagel	28.3500	1.000	Ounce	4.00	6.00	20.00	150.00	0.00	1.00	0.00	1.00
	Chips, Banana	28.3500	1.000	Ounce	0.65	9.53	16.56	147.14	0.00	2.18	0.00	8.21
	Chips, Corn	2.2310	1.000	Each	0.15	0.85	1.15	12.31	0.00	0.08	0.00	0.12
	Chips, Doritos - Cheese, Nacho	28.0000	1.000	Ounce	2.00	7.00	17.00	140.00	0.00	0.00	0.00	1.00
	Chips, Doritos - Ranch, Cool	28.0000	1.000	Ounce	2.00	7.00	18.00	140.00	0.00	0.00	0.00	1.00
	Chips, Fritos	28.0000	1.000	Ounce	2.00	10.00	15.00	160.00	0.00	0.00	0.00	1.50

Monounsaturated Fat (gm)	Polyunsaturated Fat (gm)	Vitamin D (mg)	Vitamin K (mg)	Vitamin E (mg)	Vitamin A (re)	Vitamin C (mg)	Thiamin (mg)	Riboflavin (mg)	Niacin (mg)	Vitamin B_6 (mg)	Folate (mg)	Vitamin B_{12} (mcg)	Calcium (mg)	Iron (mg)	Magnesium (mg)	Phosphorus (mg)	Potassium (mg)	Sodium (mg)	Zinc (mg)
0.26	0.56	0.00	0.00	0.87	28.05	0.00	0.05	0.12	21.91	0.58	6.60	4.93	18.15	2.52	44.55	268.95	391.05	82.50	1.27
0.25	0.52	0.00	0.00	0.82	26.18	0.00	0.05	0.11	20.45	0.54	6.16	4.60	16.94	2.36	41.58	251.02	364.98	520.52	1.19
0.37	0.62	0.00	0.00	0.00	27.72	1.54	0.06	0.18	28.89	1.51	15.40	3.37	56.98	2.46	67.76	438.90	803.88	72.38	1.62
4.41	6.02	0.00	0.00	0.00	42.72	0.00	0.04	0.14	20.83	0.77	8.19	3.92	7.12	1.16	60.52	475.26	592.74	89.00	0.84
1.34	1.91	0.00	0.00	2.73	10.32	0.00	0.02	0.07	9.98	0.38	3.44	2.01	24.08	1.67	56.76	373.24	407.64	86.00	0.83
0.17	0.31	0.00	0.00	0.00	17.00	0.85	0.43	0.05	10.15	0.88	1.70	0.51	17.85	0.80	54.40	208.25	483.65	39.95	0.57
3.94	4.25	0.00	0.00	0.00	60.06	0.00	0.26	0.23	5.93	0.54	26.18	1.48	50.82	0.72	64.68	532.84	625.24	100.10	1.96
0.38	0.39	0.00	0.00	0.27	77.52	0.00	0.04	0.14	3.26	0.53	9.93	4.43	24.48	0.68	31.28	179.52	575.28	1385.84	0.67
0.00	0.00	0.00	0.00	0.00	45.26	4.23	0.26	0.07	12.73	0.28	5.84	1.83	42.34	0.92	55.48	293.46	785.48	73.00	0.98
3.72	2.66	0.00	0.00	0.00	54.23	5.24	0.26	0.07	12.72	0.30	6.92	2.43	43.01	0.92	56.10	293.59	785.40	72.93	0.97
2.54	0.64	0.00	0.00	0.59	1.70	0.00	0.07	0.06	0.49	0.01	5.95	0.02	8.22	0.64	8.79	28.63	42.24	88.45	0.20
1.32	0.30	0.00	0.00	0.00	0.80	0.04	0.01	0.03	0.09	0.01	1.60	0.02	12.20	0.28	13.20	28.00	49.20	29.20	0.16
4.81	0.88	0.00	0.00	0.00	8.75	0.14	0.03	0.15	0.03	0.03	4.55	0.30	80.85	0.20	13.30	81.55	146.30	25.55	0.40
9.67	4.87	0.00	0.00	2.82	0.00	0.00	0.16	0.12	4.35	0.12	46.98	0.02	46.98	1.29	137.46	227.94	662.94	344.52	2.04
3.94	0.37	0.00	0.00	0.00	4.92	0.16	0.02	0.12	0.18	0.01	3.28	0.24	71.75	0.37	22.55	90.61	140.22	56.58	0.50
0.00	0.00	0.00	0.00	0.00	5.46	0.17	0.04	0.16	0.14	0.02	2.94	0.16	90.30	0.50	23.10	105.00	161.70	38.64	0.47
4.59	0.41	0.00	0.00	0.18	1.64	0.00	0.01	0.03	0.16	0.01	0.82	0.00	11.07	0.98	45.51	61.50	122.59	2.87	0.59
5.73	2.35	0.00	0.00	1.34	18.13	0.15	0.08	0.13	1.62	0.04	19.11	0.15	52.92	0.64	42.14	121.52	219.03	73.01	0.89
0.11	1.54	0.00	0.00	0.00	3.85	0.11	0.03	0.14	0.67	0.04	7.70	0.13	50.05	0.44	25.55	72.80	186.90	18.55	0.64
5.70	1.94	0.00	0.00	1.32	8.55	0.11	0.08	0.07	1.97	0.05	21.66	0.07	42.18	0.74	36.48	87.78	169.29	94.05	0.70
1.38	0.14	0.00	0.00	0.15	7.36	0.23	0.01	0.05	0.08	0.01	2.30	0.07	29.90	0.17	7.82	33.12	55.43	55.20	0.16
2.28	0.27	0.00	0.00	0.36	0.53	0.21	0.02	0.03	0.15	0.05	1.59	0.00	7.95	1.11	29.68	48.23	130.91	78.97	0.52
3.44	0.35	0.00	0.00	0.44	8.00	0.12	0.14	0.22	1.58	0.16	31.60	0.15	67.60	0.20	23.20	80.80	137.60	53.20	0.57
4.74	3.02	0.00	0.00	1.30	0.00	0.00	0.03	0.04	2.25	0.05	22.11	0.00	22.11	0.27	32.60	91.29	115.38	44.23	1.17
0.92	0.39	0.00	0.00	0.28	1.33	0.01	0.02	0.01	0.32	0.01	3.85	0.01	5.46	0.08	6.23	14.21	24.64	22.19	0.13
5.96	2.80	0.00	0.00	0.87	22.23	0.34	0.06	0.09	2.39	0.05	22.80	0.09	53.58	0.43	41.04	126.54	184.68	151.62	1.34
0.99	0.10	0.00	0.00	0.15	5.52	0.09	0.01	0.03	0.05	0.00	0.00	0.04	19.32	0.17	6.67	20.93	30.59	44.62	0.13
7.64	0.48	0.00	0.00	0.70	14.25	0.23	0.09	0.13	0.68	0.02	13.68	0.10	51.30	0.46	18.24	68.40	115.14	110.01	0.44
3.11	0.34	0.00	0.00	0.34	20.16	0.29	0.08	0.23	1.07	0.05	59.64	0.07	69.30	0.38	16.38	99.96	122.22	31.50	0.52
0.14	0.02	0.00	0.00	0.02	9.64	0.00	0.00	0.01	0.00	0.00	0.00	0.00	0.85	0.02	0.28	0.85	1.13	104.04	0.01
0.60	0.13	0.00	0.00	0.33	5.68	0.36	0.01	0.13	0.18	0.03	3.55	0.00	97.98	0.10	12.07	80.94	151.94	173.95	0.31
5.75	1.99	0.00	0.00	0.00	0.00	0.00	0.05	0.08	2.03	0.08	3.12	0.11	49.53	0.52	46.41	115.44	195.78	15.99	0.85
0.00	0.00	0.00	0.00	0.00	0.00	0.00	0.00	0.00	0.00	0.00	0.00	0.00	5.46	0.73	1.82	1.82	9.10	80.08	0.00
0.02	0.01	0.00	0.00	0.00	0.00	0.00	0.00	0.00	0.00	0.00	0.00	0.00	0.33	0.12	0.22	0.44	4.07	2.75	0.01
0.00	0.00	0.00	0.00	0.00	0.00	0.00	0.00	0.00	0.00	0.00	0.00	0.00	0.85	0.09	0.85	0.85	1.42	10.77	0.00
0.00	0.00	0.00	0.00	0.00	0.00	0.00	0.00	0.00	0.00	0.00	0.00	0.00	72.00	0.40	0.00	0.00	0.00	20.00	0.00
18.70	7.14	0.00	0.00	4.13	40.80	0.85	0.17	0.29	6.38	0.14	59.50	0.31	171.70	1.96	125.80	387.60	588.20	81.60	3.91
14.31	1.31	0.00	0.00	1.79	110.24	1.04	0.12	0.44	0.46	0.06	12.48	0.56	218.40	2.31	85.28	312.00	553.28	126.88	2.00
2.40	1.33	0.00	0.00	0.46	13.32	0.00	0.05	0.01	0.99	0.03	19.85	0.00	8.51	0.39	14.18	31.47	58.97	128.14	0.27
5.92	2.35	0.00	0.00	0.00	1.95	0.27	0.12	0.02	0.13	0.03	5.46	0.00	12.09	0.46	20.28	42.51	82.29	24.18	0.79
2.67	0.86	0.00	0.00	0.00	4.05	0.09	0.04	0.10	0.18	0.05	2.25	0.09	48.60	0.54	20.25	64.80	231.30	16.20	0.36
0.99	0.47	0.00	0.00	0.98	0.00	0.19	0.05	0.07	1.34	0.03	13.16	0.10	38.54	0.38	20.68	62.04	108.10	69.09	0.36
6.07	0.25	0.00	0.00	0.57	0.00	137.15	0.00	0.04	0.04	0.02	0.00	0.00	0.00	0.02	2.05	4.10	10.25	32.80	0.06
0.14	0.02	0.00	0.00	0.00	4.95	0.00	0.00	0.00	0.00	0.00	0.00	0.00	0.45	0.01	0.15	0.45	0.60	13.35	0.00
1.14	0.15	0.00	0.00	0.00	38.16	0.02	0.00	0.01	0.00	0.00	0.24	0.01	4.08	0.01	0.48	3.96	6.00	22.44	0.02
1.22	0.13	0.00	0.00	0.00	17.16	0.05	0.01	0.03	0.03	0.00	0.12	0.04	18.60	0.12	5.64	21.24	36.60	8.52	0.13
0.00	0.00	0.00	0.00	0.00	0.00	0.00	0.01	0.03	0.07	0.01	0.00	0.00	4.97	0.21	4.26	220.10	45.44	175.37	0.11
1.05	0.08	0.00	0.00	0.00	0.00	0.00	0.00	0.00	0.00	0.00	0.00	0.00	6.30	0.42	0.00	0.00	54.18	10.08	0.00
0.35	0.03	0.00	0.00	0.00	0.14	0.00	0.00	0.01	0.12	0.00	0.56	0.00	2.10	0.14	8.82	13.30	18.06	3.36	0.11
3.00	2.00	0.00	0.00	0.00	0.00	0.00	0.00	0.00	0.00	0.00	0.00	0.00	0.00	0.40	0.00	0.00	0.00	190.00	0.00
0.55	0.18	0.00	0.00	1.53	2.27	1.79	0.03	0.01	0.20	0.07	3.97	0.00	5.10	0.35	21.55	15.88	151.96	1.70	0.21
0.00	0.00	0.00	0.00	0.00	0.00	0.00	0.00	0.00	0.00	0.00	0.00	0.00	5.54	0.02	0.00	0.00	0.00	15.38	0.00
0.00	0.00	0.00	0.00	0.00	0.00	0.00	0.00	0.00	0.00	0.00	0.00	0.00	32.00	0.20	0.00	0.00	0.00	200.00	0.00
0.00	0.00	0.00	0.00	0.00	0.00	0.00	0.00	0.00	0.00	0.00	0.00	0.00	32.00	0.20	0.00	0.00	0.00	170.00	0.00
0.00	0.00	0.00	0.00	0.00	0.00	0.00	0.00	0.00	0.00	0.00	0.00	0.00	0.00	0.00	0.00	0.00	0.00	160.00	0.00

USDA ID Code	Food Name	Weight in Grams*	Quantity of Units	Unit of Measure	Protein (gm)	Fat (gm)	Carbohydrate (gm)	Kcalories	Caffeine (gm)	Fiber (gm)	Cholesterol (mg)	Saturated Fat (gm)
	Chips, Fritos-Barbecue	28.0000	1.000	Ounce	2.00	9.00	16.00	160.00	0.00	0.00	0.00	1.50
	Chips, Pork Skins, Barbecue-flav	28.3500	1.000	Ounce	16.41	9.02	0.45	152.52	0.00	0.00	32.60	3.28
	Chips, Pork Skins, Plain	28.3500	1.000	Ounce	17.38	8.87	0.00	154.51	0.00	0.00	26.93	3.22
	Chips, Potato - Baked Lays	28.0000	1.000	Ounce	2.00	1.50	23.00	110.00	0.00	0.00	0.00	0.00
	Chips, Potato - Barbeque	28.0000	1.000	Ounce	2.00	10.00	15.00	160.00	0.00	0.00	0.00	1.50
	Chips, Potato Sticks	28.3500	1.000	Ounce	1.90	9.75	15.11	147.99	0.00	0.96	0.00	2.52
	Chips, Potato, Barbecue-flavor	28.3500	1.000	Ounce	2.18	9.19	14.97	139.20	0.00	1.25	0.00	2.28
	Chips, Potato, Cheese-flavor	28.3500	1.000	Ounce	2.41	7.71	16.36	140.62	0.00	1.47	1.13	2.44
	Chips, Potato, Cheese-flavor - P	28.3500	1.000	Ounce	1.98	10.49	14.35	156.21	0.00	0.95	1.13	2.71
	Chips, Potato, Light	28.3500	1.000	Ounce	2.01	5.90	18.97	133.53	0.00	1.66	0.00	1.18
	Chips, Potato, Light - Pringles	28.3500	1.000	Ounce	1.59	7.29	18.40	142.03	0.00	1.02	0.00	1.45
	Chips, Potato, Plain - Pringles	28.3500	1.000	Ounce	1.67	10.89	14.46	158.19	0.00	1.02	0.00	2.68
	Chips, Potato, Plain, Salted	28.3500	1.000	Ounce	1.98	9.81	15.00	151.96	0.00	1.28	0.00	3.11
	Chips, Potato, Plain, Unsalted	28.3500	1.000	Ounce	1.98	9.81	15.00	151.96	0.00	1.36	0.00	3.11
	Chips, Potato, Reduced Fat - Ruf	28.0000	1.000	Ounce	2.00	6.70	18.00	140.00	0.00	0.00	0.00	1.00
	Chips, Potato, Sour Cream & Onio	28.3500	1.000	Ounce	1.87	10.49	14.54	155.07	0.00	0.34	0.85	2.68
	Chips, Potato, Sour Cream and On	28.3500	1.000	Ounce	2.30	9.61	14.60	150.54	0.00	1.47	1.98	2.52
	Chips, Potato, w/o Salt Added	28.3500	1.000	Ounce	1.82	10.03	14.70	148.27	0.00	1.36	0.00	2.57
	Chips, Sun, original	28.0000	1.000	Ounce	1.00	6.00	20.00	140.00	0.00	0.00	0.00	1.00
	Chips, Taro	28.3500	1.000	Ounce	0.65	7.06	19.31	141.18	0.00	2.04	0.00	1.82
	Chips, Tortilla, Low-Fat, Baked	2.1810	13.000	Chips	0.23	0.08	1.85	8.46	0.00	0.15	0.00	0.00
	Chips, Tortilla, Nacho Flavor	28.3500	1.000	Ounce	2.21	7.26	17.69	141.18	0.00	1.50	0.85	1.39
	Chips, Tortilla, Nacho-flavor, L	28.3500	1.000	Ounce	2.47	4.31	20.30	126.16	0.00	1.36	0.85	0.82
	Chips, Tortilla, Plain	28.3500	1.000	Ounce	1.98	7.43	17.83	142.03	0.00	1.84	0.00	1.42
	Chips, Tortilla, Ranch Flavor	28.3500	1.000	Ounce	2.15	6.75	18.31	138.92	0.00	1.10	0.28	1.29
	Chips, Tortilla, Taco-flavor	28.3500	1.000	Ounce	2.24	6.86	17.89	136.08	0.00	1.50	1.42	1.32
	Chips, Tostitos, Baked	28.0000	1.000	Ounce	2.00	1.00	24.00	110.00	0.00	0.00	0.00	0.00
	Chips, Tostitos, Baked, Salsa &	28.0000	1.000	Ounce	2.00	3.00	21.00	120.00	0.00	0.00	0.00	0.50
	Chocolate, Milk	168.0000	1.000	Cup	11.59	51.58	99.46	861.84	43.68	5.71	36.96	31.05
	Chocolate, Milk, w/ Almonds	41.0000	1.000	Each	3.69	14.10	21.81	215.66	9.02	2.54	7.79	6.96
191	Cliff Bar, Apple Cherry	68.0000	1.000	Each	4.00	2.00	52.00	250.00	0.00	2.00	0.00	0.50
192	Cliff Bar, Apricot	68.0000	1.000	Each	6.00	0.00	55.00	250.00	0.00	2.00	0.00	0.00
193	Cliff Bar, Berry, Real	68.0000	1.000	Each	4.00	2.00	52.00	250.00	0.00	2.00	0.00	0.50
194	Cliff Bar, Chocolate Chip	68.0000	1.000	Each	4.00	3.00	51.00	250.00	0.00	3.00	0.00	0.50
195	Cliff Bar, Chocolate Chip Peanut	68.0000	1.000	Each	12.00	6.00	40.00	250.00	0.00	5.00	0.00	1.00
196	Cliff Bar, Chocolate Espresso	68.0000	1.000	Each	4.00	2.00	52.00	250.00	0.00	2.00	0.00	0.50
197	Cliff Bar, Peanut Butter, Crunch	68.0000	1.000	Each	10.00	4.00	45.00	250.00	0.00	8.00	0.00	1.00
	Cookie Cakes, Devils Food, Fat F	16.0000	1.000	Each	1.00	0.00	13.00	50.00	0.00	0.50	0.00	0.00
	Cookie Cakes, Double Fudge, Fat	16.0000	1.000	Each	1.00	0.00	12.00	50.00	0.00	0.50	0.00	0.00
	Cookies, Butter	28.3500	1.000	Ounce	1.73	5.33	19.53	132.39	0.00	0.21	33.17	3.13
	Cookies, Chocolate Chip, Reduce	0.4480	2.000	Each	1.00	1.25	10.50	50.00	0.00	0.02	0.00	0.02
	Cookies, Chocolate Chip, Dietary	28.3500	1.000	Ounce	1.11	4.76	20.81	127.58	2.27	0.45	0.00	1.19
	Cookies, Chocolate Chip, Lower F	28.3500	1.000	Ounce	1.64	4.37	20.78	128.43	1.98	1.02	0.00	1.08
	Cookies, Chocolate Chip, Soft-ty	28.3500	1.000	Ounce	0.99	6.89	16.75	129.84	1.98	0.91	0.00	2.10
	Cookies, Chocolate Sandwich, Red	12.5000	2.000	Each	0.50	1.25	10.50	50.00	0.00	0.50	0.00	0.25
	Cookies, Creme Sandwich, Reduced	13.0000	2.000	Each	0.50	1.25	10.50	55.00	0.00	0.50	0.00	0.25
	Cookies, Fig Bars	28.3500	1.000	Ounce	1.05	2.07	20.10	98.66	0.00	1.30	0.00	0.32
	Cookies, Fig Newton, Fat Free	29.0000	2.000	Each	1.00	0.00	22.00	100.00	0.00	0.00	0.00	0.00
	Cookies, Gingersnaps	28.3500	1.000	Ounce	1.59	2.78	21.80	117.94	0.00	0.62	0.00	0.69
	Cookies, Molasses	28.3500	1.000	Ounce	1.59	3.63	20.92	121.91	0.00	0.27	0.00	0.91
	Cookies, Oatmeal Raisin, Reduced	13.5000	2.000	Each	1.00	1.25	10.00	55.00	0.00	0.50	0.00	0.00
	Cookies, Oatmeal, Dietary	28.3500	1.000	Ounce	1.36	5.10	19.82	127.29	0.00	0.81	0.00	0.76
	Cookies, Oatmeal, Regular	28.3500	1.000	Ounce	1.76	5.13	19.48	127.58	0.00	0.79	0.00	1.28
	Cookies, Oatmeal, Soft-type	28.3500	1.000	Ounce	1.73	4.17	18.63	115.95	0.00	0.77	1.42	1.03
	Cookies, Oreos, Dietary	28.3500	1.000	Ounce	1.28	6.27	19.19	130.69	0.85	1.17	0.00	1.09

Monounsaturated Fat (gm)	Polyunsaturated Fat (gm)	Vitamin D (mg)	Vitamin K (mg)	Vitamin E (mg)	Vitamin A (re)	Vitamin C (mg)	Thiamin (mg)	Riboflavin (mg)	Niacin (mg)	Vitamin B_6 (mg)	Folate (mg)	Vitamin B_{12} (mcg)	Calcium (mg)	Iron (mg)	Magnesium (mg)	Phosphorus (mg)	Potassium (mg)	Sodium (mg)	Zinc (mg)
0.00	0.00	0.00	0.00	0.00	0.00	0.00	0.00	0.00	0.00	0.00	0.00	0.00	0.00	0.00	0.00	0.00	0.00	310.00	0.00
4.26	0.98	0.00	0.00	0.00	51.60	0.43	0.02	0.12	0.95	0.05	8.79	0.04	12.19	0.29	0.00	62.37	51.03	756.09	0.20
4.19	1.03	0.00	0.00	0.17	11.06	0.14	0.03	0.08	0.44	0.01	0.00	0.18	8.51	0.25	3.12	24.10	36.00	521.07	0.16
0.00	0.00	0.00	0.00	0.00	0.00	0.00	0.00	0.00	0.00	0.00	0.00	0.00	48.00	0.40	0.00	0.00	0.00	150.00	0.00
0.00	0.00	0.00	0.00	0.00	0.00	6.40	0.00	0.00	0.00	0.00	0.00	0.00	0.00	0.20	0.00	0.00	0.00	300.00	0.00
1.75	5.07	0.00	0.00	1.38	0.00	13.41	0.03	0.03	1.36	0.09	11.34	0.00	5.10	0.64	18.14	48.76	350.69	70.88	0.28
1.85	4.64	0.00	0.00	1.42	6.24	9.61	0.06	0.06	1.33	0.18	23.53	0.00	14.18	0.55	21.26	52.73	357.49	212.63	0.27
2.19	2.71	0.00	0.00	0.00	2.27	15.34	0.05	0.05	1.42	0.10	0.00	0.00	20.41	0.52	21.26	84.77	433.19	224.82	0.26
2.02	5.29	0.00	0.00	0.00	0.00	2.41	0.05	0.03	0.74	0.15	5.10	0.00	31.19	0.45	15.03	46.21	108.01	214.04	0.18
1.36	3.10	0.00	0.00	0.82	0.00	7.29	0.06	0.08	1.98	0.19	7.65	0.00	5.95	0.38	25.23	54.72	494.42	139.48	0.02
1.68	3.82	0.00	0.00	1.42	0.00	3.40	0.05	0.02	1.19	0.22	6.52	0.00	9.64	0.43	17.86	43.66	284.92	121.34	0.17
2.06	5.66	0.00	0.00	1.38	0.00	2.32	0.06	0.03	0.89	0.04	1.98	0.00	6.80	0.43	16.44	44.51	285.77	185.98	0.17
2.79	3.45	0.00	0.00	1.38	0.00	8.82	0.05	0.06	1.09	0.19	12.76	0.00	6.80	0.46	18.99	46.78	361.46	168.40	0.31
2.79	3.45	0.00	0.00	1.38	0.00	8.82	0.05	0.06	1.09	0.19	12.76	0.00	6.80	0.46	18.99	46.78	361.46	2.27	0.31
0.00	0.00	0.00	0.00	0.00	0.00	0.00	0.00	0.00	0.00	0.00	0.00	0.00	0.00	0.20	0.00	0.00	0.00	130.00	0.00
2.02	5.32	0.00	0.00	0.00	27.78	2.69	0.05	0.03	0.71	0.14	6.52	0.00	18.14	0.40	15.59	47.91	140.62	204.12	0.20
1.74	4.94	0.00	0.00	0.00	5.95	10.57	0.05	0.06	1.14	0.19	17.58	0.28	20.41	0.45	20.98	49.90	377.34	177.19	0.28
1.77	5.15	0.00	0.00	2.23	0.00	11.79	0.04	0.01	1.19	0.14	12.81	0.00	6.80	0.34	16.73	43.38	367.98	2.27	0.30
0.00	0.00	0.00	0.00	0.00	0.00	1.20	0.00	0.00	0.00	0.00	0.00	0.00	0.00	0.00	0.00	0.00	0.00	115.00	0.00
1.26	3.65	0.00	0.00	1.39	0.00	1.42	0.05	0.01	0.15	0.12	5.67	0.00	17.01	0.34	23.81	37.14	214.04	96.96	0.11
0.00	0.00	0.00	0.00	0.00	0.00	0.00	0.00	0.00	0.00	0.00	0.00	0.00	3.69	0.00	0.00	0.00	0.00	10.77	0.00
4.28	1.00	0.00	0.00	0.00	11.62	0.51	0.04	0.05	0.41	0.08	3.97	0.01	41.67	0.41	23.25	69.17	61.24	200.72	0.34
2.54	0.60	0.00	0.00	0.00	11.91	0.06	0.06	0.08	0.12	0.07	7.37	0.00	45.08	0.46	27.50	90.15	77.11	284.35	0.00
4.38	1.03	0.00	0.00	0.39	5.67	0.00	0.02	0.05	0.36	0.08	2.84	0.00	43.66	0.43	24.95	58.12	55.85	149.69	0.43
3.98	0.94	0.00	0.00	0.00	7.65	0.26	0.03	0.07	0.41	0.06	4.82	0.00	39.97	0.41	25.23	67.76	69.17	173.50	0.35
4.05	0.95	0.00	0.00	0.00	25.80	0.26	0.07	0.06	0.57	0.09	5.95	0.00	43.94	0.57	24.95	67.76	61.52	223.11	0.36
0.00	0.00	0.00	0.00	0.00	0.00	0.00	0.00	0.00	0.00	0.00	0.00	0.00	32.00	0.20	0.00	0.00	0.00	200.00	0.00
0.00	0.00	0.00	0.00	0.00	0.00	0.00	0.00	0.00	0.00	0.00	0.00	0.00	32.00	0.20	0.00	0.00	0.00	190.00	0.00
16.75	1.78	0.00	0.00	2.08	92.40	0.67	0.13	0.50	0.54	0.07	13.44	0.66	320.88	2.34	100.80	362.88	646.80	137.76	2.32
5.53	0.93	0.00	0.00	0.77	5.74	0.08	0.02	0.18	0.30	0.02	4.92	0.14	91.84	0.67	36.90	108.24	182.04	30.34	0.55
0.00	0.00	0.00	0.00	0.00	0.00	0.00	0.00	0.00	0.00	0.00	0.00	0.00	0.00	0.00	0.00	0.00	270.00	100.00	0.00
0.00	0.00	0.00	0.00	0.00	0.00	0.00	0.00	0.00	0.00	0.00	0.00	0.00	0.00	0.00	0.00	0.00	250.00	55.00	0.00
0.00	0.00	0.00	0.00	0.00	0.00	0.00	0.00	0.00	0.00	0.00	0.00	0.00	0.00	0.00	0.00	0.00	270.00	100.00	0.00
0.00	0.00	0.00	0.00	0.00	0.00	0.00	0.00	0.00	0.00	0.00	0.00	0.00	0.00	0.00	0.00	0.00	330.00	45.00	0.00
0.00	0.00	0.00	0.00	0.00	0.00	0.00	0.00	0.00	0.00	0.00	0.00	0.00	0.00	0.00	0.00	0.00	220.00	110.00	0.00
0.00	0.00	0.00	0.00	0.00	0.00	0.00	0.00	0.00	0.00	0.00	0.00	0.00	0.00	0.00	0.00	0.00	270.00	100.00	0.00
0.00	0.00	0.00	0.00	0.00	0.00	0.00	0.00	0.00	0.00	0.00	0.00	0.00	0.00	0.00	0.00	0.00	330.00	150.00	0.00
0.00	0.00	0.00	0.00	0.00	0.00	0.00	0.00	0.00	0.00	0.00	0.00	0.00	0.00	0.00	0.00	0.00	0.00	25.00	0.00
0.00	0.00	0.00	0.00	0.00	0.00	0.00	0.00	0.00	0.00	0.00	0.00	0.00	0.00	0.20	0.00	0.00	0.00	70.00	0.00
1.56	0.28	0.00	0.00	0.15	47.63	0.00	0.10	0.10	0.90	0.01	11.06	0.10	8.22	0.63	3.40	28.92	31.47	99.51	0.11
0.02	0.00	0.00	0.00	0.00	0.00	0.00	0.00	0.00	0.00	0.00	0.00	0.00	0.00	0.01	0.00	0.00	0.00	2.63	0.00
1.91	1.43	0.00	0.00	0.70	0.00	0.00	0.10	0.05	0.81	0.01	12.76	0.00	13.04	0.99	5.95	30.90	56.42	3.12	0.13
1.73	1.32	0.00	0.00	0.00	0.00	0.00	0.08	0.08	0.79	0.07	19.85	0.00	5.39	0.87	7.94	23.81	34.87	106.88	0.20
3.69	0.99	0.00	0.00	0.00	0.00	0.00	0.03	0.06	0.46	0.05	11.06	0.00	4.25	0.68	9.92	14.18	26.37	92.42	0.13
0.25	0.00	0.00	0.00	0.00	0.00	0.00	0.00	0.00	0.00	0.00	0.00	0.00	0.00	0.20	0.00	0.00	0.00	95.00	0.00
0.50	0.00	0.00	0.00	0.00	0.00	0.00	0.00	0.00	0.00	0.00	0.00	0.00	12.00	0.10	0.00	0.00	0.00	47.50	0.00
0.85	0.79	0.00	0.00	0.35	1.13	0.09	0.05	0.06	0.53	0.02	7.65	0.03	18.14	0.82	7.65	17.58	58.68	99.22	0.11
0.00	0.00	0.00	0.00	0.00	0.00	0.00	0.00	0.00	0.00	0.00	0.00	0.00	0.00	0.00	0.00	0.00	0.00	115.00	0.00
1.52	0.39	0.00	0.00	0.37	0.00	0.00	0.06	0.08	0.92	0.03	20.41	0.00	21.83	1.81	13.89	23.53	98.09	185.41	0.16
2.02	0.49	0.00	0.00	0.48	0.00	0.00	0.10	0.07	0.86	0.03	20.98	0.00	20.98	1.82	14.74	26.93	98.09	130.13	0.13
0.25	0.25	0.00	0.00	0.00	0.00	0.00	0.00	0.00	0.00	0.00	0.00	0.00	12.00	0.20	0.00	0.00	0.00	67.50	0.00
2.14	1.92	0.00	0.00	0.91	0.28	0.09	0.13	0.06	0.92	0.01	14.74	0.00	15.31	1.15	4.82	34.59	49.61	2.55	0.14
2.84	0.72	0.00	0.00	0.71	0.57	0.14	0.08	0.07	0.63	0.02	12.76	0.00	10.49	0.73	9.36	39.12	40.26	108.58	0.22
2.27	0.62	0.00	0.00	0.00	1.42	0.06	0.05	0.07	0.52	0.03	9.64	0.00	25.52	0.79	8.51	59.25	38.27	98.94	0.12
2.62	2.25	0.00	0.00	1.07	0.00	0.00	0.15	0.08	1.13	0.01	17.58	0.01	27.78	1.34	7.37	56.70	83.63	68.89	0.16

USDA ID Code	Food Name	Weight in Grams*	Quantity of Units	Unit of Measure	Protein (gm)	Fat (gm)	Carbohydrate (gm)	Kcalories	Caffeine (gm)	Fiber (gm)	Cholesterol (mg)	Saturated Fat (gm)
	Cookies, Oreos, Regular	28.3500	1.000	Ounce	1.33	5.84	19.93	133.81	3.69	0.91	0.00	1.04
	Cookies, Oreos, w/ Extra Creme F	28.3500	1.000	Ounce	1.02	7.14	19.31	141.75	1.42	0.57	0.00	1.10
	Cookies, Peanut Butter Sandwich,	28.3500	1.000	Ounce	2.84	9.64	14.40	151.67	0.00	0.00	0.00	1.40
	Cookies, Peanut Butter Sandwich,	28.3500	1.000	Ounce	2.49	5.98	18.60	135.51	0.00	0.54	0.00	1.42
	Cookies, Peanut Butter, Regular	28.3500	1.000	Ounce	2.72	6.69	16.70	135.23	0.00	0.51	0.28	1.27
	Cookies, Peanut Butter, Soft-typ	28.3500	1.000	Ounce	1.50	6.92	16.36	129.56	0.00	0.48	0.00	1.74
	Cookies, Raisin, Soft-type	28.3500	1.000	Ounce	1.16	3.86	19.28	113.68	0.00	0.34	0.57	0.98
	Cookies, Shortbread, Pecan	28.3500	1.000	Ounce	1.39	9.21	16.53	153.66	0.00	0.51	9.36	2.32
	Cookies, Shortbread, Plain	28.3500	1.000	Ounce	1.73	6.83	18.29	142.32	0.00	0.51	5.67	1.73
	Cookies, Sugar, Dietary	28.3500	1.000	Ounce	1.16	3.69	21.77	122.19	0.00	0.25	0.00	0.53
	Cookies, Sugar, Regular (include	28.3500	1.000	Ounce	1.45	5.98	19.25	135.51	0.00	0.22	14.46	1.54
	Cookies, Vanilla Sandwich, w/ Cr	28.3500	1.000	Ounce	1.28	5.67	20.44	136.93	0.00	0.43	0.00	0.84
204	Cookies, Wafers, Chocolate	6.0000	1.000	Each	0.40	0.85	4.34	25.98	0.00	0.00	0.12	0.22
	Cookies, Wafers, Vanilla, Higher	28.3500	1.000	Ounce	1.22	5.50	20.16	134.10	0.00	0.57	0.00	1.40
205	Cookies, Wafers, Vanilla, Lower	4.0000	1.000	Each	0.20	0.61	2.94	17.64	0.00	0.00	2.32	0.14
	Cookies,Chocolate Chip, Higher F	28.3500	1.000	Ounce	1.53	6.41	18.94	136.36	3.12	0.71	0.00	2.12
	Cornnuts, Barbecue-flavor	28.3500	1.000	Ounce	2.55	4.05	20.33	123.61	0.00	2.38	0.00	0.73
	Cornnuts, Nacho-flavor	28.3500	1.000	Ounce	2.66	4.03	20.30	124.17	0.00	2.27	0.57	0.73
	Cornnuts, Plain	28.3500	1.000	Ounce	2.41	4.00	20.78	124.46	0.00	1.96	0.00	0.72
	Crackers, Animal	28.3500	1.000	Ounce	1.96	3.91	21.01	126.44	0.00	0.31	0.00	0.98
	Crackers, Classic Golden, Reduce	2.3300	6.000	Each	0.17	0.17	1.83	9.99	0.00	0.00	0.00	0.00
	Crackers, Snack, Cheese, Zesty,	0.9380	32.000	Each	0.09	0.06	0.72	3.75	0.00	0.03	0.16	0.02
	Crackers, Snack, French Onion ,	0.9380	32.000	Each	0.06	0.06	0.72	3.75	0.00	0.03	0.72	0.00
	Crackers, Triscuits	4.4290	7.000	Each	0.43	0.71	3.00	20.00	0.00	0.57	0.00	0.14
	Crackers, Triscuits, Low-Fat	4.0000	8.000	Each	0.38	0.38	3.00	16.25	0.00	0.50	0.00	0.06
	Crackers, Wheat Thins	1.8130	16.000	Each	0.13	0.38	1.19	8.75	0.00	0.13	0.00	0.06
	Crackers, Wheat Thins, Low-Fat	1.6110	18.000	Each	0.11	0.22	1.17	6.67	0.00	0.11	0.00	0.03
	Dip, Bean	15.0000	2.000	Tbsp	0.50	0.00	2.00	10.00	0.00	0.50	0.00	0.00
	Dip, Cheese, Nacho	16.5000	2.000	Tbsp	0.00	1.25	2.00	20.00	0.00	0.00	0.00	0.25
	Dip, French Onion	15.0000	2.000	Tbsp	0.50	2.50	1.00	30.00	0.00	0.00	7.50	1.50
259	Doritos, Corn, Toasted	28.0000	1.000	Ounce	2.00	7.00	18.00	140.00	0.00	1.00	0.00	1.50
260	Doritos, Flamin' Hot	28.0000	1.000	Ounce	2.00	7.00	17.00	140.00	0.00	1.00	0.00	1.50
261	Doritos, Nacho, Spicy	28.0000	1.000	Ounce	2.00	4.00	18.00	140.00	0.00	1.00	0.00	1.50
262	Doritos, Pizza Cravers	28.0000	1.000	Ounce	2.00	6.00	18.00	140.00	0.00	1.00	0.00	1.50
263	Doritos, Taco Bell Taco Supreme	28.0000	1.000	Ounce	2.00	7.00	21.00	150.00	0.00	1.00	0.00	1.50
	Doughnut Holes	15.0000	1.000	Each	0.78	3.44	7.62	63.90	0.00	0.00	4.80	0.80
	Egg Custards	282.0000	1.000	Cup	14.38	13.25	30.17	296.10	0.00	0.00	245.34	6.63
	Frostings, Chocolate, Creamy	462.0000	16.000	Ounce	5.08	81.31	291.98	1834.14	9.24	2.77	0.00	25.55
	Frostings, Cream Cheese-flavor	462.0000	16.000	Ounce	0.46	79.93	308.15	1908.06	0.00	0.00	0.00	23.28
	Frostings, Sour Cream-flavor	462.0000	16.000	Ounce	0.46	79.46	312.31	1903.44	0.00	0.46	0.00	23.15
	Frostings, Vanilla, Creamy	462.0000	16.000	Ounce	0.46	77.62	320.63	1935.78	0.00	0.46	0.00	22.59
	Frozen Bar, Fruit and Juice	77.0000	1.000	Each	0.92	0.08	15.55	63.14	0.00	0.00	0.00	0.00
	Frozen Bar, Pops, Ice	52.0000	1.000	Each	0.00	0.00	9.83	37.44	0.00	0.00	0.00	0.00
	Frozen Bar, Popsicles	56.0000	1.000	Each	0.00	0.00	11.00	40.00	0.00	0.00	0.00	0.00
	Frozen Bar, Pudding Pops, Chocol	47.0000	1.000	Each	1.88	2.21	11.94	71.91	0.00	0.19	0.94	0.00
	Frozen Bar, Pudding Pops, Vanill	47.0000	1.000	Each	1.88	2.07	12.60	74.73	0.00	0.00	0.94	0.00
	Frozen Bars, Pops, Gelatin	44.0000	1.000	Each	0.53	0.04	7.35	30.80	0.00	0.00	0.00	0.00
	Frozen Dessert, Brownie, Fudge-H	132.9690	1.000	Cup	6.00	4.00	54.00	280.00	0.00	0.00	10.00	0.00
	Frozen Dessert, Cherry, Bordeaux	132.9690	1.000	Cup	6.00	4.00	46.00	240.00	0.00	0.00	10.00	0.00
	Frozen Dessert, Chocolate Chip-H	132.9690	1.000	Cup	6.00	4.00	48.00	260.00	0.00	0.00	10.00	0.00
	Frozen Dessert, Coffee Toffee-He	132.9690	1.000	Cup	6.00	4.00	50.00	260.00	0.00	0.00	10.00	0.00
	Frozen Dessert, Cookies 'n Cream	132.9690	1.000	Cup	8.00	4.00	48.00	260.00	0.00	0.00	10.00	0.00
	Frozen Dessert, Fudge Swirl, Dou	132.9690	1.000	Cup	6.00	4.00	48.00	260.00	0.00	0.00	10.00	0.00
	Frozen Dessert, Ice Milk, Vanill	65.0000	3.500	Fl Oz	2.47	2.80	14.76	90.35	0.00	0.00	9.10	1.71
	Frozen Dessert, Ice Milk, Vanill	88.0000	0.500	Cup	4.31	2.29	19.18	110.88	0.00	0.00	10.56	1.43

Monounsaturated Fat (gm)	Polyunsaturated Fat (gm)	Vitamin D (mg)	Vitamin K (mg)	Vitamin E (mg)	Vitamin A (re)	Vitamin C (mg)	Thiamin (mg)	Riboflavin (mg)	Niacin (mg)	Vitamin B_6 (mg)	Folate (mg)	Vitamin B_{12} (mcg)	Calcium (mg)	Iron (mg)	Magnesium (mg)	Phosphorus (mg)	Potassium (mg)	Sodium (mg)	Zinc (mg)
2.43	2.06	0.00	0.00	0.98	0.00	0.00	0.02	0.05	0.59	0.01	12.19	0.01	7.37	1.10	12.76	27.78	49.61	171.23	0.23
3.03	2.66	0.00	0.00	1.27	0.00	0.00	0.02	0.04	0.45	0.01	12.19	0.01	6.80	0.81	9.64	25.80	34.59	139.77	0.18
4.36	3.41	0.00	0.00	1.63	0.00	0.00	0.10	0.04	1.49	0.02	15.31	0.00	12.19	0.72	14.46	43.66	83.35	116.80	0.29
3.17	1.08	0.00	0.00	0.92	0.28	0.03	0.09	0.07	1.06	0.04	12.47	0.07	15.03	0.74	13.89	53.30	54.43	104.33	0.30
3.51	1.56	0.00	0.00	0.96	0.85	0.00	0.05	0.05	1.21	0.03	17.58	0.01	9.92	0.71	12.76	24.38	47.34	117.65	0.15
3.92	0.90	0.00	0.00	0.00	0.00	0.00	0.07	0.05	0.61	0.01	18.99	0.00	3.40	0.25	9.07	24.66	30.33	95.26	0.16
2.17	0.50	0.00	0.00	0.54	0.28	0.11	0.06	0.06	0.56	0.01	12.47	0.01	13.04	0.65	5.95	23.53	39.69	95.82	0.09
5.28	1.17	0.00	0.00	0.00	0.28	0.00	0.08	0.06	0.70	0.01	17.86	0.00	8.51	0.69	5.10	24.10	20.70	79.66	0.16
3.80	0.92	0.00	0.00	0.91	3.40	0.00	0.09	0.09	0.95	0.02	16.73	0.03	9.92	0.78	4.82	30.62	28.35	128.99	0.15
1.49	1.35	0.00	0.00	0.63	0.00	0.00	0.14	0.07	1.04	0.01	16.44	0.00	7.09	1.14	2.55	20.70	29.48	0.85	0.10
3.36	0.75	0.00	0.00	0.80	7.65	0.03	0.07	0.06	0.76	0.02	12.76	0.05	5.95	0.61	3.40	22.68	17.86	101.21	0.12
2.39	2.14	0.00	0.00	1.02	0.00	0.00	0.07	0.07	0.76	0.01	16.73	0.00	7.65	0.63	3.97	21.26	25.80	98.94	0.11
0.45	0.10	0.00	0.00	0.00	0.12	0.00	0.01	0.02	0.17	0.00	0.66	0.00	1.86	0.24	3.18	7.92	12.60	34.80	0.07
3.14	0.69	0.00	0.00	0.00	0.00	0.00	0.10	0.06	0.84	0.01	12.19	0.01	7.09	0.63	3.40	18.14	30.33	86.75	0.09
0.24	0.15	0.00	0.00	0.00	0.72	0.00	0.01	0.01	0.12	0.00	0.36	0.00	1.92	0.10	0.56	4.16	3.88	12.48	0.01
3.31	0.67	0.00	0.00	0.73	0.00	0.00	0.06	0.08	0.77	0.02	11.91	0.00	7.09	0.80	8.79	30.62	38.27	89.30	0.18
2.09	0.91	0.00	0.00	0.00	9.64	0.11	0.10	0.04	0.43	0.05	0.00	0.00	4.82	0.48	30.90	80.23	81.08	276.70	0.53
2.07	0.91	0.00	0.00	0.00	1.13	4.39	0.10	0.02	0.34	0.06	4.25	0.00	9.92	0.48	30.90	87.60	88.17	179.74	0.51
2.06	0.90	0.00	0.00	0.29	0.00	0.00	0.01	0.04	0.48	0.07	0.00	0.00	2.55	0.47	32.04	77.96	78.81	155.64	0.50
2.17	0.53	0.00	0.00	0.52	0.00	0.00	0.10	0.09	0.98	0.01	24.10	0.01	12.19	0.78	5.10	32.32	28.35	111.42	0.18
0.00	0.00	0.00	0.00	0.00	0.00	0.00	0.00	0.00	0.00	0.00	0.00	0.00	3.99	0.07	0.00	0.00	0.00	23.30	0.00
0.02	0.00	0.00	0.00	0.00	0.00	0.00	0.00	0.00	0.00	0.00	0.00	0.00	1.50	0.02	0.00	0.00	0.00	10.94	0.00
0.02	0.00	0.00	0.00	0.00	0.00	0.00	0.00	0.00	0.00	0.00	0.00	0.00	1.50	0.02	0.00	0.00	0.00	9.06	0.00
0.07	0.21	0.00	0.00	0.00	0.00	0.00	0.00	0.00	0.00	0.00	0.00	0.00	0.00	0.11	0.00	11.43	0.00	24.29	0.00
0.00	0.13	0.00	0.00	0.00	0.00	0.00	0.00	0.00	0.00	0.00	0.00	0.00	0.00	0.13	0.00	15.00	0.00	22.50	0.00
0.03	0.16	0.00	0.00	0.00	0.00	0.00	0.00	0.00	0.00	0.00	0.00	0.00	1.50	0.03	0.00	0.00	0.00	10.63	0.00
0.00	0.08	0.00	0.00	0.00	0.00	0.00	0.00	0.00	0.00	0.00	0.00	0.00	1.33	0.02	0.00	4.44	0.00	12.22	0.00
0.00	0.00	0.00	0.00	0.00	0.00	0.00	0.00	0.00	0.00	0.00	0.00	0.00	0.00	0.10	0.00	0.00	0.00	75.00	0.00
0.00	0.00	0.00	0.00	0.00	0.00	0.00	0.00	0.00	0.00	0.00	0.00	0.00	12.00	0.00	0.00	0.00	0.00	100.00	0.00
0.00	0.00	0.00	0.00	0.00	20.00	0.60	0.00	0.00	0.00	0.00	0.00	0.00	12.00	0.00	0.00	0.00	0.00	52.50	0.00
0.00	5.50	0.00	0.00	0.00	0.00	0.00	0.00	0.00	0.00	0.00	0.00	0.00	0.00	0.00	0.00	0.00	0.00	120.00	0.00
0.00	5.50	0.00	0.00	0.00	0.00	0.00	0.00	0.00	0.00	0.00	0.00	0.00	0.00	0.00	0.00	0.00	0.00	210.00	0.00
0.00	4.50	0.00	0.00	0.00	0.00	0.00	0.00	0.00	0.00	0.00	0.00	0.00	0.00	0.00	0.00	0.00	0.00	210.00	0.00
0.00	5.50	0.00	0.00	0.00	0.00	0.00	0.00	0.00	0.00	0.00	0.00	0.00	0.00	0.00	0.00	0.00	0.00	170.00	0.00
0.00	5.50	0.00	0.00	0.00	0.00	0.00	0.00	0.00	0.00	0.00	0.00	0.00	0.00	0.00	0.00	0.00	0.00	170.00	0.00
1.79	0.39	0.00	0.00	0.00	0.45	0.02	0.03	0.03	0.23	0.00	1.80	0.03	9.00	0.16	2.55	17.55	15.30	60.30	0.07
4.26	0.99	0.00	0.00	0.00	169.20	1.41	0.09	0.64	0.24	0.14	28.20	0.87	315.84	0.85	39.48	318.66	431.46	217.14	1.49
41.67	9.84	0.00	0.00	10.95	914.76	0.00	0.05	0.09	0.55	0.05	0.00	0.00	36.96	6.56	97.02	364.98	905.52	845.46	1.34
41.72	10.86	0.00	0.00	0.00	0.00	0.00	0.00	0.05	0.05	0.00	0.00	0.00	13.86	0.74	9.24	13.86	161.70	180.18	0.00
41.53	10.81	0.00	0.00	0.00	563.64	0.00	0.05	0.09	3.10	0.00	4.62	0.05	9.24	0.32	9.24	18.48	896.28	942.48	0.05
40.52	10.53	0.00	0.00	21.81	1044.12	0.00	0.00	0.05	0.05	0.00	0.00	0.00	13.86	0.51	4.62	180.18	170.94	415.80	0.00
0.00	0.02	0.00	0.00	0.00	2.31	7.32	0.01	0.02	0.12	0.02	4.62	0.00	3.85	0.15	3.08	4.62	40.81	3.08	0.04
0.00	0.00	0.00	0.00	0.00	0.00	0.00	0.00	0.00	0.00	0.00	0.00	0.00	0.00	0.00	0.52	0.00	2.08	6.24	0.01
0.00	0.00	0.00	0.00	0.00	0.00	1.20	0.00	0.00	0.00	0.00	0.00	0.00	0.00	0.00	0.00	0.00	0.00	10.00	0.00
0.00	0.00	0.00	0.00	0.01	15.51	0.19	0.02	0.08	0.06	0.01	1.41	0.25	66.27	0.22	9.87	52.64	105.28	77.55	0.17
0.00	0.00	0.00	0.00	0.01	24.44	0.14	0.02	0.09	0.02	0.02	2.35	0.17	60.63	0.03	5.17	47.47	64.86	49.82	0.16
0.00	0.00	0.00	0.00	0.00	0.00	0.00	0.00	0.00	0.00	0.00	0.00	0.00	0.88	0.01	0.44	0.00	0.88	20.24	0.01
0.00	2.00	0.00	0.00	0.00	0.00	0.00	0.06	0.27	0.00	0.00	0.00	0.00	160.00	0.40	0.00	160.00	380.00	140.00	0.00
0.00	2.00	0.00	0.00	0.00	0.00	0.00	0.06	0.34	0.00	0.00	0.00	0.00	160.00	0.00	0.00	200.00	300.00	100.00	0.00
0.00	2.00	0.00	0.00	0.00	0.00	2.40	0.12	0.27	0.00	0.00	0.00	0.00	160.00	0.40	0.00	160.00	320.00	140.00	0.00
0.00	2.00	0.00	0.00	0.00	0.00	2.40	0.12	0.34	0.00	0.00	0.00	0.00	160.00	0.00	0.00	160.00	320.00	160.00	0.00
0.00	2.00	0.00	0.00	0.00	0.00	0.00	0.06	0.34	0.00	0.00	0.00	0.00	240.00	0.00	0.00	200.00	360.00	160.00	0.00
0.00	2.00	0.00	0.00	0.00	0.00	0.00	0.12	0.27	0.00	0.00	0.00	0.00	160.00	0.80	0.00	200.00	420.00	140.00	0.00
0.80	0.10	0.00	0.00	0.00	30.55	0.52	0.04	0.18	0.06	0.05	3.90	0.44	90.35	0.07	9.75	70.85	137.15	55.25	0.29
0.67	0.09	0.00	0.00	0.00	25.52	0.79	0.04	0.18	0.11	0.04	5.28	0.44	138.16	0.05	12.32	106.48	194.48	61.60	0.47

USDA ID Code	Food Name	Weight in Grams*	Quantity of Units	Unit of Measure	Protein (gm)	Fat (gm)	Carbohydrate (gm)	Kcalories	Caffeine (gm)	Fiber (gm)	Cholesterol (mg)	Saturated Fat (gm)
	Frozen Dessert, Mint Chocolate C	132.9690	1.000	Cup	6.00	4.00	50.00	280.00	0.00	0.00	10.00	0.00
	Frozen Dessert, Neapolitan-Healt	132.9690	1.000	Cup	6.00	4.00	44.00	240.00	0.00	0.00	10.00	0.00
	Frozen Dessert, Pecan, Butter, C	132.9690	1.000	Cup	6.00	4.00	52.00	280.00	0.00	0.00	10.00	0.00
	Frozen Dessert, Praline and Cara	132.9690	1.000	Cup	6.00	4.00	52.00	260.00	0.00	0.00	10.00	0.00
	Frozen Dessert, Rocky Road-Healt	132.9690	1.000	Cup	6.00	4.00	64.00	320.00	0.00	0.00	10.00	0.00
	Frozen Dessert, Sherbet, All Fla	74.0000	0.500	Cup	0.81	1.48	22.50	102.12	0.00	0.00	4.44	0.86
	Frozen Dessert, Sorbet, All Flav	180.0530	0.500	Cup	0.00	0.00	50.01	200.06	0.00	2.00	0.00	0.00
	Frozen Dessert, Sorbet-Ben & Jer	110.0000	0.500	Cup	0.00	0.00	32.00	130.00	0.00	0.00	0.00	0.00
	Frozen Dessert, Vanilla-Healthy	132.9690	1.000	Cup	8.00	4.00	42.00	240.00	0.00	0.00	10.00	0.00
	Frozen Desserts, Pops, Ice, w/ A	52.0000	1.000	Each	0.00	0.00	9.83	37.44	0.00	0.00	0.00	0.00
	Fudge, Brown Sugar w/ Nuts	14.0000	1.000	Piece	0.41	1.41	10.86	55.44	0.00	0.00	0.84	0.25
	Fudge, Chocolate	17.0000	1.000	Piece	0.29	1.45	13.52	64.77	2.38	0.14	2.38	0.88
	Fudge, Chocolate w/ Nuts	19.0000	1.000	Piece	0.65	3.06	13.83	80.94	2.66	0.25	2.66	1.07
	Fudge, Peanut Butter	16.0000	1.000	Piece	0.59	1.04	12.53	59.36	0.00	0.00	0.64	0.24
	Fudge, Vanilla	16.0000	1.000	Piece	0.18	0.86	13.17	59.04	0.00	0.00	2.56	0.54
	Fudge, Vanilla w/ Nuts	15.0000	1.000	Piece	0.44	2.00	11.28	62.25	0.00	0.09	2.10	0.56
	Granola Bars, Hard, Almond	28.3500	1.000	Ounce	2.18	7.23	17.58	140.33	0.00	1.36	0.00	3.55
	Granola Bars, Hard, Chocolate Ch	28.3500	1.000	Each	2.07	4.62	20.44	124.17	0.00	1.25	0.00	3.23
	Granola Bars, Hard, Peanut	28.3500	1.000	Ounce	3.12	6.07	18.06	135.80	0.00	1.22	0.00	0.71
	Granola Bars, Hard, Peanut Butte	28.3500	1.000	Ounce	2.78	6.75	17.66	136.93	0.00	0.82	0.00	0.91
	Granola Bars, Hard, Plain	24.5000	1.000	Each	2.47	4.85	15.78	115.40	0.00	1.30	0.00	0.58
	Granola Bars, Low-Fat	28.0000	1.000	Each	2.00	2.00	21.00	110.00	0.00	1.00	0.00	0.00
	Granola Bars, Soft, Chocolate Ch	42.5000	1.000	Each	3.10	7.06	29.37	178.50	0.00	2.04	0.43	4.33
	Granola Bars, Soft, Nut and Rais	28.3500	1.000	Each	2.27	5.78	18.03	128.71	0.00	1.59	0.28	2.70
	Granola Bars, Soft, Peanut Butte	28.3500	1.000	Each	2.98	4.48	18.26	120.77	0.00	1.22	0.28	1.03
	Granola Bars, Soft, Peanut Butte	28.3500	1.000	Each	2.78	5.67	17.63	122.47	0.00	1.19	0.28	1.58
	Granola Bars, Soft, Plain	28.3500	1.000	Each	2.10	4.88	19.08	125.59	0.00	1.30	0.28	2.05
	Granola Bars, Soft, Raisin	42.5000	1.000	Each	3.23	7.57	28.22	190.40	0.00	1.79	0.43	4.07
	Gum, Bubble-Carefree	3.0000	1.000	Each	0.00	0.00	2.00	10.00	0.00	0.00	0.00	0.00
	Gum, Chewing	3.0000	1.000	Stick	0.00	0.01	2.90	10.23	0.00	0.00	0.00	0.00
	Gum, Chewing, Cinnamon	3.0000	1.000	Each	0.00	0.00	2.00	10.00	0.00	0.00	0.00	0.00
	Gum, Chewing, Mint Flavors	3.0000	1.000	Each	0.00	0.00	2.00	10.00	0.00	0.00	0.00	0.00
	Gum,Chewing, Sugar-Free	1.7000	1.000	Stick	0.00	0.00	1.00	5.00	0.00	0.00	0.00	0.00
	Gum-Carefree	3.0000	1.000	Each	0.00	0.00	2.00	8.00	0.00	0.00	0.00	0.00
	Jello, Gelatin	540.0000	3.000	Ounce	6.48	0.00	75.60	318.60	0.00	0.00	0.00	0.00
	Jerky, Beef, Chopped and Formed	28.3500	1.000	Ounce	9.41	7.26	3.12	116.24	0.00	0.51	13.61	3.08
	Jerky, Slim Jims, Smoked	28.3500	1.000	Ounce	6.10	14.06	1.53	155.93	0.00	0.00	37.71	5.90
	Marshmallows	50.0000	1.000	Cup	0.90	0.10	40.65	159.00	0.00	0.05	0.00	0.03
617	Nutri-Grain Bar, Apple Cinnamon-	37.0000	1.000	Each	2.00	2.80	27.00	136.00	0.00	1.00	0.00	0.60
618	Nutri-Grain Bar, Berry, Mixed-Ke	37.0000	1.000	Each	2.00	3.00	27.00	140.00	0.00	1.00	0.00	0.50
619	Nutri-Grain Bar, Blueberry-Kello	37.0000	1.000	Each	2.00	2.80	27.00	136.00	0.00	1.00	0.00	0.60
620	Nutri-Grain Bar, Cherry-Kellogg'	37.0000	1.000	Each	2.00	2.80	27.00	136.00	0.00	1.00	0.00	6.00
621	Nutri-Grain Bar, Peach-Kellogg's	37.0000	1.000	Each	2.00	2.80	27.00	136.00	0.00	1.00	0.00	0.60
622	Nutri-Grain Bar, Raspberry-Kello	37.0000	1.000	Each	2.00	2.80	27.00	136.00	0.00	1.00	0.00	6.00
623	Nutri-Grain Bar, Strawberry-Kell	37.0000	1.000	Each	2.00	2.80	26.00	140.00	0.00	1.00	0.00	0.60
	Pastries, Toaster, Brown-sugar-c	28.3500	1.000	Ounce	1.45	4.03	19.31	116.80	0.00	0.28	0.00	1.03
	Pastries, Toaster, Fruit	28.3500	1.000	Ounce	1.33	2.89	20.16	111.42	0.00	0.59	0.00	0.43
	Peanuts, Chocolate, Milk, Coated	149.0000	1.000	Cup	19.52	49.92	73.61	773.31	32.78	7.00	13.41	21.75
	Pop Tart, Fruit, Frosted	52.0000	1.000	Each	2.00	5.00	38.00	200.00	0.00	1.00	0.00	1.50
	Popcorn, Air-popped	8.0000	1.000	Cup	0.96	0.34	6.23	30.56	0.00	1.21	0.00	0.05
	Popcorn, Air-popped, White Popco	8.0000	1.000	Cup	0.96	0.34	6.23	30.56	0.00	1.21	0.00	0.05
656	Popcorn, Butter, Golden, Fat, Re	14.0000	3.330	Cup	3.00	4.00	21.00	130.00	0.00	4.00	0.00	0.50
660	Popcorn, Butter-Smartfood	14.0000	3.000	Cup	2.00	9.00	15.00	150.00	0.00	1.00	5.00	2.00
	Popcorn, Cakes	10.0000	1.000	Cake	0.97	0.31	8.01	38.40	0.00	0.29	0.00	0.05
	Popcorn, Caramel-coated, w/ Pean	28.3500	0.660	Cup	1.81	2.21	22.88	113.40	0.00	1.08	0.00	0.29

Monounsaturated Fat (gm)	Polyunsaturated Fat (gm)	Vitamin D (mg)	Vitamin K (mg)	Vitamin E (mg)	Vitamin A (re)	Vitamin C (mg)	Thiamin (mg)	Riboflavin (mg)	Niacin (mg)	Vitamin B_6 (mg)	Folate (mg)	Vitamin B_{12} (mcg)	Calcium (mg)	Iron (mg)	Magnesium (mg)	Phosphorus (mg)	Potassium (mg)	Sodium (mg)	Zinc (mg)
0.00	4.00	0.00	0.00	0.00	0.00	0.00	0.12	0.27	0.00	0.00	0.00	0.00	160.00	0.40	0.00	0.00	340.00	160.00	0.00
0.00	2.00	0.00	0.00	0.00	0.00	0.00	0.06	0.34	0.00	0.00	0.00	0.00	160.00	0.00	0.00	200.00	320.00	120.00	0.00
0.00	2.00	0.00	0.00	0.00	0.00	2.40	0.12	0.34	0.00	0.00	0.00	0.00	160.00	0.00	0.00	160.00	300.00	160.00	0.00
0.00	2.00	0.00	0.00	0.00	0.00	0.00	0.06	0.34	0.00	0.00	0.00	0.00	160.00	0.00	0.00	200.00	320.00	140.00	0.00
0.00	2.00	0.00	0.00	0.00	0.00	0.00	0.06	0.34	0.00	0.00	0.00	0.00	160.00	0.00	0.00	200.00	380.00	140.00	0.00
0.39	0.06	0.00	0.00	0.06	10.36	2.29	0.02	0.06	0.04	0.01	3.70	0.14	39.96	0.10	5.92	29.60	71.04	34.04	0.36
0.00	0.00	0.00	0.00	0.00	0.00	24.01	0.00	0.00	0.00	0.00	0.00	0.00	0.00	0.00	0.00	0.00	0.00	20.01	0.00
0.00	0.00	0.00	0.00	0.00	0.00	0.00	0.00	0.00	0.00	0.00	0.00	0.00	80.00	0.00	0.00	0.00	0.00	10.00	0.00
0.00	2.00	0.00	0.00	0.00	0.00	0.00	0.12	0.51	0.00	0.00	0.00	0.00	240.00	0.00	0.00	200.00	360.00	120.00	0.00
0.00	0.00	0.00	0.00	0.00	0.00	5.56	0.00	0.00	0.00	0.00	0.00	0.00	0.00	0.00	0.52	0.00	2.08	6.24	0.01
0.34	0.76	0.00	0.00	0.00	2.38	0.08	0.01	0.01	0.03	0.01	1.54	0.00	15.54	0.25	6.86	12.04	52.36	13.72	0.09
0.44	0.05	0.00	0.00	0.02	7.82	0.03	0.00	0.01	0.02	0.00	0.34	0.01	7.14	0.08	4.25	9.86	17.51	10.54	0.07
0.82	1.03	0.00	0.00	0.08	8.93	0.11	0.01	0.02	0.04	0.02	1.90	0.01	9.50	0.14	8.55	17.67	30.02	11.40	0.14
0.48	0.27	0.00	0.00	0.00	1.60	0.03	0.00	0.01	0.24	0.01	1.76	0.01	6.72	0.04	3.52	10.40	20.96	11.68	0.07
0.25	0.03	0.00	0.00	0.03	8.00	0.03	0.00	0.01	0.00	0.00	0.16	0.01	6.24	0.01	0.80	5.12	8.00	10.72	0.02
0.50	0.83	0.00	0.00	0.07	6.90	0.09	0.01	0.01	0.03	0.01	1.50	0.01	7.05	0.06	4.05	10.65	16.95	9.15	0.08
2.19	1.07	0.00	0.00	0.00	1.13	0.00	0.08	0.02	0.17	0.01	3.40	0.00	9.07	0.71	22.96	64.64	77.40	72.58	0.45
0.75	0.36	0.00	0.00	0.00	1.13	0.03	0.05	0.03	0.16	0.02	3.69	0.00	21.83	0.86	20.41	57.83	71.16	97.52	0.55
1.63	3.37	0.00	0.00	0.32	0.85	0.00	0.05	0.02	0.41	0.02	6.52	0.00	11.06	0.71	31.19	85.05	86.47	78.81	0.59
1.98	3.42	0.00	0.00	0.00	0.57	0.06	0.06	0.03	0.56	0.03	5.10	0.00	11.62	0.68	15.59	39.41	82.50	80.23	0.35
1.07	2.95	0.00	0.00	0.00	3.68	0.22	0.06	0.03	0.39	0.02	5.64	0.00	14.95	0.72	23.77	67.86	82.32	72.03	0.50
0.00	0.00	0.00	0.00	0.00	0.00	0.00	0.00	0.00	0.00	0.00	0.00	0.00	0.00	0.20	0.00	0.00	0.00	70.00	0.00
1.50	0.84	0.00	0.00	0.00	2.13	0.00	0.10	0.06	0.41	0.04	9.35	0.07	39.53	1.08	33.15	97.75	144.50	115.60	0.64
1.20	1.56	0.00	0.00	0.00	1.13	0.00	0.05	0.05	0.74	0.03	8.51	0.07	23.81	0.62	25.80	68.32	111.13	72.01	0.45
1.87	1.21	0.00	0.00	0.00	0.57	0.00	0.07	0.04	0.89	0.03	9.07	0.06	25.80	0.60	24.38	70.88	82.50	115.95	0.53
2.37	1.31	0.00	0.00	0.00	0.57	0.00	0.03	0.03	0.89	0.03	9.36	0.13	22.68	0.55	24.95	74.28	106.88	92.99	0.48
1.08	1.51	0.00	0.00	0.00	0.00	0.00	0.09	0.05	0.15	0.03	6.80	0.11	29.77	0.73	20.98	65.21	92.14	78.81	0.43
1.21	1.36	0.00	0.00	0.00	0.00	0.00	0.10	0.07	0.47	0.04	8.93	0.08	42.93	1.04	30.60	93.50	153.85	119.85	0.55
0.00	0.00	0.00	0.00	0.00	0.00	0.00	0.00	0.00	0.00	0.00	0.00	0.00	0.00	0.00	0.00	0.00	0.00	0.00	0.00
0.00	0.00	0.00	0.00	0.00	0.00	0.00	0.00	0.00	0.00	0.00	0.00	0.00	0.00	0.00	0.00	0.00	0.12	0.18	0.00
0.00	0.00	0.00	0.00	0.00	0.00	0.00	0.00	0.00	0.00	0.00	0.00	0.00	0.00	0.00	0.00	0.00	0.00	0.00	0.00
0.00	0.00	0.00	0.00	0.00	0.00	0.00	0.00	0.00	0.00	0.00	0.00	0.00	0.00	0.00	0.00	0.00	0.00	0.00	0.00
0.00	0.00	0.00	0.00	0.00	0.00	0.00	0.00	0.00	0.00	0.00	0.00	0.00	0.00	0.00	0.00	0.00	0.00	0.00	0.00
0.00	0.00	0.00	0.00	0.00	0.00	0.00	0.00	0.00	0.00	0.00	0.00	0.00	0.00	0.00	0.00	0.00	0.00	0.00	0.00
0.00	0.00	0.00	0.00	0.00	0.00	0.00	0.00	0.00	0.00	0.00	0.00	0.00	10.80	0.16	5.40	118.80	5.40	226.80	0.16
3.21	0.29	0.00	0.00	0.14	0.00	0.00	0.04	0.04	0.49	0.05	37.99	0.28	5.67	1.54	14.46	115.38	169.25	627.39	2.30
5.80	1.25	0.00	0.00	0.00	47.91	1.93	0.04	0.12	1.29	0.06	0.00	0.28	19.28	0.96	5.95	51.03	72.86	419.58	0.69
0.04	0.03	0.00	0.00	0.00	0.00	0.00	0.00	0.00	0.04	0.00	0.50	0.00	1.50	0.12	1.00	4.00	2.50	23.50	0.02
1.90	0.30	0.00	0.00	0.00	750.00	0.00	0.38	0.43	5.00	0.50	40.00	0.00	14.00	1.80	8.00	40.00	73.00	110.00	1.50
0.00	0.00	0.00	0.00	0.00	750.00	0.00	0.38	0.43	5.00	0.50	40.00	0.00	0.00	1.80	8.00	40.00	0.00	110.00	1.50
1.90	0.30	0.00	0.00	0.00	750.00	0.00	0.38	0.43	5.00	0.00	40.00	0.00	18.00	1.80	8.00	40.00	73.00	110.00	1.50
1.90	0.30	0.00	0.00	0.00	750.00	0.00	0.38	0.43	5.00	0.00	40.00	0.00	18.00	1.80	8.00	40.00	73.00	110.00	1.50
1.90	0.30	0.00	0.00	0.00	750.00	0.00	0.38	0.43	5.00	0.50	40.00	0.00	18.00	1.80	8.00	40.00	73.00	110.00	1.50
1.90	0.30	0.00	0.00	0.00	750.00	0.00	0.38	0.43	5.00	0.00	4.00	0.00	18.00	1.80	8.00	4.00	73.00	110.00	1.50
1.90	0.30	0.00	0.00	0.00	750.00	0.00	0.38	0.43	5.00	0.50	40.00	0.00	17.00	1.80	0.00	40.00	56.00	110.00	1.50
2.28	0.51	0.00	0.00	0.00	63.50	0.03	0.10	0.16	1.30	0.12	8.22	0.06	9.64	1.14	6.80	37.71	32.32	120.20	0.18
1.17	1.10	0.00	0.00	0.65	0.85	0.17	0.08	0.10	1.12	0.11	18.43	0.00	7.37	0.99	5.10	31.47	31.75	118.79	0.19
19.25	6.45	0.00	0.00	3.80	0.00	0.00	0.18	0.25	6.33	0.31	11.92	0.40	154.96	1.95	140.06	315.88	747.98	61.09	2.89
0.00	0.00	0.00	0.00	0.00	100.00	0.00	0.15	0.17	1.90	0.20	20.00	0.00	0.00	1.00	0.00	16.00	0.00	170.00	0.00
0.09	0.15	0.00	0.00	0.01	1.60	0.00	0.02	0.02	0.16	0.02	1.84	0.00	0.80	0.21	10.48	24.00	24.08	0.32	0.28
0.09	0.15	0.00	0.00	0.00	0.24	0.00	0.02	0.02	0.16	0.02	1.84	0.00	0.80	0.21	10.48	24.00	24.08	0.32	0.28
0.00	0.00	0.00	0.00	0.00	0.00	0.00	0.00	0.00	0.00	0.00	0.00	0.00	0.00	0.00	0.00	0.00	0.00	410.00	0.00
0.00	0.00	0.00	0.00	0.00	0.00	0.00	0.00	0.00	0.00	0.00	0.00	0.00	0.00	0.00	0.00	0.00	0.00	240.00	0.00
0.09	0.14	0.00	0.00	0.01	0.70	0.00	0.01	0.02	0.60	0.02	1.80	0.00	0.90	0.19	15.90	27.70	32.70	28.80	0.40
0.77	0.93	0.00	0.00	0.43	1.70	0.00	0.01	0.04	0.56	0.05	4.54	0.00	18.71	1.11	22.68	36.00	100.64	83.63	0.35

USDA ID Code	Food Name	Weight in Grams*	Quantity of Units	Unit of Measure	Protein (gm)	Fat (gm)	Carbohydrate (gm)	Kcalories	Caffeine (gm)	Fiber (gm)	Cholesterol (mg)	Saturated Fat (gm)
	Popcorn, Caramel-coated, w/o Pea	28.3500	1.000	Ounce	1.08	3.63	22.42	122.19	0.00	1.47	1.42	1.02
657	Popcorn, Cheese, White Cheddar,	14.0000	3.000	Cup	4.00	6.00	19.00	140.00	0.00	4.00	0.00	1.50
658	Popcorn, Cheese, White Cheddar-S	14.0000	2.000	Cup	3.00	12.00	17.00	190.00	0.00	3.00	5.00	2.50
	Popcorn, Cheese-flavor	6.0000	1.000	Cup	1.02	3.65	5.68	57.86	0.00	1.09	1.21	0.71
	Popcorn, Microwave	14.0000	4.000	Cup	0.75	3.00	4.25	42.50	0.00	0.75	0.00	0.75
	Popcorn, Microwave, Low-Fat	14.0000	4.000	Cup	0.67	1.00	3.67	23.33	0.00	0.50	0.00	0.17
659	Popcorn, Microwave, Smart Pop-Re	15.0000	1.000	Cup	3.00	2.00	20.00	105.00	0.00	5.00	0.00	0.00
	Popcorn, Microwave-Pop Secret-94	5.0000	1.000	Serving	1.00	0.00	4.00	20.00	0.00	0.00	0.00	0.00
	Popcorn, Oil-popped	11.0000	1.000	Cup	0.99	3.09	6.29	55.00	0.00	1.10	0.00	0.54
	Popcorn, Oil-popped, White Popco	11.0000	1.000	Cup	0.99	3.09	6.29	55.00	0.00	1.10	0.00	0.54
661	Popcorn, Unpopped, Microwave, Bu	32.0000	2.000	Tbsp	2.70	5.70	19.80	122.00	0.00	4.70	0.00	1.20
662	Popcorn, Unpopped, Microwave, Li	31.0000	2.000	Tbsp	2.60	5.10	18.90	113.00	0.00	4.50	0.00	1.00
663	Popcorn, unpopped, Microwave, No	37.0000	2.000	Tbsp	2.50	12.10	18.70	176.00	0.00	4.50	0.00	2.60
664	Popcorn, Unpopped, Microwave-Sma	30.0000	2.000	Tbsp	2.80	2.10	20.30	92.00	0.00	4.90	0.00	0.40
665	Potato Chips, BBQ, Fat Free-Prin	28.0000	1.000	Ounce	1.00	0.00	15.00	70.00	0.00	1.00	0.00	0.00
666	Potato Chips, Cheezum, Right Cri	51.0000	1.800	Ounce	4.00	24.00	32.00	350.00	0.00	2.00	0.00	6.00
668	Potato Chips, Original, Fat Free	28.0000	1.000	Ounce	1.00	0.00	15.00	70.00	0.00	1.00	0.00	0.00
667	Potato Chips, Original, Right Cr	51.0000	1.800	Ounce	3.00	14.00	36.00	270.00	0.00	2.00	0.00	3.50
	Potato Chips, Pringles, Cheese F	28.3500	1.000	Ounce	1.98	10.49	14.35	156.21	0.00	0.95	1.13	2.71
669	Potato Chips, Ranch, Right Crisp	51.0000	1.800	Ounce	2.00	7.00	18.00	140.00	0.00	1.00	0.00	2.00
670	Potato Chips, S. Cream, Right Cr	51.0000	1.800	Ounce	4.00	23.00	32.00	340.00	0.00	2.00	0.00	6.00
671	Potato Chips, S. Crm/Onion, Fat	28.0000	1.000	Ounce	1.00	0.00	15.00	70.00	0.00	1.00	0.00	0.00
	Power Bar	65.0000	1.000	Each	10.00	2.50	45.00	230.00	0.00	3.00	0.00	0.50
	Pretzels, Cheddar - Combos	28.3500	1.000	Ounce	2.79	4.80	18.85	131.26	0.00	0.00	1.42	0.00
	Pretzels, Hard, Plain, Salted	28.3500	1.000	Ounce	2.58	0.99	22.45	108.01	0.00	0.91	0.00	0.21
	Pretzels, Hard, Plain, Unsalted	28.3500	1.000	Ounce	2.58	0.99	22.45	108.01	0.00	0.79	0.00	0.21
	Pretzels, Hard, Whole-wheat	28.3500	1.000	Ounce	3.15	0.74	23.02	102.63	0.00	2.19	0.00	0.16
	Pudding, Banana	28.3500	1.000	Ounce	0.68	1.02	6.01	36.00	0.00	0.03	0.00	0.16
	Pudding, Bread	252.0000	1.000	Cup	13.10	14.87	61.99	423.36	0.00	0.00	166.32	5.77
	Pudding, Chocolate	28.3500	1.000	Ounce	0.77	1.13	6.46	37.71	1.42	0.28	0.85	0.20
	Pudding, Chocolate, Fat Free	113.0000	0.500	Cup	2.83	0.45	22.71	101.70	0.00	0.90	2.26	0.34
	Pudding, Coconut Cream	140.0000	0.500	Cup	4.34	3.50	24.92	145.60	0.00	0.28	9.80	2.52
	Pudding, Lemon	28.3500	1.000	Ounce	0.03	0.85	7.09	35.44	0.00	0.03	0.00	0.13
	Pudding, Rice	28.3500	1.000	Ounce	0.57	2.13	6.24	46.21	0.00	0.03	0.28	0.33
	Pudding, Tapioca	28.3500	1.000	Ounce	0.57	1.05	5.50	33.74	0.00	0.03	0.28	0.17
	Pudding, Vanilla	28.3500	1.000	Ounce	0.65	1.02	6.21	36.86	0.00	0.03	1.98	0.16
	Pudding, Vanilla, Fat Free	113.0000	0.500	Cup	2.37	0.23	23.17	103.96	0.00	0.11	2.26	0.23
	Raisins, Chocolate, Milk, Coated	180.0000	1.000	Cup	7.38	26.64	122.94	702.00	45.00	7.56	5.40	15.84
	Rice Cakes, Brown Rice, Buckwhea	9.0000	1.000	Cake	0.81	0.32	7.21	34.20	0.00	0.34	0.00	0.06
	Rice Cakes, Brown Rice, Buckwhea	9.0000	1.000	Cake	0.81	0.32	7.21	34.20	0.00	0.00	0.00	0.06
	Rice Cakes, Brown Rice, Corn	9.0000	1.000	Cake	0.76	0.29	7.31	34.65	0.00	0.26	0.00	0.06
	Rice Cakes, Brown Rice, Multigra	9.0000	1.000	Cake	0.77	0.32	7.21	34.83	0.00	0.27	0.00	0.05
	Rice Cakes, Brown Rice, Multigra	9.0000	1.000	Cake	0.77	0.32	7.21	34.83	0.00	0.00	0.00	0.05
	Rice Cakes, Brown Rice, Plain	9.0000	1.000	Cake	0.74	0.25	7.34	34.83	0.00	0.38	0.00	0.05
	Rice Cakes, Brown Rice, Plain, U	9.0000	1.000	Cake	0.74	0.25	7.34	34.83	0.00	0.38	0.00	0.05
	Rice Cakes, Brown Rice, Rye	9.0000	1.000	Cake	0.73	0.34	7.19	34.74	0.00	0.36	0.00	0.05
	Rice Krispie Treats	40.0000	1.000	Cup	1.33	2.00	33.33	160.00	0.00	0.00	0.00	0.00
	Snack Mix, Chex Mix	28.3500	0.660	Cup	3.12	4.90	18.46	120.49	0.00	1.58	0.00	1.57
	Snack Mix, Oriental Mix, Rice-ba	28.3500	1.000	Ounce	4.91	7.25	14.63	155.64	0.00	3.74	0.00	1.07
	Snack Mix, Original Flavor- Doo	56.7000	1.000	Cup	5.84	10.49	36.46	258.55	0.00	3.86	0.57	2.00
	Trail Mix, Regular	150.0000	1.000	Cup	20.70	44.10	67.35	693.00	0.00	0.00	0.00	8.32
	Trail Mix, Regular, Unsalted	150.0000	1.000	Cup	20.70	44.10	67.35	693.00	0.00	0.00	0.00	8.32
	Trail Mix, Regular, w/ Chocolate	146.0000	1.000	Cup	20.73	46.57	65.55	706.64	0.00	0.00	5.84	8.91
	Trail Mix, Tropical	140.0000	1.000	Cup	8.82	23.94	91.84	569.80	0.00	0.00	0.00	11.87
	Soup, Asparagus, Cream Of	248.0000	1.000	Cup	6.32	8.18	16.39	161.20	0.00	0.74	22.32	3.32

Monounsaturated Fat (gm)	Polyunsaturated Fat (gm)	Vitamin D (mg)	Vitamin K (mg)	Vitamin E (mg)	Vitamin A (re)	Vitamin C (mg)	Thiamin (mg)	Riboflavin (mg)	Niacin (mg)	Vitamin B_6 (mg)	Folate (mg)	Vitamin B_{12} (mcg)	Calcium (mg)	Iron (mg)	Magnesium (mg)	Phosphorus (mg)	Potassium (mg)	Sodium (mg)	Zinc (mg)
0.82	1.27	0.00	0.00	0.34	2.84	0.00	0.02	0.02	0.62	0.01	0.57	0.00	12.19	0.49	9.92	23.53	30.90	58.40	0.16
0.00	0.00	0.00	0.00	0.00	0.00	0.00	0.00	0.00	0.00	0.00	0.00	0.00	0.00	0.00	0.00	0.00	0.00	280.00	0.00
0.00	0.00	0.00	0.00	0.00	0.00	0.00	0.00	0.00	0.00	0.00	0.00	0.00	0.00	0.00	0.00	0.00	0.00	310.00	0.00
1.07	1.69	0.00	0.00	0.01	4.84	0.06	0.01	0.03	0.16	0.03	1.21	0.06	12.43	0.25	10.01	39.71	28.71	97.79	0.22
0.00	0.00	0.00	0.00	0.00	0.00	0.00	0.00	0.00	0.00	0.00	0.00	0.00	0.00	0.05	0.00	0.00	0.00	72.50	0.00
0.00	0.00	0.00	0.00	0.00	0.00	0.00	0.00	0.00	0.00	0.00	0.00	0.00	0.00	0.07	0.00	0.00	0.00	55.00	0.00
0.00	0.00	0.00	0.00	0.00	0.00	0.00	0.00	0.00	0.00	0.00	0.00	0.00	0.00	0.00	0.00	0.00	0.00	280.00	0.00
0.00	0.00	0.00	0.00	0.00	0.00	0.00	0.00	0.00	0.00	0.00	0.00	0.00	0.00	0.00	0.00	0.00	0.00	40.00	0.00
0.90	1.48	0.00	0.00	0.01	1.65	0.03	0.01	0.02	0.17	0.02	1.87	0.00	1.10	0.31	11.88	27.50	24.75	97.24	0.29
0.90	1.48	0.00	0.00	0.00	0.22	0.03	0.01	0.02	0.17	0.02	1.87	0.00	1.10	0.31	11.88	27.50	24.75	97.24	0.29
0.00	0.00	0.00	0.00	0.00	0.00	0.00	0.00	0.00	0.00	0.00	0.00	0.00	2.00	0.66	0.00	0.00	0.00	357.00	0.00
0.00	0.00	0.00	0.00	0.00	0.00	0.00	0.00	0.00	0.00	0.00	0.00	0.00	2.00	0.63	0.00	0.00	0.00	321.00	0.00
0.00	0.00	0.00	0.00	0.00	0.00	0.00	0.00	0.00	0.00	0.00	0.00	0.00	2.00	0.62	0.00	0.00	0.00	2.00	0.00
0.00	0.00	0.00	0.00	0.00	0.00	0.00	0.00	0.00	0.00	0.00	0.00	0.00	16.00	0.12	0.00	0.00	0.00	307.00	0.00
0.00	0.00	0.00	0.00	0.00	0.00	0.00	0.00	0.00	0.00	0.00	0.00	0.00	0.00	0.00	0.00	0.00	0.00	160.00	0.00
0.00	0.00	0.00	0.00	0.00	0.00	0.00	0.00	0.00	0.00	0.00	0.00	0.00	0.00	0.00	0.00	0.00	0.00	400.00	0.00
0.00	0.00	0.00	0.00	0.00	0.00	0.00	0.00	0.00	0.00	0.00	0.00	0.00	0.00	0.00	0.00	0.00	0.00	160.00	0.00
0.00	0.00	0.00	0.00	0.00	0.00	0.00	0.00	0.00	0.00	0.00	0.00	0.00	0.00	0.00	0.00	0.00	0.00	260.00	0.00
2.02	5.29	0.00	0.00	0.00	0.00	2.41	0.05	0.03	0.74	0.15	5.10	0.00	31.19	0.45	15.03	46.21	108.01	214.04	0.18
0.00	0.00	0.00	0.00	0.00	0.00	0.00	0.00	0.00	0.00	0.00	0.00	0.00	0.00	0.00	0.00	0.00	0.00	160.00	0.00
0.00	0.00	0.00	0.00	0.00	0.00	0.00	0.00	0.00	0.00	0.00	0.00	0.00	0.00	0.00	0.00	0.00	0.00	290.00	0.00
0.00	0.00	0.00	0.00	0.00	0.00	0.00	0.00	0.00	0.00	0.00	0.00	0.00	0.00	0.00	0.00	0.00	0.00	160.00	0.00
1.50	0.50	0.00	0.00	0.00	0.00	0.00	1.50	1.70	19.00	2.00	200.00	2.00	360.00	3.50	122.50	280.00	0.00	90.00	5.25
0.00	0.00	0.00	0.00	0.00	1.98	0.00	0.09	0.16	0.90	0.01	2.27	0.03	55.85	0.26	6.24	40.54	36.86	316.67	0.21
0.39	0.35	0.00	0.00	0.06	0.00	0.00	0.13	0.18	1.49	0.03	48.48	0.00	10.21	1.22	9.92	32.04	41.39	486.20	0.24
0.39	0.35	0.00	0.00	0.06	0.00	0.00	0.13	0.18	1.49	0.03	23.53	0.00	10.21	1.22	9.92	32.04	41.39	81.93	0.24
0.29	0.24	0.00	0.00	0.00	0.00	0.28	0.12	0.08	1.85	0.08	15.31	0.00	7.94	0.76	8.51	35.44	121.91	57.55	0.18
0.43	0.38	0.00	0.00	0.00	8.51	0.14	0.01	0.04	0.05	0.01	0.57	0.05	24.10	0.04	2.27	19.56	31.19	55.57	0.08
5.42	2.39	0.00	0.00	0.00	163.80	2.02	0.23	0.56	1.58	0.19	32.76	0.00	287.28	2.77	47.88	274.68	564.48	582.12	1.31
0.48	0.41	0.00	0.00	0.04	3.12	0.51	0.01	0.05	0.10	0.01	0.85	0.00	25.52	0.14	5.95	22.68	51.03	36.57	0.12
0.00	0.00	0.00	0.00	0.00	0.00	0.34	0.00	0.00	0.00	0.00	0.00	0.00	89.27	0.60	0.00	85.88	235.04	192.10	0.00
0.73	0.10	0.00	0.00	0.10	70.00	0.98	0.04	0.21	0.13	0.21	5.60	0.36	158.20	0.28	22.40	124.60	222.60	228.20	0.52
0.37	0.32	0.00	0.00	0.00	0.00	0.03	0.00	0.00	0.00	0.00	0.00	0.00	0.57	0.02	0.28	1.42	0.28	39.69	0.01
0.91	0.79	0.00	0.00	0.39	9.92	0.14	0.01	0.02	0.05	0.01	0.85	0.06	14.74	0.09	2.27	19.28	17.01	24.10	0.14
0.45	0.39	0.00	0.00	0.03	0.00	0.20	0.01	0.03	0.09	0.01	0.85	0.06	23.81	0.07	2.27	22.40	27.50	45.08	0.08
0.44	0.38	0.00	0.00	0.04	1.70	0.00	0.01	0.04	0.07	0.00	0.00	0.03	24.95	0.04	2.27	19.28	32.04	38.27	0.07
0.00	0.00	0.00	0.00	0.00	0.00	0.34	0.00	0.00	0.00	0.00	0.00	0.00	85.88	0.05	0.00	115.26	123.17	240.69	0.00
8.53	0.92	0.00	0.00	1.75	12.60	0.36	0.14	0.29	0.72	0.14	9.00	0.32	154.80	3.08	81.00	257.40	925.20	64.80	1.46
0.10	0.10	0.00	0.00	0.00	0.00	0.00	0.01	0.01	0.73	0.01	1.89	0.00	0.99	0.10	13.59	34.20	26.91	10.44	0.23
0.10	0.10	0.00	0.00	0.00	0.00	0.00	0.01	0.01	0.73	0.01	1.89	0.00	0.99	0.10	13.59	34.20	26.91	0.36	0.23
0.10	0.10	0.00	0.00	0.00	0.00	0.00	0.01	0.01	0.58	0.01	1.71	0.00	0.81	0.11	10.26	28.80	24.75	26.19	0.20
0.10	0.13	0.00	0.00	0.00	0.00	0.00	0.01	0.02	0.59	0.01	1.80	0.00	1.89	0.18	12.33	33.30	26.46	22.68	0.23
0.10	0.13	0.00	0.00	0.00	0.00	0.00	0.01	0.02	0.59	0.01	1.80	0.00	1.89	0.18	12.33	33.30	26.46	0.36	0.23
0.09	0.09	0.00	0.00	0.06	0.45	0.00	0.01	0.02	0.70	0.01	1.89	0.00	0.99	0.13	11.79	32.40	26.10	29.34	0.27
0.09	0.09	0.00	0.00	0.01	0.45	0.00	0.01	0.02	0.70	0.01	1.89	0.00	0.99	0.13	11.79	32.40	26.10	2.34	0.27
0.12	0.14	0.00	0.00	0.00	0.00	0.00	0.01	0.01	0.63	0.01	0.45	0.00	1.89	0.16	12.96	34.20	27.99	9.90	0.27
1.33	0.00	0.02	0.00	0.00	200.00	20.00	0.50	0.57	6.33	0.67	0.00	0.67	0.00	1.33	0.00	21.33	26.67	226.67	0.00
0.00	0.00	0.00	0.00	0.00	3.97	13.47	0.44	0.14	4.77	0.44	0.00	3.52	9.92	7.00	17.86	53.01	76.26	288.32	0.59
2.80	3.02	0.00	0.00	2.39	0.00	0.09	0.09	0.04	0.87	0.02	10.77	0.00	15.31	0.69	33.45	74.28	92.99	117.09	0.75
0.00	0.00	0.00	0.00	0.00	24.38	0.06	0.20	0.15	3.04	0.11	22.68	0.01	41.96	1.42	34.02	167.83	157.06	720.66	1.28
18.80	14.48	0.00	0.00	0.00	3.00	2.10	0.69	0.30	7.07	0.45	106.50	0.00	117.00	4.58	237.00	517.50	1027.50	343.50	4.83
18.80	14.48	0.00	0.00	0.00	3.00	2.10	0.69	0.30	7.07	0.45	106.50	0.00	117.00	4.58	237.00	517.50	1027.50	15.00	4.83
19.77	16.48	0.00	0.00	0.00	7.30	1.90	0.60	0.32	6.44	0.38	94.90	0.00	159.14	4.95	235.06	565.02	946.08	176.66	4.58
3.49	7.22	0.00	0.00	0.00	7.00	10.64	0.63	0.17	2.07	0.46	58.80	0.00	79.80	3.70	134.40	260.40	992.60	14.00	1.64
2.08	2.23	0.00	0.00	0.84	84.32	3.97	0.10	0.27	0.89	0.07	29.76	0.50	173.60	0.87	19.84	153.76	359.60	1041.60	0.92

USDA ID Code	Food Name	Weight in Grams*	Quantity of Units	Unit of Measure	Protein (gm)	Fat (gm)	Carbohydrate (gm)	Kcalories	Caffeine (gm)	Fiber (gm)	Cholesterol (mg)	Saturated Fat (gm)
	Soup, Bean and Ham-Healthy Choic	212.6200	1.000	Each	12.00	4.00	35.00	220.00	0.00	0.00	5.00	1.00
	Soup, Bean w/ Bacon	264.9000	1.000	Cup	5.48	2.15	16.37	105.96	0.00	9.01	2.65	0.95
	Soup, Bean w/ Ham	243.0000	1.000	Cup	12.61	8.51	27.12	230.85	0.00	11.18	21.87	3.33
	Soup, Bean w/ Hot Dogs	250.0000	1.000	Cup	9.98	6.98	22.00	187.50	0.00	0.00	12.50	2.13
	Soup, Bean w/ Pork	253.0000	1.000	Cup	7.89	5.95	22.80	172.04	0.00	8.60	2.53	1.52
	Soup, Bean, Black	247.0000	1.000	Cup	5.63	1.51	19.81	116.09	0.00	4.45	0.00	0.40
	Soup, Bean, Navy, w/ Ham-Stouffe	283.9200	1.000	Cup	11.02	8.01	31.05	240.36	0.00	0.00	20.03	0.00
	Soup, Beef and Potato-Healthy Ch	212.6200	1.000	Each	9.00	1.00	17.00	110.00	0.00	0.00	20.00	0.00
	Soup, Beef Mushroom	244.0000	1.000	Cup	5.78	3.00	6.34	73.20	0.00	0.24	7.32	1.49
	Soup, Beef Noodle	244.0000	1.000	Cup	4.83	3.07	8.98	82.96	0.00	0.73	4.88	1.15
	Soup, Beef, Chunky	240.0000	1.000	Cup	11.74	5.14	19.56	170.40	0.00	1.44	14.40	2.54
	Soup, Beef, Hearty-Healthy Choic	212.6200	1.000	Each	9.00	1.00	17.00	120.00	0.00	0.00	20.00	0.00
	Soup, Broccoli, Cream Of,-Stouff	283.9200	1.000	Cup	12.02	21.03	16.02	300.45	0.00	0.00	60.09	0.00
	Soup, Broth or Bouillon, Beef	240.0000	1.000	Cup	2.74	0.53	0.10	16.80	0.00	0.00	0.00	0.26
	Soup, Broth or Bouillon, Chicken	244.0000	1.000	Cup	1.34	1.10	1.44	21.96	0.00	0.00	0.00	0.27
	Soup, Cauliflower	253.0000	1.000	Cup	2.89	1.72	10.73	69.15	0.00	0.00	0.00	0.26
	Soup, Celery, Cream Of	248.0000	1.000	Cup	5.68	9.70	14.53	163.68	0.00	0.74	32.24	3.94
	Soup, Cheddar Cheese, Heat'n Ser	307.5800	1.000	Cup	21.70	35.80	21.70	488.23	0.00	0.00	97.65	0.00
	Soup, Cheddar Cheese-Stouffer's	283.9200	1.000	Cup	21.03	31.05	18.03	440.66	0.00	0.00	70.11	0.00
	Soup, Cheese	247.0000	1.000	Cup	5.41	10.47	10.52	155.61	0.00	0.99	29.64	6.67
	Soup, Chicken Gumbo-Stouffer's	283.9200	1.000	Cup	7.01	5.01	9.01	110.17	0.00	0.00	20.03	0.00
	Soup, Chicken Mushroom	244.0000	1.000	Cup	4.39	9.15	9.27	131.76	0.00	0.24	9.76	2.39
	Soup, Chicken Noodle	241.0000	1.000	Cup	4.05	2.46	9.35	74.71	0.00	0.72	7.23	0.65
	Soup, Chicken Noodle, Chunky	240.0000	1.000	Cup	12.72	6.00	17.04	175.20	0.00	3.84	19.20	1.39
	Soup, Chicken Noodle, Heat'n Ser	283.9200	1.000	Cup	13.02	17.03	28.04	320.48	0.00	0.00	60.09	0.00
	Soup, Chicken Noodle, Old Fashio	212.6200	1.000	Each	5.00	2.00	11.00	90.00	0.00	0.00	20.00	0.00
	Soup, Chicken Noodle-Stouffer's	283.9200	1.000	Cup	7.01	7.01	10.02	130.20	0.00	0.00	20.03	0.00
	Soup, Chicken Pasta-Healthy Choi	212.6200	1.000	Each	7.00	2.00	13.00	100.00	0.00	0.00	15.00	0.00
	Soup, Chicken Rice	240.0000	1.000	Cup	2.33	1.37	8.78	57.60	0.00	0.72	2.40	0.31
	Soup, Chicken Rice, Chunky	240.0000	1.000	Cup	12.26	3.19	12.98	127.20	0.00	0.96	12.00	0.96
	Soup, Chicken w/ Dumplings	241.0000	1.000	Cup	5.62	5.52	6.05	96.40	0.00	0.48	33.74	1.30
	Soup, Chicken w/ Rice	241.0000	1.000	Cup	3.54	1.90	7.16	60.25	0.00	0.72	7.23	0.46
	Soup, Chicken w/ Rice-Healthy Ch	212.6200	1.000	Each	5.00	1.00	14.00	90.00	0.00	0.00	10.00	0.00
	Soup, Chicken, Chunky	240.0000	1.000	Cup	12.14	6.34	16.51	170.40	0.00	1.44	28.80	1.90
	Soup, Chicken, Cream Of	248.0000	1.000	Cup	7.46	11.46	14.98	190.96	0.00	0.25	27.28	4.64
	Soup, Chicken, Creamy-Stouffer's	283.9200	1.000	Cup	17.03	8.01	25.04	240.36	0.00	0.00	20.03	0.00
	Soup, Chicken, Hearty-Healthy Ch	212.6200	1.000	Each	7.00	2.00	17.00	110.00	0.00	0.00	25.00	0.00
	Soup, Chili Beef	250.0000	1.000	Cup	6.70	6.60	21.45	170.00	0.00	9.50	12.50	3.35
	Soup, Clam Chowder, Manhattan St	240.0000	1.000	Cup	7.25	3.38	18.82	134.40	0.00	2.88	14.40	2.11
	Soup, Clam Chowder, New England	248.0000	1.000	Cup	9.47	6.60	16.62	163.68	0.00	1.49	22.32	2.95
	Soup, Clam Chowder, New England-	283.9200	1.000	Cup	14.02	23.03	21.03	340.51	0.00	0.00	40.06	0.00
	Soup, Crab	244.0000	1.000	Cup	5.49	1.51	10.30	75.64	0.00	0.73	9.76	0.39
	Soup, Fiesta Mexicali Heat'n Ser	283.9200	1.000	Cup	3.00	3.00	18.03	110.17	0.00	0.00	10.02	0.00
	Soup, Gazpacho	244.0000	1.000	Cup	7.08	0.24	4.39	46.36	0.00	0.49	0.00	0.02
	Soup, Gumbo, Chicken	244.0000	1.000	Cup	2.64	1.44	8.37	56.12	0.00	1.95	4.88	0.32
	Soup, Hot and Sour	244.0000	1.000	Cup	15.00	8.00	5.00	162.00	0.00	0.50	34.00	3.00
	Soup, Instant	240.0000	1.000	Cup	3.00	1.00	7.00	50.00	0.00	0.70	2.00	0.00
	Soup, Lentil w/ ham	248.0000	1.000	Cup	9.28	2.78	20.24	138.88	0.00	0.00	7.44	1.12
	Soup, Lentil-Healthy Choice	212.6200	1.000	Each	8.00	1.00	23.00	140.00	0.00	0.00	0.00	0.00
	Soup, Minestrone	241.0000	1.000	Cup	4.27	2.51	11.23	81.94	0.00	0.96	2.41	0.55
	Soup, Minestrone Heat'n Serve-St	283.9200	1.000	Cup	5.01	4.01	18.03	130.20	0.00	0.00	0.00	0.00
	Soup, Minestrone, Chunky	240.0000	1.000	Cup	5.11	2.81	20.74	127.20	0.00	5.76	4.80	1.49
	Soup, Minestrone-Healthy Choice	212.6200	1.000	Each	6.00	1.00	30.00	160.00	0.00	0.00	0.00	0.00
	Soup, Minestrone-Stouffer's	283.9200	1.000	Cup	6.01	3.00	20.03	140.21	0.00	0.00	10.02	0.00
	Soup, Mushroom	253.0000	1.000	Cup	2.23	4.86	11.13	96.14	0.00	0.76	0.00	0.81

Monounsaturated Fat (gm)	Polyunsaturated Fat (gm)	Vitamin D (mg)	Vitamin K (mg)	Vitamin E (mg)	Vitamin A (re)	Vitamin C (mg)	Thiamin (mg)	Riboflavin (mg)	Niacin (mg)	Vitamin B_6 (mg)	Folate (mg)	Vitamin B_{12} (mcg)	Calcium (mg)	Iron (mg)	Magnesium (mg)	Phosphorus (mg)	Potassium (mg)	Sodium (mg)	Zinc (mg)
0.00	1.00	0.00	0.00	0.00	60.00	2.40	0.23	0.17	1.14	0.00	0.00	0.00	48.00	1.00	0.00	220.00	630.00	480.00	0.00
0.93	0.16	0.00	0.00	0.26	5.30	1.06	0.05	0.26	0.40	0.03	7.95	0.03	55.63	1.32	29.14	90.07	325.83	927.15	0.69
3.84	0.95	0.00	0.00	0.00	396.09	4.37	0.15	0.15	1.70	0.12	29.16	0.07	77.76	3.23	46.17	143.37	425.25	972.00	1.07
2.73	1.65	0.00	0.00	0.00	87.50	1.00	0.10	0.08	1.03	0.13	30.00	0.08	87.50	2.35	47.50	165.00	477.50	1092.50	1.18
2.18	1.82	0.00	0.00	0.08	88.55	1.52	0.10	0.03	0.56	0.05	31.88	0.05	80.96	2.05	45.54	131.56	402.27	951.28	1.04
0.54	0.47	0.00	0.00	0.07	49.40	0.74	0.07	0.05	0.54	0.10	24.70	0.02	44.46	2.15	41.99	106.21	274.17	1197.95	1.41
0.00	0.00	0.00	0.00	0.00	0.00	0.00	0.00	0.00	0.19	0.00	0.00	0.00	70.11	3.00	0.00	0.00	570.86	1251.88	0.00
0.00	0.00	0.00	0.00	0.00	0.00	2.40	0.03	0.00	0.38	0.00	0.00	0.00	0.00	0.20	0.00	0.00	100.00	550.00	0.00
1.24	0.12	0.00	0.00	0.00	0.00	4.64	0.05	0.05	0.95	0.05	9.76	0.20	4.88	0.88	9.76	34.16	153.72	941.84	1.46
1.24	0.49	0.00	0.00	0.00	63.44	0.24	0.07	0.05	1.07	0.05	19.52	0.20	14.64	1.10	4.88	46.36	100.04	951.60	1.54
2.14	0.22	0.00	0.00	0.17	261.60	6.96	0.05	0.14	2.71	0.14	13.44	0.62	31.20	2.33	4.80	120.00	336.00	866.40	2.64
0.00	0.00	0.00	0.00	0.00	150.00	9.00	0.06	0.10	1.90	0.00	0.00	0.00	32.00	0.40	0.00	90.00	280.00	540.00	0.00
0.00	0.00	0.00	0.00	0.00	0.00	0.00	0.00	0.01	0.00	0.00	0.00	0.00	2.48	0.00	0.00	0.00	430.64	791.19	0.00
0.22	0.02	0.00	0.00	0.00	0.00	0.00	0.00	0.05	1.87	0.02	4.80	0.17	14.40	0.41	4.80	31.20	129.60	782.40	0.00
0.41	0.37	0.00	0.00	0.02	12.20	0.00	0.00	0.02	0.20	0.00	2.44	0.02	14.64	0.07	4.88	12.20	24.40	1483.52	0.00
0.74	0.64	0.00	0.00	0.00	0.00	2.56	0.08	0.08	0.51	0.03	2.56	0.18	10.24	0.51	2.56	51.22	105.00	842.57	0.26
2.46	2.65	0.00	0.00	0.97	66.96	1.49	0.07	0.25	0.45	0.07	8.43	0.50	186.00	0.69	22.32	151.28	310.00	1009.36	0.20
0.00	0.00	0.00	0.00	0.00	0.00	0.00	0.00	0.02	0.21	0.00	0.00	0.00	4.95	0.11	0.00	0.00	553.33	770.32	0.00
0.00	0.00	0.00	0.00	0.00	0.00	0.00	0.00	0.01	0.19	0.00	0.00	0.00	4.97	0.00	0.00	0.00	510.77	681.02	0.00
2.96	0.30	0.00	0.00	0.00	108.68	0.00	0.02	0.15	0.40	0.02	4.94	0.00	140.79	0.74	4.94	135.85	153.14	958.36	0.64
0.00	0.00	0.00	0.00	0.00	0.00	0.00	0.00	0.00	0.19	0.00	0.00	0.00	160.24	0.10	0.00	0.00	180.27	1422.13	0.00
4.03	2.32	0.00	0.00	0.00	112.24	0.00	0.02	0.12	1.63	0.05	0.24	0.05	29.28	0.88	9.76	26.84	153.72	941.84	0.98
1.11	0.55	0.00	0.00	0.07	72.30	0.24	0.05	0.07	1.40	0.02	21.69	0.14	16.87	0.77	4.82	36.15	55.43	1106.19	0.39
2.66	1.51	0.00	0.00	0.79	122.40	0.00	0.07	0.17	4.32	0.05	38.40	0.31	24.00	1.44	9.60	72.00	108.00	849.60	0.96
0.00	0.00	0.00	0.00	0.00	0.00	6.01	0.00	0.00	0.57	0.00	0.00	0.00	240.36	0.20	0.00	0.00	310.46	1792.69	0.00
0.00	0.00	0.00	0.00	0.00	80.00	12.00	0.03	0.10	1.90	0.00	0.00	0.00	16.00	0.20	0.00	60.00	130.00	540.00	0.00
0.00	0.00	0.00	0.00	0.00	0.00	0.00	0.00	0.00	0.19	0.00	0.00	0.00	80.12	0.10	0.00	0.00	140.21	1281.92	0.00
0.00	0.00	0.00	0.00	0.00	60.00	0.00	0.03	0.00	0.38	0.00	0.00	0.00	0.00	0.00	0.00	0.00	70.00	560.00	0.00
0.60	0.41	0.00	0.00	0.05	0.00	0.00	0.00	0.00	0.34	0.02	0.48	0.07	7.20	0.00	0.00	9.60	9.60	931.20	0.12
1.44	0.67	0.00	0.00	0.10	585.60	3.84	0.02	0.10	4.10	0.05	3.84	0.31	33.60	1.87	9.60	72.00	108.00	888.00	0.96
2.53	1.30	0.00	0.00	0.14	53.02	0.00	0.02	0.07	1.76	0.05	2.41	0.17	14.46	0.63	4.82	60.25	115.68	860.37	0.36
0.92	0.41	0.00	0.00	0.05	65.07	0.24	0.02	0.02	1.13	0.02	0.96	0.14	16.87	0.75	0.00	21.69	101.22	814.58	0.27
0.00	0.00	0.00	0.00	0.00	80.00	6.00	0.03	0.07	1.90	0.00	0.00	0.00	16.00	0.20	0.00	70.00	140.00	510.00	0.00
2.83	1.32	0.00	0.00	0.17	124.80	1.20	0.07	0.17	4.22	0.05	4.32	0.24	24.00	1.66	7.20	108.00	168.00	849.60	0.96
4.46	1.64	0.00	0.00	0.25	94.24	1.24	0.07	0.25	0.92	0.07	7.69	0.55	181.04	0.67	17.36	151.28	272.80	1046.56	0.67
0.00	0.00	0.00	0.00	0.00	0.00	0.00	0.02	0.01	0.19	0.00	0.00	0.00	2.48	0.00	0.00	0.00	510.77	1281.92	0.00
0.00	0.00	0.00	0.00	0.00	200.00	2.40	0.09	0.17	1.90	0.00	0.00	0.00	32.00	0.40	0.00	90.00	190.00	520.00	0.00
2.80	0.28	0.00	0.00	0.18	150.00	4.00	0.05	0.08	1.08	0.15	17.50	0.33	42.50	2.13	30.00	147.50	525.00	1035.00	1.40
0.98	0.12	0.00	0.00	0.10	328.80	12.24	0.05	0.07	1.85	0.26	9.36	7.92	67.20	2.64	19.20	84.00	384.00	1000.80	1.68
2.26	1.09	0.00	0.00	0.15	39.68	3.47	0.07	0.25	1.04	0.12	9.67	10.24	186.00	1.49	22.32	156.24	300.08	992.00	0.79
0.00	0.00	0.00	0.00	0.00	0.00	0.00	0.00	0.01	0.19	0.00	0.00	0.00	2.48	0.10	0.00	0.00	570.86	961.44	0.00
0.68	0.39	0.00	0.00	0.00	51.24	0.00	0.20	0.07	1.34	0.12	14.64	0.20	65.88	1.22	14.64	87.84	326.96	1234.64	1.46
0.00	0.00	0.00	0.00	0.00	0.00	6.01	0.00	0.00	0.19	0.00	0.00	0.00	2.40	1.00	0.00	0.00	430.64	711.07	0.00
0.02	0.07	0.00	0.00	0.46	261.08	7.08	0.05	0.02	0.93	0.15	9.76	0.00	24.40	0.98	7.32	36.60	224.48	739.32	0.24
0.66	0.34	0.00	0.00	0.05	14.64	4.88	0.02	0.05	0.66	0.07	4.88	0.02	24.40	0.90	4.88	24.40	75.64	954.04	0.37
0.30	0.68	0.00	0.00	0.30	0.03	0.60	0.00	0.00	0.00	0.00	0.00	0.00	32.00	1.65	0.00	0.00	0.00	1011.00	0.00
0.00	0.00	0.00	0.00	0.00	0.03	0.03	0.00	0.00	0.00	0.00	0.00	0.00	27.00	0.45	0.00	0.00	0.00	1222.00	0.00
1.29	0.32	0.00	0.00	0.00	34.72	4.22	0.17	0.12	1.36	0.22	49.60	0.30	42.16	2.65	22.32	183.52	357.12	1319.36	0.74
0.00	0.00	0.00	0.00	0.00	60.00	2.40	0.06	0.03	0.38	0.00	0.00	0.00	0.00	0.60	0.00	0.00	160.00	480.00	0.00
0.70	1.11	0.00	0.00	0.07	233.77	1.21	0.05	0.05	0.94	0.10	36.15	0.00	33.74	0.92	7.23	55.43	313.30	910.98	0.75
0.00	0.00	0.00	0.00	0.00	0.00	0.00	0.00	0.00	0.00	0.00	0.00	0.00	0.00	0.20	0.00	0.00	310.46	1191.79	0.00
0.91	0.26	0.00	0.00	0.72	434.40	4.80	0.05	0.12	1.18	0.24	52.80	0.00	60.00	1.78	14.40	110.40	612.00	864.00	1.44
0.00	0.00	0.00	0.00	0.00	60.00	15.00	0.12	0.14	1.52	0.00	0.00	0.00	32.00	0.60	0.00	130.00	440.00	520.00	0.00
0.00	0.00	0.00	0.00	0.00	0.00	0.00	0.00	0.00	0.19	0.00	0.00	0.00	0.00	0.20	0.00	0.00	370.56	1281.92	0.00
2.25	1.54	0.00	0.00	0.63	0.00	1.01	0.28	0.10	0.51	0.03	5.06	0.25	65.78	0.51	5.06	75.90	199.87	1019.59	0.08

USDA ID Code	Food Name	Weight in Grams*	Quantity of Units	Unit of Measure	Protein (gm)	Fat (gm)	Carbohydrate (gm)	Kcalories	Caffeine (gm)	Fiber (gm)	Cholesterol (mg)	Saturated Fat (gm)
	Soup, Mushroom, Cream Of	248.0000	1.000	Cup	6.05	13.59	15.00	203.36	0.00	0.50	19.84	5.13
	Soup, Onion	241.0000	1.000	Cup	3.76	1.74	8.17	57.84	0.00	0.96	0.00	0.27
	Soup, Onion, Cream Of	248.0000	1.000	Cup	6.80	9.37	18.35	186.00	0.00	0.74	32.24	4.04
	Soup, Onion, French-Stouffer's	283.9200	1.000	Cup	4.01	4.01	10.02	100.15	0.00	0.00	0.00	0.00
	Soup, Pea, Green	254.0000	1.000	Cup	12.62	7.04	32.23	238.76	0.00	2.79	17.78	4.01
	Soup, Pea, Split w/ Ham	253.0000	1.000	Cup	10.32	4.40	27.96	189.75	0.00	2.28	7.59	1.77
	Soup, Pea, Split w/ Ham, Chunky	240.0000	1.000	Cup	11.09	3.98	26.81	184.80	0.00	4.08	7.20	1.58
	Soup, Pea, Split, and Ham-Health	212.6200	1.000	Each	10.00	3.00	25.00	170.00	0.00	0.00	10.00	1.00
	Soup, Pea, Split, and Ham-Stouff	283.9200	1.000	Cup	15.02	3.00	35.05	220.33	0.00	0.00	10.02	0.00
	Soup, Potato, Cream Of	248.0000	1.000	Cup	5.78	6.45	17.16	148.80	0.00	0.50	22.32	3.77
	Soup, Potato, Cream Of,-Stouffer	283.9200	1.000	Cup	11.02	13.02	34.05	300.45	0.00	0.00	30.04	0.00
	Soup, Shrimp, Cream Of	248.0000	1.000	Cup	6.82	9.30	13.91	163.68	0.00	0.25	34.72	5.78
	Soup, Sweet & Sour	244.0000	1.000	Cup	3.00	1.00	14.00	72.00	0.00	1.60	5.00	0.00
	Soup, Tomato	248.0000	1.000	Cup	6.10	6.00	22.30	161.20	0.00	2.73	17.36	2.90
	Soup, Tomato Beef w/ noodle	244.0000	1.000	Cup	4.47	4.29	21.15	139.08	0.00	1.46	4.88	1.59
	Soup, Tomato Garden-Healthy Choi	212.6200	1.000	Each	4.00	3.00	22.00	130.00	0.00	0.00	5.00	1.00
	Soup, Tomato Rice	247.0000	1.000	Cup	2.10	2.72	21.93	118.56	0.00	1.48	2.47	0.52
	Soup, Tomato, Garden Heat'n Serv	283.9200	1.000	Cup	4.01	3.00	16.02	110.17	0.00	0.00	10.02	0.00
	Soup, Turkey Noodle	244.0000	1.000	Cup	3.90	2.00	8.64	68.32	0.00	0.73	4.88	0.56
	Soup, Turkey, Chunky	236.0000	1.000	Cup	10.22	4.41	14.07	134.52	0.00	0.00	9.44	1.23
	Soup, Vegetable Beef	253.0000	1.000	Cup	2.93	1.11	8.02	53.13	0.00	0.51	0.00	0.56
	Soup, Vegetable, Beef w/ Barley-	283.9200	1.000	Cup	4.01	13.02	15.02	190.29	0.00	0.00	10.02	0.00
	Soup, Vegetable, Beef-Healthy Ch	212.6200	1.000	Each	8.00	1.00	21.00	130.00	0.00	0.00	15.00	0.00
	Soup, Vegetable, Chicken	241.0000	1.000	Cup	3.62	2.84	8.58	74.71	0.00	0.96	9.64	0.84
	Soup, Vegetable, Chicken, Chunky	240.0000	1.000	Cup	12.31	4.82	18.89	165.60	0.00	0.00	16.80	1.44
	Soup, Vegetable, Chunky	240.0000	1.000	Cup	3.50	3.70	19.01	122.40	0.00	1.20	0.00	0.55
	Soup, Vegetable, Country-Healthy	212.6200	1.000	Each	3.00	1.00	23.00	120.00	0.00	0.00	0.00	0.00
	Soup, Vegetable, Cream Of	260.1000	1.000	Cup	1.90	5.70	12.30	106.64	0.00	0.52	0.00	1.43
	Soup, Vegetable, Garden-Healthy	212.6200	1.000	Each	3.00	1.00	18.00	100.00	0.00	0.00	0.00	0.00
	Soup, Vegetable, Tomato	241.0000	1.000	Cup	1.90	0.82	9.74	53.02	0.00	0.48	0.00	0.36
	Soup, Vegetable, Turkey	241.0000	1.000	Cup	3.08	3.04	8.63	72.30	0.00	0.48	2.41	0.89
	Soup, Vegetable, Turkey-Healthy	212.6200	1.000	Each	4.00	3.00	17.00	110.00	0.00	0.00	15.00	1.00
	Soup, Vegetable, Vegetarian	241.0000	1.000	Cup	2.10	1.93	11.98	72.30	0.00	0.48	0.00	0.29
	Soup, Vegetable, Vegetarian-Stou	283.9200	1.000	Cup	6.01	2.00	20.03	120.18	0.00	0.00	0.00	0.00
	Soup, Won-Ton	241.0000	1.000	Cup	14.00	7.00	14.00	182.00	0.00	0.90	53.00	2.00
3	Boost Plus, Chocolate	240.0000	8.000	fl oz	14.00	14.00	45.00	360.00	0.00	0.00	0.00	2.00
4	Boost Plus, Strawberry	240.0000	8.000	fl oz	14.00	14.00	45.00	360.00	0.00	0.00	0.00	2.00
5	Boost Plus, Vanilla	240.0000	8.000	fl oz	14.00	14.00	45.00	360.00	0.00	0.00	0.00	2.00
6	Boost, Chocolate	240.0000	8.000	fl oz	10.00	4.00	40.00	240.00	0.00	0.00	5.00	0.50
7	Boost, Chocolate Mocha	240.0000	8.000	fl oz	10.00	4.00	40.00	240.00	0.00	0.00	5.00	0.50
8	Boost, Strawberry	240.0000	8.000	fl oz	10.00	4.00	40.00	240.00	0.00	0.00	5.00	0.50
9	Boost, Vanilla	240.0000	8.000	fl oz	10.00	4.00	40.00	240.00	0.00	0.00	5.00	0.50
430	Enlive-Ross Labs	243.0000	8.000	Fl Oz	10.00	0.00	65.00	300.00	0.00	0.00	3.00	0.00
431	Ensure Fiber with FOS-Ross Labs	240.0000	8.000	Fl Oz	8.80	6.10	42.00	250.00	0.00	2.80	0.00	0.00
432	Ensure Glucerna OS-Ross Labs	240.0000	8.000	Fl Oz	10.00	11.00	22.00	220.00	0.00	2.00	0.00	1.00
433	Ensure Glucerna Snack Bars-Ross	38.0000	1.000	Bar	6.00	4.00	24.00	140.00	0.00	4.00	3.00	1.00
434	Ensure High Calcium-Ross Labs	240.0000	8.000	Fl Oz	12.00	6.00	31.00	225.00	0.00	0.00	0.00	0.50
435	Ensure High Protein-Ross Labs	240.0000	8.000	Fl Oz	12.00	6.00	30.80	225.00	0.00	0.00	0.00	0.64
436	Ensure Light-Ross Labs	240.0000	8.000	Fl Oz	10.00	3.00	33.30	200.00	0.00	0.00	3.00	0.31
437	Ensure Nutrition Bars-Ross Labs	35.0000	1.000	Bar	6.00	3.00	21.00	130.00	0.00	0.00	3.00	1.00
438	Ensure Plus-Ross Labs	240.0000	8.000	Fl Oz	13.00	11.40	50.10	355.00	0.00	0.00	3.00	0.00
439	Ensure Powder-Ross Labs	240.0000	8.000	Fl Oz	9.00	9.00	34.00	250.00	0.00	0.00	0.00	0.00
440	Ensure Pudding-Ross Labs	120.0000	4.000	Ounce	4.00	5.00	27.00	170.00	0.00	0.00	0.00	0.00
441	Ensure-Ross Labs	240.0000	8.000	Fl Oz	8.80	6.10	40.00	250.00	0.00	0.00	3.00	0.00
677	Power Bar, Apple Cinnamon	65.0000	1.000	Each	10.00	2.50	45.00	230.00	0.00	3.00	0.00	0.50

Monounsaturated Fat (gm)	Polyunsaturated Fat (gm)	Vitamin D (mg)	Vitamin K (mg)	Vitamin E (mg)	Vitamin A (re)	Vitamin C (mg)	Thiamin (mg)	Riboflavin (mg)	Niacin (mg)	Vitamin B_6 (mg)	Folate (mg)	Vitamin B_{12} (mcg)	Calcium (mg)	Iron (mg)	Magnesium (mg)	Phosphorus (mg)	Potassium (mg)	Sodium (mg)	Zinc (mg)
2.98	4.61	0.00	0.00	1.34	37.20	2.23	0.07	0.27	0.92	0.07	9.92	0.50	178.56	0.60	19.84	156.24	270.32	917.60	0.64
0.75	0.65	0.00	0.00	0.29	0.00	1.21	0.02	0.02	0.60	0.05	15.18	0.00	26.51	0.67	2.41	12.05	67.48	1053.17	0.60
3.27	1.59	0.00	0.00	0.07	69.44	2.48	0.10	0.27	0.60	0.07	22.32	0.50	178.56	0.69	22.32	153.76	310.00	1004.40	0.62
0.00	0.00	0.00	0.00	0.00	0.00	0.00	0.02	0.02	0.00	0.00	0.00	0.00	240.36	0.00	0.00	0.00	170.26	2073.11	0.00
2.18	0.53	0.00	0.00	0.18	58.42	2.79	0.15	0.28	1.35	0.10	7.87	0.43	172.72	2.01	55.88	238.76	375.92	970.28	1.75
1.80	0.63	0.00	0.00	0.00	45.54	1.52	0.15	0.08	1.47	0.08	2.53	0.25	22.77	2.28	48.07	212.52	399.74	1006.94	1.32
1.63	0.58	0.00	0.00	0.14	487.20	6.96	0.12	0.10	2.52	0.22	4.56	0.24	33.60	2.14	38.40	177.60	304.80	964.80	3.12
0.00	0.00	0.00	0.00	0.00	100.00	6.00	0.15	0.14	1.90	0.00	0.00	0.00	16.00	0.60	0.00	190.00	450.00	460.00	0.00
0.00	0.00	0.00	0.00	0.00	0.00	0.00	0.01	0.00	0.38	0.00	0.00	0.00	240.36	0.20	0.00	0.00	570.86	1191.79	0.00
1.74	0.57	0.00	0.00	0.10	66.96	1.24	0.07	0.25	0.64	0.10	9.18	0.50	166.16	0.55	17.36	161.20	322.40	1061.44	0.67
0.00	0.00	0.00	0.00	0.00	0.00	0.00	0.00	0.01	0.19	0.00	0.00	0.00	2.08	0.10	0.00	0.00	791.19	1422.13	0.00
2.68	0.35	0.00	0.00	0.87	54.56	1.24	0.07	0.22	0.52	0.45	9.92	1.04	163.68	0.60	22.32	146.32	248.00	1036.64	0.79
0.00	0.00	0.00	0.00	0.00	30.00	16.80	0.00	0.00	0.00	0.00	0.00	0.00	27.00	0.45	0.00	0.00	0.00	1292.00	0.00
1.61	1.12	0.00	0.00	2.60	109.12	67.70	0.12	0.25	1.51	0.17	20.83	0.45	158.72	1.81	22.32	148.80	448.88	744.00	0.30
1.73	0.68	0.00	0.00	0.78	53.68	0.00	0.07	0.10	1.88	0.10	19.52	0.20	17.08	1.12	7.32	56.12	219.60	917.44	0.76
0.00	0.00	0.00	0.00	0.00	100.00	6.00	0.06	0.10	1.14	0.00	0.00	0.00	32.00	0.40	0.00	70.00	440.00	510.00	0.00
0.59	1.36	0.00	0.00	0.79	76.57	14.82	0.07	0.05	1.06	0.07	13.59	0.00	22.23	0.79	4.94	34.58	330.98	815.10	0.52
0.00	0.00	0.00	0.00	0.00	0.00	0.00	0.00	0.00	0.19	0.00	0.00	0.00	240.36	0.30	0.00	0.00	430.64	1051.58	0.00
0.81	0.49	0.00	0.00	0.05	29.28	0.24	0.07	0.07	1.39	0.05	19.52	0.15	12.20	0.95	4.88	48.80	75.64	814.96	0.59
1.77	1.09	0.00	0.00	0.00	715.08	6.37	0.05	0.12	3.59	0.31	11.09	2.12	49.56	1.91	23.60	103.84	361.08	922.76	2.12
0.46	0.05	0.00	0.00	0.03	22.77	1.27	0.03	0.03	0.46	0.05	7.59	0.25	12.65	0.86	22.77	35.42	75.90	1001.88	0.28
0.00	0.00	0.00	0.00	0.00	0.00	0.00	0.00	0.00	0.19	0.00	0.00	0.00	240.36	0.10	0.00	0.00	340.51	1251.88	0.00
0.00	0.00	0.00	0.00	0.00	150.00	15.00	0.09	0.10	1.90	0.00	0.00	0.00	32.00	0.40	0.00	120.00	360.00	530.00	0.00
1.28	0.60	0.00	0.00	0.07	265.10	0.96	0.05	0.05	1.23	0.05	4.82	0.12	16.87	0.87	7.23	40.97	154.24	944.72	0.36
2.16	1.01	0.00	0.00	0.00	600.00	5.52	0.05	0.17	3.29	0.10	12.00	0.24	26.40	1.46	9.60	105.60	367.20	1068.00	2.16
1.58	1.39	0.00	0.00	0.60	588.00	6.00	0.07	0.07	1.20	0.19	16.56	0.00	55.20	1.63	7.20	72.00	396.00	1010.40	3.12
0.00	0.00	0.00	0.00	0.00	200.00	6.00	0.06	0.07	1.52	0.00	0.00	0.00	32.00	0.40	0.00	100.00	380.00	540.00	0.00
2.55	1.48	0.00	0.00	1.25	2.60	3.90	1.22	0.10	0.52	0.03	7.80	0.13	31.21	0.52	10.40	54.62	96.24	1170.45	0.26
0.00	0.00	0.00	0.00	0.00	350.00	9.00	0.09	0.07	0.76	0.00	0.00	0.00	16.00	0.40	0.00	0.00	230.00	560.00	0.00
0.29	0.07	0.00	0.00	0.77	19.28	5.78	0.05	0.05	0.75	0.05	9.64	0.00	7.23	0.60	19.28	28.92	98.81	1091.73	0.17
1.33	0.67	0.00	0.00	0.14	243.41	0.00	0.02	0.05	1.01	0.05	4.82	0.17	16.87	0.77	4.82	40.97	175.93	906.16	0.60
0.00	1.00	0.00	0.00	0.00	150.00	4.80	0.03	0.03	0.38	0.00	0.00	0.00	16.00	0.20	0.00	0.00	140.00	540.00	0.00
0.82	0.72	0.00	0.00	0.80	301.25	1.45	0.05	0.05	0.92	0.05	10.60	0.00	21.69	1.08	7.23	33.74	209.67	821.81	0.46
0.00	0.00	0.00	0.00	0.00	0.00	0.00	0.00	0.00	0.19	0.00	0.00	0.00	0.00	0.10	0.00	0.00	400.60	911.37	0.00
0.00	0.00	0.00	0.00	0.00	100.00	3.60	0.00	0.00	0.00	0.00	0.00	0.00	29.00	1.50	0.00	0.00	0.00	543.00	0.00
0.00	0.00	0.00	0.00	0.00	0.00	0.00	0.00	0.00	0.00	0.00	0.00	0.00	0.00	0.00	0.00	0.00	350.00	200.00	0.00
0.00	0.00	0.00	0.00	0.00	0.00	0.00	0.00	0.00	0.00	0.00	0.00	0.00	0.00	0.00	0.00	0.00	350.00	200.00	0.00
0.00	0.00	0.00	0.00	0.00	0.00	0.00	0.00	0.00	0.00	0.00	0.00	0.00	0.00	0.00	0.00	0.00	350.00	200.00	0.00
0.00	0.00	0.00	0.00	0.00	0.00	0.00	0.00	0.00	0.00	0.00	0.00	0.00	0.00	0.00	0.00	0.00	400.00	130.00	0.00
0.00	0.00	0.00	0.00	0.00	0.00	0.00	0.00	0.00	0.00	0.00	0.00	0.00	0.00	0.00	0.00	0.00	400.00	130.00	0.00
0.00	0.00	0.00	0.00	0.00	0.00	0.00	0.00	0.00	0.00	0.00	0.00	0.00	0.00	0.00	0.00	0.00	400.00	130.00	0.00
0.00	0.00	0.00	0.00	0.00	0.00	0.00	0.00	0.00	0.00	0.00	0.00	0.00	0.00	0.00	0.00	0.00	400.00	130.00	0.00
0.00	0.00	1.50	20.00	3.00	118.12	24.00	0.38	0.34	2.00	0.40	80.00	1.20	60.00	2.70	8.00	20.00	40.00	65.00	3.80
0.00	0.00	2.50	20.00	2.50	118.12	30.00	0.38	0.43	5.00	0.50	100.00	1.50	350.00	4.50	100.00	300.00	370.00	200.00	3.80
0.00	0.00	2.50	20.00	10.00	118.12	60.00	0.38	0.43	5.00	0.50	100.00	1.50	250.00	4.50	100.00	250.00	370.00	210.00	3.80
0.00	0.00	1.50	12.00	10.00	118.12	60.00	0.23	0.26	3.00	0.30	60.00	0.90	250.00	2.70	60.00	150.00	60.00	75.00	2.25
0.00	0.00	3.50	28.00	5.00	118.12	42.00	0.38	0.43	5.00	0.50	120.00	1.80	400.00	4.50	100.00	250.00	500.00	290.00	6.00
0.00	0.00	2.50	20.00	4.00	118.12	30.00	0.38	0.43	5.00	0.50	100.00	1.50	300.00	4.50	100.00	250.00	500.00	290.00	5.70
0.00	0.00	2.50	20.00	2.50	118.12	30.00	0.38	0.43	5.00	0.50	100.00	1.50	250.00	4.50	100.00	250.00	370.00	200.00	3.80
0.00	0.00	1.50	10.00	2.00	67.64	21.00	0.23	0.26	3.00	0.30	60.00	0.90	250.00	2.70	60.00	150.00	200.00	115.00	2.30
0.00	0.00	2.50	20.00	2.50	118.12	30.00	0.38	0.43	5.00	0.50	100.00	1.50	200.00	4.50	100.00	200.00	440.00	240.00	3.80
0.00	0.00	1.25	10.00	1.88	58.62	37.50	0.38	0.43	5.00	0.50	100.00	1.50	125.00	2.25	50.00	125.00	370.00	200.00	2.82
0.00	0.00	1.00	12.00	2.00	45.09	9.00	0.23	0.26	3.00	0.30	60.00	1.20	100.00	2.70	40.00	100.00	180.00	135.00	3.00
0.00	0.00	2.50	20.00	2.50	118.12	30.00	0.38	0.43	5.00	0.50	100.00	1.50	300.00	4.50	100.00	300.00	370.00	200.00	3.80
1.50	0.50	0.00	0.00	0.00	0.00	0.00	0.00	0.00	0.00	0.00	0.00	0.00	0.00	0.00	0.00	0.00	110.00	90.00	0.00

USDA ID Code	Food Name	Weight in Grams*	Quantity of Units	Unit of Measure	Protein (gm)	Fat (gm)	Carbohydrate (gm)	Kcalories	Caffeine (gm)	Fiber (gm)	Cholesterol (mg)	Saturated Fat (gm)
678	Power Bar, Banana	65.0000	1.000	Each	9.00	2.00	45.00	230.00	0.00	3.00	0.00	0.50
679	Power Bar, Berry, Wild	65.0000	1.000	Each	10.00	2.50	45.00	230.00	0.00	3.00	0.00	0.50
680	Power Bar, Chocolate	65.0000	1.000	Each	10.00	2.00	45.00	230.00	0.00	3.00	0.00	0.50
681	Power Bar, Harvest, Apple Crisp	65.0000	1.000	Each	7.00	4.00	45.00	240.00	0.00	4.00	0.00	0.50
682	Power Bar, Harvest, Cherry Crunc	65.0000	1.000	Each	7.00	4.00	45.00	240.00	0.00	4.00	0.00	0.50
683	Power Bar, Harvest, Chocolate	65.0000	1.000	Each	7.00	4.00	45.00	240.00	0.00	4.00	0.00	1.00
684	Power Bar, Harvest, Strawberry	65.0000	1.000	Each	7.00	4.00	45.00	240.00	0.00	4.00	0.00	0.50
685	Power Bar, Malt Nut	65.0000	1.000	Each	10.00	2.50	45.00	230.00	0.00	3.00	0.00	0.50
686	Power Bar, Mocha	65.0000	1.000	Each	10.00	2.50	45.00	230.00	0.00	3.00	0.00	1.00
687	Power Bar, Oatmeal Raisin	65.0000	1.000	Each	10.00	2.50	45.00	230.00	0.00	3.00	0.00	0.50
688	Power Bar, Peanut Butter	65.0000	1.000	Each	10.00	2.50	45.00	230.00	0.00	3.00	0.00	0.50
673	Power Bar, Power Gel, Fruit, Tro	41.0000	1.400	Ounce	0.00	0.00	28.00	110.00	0.00	0.00	0.00	0.00
674	Power Bar, Power Gel, Lemon Lime	41.0000	1.400	Ounce	0.00	0.00	28.00	110.00	0.00	0.00	0.00	0.00
675	Power Bar, Power Gel, Straw-Bana	41.0000	1.400	Ounce	0.00	0.00	28.00	110.00	0.00	0.00	0.00	0.00
676	Power Bar, Power Gel, Vanilla	41.0000	1.400	Ounce	0.00	0.00	28.00	110.00	0.00	0.00	0.00	0.00
698	Slim-Fast Bar, Chocolate, Dutch	34.0000	1.200	Ounce	5.00	5.00	20.00	140.00	0.00	2.00	1250.00	2.00
699	Slim-Fast Bar, Peanut Butter	34.0000	1.200	Ounce	6.00	5.00	19.00	150.00	0.00	2.00	1250.00	3.00
700	Slim-Fast Powder, Chocolate	28.0000	1.000	Ounce	5.00	1.00	20.00	100.00	0.00	2.00	750.00	0.50
701	Slim-Fast Powder, Chocolate Malt	28.0000	1.000	Ounce	5.00	1.00	20.00	100.00	0.00	2.00	750.00	0.50
702	Slim-Fast Powder, Strawberry	28.0000	1.000	Ounce	5.00	0.50	20.00	100.00	0.00	2.00	750.00	0.00
703	Slim-Fast Powder, Vanilla	28.0000	1.000	Ounce	5.00	0.50	20.00	100.00	0.00	2.00	750.00	0.00
740	Tiger Bar, Caf_ Mocha	65.0000	1.000	Each	10.00	2.00	43.00	200.00	0.00	3.00	0.00	0.50
741	Tiger Bar, Chocolate	65.0000	1.000	Each	10.00	2.00	43.00	200.00	0.00	3.00	0.00	0.50
742	Tiger Bar, Vanilla	65.0000	1.000	Each	10.00	2.00	43.00	200.00	0.00	3.00	0.00	0.50
751	Ultra Slim-Fast Bar, Choc Chip C	28.0000	1.000	Ounce	1.00	4.00	16.00	120.00	0.00	2.00	0.00	2.00
752	Ultra Slim-Fast Bar, Peanut Butt	28.0000	1.000	Ounce	2.00	4.00	19.00	120.00	0.00	2.00	0.00	2.00
753	Ultra Slim-Fast Bar, Peanut Cara	28.0000	1.000	Ounce	1.00	4.00	22.00	120.00	0.00	2.00	500.00	2.00
754	Ultra Slim-Fast Powder, Caf_ Moc	33.0000	1.200	Ounce	5.00	1.00	24.00	120.00	0.00	5.00	5.00	0.50
755	Ultra Slim-Fast Powder, Chocolat	33.0000	1.200	Ounce	5.00	2.00	24.00	120.00	0.00	5.00	5.00	1.00
756	Ultra Slim-Fast Powder, Chocolat	33.0000	1.200	Ounce	5.00	1.00	24.00	120.00	0.00	5.00	5.00	0.50
757	Ultra Slim-Fast Powder, Chocolat	33.0000	1.200	Ounce	5.00	1.00	24.00	110.00	0.00	5.00	5.00	0.50
758	Ultra Slim-Fast Powder, Chocolat	33.0000	1.200	Ounce	5.00	1.00	24.00	120.00	0.00	6.00	750.00	0.00
759	Ultra Slim-Fast Powder, Fruit Ju	31.0000	1.100	Ounce	5.00	1.00	24.00	120.00	0.00	5.00	4.00	0.00
760	Ultra Slim-Fast Powder, Strawber	33.0000	1.200	Ounce	5.00	0.50	25.00	120.00	0.00	4.00	5.00	0.00
761	Ultra Slim-Fast Powder, Vanilla	33.0000	1.200	Ounce	5.00	0.50	22.00	110.00	0.00	6.00	5.00	0.00
762	Ultra Slim-Fast, Juice Base, Rtd	350.0000	11.500	Fl Oz	7.00	1.50	46.00	220.00	0.00	5.00	10.00	0.50
763	Ultra Slim-Fast, Juice Base, Rtd	350.0000	11.500	Fl Oz	7.00	1.50	48.00	220.00	0.00	5.00	10.00	0.50
764	Ultra Slim-Fast, Juice Base, Rtd	350.0000	11.500	Fl Oz	7.00	1.50	47.00	220.00	0.00	5.00	10.00	0.50
765	Ultra Slim-Fast, Rtd, Choc Fudge	350.0000	11.000	Fl Oz	10.00	3.00	42.00	220.00	0.00	5.00	5.00	1.00
766	Ultra Slim-Fast, Rtd, Choc Royal	350.0000	11.000	Fl Oz	10.00	3.00	38.00	220.00	0.00	5.00	5.00	1.00
770	Ultra Slim-Fast, Rtd, Chocolate,	350.0000	11.000	Fl Oz	10.00	3.00	42.00	220.00	0.00	5.00	5.00	1.00
767	Ultra Slim-Fast, Rtd, Coffee	350.0000	11.000	Fl Oz	10.00	3.00	38.00	220.00	0.00	5.00	5.00	0.50
768	Ultra Slim-Fast, Rtd, Strawberry	350.0000	11.000	Fl Oz	10.00	3.00	42.00	220.00	0.00	5.00	5.00	1.00
769	Ultra Slim-Fast, Rtd, Vanilla	350.0000	11.000	Fl Oz	10.00	3.00	38.00	220.00	0.00	5.00	5.00	1.00
771	Viactiv-Calcium Chew, Caramel	2.0000	1.000	Each	0.00	0.50	4.00	20.00	0.00	0.00	0.00	0.00
772	Viactiv-Calcium Chew, Chocolate	2.0000	1.000	Each	0.00	0.50	4.00	20.00	0.00	0.00	0.00	0.00
773	Viactiv-Calcium Chew, Mochaccino	2.0000	1.000	Each	0.00	0.50	4.00	20.00	0.00	0.00	0.00	0.00
774	Viactiv-Energy Bar, Fruit Crispy	30.0000	1.000	Each	4.00	2.00	22.00	120.00	0.00	0.00	0.00	0.00
775	Viactiv-Energy Bar, Fruit Crispy	30.0000	1.000	Each	4.00	2.00	20.00	120.00	0.00	0.00	0.00	0.00
776	Viactiv-Energy Bar, Hearty, Appl	45.0000	1.000	Each	6.00	4.50	29.00	180.00	0.00	0.00	0.00	3.50
777	Viactiv-Energy Bar, Hearty, Choc	45.0000	1.000	Each	6.00	4.50	29.00	180.00	0.00	0.00	0.00	3.50
778	Viactiv-Energy Fruit Smoothie, F	240.0000	8.000	Fl Oz	0.00	0.00	37.00	150.00	0.00	0.00	0.00	0.00
779	Viactiv-Energy Fruit Smoothie, S	240.0000	8.000	Fl Oz	0.00	0.00	28.00	110.00	0.00	0.00	0.00	0.00
780	Viactiv-Energy Fruit Spritzer, C	240.0000	8.000	fl oz	0.00	0.00	22.00	90.00	0.00	0.00	0.00	0.00
781	Viactiv-Energy Fruit Spritzer, C	240.0000	8.000	fl oz	0.00	0.00	22.00	90.00	0.00	0.00	0.00	0.00

Monounsaturated Fat (gm)	Polyunsaturated Fat (gm)	Vitamin D (mg)	Vitamin K (mg)	Vitamin E (mg)	Vitamin A (re)	Vitamin C (mg)	Thiamin (mg)	Riboflavin (mg)	Niacin (mg)	Vitamin B_6 (mg)	Folate (mg)	Vitamin B_{12} (mcg)	Calcium (mg)	Iron (mg)	Magnesium (mg)	Phosphorus (mg)	Potassium (mg)	Sodium (mg)	Zinc (mg)
1.00	0.50	0.00	0.00	0.00	0.00	0.00	0.00	0.00	0.00	0.00	0.00	0.00	0.00	0.00	0.00	0.00	200.00	90.00	0.00
1.50	0.50	0.00	0.00	0.00	0.00	0.00	0.00	0.00	0.00	0.00	0.00	0.00	0.00	0.00	0.00	0.00	110.00	90.00	0.00
0.50	1.00	0.00	0.00	0.00	0.00	0.00	0.00	0.00	0.00	0.00	0.00	0.00	0.00	0.00	0.00	0.00	145.00	90.00	0.00
0.00	0.00	0.00	0.00	0.00	0.00	0.00	0.00	0.00	0.00	0.00	0.00	0.00	0.00	0.00	0.00	0.00	0.00	80.00	0.00
0.00	0.00	0.00	0.00	0.00	0.00	0.00	0.00	0.00	0.00	0.00	0.00	0.00	0.00	0.00	0.00	0.00	0.00	80.00	0.00
0.00	0.00	0.00	0.00	0.00	0.00	0.00	0.00	0.00	0.00	0.00	0.00	0.00	0.00	0.00	0.00	0.00	0.00	80.00	0.00
0.00	0.00	0.00	0.00	0.00	0.00	0.00	0.00	0.00	0.00	0.00	0.00	0.00	0.00	0.00	0.00	0.00	0.00	80.00	0.00
1.00	1.00	0.00	0.00	0.00	0.00	0.00	0.00	0.00	0.00	0.00	0.00	0.00	0.00	0.00	0.00	0.00	110.00	90.00	0.00
1.50	0.50	0.00	0.00	0.00	0.00	0.00	0.00	0.00	0.00	0.00	0.00	0.00	0.00	0.00	0.00	0.00	145.00	90.00	0.00
1.00	1.00	0.00	0.00	0.00	0.00	0.00	0.00	0.00	0.00	0.00	0.00	0.00	0.00	0.00	0.00	0.00	180.00	120.00	0.00
1.00	1.00	0.00	0.00	0.00	0.00	0.00	0.00	0.00	0.00	0.00	0.00	0.00	0.00	0.00	0.00	0.00	150.00	110.00	0.00
0.00	0.00	0.00	0.00	0.00	0.00	0.00	0.00	0.00	0.00	0.00	0.00	0.00	0.00	0.00	0.00	0.00	40.00	50.00	0.00
0.00	0.00	0.00	0.00	0.00	0.00	0.00	0.00	0.00	0.00	0.00	0.00	0.00	0.00	0.00	0.00	0.00	40.00	50.00	0.00
0.00	0.00	0.00	0.00	0.00	0.00	0.00	0.00	0.00	0.00	0.00	0.00	0.00	0.00	0.00	0.00	0.00	40.00	50.00	0.00
0.00	0.00	0.00	0.00	0.00	0.00	0.00	0.00	0.00	0.00	0.00	0.00	0.00	0.00	0.00	0.00	0.00	40.00	50.00	0.00
0.00	0.00	0.00	0.00	0.00	0.38	15.00	5.00	0.43	1.50	0.40	40.00	2.50	40.00	0.50	16.00	4.50	40.00	80.00	3.75
0.00	0.00	0.00	0.00	0.00	0.38	15.00	1.50	0.40	1.50	0.40	40.00	2.50	40.00	0.50	16.00	4.50	40.00	80.00	3.75
0.00	0.00	0.00	0.00	0.00	0.45	18.00	7.00	0.26	1.20	0.60	100.00	2.50	150.00	0.40	100.00	6.30	100.00	110.00	4.50
0.00	0.00	0.00	0.00	0.00	0.45	18.00	7.00	0.26	1.20	0.60	100.00	2.50	150.00	0.40	100.00	6.30	100.00	120.00	4.50
0.00	0.00	0.00	0.00	0.00	0.45	18.00	7.00	0.26	1.20	0.60	100.00	2.50	150.00	0.40	100.00	6.30	100.00	130.00	4.50
0.00	0.00	0.00	0.00	0.00	0.45	18.00	7.00	0.26	1.20	0.60	100.00	2.50	150.00	0.40	100.00	6.30	100.00	130.00	4.50
0.00	0.00	0.00	0.00	0.00	0.00	0.00	0.00	0.00	0.00	0.00	0.00	0.00	0.00	0.00	0.00	0.00	0.00	90.00	0.00
0.00	0.00	0.00	0.00	0.00	0.00	0.00	0.00	0.00	0.00	0.00	0.00	0.00	0.00	0.00	0.00	0.00	0.00	90.00	0.00
0.00	0.00	0.00	0.00	0.00	0.00	0.00	0.00	0.00	0.00	0.00	0.00	0.00	0.00	0.00	0.00	0.00	0.00	90.00	0.00
0.00	0.00	0.00	0.00	0.00	750.00	9.00	0.15	0.26	3.00	0.30	60.00	0.90	150.00	2.70	0.00	150.00	110.00	40.00	0.60
0.00	0.00	0.00	0.00	0.00	750.00	9.00	0.23	0.26	3.00	0.30	60.00	0.90	150.00	2.70	16.00	150.00	100.00	45.00	0.60
0.00	0.00	0.00	0.00	0.00	0.23	6.00	3.00	0.26	0.90	0.30	60.00	1.00	150.00	0.00	0.00	2.70	150.00	35.00	0.60
0.00	0.00	0.00	0.00	0.00	750.00	27.00	0.45	0.17	10.00	0.60	100.00	2.10	150.00	6.30	100.00	100.00	210.00	110.00	4.50
0.00	0.00	0.00	0.00	0.00	750.00	27.00	0.45	0.17	10.00	0.60	100.00	2.10	150.00	6.30	100.00	100.00	340.00	100.00	4.50
0.00	0.00	0.00	0.00	0.00	750.00	27.00	0.45	0.17	10.00	0.60	100.00	2.10	150.00	6.30	100.00	100.00	220.00	100.00	4.50
0.00	0.00	0.00	0.00	0.00	750.00	27.00	0.45	0.17	10.00	0.60	100.00	2.10	150.00	6.30	100.00	100.00	280.00	130.00	4.50
0.00	0.00	0.00	0.00	0.00	0.45	27.00	10.00	0.17	2.10	0.60	100.00	4.00	150.00	0.50	100.00	100.00	100.00	120.00	4.50
0.00	0.00	0.00	0.00	0.00	750.00	27.00	0.45	0.17	10.00	0.60	100.00	2.10	150.00	6.30	100.00	200.00	210.00	110.00	4.50
0.00	0.00	0.00	0.00	0.00	750.00	27.00	0.45	0.17	10.00	0.60	100.00	2.10	150.00	6.30	100.00	100.00	170.00	130.00	4.50
0.00	0.00	0.00	0.00	0.00	750.00	27.00	0.45	0.17	10.00	0.60	100.00	2.10	150.00	6.30	100.00	100.00	140.00	130.00	4.50
0.00	0.00	0.00	0.00	0.00	2500.00	60.00	0.38	0.43	5.00	0.50	100.00	1.50	250.00	4.50	100.00	250.00	200.00	240.00	3.75
0.00	0.00	0.00	0.00	0.00	2500.00	60.00	0.38	0.43	5.00	0.50	100.00	1.50	250.00	4.50	100.00	250.00	190.00	260.00	3.75
0.00	0.00	0.00	0.00	0.00	2500.00	60.00	0.38	0.43	5.00	0.50	100.00	1.50	250.00	4.50	100.00	250.00	200.00	240.00	3.75
0.00	0.00	0.00	0.00	0.00	1750.00	21.00	0.53	0.60	7.00	0.70	120.00	2.10	400.00	2.70	140.00	350.00	530.00	300.00	2.25
0.00	0.00	0.00	0.00	0.00	1750.00	21.00	0.53	0.60	7.00	0.70	120.00	2.10	400.00	2.70	140.00	350.00	530.00	220.00	2.25
0.00	0.00	0.00	0.00	0.00	1750.00	21.00	0.53	0.60	7.00	0.70	120.00	2.10	400.00	2.70	140.00	350.00	530.00	220.00	2.25
0.00	0.00	0.00	0.00	0.00	1750.00	21.00	0.53	0.60	7.00	0.70	120.00	2.10	400.00	2.70	140.00	350.00	500.00	300.00	2.25
0.00	0.00	0.00	0.00	0.00	1750.00	21.00	0.53	0.60	7.00	0.70	120.00	2.10	400.00	2.70	140.00	350.00	450.00	460.00	2.25
0.00	0.00	0.00	0.00	0.00	1750.00	21.00	0.53	0.60	7.00	0.70	120.00	2.10	400.00	2.70	140.00	350.00	450.00	460.00	2.25
0.00	0.00	2.50	40.00	0.00	0.00	0.00	0.00	0.00	0.00	0.00	0.00	0.00	500.00	0.00	0.00	0.00	0.00	10.00	0.00
0.00	0.00	2.50	40.00	0.00	0.00	0.00	0.00	0.00	0.00	0.00	0.00	0.00	500.00	0.00	0.00	0.00	0.00	10.00	0.00
0.00	0.00	2.50	40.00	0.00	0.00	0.00	0.00	0.00	0.00	0.00	0.00	0.00	500.00	0.00	0.00	0.00	0.00	10.00	0.00
0.00	0.00	0.00	0.00	33.00	0.00	120.00	0.00	0.00	0.00	2.00	400.00	6.00	0.00	0.00	0.00	0.00	0.00	65.00	0.00
0.00	0.00	0.00	0.00	33.00	0.00	120.00	0.00	0.00	0.00	2.00	400.00	6.00	0.00	0.00	0.00	0.00	0.00	80.00	0.00
0.00	0.00	2.50	40.00	0.00	0.00	0.00	0.00	0.00	0.00	2.00	400.00	6.00	330.00	1.80	0.00	66.66	0.00	90.00	15.00
0.00	0.00	2.50	40.00	0.00	0.00	0.00	0.00	0.00	0.00	2.00	400.00	6.00	330.00	1.80	0.00	66.66	0.00	90.00	15.00
0.00	0.00	0.00	0.00	0.00	0.00	60.00	0.00	0.00	0.00	2.00	400.00	6.00	300.00	0.00	0.00	0.00	0.00	15.00	0.00
0.00	0.00	0.00	0.00	0.00	0.00	60.00	0.00	0.00	0.00	2.00	400.00	6.00	300.00	0.00	0.00	0.00	0.00	5.00	0.00
0.00	0.00	0.00	0.00	0.00	0.00	60.00	0.00	0.00	0.00	2.00	400.00	6.00	0.00	0.00	0.00	0.00	0.00	70.00	0.00
0.00	0.00	0.00	0.00	0.00	0.00	60.00	0.00	0.00	0.00	2.00	400.00	6.00	0.00	0.00	0.00	0.00	0.00	70.00	0.00

USDA ID Code	Food Name	Weight in Grams*	Quantity of Units	Unit of Measure	Protein (gm)	Fat (gm)	Carbohydrate (gm)	Kcalories	Caffeine (gm)	Fiber (gm)	Cholesterol (mg)	Saturated Fat (gm)
	Vitamin Supplement, Centrum	1.0000	1.000	Each	0.00	0.00	0.00	0.00	0.00	0.00	0.00	0.00
782	Vitamin Supplement, Maximum One-	2.0000	1.000	Each	0.00	0.00	0.00	0.00	0.00	0.00	0.00	0.00
	Vitamin Supplement, One-A-Day	1.0000	1.000	Each	0.00	0.00	0.00	0.00	0.00	0.00	0.00	0.00
	Vitamin Supplement, StressTab	1.0000	1.000	Each	0.00	0.00	0.00	0.00	0.00	0.00	0.00	0.00
783	Vitamin Supplement, Theragram	2.0000	1.000	Each	0.00	0.00	0.00	0.00	0.00	0.00	0.00	0.00
784	Vitamite	240.0000	1.000	Cup	3.00	5.00	14.00	110.00	0.00	0.00	0.00	1.50
	Apple Butter	282.0000	1.000	Cup	1.10	0.00	120.61	487.86	0.00	4.23	0.00	0.00
	Catsup	240.0000	1.000	Cup	3.65	0.86	65.50	249.60	0.00	3.12	0.00	0.12
	Catsup, Low Sodium	240.0000	1.000	Cup	3.65	0.86	65.50	249.60	0.00	3.12	0.00	0.12
	Gravy, Au Jus, Cnd	149.0000	0.250	Cup	2.86	0.48	5.96	38.14	0.00	0.00	0.00	0.24
	Gravy, Beef, Cnd	233.0000	1.000	Cup	8.74	5.50	11.21	123.49	0.00	0.93	6.99	2.68
	Gravy, Chicken, Cnd	238.0000	1.000	Cup	4.59	13.59	12.90	188.02	0.00	0.95	4.76	3.36
	Gravy, Mushroom, Cnd	238.4000	1.000	Cup	3.00	6.46	13.04	119.20	0.00	0.95	0.00	0.95
	Gravy, Turkey, Cnd	298.0000	0.250	Cup	6.20	5.01	12.16	121.58	0.00	0.95	4.77	1.48
	Gravy, Unspecified Type	298.0000	0.250	Cup	3.22	1.99	14.38	86.26	0.00	0.00	0.00	0.71
	Honey	339.0000	1.000	Cup	1.02	0.00	279.34	1030.56	0.00	0.68	0.00	0.00
	Jams and Preserves	20.0000	1.000	Tbsp	0.07	0.01	13.77	55.60	0.00	0.22	0.00	0.00
	Jellies	300.0000	1.000	Cup	0.60	0.09	211.41	849.00	0.00	3.00	0.00	0.06
	Marmalade, Orange	320.0000	1.000	Cup	0.96	0.00	212.16	787.20	0.00	0.64	0.00	0.00
	Mustard	5.0000	1.000	Tbsp	0.00	0.00	0.00	0.00	0.00	0.00	0.00	0.00
	Relish, Pickle, Hamburger	15.0000	1.000	Tbsp	0.09	0.08	5.17	19.35	0.00	0.48	0.00	0.01
	Relish, Pickle, Hot Dog	15.0000	1.000	Tbsp	0.23	0.07	3.50	13.65	0.00	0.23	0.00	0.01
	Relish, Pickle, Sweet	245.0000	1.000	Cup	0.91	1.15	85.87	318.50	0.00	2.70	0.00	0.15
	Salsa	16.5170	2.000	Tbsp	0.00	0.00	2.50	10.01	0.00	0.00	0.00	0.00
	Salt Substitute	4.8000	0.250	Tsp	0.00	0.00	0.00	0.00	0.00	0.00	0.00	0.00
	Salt, Table	292.0000	1.000	Cup	0.00	0.00	0.00	0.00	0.00	0.00	0.00	0.00
	Sauce, A-1 Steak	31.3000	2.000	Tbsp	0.00	0.01	5.00	19.00	0.00	0.50	0.00	0.00
	Sauce, Barbecue	250.0000	1.000	Cup	4.50	4.50	32.00	187.50	0.00	3.00	0.00	0.68
	Sauce, Marinara	250.0000	0.500	Cup	4.00	8.37	25.45	170.00	0.00	0.00	0.00	1.20
	Sauce, Mustard, Chinese	15.0000	1.000	Tbsp	1.00	1.00	1.00	11.00	0.00	0.40	0.00	0.00
	Sauce, Soy (Tamari)	18.0000	1.000	Tbsp	0.93	0.01	1.53	9.54	0.00	0.00	0.00	0.00
	Sauce, Spaghetti	249.0000	0.500	Cup	4.53	11.88	39.67	271.41	0.00	8.47	0.00	1.70
	Sauce, Spaghetti, w/ Garlic & He	113.0000	1.000	Cup	2.00	0.59	9.00	40.00	0.00	0.00	0.00	0.00
	Sauce, Spaghetti-Prego	146.0000	1.000	Cup	3.56	4.15	26.11	154.31	0.00	3.56	0.00	1.19
	Sauce, Spaghetti-Ragu	146.0000	1.000	Cup	3.56	4.75	20.18	130.57	0.00	3.56	0.00	1.78
	Sauce, Teriyaki	288.0000	1.000	Cup	17.08	0.00	45.94	241.92	0.00	0.29	0.00	0.00
	Sauce, White	263.8000	0.500	Cup	10.21	13.45	21.39	240.06	0.00	0.00	34.29	6.41
	Sauce, Worcestershire	34.0000	2.000	Tbsp	0.00	0.00	6.00	23.00	0.00	0.00	0.00	0.00
	Sugar, Brown	220.0000	1.000	Cup	0.00	0.00	214.06	827.20	0.00	0.00	0.00	0.00
	Sugar, Granulated	200.0000	1.000	Cup	0.00	0.00	199.80	774.00	0.00	0.00	0.00	0.00
	Sugar, Powdered	120.0000	1.000	Cup	0.00	0.12	119.40	466.80	0.00	0.00	0.00	0.02
	Syrup, Corn, Dark	328.0000	1.000	Cup	0.00	0.00	251.25	924.96	0.00	0.00	0.00	0.00
	Syrup, Corn, High-fructose	310.0000	1.000	Cup	0.00	0.00	235.60	871.10	0.00	0.00	0.00	0.00
	Syrup, Corn, Light	328.0000	1.000	Cup	0.00	0.00	251.25	924.96	0.00	0.00	0.00	0.00
	Syrup, Malt	384.0000	1.000	Cup	23.81	0.00	273.79	1221.12	0.00	0.00	0.00	0.00
	Syrup, Maple	315.0000	1.000	Cup	0.00	0.63	211.68	825.30	0.00	0.00	0.00	0.13
	Syrup, Pancake, Lo Cal	240.0000	1.000	Cup	0.00	0.00	106.32	393.60	0.00	0.00	0.00	0.00
	Syrup, Pancake, w/ 2% Maple	315.0000	1.000	Cup	0.00	0.32	219.24	834.75	0.00	0.00	0.00	0.06
	Syrup, Pancake, w/ Butter	315.0000	1.000	Cup	0.00	5.04	233.42	932.40	0.00	0.00	12.60	3.18
	Toppings, Butterscotch or Carame	41.0000	2.000	Tbsp	0.62	0.04	27.02	103.32	0.00	0.37	0.41	0.05
	Toppings, Caramel	16.6800	1.000	Tbsp	0.27	0.00	13.01	51.71	0.00	0.00	0.00	0.00
	Toppings, Chocolate	304.0000	1.000	Cup	13.98	27.06	191.22	1064.00	18.24	8.51	6.08	12.10
	Toppings, Fudge, Hot	19.0180	1.000	Tbsp	1.00	2.00	11.01	70.07	0.00	0.00	0.00	0.50
	Toppings, Marshmallow Cream	28.3500	1.000	Ounce	0.23	0.09	22.40	91.29	0.00	0.03	0.00	0.02
	Toppings, Nuts in Syrup	328.0000	1.000	Cup	14.76	72.16	175.15	1338.24	0.00	5.25	0.00	6.43
	Toppings, Pineapple	340.0000	1.000	Cup	0.34	0.34	225.76	860.20	0.00	3.40	0.00	0.07
	Toppings, Strawberry	340.0000	1.000	Cup	0.68	0.34	225.42	863.60	0.00	3.40	0.00	0.03

Monounsaturated Fat (gm)	Polyunsaturated Fat (gm)	Vitamin D (mg)	Vitamin K (mg)	Vitamin E (mg)	Vitamin A (re)	Vitamin C (mg)	Thiamin (mg)	Riboflavin (mg)	Niacin (mg)	Vitamin B_6 (mg)	Folate (mg)	Vitamin B_{12} (mcg)	Calcium (mg)	Iron (mg)	Magnesium (mg)	Phosphorus (mg)	Potassium (mg)	Sodium (mg)	Zinc (mg)
0.00	0.00	5.00	0.00	10.00	1000.00	60.00	1.50	1.70	20.00	2.00	400.00	6.00	162.00	18.00	100.00	109.00	40.00	0.00	15.00
0.00	0.00	0.25	0.00	20.00	1000.00	60.00	1.50	1.70	20.00	2.00	400.00	6.00	130.00	18.00	100.00	0.00	37.50	0.00	15.00
0.00	0.00	5.00	0.00	10.00	1000.00	60.00	1.50	1.70	20.00	2.00	400.00	6.00	0.00	0.00	0.00	0.00	0.00	0.00	0.00
0.00	0.00	0.00	0.00	10.00	0.00	500.00	10.00	0.00	100.00	5.00	400.00	12.00	0.00	18.00	0.00	0.00	0.00	0.00	0.00
0.00	0.00	0.25	0.00	20.00	1100.00	120.00	3.00	3.40	30.00	3.00	400.00	9.00	40.00	27.00	100.00	0.00	7.50	0.00	15.00
0.00	0.00	0.00	0.00	0.00	0.00	0.00	0.00	0.00	0.00	0.00	0.00	0.00	0.00	0.00	0.00	0.00	110.00	120.00	0.00
0.00	0.00	0.00	0.00	0.03	33.84	1.97	0.06	0.06	0.31	0.14	2.82	0.00	39.48	0.87	14.10	28.20	256.62	11.28	0.17
0.14	0.36	0.00	0.00	3.53	244.80	36.24	0.22	0.17	3.29	0.43	36.00	0.00	45.60	1.68	52.80	93.60	1154.40	2846.40	0.55
0.14	0.36	0.00	0.00	3.53	244.80	36.24	0.22	0.17	3.29	0.43	36.00	0.00	45.60	1.68	52.80	93.60	1154.40	48.00	0.55
0.19	0.02	0.00	0.00	0.00	0.00	2.38	0.05	0.14	2.15	0.02	4.77	0.24	9.54	1.43	4.77	71.52	193.10	119.20	2.38
2.24	0.19	0.00	0.00	0.14	0.00	0.00	0.07	0.09	1.54	0.02	4.66	0.23	13.98	1.63	4.66	69.90	188.73	1304.80	2.33
6.07	3.57	0.00	0.00	0.38	264.18	0.00	0.05	0.10	1.05	0.02	4.76	0.24	47.60	1.12	4.76	69.02	259.42	1373.26	1.90
2.79	2.43	0.00	0.00	0.00	0.00	0.00	0.07	0.14	1.60	0.05	28.61	0.00	16.69	1.57	4.77	35.76	252.70	1358.88	1.67
2.15	1.17	0.00	0.00	0.14	0.00	0.00	0.05	0.19	3.10	0.02	4.77	0.24	9.54	1.67	4.77	69.14	259.86	1375.57	1.91
0.78	0.39	0.00	0.00	0.00	0.00	1.83	0.05	0.11	0.78	0.03	3.40	0.18	36.60	0.26	10.46	49.67	65.35	1422.02	0.26
0.00	0.00	0.00	0.00	0.00	0.00	1.70	0.00	0.14	0.41	0.07	6.78	0.00	20.34	1.42	6.78	13.56	176.28	13.56	0.75
0.01	0.00	0.00	0.00	0.00	0.20	1.76	0.00	0.00	0.01	0.00	6.60	0.00	4.00	0.10	0.80	2.20	15.40	6.40	0.01
0.03	0.06	0.00	0.00	0.00	6.00	2.70	0.00	0.09	0.12	0.06	3.00	0.00	24.00	0.60	18.00	15.00	192.00	84.00	0.12
0.00	0.00	0.00	0.00	0.00	16.00	15.36	0.03	0.03	0.16	0.03	115.20	0.00	121.60	0.48	6.40	19.20	118.40	179.20	0.13
0.00	0.00	0.00	0.00	0.00	0.00	0.00	0.00	0.00	0.00	0.00	0.00	0.00	0.00	0.00	0.00	0.00	0.00	75.00	0.00
0.04	0.02	0.00	0.00	0.00	4.05	0.35	0.00	0.01	0.09	0.00	0.15	0.00	0.60	0.17	1.05	2.55	11.40	164.40	0.02
0.03	0.02	0.00	0.00	0.00	2.55	0.15	0.01	0.01	0.08	0.00	0.15	0.00	0.75	0.19	2.85	6.00	11.70	163.65	0.03
0.51	0.29	0.00	0.00	0.10	39.20	2.45	0.00	0.07	0.56	0.05	2.45	0.00	7.35	2.13	12.25	34.30	61.25	1986.95	0.34
0.00	0.00	0.00	0.00	0.00	40.04	1.80	0.00	0.00	0.00	0.00	0.00	0.00	0.00	0.00	0.00	0.00	0.00	120.12	0.00
0.00	0.00	0.00	0.00	0.00	0.00	0.00	0.00	0.00	0.00	0.00	0.00	0.00	0.00	0.00	0.00	0.00	2440.00	0.00	0.00
0.00	0.00	0.00	0.00	0.00	0.00	0.00	0.00	0.00	0.00	0.00	0.00	0.00	70.08	0.96	2.92	0.00	23.36	113173.36	0.29
0.00	0.00	0.00	0.00	0.00	32.00	4.80	0.00	0.00	0.00	0.00	0.00	0.00	12.00	0.30	0.00	0.00	0.00	454.00	0.00
1.93	1.70	0.00	0.00	2.78	217.50	17.50	0.08	0.05	2.25	0.20	10.00	0.00	47.50	2.25	45.00	50.00	435.00	2037.50	0.50
4.28	2.29	0.00	0.00	0.00	240.00	32.00	0.11	0.15	3.97	0.62	33.75	0.00	45.00	2.00	60.00	87.50	1060.00	1572.50	0.67
0.00	0.00	0.00	0.00	0.00	0.00	0.00	0.00	0.00	0.00	0.00	0.00	0.00	12.00	0.30	0.00	0.00	0.00	188.00	0.00
0.00	0.01	0.00	0.00	0.00	0.00	0.00	0.01	0.02	0.60	0.03	2.79	0.00	3.06	0.36	6.12	19.80	32.40	1028.70	0.07
6.07	3.25	0.00	0.00	6.22	306.27	27.89	0.14	0.15	3.75	0.88	53.78	0.00	69.72	1.62	59.76	89.64	956.16	1235.04	0.52
0.00	0.00	0.00	0.00	0.00	56.00	18.00	0.00	0.00	0.00	0.00	0.00	0.00	24.00	0.80	0.00	0.00	0.00	390.00	0.00
0.00	0.00	0.00	0.00	0.00	356.10	21.37	0.00	0.00	0.00	0.00	0.00	0.00	85.46	0.71	0.00	0.00	0.00	724.07	0.00
0.00	0.00	0.00	0.00	0.00	178.05	1.42	0.00	0.00	0.00	0.00	0.00	0.00	56.98	0.71	0.00	0.00	0.00	652.85	0.00
0.00	0.00	0.00	0.00	0.00	0.00	0.00	0.09	0.20	3.66	0.29	57.60	0.00	72.00	4.90	175.68	443.52	648.00	11039.04	0.29
4.70	1.69	0.00	0.00	0.00	92.33	2.64	0.08	0.45	0.53	0.07	15.83	1.06	424.72	0.26	263.80	255.89	443.18	796.68	0.55
0.00	0.00	0.00	0.00	0.00	0.00	4.20	0.00	0.00	0.00	0.00	0.00	0.00	43.00	1.50	0.00	0.00	0.00	333.00	0.00
0.00	0.00	0.00	0.00	0.00	0.00	0.00	0.02	0.02	0.18	0.07	2.20	0.00	187.00	4.20	63.80	48.40	761.20	85.80	0.40
0.00	0.00	0.00	0.00	0.00	0.00	0.00	0.00	0.04	0.00	0.00	0.00	0.00	2.00	0.12	0.00	4.00	4.00	2.00	0.06
0.04	0.06	0.00	0.00	0.00	0.00	0.00	0.00	0.00	0.00	0.00	0.00	0.00	1.20	0.07	0.00	2.40	2.40	1.20	0.04
0.00	0.00	0.00	0.00	0.00	0.00	0.00	0.03	0.03	0.07	0.03	0.00	0.00	59.04	1.21	26.24	36.08	144.32	508.40	0.13
0.00	0.00	0.00	0.00	0.00	0.00	0.00	0.00	0.06	0.00	0.00	0.00	0.00	0.00	0.09	0.00	0.00	0.00	6.20	0.06
0.00	0.00	0.00	0.00	0.00	0.00	0.00	0.03	0.03	0.07	0.03	0.00	0.00	9.84	0.16	6.56	6.56	13.12	396.88	0.07
0.00	0.00	0.00	0.00	0.00	0.00	0.00	0.04	1.50	31.18	1.92	46.08	0.00	234.24	3.69	276.48	906.24	1228.80	134.40	0.54
0.19	0.32	0.00	0.00	0.00	0.00	0.00	0.03	0.03	0.09	0.00	0.00	0.00	211.05	3.78	44.10	6.30	642.60	28.35	13.10
0.00	0.00	0.00	0.00	0.00	0.00	0.00	0.02	0.02	0.05	0.00	0.00	0.00	2.40	0.05	0.00	103.20	7.20	480.00	0.05
0.09	0.16	0.00	0.00	0.00	0.00	0.00	0.03	0.06	0.06	0.00	0.00	0.00	15.75	0.22	6.30	31.50	18.90	192.15	0.72
1.48	0.19	0.00	0.00	0.09	47.25	0.00	0.03	0.03	0.06	0.00	0.00	0.00	6.30	0.28	6.30	31.50	9.45	308.70	0.13
0.01	0.00	0.00	0.00	0.00	11.07	0.12	0.00	0.04	0.02	0.00	0.82	0.04	21.73	0.08	2.87	19.27	34.44	143.09	0.08
0.00	0.00	0.00	0.00	0.00	0.00	0.00	0.00	0.00	0.00	0.00	0.00	0.00	2.34	0.00	0.00	4.67	5.67	11.01	0.03
11.73	0.85	0.00	0.00	8.88	12.16	0.61	0.18	0.67	0.91	0.18	12.16	0.64	246.24	3.95	155.04	410.40	1100.48	1051.84	2.07
0.00	0.00	0.00	0.00	0.00	0.00	0.00	0.00	0.00	0.00	0.00	0.00	0.00	36.03	0.20	0.00	0.00	0.00	35.03	0.00
0.02	0.01	0.00	0.00	0.00	0.00	0.00	0.00	0.00	0.02	0.00	0.28	0.00	0.85	0.06	0.57	2.27	1.42	13.89	0.01
16.30	45.03	0.00	0.00	2.85	13.12	3.61	0.59	0.39	1.34	0.62	68.88	0.00	131.20	3.44	206.64	364.08	685.52	137.76	3.41
0.10	0.17	0.00	0.00	0.00	6.80	199.24	0.10	0.03	0.31	0.07	10.20	0.00	74.80	1.63	6.80	27.20	1077.80	214.20	1.63
0.03	0.17	0.00	0.00	0.48	6.80	84.66	0.03	0.07	0.85	0.07	6.80	0.00	81.60	3.30	13.60	44.20	248.20	71.40	1.67

Appendix

B Amino Acid Content of Foods, 100 g, Edible Portion

Protein Content and Nitrogen Conversion Factor	Tryptophan (g)	Threonine (g)	Isoleucine (g)	Leucine (g)	Lysine (g)	Methionine (g)	Cystine (g)	Phenylalanine (g)	Tyrosine (g)	Valine (g)	Arginine (g)	Histidine (g)
Milk, Milk Products												
Milk (Protein, N × 6.38)												
Cow												
Fluid, whole and nonfat (3.5% protein)	0.049	0.161	0.223	0.344	0.272	0.086	0.031	0.170	0.178	0.240	0.128	0.092
Canned												
Evaporated, unsweetened (7.0% protein)	0.099	0.323	0.447	0.688	0.545	0.171	0.063	0.340	0.357	0.481	0.256	0.185
Condensed, sweetened (8.1% protein)	0.114	0.374	0.518	0.796	0.631	0.198	0.072	0.393	0.413	0.557	0.296	0.214
Dried												
Whole (25.8% protein)	0.364	1.191	1.648	2.535	2.009	0.632	0.231	1.251	1.316	1.774	0.944	0.680
Nonfat (35.6% protein)	0.502	1.641	2.271	3.493	2.768	0.870	0.318	1.724	1.814	2.444	1.300	0.937
Goat (3.3% protein)	0.039	0.217	0.087	0.278	0.312	0.065	—	0.121	—	0.139	0.174	0.068
Human (1.4% protein)	0.023	0.062	0.075	0.124	0.090	0.028	0.027	0.060	0.071	0.086	0.055	0.030
Milk Products												
Buttermilk (3.5% protein, N × 6.38)	0.038	0.165	0.219	0.346	0.291	0.082	0.032	0.186	0.137	0.262	0.168	0.099
Casein (100% protein, N × 6.29)	1.335	4.277	6.550	10.048	8.013	3.084	0.382	5.389	5.819	7.393	4.070	3.021
Cheese (protein, N × 6.38)												
Blue mold (21.5% protein)	0.293	0.799	1.449	2.096	1.577	0.559	0.121	1.153	1.028	1.543	0.785	0.701
Camembert (17.5% protein)	0.239	0.650	1.179	1.706	1.284	0.455	0.099	0.938	0.837	1.256	0.639	0.571
Cheddar processed (23.2% protein)	0.316	0.862	1.563	2.262	1.702	0.604	0.131	1.244	1.109	1.665	0.847	0.756
Cheese foods, Cheddar (20.5% protein)	0.280	0.761	1.382	1.998	1.504	0.533	0.116	1.099	0.980	1.472	0.749	0.668
Cottage (17.0% protein)	0.179	0.794	0.989	1.826	1.428	0.469	0.147	0.917	0.917	0.978	0.802	0.549
Cream cheese (9.0% protein)	0.080	0.408	0.519	0.923	0.721	0.229	0.085	0.547	0.408	0.538	0.313	0.278
Limburger (21.2% protein)	0.289	0.788	1.429	2.067	1.555	0.552	0.120	1.136	1.014	1.522	0.774	0.691

Protein Content and Nitrogen Conversion Factor	Tryptophan (g)	Threonine (g)	Isoleucine (g)	Leucine (g)	Lysine (g)	Methionine (g)	Cystine (g)	Phenylalanine (g)	Tyrosine (g)	Valine (g)	Arginine (g)	Histidine (g)
Milk, Milk Products—cont'd												
Cheese—cont'd												
Parmesan (36.0% protein)	0.491	1.337	2.426	3.510	2.641	0.937	0.203	1.930	1.721	2.584	1.315	1.174
Swiss (27.5% protein)	0.375	1.021	1.853	2.681	2.017	0.715	0.155	1.474	1.315	1.974	1.004	0.896
Swiss processed (26.4% protein)	0.360	0.981	1.779	2.574	1.937	0.687	0.149	1.415	1.262	1.895	0.964	0.861
Eggs, Chicken (Protein, N × 6.25)												
Fresh or Stored												
Whole (12.8% protein)	0.211	0.637	0.850	1.126	0.819	0.401	0.299	0.739	0.551	0.950	0.840	0.307
Whites (10.8% protein)	0.164	0.477	0.698	0.950	0.648	0.420	0.263	0.689	0.449	0.842	0.634	0.233
Yolks (16.3% protein)	0.235	0.827	0.996	1.372	1.074	0.417	0.274	0.717	0.756	1.121	1.132	0.368
Dried												
Whole (46.8% protein)	0.771	2.329	3.108	4.118	2.995	1.468	1.093	2.703	2.014	3.474	3.070	1.123
Whites (85.9% protein)	1.306	3.793	5.553	7.559	5.154	3.340	3.089	5.484	3.573	6.693	5.044	1.855
Yolks (31.2% protein)	0.449	1.582	1.907	2.626	2.057	0.799	0.524	1.373	1.448	2.147	2.167	0.704
Meat, Poultry, Fish, and Shellfish (Their Products)												
Meat (Protein, N × 6.25)												
Beef cuts, medium fat												
Chuck (18.6% protein)	0.217	0.821	0.973	1.524	1.625	0.461	0.235	0.765	0.631	1.033	1.199	0.646
Flank (19.9% protein)	0.232	0.879	1.041	1.630	1.738	0.494	0.252	0.818	0.675	1.105	1.283	0.691
Hamburger (16.0% protein)	0.187	0.707	0.837	1.311	1.398	0.397	0.202	0.658	0.543	0.888	1.032	0.556
Porterhouse (16.4% protein)	0.192	0.724	0.858	1.343	1.433	0.407	0.207	0.674	0.556	0.911	1.057	0.569
Rib roast (17.4% protein)	0.203	0.768	0.910	1.425	1.520	0.432	0.220	0.715	0.590	0.966	1.122	0.604
Round (19.5% protein)	0.228	0.861	1.020	1.597	1.704	0.484	0.246	0.802	0.661	1.083	1.257	0.677
Rump (16.2% protein)	0.189	0.715	0.848	1.327	1.415	0.402	0.205	0.666	0.550	0.899	1.045	0.562
Sirloin (17.3% protein)	0.202	0.764	0.905	1.417	1.511	0.429	0.219	0.711	0.587	0.960	1.116	0.601
Beef, canned (25.0% protein)	0.292	1.104	1.308	2.048	2.184	0.620	0.316	1.028	0.848	1.388	1.612	0.868
Beef, dried or chipped (34.3% protein)	0.401	1.515	1.795	2.810	2.996	0.851	0.434	1.410	1.163	1.904	2.212	1.191
Lamb cuts, medium fat												
Leg (18.0% protein)	0.233	0.824	0.933	1.394	1.457	0.432	0.236	0.732	0.625	0.887	1.172	0.501
Rib (14.9% protein)	0.193	0.682	0.772	1.154	1.206	0.358	0.195	0.606	0.517	0.734	0.970	0.415
Shoulder (15.6% protein)	0.202	0.714	0.809	1.208	1.263	0.374	0.205	0.634	0.542	0.769	1.016	0.434
Pork cuts, medium fat, fresh												
Ham (15.2% protein)	0.197	0.705	0.781	1.119	1.248	0.379	0.178	0.598	0.542	0.790	0.931	0.525
Loin (16.4% protein)	0.213	0.761	0.842	1.207	1.346	0.409	0.192	0.646	0.585	0.853	1.005	0.567
Miscellaneous lean cuts (14.5% protein)	0.188	0.673	0.745	1.067	1.190	0.362	0.169	0.571	0.517	0.754	0.889	0.501
Pork, cured												
Bacon, medium fat (9.1% protein)	0.095	0.306	0.399	0.728	0.587	0.141	0.106	0.434	0.234	0.434	0.622	0.246
Fat back or salt pork (3.9% protein)	0.006	0.141	0.110	0.367	0.317	0.055	0.043	0.157	0.052	0.168	0.379	0.035
Ham (16.9% protein)	0.162	0.692	0.841	1.306	1.420	0.411	0.273	0.646	0.652	0.879	1.068	0.544
Luncheon meat												
Boiled ham (22.8% protein)	0.219	0.934	1.135	1.762	1.915	0.554	0.368	0.872	0.879	1.186	1.441	0.733
Canned, spiced (14.9% protein)	0.143	0.610	0.741	1.161	1.252	0.362	0.241	0.570	0.575	0.775	0.942	0.479

Protein Content and Nitrogen Conversion Factor	Trypto-phan (g)	Threo-nine (g)	Iso-leucine (g)	Leucine (g)	Lysine (g)	Methi-onine (g)	Cystine (g)	Phenyl-alanine (g)	Tyro-sine (g)	Valine (g)	Argi-nine (g)	Histi-dine (g)
Meat, Poultry, Fish, and Shellfish (Their Products)—cont'd												
Meat (Protein, N × 6.25)—cont'd												
Rabbit, domesticated, flesh only (21.9% protein)	—	1.021	1.082	1.636	1.818	0.541	—	0.793	—	1.021	1.176	0.474
Veal cuts, medium fat												
Round (19.5% protein)	0.256	0.846	1.030	1.429	1.629	0.446	0.231	0.792	0.702	1.008	1.270	0.627
Shoulder (19.4% protein)	0.255	0.841	1.024	1.422	1.620	0.444	0.230	0.788	0.698	1.003	1.263	0.624
Stew meat (18.3% protein)	0.240	0.793	0.966	1.341	1.528	0.419	0.217	0.744	0.659	0.946	1.192	0.589
Poultry (Protein, N × 6.25)												
Chicken, flesh only												
Broilers or fryers (20.6% protein)	0.250	0.877	1.088	1.490	1.810	0.537	0.277	0.811	0.725	1.012	1.302	0.593
Hens (21.3% protein)	0.259	0.907	1.125	1.540	1.871	0.556	0.286	0.838	0.750	1.046	1.346	0.613
Ducks, domesticated, flesh only (21.4% protein)	—	0.935	1.109	1.657	1.842	0.531	—	0.842	—	1.027	1.301	0.486
Turkey, flesh only (24.0% protein)	—	1.014	1.260	1.836	2.173	0.664	0.330	0.960	—	1.187	1.513	0.649
Fish and Shellfish (Protein, N × 6.25)												
Bluefish (20.5% protein)	0.203	0.889	1.040	1.548	1.797	0.597	0.276	0.761	0.554	1.092	1.155	—
Cod												
Fresh (16.5% protein)	0.164	0.715	0.837	1.246	1.447	0.480	0.222	0.612	0.446	0.879	0.929	—
Dried (81.8% protein)	0.811	3.547	4.149	6.178	7.172	2.382	1.099	3.036	2.212	4.358	4.607	—
Croaker (17.8% protein)	0.177	0.772	0.903	1.344	1.561	0.518	0.239	0.661	0.481	0.948	1.002	—
Eel (18.6% protein)	0.185	0.806	0.943	1.405	1.631	0.542	0.250	0.690	0.503	0.991	1.048	—
Flounder (14.9% protein)	0.148	0.646	0.756	1.125	1.306	0.434	0.200	0.553	0.403	0.794	0.839	—
Haddock (18.2% protein)	0.181	0.789	0.923	1.374	1.596	0.530	0.245	0.676	0.492	0.970	1.025	—
Halibut (18.6% protein)	0.185	0.806	0.943	1.405	1.631	0.542	0.250	0.690	0.503	0.991	1.048	—
Herring												
Atlantic (18.3% protein)	0.182	0.793	0.928	1.382	1.605	0.533	0.246	0.679	0.495	0.975	1.031	—
Mackerel, canned, solids and liquid												
Pacific (21.1% protein)	0.209	0.915	1.070	1.593	1.850	0.614	0.284	0.783	0.571	1.124	1.118	—
Salmon												
Raw, Pacific (Chinook or King) (17.4% protein)	0.173	0.754	0.883	1.314	1.526	0.507	0.234	0.646	0.470	0.927	0.980	—
Canned, solids and liquid (sockeye or red) (20.2% protein)	0.200	0.876	1.025	1.526	1.771	0.588	0.271	0.750	0.546	1.076	1.138	—
Sardines, canned, solids and liquid												
Atlantic type (21.1% protein)	0.209	0.915	1.070	1.593	1.850	0.614	0.284	0.783	0.571	1.124	1.188	—
Shrimp, canned, solids and liquid (18.7% protein)	0.186	0.811	0.948	1.412	1.640	0.545	0.251	0.694	0.506	0.996	1.053	—
Products From Meat, Poultry, and Fish (Protein, N × 6.25)												
Brains (10.4% protein)	0.138	0.494	0.504	0.845	0.760	0.220	0.145	0.506	0.433	0.536	0.614	0.278
Chitterlings (8.6% protein)	0.094	0.398	0.308	0.457	0.670	0.193	0.109	0.359	0.228	0.462	1.406	0.169
Gizzard, chicken (23.1% protein)	0.207	1.072	1.094	1.689	1.567	0.554	0.218	0.968	0.680	1.116	1.741	0.480
Heart												
Beef or pork (16.9% protein)	0.219	0.776	0.857	1.509	1.387	0.403	0.168	0.765	0.627	0.973	1.068	0.433

Protein Content and Nitrogen Conversion Factor	Trypto-phan (g)	Threo-nine (g)	Iso-leucine (g)	Leucine (g)	Lysine (g)	Methi-onine (g)	Cystine (g)	Phenyl-alanine (g)	Tyro-sine (g)	Valine (g)	Argi-nine (g)	Histi-dine (g)
Meat, Poultry, Fish, and Shellfish (Their Products)—cont'd												
Products From Meat, Poultry, and Fish (Protein, N × 6.25)—cont'd												
Kidney												
Beef (15.0% protein)	0.221	0.665	0.730	1.301	1.087	0.307	0.182	0.706	0.557	0.876	0.934	0.377
Liver												
Beef or pork (19.7% protein)	0.296	0.936	1.031	1.819	1.475	0.463	0.243	0.993	0.738	1.239	1.201	0.523
Calf (19.0% protein)	0.286	0.903	0.994	1.754	1.423	0.447	0.234	0.958	0.711	1.195	1.158	0.505
Chicken (22.1% protein)	0.332	1.050	1.156	2.040	1.655	0.520	0.272	1.114	0.827	1.390	1.347	0.587
Sausage												
Bologna (14.8% protein)	0.126	0.606	0.718	1.061	1.191	0.313	0.185	0.540	0.481	0.744	1.028	0.398
Braunschweiger (15.4% protein)	0.172	0.668	0.754	1.291	1.200	0.320	0.187	0.700	0.471	0.956	0.954	0.458
Frankfurters (14.2% protein)	0.120	0.582	0.688	1.018	1.143	0.300	0.177	0.518	0.461	0.713	0.986	0.382
Head cheese (15.0% protein)	0.079	0.418	0.509	0.946	0.907	0.250	0.209	0.569	0.569	0.617	1.075	0.278
Liverwurst (16.7% protein)	0.187	0.724	0.818	1.400	1.301	0.347	0.203	0.759	0.510	1.037	1.034	0.497
Pork, links or bulk, raw (10.8% protein)	0.092	0.442	0.524	0.774	0.869	0.228	0.135	0.394	0.351	0.543	0.750	0.290
Salami (23.9% protein)	0.023	0.979	1.159	1.713	1.923	0.505	0.298	0.872	0.776	1.201	1.660	0.642
Vienna sausage, canned (15.8% protein)	0.134	0.647	0.766	1.133	1.272	0.334	0.197	0.576	0.513	0.794	1.097	0.425
Tongue												
Beef (16.4% protein)	0.197	0.708	0.792	1.286	1.364	0.357	0.207	0.661	0.548	0.840	1.065	0.412
Pork (16.8% protein)	0.202	0.726	0.812	1.317	1.398	0.366	0.212	0.677	0.562	0.860	1.091	0.422
Veal and pork loaf, canned (17.2% protein)	0.198	0.627	0.859	1.236	1.258	0.418	0.209	0.619	0.468	0.958	0.916	0.388
Legumes (Dry Seed), Common Nuts, Other Nuts, and Dry Seeds (Their Products)												
Legume Seeds and Their Products												
Beans (*Phaseolus vulgaris*) (Protein, N × 6.25)												
Pinto and red Mexican (23.0% protein)	0.213	0.997	1.306	1.976	1.708	0.232	0.228	1.270	0.887	1.395	1.384	0.655
Red kidney												
Raw (23.1% protein)	0.214	1.002	1.312	1.985	1.715	0.233	0.229	1.275	0.891	1.401	1.390	0.658
Canned, solids and liquid (5.7% protein)	0.053	0.247	0.324	0.490	0.423	0.057	0.057	0.315	0.220	0.346	0.343	0.162
Other common beans, including navy, peabean, white marrow												
Raw (21.4% protein)	0.199	0.928	1.216	1.839	1.589	0.216	0.212	1.181	0.825	1.298	1.287	0.609
Baked with pork, canned (5.8% protein)	0.057	0.274	0.291	0.486	0.354	0.059	0.018	0.333	0.165	0.312	0.251	0.186
Broadbeans, raw (25.4% protein, N × 6.25)	0.236	0.829	1.593	2.211	1.426	0.106	0.179	1.057	0.687	1.276	1.780	0.748

Protein Content and Nitrogen Conversion Factor	Tryptophan (g)	Threonine (g)	Isoleucine (g)	Leucine (g)	Lysine (g)	Methionine (g)	Cystine (g)	Phenylalanine (g)	Tyrosine (g)	Valine (g)	Arginine (g)	Histidine (g)
Legumes (Dry Seed), Common Nuts, Other Nuts, and Dry Seeds (Their Products)—cont'd												
Legume Seeds and Their Products—cont'd												
Chickpeas (20.8% protein, N × 6.25)	0.170	0.739	1.195	1.538	1.434	0.276	0.296	1.012	0.692	1.025	1.551	0.559
Cowpeas (22.9% protein, N × 6.25)	0.220	0.901	1.110	1.715	1.491	0.352	0.297	1.198	0.678	1.293	1.473	0.692
Lentils, whole (25.0% protein, N × 6.25)	0.216	0.896	1.316	1.760	1.528	0.180	0.294	1.104	0.664	1.360	1.908	0.548
Lima beans (20.7% protein, N × 6.25)	0.195	0.980	1.199	1.722	1.378	0.331	0.311	1.222	0.543	1.298	1.315	0.669
Lupine (32.3% protein, N × 6.25)	—	1.101	1.618	1.964	1.447	0.114	—	1.271	—	1.328	2.718	0.811
Mung beans (24.4% protein, N × 6.25)	0.180	0.765	1.351	2.202	1.667	0.265	0.152	1.167	0.390	1.444	1.370	0.543
Peas *(Pisum sativum)* (protein, N × 6.25)												
Entire seeds (23.8% protein)	0.251	0.918	1.340	1.969	1.744	0.286	0.308	1.200	0.960	1.333	2.102	0.651
Split (24.5% protein)	0.259	0.945	1.380	2.027	1.795	0.294	0.318	1.235	0.988	1.372	2.164	0.670
Soybeans, whole (34.9% protein, N × 5.71)	0.526	1.504	2.054	2.946	2.414	0.513	0.678	1.889	1.216	2.005	2.763	0.911
Soybean flour, flakes, and grits (protein, N × 5.71)												
Low fat (44.7% protein)	0.673	1.926	2.630	3.773	3.092	0.658	0.869	2.419	1.558	2.568	3.538	1.166
Medium fat (42.5% protein)	0.640	1.831	2.501	3.588	2.940	0.625	0.826	2.300	1.481	2.441	3.364	1.109
Full fat (35.9% protein)	0.541	1.547	2.112	3.030	2.483	0.528	0.698	1.943	1.251	2.062	2.842	0.937
Soybean curd (7.0% protein, N × 5.71)	—	—	—	—	—	0.081	0.091	—	—	—	—	—
Soybean milk (3.4% protein, N × 5.71)	0.051	0.176	0.175	0.305	0.269	0.054	0.071	0.195	0.193	0.186	0.302	0.121
Common Nuts and Their Products												
Almonds (18.6% protein, N × 5.18)	0.176	0.610	0.873	1.454	0.582	0.259	0.377	1.146	0.618	1.124	2.729	0.517
Brazil nuts (14.4% protein, N × 5.46)	0.187	0.422	0.593	1.129	0.443	0.941	0.504	0.617	0.483	0.823	2.247	0.367
Cashews (18.5% protein, N × 5.30)	0.471	0.737	1.222	1.522	0.792	0.353	0.527	0.946	0.712	1.592	2.098	0.415
Coconut (3.4% protein, N × 5.30)	0.033	0.129	0.180	0.269	0.152	0.071	0.062	0.174	0.101	0.212	0.486	0.069
Coconut meal (20.3% protein, N × 5.30)	0.199	0.770	1.076	1.605	0.908	0.421	0.372	1.038	0.605	1.268	2.899	0.414
Filberts (12.7% protein, N × 5.30)	0.211	0.415	0.853	0.939	0.417	0.139	0.165	0.537	0.434	0.934	2.171	0.288
Peanuts (26.9% protein, N × 5.46)	0.340	0.828	1.266	1.872	1.099	0.271	0.463	1.557	1.104	1.532	3.296	0.749
Pecans (9.4% protein, N × 5.30)	0.138	0.389	0.553	0.773	0.435	0.153	0.216	0.564	0.316	0.525	1.185	0.273
Walnuts (15.0% protein, N × 5.30)	0.175	0.589	0.767	1.228	0.441	0.306	0.320	0.767	0.583	0.974	2.287	0.405

Protein Content and Nitrogen Conversion Factor	Tryptophan (g)	Threonine (g)	Isoleucine (g)	Leucine (g)	Lysine (g)	Methionine (g)	Cystine (g)	Phenylalanine (g)	Tyrosine (g)	Valine (g)	Arginine (g)	Histidine (g)
Legumes (Dry Seed), Common Nuts, Other Nuts, and Dry Seeds (Their Products)—cont'd												
Other Nuts and Seeds and Their Products (Protien N × 5.30)												
Acorns (10.4% protein)	0.126	0.434	0.561	0.808	0.636	0.139	0.184	0.473	—	0.718	0.722	0.251
Amaranth (14.6% protein)	0.149	0.832	0.882	1.209	1.074	0.372	0.521	1.141	—	0.849	1.747	0.441
Cottonseed flour and meal (42.3% protein)	0.591	1.764	1.884	2.945	2.139	0.686	0.814	2.610	1.365	2.458	5.603	1.325
Pumpkin seed (30.9% protein)	0.560	0.933	1.737	2.437	1.411	0.577	—	1.749	—	1.679	4.810	0.711
Safflower seed meal (42.1% protein)	0.675	1.462	1.914	2.740	1.525	0.731	—	2.605	—	2.446	4.623	0.985
Sesame seed (19.3% protein)	0.331	0.707	0.951	1.679	0.583	0.637	0.495	1.457	0.951	0.885	1.992	0.441
Sunflower kernel (23.0% protein)	0.343	0.911	1.276	1.736	0.868	0.443	0.464	1.220	0.647	1.354	2.370	0.586
Grains and Their Products												
Barley (12.8% protein, N × 5.83)	0.160	0.433	0.545	0.889	0.433	0.184	0.257	0.661	0.466	0.643	0.659	0.239
Bread, white (4% nonfat dry milk, flour basis) (8.5% protein, N × 5.70)	0.091	0.282	0.429	0.668	0.225	0.142	0.200	0.465	0.243	0.435	0.340	0.192
Buckwheat flour, dark (11.7 % protein, N × 6.25)	0.165	0.461	0.440	0.683	0.687	0.206	0.228	0.442	0.240	0.607	0.930	0.256
Cereal combinations												
Corn and soy grits (18.0% protein, N × 6.25)	0.161	0.792	0.841	1.656	0.772	0.271	0.311	0.832	0.562	1.054	0.982	0.472
Infants' food, precooked, mixed cereals with nonfat dry milk and yeast (19.4% protein, N × 6.25)	0.118	—	—	—	0.273	0.310	0.137	0.543	0.447	—	0.447	0.233
Oat-corn-rye mixture, puffed (14.5% protein, N × 5.83)	0.172	0.545	0.841	1.368	0.343	0.388	0.234	0.933	0.622	0.900	0.776	0.326
Corn, field (10.0% protein, N × 6.25)	0.061	0.398	0.462	1.296	0.288	0.186	0.130	0.454	0.611	0.510	0.352	0.206
Cornmeal												
Whole ground (9.2% protein, N × 6.25)	0.056	0.367	0.425	1.192	0.265	0.171	0.119	0.418	0.562	0.470	0.324	0.190
Degermed (7.9% protein, N × 6.25)	0.048	0.315	0.365	1.024	0.228	0.147	0.102	0.359	0.483	0.403	0.278	0.163
Corn products												
Flakes (8.1% protein, N × 6.25)	0.052	0.275	0.306	1.047	0.154	0.135	0.152	0.354	0.283	0.386	0.231	0.226
Germ (14.5% protein, N × 6.25)	0.144	0.622	0.578	1.030	0.791	0.232	0.130	0.483	0.343	0.789	1.134	0.464
Gluten (10.0% protein, N × 6.25)	0.059	0.344	0.443	1.563	0.179	0.282	0.141	0.558	0.582	0.512	0.322	0.200
Grits (8.7% protein, N × 6.25)	0.053	0.347	0.402	1.128	0.251	0.161	0.113	0.395	0.532	0.444	0.306	0.180

Protein Content and Nitrogen Conversion Factor	Tryptophan (g)	Threonine (g)	Isoleucine (g)	Leucine (g)	Lysine (g)	Methionine (g)	Cystine (g)	Phenylalanine (g)	Tyrosine (g)	Valine (g)	Arginine (g)	Histidine (g)
Grains and Their Products—cont'd												
Corn products—cont'd												
Hominy (8.7% protein, N × 6.25)	0.084	0.316	0.349	0.810	0.358	0.099	—	0.333	0.331	0.398	0.444	0.203
Masa (2.8% protein, N × 6.25)	0.010	—	—	—	0.103	0.108	0.030	—	—	—	—	—
Pozole (5.9% protein, N × 6.25)	0.042	0.336	0.304	0.591	0.234	0.087	—	0.254	—	0.267	0.197	0.122
Tortilla (5.8% protein, N × 6.25)	0.031	0.235	0.345	0.939	0.145	0.111	—	0.252	—	0.304	0.223	0.128
Zein (16.1% protein, N × 6.25)	0.010	0.495	0.822	3.184	—	0.281	0.162	1.664	0.981	0.654	0.286	0.216
Millet												
Pearl millet (11.4% protein, N × 5.83)	0.248	0.456	0.635	1.746	0.383	0.270	0.152	0.506	—	0.682	0.524	0.240
Ragimillet (6.2% protein, N × 5.83)	0.085	0.270	0.398	0.620	0.202	0.270	0.187	0.263	—	0.473	0.100	0.079
Oatmeal and rolled oats (14.2% protein, N × 5.83)	0.183	0.470	0.733	1.065	0.521	0.209	0.309	0.758	0.524	0.845	0.935	0.261
Quinoa (11.0% protein, N × 6.25)	0.120	0.523	0.722	0.781	0.729	0.278	0.107	0.394	0.253	0.447	0.820	0.297
Rice												
Brown (7.5% protein, N × 5.95)	0.081	0.294	0.352	0.646	0.296	0.135	0.102	0.377	0.343	0.524	0.432	0.126
White and converted (7.6% protein, N × 5.95)	0.082	0.298	0.356	0.655	0.300	0.137	0.103	0.382	0.347	0.531	0.438	0.128
Rice products												
Flakes or puffed (5.9% protein, N × 5.95)	0.046	—	—	—	0.056	—	0.044	0.286	0.124	—	0.137	0.137
Germ (14.2% protein, N × 5.95)	0.270	2.177	0.630	0.838	1.707	0.420	0.169	0.750	0.929	0.938	1.559	0.430
Rye (12.1% protein, N × 5.83)	0.137	0.448	0.515	0.813	0.494	0.191	0.241	0.571	0.390	0.631	0.591	0.276
Rye flour, medium (11.4% protein, N × 5.83)	0.129	0.422	0.485	0.766	0.465	0.180	0.227	0.538	0.368	0.594	0.557	0.260
Sorghum (11.0% protein, N × 6.25)	0.123	0.394	0.598	1.767	0.299	0.190	0.183	0.547	0.303	0.628	0.417	0.211
Teosinte (22.0% protein, N × 6.25)	0.049	—	—	—	0.348	0.496	—	—	—	—	—	—
Wheat flour												
Whole grain (13.3% protein, N × 5.83)	0.164	0.383	0.577	0.892	0.365	0.203	0.292	0.657	0.497	0.616	0.636	0.271
White (10.5% protein, N × 5.70)	0.129	0.302	0.483	0.809	0.239	0.138	0.210	0.577	0.539	0.453	0.466	0.210
Wheat products												
Bran (12.0% protein, N × 6.31)	0.196	0.342	0.485	0.717	0.491	0.145	0.270	0.434	0.259	0.552	0.742	0.280
Bulgur (12.4% protein, N × 5.83)	0.070	—	—	—	0.430	0.300	0.319	—	—	—	—	—
Farina (10.9% protein, N × 5.70)	0.124	—	—	—	0.199	0.143	0.184	0.579	0.447	—	0.424	0.268
Flakes (10.8% protein, N × 5.70)	0.121	0.356	0.496	0.891	0.360	0.127	0.191	0.478	0.311	0.572	0.559	0.231

Protein Content and Nitrogen Conversion Factor	Tryptophan (g)	Threonine (g)	Isoleucine (g)	Leucine (g)	Lysine (g)	Methionine (g)	Cystine (g)	Phenylalanine (g)	Tyrosine (g)	Valine (g)	Arginine (g)	Histidine (g)
Grains and Their Products—cont'd												
Wheat products—cont'd												
Germ (25.2% protein, N × 5.80)	0.265	1.343	1.177	1.708	1.534	0.404	0.287	0.908	0.882	1.364	1.825	0.687
Macaroni or spaghetti (12.8% protein, N × 5.70)	0.150	0.499	0.642	0.849	0.413	0.193	0.243	0.669	0.422	0.728	0.582	0.303
Noodles, containing egg solids (12.6% protein, N × 5.70)	0.133	0.533	0.621	0.834	0.411	0.212	0.245	0.610	0.312	0.745	0.621	0.301
Shredded Wheat (10.1% protein, N × 5.83)	0.085	0.405	0.449	0.684	0.331	0.139	0.204	0.481	0.236	0.577	0.523	0.236
Whole wheat with added germ (12.8% protein, N × 5.83)	0.136	—	—	—	0.466	—	0.246	0.755	0.481	—	0.742	0.371
Fruits												
Fruits are not a significant source of amino acids												
Vegetables												
Immature Seeds (Protein, N × 6.25)												
Corn, sweet, white or yellow												
Raw (3.7% protein)	0.023	0.151	0.137	0.407	0.137	0.072	0.062	0.207	0.124	0.231	0.174	0.095
Canned, solids and liquid (2.0% protein)	0.012	0.082	0.074	0.220	0.074	0.039	0.033	0.112	0.067	0.125	0.094	0.052
Cowpeas (9.4% protein)	0.099	0.353	0.465	0.653	0.617	0.131	—	0.523	—	0.513	0.615	0.310
Lima beans												
Raw (7.5% protein)	0.097	0.338	0.460	0.605	0.474	0.080	0.083	0.389	0.259	0.485	0.454	0.247
Canned, solids and liquid (3.8% protein)	0.049	0.171	0.233	0.306	0.240	0.041	0.042	0.197	0.131	0.246	0.230	0.125
Peas												
Raw (6.7% protein)	0.056	0.245	0.308	0.418	0.316	0.054	0.073	0.257	0.163	0.274	0.595	0.109
Canned, solids and liquid (3.4% protein)	0.028	0.125	0.156	0.212	0.160	0.027	0.037	0.131	0.083	0.139	0.302	0.055
Leafy Vegetables, Raw (Protein, N × 6.25)												
Amaranth (3.5% protein)	0.038	0.056	0.164	0.206	0.141	0.025	0.024	0.096	0.105	0.136	0.134	0.069
Beet greens (2.0% protein)	0.024	0.076	0.084	0.129	0.108	0.034	—	0.116	—	0.101	0.083	0.026
Brussels sprouts (4.4% protein)	0.044	0.153	0.186	0.194	0.197	0.046	—	0.148	—	0.193	0.279	0.106
Cabbage (1.4% protein)	0.011	0.039	0.040	0.057	0.066	0.013	0.028	0.030	0.030	0.043	0.105	0.025
Chard (1.4% protein)	0.014	0.058	0.060	0.076	0.055	0.004	—	0.046	—	0.055	0.035	0.018
Chicory (1.6% protein)	0.024	—	—	—	0.052	0.016	0.006	—	0.040	—	—	0.024
Collards (3.9% protein)	0.055	0.114	0.121	0.218	0.202	0.046	0.059	0.124	0.151	0.195	0.258	0.087
Kale (3.9% protein)	0.042	0.139	0.133	0.252	0.121	0.035	0.036	0.158	—	0.184	0.202	0.062
Lettuce (1.2% protein)	0.012	—	—	—	0.070	0.004	—	—	—	—	—	—
Mustard greens (2.3% protein)	0.037	0.060	0.075	0.062	0.111	0.024	0.035	0.074	0.121	0.108	0.167	0.041
Parsley, curly garden	0.050	—	—	—	0.160	0.012	—	—	—	—	—	—
(2.5% protein)	0.037	0.102	0.107	0.176	0.142	0.039	0.046	0.099	0.073	0.126	0.116	0.049

Protein Content and Nitrogen Conversion Factor	Trypto-phan (g)	Threo-nine (g)	Iso-leucine (g)	Leucine (g)	Lysine (g)	Methi-onine (g)	Cystine (g)	Phenyl-alanine (g)	Tyro-sine (g)	Valine (g)	Argi-nine (g)	Histi-dine (g)
Vegetables—cont'd												
Leafy Vegetables, Raw (Protein, N × 6.25)—cont'd												
Spinach (2.3% protein)	0.045	0.125	0.107	0.207	0.129	0.052	0.045	0.146	0.105	0.149	0.167	0.051
Turnip greens (2.9% protein)	0.028	0.084	0.076	0.131	0.091	0.010	—	0.062	0.036	0.084	0.053	0.034
Watercress (1.7% protein)												
Starchy Roots and Tubers (Protein, N × 6.25)												
Cassava	0.021	0.044	0.045	0.066	0.066	0.010	0.018	0.045	0.030	0.049	0.159	0.025
Flour (1.6% protein)	0.014	0.030	0.031	0.045	0.045	0.007	0.012	0.031	0.021	0.033	0.110	0.017
Root (1.1% protein)												
Potatoes	0.021	0.079	0.088	0.100	0.107	0.025	0.019	0.088	0.036	0.107	0.099	0.029
Raw (2.0% protein)	0.018	0.067	0.075	0.085	0.091	0.021	0.016	0.075	0.030	0.091	0.084	0.024
Canned, solids and liquid (1.7% protein)	0.031	0.085	0.087	0.103	0.085	0.033	0.029	0.100	0.081	0.135	0.094	0.036
Sweet potatoes (*Ipomoea batatas*), raw (1.8% protein)	0.035	0.089	0.099	0.169	0.110	0.021	—	0.099	—	0.114	0.118	0.032
Taro (1.9% protein)	0.035	—	—	—	0.110	0.034	—	—	—	—	—	—
Yam (*Dioscorea* spp.) (2.1% protein)												
Other Vegetables (Protein, N × 6.25)												
Asparagus	0.027	0.066	0.080	0.096	0.103	0.032	—	0.069	—	0.106	0.123	0.036
Raw (2.2% protein)	0.023	0.057	0.069	0.083	0.089	0.027	—	0.060	—	0.092	0.106	0.031
Canned, solids and liquid (1.9% protein)												
Beans, snap	0.033	0.091	0.109	0.139	0.126	0.035	0.024	0.057	0.050	0.115	0.101	0.045
Raw (2.4% protein)	0.014	0.038	0.045	0.058	0.052	0.014	0.010	0.024	0.021	0.048	0.042	0.019
Canned, solids and liquid (1.0% protein)												
Beets	0.014	0.034	0.051	0.055	0.086	0.006	—	0.027	—	0.049	0.028	0.022
Raw (1.6% protein)	0.0008	0.019	0.029	0.031	0.048	0.003	—	0.015	—	0.028	0.016	0.012
Canned, solids and liquid (0.9% protein)	0.037	0.122	0.126	0.163	0.147	0.050	—	0.119	—	0.170	0.192	0.063
Broccoli (3.3% protein)												
Carrots	0.010	0.043	0.046	0.065	0.052	0.010	0.029	0.042	0.020	0.056	0.041	0.017
Raw (1.2% protein)	0.004	0.018	0.019	0.027	0.022	0.004	0.012	0.018	0.008	0.023	0.017	0.007
Canned, solids and liquid (0.5% protein)	0.033	0.102	0.104	0.162	0.134	0.047	—	0.075	0.034	0.144	0.110	0.048

Protein Content and Nitrogen Conversion Factor	Tryptophan (g)	Threonine (g)	Isoleucine (g)	Leucine (g)	Lysine (g)	Methionine (g)	Cystine (g)	Phenylalanine (g)	Tyrosine (g)	Valine (g)	Arginine (g)	Histidine (g)
Vegetables—cont'd												
Other Vegetables (Protein, N × 6.25)—cont'd												
Cauliflower (2.4% protein)	0.012	—	—	—	0.021	0.015	0.006	—	0.016	—	—	—
Celery (1.3% protein)	0.008	—	—	—	0.038	0.001	—	—	—	—	—	—
Chayote (0.6% protein)	0.034	—	—	—	0.203	0.021	—	—	—	—	—	—
Cowpeas, yardlong, immature pod (3.4% protein)	0.005	0.019	0.022	0.030	0.031	0.007	—	0.016	—	0.024	0.053	0.001
Cucumbers (0.7% protein)	0.014	—	—	—	0.044	0.008	—	—	—	—	—	—
Cushaw (1.5% protein)	0.010	0.038	0.056	0.068	0.030	0.006	—	0.048	—	0.065	0.037	0.019
Eggplant (1.1% protein)	0.144	0.155	—	0.259	0.155	0.030	—	0.166	—	0.181	0.189	0.063
Mallow (3.7% protein)												
Mushrooms	0.006	—	0.532	0.281	—	0.167	—	—	—	0.378	0.235	—
*Agaricus campestris**	0.006	0.156	0.201	0.139	0.088	0.021	—	0.018	—	0.116	0.021	0.027
Lactarius spp.†	0.018	0.066	0.069	0.101	0.076	0.022	0.017	0.065	0.079	0.091	0.093	0.030
Okra (1.8% protein)	0.021	0.022	0.021	0.037	0.064	0.013	—	0.039	0.046	0.031	0.180	0.014
Onions, mature (1.4% protein)	0.009	0.050	0.046	0.046	0.051	0.016	—	0.055	—	0.033	0.024	0.014
Peppers (1.2% protein)	0.009	0.053	0.044	0.057	0.044	0.008	—	0.059	—	0.041	0.032	0.016
Prickly pears (1.1% protein)	0.016	0.028	0.044	0.063	0.058	0.011	—	0.032	0.016	0.045	0.043	0.019
Pumpkin (1.2% protein)	0.005	0.059	—	—	0.034	0.002	—	—	—	0.030	—	—
Radishes (1.2% protein)	—	0.159	0.225	0.265	0.211	0.045	—	0.186	—	0.225	0.225	0.133
Soybean sprouts (6.2% protein)	0.005	0.014	0.019	0.027	0.023	0.008	—	0.016	—	0.022	0.027	0.009
Squash, summer (0.6% protein)	0.009	0.033	0.029	0.041	0.042	0.007	—	0.028	0.014	0.028	0.029	0.015
Tomatoes and cherry tomatoes (1.0% protein)	—	—	0.020	—	0.057	0.012	—	0.020	0.029	—	—	—
Turnips (1.1% protein)												
Miscellaneous Food Items	0.142	0.411	0.884	1.079	0.321	0.253	—	0.811	—	0.705	0.597	0.321
Vegetable patty or steak (principally wheat protein) (15% protein, N × 5.70)												
Yeast	0.122	0.655	0.655	1.151	0.914	0.248	0.120	0.607	0.580	0.840	0.536	0.353
Baker's, compressed (N × 6.25)	0.710	2.353	2.398	3.226	3.300	0.836	0.548	1.902	1.902	2.723	2.250	1.251
Brewer's dried (N × 6.25)												

*Total nitrogen is 0.58%. This is equivalent to 2.4% protein on the basis that two thirds of the nitrogen is protein nitrogen. If total nitrogen is used for the calculation, the protein content is 3.6%.

†Total nitrogen is 0.69%. This is equivalent to 2.9% protein on the basis that two thirds of the nitrogen is protein nitrogen. If total nitrogen is used for the calculation, the protein content is 4.3%.

Appendix

C Fatty Acid Content of Common Vegetable Oils

Vegetable Oil	Polyunsaturated (%)	Monounsaturated (%)	Saturated (%)
Safflower	74	12	9
Walnut	66	15	11
Sunflower	64	21	10
Wheat germ	61	16	17
Corn	58	25	13
Soybean (unhydrogenated)	58	23	15
Cottonseed	51	19	26
Sesame seed	40	40	15
Soybean (partially hydrogenated)	40	47	13
Peanut	30	46	19
Olive	9	72	14
Palm	9	38	48
Coconut	2	6	86

Modified from Brown HB: Current focus on fat in the diet, ADA White Paper, *J Am Diet Assoc* 68:25, 1977.

NOTE: Other substances in the oils that make up total composition (100%) include such materials as sterols, vitamins, phospholipids, and water.

Appendix D Relative Ratios of Polyunsaturated Fat and Saturated Fat (P/S Ratio) in Representative Foods

P/S Ratio	Foods
High >2.5:1	Almonds Corn oil Cottonseed oil Mayonnaise (made with oils in this group) Safflower oil Sesame oil Soft margarines Soybean oil Sunflower oil Walnuts
Medium high 2:1	Chicken Fish Peanut oil Semisolid margarines
Medium 1:1	Beef heart, liver Hydrogenated or hardened vegetable oils (shortenings, special products) Peanuts, peanut butter Pecans Solid margarines
Low 0.1-0.5:1	Chicken liver Lamb Lard Olive oil Palm oil Pork Veal
Very low <0.1:1	Beef Butter, cream Coconut oil Egg yolk Whole milk, milk products

Appendix E

Caffeine Content of Common Beverages and Drugs

Source	Caffeine (mg)
Beverages (180 ml cup)	
Brewed coffee	80-140
Instant coffee	60-100
Decaffeinated coffee	1-6
Leaf tea	30-80
Tea bags	25-75
Instant tea	30-60
Cocoa	10-50
Cola drinks (8 oz)	15-50
Candy bar, chocolate (1 oz)	20
Caffeine-containing analgesics	
General	30 (per unit)
Excedrin	60 (per unit)
Cafergot	100 (per unit)

Appendix

F Dietary Fiber in Selected Plant Foods

Food	Amount	Weight (g)	Total Dietary Fiber (g)	Noncellulose Polysaccharides (g)	Cellulose (g)	Lignin (g)
Apple	1 med					
Flesh		138	1.96	1.29	0.66	0.01
Skin		100	3.71	2.21	1.01	0.49
Banana	1 small	119	2.08	1.33	0.44	0.31
Beans						
Baked	1 cup	255	18.53	14.45	3.59	0.48
Green, cooked	1 cup	125	4.19	2.31	1.61	0.26
Bread						
White	1 slice	25	0.68	0.50	0.18	Trace
Whole meal	1 slice	25	2.13	1.49	0.33	0.31
Broccoli, cooked	1 cup	155	6.36	4.53	1.78	0.05
Brussels sprouts, cooked	1 cup	155	4.43	3.08	1.24	0.11
Cabbage, cooked	1 cup	145	4.10	2.55	1.00	0.55
Carrots, cooked	1 cup	155	5.74	3.44	2.29	Trace
Cauliflower, cooked	1 cup	125	2.25	0.84	1.41	Trace
Cereals						
All-Bran	1 oz	30	8.01	5.35	1.80	0.86
Corn Flakes	1 cup	25	2.75	1.82	0.61	0.33
Grapenuts	¼ cup	30	2.10	1.54	0.38	0.17
Puffed Wheat	1 cup	15	2.31	1.55	0.39	0.37
Rice Krispies	1 cup	30	1.34	1.04	0.23	0.07
Shredded Wheat	1 biscuit	25	3.07	2.20	0.66	0.21
Special K	1 cup	30	1.64	1.10	0.22	0.32
Cherries	10 cherries	68	0.84	0.63	0.17	0.05
Cookies						
Ginger	4 snaps	28	0.56	0.41	0.08	0.07
Oatmeal	4 cookies	52	2.08	1.64	0.21	0.22
Plain	4 cookies	48	0.80	0.68	0.05	0.06
Corn	1 cup	165	7.82	7.11	0.51	0.20
Canned	1 cup	165	9.39	8.20	1.06	0.13
Flour						
Bran	1 cup	100	44.00	32.70	8.05	3.23
White	1 cup	115	3.62	2.90	0.69	0.03
Whole meal	1 cup	120	11.41	7.50	2.95	0.96
Grapefruit	½ cup	100	0.44	0.34	0.04	0.06

Continued

Food	Amount	Weight (g)	Total Dietary Fiber (g)	Noncellulose Polysaccharides (g)	Cellulose (g)	Lignin (g)
Jam, strawberry	1 tbsp	20	0.22	0.17	0.02	0.03
Lettuce	⅙ head	100	1.53	0.47	1.06	Trace
Marmalade, orange	1 tbsp	20	0.14	0.13	0.01	Trace
Onions, raw, sliced	1 cup	100	2.10	1.55	0.55	Trace
Orange	1 cup	200	0.58	0.44	0.08	0.06
Parsnips, raw, diced	1 cup	100	4.90	3.77	1.13	Trace
Peach, flesh and skin	1 med	100	2.28	1.46	0.20	0.62
Peanuts	1 oz	30	2.79	1.92	0.51	0.36
Peanut butter	1 tbsp	16	1.21	0.90	0.31	Trace
Pear	1 med					
Flesh		164	4.00	2.16	1.10	0.74
Skin		100	8.59	3.72	2.18	2.67
Peas, canned	1 cup	170	13.35	8.84	3.91	0.60
Peas, raw or frozen	1 cup	100	7.75	5.48	2.09	0.18
Plums	1 plum	66	1.00	0.65	0.15	0.20
Potato, raw	1 med	135	4.73	3.36	1.38	Trace
Raisins	1 oz	30	1.32	0.72	0.25	0.35
Strawberries	1 cup	149	2.65	1.39	1.04	0.22
Tomato						
Raw	1 med	135	1.89	0.88	0.61	0.41
Canned, drained	1 cup	240	2.04	1.08	0.89	0.07
Turnips, raw	1 med	100	2.20	1.50	0.70	Trace

Modified from Southgate DAT et al: A guide to calculating intakes of dietary fiber, *J Hum Nutr* 30:303, 1976.

Appendix

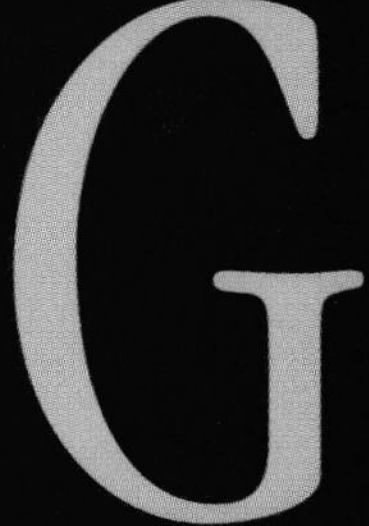

Sodium Content of Popular Condiments, Fats, and Oils

Product	Portion Size	Sodium (mg)	Product	Portion Size	Sodium (mg)
Salt	1 tsp	1938	Pickle, sweet	1 pickle	128
Garlic salt	1 tsp	1850	Relish, sweet	1 tbsp	124
Meat tenderizer (regular)	1 tsp	1750	Italian dressing (bottled, store bought)	1 tbsp	116
Onion salt	1 tsp	1620	Butter (regular)	1 tbsp	116
Soy sauce	1 tbsp	1029	Thousand island dressing (regular)	1 tbsp	109
Pickle, dill	1 pickle	928	Pickles, bread and butter	2 slices	101
Baking soda	1 tsp	821	Olives, mission, ripe	3 olives	96
Teriyaki sauce	1 tbsp	690	French dressing (home recipe)	1 tbsp	92
Monosodium glutamate (MSG)	1 tsp	492	Mayonnaise	1 tbsp	78
Baking powder	1 tsp	339	Butter (whipped)	1 tbsp	74
Olives, green	4 olives	323	Mustard (prepared)	1 tsp	65
A-1 Steak Sauce	1 tbsp	275	Chili powder	1 tsp	26
French dressing (dry mix, prepared)	1 tbsp	253	Tabasco sauce	1 tsp	24
Chili sauce (regular)	1 tbsp	227	Chili sauce (low sodium)	1 tbsp	11
French dressing (bottled, store bought)	1 tbsp	214	Parsley, dried	1 tbsp	6
Worcestershire sauce	1 tbsp	206	Catsup (low sodium)	1 tbsp	3
Horseradish (prepared)	1 tbsp	198	French dressing (low sodium)	1 tbsp	3
Tartar sauce	1 tbsp	182	Butter (unsalted)	1 tbsp	2
Italian dressing (dry mix, prepared)	1 tbsp	172	Meat tenderizer (low sodium)	1 tsp	1
Catsup (regular)	1 tbsp	156	Onion powder	1 tsp	1
Thousand island dressing (low calorie)	1 tbsp	153	Black pepper	1 tsp	1
Blue cheese dressing	1 tbsp	153	Vinegar	½ cup	1
Margarine (regular)	1 tbsp	140	Margarine (unsalted)	1 tbsp	1
Russian dressing	1 tbsp	133	Oil, vegetable (corn, olive, soybean)	1 tbsp	0
Barbecue sauce	1 tbsp	130			

Modified from *The sodium content of your food,* Home and Garden Bulletin No 233, U.S. Department of Agriculture, Washington, DC, Aug 1980, U.S. Government Printing Office.

Appendix H

Salt-Free Seasoning Guide

Fish	Beef	Poultry and Veal	Gravies and Sauces
Breaded, battered fillets Dry mustard, onion; oregano, basil, garlic; thyme Broiled steaks or fillets Chili or curry powder; tarragon Fillets in butter sauce Thyme, chervil; dill; fennel Fish soup Italian seasoning; bay leaf, thyme, tarragon Fish cakes Tarragon, savory; dry mustard, white pepper; red pepper, oregano	Swiss steak Rosemary, black pepper; bay leaf, thyme; clove Roast beef Basil, oregano; bay leaf; nutmeg; tarragon, marjoram Beef stew Chili powder; bay leaf, tarragon; caraway; marjoram Meatballs Garlic, thyme; basil, oregano, onion; thyme, garlic; black pepper, dry mustard Beef stroganoff Red pepper, onion, garlic; nutmeg, onion; curry powder	Fried chicken Basil, oregano, garlic; onion, dill; sesame seed, nutmeg Roast chicken or turkey Ginger, garlic; onion, thyme, tarragon Chicken croquettes Dill, curry; chili powder, cumin; tarragon, oregano Veal patties Italian seasoning; tarragon; dill, onion, sesame seed Barbecue chicken Garlic, dry mustard; clove, allspice, dry mustard; basil, garlic, oregano	Barbecue Bay leaf, thyme, red pepper; cinnamon, ginger allspice, dry mustard, red pepper; chili powder Brown Chervil, onion; onion, bay leaf, thyme; onion, nutmeg; tarragon Chicken Dry mustard; ginger, garlic; marjoram, thyme, bay leaf Cream White pepper, dry mustard; curry powder; dill, onion, paprika; tarragon, thyme
Soups	**Salads**	**Pasta, Beans, and Rice**	**Vegetables**
Chicken Thyme, savory; ginger; clove, white pepper, allspice Clam chowder Basil, oregano; nutmeg, white pepper; thyme, garlic powder Mushroom Ginger; oregano; thyme, tarragon; bay leaf, black pepper; chili powder Onion Curry, caraway; marjoram, garlic; cloves Tomato Bay leaf, thyme; Italian seasoning; oregano, onion; nutmeg Vegetable Italian seasoning; paprika, caraway; rosemary, thyme; fennel, thyme	Chicken Curry or chili powder; Italian seasoning; thyme, tarragon Coleslaw Dill; caraway; poppy; dry mustard, ginger Fish or seafood Dill; tarragon, ginger, dry mustard, red pepper; ginger, onion, garlic Macaroni Dill; basil, thyme, oregano; dry mustard, garlic Potato Chili powder; curry; dry mustard, onion	Baked beans Dry mustard; chili powder; clove, onion; ginger, dry mustard Rice and vegetables Curry; thyme, onion, paprika; rosemary, garlic; ginger, onion, garlic Spanish rice Cumin, oregano, basil; Italian seasoning Spaghetti Italian seasoning, nutmeg; oregano, basil, nutmeg; red pepper, tarragon Rice pilaf Dill; thyme; savory, black pepper	Asparagus Ginger; sesame seed; basil, onion Broccoli Italian seasoning; marjoram, basil; nutmeg, onion; sesame seed Cabbage Caraway; onion, nutmeg; allspice, clove Carrots Ginger; nutmeg; onion, dill Cauliflower Dry mustard; basil; paprika, onion Tomatoes Oregano; chili powder; dill, onion Spinach Savory, thyme; nutmeg; garlic, onion

Appendix I

CDC Growth Charts: United States

CDC Growth Charts: United States

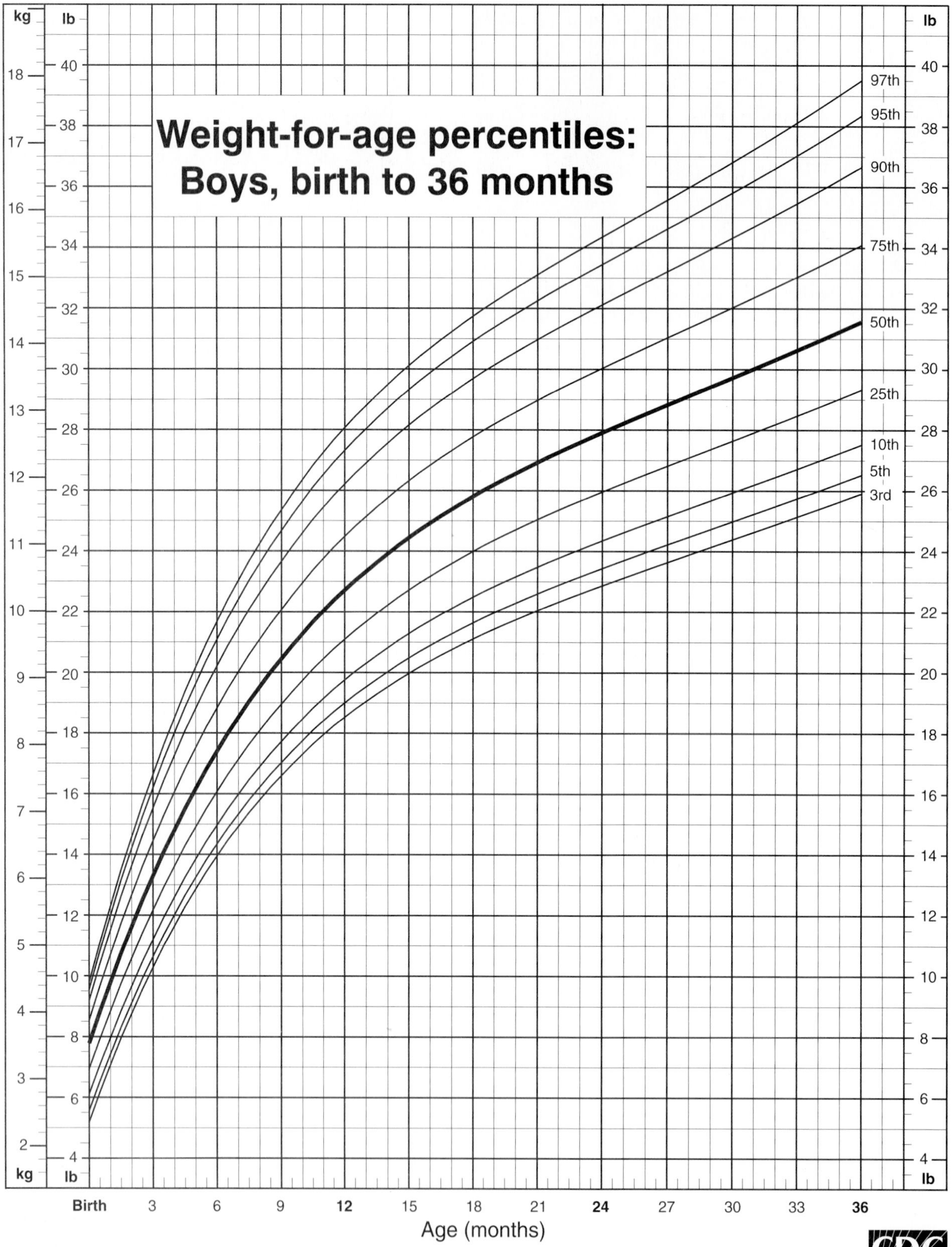

Weight-for-age percentiles: Boys, birth to 36 months

kg lb

97th
95th
90th
75th
50th
25th
10th
5th
3rd

Birth 3 6 9 12 15 18 21 24 27 30 33 36

Age (months)

Published May 30, 2000.

SOURCE: Developed by the National Center for Health Statistics in collaboration with the National Center for Chronic Disease Prevention and Health Promotion (2000).

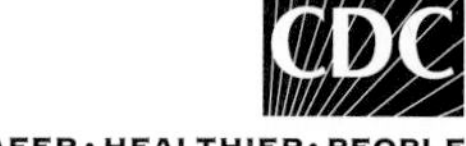

CDC Growth Charts: United States

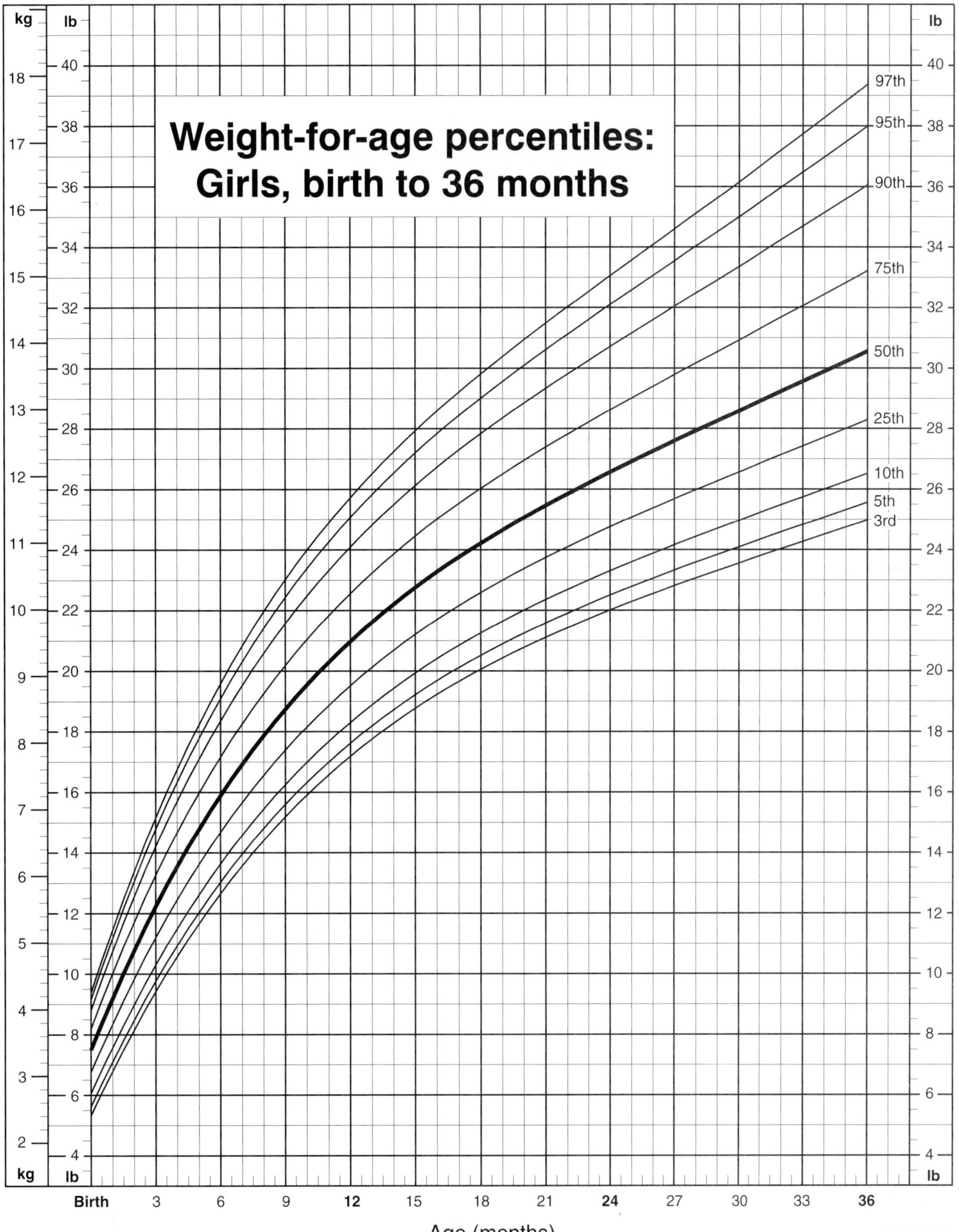

Weight-for-age percentiles: Girls, birth to 36 months

kg | lb

97th
95th
90th
75th
50th
25th
10th
5th
3rd

Birth 3 6 9 12 15 18 21 24 27 30 33 36

Age (months)

Published May 30, 2000.
SOURCE: Developed by the National Center for Health Statistics in collaboration with the National Center for Chronic Disease Prevention and Health Promotion (2000).

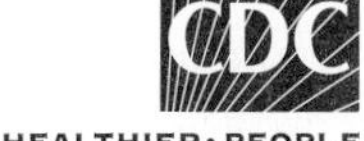

SAFER • HEALTHIER • PEOPLE™

CDC Growth Charts: United States

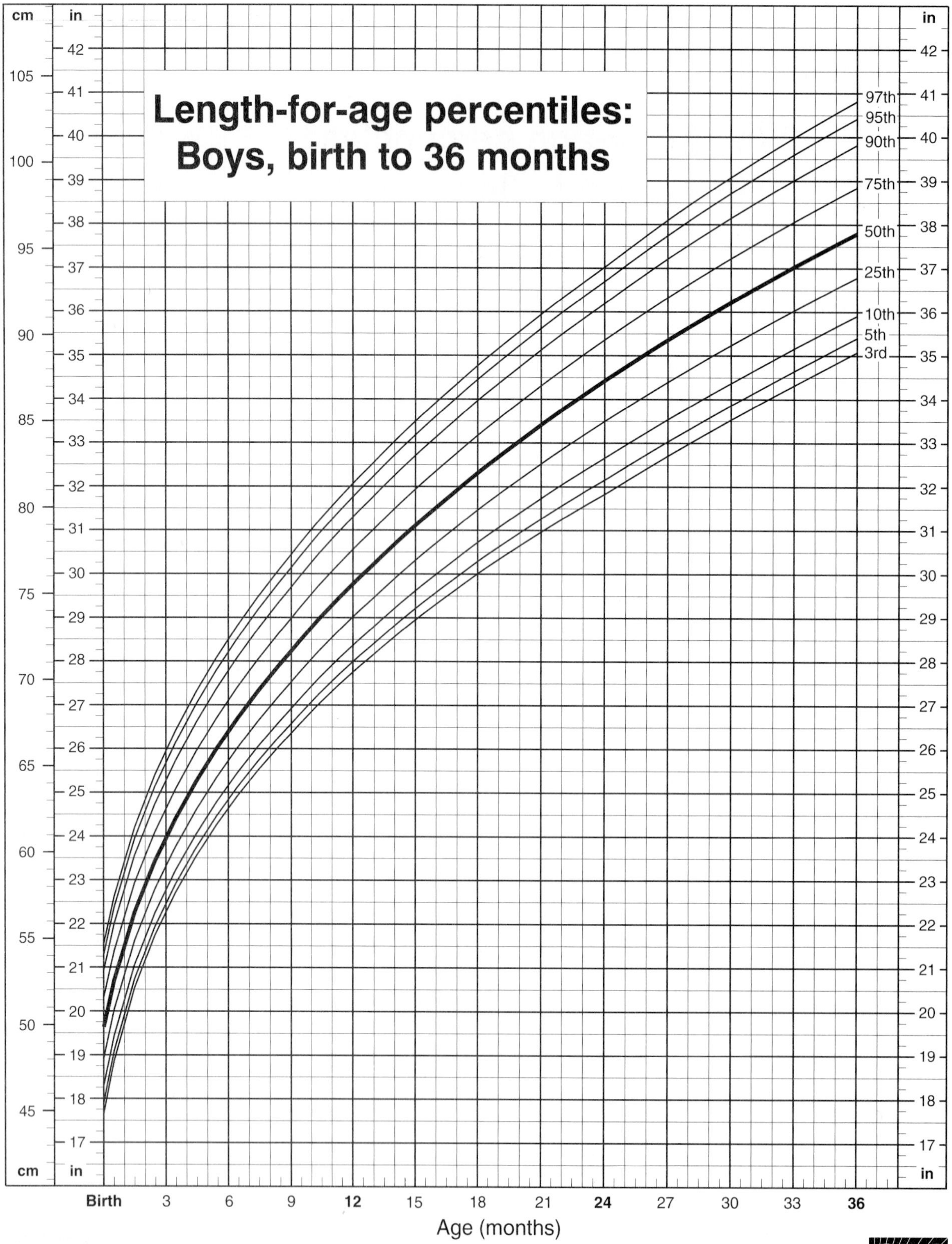

Length-for-age percentiles: Boys, birth to 36 months

cm | in

97th
95th
90th
75th
50th
25th
10th
5th
3rd

Birth 3 6 9 12 15 18 21 24 27 30 33 36

Age (months)

Published May 30, 2000.
SOURCE: Developed by the National Center for Health Statistics in collaboration with the National Center for Chronic Disease Prevention and Health Promotion (2000).

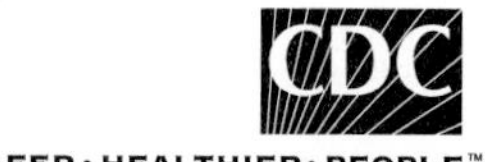

CDC Growth Charts: United States

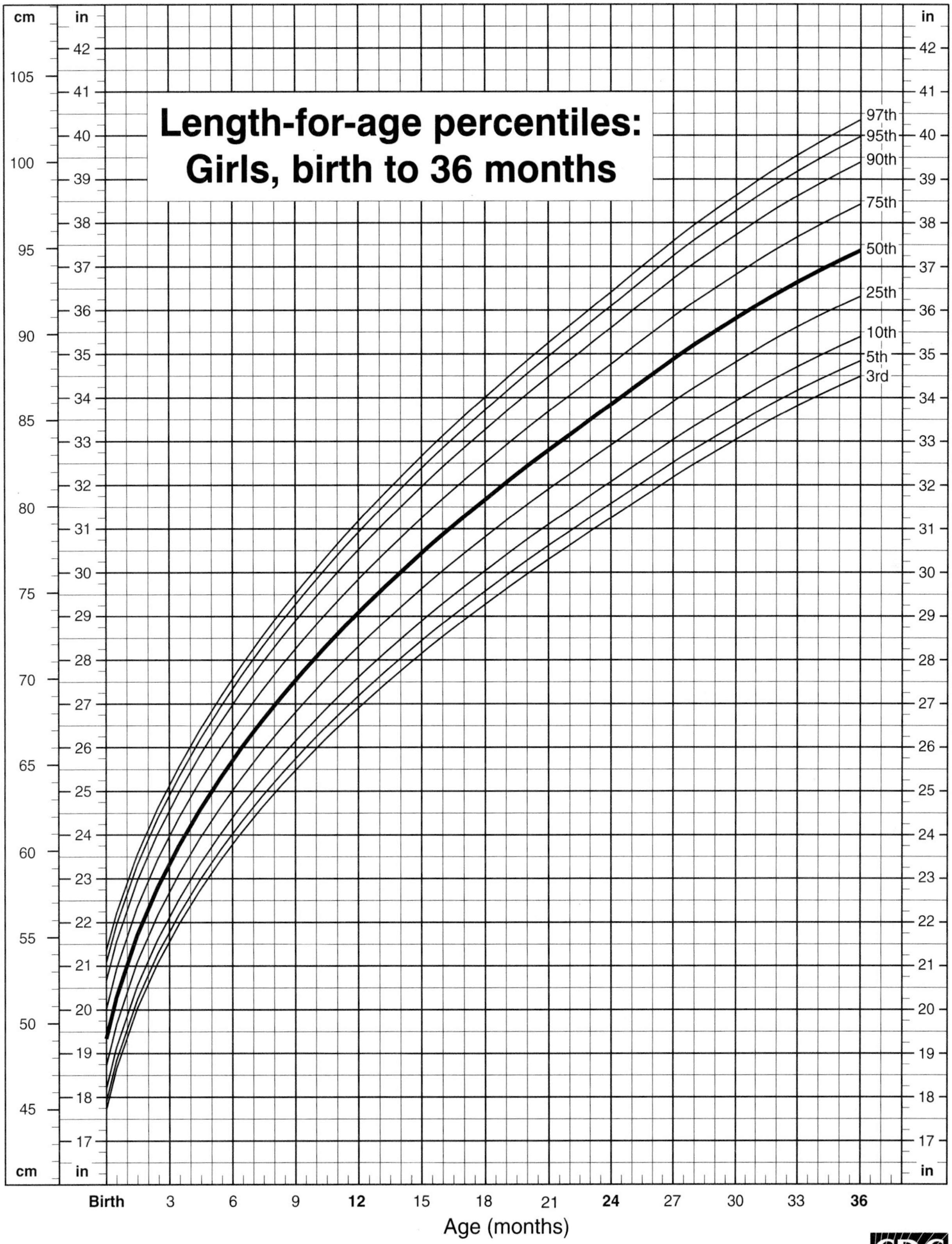

Length-for-age percentiles: Girls, birth to 36 months

Published May 30, 2000.
SOURCE: Developed by the National Center for Health Statistics in collaboration with the National Center for Chronic Disease Prevention and Health Promotion (2000).

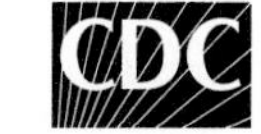

SAFER • HEALTHIER • PEOPLE™

CDC Growth Charts: United States

Weight-for-length percentiles: Boys, birth to 36 months

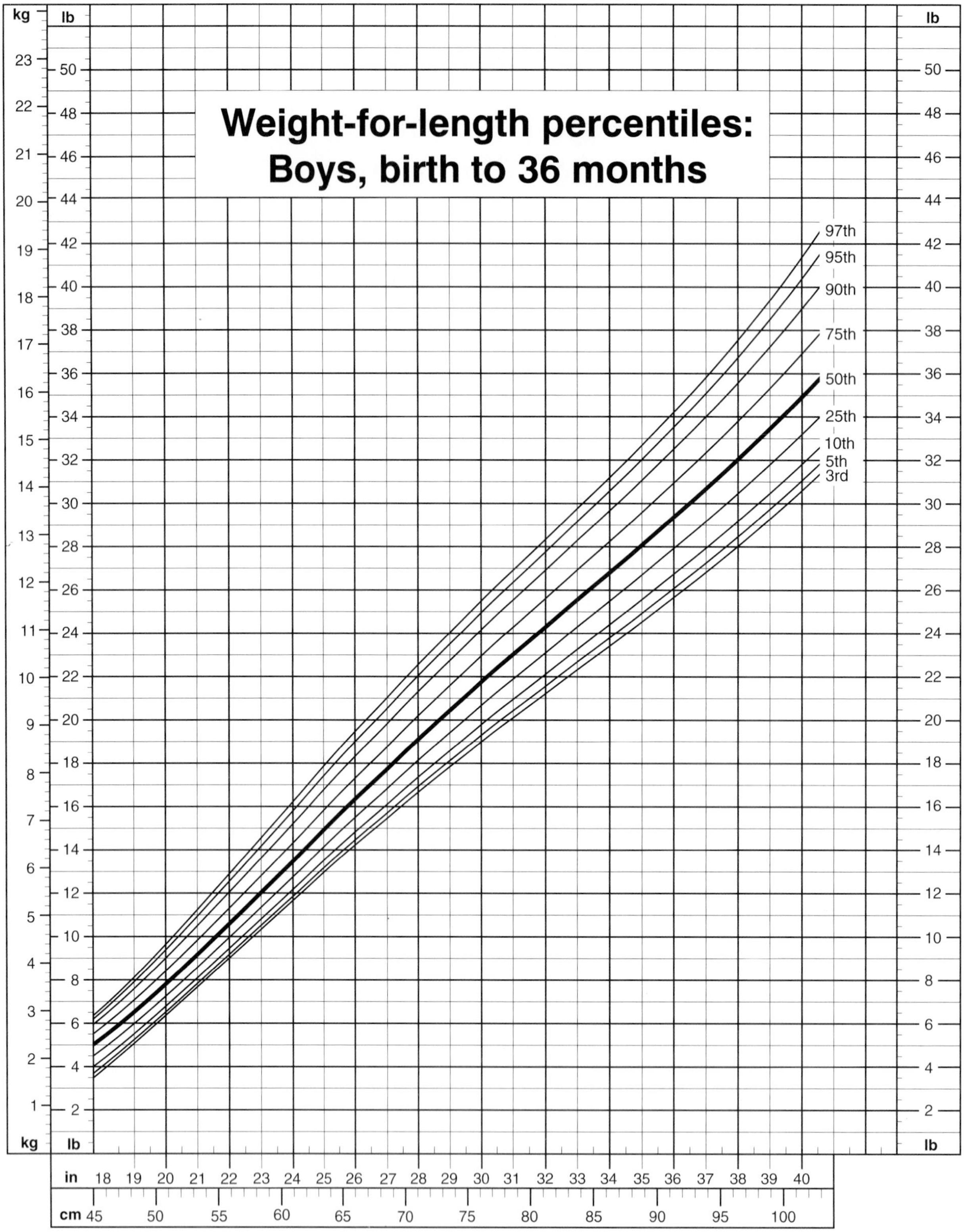

kg lb

23 50
22 48
21 46
20 44
19 42
18 40
17 38
16 36
15 34
14 32
13 30
12 28
11 26
10 24
9 22
8 20
7 18
6 16
5 14
4 12
3 10
2 8
1 6

97th
95th
90th
75th
50th
25th
10th
5th
3rd

in 18 19 20 21 22 23 24 25 26 27 28 29 30 31 32 33 34 35 36 37 38 39 40

cm 45 50 55 60 65 70 75 80 85 90 95 100

Length

Published May 30, 2000. (modified 6/8/00).
SOURCE: Developed by the National Center for Health Statistics in collaboration with the National Center for Chronic Disease Prevention and Health Promotion (2000).

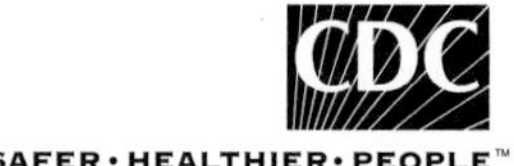

CDC Growth Charts: United States

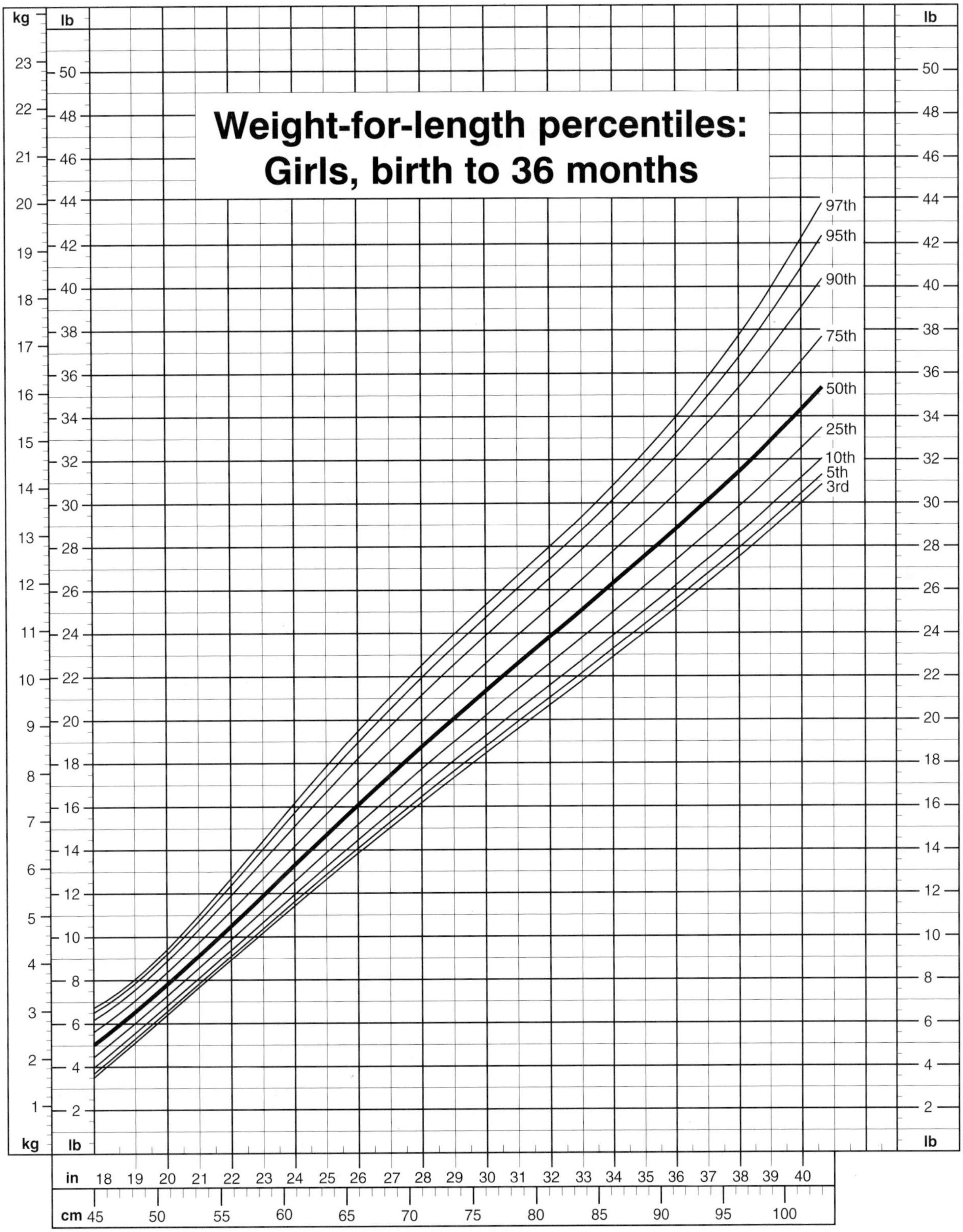

Weight-for-length percentiles: Girls, birth to 36 months

97th
95th
90th
75th
50th
25th
10th
5th
3rd

kg: 1 2 3 4 5 6 7 8 9 10 11 12 13 14 15 16 17 18 19 20 21 22 23

lb: 2 4 6 8 10 12 14 16 18 20 22 24 26 28 30 32 34 36 38 40 42 44 46 48 50

in: 18 19 20 21 22 23 24 25 26 27 28 29 30 31 32 33 34 35 36 37 38 39 40

cm: 45 50 55 60 65 70 75 80 85 90 95 100

Length

Published May 30, 2000. (modified 6/8/00).
SOURCE: Developed by the National Center for Health Statistics in collaboration with the National Center for Chronic Disease Prevention and Health Promotion (2000).

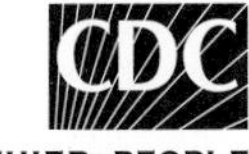

SAFER • HEALTHIER • PEOPLE™

CDC Growth Charts: United States

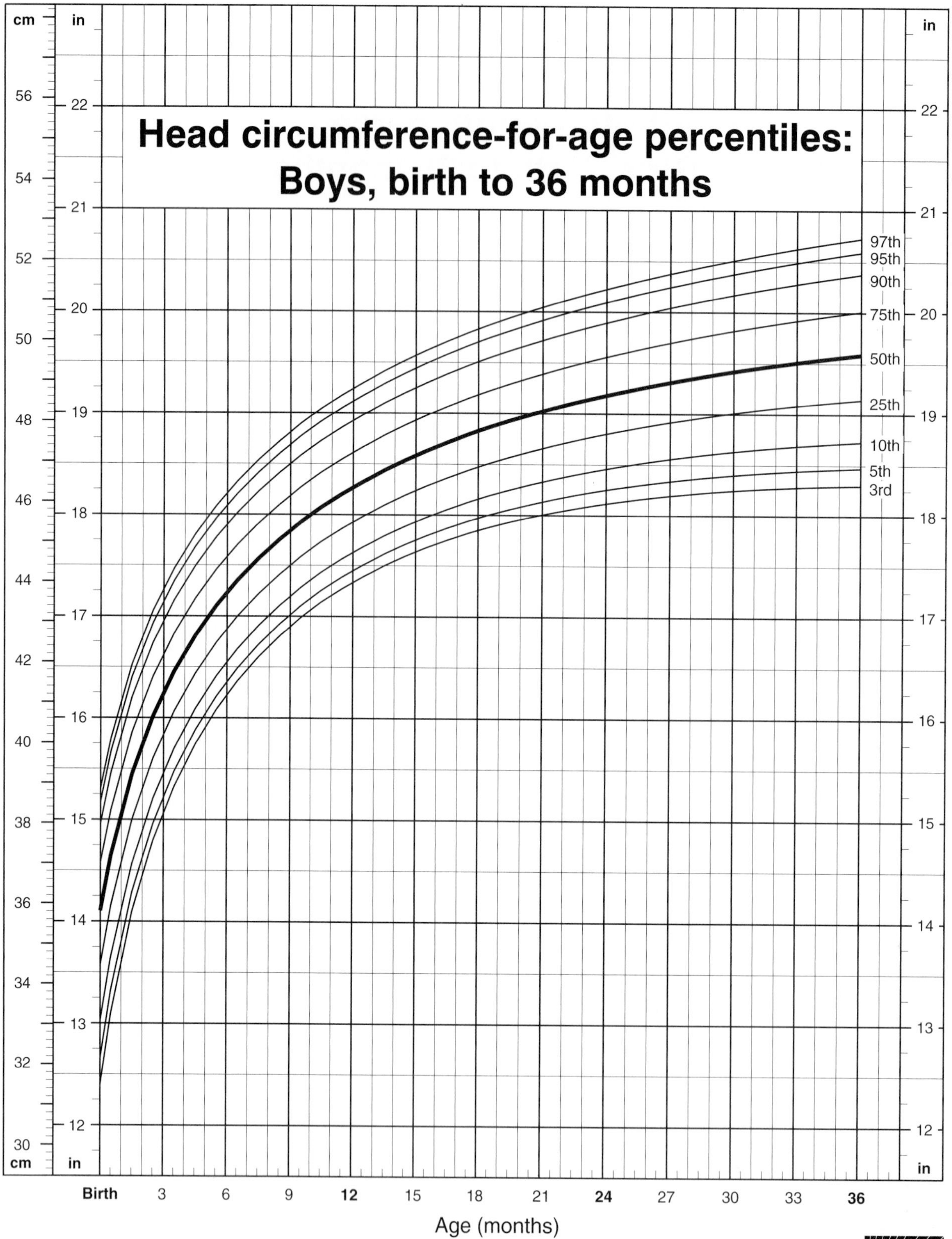

Head circumference-for-age percentiles: Boys, birth to 36 months

cm | in | in

56 | 22 | 22
54 | 21 | 21
52 | 20 | 20
50 | 19 | 19
48 | 18 | 18
46 | 17 | 17
44 | 16 | 16
42 | 15 | 15
40 | 14 | 14
38 | 13 | 13
36 | 12 | 12
34
32
30
cm | in | in

97th
95th
90th
75th
50th
25th
10th
5th
3rd

Birth 3 6 9 12 15 18 21 24 27 30 33 36

Age (months)

Published May 30, 2000.
SOURCE: Developed by the National Center for Health Statistics in collaboration with the National Center for Chronic Disease Prevention and Health Promotion (2000).

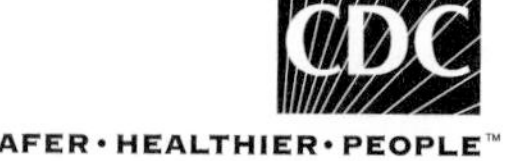

SAFER • HEALTHIER • PEOPLE™

CDC Growth Charts: United States

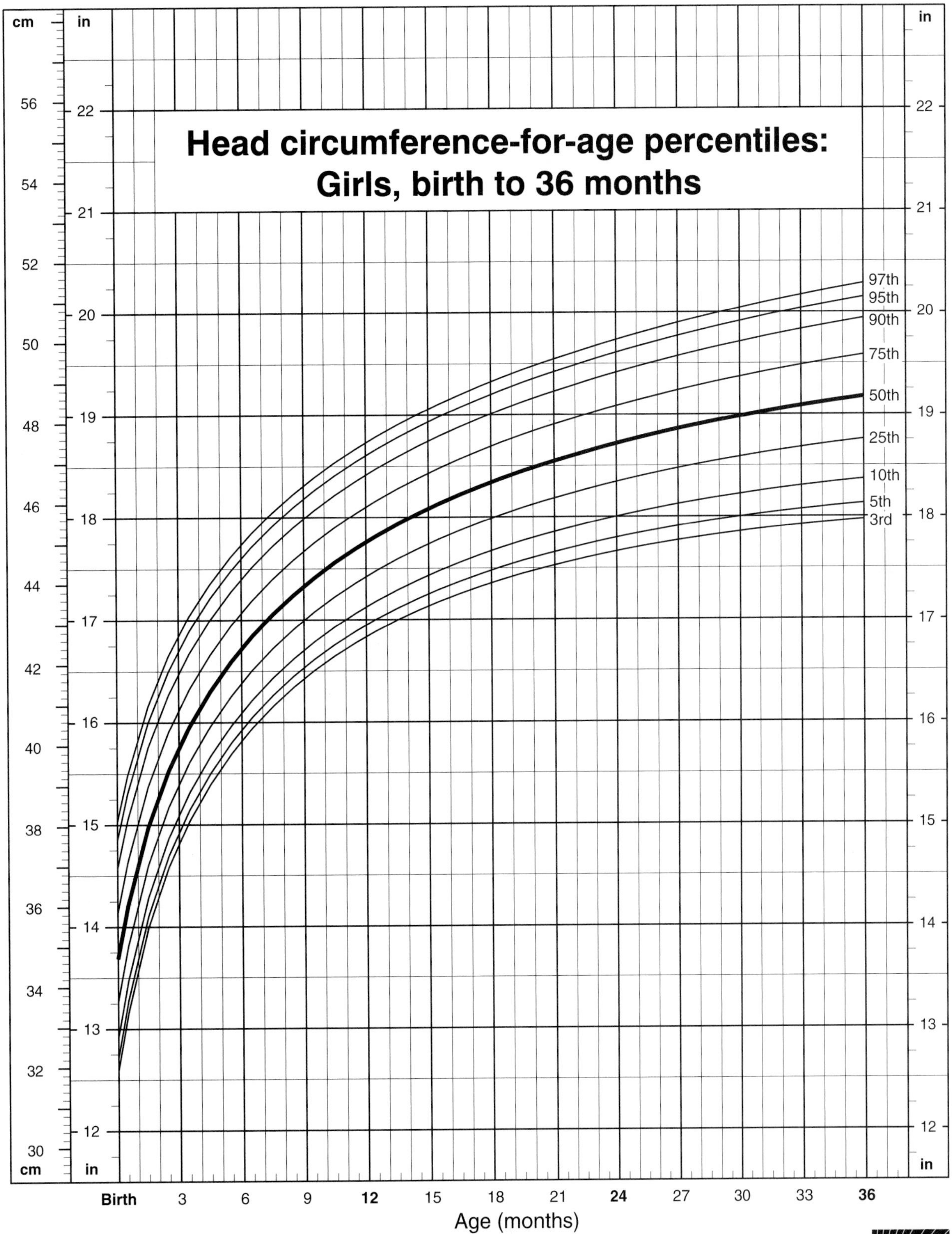

Head circumference-for-age percentiles: Girls, birth to 36 months

cm: 56, 54, 52, 50, 48, 46, 44, 42, 40, 38, 36, 34, 32, 30 cm

in: 22, 21, 20, 19, 18, 17, 16, 15, 14, 13, 12 in

97th
95th
90th
75th
50th
25th
10th
5th
3rd

Birth 3 6 9 **12** 15 18 21 **24** 27 30 33 **36**

Age (months)

Published May 30, 2000.
SOURCE: Developed by the National Center for Health Statistics in collaboration with the National Center for Chronic Disease Prevention and Health Promotion (2000).

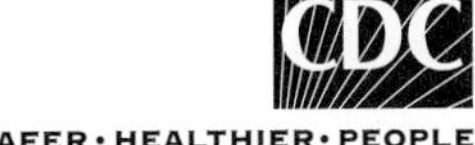

CDC Growth Charts: United States

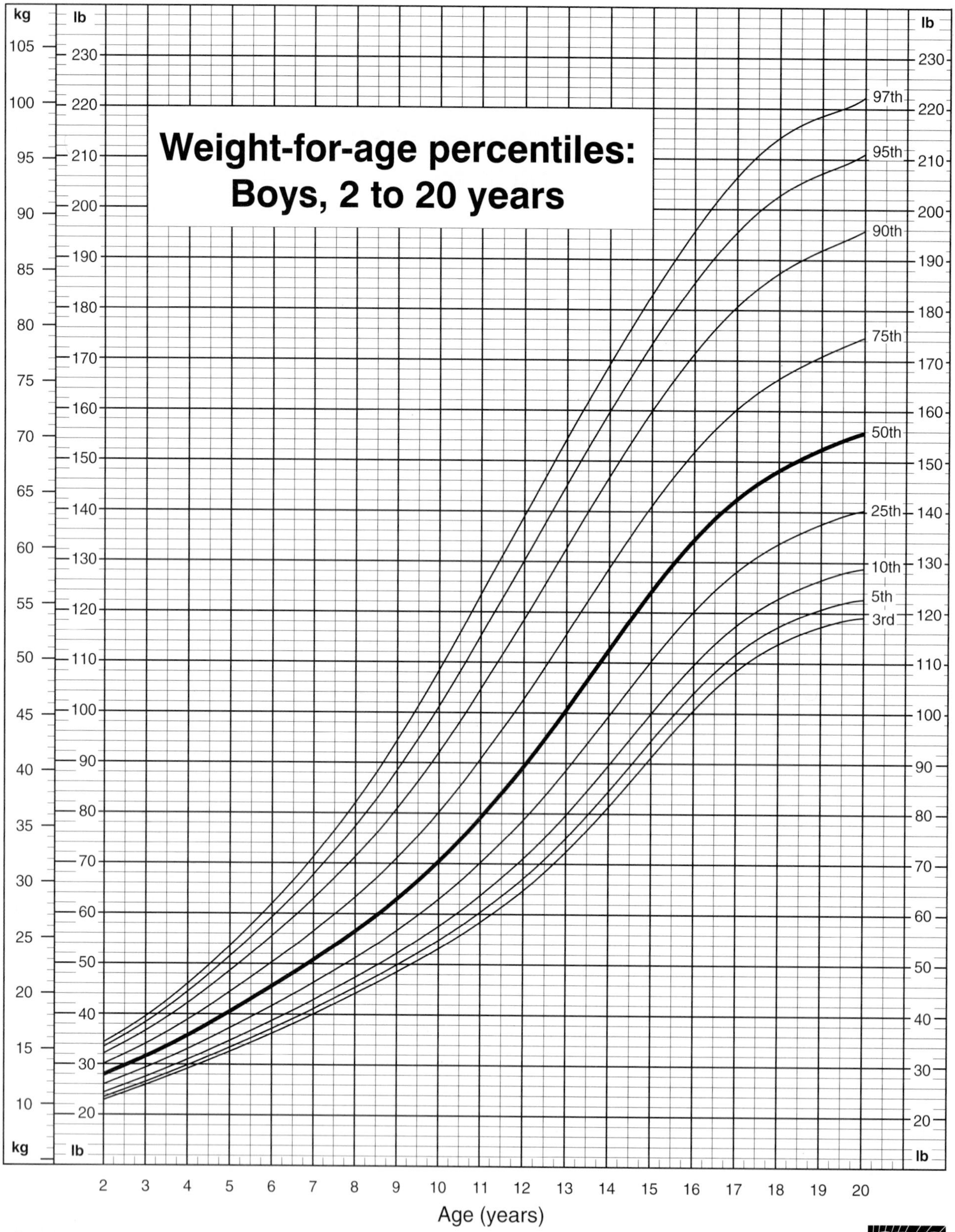

Weight-for-age percentiles: Boys, 2 to 20 years

kg | lb

97th
95th
90th
75th
50th
25th
10th
5th
3rd

Age (years): 2 3 4 5 6 7 8 9 10 11 12 13 14 15 16 17 18 19 20

Published May 30, 2000.

SOURCE: Developed by the National Center for Health Statistics in collaboration with the National Center for Chronic Disease Prevention and Health Promotion (2000).

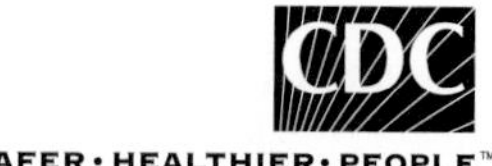

CDC Growth Charts: United States

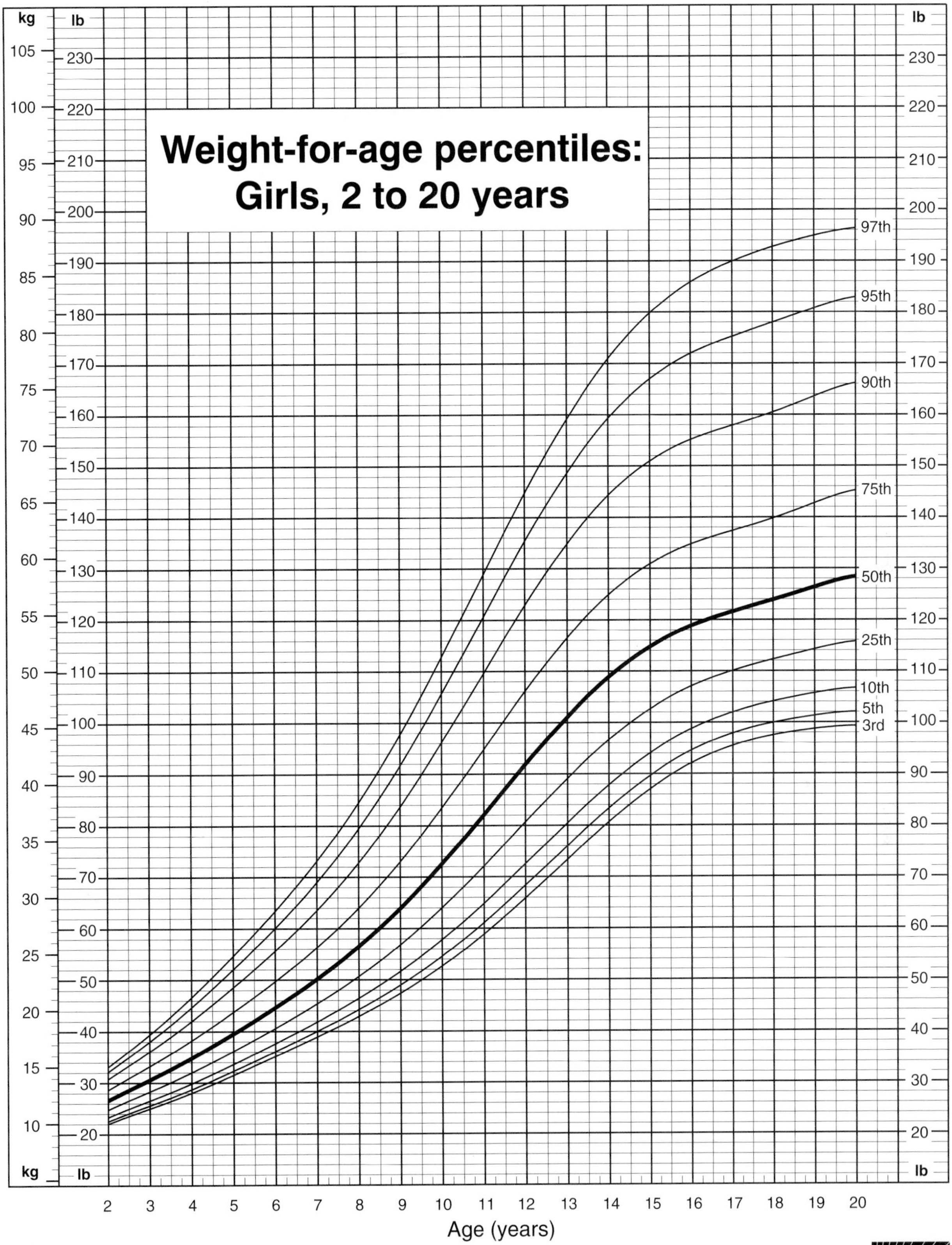

Weight-for-age percentiles: Girls, 2 to 20 years

kg | lb | lb
105 | 230 | 230
100 | 220 | 220
95 | 210 | 210
90 | 200 | 200
85 | 190 | 190
80 | 180 | 180
75 | 170 | 170
70 | 160 | 160
65 | 150 | 150
60 | 140 | 140
55 | 130 | 130
50 | 120 | 120
45 | 110 | 110
40 | 100 | 100
35 | 90 | 90
30 | 80 | 80
25 | 70 | 70
20 | 60 | 60
15 | 50 | 50
10 | 40 | 40
30 | 30
20 | 20
kg | lb | lb

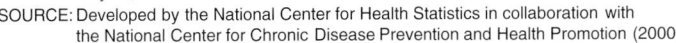

97th
95th
90th
75th
50th
25th
10th
5th
3rd

2 3 4 5 6 7 8 9 10 11 12 13 14 15 16 17 18 19 20

Age (years)

Published May 30, 2000.

SOURCE: Developed by the National Center for Health Statistics in collaboration with the National Center for Chronic Disease Prevention and Health Promotion (2000).

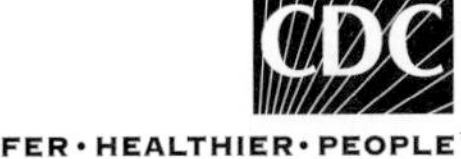

CDC Growth Charts: United States

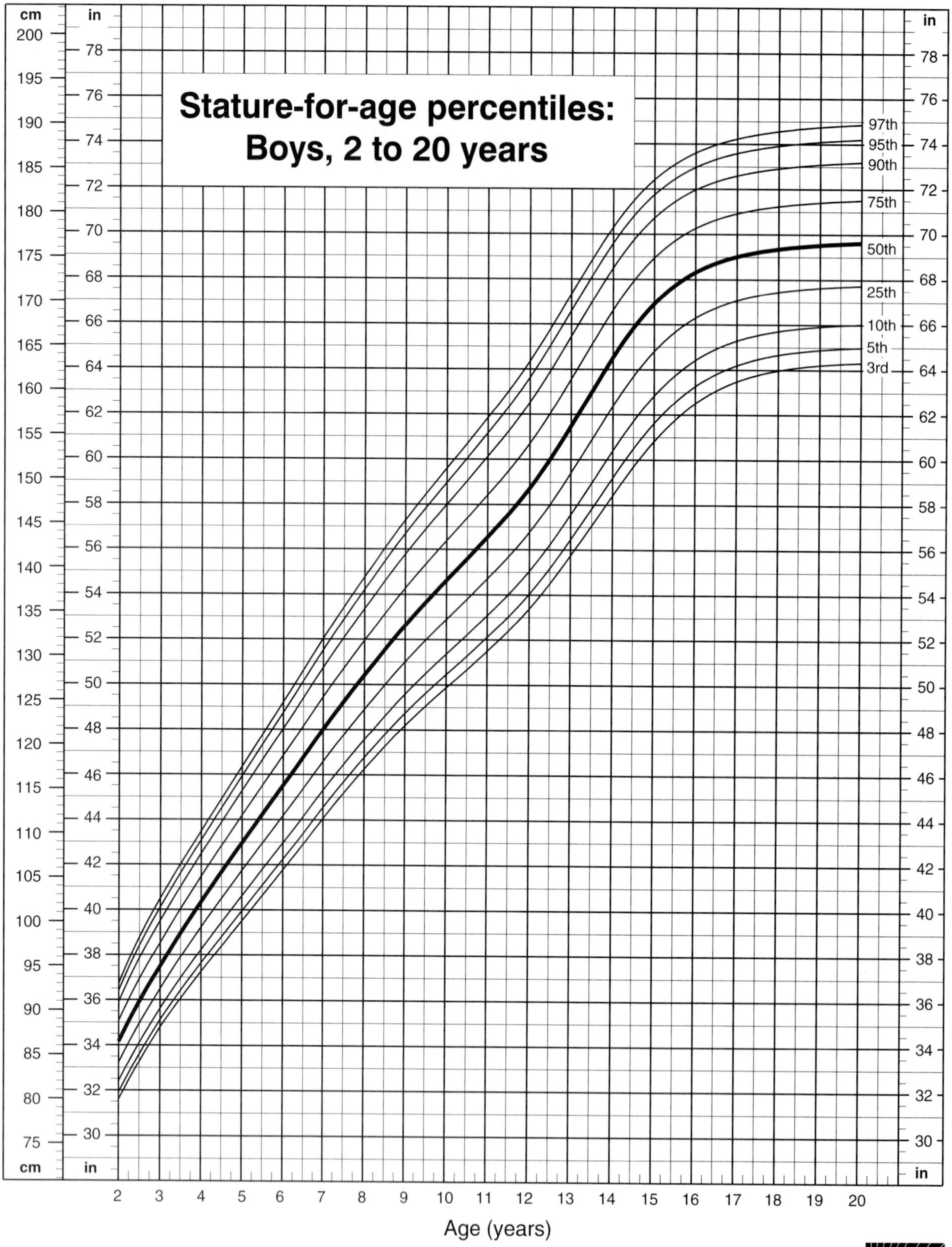

Stature-for-age percentiles: Boys, 2 to 20 years

97th
95th
90th
75th
50th
25th
10th
5th
3rd

Age (years)

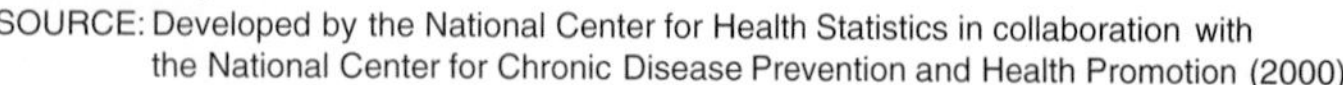
Published May 30, 2000.
SOURCE: Developed by the National Center for Health Statistics in collaboration with the National Center for Chronic Disease Prevention and Health Promotion (2000).

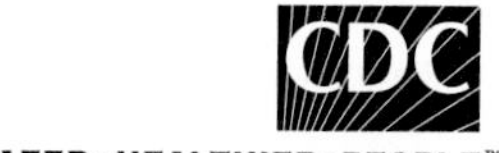

CDC Growth Charts: United States

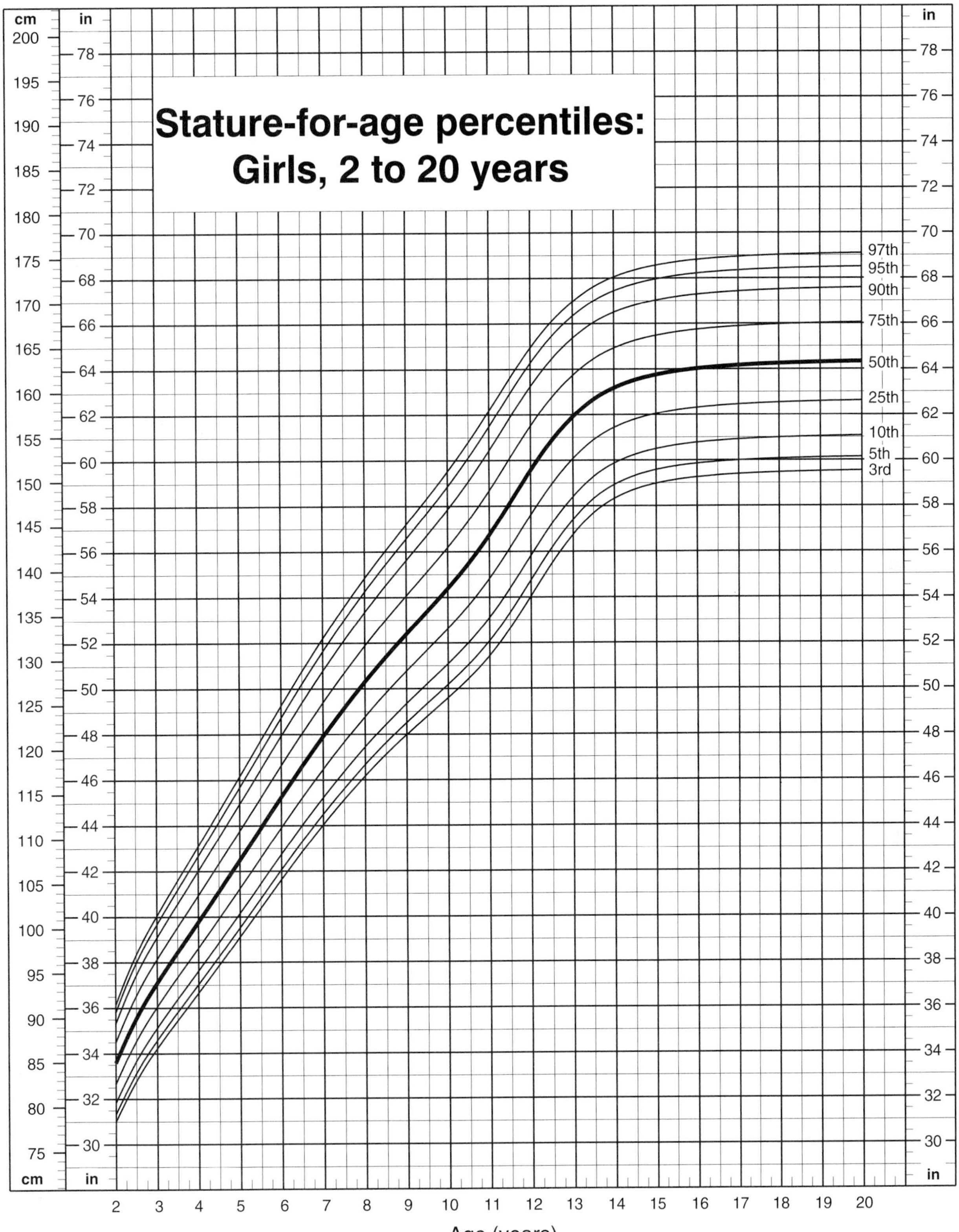

Stature-for-age percentiles: Girls, 2 to 20 years

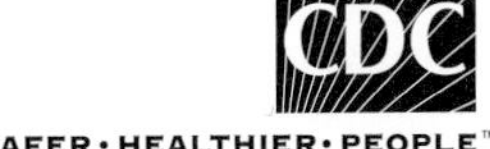

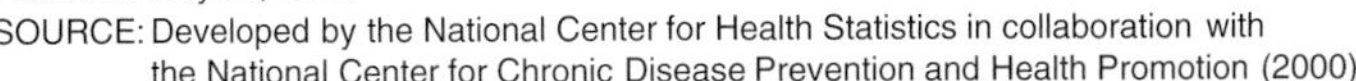
Published May 30, 2000.
SOURCE: Developed by the National Center for Health Statistics in collaboration with the National Center for Chronic Disease Prevention and Health Promotion (2000).

CDC Growth Charts: United States

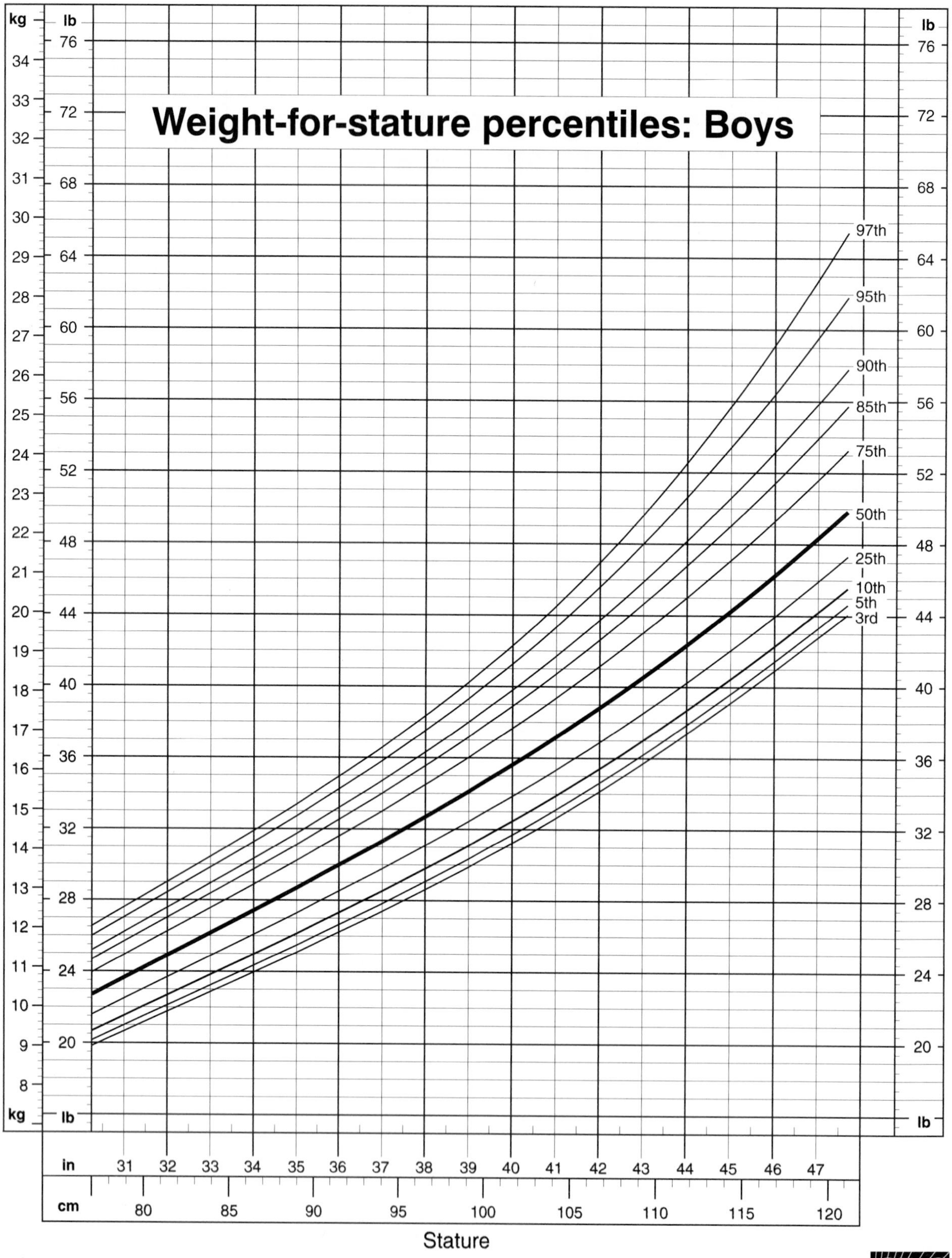

Weight-for-stature percentiles: Boys

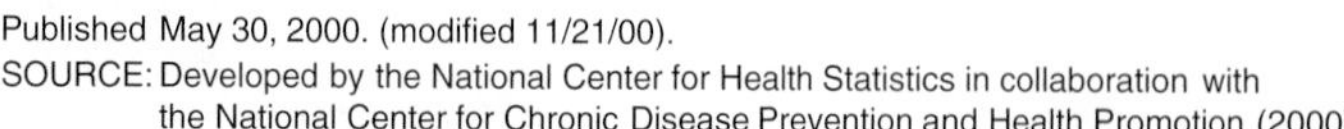

Published May 30, 2000. (modified 11/21/00).
SOURCE: Developed by the National Center for Health Statistics in collaboration with the National Center for Chronic Disease Prevention and Health Promotion (2000).

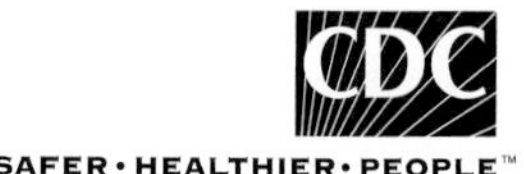

CDC Growth Charts: United States

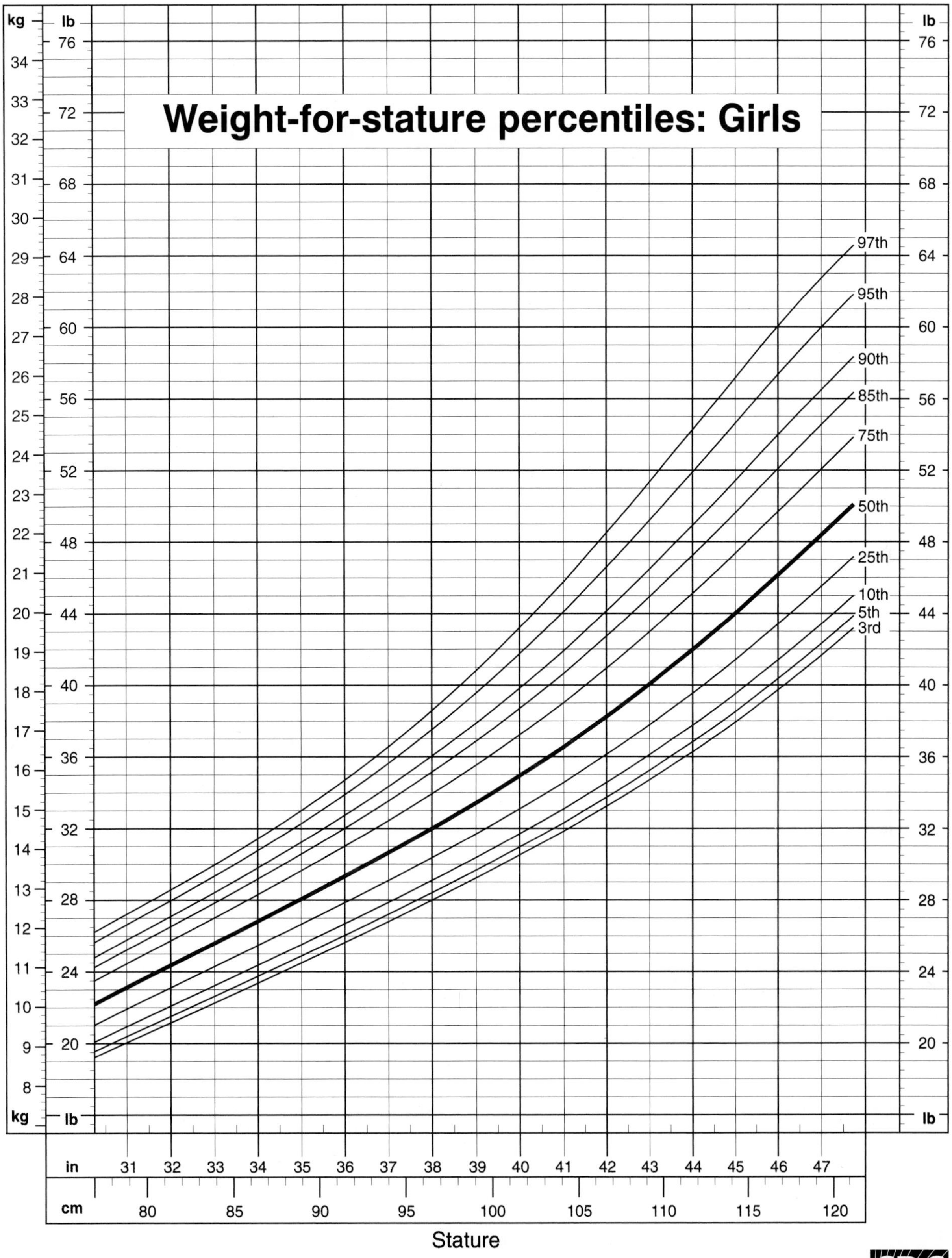

Weight-for-stature percentiles: Girls

kg | lb

97th
95th
90th
85th
75th
50th
25th
10th
5th
3rd

in: 31 32 33 34 35 36 37 38 39 40 41 42 43 44 45 46 47

cm: 80 85 90 95 100 105 110 115 120

Stature

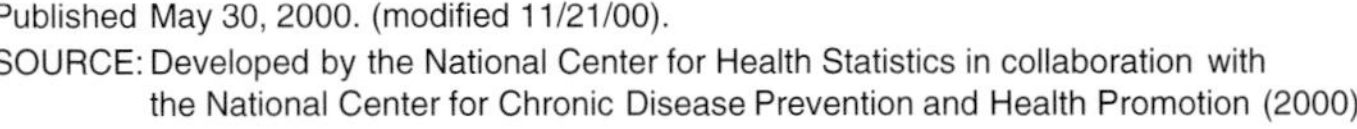
Published May 30, 2000. (modified 11/21/00).
SOURCE: Developed by the National Center for Health Statistics in collaboration with the National Center for Chronic Disease Prevention and Health Promotion (2000).

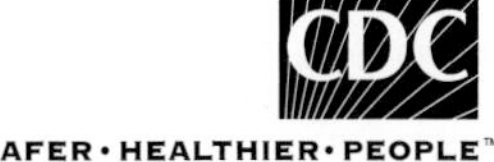

CDC Growth Charts: United States

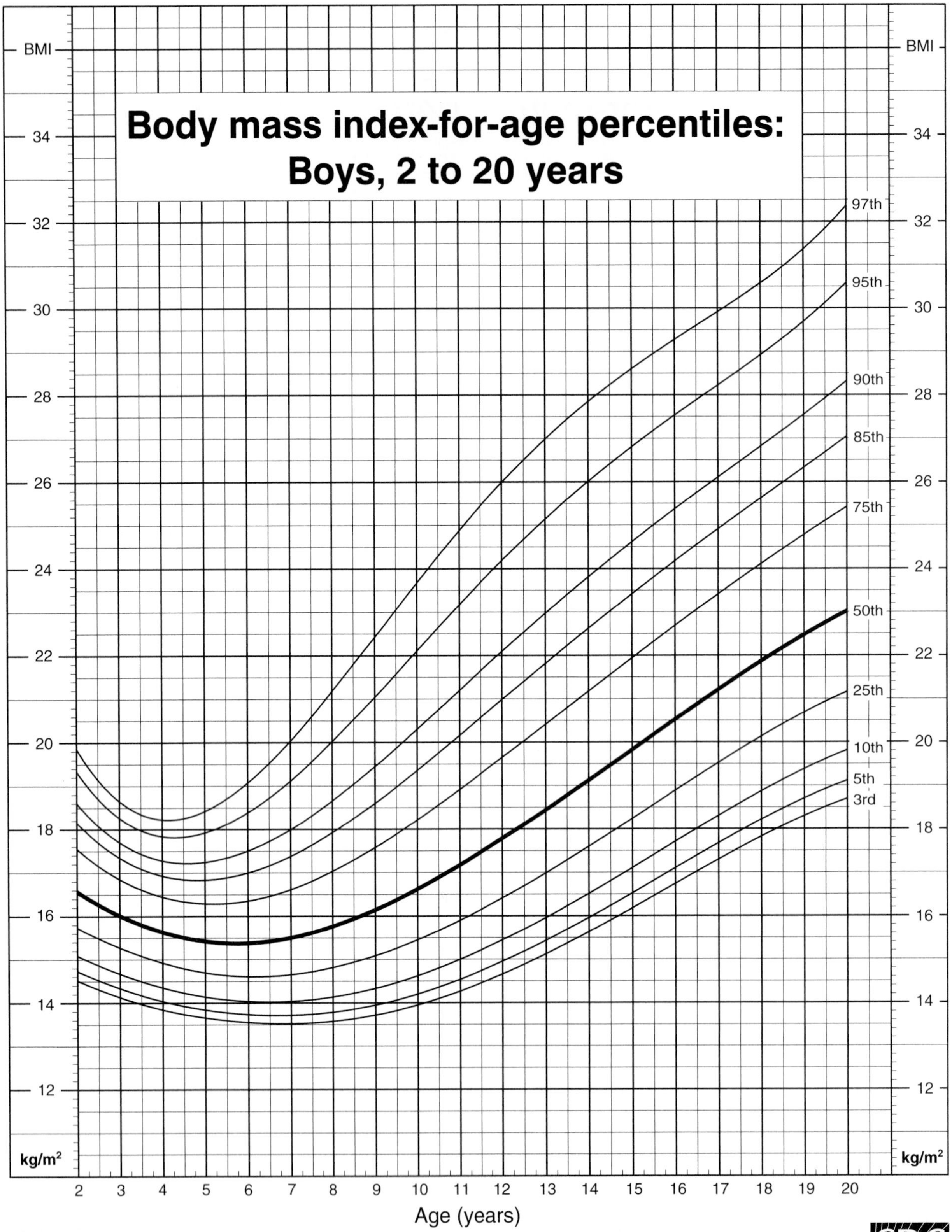

Body mass index-for-age percentiles: Boys, 2 to 20 years

BMI

34
32
30
28
26
24
22
20
18
16
14
12

kg/m²

97th
95th
90th
85th
75th
50th
25th
10th
5th
3rd

2 3 4 5 6 7 8 9 10 11 12 13 14 15 16 17 18 19 20

Age (years)

Published May 30, 2000.
SOURCE: Developed by the National Center for Health Statistics in collaboration with the National Center for Chronic Disease Prevention and Health Promotion (2000).

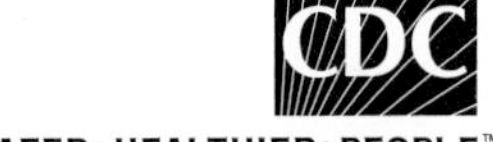

SAFER • HEALTHIER • PEOPLE™

CDC Growth Charts: United States

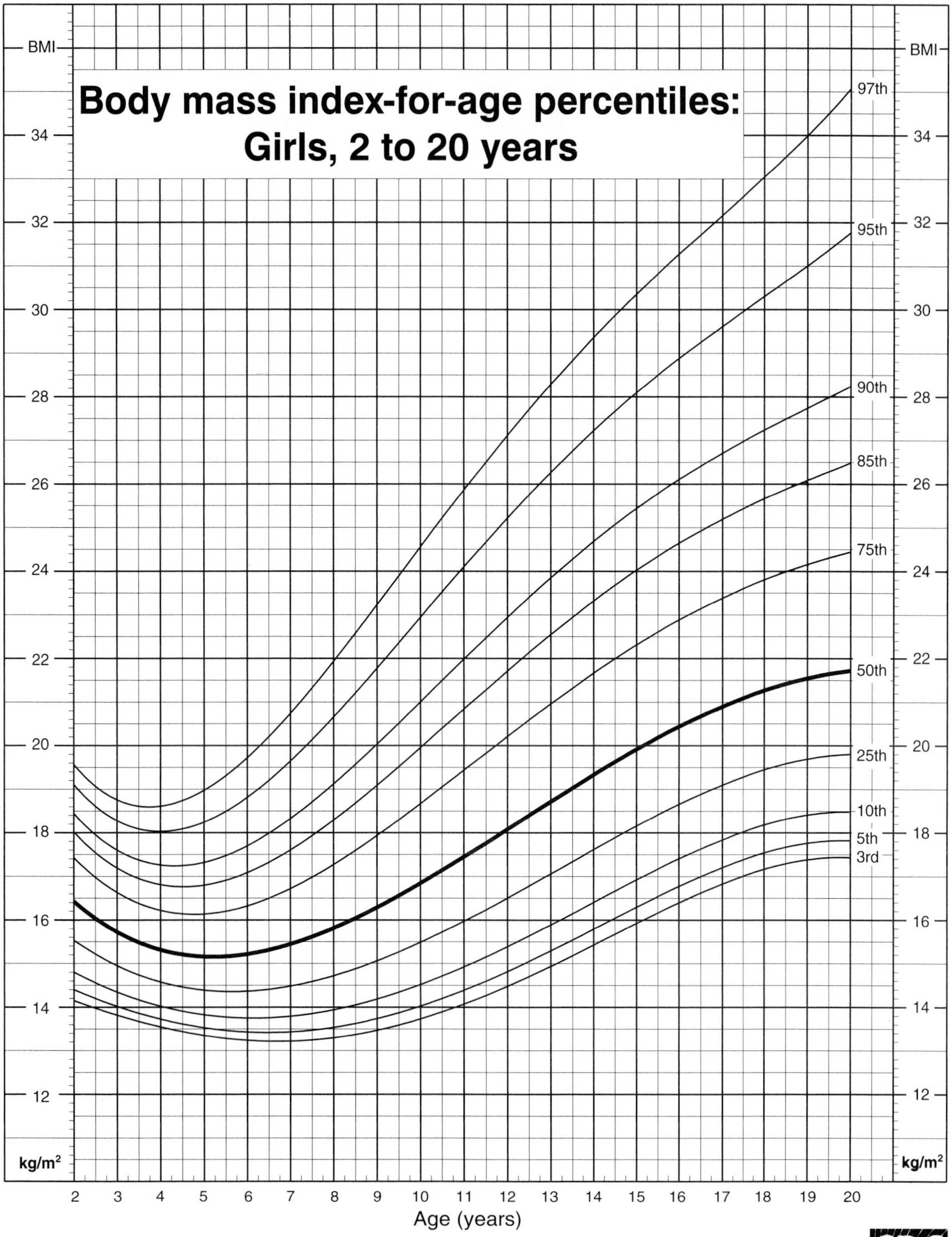

Body mass index-for-age percentiles: Girls, 2 to 20 years

Published May 30, 2000.
SOURCE: Developed by the National Center for Health Statistics in collaboration with the National Center for Chronic Disease Prevention and Health Promotion (2000).

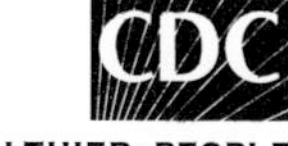

SAFER • HEALTHIER • PEOPLE™

Appendix

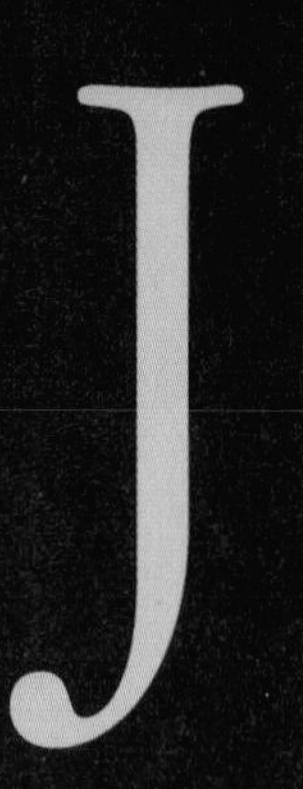

Assessment of Nutritional Status: Percentiles

Mid-Upper-Arm Circumference Percentiles (cm)

	Female Percentiles					Male Percentiles				
Age (yr)	5th	25th	50th	75th	95th	5th	25th	50th	75th	95th
1	13.8	14.8	15.6	16.4	17.7	14.2	15.0	15.9	17.0	18.3
2	14.2	15.2	16.0	16.7	18.4	14.1	15.3	16.2	17.0	18.5
3	14.3	15.8	16.7	17.5	18.9	15.0	16.0	16.7	17.5	19.0
4	14.9	16.0	16.9	17.7	19.1	14.9	16.2	17.1	18.0	19.2
5	15.3	16.5	17.5	18.5	21.1	15.3	16.7	17.5	18.5	20.4
6	15.6	17.0	17.6	18.7	21.1	15.5	16.7	17.9	18.8	22.8
7	16.4	17.4	18.3	19.9	23.1	16.2	17.7	18.7	20.1	23.0
8	16.8	18.3	19.5	21.4	26.1	16.2	17.7	19.0	20.2	24.5
9	17.8	19.4	21.1	22.4	26.0	17.5	18.7	20.0	21.7	25.7
10	17.4	19.3	21.0	22.8	26.5	18.1	19.6	21.0	23.1	27.4
11	18.5	20.8	22.4	24.8	30.3	18.6	20.2	22.3	24.4	28.0
12	19.4	21.6	23.7	25.6	29.4	19.3	21.4	23.2	25.4	30.3
13	20.2	22.3	24.3	27.1	33.8	19.4	22.8	24.7	26.3	30.1
14	21.4	23.7	25.2	27.2	32.2	22.0	23.7	25.3	28.3	32.3
15	20.8	23.9	25.4	27.9	32.2	22.2	24.4	26.4	28.4	32.0
16	21.8	24.1	25.8	28.3	32.4	24.4	26.2	27.8	30.3	34.3
17	22.0	24.1	26.4	29.5	35.0	24.6	26.7	28.5	30.8	34.7
18	22.2	24.1	25.8	28.1	32.5	24.5	27.6	29.7	32.1	37.9
19-25	21.1	24.7	26.5	29.0	34.5	26.2	28.8	30.8	33.1	37.2
25-35	23.3	25.6	27.7	30.4	36.8	27.1	30.0	31.9	34.2	37.5
35-45	24.1	26.7	29.0	31.7	37.8	27.8	30.5	32.6	34.5	37.4
45-55	24.2	27.4	29.9	32.8	38.4	26.7	30.1	32.2	34.2	37.6
55-65	24.3	28.0	30.3	33.5	38.5	25.8	29.6	31.7	33.6	36.9
65-75	24.0	27.4	29.9	32.6	37.3	24.8	28.5	30.7	32.5	35.5

Data derived from the Health and Nutrition Examination Survey data of 1971-1974, using same population samples as those of the National Center for Health Statistics (NCHS) growth percentiles for children. Modified from Frisancho AR: New norms of upper limb fat and muscle areas for assessment of nutritional status, *Am J Clin Nutr* 34:2540, 1981.

Triceps Skinfold Percentiles (mm)

	Female Percentiles					Male Percentiles				
Age (yr)	5th	25th	50th	75th	95th	5th	25th	50th	75th	95th
1	6	8	10	12	16	6	8	10	12	16
2	6	9	10	12	16	6	8	10	12	15
3	7	9	11	12	15	6	8	10	11	15
4	7	8	10	12	16	6	8	9	11	14
5	6	8	10	12	18	6	8	9	11	15
6	6	8	10	12	16	5	7	8	10	16
7	6	9	11	13	18	5	7	9	12	17
8	6	9	12	15	24	5	7	8	10	16
9	8	10	13	16	22	6	7	10	13	18
10	7	10	12	17	27	6	8	10	14	21
11	7	10	13	18	28	6	8	11	16	24
12	8	11	14	18	27	6	8	11	14	28
13	8	12	15	21	30	5	7	10	14	26
14	9	13	16	21	28	4	7	9	14	24
15	8	12	17	21	32	4	6	8	11	24
16	10	15	18	22	31	4	6	8	12	22
17	10	13	19	24	37	5	6	8	12	19
18	10	15	18	22	30	4	6	9	13	24
19-25	10	14	18	24	34	4	7	10	15	22
25-35	10	16	21	27	37	5	8	12	16	24
35-45	12	18	23	29	38	5	8	12	16	23
45-55	12	20	25	30	40	6	8	12	15	25
55-65	12	20	25	31	38	5	8	11	14	22
65-75	12	18	24	29	36	4	8	11	15	22

Mid-Upper-Arm Muscle Circumference Percentiles (cm)

	Female Percentiles					Male Percentiles				
Age (yr)	5th	25th	50th	75th	95th	5th	25th	50th	75th	95th
1	10.5	11.7	12.4	13.9	14.3	11.0	11.9	12.7	13.5	14.7
2	11.1	11.9	12.6	13.3	14.7	11.1	12.2	13.0	14.0	15.0
3	11.3	12.4	13.2	14.0	15.2	11.7	13.1	13.7	14.3	15.3
4	11.5	12.8	13.8	14.4	15.7	12.3	13.3	14.1	14.8	15.9
5	12.5	13.4	14.2	15.1	16.5	12.8	14.0	14.7	15.4	16.9
6	13.0	13.8	14.5	15.4	17.1	13.1	14.2	15.1	16.1	17.1
7	12.9	14.2	15.1	16.0	17.6	13.7	15.1	16.0	16.8	19.0
8	13.8	15.1	16.0	17.1	19.4	14.0	15.4	16.2	17.0	18.7
9	14.7	15.8	16.7	18.0	19.8	15.1	16.1	17.0	18.3	20.2
10	17.8	15.9	17.0	18.0	19.7	15.6	16.6	18.0	19.1	22.1
11	15.0	17.1	18.1	19.6	22.3	15.9	17.3	18.3	19.5	23.0
12	16.2	18.0	19.1	20.1	22.0	16.7	18.2	19.5	21.0	24.1
13	16.9	18.3	19.8	21.1	24.0	17.2	19.6	21.1	22.6	24.5
14	17.4	19.0	20.1	21.6	24.7	18.9	21.2	22.3	24.0	26.4
15	17.5	18.9	20.2	21.5	24.4	19.9	21.8	23.7	25.4	27.2
16	17.0	19.0	20.2	21.6	24.9	21.3	23.4	24.9	26.9	29.6
17	17.5	19.4	20.5	22.1	25.7	22.4	24.5	25.8	27.3	31.2
18	17.4	19.1	20.2	21.5	24.5	22.6	25.2	26.4	28.3	32.4
19-25	17.9	19.5	20.7	22.1	24.9	23.8	25.7	27.3	28.9	32.1
25-35	18.3	19.9	21.2	22.8	26.4	24.3	26.4	27.9	29.8	32.6
35-45	18.6	20.5	21.8	23.6	27.2	24.7	26.9	28.6	30.2	32.7
45-55	18.7	20.6	22.0	23.8	27.4	23.9	26.5	28.1	30.0	32.6
55-65	18.7	20.9	22.5	24.4	28.0	23.6	26.0	27.8	29.5	32.0
65-75	18.5	20.8	22.5	24.4	27.9	22.3	25.1	26.8	28.4	30.6

Values derived by formula calculation. Data derived from the Health and Nutrition Examination Survey data of 1971-1974, using same population samples as those of the National Center for Health Statistics (NCHS) growth percentiles for children. Modified from Frisancho AR: New norms of upper limb fat and muscle areas for assessment of nutritional status, *Am J Clin Nutr* 34:2540, 1981.

Appendix

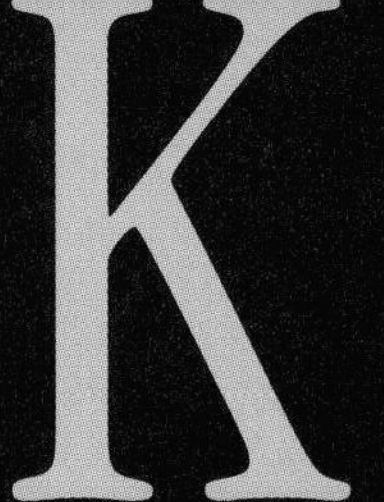

K Normal Constituents of Blood and Urine in Adults

Normal Constituents of Blood in the Adult

Physical Measurements		
Specific gravity		1.025-1.029
Viscosity (water as unity)		4.5
Bleeding time (capillary)	Minutes	1-3
Prothrombin time (plasma) (Quick)	Seconds	10-20
Sedimentation rate (Wintrobe method)		
Men	mm/hr	0-9
Women	mm/hr	0-20
Hemologic Studies		
Cell volume	%	39-50
Red blood cells	Million per mm^3	4.25-5.25
White blood cells	Per mm^3	5000-9000
Lymphocytes	%	25-30
Neutrophils	%	60-65
Monocytes	%	4-8
Eosinophils	%	0.5-4
Basophils	%	0-1.5
Platelets	Per mm^3	125,000-300,000
Proteins		
Total protein (serum)	g/dl	6.5-7.5
Albumin (serum)	g/dl	4.5-5.5
Globulin (serum)	g/dl	1.5-2.5
Albumin:globulin ratio		1.8-2.5
Fibrinogen (plasma)	g/dl	0.2-0.5
Hemoglobin		
Males	g/dl	14-17
Females	g/dl	13-16

Nitrogen Constituents		
Nonprotein N (serum)	mg/dl	20-36
(whole blood)	mg/dl	25-40
Urea (whole blood)	mg/dl	18-38
Urea N (whole blood)	mg/dl	8-18
Creatinine (whole blood)	mg/dl	1-2
Uric acid (whole blood)	mg/dl	2.5-5.0
Amino acid N (whole blood)	mg/dl	3-6
Carbohydrates and Lipids		
Glucose (whole blood)	mg/dl	70-90
Ketones—as acetone (whole blood)	mg/dl	1.5-2
Fats (total lipids) (serum)	mg/dl	570-820
Cholesterol (serum)	mg/dl	100-230
Bilirubin (serum)	mg/dl	0.1-0.25
Icteric index (serum)	Units	4-6
Blood Gases		
CO_2 content (serum)	vol %	55-75
	mmol/L	24.5-33.5
CO_2 content (whole blood)	vol %	40-60
	mmol/L	18.0-27.0
Oxygen capacity (whole blood)		
Males	vol %	18.7-22.7
Females	vol %	17.0-21.0
Oxygen saturation		
Arterial blood	%	94-96
Venous blood	%	60-85

Abbreviations and conversion factors:

- dl = deciliter
- ml = milliliter
- μg = microgram
- mEq/L $= \frac{\text{mg/L}}{\text{Equivalent weight}}$
- Equivalent weight $= \frac{\text{Atomic weight}}{\text{Valence of element}}$
- g = gram
- mm^3 = cubic millimeter
- mEq = milliequivalent
- mmol (millimole)/L $= \frac{\text{mg/L}}{\text{Molecular weight}}$
- vol % (volumes percent) = mmol/L × 2.24

Normal Constituents of Blood in the Adult—cont'd

Acid-Base Constituents		
Base, total fixed (serum)	mEq/L	142-150
Sodium (serum)	mg/dl	320-335
	mEq/L	139-146
Potassium (serum)	mg/dl	16-22
	mEq/L	4.1-5.6
Calcium (serum)	mg/dl	9.0-11.5
	mEq/L	4.5-5.8
Magnesium (serum)	mg/dl	1.0-3.0
	mEq/L	1.0-2.5
Phosphorus, inorganic (serum)	mg/dl	3.0-5.0
	mEq/L	1.0-1.6
Chlorides, expressed		
as Cl (serum)	mg/dl	352-383
	mEq/L	99-108
as NaCl (serum)	mg/dl	580-630
	mEq/L	99-108

Acid-Base Constituents—cont'd		
Sulfates, inorganic as SO_4 (serum)	mg/dl	2.5-5.0
	mEq/L	0.5-1.0
Lactic acid (venous blood)	mg/dl	10-20
	mEq/L	1.1-2.2
Serum protein base binding power	mEq/L	15.5-18.0
Base bicarbonate HCO_3 (serum)	mEq/L	19-30
pH (blood or plasma at 38° C)		7.3-7.45
Miscellaneous		
Phosphatase (serum)	Bodansky units/dl	5
Iron (whole blood)	mg/dl	46-55
Ascorbic acid (whole blood)	mg/dl	0.75-1.50
Carotene (serum)	μg/dl	75-125

Normal Constituents of Urine in the Adult

Urine Constituents	g/24 hr
Total solids	55-70
Nitrogenous constituents	
Total nitrogen	10-17
Ammonia	0.5-1.0
Amino acid N	0.4-1
Creatine	None
Creatinine	1-1.5
Protein	None
Purine bases	0.016-0.060
Urea	20-35
Uric acid	0.5-0.7
Acetone bodies	0.003-0.015
Bile	None
Calcium	0.2-0.4
Chloride (as NaCl)	10-15
Glucose	None
Indican	0-0.030
Iron	0.001-0.005
Magnesium (as MgO)	0.15-0.30
Phosphate, total (as phosphoric acid)	2.5-3.5
Potassium (as K_2O)	2.0-3.0
Sodium (as Na_2O)	4.0-5.0
Sulfates, total (as sulfuric acid)	1.5-3.0
Physical Measurements	
Specific gravity	1.010-1.025
Reaction (pH)	5.5-8.0
Volume (ml/24 hr)	800-1600

Appendix L

Exchange Lists for Meal Planning

Starch Exchange List

(One exchange = 15 g carbohydrate, 3 g protein, 0-1 g fat, 80 calories)

Bread

Bagel	½ (1 oz)
Bread, reduced calorie	2 slices (1½ oz)
Bread, white, whole wheat, pumpernickel, rye	1 slice (1 oz)
Bread sticks, crisp, 4 in × ½ in	2 (⅔ oz)
English muffin	½
Hot dog or hamburger bun	½ (1 oz)
Pita, 6 in across	½
Roll, plain, small	1 (1 oz)
Raisin bread, unfrosted	1 slice (1 oz)
Tortilla, corn, 6 in across	1
Tortilla, flour, 7-8 in across	1
Waffle, 4½ in square, reduced fat	1

Cereals and Grains

Bran cereals	½ cup
Bulgur	½ cup
Cereals	½ cup
Cereals, unsweetened, ready to eat	¾ cup
Cornmeal (dry)	3 tbsp
Couscous	⅓ cup
Flour (dry)	3 tbsp
Granola, low-fat	¼ cup
Grape-Nuts	¼ cup
Grits	½ cup
Kasha	½ cup
Millet	¼ cup
Muesli	¼ cup
Oats	½ cup
Pasta	½ cup
Puffed cereal	1½ cups
Rice milk	½ cup
Rice, white or brown	⅓ cup
Shredded Wheat	½ cup
Sugar-frosted cereal	½ cup
Wheat germ	3 tbsp

Starchy Vegetables

Baked beans	⅓ cup
Corn	½ cup
Corn on cob, medium	1 (5 oz)
Mixed vegetables with corn, peas, or pasta	1 cup
Peas, green	½ cup
Plantain	½ cup
Potato, baked or boiled	1 small (3 oz)
Potato, mashed	½ cup
Squash, winter (acorn, butternut)	1 cup
Yam, sweet potato, plain	½ cup

Crackers and Snacks

Animal crackers	8
Graham crackers, 2½ in square	3
Matzoh	¾ oz
Melba toast	4 slices
Oyster crackers	24
Popcorn (popped, no fat added or low-fat microwave)	3 cups
Pretzels	¾ oz
Rice cakes, 4 in across	2
Saltine-type crackers	6
Snack chips, fat-free (tortilla, potato)	15-20 (¾ oz)
Whole-wheat crackers, no fat added	2-5 (¾ oz)

Beans, Peas, and Lentils

(Count as 1 starch exchange, plus 1 very lean meat exchange)

Beans and peas (garbanzo, pinto, kidney, white, split, black-eyed)	½ cup
Lima beans	⅔ cup
Lentils	½ cup
Miso*	3 tbsp

Starchy Foods Prepared With Fat

(Count as 1 starch exchange, plus 1 fat exchange)

Biscuit, 2½ in across	1
Chow mein noodles	½ cup
Cornbread, 2-in cube	1 (2 oz)
Crackers, round butter type	6
Croutons	1 cup

* = 400 mg or more sodium per exchange.

Starch Exchange List

Starchy Foods Prepared With Fat—cont'd

French-fried potatoes	16-25 (3 oz)
Granola	¼ cup
Muffin, small	1 (1½ oz)
Pancake, 4 in across	2
Popcorn, microwave	3 cups
Sandwich crackers, cheese or peanut butter filling	3
Stuffing, bread (prepared)	⅓ cup
Taco shell, 6 in across	2
Waffle, 4½ in square	1
Whole-wheat crackers, fat added	4-6 (1 oz)

Fruit Exchange List

(One exchange = 15 g carbohydrate, 60 calories; weight includes skin, core, seeds, and rind)

Fruit

Apple, unpeeled, small	1 (4 oz)
Applesauce, unsweetened	½ cup
Apples, dried	4 rings
Apricots, fresh	4 whole (5½ oz)
Apricots, dried	8 halves
Apricots, canned	½ cup
Banana, small	1 (4 oz)
Blackberries	¾ cup
Blueberries	¾ cup
Cantaloupe, small	⅓ melon (11 oz) or 1 cup cubes
Cherries, sweet, fresh	12 (3 oz)
Cherries, sweet, canned	½ cup
Dates	3
Figs, fresh	1½ large or 2 medium
Figs, dried	1½
Fruit cocktail	½ cup
Grapefruit, large	½ (11 oz)
Grapefruit sections, canned	¾ cup
Grapes, small	17 (3 oz)
Honeydew melon	1 slice (10 oz) or 1 cup cubes
Kiwi	1 (3½ oz)
Mandarin oranges, canned	¾ cup
Mango, small	½ fruit (5½ oz) or ½ cup
Nectarine, small	1 (5 oz)
Orange, small	1 (6½ oz)
Papaya	½ fruit (8 oz) or 1 cup cubes
Peach, medium, fresh	1 (6 oz)
Peaches, canned	½ cup

Fruit—cont'd

Pear, large, fresh	½ (4 oz)
Pears, canned	½ cup
Pineapple, fresh	¾ cup
Pineapple, canned	½ cup
Plums, small	2 (5 oz)
Plums, canned	½ cup
Prunes, dried	3
Raisins	2 tbsp
Raspberries	1 cup
Strawberries	1¼ cup whole berries
Tangerines, small	2 (8 oz)
Watermelon	1 slice (13½ oz) or 1¼ cup cubes

Fruit Juice

Apple juice/cider	½ cup
Cranberry juice cocktail	⅓ cup
Cranberry juice cocktail, reduced-calorie	1 cup
Fruit juice blends, 100% juice	⅓ cup
Grape juice	⅓ cup
Grapefruit juice	½ cup
Orange juice	½ cup
Pineapple juice	½ cup
Prune juice	⅓ cup

Milk Exchange List

(One exchange = 12 g carbohydrate, 8 g protein)

Fat-Free and Low-Fat Milk

(0-3 g fat per serving)

Skim milk	1 cup
½% milk	1 cup
1% milk	1 cup
Nonfat or low-fat buttermilk	1 cup
Evaporated skim milk	½ cup
Nonfat dry milk	⅓ cup dry
Plain nonfat yogurt	¾ cup
Nonfat or low-fat fruit-flavored yogurt sweetened with aspartame or with a nonnutritive sweetener	1 cup

Reduced Fat Milk

(5 g fat per serving)

2% milk	1 cup
Plain low-fat yogurt	¾ cup
Sweet acidophilus milk	1 cup

Whole Milk

(8 g fat per serving)

Whole milk	1 cup
Evaporated whole milk	½ cup
Goat's milk	1 cup
Kefir	1 cup

Other Carbohydrates List

(One exchange = 15 g carbohydrate, or 1 starch, 1 fruit, or 1 milk)

Food	*Serving Size*	*Exchanges Per Serving*
Angel food cake, unfrosted	1/12 cake	2 carbohydrates
Brownie, small, unfrosted	2 in square	1 carbohydrate, 1 fat
Cake, unfrosted	2 in square	1 carbohydrate, 1 fat
Cake, frosted	2 in square	2 carbohydrates, 1 fat
Cookie, fat-free	2 small	1 carbohydrate
Cookie or sandwich cookie with creme filling	2 small	1 carbohydrate, 1 fat
Cupcake, frosted	1 small	2 carbohydrates, 1 fat
Cranberry sauce, jellied	¼ cup	2 carbohydrates
Doughnut, plain cake	1 medium (1½ oz)	1½ carbohydrates, 2 fats
Doughnut, glazed	3¾ in across (2 oz)	2 carbohydrates, 2 fats
Fruit juice bars, frozen, 100% juice	1 bar (3 oz)	1 carbohydrate
Fruit snacks, chewy (pureed fruit concentrate)	1 roll (¾ oz)	1 carbohydrate
Fruit spreads, 100% fruit	1 tbsp	1 carbohydrate
Gelatin, regular	½ cup	1 carbohydrate
Gingersnaps	3	1 carbohydrate
Granola bar	1 bar	1 carbohydrate, 1 fat
Granola bar, fat-free	1 bar	2 carbohydrates
Hummus	⅓ cup	1 carbohydrate, 1 fat
Ice cream	½ cup	1 carbohydrate, 2 fats
Ice cream, light	½ cup	1 carbohydrate, 1 fat
Ice cream, fat-free, no sugar added	½ cup	1 carbohydrate
Jam or jelly, regular	1 tbsp	1 carbohydrate
Milk, chocolate, whole	1 cup	2 carbohydrates, 1 fat
Pie, fruit, 2 crusts	⅙ pie	3 carbohydrates, 2 fats
Pie, pumpkin or custard	⅛ pie	1 carbohydrate, 2 fats
Potato chips	12-18 (1 oz)	1 carbohydrate, 2 fats
Pudding, regular (made with low-fat milk)	½ cup	2 carbohydrates
Pudding, sugar-free (made with low-fat milk)	½ cup	1 carbohydrate
Salad dressing, fat-free*	¼ cup	1 carbohydrate
Sherbet, sorbet	½ cup	2 carbohydrates
Spaghetti or pasta sauce, canned*	½ cup	1 carbohydrate, 1 fat
Sweet roll or Danish	1 (2½ oz)	2½ carbohydrates, 2 fats
Syrup, light	2 tbsp	1 carbohydrate
Syrup, regular	1 tbsp	1 carbohydrate
Syrup, regular	¼ cup	4 carbohydrates
Tortilla chips	6-12 (1 oz)	1 carbohydrate, 2 fats
Vanilla Wafers	5	1 carbohydrate, 1 fat
Yogurt, frozen, low-fat, fat-free	⅓ cup	1 carbohydrate, 0-1 fat
Yogurt, frozen, fat-free, no sugar added	½ cup	1 carbohydrate
Yogurt, low-fat with fruit	1 cup	3 carbohydrates, 0-1 fat

Vegetable Exchange List

(One exchange = 5 g carbohydrate, 2 g protein, 0 g fat, 25 calories)

One exchange = ½ cup of cooked vegetables or vegetable juice, or 1 cup of raw vegetables

Artichoke
Artichoke hearts
Asparagus
Beans (green, wax, Italian)
Bean sprouts
Beets
Broccoli
Brussels sprouts
Cabbage
Carrots
Cauliflower
Celery
Cucumber
Eggplant
Green onions or scallions
Greens (collard, kale, mustard, turnip)
Kohlrabi
Leeks
Mixed vegetables (without corn, peas, or pasta)
Mushrooms
Okra
Onions

Continued

* = 400 mg or more sodium per exchange.

Vegetable Exchange List—cont'd

Pea pods
Radishes
Salad greens
Sauerkraut*
Spinach
Summer squash
Tomato
Tomatoes, canned
Tomato sauce*
Tomato/vegetable juice*
Turnips
Water chestnuts
Watercress
Zucchini

Meat Exchange List

Very Lean Meat and Substitutes	
(One exchange = 0 g carbohydrate, 7 g protein, 0-1 g fat, 35 calories)	
Poultry: Chicken or turkey (white meat, no skin), Cornish game hen (no skin)	1 oz
Fish: Fresh or frozen cod, flounder, haddock, trout; tuna fresh or canned in water	1 oz
Shellfish: Clams, crab, lobster, scallops, shrimp, imitation shellfish	1 oz
Game: Duck or pheasant (no skin), venison, buffalo, ostrich	1 oz
Cheese with 1 g or less fat per ounce:	
Nonfat or low-fat cottage cheese	¼ cup
Fat-free cheese	1 oz
Other:	
Processed sandwich meats with 1 g or less fat per ounce, such as deli thin, shaved meats, chipped beef*, turkey ham	1 oz
Egg whites	2
Egg substitutes, plain	¼ cup
Hot dogs with 1 g or less fat per ounce*	1 oz
Kidney (high in cholesterol)	1 oz
Sausage with 1 g or less fat per ounce	1 oz
Count as one very lean meat and one starch exchange:	
Dried beans, peas, lentils (cooked)	½ cup
Lean Meat and Substitutes	
(One exchange = 0 g carbohydrate, 7 g protein, 3 g fat, 55 calories)	
Beef: USDA Select or Choice grades of lean beef trimmed of fat, such as round, sirloin, and flank steak; tenderloin; roast (rib, chuck, rump); steak (T-bone, porterhouse, cubed); ground round	1 oz
Pork: Lean pork, such as fresh ham; canned, cured, or boiled ham; Canadian bacon*; tenderloin, center loin chop	
Lamb: Roast, chop, leg	1 oz
Veal: Lean chop, roast	
Poultry: Chicken, turkey (dark meat, no skin), chicken white meat (with skin), domestic duck or goose (well-drained of fat, no skin)	1 oz
Fish: Herring (uncreamed or smoked)	1 oz
Oysters	6 medium
Salmon (fresh or canned), catfish	1 oz
Sardines (canned)	2 medium
Tuna (canned in oil, drained)	1 oz
Game: Goose (no skin), rabbit	1 oz
Cheese: 4.5% fat cottage cheese	¼ cup
Grated parmesan	2 tbsp
Cheeses with 3 g or less fat per ounce	1 oz
Other: Hot dogs with 3 g or less fat per ounce	1½ oz
Processed sandwich meat with 3 g or less fat per ounce, such as turkey pastrami or kielbasa	1 oz
Liver, heart (high in cholesterol)	1 oz
Medium-Fat Meat and Substitutes	
(One exchange = 0 g carbohydrate, 7 g protein, 5 g fat, 75 calories)	
Beef: Most beef products fall into this category (ground beef, meat loaf, corned beef, short ribs, prime grades of meat trimmed of fat, such as prime rib)	1 oz
Pork: Top loin, chop, Boston butt, cutlet	1 oz

* = 400 mg or more sodium per exchange.

Medium-Fat Meat and Substitutes—cont'd	
Lamb: Rib roast, ground	1 oz
Veal: Cutlet (ground or cubed, unbreaded)	1 oz
Poultry: Chicken dark meat (with skin), ground turkey or ground chicken, fried chicken (with skin)	1 oz
Fish: Any fried fish product	1 oz
Cheese: With 5 g or less fat per ounce	
Feta	1 oz
Mozzarella	1 oz
Ricotta	¼ cup (2 oz)
Other: Egg (high in cholesterol, limit to 3 per week)	1
Sausage with 5 g or less fat per ounce	1 oz
Soy milk	1 cup
Tempeh	¼ cup
Tofu	4 oz or ½ cup
High-Fat Meat and Substitutes	
(One exchange = 0 g carbohydrate, 7 g protein, 8 g fat, 100 calories)	
Remember these items are high in saturated fat, cholesterol, and calories and may raise blood cholesterol levels if eaten on a regular basis.	
Pork: Spareribs, ground pork, pork sausage	1 oz
Cheese: All regular cheeses, such as American,* cheddar, Monterey Jack, Swiss	1 oz
Other: Processed sandwich meats with 8 g or less fat per ounce, such as bologna, pimento loaf, salami	1 oz
Sausage, such as bratwurst, Italian, knockwurst, Polish, smoked	1 oz
Hot dog (turkey or chicken)*	1 (10 per lb)
Bacon	3 slices (20 slices per lb)
Count as 1 high-fat meat plus 1 fat exchange:	
Hot dog (beef, pork, or combination)*	1 (10 per lb)
Count as 1 high-fat meat plus 2 fat exchanges:	
Peanut butter (contains unsaturated fat)	2 tbsp

Fat Exchange List	
(One exchange = 5 g fat, 45 calories)	
Monounsaturated Fats	
Avocado, medium	⅛ (1 oz)
Oil (canola, olive, peanut)	1 tsp
Olives: ripe (black)	8 large
Green, stuffed*	10 large
Nuts: almonds, cashews	6 nuts
Mixed (50% peanuts)	6 nuts
Peanuts	10 nuts
Pecans	4 halves
Peanut butter, smooth or crunchy	2 tsp
Sesame seeds	1 tbsp
Tahini paste	2 tsp
Polyunsaturated Fats	
Margarine: stick, tube, or squeeze	1 tsp
Margarine: lower-fat (30% to 50% vegetable oil)	1 tbsp
Mayonnaise: regular	1 tsp
Mayonnaise: reduced-fat	1 tbsp
Nuts: walnuts, English	4 halves
Oil (corn, safflower, soybean)	1 tsp
Salad dressing: regular*	1 tbsp
Salad dressing: reduced-fat	2 tbsp
Polyunsaturated Fats—cont'd	
Miracle Whip salad dressing: regular	2 tsp
Miracle Whip salad dressing: reduced-fat	1 tbsp
Seeds: pumpkin, sunflower	1 tbsp
Saturated Fats	
Saturated fats can raise blood cholesterol levels.	
Bacon, cooked	1 slice (20 slices per lb)
Bacon grease	1 tsp
Butter, stick	2 tsp
Butter, whipped	2 tsp
Butter, reduced-fat	1 tbsp
Chitterlings, boiled	2 tbsp (½ oz)
Coconut, sweetened, shredded	2 tbsp
Cream, half and half	2 tbsp
Cream cheese, regular	1 tbsp (½ oz)
Cream cheese, reduced-fat	2 tbsp (½ oz)
Fatback or salt pork†	
Shortening or lard	1 tsp
Sour cream, regular	2 tbsp
Sour cream, reduced-fat	3 tbsp

* = 400 mg or more sodium per exchange.

† Use a piece 1 in × 1 in × ¼ in if you plan to eat the fatback cooked with vegetables.
Use a piece 2 in × 1 in × ½ in when eating only the vegetables with the fatback removed.

Free Foods List

A *free food* is any food or drink that contains less than 20 calories or less than 5 grams of carbohydrate per serving. Foods with a serving size listed should be limited to three servings per day. Be sure to spread them out throughout the day. If you eat all three servings at one time, it could affect your blood glucose level. Food listed without a serving size can be eaten as often as you like.

Fat-Free or Reduced-Fat Foods	
Cream cheese, fat-free	1 tbsp
Creamers, nondairy, liquid	1 tbsp
Creamers, nondairy, powdered	2 tsp
Mayonnaise, fat-free	1 tbsp
Mayonnaise, reduced-fat	1 tsp
Margarine, fat-free	4 tbsp
Margarine, reduced-fat	1 tsp
Miracle Whip, nonfat	1 tbsp
Miracle Whip, reduced-fat	1 tsp
Nonstick cooking spray	
Salad dressing, fat-free	1 tbsp
Salad dressing, fat-free, Italian	2 tbsp
Salsa	¼ cup
Sour cream, fat-free, reduced-fat	1 tbsp
Whipped topping, regular or light	2 tbsp
Sugar-Free or Low-Sugar Foods	
Candy, hard, sugar-free	1 candy
Gelatin dessert, sugar-free	
Gelatin, unflavored	
Gum, sugar-free	
Jam or jelly, low-sugar or light	2 tsp
Sugar substitutes‡	
Syrup, sugar-free	2 tbsp
Sprinkle Sweet® (saccharin)	
Sweet One® (acesulfame K)	
Sweet-10® (saccharin)	
Sugar-Free or Low-Sugar Foods—cont'd	
Sugar Twin® (saccharin)	
Sweet 'n Low® (saccharin)	
Drinks	
Bouillon, broth, consomme*	
Bouillon or broth, low-sodium	
Carbonated or mineral water	
Cocoa powder, unsweetened	1 tbsp
Coffee	
Club soda	
Diet soft drinks, sugar-free	
Drink mixes, sugar-free	
Tea	
Tonic water, sugar-free	
Condiments	
Catsup	1 tbsp
Horseradish	
Lemon juice	
Lime juice	
Mustard	
Pickles, dill*	1½ large
Soy sauce, regular or light*	
Taco sauce	1 tbsp
Vinegar	

Seasonings

Be careful with seasonings that contain sodium or are salts, such as garlic or celery salt, and lemon pepper.

Flavoring extracts
Garlic
Herbs, fresh or dried
Pimento
Spices
Tabasco® or hot pepper sauce
Wine, used in cooking
Worcestershire sauce

Combination Foods List

Many of the foods we eat are mixed together in various combinations. These combination foods do not fit into any one exchange list. Often it is hard to tell what is in a casserole dish or prepared food item. This is a list of exchanges for some typical combination foods. This list will help you fit these foods into your meal plan. Ask your dietitian for information about any other combination foods you would like to eat.

Food	***Serving Size***	***Exchanges Per Serving***
Entrees		
Tuna noodle casserole, lasagna, spaghetti with meatballs, chili with beans, macaroni and cheese*	1 cup (8 oz)	2 carbohydrates, 2 medium-fat meats
Chow mein (without noodles or rice)*	1 cup (16 oz)	1 carbohydrate, 2 lean meats
Pizza, cheese, thin crust*	¼ of 10 inch (5 oz)	2 carbohydrates, 2 medium-fat meats, 1 fat
Pizza, meat topping, thin crust*	¼ of 10 inch (5 oz)	2 carbohydrates, 2 medium-fat meats, 2 fats
Pot pie*	1 (7 oz)	2 carbohydrates, 1 medium-fat meat, 4 fats
Frozen Entrees		
Salisbury steak with gravy, mashed potato*	1 (11 oz)	2 carbohydrates, 3 medium-fat meats, 3-4 fats
Turkey with gravy, mashed potato, dressing*	1 (11 oz)	2 carbohydrates, 2 medium-fat meats, 2 fats
Entree with less than 300 calories*	1 (8 oz)	2 carbohydrates, 3 lean meats

* = 400 mg or more of sodium per exchange.

‡Sugar substitutes, alternatives, or replacements that are approved by the Food and Drug Administration (FDA) are safe to use. Common brand names include: Equal® (aspartame).

Soups		
Bean*	1 cup	1 carbohydrate, 1 very lean meat
Cream (made with water)*	1 cup (8 oz)	1 carbohydrate, 1 fat
Split pea (made with water)*	½ cup (4 oz)	1 carbohydrate
Tomato (made with water)*	1 cup (8 oz)	1 carbohydrate
Vegetable beef, chicken noodle, or other broth-type*	1 cup (8 oz)	1 carbohydrate

Fast Foods

Ask at your fast-food restaurant for nutrition information about your favorite fast foods.

Food	*Serving Size*	*Exchanges Per Serving*
Burritos with beef*	2	4 carbohydrates, 2 medium-fat meats, 2 fats
Chicken nuggets*	6	1 carbohydrate, 2 medium-fat meats, 1 fat
Chicken breast and wing, breaded and fried*	1 each	1 carbohydrate, 4 medium-fat meats, 2 fats
Fish sandwich with tarter sauce*	1	3 carbohydrates, 1 medium-fat meat, 3 fats
French fries, thin*	20-25	2 carbohydrates, 2 fats
Hamburger, regular	1	2 carbohydrates, 2 medium-fat meats
Hamburger, large*	1	2 carbohydrates, 3 medium-fat meats, 1 fat
Hot dog with bun*	1	1 carbohydrate, 1 high-fat meat, 1 fat
Individual pan pizza*	1	5 carbohydrates, 3 medium-fat meats, 3 fats
Soft-serve cone	1 medium	2 carbohydrates, 1 fat
Submarine sandwich*	1 sub (6 inch)	3 carbohydrates, 1 vegetable, 2 medium-fat meats, 1 fat
Taco, hard shell*	1 (6 oz)	2 carbohydrates, 2 medium-fat meats, 2 fats
Taco, soft shell*	1 (3 oz)	1 carbohydrate, 1 medium-fat meat, 1 fat

The Exchange Lists are the basis of a meal planning system designed by a committee of the American Diabetes Association and The American Dietetic Association. While designed primarily for people with diabetes and others who must follow special diets, the Exchange Lists are based on principles of good nutrition that apply to everyone.

* = 400 mg or more of sodium per exchange.

Appendix

M Dietary Guidelines for Americans 2000

"Aim, Build, and Choose—for Good Health." This is the slogan of the most recent *Dietary Guidelines for Americans* (5th edition, 2000), developed by the U.S. Department of Agriculture's Center for Nutrition Policy and Promotion. The guidelines are easily remembered through their creative use of an A—B—C approach: Aim for fitness; Build a healthy base; and Choose sensibly. These ten important guidelines help people build healthy eating patterns and take action for good health. The dietary guidelines are intended for healthy children aged 2 years and older and adults of all ages.

Aim for Fitness

The following two guidelines help keep everyone healthy and fit, which enables people of all ages to work productively, enjoy life, and feel their best. They help children grow, develop, and do well in school.

AIM FOR A HEALTHY WEIGHT

A healthy weight is the key to a long, healthy life. Adults can evaluate their weight in relation to their height using the Body Mass Index (BMI) scale. A person with a BMI above 25 usually will benefit from weight loss. Weight loss that is done gradually will be more likely to last. Choosing sensible food portion sizes will help maintain healthy weight. Control of portion size is especially important when eating out and when eating foods high in calories. A healthy weight is important for children also; they need encouragement and guidance to develop healthy eating habits and to participate in vigorous physical activity.

BE PHYSICALLY ACTIVE EACH DAY

Adults and children alike should balance the calories they eat with physical activity each day. Being physically active benefits both health and a person's sense of well-being. All adults, including older persons, should aim to accumulate at least 30 minutes of moderate physical activity each day, especially through activities that are enjoyable and that can be done regularly. Aerobic activities that speed up heart rate and breathing will help cardiovascular fitness. Activities that develop strength and bodily flexibility can help build and maintain sound bones. Adults should set a good example for children, who need at least 60 minutes of physical activity daily.

Build a Healthy Base

The following four guidelines build a base for healthy eating. Make grains, fruits, and vegetables the foundation of your meals. Be flexible and adventurous and try new choices from these three food groups instead of less nutritious and higher calorie foods.

LET THE FOOD GUIDE PYRAMID GUIDE YOUR FOOD CHOICES

No single food can supply all of the nutrients that people need in the amounts that are needed. The Food Guide Pyramid helps in building a healthy base in food choices. The Pyramid displays the recommended number of daily servings from each of the five major food groups: the Grains Group (bread, cereal, rice, and pasta), 6 to 11 servings; the Vegetable Group, 3 to 5 servings; the Fruit Group, 2 to 4 servings; the Milk Group (milk, yogurt, and cheese), 2 to 3 servings; and the Meat and Beans Group (meat, poultry, fish, dry beans, eggs, and nuts), 2 to 3 servings. Fats, Oils, and Sweets, the small group at the top of the Pyramid, should be used sparingly. Choosing a variety of foods, with the amount varying according to age and activity level, will result in good nutrition.

CHOOSE A VARIETY OF GRAINS DAILY, ESPECIALLY WHOLE GRAINS

Foods made from grains (like wheat, rice, and oats) provide the foundation of a nutritious diet. They provide carbohydrates, vitamins, minerals, and other nutrients important for good health. Usually grain products are low in fat. Products made with whole grains (such as whole wheat, oatmeal, or brown rice) are rich in healthy dietary fiber, vitamins, and minerals. The *Healthy People 2010* program of the U.S. Department of Health and Human Services gives national objectives for persons aged 2 years and older. For grains, the target objective is to increase the proportion of people who eat at least six daily servings of grain products, with at least three being whole grains, to 50%.

CHOOSE A VARIETY OF FRUITS AND VEGETABLES DAILY

Eating plenty of fruits and vegetables of different kinds provides essential vitamins and minerals and may help protect against many chronic diseases. Different fruits and vegetables are sources of vital nutrients, such as vitamin A (carotenoids), vitamin C, folate, and potassium; therefore eating a variety of kinds and colors is best. Most fruits and vegetables are naturally low in fat and calories, and many are high in fiber. The *Healthy People 2010* program of the U.S. Department of Health and Human Services gives national objectives for persons aged 2 years and older. For fruit, the target objective is to increase the proportion of people who eat at least two daily servings of fruit to 75%. For vegetables, the target objective is to increase the proportion of people who eat at least three daily servings of vegetables, with at least one third being dark green or orange vegetables, to 50%.

KEEP FOOD SAFE TO EAT

Safe food is food that is free from harmful bacteria, viruses, toxins, parasites, and chemical contaminants and that therefore poses little risk of foodborne illness. Eating even a small portion of an unsafe food can make a person sick. Those at a high risk of foodborne illness—pregnant women, young women, older persons, and people with weakened immune systems or some chronic illnesses—should be extra cautious. The most current information on food safety can be found at the U.S. government's special website: *http://www.FoodSafety.gov.* Everyone should practice safe food techniques.

- *Clean:* Wash hands and surfaces often.
- *Separate:* Separate raw, cooked, and ready-to-eat foods while shopping for, preparing, or storing food.
- *Cook:* Cook foods to a safe temperature.
- *Chill:* Refrigerate perishable foods promptly.
- *Check:* Read and follow the safe handling instructions on the package.
- *Serve safely:* Keep hot foods hot and cold foods cold.

When in doubt, throw it out.

Choose Sensibly

The following four guidelines help people make sensible choices that promote health and reduce the risk of certain chronic diseases. All foods can be enjoyed as part of a healthy diet as long as fat (especially saturated fat), sugars, salt, and alcohol are not consumed in excess amounts.

CHOOSE A DIET THAT IS LOW IN SATURATED FAT AND CHOLESTEROL AND MODERATE IN TOTAL FAT

Some fat is needed in food. Fats in food supply energy and essential fatty acids, and they help absorb the fat-soluble vitamins A, D, E, and K, and carotenoids. Excess fat of any type in the diet supplies unnecessary calories, and a diet low in saturated fat is the healthiest. Saturated fat increases the risk of coronary heart disease by raising the blood cholesterol level. Unsaturated fats, which are found mostly in vegetable oils, do not raise blood cholesterol. Limiting the use of solid fats, such as butter and hard margarine, and choosing fat-free or low-fat dairy products helps reduce saturated fat and cholesterol in the diet. Sensible diet choices are plenty of grains, vegetables, and fruits, along with beans and peas, fish, and lean meats and poultry. The *Healthy People 2010* program of the U.S. Department of Health and Human Services gives national objectives for persons aged 2 years and older. For fats, the target objectives are to increase to 75% both the proportion of people who consume less than 10% of calories from saturated fat and the proportion who consume no more than 30% of calories from total fat.

CHOOSE BEVERAGES AND FOODS TO MODERATE YOUR INTAKE OF SUGARS

Sugars are carbohydrates and a source of energy. During digestion all carbohydrates in food break down into sugars. Many nutritious foods contain naturally occurring sugars and starches, such as milk, fruits, some vegetables, breads, cereals, and grains. Many foods today contain added sugars and syrups put in during processing or preparation. The body cannot distinguish between natural and added sugars; therefore consumption of foods high in added sugars should be monitored closely. The major sources of added sugars are nondiet soft drinks, fruit drinks, cakes and cookies, ice cream, and candy. A lot of sugar in the diet is a major cause of tooth decay. The excess calories in foods high in added sugar can contribute to weight gain or displace more nutritious foods in the diet.

CHOOSE AND PREPARE FOODS WITH LESS SALT

The link between salt intake and health relates to blood pressure. A high intake of sodium, which primarily comes from salt, is associated with higher blood pressure. Most people consume much more salt than the body needs; therefore reducing salt intake is wise. Most of the salt that people eat comes from salt added to food during processing or during preparation in a restaurant or at home. Salt consumption can be reduced by choosing fruits and vegetables often; using herbs, spices, and fruits to flavor food; and cutting in half the use of salty seasonings. The *Healthy People 2010* program of the U.S. Department of Health and Human Services gives national objectives for persons aged 2 years and older. For sodium, the target objective is to increase to 65% the proportion of people who consume 2400 mg or less of sodium daily.

IF YOU DRINK ALCOHOLIC BEVERAGES, DO SO IN MODERATION

Alcoholic beverages contain calories but few nutrients. Excess alcohol consumption impairs judgment and can lead to alcohol dependency and increased risk of serious health problems such as high blood pressure, stroke, and certain types of cancer. Alcohol use is a major factor in motor vehicle accidents and other injuries. Some people should not drink alcoholic beverages at all: children and adolescents, those who cannot restrict their drinking to moderate levels, pregnant women, those who plan to drive or operate equipment, and those who are taking medications that may interact with alcohol. Adults who do choose to drink alcoholic beverages should do so sensibly and in moderation. Alcohol consumption should be limited to one drink per day for women and two per day for men.

■ References

U.S. Department of Agriculture Center for Nutrition Policy and Promotion: *The food guide pyramid,* USDA Home and Garden Bulletin No. 252, Washington, DC, 1996, U.S. Government Printing Office.

U.S. Department of Agriculture Center for Nutrition Policy and Promotion and U.S. Department of Health and Human Services: *Dietary guidelines for Americans, 2000,* ed 5, USDA Home and Garden Bulletin No. 232, Washington, DC, 2000, U.S. Government Printing Office.

U.S. Department of Health and Human Services: *Healthy People 2010,* ed 2. With Understanding and Improving Health and Objectives for Improving Health, 2 vols. Washington, DC, 2000, U.S. Government Printing Office.

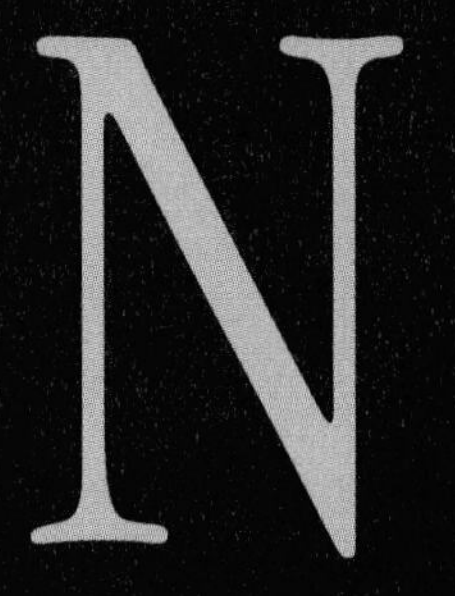

Appendix N Guidelines for Nutritional Assessment and Care of Cystic Fibrosis

Step One: Calculation of Basal Metabolic Rate (BMR)

In cystic fibrosis care, if a patient fails to grow adequately while receiving kilocalorie (kcalorie) intake based on Recommended Daily Allowances (RDAs), use this table to calculate BMR daily energy requirement.

World Health Organization Equations for Calculating BMR (Kcalories) From Body Weight (kg)

Age (yr)	BMR (Kcalories) Females	Males
0-3	61.0 × (wt kg) − 51	60.9 × (wt kg) − 54
3-10	22.5 × (wt kg) + 499	22.7 × (wt kg) + 495
10-18	12.2 × (wt kg) + 746	17.5 × (wt kg) + 651
18-30	14.7 × (wt kg) + 496	15.3 × (wt kg) + 679
30-60	8.7 × (wt kg) + 829	11.6 × (wt kg) + 879

Adapted from World Health Organization *Energy and protein requirements,* WHO Technical Report Series, vol 924, No 724, 1985; Ramsey BW et al: Nutritional assessment and management in cystic fibrosis, *Am J Clin Nutr* 55:108, 1992, and Cystic Fibrosis Foundation guidelines.

Step Two: Calculation of Daily Energy Expenditure (DEE) in Therapy

$$\text{DEE} = \text{BMR} \times (\text{AC} + \text{DC})$$

Abbreviations

DEE	=	daily energy expenditure (kcalories)
BMR	=	basal metabolic rate (kcalories)
AC	=	activity coefficient
DC	=	disease coefficient

GUIDELINES FOR AC AND DC VALUES

Use the following tables to establish the appropriate activity coefficient and disease coefficient values.

Activity Coefficients (AC)

Activity Level of Patient	AC Value
Confined to bed	1.3
Sedentary	1.5
Active	1.7

Disease Coefficients (DC)

Lung Functioning Level in Cystic Fibrosis	Forced Air Expiration Volume in 1 Second ($FEV_{1.0}$) (100% = Normal FEV)	DC Value
Close to normal lung function	>80%	0.0
Moderate lung disease	40%-79%	0.2
Severe lung disease	<40%	0.3
Very severe lung disease	<40%	0.5

Modified from Ramsey BW et al: Nutritional assessment and management in cystic fibrosis, *Am J Clin Nutr* 55:108, 1992, and Cystic Fibrosis Foundation guidelines.

DEE CALCULATION

Determine the DEE for a school-age child with cystic fibrosis who is attending school, is relatively sedentary, and has a measured $FEV_{1.0}$ of 50% of predicted normal value.

$$\begin{aligned} DEE &= BMR \times (AC + DC) \\ &= BMR \times (1.5 + 0.2) \\ &= BMR \times 1.7 \end{aligned}$$

Step Three: Calculation of Daily Energy Requirement (DER) From Daily Energy Expenditure (DEE)

CALCULATION METHOD

1. Calculate the coefficient of fat absorption (CFA):

$$CFA = \frac{\text{Fat absorption (FA)}}{\text{Fat intake (FI)}} = \text{Fat absorption } \%*$$

2. Use one of the following guideline formulas for DER:

$$\text{If } CFA > 0.93, \text{ then } DER = DEE$$

or

$$\text{If } CFA \leq 0.93, \text{ then } DER = DEE \times \frac{0.93}{CFA}$$

Abbreviations

CFA	=	coefficient of fat absorption
FA	=	fat absorption (kcalorie)
FI	=	fat intake (kcalorie)
DEE	=	daily energy expenditure (kcalorie)
DER	=	daily energy requirement (kcalorie)

DER CALCULATION EXAMPLE

The fat absorption of a cystic fibrosis patient on enzyme therapy has been determined by laboratory analysis to be 78% of normal. Therefore the CFA for this patient is 0.78. The DEE for this same patient is calculated to be 2000 kcalories. Therefore the DER for this patient is as follows:

$$DER = DEE \times \frac{0.93}{CFA}$$

$$DER = 2000 \text{ kcalories} \times \frac{0.93}{0.78}$$

$$DER = 2384 \text{ kcalories/day}$$

Modified from Ramsey BW et al: Nutritional assessment and management in cystic fibrosis, *Am J Clin Nutr* 55:108, 1992, and Cystic Fibrosis Foundation guidelines.

*NOTE 1: The fat absorption % (CFA) is usually calculated in a clinical setting by medical laboratory analysis from a patient stool sample.

NOTE 2: If no laboratory analysis report is available, then use CFA = 0.85 as an approximation value in the DER calculation.

Appendix

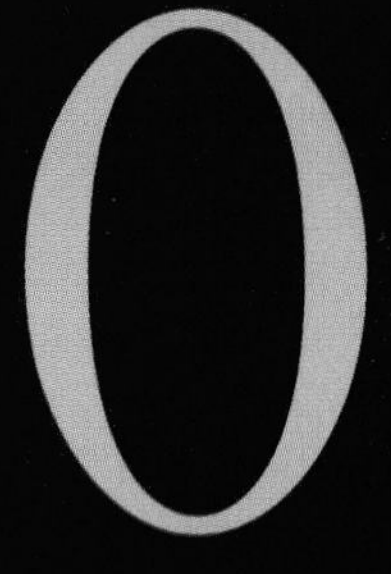

Diets for Nutritional Management of Renal Calculi

Low-Calcium Diet (approximately 400 mg calcium)

	Foods Allowed	Foods Not Allowed
Beverage*	Carbonated beverage, coffee, tea	Chocolate-flavored drinks, milk, milk drinks
Bread	White, light rye bread, crackers	
Cereals	Refined cereals	Oatmeal, whole-grain cereals
Desserts	Cake, cookies, gelatin desserts, pastries, pudding, sherbets, all made without chocolate, milk, or nuts; if egg yolk is used, it must be from one egg allowance	
Fat	Butter, cream, 2 tbsp/day; French dressing, margarine, salad oil, shortening	Cream (except in amount allowed), mayonnaise
Fruits	Canned, cooked, or fresh fruits or juice except rhubarb	Dried fruit, rhubarb
Meat, eggs	224 g (8 oz) daily of any meat, fowl, fish except clams, oysters, shrimp; not more than one egg daily, including those used in cooking	Clams, oysters, shrimp, cheese
Potato or substitute	Potato, hominy, macaroni, noodles, refined rice, spaghetti	Whole-grain rice
Soup	Broth, vegetable soup made from vegetables allowed	Bean or pea soup, cream or milk soup
Sweets	Honey, jam, jelly, sugar	
Vegetables	Any canned, cooked, fresh vegetables or juice except those listed	Dried beans, broccoli, green cabbage, celery, chard, collards, endive, greens, lettuce, lentils, okra, parsley, parsnips, dried peas, rutabagas
Miscellaneous	Herbs, pickles, popcorn, relishes, salt, spices, vinegar	Chocolate, cocoa, milk gravy, nuts, olives, white sauce

*Depending on calcium content of local water supply. In instances of high calcium content, distilled water may be indicated.

Low-Phosphorus Diet (approximately 1 g phosphorous and 40 g protein)

	Foods Allowed	Foods Not Allowed
Milk	Not more than 1 cup daily; whole, skim, buttermilk, or 3 tbsp powdered, including the amount used in cooking	
Beverages	Fruit juices, tea, coffee, carbonated drinks, Postum	Milk and milk drinks except as allowed
Bread	White only; enriched commercial, French, hard rolls, soda crackers, rusk	Rye and whole-grain breads, cornbread, biscuits, muffins, waffles
Cereals	Refined cereals, such as Cream of Wheat, Cream of Rice, rice, cornmeal, dry cereals, cornflakes, spaghetti, noodles	All whole-grain cereals
Desserts	Berry or fruit pies, cookies, cakes in average amounts; Jell-O, gelatin, angel food cake, sherbet, meringues made with egg whites, puddings if made with one egg or milk allowance	Desserts with milk and eggs, unless made with the daily allowance
Eggs	Not more than one egg daily, including those used in cooking; extra egg whites may be used	
Fats	Butter, margarine, oils, shortening	
Fruits	Fresh, frozen, canned, as desired	Dried fruits such as raisins, prunes, dates, figs, apricots
Meat	One large serving or two small servings daily of beef, lamb, veal, pork, rabbit, chicken, turkey	Fish, shellfish (crab, oyster, shrimp, lobster), dried and cured meats (bacon, ham, chipped beef), liver, kidney, sweetbreads, brains
Cheese	None	Avoid all cheeses and cheese spreads
Vegetables	Potatoes as desired; at least two servings per day of any of the following: asparagus, carrots, beets, green beans, squash, lettuce, rutabagas, tomatoes, celery, peas, onions, cucumber, corn; no more than 1 serving daily of either cabbage, spinach, broccoli, cauliflower, brussels sprouts, artichokes	Dried vegetables such as peas, mushrooms, lima beans
Miscellaneous	Sugar, jams, jellies, syrups, salt, spices, seasonings; condiments in moderation	Chocolate, nuts, nut products such as peanut butter, cream sauces

Sample Menu Pattern

Breakfast	Lunch	Dinner
Fruit juice	Meat, 56 g (2 oz)	Meat, 56 g (2 oz)
Refined cereal	Potato	Potato
Egg	Vegetable	Vegetable
White toast	Salad	Salad
Butter	Bread, white	Bread, white
½ cup milk	Butter	Butter
Coffee or tea	½ cup milk	Dessert
	Dessert	Coffee or tea
	Coffee or tea	

Low-Calcium Test Diet (200 mg calcium)

	Grams	Calcium (mg)
Breakfast		
Orange juice, fresh	100	19.00
Bread (toast), white	25	19.57
Butter	15	3.00
Rice Krispies	15	3.70
Cream, 20% butterfat	35	33.95
Sugar	7	0.00
Jam	20	2.00
Distilled water, coffee, or tea*		0.00
TOTAL		81.22
Lunch		
Beef steak, cooked	100	10.00
Potato	100	11.00
Tomatoes	100	11.00
Bread	25	19.57
Butter	15	3.00
Honey	20	1.00
Applesauce	20	1.00
Distilled water, coffee, or tea		0.00
TOTAL		56.57
Dinner		
Lamb chop, cooked	90	10.00
Potato	100	11.00
Frozen green peas	80	10.32
Bread	25	19.57
Butter	15	3.00
Jam	20	2.00
Peach sauce	100	5.00
Distilled water, coffee, or tea		0.00
TOTAL		60.89
TOTAL MILLIGRAMS CALCIUM		198.68

*Use distilled water only for cooking and for beverages.

Acid Ash Diet

The purpose of this diet is to furnish a well-balanced diet in which the total acid ash is greater than the total alkaline ash each day. It lists (1) unrestricted food, (2) restricted foods, (3) foods not allowed, and (4) sample of a day's diet.

Unrestricted Foods

Eat as much as desired of the following foods:

- Bread: any, preferably whole grain; crackers, rolls
- Cereals: any, preferably whole grain
- Desserts: angel food or sunshine cake; cookies made without baking powder or baking soda; cornstarch pudding, cranberry desserts, custards, gelatin desserts, ice cream, sherbet, plum or prune desserts; rice or tapioca pudding
- Fats: any, as butter, margarine, salad dressings, shortening, lard, salad oils, olive oil
- Fruits: cranberries, plums, prunes
- Meat, eggs, cheese; any meat, fish, or fowl, two servings daily; at least one egg daily
- Potato substitutes: corn, hominy, lentils, macaroni, noodles, rice, spaghetti, vermicelli
- Soup: broth as desired; other soups from foods allowed
- Sweets: cranberry or plum jelly; sugar, plain sugar candy
- Miscellaneous: cream sauce, gravy, peanut butter, peanuts, popcorn, salt, spices, vinegar, walnuts

Restricted Foods

Do not eat any more than the amount allowed each day.

- Milk: 2 cups daily (may be used in other ways than as beverage)
- Cream: ⅓ cup or less daily
- Fruits: one serving of fruit daily (in addition to prunes, plums, cranberries); certain fruits listed under "Foods Not Allowed" are not allowed at any time
- Vegetables including potato: two servings daily; certain vegetables listed under "Foods Not Allowed" are not allowed at any time

Foods Not Allowed

- Carbonated beverages, such as ginger ale, cola, root beer
- Cakes or cookies made with baking powder or soda
- Fruits: dried apricots, bananas, dates, figs, raisins, rhubarb
- Vegetables: dried beans, beet greens, dandelion greens, carrots, chard, lima beans
- Sweets: chocolate or candies other than those under "Unrestricted Foods"; syrups
- Miscellaneous: other nuts, olives, pickles

Sample Menu

Breakfast	Lunch	Dinner
Grapefruit	Creamed chicken	Broth
Wheatena	Steamed rice	Roast beef, gravy
Scrambled eggs	Green beans	Buttered noodles
Toast, butter, plum jam	Stewed prunes	Sliced tomato
Coffee, cream, sugar	Bread, butter	Mayonnaise
	Milk	Vanilla ice cream
		Bread, butter

Low-Purine Diet (approximately 125 mg purine)

General Directions

- During acute stages use only list 1.
- After acute stage subsides and for chronic conditions, use the following schedule:
  Two days a week, not consecutive, use list 1 entirely.
  The remaining days add foods from list 2 and 3, as indicated.
  Avoid list 4 entirely.
- Keep diet moderately low in fat.

Typical Meal Pattern

Breakfast	Lunch	Dinner
Fruit	Egg or cheese dish	Egg or cheese dish
Refined cereal and/or egg	Vegetables, as allowed (cooked or salad)	Cream of vegetable soup, if desired
White toast	Potato or substitute	Starch (potato or substitute)
Butter, 1 tsp	White bread	Colored vegetable, as allowed
Sugar	Butter, 1 tsp	White bread, butter, 1 tsp, if desired
Coffee	Fruit or simple dessert	Salad, as allowed
Milk, if desired	Milk	Fruit or simple dessert
		Milk

Food List 1: may be used as desired; foods that contain an insignificant amount of purine bodies

Beverages
- Carbonated
- Chocolate
- Cocoa
- Coffee
- Fruit juices
- Postum
- Tea

Butter*

Bread: white and crackers, cornbread

Cereals and cereal products
- Corn
- Rice
- Tapioca
- Refined wheat
- Macaroni
- Noodles

Cheese of all kinds*

Eggs

Fats of all kinds* (moderation)

Fruits of all kinds

Gelatin, Jell-O

Milk: buttermilk, evaporated, malted, sweet

Nuts of all kinds,* peanut butter*

Pies* (except mincemeat)

Sugar and sweets

Vegetables
- Artichokes
- Beets
- Beet greens
- Broccoli
- Brussels sprouts
- Cabbage
- Carrots
- Celery
- Corn
- Cucumber
- Eggplant
- Endive
- Kohlrabi
- Lettuce
- Okra
- Parsnips
- Potato, white and sweet
- Pumpkin
- Rutabagas
- Sauerkraut
- String beans
- Summer squash
- Swiss chard
- Tomato
- Turnips

*High in fat.

Low-Purine Diet (approximately 125 mg purine)—cont'd

Food List 2: one item four times a week; foods that contain a moderate amount (up to 75 mg) of purine bodies in 100 g serving			
Asparagus	Finnan haddie	Mushrooms	Salmon
Bluefish	Ham	Mutton	Shad
Bouillon	Herring	Navy beans	Spinach
Cauliflower	Kidney beans	Oatmeal	Tripe
Chicken	Lima beans	Oysters	Tuna fish
Crab	Lobster	Peas	Whitefish
Food List 3: one item once a week; foods that contain a large amount (75-150 mg) of purine bodies in 100 g serving			
Bacon	Duck	Perch	Sheep
Beef	Goose	Pheasant	Shellfish
Calf tongue	Halibut	Pigeon	Squab
Carp	Lentils	Pike	Trout
Chicken soup	Liver sausage	Pork	Turkey
Codfish	Meat soups	Quail	Veal
	Partridge	Rabbit	Venison

Food List 4: avoid entirely; foods that contain large amounts (150-1000 mg) of purine bodies in 100 g serving					
Sweetbreads	825 mg	Liver (calf, beef)	233 mg	Meat extracts	160-400 mg
Anchovies	363 mg	Kidneys (beef)	200 mg	Gravies	Variable
Sardines (in oil)	295 mg	Brains	195 mg		

Low-Methionine Diet

	Foods Allowed	Foods Not Allowed
Soup	Any soup made without meat stock or addition of milk	Rich meat soups, broths, canned soups made with meat broth
Meat or meat substitute	Peanut butter sandwich; spaghetti, or macaroni dish made without addition of meat, cheese, or milk; one serving per day: chicken, lamb, veal, beef, pork, crab, or bacon (3)	Fish and those not listed above
Beverages	Soy milk, tea, coffee	Milk in any form
Vegetables	Asparagus, artichoke, beans, beets, carrots, chicory, cucumber, eggplant, escarole, lettuce, onions, parsnips, potatoes, pumpkin, rhubarb, tomatoes, turnips	Those not listed as allowed
Fruits	Apples, apricots, bananas, berries, cherries, fruit cocktail, grapefruit, grapes, lemon juice, nectarines, oranges, peaches, pears, pineapple, plums, tangerines, watermelon, cantaloupe	Those not listed as allowed
Salads	Raw or cooked vegetable or fruit salad	
Cereals	Macaroni, spaghetti, noodles	
Bread	Whole wheat, rye, white	
Nuts	Peanuts	
Desserts	Fresh or cooked fruit, ices, fruit pies	
Eggs		In any form
Cheese		All varieties
Concentrated sweets	Sugar, jams, jellies, syrup, honey, hard candy	
Concentrated fats	Butter, margarine, cream	
Miscellaneous	Pepper, mustard, vinegar, garlic, oil, herbs, spices	

Meal pattern

Breakfast	Lunch	Dinner
1 cup fruit juice	1 serving soup	56 g (2 oz) meat
½ cup fruit	1 serving sandwich	1 med starch
1 slice toast	1 cup fruit	½ cup vegetable
1½ pats butter	240 ml (8 oz) soy milk*	1 serving salad
2 tsp jelly	3 tsp sugar	1 tbsp dressing
1 tbsp sugar	1 tbsp cream	1 slice bread
Beverage	Beverage	1 serving dessert
1 tbsp cream		1 tbsp sugar
		1 tbsp cream
		1½ pats butter
		Beverage

Sample Menu

Breakfast	Lunch	Dinner
Orange juice	Vegetable soup, vegetarian	Chicken, roast
Applesauce	Peanut butter sandwich	Baked potato
Whole-wheat toast	Canned peaches	Artichoke
Butter	Soy milk*	Sliced tomatoes
Jelly	Sugar	French dressing
Sugar	Cream	Whole-wheat bread
Coffee	Coffee or tea	Fruit ice
Cream		Sugar
		Cream
		Butter
		Coffee or tea

Modified from Smith DR, Kolb FO, and Harper HA: The management of cystinuria and cystine-stone disease, *J Urol* 81:61, 1959.
*Optional: use in children to include protein intake. Omit if urine calcium level is elevated in adults.

Appendix

P Calculation Aids and Conversion Tables

In 1799 a group of French scientists set up the metric system of weights and measures. Today, with refinements over years of use, it is called the "Système International" (SI). In 1975 the United States Congress passed the Metric Conversion Act, which provides for conversion of our customary British/American system to the simpler metric system used by the rest of the world. We are now in the midst of this conversion, as evidenced by distance signs along highways and labels on many packaged foods in supermarkets. Here are a few conversion factors to help you make these transitions in your necessary calculations.

Metric System of Measurement

Like our money system, this is a simple decimal system based on units of 10. It is uniform and used internationally.

Weight units: 1 kilogram (kg) = 1000 grams (gm or g)
1 g = 1000 milligrams (mg)
1 mg = 1000 micrograms (mcg or μg)

Length units: 1 meter (m) = 100 centimeters (cm)
1000 meters = 1 kilometer

Volume units: 1 liter (L) = 1000 milliliters (ml)
1 milliliter = 1 cubic centimeter (cc)

Temperature units: Celsius (C) scale, based on 100 equal units between 0° C (freezing point of water) and 100° C (boiling point of water); this scale is used in all scientific work.

Energy units: Kilocalorie (kcal) = Amount of energy required to raise 1 kg water 1° C
Kilojoule (kJ) = Amount of energy required to move 1 kg mass 1 m by a force of 1 newton
1 kcal = 4.184 kJ

In 1970 the American Institute of Nutrition's Committee on Nomenclature recommended that the term *Kilojoule* (kJ) replace the kilocalorie (kcal).

British/American System of Measurement

This system is a confusion of units with no uniform relationships. It is not a decimal system, but rather a jumbled collection of different units collected in usage and language over time. It is used mainly in America.

Weight units: 1 pound (lb) = 16 ounces (oz)

Length units: 1 foot (ft) = 12 inches (in)
1 yard (yd) = 3 feet (ft)

Volume units: 3 teaspoons (tsp) = 1 tablespoon (tbsp)
16 tbsp = 1 cup
1 cup = 8 fluid ounces (fl oz)
4 cups = 1 quart (qt)
5 cups = 1 imperial quart (qt), Canada

Temperature units: Fahrenheit (F) scale, based on 180 equal units between 32° F (freezing point of water) and 212° F (boiling point of water) at standard atmospheric pressure

Conversions Between Measurement Systems

Weight: 1 oz = 28.35 g (usually used as 28 or 30 g)
2.2 lb = 1 kg

Length: 1 in = 2.54 cm
1 ft = 30.48 cm
39.37 in = 1 m

Volume: 1.06 qt = 1 L
0.85 imperial qt = 1 L (Canada)

Temperature:

Boiling point of water	100° C	212° F
Body temperature	37° C	98.6° F
Freezing point of water	0° C	32° F

Interconversion formulas:

Fahrenheit temperature (°F) = ⁹⁄₅ (°C + 32)

Celsius temperature (°C) = ⁵⁄₉ (°F − 32)

Retinol Equivalents

The following internationally agreed on definitions and equivalences provide a basis for calculating retinol equivalent conversions.

DEFINITIONS

International units (IU) and retinol equivalents (RE) are defined as follows:

1 IU = 0.3 μg retinol (0.0003 mg)
1 IU = 0.6 μg beta-carotene (0.0006 mg)
1 RE = 6 μg retinol
1 RE = 6 μg beta-carotene
1 RE = 12 μg other provitamin A carotenoids
1 RE = 3.33 IU retinol
1 RE = 10 IU beta-carotene

CONVERSION FORMULAS

On the basis of weight, beta-carotene is ½ as active as retinol; on the basis of structure the other provitamin carotenoids are ¼ as active as retinol. In addition, retinol is more completely absorbed in the intestine, whereas the provitamin carotenoids are much less well utilized, with an average absorption of about ⅓. Therefore in overall activity, beta-carotene is ⅙ as active as retinol and the other carotenoids are 1⁄12 as active. These differences in utilization provide the basis for the 1:6:12 relationship shown in the equivalences given and in the following formulas for calculating retinol equivalents from values of vitamin A, beta-carotene, and other active carotenoids, expressed either as international units or micrograms:

If retinol and beta-carotene are given in micrograms:

Micrograms of retinol + (Micrograms of beta-carotene ÷ 6) = RE

If both are given as IU:

(International units of retinol ÷ 3.33) + (International units of beta-carotene ÷ 10) = RE

If beta-carotene and other carotenoids are given in micrograms:

(Micrograms of beta-carotene ÷ 6) + (Micrograms of other carotenoids ÷ 12) = RE

Approximate Metric Conversions

When You Know	Multiple By	To Find
Weight		
Ounces	28	Grams
Pounds	0.45	Kilograms
Length		
Inches	2.5	Centimeters
Feet	30	Centimeters
Yards	0.9	Meters
Miles	1.6	Kilometers
Volume		
Teaspoons	5	Millimeters
Tablespoons	15	Millimeters
Fluid ounces	30	Millimeters
Cups	0.24	Liters
Pints	0.47	Liters
Quarts	0.95	Liters
Temperature		
Fahrenheit temperature	5/9 (after subtracting 32)	Celsius temperature

Appendix Q

Cultural Dietary Patterns

Only foods that are specifically associated with these cultural groups are noted. Individuals may also consume typical American foods as well; assumptions of dietary patterns cannot be made, but knowledge of these unique foods provides a common understanding of the range of possible food choices.

Native American

Each tribe may have specific foods; listed here are commonly consumed foods.

1. BREAD, CEREAL, RICE, AND PASTA GROUP

Blue corn flour (ground dried blue corn kernels) used to make cornbread, mush dumplings; fruit dumplings (walakshi); fry bread (biscuit dough deep fried); ground sweet acorn; tortillas; wheat or rye used to make cornmeal and flours.

2. VEGETABLE GROUP

Cabbage, carrots, cassava, dandelion greens, eggplant, milkweed, onions, pumpkin, squash (all varieties), sweet and white potatoes, turnips, wild tullies (a tuber), yellow corn.

3. FRUIT GROUP

Dried wild cherries and grapes; wild banana, berries, and yucca.

4. MILK, YOGURT, AND CHEESE GROUP

None.

5. MEAT, POULTRY, FISH, DRY BEANS, EGGS, AND NUTS GROUP

Duck, eggs, fish eggs (roe), geese, groundhog, kidney beans, lentils, peanuts, pinenuts, pinto beans, all nuts, venison, wild rabbit.

6. FATS, OILS, AND SWEETS

None.

African American

1. BREAD, CEREAL, RICE, AND PASTA GROUP

Biscuits, cornbread as spoon bread, cornpone or hush puppies, grits.

2. VEGETABLE GROUP

Leafy greens including dandelion greens, kale, mustard greens, collard greens, turnips.

3. FRUIT GROUP

None.

4. MILK, YOGURT, AND CHEESE GROUP

Buttermilk.

From Grodner M, Anderson SL, DeYoung S: *Foundations and clinical applications of nutrition: a nursing approach,* ed 2, St Louis, 2000, Mosby.

5. MEAT, POULTRY, FISH, DRY BEANS, EGGS, AND NUTS GROUP

Pork and pork products, scrapple (cornmeal and pork), chitterlings (pork intestines), bacon, pig's feet, pig ears, souse, pork neck bones, fried meats and poultry, organ meats (kidney, liver, tongue, tripe), venison, rabbit, catfish, buffalo fish, mackerel, legumes (black-eyed peas, kidney, navy, chickpeas).

6. FATS, OILS, AND SWEETS

Lard.

Japanese

1. BREAD, CEREAL, RICE, AND PASTA GROUP

Rice and rice products, rice flour (mochiko), noodles (comen/soba), seaweed around rice with or without fish (sushi).

2. VEGETABLE GROUP

Bamboo shoots (takenoko), burdock (gobo), cabbage (nappa), dried mushrooms (shiitake), eggplant, horseradish (wasabi), Japanese parsley (seri), lotus root (renkon), mustard greens, pickled cabbage (kimchee), pickled vegetables, seaweed (laver, nori, wakame, kombu), vegetable soup (mizutaki), white radish (daikon)

3. FRUIT GROUP

Pear-like apple (nasi), persimmons.

4. MILK, YOGURT, AND CHEESE GROUP

None.

5. MEAT, POULTRY, FISH, DRY BEANS, EGGS, AND NUTS GROUP

Fish and shellfish including dried fish with bones, raw fish (sashimi), and fish cake (kamaboko); soybeans as soybean curd (tofu), fermented soybean paste (miso), and sprouts; red beans (azuki).

6. FATS, OILS, AND SWEETS

Soy and rice oil.

Chinese

1. BREAD, CEREAL, RICE, AND PASTA GROUP

Rice and related products (flour, cakes, and noodles); noodles made from barley, corn, and millet; wheat and related products (breads, noodles, spaghetti, stuffed noodles [won ton] and filled buns [bow]).

2. VEGETABLE GROUP

Bamboo shoots; cabbage (napa); Chinese celery; Chinese parsley (coriander); Chinese turnips (lo bok); dried day lilies; dry fungus (black Juda's ear); leafy green vegetables including kale, Chinese cress, Chinese mustard greens (gai choy), Chinese chard (bok choy), amaranth greens (yin choy), wolfberry leaves (gou gay), and Chinese broccoli (gai lan); lotus tubers; okra; snow peas; stir-fried vegetables (chow yuk); taro roots, white radish (daikon).

3. FRUIT GROUP

Kumquat.

4. MILK, YOGURT, AND CHEESE GROUP

None.

5. MEAT, POULTRY, FISH, DRY BEANS, EGGS, AND NUTS GROUP

Fish and seafood (all kinds, dried and fresh), hen, legumes, nuts, organ meats, pigeon eggs, pork and pork products, soybean curd (tofu), steamed stuffed dumplings (dim sum).

6. FATS, OILS, AND SWEETS

Peanut, soy, sesame and rice oil; lard.

Filipino

1. BREAD, CEREAL, RICE, AND PASTA GROUP

Noodles, rice, rice flour (mochiko), stuffed noodles (won ton), white bread (pan de sal).

2. VEGETABLE GROUP

Bamboo shoots, dark green leafy vegetables (malunggay and salvyot), eggplant, sweet potatoes (camotes), okra, palm, peppers, turnips, root crop (gabi).

3. FRUIT GROUP

Avocado, bitter melon (ampalaya), guavas, jackfruit, limes, mangoes, papaya, pod fruit (tamarind), pomelos, tangelo (naranghita).

4. MILK, YOGURT, AND CHEESE GROUP

Custards.

5. MEAT, POULTRY, FISH, DRY BEANS, EGGS, AND NUTS GROUP

Fish in all forms; dried fish (dilis); egg roll (lumpia); fish sauce (alamang and bagoong); legumes such as mung beans, bean sprouts, chickpeas, organ meats (liver, heart, intestines); pork with chicken in soy sauce (adobo); pork sausage; soybean curd (tofu).

6. FATS, OILS, AND SWEETS

None.

Southeastern Asians: (Laos, Cambodia, Thailand, Vietnam, the Hmong and the Mien)

1. BREAD, CEREAL, RICE, AND PASTA GROUP

Rice (long and short grain) and related products such as noodles; Hmong cornbread or cake.

2. VEGETABLE GROUP

Bamboo shoots, broccoli, Chinese parsley (coriander), mustard greens, pickled vegetables, water chestnuts, Thai chili peppers.

3. FRUIT GROUP

Apple pear (Asian pear), bitter melon, coconut cream and milk, guava, jackfruit, mango.

4. MILK, YOGURT, AND CHEESE GROUP

Sweetened condensed milk.

5. MEAT, POULTRY, FISH, DRY BEANS, EGGS, AND NUTS GROUP

Beef; chicken; deer; eggs; fish and shellfish (all kinds of freshwater and saltwater); legumes including black-eyed peas, peanuts, kidney beans, and soybeans; organ meats (liver, stomach); pork; rabbit; soybean curd (tofu).

6. FATS, OILS, AND SWEETS

Lard, peanut oil.

Mexican

1. BREAD, CEREAL, RICE, AND PASTA GROUP

Corn and related products; taco shells (fried corn tortillas); tortillas (corn and flour); white bread.

2. VEGETABLE GROUP

Cactus (nopoles), chili peppers, salsa, tomatoes, yambean root (jicama), yucca root (cassava or manioc).

3. FRUIT GROUP

Avocado, guacamole (mashed avocado, onion, cilantro [coriander], and chilis), papaya.

4. MILK, YOGURT, AND CHEESE GROUP

Cheese, flan, sour cream.

5. MEAT, POULTRY, FISH, DRY BEANS, EGGS, AND NUTS GROUP

Black or pinto beans (reijoles); refried beans (frijoles refritos); flour tortilla stuffed with beef, chicken, eggs, or beans (burrito); corn tortilla stuffed with chicken, cheese, or beef topped with chili sauce (enchilada); Mexican sausage (chorizo).

6. FATS, OILS, AND SWEETS

Bacon fat, lard (manteca), salt pork.

Puerto Rican and Cuban

1. BREAD, CEREAL, RICE, AND PASTA GROUP

Rice; starchy green bananas, usually fried (plantain).

2. VEGETABLE GROUP

Beets; eggplant; tubers (yucca); white yams (boniato).

3. FRUIT GROUP

Coconuts, guava, mango, oranges (sweet and sour), prune and mango paste.

4. MILK, YOGURT, AND CHEESE GROUP

Flan, hard cheese (queso de mano).

5. MEAT, POULTRY, FISH, DRY BEANS, EGGS, AND NUTS GROUP

Chicken, fish (all kinds and preparations including smoked, salted, canned, and fresh), legumes (all kinds especially black beans), pork (fried), sausage (chorizo).

6. FATS, OILS, AND SWEETS

Olive and peanut oil, lard.

Jewish

The foods below reflect both religious and cultural customs of Jewish people. Adherence to religious dietary patterns by followers of the different forms of Judaism (Orthodox, Conservative, Reform, and Reconstructionist) vary. Generally, Orthodox Jews and many Conservative Jews follow kosher dietary rules both at home and when out. Others may only observe when in their own homes. These rules of "keeping kosher" are reviewed in the next section on religious dietary patterns.

1. BREAD, CEREAL, RICE, AND PASTA GROUP

Bagel, buckwheat groats (kasha), dumplings made with matzoh meal (matzoh balls or knaidelach), egg bread (challah), noodle or potato pudding (kugel), crepe filled with farmer cheese and/or fruit (blintz), unleavened bread or large cracker made with wheat flour and water (matzoh).

2. VEGETABLE GROUP

Potato pancakes (latkes); a vegetable stew made with sweet potatoes, carrots, prunes, and sometimes brisket (tzimmes); beet soup (borscht).

3. FRUIT GROUP

None.

4. MILK, YOGURT, AND CHEESE GROUP

None.

5. MEAT, POULTRY, FISH, DRY BEANS, EGGS, AND NUTS GROUP

A mixture of fish formed into balls and poached (gefilte fish); smoked salmon (lox).

6. FATS, OILS, AND SWEETS

Chicken fat.

Religious Dietary Patterns

Beliefs of several major religions include practices that affect or prescribe specific dietary patterns or prohibit consumption of certain types of foods. Individuals practicing these religions may or may not adhere to all of the prescribed customs. Following is a brief review of some of these practices.

MOSLEM

Pork and pork-related products are not eaten. Meats that are consumed must be slaughtered by prescribed rituals; these procedures are similar to the Judaic kosher slaughtering of animals, so Moslems may eat kosher meats. Coffee, tea, and alcohol are not consumed. During the month of Ramadan, Muslims fast during the day from dawn to sunset.

CHRISTIANITY

Some sects may not eat meats on holy days; others prohibit alcohol consumption.

HINDUISM

Animal foods of beef, pork, lamb, and poultry are not eaten. Followers are lacto-vegetarians or vegans.

JUDAISM

Food consumption is guided by religious doctrines; no pork or pork-related products nor seafood or fish without scales and fins are eaten. Dairy foods are not consumed with meat or animal-related foods (excludes fish). If meat or dairy is eaten, 6 hours must pass for the other to be acceptable for consumption. Animals are slaughtered according to a ritual in which blood is drained and the carcass is salted and rinsed; meat prepared in this manner is "kosher." The preparation of all processed foods eaten must also adhere to these guidelines. Because meat and dairy must not mix, two sets of dishes and utensils are used at home and in kosher restaurants. Foods that are neither meat nor dairy are called parve and are often so labeled by food manufacturers. Additional customs affect food consumption on Saturday, the Sabbath, during which no cooking occurs. Special foods are associated with each religious holiday. Fasting (no water or food) for 24 hours occurs during Yom Kippur (Day of Atonement). During Passover, an 8-day holiday, no leavened bread is consumed, only matzoh (made from flour and water) and products made from matzoh flour; other symbolic food restrictions are also observed.

SEVENTH DAY ADVENTIST

General restrictions of pork and pork-related products, shellfish, alcohol, coffee, and tea are followed. Some followers are ovo-lacto-vegetarians, whereas others are vegans.

From Grodner M, Anderson SL, DeYoung S: *Foundations and clinical applications of nutrition: a nursing approach,* ed 2, St Louis, 2000, Mosby.

Appendix

R Activities Expenditure Table

Total Kcalories Burned for Each 1 Hour of Expenditure Item Using Body Weight Shown

	Body Weight (lb)						
Expenditure Description	**100**	**125**	**150**	**175**	**200**	**225**	**250**
Aerobics, easy	269	336	403	470	538	605	672
Aerobics, medium	278	348	418	487	557	626	696
Aerobics, hard	360	450	540	630	720	810	900
Archery	216	270	324	378	432	486	540
Assembly work, standing	132	164	197	230	263	296	329
Badminton, competition	389	486	583	680	778	875	972
Badminton, recreation	230	288	346	403	461	518	576
Bartending, standing	115	144	173	201	230	259	288
Baseball, pitcher	240	300	360	420	480	540	600
Baseball, player	187	234	281	328	374	421	468
Basketball, competition	394	492	591	689	787	886	984
Basketball, half-court	197	246	295	344	394	443	492
Basketball, moderate	283	354	425	496	566	637	708
Bathing, in tub	96	120	144	168	192	216	240
Bicycling (level) 13 mph	427	534	641	748	855	962	1068
Bicycling (level) 5.5 mph	202	252	302	353	403	454	504
Bowling, nonstop	269	336	403	470	538	605	672
Boxing, sparring	202	252	302	353	403	454	504
Calisthenics	202	252	302	353	403	454	504
Canoeing, 2.5 mph	110	138	166	193	221	248	276
Canoeing, 4.0 mph	283	354	425	496	566	637	708
Chambermaid	110	137	164	192	219	247	274
Childcare, general	138	173	207	242	276	311	345
Computer work, emailing, etc.	77	96	115	134	154	173	192
Construction, brick layer	359	449	539	628	718	808	898
Construction, carpentry	155	194	233	272	311	349	388
Construction, electrical/plumbing	150	187	224	262	299	336	374
Construction, painting, papering, etc.	169	212	254	297	339	381	424
Construction, remodeling, etc.	243	304	364	425	486	546	607
Construction, road building, laborers	276	345	415	484	553	622	691
Construction, shoveling, digging ditches	379	473	568	663	758	852	947
Cooking	86	108	130	151	173	194	216
Dance, fox-trot	178	222	266	311	355	400	444
Dance, modern, moderate	168	210	252	294	336	378	420

Developed by SureQuest Systems, Inc., and includes all of the activities listed in *Mosby's NutriTrac Nutrition Analysis CD-ROM, Version III,* which accompanies every copy of this text.

Total Kcalories Burned for Each 1 Hour of Expenditure Item Using Body Weight Shown—cont'd

	Body Weight (lb)						
Expenditure Description	100	125	150	175	200	225	250
Dance, modern, vigorous	226	282	338	395	451	508	564
Dance, rumba	278	348	418	487	557	626	696
Dance, square	274	342	410	479	547	616	684
Dance, waltz	206	258	310	361	413	464	516
Driving	62	78	94	109	125	140	156
Eating	62	78	94	109	125	140	156
Elliptical machine, moderate	303	379	455	531	607	683	758
Fencing, moderate	202	252	302	353	403	454	504
Fencing, vigorous	413	516	619	723	826	929	1032
Firefighter, fighting fires	517	646	775	904	1034	1163	1292
Fishing, general	157	196	235	274	313	352	391
Football, moderate	202	252	302	353	403	454	504
Football, vigorous	331	414	497	579	662	745	828
Frisbee	264	330	396	462	528	594	660
Golf, 2-some	216	270	324	378	432	486	540
Golf, 4-some	163	204	245	286	326	367	408
Hacky sack	158	197	237	276	316	355	395
Handball	389	486	583	680	778	875	972
Hiking, 40 lb pack, 3.0 mph	274	342	410	479	547	616	684
Hockey, field	360	450	540	630	720	810	900
Hockey, ice	380	475	570	665	760	855	950
Home gym equipment, general	267	334	401	468	535	602	669
Horseback riding, trot	269	336	403	470	538	605	672
Horseback riding, walk	134	168	202	235	269	302	336
Horseshoe pitching	144	180	216	252	288	324	360
Housecleaning	144	180	216	252	288	324	360
Hunting, general	201	251	301	351	402	452	502
Ironing, standing	103	128	154	180	205	231	256
Jai Alai	544	680	816	952	1088	1224	1360
Jazzercise	283	353	424	495	566	636	707
Jet skiing	199	249	299	349	399	449	499
Jogging, 4.0-5.0 mph	302	377	453	528	604	679	755
Judo, karate	514	642	771	899	1027	1156	1284
Lacrosse	398	498	598	697	797	896	996
Lying at ease	58	72	86	101	115	130	144
Machine operator, standing	110	137	164	192	219	247	274
Marching band, drum major	164	205	245	286	327	368	409
Marching band, playing instrument	188	234	281	328	375	422	469
Marching, general	210	262	314	367	419	472	524
Masseuse	161	202	242	282	323	363	403
Meditation	62	78	94	109	125	140	156
Mountain climbing	403	504	605	706	806	907	1008
Movers, furniture, boxes, etc.	331	414	497	579	662	745	828
Mowing lawn, riding mower	115	144	173	202	231	260	288
Mowing lawn, walking, power mower	199	249	299	349	399	449	499
Office work, at desk	77	96	115	134	154	173	192
Paddle ball, racquetball	389	486	583	680	778	875	972
Playing instrument, drums	158	197	237	276	316	355	395
Playing instrument, general	113	141	170	198	226	255	283
Playing instrument, guitar	113	141	170	198	226	255	283
Playing instrument, piano	113	141	170	198	226	255	283
Police work, driving squad car	101	127	152	178	203	228	254
Pool, billiards	72	90	108	126	144	162	180
Racquetball	480	600	720	840	960	1080	1200
Raking leaves	170	213	255	298	341	383	426
Reading, sitting	70	87	105	122	140	157	175

Continued

Total Kcalories Burned for Each 1 Hour of Expenditure Item Using Body Weight Shown—cont'd

	Body Weight (lb)						
Expenditure Description	100	125	150	175	200	225	250
Rollerblading	312	390	468	546	624	702	780
Rope jumping, 110 rpm	389	486	583	680	778	875	972
Rope jumping, 120 rpm	370	462	555	647	739	832	924
Rope jumping, 130 rpm	346	432	518	605	691	778	864
Rowing, machine	547	684	821	958	1095	1232	1369
Rowing, recreation	202	252	302	353	403	454	504
Rugby	355	444	533	622	710	799	888
Running, 5-min mile, 12 mph	787	984	1181	1378	1575	1772	1969
Running, 7-min mile, 9 mph	629	786	943	1101	1258	1415	1572
Running, 8.5-min mile, 7 mph	562	702	843	983	1124	1264	1404
Running, 11-min mile, 5.5 mph	432	540	648	756	864	972	1080
Sailing	115	144	173	202	230	259	288
Scuba diving	320	400	479	559	639	719	799
Shopping, grocery w/cart	153	192	230	268	306	345	383
Shopping, walking, non-grocery	108	136	163	190	217	244	271
Showering, towel drying	135	169	203	237	271	305	338
Sitting quietly	62	78	94	109	125	140	156
Skateboarding/scooter	202	252	302	353	403	454	504
Skating, ice	230	288	346	403	461	518	576
Skating, roller	413	516	619	723	826	929	1032
Skiing, downhill	389	486	583	680	778	875	972
Skiing, level, 5 mph	470	588	705	823	940	1058	1176
Skiing, racing downhill	658	822	987	1151	1316	1480	1645
Sleeping	48	60	72	84	96	108	120
Snorkeling	224	280	336	392	448	504	560
Snow shoeing, 2.3 mph	250	312	374	437	499	562	624
Snow shoeing, 2.5 mph	360	450	540	630	720	810	900
Snowboarding	261	326	391	457	522	587	652
Soccer	360	450	540	630	720	810	900
Softball	187	234	281	328	374	421	468
Sprinting	922	1152	1382	1613	1843	2074	2304
Squash	418	522	626	731	835	939	1044
Stair climbing and descending	384	480	576	672	768	864	960
Standing	72	90	108	126	144	162	180
Stationary running, 140 counts/min	979	1223	1468	1713	1958	2202	2447
Stretching, hatha yoga	158	197	237	276	316	355	395
Surfing	288	360	432	504	576	648	720
Swimming, back 20 yds/min	154	192	230	269	307	346	384
Swimming, back 30 yds/min	211	264	317	370	422	475	528

Total Kcalories Burned for Each 1 Hour of Expenditure Item Using Body Weight Shown—cont'd

	Body Weight (lb)						
Expenditure Description	100	125	150	175	200	225	250
Swimming, back 40 yds/min	336	420	504	588	672	756	840
Swimming, breast 20 yds/min	192	240	288	336	384	432	480
Swimming, breast 30 yds/min	288	360	432	504	576	648	720
Swimming, breast 40 yds/min	384	480	576	672	768	864	960
Swimming, butterfly 50 yds/min	470	588	705	823	940	1058	1176
Swimming, crawl 20 yds/min	192	240	288	336	384	432	480
Swimming, crawl 45 yds/min	350	438	526	613	701	789	876
Swimming, crawl 50 yds/min	427	534	641	748	855	962	1068
Swimming, pleasure 25 yds/min	240	300	360	420	480	540	600
Synchronized swimming	378	473	567	662	756	851	945
Table tennis, ping-pong	154	192	230	269	307	346	384
Talking, sitting	70	87	105	122	140	157	175
Tennis, competition	389	486	583	680	778	875	972
Tennis, recreation	278	348	418	487	557	626	696
Timed calisthenics	585	732	878	1024	1171	1317	1463
Volleyball, beach	389	486	583	680	778	875	972
Volleyball, casual, 6-9 team members	152	190	228	265	303	341	379
Volleyball, competitive, in gym	230	288	346	403	461	518	576
Walking, 110-120 steps/min	206	258	310	361	413	464	516
Walking, 2.0 mph	139	174	209	244	278	313	348
Walking, 4.5 mph	264	330	396	462	528	594	660
Walking, to work or class	158	197	237	276	316	355	395
Walking, with stroller	109	136	164	191	218	245	273
Washing car	199	249	299	349	399	449	499
Washing dishes, standing	103	128	154	180	205	231	256
Water aerobics	158	197	237	276	316	355	395
Water polo	454	567	681	794	908	1021	1135
Water skiing	312	390	468	546	624	702	780
Weight training	322	402	482	563	643	723	804
Wrestling	514	642	771	899	1027	1156	1284
Writing, sitting	77	96	115	134	154	173	192

Developed by SureQuest Systems, Inc., and includes all of the activities listed in *Mosby's NutriTrac Nutrition Analysis CD-ROM, Version III*, which accompanies every copy of this text.

NOTE: To determine kcalories used for more or less than one hour use the following formula:

Actual min/60 × Total kcalories used (from table above) = Actual kcalories burned

Example: Using "Aerobics, easy" for 150 lb body weight from table above

Actual minutes = 45

(45/60) × 403 = Total kcalories burned

.75 × 403 = 302 Total kcalories burned

Glossary

absorption Transport of digested nutrients across the intestinal wall into the body circulation.

achlasia (Gr *a-*, negative, without; *cholasis*, relaxation) Failure to relax the smooth muscle fibers of the gastrointestinal tract at any point of juncture of its parts, especially failure of the esophagogastric sphincter to relax when swallowing, as a result of degeneration of ganglion cells in the wall of the organ. The lower esophagus also loses its normal peristaltic activity. Also called cardiospasm.

actin (Gr *aktis*, a radiating activating substance) Myofibril protein whose synchronized meshing action in conjunction with **myosin** causes muscles to contract and relax.

adenosine triphosphate (ATP) The high-energy compound formed in the cell and called the "energy currency" of the cell because of the binding of energy in its high-energy phosphate bonds for release for cell work as these bonds are split. A compound of adenosine (a nucleotide containing adenine and ribose) that has three phosphoric acid groups. ATP is a high-energy phosphate compound important in energy exchange for cellular activity. The splitting off of the terminal phosphate bond (PO_4) of ATP to produce adenosine diphosphate (ADP) releases bound energy and transfers it to free energy available for body work. The reforming of ATP in cell oxidation again stores energy in high-energy phosphate bonds for use as needed.

Adequate Intake (AI) Suggested daily intake of a nutrient to meet daily needs and support health; AIs have a more limited research base than do the RDAs but were developed to address current health concerns; the AI for calcium is expected to reduce the risk of bone loss and bone fractures in older adults.

adipocyte (L *adipis*, fat; Gr *kytos*, hollow vessel) A fat cell. All cell names end in the suffix *-cyte*, with the type of cell indicated by the root word to which it is added.

adipose (L *adeps*, fat; *adiposus*, fatty) Fat present in cells of adipose (fatty) tissue.

admixture (L *admixtus*, admixture) A mixture of ingredients that each retain their own physical properties; a combination of two or more substances that are not chemically united or that exist in no fixed proportion to each other.

advance directives Instructions for medical treatment given by a patient while he or she has decisional capacity to do so.

aerobic capacity (Gr *aer*, air or gas) Milliliters of oxygen consumed per kilogram of body weight per minute; influenced by body composition.

aldosterone Potent hormone of the cortex of the adrenal glands, which acts on the distal renal tubule to cause reabsorption of sodium in an ion exchange with potassium. The aldosterone mechanism is essentially a sodium-conserving mechanism but indirectly also conserves water, since water absorption follows the sodium reabsorption.

alpha-fetoprotein A fetal antigen in amniotic fluid that provides an early pregnancy test for fetal malformations such as neural tube defect.

amine An organic compound containing nitrogen. Amino acids and pyridoxine are examples of amines.

amino acid (*amino*, the monovalent chemical group NH_2) An acid containing the essential element nitrogen (in the chemical group NH_2). Amino acids are the structural units of protein and the basic building blocks of the body.

aminopeptidase (Chemistry: *amino*, nitrogen-containing; Gr *pepsis*, digestion) Protein-splitting enzyme that cuts the peptide bond (linkage) at the amino end of amino acids, splitting off the amino group NH_2.

amniotic fluid (Gr *amnion*, bowl) The watery fluid within the membrane enveloping the fetus, in which the fetus is suspended.

amphoteric (Gr *amphoteros,* both) Having opposite characteristics; capable of acting either as an acid or a base, combining with both acids and bases.

ampullae (L *ampulla,* a jug) A general term for flasklike wider portion of a tubular structure; spaces under the nipple of the breast for storing milk.

amyloid (Gr *amylon,* starch; *-oid, eidos,* form, shape) A glycoprotein substance having a relation to starchlike structure but more a protein compound; an abnormal complex material forming characteristic brain deposits of fibrillary tangles always found in postmortem examinations of patients with Alzheimer's disease, the only means of definitive diagnosis; found in various body tissues that, when advanced, form lesions that destroy functional cells and injure the organ.

amyotrophic lateral sclerosis (ALS) (Gr *a-,* negative; *mys,* muscle; *trophē,* nourishment; L *lateralis,* to the side; *sklērōis,* hardness) A progressive neuromuscular disease characterized by the degeneration of the neurons of the spinal cord and the motor cells of the brain stem, causing a deficit of upper and lower motor neurons; death usually occurs in 2 to 3 years.

anabolism (Gr *anabole,* a building up) Metabolic process by which body tissues are built.

anastomosis A surgical joining of two ducts to allow flow from one to the other.

anemia (Gr *an-,* negative prefix; *haima,* blood) Blood condition characterized by decreased number of circulating red blood cells, hemoglobin, or both.

anorexia nervosa (Gr "want of appetite") Extreme psychophysiologic aversion to food, resulting in life-threatening weight loss; a psychiatric eating disorder caused by a morbid fear of fat, in which the person's distorted body image is reflected as fat when the body is actually malnourished and extremely thin from self-starvation.

anthropometry (Gr *anthropos,* man; *metron,* measure) The science of measuring the size, weight, and proportions of the human body.

antibody Any of numerous protein molecules produced by B cells as a primary immune defense for attaching to specific related **antigens;** animal protein made up of a specific sequence of amino acids that is designed to interact with its specific antigen during an allergic response or to prevent infection.

antidiuretic hormone (ADH) Water-conserving hormone from posterior lobe of pituitary gland; causes resorption of water by kidney nephrons according to body need.

antigen (antibody + Gr *gennan,* to produce) Any foreign or "non-self" substances, such as toxins, viruses, bacteria, and foreign proteins, that stimulate the production of **antibodies** specifically designed to interact with them.

antimetabolite A substance bearing a close structural resemblance to one required for normal physiologic functioning that exerts its effect by interfering with the utilization of the essential metabolite.

antioxidant (Gr *anti,* against; *oxys* keen) A substance that inhibits oxidation of polyunsaturated fatty acids and formation of free radicals in the cells.

apolipoprotein A separate protein compound that attaches to its specific receptor site on a particular lipoprotein and activates certain functions, such as synthesis of a related enzyme. An example is apolipoprotein C-II, an apolipoprotein of chylomicrons and very low-density lipoprotein that functions to activate the enzyme lipoprotein lipase.

areola (L *areola,* area, space) A defined space; a circular area of different color surrounding a central point, such as the darkened pigmented ring surrounding the nipple of the breast.

ariboflavinosis Group of clinical manifestations of riboflavin deficiency.

arteriosclerosis (Gr *arteria,* from *aēr,* air, and *tērein,* to keep, because of the ancient belief that the arteries contained vital air; *sklēros,* hard) Blood vessel disease characterized by thickening and hardening of artery walls, with loss of functional elasticity, mainly affecting the intima (inner lining) of the arteries.

arthroplasty (Gr *arthron,* joint; *plassein,* to form) Plastic surgery of nonfunctioning body joints to form movable joints with replacement metal or plastic materials.

atheroma (Gr *athērē,* gruel; *-oma,* a mass or body of tissue) A mass of fatty plaque formed in inner arterial walls in atherosclerosis.

atherosclerosis (Gr *athērē,* gruel; *sklēros,* hard) Common form of arteriosclerosis, characterized by the gradual formation—beginning in childhood in genetically predisposed individuals—of yellow cheeselike streaks of cholesterol and fatty material that develop into hardened plaques in the intima or inner lining of major blood vessels, such as coronary arteries, eventually in adulthood cutting off blood supply to the tissue served by the vessels; the underlying pathology of coronary heart disease.

autonomy (Gr *autos,* self; *nomos,* law) The state of functioning independently, without extraneous influence.

bariatrics The field of medicine that focuses on the treatment and the control of obesity and diseases associated with obesity.

basal metabolic rate (BMR) Amount of energy required to maintain the resting body's internal activities after an overnight fast with the subject awake. See also **resting metabolic rate (RMR).**

beriberi (Singhalese "I cannot, I cannot") A disease of the peripheral nerves caused by a deficiency of thiamin (vitamin B_1). It is characterized by pain (neuritis) and paralysis of the extremities, cardiovascular changes, and edema. Beriberi is common in the Orient, where diets consist largely of milled rice with little protein.

bezoar A hard ball of hair or vegetable fiber that may develop within the stomach and intestines; can cause an obstruction, requiring removal. Formed because of reduced gastric motility, decreased gastric mixing and churning, and reduced gastric secretions.

bile (L *bilis,* bile) A fluid secreted by the liver and transported to the gallbladder for concentration and storage. It is released into the duodenum upon entry of fat to facilitate enzymatic fat digestion by acting as an emulsifying agent.

bilirubin (L *bilis,* bile; *ruber,* red) A reddish bile pigment resulting from the degradation of heme by reticuloendothelial cells in the liver; a high level in the blood produces the yellow skin symptomatic of jaundice.

binge eating An eating disorder that includes binge eating episodes, but without the purging behavior of persons with bulimia nervosa. This is an emotional, reactive eating pattern occurring in response to stress or anxiety and used to soothe painful feelings.

bioavailability Amount of a nutrient ingested in food that is absorbed and thus available to the body for metabolic use.

blood urea nitrogen (BUN) The nitrogen component of urea in the blood; a measure of kidney function; elevated levels of BUN indicate a disorder of kidney function.

body composition The relative sizes of the four basic body compartments that make up the total body: lean body mass (muscle and vital organs), fat, water, and bone.

bolus (Gr *bolos,* lump) Rounded mass of food formed in the mouth and ready to be swallowed.

buffer Mixture of acidic and alkaline components that, when added to a solution, is able to protect the solution against wide variations in its pH, even when strong acids and bases are added to it. If an acid is added, the alkaline partner reacts to counteract the acidic effect. If a base is added, the acid partner reacts to counteract the alkalizing effect. A solution to which a buffer has been added is called a buffered solution.

bulimia nervosa (L *bous,* ox; *limos,* hunger) A psychiatric eating disorder in which cycles of gorging on large quantities of food are followed by self-induced vomiting and use of diuretics and laxatives to maintain a "normal" body weight.

calcitonin (L *calx,* lime, calcium; *tonus,* balance) A polypeptide hormone secreted by the thyroid gland in response to hypercalcemia, which acts to lower both calcium and phosphate in the blood.

calcitriol Activated hormone form of vitamin D [1,25$(OH)_2D_3$]-1,25-dihydroxycholecalciferol.

callus (L *callositis,* callus, bone) Unorganized meshwork of newly grown, woven bone developed on pattern of original fibrin clot (formed after fracture or surgery) and normally replaced in the healing process by hard adult bone.

calorie (L *calor,* heat) A unit of heat energy. The calorie used in the study of metabolism is the large calorie, or *kilocalorie,* defined as the amount of heat required to raise the temperature of 1 kg of water 1° Celsius (centigrade).

calorimetry (L *calor,* heat; Gr *metron,* measure) Measurement of amounts of heat absorbed or given out. *Direct method:* measurement of amount of heat produced by a subject enclosed in a small chamber. *Indirect method:* measurement of amount of heat produced by a subject by the quantity of nitrogen and carbon dioxide eliminated.

cancer (L *cancer,* crab) A malignant cellular tumor with properties of tissue invasion and spread to other parts of the body.

candidiasis (L *candidus,* glowing white) Infection with the fungus of the genus *Candida,* generally caused by *C. albicans,* so-named for the whitish appearance of its small lesions; usually a superficial infection in moist areas of the skin or inner mucous membranes.

capillary fluid shift mechanism Process that controls the movement of water and small molecules in solution (electrolytes, nutrients) between the blood in the capillary and the surrounding interstitial area. Filtration of water and solutes out of the capillary at the arteriole end and reabsorption at the venule end are accomplished by shifts in balance between the intracapillary hydrostatic blood pressure and the colloidal osmotic pressure exerted by the plasma proteins.

carbohydrate Compound of carbon, hydrogen, and oxygen; starches, sugars, and dietary fiber made and stored in plants; major energy source in the human diet.

carboxyl (COOH) The monovalent radical, COOH, occurring in those organic acids termed carboxylic acids.

carboxypeptidase (L *carbo-,* carbon; *oxy,* oxygen) A protein enzyme that splits off the chemical group *carboxyl* (COOH) at the end of peptide chains, acting on the peptide bond of the terminal amino acid having a free-end carboxyl group.

carcinoma (Gr *karkinos,* crab; *onkoma,* a swelling) A malignant new growth made up of epithelial cells, infiltrating the surrounding tissue and spreading to other parts of the body.

cardiac output (Gr *kardia,* heart) Total volume of blood propelled from the heart with each contraction; equal to the stroke output multiplied by the number of beats per the time unit used in the calculation.

carnitine A naturally occurring amino acid ($C_{17}H_{15}NO_3$) formed from methionine and lysine, required for transport of long-chain fatty acids across the mitochondrial membrane, where they are oxidized as fuel substrate for metabolic energy.

casein hydrolysate formula (L *caseus,* cheese) Infant formula with base of hydrolyzed casein, major milk protein, produced by partially breaking down the casein into smaller peptide fragments, making a product that is more easily digested.

catabolism (Gr *katabole,* a throwing down) The breaking-down phase of metabolism, the opposite of anabolism. Catabolism includes all the processes in which complex substances are progressively broken down into simpler ones. Catabolism usually involves the release of energy. Together, anabolism and catabolism constitute metabolism, which is the coordinated operation of anabolic and catabolic processes into a dynamic balance of energy and substance.

chemical bonding Process of linking the radicals, chemical elements, or groups of a chemical compound.

cholecalciferol Chemical name for vitamin D in its inactive dietary form (D_3). When the inactive cholecalciferol is consumed or its counterpart cholesterol compound is developed in the skin, its first stage of activation occurs in the liver and then is completed in the kidney to the active vitamin D hormone *calcitriol* 1,25-dihydroxycholecalciferol, or $1,25(OH)_2D_3$.

cholecystokinin (CCK) (Gr *chole,* bile or gall; *kystis,* bladder, *kinein,* to move) A peptide hormone secreted by the mucosa of the duodenum in response to the presence of fat. Cholecystokinin causes the gallbladder to contract and propel bile into the duodenum, where it is needed to emulsify the fat. The fat is thus prepared for digestion and absorption.

cholesterol A fat-related compound, a sterol ($C_{27}H_{45}OH$). It is a normal constituent of bile and a principal constituent of gallstones. In body metabolism cholesterol is important as a precursor of various steroid hormones, such as sex hormones and adrenal corticoids. Cholesterol is synthesized by the liver. It is widely distributed in nature, especially in animal tissue such as glandular meats and egg yolk.

chorea (L *choreia,* dance) A wide variety of ceaseless involuntary movements that are rapid, complex, and jerky, yet appear to be well coordinated; characteristic movements of Huntington's disease.

chyle The fat-containing, creamy white fluid that is formed in the lacteals of the intestine during digestion, transported through the lymphatics, and enters the venous circulation via the thoracic duct.

chylomicrons (L *chylus,* juice, milky fluid taken up by lacteals of the intestinal villi; Gr *mikros,* small) Initial lipoproteins formed in the intestinal wall after a meal for absorption of the food fats into circulation.

chyme (Gr *chymos,* juice) Semifluid food mass in the gastrointestinal tract after gastric digestion.

chymotrypsin (Gr *chymos,* chyme, creamy gruel-like material produced by gastric digestion of food) One of the protein-splitting and milk-curdling pancreatic enzymes, activated in the intestine from precursor chymotrypsinogen. It breaks peptide linkages of the amino acids phenylalanine and tyrosine.

cirrhosis (Gr *kirrhos,* orange-yellow) Chronic liver disease, characterized by loss of functional cells, with fibrous and nodular regeneration.

cisterni chyli Cistern or receptacle of the chyle; a dilated sac at the origin of the thoracic duct, which is the common truck that receives all the lymphatic vessels. The cisterna chyli lies in the abdomen between the second lumbar vertebra and the aorta. It receives the lymph from the intestinal trunk, the right and left lumbar lymphatic trunks, and two descending lymphatic trunks. The chyle, after passing through the cisterna chyli, is carried upward into the chest through the thoracic duct and empties into the venous blood at the point where the left subclavian vein joins the left internal jugular vein. This is the way absorbed fats enter the general circulation.

clinical pathways Clear standards or protocols for patient care that are designed to promote cost efficiency, better outcomes, and faster recovery.

coenzyme A major metabolic role of the micronutrients, vitamins and minerals, as essential partners with cell enzymes in a variety of reactions in energy, lipid, and protein metabolism.

cognitive (L *cognoscere,* to know) Pertaining to the mental processes of perceptions, memory, judgment, and reasoning, as contrasted with emotional and volitional processes.

collagen (Gr *kolla,* glue; *gennan,* to produce) The protein substance of the white collagen fibers of skin, tendon, bone, cartilage, and all other connective tissue.

colloidal osmotic pressure (COP) Pressure produced by the protein molecules in the plasma and in the cell. Because proteins are large molecules, they do not pass through the separating membranes of the capillary cells. Thus they remain in their respective compartments, exerting a constant osmotic pull that protects vital plasma and cell fluid volumes in these compartments.

colon (Gr *kolon,* colon) The large intestine extending from the cecum to the rectum.

colostrum (L *colostrum,* premilk) Thin yellow fluid first secreted by the mammary gland a few days before and after childbirth, preceding the mature breast milk. It contains up to 20% protein including a large amount of lactalbumin, more minerals and less lactose and fat than does mature milk, and immunoglobulins representing the antibodies found in maternal blood.

compartment The collective quantity of material of a given type in the body. The four body compartments are *lean body mass* (muscle), *bone, fat,* and *water.*

complement (L *complere,* to fill) A complex series of enzymatic proteins occurring in normal serum that interact to combine with and augment (fill out, complete) the antigen-antibody complex of the body's immune system, producing lysis when the antigen is an intact cell; composed of 11 discrete proteins or functioning components, activated by the immunoglobulin factors IgG and IgM.

constitutive proteins Albumin, prealbumin, transferrin. Plasma proteins often used to assess the response to nutrition support. Serum levels are nonspecific and nonsensitive to the nutritional care or requirements of critically ill patients.

cretinism (F *cretinisine*) A congenital disease resulting from absence or deficiency of normal thyroid secretion, characterized by physical deformity, dwarfism, mental retardation, and often goiters.

cruciferous (L *cruces,* cross; *forma,* form) Bearing a cross; botanical term for plants belonging to the botanical family Cruciferae or Brassicaceae, the mustard family, so-called because of cross-like, four-petaled flowers; name given to certain vegetables of this family, such as broccoli, cabbage, brussels sprouts, and cauliflower.

cytokines (Gr *kytos,* hollow vessel, cell; *kinētos,* movable, changing) Substances, produced in tissues, that can cause inflammatory changes in tissue cells (e.g., tumor necrosis factor and interleukin-1).

deamination Removal of an amino group (NH_2) from an amino acid.

decubitus ulcer (L *decubitus,* lying down; *ulcus,* ulcer) Pressure sores in long-term bed-bound or immobile patients at points of bony protuberances, where prolonged pressure of body weight in one position cuts off adequate blood circulation to that area, causing tissue death and ulceration.

dehydrocholesterol A precursor cholesterol compound in the skin that is irradiated by sunlight to produce cholecalciferol (D_3).

demographic (Gr *demos,* people; *graphein,* to write) The statistical data of a population, especially those showing average age, income, education, births, and deaths.

diabetes insipidus (Gr *dia,* through; *bainein,* to go; *diabetes,* siphon; L *insipidus,* tasteless, not sweet, as compared to diabetes *mellitus,* L honey) A condition of the pituitary gland and insufficiency of one of its hormones, vasopressin or antidiuretic hormone; characterized by a copious output of a nonsweet urine, great thirst, and sometimes a large appetite. In diabetes insipidus these symptoms result from a specific injury to the pituitary gland, not a collection of metabolic disorders as in diabetes mellitus. The injured pituitary gland produces less vasopressin, a hormone that normally helps the kidneys reabsorb adequate water.

dialysis (Gr *dia,* through; *lysis,* dissolution) Process of separating crystalloids and colloids in solution by the difference in their rates of diffusion through a semipermeable membrane; crystalloids pass through readily and colloids very slowly or not at all.

dietary fiber Nondigestible carbohydrates and lignin found in plants; the plant foods supplying fiber also contain other macronutrients and vitamins and minerals; plant foods containing dietary fiber have nutritional benefits such as preventing gastrointestinal disease like diverticulosis or reducing serum lipid and glucose levels that are related to the chronic conditions of heart disease and diabetes.

Dietary Reference Intakes (DRIs) Term referring to the framework of nutrient standards now in place in the United States; this includes the Recommended Dietary Allowances, Adequate Intakes, and Tolerable Upper Intake Level.

dietetics Management of diet and the use of food; the science concerned with the nutritional planning and preparation of foods.

digestion The process of breaking down food to release its nutrients for absorption and transport to the cells for use in body functions.

disability A mental or physical impairment that prevents an individual from performing one or more gainful activities; not synonymous with handicap, which implies serious disadvantage.

disaccharides (Gr *di,* two; *saccharide,* sugar) Class of compound sugars composed of two molecules of monosaccharide. The three most common are sucrose, lactose, and maltose.

disulfiram White to off-white crystalline antioxidant; inhibits oxidation of the acetaldehyde metabolized from alcohol. It is used in the treatment of alcoholism, producing extremely uncomfortable symptoms when alcohol is ingested after oral administration of the drug.

dumping syndrome Constellation of postprandial symptoms that result from rapid emptying of hyperosmolar gastric contents into the duodenum. The hypertonic load in the small intestine promotes reflux of vascular fluid into the bowel lumen, causing a rapid decrease in the circulating blood volume. Rapid symptoms of abdominal cramping, nausea, vomiting, palpitations, sweating, weakness, reduced blood pressure, tremors, and osmotic diarrhea occur. Symptoms of early dumping begin 10 to 30 minutes after eating; late dumping occurs 1 to 4 hours after a meal. Late dumping is a result of insulin hypersecretion in response to the carbohydrate load dumped into the small intestine. Once the carbohydrate is absorbed, the hyperinsulinemia causes hypoglycemia, which results in vasomotor symptoms such as diaphoresis, weakness, flushing, and palpitations. Individuals who have undergone gastrointestinal surgery resulting in a reduced or absent gastric pouch are more prone to dumping syndrome.

dysentery (Gr *dys,* painful, bad; *enteron,* intestine) A general term given to a number of disorders marked by inflammation of the intestines, especially of the colon, and attended by abdominal pain and frequent stools containing blood and mucus. The causative agent may be chemical irritants, bacteria, protozoa, or parasites.

dyspnea (Gr *dysnoia,* difficulty of breathing) Labored, difficult breathing.

eclampsia (Gr *eklampein,* to shine forth) Advanced pregnancy-induced hypertension (PIH), manifested by convulsions.

ecology (Gr *oikos,* house) Relations between organisms and their environments.

eicosanoids (Gr *eikosa,* twenty) Long-chain fatty acids composed of 20 carbon atoms.

electrolytes (Gr *electron,* amber [which emits electricity when rubbed]; *lytos,* soluble) A chemical element or compound that in solution dissociates as ions carrying a positive or negative charge (for example, H^+, Na^+, K^+, Ca^{++}, Mg^{++}, and Cl^- , HCO_3^-, HPO_4^{2-}, SO_4^{2-}. Electrolytes constitute a major force controlling fluid balances within the body through their concentrations and shifts from one place to another to restore and maintain balance—*homeostasis.*

elemental formula A nutrition support formula composed of simple elemental nutrient components that require no further digestive breakdown and are thus readily absorbed; infant formula produced with elemental ready-to-be-absorbed components of free amino acids and carbohydrate as simple sugars.

emulsifier An agent that breaks down large fat globules to smaller, uniformly distributed particles. This action is accomplished in the intestine chiefly by the bile acids, which lower surface tension of the fat particles. Emulsification greatly increases the surface area of fat, facilitating contact with fat-digesting enzymes.

endemic (Gr *endemos,* dwelling in a place) Characterizing a disease of low morbidity that remains constantly in a human community but is clinically recognizable in only a few.

endocarditis (Gr *endon,* within; *kardia,* heart) Inflammation of the endocardium, the serous membrane that lines the cavities of the heart.

energy (Gr *en,* in, with; *ergon,* work) The capacity of a system for doing work; available power. Energy is manifest in various forms—motion, position, light, heat, and sound. Energy is interchangeable among these various forms and is constantly being transformed and transferred among them.

enteral (Gr *enteron,* intestine) A feeding modality that provides nutrients, either orally or by tube feeding through the gastrointestinal tract.

enterogastrone (Gr *enteron,* intestine; *gaster,* stomach; *-one,* suffix for hormones) A duodenal peptide hormone that inhibits gastric hydrochloric acid secretion and motility.

enzyme (Gr *en,* in; *zyme,* leaven) Various complex proteins produced by living cells that act independently of these cells. Enzymes are capable of producing certain chemical changes in other substances without themselves being changed in the process. Their action is therefore that of a catalyst. Digestive enzymes of the gastrointestinal secretions act on food substances to break them down into simpler compounds and greatly accelerate the speed of these chemical reactions. An enzyme is usually named according to the substance (substrate) on which it acts, with the common suffix -ase; for example, sucrase is the specific enzyme for sucrose and breaks it down to glucose and fructose.

ergogenic (Gr *ergo,* work; *gennan,* to produce) Tendency to increase work output; various substances that increase work or exercise capacity and output.

erythema (Gr *erythros,* red; *erythema,* flush upon the skin) Redness of the skin produced by coagulation of the capillaries.

essential fatty acid (EFA) (L *essentialis,* necessary or inherent) A fatty acid required in the diet because the body cannot synthesize it or synthesize it in adequate amounts.

essential hypertension An inherent form of hypertension with no specific discoverable cause and considered to be familial; also called primary hypertension.

ester A compound produced by the reaction between an acid and an alcohol with elimination of a molecule of water. This process is called esterification. For example, a triglyceride is a glycerol ester. Cholesterol esters are formed in the mucosal cells by combination with fatty acids, largely linoleic acid.

fasciculi (L *fascis,* bundle) A general term for a small bundle or cluster of muscle, tendon, or nerve fibers.

fatty acid The structural components of fats.

ferritin Protein-iron compound in which iron is stored in tissues; the storage form of iron in the body.

fetus (L *fetus,* unborn offspring) The unborn offspring in the postembryonic period, after major structures have been outlined; in humans the growing offspring from 7 to 8 weeks after fertilization until birth.

fistula (L *fistula,* pipe) Abnormal connection between two internal organs, an internal organ and the skin, or an internal organ and a body cavity.

flushing reaction Short-term reaction resulting in redness of neck and face.

fuel factor The kilocalorie value (energy potential) of food nutrients; that is, the number of kilocalories that 1 g of the nutrient yields when oxidized. The kilocalorie fuel factor for carbohydrate is 4; for protein, 4; and for fat, 9. The basic figures are used in computing diets and energy values of foods. (For example, 10 g of fat yields 90 kcal.)

functional fiber Nondigestible carbohydrates isolated from plant foods or manufactured that have been individually tested and found to have beneficial physiologic effects in the body; these substances may be added to natural foods to increase their fiber content.

gastric polyposis An abnormal condition characterized by the presence of numerous polyps in the stomach.

gastrin Hormone secreted by mucosal cells in the antrum of the stomach that stimulates the parietal cells to produce hydrochloric acid. Gastrin is released into the stomach in response to stimulants, especially coffee, alcohol, and meat extractives. When the gastric pH falls below 3, a feedback mechanism cuts off gastrin secretion and prevents excess acid formation.

gastritis (Gr *gaster,* stomach) Inflammation of the stomach.

gastroesophageal reflux disease (GERD) Describes symptoms that result from reflux of gastric juices, and sometimes duodenal juices, into the esophagus. Symptoms include substernal burning (heartburn), epigastric pressure sensation, and severe epigastric pain. Prolonged and severe GERD can lead to esophageal bleeding, perforation, strictures, Barrett's epithelium, adenocarcinoma, and pulmonary fibrosis (from aspiration). Conservative dietary therapy involves weight reduction; restriction of carbonated beverages, caffeine, fatty foods, peppermint, chocolate, and ethanol; small frequent meals; and wearing of loose clothing to promote symptomatic relief.

geriatrics (Gr *geras,* old age; *iatrike,* surgery, medicine) Branch of medicine specializing in medical problems associated with old age.

gerontology (Gr *geronto,* old man; *logy,* work, reason, study) Study of the aging process and its remarkable progressive events.

gestation (L *gestatio,* from; *gestare,* to bear) The period of embryonic and fetal development from fertilization to birth; pregnancy.

glomerulonephritis A form of nephritis affecting the capillary loops in an acute short-term infection. It may progress to a more serious chronic condition leading to irreversible renal failure.

glossitis (Gr *glossa,* tongue + *itis*) Swollen, reddened tongue; riboflavin deficiency symptom.

glucagon (Gr *glykys,* sweet; *gonē,* seed) A polypeptide hormone secreted by the A cells of the pancreatic islets of Langerhans in response to hypoglycemia; has an opposite balancing effect to that of insulin, raising the blood sugar, thus is used as a quick-acting antidote for the hypoglycemic reaction of insulin. It stimulates the breakdown of glycogen (glycogenolysis) in the liver by activating the liver enzyme phosphorylase and thus raises blood sugar levels during fasting states to ensure adequate levels for normal nerve and brain function.

gluconeogenesis (Gr *gleukos,* sweetness; *neos,* new; *genesis,* production, generation) Production of glucose from keto acid carbon skeletons from deaminated amino acids and the glycerol portion of fatty acids.

glyceride Group name for fats; any of a group of esters obtained from glycerol by the replacement of one, two, or three hydroxyl (OH) groups with a fatty acid. Monoglycerides contain one fatty acid; diglycerides contain two fatty acids; triglycerides contain three fatty acids. Glycerides are the principal constituent of adipose tissue and are found in animal and vegetable fats and oils.

glycerol A colorless, odorless, syrupy, sweet liquid; a constituent of fats usually obtained by the hydrolysis of fats. Chemically glycerol is an alcohol; it is esterified with fatty acids to produce fats.

glycogen (Gr *glykys,* sweet; *genes,* born, produced) A polysaccharide, that is, a large compound of many saccharide (i.e., sugar) units. It is the main body storage form of carbohydrate, largely stored in the liver, with lesser amounts stored in muscle tissue.

glycogenesis Synthesis of glycogen from blood glucose.

glycogenolysis (*glycogen* + Gr *lysis,* dissolution) Specific term for conversion of glycogen into glucose in the liver; chemical process of enzymatic hydrolysis or breakdown by which this conversion is accomplished.

glycolysis Cell oxidation of glucose for energy.

goiter (L *guttur,* throat) Enlargement of the thyroid gland caused by lack of sufficient available iodine to produce the thyroid hormone thyroxine.

gravida (L *gravida,* heavy, loaded) A pregnant woman.

growth acceleration (L *celerare,* to quicken) Period of increased speed of growth at different points of childhood development.

growth channel The progressive regular growth pattern of children, guided along individual genetically controlled channels, influenced by nutritional and health status.

growth chart grids Grids comparing stature (length), weight, and age of children by percentile; used for nutritional assessment to determine how their growth is progressing. The most commonly used grids are those of the National Center for Health Statistics (NCHS).

growth deceleration (L *de,* from; *celerare,* to quicken) Period of decreased speed of growth at different points of childhood development.

growth velocity (L *velocitas,* speed) Rapidity of motion or movement; rate of childhood growth over normal periods of development, as compared with a population standard.

handicap A mental or physical defect that may or may not be congenital that prevents the individual from participating in normal life activities; implies disadvantage.

Heimlich maneuver A first-aid maneuver to relieve a person who is choking from blockage of the breathing passageway by a swallowed foreign object or food particle. Standing behind the person, clasp the victim around the waist, placing one fist under the sternum (breastbone) and grasping the fist with the other hand. Then make a quick, hard, thrusting movement inward and upward.

helix A coiled structure as found in protein. Some are simple chain coils; others are made of several coils, as in a triple helix.

hematuria (Gr *haima,* blood; *ouron,* urine) The abnormal presence of blood in the urine.

heme iron Dietary iron from animal sources, from the heme portion of hemoglobin in red blood cells. Heme iron is more easily absorbed and transported in the body than nonheme iron from plant sources, but it supplies the smaller portion of the body's total dietary iron intake.

hemodialysis (Gr *haima,* blood; *dia,* through; *lysis,* dissolution) Removal of certain elements from the blood according to their rates of diffusion through a semipermeable membrane—e.g., by a hemodialysis machine.

hemoglobin (Gr *haima, blood; L globus,* a ball) Oxygen-carrying pigment in red blood cells; a conjugated protein containing four heme groups combined with iron and four long polypeptide chains forming the protein globin, named for its ball-like form; made by the developing red blood cells in bone marrow. Hemoglobin carries oxygen in the blood to body cells.

hemolytic anemia (Gr *haima,* blood; *lysis,* dissolution) An anemia (reduced number of red blood cells) caused by breakdown of the outer membrane of red blood cells and loss of their hemoglobin.

hemosiderin (Gr *haima,* blood; *sideros,* iron) Insoluble iron oxide–protein compound in which iron is stored in the liver if the amount of iron in the blood exceeds the storage capacity of ferritin, for example, during rapid destruction of red blood cells (malaria, hemolytic anemia).

herpes zoster (Gr *herpēs,* herpes; *zoster,* a girdle or encircling structure or pattern) An acute self-limiting viral inflammatory disease of posterior nerve roots causing skin eruptions in a lateral pattern across the back of the torso served by these nerves, accompanied by neuralgic pain; caused by the virus of chickenpox and commonly called *shingles.*

homeostasis (Gr *homoios,* like, unchanging; *stasis,* standing, stable) State of relative dynamic equilibrium within the body's internal environment; a balance achieved through the operation of various interrelated physiologic mechanisms.

hormones Various internally secreted substances from the endocrine organs, which are conveyed by the blood to another organ or tissue on which they act to stimulate increased functional activity or secretion. This tissue or substance is called its target organ or substance.

hydrogenation Process of hardening liquid vegetable oils by injecting hydrogen gas to produce margarines and shortenings.

hydrolysis (Gr *hydro,* water; *lysis,* dissolution) Process by which a chemical compound is split into other simpler compounds by taking up the elements of water, as in the manufacture of infant formulas to produce easier-to-digest derivatives of the main protein casein in the cow's milk base. This process occurs naturally in digestion.

25-hydroxycholecalciferol [25, (OH)D_3] Initial product formed in the liver in the process of developing the active vitamin D hormone.

hygroscopic (Gr *hygros,* moist) Taking up and retaining moisture readily.

hypercapnia (Gr *hyper,* above; *kapnos,* smoke) Excess CO_2 in the blood.

hyperemesis gravidarum (Gr *hyper,* above, excessive; *emesis,* vomiting; L *gravida,* heavy loaded) Severe vomiting during pregnancy, which is potentially fatal.

hyperlipoproteinemia (Gr *hyper,* above; *lipoprotein,* fat-protein compound; *-emia,* suffix referring to *haima,* blood) Elevated level of lipoproteins in the blood.

hyperthyroidism (Gr *hyper,* above; *thyroidism,* thyroid gland function) Abnormally increased activity of the parathyroid gland, resulting in excessive secretion of parathyroid hormone, which normally helps regulate serum calcium levels in balance with vitamin D hormone; excess secretion occurs when the serum calcium level falls below normal, as in chronic renal disease or in vitamin D deficiency.

hypovolemia (Gr *hypo,* under; *haima,* blood) Abnormally decreased volume of circulating blood in the body.

hypoxemia (Gr *hypo,* under; *-ox-,* oxygen; *emia (haima),* blood) Deficient oxygenation of the blood, resulting in hypoxia, reduced O_2 supply to tissue.

iatrogenic (Gr *iatros,* healer; *genesis,* origin or source) Describing a medical disorder caused by physician diagnosis, manner, or treatment.

icteric (Gr *ikteros,* jaundice) Alternate term for jaundice: nonicteric indicates absence of jaundice; preicteric indicates a state prior to development of icterus, or jaundice.

immunocompetence (L *immunis,* free, exempt) The ability or capacity to develop an immune response, that is, antibody production and/or cell-mediated immunity, following exposure to antigen.

incomplete protein food A protein food having a ratio of amino acids different from that of the average body protein and therefore less valuable for nutrition than complete protein food.

indispensable (essential) amino acid Any one of nine amino acids that the body cannot synthesize at all or in sufficient amounts to meet body needs and that therefore must be supplied by the diet and is hence a *dietary* essential. These nine specific amino acids are histidine, isoleucine, leucine, lysine, methionine, phenylalanine, threonine, tryptophan, and valine. Two amino acids—cysteine and tyrosine—are called conditionally essential amino acids because the body cannot synthesize sufficient amounts under certain conditions.

indole A compound produced in the intestines by the decomposition of tryptophan; also found in the oil of jasmine and clove.

infarct (L *infarcire,* to stuff in) An area of tissue necrosis caused by local ischemia, resulting from obstruction of blood circulation to that area.

insulin (L *insula,* island) Hormone formed in the B cells of the islets of Langerhans in the pancreas. Insulin is secreted when blood glucose and amino acid levels rise and assists their entry into body cells. It also promotes glycogenesis and conversion of glucose into fat and inhibits lipolysis and gluconeogenesis (protein breakdown). Commercial insulin is manufactured from pigs and cows; new "artificial" human insulin products have recently been made available.

intermittent claudication (L *claudicatio,* limping or lameness) A symptomatic pattern of peripheral vascular disease, characterized by absence of pain or discomfort in a limb, usually the legs, when at rest, which is followed by pain and weakness when walking, intensifying until walking becomes impossible, and then disappearing again after a rest period; seen in occlusive arterial disease.

interstitial fluid (L *inter,* between; *sistere,* to set) The fluid situated between parts or in the interspaces of a tissue.

intima (L *intima,* inner area) General term indicating an innermost part of a structure or vessel; inner layer of the blood vessel wall.

intramural nerve plexus (L *intra,* within; *murus,* wall; plexus, plait or network) Network of nerves in the walls of the intestine that make up the intramural nervous system, controlling muscle action and secretions for digestion and absorption.

ischemia (Gr *ischein,* to suppress; *haima,* blood) Deficiency of blood to a particular tissue, resulting from functional blood vessel constriction or actual obstruction walls in atherosclerosis.

jaundice (Fr *jaune,* yellow) A syndrome characterized by hyperbilirubinemia and deposits of bile pigment in the skin, mucous membranes, and sclera, giving a yellow appearance to the patient.

joule (James Prescott Joule, 1818-1889, English physicist) The international (SI) unit of energy and heat, defined as the work done by the force of 1 newton acting over the distance of 1 meter. A newton (named for Sir Isaac Newton, 1643-1727, English mathematician, physicist, and astronomer) is the international unit of force, defined as the amount of force that, when applied in a vacuum to a body having a mass of 1 kg, accelerates it at the rate of 1 meter per second. These are examples of the exactness with which terms and values used by the world's scientific community must be defined, as illustrated in the *Systēme International d'Unitēs (SI).*

keratinization The process of creating the protein keratin, which is the principal constituent of skin, hair, nails, and the organizing matrix of the enamel of the teeth. It is a very insoluble protein.

keto acid Amino acid residue after deamination. The glycogenic keto acids are used to form carbohydrates.

kilocalorie (Fr *chilioi,* thousand; L *calor,* heat) The general term *calorie* refers to a unit of heat measure and is used alone to designate the *small calorie.* The calorie used in nutritional science and the study of metabolism is the *large calorie,* 1000 calories, or kilocalorie, to be more accurate and to avoid the use of very large numbers in calculations.

kinetic (Gr *kinetikos,* moving) Energy released from body fuels by cell metabolism and now active in moving muscles and energizing all body activities.

kyphosis (Gr *hyphos,* a hump) Increased, abnormal convexity of the upper part of the spine; hunchback.

lactase Enzyme that splits the disaccharide lactose into its two monosaccharides: glucose and galactose.

lactated Ringer's solution Sterile solution of calcium chloride, potassium chloride, sodium chloride, and sodium lactate in water given to replenish fluid and electrolytes.

lactiferous ducts (L *lac,* milk; *ferre,* to bear) Branching channels in the mammary gland that carry breast milk to holding spaces near the nipple, ready for the infant's feeding.

limiting amino acid The amino acid in foods occurring in the smallest amount, thus limiting its availability for tissue structure.

linoleic acid An essential fatty acid for humans; an n-6 polyunsaturated fatty acid.

linolenic acid An essential fatty acid for humans; an n-3 polyunsaturated fatty acid.

lipase (Gr *lipos,* fat; *-ase,* enzyme) Group of fat enzymes that cut the ester linkages between the fatty acids and glycerol of triglycerides (fats).

lipids (Gr *lipos,* fat) Chemical group name for fats and fat-related compounds such as cholesterol, lipoproteins, and phospholipids; general group name for organic substances of a fatty nature, including fats, oils, waxes, and related compounds.

lipogenesis Synthesis of fat from blood glucose.

lipoprotein Noncovalent complexes of fat with protein. The lipoproteins function as major carriers of lipids in the plasma because most of the plasma fat is associated with them. Such a combination makes possible the transport of fatty substances in a water medium such as plasma.

low molecular weight chromium complex (previously referred to as glucose tolerance factor) A biologically active complex of chromium that facilitates the reaction of insulin with receptor sites on tissues.

lumen (L *lumen,* light) The cavity or channel within a tube or tubular organ, such as the intestines.

lymphocytes (L *lympho-,* water; Gr *kytos,* hollow vessel, suffix for a cell type of the root to which it is designated or attached) Special white cells from lymphoid tissue that participate in humeral and cell-mediated immunity.

lymphoma (L *lympha,* water; Gr *sōma,* body) General term applied to any neoplastic disorder (cancer) of the lymphoid tissue.

macronutrients (Gr *makros,* large; L *nutriens,* nourishment) The three large energy-yielding nutrients: carbohydrates, fats, and proteins.

macrosomia Unusually large size.

malabsorption and **maldigestion** Malabsorption is a syndrome in which normal products of digestion do not traverse the intestinal mucosa and enter the lymphatic or portal venous branches. Maldigestion, which may be clinically similar to malabsorption, describes defects in the intraluminal phase of the digestive process caused by inadequate exposure of chyme to bile salts and pancreatic enzymes. Clinical symptoms of malabsorption include diarrhea, steatorrhea, and weight loss. Laboratory signs include depressed serum fat-soluble vitamin levels, accelerated prothrombin time, hypomagnesemia, and hypocholesterolemia. Patients with symptoms of malabsorption should have a laboratory work-up to determine the presence and degree of nutrient loss.

malignant melanoma (L *malignans,* acting maliciously; Gr *melos,* black) A tumor tending to become progressively worse, composed of melanin, the dark pigment of the skin and other body tissues, usually arising from the skin and aggravated by excessive sun exposure.

maltase Enzyme that breaks down the disaccharide maltose into two units of glucose; a monosaccharide.

median (L *medianus,* middle, midpoint) In statistics, the middle number in a sequence such that half of the numbers are higher and half of the numbers are lower.

medical foods Specially formulated nutrient mixtures for use under medical supervision to treat various metabolic diseases.

medulla (L *medulla,* marrow, center) Inner tissue substance of the kidney.

megaloblastic anemia (Gr *mega,* great size; *blastos,* embryo, germ) Anemia resulting from faulty production of abnormally large immature red blood cells, caused by a deficiency of vitamin B_{12} or folate.

menadione The parent compound of vitamin K in the body; called also *vitamin* K_3.

menaquinone Form of vitamin K synthesized by intestinal bacteria; called also *vitamin* K_2.

menarche (Gr *men,* month; *arche,* beginning) The beginning of first menstruation with the onset of puberty.

Menetrier's disease (giant hypertrophic gastritis) Rare disease characterized by large folds of nodular gastric rugae that may cover the wall of the stomach, causing anorexia, nausea, vomiting, and abdominal distress.

meningitis (Gr *meninx,* membrane) Inflammation of the *meninges,* the three membranes that envelop the brain and spinal cord, caused by a bacterial or viral infection and characterized by high fever, severe headache, and stiff neck or back muscles.

metabolic syndrome Multiple metabolic risk factors in one individual: overweight/obesity, physical inactivity, and genetic factors.

metabolism (Gr *metaballein,* to change, alter) Sum of all the various biochemical and physiologic processes by which the body grows and maintains itself (anabolism), breaks down and reshapes tissue (catabolism), and transforms energy to do its work. Products of these various reactions are called *metabolites.*

metabolites Any substance produced by metabolism or by a metabolic process.

micellar bile-lipid complex (L *mica,* crumb, particle) A combination of bile and fat in which the bile emulsifies fat into very minute globules or particles that can be absorbed easily into the small intestine wall in preparation for the final stage of absorption into circulation to the cells.

micronutrients (Gr *mikros,* small; L *nutriens,* nourishment) The two classes of small non–energy-yielding elements and compounds: minerals and vitamins are essential for regulation and control functions in cell metabolism and for building certain body structures.

microvilli (Gr *mikros,* small; L *villus,* tuft of hair) Minute vascular structures protruding from the surface of villi covering the inner surface of the small intestine, forming a "brush border" that facilitates absorption of nutrients.

monosaccharide (Gr *mono,* single; *sakcharon,* sugar) Simple single sugar; a carbohydrate containing a single saccharide (sugar) unit.

motivation Forces that affect individual goal-directed behavior toward satisfying needs or achieving personal goals.

mucosa (L *mucus*) The mucous membrane comprising the inner surface layer of the gastrointestinal tract, providing extensive nutrient absorption and transport functions.

mucus Viscous fluid secreted by mucous membranes and glands, consisting mainly of mucin (a glycoprotein), inorganic salts, and water. Mucus lubricates and protects the gastrointestinal mucosa and helps move the food mass along the digestive tract.

myasthenia gravis (MG) (Gr *mys,* muscle; *asthenia,* weakness; L *gravis,* heavy, weighty, grave) A progressive neuromuscular disease caused by faulty nerve conduction resulting from the presence of antibodies to acetylcholine receptors at the neuromuscular junction.

myelin (Gr *myelos,* marrow) Substance with a high lipid-to-protein composition forming a fatty sheath to insulate and protect neuron axons and facilitate their neuromuscular impulses.

myelin sheath (Gr *myelos,* marrow; *thēkē,* sheath) Covering of myelin, a lipid-protein substance with a high fat proportion to protein, surrounding nerve axons; serves as electrical insulator and speeds the conduction of nerve impulses; interrupted at intervals along the length of the axon by gaps known as Ranvier's nodes.

myofibril (Gr mys, muscle; L *fibrilla,* very small fiber) Slender thread of muscle; runs parallel to the muscle fiber's long axis.

myofilaments (Gr *mys,* muscle; L *filare,* to wind thread, spin) Threadlike filaments of actin or myosin, which are components of myofibrils.

myosin (Gr *mys,* muscle) Myofibril protein whose synchronized meshing action in conjunction with **actin** causes muscles to contract and relax.

necrosis (Gr *nekrosis,* deadness) Cell death caused by progressive enzyme breakdown.

neoplasm (Gr *neos,* new; *plasma,* formation) Any new or abnormal cellular growth that is abnormal, uncontrolled, and progressive.

nephron (Gr *nephros,* kidney) Microscopic anatomic and functional unit of the kidney that selectively filters and reabsorbs essential blood factors, secretes hydrogen ions as needed for maintaining acid-base balance, then reabsorbs water to protect body fluids, and forms and excretes a concentrated urine for elimination of wastes. The nephron includes the renal corpuscle (glomerulus), the proximal convoluted tubule, the loop of Henle, the distal convoluted tubule, and the collecting tubule, which empties the urine into the renal medulla. The urine passes into the papilla and then to the pelvis of the kidney. Urine is formed by filtration of blood in the glomerulus and by the selective reabsorption and secretion of solutes by cells that comprise the walls of the renal tubules. There are approximately 1 million nephrons in each kidney.

nephropathy (Gr *nephros,* kidney; *pathos,* disease) Disease of the kidneys; in diabetes, renal damage associated with functional and pathologic changes in the nephrons, which can lead to glomerulosclerosis and chronic renal failure.

neuropathy (Gr *neuron,* nerve; *pathos,* disease) General term for functional and pathologic changes in the peripheral nervous system; in diabetes, a chronic sensory condition affecting mainly the nerves of the legs, marked by numbness from sensory impairment, loss of tendon reflexes, severe pain, weakness, and wasting of muscles involved.

niacin equivalent (NE) A measure of the total dietary sources of niacin equivalent to 1 mg of niacin. Thus an NE is 1 mg of niacin or 60 mg of tryptophan.

night blindness Inability to see well at night in diminished light, resulting from lack of required vitamin A.

nitrogen balance The metabolic balance between nitrogen intake in dietary protein and output in urinary nitrogen compounds such as urea and creatinine. For every 6.25 g dietary protein consumed, 1 g nitrogen is excreted.

nonheme iron The larger portion of dietary iron, including all the plant food sources and 60% of the animal food sources. This form of iron is not part of a heme complex and is less easily absorbed.

nulligravida (L *nullus,* none; *gravida,* pregnant) A woman who has never been pregnant.

nutrients (L *nutriens,* nourishment) Substances in food that are essential for energy, growth, normal functioning of the body, and maintenance of life.

nutrition (L *nutritio,* nourishment) The sum of the processes involved in taking in food nutrients, assimilating and using them to maintain body tissue and provide energy; a foundation for life and health.

nutritional science The body of scientific knowledge, developed through controlled research, that relates to the processes involved in nutrition—national, international, community, and clinical.

obesity (L *obesus,* excessively fat) Fatness; an excessive accumulation of fat in the body.

oligosaccharides (Gr *oligos,* little; *saccharide,* sugar) Intermediate products of polysaccharide breakdown that contain a small number (from 3 to 10) of single sugar units of the monosaccharide glucose.

oliguria (Gr *oligos,* little; *ouron,* urine) Secretion of a very small amount of urine in relation to fluid intake.

oncogene (Gr *onkos,* mass; *genesis,* generation, production) Any of various genes that, when activated as by radiation or a virus, may cause a normal cell to become cancerous; viral genetic material carrying the potential of cancer and passed from parent to offspring.

organic (Gr *organikos,* organ) Carbon-based chemical compounds.

osmolality (Gr *osmos,* impulse, osmotic force) The ability of a solution to create osmotic pressure and determine the movement of water between fluid compartments, determined by the number of osmotically active particles per kilogram of solvent; serum osmolality is 280 to 300 mOsm/kg.

osmolarity The number of millimoles of liquid or solid in a liter of solution; parenteral nutrition solutions given by central vein have an osmolarity around 1800 mOsm/L; peripheral parenteral solutions are limited to 600 to 900 mOsm/L (dextrose and amino acids have the greatest impact on a solution's osmolarity).

osteodystrophy (Gr *osteon,* bone) Defective bone formation.

osteopenia Below normal level of bone mineral density, which increases the risk of stress fractures; the bone thinning is not as severe as that found in osteoporosis.

osteoporosis (Gr *osteon,* bone; *poros,* passage, pore) Abnormal thinning of bone, producing a porous, fragile bone tissue of enlarged spaces prone to fracture or deformity, associated with the aging process in older men and women.

palliative (L *palliatus,* cloaked) Care affording relief but not cure; useful for comfort when cure is still unknown or obscure.

palmar grasp (L *palma,* palm) Early grasp of the young infant, clasping an object in the palm and wrapping the whole hand around it.

pandemic (Gr *pan,* all; *dēmos,* people) A widespread epidemic, distributed through a region, continent, or the world.

pantothenic acid (Gr *pantothen,* "from all sides" or "in every corner") A B vitamin found widely distributed in nature and occurring throughout the body tissues. Pantothenic acid is an essential constituent of coenzyme A, which has extensive metabolic responsibility as an activating agent of a number of compounds in many tissues.

paradigm (Gr *para,* side-by-side; *deiknynai,* to show) A pattern or model serving as an example; a standard or ideal for practice or behavior based on a fundamental value or theme.

parasite (Gr *para,* along side; *sitos,* food, grain; *parasitos,* one who eats at another's table; in ancient Greece, a term for a person who received free meals in return for amusing or flattering conversation) An organism that lives on or in an organism of another species, known as the host, from whom all life cycle nourishment is obtained.

parenchymal cells (Gr *parenchyma,* "anything poured in beside") Functional cells of an organ, as distinguished from the cells comprising its structure or framework.

parenteral (Gr *para,* along side, beyond, accessory; *enteron,* intestine) A feeding modality that provides nutrient solutions intravenously rather than through the gastrointestinal tract.

paresthesia (Gr *para,* beyond; *aisthesis,* perception) Abnormal sensations such as prickling, burning, and crawling of skin.

parity (L *parere,* to bring forth, produce) The condition of a woman with respect to having borne viable offspring.

pepsin The main gastric enzyme specific for proteins. Pepsin begins breaking large protein molecules into shorter chain polypeptides, proteoses, and peptones. Gastric hydrochloric acid is necessary to activate pepsin.

peptide bond The characteristic joining of amino acids to form proteins. Such a chain of amino acids is termed a peptide. Depending on its size, it may be a dipeptide fragment of protein digestion or a large polypeptide.

percentile (L *per,* throughout, in space or time; *centrum,* a hundred) One of 100 equal parts of a measured series of values; rate or proportion per hundred.

peristalsis (Gr *peri,* around; *stalsis,* contraction) A wavelike progression of alternate contraction and relaxation of the muscle fibers of the gastrointestinal tract.

peritoneal dialysis Dialysis through the peritoneum into and out of the peritoneal cavity.

peritoneum (Gr *per,* around; *teinein,* to stretch) A strong smooth surface—a serous membrane—lining the abdominal/pelvic walls and the undersurface of the diaphragm, forming a sac enclosing the body's vital visceral organs within the peritoneal cavity.

pernicious anemia A chronic macrocytic anemia occurring most commonly after age 40. It is caused by absence of the intrinsic factor normally present in the gastric juices and necessary for the absorption of cobalamin vitamin B_{12} and controlled by intramuscular injections of vitamin B_{12}.

phagocytes (Gr *phagein,* to eat; *kytos,* hollow vessel, cell) Cells that ingest microorganisms, other cells, or foreign particles; macrophages.

phospholipid Any of a class of fat-related substances that contain phosphorus, fatty acids, and a nitrogenous base. The phospholipids are essential elements in every cell.

photosynthesis (Gr *photos,* light; *synthesis,* putting together) Process by which plants containing chlorophyll are able to manufacture carbohydrate by combining CO_2 from air and water from soil. Sunlight is used as energy; chlorophyll is a catalyst. $6\ CO_2 + 6\ H_2O + \text{Energy} + \text{Chlorophyll} \rightarrow C_6H_{12}O_6 + 6\ O_2$.

phylloquinone A fat-soluble vitamin of the K group (K_1), $C_3,H_{46}O_2$, found in green plants or prepared synthetically.

physiologic age (Gr *physis,* nature; *logikos,* or speech or reason) Rate of biologic maturation in individual adolescents that varies widely and accounts more for wide and changing differences in their metabolic rates, nutritional needs, and food requirements than does chronologic age.

pincer grasp Later digital grasp of the older infant, usually picking up smaller objects with a precise grip between thumb and forefinger.

placenta (L *placenta,* a flat cake) Special organ developed in early pregnancy that provides nutrients to the fetus and removes metabolic waste.

plaque (Fr *plaque,* patch or flat area) Thickened deposits of fatty material, largely cholesterol, within the arterial wall that eventually may fill the lumen and cut off blood supply to the tissue served by the damaged vessel.

polysaccharides (Gr *poly,* many; *saccharide,* sugar) Class of complex carbohydrates composed of many monosaccharide units. Common members are starch, dextrins, dietary fiber, and glycogen.

portal An entryway, usually referring to the portal circulation of blood through the liver. Blood is brought into the liver via the portal vein and out via the hepatic vein.

potential (L *potentia,* power) Energy existing in stored fuels and ready for action, but not yet released and active.

precursor (L *praecursor,* a forerunner) Something that precedes; in biology, a substance from which another substance is derived.

pressure sores Long-term bed-bound or immobile patients risk the development of pressure sores at points of bony protuberances, where prolonged pressure of body weight in one position cuts off adequate blood circulation to that area, causing tissue death and ulceration.

primigravida (L *prima,* first; *gravida,* pregnant) A woman pregnant for the first time.

proenzyme An inactive precursor converted to the active enzyme by the action of an acid, another enzyme, or other means. Also called zymogen.

prostaglandins (Gr *prostates,* standing before; L *glans,* acorn; hence, male prostate gland) Group of naturally occurring substances, first discovered in semen, derived from long-chain fatty acids that have multiple local hormone-like actions; these include regulation of gastric acid secretion, blood platelet aggregation, body temperature, and tissue inflammation.

protein balance (Gr *protos,* first) Body tissue protein balance between building up tissue (anabolism) and breaking down tissue (catabolism) to maintain healthy body growth and maintenance.

proteinuria (Gr *protos,* first, protein; *ouron,* urine) The presence of an excess of serum proteins, such as albumin, in the urine.

prothrombin (Gr *pro,* before; *thrombos,* clot) Blood-clotting factor (number II) synthesized in the liver from glutamic acid and carbon dioxide, catalyzed by vitamin K.

public health nutritionist A professional nutritionist who has completed an academic university program and special graduate study (MPH, DrPH) in a school of public health accredited by the American Association of Public Health and is responsible for nutrition components of public health programs in varied community settings—county, state, national, international.

pulmonary edema Accumulation of fluid in tissues of the lung.

pyrosis (Gr *pyro,* fire, burning) Heartburn.

radiation A highly controlled treatment for cancer, using radioactive substances in limited, controlled exposure to kill cancerous cells.

raffinose (Fr *raffin,* to refine) A colorless crystalline trisaccharide found in legumes, composed of galactose and sucrose connected by bonds that human enzymes cannot break; thus it remains whole in the intestines and produces gas as bacteria attack it.

Recommended Dietary Allowances (RDAs) Recommended daily allowances of nutrients and energy intake for population groups according to age and sex, with defined weight and height. The RDAs are established and reviewed periodically by a representative group of nutritional scientists in response to current research. These standards are very similar among the developed countries.

registered dietitian (RD) A professional dietitian who has completed an accredited academic program and 900 hours of postbaccalaureate supervised professional practice and has passed the National Registration Examination for Dietitians administered by the American Dietetic Association.

renal solute load (L *ren,* kidney) Collective number and concentration of solute particles in a solution, carried by the blood to the kidney nephrons for excretion in the urine. These particles are usually nitrogenous products from protein metabolism and the electrolyte sodium.

renin-angiotensin-aldosterone mechanism Three-stage system of sodium conservation, hence control of water loss, in response to diminished filtration pressure in the kidney nephrons: (1) pressure loss causes kidney to secrete the enzyme renin, which combines with and activates angiotensinogen from the liver; (2) active angiotensin stimulates of the adjacent adrenal gland to release the hormone aldosterone; (3) the hormone causes reabsorption of sodium from the kidney nephrons and water follows.

replication (L *replicare,* to fold back) Making an exact copy; to repeat, duplicate, or reproduce. In genetics, replication is the process by which double-stranded DNA makes copies of itself, each separating strand synthesizing a complementary strand. Cell replication is the process by which living cells, under gene control, make exact copies of themselves a programmed number of times during the life span of the organism. The process can be reproduced in the laboratory with cultured cell lines for special studies in cell biology.

resting metabolic rate (RMR) Amount of energy required to maintain the resting body's internal activities when in a normal environmental temperature and awake. Because of small differences in measuring techniques, RMR may be slightly different from the same person's **basal metabolic rate (BMR).** In practice, however, RMR and BMR measurements may be used interchangeably.

retinal Organic compound that is the aldehyde form of **retinol,** derived by the enzymatic splitting of absorbed carotene. It performs vitamin A activity. In the retina of the eye, retinal combines with opsins to form visual pigments. In the rods it combines with scotopsin to form rhodopsin (visual purple). In the cones it combines with photopsin to form the three pigments responsible for color vision.

retinol Chemical name for vitamin A, derived from its function relating to the retina of the eye and light-dark adaptation. Daily RDA standards are stated in retinol equivalents (RE) to account for sources of the preformed vitamin A and its precursor provitamin A, beta-carotene.

retinol equivalent (RE) Unit of measure for dietary sources of vitamin A, both preformed vitamin, retinol, and the precursor provitamin, beta-carotene. 1 RE = 1 μg retinol or 6 μg beta-carotene.

retinopathy (L *rete,* net, network; *retina,* innermost layer covering the eyeball; *pathos,* disease) Noninflammatory disease of the retina—the visual tissue of the eye—characterized by microaneurysms, intraretinal hemorrhages, waxy yellow exudates, "cotton wool" patches, and macular edema; a complication of diabetes that may lead to proliferation of fibrous tissue, retinal detachment, and blindness.

retrovirus (L *retro-,* backward) Any of a family of single-strand RNA viruses having an envelope and containing a reverse coding enzyme that allows for a reversal of genetic transcription from RNA to DNA rather than the usual DNA to RNA, the newly transcribed viral DNA then being incorporated into the host cell's DNA strand for the production of new RNA retroviruses.

rooting reflex A reflex in a newborn in which stimulation of the side of the cheek or the upper or lower lip causes the infant to turn its mouth and face to the stimulus.

rule of nines Describes the percentage of the body surface represented by various anatomic areas. For example: each upper limb, 9%; each lower limb, 18%; anterior and posterior trunk, each 18%; head and neck, 9%; and perineum and genitalia, 1%.

sarcoma (Gr *sarkos,* flesh; *onkoma,* a swelling) A tumor, usually malignant, arising from connective tissue.

saturated (L *saturare,* to fill) Term used for a substance that is united with the greatest possible amount of another substance through solution, chemical combination, or the like. A saturated fat, for example, is one in which the component fatty acids are filled with hydrogen atoms. A fatty acid is said to be saturated if all available chemical bonds of its carbon chain are filled with hydrogen. If one bond remains unfilled, it is a monounsaturated fatty acid. If two or more bonds remain unfilled, it is a polyunsaturated fatty acid. Fats of animal sources are more saturated. Fats of plant sources are unsaturated.

scurvy A hemorrhagic disease caused by lack of vitamin C. Diffuse tissue bleeding occurs, limbs and joints are painful and swollen, bones thicken as a result of subperiosteal hemorrhage, ecchymoses (large irregular discolored skin areas caused by tissue hemorrhages) form, bones fracture easily, wounds do not heal well, gums are swollen and bleeding, and teeth loosen.

secretin Hormone produced in the mucous membrane of the duodenum in response to the entrance of acid contents from the stomach into the duodenum. Secretin in turn stimulates the flow of pancreatic juices, providing needed enzymes and the proper alkalinity for their action.

sepsis (Gr *sēpsis,* decay) Presence in the blood or other tissues of pathogenic microorganisms or their toxins; conditions associated with such pathogens.

serosa Outer surface layer of the intestines interfacing with the blood vessels of the portal system going to the liver.

solutes (Gr *solvere,* to solve) Particles of a substance in solution; a solution consists of solutes and a dissolving medium (solvent), usually a liquid.

somatostatin (Gr *soma,* body; *stasis,* standing still, maintaining a constant level) A hormone formed in the D cells of the pancreatic islets of Langerhans and the hypothalamus. It is a balancing factor in maintaining normal blood glucose levels by inhibiting insulin and glucagon production in the pancreas as needed.

spina bifida (L *spina,* spine; *bifidus,* cleft into two parts or branches) A congenital defect in the fetal closing of the neural tube to form a portion of the lower spine, leaving the spine unclosed and the spinal cord open in various degrees of exposure and damage.

sphincter A circular band of muscle fibers that constricts a passage or closes a natural opening in the body (e.g., lower esophageal sphincter, pyloric sphincter).

steroids (Gr *stereos,* solid; L *-ol, oleum,* oil) Group name for lipid-based sterols, including hormones, bile acids, and cholesterol.

stomatitis (Gr *stoma,* mouth; *-itis,* inflammation) Inflammation of the oral mucosa, especially the buccal tissue lining the inside of the cheeks, but also it may involve the tongue, palate, floor of mouth, and the gums.

stroke volume (Gr *streich,* to strike or stretch) The amount of blood pumped from a ventricle (chamber of the heart releasing blood to body circulations) with each beat of the heart.

substrate (L *sub,* under; *stratum,* layer) The specific organic substance on which a particular enzyme acts to produce new metabolic products.

sucrase Enzyme splitting the disaccharide sucrose into its two monosaccharides of glucose and fructose.

synergism (Gr *syn,* with or together; *ergon,* work) The joint action of separate agents in which the total effect of their combined action is greater than the sum of their separate actions. (Adjective: **synergistic.**)

synosheath (Gr syno-, with, together; *thēkē,* sheath) Protective pliable connective tissue surrounding the bony-collagen meshwork and fluid that come together in the synovial area between major bone heads in joints, allows normal padded and lubricated joint movement and motion.

taurine A sulfur-containing amino acid, $NH_2(CH_2)_2 \cdot SO_2OH$, formed from the indispensable amino acid methionine. It is found in various body tissues, such as lungs and muscles, and in bile and breast milk.

thermic effect of food (TEF) (Gr *therme,* heat, of or pertaining to heat) Body heat produced by food; amount of energy required to digest and absorb food and transport nutrients to the cells. This basic preparatory work accounts for about 10% of the day's total energy (kcalories) requirement.

thiamin pyrophosphate (TPP) Activating coenzyme form of thiamin that plays a key role in carbohydrate metabolism.

tocopherol (Gr *tokos,* childbirth; *pherein,* to carry) Chemical name for vitamin E. In humans it functions as a strong antioxidant to preserve structural membranes, such as cell walls.

Tolerable Upper Intake Level (UL) The highest amount of a vitamin or mineral that can be consumed with safety; this standard was developed to advise people regarding inappropriate intakes of nutrient supplements.

total fiber Dietary fiber plus functional fiber; the total amount of fiber in an individual's diet from all sources.

***trans* fatty acids** Fatty acids that have been hydrogenated to be used in margarine and in the food industry; have been shown to increase LDL cholesterol and lower HDL cholesterol.

triglyceride (Gr *tri,* three) Chemical name for fat, indicating structure; attachment of three fatty acids to a glycerol base. A neutral fat, synthesized from carbohydrate and stored in adipose tissue, it releases free fatty acids into the blood when hydrolyzed by enzymes.

trypsin (Gr *trypein,* to rub; *pepsis,* digestion) A protein-splitting enzyme formed in the intestine by action of enterokinase on the inactive precursor trypsinogen.

vagotomy (L *vagus,* wandering; Gr *tomē,* a cutting) Cutting of certain branches of the vagus nerve, performed with gastric surgery, to reduce the amount of gastric acid secreted and lessen the chance of recurrence of a gastric ulcer.

valence (L *valens,* powerful) Power of an element or a radical to combine with or to replace other elements or radicals. Atoms of various elements combine in definite proportions. The valence number of an element is the number of atoms of hydrogen with which one atom of the element can combine.

vasoactive (L *vas,* vessel) Having an effect on the diameter of blood vessels.

vasopressin Alternate name of antidiuretic hormone (ADH).

villi (L *villus,* "tuft of hair") Small protrusions from the surface of a membrane; fingerlike projections covering the mucosal surfaces of the small intestine.

virus (L *virus,* poison; *virion,* individual virus particle) Minute infectious agent, characterized by lack of independent metabolism and by the ability to reproduce with genetic continuity only within living host cells. Viruses range in decreasing size from about 200 nanometers (nm) down to only 15 nm. (A nanometer is a linear measure equal to one-billionth of a meter; it is also called a millimicron.) Each particle (virion) consists basically of nucleic acids (genetic material) and a protein shell that protects and contains the genetic material and any enzymes present.

viscous (L *viscidus,* glutinous or sticky) Physical property of a substance dependent on the friction of its component molecules as they slide by one another; viscosity.

VO_2max Maximum uptake volume of oxygen during exercise; used to measure the intensity and duration of exercise a person can perform.

Zollinger-Ellison syndrome A condition characterized by severe peptic ulceration, gastric hypersecretion, elevated serum gastrin, and gastrinoma of the pancreas or the duodenum. Total gastrectomy may be necessary.

Index

Page numbers followed by b indicate boxed material (numbered and unnumbered); page numbers followed by f indicate figures; page numbers followed by t indicate tables.

F

M

W

Estimated Sodium, Chloride, and Potassium Minimum Requirements of Healthy Persons*

Age	Weight (kg)	Sodium (mg)*†	Chloride (mg)*†	Potassium (mg)‡
Months				
0-5	4.5	120	180	500
6-11	8.9	200	300	700
Years				
1	11.0	225	350	1000
2-5	16.0	300	500	1400
6-9	25.0	400	600	1600
10-18	50.0	500	750	2000
>18§	70.0	500	750	2000

Reprinted with permission from *Recommended Dietary Allowances,* 10th ed., © 1989 by the National Academy of Sciences. Published by National Academy Press.

*No allowance has been included for large, prolonged losses from the skin through sweat.

†There is no evidence that higher intakes confer any health benefit.

‡Desirable intakes of potassium may considerably exceed these values (~3500 mg for adults).

§No allowance included for growth. Values for those below 18 years assume a growth rate at the 50th percentile reported by the National Center for Health Statistics and averaged for males and females.

Median Height and Weight and Recommended Energy Intake

		Weight		Height			Average Energy Allowance (kcal)		
Category	Age (years) or Condition	(kg)	(lb)	(cm)	(in)	REE* (kcal/day)	Multiples of REE	Per kg	Per Day†
Infants	0-0.5	6	13	60	24	320		108	650
	0.5-1	9	20	71	28	500		98	850
Children	1-3	13	29	90	56	740		102	1300
	4-6	20	44	112	44	950		90	1800
	7-10	28	62	132	52	1130		70	2000
Men	11-14	45	99	157	62	1440	1.70	55	2500
	15-18	66	145	176	69	1760	1.67	45	3000
	19-24	72	160	177	70	1780	1.67	40	2900
	25-50	79	174	176	70	1800	1.60	37	2900
	51+	77	170	173	68	1530	1.50	30	2300
Women	11-14	46	101	157	62	1310	1.67	47	2200
	15-18	55	120	163	64	1370	1.60	40	2200
	19-24	58	128	164	65	1350	1.60	38	2200
	25-50	63	138	163	64	1380	1.55	36	2200
	51+	65	143	160	63	1280	1.50	30	1900
Pregnant	1st trimester								+0
	2nd trimester								+300
	3rd trimester								+300
Lactating	1st 6 months								+500
	2nd 6 months								+500

Reprinted with permission from *Recommended Dietary Allowances,* 10th ed., © 1989 by the National Academy of Sciences. Published by National Academy Press.

*Resting energy expenditure (REE); calculation based on FAQ equations and then rounded. This is the same as RMR (resting metabolic rate).

†Figure is rounded.